Imaging *of* Arthritis *and* Metabolic Bone Disease

Imaging *of* Arthritis *and* Metabolic Bone Disease

Barbara N. Weissman, MD
Professor of Radiology
Harvard Medical School
Vice Chair, Department of Radiology
Director, Radiology Residency Program
Section Head Emeritus, Musculoskeletal Imaging
Brigham and Women's Hospital
Boston, Massachusetts

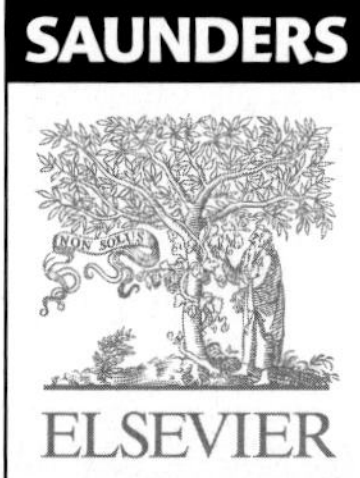

SAUNDERS
ELSEVIER

1600 John F. Kennedy Blvd.
Ste 1800
Philadelphia, PA 19103-2899

IMAGING OF ARTHRITIS AND METABOLIC BONE DISEASE ISBN: 978-0-323-04177-5

Library of Congress Cataloging-in-Publication Data

Imaging of arthritis and metabolic bone disease / [edited by] Barbara N. Weissman.
p. ; cm.
Includes bibliographical references.
ISBN 978-0-323-04177-5
1. Arthritis–Imaging. 2. Bones–Metabolism–Disorders–Imaging. I. Weissman, Barbara N. W. (Barbara N. Warren)
[DNLM: 1. Arthritis–diagnosis. 2. Bone Diseases, Metabolic–diagnosis. 3. Diagnostic Imaging. WE 346 I31 2009]
RC933.I423 2009
616.7′220754–dc22

2008027097

Publishing Director: Kim Murphy
Developmental Editor: Cathy Carroll
Project Manager: Bryan Hayward
Design Direction: Karen O'Keefe Owens

Printed in China

Last digit is the print number: 9 8 7 6 5 4 3 2 1

Dedication

This book is dedicated to my wonderful family,
Abigail, Matthew, Juliet, and my granddaughter Liana Weissman;
Nana Lillian Warren; and especially to my husband,
Irving, whose support, encouragement, and sense of humor made it possible.

CONTRIBUTORS

Judith E. Adams, MBBS, FRCR, FRCP
Professor of Diagnostic Radiology
Imaging Science and Biomedical Engineering
University of Manchester
Honorary Consultant Radiologist
Manchester Royal Infirmary
Central Manchester and Manchester Children's University Hospitals
Manchester, England, United Kingdom
Imaging Evaluation of Osteoporosis

Piran Aliabadi, MD
Associate Professor of Radiology
Staff Radiologist
Brigham and Women's Hospital
Harvard Medical School
Boston, Massachusetts
Imaging of Infection

Leyla H. Alparslan, MD
Överläkare
Akademiska Sjukhuset
Uppsala University
Uppsala, Sweden
Imaging Findings of Drug-Related Musculoskeletal Disorders
Scleroderma and Related Disorders

Paul Babyn, MDCM
Radiologist in Chief
Hospital for Sick Children
Associate Professor of Medical Imaging
University of Toronto
Toronto, Ontario, Canada
Imaging Investigation of Arthritis in Children

D. Lee Bennett, MD, MA
Assistant Professor of Radiology
University of Iowa Roy J. and Lucille A. Carver College of Medicine
Iowa City, Iowa
Imaging Hyperparathyroidism and Renal Osteodystrophy

Melissa Birnbaum, MD
Resident
Department of Radiology
New York Presbyterian–Weill Cornell
New York, New York
Imaging of Diabetes Mellitus and Neuropathic Arthropathy: The Diabetic Foot

Bernd Bittersohl, MD
Department of Radiology
Brigham and Women's Hospital
Harvard Medical School
Boston, Massachusetts
Magnetic Resonance Imaging of Articular Cartilage

Carolyn Boltin, MD
Assistant Professor
Department of Radiology
New York University
New York, New York
Bone Disease Following Organ Transplantation

Ethan M. Braunstein, MD
Professor of Radiology
Consultant in Radiology
Mayo College of Medicine
Scottsdale, Arizona
Crystal Diseases

John Braver, MD
Assistant Professor
Department of Radiology
Brigham and Women's Hospital
Harvard Medical School
Boston, Massachusetts
Systemic Lupus Erythematosus and Related Conditions and Vasculitic Syndromes

Mathias Brem, MD
Department of Radiology
Brigham and Women's Hospital
Harvard Medical School
Boston, Massachusetts
Magnetic Resonance Imaging of Articular Cartilage

John A. Carrino, MD, MPH
Associate Professor of Radiology and Orthopaedic Surgery
Johns Hopkins University School of Medicine
Section Chief, Musculoskeletal Radiology
Russell H. Morgan Department of Radiology and Radiological Science
Johns Hopkins Outpatient Center
Baltimore, Maryland
Degenerative Disorders of the Spine
Hypoparathyroidism and PTH Resistance
Rickets and Osteomalacia
Hypophosphatasia
Fanconi Syndrome and Renal Tubular Acidosis
Percutaneous Spine Interventions: Discography, Injection Procedures (Epidural Corticosteroids and Facet Joint and Sacroiliac Joint Injections), and Vertebral Augmentation (Vertebroplasty and Kyphoplasty)

Kevin Carter, DO
Fellow of Musculoskeletal Imaging
Brigham and Women's Hospital
Boston, Massachusetts
Arthrography and Injection Procedures
Reflex Sympathetic Dystrophy, Migratory Osteoporosis, and Osteogenesis Imperfecta

Anil K. Chandraker, MB, FRCP
Assistant Professor of Medicine
Harvard Medical School
Medical Director of Kidney Transplantation
Renal Division
Brigham and Women's Hospital
Boston, Massachusetts
Bone Disease Following Organ Transplantation

Richard H. Daffner, MD, FACR
Professor of Radiological Science
Drexel University College of Medicine
Allegheny General Hospital
Allegheny, Pennsylvania
Stress Injuries to Bone

Murray K. Dalinka, MD
Professor of Radiology
Chief, Musculoskeletal Section
Department of Musculoskeletal Radiology
Hospital of the University of Pennsylvania
Philadelphia, Pennsylvania
Infarction and Osteonecrosis

Andrea Schwartz Doria, MD, PhD, MSc
Associate Professor
Department of Diagnostic Imaging
Hospital for Sick Children
Toronto, Ontario, Canada
Imaging Investigation of Arthritis in Children

Jeff Duryea, PhD
Assistant Professor
Departments of Radiology
Brigham and Women's Hospital
Harvard Medical School
Boston, Massachusetts
Magnetic Resonance Imaging of Articular Cartilage

Georges Y. El-Khoury, MD
Professor of Radiology and Orthopedic Surgery
University of Iowa Roy J. and Lucille A. Carver College of Medicine
Iowa City, Iowa
Imaging Hyperparathyroidism and Renal Osteodystrophy

Hale Ersoy, MD
Assistant Professor of Radiology
Harvard Medical School
Department of Radiology
Brigham and Women's Hospital
Boston, Massachusetts
Systemic Lupus Erythematosus and Related Conditions and Vasculitic Syndromes

Joshua M. Farber, MD
Director, MRI
Vascular Interventional Radiology Associates of Northern Kentucky
Crestview Hills, Kentucky
Clinical Applications of Multidetector Computed Tomography in Musculoskeletal Imaging

Stephen W. Farraher, MD
Clinical Assistant Professor of Radiology
University of Vermont School of Medicine
Diagnostic Radiologist
Maine Medical Center
Scarborough, Maine
Imaging of Tendons and Bursae

Frieda Feldman, MD, FACR
Professor of Radiology and Orthopaedics
Columbia University College of Physicians and Surgeons
Attending Radiologist
Chief, Musculoskeletal Radiology
New York Presbyterian Hospital
New York, New York
Oncogenic Osteomalacia

Raul Galvez-Trevino, MD
Research Fellow Radiology Resident
Department of Radiology
Harvard Medical School
Brigham and Women's Hospital
Boston, Massachusetts
Bone Disease Following Organ Transplantation

Gandikota Girish, MBBS, FRCS(ed), FRCR
Assistant Professor
Musculoskeletal Radiology
University of Michigan Hospital
Ann Arbor, Michigan
Ultrasound

Christian Glaser, MD
Klinikum Grosshadern
Ludwig Maximilian University Munich
Munich, Germany
Magnetic Resonance Imaging of Articular Cartilage

Mary G. Hochman, MD
Chief, Musculoskeletal Imaging
Department of Radiology
Beth Israel Deaconess Medical Center
Assistant Professor, Radiology
Harvard Medical School
Boston, Massachusetts
Imaging of Tendons and Bursae
Entrapment Syndromes

Liangge Hsu, MD
Assistant Professor of Radiology
Harvard Medical School
Brigham and Women's Hospital
Boston, Massachusetts
Systemic Lupus Erythematosus and Related Conditions and Vasculitic Syndromes

Andetta Hunsaker, MD
Assistant Professor of Radiology
Harvard Medical School
Director of Thoracic Imaging
Brigham and Women's Hospital
Boston, Massachusetts
Systemic Lupus Erythematosus and Related Conditions and Vasculitic Syndromes

Hakan Ilaslan, MD
Assistant Professor of Radiology
Staff Radiologist
Department of Diagnostic Radiology
Cleveland Clinic
Cleveland, Ohio
Paget's Disease, Fibrous Dysplasia, Sarcoidosis, and Amyloidosis of Bone

Jon A. Jacobson, MD
Professor of Radiology
Director, Division of Musculoskeletal Radiology
University of Michigan
Ann Arbor, Michigan
Ultrasound

David Karasick, MD, FACR
Department of Radiology
Thomas Jefferson University
Jefferson Medical College
Philadelphia, Pennsylvania
Imaging of Rheumatoid Arthritis

Katsumi Kose, PhD
Professor
Institute of Applied Physics
University of Tsukuba
Tsukuba, Ibaraki, Japan
Magnetic Resonance Imaging

Philipp Lang, MD, MBA
Associate Professor
Departments of Radiology
Brigham and Women's Hospital
Harvard Medical School
Boston, Massachusetts
Magnetic Resonance Imaging of Articular Cartilage

Tara Lawrimore, MD, FRCPC
Department of Radiology
Musculoskeletal Division
Massachusetts General Hospital
Boston, Massachusetts
Traumatic Muscle Injuries

Amy Rosen Lecomte, MD
Instructor in Radiology
Harvard Medical School
Staff Radiologist
Brigham and Women's Hospital
Boston, Massachusetts
Imaging of Infection

Marc J. Lee, MD
Department of Imaging Services
Providence St. Joseph's Medical Center
Burbank, California
Pediatric Developmental and Chronic Traumatic Conditions, the Osteochondroses, and Childhood Osteoporosis

Leon Lenchik, MD
Associate Professor
Department of Radiology
Wake Forest University School of Medicine
Winston-Salem, North Carolina
Dual X-Ray Absorptiometry

John D. MacKenzie, MD
Assistant Professor of Radiology
Stanford University School of Medicine
Stanford, California
Infarction and Osteonecrosis
Imaging of Rheumatoid Arthritis

Sanjay Mudigonda, MD
Instructor in Radiology
Staff Radiologist
Newton-Wellesley Hospital
Newton, Massachusetts
Arthrography and Injection Procedures

Gesa Neumann, MD
Department of Radiology
Brigham and Women's Hospital
Harvard Medical School
Boston, Massachusetts
Magnetic Resonance Imaging of Articular Cartilage

Arthur H. Newberg, MD, FACR
Professor of Radiology and Orthopaedics
Tufts University School of Medicine
Chief, Musculoskeletal Imaging
New England Baptist Hospital
Boston, Massachusetts
Soft Tissue Calcification and Ossification

Joel S. Newman, MD
Chairman
Department of Radiology
New England Baptist Hospital
Associate Clinical Professor of Radiology
Tufts University School of Medicine
Boston, Massachusetts
Imaging of Tendons and Bursae
Juxtaarticular Cysts and Fluid Collections: Imaging and Intervention

Joel Nielsen, DO
Musculoskeletal Radiologist
Marshfield Clinic
Weston, Wisconsin
Reflex Sympathetic Dystrophy, Migratory Osteoporosis, and Osteogenesis Imperfecta

Nayer Nikpoor, MD
Assistant Professor of Radiology
Director of Nuclear Medicine
Tufts Medical Center
Boston, Massachusetts
Scintigraphy of the Musculoskeletal System

Mohamad Ossiani, MD
Staff Radiologist
Instructor of Radiology
Brigham and Women's Hospital
Boston, Massachusetts
Imaging of Infection

William Palmer, MD
Director, Musculoskeletal Imaging
Massachusetts General Hospital
Harvard Medical School
Boston, Massachusetts
Traumatic Muscle Injuries

Tarak H. Patel, MD
Johns Hopkins University School of Medicine
Russell H. Morgan Department of Radiology and Radiological Science
Baltimore, Maryland
Degenerative Disorders of the Spine
Percutaneous Spine Interventions: Discography, Injection Procedures (Epidural Corticosteroids and Facet Joint and Sacroiliac Joint Injections), and Vertebral Augmentation (Vertebroplasty and Kyphoplasty)

Jeannette M. Perez-Rossello, MD
Instructor in Radiology
Harvard Medical School
Children's Hospital Boston
Boston, Massachusetts
Pediatric Developmental and Chronic Traumatic Conditions, the Osteochondroses, and Childhood Osteoporosis

Parham Pezeshk, MD
Research Fellow Radiology Resident
Department of Radiology
Harvard Medical School
Brigham and Women's Hospital
Boston, Massachusetts
Hypoparathyroidism and PTH Resistance
Rickets and Osteomalacia
Hypophosphatasia
Fanconi Syndrome and Renal Tubular Acidosis
Bone Disease Following Organ Transplantation

Arun J. Ramappa, MD
Department of Orthopedics
Beth Israel Deaconess Medical Center
Instructor, Orthopedic Surgery
Harvard Medical School
Boston, Massachusetts
Imaging of Tendons and Bursae

Catherine C. Roberts, MD
Consultant Radiologist
Department of Diagnostic Radiology
Mayo Clinic
Phoenix, Arizona
Associate Professor of Radiology
Mayo Clinic College of Medicine
Rochester, Minnesota
Crystal Diseases

Daniel I. Rosenthal, MD
Professor of Radiology
Harvard Medical School
Associate Radiologist-in-Chief
Musculoskeletal Radiology
Massachusetts General Hospital
Boston, Massachusetts
Gaucher's Disease

Joel Rubenstein, MD, FRCPC
Department of Medical Imaging
University of Toronto
Sunnybrook and Women's College Health Sciences Center
Toronto, Ontario, Canada
Seronegative Spondyloarthropathies and SAPHO Syndrome

Philipp M. Schlechtweg, MD
Research Fellow
Harvard Medical School
Department of Radiology
Brigham and Women's Hospital
Boston, Massachusetts
Magnetic Resonance Imaging

Mark E. Schweitzer, MD
Chief of Diagnostic Imaging
The Ottawa Hospital
Professor of Radiology
University of Ottawa
Ottawa, Ontario, Canada
Imaging of Diabetes Mellitus and Neuropathic Arthropathy: The Diabetic Foot

Murali Sundaram, MD, FRCR
Professor of Radiology
Section of Musculoskeletal Radiology
Cleveland Clinic
Cleveland, Ohio
Paget's Disease, Fibrous Dysplasia, Sarcoidosis, and Amyloidosis of Bone

Andrew A. Wade, MD
Resident
Department of Radiology
Harvard Medical School
Massachusetts General Hospital
Boston, Massachusetts
Gaucher's Disease

Barbara N. Weissman, MD

Professor of Radiology
Harvard Medical School
Vice Chair, Department of Radiology
Director, Radiology Residency Program
Section Head Emeritus, Musculoskeletal Imaging
Brigham and Women's Hospital
Boston, Massachusetts

Osteoarthritis
Imaging Findings of Drug-Related Musculoskeletal Disorders
Imaging Arthropathies Associated with Malignant Disorders
Systemic Lupus Erythematosus and Related Conditions and Vasculitic Syndromes
Pediatric Developmental and Chronic Traumatic Conditions, the Osteochondroses, and Childhood Osteoporosis
Hemochromatosis, Wilson's Disease, Ochronosis, Fabry Disease, and Multicentric Reticulohistiocytosis
Imaging of Total Joint Replacement

Hiroshi Yoshioka, MD, PhD

Associate Professor of Radiology
Harvard Medical School
Associate Radiologist
Department of Radiology
Brigham and Women's Hospital
Boston, Massachusetts

Magnetic Resonance Imaging
Magnetic Resonance Imaging of Articular Cartilage

PREFACE

The conditions described in this textbook range from the most common disorders affecting the musculoskeletal system, such as osteoarthritis and osteoporosis, to some of the most rare. Imaging has become an integral part of the evaluation of patients with arthritis and metabolic diseases, and it often provides the standard method for diagnosing, classifying, and following these conditions. Examples include the use of the radiographic Kellgren-Lawrence grading system for osteoarthritis and DXA scanning for the diagnosis of osteoporosis. Advanced imaging techniques have been developed that can provide information in addition to that available from the radiograph. Thus, for example, while radiographs provide an indirect measure of cartilage damage by assessing the width of the joint space, magnetic resonance imaging (MRI) provides direct anatomical information regarding cartilage thickness and structure and delayed gadolinium-enhanced MRI of cartilage (dGEMRIC) adds information regarding its glycosaminoglycan content.

In the face of current imaging options, the question of test ordering becomes not *could we order this test*, but *should we?* What can be gleaned from the radiograph alone? What options are available? Which is the best examination, and how is it optimally performed? What information should we expect from advanced imaging studies in the various arthritic and metabolic conditions? This book is written specifically to help both the radiologist and the nonradiologist answer these questions.

Introductory chapters review the principles of pertinent imaging techniques and are primarily designed for nonradiologists. They provide a background for understanding these techniques, their uses, and their limitations. Vocabulary specific to these studies is provided in order to aid understanding of the tests themselves and to facilitate communication of results and image review with radiologists and other practitioners.

Chapters devoted to the various disorders are structured in a uniform format. Discussion of the disease process is followed by its general musculoskeletal manifestations, specific features in various locations, and then by extraskeletal manifestations. While musculoskeletal involvement by these disorders is emphasized, other important manifestations of these conditions are included at the discretion of the authors and editor. It is hoped that this more comprehensive approach provides a clinically useful picture of these conditions. When possible, algorithms or specific discussions are provided at the end of each chapter to clarify the indications for the various imaging studies.

It is acknowledged that the topics included in these chapters were selected to be the most useful clinically and that topics may be included that are not specifically either arthritis or metabolic bone disease (such as stress fractures) and that some conditions may have been omitted. It is hoped that the basic principles presented here will allow any such omissions to be of minimal consequence and that readers will provide feedback to allow ongoing improvement of this product.

Multiauthored textbooks have the advantage of permitting experts in the various areas to participate but engender logistical and editorial challenges. Success of the final product depends on the work of a large number of professionals who deserve credit and accolades. Mrs. Nena Andrade-Karama provided expert support in data gathering, manuscript preparation, tracking, and communication. Mrs. Reiko O'Brien prepared images for many of the chapters to provide optimal clarity. Mr. Calvin Brown provided support for image retrieval. I am deeply grateful for the guidance, support, and expertise of those at Elsevier who have made this book possible, most especially Mrs. Karen Carter, whose encouragement, patience, flexibility, and expertise were invaluable. Kim Murphy, Amy Cannon, and Janine Kusza of Elsevier and Megan Greiner of Graphic World Inc. were all instrumental in guiding this book from concept to completion. Special heartfelt thanks go to the authors who agreed to participate so fully to realize these goals.

ACKNOWLEDGMENTS

The reviews by Simon M. Helfgott, MD, and Derrick J. Todd, MD, PhD, of the Department of Rheumatology at Brigham and Women's Hospital were invaluable in ensuring the relevance of the chapters on arthritis to current practice.

CONTENTS

SECTION I

GENERAL IMAGING PRINCIPLES

CHAPTER 1

Clinical Applications of Multidetector Computed Tomography in Musculoskeletal Imaging

JOSHUA M. FARBER, MD

KEY FACTS

- MRI has superior contrast resolution to CT.
- CT, unlike MRI, can directly image trabecular and cortical bone.
- Computed tomography (CT) has greater spatial resolution than magnetic resonance imaging (MRI), so very small structures can be examined with excellent detail.
- Multidetector CT (MDCT) scanners are fast, producing image data sets of a body part in seconds.
- Isotropic imaging, in which all dimensions of the volume elements of the image are equal in size, allows production of high-resolution images in any plane after the initial source images are obtained.
- Intraarticular contrast injection (arthroCT) can evaluate internal derangement and is particularly useful in patients who cannot undergo MRI examination or have undergone joint surgery (e.g., articular cartilage or meniscal surgery).
- The radiation dose from MDCT can be relatively high.
- Three-dimensional displays may be helpful especially for analyzing complex fractures and lessening artifact accompanying orthopedic hardware.

Recent advances in multidetector computed tomography (MDCT) greatly affect musculoskeletal imaging[4]. Current MDCT systems have unsurpassed spatial resolution, are capable of scanning through metal, and are lightning-fast. These attributes make the modality ideally suited for, among other things, assessing bone surfaces, the integrity of orthopedic hardware, and trauma patients.[1,2] When used in combination with arthrography, MDCT is often preferable to magnetic resonance imaging (MRI) for evaluating internal derangement, especially in the postoperative setting. The essential features of these new systems that allow such imaging are the new detector arrays, improved software, and variable scan speed. This chapter will briefly address some of the technical aspects of MDCT and illustrate how this new technology contributes to patient care. MDCT radiation dose issues will be addressed as well.

MDCT TECHNOLOGY

All computed tomography (CT) relies on a photon beam passing through a patient and being detected after the passage by a detector; hence the circular, or doughnut, shape of CT systems. If the photon beam passes through dense material, such as bone, the detector senses a faint signal. Conversely, if the beam passes through mostly air, such as in the lungs, the detector senses a strong signal. After a scan is complete, a computer sorts out the various signals, or attenuation values, and constructs an image. Prior to MDCT, CT systems generated a single beam, which passed through the patient and was sensed by a single detector. Current MDCT systems generate multiple photon beams simultaneously that are sensed by broad detector arrays. Thus many slices may be obtained at once.

Current MDCT systems generate multiple photon beams simultaneously that are sensed by broad detector arrays. Thus many slices may be obtained at once.

In addition, the new detector arrays may be adjusted, or collimated, to select a greater variety of slice thicknesses. Another feature of MDCT systems that warrants mention is the table that the patient lies on. The speed of this table may be varied. For trauma imaging of an uncooperative patient, a fast table speed is desirable to minimize patient motion. Sometimes, such as when scanning through orthopedic hardware, a slow table speed is desired to scan through metal. These features of MDCT make the systems extremely versatile.

Current MDCT systems typically have matrix sizes of 512 × 512 or 1024 × 1024. The higher the matrix is, the greater the spatial resolution. For example, a scan with a field of view of 30 cm and a 512 × 512 matrix is made of a grid with squares that are less than 0.06 cm on each side. This defines the resolution in two planes, height (anteroposterior) and width (mediolateral). The resolution in the third plane (depth) is defined by the slice thickness. Current MDCT scanners produce slices as thin as 0.5 or 0.6 mm. The result is that MDCT systems can collect data in true cubes. More precisely, MDCT scanners can produce *isometric* data sets that have the same dimensions in all three

TABLE 1-1. Hounsfield Units and Appearance of Various Tissues

Tissue	Appearance	Hounsfield units
Air	Black	−1000
Fat		−60 to −100
Soft tissue		+40 to +80
Bone	White (cortex)	+400 to +1000

The circle represents the region of interest.

planes.[3] In turn, isometric data sets allow reformatted images to be produced in any plane without image degradation. Hence two-dimensional (2D) multiplanar reformatted (MPR) images look as though they were acquired directly and three-dimensional (3D) images have exquisite detail. Current software allows quick and easy data manipulation to produce reformatted images in any plane and angle.

> The production of isometric data sets (identical length, width, and depth image information) allows images to be reformatted in any plane without image degradation and the production of exquisite 3D images.

To produce robust image data sets, overlapped slices are obtained during scanning. For example, a wrist scan, which requires high detail, will be obtained, using 0.6-mm slices at 0.2-mm or 0.3-mm intervals. Such scan overlap acquires data sets that produce seamless reformatted images. Another consequence of overlapping slices is increased mAs, or simply the number of photons that pass through a body part.

> Overlapping slices, useful when imaging small structures, increase the number of photons that pass through a body part and therefore increase the radiation dose.

Large orthopedic devices can be scanned through using thick slices with 50% to 60% slice overlap. For example, a total hip prosthesis can be scanned through to evaluate for loosening. Such a scan might use 3-mm slices with 2-mm overlap and generate more than 500 mAs. Fortunately, new MDCT systems are increasingly efficient and reduce radiation dose to the patient. In addition, such a scan should be performed only in an older patient.

Many parameters can be manipulated in current MDCT systems. The result is an extremely versatile technology that can scan small body parts with high resolution as well as large body parts that may contain large orthopedic devices. If proper scanning technique is used, MPR or 3D images may be obtained in all cases. Examples of this technology's clinical versatility and utility are presented below.

HOUNSFIELD UNITS

As noted earlier, computers generate MDCT images from the differing attenuation values of tissues. These attenuation values are measured in Hounsfield units. Dense tissues, like bone, have high Hounsfield unit values. Air, which has relatively low density, has an extremely low Hounsfield unit value. Tissues such as fat and muscle have intermediate values and vary according to their density (Table 1-1; see Glossary). Cortical bone typically has values of 400 to 1000, while traebecular bone has values of 100 to 300. By contrast, air measures -400 to -600. An intermediate tissue like muscle typically has values of 40 to 80. Fat, which is less dense then muscle, has values of -60 to -100. Simple fluid, such as may be found in a simple renal cyst or uncomplicated joint effusion, has a density between muscle and fat. Accordingly, fluid has Hounsfield values of 10 to 20 or 30.

The Hounsfield values for blood vary depending on the age and location of the blood. Extravascular blood from an acute bleed typically will have values of 50 to 90. As a hematoma forms, portions of the clot may liquefy and have Hounsfield values that approach fluid (20 to 30). However, some portions may contain hemosiderin or dystrophic calcification and have Hounsfield values in the 90s or low 100s. Intravascular blood typically has Hounsfield values around 90, unless the patient has been given intravenous contrast. Many factors influence the Hounsfield value of contrast-enhanced blood, including the timing of the image acquisition relative to the injection and whether the blood is venous or arterial. In general, arterial blood has higher Hounsfield values (low to mid or high hundreds) than venous blood (low hundreds).

Assessing Cortical Surfaces

Radiographs are used first in the workup of cortical surfaces; they are an excellent first step and often all that is required.

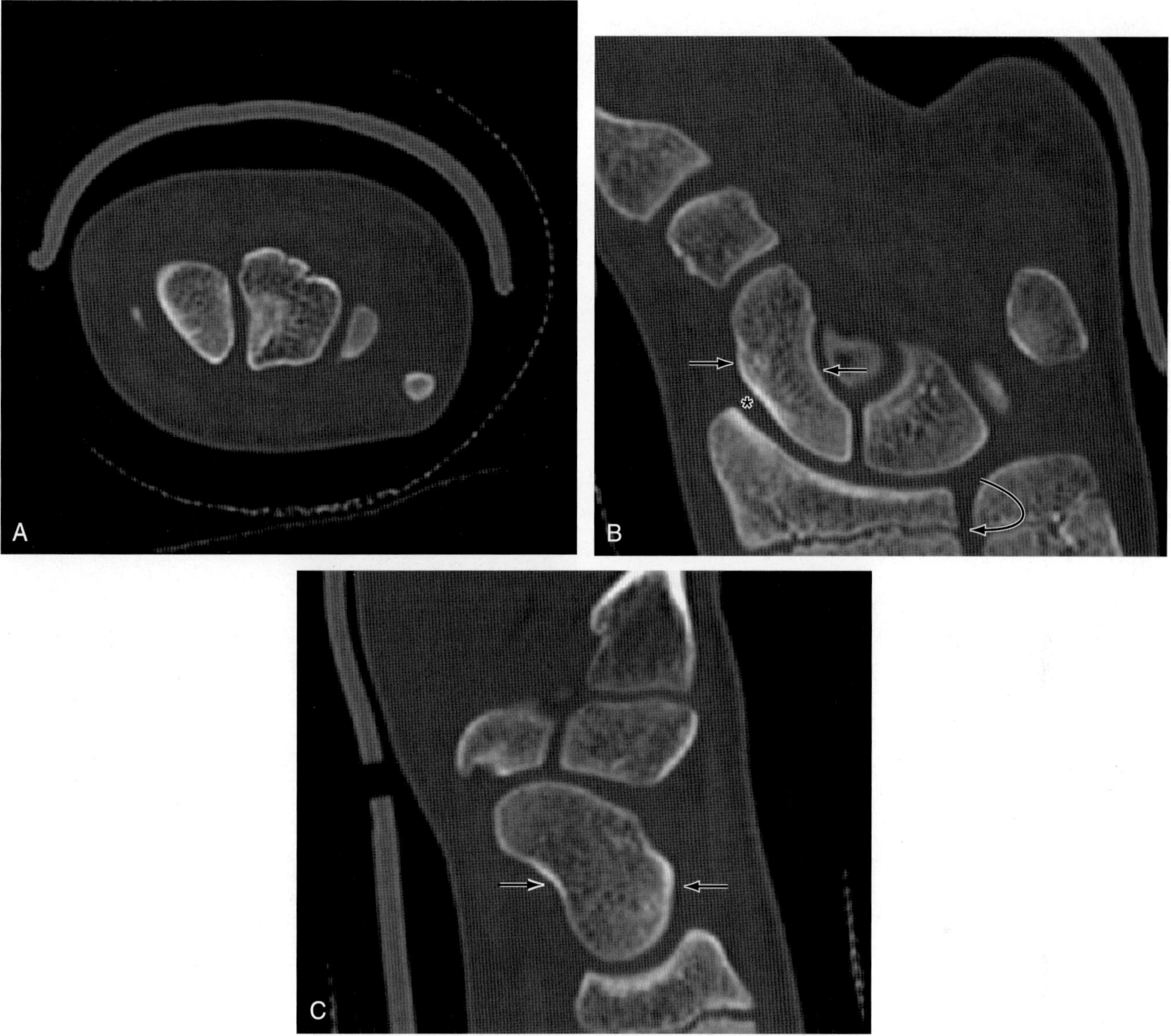

FIGURE 1-1. Normal MDCT of the right wrist in a 12-year-old female with a suspected scaphoid fracture. The patient's wrist was in a splint. **A,** Source axial image through the wrist. Thin (0.6 mm) slices obtained at 0.2-mm intervals provide excellent bone detail and allow for excellent image reformatting. **B,** Coronal MPRs through the wrist and **C,** oblique sagittal MPRs through the scaphoid demonstrate intact cortical margins of the scaphoid *(arrows)*. Note that the distal radius growth plate is intact *(curved arrow)* and that the radiocarpal joint space is preserved *(asterisk)*. All of these structures, which may mimic scaphoid pathology when injured, are nicely imaged on a routine exam.

Radiographs can diagnose fractures, dislocations, erosions, osteomyelitis, and a host of other disorders. In addition, radiography is inexpensive and widely available. Unfortunately radiographs suffer limitations and sometimes fail to diagnose the abnormality in question. For example, scaphoid fractures are frequently missed with radiographs. Radiographs also can misdiagnose femoral head collapse in patients with osteonecrosis.

Scaphoid wrist fractures can have poor outcomes if they are not recognized and treated. Fractures of the waist or proximal pole of the bone can disrupt the blood supply and lead to osteonecrosis of the proximal pole. Because the scaphoid has cortical surfaces that run in many planes and at various angles, fractures of the bone may be radiographically occult. In patients with persistent symptoms but negative or equivocal radiographs, MDCT or MRI can be used to diagnose a radiographically occult fracture. Theoretically MRI may be more sensitive than MDCT for detecting occult fractures because of superior contrast resolution that allows edema and hemorrhage and the fracture line to be identified. Currently, however, MDCT has superior spatial resolution and can visualize directly the cortical surfaces. Because the management of scaphoid injury requires visualization of the cortical surfaces and any cortical offset or discontinuity, MDCT is frequently ordered to diagnose radiographically occult fractures. Our hand surgeons reserve MRI for cases where MDCT is negative and concern for fracture persists or if there is concern for soft tissue damage.

> Because of its availability and ability to define cortical discontinuity and deformity, MDCT may be the imaging modality of choice for identifying acute, radiographically occult scaphoid fractures.

MDCT scanning for scaphoid fractures uses thin slices with overlap and a high-resolution filter for extreme bone detail. The images are acquired axially or oblique axially, and then MPRs are produced in the coronal and oblique sagittal planes, the latter along the long axis of the scaphoid (Figures 1-1 and 1-2). If necessary, patients can be scanned without removing their casts or splints.[7]

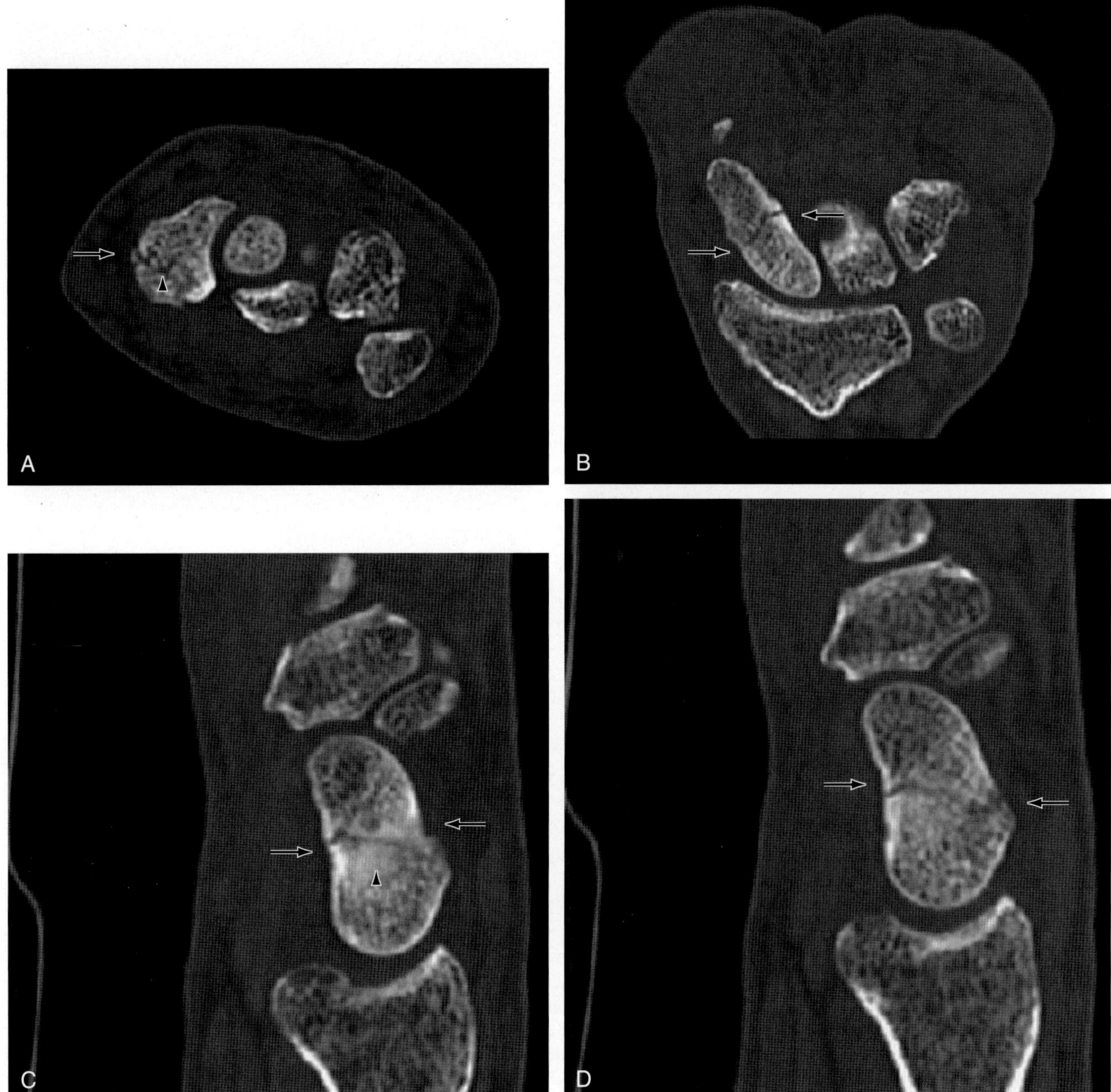

FIGURE 1-2. MDCT of the right wrist in a 22-year-old male with a scaphoid fracture. **A,** Thin slice source axial image demonstrates cortical disruption of the scaphoid bone *(arrow)* that extends through the trabecular bone *(arrowhead).* **B,** Coronal reformatted image through the wrist demonstrates the scaphoid waist fracture *(arrows).* **C** and **D,** Oblique sagittal reformatted images along the long axis of the scaphoid demonstrate the fracture most clearly. The fracture is seen extending through the entire bone *(arrows)* and early sclerosis is seen proximal to the fracture line *(arrowhead).* This sclerosis may reflect early osteonecrosis. Because thin slices with extensive overlap were used to obtain the source images, MPRs may be obtained in any plane with no loss of resolution.

A CT scan can be obtained with the extremity in a cast or splint.

The management of osteonecrosis of the femoral head relies on cortical integrity as well. Some surgeons will consider core decompression or free fibular graft transplant in young patients with stage III disease. However, once the femoral head collapses, those interventions are no longer tenable. Frequently, femoral head collapse is difficult to see with radiography, but MDCT can detect collapse easily. Moderately thick slices with 50% overlap are obtained in the axial orientation. Subsequently, coronal and sagittal MPRs are obtained. Even large patients or patients with prosthetic devices in the contralateral hip can be scanned, although the slice thickness and other parameters may require adjustment to increase mAs (Figure 1-3).

Imaging Patients with Orthopedic Hardware

Patients with orthopedic hardware devices frequently require imaging to evaluate the status of the device as well as the surrounding bone. For example, fixation devices for fractures can fail, and sometimes, even if the fixation device maintains its integrity, nonunion of

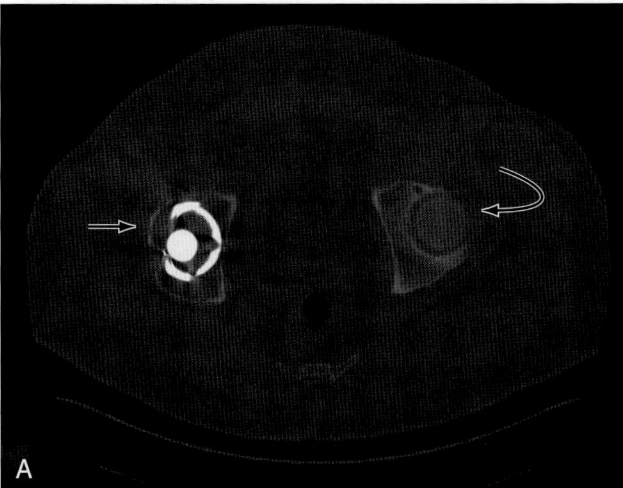

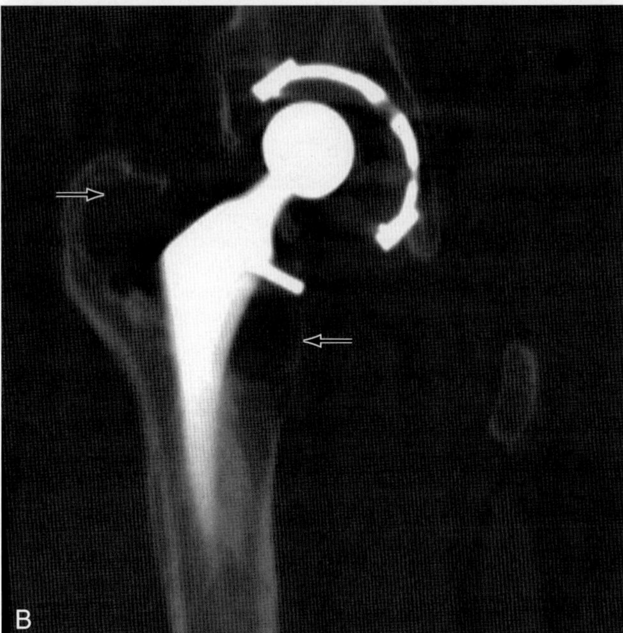

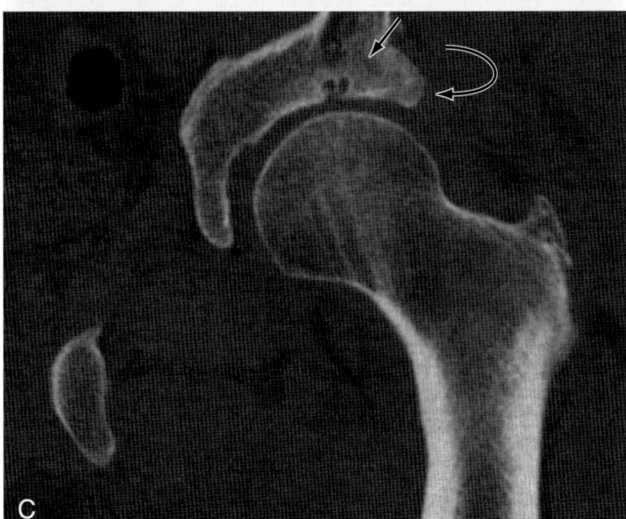

FIGURE 1-3. MDCT of both hips in a patient with a total hip replacement on the right and concern for loosening. **A,** Axial source image at the level of the femoral heads demonstrates the femoral head prosthesis on the right *(arrow)* and the native hip on the left *(curved arrow)*. **B,** Coronal multiplane reformatted image (MPR) of the right hip demonstrates the prosthesis in situ. There is cystic lucency about the proximal portion of the femoral component consistent with particle disease *(arrows)*. The eccentric position of the prosthetic femoral head within the acetabular component is due to the wear of the acetabular liner. **C,** Coronal MPR of the left hip shows mild to moderate degenerative changes. There is cyst formation and sclerosis in the superior acetabulum *(arrow)*, and the joint space is mildly narrowed in a superior-lateral orientation *(curved arrow)*. The high-mAs technique used in this exam allows scanning through the prosthesis, and the overlapping slices provide the data for excellent reformatted images. Note that the MPRs of each hip can be done separately from the source axial images through the pelvis. The separate MPR construction allows for optimal imaging of each hip. Despite the large prosthesis on the right side, fine bone detail can be visualized on the left side. (Images courtesy of the Department of Radiology, Indiana University School of Medicine, Indianapolis.)

the fracture can occur. Radiographs are frequently inconclusive, and magnetic resonance (MR) images can become badly degraded in the presence of metal. MDCT easily scans through such devices and can assess bone healing as well as the integrity of the device.

Small fixation devices require relatively high-resolution MDCT scans. Scans to evaluate scaphoid fracture fixation screws, for example, use thin, overlapping slices and high-resolution filters. The wrist is scanned axially or oblique axially, and MPRs are obtained coronally to the wrist and oblique sagittally to the long axis of the scaphoid or the fixation screw. Bony union or nonunion can be determined, and the status of the fixation screw can be assessed as well (Figures 1-4 and 1-5).

Large fixation devices can be scanned as well, but these scans require imaging parameters, such as thicker slices, that produce higher mAs.[9] A relatively low-resolution or soft-tissue filter is used. Again, the image data acquisition is axial, and MPR images are obtained in any desired plane. Because the scans are nearly isotropic and overlapping slices are used, the MPRs can be obliqued in any orientation without significant loss of spatial resolution (Figure 1-6).

The total hip prosthesis presents perhaps the most difficult situation for imaging. These implants are made of dense metal, are thick, have an interface to allow movement, and have a curved geometry. Despite the problems that such devices present, the need for imaging is increasing because the use of these devices increases each year for indications such as end-stage osteoarthritis or inflammatory disorders, osteonecrosis, and trauma. Indications for imaging patients with total hip implants include suspected loosening, infection, particle disease, and fracture.[6]

The nature of total hip prostheses necessitates high-mAs technique for adequate scanning. Relatively thick, overlapped slices are obtained axially with a low-resolution filter. However, with proper MDCT scanning parameters, high-quality source images and MPRs can be obtained, and the numerous causes of pain and failed hip prostheses can be evaluated (Figures 1-7 and 1-8). Because of the high-mAs technique (and therefore high radiation dose), such scanning should be reserved for an appropriate patient population.

Imaging Trauma Patients

Trauma patients present many difficulties for imaging. Injured patients more often than not are in pain. Because of the pain, they may not remain still and may not assume ideal positions for imaging. If they have suffered head trauma, they may not be able to cooperate. In fact, they may be combative. Frequently they are on trauma boards and may have their injured limbs in slings or external fixation devices. These factors may create patient movement and difficulty in positioning body parts.

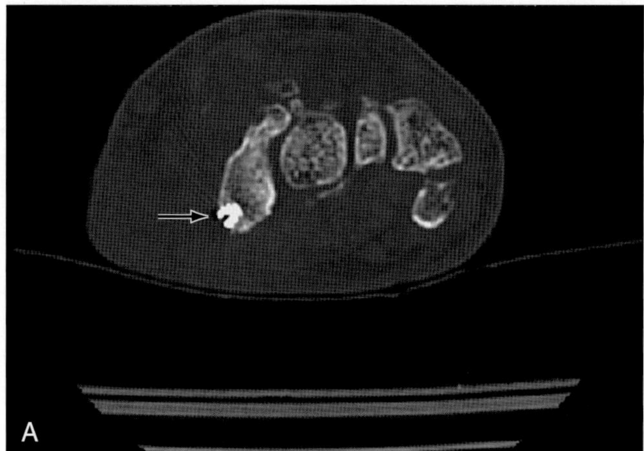

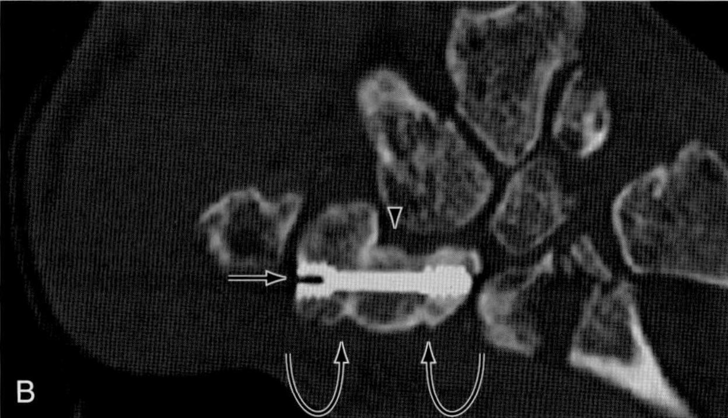

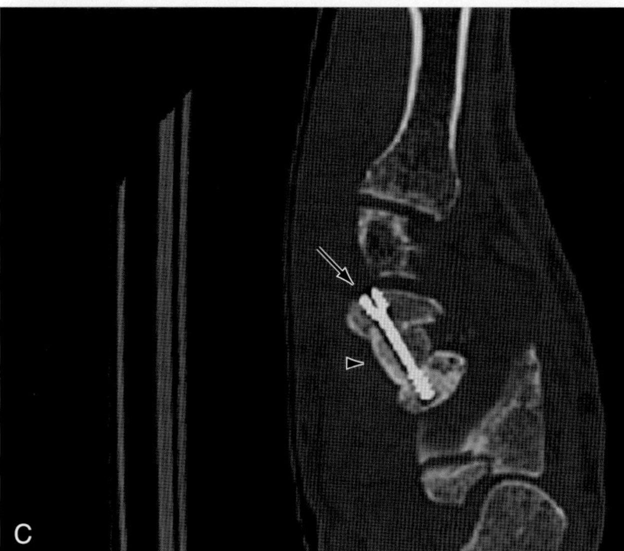

FIGURE 1-4. MDCT of the wrist in a 25-year-old male who is status-post successful bone grafting and Herbert screw placement for a scaphoid fracture. **A,** Source axial image through the wrist at the level of the scaphoid demonstrates the Herbert screw in situ *(arrow)*. **B,** Coronal MPR of the wrist oriented along the long axis of the Herbert screw *(arrow)* demonstrates the bone graft *(arrowhead)*. Bone healing has occurred on both sides of the graft *(curved arrows)*. **C,** Oblique sagittal images oriented along the long axis of the Herbert screw *(arrow)* also demonstrate the bone graft *(arrowhead)* and healing on both sides of the graft. The thin overlapping slices obtained in this scan allow for MPRs with incredible detail to be constructed even though orthopedic hardware is present.

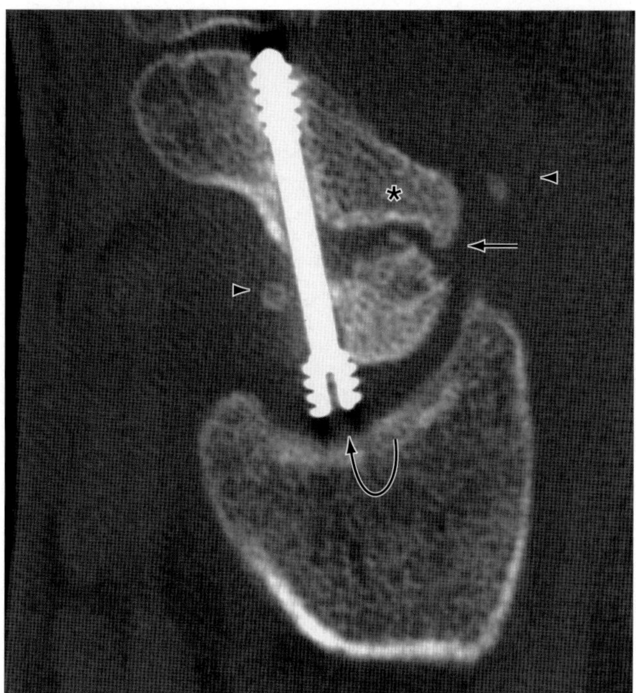

FIGURE 1-5. MDCT of the wrist in a patient with nonunion of a scaphoid fracture after Herbert screw placement. Oblique coronal MPR oriented along the long axis of the Herbert screw *(curved arrow)* demonstrates nonunion of the scaphoid at the fracture site *(arrow)*. Note the sclerosis along the distal portion of the fracture line *(asterisk)*. Bone fragments are seen *(arrowheads)*. Thin axial slices with 60% overlap were obtained to create this scan. The result is MPR images with incredible detail despite the presence of orthopedic hardware. Note that the screw threads are visible. (Image courtesy of the Department of Radiology, Indiana University School of Medicine, Indianapolis.)

MDCT is ideally suited to image these patients. As noted previously, the patient table on these systems has a variable speed. By increasing table speed, scans may be acquired more quickly and the effect of patient movement minimized. Likewise, scan time can be shortened by decreasing slice overlap and increasing slice thickness. The effect of increasing table speed and decreasing slice overlap is loss of mAs. The effect of increasing slice thickness is loss of spatial resolution. These trade-offs are manageable and acceptable to obtain a diagnostic scan in a badly hurt or uncooperative patient. Using these strategies, injuries that require immediate attention can be identified.

MDCT deals with the difficulty of positioning trauma patients through the use of isotropic or nearly isotropic imaging. Even if the obliquity used to scan a limb is not ideal, MPRs can be obtained. Because relatively thicker slices with little or no overlap may be used on a trauma patient, the data set may not be isotropic. Nonetheless, MPRs of some sort should be obtainable for initial evaluation. Once the patient is stable, more definitive scans may be obtained if indicated.

Even with trauma boards, splints, and external fixation devices in place, scans of injured limbs and joints may be obtained with appropriate MDCT technique. These scans are particularly valuable when assessing comminuted fractures around complex joints such as the shoulder, elbow, wrist, knee, and ankle. Spine trauma may be assessed as well. Again, the scanner's ability to obtain isometric or nearly isometric data sets overcomes problems with patient positioning. The ability to concurrently generate high mAs overcomes the issue of external fixation devices and other orthopaedic hardware (Figures 1-9 to 1-11).

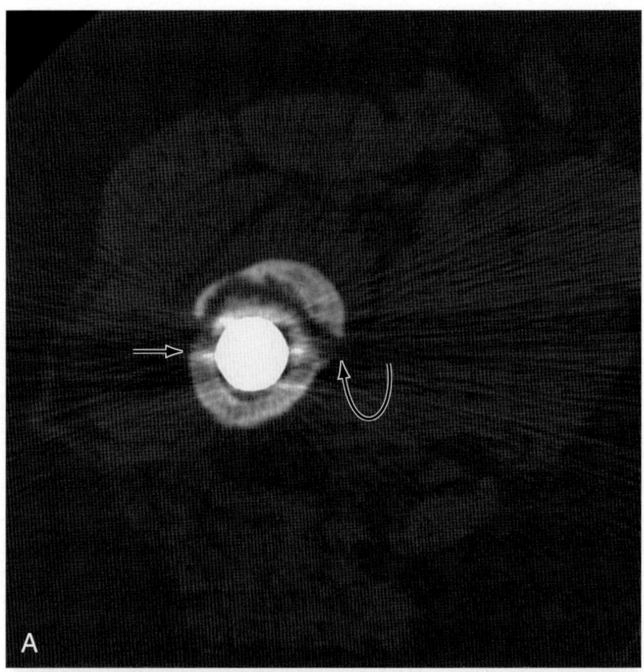

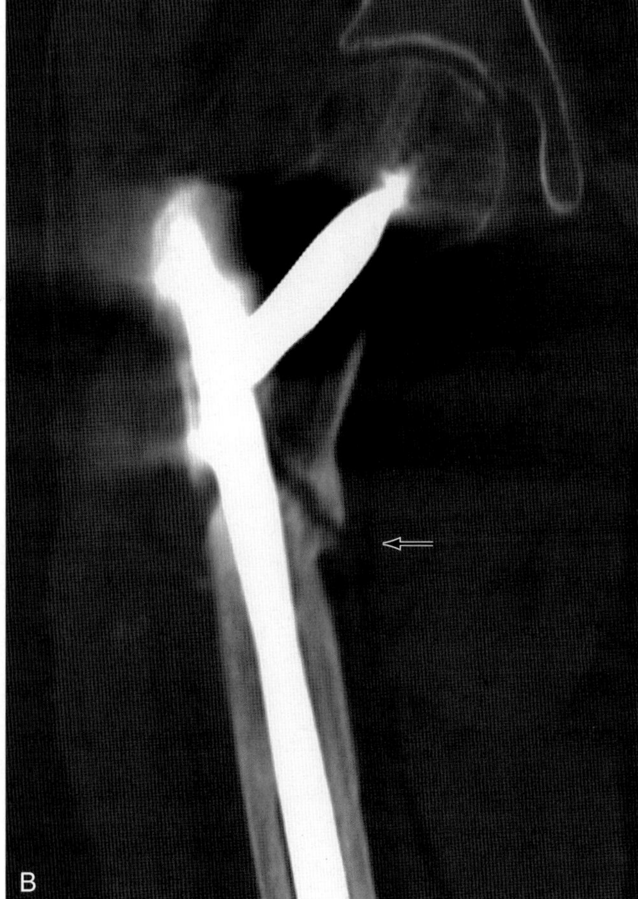

FIGURE 1-6. MDCT of a femoral nonunion after intramedullary (IM) rod placement. **A,** Source axial image through the right femur in a patient with an IM rod *(arrow)* in place for a proximal femoral fracture *(curved arrow)*. **B,** Coronal MPR image demonstrates the persistent fracture line *(arrow)* with sclerotic borders. MDCT imaging with high-mAs technique allows scanning through a large prosthesis and easy visualization of the surrounding osseous structures. (Images courtesy of the Department of Radiology, Indiana University School of Medicine, Indianapolis.)

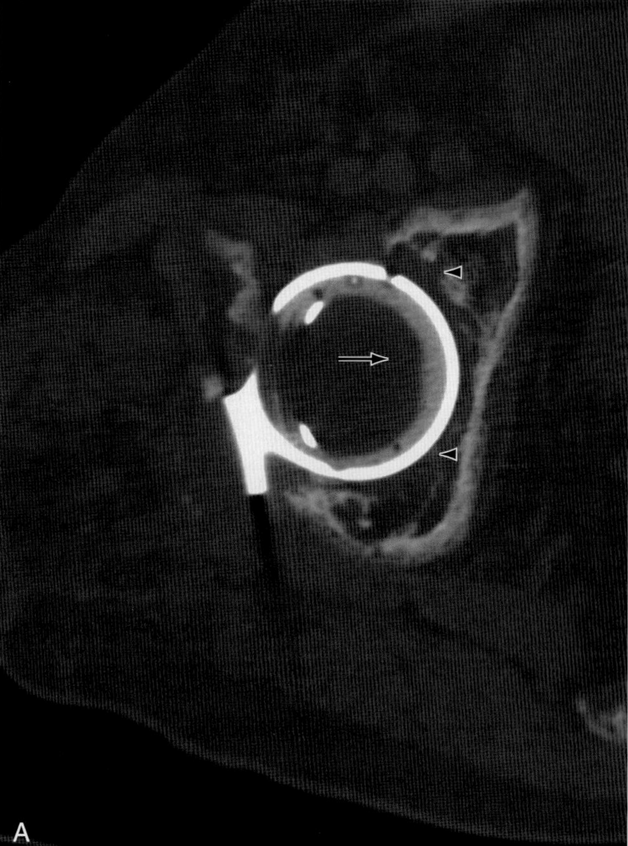

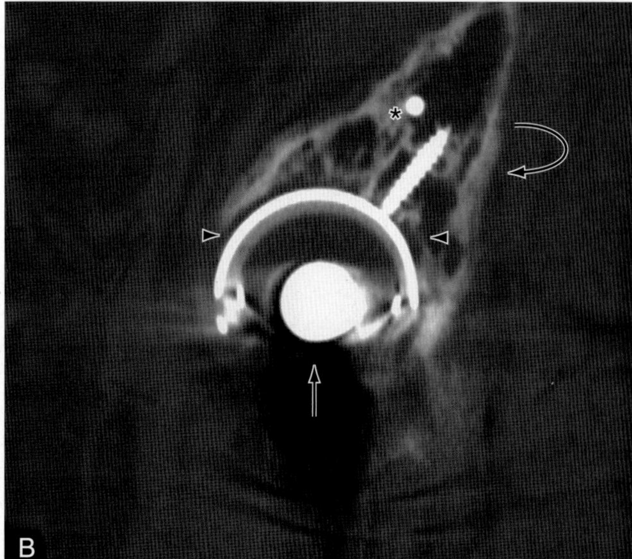

FIGURE 1-7. MDCT of a failed acetabular component in a patient with Paget's disease and a total hip replacement of the right hip. **A,** Source axial image with high-mAs technique demonstrates an acetabular component *(arrow)* with linear lucency between the prosthesis and the acetabular bone *(arrowheads)*. The circumferential lucency indicates loosening. **B,** Sagittal MPR image also shows the circumferential lucency *(arrowheads)*. The femoral component is seen on this image as well *(arrow)*. Despite the presence of a large metallic prosthesis, excellent bony detail is obtained. Note the thickened cortex *(curved arrow)* and trabeculae *(black asterisk)* in this patient with Paget's disease. Even though this scan utilized relatively thick slices, the threads of the acetabular fixation screw are visible. (Images courtesy of the Department of Radiology, Indiana University School of Medicine, Indianapolis.)

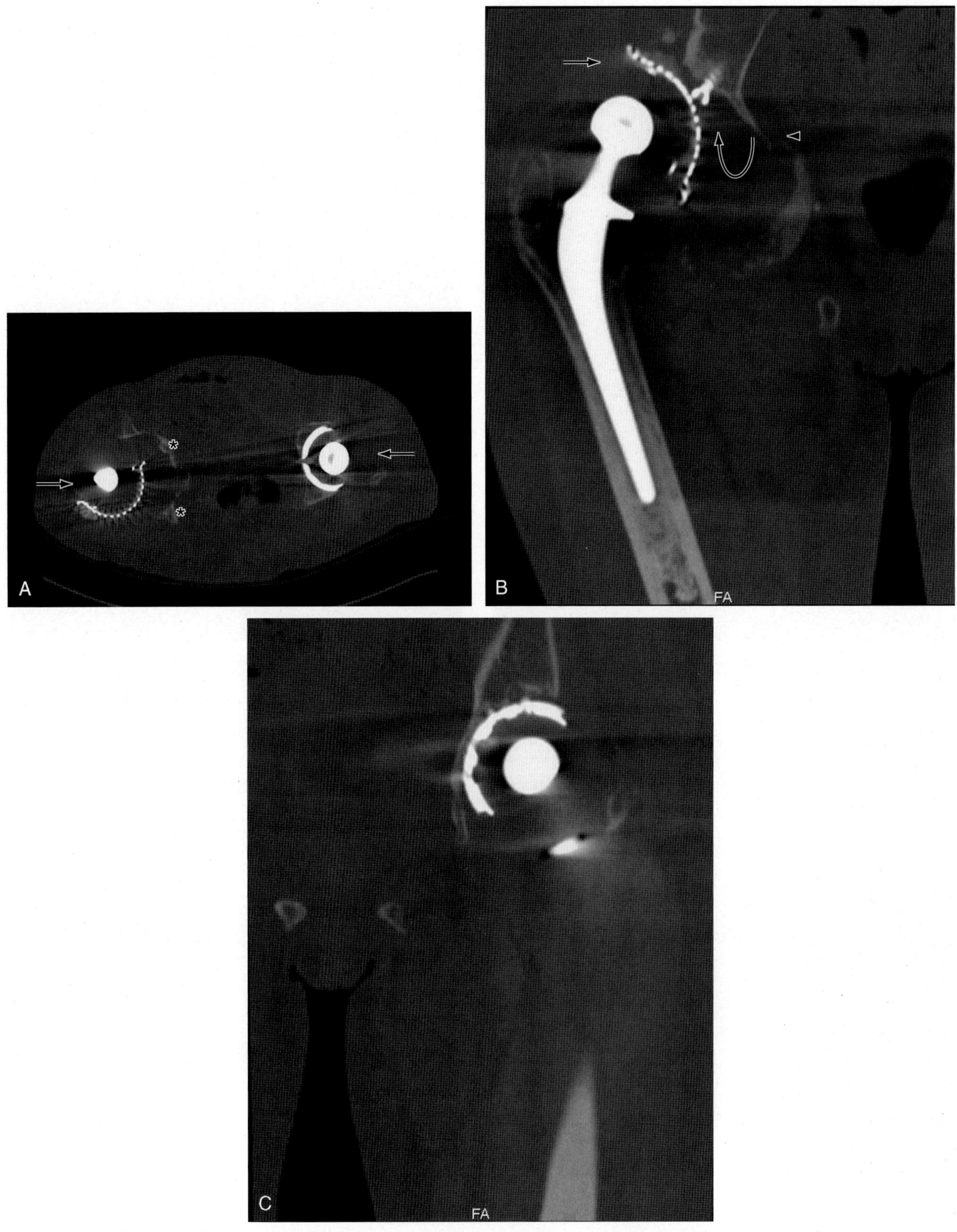

FIGURE 1-8. MDCT of a failed right hip prosthesis in a patient with bilateral hip replacements. **A,** Axial source image demonstrates a well-seated left hip prosthesis *(arrow)* but a poorly seated right hip prosthesis *(curved arrow)*. The right acetabular component is posteriorly rotated and is not in contact with the bony acetabulum *(asterisks)*. **B,** Coronal MPR of the right prosthesis demonstrates superior subluxation of the acetabular component *(arrow)* relative to the native joint. The acetabular fixation screw has no purchase of the acetabular component *(curved arrow)*. The native acetabulum is fractured *(arrowhead)*. **C,** Coronal MPR of the left hip demonstrates good alignment of the prosthesis. With the proper technique, MDCT allows clinically useful scanning despite the presence of two hip prostheses, each of which contains a large amount of dense metal. (Images courtesy of the Department of Radiology, Indiana University School of Medicine, Indianapolis.)

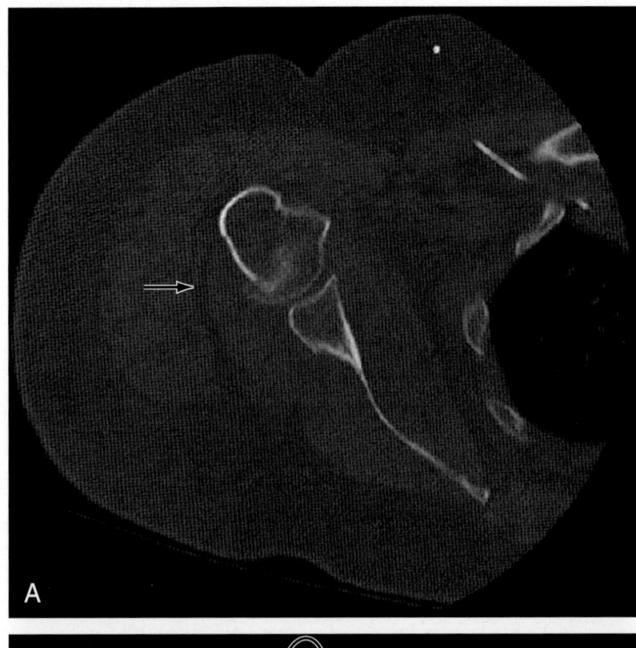

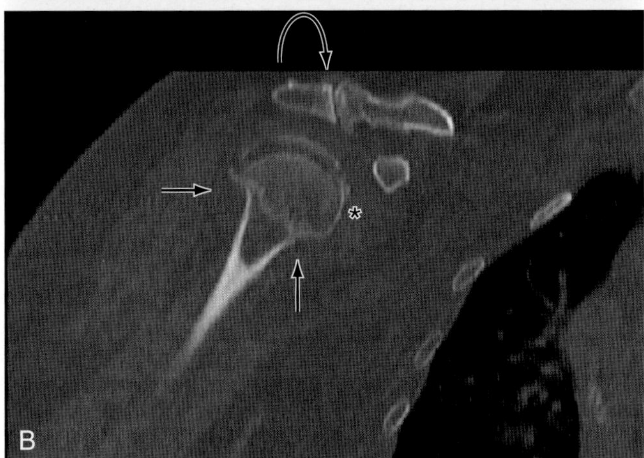

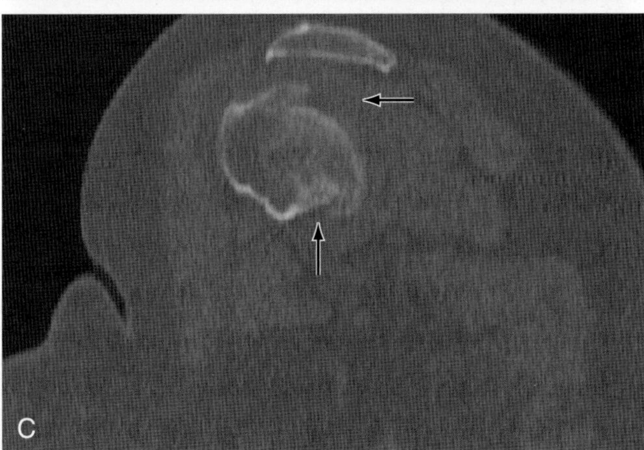

FIGURE 1-9. MDCT of a right humeral head fracture in a 62-year-old female. **A,** Source axial image through the humeral head demonstrates cortical disruption *(arrow)*. **B,** Coronal MPR image demonstrates the proximal humeral head fracture as well as impaction *(arrows)*. Note the effusion *(asterisk)* and the acromioclavicular degenerative disease *(curved arrow)*. **C,** Sagittal MPR image (anterior on the left) further demonstrates the degree of fracture and impaction *(arrows)*. The heavily overlapped source images allow construction of MPR images in any plane while maintaining excellent bone detail. This technique is useful in trauma patients who cannot move or position the injured body part.

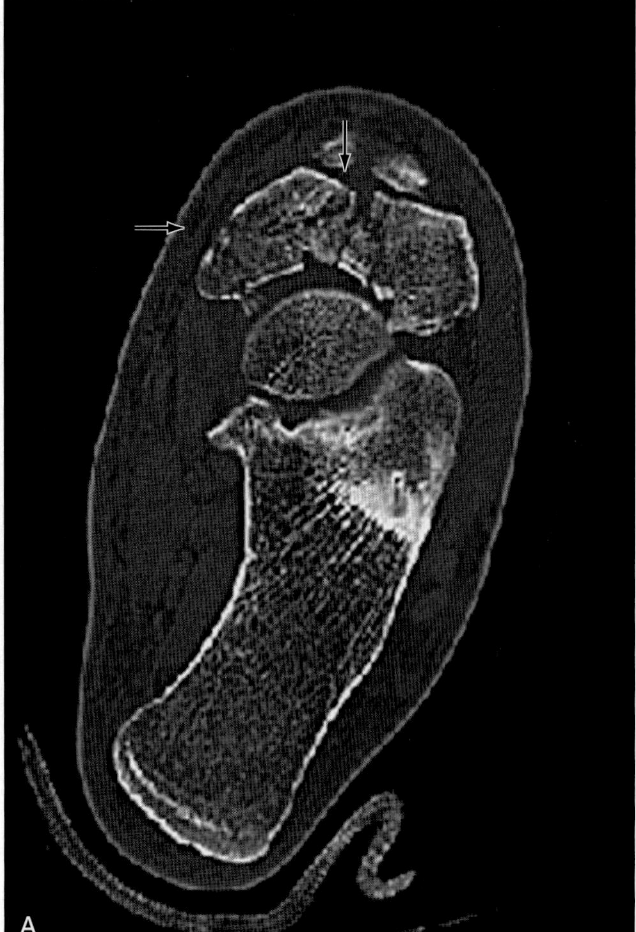

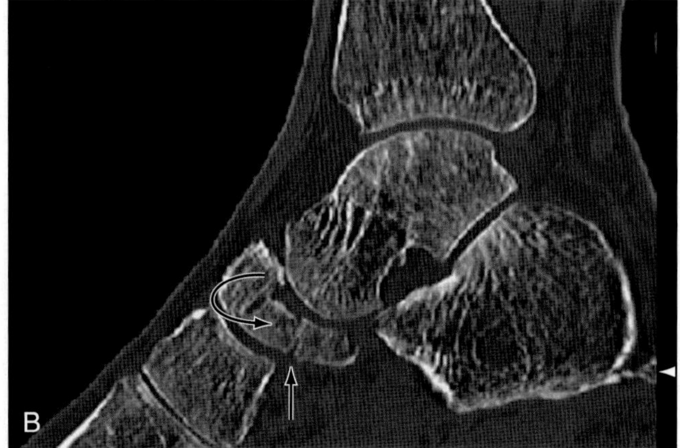

FIGURE 1-10. MDCT of an tarsal navicular fracture in a 41-year-old male. **A,** Axial source image demonstrates a badly comminuted navicular fracture *(arrows)*. **B,** Sagittal MPR image also shows the comminuted fracture *(arrow)* and the intraarticular extension *(curved arrow)*. Note also the calcaneal spur *(arrowhead)*. With proper scanning technique, such high-resolution scans may be obtained routinely despite the presence of splinting material.

MDCT ARTHROGRAPHY

The usual indications for CT or MDCT arthrography include patient contraindications to MRI and prior surgery in the area to be scanned (Box 1-1). The former indication follows from patient safety considerations. The latter follows from concerns

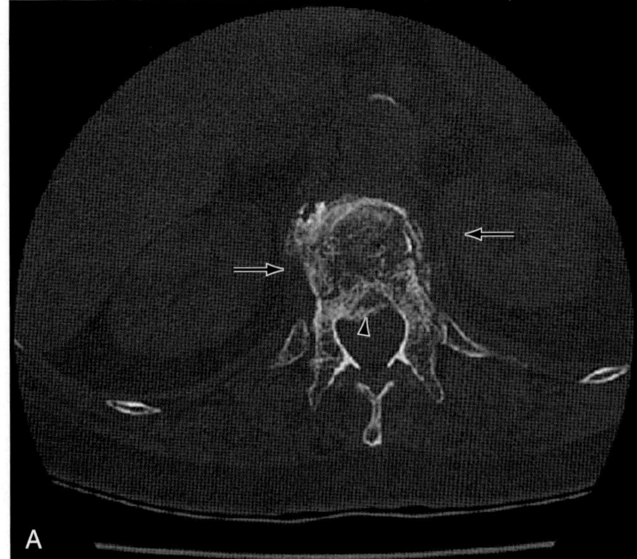

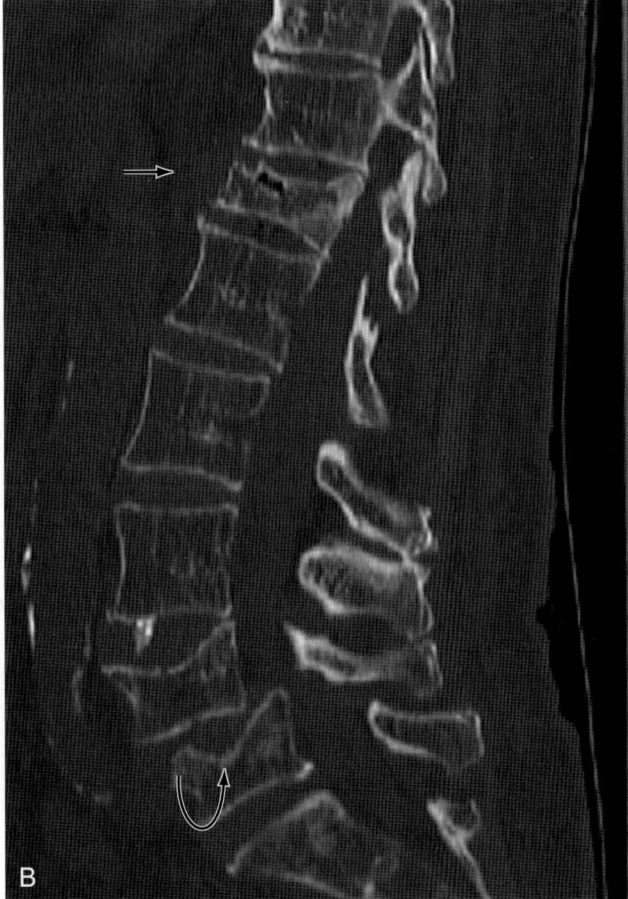

FIGURE 1-11. MDCT of the spine in an 83-year-old female with vertebral body fractures suffered in a motor vehicle accident. **A,** Source axial image through the T12 vertebral body demonstrates a fracture through the vertebral body *(arrows)* with retropulsion of bone fragments into the spinal canal *(arrowhead)*. **B,** Sagittal MPR image demonstrates compression of the superior end plate of the T12 vertebral body *(arrow)* with gas in the fracture. The gas indicates a chronic component to the endplate abnormality and a benign process (Kummell's disease). Note the increased bone density in this vertebral body, which may indicate a superimposed acute component to the endplate compression. The sagittal image also demonstrates a fracture involving the superior end plate of the L4 vertebral body *(curved arrow)*. This fracture is also associated with increased bone density. A subluxation is present at the L4-L5 level *(arrowhead)*. The bones appear osteopenic. This patient had pain relief from vertebroplasty at T12 and L4.

BOX 1-1. Indications for CT Arthrography

Contraindications to MR arthrography
Postoperative evaluations of joints
Equivocal cases of prosthetic loosening

for scan quality; postarthroscopic and postsurgical joints contain tiny pieces of metal that cause metallic dephasing artifact. This artifact can render MR and MR arthrographic scans nondiagnostic.

Fortunately, MDCT arthrography offers an excellent alternative.[8] In fact, in the postprocedural setting, even in the absence of metallic dephasing artifact, MDCT arthrography may be superior to MR arthrography for some indications. For example, MDCT arthrography may be superior to MR arthrography in diagnosing new tears in patients who are status postpartial meniscectomy. Likewise, the postsurgical shoulder labrum may be better assessed with MDCT arthrography. This debate is currently unsettled and certainly beyond the scope of this chapter. Nonetheless, it is important to emphasize that MDCT arthrography is an elegant imaging modality and highly accurate.

The features of MDCT that contribute to the production of excellent arthrographic images include excellent spatial resolution and isometric imaging, which in turn allows for MPRs in any plane, and speed, which minimizes the effect of patient motion.[5] With the addition of iodinated contrast into a joint, MDCT arthrography offers outstanding contrast resolution as well. In general, arthrography is simple and quick and has low morbidity.

An excellent use of MDCT arthrography is for evaluating possible internal derangement of the knee. The scans are obtained with thin overlapping slices. The combination of high spatial resolution and the addition of contrast into the knee joint allows outstanding visualization of the menisci and articular surfaces. Ligaments may be assessed as well, and the exam may be performed even with large orthopedic hardware in situ (Figures 1-12 and 1-13).

The high spatial resolution combined with intraarticular contrast (creating high-contrast resolution) makes the exam excellent for evaluating ligaments and articular surfaces of the wrist as well. In this case the thinnest slices possible are obtained with 50% to 60% overlap. MPR images can be produced in any plane after the source axial images are obtained (Figure 1-14). MDCT arthrography may be useful in equivocal cases of prosthesis loosening as well (Figure 1-15).

MDCT AND ARTHRITIS

Arthritis patients unfortunately suffer a host of ailments. Many of these involve the soft tissues around a joint. Patients may suffer from tenosynovitis, synovitis, and debris in joint spaces. MRI, under most circumstances, best images these abnormalities because of its unsurpassed tissue contrast resolution. For similar reasons, MRI is the modality of choice for detecting early erosions.

> MRI is the modality of choice for detecting early erosions in rheumatoid arthritis patients.

MDCT, as previously discussed, is useful in arthritis patients who have prostheses that may be problematic. The indications for MDCT in arthritis patients are the same for the population at large.

MDCT is also useful in arthritis patients to diagnose systemic manifestations of the disease. Rheumatoid patients, for example,

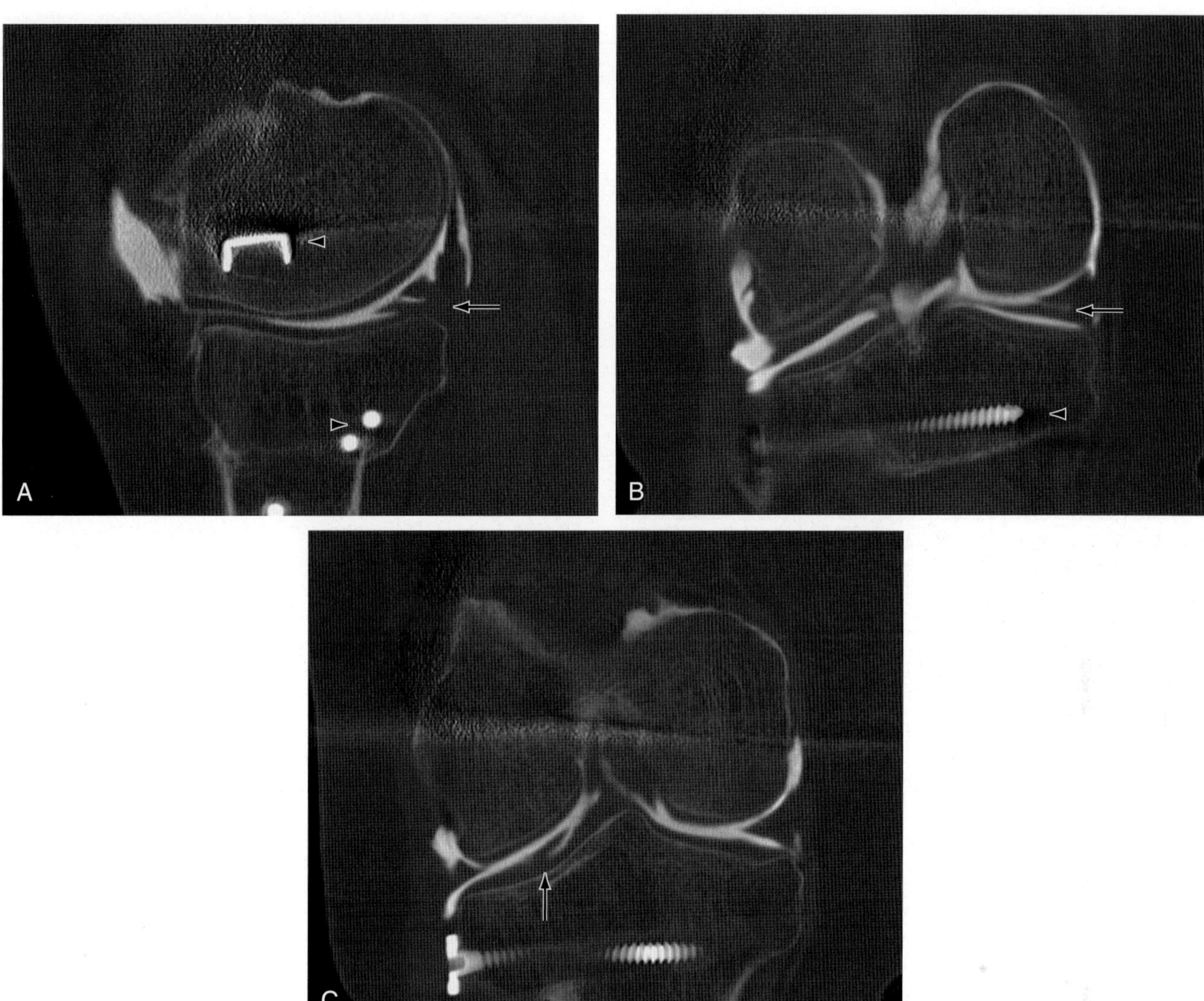

FIGURE 1-12. MDCT arthrogram of a medial meniscus tear in the right knee in a postoperative patient. **A,** Sagittal MPR image demonstrates the (white) contrast material injected into the joint extending into a tear of the posterior horn of the medial meniscus *(arrow)*. The menisci and articular cartilage are gray. Note the orthopedic hardware from prior surgery *(arrowheads)*. **B,** Coronal MPR also shows the medial meniscal tear *(arrow)* and orthopedic hardware *(arrowhead)*. **C,** Coronal MPR image at a different level demonstrates an articular cartilage fissure in the lateral tibial plateau *(arrow)* that has filled with the contrast. The source axial images were 2 mm thick and were obtained at 1-mm intervals. This data set allows high-resolution MPR images to be constructed despite the presence of orthopedic hardware. (Images courtesy of the Department of Radiology, Indiana University School of Medicine, Indianapolis.)

may have manifestations of the disease in a variety of organs. Because of its speed, scans of the lungs and of solid organs after contrast administration can be obtained in a few seconds. Such short scan time allows breath-hold exams even in debilitated patients, which result in exquisite images for accurate diagnoses (Figure 1-16). As 64-slice scanners become prevalent, MDCT angiography may be used routinely to screen high-risk patients for coronary artery disease.

MDCT AND PATIENT RADIATION DOSE

The dose effect on patients with MDCT is a complicated issue. On one hand, MDCT systems reduce patient radiation dose compared with older, single-beam CT systems because the newer scanners have more efficient beams (smaller penumbra) and less scatter for a given slice, given the same parameters. However, MDCT systems generally create more slices per scan with more overlap than single-slice systems, which increases dose. For musculoskeletal imaging, MDCT systems require scanning in one plane only; direct coronal and sagittal scans are replaced by MPRs, which decreases dose. Further complicating matters is the proliferation of new scanners with ever broader detector rows. The dose to the patient has not been measured for all of these systems for all types of scans.

Despite these confounding factors, some comments about patient dose from MDCT may be made to put radiation exposure in perspective. According to the U.S. Food and Drug Administration (FDA), a clinical CT scan of the head produces an effective dose of 2.0 millisieverts (mSv) and a clinical CT of the abdomen produces an effective dose of 10 mSv.[10] These numbers are comparable to 100 and 500 frontal-view chest x-rays. The radiation from a single frontal chest radiograph is equivalent to the effective

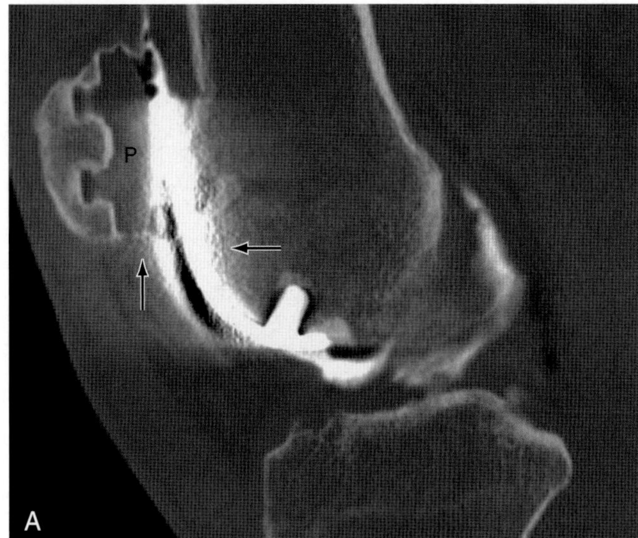

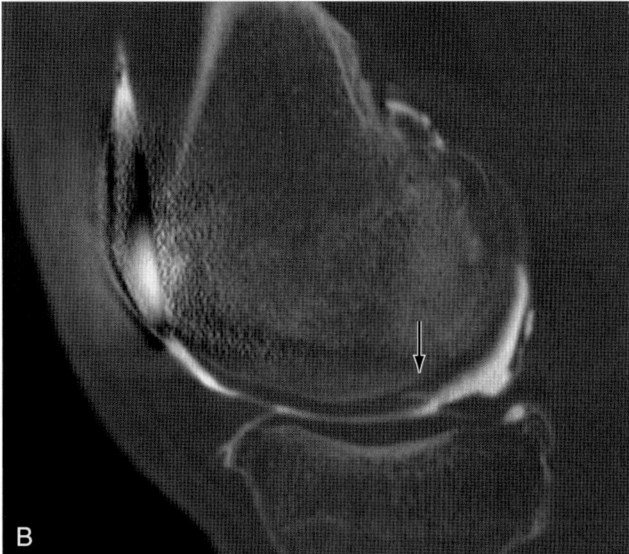

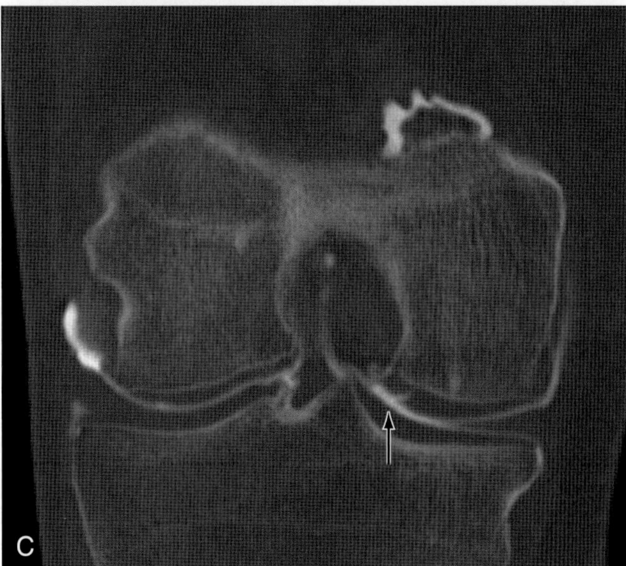

FIGURE 1-13. MDCT arthrogram of an articular cartilage fissure in a patient with a patellofemoral joint prosthesis. **A,** Sagittal MPR image demonstrates a patellofemoral prosthesis *(arrows)*. The femoral resurfacing component is made of dense metal, but the patellar component *(p)* is made of polyethylene that is nearly the density of soft tissue. **B,** Sagittal MPR image at a different level demonstrates an articular cartilage fissure in the medial femoral condyle *(arrow)*. **C,** Coronal MPR image demonstrates the articular cartilage fissure as well *(arrow)*. The triangular shapes of the normal menisci are clearly visible, outlined by the intraarticular contrast. These high-resolution images offer fine detail despite the presence of bulky orthopedic hardware. (Images courtesy of the Department of Radiology, Indiana University School of Medicine, Indianapolis.)

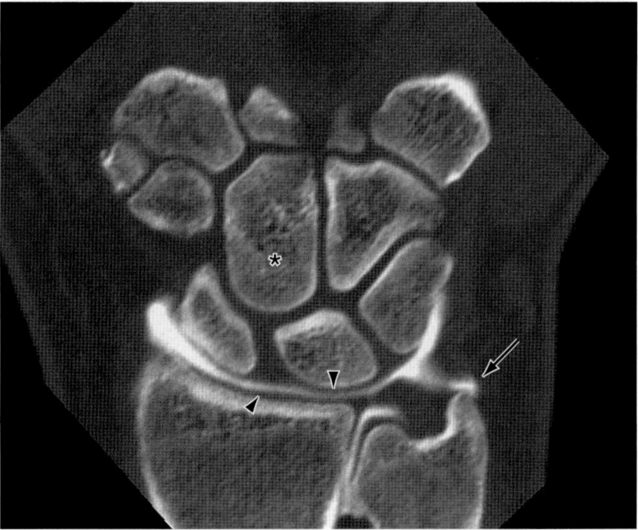

FIGURE 1-14. MDCT arthrogram of a triangular fibrocartilage complex (TFCC) tear of the wrist. Coronal MPR image from an MDCT arthrogram demonstrates contrast extending to the ulna styloid *(arrow)*. The contrast extension is abnormal and irregular and indicates a tear of the proximal ulnar limb of the TFCC. The combination of contrast material in the joint and high spatial resolution provides fine detail of the articular surfaces *(arrowheads)*. Note also the exquisite bone detail. For example, the trabecular pattern in the capitate is seen easily *(asterisk)*. (Image courtesy of the Department of Radiology, Indiana University School of Medicine, Indianapolis.)

dose of 2.4 days of natural background radiation. The number equivalent for a head CT is 243 days, and the number for an abdomen CT is 3.3 years. Also, according to the FDA, a CT exam with an effective dose of 10 mSv may be associated with an increase in the possibility of a fatal cancer of 1 in 2000 individuals. The natural incidence of fatal cancer risk in the United States is 1 in 5 individuals.

Although musculoskeletal MDCT scanning sometimes involves high effective dose, the scanned body part is often placed away from radiosensitive tissues in the brain, neck, chest, and abdomen. As with all exams that involve ionizing radiation, relative risk is involved. These relative risks must be weighed against the benefits derived from obtaining the scan and the natural incidence of fatal cancer, which is almost three orders of magnitude higher than the risk associated with a high-dose CT exam. Obviously, scan parameters should be optimized to minimize effective patient dose. As new MDCT systems enter clinical practice, the optimization process needs continuous attention. Attention should also be given to the number of repeat examinations patients undergo, which should be minimized, especially in sensitive areas, if possible.

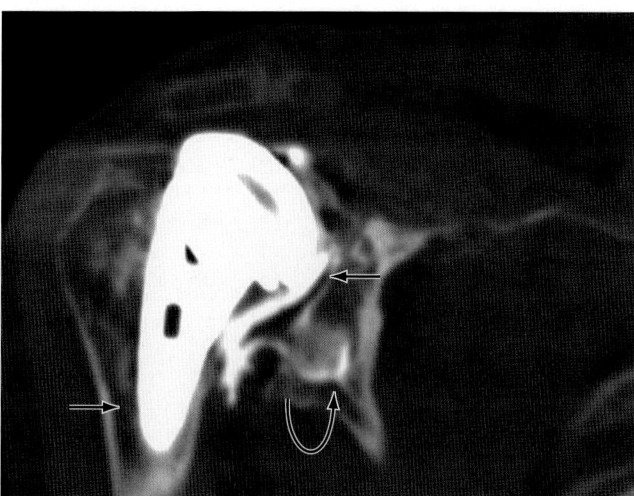

FIGURE 1-15. MDCT arthrogram of total shoulder prosthesis with glenoid component loosening. Coronal MPR image demonstrates total shoulder prosthesis of the right shoulder *(arrows)*. The humeral component appears well seated. However, contrast material extends deep to the glenoid component, between the cement-bone interface *(curved arrow)*. This contrast extension indicates loosening of the glenoid component. Because of the presence of the large humeral component, relatively thick source axial slices (3 mm) were used to achieve high-mAs technique. Nonetheless, the MPR images have acceptable spatial resolution and are diagnostic. (Image courtesy of the Department of Radiology, Indiana University School of Medicine, Indianapolis.)

3D IMAGES

3D image display may be particularly useful for analysis of complex fractures and curved surfaces and is used in cases of trauma, congenital abnormality, and arthritis. Three primary methods are used for rendering a volume of CT data to create 3D images: volume rendering (VR), shaded surface display (SSD), and maximum intensity projection (MIP). These techniques are well described in Choplin, Buckwalter, and Rydberg, et al.[11] Each has advantages and disadvantages, and the fine detail (e.g., a thin fracture line) seen on 2D images may be lost on the 3D display. VR programs may be helpful for displaying relationships of bone to soft tissue. MIP does not display the soft tissues well but is very useful when metal is present because of the decreased artifacts associated with this rendering technique.[11] MIP is frequently used to display contrast-enhanced blood vessels on CT or the high signal intensity of vessels on MRI. SSD is used when the analysis of the 3D shape of only one tissue type is desired. This method can produce a disarticulated view, which may be useful to understand fractures that extend to the articular cortex.[11]

CONCLUSION

MDCT is a versatile modality that complements existing imaging choices for the musculoskeletal system in some cases and replaces them in others. With appropriate scanning parameters, MDCT can produce high-resolution images that are extremely accurate. Current MDCT systems greatly enhance patient care, especially when high spatial resolution is required, a prosthesis is in place, or imaging is required in a postoperative setting. In conjunction with arthrography, MDCT can evaluate internal derangement as well.

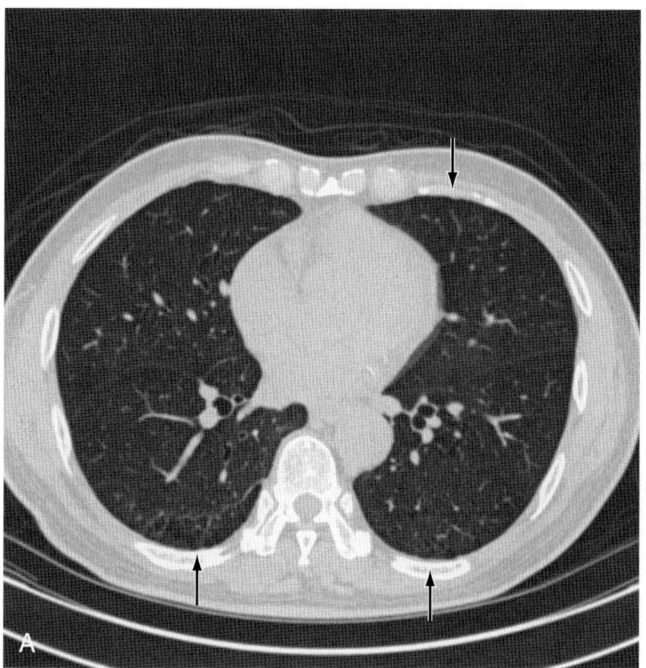

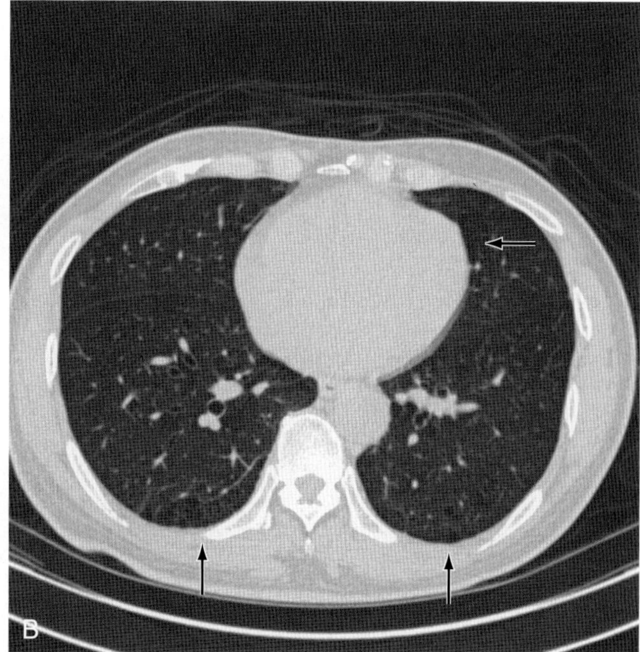

FIGURE 1-16. MDCT of the chest in a patient with rheumatoid arthritis. **A** and **B,** Axial MDCT images through the chest in a patient with rheumatoid arthritis show manifestations of rheumatoid lung, specifically honeycombing in a peripheral, basilar distribution *(arrows)*. MDCT allows images such as these to be obtained with a single breath hold, which creates sharp images of the lungs with high detail. The findings seen on this patient's CT were inconspicuous on radiographs of the chest. (Images courtesy of Dr. Francine Jacobson, Department of Radiology, Brigham and Women's Hospital, Boston.)

REFERENCES

1. Farber JM: Musculoskeletal applications of multichannel computed tomography, *Semin Musculoskelet Radiol* 8(2):135, 2004.
2. Rydberg J, Buckwalter KA, Caldemeyer KS et al: Multisection CT: scanning techniques and clinical applications, *Radiographics* 20(6):1787-1806, 2000.
3. Crow K, Buckwalter KA, Farber JM et al: *Isotropic imaging of the wrist with multidetector CT; a comparison of direct versus isotropic MPR imaging,* Radiologic Society of North America 87th Scientific Assembly and Annual Meeting poster presentation, Chicago, 2001.
4. Buckwalter KA, Rydberg J, Kopecky KK et al: Musculoskeletal imaging with multislice computed tomography, *Am J Roentgenol* 176(4):979-986, 2001.
5. Farber J. *CT arthrography and postoperative musculoskeletal imaging with current multichannel CT systems,* RSNA Categorical Course in Diagnostic Radiology: Musculoskeletal Imaging—Exploring New Limits 119-126, 2003.
6. Farber J, Buckwalter KM et al: *The role of multislice CT in evaluating particle disease of the hip: initial experience,* Society of Skeletal Radiogy 25th Annual Meeting oral presentation, Ponte Verde, Fla., 2002.
7. Farber J, Brandser E, Sommerkamp C et al: *The effect of wrist positioning on MDCT multiplanar image quality when evaluating acute, chronic and fixated scaphoid fractures,* Society of Skeletal Radiogy 29th Annual Meeting oral presentation, Tucson, Ariz., 2006.
8. Vande Berg BC, Lecouvet FE, Poilvache P et al: Dual-detector spiral CT arthrography of the knee: accuracy for detection of meniscal abnormalities and unstable meniscal tears, *Radiology* 216:851-857, 2000.
9. Fishman EK, Magid D, Robertson DD et al: Metallic hip implants: CT with multiplanar reconstruction, *Radiology* 160:675-681, 1986.
10. U.S. Food and Drug Administration, Centers for Devices and Radiological Health. Whole body scanning using computed tomography (CT): what are the radiation risks from CT?.

CHAPTER 2

Scintigraphy of the Musculoskeletal System

NAYER NIKPOOR, MD

KEY FACTS

- The three-phase bone scan consists of (1) an early blood flow phase that reflects vascularity, (2) a blood pool phase that shows the level of soft tissue involvement, and (3) delayed images (2 to 4 hours after injection) that reflect the osteoblastic response to the underlying disease.
- A normal bone scan essentially excludes osteomyelitis.
- Indium white blood cell scanning requires in vitro labeling of 40 mL of the patient's blood for imaging.
- Gallium scans are interpreted by comparison to bone scan images; if gallium uptake exceeds that of the bone scan uptake or differs in distribution from the area of bone scan uptake (termed *incongruent uptake*), then osteomyelitis is likely.
- Unlike the bone scan, Gallum-67 citrate activity returns to baseline approximately 6 weeks after successful treatment of osteomyelitis and can therefore be used to monitor the clinical course of the disease.
- Indium scanning may be falsely negative in patients with vertebral osteomyelitis and discitis.
- Magnetic resonance imaging (MRI) is more sensitive and specific than scintigraphy for identifying radiographically occult scaphoid fractures.
- In elderly patients, it may take several days for an acute fracture to be seen on a bone scan.
- After a fracture, the delayed images of a bone scan may remain positive for years; an abnormal scan has been reported as long as 40 years.
- A healing "flare phenomenon" has been described as increased radiotracer uptake in an area of previously noted skeletal metastasis on a bone scan associated with increased sclerosis on radiographs or CT scan. A flare phenomenon is usually seen during the first 3 months after chemotherapy and represents a favourable response to therapy.

PRINCIPLES OF MUSCULOSKELETAL SCINTIGRAPHY

Nuclear medicine plays an important role in the diagnosis and management of various skeletal diseases. Bone scanning reflects changes in bone physiology in response to underlying disease. Diphosphonate compounds (methylene diphosphonate [MDP], hydroxymethylene diphosphonate [HDP]) labeled with technetium-99 (Tc-99m) are the radiotracers of choice for routine bone scintigraphy. In addition to diphosphonates, other radiopharmaceuticals are useful for skeletal imaging (Table 2-1).

Technical Considerations

Radiopharmaceuticals such as Tc-99m MDP or Tc-99m HDP should be used within 2 hours and no later than 6 hours after preparation. These compounds decompose with time due to the oxidation-reduction process and result in excess free pertechnetate that may degrade the image. The recommended dose of Tc-99m MDP is 20 to 25 millicurie (mCi) (750 to 900 megabecquerel [MBQ]). Hydration of the patient before imaging is useful; it is suggested that the patient drink 4 to 6 glasses of water between injection of the isotope and imaging. The time of imaging depends on age; in patients younger than 20 years, imaging is done 2 hours after injection, and in older patients, a 3- to 4-hour delay is recommended to provide better image quality.

Imaging Technique

Whole body anterior and posterior images are routinely performed. These may be supplemented by single photon emission computed tomography (SPECT) images or pinhole (high resolution) views of a hip, wrist, or ankle for further evaluation of an area of interest. Sedation for patients younger than 4 years or older patients who are mentally challenged is recommended. When scans are interpreted, consideration is given to the positioning of the patient under the camera, the clinical information, and the biodistribution of the radiotracer; lack of knowledge about any of these factors may lead to false-positive or false-negative readings.

What Is SPECT?

SPECT (SPET in Europe) is a routine technique used in nearly any nuclear medicine department. With SPECT, the gamma camera (either single- or multi-head camera) moves around, viewing the patient from at least 180 degrees. For musculoskeletal imaging, 360 degrees of rotation is required for accurate image reconstruction; 180 degrees of rotation is usually used for cardiac imaging. The data set after SPECT imaging is reconstructed by filtered-back projection methods. The SPECT slices are viewed in the transverse, sagittal, or coronal planes or as three-dimensional (3D) representation of the organ. The main advantage of SPECT is the ability to view the reconstructed image in multiple planes and to separate overlapping structures. As much as a sixfold increase in image contrast can be obtained with SPECT. The anatomic location of various areas of increased or decreased radiopharmaceutical uptake can be better defined spatially. Recent technologic advances of SPECT imaging provide fusion of SPECT images with computed tomography (CT) or magnetic resonance imaging (MRI) to better identify the location of lesions.

TABLE 2-1. Common Radiopharmaceuticals for Skeletal Imaging

Radiotracer	Physiologic Half-Life	Mode of Photon Decay	Energy (kev)	Mode of Production	Critical Organ
Tc-99m diphosphonate MDP/HDP	6.0 hours	IT	140	Reactor	Bladder
In-111 oxine	2.81 days	EC	172, 247	Accelerator	Spleen
Gallium-67 citrate	78.1 hours	EC	93,185, 300, 394	Accelerator	Large bowel
F-18 FDG	110 minutes	B+	511	Accelerator	Bladder
Thallium 201 chloride	73.1 hours	EC	81	Accelerator	Renal cortex

Bt, Positron; *EC*, electron capture; *IT*, isomeric transformation.
Total body radiation dose from radiopharmaceuticals commonly used for skeletal imaging is less than 1 RAD per scan.

What Is a Pinhole Collimator?

The selection of a particular type of collimator is made primarily on the basis of the size or area of the organ to be imaged and on the degree of detail desired in the anatomy. When the target area is not too large and higher-resolution scintigraphy and greater detail are desired, the pinhole collimator is used. A pinhole collimator is a cone-shaped lead shield, which tapers into a small aperture perforated at the center of the tip at a distance from the detector face. The geometry of the pinhole creates an inverted image of the target organ in the detector from the photons traveling through a small aperture. Any change in pinhole collimator design can affect lesion detectability by altering the spatial resolution and sensitivity. Common indications for pinhole imaging of the skeleton are the evaluation of Legg-Perthes disease (osteonecrosis of the hip in children) and better localization of fractures of the small bones in the wrist or ankle. In general nuclear medicine, the pinhole collimator is used routinely for imaging the thyroid or for renal cortical scintigraphy using technetium (dimercaptosuccinic acid) (Tc-DMSA) in cases of pyelonephritis.

What Is a Three-Phase Bone Scan?

The three-phase bone scan is primarily used to differentiate cellulitis from osteomyelitis. It can also be used for the diagnosis of osteoid osteoma, acute stress fracture, and reflex sympathetic dystrophy (RSD) (Box 2-1).

Acquisition

Images are obtained at specific time periods after isotope injection to demonstrate different physiologic information. Three phases are usually described (Table 2-2).

Phase one: A dynamic flow study (radionuclide angiogram) consists of images obtained at 1-second intervals for 60 seconds after the intravenous injection of the radiopharmaceutical. The egion of interest should be within the camera's field of view.

Phase two: Immediately following the angiogram, static ("blood pool") images are obtained of the specific area or, when the localization of a lesion is not clear, a whole body image can be acquired.

Phase three: Delayed images are acquired 2 to 4 hours after injection of radiopharmaceutical.

BOX 2-1. Indications for a Three-Phase Bone Scan

Cellulitis versus osteomyelitis
Suspected osteoid osteoma
Suspected acute stress fracture
Suspected reflex sympathetic dystrophy

TABLE 2-2. The Three-Phase Bone Scan

Phase	Name	Time after Injection	Purpose
One	Radionuclide angiogram (Blood flow)	2 to 4 hours	Reflects vascularity
Two	Blood pool	Few minutes	Reflects soft tissue involvement
Three	Delayed	Immediate	Reflects osteoblastic response

Interpretation

Blood flow images reflect the vascular supply (vascularity), blood pool images show the level of soft tissue involvement, and delayed images indicate osteoblastic response to the underlying disease (Figure 2-1, *A* to *C*).

What Is PET Imaging?

Positron emission tomography (PET) is a functional imaging technique using radionuclides (frequently F-18 FDG [fluoro-2-deoxy-D-glucose]) that measure the metabolic activity of the cell. This technique has broad clinical applications in oncology as well as for evaluation of neurologic and cardiac disorders. Oncology patients are asked to fast 4 to 6 hours prior to the examination.

A recent advance that combines functional imaging and CT, the PET/CT scanner, has reduced the study duration by eliminating the lengthy PET transmission scan and also provides accurate anatomic localization of functional abnormalities. A PET scanner provides resolution in the 7-mm to 10-mm range. Because the urinary bladder wall is the critical organ, hydration and frequent emptying of the bladder are recommended practices.

There are no absolute contraindications for PET imaging. A relative contraindication is pregnancy. Breastfeeding can resume 24 hours after isotope injection.

SCINTIGRAPHY OF INFLAMMATORY BONE DISEASES

Rheumatoid Arthritis

Accurate detection of the early synovitis in rheumatoid arthritis (RA) and other destructive inflammatory joint diseases is important to establish the most appropriate treatment and indicate prognosis. There has been no gold-standard study for the detection of synovitis activity[1]; MRI may be developing into a gold standard, but it is limited in the number of joints that can be assessed at

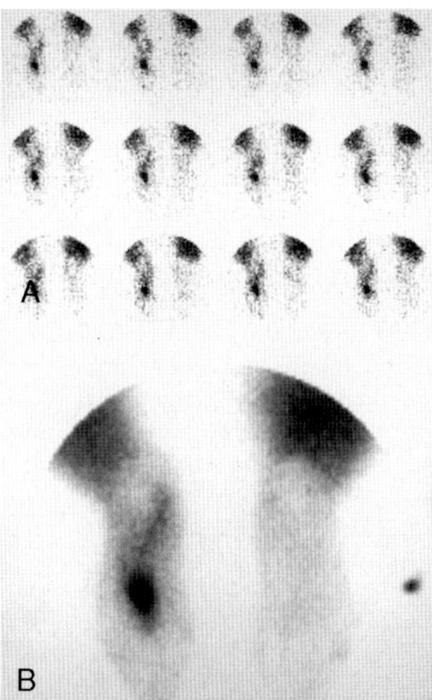

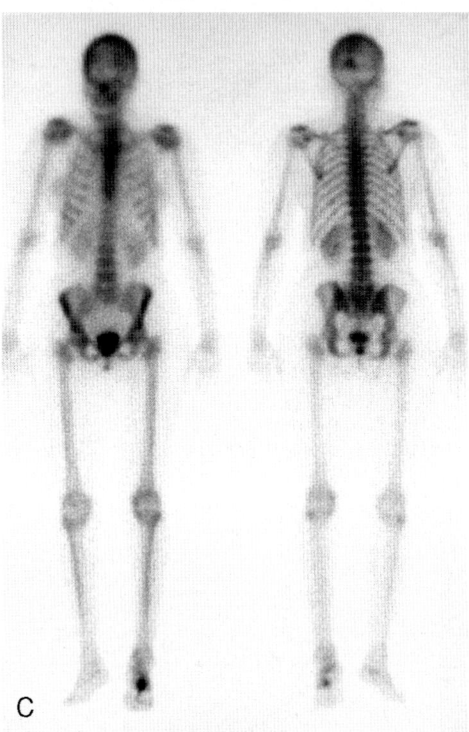

FIGURE 2-1. Osteomyelitis. Dynamic blood flow **(A)**, static blood pool **(B)**, and delayed **(C)** images of a three-phase bone scan show focal increased uptake in the left second metatarsal in a patient with osteomyelitis. The findings are not specific, and a similar pattern of uptake could indicate an acute fracture. Clinical and imaging correlations are therefore necessary.

one time. Bone scintigraphy is sensitive but not specific for the diagnosis of RA. In the acute stage of RA, the three-phase bone scan is positive. In the subacute and chronic stages of the disease, there is symmetric increased uptake, especially on delayed images, around affected joints (Figure 2-2).

Labeled leukocytes are a promising method to evaluate the activity of the disease. The applicability of Tc-99m hexamethylpropylene amine oxime (HMPAO) labeled leukocyte scintigraphy in assessment of disease activity was tested in 21 patients with RA by Goal et al.[2] In this study, significant correlation was found between labeled leukocyte accumulation in the hands and feet and clinical assessment of joint activity. F-18 FDG PET as a metabolic imaging device might be able to detect early inflammation. In addition, PET allows quantitation of F-18 FDG uptake, by which means disease activity can be assessed.[3]

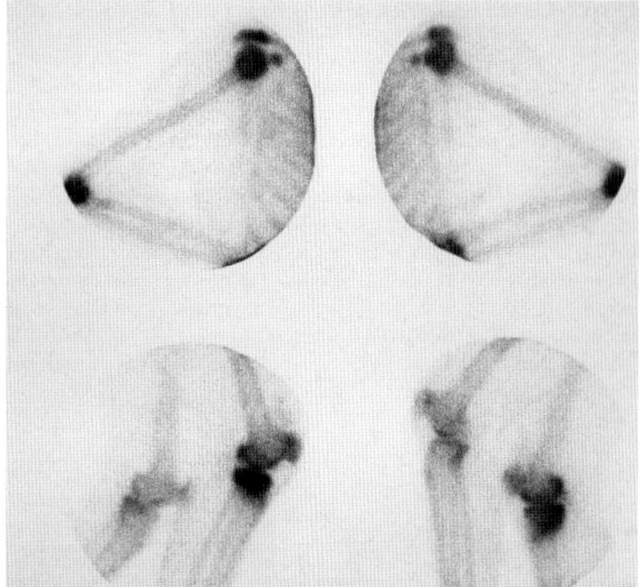

FIGURE 2-2. Rheumatoid arthritis (RA) in a 45-year-old female. Multiple spot views from a bone scan show bilateral, symmetric radiotracer uptake in the elbows and shoulders and unilateral uptake in the left knee. Symmetric uptake is a typical finding in RA.

Osteoarthritis

Osteoarthritic changes can usually be demonstrated on standard radiographs. The blood flow and blood pool images of the bone scan usually do not show significant uptake. Delayed images, however, show increased periarticular uptake in a distribution typical of osteoarthritis (e.g., the thumb bases). Such findings are often incidentally seen on bone scans. The degree of uptake is proportional to the severity of disease.

Sacroiliitis

The role of scintigraphy in the evaluation of patients with sacroiliitis is controversial. Planar and SPECT bone scintigraphy and Tc-99m sulfur colloid scanning with quantitative methods have all been used for the diagnosis. A combination of bone (Tc-99m MDP) and bone marrow (Tc-99m sulfur colloid) scanning may be useful in patients with active sacroiliitis.[4] Increased Tc-99m MDP uptake with decreased or normal sulfur colloid uptake was the most common scintigraphic pattern in the acute phase of sacroiliitis in one study in which radiographic findings were normal or only slightly abnormal. SPECT bone scan was found to have the best accuracy (97% sensitivity, 90% specificity).[5]

SCINTIGRAPHY IN SKELETAL INFECTION

When confronted with the potential diagnosis of an early skeletal infection, both morphologic and functional imaging modalities are frequently employed. The choice of imaging modality often depends mainly on whether or not the bone has been previously affected by another disease or surgery.

Ga67-Citrate Imaging

Unlike the bone scan, Ga-67 citrate activity returns to baseline approximately 6 weeks after successful treatment of osteomyelitis and can therefore be used to monitor the clinical course of the disease.[6,7] The sensitivity of Ga-67 for acute osteomyelitis is 80% to 85%. Positive gallium scans may also be seen with primary skeletal tumor, skeletal metastasis, chronic infection, and septic inflammatory and traumatic lesions[8]; therefore specificity is low, approximately 70%. To improve the specificity, Tumeh et al.[9] suggested that osteomyelitis is more likely to be present when gallium uptake exceeds that of Tc-99m MDP (bone scan) uptake or differs in distribution (termed *incongruent* uptake) (Figure 2-3, *A* to *C*). If gallium uptake is less than that of Tc-99m MDP uptake, infection is unlikely. If uptake on both exams is equivalent, the finding may be indeterminant, a circumstance seen mainly with preexisting abnormalities such as diabetes or posttraumatic changes. Gallium scanning may not be able to differentiate osteomyelitis from neuropathy or healing fracture[10]; in these conditions, In-111 white blood cell (WBC) scanning is useful. SPECT gallium and SPECT bone scans are more sensitive than planar gallium and planar bone scans specifically for vertebral osteomyelitis.[11,12]

In-111 Leukocyte Imaging

In-111 oxine and Tc-99m HMPAO labeled leukocyte imaging are widely used in the diagnosis of osteomyelitis. An overall sensitivity of 88% and specificity of 91% are reported for osteomyelitis.[13] These studies are especially useful in excluding infection in a previously violated bone such as may occur from prior trauma,

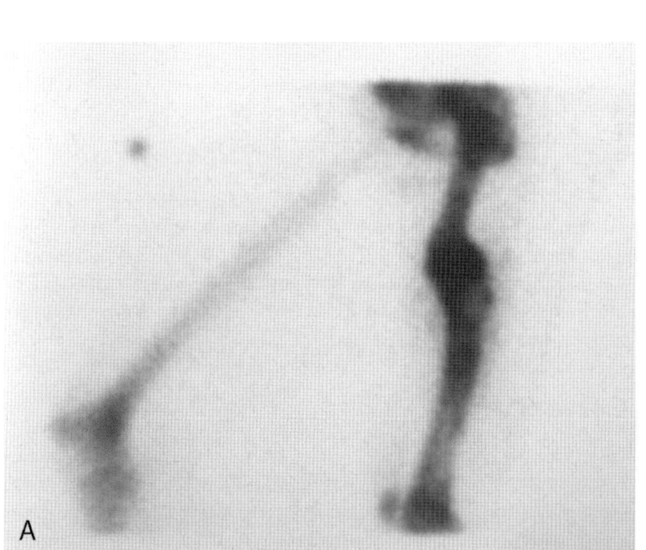

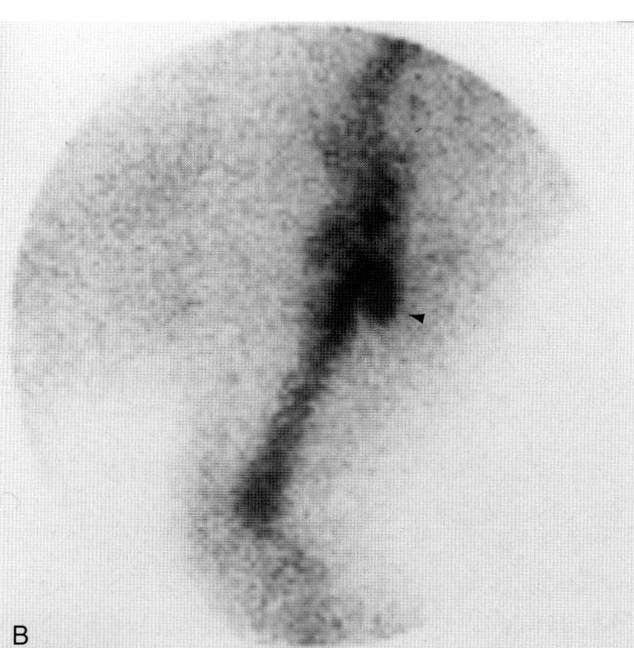

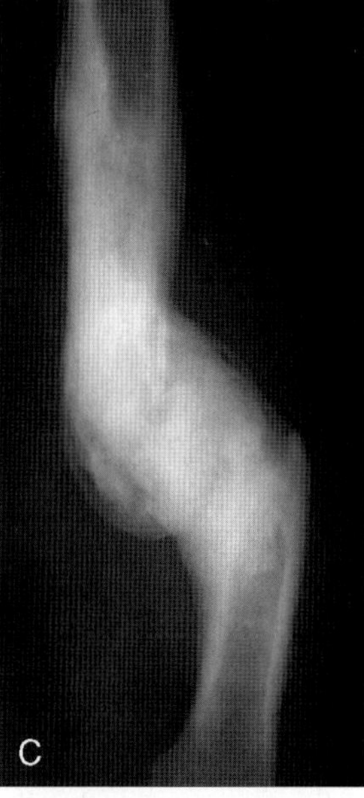

FIGURE 2-3. Fracture and osteomyelitis. **A,** A bone scan of the lower extremities shows increased uptake and deformity of the left femur in a patient with a prior history of fracture. **B,** In addition to the diffuse gallium uptake, there is a focal area of intense uptake that is incongruent with the bone scan *(arrowhead)* and therefore consistent with osteomyelitis. **C,** The radiograph shows sclerosis and malunion, but is nonspecific for infection.

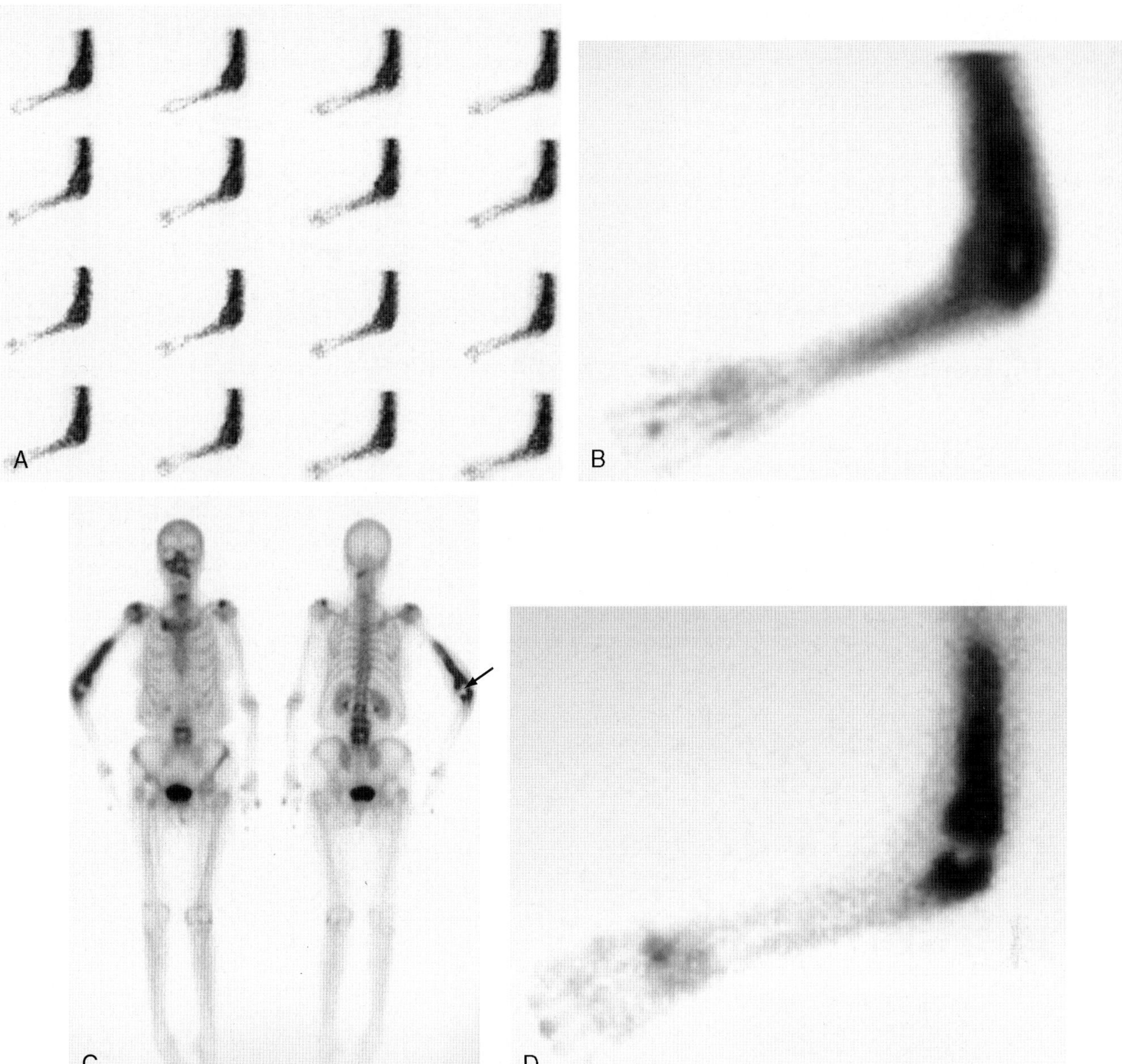

FIGURE 2-4. Combined bone scan and WBC scan demonstrating an infected right total elbow prosthesis. Dynamic blood flow **(A)** and blood pool **(B)** images show significant diffuse tracer uptake in the upper arm and elbow. **C,** The delayed whole body bone scan shows significant increased uptake in the elbow and distal upper arm around the prosthesis. The area of the prosthesis *(arrow)* and its stems show no isotope activity. **D,** The In-111 WBC scan shows marked tracer uptake in a distribution matching that of the bone scan, consistent with infection.

postsurgery, or with diabetes (Figure 2-4, *A* to *D*). False-positive scans have been reported with recent trauma or acute fracture or following arthroplasty, and the addition of bone marrow scanning may be needed in these situations.[14] Delay in the injection of the labeled leukocytes may cause false-negative results mainly due to decreased leukocyte viability when out of the body for a prolonged time.

Bone scanning should be performed in conjunction with labeled leukocyte imaging for anatomic localization. Because a negative bone scan essentially rules out osteomyelitis, there is no need to proceed with WBC scan if the bone scan is normal. Tc-99m HMPAO labeled leukocyte scanning has been reported to yield an accuracy similar to that of In-111 WBC scanning in the diagnosis of osteomyelitis but has the additional benefit of providing same-day results.[15] This technique may be particularly useful in children, as the radiation dose is much lower than that of the In-111 leukocyte technique. A disadvantage of the Tc-99m HMPAO scan is the inability to acquire dual Tc-99m MDP and Tc-HMPAO leukocyte scans simultaneously.

> A negative bone scan essentially rules out osteomyelitis; there is no need to proceed with a WBC scan if the bone scan is normal.

In-111 leukocyte scanning is not generally useful in the diagnosis of vertebral osteomyelitis; the images may show normal or decreased uptake even when osteomyelitis is present. This may be related to the chronic nature of the disease due to delayed diagnosis. Gallium scanning is the modality of choice for vertebral osteomyelitis and discitis.

Tc-99m Bone Marrow Scintigraphy

The addition of Tc-99m sulfur colloid scanning to the WBC scan protocol improves specificity for infection in complicated cases such as postarthroplasty infections. Infection is confirmed when there is less or no bone marrow activity on the sulfur colloid scan in areas with increased uptake on the labeled WBC scan. Activity present on bone marrow scans equal to or greater than that of the WBC scan indicates physiologic bone marrow activity and rules out infection (Figure 2-5, *A* to *C*).

> Infection is confirmed when there is no activity or less bone marrow activity on the sulfur colloid scan in areas in which there is increased uptake on the labeled WBC scan.

Tc-99m Diphosphonate Imaging (Tc-99m MDP or HDP)

Three-phase bone scanning is the imaging modality of choice for suspected osteomyelitis. This examination becomes positive within 24 hours after onset of symptoms. The classic findings of osteomyelitis on three-phase bone scan are increased regional perfusion as seen in blood flow (phase 1) and blood pool (phase 2) and corresponding focal increased uptake on delayed images (see Figure 2-1). Pinhole imaging can be of value in children for better characterization of delayed focal uptake or for the small bones in adults, such as the wrist and ankle. This uptake pattern is different from cellulitis, which shows regional or diffusely increased uptake in the area involved on phase 1 and phase 2 but either no corresponding uptake on delayed images or only mildly increased uptake secondary to the hyperemia of adjacent or surrounding soft tissue infection.

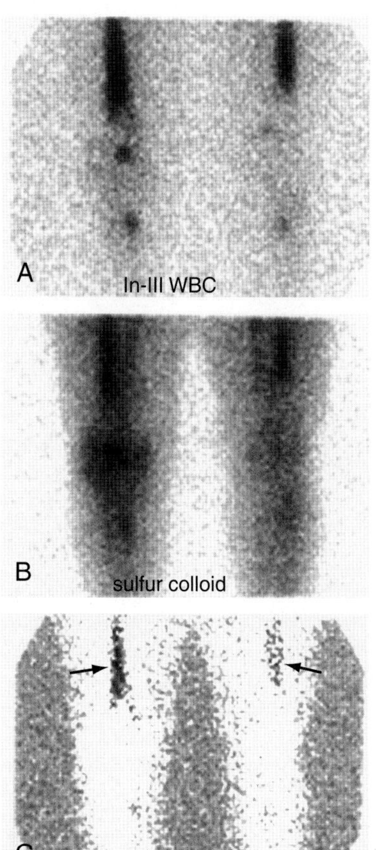

FIGURE 2-5. Infection. In-111 WBC scan **(A)**, Tc-99m sulfur colloid scan **(B)**, and a subtraction image **(C)** show asymmetric uptake in the distal femurs (right greater than left) *(arrows)* indicating infection of the distal right femur.

> Cellulitis shows regional or diffusely increased uptake in the area involved on phase 1 and phase 2 with either no corresponding uptake on delayed images or only mildly increased uptake secondary to the hyperemia. Osteomyelitis shows increased uptake in all three phases of the bone scan.

Bone scanning is very specific for the early diagnosis of osteomyelitis when the bone is not previously affected by other pathologic conditions (nonviolated) and is an efficient and cost-effective modality in the diagnosis. Overall sensitivity and specificity of bone scan for osteomyelitis in nonviolated bone are 90% and 95%, respectively. However, there have been some reports of false-negative scans in cases with proven early acute osteomyelitis, demonstrating either reduced or normal accumulation of the radiotracer, particularly in neonates. Cold lesions on bone scan may indicate a more virulent infectious process and are thought to be secondary to increased intraosseous and subperiosteal pressure, likely due to edema. Tuson et al.[16] found that the positive predictive value of reduced uptake (cold lesion) in a selected group of patients was higher (100%) than that of a hot lesion (82%). Gallium scan or indium WBC scan may be helpful.[16,17] A normal-appearing bone scan at a region of osteomyelitis may be due to its being obtained during the transition from cold to hot phases; otherwise, a negative three-phase bone scan can rule out osteomyelitis, and no further imaging is required. In violated bone, the bone scan alone may not establish the diagnosis, requiring complementary radionuclide imaging such as gallium or In-111 WBC scanning to improve the specificity.

F-18 FDG PET

F-18 FDG PET plays a major role in the field of oncology; however, its utility in infection and inflammatory lesions has also been described. Love et al. compared F-18 FDG with WBC/bone marrow scan (BMS) imaging. PET was 100% sensitive (94% for WBC/BMS) but its specificity was very low at 11% (100% for WBC/BMS). Further studies are needed to evaluate the efficiency of PET imaging in osteomyelitis. Thus far, the In-111 WBC/BMS combination remains the gold standard for the diagnosis of osteomyelitis.

Scintigraphy of Infected Prostheses

The distinction between mechanical failure of a prosthesis and infection may be difficult clinically, radiographically, and on scintigraphy. There is no specific scintigraphic pattern that indicates infection versus loosening. Furthermore, the pattern of normal postoperative increased uptake that occurs due to bone remodeling varies considerably depending on the type of prosthesis used and the time since surgery.

In the case of total hip arthroplasty (THA), knowledge of the type of implant and implant fixation are important to plan a diagnostic strategy. In cemented THAs, most asymptomatic patients show no significant periprosthetic uptake 6 months or more after operation. Focal uptake at the tip of a femoral component after 6 months indicates loosening. In a symptomatic patient, diffuse uptake around the shaft is thought to be more in favor of infection, and further evaluation with In-111 WBC is needed.[18] In noncemented THA, postoperative periprosthetic uptake may continue for 2 years or longer in asymptomatic patients[18] (Figure 2-6, *A, B*). In these noncemented THAs, focal uptake at

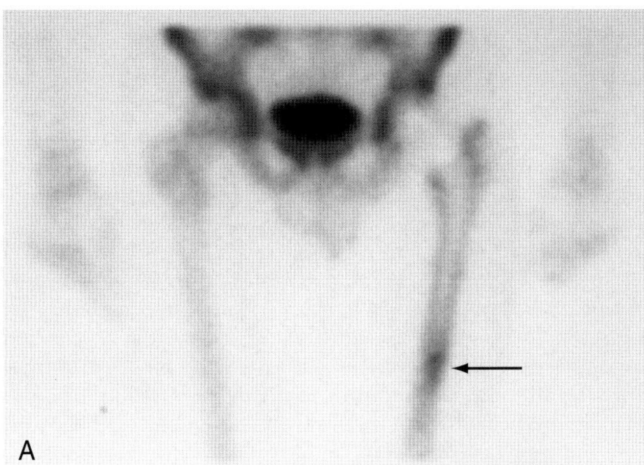

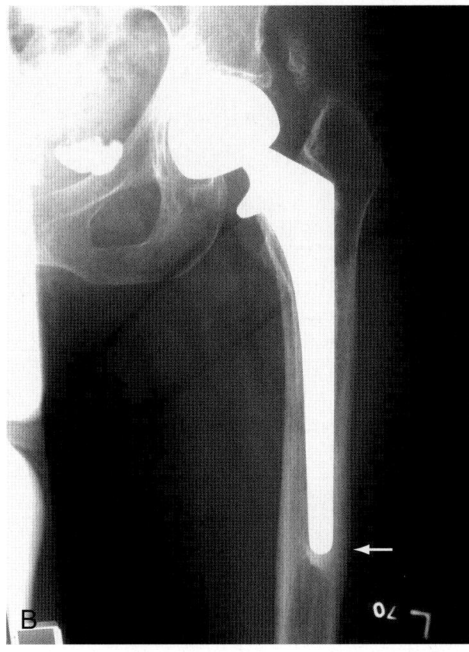

FIGURE 2-6. Bone ingrowth prosthesis with increased uptake on bone scan due to bone remodeling. **A,** This scan was obtained to exclude prosthetic loosening. The anterior view of the left hip shows focal mild increased uptake at the tip of the femoral component *(arrow)* and even milder uptake proximally near the greater and lesser trochanters. **B,** The radiograph shows that the increased uptake corresponds to sclerotic changes and cortical thickening seen at the tip of the femoral component *(arrow)*. Prior settling of the prosthesis into rarus is suggested, but there is no lucency in bone in growth areas. Uptake at the tip of the femoral stem may be seen in uncemented prostheses that are not loose. Radiographic correlation is therefore necessary.

the tip of a femoral component may indicate remodeling due to mechanical changes in the adjacent bone rather than loosening (see Figure 2-6).

After total knee replacement, bone scan may show increased uptake around the femoral (60%) and tibial (75% to 90%) components for 1 year after surgery in asymptomatic patients, usually due to postsurgical remodeling. When a bone scan is clearly negative, it excludes infection and/or loosening.

> A negative bone scan usually excludes prosthetic loosening or infection.

Combined gallium scan and bone scan have better specificity than either scan alone for assessing possible infection. An In-111 WBC scan has proven to be more accurate than combined bone scan and gallium scans, although false-positive In-111 WBC scanning may occur as a result of physiologic uptake by cellular bone marrow. To correct for this marrow uptake, a combination of In-111 WBC and sulfur colloid (marrow) scan subtraction either visually or by computer is helpful and highly specific. A study is considered to be positive for infection if the In-111 WBC leukocyte uptake exceeds that of the Tc-99m sulfur colloid BMS in extent or intensity (discordant pattern) (see Figure 2-5). If the relative intensity and distribution of In-111 leukocytes are equal to or less than that of Tc-99m sulfur colloid (concordant pattern), the study should be considered negative for infection.[19]

Antibody imaging has been used to diagnose infection in patients with hip and knee prostheses.[20] FDG-PET has recently been used to detect both infection and loosening. The results seem promising and appear to be more accurate for hip than for knee prostheses.[21] Sensitivity and specificity for detection of hip infection are 90% and 89%, respectively, and 90% and 72%, respectively, for knee infection. Further studies are required for evaluation of PET in infected prosthesis.

SCINTIGRAPHY OF METABOLIC AND ENDOCRINE DISEASES

The most important advantage of bone scintigraphy in metabolic bone disease is its high sensitivity and its capacity to easily image the whole body. Important practical applications of bone scanning in metabolic bone disease are the detection of a bone abnormality or the detection of focal complications of generalized diseases. Examples include detection of fractures in osteoporosis, pseudofracture in osteomalacia, and evaluation of Paget's disease including assessing disease activity.

Paget's Disease

Paget's disease begins with a phase of active and excessive bone resorption (lytic or resorption phase), which may progress rapidly. The term *mixed* is used when resorption and bone formation are approximately equal. The final sclerotic, or burned out, phase is characterized predominantly by new bone formation.[22] Using three-phase bone scanning, the dynamic flow and blood pool images show varying degrees of hyperemia and uptake at sites of involvement, depending on the stage of the disease; the earlier the phase, the higher degree of hyperemia and uptake. During the active lytic phase (phase one), intensely increased uptake is characteristically seen and uniformly distributed throughout the affected region. An exception to this is the early phase in the skull, osteoporosis circumscripta, which shows intense uptake at the periphery of the lesion while the center is cold (Figure 2-7). Phase two usually shows increased uptake (Figure 2-8, *A, B*), and in the third phase (sclerotic phase), the uptake of bone imaging agent decreases. With time the sclerotic phase may show no abnormal uptake of radiotracer, and these cases will be missed by bone scan and detected by radiographs. Bone scan detects abnormalities in bones that are difficult to explore by radiography, such as the sternum, ribs, and scapulae. Because In-111 WBCs are taken up by hematopoietic bone marrow, uptake is seen in areas of Paget's disease with active marrow; this can mimic infection, particularly when it is focal. The bone scan can be used for assessment of the activity of Paget's disease, for follow-up, and for evaluating response to treatment.[22] Bisphosphonates decrease bone resorption by inhibiting osteoclasts. Successful response to treatment causes

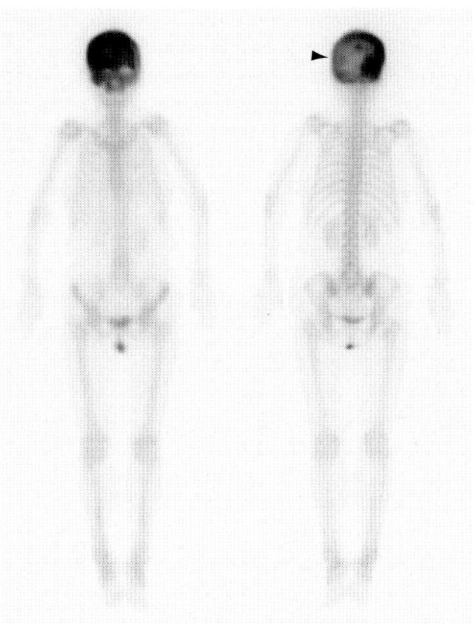

FIGURE 2-7. Lytic phase of Paget's disease (osteoporosis circumscripta). Anterior *(left image)* and posterior views of a Tc-99m bone scan show marked increased uptake in the skull as compared with the skeleton in general. A large photopenic area *(arrowhead)* posteriorly is consistent with osteoporosis circumscripta with a peripherally active border.

normalization of the bone scan, although there are cases of Paget's disease remission with active bone scans.

Renal Osteodystrophy

Renal osteodystrophy is a metabolic bone condition associated with chronic renal failure. The pathogenesis of renal osteodystrophy is not completely understood. Two mechanisms predominate are secondary hyperparathyroidism and abnormal vitamin D metabolism following reduced renal function.[23] Scintigraphically symmetric increased activity is mainly seen in the calvaria, sternum, shoulders, vertebrae, and distal aspects of the femurs and tibias (Figure 2-9). The degree and extent of abnormal activity correlates with the length of dialysis and the level of alkaline phosphatase. In hemodialysis patients with symptomatic bone disease, the Tc-99m MDP scan can provide useful information for differential diagnosis between dialysis-related osteomalacia, which shows decreased tracer uptake, and secondary hyperparathyroidism, which shows increased tracer uptake in the skeleton.

Complex Regional Pain Syndrome (Reflex Sympathetic Dystrophy [RSD])

RSD is defined as a pain syndrome that usually develops after an initiating noxious event with no identifiable major nerve injury. It is not limited to the distribution of a single peripheral nerve, and the level of pain is out of proportion to the inciting event or the expected healing response. It is associated during its course with edema, change in skin blood flow, and abnormal vasomotor activity in the region of the pain. The distal aspect of an affected extremity is usually involved.[24] The pathophysiology of RSD is not known. The scintigraphic pattern depends on the duration

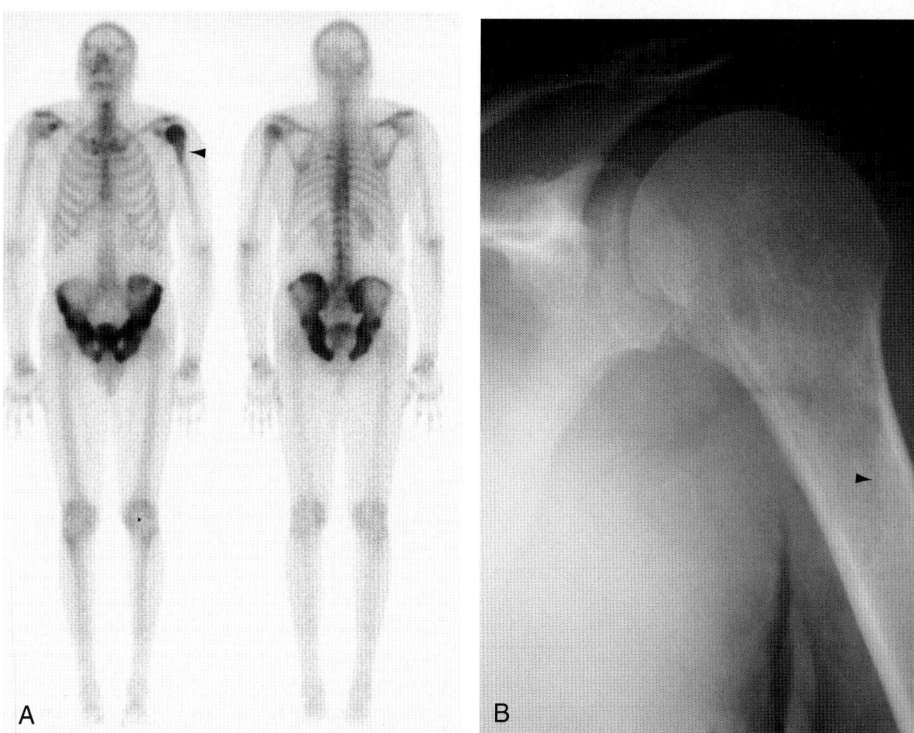

FIGURE 2-8. Paget's disease. **A,** Anterior *(left image)* and posterior images of a Technetium-99m labeled bone scan show striking and extensive increased uptake in the pelvis and the left humeral head and neck *(arrowhead)*. **B,** The radiograph of left shoulder shows the lytic phase of Paget's disease (the "blade of grass" sign; *arrowhead*).

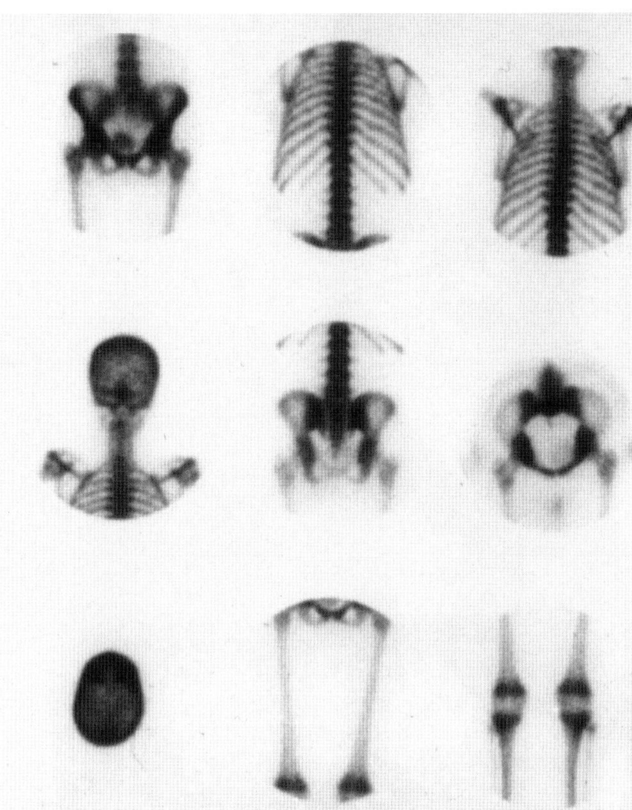

FIGURE 2-9. Renal osteodystrophy. The Technetium-99m labeled bone scan shows no excretion of isotope in the kidneys consistent with renal failure. Increased uptake in the skull, spine, pelvis, and tibias is due to secondary hyperparathyroidism. This appearance of extensive bone uptake without renal uptake is termed a *super scan*. Other causes of a *super scan* include extensive metastatic disease or Paget's disease.

of the disease, the age of the patient, the predisposing injury, and the location of the disease.[24] In the acute stage (before 20 weeks) all three phases of the bone scan show increased uptake; typically there is diffuse hyperemia of the affected hand or foot and periarticular increased uptake of the affected region on delayed images (Figure 2-10, *A* to *C*). Between 20 and 60 weeks, phase one and two of the bone scan may be normal, but phase three continues to show periarticular uptake. After 60 weeks (atrophic phase), phase two of the bone scan shows decreased uptake with normal uptake on delayed or early images. The multiphase bone scan is sensitive for detecting the early phase of RSD[25]; the sensitivity ranges between 73% and 96%, whereas the specificity is between 86% and 100%. The bone scan has a high negative predictive value. Bone scan is useful in determining the stage of RSD and in predicting the response to therapy.[26]

> In the acute stage of RSD (before 20 weeks) all three phases of the bone scan show increased uptake; typically there is diffuse hyperemia of the affected hand or foot and periarticular increased uptake of the affected region on delayed images.

Hypertrophic Osteoarthropathy

Two types of hypertrophic osteoarthropathy (HOA) are recognized: Primary HOA, also called *pachydermoperiostosis*, is less common. The secondary form follows a variety of pathologic conditions predominantly in the thorax, mainly lung cancer or other intrathoracic malignancies or cyanotic heart disease. HOA is also seen in hepatic biliary cirrhosis and inflammatory bowel disease.[27]

Scintigraphy shows diffusely increased uptake along the cortical margins of the long bones, giving the appearance of parallel tracks. The scintigraphic abnormalities are usually bilateral and confined to the diaphyseal regions but may also occur in the epiphyses. In approximately 15% of cases, the abnormalities may be unilateral.[27] The tibias and fibulas are affected most commonly, followed by the distal femurs, radii, ulnas, hands, feet, and distal humeri (Figure 2-11). The scapulae, patellae, maxilla, mandible, and clavicles are less commonly affected. The ribs and pelvis are rarely affected.

> Scintigraphy of HOA shows diffusely increased, bilateral, primarily diaphyseal uptake along the cortical margins of the long bones, giving the appearance of parallel tracks.

Fibrous Dysplasia

Fibrous dysplasia is a benign bone disorder characterized by the presence of fibrous tissue containing trabeculae composed of nonlamellar bone. The condition presents as a solitary lesion (monostotic) or with multiple foci (polyostotic). The etiology of fibrous dysplasia is not entirely clear, but there is growing evidence of a genetic mechanism. Fibrous dysplasia generally appears as an area of markedly increased uptake on bone scintigraphy (Figure 2-12, *A* to *C*). The possibility of fibrous dysplasia is unlikely when the lesion shows no uptake.[28] Fibrous dysplasia is commonly seen in the craniofacial bones, scapula, ribs, pelvis, spine, and extremities, usually in an asymmetric pattern; it may be unilateral in the polyostotic variant. Bone scan is useful for confirming the diagnosis and establishing the extent of bone involvement. SPECT has been reported to provide additional information, particularly for lesions in cranial bones. A report on the use of PET scanning in fibrous dysplasia of the craniofacial bones showed signs of accelerated bone mineral turnover with increased uptake on bone scintigraphy without elevated glucose metabolism on F-18 FDG PET scanning.[29]

> Fibrous dysplasia generally appears as an area of markedly increased uptake on bone scintigraphy; fibrous dysplasia is an unlikely diagnosis when a lesion shows no uptake.

Scintigraphy of Traumatic Disorders

Nuclear medicine has a limited but important role in trauma and its complications. It is particularly useful and indicated in radiographically occult acute fractures, including those in children who are the victims of physical abuse, and in stress fractures. It is also used in the assessment of physeal closure and stimulation after trauma and to predict the outcome of leg length by semiquantitative analysis.

Acute Fracture

Most fractures show increased uptake on bone scintigraphy within hours after trauma.[30] In elderly patients, however, fractures may take several days to be seen on bone scan. The optimal timing for imaging of a fracture is unclear. Holder et al.[31] reported a sensitivity of 93% and specificity of 95% for fracture identification if the bone scan is performed within 72 hours and 100% sensitivity if performed 72 hours or longer after injury. In addition to patient age, the bone metabolic activity, mineral content, and imaging technique are all factors that can significantly affect the ability to detect a fracture. The scintigraphic appearance of fractures depends on the time elapsed since injury.[30] Acute fractures show

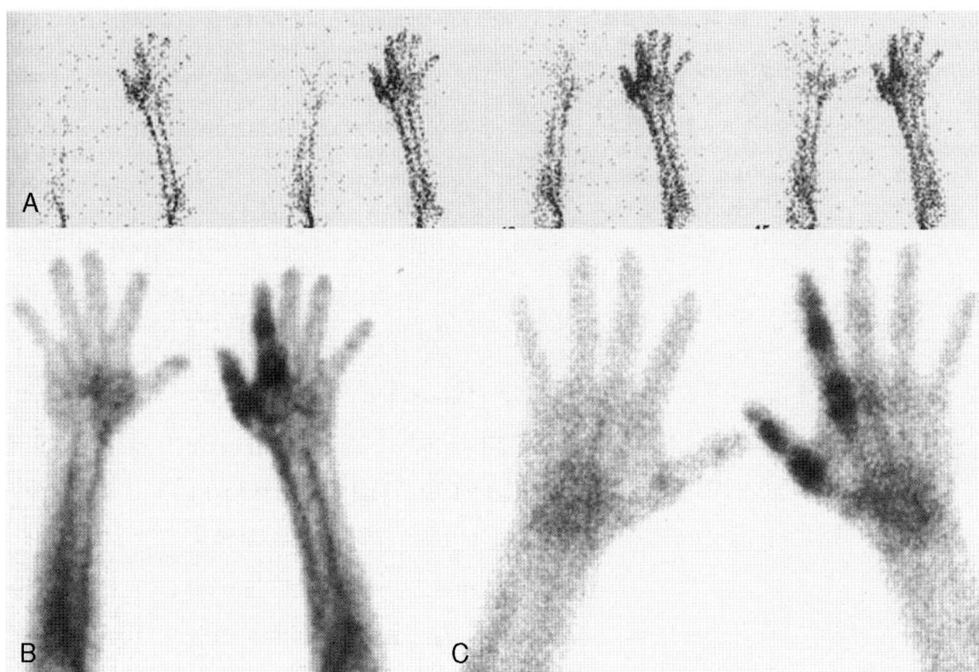

FIGURE 2-10. RSD (chronic regional pain syndrome) in a 32-year-old man with right hand pain after elbow surgery. A three-phase bone scan of the hands (palmar view) was obtained. Blood flow **(A)** and blood pool **(B)** images of both hands show increased uptake in the radial aspect of the right hand. **C,** Delayed images show periarticular uptake, mainly in the first and second fingers, consistent with RSD.

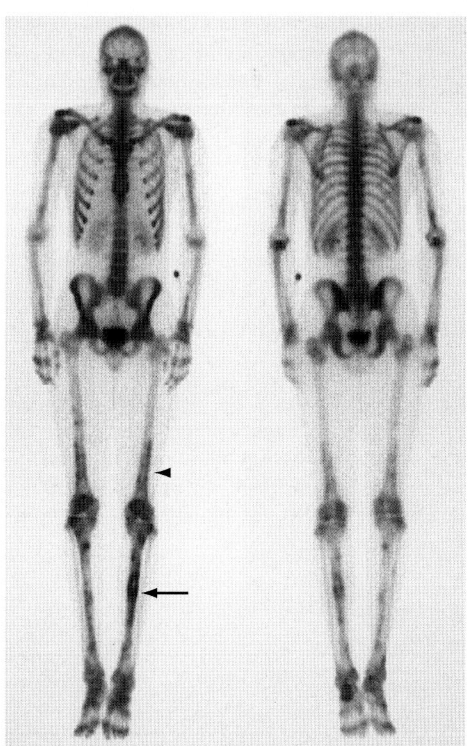

FIGURE 2-11. Hypertrophic osteoarthropathy in a patient with lung cancer. Anterior *(left)* and posterior bone scan images show increased tracer uptake in the upper and lower extremities. The parallel track of uptake ("tram sign"; *open arrow*) in the distal femurs indicates hypertrophic osteoarthropathy. Also noted is a photopenic focal area with a peripheral rim of uptake *(arrow)* due to a skeletal metastasis (as proven by radiography).

focally increased flow, increased blood pool activity, and a corresponding increased uptake on delayed images. Later, blood flow and blood pool activity decrease progressively until they become normal. This may take as long as 6 months.[32] Uptake on delayed images remains positive for a longer time and has been reported as long as 40 years after injury depending on the age and healing status of the patient.[30]

> 100% sensitivity for fracture identification has been found if the bone scan is performed 72 hours or longer after recent injury.

Specific fractures such as sternal fractures are difficult to detect by radiography, and bone scintigraphy may play a role in their diagnosis. Multiphase bone scan is considered very useful in detecting a scaphoid fracture when radiographs are negative. Pinhole imaging is particularly useful in localizing these fractures. Initial experience with MRI, however, suggests that it is sensitive and more specific than scintigraphy for scaphoid fracture, and ligamentous injury and carpal instability that may be seen by MRI are not evident on scintigraphy.[33]

Stress Fracture

Scintigraphy has a major role in the diagnosis of stress fracture, whether due to fatigue or insufficiency. (A fatigue fracture is due to increased repeated stress on normal bone, such as training for a race, whereas an insufficiency fracture is due to usual stress on abnormal bone, such as is seen in osteoporosis.) Scintigraphy can differentiate between recent and old fractures. Bone scintigraphy has been recommended as the initial imaging modality of choice in patients with a clinical suspicion of stress fracture. In the acute fracture, all phases of the bone scan show increased uptake; in a chronic stress fracture, only the delayed phase shows increased

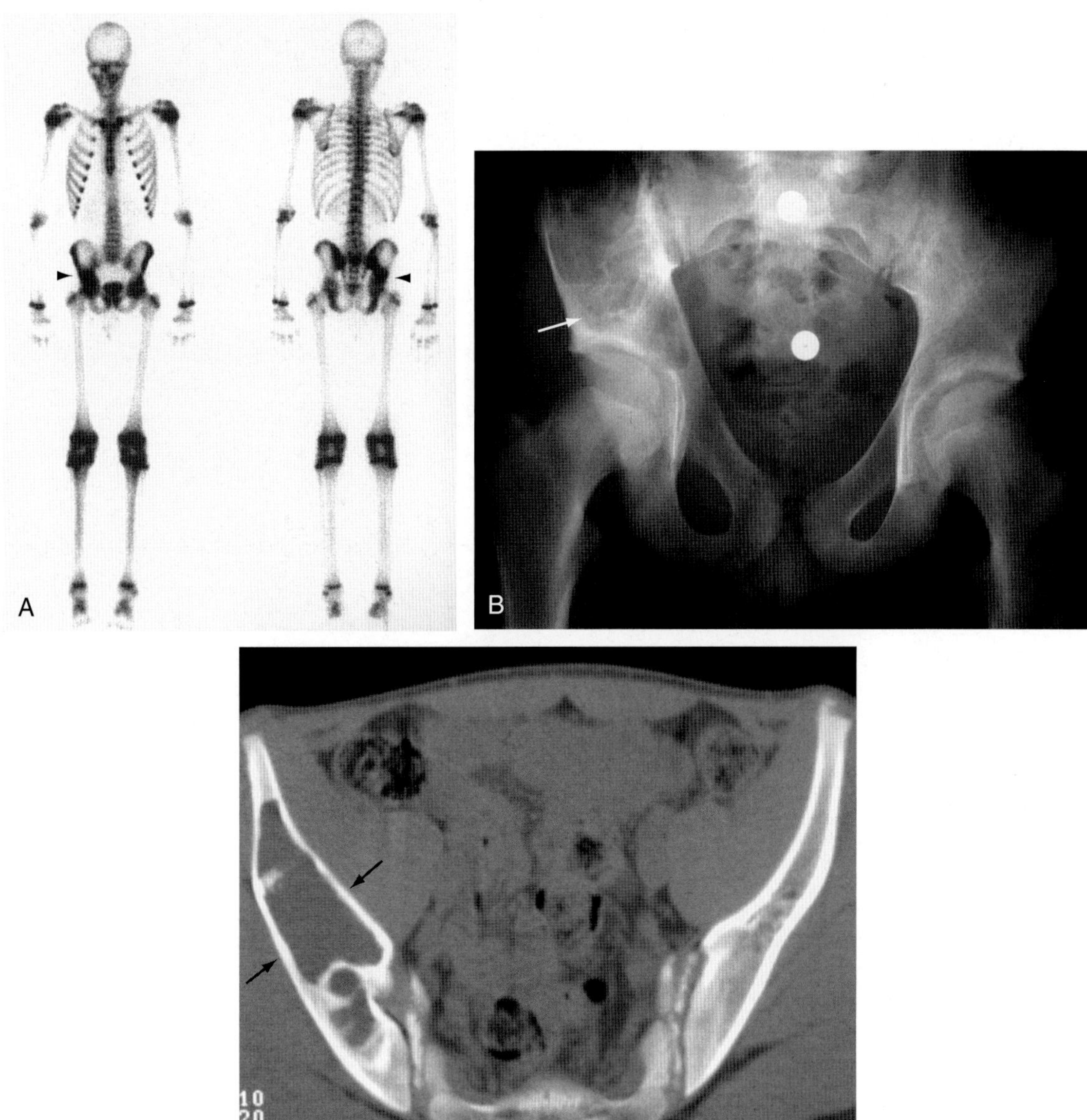

FIGURE 2-12. Fibrous dysplasia in a 17-year-old male. **A,** A bone scan shows increased uptake in the right iliac bone *(arrowhead)*. The linear areas of increased uptake in the physes are normal. **B,** The radiograph of the pelvis shows an expansile lesion with typical "ground glass" density centrally *(arrow)*. **C,** CT of the same patient shows the septated expansile lesion *(arrows)* with intact cortex.

activity (Figure 2-13). In general, three patterns of uptake on delayed images can be recognized in fracture: a focal band of uptake, diffuse uptake, or peripheral linear uptake parallel to the periosteum.[34] Complete or partial scintigraphic resolution occurs within 4 to 6 months in the presence of normal healing.[34]

Insufficiency Fractures

Insufficiency fractures usually occur in the sacroiliac region and the pubis and can mimic bone metastasis. Bone scintigraphy is an excellent method for diagnosis. An MRI or CT scan provides a definitive diagnosis in many cases. The typical (but uncommon) scintigraphic pattern is H-shaped uptake in the sacrum, called the *Honda sign* (Figure 2-14).

> H-shaped uptake in the sacrum, called the *Honda sign*, is characteristic of sacral insufficiency fractures.

The Honda sign is seen in approximately 20% of cases. The most common pattern of a sacral insufficiency fracture is unilateral vertical uptake in a sacral ala; this is present in approximately 32% of cases. Horizontal uptake is seen in 27% of cases.[36] Bone scintigraphy is not only an adequate procedure for the detection of radiographically occult sacral fractures but also reveals the often coexisting fractures in the pubic bone, spine, or ribs.[36]

Scintigraphic Evaluation of Fracture and Bone Graft Healing

Approximately 60% of fractures heal scintigraphically within 1 year and 90% by 2 years.[37] Healing depends on the location of the fracture.

Bone scans can be used for evaluation of nonunion. In hypervascular nonunion the three-phase bone scan is positive, whereas in avascular (atrophic) nonunion there is no activity.[38] The gap

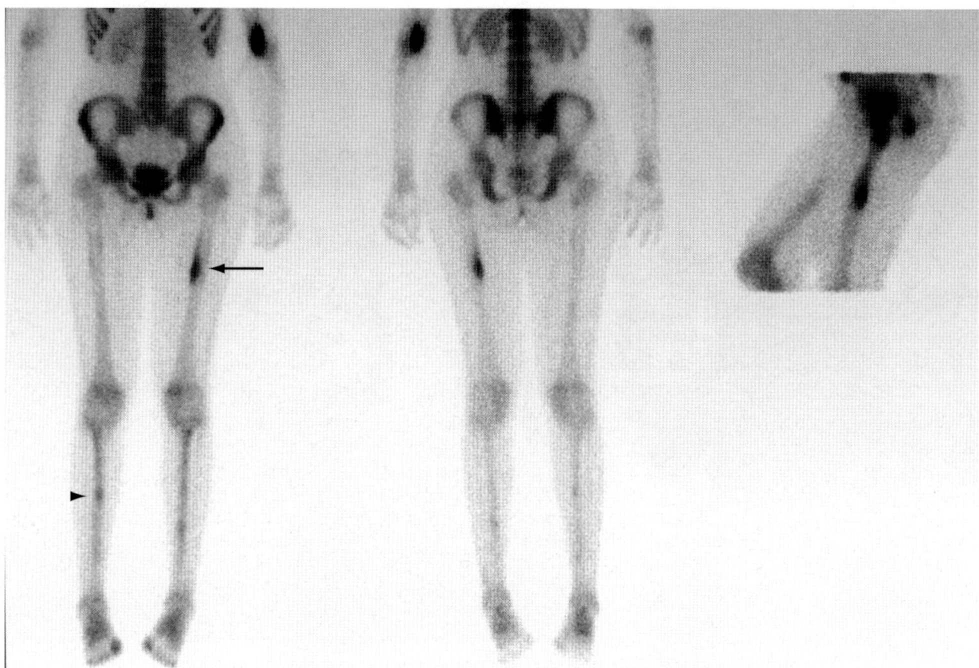

FIGURE 2-13. Stress fractures. Whole body bone scan (anterior and posterior projections) and a lateral scan show increased uptake at the site of a left femoral stress fracture *(arrow)*. Mild uptake in the mid shafts of both tibias indicates early stress fractures *(arrowhead)*.

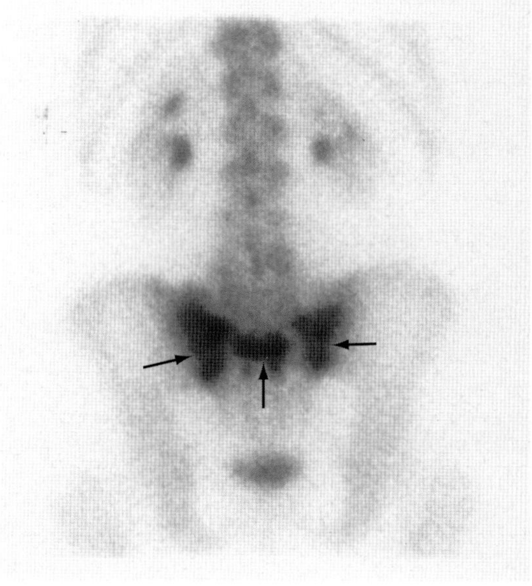

FIGURE 2-14. Insufficiency fractures of the sacrum in a 76-year-old female with a history of osteoporosis. A bone scan shows H-shaped sacral uptake (the Honda sign; *arrows*) characteristic of an insufficiency fracture of the sacrum.

between the fracture margins could indicate a pseudarthrosis. Bone scan can also be used for evaluation of bone graft viability. Autologous graft revascularization shows increased uptake on all phases of the bone scan that eventually extends to adjacent bone as it is incorporated. Allografts initially show a photon deficient area and gradually show uptake on serial scans.[39] Serial three-phase bone scanning not only permits assessment of vascular patency at an early stage but also allows continuing observation of any complications. The sensitivity and positive predictive value of bone scan are low for evaluation of stability of spinal fusion.[40]

Shin Splints

Shin splints are painful conditions that result from extreme tension on the muscles inserting on the tibia and, to a lesser extent, the femur. This tension leads to periosteal elevation and reactive bone formation. Differentiating shin splints from stress fracture is crucial because the management is different. Radiographs are normal in patients with shin splints. Scintigraphically the blood flow and blood pool images are typically normal. On delayed images there is characteristically longitudinal increased uptake (which may be faint) along the diaphyses of the posteromedial and anterolateral aspects of the tibial cortex, affecting usually one third of the length of the bone, or the anteromedial border of the femur, affecting usually the proximal or mid-portion of the bone (Figure 2-15). Both posterior and anterior tibial changes may be present in the same individual.[35] Shin splints also occur in upper extremity bones.

> On delayed images, shin splints are seen as longitudinal increased uptake along the diaphyses of the posteromedial and anterolateral aspects of the tibial cortex, affecting usually one third of the length of the bone, or the anteromedial border of the femur, affecting usually the proximal or mid-portion of the bone.

DISORDERS OF CIRCULATION: OSTEONECROSIS: SCINTIGRAPHIC FEATURES AND STAGING

Osteonecrosis is a common condition that is believed to develop after an ischemic event in bone and bone marrow. The resulting vascular compromise leads to imbalance between the demand and supply of oxygen to osseous tissue and consequently

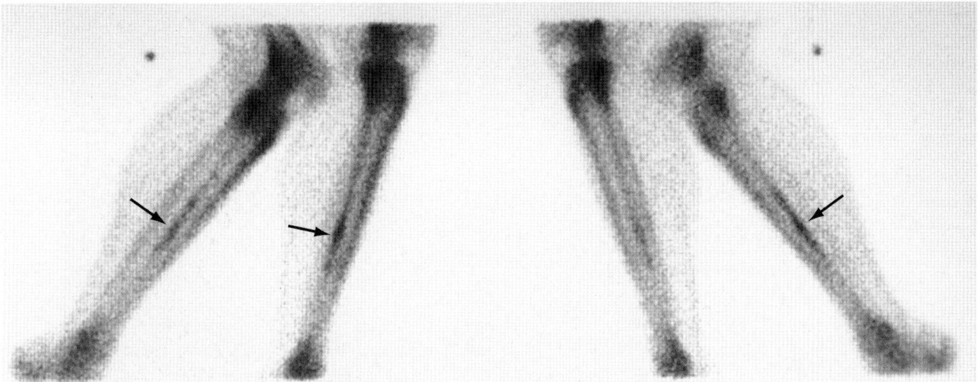

FIGURE 2-15. Shin splints. Lateral views of the legs obtained to augment the standard views of the bone scan show mild linear uptake along the posterior aspect of each tibia, consistent with shin splints. The linear anterior cortical uptake is normal.

osteonecrosis (avascular necrosis) of bone. The different scintigraphic patterns of femoral head avascular necrosis correlate with the sequence of pathological events (Table 2-3). During the first 48 hours (stage I) the morphology of bone is preserved and the radiographs are normal; however, a cold area may be seen on bone scan. This avascular pattern will be seen immediately if interruption of the blood supply is abrupt and severe. The next stage (stage II) begins with the reparative process; in this stage, hyperemia is frequent and there is diffuse osteopenia of the area surrounding the necrotic tissue. This stage is characterized scintigraphically by progressively increased radiotracer uptake starting at the boundaries usually beginning after 1 to 3 weeks. SPECT should be used in the diagnosis of femoral head avascular necrosis to show the central photopenic area surrounded by a rim of activity (termed the *doughnut pattern*). If repair and ischemia are balanced, the bone scan may appear normal. If bone collapse (stage III) occurs, increased uptake may persist indefinitely. Stage IV is characterized by collapse of the articular surface with degenerative changes on both sides of the joint with resultant increased periarticular uptake[41] (Figure 2-16, *A* to *C*).

Bone scan and MRI are the most valuable imaging modalities in the diagnosis and follow-up of avascular necrosis. The multiphase bone scan is reported to be 98% sensitive and 96% specific.[42] In children with Legg-Calvé-Perthes disease, the bone scan is both a sensitive and specific modality for diagnosis of this condition, showing a cold area with or without a rim of increased uptake (Figure 2-17). Pinhole imaging has proved to be valuable in the evaluation of this condition and is preferred to SPECT in the pediatric age group. Progressive degenerative changes may develop in subsequent years with nonspecific increased uptake in the area of the femoral head.

TABLE 2-3. Scintigraphic Findings in Osteonecrosis

Stage	Time after Insult	Scintigraphic Findings
I: Ischemia	48 hours	Decreased uptake (photopenia)
II: Early repair begins	1–3 weeks	Doughnut sign
III: Collapse	Weeks	Increased uptake in affected bone
IV: Degenerative	Months	Periarticular uptake change

The femoral head is a common site of osteonecrosis in adults and in children. In adults the condition commonly occurs secondary to trauma, renal transplantation, systemic lupus erythematosus or following corticosteroid medication. Bone scanning is useful for early diagnosis and follow-up of osteonecrosis. SPECT has been found to be more sensitive than MRI for the detection of femoral head osteonecrosis in patients who have had renal transplants.[43] Bone scan with SPECT is particularly necessary for the diagnosis of osteonecrosis in adults with this disorder. Phase one (blood flow) and two (blood pool) of the bone scan may be normal or show decreased uptake in the area of necrosis, although phase three (delayed scan) usually shows increased uptake.

Scintigraphy in Primary Bone Tumors

Primary bone tumors are rare, whereas metastatic bone tumors are common and have a significant impact on decision-making regarding choice of therapy.

A healing "flare phenomenon" has been characterised by increased radiotracer uptake in an area of previously noted skeletal metastasis on a bone scan associated with increased sclerosis on radiographs or CT scan.

> A flare phenomenon is usually seen during the first 3 months after chemotherapy and represents a favorable response to therapy.

Functional nuclear medicine modalities generally have a limited role in the imaging of primary bone tumors but are very useful in the initial detection of metastases, gauging the response to therapy and estimating the prognosis. Various other radiopharmaceuticals such as I-123 MIBG, Thallium-201 chloride, Tc-99m MIBI, and F-18 FDG are all used for bone tumor imaging, mainly to rule out metastases. Bone scan with planar images may detect metastases and other lesions as small as 2 cm. SPECT images are able to detect lesions as small as 1 cm.[44] Sensitivity depends on the size and location of the tumor; the specificity of bone scan is very low.

> Bone scan with planar images may detect lesions as small as 2 cm, whereas SPECT images are able to detect lesions as small as 1 cm.

The Role of PET in Bone Tumors

F-18 FDG PET imaging has several roles in malignant bone disease:

1. Evaluation of the response to treatment of primary or metastatic bone disease

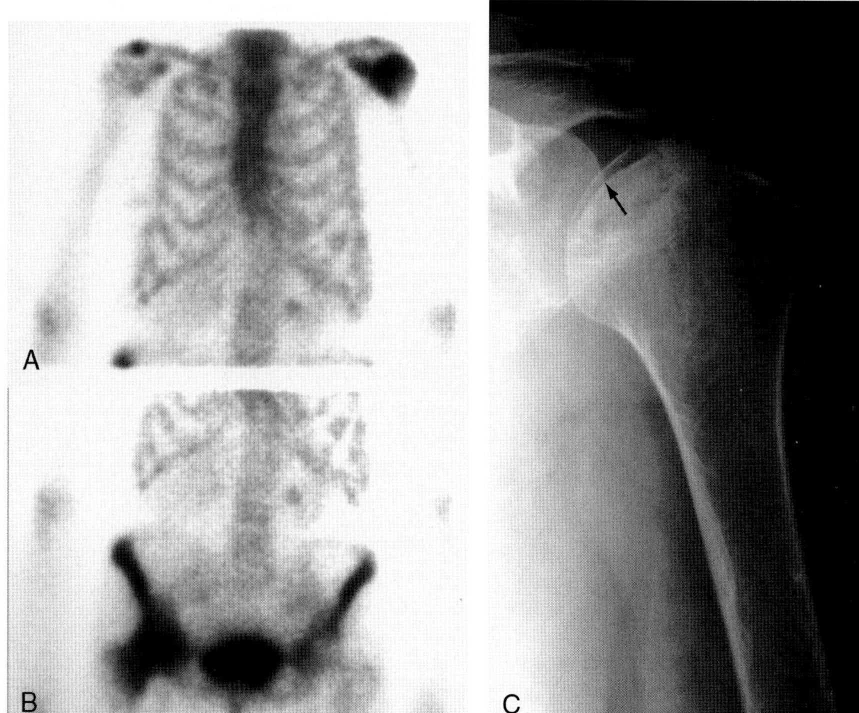

FIGURE 2-16. Osteonecrosis in a 65-year-old female with systemic lupus erythematosus on corticosteroids. Bone scan images of the thorax **(A)** and pelvis **(B)** show increased radiotracer uptake in the head of the left humerus and head of the right femur, consistent with osteonecrosis. **C,** A radiograph of the left shoulder shows lucency in the humeral head with a subchondral fracture (crescent sign; *arrow*), diagnostic of the condition.

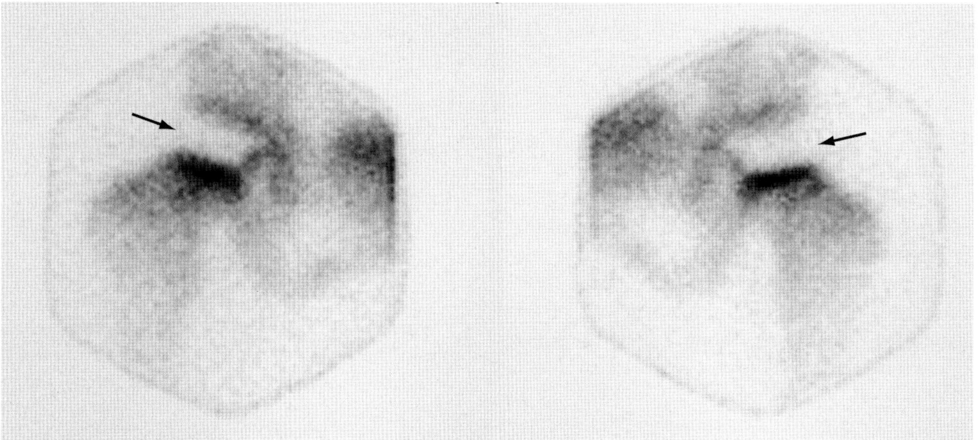

FIGURE 2-17. Legg-Calvé-Perthes disease. Pinhole views of each hip from a bone scan clearly show photopenia of each femoral head *(arrows)* consistent with Legg-Calve-Perthes disease. Distal to these areas is the increased uptake in the physes.

2. Detection of recurrence of primary bone malignancies
3. Early differentiation between progression and flare of metastatic bone disease seen on bone scan
4. Evaluation of a solitary bone lesion seen on radiographs
5. Detection of metastasis in bone and soft tissue

PET is increasingly used to evaluate tumor response to therapy[45] and is considered the modality of choice for this purpose. PET also has a significant role in detecting distant metastases of primary bone tumors; accuracy depends on tumor type and location. FDG-PET was compared with Tc-99m MDP bone scintigraphy for the detection of osseous metastases from osteogenic sarcoma and Ewing's sarcoma.[45] FDG had a sensitivity of 90%, specificity of 96%, and accuracy of 95% for osteogenic sarcoma compared with 92%, 71%, and 88%, respectively for bone scan. For Ewing's sarcoma, PET showed sensitivity, specificity, and accuracy of 100%, 96%, and 97%, respectively compared with 68%, 87%, and 82%, respectively for bone scan. Statistically significant standard uptake value (SUV) differences between benign (2.18) and malignant (4.34) lesions were found by Aoki et al.[46] in 52 primary bone lesions. There was no significant difference in SUV value among benign lesions including fibrous dysplasia, chondroblastoma, and sarcoid.

SUV refers to a standard uptake value: a semiquantitative measure of F-18 FDG uptake either in bone or soft tissue.

Osteoid Osteoma

Osteoid osteoma is a primary bone tumor arising from osteoblasts that affects mainly young people. The lesion is small (less than 2 cm) and growth is self-limited, although extensive reactive changes may be produced in the surrounding bone. Most often the proximal femur or the diaphyses of long bones are involved; less common sites of involvement are the foot or hand and the posterior elements of the spine.

Osteoid osteoma may cause a painful scoliosis in a child.

Pain at night, relieved by salicylates is the classic history. Cyclooxygenase (cox-2) is present in the nidus of the osteoid osteoma and is a mediator of increased production of prostaglandins in the tumor; this may be the cause of the pain and also the secondary changes shown by MRI.[47]

Osteoid osteomas that are located within or near a joint may produce synovitis that can be confused with other causes of monarticular arthritis.

If osteoid osteoma is suspected and the radiograph is negative, bone scintigraphy would be useful because it has a sensitivity of 100%. Phase one and two often, but not always, show prominent uptake and allow early localization of tumor. Delayed skeletal images (phase three) show focal intense tracer uptake at the periphery of the lesion (the so-called double density pattern), which can be better seen by a pinhole magnification technique (Figure 2-18). SPECT is useful in areas with complex anatomy, such as the spine. Radionuclide imaging also may be used preoperatively and intraoperatively to localize the tumor and establish complete removal of the nidus using a handheld radioactivity detector. Recently F-18 FDG has been used in the diagnosis of osteoid osteoma.

Osteogenic Sarcoma

Scintigraphically, osteogenic sarcoma presents as an area of intense isotope uptake (Figure 2-19). Bone scan usually overestimates the size of the lesion,[48] and MRI is superior to bone scan for evaluating the size and extent of the tumor. Mckillop et al.[49] have investigated the value of bone scan at the time of presentation and during follow-up. Although at presentation the chance of metastasis to the skeleton is low, the author concluded that performing a bone scan is justified because the result may profoundly alter the treatment plan even if the patient is asymptomatic. Thallium-201 and Tc-99m MIBI imaging are useful for evaluation of recurrence of disease and response to treatment. The glucose metabolism of osteogenic sarcoma can be assessed by F-18 FDG, and the use of a tumor to non-tumor ratio provides prognostic information related to the grading and biologic aggressiveness of the tumor. High F-18 FDG uptake correlates with poor outcome. F-18 FDG uptake may be complementary to other factors in judging the prognosis in osteogenic sarcoma.[50,51]

Ewing's Sarcoma

Bone scintigraphy is indicated in patients with Ewing's sarcoma mainly to rule out metastasis. Primary bone lesions with central necrosis may show a central area of decreased activity (photopenia) with a peripheral rim of tracer uptake (Figure 2-20). As with osteogenic sarcoma, CT and MRI are the primary imaging modalities for assessing the local extent of the tumor.

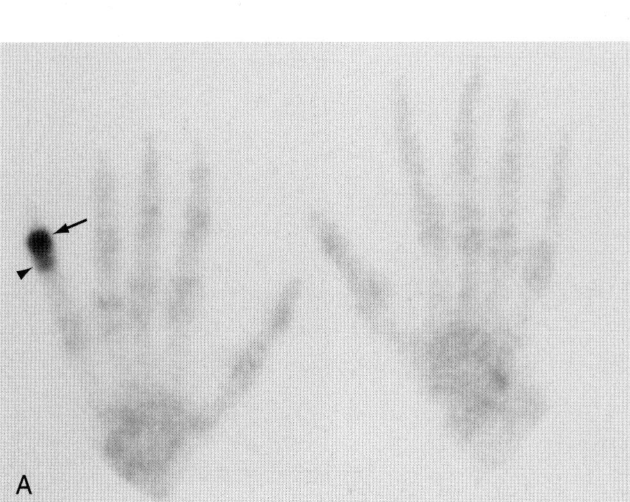

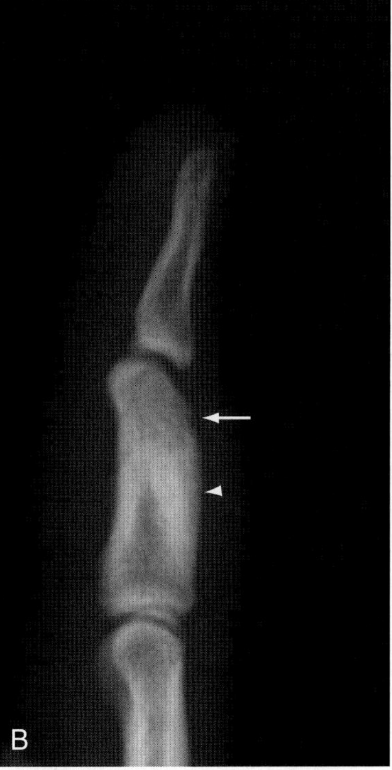

FIGURE 2-18. Osteoid osteoma. **A,** A palmar image from a bone scan of both hands shows focal intense uptake in the left fifth digit *(arrow)* with milder uptake at the periphery *(arrowhead)*. This "double density sign" is primarily seen in osteoid osteoma. **B,** The radiograph shows a lucent area (nidus; *arrow*) with reactive sclerotic changes *(arrowhead)* in the middle phalanx.

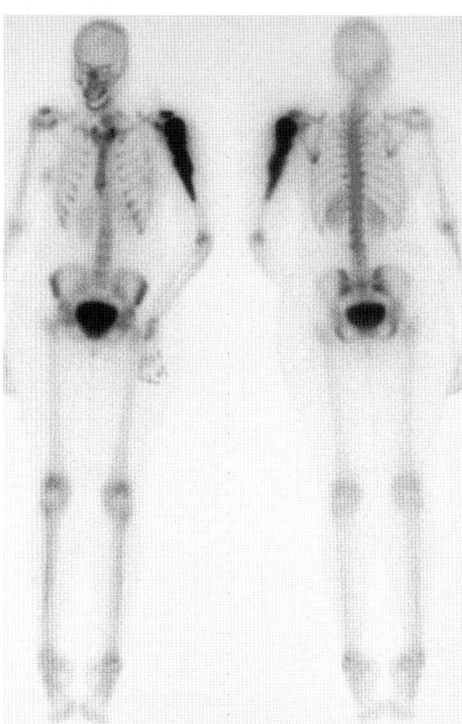

FIGURE 2-19. Bone scan findings in osteogenic sarcoma. The anterior and posterior views of a whole body bone scan in a patient with osteogenic sarcoma of the humerus show increased uptake in the left humeral head extending to the humeral shaft.

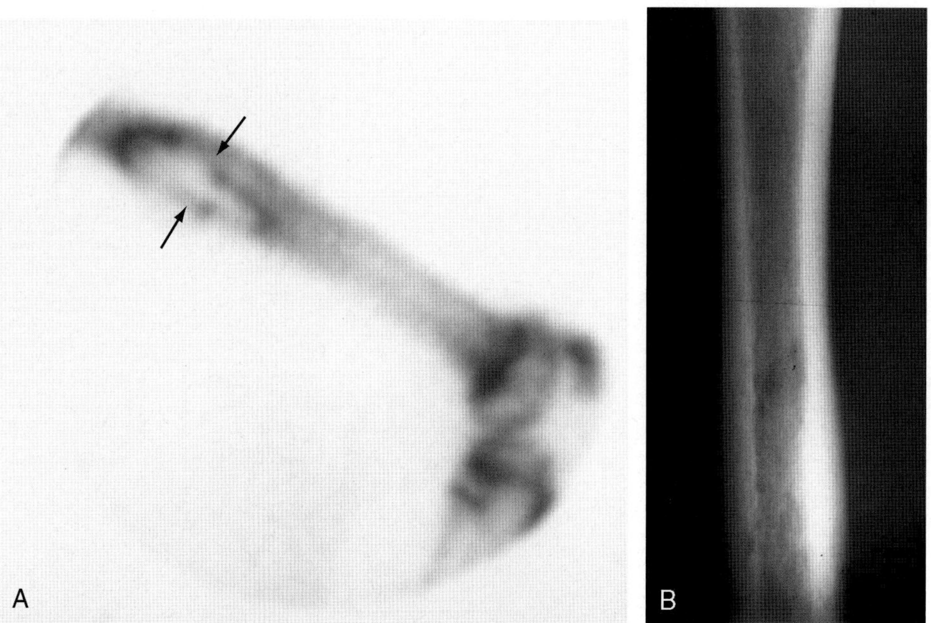

FIGURE 2-20. Bone scan findings in Ewing's sarcoma. **A,** Planar lateral view of the right femur in a patient with Ewing's sarcoma shows a photopenic area in the center of the lesion (due to necrosis within the tumor) and a peripheral rim of increased activity. Differential for this appearance includes aggressive infection or fracture with hematoma. **B,** The corresponding radiograph shows lytic changes in the diaphysis and cortical thickening consistent with Ewing's sarcoma.

FDG-PET is useful for the detection of osseous metastasis of Ewing's sarcoma, therapy monitoring, and evaluation of recurrence of disease. FDG-PET has been reported to detect a greater number of metastatic lesions in patients with Ewing's sarcoma than are found by bone scan and gallium scan, especially for those patients with bone marrow involvement.[52]

REFERENCES

1. Vos K, Vander Linden E, Pauwels EK: The clinical role of nuclear medicine in rheumatoid arthritis patients. A comparison with other diagnostic imaging modalities, *Quart J Nucl Med* 43:38-45, 1999.
2. Goal J, Mezes A, Siro B et al: Tc-99m HMPAO labeled leukocyte scintigraphy in patients with rheumatoid arthritis. A comparison with disease activity, *Nucl Med Commun* 23:39-46, 2002.
3. Bekers C, Ribbons C, Andre B et al: Assessment of disease activity in rheumatoid arthritis with F-18 FDG PET, *J Nucl Med* 45:956-964, 2002.
4. Bozhurt MF, Ugur O, Ertenli I et al: Combined use of bone and bone marrow scintigraphy for the diagnosis of active sacroiliitis: a new approach, *Ann Nucl Med* 15:117-121, 2001.
5. Yildiz A, Gungor F, Tuner T et al: Evaluation of sacroiliitis using Tc-99m nano colloid and Tc-99m MDP scintigraphy, *Nucl Med Commun* 22:785-794, 2001.
6. Handmaker H, Leonards R: The bone scan in inflammatory osseous disease, *Semin Nucl Med* 6:95-205, 1967.
7. Scoles PV, Hilty MD, Sfakianakis GN: Bone scan patterns in acute osteomyelitis, *Clin Orthop* 153:210-217, 1980.
8. Rosenthal L, Kloiber R, Damtew B et al: Sequential use of radiophosphate and radiogallium imaging in the differential diagnosis of bone and joint and soft tissue infection: quantitative analysis, *Diagn Imag* 51:249-258, 1982.
9. Tumeh SS, Aliabadi P, Weissman BN et al: Chronic osteomyelitis: bone and gallium scan patterns associated with active disease, *Radiology* 158:685-688, 1986.
10. Elgazzar AH, Abdel Dayem HM, Clark J et al: Multimodality imaging of osteomyelitis, *Eur J Nucl Med* 22:1043-1063, 1995.
11. Knight D, Gary HW, Bessent RG: Imaging for infection: caution required with the Charcot joint, *Eur J Nucl Med* 13:523-526, 1988.
12. Love C, Petel M, Loner BS et al: Diagnosing spinal osteomyelitis: a comparison of bone and gallium scintigraphy and magnetic resonance imaging, *Clin Nucl Med* 25:963-977, 2000.
13. Kolindou A, Liug Y, Ozker K et al: In-111 leukocyte imaging of osteomyelitis in patient with underlying bone scan abnormalities, *Clin Nucl Med* 21:83-191, 1996.
14. Seabald JE, Ferlic RJ, Marsh JL et al: Peri-articular bone uptake associated with traumatic injury: false positive findings with In-111 WBC and Tc-99m MDP scintigraphy, *Radiology* 186:845-849, 1993.
15. Ivanovic V, Dodig D, Livakovic M et al: Comparison of three phase bone scan, Tc-99m HMPAO and gallium scan in chronic bone infection, *Pro Clin Biol Res* 355:189-198, 1990.
16. Tuson GE, Hoffman EB, Mann MD: Isotope bone scanning for acute osteomyelitis and septic arthritis in children, *J Bone Joint Surg (Br)* 76B:306-310, 1994.
17. Demopulos GA, Black EE, Mcdougall R et al: Role of radionuclide imaging in the diagnosis of acute osteomelitis, *J Pedistr Orthop* 8:558-565, 1988.
18. Oswald SG, Vannostrand D, Savory CG et al: The acetabulum, a prospective study of three phase bone and indium white blood cell scintigraphy following coated hip arthroplasty, *J Nucl Med* 31:274-280, 1990.
19. Seabald JE, Nepola JV, Marsh JL et al: Post operative bone marrow alteration, potential pitfalls in the diagnosis of osteomyelitis with In-111 labeled leukocyte scintigraphy, *Radiology* 180:741-747, 1991.
20. Oyen WJG, Vanhorn JR, Claessens RAMJ et al: Diagnosis of bone, joint and joint prosthesis infection with IN-111 labeled nonspecific human immunoglobulin G scintigraphy, *Radiology* 182:195-199, 1992.
21. Zhuang H, Durate PS, Pourdehnad M et al: The promising role of F-18 FDG PET in detecting infected lower limb prosthesis implants, *J Nucl Med* 42:44-48, 2001.
22. Lander PH, Hadjipavlou AG: A dynamic classification of Paget's disease, *J Bone Joint Surg (Br)* 686:431-438, 1986.
23. Goen G, Mazzaferro S: Bone metabolism and its assessment in renal failure, *Nephron J* 67:383-401, 1994.
24. Fourier RS, Holder LE: Reflex sympathetic dystrophy, diagnostic controversies, *Semin Nucl Med* 28:116-123, 1998.
25. Zyluk A, Birkinfeed B: Quantitative evaluation of three phase bone scintigraphy before and after the treatment of post-traumatic RSD, *Nucl Med Commun* 20: 327-333, 1999.
26. Schiepers C: Clinical value of dynamic bone and vascular scintigraphy in diagnosing reflex sympathetic dystrophy of the upper extremity, *Hand Clin* 13:423-429, 1997.
27. Ali A, Telaman MR, Fordham EW et al: Distribution of hypertrophic pulmonary osteoarthropathy, *Amer J Roentger* 134:771-780, 1980.
28. Hans J, Ryu JS, Shin MS et al: Fibrous dysplasia with barely increased uptake on bone scan: a case report, *Clin Nucl Med* 25:785-788, 2000.
29. Toba M, Hayashida K, Imakita S et al: Increased bone mineral turn over without increased glucose utilization in sclerotic and hyperplastic change in fibrous dysplasia, *Ann Nucl Med* 12:153-155, 1968.
30. Matin P: The appearance of bone scan following fractures including intermediate and long term studies, *J Nucl Med* 20:1227-1231, 1979.
31. Holder LE, Schwarz C, Wernicke PG et al: Radiographic bone imaging in early detection of fractures of the proximal femur. Multifactorial analysis, *Radiology* 152: 509-515, 1990.
32. Elsaid M, Hamada A, Elgazzar A et al: When do flow and blood pool activity at fracture sites on bone scintigraphy normalize? *J Nucl Med* 41:327p, 2000.
33. Fowler C, Sullivan B, William LA et al: A comparison of bone scintigraphy and MRI in the diagnosis of the occult scaphoid fracture, *Skeletal Radiol* 27:683-687, 1998.
34. Zwas ST, Elkanovitch R, Frank G: Interpretation and classification of bone scintigraphic findings in stress fractures, *J Nucl Med* 28:452-457, 1987.
35. Holder LE, Michael RH: The scintigraphic pattern of shin splint in the lower leg concise communication, *J Nucl Med* 25:865-869, 1984.
36. Hatzl GM, Pichler R, Huber H et al: The insufficiency fracture of the sacrum. An often unrecognized cause of low back pain. Results of bone scanning in a major hospital, *Nuklearmedizin* 40:221-227, 2001.
37. Pavlov H: Imaging of the foot and ankle, *Radiol Clin Am* 28:991-1017, 1990.
38. Etchebehere EC, Etchebahere M, Gamba R et al: Orthopedic pathology of the lower extremities: scintigraphic evaluation in the thigh, knee and leg, *Semin Nucl Med* 28:41-61, 1998.
39. Stevenson JS, Right RW, Dunson GL et al: Tc-99m phosphonate bone imaging: a method of assessing bone graft healing, *Radiology* 110:391-396, 1974.
40. Bohnsack M, Gosse F, Ruhmann O et al: The value of scintigraphy in the diagnosis of pseudoarthrosis after fusion surgery, *J Spine Disord* 12:482-484, 1999.
41. Enneking WF: *Classification of nontraumatic osteonecrosis of the femoral head*, Rosemont, Ill., 1997, American Academy of Orthopaedic Surgeons, pp 269-275.
42. Macleod MA, Houston AS: Functional bone imaging in the detection of ischemic osteopathies, *Clin Nucl Med* 22:1-5, 1997.
43. Jin Sook R, Jae KS, Dae MH et al: Bone SPECT is more sensitive than MRI in the detection of early osteonecrosis of the femoral head after renal transplantation, *J Nucl Med* 43:1008-1011, 2002.
44. Schutle M, Brecht KD, Werner M et al: Evaluation of neoadjuvant therapy response of osteogenic sarcoma using FDG-PET, *J Nucl Med* 40:1637-1643, 2000.
45. Franzius C, Sciuk J, Daldrup HE et al: FDG PET for detection of osseous metastasis from malignant primary bone tumors; comparison with bone scintigraphy, *Eur J Nucl Med* 27:1305-1311, 2000.
46. Aoki J, Watanabe H, Shinoza K et al: FDG-PET of primary benign and malignant bone tumors standard uptake value (SUV) in 52 lesions, *Radiology* 219:774-777, 2001.
47. Mungo DV, Zhang X, O'Keefe RJ et al: Cox-1 and Cox-2 expression in osteoid osteoma, *J Orthop Res* 20:159-162, 2002.
48. Dablin DC, Conventry MB: Osteogenic sarcoma; a study of 600 cases, *J Bone Joint Surg (Am)* 49:101-110, 1967.
49. Mckillop JH, Etcubanas E, Goris ML: The indications for and limitation of bone scintigraphy in osteogenic sarcoma, *Cancer* 48:1133-1138, 1981.
50. Franzius F, Bielack S, Flege S et al: Prognostic significance of F-18 FDG and Tc-99m MDP uptake in primary osteogenic sarcoma, *J Nucl Med* 43:1012-1017, 2002.
51. Kile AC, Nieweg OE, Hoekstra HS et al: F-18 FDG assessment of glucose metabolism in bone tumors, *J Nucl Med* 39:810-815, 1998.
52. Hung GU, Tan TS, Kao CH et al: Multiple skeletal metastasis of Ewing's sarcoma demonstrated on FDG-PET and compared with bone and gallium scans, *Kaohsing J Med Sci* 16:315-318, 2000.

CHAPTER 3

Magnetic Resonance Imaging

HIROSHI YOSHIOKA, MD, PHD, PHILIPP M. SCHLECHTWEG, MD, *and* KATSUMI KOSE, PHD

KEY FACTS

- Clinical magnetic resonance imaging (MRI) measures the spatial distribution of protons in the body.
- Gradient coils are used to provide spatial information. The changing gradients are associated with noise produced during imaging.
- Relaxation times T1, T2, and T2* are important tissue characteristics for imaging.
- Low-field magnets have lower signal to noise ratio (SNR); longer scan times, making patient motion a potential problem; decreased resolution; decreased sensitivity to old blood and calcified lesions; lower gadolinium enhancement; and difficulty in spectral fat suppression.
- Gadolinium contrast medium is often used combined with fat-suppressed T1-weighted imaging to increase contrast between enhanced tissue and surrounding tissue.
- Artifacts are numerous in MRI and can lead to erroneous diagnosis if not understood or eliminated. The magic angle phenomenon produces increased signal in portions of tendons oriented at approximately 55 degrees to the main magnetic field. These areas will appear bright on short TE sequences (e.g., T1) and can lead to an erroneous diagnosis of degeneration or tear.
- Patient safety is paramount and can be maximized by thorough prescreening and other safety measures.

GENERAL PRINCIPLES

Imaging Principles

Magnetic resonance imaging (MRI) measures the spatial distribution of specific nuclear spins (usually those of protons) in the body. Electric signals from the spins are measured using precessional motion of the proton spins after they are excited by radiofrequency (RF) pulses irradiated in a static magnetic field.

> *Precession* refers to a change in the direction of the axis of a rotating object.

The phenomenon in which the nuclear spins generate or emit electric signals of a specific frequency (Larmor frequency) in a static magnetic field is called *nuclear magnetic resonance* (NMR).

The electric signal (NMR signal) itself carries no spatial information. The spatial information necessary to generate an image is given by magnetic field gradients that are generated by gradient coils. Because they are driven by pulsed electric currents in a strong magnetic field, the coils receive a repetitive strong force, and a loud sound is produced during the MRI scan.

NMR Signal: Free Induction Decay and Spin Echo

Two kinds of NMR signal are generally used in MRI: free induction decay (FID) and spin echo. FID is elicited by a single RF pulse (e.g., 90 degrees) (Figure 3-1). The FID decays with the time constant T2*. The decay of the NMR signal can be recovered by applying a second RF pulse, called a *180-degree pulse.* At a specific time (TE/2) after the second RF pulse, the spin echo signal is observed. The intensity of the spin echo signal decays with the time constant T2.

Relaxation Times

The relaxation times of proton spins are the most important parameters in MRI. Three kinds of relaxation times are generally used: T1, T2, and T2*. T1 or longitudinal relaxation time is the time by which nuclear spins return to thermal equilibrium (initial state) after irradiation by an RF pulse(s). T1 is generally used to visualize the degree of saturation or suppression of NMR signal or image intensity because tissues with longer T1 give suppressed NMR signal in T1-weighted sequences, as described below.

> Tissues with long T1 are dark on T1-weighted images.

T2, or transverse relaxation time, describes the lifetime of spin echo signal, as shown in Figure 3-1. T2 is generally used to distinguish pathologic tissues from normal tissues, because proton spins of pathologic tissues usually have longer T2.

> Tissues with a long T2 appear bright on T2-weighted images.

T2* describes the decay rate of FID signal, as shown in Figure 3-1. Although T1 and T2 depend on NMR frequency (magnetic field strength), typical T1 and T2 values of water content in normal tissues are roughly 1000 ms and 50 ms, respectively. T1 and T2 of pathologic tissues usually become longer than those of normal tissues, making MRI very useful in diagnosis of various diseases.

PULSE SEQUENCES AND IMAGE CONTRAST

The contrast of magnetic resonance (MR) images is determined by combinations of relaxation times and pulse sequences. The pulse sequences are divided into two major categories: spin echo and gradient echo sequences.

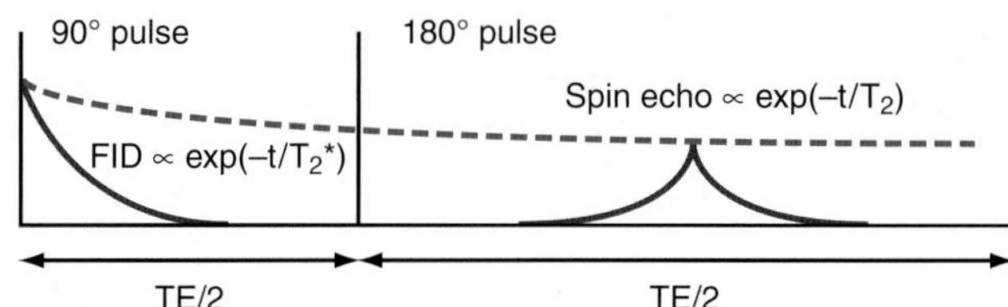

FIGURE 3-1. FID and spin echo. The spin echo signals decay exponentially. The time constant of this decay curve is called *T2 relaxation time.* The faster decay due to non-uniformities in the main magnetic field is called a *free induction decay* (FID) with a time constant of T2*.

Spin Echo Sequence

Spin echo (SE) sequences utilize spin echo signal and produce spin echo images, in which image intensity, $I(x,y)$, is expressed as:

$$I(x,y) = k\rho(x,y)\{1 - \exp(-TR/T1(x,y))\}\ \exp(-TE/T2(x,y)),$$

where k, ρ (x,y), TR, and TE are a constant, proton density, repetition time of the pulse sequence, and spin echo time, respectively (see Figure 3-1). This equation shows that spin echo images are proton density images modified by the ratios of TR/T1 and TE/T2. Although $\rho(x,y)$, $T1(x,y)$, and $T2(x,y)$ can be computed by combinations of several spin echo images, three practically useful images are widely used: T1-weighted images (T1WI), T2-weighted images (T2WI), and proton density weighted images (PDWI). Because T1 and T2 of water-content normal tissues are roughly 1000 ms and 50 ms, respectively, the pulse sequences shown in Table 3-1 are used for T1WI, T2WI, and PDWI acquisition. Typical and instructive T1WI, T2WI, and PDWI of a chicken egg are shown in Figure 3-2. The yolk and white of the egg are visualized with various image contrasts because they have different T1, T2, and proton densities.

Because imaging appearances vary depending on the imaging parameters used, attention should be directed to the parameters listed on the image itself. The TR and TE, among other parameters, are indicated adjacent to the MR image (Figure 3-3).

TABLE 3-1. Parameter-Weighted Spin Echo Sequences

	TR << 1000 ms	1000 ms << TR
TE << 50 ms	T1WI	PDWI
50 ms << TE	Not used	T2WI

Table 3-2 explains the appearance of common tissues on SE imaging. The signal may change depending on the combination of the TR, TE, and inversion time (TI) used for obtaining the sequence.

In actual clinical settings, SE sequences are usually performed as fast spin echo (FSE) sequences to shorten the imaging time by using multiple spin echoes. Basic image contrasts are similar to those obtained by the traditional or conventional spin echo sequences described above. However, fat tissue is of higher signal on FSE T2-weighted imaging than on spin echo T2-weighted imaging.

Gradient Echo Sequence

Gradient echo (GRE) sequences utilize FID signal and are characterized by sequence parameters TR, TE, and FA (flip angle). The FA is the angle by which nuclear spins are rotated from the direction of the static magnetic field. However, the image contrasts of GRE images are not determined solely by the sequence parameters but are strongly affected by the pulse sequence design.

Regarding the pulse sequence design, GRE sequences are categorized into three groups: incoherent acquisition sequence (e.g., FLASH, SPGR), partially coherent acquisition sequence (e.g., GRASS, FISP), and coherent acquisition sequence (e.g., TrueFISP, SSFP). MRI manufacturers use different names for their own GRE sequences. However, for simplicity, we use the terms FLASH, GRASS, and TrueFISP to represent the three acquisition methods described above. FLASH is mainly used as a T1-weighted sequence. GRASS is used as a T2*-weighted or T1-weighted sequence. FLASH and GRASS are faster than the spin echo T1-weighted sequence, but the image contrasts are slightly different (Figure 3-4). TrueFISP is a very fast sequence and is mainly used for visualization of fluids such as blood.

VARIOUS TECHNIQUES

Multislice and Three-Dimensional Imaging

As shown in Table 3-1, TR is usually much longer than TE or T2 because T1 recovery of proton spins takes longer than T2 decay. To shorten the scan time for an imaging volume, the pulse sequences are designed to excite multiple planes successively during the repetition time. This technique is called *multislice imaging.*

Three-dimensional (3D) imaging is another solution for shortening the scan time. 3D imaging is usually performed with short TR gradient echo sequences because long TR requires a long acquisition time. 3D imaging has several advantages over multislice imaging, including thin slices, no slice gap, and isotropic voxel.

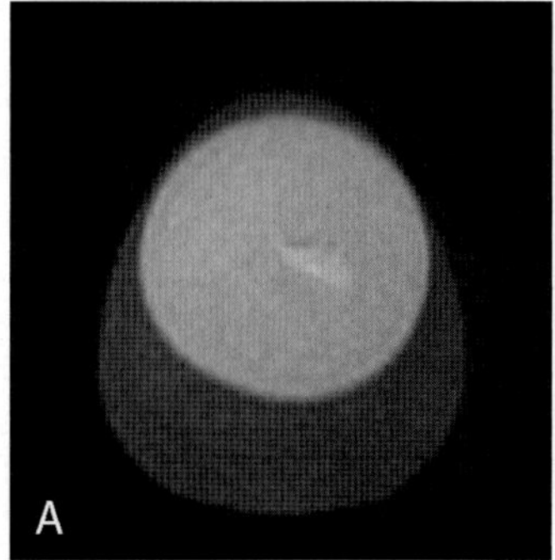

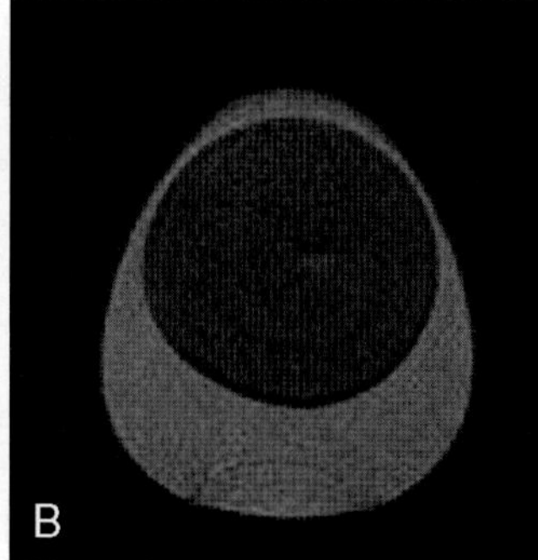

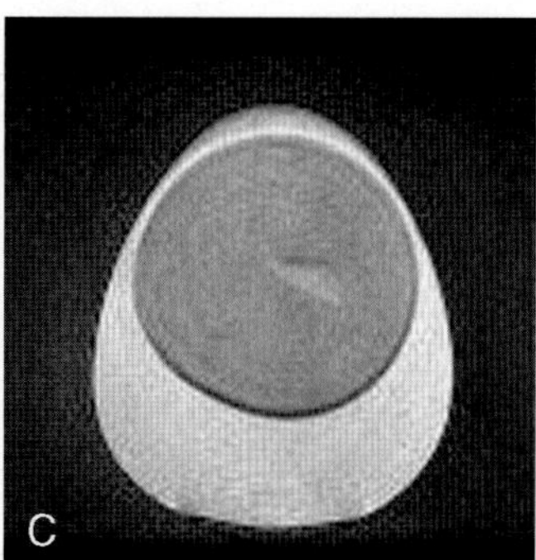

FIGURE 3-2. Spin echo images of an egg show different contrast among **(A)** T1-weighted image (TR/TE = 400/6 msec), **(B)** T2-weighted image (TR/TE = 1000/48 msec), and **(C)** Proton density weighted image (PDWI) (TR/TE = 4000/6 msec). Note the bright appearance of the fatty yolk on the T1-weighted image.

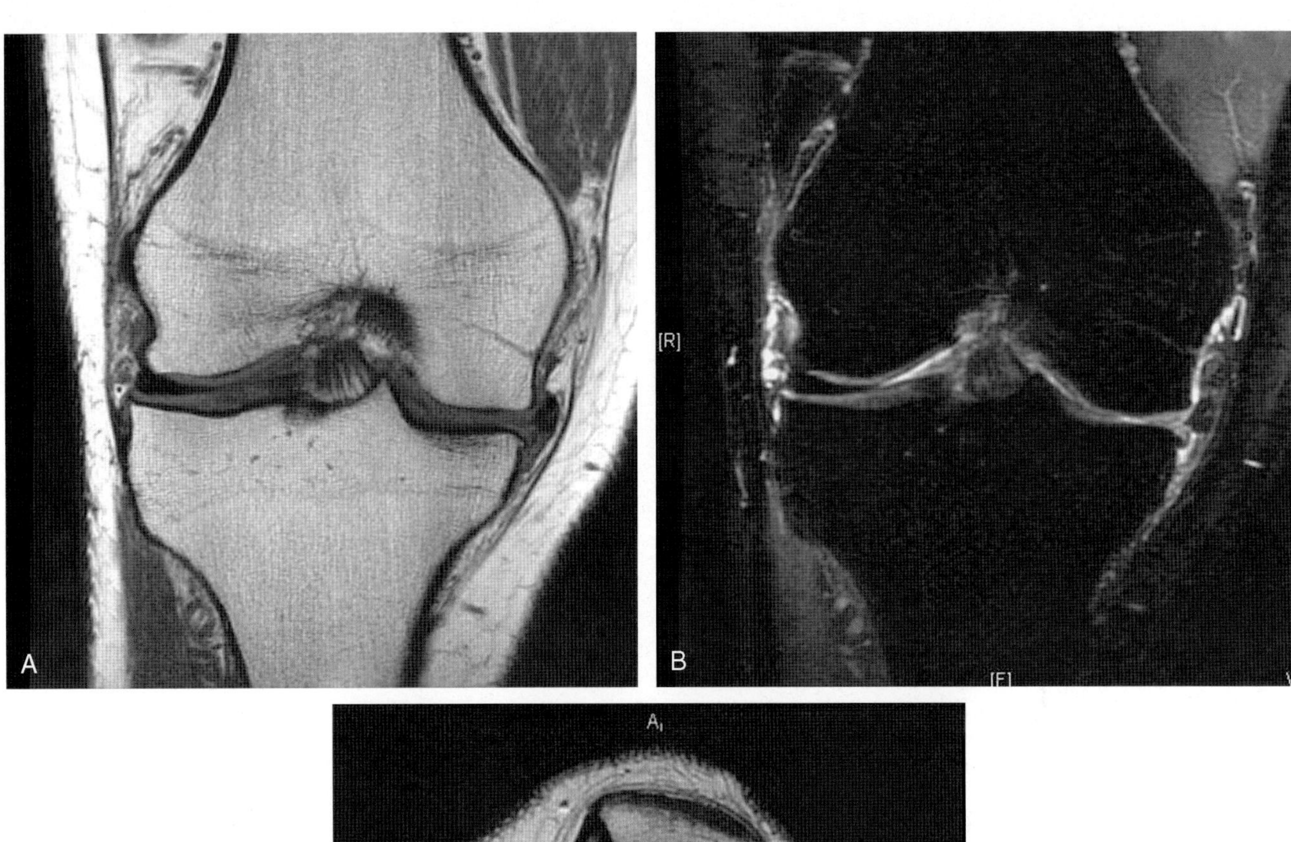

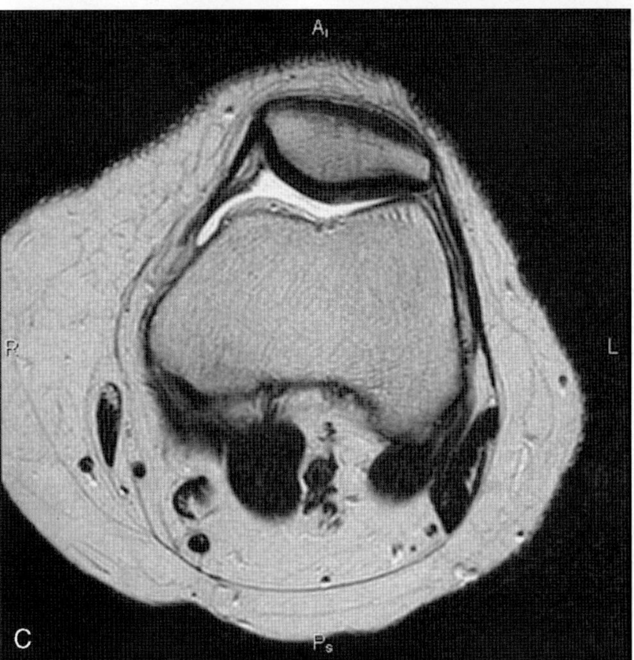

FIGURE 3-3. MRI appearances of the knee on **(A)** coronal T1-weighted image, **(B)** coronal STIR image, and **(C)** axial T2-weighted image. MR parameters are indicated adjacent to the MR image. Note that the appearance of fat is bright on the T1-weighted image and dark on the STIR image. Fluid signal is bright on the STIR sequence, making this sequence useful for identifying conditions with increased fluid such as tumor or edema. On the T2-weighted fast spin echo sequence **(C)** the joint fluid is bright. In fast spin echo images, fat is also bright, which sometimes limits the distinction between these two tissues.

A voxel is a volume element that forms a small portion of the image.

Fat Suppression

Fat is visualized as a high-intensity signal on T1WI, PDWI, and even in T2WI. Fat signal therefore frequently conceals slight contrast differences between water-content tissues near the fatty tissues. In this situation, fat suppression techniques are used, either by utilizing Larmor frequency difference (~220 Hz at 1.5T) between water and fat signals or by using T1 difference between fat and other tissues. The former technique is the "chemical shift selective" method and is used in high-field MRI machines. The latter technique is one of the inversion recovery methods in which image acquisition is performed when the fat signal becomes zero after the fat proton spins are inverted from the direction of the static magnetic field. This technique is called *short tau inversion recovery* (STIR) and is used mainly in low-field MRI machines.

TABLE 3-2. Examples of Tissue Appearance on Common Imaging Sequences

	T1 weighted	T2 weighted	STIR
Bone cortex, calcification	Very low signal	Very low signal	Very low signal
Bone marrow	High signal	High signal	Low signal
Cartilage	Iso-signal	Slightly low signal	Iso-signal
Joint effusion	Iso-signal	High signal	High signal
Acute hemorrhage	Low to iso-signal	Low to iso-signal	Low to iso-signal
Subacute hemorrhage	High signal	High signal	Various signal
Hemosiderin	Very low signal	Very low signal	Very low signal
Fat	High signal	High signal if FSE	Low signal

Comparison is made to the signal of muscle. FSE, Fast spin echo.

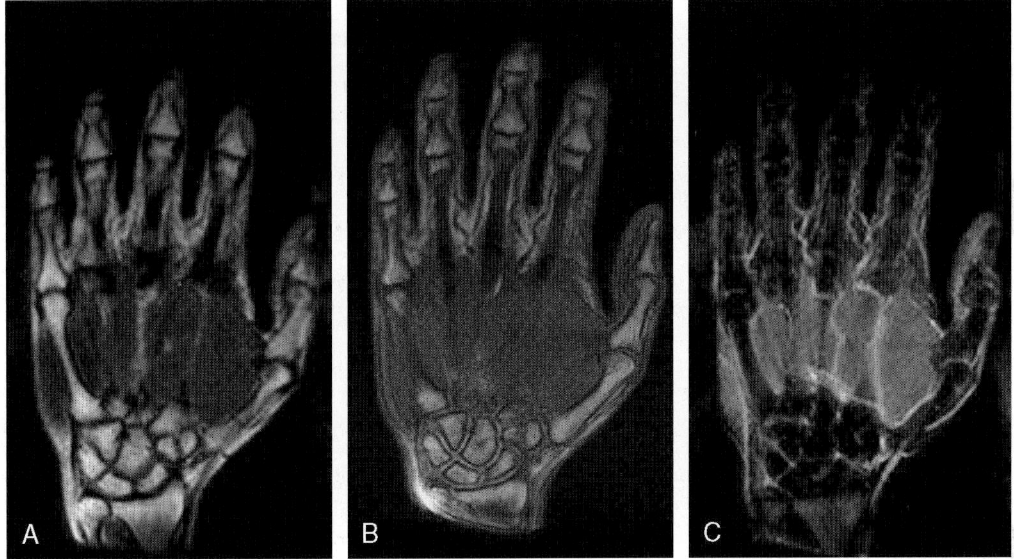

FIGURE 3-4. MR images of a hand at 0.2T: **(A)** fast spin echo T1WI (TR/TE = 200/20), **(B)** GRASS (TR/TE/flip angle = 50/9/60 degrees), and **(C)** STIR (TR/inversion time/TE = 1000/120/40). Note the bright fat in the bone marrow on the T1-weighted image, the dark fat on the STIR image, and the bright fluid within vessels on the STIR image.

Figure 3-4, *C*, shows a STIR image of a hand acquired at 0.2T. Bone marrow and subcutaneous fat signals are well suppressed.

> STIR images are clinically useful because the fat signal is suppressed (black) and fluid (e.g., edema) becomes easier to identify (white).

MRI SYSTEM: FIELD STRENGTH AND MAGNET CONFIGURATION

Field Strength

A variety of magnetic field strengths from 0.2T to 3.0T are used for clinical MRI of arthritis and bone lesions.

> T (Tesla) is a measure of magnetic field strength; 1 Tesla is approximately 20,000 times the Earth's magnetic force.

The major advantage of high-field MRI is the increase in SNR, which improves spatial and/or temporal resolution and reduces scan time while preserving image quality. On the other hand, a low-field magnet allows a variety of configurations, increases the patient's comfort by using an open magnet and dedicated MRI system for extremities, and makes possible isocenter imaging even for off-center anatomic sites. The open MRI magnets usually have field strength in the range of 0.2T to 0.7T. Disadvantages of low-field magnets are lower SNR, increased acquisition time, decreased resolution, decreased sensitivity to old blood and calcified lesions, lower gadolinium enhancement, and difficulty of spectral fat suppression (Table 3-3).

Closed Magnet MRI

The closed magnet configuration refers to the original tube shape of most MRI scanners (Figure 3-5, *A*). All high-field superconducting MRI scanners are of the closed configuration type. Currently, 90% of MRI machines are traditional closed MRIs. As mentioned previously, high-field MRIs produce higher SNR and superior quality imaging. Therefore MRI with a closed magnet would be the first choice in many cases. Problems arise with claustrophobic patients and overweight (over 350 lb) patients, for whom open magnet or extremity MRI would be the next choice.

TABLE 3-3. Advantages and Disadvantages of Low-Field MRI

	Advantages*	Disadvantages*
Length of exam		Longer scan times
Patient comfort	"Open" magnets may be more comfortable	
Large or claustrophobic patients	May be scanned on open or extremity scanners	
Signal to noise ratio		Lower
Resolution		Decreased
Fat suppression		Limited
Gadolinium		May need higher dose
Cost of unit	Relatively less expensive	
Size of unit	Extremity units are smaller	

*In comparison to high-field units.

Extremity and Open Magnet MRI

Despite the previous considerations, the use of dedicated extremity and open magnet MRI for the evaluation of arthritis and other musculoskeletal pathologic conditions has several advantages over the use of whole body MRI.

Dedicated extremity MRI requires less space than a whole body MRI system, is less expensive, offers greater patient comfort, avoids claustrophobia, and minimizes potential biohazards associated with the presence of metal in or on the patient by placing only the limb of interest in the magnet bore (Figure 3-5, *B*). It has been reported that 64% of patients with arthritis of the hand and wrist preferred 0.2T extremity MRI to 1.5T high-field MRI because it was more comfortable, less claustrophobic, and quieter.[1] Recently, low-field dedicated extremity MRI has been used for the evaluation of rheumatoid arthritis (RA) of the hand and wrist. Low-field MRI performed well for cross-sectional grading of bone erosions, joint space narrowing, and synovitis in RA. Even low-field MRI detected approximately twice as many erosions as radiography.[2] The volume of synovial membrane determined with extremity MRI was significantly correlated with and not significantly different from that determined with high-field MRI with gadolinium injection.[1] Therefore low-field dedicated extremity MRI may be useful for the evaluation of RA.

Open MRI allows easy access to patients (Figure 3-5, *C*), making it well suited for patients who are very large, severely anxious, claustrophobic, or in need of constant support during an exam (e.g., children). In addition, open MRI makes it possible to perform interventional MRI, which requires open magnet technology and real-time imaging. There are two types of open magnet MRI: vertically and horizontally open magnets. The vertically open MRI system (Signa SP, GE Medical Systems, Milwaukee) allows radiologists and surgeons direct vertical access to the patient through an opening, with near real-time imaging. This system is a whole body scanner operating with a 0.5T-superconducting magnet with actively shielded gradients. The flexible RF coil with sterile covers is placed on the patient during an intervention. MRI has several advantages over other equipment for interventional guidance. MRI does not expose patients, radiologists, or surgeons to ionizing radiation. Excellent soft tissue contrast aids in selecting a biopsy site with multiplanar imaging capability.

MRI ARTIFACT

MRI produces several specific artifacts; familiarity with them is essential for a correct diagnosis.

Motion Artifact

Motion artifact is presumably the most common artifact in MRI. It causes ghosts and blurring on MR images, as the phase gradient cannot anticipate and encode signals from moving structures. Its sources are voluntary motions, involuntary motions, and physiologic motions.[3] Voluntary motions by the patient can be minimized by explaining the importance of keeping still. Children may have lower compliance, and sedation might be necessary. Involuntary motions are more difficult to handle, as they cannot be suppressed through the patient's own will. There is a broad range of causes, from mental illness to neurodegenerative processes such as Parkinson's disease or Huntington's chorea. Physiologic motions in the patient's body are multifactorial. For example, great difficulties in thoracic imaging have been caused by respiration and cardiac action. Shorter sequences and electrocardiogram (ECG)-controlled picture acquisition help counteract these problems.[4] Other physiologic motions such as pulsation in arteries or bowel peristalsis are more difficult to handle.[5,6] At least the latter can be controlled to a certain extent by antispasmodics. Using short sequences such as single shot fast spin echo (SSFSE) helps reduce the likelihood of motion artifacts.[7]

Flow Artifact

Flow artifact is one type of motion artifact caused by motion of liquids within the human body, usually blood or cerebrospinal fluid (CSF). Arterial flow artifact has not only a flowing component but also a pulsating one. The reasons for flow artifacts are multiple, and their appearance varies. Blood flowing through a slice can undergo excitation from an incoming RF pulse but might already have left the slice before readout. As a result, the vessel would appear empty or at least less bright than expected. It is more difficult to record an adequate signal from within vessels with a laminar pulsatile flow. Possible reasons for low signal intensity are: (1) fast flow, (2) intravoxel phase dispersion from different velocities in the voxel, (3) odd-ordered echo dephasing, (4) displacement effects related to in-plane flow during acquisition, and (5) saturation from prior RF pulse.[3]

The artifacts caused by flow might even appear bright. If blood flow is slow, a certain amount of unsaturated blood might follow the saturated blood, which has experienced a prior RF pulse. When the unsaturated volume flows into the slice just in time to experience the 90-degree pulse, it creates a stronger signal than expected. Hence possible reasons for high signal intensity are: (1) slice-related

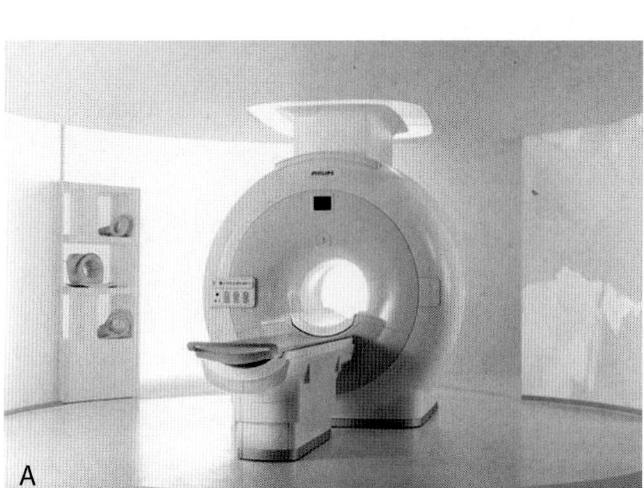

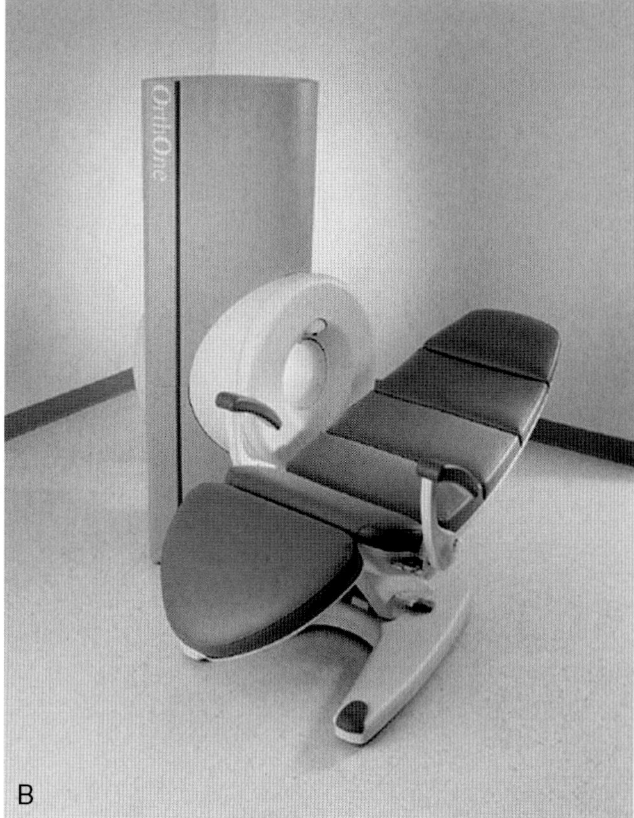

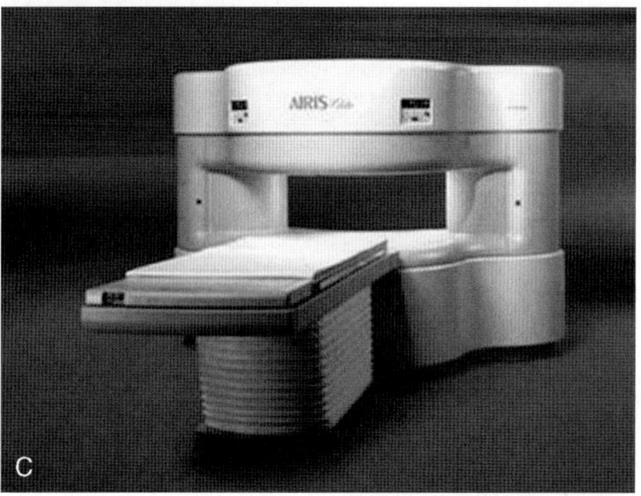

FIGURE 3-5. Various magnets used for MRI: **(A)** 1.5T closed magnet MRI system; **(B)** 1T high-field dedicated extremity MRI system, and **(C)** 0.3T open MRI system. (**A,** Courtesy of Philips Medical Systems; **B,** courtesy of ONI Medical Systems; **C,** courtesy of Hitachi Medical Corporation.)

inflow enhancement, (2) even-echo rephrasing, (3) diastolic pseudogating, and (4) pseudoflow related to methemoglobin.[3]

Possible techniques to reduce artifacts include flow compensation, saturation pulses, and cardiac triggering.[4,8] Flow compensation uses a series of gradient pulse sequences to eliminate the interfering effects of fluids in motion. With saturation pulses, signals are added parallel to slices to suppress the blood signal.[8] Cardiac triggering works by synchronizing the imaging sequences with cardiac action.[4] Sometimes this artifact overlies normal or pathologic structures, making diagnosis difficult. The switching of phase and frequency direction may help in such cases[9] (Figure 3-6).

Flow artifacts may overlie normal tissues and lead to diagnostic errors.

Wrap-Around Artifact

Wrap-around is a preventable artifact caused by improper choice of parameters in an MRI scan. If the field of view (FOV) is made too small, the tissue surrounding the FOV might become excited and produce interference signals during readout. As phase encoding gradients are gauged for the FOV alone, they cannot integrate this "external"

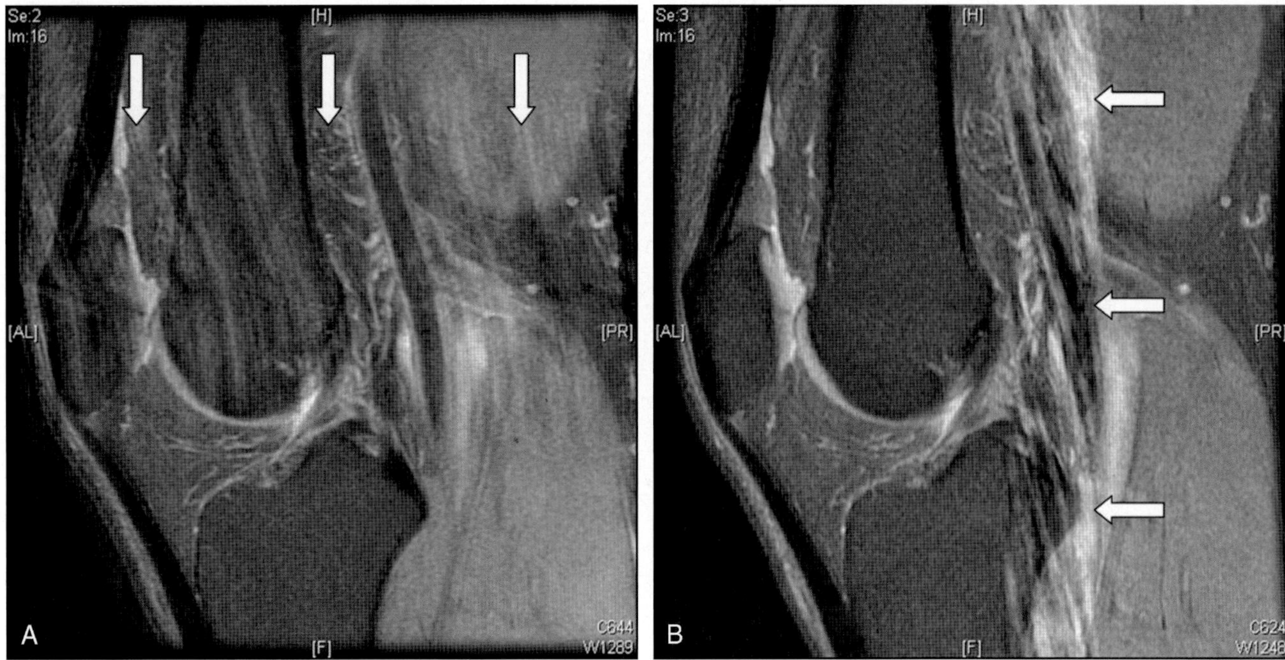

FIGURE 3-6. Flow artifact. The direction of the flow artifact *(arrows)* from the popliteal artery occurs along with phase-encoding direction: **A,** anterior-posterior; **B,** superior-inferior (head-feet). Note that in **A,** the bone detail is obscured by artifact.

signal. Thus the signal is not correctly registered as to location, but instead gets wrapped around to the opposite side of the FOV (Figure 3-7). This phenomenon is also called "aliasing." In a clinical setting, the frequency direction is usually chosen along the long axis of the object to be scanned to avoid wrap-around artifacts. There are other approaches to avoid this common artifact. The simplest way is to add presaturation pulses to tissue you do not want to image before applying the pulses for excitation.[10] Another solution is the use of low-pass and high-pass RF filters, which filter out initial signals that exceed the bandwidth. Increasing the FOV is a possible solution, with the caveat that it decreases spatial resolution of images.[3] Finally, a "no phase wrap" option is provided by some manufacturers.[9] This doubles the FOV, thereby doubling the phase encoding steps (phase oversampling) to keep resolution at the same level while halving the number of excitations to keep scan time constant.

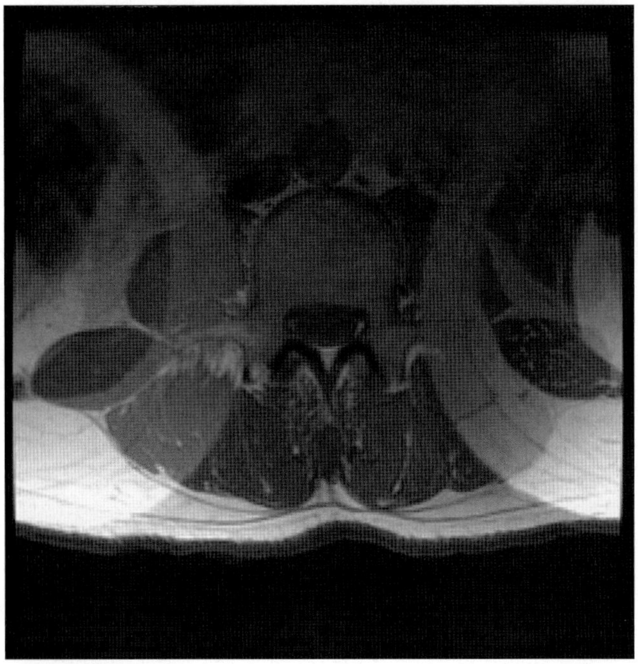

FIGURE 3-7. Wrap-around artifact. Small FOV and anterior-posterior frequency encoding lead to wrap-around artifact on axial MR images of the lumbar spine.

Chemical Shift Artifact

At the boundary between tissues high in fat and those high in water, protons of fat can be incorrectly imaged, an effect called *chemical shift artifact.* It can occur in MRI because of slight differences in the precession frequency (also known as *Lamor frequency;* $\nu = \gamma * B0$) of these protons. These different frequencies are caused by slight inhomogeneities of the main magnetic field ($\Delta\ \nu = \gamma * \Delta B0$) and get worse with increasing field strengths. In a 1T magnet, the difference in frequency is 147 Hz, whereas in a 1.5-T magnetic field the difference is 224 Hz.[11]

> Hertz (Hz) is the SI unit (International System of Units) of frequency. One Hertz is defined as the reciprocal second: $1\ \text{Hz} = 1\ \text{s}^{-1}$.

Because the computer assumes all protons precess at the same frequency, the signal from fat is mapped to a different location corresponding to the frequency at which it is processing. Narrow receive bandwidths accentuate this by assigning a smaller number of frequencies across the image (Figure 3-8). This artifact may appear as high-intensity areas when signals of water and fat overlap and low-intensity areas when their signals spread apart.[12] As a result, the affected structures may be incorrectly imaged and thereby misinterpreted. The chemical shift artifacts in musculoskeletal imaging are seen in vertebral end plates, fluid-filled cysts, fat containing tumors, and at the cartilage–bone marrow interface.[13,14]

Increasing bandwidth and using low-field magnets are options to reduce chemical shift artifact. Other feasible solutions to reduce

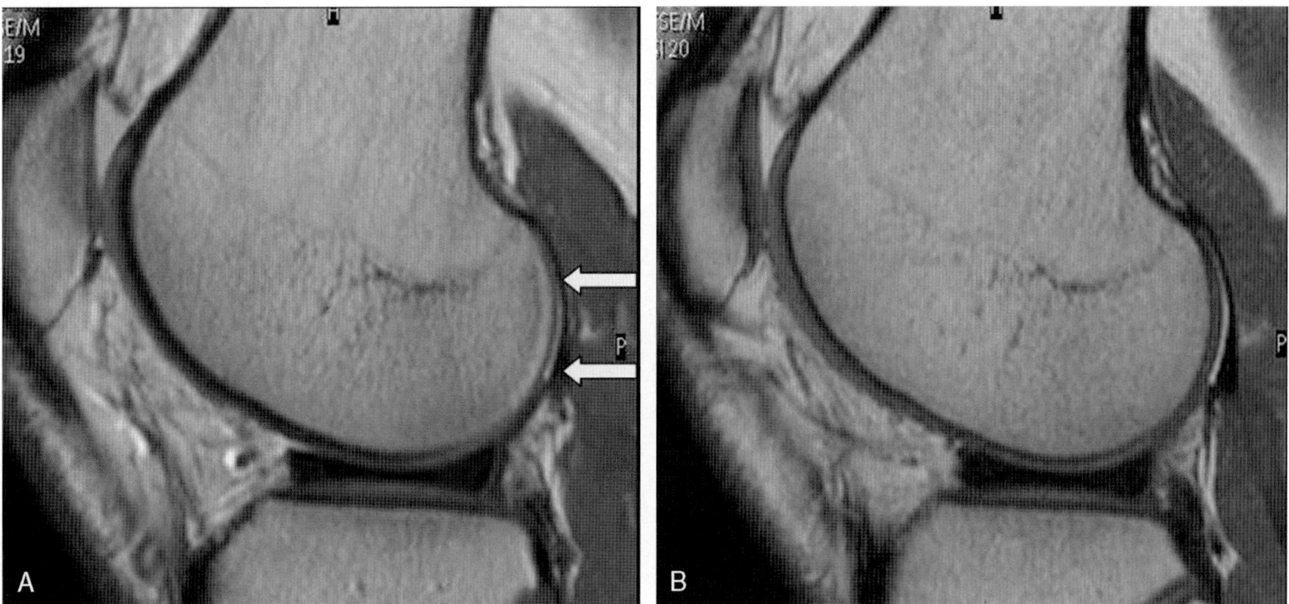

FIGURE 3-8. Chemical shift artifact. **A,** MR image with narrow bandwidth (72.4 Hz) shows more prominent chemical shift artifact than **(B)** that with wide bandwidth (446.4 kHz). The chemical shift artifact makes it difficult to evaluate cartilage *(arrows)*. Note the apparent change in the thickness of the anterior femoral cortex on the two images. (Courtesy of Philips Medical Systems.)

this artifact include fat suppression techniques or switching phase and frequency encoding directions.[15-17]

Susceptibility Artifact

Susceptibility artifacts are caused by microscopic gradients or by substances with different magnetic susceptibilities at the boundary between contiguous tissues. The difference in magnetic susceptibility can lead to minor inhomogeneities in the magnetic field strength, which in turn cause distortion in terms of spatial frequency or signal intensity. A ferromagnetic object residing in a diamagnetic structure like the human body is sensitive to magnetic susceptibility. This object induces eddy current due to the incident RF magnetic field, altering the RF field near itself and thereby causing distortion. This in turn creates gradients that produce dephasing of spins and frequency shifts in surrounding tissue.[18] Susceptibility artifacts on MR images appear as areas with profuse signal intensity or are totally devoid of signal.

Susceptibility artifacts obscure surrounding normal structures and may also mask areas of abnormality (Figure 3-9). Large susceptibility artifacts can be seen around prosthetic joints with GRE sequences.[19] Long echo times also exacerbate these artifacts[18];

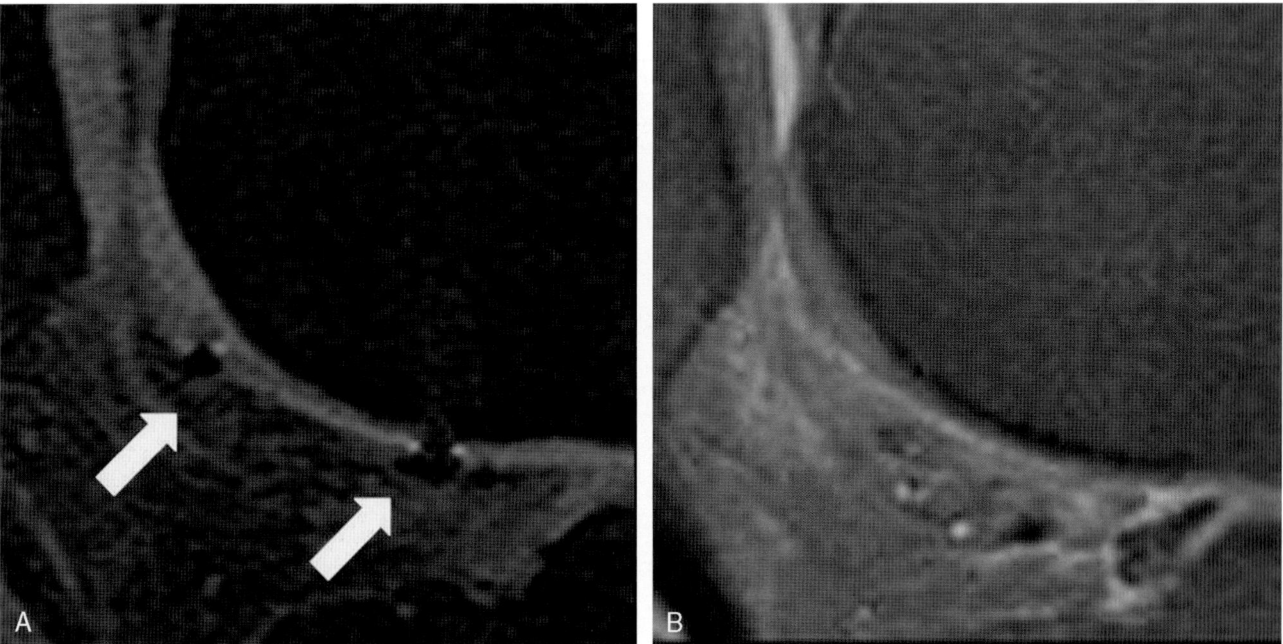

FIGURE 3-9. Magnetic susceptibility artifact over the cartilage surface of the knee *(arrows)*. **A,** GRE image is more sensitive to difference in the magnetic susceptibility than **(B)** FSE image. These artifacts *(arrows)* typically result from prior surgery and may not be visible on radiographs.

SE or FSE may help minimize these artifacts, as do high bandwidth and short echo times.

Magic Angle Effect

This effect is responsible for producing increased signal (and therefore possible erroneus diagnosis) in certain tissues such as tendons. The magic angle effect is a phenomenon related to collagen anisotropy in MRI.[20]

Anisotropy is the property of being directionally dependent.

If the angle between the main magnetic field (B0) direction and the collagen fiber increases from 0 degrees, the signal intensity on short TE sequence changes as a result of increasing T2 relaxation time.[21] T2 relaxation time is at its maximum at an angle of almost 55 degrees relative to B0.[20,22-24] It occurs in any tissue that contains anisotropically arranged collagen fibres such as tendons, menisci, and hyaline cartilage.[22,25,26]

The water content of cartilage varies from 76% in deep layers to 84% in superficial layers.[27,28] The short T2 relaxation time in cartilage depends on the dipolar orientation of water molecules, which are linked to collagen macromolecules. Histologically, hyaline cartilage has multiple layers (superficial, transitional, deep radial, calcified cartilage) that are distinct from the layers seen on high-resolution MRI.[29] Microscopy studies reveal that collagen fibrils in the deep radial layer of cartilage are arranged perpendicular to the subchondral bone, but more superficially, fiber orientation parallels the articular surface.[24] This arrangement induces the magic angle effect. If cartilage is placed in the magnet, the area of anisotropic arrangement of collagen fibers increases signal intensity at magic angle.[20,22,23] It can occur in any depth of cartilage.[30] The increased signal and inhomogeneity of signal in the articular cartilage created by this artifact should not be confused with early degenerative changes in the cartilage substance.

The magic angle effect is also seen in various tendons. The rotator cuff, in particular the supraspinatus tendon, is frequently examined in MRI (Figure 3-10).[31,32] Magic angle effects in healthy tissue can look similar to signal abnormalities caused by degenerative processes or a partial tear and can lead to difficulties in diagnosis. To avoid the magic angle effect, long TE sequences with and without fat suppression may help or, if necessary, repositioning of the patient may be tried.[21,33]

Truncation Artifact

Truncation artifacts are also known as *Gibbs ringing artifacts* (in honor of Josiah W. Gibbs). They appear in MR images as alternating dark and bright lines that run parallel to a sharp change in signal intensity.[34] For example, this change can be produced at the boundary between layers of fat and muscle tissue. Truncation artifact was also frequently observed in the cartilage of both the patellofemoral compartment and the posterior region of the femoral condyles on fat-suppressed 3D SPGR images. This laminar appearance does not indicate degenerative change of the articular cartilage, nor does it reflect the anatomic layers of the cartilage; it is merely an artifact (Figure 3-11).[35-37]

Truncation artifact occurs when the echo at the edges of the acquisition window does not return to 0. This happens especially when a small acquisition matrix is used. One way to reduce the severity of this effect is to increase the resolution of image, but this reduces the SNR or extends the imaging time. Another possibility is to use filters on images, although this can be associated with decreased image resolution. Changing the frequency and phase encoding directions may help to reduce truncation artifact.[38-40]

CLINICAL APPLICATIONS

Osteoarthritis

MRI is increasingly being utilized to evaluate lesions of the articular cartilage, and numerous imaging sequences have been advocated for this purpose. Early studies suggested that T1-weighted and T2-weighted images were indispensable for detailed evaluation of articular cartilage degeneration.[41] Subsequently, several new imaging sequences have been developed. Magnetization transfer contrast (MTC) imaging can separate articular cartilage from adjacent joint fluid by suppressing the signal produced from cartilage.[42-44] FSE imaging with fat suppression for proton density weighted images and T2-weighted images can depict articular cartilage abnormalities in osteoarthrits with higher accuracy than arthroscopic grading[45,46] (Figure 3-12). Fat-suppressed 3D spoiled gradient-recalled acquisition in the steady state (SPGR) has been reported as a more sensitive imaging sequence for the detection of articular cartilage defects in the knee.[47-49] In recent studies, driven equilibrium Fourier transform (DEFT) imaging has been shown to provide contrast between cartilage and joint fluid by enhancing the signal from joint fluid, rather than by suppressing the signal from cartilage as other sequences do.[50] Delayed gadolinium-DTPA[2] enhanced MR imaging is also a promising method that has potential for monitoring the glycosaminoglycan content of cartilage in vivo.[51,52]

The relative signal intensity of the normal articular cartilage is dependent on the pulse sequences used. T2-weighted SE imaging, proton density weighted and T2-weighted FSE imaging, MTC imaging, and DEFT imaging can show synovial fluid of high signal intensity (bright) and cartilage of intermediate to low signal intensity (dark), whereas fat-suppressed 3D SPGR sequences produce bright cartilage and dark synovial fluid. However, the signal intensity of the normal articular cartilage may not be uniform due to artifacts and other phenomena such as magic angle effect, truncation artifact, chemical shift artifact, magnetic susceptibility effect, and regional anatomic variations.[37,53] The laminar appearance within the articular cartilage on fat-suppressed 3D SPGR images is predominantly attributable to truncation artifact rather than to histologic zonal anatomy, as mentioned above.[35,36] Thus the MR appearance of the articular cartilage is highly variable, and understanding normal variations is clinically important in order to improve diagnostic accuracy and avoid misdiagnoses.[54]

Rheumatoid Arthritis

MRI is much more sensitive than radiography or ultrasonography for the diagnosis of rheumatoid arthritis (RA) especially in its early stages. Previous studies have reported MRI is seven- to nine-fold more sensitive than radiography for detecting erosions in early disease and is able to detect lesions 6 to 12 months before they appear on radiographs.[55-59] MRI identified more than twice as many erosions than did ultrasonography and radiography and was more sensitive than ultrasonography for detecting synovial disease.[60]

Because MRI can provide excellent soft tissue contrast, it can detect synovitis, erosions, and bone marrow edema due to RA very well. Previous studies comparing various imaging sequences found that dynamic imaging or fat-suppressed T1-weighted imaging with gadolinium contrast medium was useful in diagnosing synovial inflammation of early-stage RA[58,61-65] (Figure 3-13). However, enhancement of synovium in patients with RA is time dependent, and it is necessary that MR images be acquired within 5 minutes following contrast medium administration to differentiate active synovitis from fibrosis or joint effusion.[62,65-67]

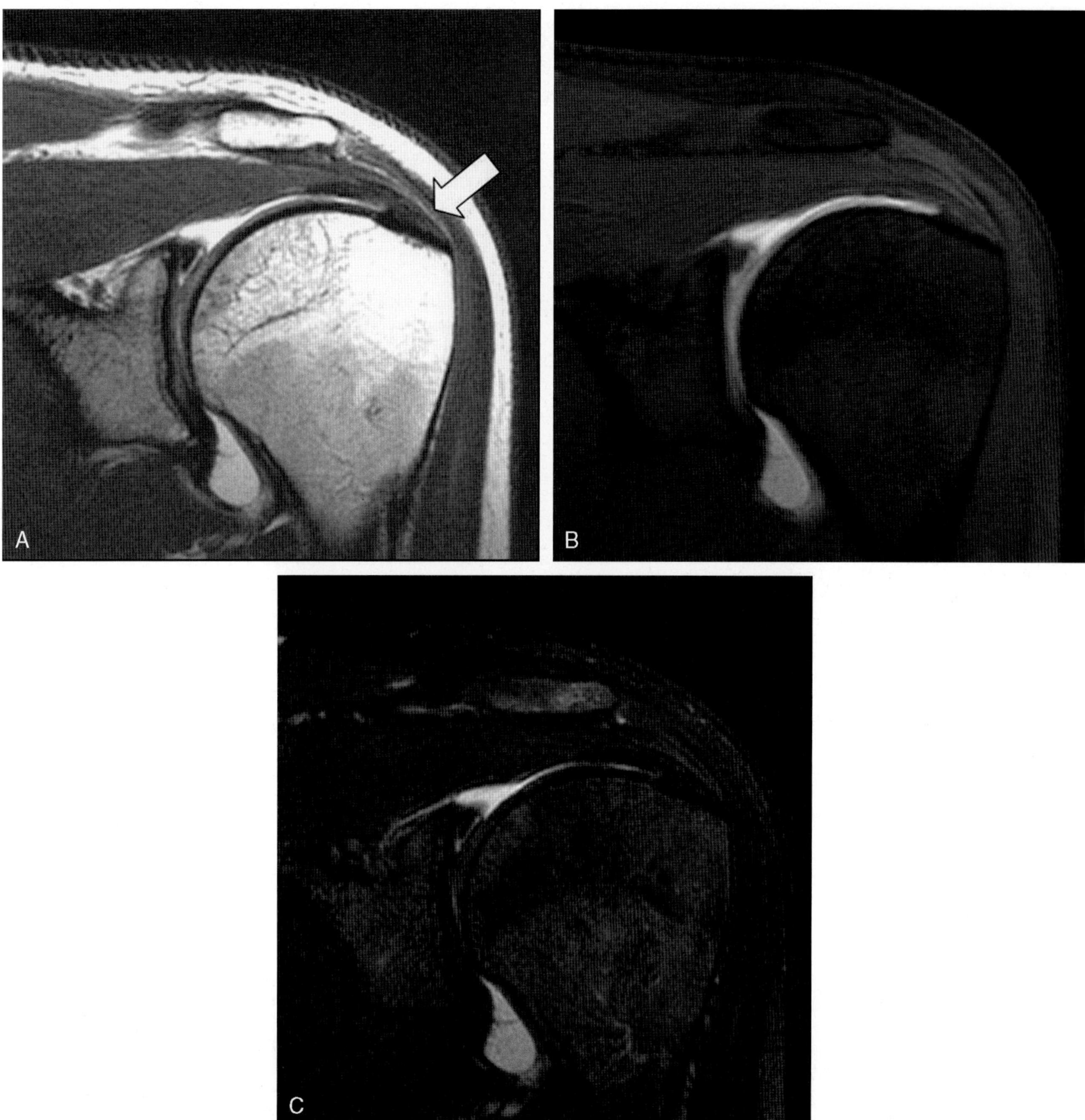

FIGURE 3-10. Magic angle effect. The supraspinatus tendon of the shoulder on this MR arthrogram shows slightly high signal intensity on **(A)** PD-weighted image due to magic angle effect *(arrow)*, whereas **(B)** fat-suppressed T1-weighted image and **(C)** fat-suppressed T2-weighted image show no abnormality. Note that the joint fluid appears bright even on the T1-weighted sequences due to the instillation of a dilute gadolinium solution into the joint for MR arthrography.

Extremity MRI may play an important role in the diagnosis of RA. Conventional whole body high-field MRI is expensive and inconvenient for patients and has some contraindications, such as implanted metal objects (pacemakers, aneurysm clips, and cochlear implants) and claustrophobia. Low-field dedicated extremity MR machines are now commercially available and have been applied to the evaluation of RA. In some reports, the diagnostic accuracy of low-field dedicated extremity MRI for synovitis, bone marrow edema, joint effusion, and bone erosion accompanying RA is comparable to that of the high-field MRI.[1,2] Even at low field, the sensitivity to bone damage of a portable MRI system was superior to that of radiographs of the wrists and metacarpophalangeal joints.[68] MRI identified bony erosion in 95% of patients with inflammatory arthritis, whereas radiographs identified only 59%. The introduction of effective therapies for RA has increased the importance of imaging in rheumatology, and low-field extremity MRI offers adequate performance but at lower cost and with greater comfort and convenience for the patient.[69] However, a recent review of in-office MRI scanning concluded that additional study is warranted.[70]

Osteoporosis

Osteoporosis is a metabolic bone disease characterized by bone loss and structural deterioration of bone tissue, leading to bone fragility

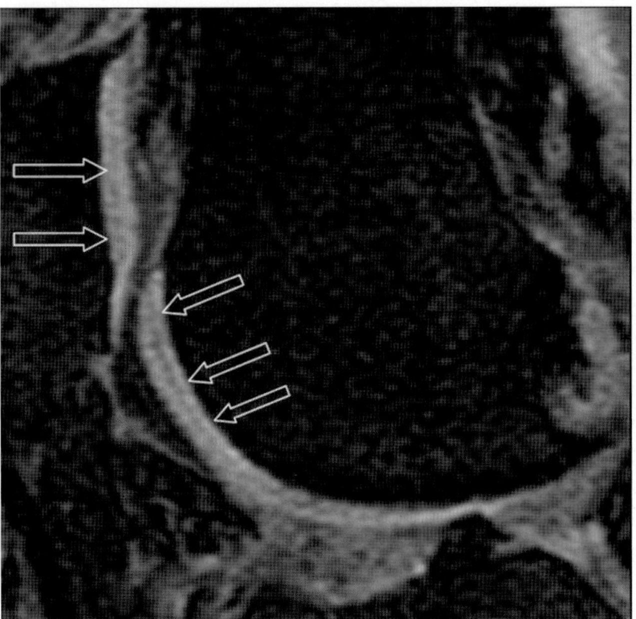

FIGURE 3-11. Truncation artifact. Linear low-signal intensity in the cartilage of the femoral trochlea and patellar facet is seen due to truncation artifact on fat-suppressed SPGR image.

and increased susceptibility to fractures, especially of the hip, spine, or wrist. According to National Osteoporosis Foundation estimates, osteoporosis is a major public health threat for an estimated 44 million Americans, or 55% of people 50 years of age and older. In the United States today, 10 million individuals are estimated to already have the disease.[71] Radiographs or MRI may be used for diagnosis of fractures secondary to osteoporosis. Critical to the evaluation of vertebral fractures on imaging studies is the fact that not all vertebral fractures are due to osteoporosis. In particular, antecedent trauma, infection, and tumor must be excluded. In many cases, MRI is useful for differentiating osteoporotic fractures from pathologic fractures by showing abnormal contrast enhancement of bone marrow and adjacent soft tissues in pathologic fractures.[72]

> MRI may allow compression fractures due to osteoporosis to be distinguished from fractures due to tumor.

Osteoporosis screening with MRI is a challenging area. Dual x-ray absorptiometry (DXA) scanning is used for screening but does not allow determination of the microstructure of bone. The methods available for quantitatively assessing microstructure of trabecular bone noninvasively include high-resolution or micro-computed tomography (CT) and high-resolution or micro-MRI. MRI can be used to assess the properties of trabecular bone in two different ways. The first is an indirect measure, often termed *relaxometry* or *quantitative magnetic resonance* (QMR). This method takes advantage of the fact that trabecular bone alters the adjoining marrow relaxation properties in proportion to bone density and structure. The second is the direct visualization of the dark trabecular bone, which, because of its low water content and short MR relaxation times, appears in stark contrast to the bright marrow fat and water in high-resolution MRI.[73] Currently two primary sequences used for micro-MRI of trabecular bone are variants of the basic GRE and SE-based fast large angle spin echo (FLASE) sequences.[74]

MR SAFETY

MRI is noninvasive and does not involve radiation. However, special safety issues have to be considered. The main risk associated with MRI is the effect of the strong magnetic field on ferromagnetic objects on or inside a patient's body, such as pacemakers, aneurysm clips, cochlear implants, neurostimulators, metal implants, surgical staples, some artificial heart valves, and foreign metal objects in the eye. Most orthopedic implants such as total joint prostheses do not present a hazard for MRI, although they do distort the magnetic field, potentially limiting the delineation of tissues near the implant.

The safety of pregnant patients should be considered. In 1997, the American College of Radiology issued a statement on the safety of MRI in pregnant patients. The statement is that in light of the

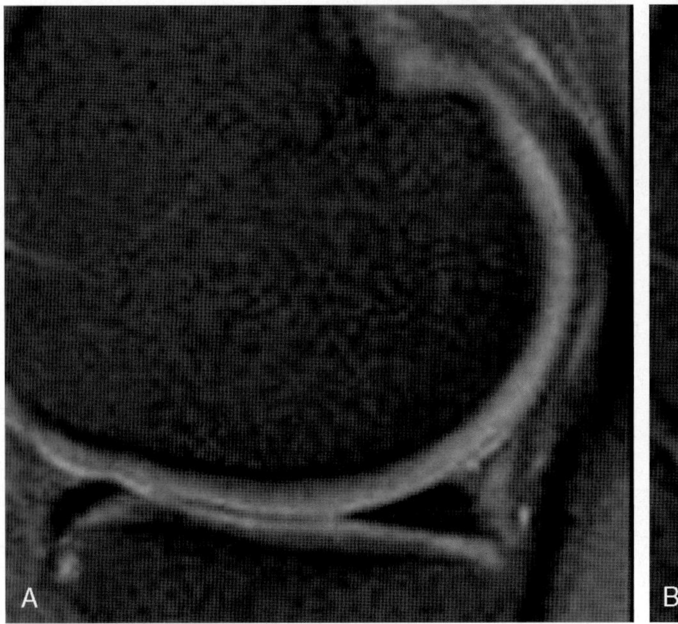

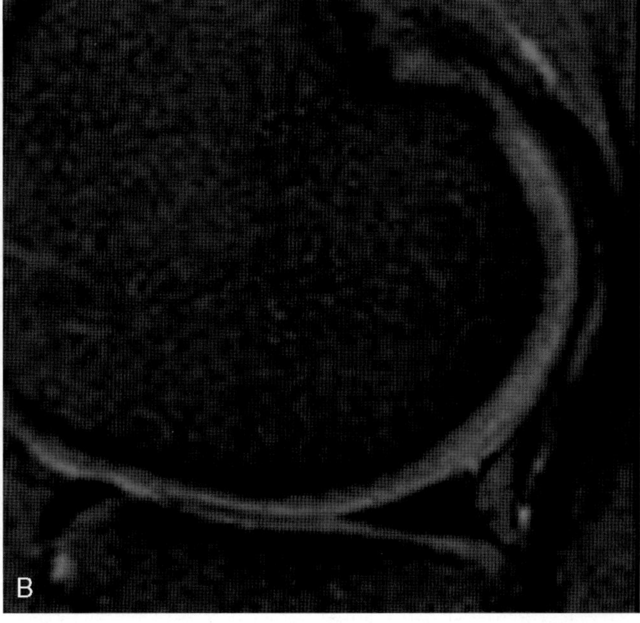

FIGURE 3-12. Normal MRI of the knee cartilage: **A,** fat-suppressed FSE PDW image; **B,** fat-suppressed FSE T2-weighted image; and

(Continued)

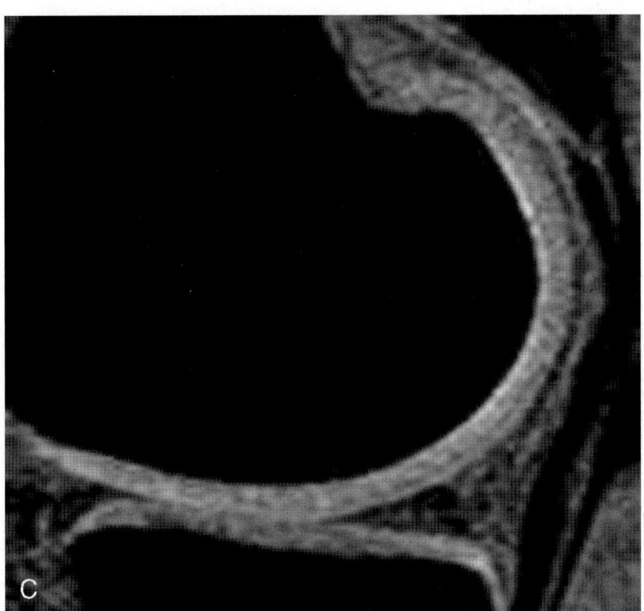

FIGURE 3-12—cont'd. **C,** fat-suppressed SPGR image.

lack of data demonstrating deleterious effects of MR on the developing human fetus, MRI should be recommenced for evaluating pregnant patients when any alternative imaging procedure involves ionizing radiation.[75] The question also arises about how to advise pregnant health care practitioners appropriately regarding exposures related to the MRI environment.[76] One survey of reproductive health among female MR workers suggested that the data do not demonstrate a correlation between working in the MR environment and offspring gender or changes in the prevalence of premature delivery, infertility, low birth weight, or spontaneous abortion.[76] However, sufficient safety has not been fully proven at this time.

In addition, certain metallic objects are not allowed into the examination room. Items such as jewelry, watches, credit cards, and hearing aids can be damaged (Box 3-1). Pins, hairpins, metal zippers, and similar metallic items can distort the images. Patients with a history of potential exposure to small metal fragments will be screened for metal shards within the eyes by orbit radiographs or by a radiologist's review and assessment of contiguous-cut CT. For patients with tattoos, it is recommended that cold compresses or ice packs be placed onto the tattooed areas in order to decrease the potential for RF heating of the tattooed tissue.[77] Several websites are available for reference. These include http://www.mrisafety.com, which includes a listing of implants, materials, and medical devices that can be referred to for screening patients prior to MRI, http://www.radiology.upmc.edu/MRsafety, and http://www.ismrm.org.

Time-varying gradient magnetic fields may have biologic effects with the introduction of rapid echo planar imaging and the use of high-performance gradient systems, as it is known that rapidly switching magnetic fields can stimulate muscle and nerve tissue.[75] At present, however, there is no known mechanism that would suggest an irreversible biologic effect caused by rapidly switching magnetic fields.[75]

RF burns are related to contact between electrically conductive materials such as wires, leads, and implants and the patient's bare skin during an MRI procedure. Care should be taken to place thermal insulation between the patient and the electrically conductive material during imaging.[77] The rapidly changing magnetic field will induce an electromotive force or voltage in the conductor that causes a flow of current.[75] The flowing current in a conductor with electrical resistance will result in heating the conductor, thus causing a burn if it contacts the skin.[75] Heating also occurs at the point of skin-to-skin contact. The patient's bare skin should not be allowed to form a large conductive loop, as occurs when crossing arms and legs while in the magnet.

The specific absorption rate (SAR) is a measure of the absorption of electromagnetic energy in the body (in watts per kilogram

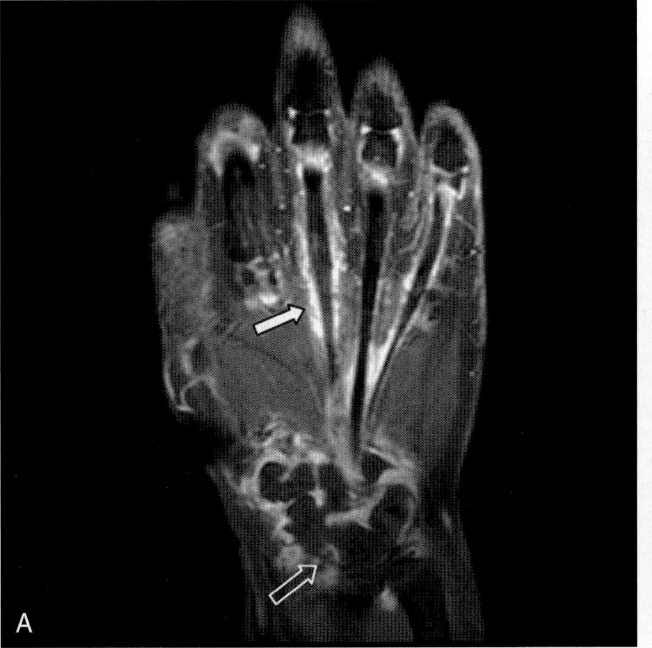

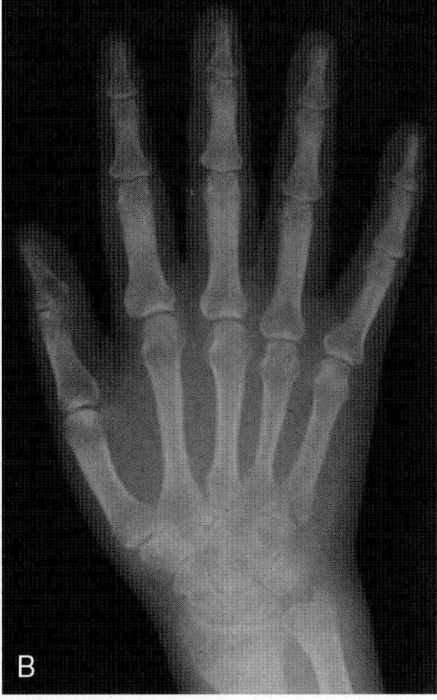

FIGURE 3-13. MRI in early-stage rheumatoid arthritis. **A,** Fat-suppressed T1-weighted image with gadolinium is more sensitive to early-stage rheumatoid arthritis than **(B)** radiograph. Note the bright signal fluid within tendon sheaths owing to tenosynovitis, small bright areas in the carpal bones *(arrow)* due to erosion, and bright joint fluid.

BOX 3-1 Contraindications for MRI*

ABSOLUTE CONTRAINDICATION:
Pacemaker
Otic implant
Metal in eye or orbit
Implanted cardiac defibrillator

LIKELY CONTRAINDICATION:
Heart valve or aneurysm clip installed before 1996

POSSIBLE CONTRAINDICATION:
Heart valve or aneurysm clip installed after 1996

USUALLY ALLOWABLE 6-8 WEEKS AFTER IMPLANTATION:
Passive implants, weakly ferromagnetic (e.g., coils, filters, and stents; metal sutures or staples)[78]

USUALLY ALLOWABLE IMMEDIATELY AFTER IMPLANTATION:
Passive implants, nonferromagnetic (e.g., bone/joint pins, screws, or rods; coils, filters, and stents; metal sutures or staples)
Rigidly fixed passive implants, weakly ferromagnetic (e.g., bone/joint pins, screws, rods)

CAUTION:
Tattoos

Modified from http://mghradrounds.org/clientuploads/february_2005/february_2005.pdf. Copyright 2005 MGH Department of Radiology.

[W/kg]). The SAR describes the potential for heating of the patient's tissue due to the application of the RF energy to produce the MR signal. It increases with field strength, RF power and duty cycle, transmitter coil type, and body size. In a high-field magnet, FSE sequences may create a higher SAR than is recommended by the U.S. Food and Drug Administration (FDA). The FDA limits SAR to 4 W/kg averaged over the whole body for any 15-minute period, 3 W/kg averaged over the head for any 10-minute period, or 8 W/kg in any gram of tissue in the extremities for any period of 5 minutes (http://www.fda.gov/cdrh/safety/mrisafety.html).

Commonly Used MR Terms

Term	Definition
Field strength	Static magnetic field within the scanner, measured in Tesla (T).
Field of view (FOV)	The distance of anatomic coverage in a given imaging direction.
Fringe field	"Stray" magnetic field extending outside the imaging bore of the magnet. The distance this field extends outside the bore is a major safety consideration in designing the size and shielding requirements of MRI rooms.
Gradient	Variation in magnetic field strength with change in distance, used to determine voxel location when making an image. Measured in milli-Tesla per meter (mT/m).
Image plane	May be selected based on anatomic considerations. The most common imaging planes are axial, coronal, and sagittal.
Matrix	The number of "in-plane" pixels along each given image direction. In combination with FOV, determines the in-plane image resolution.
Pulse sequences	Timing of MRI parameters (RF pulse strength and spacing, magnetic field gradients, and signal collection) used to create MR images with varying degrees of tissue contrast.
Radiofrequency (RF)	Energy deposited in the patient in order to produce MRI signals (usually in the megahertz frequency range at typical magnetic field strengths used). A side effect is unwanted heating of tissues, which limits the amount of allowable energy deposition.
Selective fat saturation	Also known as *chemical shift fat saturation,* a method of removing fat signal based on the different signal frequencies of fat and water. More subject to non-uniform fat suppression than STIR imaging.
Signal to noise ratio (SNR)	Quantitative value to describe the image quality of a detected signal relating the true signal and superimposed background noise signal.
Slice thickness	The through-plane voxel dimension.
Spatial resolution	Definition of the smallest structures that can be differentiated on an image, generally related to pixel or voxel dimensions, although voxels can be interpolated to artificially increase display resolution from the true image resolution. True in-plane resolution equals field of view divided by matrix.
STIR	"Short Tau Inversion Recovery" pulse sequence; a popular and robust method used for suppression of MRI signal from fat.
Slice thickness	The through-plane voxel dimension.
Tesla (T)	Unit of magnetic field strength. 1 Tesla equals 10,000 Gauss (the earth's magnetic field strength is approximately 0.5 Gauss).
TR	Repetition time; the time between successive pulse sequences applied to the same slice. TR controls image contrast characteristics.
TE	Echo time; the time between the initial pulse and the peak of the echo signal.
T1 weighted	Represents image contrast due to differences in T1 relaxation time. T1-weighted image is created by using short TR and TE (see Table 3-1).
T2 weighted	Represents image contrast due to differences in T2 relaxation time. T2-weighted image is created by using long TR and TE (see Table 3-1).
T1 relaxation time	Time constant that the longitudinal magnetization returns toward equilibrium after RF excitation. Each tissue has a characteristic T1 time.
T2 relaxation time	Time constant that the transverse magnetization decays toward zero after RF excitation. Each tissue has a characteristic T2 time.
Voxel	"Volume element," the 3D size of each point in an image, generally determined by two in-plane pixel dimensions (in turn determined by FOV and matrix) and the slice thickness.

Portions of this table are courtesy of Aaron D. Sodickson, MD, PhD, Brigham and Women's Hospital, Boston, MA and were borrowed with permission from American College of Rheumatology Extremity Magnetic Resonance Imaging Task Force: extremity magnetic resonance imaging in rheumatoid arthritis, *Arthritis Rheum* 54:1034–1047, 2006.

REFERENCES

1. Savnik A, Malmskov H, Thomsen HS et al: MRI of the arthritic small joints: comparison of extremity MRI (0.2 T) vs high-field MRI (1.5 T), *Eur Radiol* 11:1030-1038, 2001.
2. Taouli B, Zaim S, Peterfy CG et al: Rheumatoid arthritis of the hand and wrist: comparison of three imaging techniques, *AJR Am J Roentgenol* 182:937-943, 2004.
3. Schiebler ML, Listerud J: Common artifacts encountered in thoracic magnetic resonance imaging: recognition, derivation, and solutions, *Top Magn Reson Imaging* 4:1-17, 1992.
4. Meaney JF, Johansson LO, Ahlstrom H et al: Pulmonary magnetic resonance angiography, *J Magn Reson Imaging* 10:326-338, 1999.
5. Wood ML, Henkelman RM: MR image artifacts from periodic motion, *Med Phys* 12:143-151, 1985.
6. Wood ML, Runge VM, Henkelman RM: Overcoming motion in abdominal MR imaging, *AJR Am J Roentgenol* 150:513-522, 1988.
7. Nozaki A: [Single shot fast spin echo (SSFSE)], *Nippon Rinsho* 56:2792-2797, 1998.
8. Taber KH, Herrick RC, Weathers SW et al: Pitfalls and artifacts encountered in clinical MR imaging of the spine, *Radiographics* 18:1499-1521, 1998.
9. Peh WC, Chan JH: Artifacts in musculoskeletal magnetic resonance imaging: identification and correction, *Skeletal Radiol* 30:179-191, 2001.
10. Edelman RR, Atkinson DJ, Silver MS et al: FRODO pulse sequences: a new means of eliminating motion, flow, and wraparound artifacts, *Radiology* 166:231-236, 1988.
11. Lufkin R, Anselmo M, Crues J et al: Magnetic field strength dependence of chemical shift artifacts, *Comput Med Imaging Graph* 12:89-96, 1988.
12. Soila KP, Viamonte M Jr, Starewicz PM: Chemical shift misregistration effect in magnetic resonance imaging, *Radiology* 153:819-820, 1984.
13. Dwyer AJ, Knop RH, Hoult DI: Frequency shift artifacts in MR imaging, *J Comput Assist Tomogr* 9:16-18, 1985.
14. Whitehouse RW, Hutchinson CE, Laitt R et al: The influence of chemical shift artifact on magnetic resonance imaging of the ligamentum flavum at 0.5 tesla, *Spine* 22:200-202, 1997.
15. Rosen BR, Wedeen VJ, Brady TJ: Selective saturation NMR imaging, *J Comput Assist Tomogr* 8:813-818, 1984.
16. Haase A, Frahm J, Hanicke W et al: 1H NMR chemical shift selective (CHESS) imaging, *Phys Med Biol* 30:341-344, 1985.
17. Frahm J, Haase A, Hanicke W et al: Chemical shift selective MR imaging using a whole-body magnet, *Radiology* 156:441-444, 1985.
18. Arena L, Morehouse HT, Safir J: MR imaging artifacts that simulate disease: how to recognize and eliminate them, *Radiographics* 15:1373-1394, 1995.
19. Czervionke LF, Daniels DL, Wehrli FW et al: Magnetic susceptibility artifacts in gradient-recalled echo MR imaging, *AJNR Am J Neuroradiol* 9:1149-1155, 1988.
20. Henkelman RM, Stanisz GJ, Kim JK et al: Anisotropy of NMR properties of tissues, *Magn Reson Med* 32:592-601, 1994.
21. Peh WC, Chan JH: The magic angle phenomenon in tendons: effect of varying the MR echo time, *Br J Radiol* 71:31-36, 1998.
22. Fullerton GD, Cameron IL, Ord VA: Orientation of tendons in the magnetic field and its effect on T2 relaxation times, *Radiology* 155:433-435, 1985.
23. Mlynarik V, Trattnig S: Physicochemical properties of normal articular cartilage and its MR appearance, *Invest Radiol* 35:589-594, 2000.
24. Rubenstein JD, Kim JK, Morova-Protzner I et al: Effects of collagen orientation on MR imaging characteristics of bovine articular cartilage, *Radiology* 188:219-226, 1993.
25. Erickson SJ, Cox IH, Hyde JS et al: Effect of tendon orientation on MR imaging signal intensity: a manifestation of the "magic angle" phenomenon, *Radiology* 181:389-392, 1991.
26. Erickson SJ, Prost RW, Timins ME: The "magic angle" effect: background physics and clinical relevance, *Radiology* 188:23-25, 1993.
27. Mow VC, Fithian DC, Kelly M: Fundamentals of articular cartilage and meniscus biomechanics. In: Ewing JW, ed. *Articular cartilage and knee joint function*, New York, 1990, Raven Press, pp 1-18.
28. Akeson WH, Amiel D, Gershuni DH: Articular cartilage physiology and metabolism. In: Resnick D, ed. *Diagnosis of bone and joint disorders*, ed 3, Philadelphia, 1995, Saunders.
29. Xia Y, Farquhar T, Burton-Wurster N et al: Origin of cartilage laminae in MRI, *J Magn Reson Imaging* 7:887-894, 1997.
30. Goodwin DW, Zhu H, Dunn JF: In vitro MR imaging of hyaline cartilage: correlation with scanning electron microscopy, *AJR Am J Roentgenol* 174:405-409, 2000.
31. Timins ME, Erickson SJ, Estkowski LD et al: Increased signal in the normal supraspinatus tendon on MR imaging: diagnostic pitfall caused by the magic-angle effect, *AJR Am J Roentgenol* 165:109-114, 1995.
32. Seibold CJ, Mallisee TA, Erickson SJ et al: Rotator cuff: evaluation with US and MR imaging, *Radiographics* 19:685-705, 1999.
33. Peh WC, Chan JH, Shek TW et al: The effect of using shorter echo times in MR imaging of knee menisci: a study using a porcine model, *AJR Am J Roentgenol* 172:485-488, 1999.
34. Czervionke LF, Czervionke JM, Daniels DL et al: Characteristic features of MR truncation artifacts, *AJR Am J Roentgenol* 151:1219-1228, 1988.
35. Erickson SJ, Waldschmidt JG, Czervionke LF et al: Hyaline cartilage: truncation artifact as a cause of trilaminar appearance with fat-suppressed three-dimensional spoiled gradient-recalled sequences, *Radiology* 201:260-264, 1996.
36. Frank LR, Brossmann J, Buxton RB et al: MR imaging truncation artifacts can create a false laminar appearance in cartilage, *AJR Am J Roentgenol* 168:547-554, 1997.
37. Waldschmidt JG, Rilling RJ, Kajdacsy-Balla AA et al: In vitro and in vivo MR imaging of hyaline cartilage: zonal anatomy, imaging pitfalls, and pathologic conditions, *Radiographics* 17:1387-1402, 1997.
38. Bronskill MJ, McVeigh ER, Kucharczyk W et al: Syrinx-like artifacts on MR images of the spinal cord, *Radiology* 166:485-488, 1988.
39. Breger RK, Czervionke LF, Kass EG et al: Truncation artifact in MR images of the intervertebral disk, *AJNR Am J Neuroradiol* 9:825-828, 1988.
40. Levy LM, Di Chiro G, Brooks RA et al: Spinal cord artifacts from truncation errors during MR imaging, *Radiology* 166:479-483, 1988.
41. Lehner KB, Rechl HP, Gmeinwieser JK et al: Structure, function, and degeneration of bovine hyaline cartilage: assessment with MR imaging in vitro, *Radiology* 170:495-499, 1989.
42. Peterfy CG, Majumdar S, Lang P et al: MR imaging of the arthritic knee: improved discrimination of cartilage, synovium, and effusion with pulsed saturation transfer and fat-suppressed T1-weighted sequences, *Radiology* 191:413-419, 1994.
43. Peterfy CG, van Dijke CF, Janzen DL et al: Quantification of articular cartilage in the knee with pulsed saturation transfer subtraction and fat-suppressed MR imaging: optimization and validation, *Radiology* 192:485-491, 1994.
44. Wolff SD, Chesnick S, Frank JA et al: Magnetization transfer contrast: MR imaging of the knee, *Radiology* 179:623-628, 1991.
45. Broderick LS, Turner DA, Renfrew DL et al: Severity of articular cartilage abnormality in patients with osteoarthritis: evaluation with fast spin-echo MR vs arthroscopy, *AJR Am J Roentgenol* 162:99-103, 1994.
46. Potter HG, Linklater JM, Allen AA et al: Magnetic resonance imaging of articular cartilage in the knee. An evaluation with use of fast-spin-echo imaging, *J Bone Joint Surg (Am)* 80:1276-1284, 1998.
47. Recht MP, Piraino DW, Paletta GA et al: Accuracy of fat-suppressed three-dimensional spoiled gradient-echo FLASH MR imaging in the detection of patellofemoral articular cartilage abnormalities, *Radiology* 198:209-212, 1996.
48. Disler DG: Fat-suppressed three-dimensional spoiled gradient-recalled MR imaging: assessment of articular and physeal hyaline cartilage, *AJR Am J Roentgenol* 169:1117-1123, 1997.
49. Disler DG, McCauley TR, Kelman CG et al: Fat-suppressed three-dimensional spoiled gradient-echo MR imaging of hyaline cartilage defects in the knee: comparison with standard MR imaging and arthroscopy, *AJR Am J Roentgenol* 167:127-132, 1996.
50. Hargreaves BA, Gold GE, Lang PK et al: MR imaging of articular cartilage using driven equilibrium, *Magn Reson Med* 42:695-703, 1999.
51. Bashir A, Gray ML, Boutin RD et al: Glycosaminoglycan in articular cartilage: in vivo assessment with delayed Gd(DTPA)(2-)-enhanced MR imaging, *Radiology* 205:551-558, 1997.
52. Bashir A, Gray ML, Burstein D: Gd-DTPA2- as a measure of cartilage degradation, *Magn Reson Med* 36:665-673, 1996.
53. Waldschmidt JG, Braunstein EM, Buckwalter KA: Magnetic resonance imaging of osteoarthritis, *Rheum Dis Clin North Am* 25:451-465, 1999.
54. Yoshioka H, Stevens K, Genovese M et al: Articular cartilage of knee: normal patterns at MR imaging that mimic disease in healthy subjects and patients with osteoarthritis, *Radiology* 231:31-38, 2004.
55. McQueen FM, Benton N, Crabbe J et al: What is the fate of erosions in early rheumatoid arthritis? Tracking individual lesions using x rays and magnetic resonance imaging over the first two years of disease, *Ann Rheum Dis* 60:859-868, 2001.
56. Lindegaard H, Vallo J, Horslev-Petersen K et al: Low field dedicated magnetic resonance imaging in untreated rheumatoid arthritis of recent onset, *Ann Rheum Dis* 60:770-776, 2001.
57. McQueen F, Lassere M, Edmonds J et al: OMERACT Rheumatoid Arthritis Magnetic Resonance Imaging Studies. Summary of OMERACT 6 MR Imaging Module, *J Rheumatol* 30:1387-1392, 2003.
58. McQueen FM, Stewart N, Crabbe J et al: Magnetic resonance imaging of the wrist in early rheumatoid arthritis reveals a high prevalence of erosions at four months after symptom onset, *Ann Rheum Dis* 57:350-356, 1998.
59. Klarlund M, Ostergaard M, Jensen KE et al: Magnetic resonance imaging, radiography, and scintigraphy of the finger joints: one year follow up of patients with early arthritis. The TIRA Group, *Ann Rheum Dis* 59:521-528, 2000.
60. Hoving JL, Buchbinder R, Hall S et al: A comparison of magnetic resonance imaging, sonography, and radiography of the hand in patients with early rheumatoid arthritis, *J Rheumatol* 31:663-675, 2004.
61. Konig H, Sieper J, Wolf KJ: Rheumatoid arthritis: evaluation of hypervascular and fibrous pannus with dynamic MR imaging enhanced with Gd-DTPA, *Radiology* 176:473-477, 1990.
62. Nakahara N, Uetani M, Hayashi K et al: Gadolinium-enhanced MR imaging of the wrist in rheumatoid arthritis: value of fat suppression pulse sequences, *Skeletal Radiol* 25:639-647, 1996.
63. Klarlund M, Ostergaard M, Rostrup E et al: Dynamic magnetic resonance imaging of the metacarpophalangeal joints in rheumatoid arthritis, early unclassified polyarthritis, and healthy controls, *Scand J Rheumatol* 29:108-115, 2000.
64. McQueen FM: Magnetic resonance imaging in early inflammatory arthritis: what is its role? *Rheumatology (Oxford)* 39:700-706, 2000.
65. Sugimoto H, Takeda A, Masuyama J et al: Early-stage rheumatoid arthritis: diagnostic accuracy of MR imaging, *Radiology* 198:185-192, 1996.
66. Tamai K, Yamato M, Yamaguchi T et al: Dynamic magnetic resonance imaging for the evaluation of synovitis in patients with rheumatoid arthritis, *Arthritis Rheum* 37:1151-1157, 1994.
67. Yamato M, Tamai K, Yamaguchi T et al: MRI of the knee in rheumatoid arthritis: Gd-DTPA perfusion dynamics, *J Comput Assist Tomogr* 17:781-785, 1993.

68. Crues JV, Shellock FG, Dardashti S et al: Identification of wrist and metacarpophalangeal joint erosions using a portable magnetic resonance imaging system compared to conventional radiographs, *J Rheumatol* 31:676-685, 2004.
69. Peterfy CG: Is there a role for extremity magnetic resonance imaging in routine clinical management of rheumatoid arthritis? *J Rheumatol* 31:640-644, 2004.
70. American College of Rheumatology Extremity Magnetic Resonance Imaging Task Force: extremity magnetic resonance imaging in rheumatoid arthritis report of the American College of Rheumatology. Extremity magnetic resonance imaging task force, *Arthritis Rheumatism* 54:1034-1047, 2006.
71. National osteoporosis Foundation: NOF's 2003 annual report, Washington, DC, 2004.
72. Lenchik L, Rogers LF, Delmas PD et al: Diagnosis of osteoporotic vertebral fractures: importance of recognition and description by radiologists, *AJR Am J Roentgenol* 183:949-958, 2004.
73. Majumdar S: Magnetic resonance imaging of trabecular bone structure, *Top Magn Reson Imaging* 13:323-334, 2002.
74. Techawiboonwong A, Song HK, Magland JF et al: Implications of pulse sequence in structural imaging of trabecular bone, *J Magn Reson Imaging* 22:647-655, 2005.
75. Price RR: The AAPM/RSNA physics tutorial for residents. MR imaging safety considerations. Radiological Society of North America, *Radiographics* 19:1641-1651, 1999.
76. Kanal E, Gillen J, Evans JA et al: Survey of reproductive health among female MR workers, *Radiology* 187:395-399, 1993.
77. Kanal E, Borgstede JP, Barkovich AJ et al: American College of Radiology White Paper on MR Safety, *AJR Am J Roentgenol* 178:1335-1347, 2002.
78. Shellock FG, Crues JV: MR procedures: biologic effects, safety, and patient care, *Radiology* 232:635-652, 2004.

CHAPTER 4

Magnetic Resonance Imaging of Articular Cartilage

PHILIPP LANG, MD, MBA, MATHIAS BREM, MD, GESA NEUMANN, MD, HIROSHI YOSHIOKA, MD, PHD, CHRISTIAN GLASER, MD, BERND BITTERSOHL, MD, *and* JEFF DURYEA, PHD

KEY FACTS

- Magnetic resonance imaging (MRI) has the capability of defining normal and abnormal articular cartilage morphology. Imaging at high-field strength (such as 3T) aids in the resolution of articular cartilage.
- MRI can evaluate the structure as well as the thickness of articular cartilage.

Osteoarthritis (OA) is the most common condition to affect human joints as well as a frequent cause of locomotor pain and disability.[1] Despite its societal impact and prevalence, there is a paucity of information on the factors that cause OA to progress. Previously considered a "wear and tear" degenerative disease with little opportunity for therapeutic intervention, OA is now increasingly viewed as a dynamic process with exciting potential for new pharmacologic and surgical treatment modalities such as cartilage transplantation,[2,3] osteochondral allografting[4,5] or autografting,[6] osteotomies,[7] and tibial corticotomies with angular distraction.[8,9] The appropriate deployment and selection of newer treatment interventions for OA is dependent on the development of better methods for the assessment of the disease process. Degenerative changes to articular cartilage can be described in biologic, mechanical, and morphologic terms. From a morphologic viewpoint there has been substantial progress in our ability to study cartilage using magnetic resonance imaging (MRI).

MRI, with its superior soft tissue contrast, is the best technique available for assessment of normal articular cartilage and cartilage lesions.[10] MRI can provide morphologic information about the area of damage. Specifically, changes such as fissuring, partial- or full-thickness cartilage loss, and signal changes within residual cartilage can be detected. The ideal MRI technique for cartilage will provide accurate assessment of cartilage thickness, demonstrate internal cartilage signal changes, evaluate the subchondral bone for signal abnormalities, and demonstrate morphologic changes of the cartilage surface.[11]

MRI PULSE SEQUENCES

Routine MRI pulse sequences available for imaging of articular cartilage include conventional T1- and T2-weighted spin echo techniques,[12] gradient recalled echo imaging,[13-15] magnetization transfer contrast imaging,[16,17] and fast spin echo sequences.[16]

Conventional T1-Weighted and T2-Weighted Imaging

Conventional T1-weighted and T2-weighted MRI do depict articular cartilage and can demonstrate defects and gross morphologic changes. T1-weighted images show excellent intrasubstance anatomic detail of hyaline cartilage.[12] However, T1-weighted imaging does not show significant contrast between joint effusions and the cartilage surface, making surface irregularities difficult to detect. T2-weighted imaging demonstrates joint effusion and thus surface cartilage abnormalities, but because some components of cartilage have relatively short T2 relaxation times,[17,18] these are not well depicted.

Gradient Recalled Echo Imaging

Gradient recalled echo imaging has been employed because of its three-dimensional (3D) capability and ability to provide high-resolution images with relatively short scan times.[13,14,19] Fat-suppressed 3D spoiled gradient echo (FS-3D-SPGR) imaging has been shown to be more sensitive than standard MRI for the detection of hyaline cartilage defects in the knee.[13,14,19] FS-3D-SPGR imaging can be, however, subject to image artifacts and ambiguity in cartilage contour (Figure 4-1).

Fast Spin Echo Imaging

Fast spin echo imaging is another useful pulse sequence to evaluate articular cartilage[20] (Figure 4-2). Incidental magnetization transfer contrast contributes to the signal characteristics of articular cartilage on fast spin echo images and can enhance the contrast between cartilage and joint fluid.[21] Sensitivity and specificity of fast spin echo imaging have been reported to be 87% and 94% in a study with arthroscopic correlation.[16]

Many other MRI sequences have been proposed for cartilage imaging but have not found widespread acceptance. These include T1-weighted proton,[22-25] density-weighted and T2-weighted spin echo (SE) sequences,[16,26] inversion recovery (IR) sequences,[27] two-dimensional (2D) and 3D magnetization transfer contrast (MTC) sequences[28,29] projection reconstruction spectroscopic imaging (PRSI)[30-32] and 2D- and 3D-driven equilibrium Fourier transform (DEFT).[33-35]

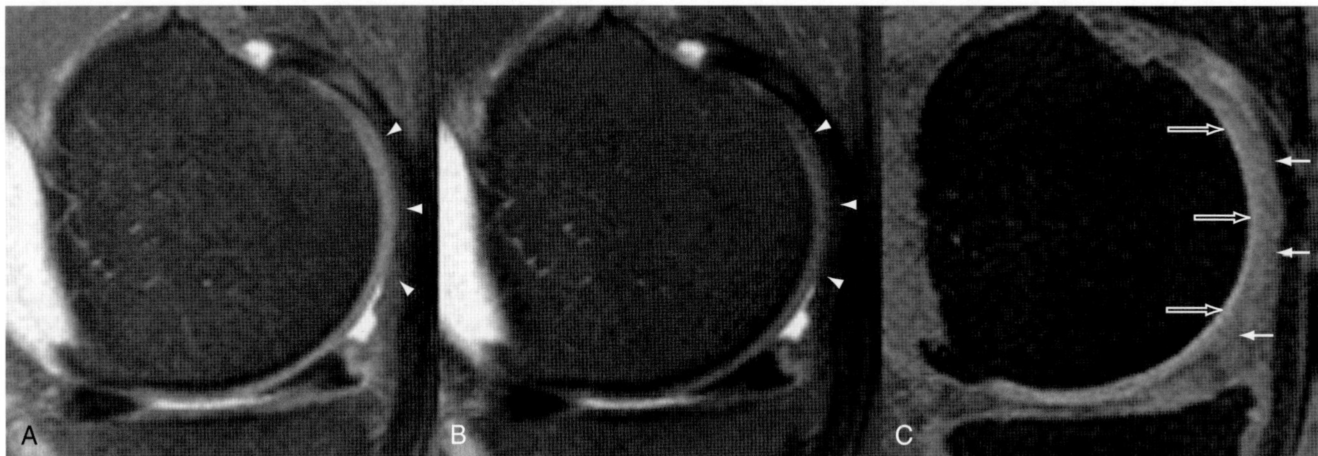

FIGURE 4-1. Ambiguity of cartilage surface contour on 3D SPGR image. MR images in a 60-year-old man. **A,** Sagittal short TE FSE image (4000/13) and **(B)** long TE FSE image (4000/39) with fat suppression showing clearly defined cartilage contour *(arrowheads)* in the region of the posterior femoral condyle. **C,** Sagittal fat-suppressed 3D SPGR image (60/5, 40-degree flip angle) shows difficulty in identifying the surface contour *(arrows)* of the posterior femoral condylar cartilage.

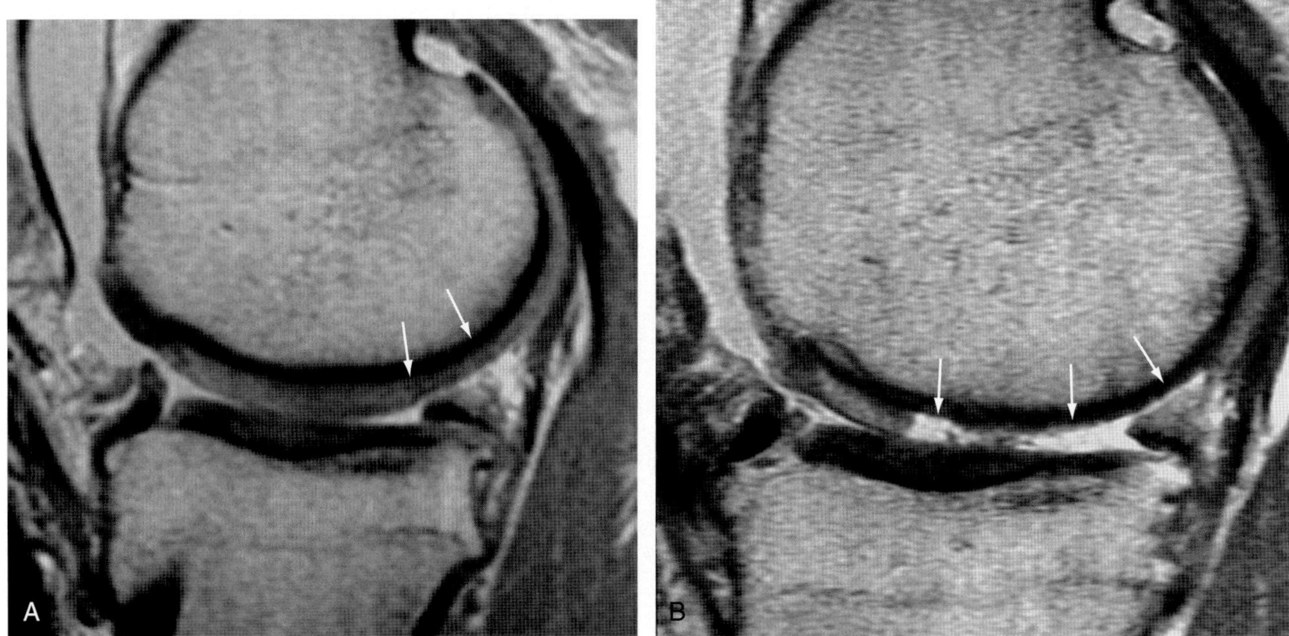

FIGURE 4-2. Progression of cartilage loss demonstrated on MR images. **A,** A baseline MRI (sagittal 2D FSE) shows thinning of less than 50% of normal cartilage thickness in the medial compartment with greater than 1 cm^2 involvement (grade 4B). **B,** Follow-up MRI shows that the region of thinning has progressed to full-thickness cartilage loss *(arrows)* over a larger area (grade 6B).

Novel MRI Pulse Sequences

Cartilage, as an ordered tissue, demonstrates the effects of magnetization transfer.[36,37] Several studies have demonstrated that the magnetization transfer effect can be used to separate articular cartilage from adjacent joint fluid and inflamed synovium.[16,17]

Poor cartilage signal-to-noise ratio (SNR) and contrast-to-noise ratio (CNR) (SE, IR sequences), limited SNR efficiency (SE, IR), need for offline reconstruction (PRSI) or for image subtraction (MTC), and unstable sequence performance (DEFT) are among the factors that have prevented the broad dissemination and acceptance of these techniques for cartilage MRI.

The most promising novel MRI pulse sequences for cartilage imaging are water-selective excitation techniques such as 3D spoiled gradient echo with spectral spatial pulses (3D SS-SPGR),[38,39] 3D steady state free precession (3D SSFP),[40,41] 3D DESS and 3D fast spin echo (3D FSE) techniques.[42] These fast sequences hold the promise of providing 3D coverage (unlike 2FSE) while yielding superior CNR between cartilage and surrounding tissues (unlike 3D SPGR) and are likely to improve the accuracy and reproducibility of cartilage MRI.

The 3D SSFP sequence is a fully balanced steady-state coherent imaging pulse sequence designed to produce high SNR images at very short sequence times (TR) (Figure 4-3). The pulse sequence uses fully balanced gradients to rephase the transverse magnetization at the end of each TR interval. To achieve fat saturation in a steady state, it is important to bring the magnetization back to the steady state as quickly as possible to avoid artifacts. Therefore a half-alpha technique is used to store magnetization and then return it to steady state relatively quickly. This is repeated

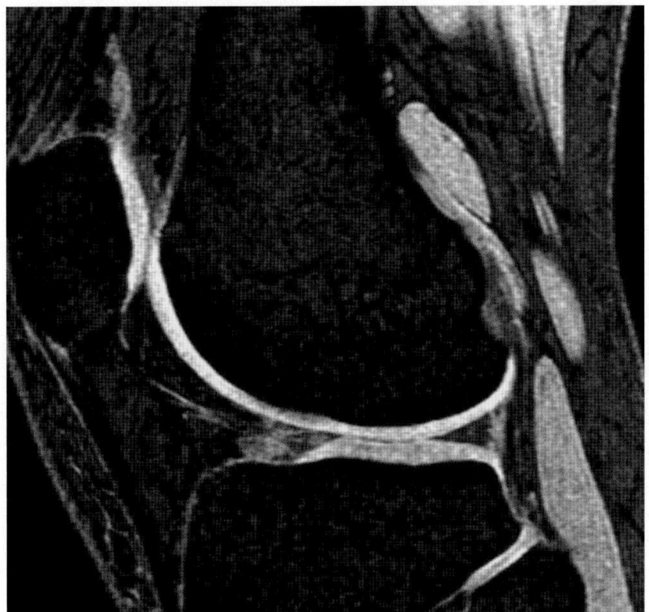

FIGURE 4-3. Cartilage imaging on a 3D FIESTA or 3D SSFP sequence. The cartilage contrast is excellent, with the bright signal cartilage able to be distinguished from the underlying bone and the joint fluid. The acquisition is near isotropic, with an acquisition time that is 30% to 40% less than that required for 3D SPGR (TR/TE/TI 6.6/1.2/20, flip 10 degrees, 128 slices, 0.8 mm thick, 2 NA, matrix 256 × 256, FOV 14 cm, acquisition time 8 min).

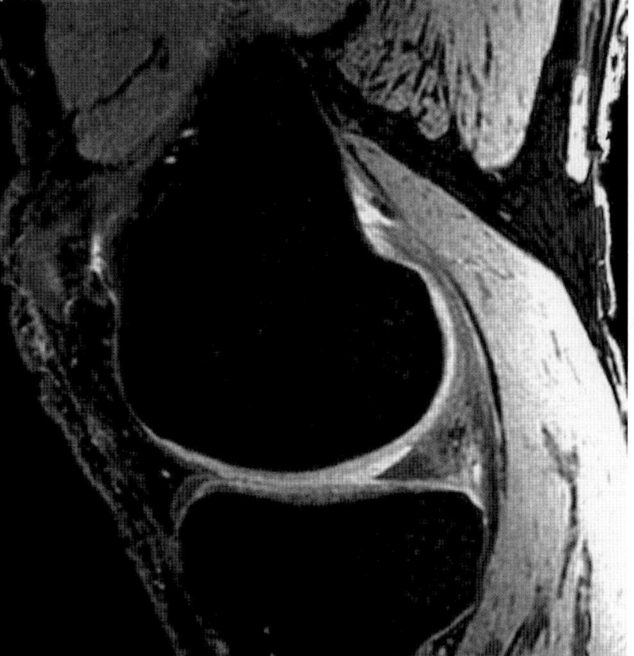

FIGURE 4-4. Cartilage imaging with 3D DESS sequence with voxel size of 0.7 × 0.55 × 0.55 mm. This sequence can provide near-isotropic resolution with strong T2 weighting. Cartilage fluid contrast is excellent.

throughout the sequence at regular intervals. Figure 4-7 shows the sequence diagram.

3D DESS is a steady-state pulse sequence where both SSFP and time-reversed SSFP signals are acquired within the same repetition time[43] (Figure 4-4). A second gradient echo is added immediately before each radiofrequency (RF) in a 3D SSFP sequence. This additional strong T2W time-reversed SSFP signal adds onto the regular SSFP signal, resulting in improved SNR and stronger T2 contrast (see Figure 4-4).

3D FSE provides SE contrast. SE sequences are resistant to image artifacts from a variety of sources such as RF or static field inhomogeneity and susceptibility. Recently a single-slab version of 3D FSE has been reported (Figure 4-5). Compared with conventional multi-slab 3D FSE sequences, a single-slab sequence can improve SNR, reduce total power deposition, and avoid slab-to-slab difference in image contrast. In order to reduce acquisition time, effective echo time and echo spacing, all the RF pulses are nonselective hard pulses. The duration of the excitation RF pulse is 400 μs whereas the refocusing pulse is only 500 μs. Such short pulses result in effective echo time and echo spacing of about 3 to 5 msec. The short echo time enhances T1 contrast and improves SNR; the short echo spacing reduces blurring artifact. With short echo spacing, more echoes can be acquired after each excitation, thus reducing scan time.

The basic promise of these isotropic and near-isotropic 3D imaging sequences is to provide T1- and T2-weighted contrast with unprecedented resolution in three dimensions, thereby obviating the need for acquisition of 2D sequences in the coronal, sagittal, and axial planes. In the future, 3D volume data generated in this manner can be viewed on an interactive workstation with real-time interactive display of any desired imaging plane, without loss or without significant loss in in-plane resolution.

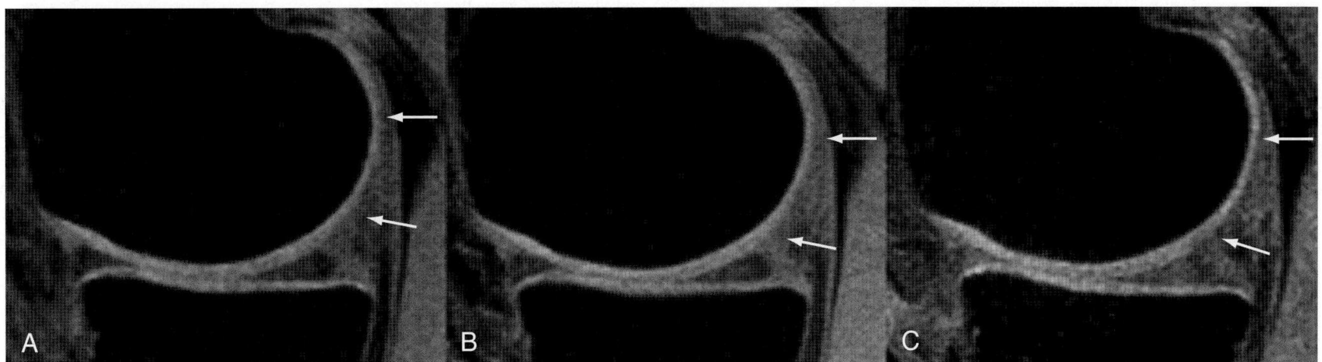

FIGURE 4-5. Comparison of MRI sequences for cartilage imaging. **A,** 3D SPGR; **B,** 3D SS-SPGR; **C,** 3D FSE images. Contrast between the cartilage and posterior capsule *(arrows)* is best seen in this patient with 3D FSE. This is a problem area for automated or semiautomated segmentation of cartilage for subsequent quantitative analysis such as measurements of volume and thickness. Blurring is not a problem with this sequence due to its short echo times.

Multiple MRI sequences have been investigated for evaluation of articular cartilage. Sequences in which the voxels (volume elements) are isotropic (the same size in each dimension) can provide images in any plane without loss of resolution, as well as provide 3D imaging.

MRI SENSITIVITY AND SPECIFICITY: CORRELATION TO ARTHROSCOPY

The sensitivity and specificity of standard MRI in detecting cartilage loss has been examined by correlating 2D FSE and/or 3D SPGR sequences with arthroscopic findings.* The specificity of standard 2D FSE and 3D SPGR sequences is excellent, ranging between 81% and 97%.* The data reported on the sensitivity of 2D FSE[16,44] and 3D SPGR[13-15,24] sequences are inconsistent, ranging between 60% and 94%.*

The sensitivity of standard MRI sequences for cartilage defects is between 60% and 94%, with a specificity between 81% and 97%. The sensitivity is greater for more severe lesions.

The severity of cartilage loss and the grade of OA is important: Kawahara et al.[28] reported that the sensitivity of 2D FSE improved with higher grades of cartilage loss; the sensitivity reported for early, superficial cartilage lesions was only 31.8%, whereas the sensitivity for full-thickness defects was greater than 90%.[28] Limited spatial resolution of the 2D FSE sequence in the slice direction may be the cause for this observation. Bredella et al. reported a sensitivity of only 61% for single-plane 2D FSE sequences; when two or more planes were combined in the interpretation, the sensitivity increased to 93%.[44] These data along with the limited sensitivity observed for superficial cartilage lesions in the study by Kawahara et al.[28] provide a strong indication that novel pulse sequences with near-isotropic resolution, such as 3D SSFP or 3D FSE, are needed in order to achieve sensitivities of cartilage MRI that are consistently greater than 90%.

QUANTITATIVE IMAGE PROCESSING AND IMAGE ANALYSIS

Quantitative image processing techniques are increasingly important for the detection and monitoring of cartilage volume, thickness, and surface, especially when the success of surgical procedures or response of medical treatment is being evaluated.

*References 13, 15, 16, 19, 20, 24, 28, 44.

Therefore a 3D model of cartilage can be generated by segmenting it from surrounding tissue by either manual or semiautomatic segmentation based on threshold techniques (Figure 4-6). With manual segmentation, the reader draws a line around the borders of femoral and tibial cartilage on every single MRI slice with a computer mouse. The semiautomatic method is similar to the manual one, with the difference that the computer generates, according to a mathematical algorithm, an estimation of the cartilage borders, which have to be controlled and eventually changed by the reader. The resultant 3D models can be used to calculate the volume, thickness (Figure 4-7), and surface area of the segmented cartilage. The interreader and intrareader reproducibility of these methods has been evaluated by reading MRI data acquired from healthy volunteers or patients with mild OA.[45-47]

3D measurements of total cartilage volume and cartilage thickness have evolved as the standard for quantitative MRI-based assessment of cartilage loss.* Both measurements require segmentation of the cartilage from the surrounding tissue using techniques such as manual segmentation,[42,49,51] intensity-based thresholding,[42,49,51] filtering,[59-61] watershed,[32] and live wire approaches[56,57,62,63] or model-based segmentation.[25,64-66]

3D measurements of total cartilage volume and cartilage thickness have evolved as the standard for quantitative MRI assessment of articular cartilage but require considerable time for evaluation, making them most useful currently for research purposes.

The ability to distinguish changes of cartilage volume and thickness over time, which is determined by the reproducibility of the technique, is a critical component of any OA outcome measure. There is significant disagreement in the literature as to the reproducibility of MRI derived measurements of cartilage loss in the knee. Coefficients of variation (COV) for repeated measurements of total cartilage volume derived from standard 3D SPGR sequences ranged from 1.8%[22,45,67] to 8.2%[47,51,68,69] and were as high as 10% to 15% in one study.[52]

MEASUREMENT OF LONGITUDINAL PROGRESSION, IMPACT OF REPRODUCIBILITY

Wluka et al.[70] reported that the annual rate of total tibial cartilage loss in a longitudinal study in OA patients amounted to 5.3 ± 5.2% (mean ± 1 standard deviation [SD]) (95% confidence interval [95% CI] 4.4%, 6.2%) per year, a value only slightly above most of the published reproducibility errors. The annual

*References 25, 29, 42, 47-58.

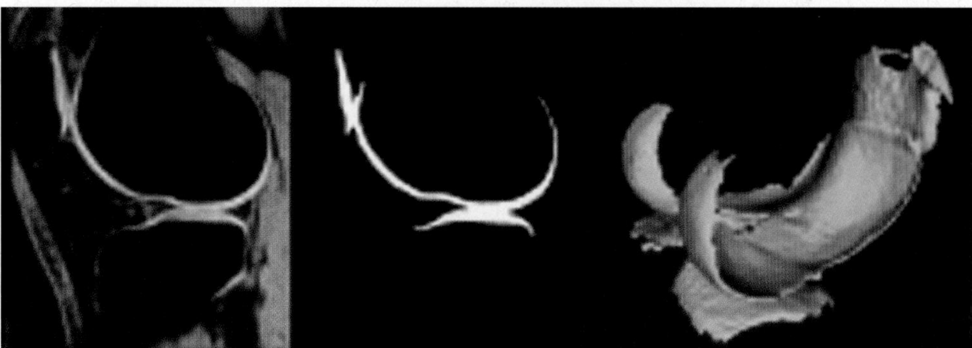

FIGURE 4-6. Cartilage segmentation. *Left,* 3D SSFP image; *middle,* result of cartilage segmentation; *right,* 3D view of segmented cartilage.

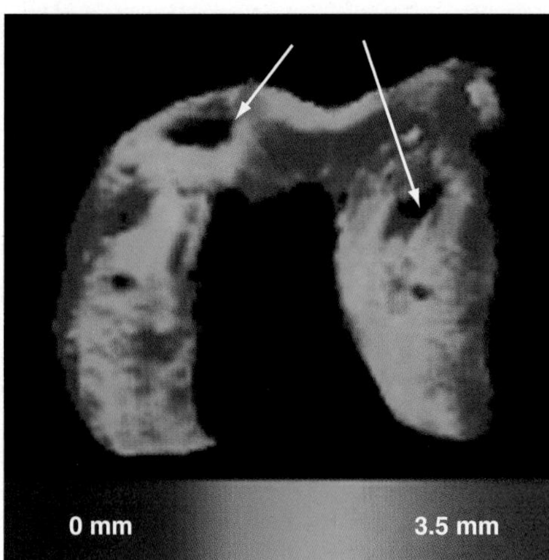

FIGURE 4-7. 3D MRI–derived map of cartilage thickness. The cartilage thickness map was generated using a 3D euclidean distance transformation. Full-thickness defects are seen *(arrows)*. Multiple areas of severe cartilage thinning *(dark blue)* are also present, particularly in the trochlea and medial femoral condyle.

percentages of loss of medial and lateral tibial cartilage were 4.7 ± 6.5% and 5.3 ± 7.2%, respectively[70] (see Figure 4-2). Gandy et al.[49] did not see any discernable change in cartilage volume in OA cases that were followed with MRI for 3 years. Remarkably, radiologists' visual readings showed progression of cartilage loss in the same cohort.[71] Difficulties in cartilage segmentation caused by low cartilage contrast in the 3D SPGR sequence appeared to be responsible for the problems noted with quantitative cartilage measurement.[49] This is a fundamental problem affecting all OA studies that utilize standard technology; in other words, standard 2D FSE and 3D SPGR sequences.

Hardy et al.[50] showed that the spatial resolution of the imaging sequence is of critical importance for reducing partial volume artifacts in cartilage MRI and for improving the reproducibility of quantitative measurements of cartilage loss. Changing the slice thickness from 1.0 to 0.5 mm resulted on average in a 2% decrease in COV in the tibiofemoral compartments.[50] Similarly, a change in in-plane resolution from 0.55 to 0.275 mm caused a threefold decrease in COV of repeated cartilage volume measurements. In addition to the high variability in published reproducibility errors[22,67] and the difficulties encountered by some investigators in segmenting the articular cartilage in OA patients,[24,43,49,71-74] the results of Hardy et al.[69] emphasize the need for novel 3D imaging techniques with high contrast and high spatial resolution, such as the new 3D SSFP, 3D DESS, and 3D FSE sequences.

THE NATIONAL INSTITUTES OF HEALTH OSTEOARTHRITIS INITIATIVE

The National Institutes of Health (NIH) Osteoarthritis Initiative (OAI) is a public-private partnership that aims to find biologic markers for the progression of OA. For 5 to 7 years, the OAI will collect information and define disease standards on 5000 people at high risk for OA and at high risk of progressing to severe OA during the study. Efforts to develop novel therapies for OA have been frustrated by the lack of objective and measurable standards for disease progression by which new drugs can be evaluated. It is hoped that the OAI will speed progress toward better drugs. The OAI will establish and maintain a natural history database for OA that will include clinical evaluation data, radiographic and MRI images, and a biospecimen repository. Recognizing the limitations of current MRI technology, the NIH OAI has decided to invest in new hardware technology by purchasing novel 3.0T MRI systems rather than standard 1.5T MRI systems. Imaging arthritic joints at 3.0T offers the unique opportunity to image articular cartilage with unprecedented signal, thereby providing the opportunity for high-resolution, near-isotropic imaging. Exciting new technologies such as 3D SS-SPGR, 3D SSFP, 3D DESS, and 3D FSE can be brought to their full potential at 3.0T and can be combined with other novel approaches such as parallel imaging.

> MRI at 3T allows improved resolution of articular cartilage and near-isotropic imaging.

T2 RELAXATION MAPPING

The biochemical and physiologic composition of cartilage offers the possibility of noninvasive MRI detection of molecular changes that may lead to cartilage destruction and OA. The transverse relaxation time (T2), which is sensitive to changes of water and collagen content of the cartilage tissue,[75] and the anisotropy (a state in which a physical characteristic varies in value along axes in different directions) of the tissue matrix[76] are especially useful for the early detection of cartilage changes. T2 is the time it takes for spinning protons to lose phase coherence among the nuclei spinning perpendicular to the main magnetic field. This interaction between spins results in a reduction in the transverse magnetization (T2). The decay of T2 is tissue specific, as tissue with high proton mobility has a longer T2 period than tissue with lower proton mobility.

A high correlation between water content and T2 of the cartilage[77] allows one to generate T2 maps of the cartilage with an estimated weight error of only 2%[78] (Figure 4-8). The freedom of movement of the water is restricted by the anisotropic extracellular matrix of the cartilage tissue. The matrix differences in the particular histologic zones (superficial, transitional, and radial) lead to variable concentrations of water in the cartilage tissue. The water content decreases from the cartilage surface to the deeper zones.[79] As a result of water distribution, the T2 values appear in different phases. Some in vitro studies on cartilage samples have shown T2 values to measure from 10 ms near subchondral bone to 50 to 60 ms at the cartilage surface.[17,78,80-82] The tendency to exhibit lower T2 values in the deep radial zone has been confirmed in in vivo studies showing T2 values of 30 to 46 ms in the deeper radial zone and 55 to 65 ms at the cartilage surface.[83-85]

The intactness of the collagen fibers is also an important factor in T2. Different studies have shown that the collagen content influences the MRI appearance. Damage to the network integrity leads to an increased cartilage T2.[81,86,87] In contrast to the influence of collagen, the impact of proteoglycan (PG) loss appears to be low in terms of cartilage T2.[81,87] In in vitro studies a single component of the cartilage was enzymatically erased. This is a finding unlikely to be seen in vivo in OA. Rather, a multifactor event leads to cartilage destruction. Menezes suggested that both hydration and structure are important factors.[88]

In OA the cartilage structure is damaged, and cartilage T2 values increase because of an increase in the relative water content. A recent study has shown that in mild OA the cartilage T2 (34.4 to 41.0 ms) is significantly greater than the healthy values (32.1 to 35.0 ms), but a further increase of T2 in severe OA could not be found.[89]

In many in vitro studies using cartilage/bone samples for creating a T2 map, magnetic fields at 7T or higher have been used.[17,87,90,91] These studies used pixel resolution ranging from

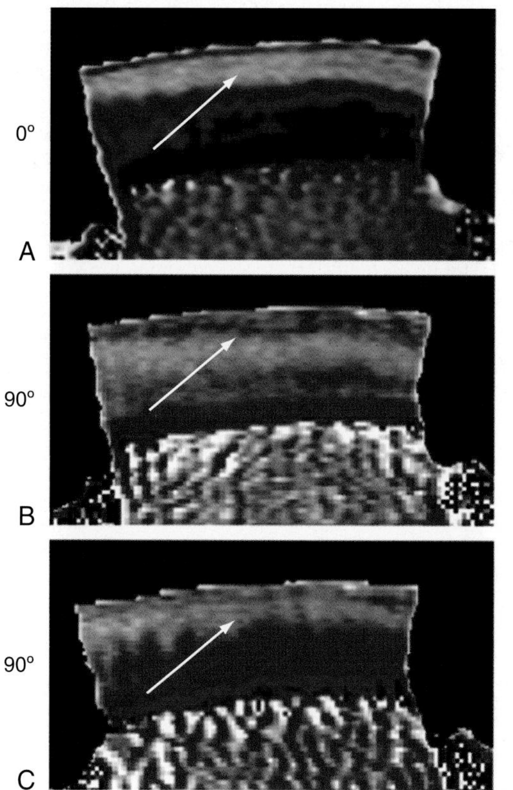

FIGURE 4-8. T2 relaxation maps of bone cartilage plugs. The bone cartilage plugs were imaged at different orientations relative to B0 (the main magnetic field). Note that T2 relaxation changes when the orientation of the articular cartilage is altered relative to B0. In this example, the relaxation time of the transitional layer *(arrow)* changes from 61.7 ms **(A)** at 0 degrees to 29.2 ms **(B)** at 90 degrees to 34.5 ms **(C)** at −90 degrees of rotation of the bone cartilage plug. This is important in conducting longitudinal MRI studies using T2 relaxation and may require the use of a leg holder in order to achieve higher reproducibility of measurements. (Courtesy Doug Goodwin, MD.)

30 to 78 μm. In the in vivo studies evaluating the knee cartilage, either a 1.5T[92,93] or 3T[83,94] magnet was used, with pixel resolution ranging from 100 to 547 μm.

For T2 cartilage mapping of the knee, multiecho is preferable to single echo data acquisition with a TE range of 10 to 100 ms. A short interecho spacing is dictated by the fast decay of cartilage T2. A decreasing SNR has to be taken into account by utilizing large bandwidth for registration of these short echo signals. A further method of reducing the interecho spacing is the use of extremity transmit/receive coils. The difficulty of reducing interecho spacing and otherwise keeping high resolution can be solved on the one hand by using a small field of view and on the other hand by larger matrix places demanding high gradient strength and rise time.[95]

Mosher et al. described in several publications a method for calculating cartilage T2 maps by fitting the signal intensity for different pixels as a function of time, including constants as pixel intensity and T2. He furthermore suggested fitting the signal intensity of every pixel to a single exponential decay.[94-96] In another report, Dardzinski et al. suggested that a better fit could be achieved if the first echo time, which includes a combination of T1 and T2 signal, is excluded.[97] Color-coded maps of every single cartilage region can be generated from the calculated T2 signals.

A pitfall of this technique is a phenomenon called "magic angle effect," related to the collagen anisotropy in MRI. In addition to the orientation of cartilage collagen fibers in the magnetic field, the cartilage T2 values are influenced by this phenomenon. This effect is described in different in vitro studies using cartilage samples.[91,98] When the collagen fibers are aligned 55 degrees to the applied static magnetic field (B0), longer cartilage T2 results[96,99] and leads to higher apparent imaging signal. The increased signal and inhomogeneous signal in the articular cartilage created by this artifact should not be confused with early degenerative changes in the cartilage substance. In daily clinical application this increased signal intensity can cause diagnostic mistakes, especially along curved surfaces.[100] This phenomenon was evaluated in in vitro studies that showed strong influence on the MRI appearance in the radial zone, where the collagen fibrils are perpendicular to the articular surface of cartilage.[91,101] Mosher et al. showed in an in vivo study that the transitional zone also influences the T2 and suggested a regional difference of cartilage tissue and fiber orientation in weight-bearing and non–weight-bearing areas.[96] Xia et al. reported a complicated multizone structure found in the cartilage of the peripheral humerus head with a second transitional zone and a second tangential zone located at the deep part of the tissue.[102] Not only does the orientation of collagen fibers in the magnetic field determine the increased signal, but the arrangement of PGs on the collagen frame as a structural component of the cartilage and their variable distribution influence the dipolar interactions of the water molecules.[91,101,103]

> Magic angle artifact, which occurs when the tissue is oriented at approximately 55 degrees to the main magnetic field, causes that portion of the articular cartilage to appear brighter than the other areas, potentially simulating a cartilage lesion.

T1ρ RELAXATION MAPPING

T1ρ imaging is based on spin lock MRI studies. The basic premise of this technique is that T1ρ is correlated with proteoglycan content ($R^2 = 0.926$).[104] Unlike dGEMRIC studies (see later section), it does not require the use of a contrast agent but is based on an inherent tissue specific relaxation phenomenon. Greater dispersion of values between normal and OA cartilage has been reported with this technique when compared with T2 measurements.[105] Thus T1ρ may be more sensitive for detecting earlier biochemical alterations when compared with T2 relaxation imaging. However, T1ρ in the deep radial zone depends on cartilage orientation[106] and, similar to T2 measurements,[107] may be subject to position-dependent changes.

SODIUM MR IMAGING (23Na MRI)

One of the early events in OA is the loss of PG content or fixed charge density (FCD) in the cartilage tissue. Sodium (23Na) MRI is described as another method for early detection of OA. It is concerned with displaying cartilage regions with reduced PG.[108,109] The PGs serve as a connective and stabilizing component between collagen fibers and are surrounded by glycosaminoglycans (GAGs). The molecular composition of the GAG induces a negative FCD to which the positively charged 23Na is attracted. To maintain a state of electroneutrality, a direct relationship between the concentrations of 23Na and GAG appears to exist.[109,110] In the early stages of OA, GAGs are reduced, resulting in decreased 23Na concentration.

Different investigators have analyzed cartilage with Na spectroscopy and shown that the 23Na image is modified in degraded cartilage.[111-114] These in vitro studies show the sensitivity of sodium MRI as a function of cartilage depletion and show that the relaxation times of 23Na change in combination with progressive loss of PGs. A 100% visibility of 23Na in cartilage and the spatial distribution of sodium in healthy cartilage have also been reported.[115] These findings could be transferred to in vivo investigations of 23Na and calculation of FCD. Shapiro et al. reported an in vivo examination of human patellar cartilage FCD in which 23Na ranging from 140 to 350 mM corresponded to a maximum FCD of −270 mM, with lower values at the edges of the cartilage.[108] An in vivo examination of patella cartilage in healthy volunteers and patients with symptoms of early OA reported a significantly lower FCD in the symptomatic group.[109] These results indicate a possible method of noninvasive determination of early cartilage changes, even if further investigations are necessary to introduce it to clinical routine.

DELAYED GADOLINIUM-ENHANCED MRI OF CARTILAGE

Delayed gadolinium-enhanced MRI of cartilage or delayed contrast-enhanced MRI of cartilage (dGEMRIC) is another imaging method analyzing the GAG content of the cartilage, in this case after penetration of the hydrophilic contrast agent Gd-DTPA2-. The term *delayed* refers to the interval required for the contrast agent to penetrate after injection into the cartilage. The negatively charged contrast medium (Gd-DTPA2-) distributes in damaged cartilage with reduced GAG content more than in healthy cartilage because it is rejected by the negative charge of the GAG. Thus areas with significant T1 shortening reflect areas of GAG loss. The higher the concentration of contrast medium—in other words, the greater the T1 shortening in the cartilage—the higher the apparent loss of GAG. The concentration of the Gd-DTPA2- can be optionally calculated by the difference between precontrast and postcontrast T1 values.[116-119] The technique provides noninvasive in vivo mapping of GAG content, similar to a noninvasive safranin-O stain (Figure 4-9).

> The negatively charged contrast medium (Gd-DTPA2-) is distributed in damaged cartilage (with reduced GAG content) more than in healthy cartilage because normally the contrast is repelled by the negative charge of the GAG. This technique provides noninvasive in vivo mapping of GAG content.

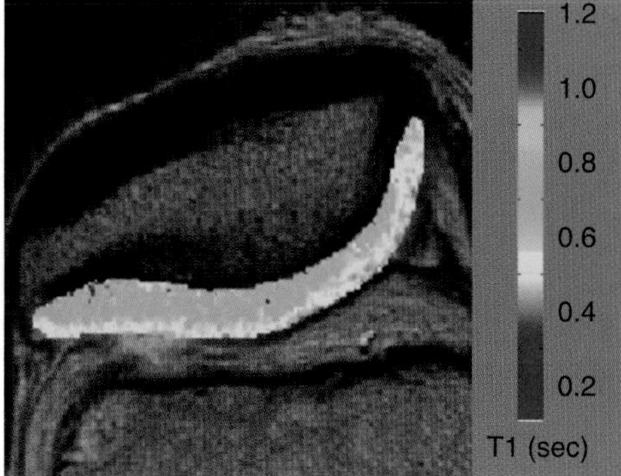

FIGURE 4-9. dGEMRIC map of the patellar cartilage. T1 relaxation time changes from the deep to the superficial cartilage layers. The dGEMRIC scan provides information on GAG content similar to a safranin-O stain, in a completely noninvasive fashion using contrast-enhanced MRI. (Courtesy Deborah Burstein, Beth Israel Hospital, Harvard Medical School, Boston.)

This method was investigated by several in vitro studies.[119-121] One study showed, after in vivo intravenous application and ex vivo examination, agreement between MRI and histologic findings.[122] It was also reported that regional differences of Gd-DTPA2- uptake depend on cartilage thickness. The thicker the cartilage, the longer it takes to reach maximal and optimal distribution within the cartilage.[122] To ameliorate the contrast distribution in the cartilage, physical exercise after the intravenous application of Gd-DTPA2- is recommended.[122-124] To assess all cartilage compartments of the knee, a time window of 2 hours is suggested between intravenous application and MR image acquisition.[122-124]

Tiderius et al. reported a change of T1 values that indicated an adaptation of the cartilage GAG content after physical exercise. He evaluated T1 in three groups of volunteers who underwent different levels of physical exercise. The T1 values ranged from 382 ± 33 ms for a sedentary group to 476 ± 36 ms for the elite, heavily exercising group.[125]

A study of T1 in diseased areas of the knee showed decreased T1 values with progression of OA. Thirty-one patients with different stages of OA were evaluated with dGEMRIC and results were compared with radiologic findings on weight-bearing radiographs. In patients without joint space narrowing, the T1 mean value was 408 ms and decreased to a mean value of 369 ms in patients with joint space narrowing.[126] Another study compared dGEMRIC findings with those in arthroscopy and reported a decrease of T1 in more-diseased knees. Using the arthroscopic Outerbridge Classification, which defines successive stages of cartilage loss, T1 decreased from 35 1 ± 28.2 ms for grade I to 297 ± 54.1 ms for grade IV.[122-124,127]

DIFFUSION-WEIGHTED AND DIFFUSION TENSOR IMAGING

The motivation for diffusion-weighted and diffusion tensor imaging of articular cartilage as new techniques is to directly obtain additional architectural and directional information regarding the cartilage matrix. Directional information on alignment of collagenous fibers may help to differentiate potentially reversible loss of PG content and irreversible disruption of the collagenous fiber network in cartilage.

Diffusion-weighted and diffusion-tensor imaging are used to study the direction of articular cartilage collagen fibers to help differentiate potentially reversible loss of proteoglycan from irreversible disruption of the collagen framework.

Tissue analysis using diffusion-weighted imaging is based on the assumption that the magnitude and direction of local diffusivity are influenced by the macromolecular environment of the diffusing bulk water. Measuring the spatial restriction of diffusivity in any tissue (in contrast to unrestricted diffusion in free water) gives information on the tissue's (ultra)structural properties.

The most commonly applied technique of measuring diffusion is the pulsed gradient spin echo (PGSE) method, according to Stejskal and Tanner.[128] It applies a pair of additional (diffusion-sensitizing) gradients before and after the refocusing pulse. The concomitant signal (S) attenuation is related to additional spin dephasing due to diffusional movement of the water protons, which cannot be refocused prior to read-out. The amount of this signal attenuation is expressed as the apparent diffusion coefficient (ADC) and depends on both the amount of diffusion in the tissue and the diffusion weighting (b) of the sequence: $S(b) = S0 \exp(-b \times ADC)$. The degree of diffusion weighting depends on the strength (i.e., amplitude and duration) of the diffusion gradients and on the time interval (Δ, the so-called diffusion time) between these gradients (allowing for diffusion-related dephasing to occur). Pixelwise calculation of the ADC results in an ADC map that reflects local diffusional properties throughout the cross-section of the tissue analyzed.

In conventional diffusion-weighted imaging, the diffusion-sensitizing gradients are applied in only one direction; consequently, only the component of the total diffusional movement in this direction can be registered. This restriction in view of the directional information desired is overcome with diffusion tensor imaging (DTI) by applying several diffusion-sensitizing gradient pairs in different non-coplanar directions (Figure 4-10). If six or more gradient directions are available, enough information can be obtained to completely evaluate the various directional components of the diffusion pathway.[27,51] This spatially oriented information can be obtained pixelwise and collected in a 3×3 data matrix, the diffusion tensor. Diagonalization of this tensor permits calculation of the three orthogonal "eigenvectors" and their absolute values, the "eigenvalues," of the tensor. They represent the three main axes of diffusion and correspond to the three main axes of anisotropy in the tissue. Going beyond T2, these eigenvectors are able to provide directional information in various orientations in addition to nondirectional anisotropy without the necessity to manipulate the probe relative to B0. The largest eigenvector would represent the predominant local (voxel) direction of diffusion as related to the structural anisotropy in the probe. As the strongly anisotropic zonal alignment of the collagen fibers determines the architecture and, to a large extent, the functional integrity of the cartilage matrix, such an access to directional information would help to overcome current MRI limitations in tissue analysis and may indeed be valuable for detecting early degenerative change in cartilage. From the diffusion tensor the ADC can be calculated as a scalar quantity, defined as the mean of the three eigenvalues. ADC then would correspond to the overall amount of diffusivity (independent of its direction) in cartilage. As a measure of anisotropy, parameters such as the fractional anisotropy (FA) can be calculated as the amount of anisotropic diffusion within the tensor normalized to the modulus of the tensor with values in the interval [0,1]. Thus, going beyond conventional diffusion-weighted MR imaging, DTI allows us to determine the degree of diffusional anisotropy and the main directions of local diffusion in a tissue.[129]

Application of diffusion-weighted imaging to cartilage requires low sensitivity to susceptibility differences (e.g., cartilage-bone interface), which is provided by PGSE sequences. However, PGSE sequences require acquisition times of several minutes for each diffusion-sensitizing gradient direction in order to obtain sufficient SNRs (by applying TRs that are not too short) and are very sensitive to motion. One way to overcome this sensitivity to motion is to acquire additional echoes, navigator echoes, which are used to adjust for inconsistent phase information.[130-133] The first in vivo measurements at 1.5T of patellar cartilage ADC (one direction; $0.5 \times 0.7 \times 3$ mm^3 spatial resolution applying a $256 \times 192 \times 16$ matrix) using a 3D steady-state sequence[134] with a nonlinear 3D navigator technique have been presented. In addition, Brihuega-Moreno et al.[135] have proposed a theoretic approach to optimize the b-value scheme with regard to acquisition time and precision of ADC calculation in cartilage.

For the analysis of a tissue's structural anisotropy, the diffusion time (Δ) may play an important role. Burstein described a 40% reduction of diffusivity in intact, trypsin-treated, and compressed cartilage samples due to increased (from 25 to 2000 ms) diffusion times.[136] Whereas diffusivity in cartilage was restricted to 60% of the diffusivity of free water at short diffusion times, it was restricted to only 40% of the diffusivity of free water at long diffusion times, which indicates that diffusion-restricting structural properties of the cartilage matrix can be emphasized in imaging and thus can be better visualized when longer diffusion times are used. Knauss et al. suggested that short and long diffusion times may primarily reflect water content and properties of the collagenous matrix component of cartilage, respectively.[137]

The ADC of cartilage has been reported to increase from between 0.68 and 0.75×10^{-3} mm^2/s close to the tide mark to between 1.20 and 1.45×10^{-3} mm^2/s close to the cartilage surface in excised plugs of calf, canine humeral head, and human patellar and femoral condyle cartilage.[17,45,136,138] In vivo diffusion measurements are expected to yield higher ADC values because they are conducted at higher temperatures (37° C body temperature as opposed to 20° C to 25° C room temperature) than ex vivo experiments.[139] Budinsky demonstrated a linear relationship between (not spatially resolved) cartilage water content of 60% to 80% and cartilage diffusivity as normalized to free water diffusivity.[139] According to Burstein et al.,[136] matrix charge did not affect diffusivity, whereas compression (35% strain) led to a 19% decrease of cartilage diffusivity.

Trypsin digestion,[136,140,141] hyaluronidase, and collagenase digestion[140] led to an increase (10% to 30%) of bulk ADC in contrast to retinoic acid digestion.[140] Xia reported on concomitant PG loss measured by the DMMB assay[142] in cartilage exclusively treated with collagenase.[85] However, according to Toffanin et al.,[143]

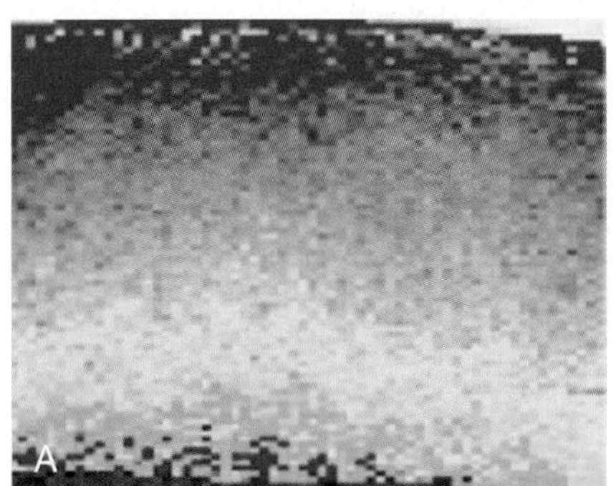

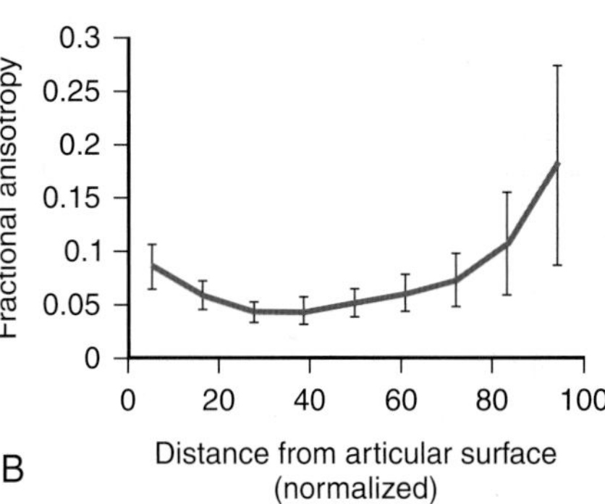

FIGURE 4-10. Diffusion tensor imaging of excised human patellar cartilage-on-bone plug. **A,** In the ADC map, a gradual decrease of ADC from the surface down to the tidemark can be observed. On the contrary, there is no such gradient in the horizontal plane. **B,** The fractional anisotropy (profile across the cartilage, depth normalized to total height from the surface) is minimal at a depth of 20%, indicating an almost isotropic architecture. There is only minimal increase toward the cartilage surface. In the lower 50% of the cartilage there is a marked increase in fractional anisotropy. **C,** The projection of the largest eigenvector on the image plane visualizes the pixelwise distribution of the predominant direction of diffusion. It shows a layer with predominance of tangential orientation in the upper portion and a predominance of a more radial alignment in the lower portion of the cartilage. This distribution is consistent with the alignment of the collagen fibers.

diffusivity in cartilage was reduced by applying PG extracting agents. One theory to explain the observed increase of ADC subsequent to enzymatic treatment is that removal of macromolecules from the cartilage matrix may create pores at the molecular level in the tissue, facilitating diffusional movement.[140,141]

Qualitatively, in a cadaveric specimen, ADC was increased at 1.5T in an area of softening compared with adjacent normal patellar cartilage.[144] In an experimental scanner (7T), ADC was found to be elevated by 10% throughout the whole depth of cartilage in osteoarthritic compared with normal canine humeral cartilage samples.[140] Recently, Mlynarik and colleagues showed an increase of ADC by 30% to 40% in regions of short T1 and low PG staining from osteoarthritic cartilage compared with adjacent normal cartilage.[138] However, this relationship could only be observed in two thirds of their samples, whereas in the remaining third no differences in ADC could be observed in the areas of PG loss. This finding is consistent with the assumption that, in addition to compositional changes, altered ADC values reflect structural degradation of the cartilage matrix.

Going beyond the assessment of the spatial distribution of (nondirectional) ADC in cartilage, Wentorf applied diffusion-sensitizing gradients parallel and perpendicular to the cartilage surface in human femoral and bovine patellar cartilage samples,[145] indicating variations of ADC in both directions with increasing distance from the cartilage surface. Variation of ADC was between 1.1×10^{-3} mm^2/s and 0.8×10^{-3} mm^2/s. In an early study in which DTI was applied to cartilage specimen, Filidoro et al. demonstrated lowest fractional anisotropy (0.04 mm^2/s) at a depth of 20% from the surface, clearly increasing (to 0.27 mm^2/s) close to the tide mark.[146] Mean diffusivity decreased from the surface ($1.28 \times 10^{-3} \pm 0.14$ mm^2/s) to the tide mark ($0.74 \times 10^{-3} \pm 0.19$ mm^2/s). The alignment of the largest eigenvector showed high similarity to the zonal alignment of the collagenous fibers as reported from scanning electron microscopy data. Thus, given the high degree of internal structural anisotropy of articular cartilage, DTI appears to be a potentially rewarding technique for the analysis of the spatial organization of its matrix and as an imaging tool may contribute to assessment of matrix properties related to cartilage biomechanics.[147]

References

1. Doherty M, Hutton C, Bayliss MT: Osteoarthritis. In Maddison PJ, Issenberg DA, Woo P et al, editors: *Oxford textbook of rheumatology*, Oxford, 1993, Oxford University Press, pp 959-983.
2. Brittberg M, Lindahl A, Nilsson A et al: Treatment of deep cartilage defects in the knee with autologous chondrocyte transplantation, *N Engl J Med* 331:889-895, 1994.
3. Brittberg M, Lindahl A, Homminga G et al: A critical analysis of cartilage repair, *Acta Orthop Scand* 68:186-191, 1997.
4. Garrett JC: Osteochondral allografts for reconstruction of articular defects of the knee, *Instr Course Lect* 47:517-522, 1998.
5. Stevenson S, Li XQ, Martin B: The fate of articular cartilage after transplantation of fresh and cryopreserved tissue-antigen-matched and mismatched osteochondral allografts in dogs, *J Bone Joint Surg (Am)* 71:1297-1307, 1989.
6. Bobic V: Arthroscopic osteochondral autograft transplantation in anterior cruciate ligament reconstruction: a preliminary clinical study, *Knee Surg Sports Traumatol Arthrosc* 3:262-264, 1996.
7. Nizard RS: Role of tibial osteotomy in the treatment of medial femorotibial osteoarthritis, *Rev Rhum Engl Ed* 65:443-446, 1998.
8. Elting JJ, Hubbell JC: Unilateral frame distraction: proximal tibial valgus osteotomy for medial gonarthritis, *Contemp Orthop* 27:522-524, 1993.
9. Mollica Q, Leonardi W, Longo G et al: Surgical treatment of arthritic varus knee by tibial corticotomy and angular distraction with an external fixator, *Ital J Orthop Traumatol* 18:7-23, 1992.
10. Recht MP, Resnick D: MR imaging of articular cartilage: current status and future directions, *AJR Am J Roentgenol* 163:283-290, 1994.
11. Hayes C, Conway W: Evaluation of articular cartilage: radiographic and cross-sectional imaging techniques, *Radiographics* 12:409-428, 1992.
12. Hayes C, Sawyer R, Conway W: Patellar cartilage lesions: in vitro detection and staging with MR imaging and pathologic correlation, *Radiology* 176:763-766, 1990.
13. Disler DG: Fat-suppressed three-dimensional spoiled gradient-recalled MR imaging: assessment of articular and physeal hyaline cartilage, *AJR Am J Roentgenol* 169:1117-1123, 1997.
14. Disler DG, McCauley TR, Kelman CG et al: Fat-suppressed three-dimensional spoiled gradient-echo MR imaging of hyaline cartilage defects in the knee: comparison with standard MR imaging and arthroscopy, *AJR Am J Roentgenol* 167:127-132, 1996.
15. Disler DG, McCauley TR, Wirth CR et al: Detection of knee hyaline cartilage defects using fat-suppressed three-dimensional spoiled gradient-echo MR imaging: comparison with standard MR imaging and correlation with arthroscopy, *AJR Am J Roentgenol* 165:377-382, 1995.
16. Potter HG, Linklater JM, Allen AA et al: Magnetic resonance imaging of articular cartilage in the knee: an evaluation with use of fast-spin echo imaging, *J Bone Joint Surg (Am)* 80:1276-1284, 1998.
17. Xia, Y, Farquhar T, Burton-Wurster N et al: Diffusion and relaxation mapping of cartilage-bone plugs and excised disks using microscopic magnetic resonance imaging, *Magn Res Med* 31:273-282, 1994.
18. Freeman D, Bergman G, Glover G: Short TE MR microscopy: accurate measurement and zonal differentiation of normal hyaline cartilage, *Magn Res Med* 38:72-81, 1997.
19. Recht MP, Piraino DW, Paletta GA et al: Accuracy of fat-suppressed three-dimensional spoiled gradient-echo FLASH MR imaging in the detection of patellofemoral articular cartilage abnormalities, *Radiology* 198:209-212, 1996.
20. Broderick LS, Turner DA, Renfrew DL et al: Severity of articular cartilage abnormality in patients with osteoarthritis: evaluation with fast spin echo MR vs arthroscopy, *AJR Am J Roentgenol* 162:99-103, 1994.
21. Yao L, Gentili A, Thomas A: Incidental magnetization transfer contrast in fast spin echo imaging of cartilage, *J Magn Reson Imaging* 6:180-184, 1996.
22. Eckstein F, Gavazzeni A, Sittek H et al: Determination of knee joint cartilage thickness using three-dimensional magnetic resonance chondro-crassometry (3D MR-CCM), *Magn Reson Med* 36:256-265, 1996.
23. Kapur T, Bearrlsly P, Gibson S et al. Model based segmentation of clinical knee MRI. in Model-based 3D Image Analysis (in conjunction with ICCV). Workshop presentation, Bombay, India. 1998.
24. McCauley TR, Kier R, Lynch KJ et al: Chondromalacia patellae: diagnosis with MR imaging, *AJR Am J Roentgenol* 158:101-105, 1992.
25. Warfield S: Fast k-NN classification for multichannel image data, *Pattern Recognition Lett* 17:713-721, 1996.
26. Walter SD, Eliasziw M, Donner A: Sample size and optimal designs for reliability studies, *Statistics Med* 17:101-110, 1998.
27. Peterfy CG, Majumdar S, Lang P et al: MR imaging of the arthritic knee: improved discrimination of cartilage, synovium, and effusion with pulsed saturation transfer and fat-suppressed T1-weighted sequences, *Radiology* 191:413-419, 1994.
28. Kawahara Y, Uetani M, Nakahara N et al: Fast spin echo MR of the articular cartilage in the osteoarthrotic knee. Correlation of MR and arthroscopic findings, *Acta Radiol* 39:120-125, 1998.
29. Stammberger T, Eckstein F, Michaelis M et al: Interobserver reproducibility of quantitative cartilage measurements: comparison of B-spline snakes and manual segmentation, *Magn Reson Imaging* 17:1033-1042, 1999.
30. Diamond WJ: *Practical experiment designs*, New York, 1989, Van-Nostrand Reinhold.
31. Hargreaves BA, Gold GE, Lang PK et al: Imaging of articular cartilage using driven equilibrium, *Magn Reson Med* 42:695-703, 1999.
32. Sijbers J., Scheunders P, Verhoye M et al: Watershed-based segmentation of 3D MR data for volume quantization, *Magn Reson Imaging* 15:679-688, 1997.
33. Jaume S, Ferrant M, Macq B et al: Tumor detection in the bladder wall with a measurement of abnormal thickness, *IEEE Trans Biomed Eng*, 2003.
34. Kallman DA, Wigley FM, Scott WW Jr et al: New radiographic grading scales for osteoarthritis of the hand. Reliability for determining prevalence and progression, *Arthritis Rheum* 32:1584-1591, 1989.
35. Pessis E, Drapé JL, Ravaud P et al: Assessment of progression in knee osteoarthritis: results of a 1 year study comparing arthroscopy and MRI, *Osteoarthritis Cartilage* 11:361-369, 2003.
36. Felson DT, Chaisson CE, Hill CL et al: The association of bone marrow lesions with pain in knee osteoarthritis, *Ann Intern Med* 134:541-549, 2001.
37. Fielding JR: Practical MR imaging of female pelvic floor weakness, *Radiographics* 22:295-304, 2002.
38. Helm PA, Eckel TS: Accuracy of registration methods in frameless stereotaxis, *Comput Aided Surg* 3:51-56, 1998.
39. Landis JR, Koch GG: The measurement of observer agreement for categorical data, *Biometrics* 33:159-174, 1977.
40. Iosifescu DV, Shenton ME, Warfield SK et al: An automated registration algorithm for measuring MRI subcortical brain structures, *Neuroimage* 6:13-25, 1997.
41. Warfield S, Dengler J, Zaers J et al: Automatic identification of gray matter structures from MRI to improve the segmentation of white matter lesions, *J Image Guid Surg* 1:326-338, 1995.
42. Peterfy C, van Dijke CF, Lu Y et al: Quantification of the volume of articular cartilage in the metacarpophalangeal joints of the hand: accuracy and precision of three-dimensional MR imaging, *AJR Am J Roentgenol* 165:371-375, 1995.
43. Hargreaves BA, Gold G, Conolly S et al: Technical considerations for DEFT imaging. In *International Society for Magnetic Resonance in Medicine*. 1998. Scientif Meeting, Sydney, Australia.
44. Bredella MA, Tirman PF, Peterfy CG et al: Accuracy of T2-weighted fast spin echo MR imaging with fat saturation in detecting cartilage defects in the knee: comparison with arthroscopy in 130 patients, *AJR Am J Roentgenol* 172:1073-1080, 1999.

45. Eckstein F, Heudorfer L, Faber SC et al: Long-term and resegmentation precision of quantitative cartilage MR imaging (qMRI), *Osteoarthritis Cartilage* 10:922-928, 2002.
46. Cicuttini F, Wluka A, Hankin J et al: Longitudinal study of the relationship between knee angle and tibiofemoral cartilage volume in subjects with knee osteoarthritis, *Rheumatology (Oxford)* 43:321-324, 2004.
47. Eckstein F, Westhoff J, Sittek H et al: In vivo reproducibility of three-dimensional cartilage volume and thickness measurements with MR imaging, *AJR Am J Roentgenol* 170:593-597, 1998.
48. Eckstein, F., Sittek H, Gavazzeni A et al: Magnetic resonance chondro-crassometry (MR CCM): a method for accurate determination of articular cartilage thickness? *Magn Reson Med* 35:89-96, 1996.
49. Gandy SJ, Dieppe PA, Keen MC et al: No loss of cartilage volume over three years in patients with knee osteoarthritis as assessed by magnetic resonance imaging, *Osteoarthritis Cartilage* 10:929-937, 2002.
50. Hardy PA, Nammalwar P, Kuo S: Measuring the thickness of articular cartilage from MR images, *J Magn Reson Imaging* 13:120-126, 2001.
51. Peterfy CG, van Dijke CF, Janzen DL et al: Quantification of articular cartilage in the knee with pulsed saturation transfer subtraction and fat-suppressed MR imaging: optimization and validation, *Radiology* 192:485-491, 1994.
52. Pilch L, Stewart C, Gordon D et al: Assessment of cartilage volume in the femorotibial joint with magnetic resonance imaging and 3D computer reconstruction, *J Rheumatol* 21:2307-2321, 1994.
53. Piplani MA, Disler DG, McCauley TR et al: Articular cartilage volume in the knee: semiautomated determination from three-dimensional reformations of MR images, *Radiology* 198:855-859, 1996.
54. Stammberger T, Eckstein F, Englmeier KH et al: Determination of 3D cartilage thickness data from MR imaging: computational method and reproducibility in the living, *Magn Reson Med* 41:529-536, 1999.
55. Stammberger T et al: Patellofemoral joint cartilage thickness and contact areas from MRI in patients with osteoarthritis. In *Int Soc Magn Res Med*, 1998. Sydney, Australia.
56. Steines D, et al: Segmentation of osteoarthritic femoral cartilage using live wire. In *ISMRM Eighth Scientific Meeting*. 2000. Denver.
57. Steines D, Napel S, Lang P: Measuring volume of articular cartilage defects in osteoarthritis using MRI: validation of a new method. In Radiological Society of North America. Chicago, IL, 2000.
58. Tieschky M, Faber S, Haubner M et al: Repeatability of patellar cartilage thickness patterns in the living, using a fat-suppressed magnetic resonance imaging sequence with short acquisition time and three-dimensional data processing, *J Orthop Res* 15:808-813, 1997.
59. Rodrigues-Florido MA, Krissian K, Ruiz-Aloza J et al: Comparison of two restoration techniques in the context of 3D medical imaging. In MICCAI 2000: Fourth International Conference on Medical Image Computing and Computer-Assisted Intervention. 2000. Utrecht, 2000, Springer-Verlag.
60. Westin CF, Richolt J, Moharir V et al: Affine adaptive filtering of CT data, *Med Image Anal* 4:161-177, 2000.
61. Westin CF, Wigström L, Loock T et al: Three-dimensional adaptive filtering in magnetic resonance angiography, *J Magn Reson Imaging* 14:63-71, 2001.
62. Falcão AX, Udupa JK: Segmentation of 3D objects using live wire. In SPIE Medical Imaging. 1997. San Diego.
63. Falcão AX, Udupa JK: User-steered image segmentation paradigms: live wire and live lane, *GMIP* 60:233-260, 1998.
64. Iosifescu DV, Shenton ME, Warfield SK et al: An automated registration algorithm for measuring MRI subcortical brain structures, *Neuroimage* 6:13-25, 1997.
65. Warfield S, Winalski C, Jolesz F et al. Automatic segmentation of MRI of the knee. In International Society for Magnetic Resonance in Medicine. 1998. Sydney, Australia.
66. Warfield SK, Kaus M, Jolesz FA et al: Adaptive, template moderated, spatially varying statistical classification, *Med Image Anal* 4(1):43-45, 2000.
67. Burgkart R, Glaser C, Hyhlik-Dürr A et al: Magnetic resonance imaging-based assessment of cartilage loss in severe osteoarthritis: accuracy, precision, and diagnostic value, *Arthritis Rheum* 44:2072-2077, 2001.
68. Glaser C, Draeger M, Englmeier KH et al: Cartilage loss over two years in femorotibial osteoarthritis. In Radiological Society of North America. Chicago, 2002.
69. Hardy PA, Newmark R, Liu YM et al: The influence of the resolution and contrast on measuring the articular cartilage volume in magnetic resonance images, *Magn Reson Imaging* 18:965-972, 2000.
70. Wluka AE, Stuckey S, Snaddon J et al: The determinants of change in tibial cartilage volume in osteoarthritic knees, *Arthritis Rheum* 46:2065-2072, 2002.
71. Gandy SJ et al: No apparent progressive change to knee cartilage volumes over one year in rheumatoid and osteoarthritis. In Proc Intl Soc Magn Reson Med, Denver, 2000.
72. Higgins W, Ojard E: Interactive morphological watershed analysis for 3D medical images, *Computer Med Imaging Graphics* 17:387-395, 1993.
73. Kaus MR, Warfield SK, Nabavi A et al: Automated segmentation of MR images of brain tumors, *Radiology* 218:586-591, 2001.
74. Margosian P, Schmitt F, Purdy P: Faster MR imaging: imaging with half the data, *Health Care Instrum* 1:195-197, 1986.
75. Harrison R, Bronskill MJ, Henkelman RM: Magnetization transfer and T2 relaxation components in tissue, *Magn Reson Med* 33:490-496, 1995.
76. Henkelman RM, Stanisz GJ, Kim JK et al: Anisotropy of NMR properties of tissues, *Magn Reson Med* 32:592-601, 1994.
77. Lusse S, Knauss R, Werner A et al: Action of compression and cations on the proton and deuterium relaxation in cartilage, *Magn Reson Med* 33:483-489, 1995.
78. Lusse S, Claassen H, Gehrke T et al: Evaluation of water content by spatially resolved transverse relaxation times of human articular cartilage, *Magn Reson Imaging* 18:423-430, 2000.
79. Venn M, Maroudas A: Chemical composition and swelling of normal and osteoarthrotic femoral head cartilage. I. Chemical composition, *Ann Rheum Dis* 36:121-129, 1977.
80. Mlynarik V, Degrassi A, Toffanin R et al: Investigation of laminar appearance of articular cartilage by means of magnetic resonance microscopy, *Magn Reson Imaging* 14:435-442, 1996.
81. Watrin A, Ruaud JP, Olivier PT et al: T2 mapping of rat patellar cartilage, *Radiology* 219:395-402, 2001.
82. Freeman DM, Bergman G, Glover G: Short TE MR microscopy: accurate measurement and zonal differentiation of normal hyaline cartilage, *Magn Reson Med* 38:72-81, 1997.
83. Smith HE, Mosher TJ, Dardzinski BJ et al: Spatial variation in cartilage T2 of the knee, *J Magn Reson Imaging* 14:50-55, 2001.
84. Dardzinski BJ, Laor T, Schmithorst L et al: Mapping T2 relaxation time in the pediatric knee: feasibility with a clinical 1.5-T MR imaging system, *Radiology* 225:233-239, 2002.
85. Liess C, Lüsse J, Karger N et al: Detection of changes in cartilage water content using MRI T2-mapping in vivo, *Osteoarthritis Cartilage* 10:907-913, 2002.
86. Fragonas E, Mlynárik V, Jellús V et al: Correlation between biochemical composition and magnetic resonance appearance of articular cartilage, *Osteoarthritis Cartilage* 6:24-32, 1998.
87. Nieminen MT, Töyräs J, Rieppo J et al: Quantitative MR microscopy of enzymatically degraded articular cartilage, *Magn Reson Med* 43:676-681, 2000.
88. Menezes NM, Gray ML, Hartke JR et al: T2 and T1rho MRI in articular cartilage systems, *Magn Reson Med* 51:503-509, 2004.
89. Dunn TC, Lu Y, Jin H et al: T2 relaxation time of cartilage at MR imaging: comparison with severity of knee osteoarthritis, *Radiology* 232:592-598, 2004.
90. Mlynarik V, Degrassi A, Toffanin R et al: A method for generating magnetic resonance microimaging T2 maps with low sensitivity to diffusion, *Magn Reson Med* 35:423-425, 1996.
91. Goodwin DW, Wadghiri YZ, Dunn JF: Micro-imaging of articular cartilage: T2, proton density, and the magic angle effect, *Acad Radiol* 5:790-798, 1998.
92. Van Breuseghem I, Bosmans HT, Elst LV et al: T2 mapping of human femorotibial cartilage with turbo mixed MR imaging at 1.5 T: feasibility, *Radiology* 233:609-614, 2004.
93. Frank LR, Wong EC, Luh WM et al: Articular cartilage in the knee: mapping of the physiologic parameters at MR imaging with a local gradient coil—preliminary results, *Radiology* 210:241-246, 1999.
94. Mosher TJ, Dardzinski BJ, Smith MB: Human articular cartilage: influence of aging and early symptomatic degeneration on the spatial variation of T2—preliminary findings at 3 T, *Radiology* 214:259-266, 2000.
95. Mosher TJ, Dardzinski BJ: Cartilage MRI T2 relaxation time mapping: overview and applications, *Semin Musculoskelet Radiol* 8:355-368, 2004.
96. Mosher TJ, Smith H, Dardzinski BJ et al: MR imaging and T2 mapping of femoral cartilage: in vivo determination of the magic angle effect, *AJR Am J Roentgenol* 177:665-669, 2001.
97. Dardzinski BJ, Mosher TJ, Li S et al: Spatial variation of T2 in human articular cartilage, *Radiology* 205:546-550, 1997.
98. Rubenstein JD, Kim JK, Morova-Protzner I et al: Effects of collagen orientation on MR imaging characteristics of bovine articular cartilage, *Radiology* 188:219-226, 1993.
99. Xia Y, Moody JB, Alhadlaq H: Orientational dependence of T2 relaxation in articular cartilage: a microscopic MRI (microMRI) study, *Magn Reson Med* 48:460-469, 2002.
100. Wacker FK, Bolze X, Felsenberg D et al: Orientation-dependent changes in MR signal intensity of articular cartilage: a manifestation of the "magic angle" effect, *Skeletal Radiol* 27:306-310, 1998.
101. Xia Y: Relaxation anisotropy in cartilage by NMR microscopy (muMRI) at 14–microm resolution, *Magn Reson Med* 39:941-949, 1998.
102. Xia Y, Moody JB, Alhadlaq H et al: Imaging the physical and morphological properties of a multi-zone young articular cartilage at microscopic resolution, *J Magn Reson Imaging* 17:365-374, 2003.
103. Goodwin DW, Zhu H, Dunn JF: In vitro MR imaging of hyaline cartilage: correlation with scanning electron microscopy, *AJR Am J Roentgenol* 174:405-409, 2000.
104. Wheaton AJ, Dodge GR, Elliott DM et al: Quantification of cartilage biomechanical and biochemical properties via T1rho magnetic resonance imaging, *Magn Reson Med* 54:1087-1093, 2005.
105. Regatte RR, Akella SV, Lonner JH et al: T1rho relaxation mapping in human osteoarthritis (OA) cartilage: comparison of T1rho with T2, *J Magn Reson Imaging* 23:547-553, 2006.
106. Mlynárik V, Szomolányi P, Toffanin R et al., Transverse relaxation mechanisms in articular cartilage, *J Magn Reson* 169:300-307, 2004.
107. Goodwin DW, Wadghiri YZ, Zhu H et al: Macroscopic structure of articular cartilage of the tibial plateau: influence of a characteristic matrix architecture on MRI appearance, *AJR Am J Roentgenol* 182:311-318, 2004.
108. Shapiro EM, Borthakur A, Gougoutas A et al: 23Na MRI accurately measures fixed charge density in articular cartilage, *Magn Reson Med* 47:284-291, 2002.
109. Wheaton AJ, Borthakur A, Shapiro EM et al: Proteoglycan loss in human knee cartilage: quantitation with sodium MR imaging—feasibility study, *Radiology* 231:900-905, 2004.
110. Van Breuseghem I: Ultrastructural MR imaging techniques of the knee articular cartilage: problems for routine clinical application, *Eur Radiol* 14:184-192, 2004.
111. Insko EK, Kaufman JH, Leigh J et al: Sodium NMR evaluation of articular cartilage degradation, *Magn Reson Med* 41:30-34, 1999.
112. Lesperance LM, Gray ML, Burstein D: Determination of fixed charge density in cartilage using nuclear magnetic resonance, *J Orthop Res* 10:1-13, 1992.

113. Regatte RR, Kaufman JH, Noyszewski EA et al: Sodium and proton MR properties of cartilage during compression, *J Magn Reson Imaging* 10:961-967, 1999.
114. Jelicks LA: Hydrogen-1, sodium-23, and carbon-13 MR spectroscopy of cartilage degeneration in vitro, *J Magn Reson Imaging* 3:565-568, 1993.
115. Shapiro EM, Borthakur A, Dandora R et al: Sodium visibility and quantitation in intact bovine articular cartilage using high field (23)Na MRI and MRS, *J Magn Reson* 142:24-31, 2000.
116. Tiderius CJ, Olsson LE, Leander P et al: Delayed gadolinium-enhanced MRI of cartilage (dGEMRIC) in early knee osteoarthritis, *Magn Reson Med* 49:488-492, 2003.
117. Kim YJ, Jaramillo D, Millis MB et al: Assessment of early osteoarthritis in hip dysplasia with delayed gadolinium-enhanced magnetic resonance imaging of cartilage, *J Bone Joint Surg (Am)* 85:1987-1992, 2003.
118. Bashir A, Gray ML, Boutin RD et al: Glycosaminoglycan in articular cartilage: in vivo assessment with delayed Gd(DTPA)(2-)-enhanced MR imaging, *Radiology* 205:551-558, 1997.
119. Bashir A, Gray ML, Hartke J et al: Nondestructive imaging of human cartilage glycosaminoglycan concentration by MRI, *Magn Res Med* 41:857-865, 1999.
120. Nieminen MT, Rieppo J, Silvennoinen J et al: Spatial assessment of articular cartilage proteoglycans with Gd-DTPA-enhanced T1 imaging, *Magn Reson Med* 48:640-648, 2002.
121. Allen RG, Burstein D, Gray ML: Monitoring glycosaminoglycan replenishment in cartilage explants with gadolinium-enhanced magnetic resonance imaging, *J Orthop Res* 17:430-436, 1999.
122. Trattnig S, Mlynárik V, Breitenseher M et al: MRI visualization of proteoglycan depletion in articular cartilage via intravenous administration of Gd-DTPA, *Magn Reson Imaging* 17:577-583, 1999.
123. Tiderius CJ, Olsson LE, de Verdier H et al: Gd-DTPA2)-enhanced MRI of femoral knee cartilage: a dose-response study in healthy volunteers, *Magn Reson Med* 46:1067-1071, 2001.
124. Burstein D, Velyvis J, Scott KT et al: Protocol issues for delayed Gd(DTPA)(2-)-enhanced MRI (dGEMRIC) for clinical evaluation of articular cartilage, *Magn Reson Med* 45:36-41, 2001.
125. Tiderius CJ, Svensson J, Leander P et al: dGEMRIC (delayed gadolinium-enhanced MRI of cartilage) indicates adaptive capacity of human knee cartilage, *Magn Reson Med* 51:286-290, 2004.
126. Williams A, Sharma L, McKenzie CA et al: Delayed gadolinium-enhanced magnetic resonance imaging of cartilage in knee osteoarthritis: findings at different radiographic stages of disease and relationship to malalignment, *Arthritis Rheum* 52:3528-3535, 2005.
127. Nojiri T, Watanabe N, Namura T et al: Utility of delayed gadolinium-enhanced MRI (dGEMRIC) for qualitative evaluation of articular cartilage of patellofemoral joint, *Knee Surg Sports Traumatol Arthrosc* 14:718-723, 2006.
128. Stejskal E: Spin diffusion measurements: spin echoes in presence of a time-dependent field gradient, *J Chem Phys* 42:288-292, 1965.
129. Le Bihan D, Mangin JF, Poupon C et al: Diffusion tensor imaging: concepts and applications, *J Magn Reson Imaging* 13:534-546, 2001.
130. Basser PJ, Pierpaoli C: A simplified method to measure the diffusion tensor from seven MR images, *Magn Reson Med* 39:928-934, 1998.
131. Ordidge RJ, Helpern JA, Qing ZX et al: Correction of motional artifacts in diffusion-weighted MR images using navigator echoes, *Magn Reson Imaging* 12:455-460, 1994.
132. Anderson AW, Gore JC: Analysis and correction of motion artifacts in diffusion weighted imaging, *Magn Reson Med* 32:379-387, 1994.
133. Dietrich O, Heiland S, Benner T et al: Reducing motion artifacts in diffusion-weighted MRI of the brain: efficacy of navigator echo correction and pulse triggering, *Neuroradiology* 42:85-91, 2000.
134. Miller KL, Hargreave BA, Gold GE et al: Steady-state diffusion-weighted imaging of in vivo knee cartilage, *Magn Reson Med* 51:394-398, 2004.
135. Brihuega-Moreno O, Heese FP, Hall LD: Optimization of diffusion measurements using Cramer-Rao lower bound theory and its application to articular cartilage, *Magn Reson Med* 50:1069-1076, 2003.
136. Burstein D: Diffusion of small solutes in cartilage as measured by nuclear magnetic resonance (NMR) spectroscopy and imaging, *J Orthop Res* 11:465-478, 1993.
137. Knauss R, Schiller J, Fleischer G et al: Self-diffusion of water in cartilage and cartilage components as studied by pulsed field gradient NMR, *Magn Reson Med* 41:285-292, 1999.
138. Mlynarik V, Sulzbacher I, Bittsanský M et al: Investigation of apparent diffusion constant as an indicator of early degenerative disease in articular cartilage, *J Magn Reson Imaging* 17:440-444, 2003.
139. Budinsky L: Navigator echo based motion corrected diffusion imaging of articular cartilage in vivo at 1,5 T. In: *Proc Intl Soc Mag Reson Med*, 2001.
140. Xia Y, Farquhar T, Burton-Wur et al: Self-diffusion monitors degraded cartilage, *Arch Biochem Biophys* 323:323-328, 1995.
141. Berg A, Singer T, Moser E: High-resolution diffusivity imaging at 3.0 T for the detection of degenerative changes: a trypsin-based arthritis model, *Invest Radiol* 38:460-466, 2003.
142. Farndale RW, Sayers CA, Barrett AJ: A direct spectrophotometric microassay for sulfated glycosaminoglycans in cartilage cultures, *Connect Tissue Res* 9:247-248, 1982.
143. Toffanin, R., Mlynárik V, Russo S et al: Proteoglycan depletion and magnetic resonance parameters of articular cartilage, *Arch Biochem Biophys* 390:235-242, 2001.
144. Frank LR, Wong EC, Buxton RB et al: Mapping the physiological parameters of articular cartilage with magnetic resonance imaging, *Top Magn Reson Imaging* 10:153-179, 1999.
145. Wentorf F: Initial findings of diffusion tensor imaging of human patellar cartilage: feasibility and preliminary findings, *Magn Reson Imaging* 53:993-998, 2003.
146. Filidoro L, Dietrich O, Weber J et al: High-resolution diffusion tensor imaging of human patellar cartilage: feasibility and preliminary findings, *Magn Reson Med* 53:993-998, 2005.
147. Evans RC, Quinn TM: Solute diffusivity correlates with mechanical properties and matrix density of compressed articular cartilage, *Arch Biochem Biophys* 442:1-10, 2005.

CHAPTER 5

Arthrography and Injection Procedures

KEVIN CARTER, DO, *and* SANJAY MUDIGONDA, MD

KEY FACTS

- Intraarticular contrast injection under image guidance can be combined with radiography to evaluate intraarticular structures or with computed tomography (CT) or magnetic resonance imaging (MRI) to provide detailed assessment of both intraarticular and extraarticular structures.
- Magnetic resonance arthrography involves injection of a dilute gadolinium solution into the joint, but iodinated contrast is usually also injected to confirm intraarticular needle position.
- CT arthrography is performed using iodinated contrast and/or air to outline articular structures.
- These procedures are generally safe; uncommon complications include infection and bleeding.
- Injection under image guidance, usually fluoroscopy, is of benefit in deeper joints (e.g., the hip, sacroiliac joints), in the midfoot and subtalar joints, and in larger patients.

Arthrography is the intraarticular injection of contrast usually under image guidance to improve the visualization of intraarticular structures (e.g., ligaments, cartilaginous surfaces, free bodies). The type of contrast that is delivered into the joint will vary depending upon the patient's presenting symptoms and the subsequent imaging modality chosen. Other applications of contrast injection into a joint include confirmation of intraarticular needle placement at the time of joint aspiration or prior to intraarticular delivery of medications. When performed with proper technique, under image guidance, arthrography is relatively safe with few contraindications.

For many years arthrography was performed using fluoroscopic guidance to monitor contrast injection and provide postinjection radiographs for evaluation of intraarticular structures. This procedure coated the articular structures and filled the joint, providing limited evaluation of the joint capsule, articular cartilage, menisci, intraarticular bodies, and immediate surrounding structures. With advances in imaging technology, arthrography is now often performed followed by magnetic resonance (MR arthrography) or computed tomography (CT arthrography) for a complete evaluation of the joint and the surrounding structures. Imaging with either magnetic resonance imaging (MRI) or CT following arthrography improves both the sensitivity and specificity of these individual imaging modalities for evaluation of the intrinsic structures of a joint.[1-3] By distending the joint capsule with contrast, the intrinsic redundancy is reduced, allowing specific structures to be assessed that would normally not be as well seen on the standard MR or CT examinations. This is especially true when evaluating the shoulder or hip for labral abnormalities, the wrist for ligamentous injury, and the elbow for intraarticular bodies. These techniques can be applied to virtually any joint; additional indications are discussed below.

It is important to specify the type of examination (MR or CT) required because this will determine the type of contrast that will be instilled into the joint. MR arthrography allows for multiplanar imaging of an articulation with no radiation exposure (except that incurred during fluoroscopy for contrast instillation). MR arthrography usually requires the intraarticular administration of a mixture of gadolinium, saline, and non-ionic iodinated contrast. This combination allows visualization of the contrast both at fluoroscopy and at MRI. Optimal technique must be followed when performing MR arthrography to prevent the intraarticular injection of air bubbles, which may result in artifacts that could simulate intraarticular bodies.[4] Because of the broad capabilities of MRI and the intraarticular contrast, MR arthrography has the advantage of being able to evaluate not only the intraarticular structures but also the adjacent soft tissues and extraarticular structures including the adjacent osseous marrow. MR arthrography cannot be performed in patients who have contraindications to MRI and may be limited in those who have surgical metal in the area (e.g., fracture fixation hardware), which may affect the visualization of adjacent structures. MRI examinations are contraindicated in those patients with various surgical implants such as pacemakers, defibrillators, and spinal electronic stimulators.[5] Occasionally, an MR arthrogram my fail due to equipment problems, a claustrophobic or uncooperative patient, or an unusually large patient. In these cases, a CT arthrogram is a good alternative examination.

CT arthrography usually requires the intraarticular administration of non-ionic iodinated contrast material to distend the joint and coat articular structures. Current multidetector CT technology allows for submillimeter-thick slices to examine the joint with high spatial resolution. Through the use of multiplanar reconstructions (MPRs), many of the imaging planes traditionally utilized on MR examinations (axial, sagittal, and coronal) can be duplicated on CT examination for excellent visual evaluation of the articulation. The most important indications for this technique over MR arthrography include a failed MR arthrogram, an obese or severely claustrophobic patient, a patient with an MR-incompatible implanted medical device, or a postoperative patient with metal hardware in close proximity to the joint[5] (Box 5-1). In addition, in locations without access to an MR scanner, CT arthrography can serve as a reasonable alternative imaging modality. The limitations of CT arthrography include exposure to ionizing radiation, the necessity

BOX 5-1. General Indications for CT Arthrography

Failed or contraindicated MRI examination
Claustrophobic patient
Obese patient
Metallic hardware near the joint
MRI scanner not available

for intraarticular administration of iodinated contrast, and the more limited soft tissue contrast when compared with MRI, potentially compromising evaluation of structures adjacent to the joint (e.g., the bursal side of the rotator cuff).

If proper technique is followed and image guidance is utilized, there are few contraindications to either CT or MR arthrography (Box 5-2). One contraindication occurs when the superficial tissues overlying the joint are infected, because entering the joint through these infected tissues could introduce bacteria into the articulation. If a safe alternative approach to the joint cannot be identified, then the exam should not be performed.

Joint aspiration/arthrography should not be performed through an area of infected soft tissue.

Other skin abnormalities such as psoriatic involvement should also be avoided.[6] Patients with anticoagulation or elevated clotting times should be aware of the risks associated with this procedure, and consultation should be made with the ordering physician to discuss alternatives or medical management of the anticoagulation prior to proceeding with the examination. Although Thumboo et al. indicate that joint aspiration is safe if the international normalized ratio (INR) is less than 4.5, it is the practice at our institution to perform these procedures only with an INR of 2 or less.[7]

There are numerous relative contraindications. The most significant of these to consider when performing MR or CT arthrography is an allergy to iodinated contrast. Even though there is only a small amount of iodinated contrast administered during MR arthrography (to confirm needle position), the possible risk for a serious reaction is still present. These patients can be premedicated with corticosteroids and diphenhydramine according to the American College of Radiology guidelines prior to the initiation of the examination.* More often, however, if iodinated contrast cannot be used to confirm correct intraarticular needle placement, needle position can be confirmed by test injection of normal saline when the needle seems to be in correct position. If reaspiration indicates that the needle is not in a vessel and the saline advances without resistance, the needle can be assumed to be positioned in

BOX 5-2. Contraindications to Arthrography at the Brigham and Women's Hospital

Infected or damaged soft tissue over the injection site
Anticoagulation (INR > 2)*
Prior allergic reaction to contrast or anesthetic (another contrast can sometimes be substituted)
Inability to lie flat or remain still

*Higher levels have been shown in the literature to be safe.[7]

*See http://www.acr.org/Secondary/MainMenuCategories/quality_safety/contrast_manuel. aspx.

the joint and the gadolinium contrast can then be instilled. Aspiration of joint fluid prior to injection is reassuring but has been shown to be an imperfect indicator that subsequent injection will be intraarticular.[8] In patients with absolute contraindications to gadolinium and iodinated contrast, air can be injected into the joint followed by CT. Claustrophobia is also a relative contraindication for the performance of MR arthrography, and in these cases either a mild sedative can be administered to the patient or a CT arthrogram can be performed.

As with any invasive procedure, it is important to consider the benefits for the patient compared with the potential risks involved from the examination. The utilization of iodinated contrast material for either MR or CT arthrography carries a small risk of a reaction in all patients. Initially, for the first few hours following injection, slight joint discomfort may be present, but this will usually resolve as the instilled contrast is reabsorbed. Vasovagal reactions are rare and are usually managed in the fluoroscopy suite. The most serious (and fortunately rare) risk associated with arthrography is the development of a joint infection.[9] This risk can be minimized through adherence to a strict aseptic protocol. There are no reports of serious adverse events such as anaphylactic shock or other events requiring treatment in the intensive care unit or hospitalization as a result of intraarticular gadolinium for MR arthrography.[9]

Contrast reaction and the introduction of infection are rare but potentially serious complications of arthrography.

SHOULDER ARTHROGRAPHY

Ultrasound and noncontrast MRI examinations are the primary modalities currently utilized to evaluate shoulder problems, especially rotator cuff tears. These methods have largely supplanted "conventional" arthrography in which radiographs are obtained following intraarticular contrast administration. Arthrography in conjunction with MRI or CT is used most often to evaluate the intraarticular structures (e.g., glenoid labrum, synovial disorders) that are not as easily seen without intraarticular contrast. Other applications of shoulder arthrography include the treatment of adhesive capsulitis, as well as the intraarticular delivery of corticosteroids.[10]

Arthrography Technique

The intraarticular injection of contrast is usually performed under fluoroscopic guidance. The patient is then transferred to either the CT or MRI scanner for the completion of the imaging portion of the procedure. Ideally, the patient should be imaged within the 30 minutes following contrast injection; therefore coordination in the scheduling of fluoroscopy and MRI or CT is important.

Placement of the needle within the joint must avoid contrast injection into the cartilage, labrum, or capsular attachments to be of maximal diagnostic benefit. Many injection techniques have been described; the anterior approach is the most commonly utilized.[11-15] For injection using the anterior approach, the patient in placed in the supine position with the humerus in external rotation. External rotation results in exposure of more of the articular surface of the humeral head anteriorly and also increases the intraarticular area for needle insertion. The area of desired needle placement (either on the medial, superior third of the humeral head [the rotator cuff interval], or the inferior third of the humeral head) is visualized under fluoroscopy and marked on the patient's skin (Figure 5-1). This area is then prepared and draped in a sterile fashion. The subcutaneous tissues are anesthetized. A 22-gauge (G), 3.5-cm spinal needle is advanced in an anteroposterior direction until it contacts the

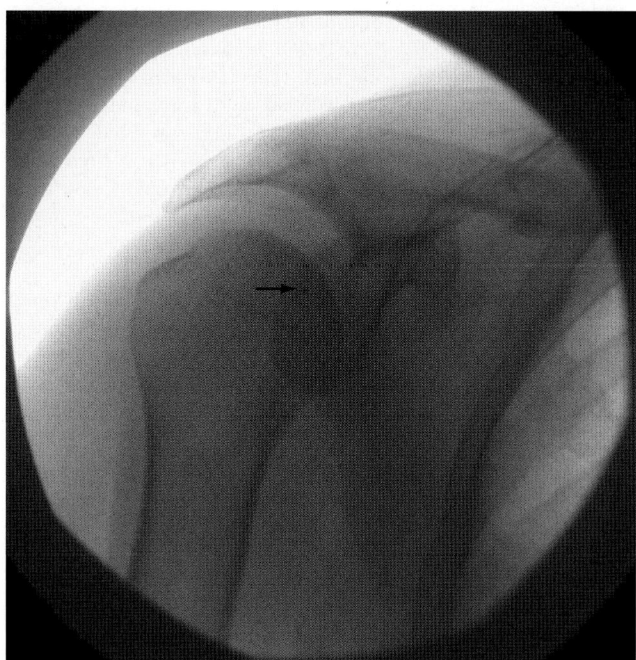

FIGURE 5-1. Normal positioning of shoulder prior to arthrography. The right humerus is externally rotated to maximize to exposure of the anterior articular surface of the humeral head. The planned site for needle placement in this case is in the medial aspect of the upper third of the humeral head. A BB *(arrow)* placed on the skin marks the desired location.

humeral head.[11] Once the needle tip contacts the cortex of the humeral head, confirmation of intraarticular needle position is made by injecting contrast, which should immediately flow away from the needle tip if it is within the joint. Ten to 15 mL (usually about 14 mL) of contrast is then injected until the patient feels full or injection becomes more difficult.[1] Injections of less than 15 mL will decrease the likelihood of extraarticular leakage, which could lead to failure to diagnose a full-thickness rotator cuff tear. Overdistension may lead to capsular rupture and contrast extravasation, which could limit joint distension.

The type of contrast utilized will depend on the imaging that the patient will have following the procedure. If the patient is having a CT exam, a non-ionic iodinated agent will be utilized. If MRI is to follow, a dilute solution of gadopentetate dimeglumine mixed with a small amount of iodinated contrast will be injected[4] (10 mL saline, 0.1 mL gadopentetate, and 10 mL non-ionic iodinated contrast). Following the injection, the patient will be moved through a full range of motion to coat the articular structures. Various fluoroscopic images are usually obtained before the patient is taken for the MRI or CT portion of the examination.

Indications

Many factors are considered when deciding which patients should undergo arthrography as part of their evaluation. Instability of the shoulder is a common clinical problem, especially in young active individuals. The glenoid labrum, the glenohumeral ligaments, and the muscles of the rotator cuff all contribute to stability. The diagnosis of abnormality of these structures, especially the labrum, on a nonarthrographic study may be difficult because of the redundancy of the axillary recess and the presence of clefts and overlying structures that may mimic abnormalities.[1] By distending the capsule with contrast, these structures can be more fully evaluated (Figure 5-2). The use of MR or CT arthrography allows for better detection of capsulolabral abnormalities and partial thickness rotator cuff tears (Figure 5-3). Distension of the joint capsule allows differentiation between irregular tears of the labrum and normal anatomic variants such as the sublabral sulcus and foramen (Figure 5-4). The glenohumeral ligaments are routinely visualized on MR or CT arthrography exams owing to the joint distension. Abnormalities of these ligaments can more easily be identified on MR or CT arthrography than on noncontrast studies[16] (Figure 5-5) (Table 5-1).

Findings

The normal shoulder joint capsule is smooth; irregularity or filling defects suggest synovitis. Normally the biceps tendon sheath and axillary recess fill with contrast. A small joint volume and nonfilling of these structures can be seen in adhesive capsulitis.

> Adhesive capsulitis can be apparent on arthrography if the joint capacity is unusually small with absent filling of the biceps sheath and axillary recess and high injection pressure.

Articular-sided rotator cuff tears will show contrast extending from the joint into the substance of the rotator cuff (partial tear) or through the entire thickness of the cuff into the subacromial subdeltoid bursa (full thickness, complete tears). Sometimes complete tears can allow contrast to communicate with the acromioclavicular (AC) joint (termed the *geyser sign*) (Figure 5-6). Not only can the tear be recognized, but the size of the tear, quality of the torn edges, and any atrophy or fatty replacement of the muscles can be assessed. These are important surgical considerations.

> Some full-thickness rotator cuff tears are accompanied by chronic fluid extravasation into the AC joint. This produces a fluid mass on clinical examination that corresponds to the contrast extravasation seen on arthrography, termed the *geyser sign*.

Labral tears can be identified by abnormalities in the shape of the labrum or contrast extravasation into labral tissue. Sometimes additional maneuvers, such as having the patient imaged while in external rotation and abduction (the ABER position), can be helpful for labral assessment. These supplemental images may be added to the protocol at the MRI facility where the study is planned, depending on the clinical indications for examination.

> MRI examination protocols are tailored to the specific clinical question.

HIP ARTHROGRAPHY

The initial imaging for the evaluation of hip pain should be radiographs to exclude etiologies such as fractures and avascular necrosis (AVN). Noncontrast MRI is effective in the evaluation of hip pain with normal radiographs, showing acute fractures as well as confirming cases of AVN that are not visible or are atypical on radiographic examination. Unless a large joint effusion is present, evaluation of the intrinsic structures of the hip joint (e.g., the labrum) is limited on MRI due to redundancy within the capsule. MR and CT arthrography are effective in the evaluation of these structures including the labrum, ligaments, and articular cartilage.

Technique

When performing hip arthrography, the patient should be lying supine on the fluoroscopy table with the hip to be injected in neutral position. External rotation of the femur should be avoided

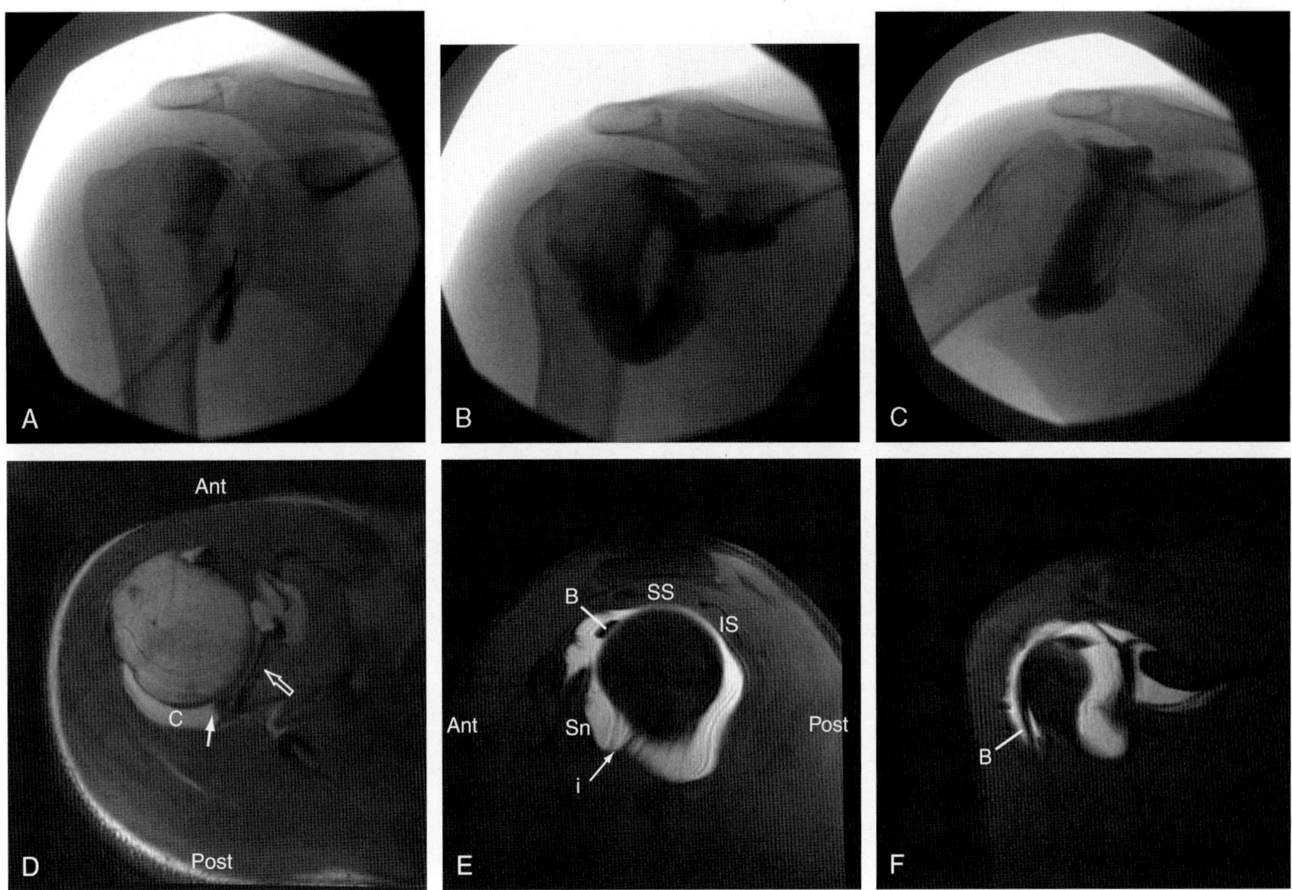

FIGURE 5-2. Normal shoulder arthrogram. This 38-year-old male presented with shoulder pain. **A** to **C**, Three fluoroscopic views of the right shoulder during **(A)** and immediately following injection of contrast (**B**, internal rotation; **C**, external rotation) display a normal-appearing arthrogram with no extravasation of contrast or contrast filling the subacromial bursa. The contrast is smooth in outline and no filling defects are present to indicate intraarticular bodies or synovitis. **D**, An axial T1-weighted MR image shows how the intraarticular contrast *(c)* distends the joint and allows easy evaluation of the labrum *(arrow)*, cartilage *(open arrow)*, and glenohumeral ligaments (*Ant*, anterior; *Post*, posterior). **E**, An oblique sagittal T1-weighted fat-saturated image shows contrast within the joint outlining the long head of the biceps tendon *(B)*. The dark tendons and gray muscles of the supraspinatus *(SS)* and infraspinatus *(IS)* and subscapularis *(Sn)* are seen adjacent to the contrast filled joint (*ant*, anterior; *post*, posterior). **F**, An oblique coronal T1-weighted fat saturated image shows contrast outlining *(B)*. The tendon of the long head of the biceps brachi; *i*, inferior glenohumeral ligaments; *IS*, infraspinatus; *SS*, supraspinatus; *Su*, subscapularis.

because this moves the femoral vessels and nerves laterally, potentially in the path of the needle. A small pillow may be placed under the knee to not only make the patient more comfortable but also to relax the anterior joint capsule. Multiple injection approaches have been described.[17] Initially, the femoral artery is palpated and marked to avoid injury during the needle placement. The overlying tissues are then prepared with alcohol and Betadine and draped in a sterile fashion. The skin and subcutaneous tissues are anesthetized. A common approach involves advancing a 22 G spinal needle under fluoroscopic guidance to the lateral aspect of the superolateral femoral head-neck junction until the cartilage is reached (Figure 5-7). A different technique involves advancing the needle straight down to the femoral neck at the midpoint between the base of the femoral head and the intertrochanteric line. The latter approach has been shown to produce less patient discomfort but does have a higher rate of extravasation of contrast from the joint capsule.[18] After placing the needle within the joint, the joint should be aspirated, especially if administering gadolinium contrast to prevent its dilution. Joint fluid is sent for culture and crystals depending on the clinical circumstance. In all techniques, a small amount of non-ionic iodinated contrast material should be injected to confirm location of the needle within the joint capsule. Then between 8 and 20 mL of contrast should be injected into the joint for good distension.[1] The administration of 0.3 mL of 1:1000 epinephrine into the hip joint can also be performed to slow the absorption of the contrast agent to allow clarity of images if there is an imaging delay.[1] Fluoroscopic images will be obtained throughout the procedure to confirm needle placement and immediately after injection of the contrast into the joint to document intraarticular injection and delineate gross joint anatomy. Following this, the patient will be transferred to the MRI or CT suite via wheelchair for the completion of the examination.

Indications

Hip pain has numerous etiologies including both intrinsic abnormalities and pain referred from remote sites. When encountered in the young patient or athlete, concern for the intrinsic structures should be the primary consideration. The use of conventional radiographs is not reliable in identifying all abnormalities, but radiographs should be obtained prior to other imaging tests. As in the shoulder, the joint capsule of the hip has intrinsic redundancy that limits evaluation of the internal structures. In the absence of preexisting joint fluid, the evaluation of the acetabular

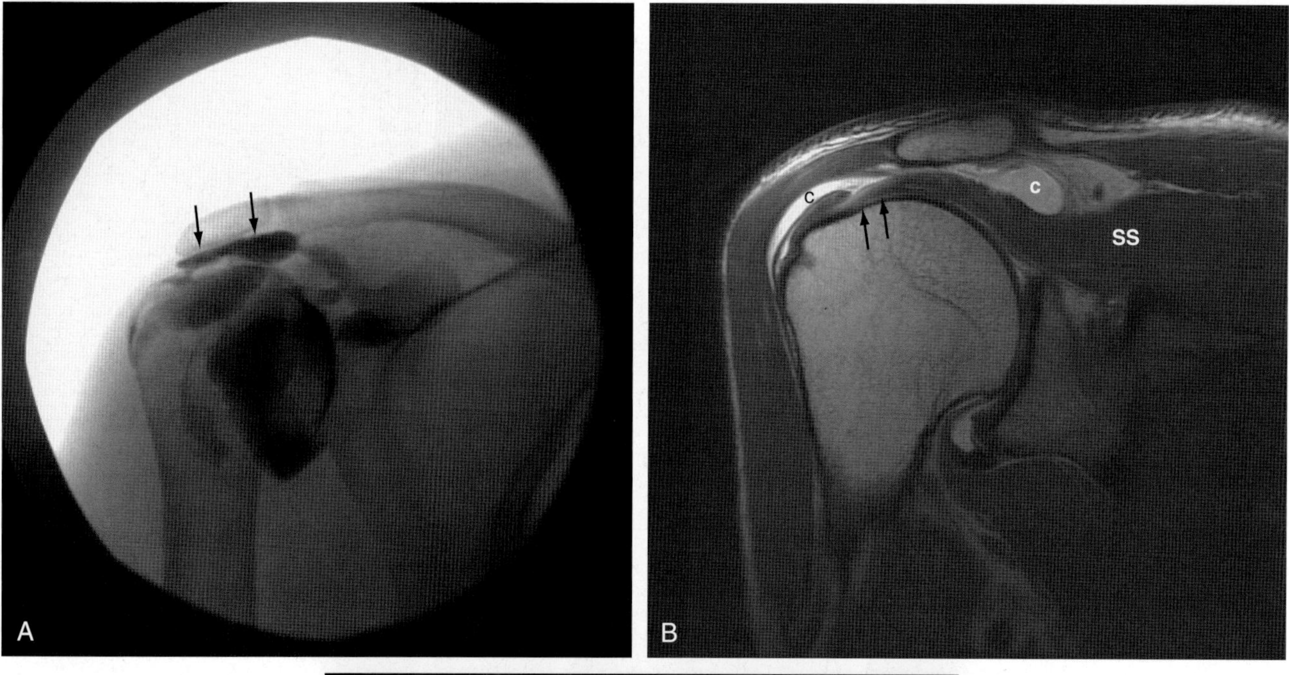

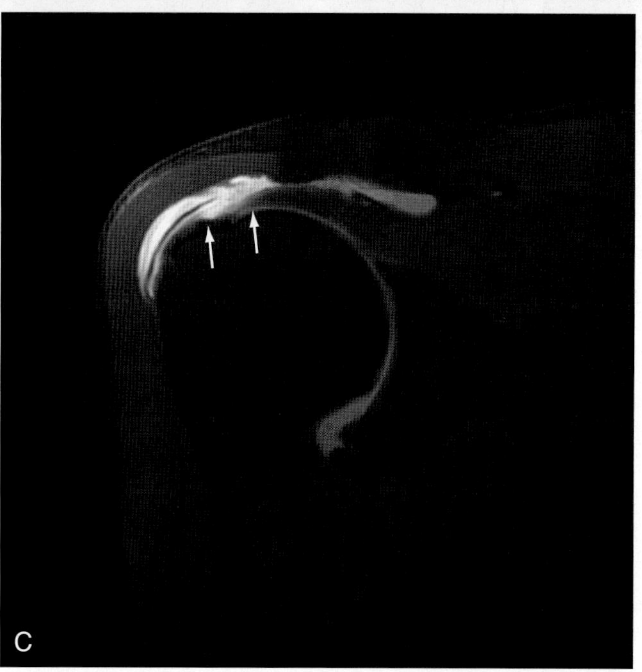

FIGURE 5-3. Large rotator cuff tear. This 65-year-old female presented with shoulder pain and decreased range of motion. **A,** The arthrogram shows that contrast from the intraarticular injection has entered the subacromial/subdeltoid bursa *(arrows)*, indicating a full thickness rotator cuff tear. **B,** Coronal oblique T1-weighted MR image displays discontinuity *(arrows)* in the tendon of the supraspinatus muscle *(SS)* with contrast *(c)* extending into the subacromial/subdeltoid bursa, confirming a large rotator cuff tear. **C,** Coronal oblique T1-weighted fat-saturated MR image confirms the large rotator cuff tear *(arrows)*. The fat-suppression technique allows the bright contrast to be better seen, as the adjacent fat is now dark.

labral complex is difficult on conventional MR and CT examinations.[16] Distension of the joint capsule following the addition of contrast into the joint allows for easier evaluation of the intrinsic structures[1] (Figures 5-8 and 5-9). In addition, intraarticular bodies[17] and the articular cartilage can be evaluated[18] (Figure 5-10). Patients with a history of acetabular dysplasia can be routinely evaluated utilizing MR or CT arthrography to monitor the progression of osteoarthritis and to determine when surgical treatment should be considered[19] (Table 5-2). Detailed imaging of the joint may be difficult with MR arthrography in those patients who are large or obese; in these situations, CT arthrography should be considered as an alternative imaging modality.[5]

Findings

Detailed MR images of the hip are performed after contrast injection. Ideally, these include at least one series that allows evaluation of bone marrow, as well as the fat-suppressed images usually obtained for evaluation of the joint. Joint contour, communication with a psoas bursa, or synovitis can be detected (Figure 5-11). Hip

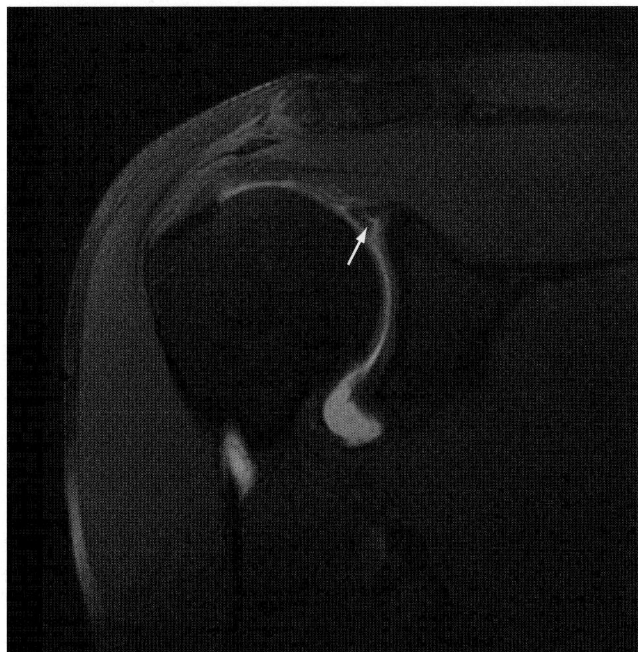

FIGURE 5-4. Superior labral tear with anterior-posterior extension (SLAP tear). This patient presented with shoulder pain. Oblique coronal T1-weighted MR image with fat suppression displays contrast extending superiorly and laterally into the normally dark glenoid labrum, consistent with a SLAP tear *(arrow)*.

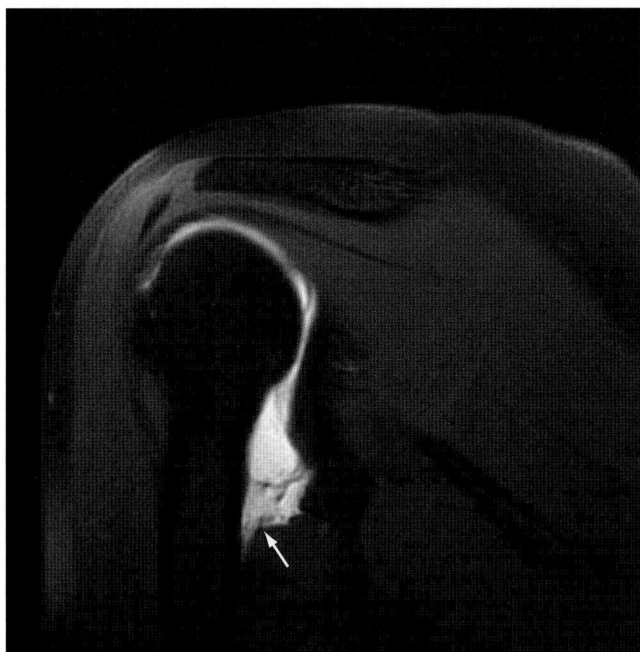

FIGURE 5-5. Humeral avulsion of the glenohumeral ligament (HAGL). This patient presented after reduction of a traumatic dislocation of the right shoulder. The T1-weighted fat-saturated oblique coronal image from the MR arthrogram shows contrast extending along the humeral shaft *(arrow)*, indicating disruption of the attachment of the axillary recess (the anterior inferior glenohumeral ligament).

TABLE 5-1. Potential Uses for MR or CT Arthrography of the Shoulder

Imaging Technique	Uses
MR arthrography	Athletes with chronic injuries
	Instability (patient < 40 years old)
	Rotator cuff tears
	Biceps anchor evaluation
	Labral evaluation
	Identification of intraarticular loose bodies
	Postoperative evaluation of the labrum or rotator cuff
CT arthrography	Postoperative rotator cuff evaluation
	Any of the above indications if contraindications exist for MRI

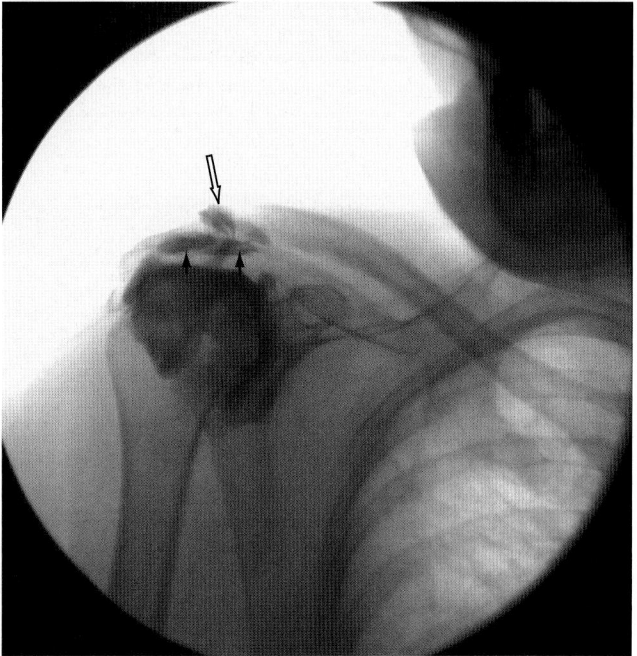

FIGURE 5-6. Geyser sign in a 57-year-old female with recurrent shoulder pain. Fluoroscopic image after intraarticular injection of 14 mL of 50% Ultravist 300. Contrast in the subacromial subdeltoid bursa *(arrows)* of a full thickness rotator cuff tear. There is a "geyser sign" confirms contrast filling the AC joint *(open arrow)*.

labral tears are typically anteriorly located and seen as contrast-filled defects in the labrum or as an abnormal labral shape (see Figure 5-8). Tears must be distinguished from normally occurring recesses. Periarticular labral cysts or subchondral cysts may fill with injected contrast (see Figure 5-9). The articular cartilage should be smooth. Focal areas of thinning or irregularity can be detected. Recently, hip arthrography has been used to assess possible femoroacetabular impingement. Anterosuperior cartilage lesions may be prominent in patients with cam-type impingement. Cam-type impingement is a congenital disorder usually seen in young men characterized by an increase in the size of the femoral head that results in a mismatch between the femoral head and acetabulum. This may result in cartilage damage and premature

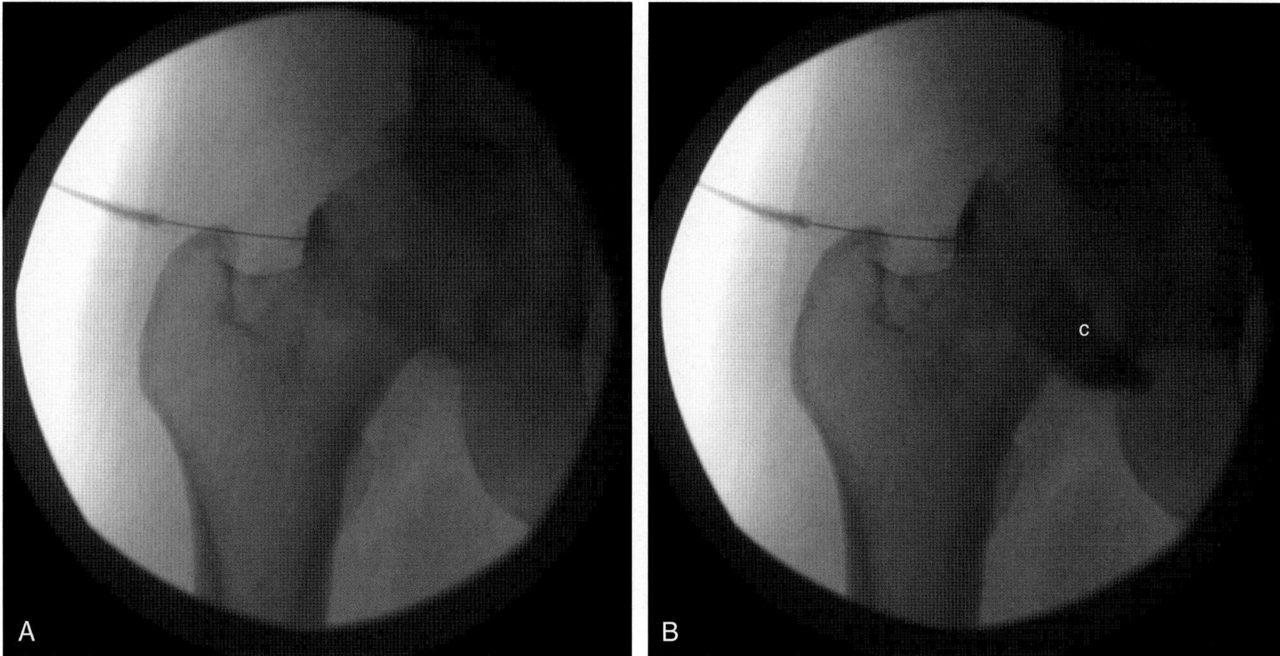

FIGURE 5-7. Normal hip arthrography. The lateral approach was utilized with the needle being advanced into the joint capsule at the lateral aspect of the femoral head. Early **(A)** and later **(B)** fluoroscopic images during contrast injection show the contrast *(c)* filling the posterior recess of the joint capsule, confirming the intraarticular position of the needle tip.

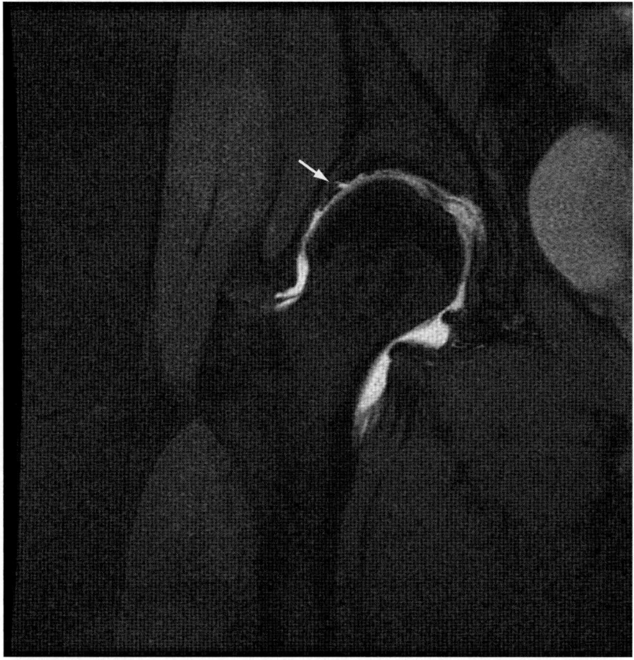

FIGURE 5-8. MR arthrography demonstrating an anterior superior labral tear. This 24-year-old athlete presented with chronic hip pain and the sensation of "clicking" with movement. Coronal T1-weighted fat-suppressed image reveals contrast extending into the superior labrum *(arrow)*, consistent with a labral tear. This abnormality was not identified on the patient's previous MR examination of the hip performed without arthrography.

osteoarthritis. Posteroinferior cartilage loss and labral lesions are seen in so-called pincer impingement due to acetabular deformity.[20] In addition, the contours of the bony structures and measurement of the alpha angle that could indicate impingement can be evaluated on MRI. Filling defects in the contrast may be the result of intraarticular bodies (cartilage or cartilage and bone), synovitis, or air bubbles (see Figure 5-11).

KNEE ARTHROGRAPHY

Conventional MRI is currently the most widely utilized noninvasive, cross-sectional imaging technique to evaluate the knee, and it is extremely reliable in making the diagnosis of meniscal tears or in evaluating the intrinsic ligaments of the knee.[1] Although arthrography introduces an invasive component to the imaging evaluation, it is an established method for optimizing diagnostic accuracy.[21] Arthrography is well tolerated by most patients and has proven to be useful when considering treatment planning.[22] This technique is most accurate and precise when internal derangement is present based on the clinical history, the patient's symptoms, and the physical examination.

MR arthrography or CT arthrography should be strongly considered in the evaluation of patients after surgical meniscectomy if there is concern for a recurrent tear.[23] MR and CT arthrography are also excellent for detection of cartilage defects (Table 5-3).

Technique

Classically performed under fluoroscopic guidance, the injection of the knee could also be performed without any imaging guidance due to the superficial nature of this joint. The patient is placed in the supine position with a small pillow or towel placed under the knee. This will produce slight flexion to the hip and knee and results in relaxation of the extensor muscles. Several routes of injection (lateral, medial, anterior) have been proposed, but the lateral route is most often utilized and has been shown to be most accurate.[24] After sterile preparation and draping of the skin along the lateral aspect of the patella, the patella is pushed slightly laterally to open the joint. The soft tissues just inferior (posterior) to the lateral patella and at its midportion are anesthetized. A 22 G needle is directed anteriorly and cephalad (at about 45 degrees in

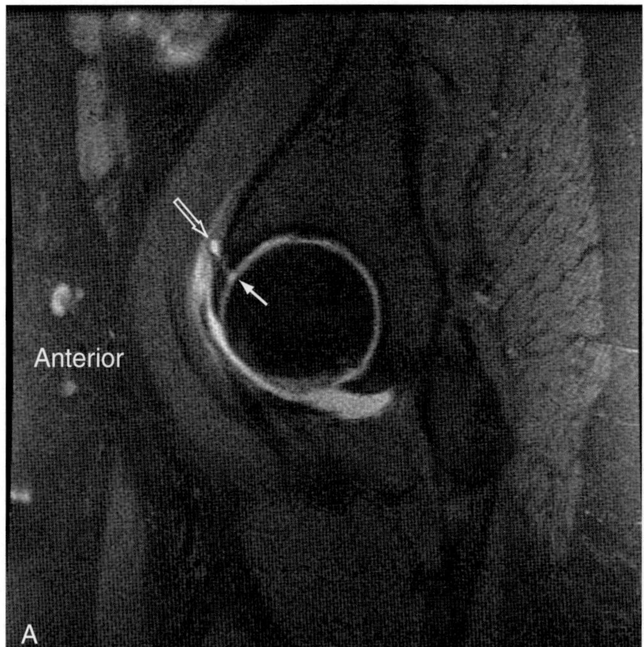

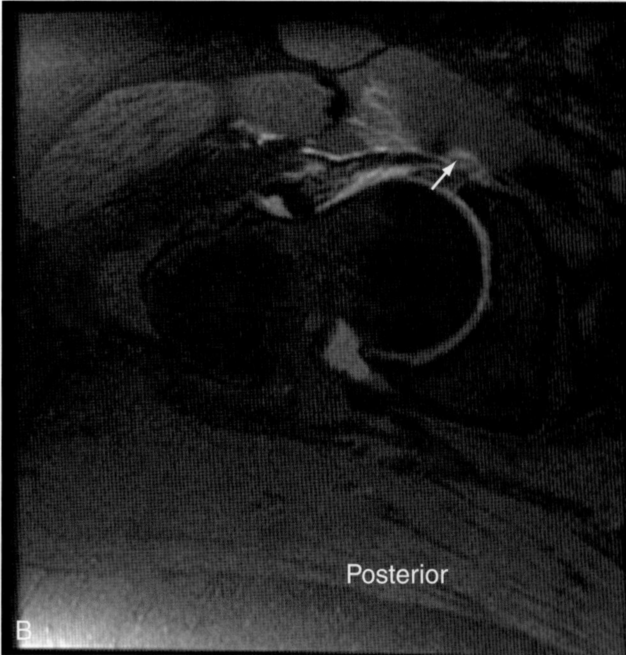

FIGURE 5-9. A 48-year-old female with right hip pain. Sagittal **(A)** and oblique **(B)** axial T1 fat-saturated MR arthrographic images show contrast extending into the anterior superior labrum indicating a tear *(arrows)*. Additionally there is filling of contrast in an associated small anterior superior paralabral cyst *(open arrow)*.

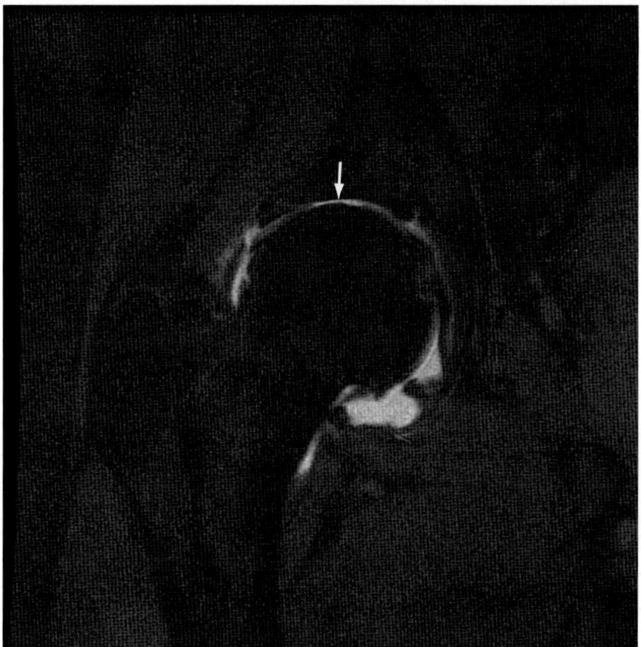

FIGURE 5-10. MR arthrography of osteoarthritis in a 56-year-old male with chronic hip pain. The T1-weighted fat- suppressed coronal image from MR arthrogram displays contrast between the cartilaginous surfaces outlining the irregularly thinned articular cartilage along the superior aspect of the femoral head *(arrow)* consistent with osteoarthritis. The remainder of the intrinsic structures of the hip were normal.

each direction) until the patella is contacted. Aspiration of joint fluid is then attempted (Figure 5-12). As much fluid as possible is removed, especially if gadolinium is to be administered, so that a standard concentration of the contrast will be maintained.[4] The intraarticular position of the needle tip is confirmed before contrast is injected with a test injection of iodinated contrast even if joint fluid has been obtained. Contrast for the arthrogram can then be instilled until slight resistance is felt; this may require 20 to 40 mL.[1] MR imaging should be performed within 1 hour of injection to prevent synovial resorption of the contrast that would limit the examination. If imaging will be delayed, intraarticular epinephrine can be administered with the contrast to prevent rapid resorption.[1]

TABLE 5-2. Possible Uses of Hip Arthrography

Imaging Technique	Uses
MR or CT arthrography	Labral tears
	Cartilage defects
	Osteochondral bodies
	Ligamentum teres injuries
	Monitoring of hip dysplasia
Only CT arthrography	Consider in large or obese patients for the above indications
	Postoperative evaluation of labral tears
	All other patients with contraindications for MRI

Indications

In the postoperative knee, the presence of redundant capsular tissue, synovial hypertrophy, soft tissue deformity, and artifact make evaluation of intraarticular abnormalities difficult. Through the addition of intraarticular contrast there is separation of tissues, making delineation of individual structures on either CT or MRI much easier. Postoperative patients may be assessed, including those with suspected recurrent meniscal tears. Other indications include the evaluation of the integrity of the ligaments of the knee

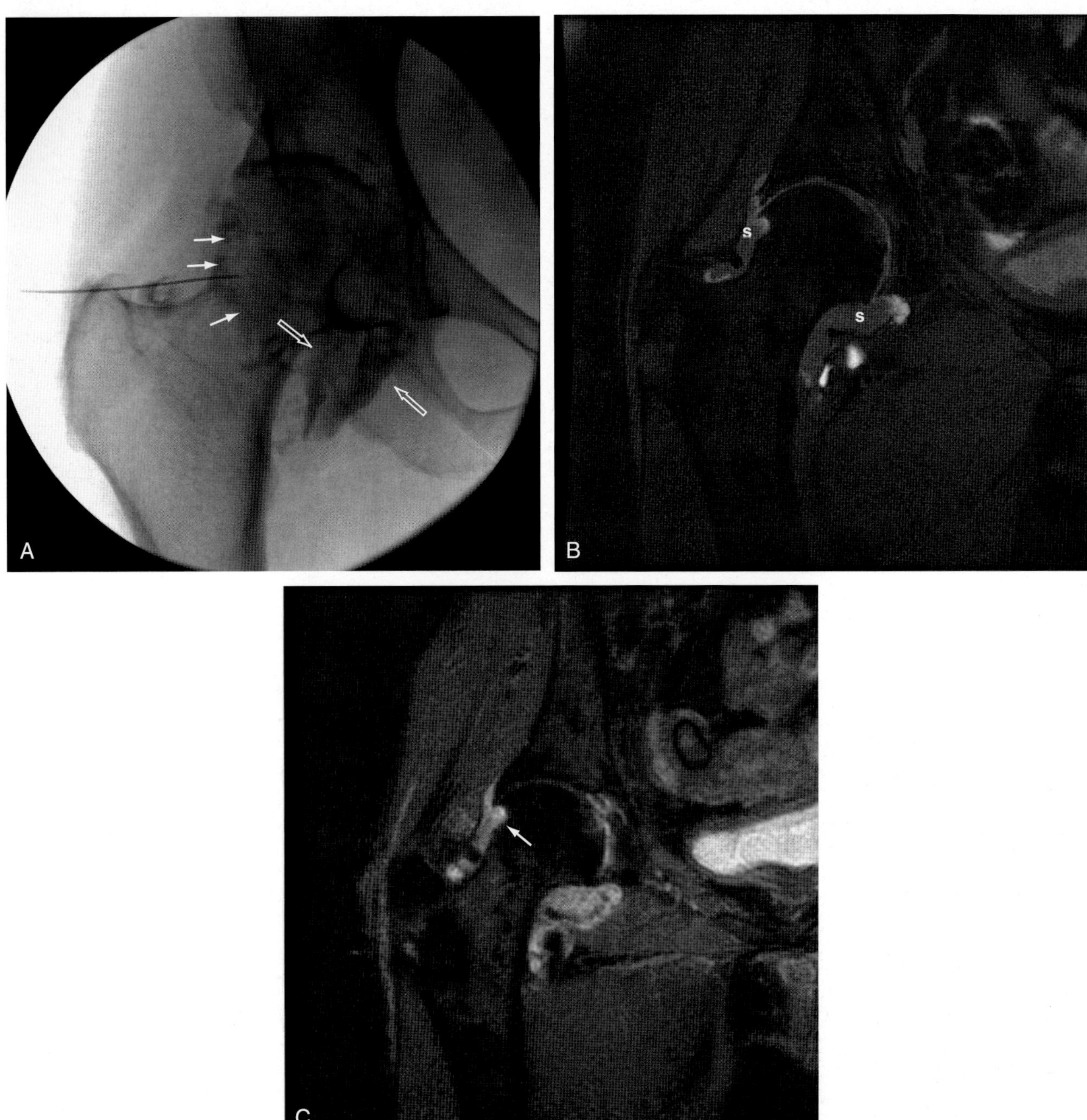

FIGURE 5-11. Rheumatoid synovitis. This 54-year-old female had a known diagnosis of rheumatoid arthritis. **A,** Fluoroscopic spot film, obtained during instillation of contrast, shows multiple filling defects and an irregular contour of the capsule *(arrows)* consistent with synovitis (pannus). There is filling of the iliopsoas bursa *(open arrows)*, which also demonstrates filling defects. The iliopsoas tendon is visible because of the bursal contrast material. **B,** Coronal T1-weighted MR image after intraarticular instillation of dilute gadolinium shows intermediate intensity in the joint consistent with synovitis *(s)*. Note the cartilage space narrowing. **C,** Coronal STIR MR image shows the intermediate signal material in the joint corresponding to the synovitis. An erosion *(arrow)* of the femoral head is present and is seen on all images to be filled with fluid and pannus.

(anterior cruciate ligament, posterior cruciate ligament) in patients who have had these structures repaired.[5,25] Additionally, arthrography allows evaluation of the chondral surfaces, which aids in grading chondral defects and is also beneficial in the evaluation of the stability of osteochondral lesions[26,27] (see Table 5-3). CT arthrography is also indicated in the evaluation of any patient with contraindications for MRI[5] (Figure 5-13).

Findings

MR arthrography may be especially useful for evaluating the patient who has recurrent symptoms after partial meniscectomy. In these patients, it is thought that contrast extending into an area of signal abnormality in the meniscal remnant confirms the presence of a recurrent tear, whereas a meniscal signal abnormality that does not fill with contrast suggests a postoperative abnormality

TABLE 5-3. Potential Uses of Knee Arthrography

Imaging Technique	Uses
MR or CT arthrography	Meniscal tears
	Cartilage defects
	Postoperative cartilage repair procedure
Only CT arthrography	Consider in bulky or obese patients for the above indications
	Patients with contraindications for MRI

(residual tear containing granulation tissue).[23] In the evaluation of osteochondral lesions, contrast extending beneath an osteochondral abnormality suggests that it is unstable. As in other joints, synovitis can be indicated by the presence of filling defects, capsular irregularity, and, in rheumatoid arthritis, lymphatic filling.[28]

WRIST ARTHROGRAPHY

Conventional wrist arthrography is adequate for the evaluation of various causes of wrist pain, allowing assessment of the intrinsic ligaments of the proximal carpal row and the triangular fibrocartilage complex (TFCC). The application of MR arthrography and CT arthrography allows visualization of the soft tissue structures that stabilize the wrist and simultaneous evaluation of the adjacent osseous structures and tendons. These combined techniques result in a complete evaluation to determine the underlying etiology of the patient's symptoms.

Technique

Multiple approaches for performing wrist arthrography exist including single compartment (radiocarpal) injection, double compartment (radiocarpal and midcarpal or radiocarpal and distal radioulnar joint) injections, and triple compartment (midcarpal, radiocarpal, and distal radioulnar joint) injections.[28-30] Some have advocated bilateral studies for comparison. When more than one compartment is injected, digital subtraction technique is helpful to avoid confusion between previously injected and newly injected contrast. The intraarticular administration of contrast is usually performed under fluoroscopic guidance, but arthrography utilizing CT, MRI, or ultrasound guidance or palpation alone has also been described.[4] At our institution, the single compartment (radiocarpal) injection is most often performed.

When performing wrist arthrography, the patient is positioned prone on the fluoroscopic table with the wrist in neutral rotation and slight volar flexion over a bolster. Multiple sites can be selected to inject the radiocarpal joint. Some authors advocate injecting a site on the side of the patient's wrist opposite the symptoms to aid in distinguishing iatrogenic leakage of contrast from actual capsular disruption.[28] The site of injection is identified on fluoroscopic examination, and the skin is marked. After sterile preparation of the skin and anesthetizing the overlying soft tissues, a 25 G needle is advanced through the skin into the expected area of the joint. Small needles are utilized to limit tissue trauma and postinjection leakage of contrast. For radial-sided injections, the needle should be directed to the radioscaphoid space away from the scapholunate joint. Due to the natural volar tilt of the distal radius, a slight angulation of the image intensifier in the cranial direction will better profile the radioscaphoid space and prevent the needle tip from striking the dorsal tip of the radius, which could interfere with completion of the procedure.[28] The injection needle typically requires insertion to a depth of 0.5 to 1.5 cm.[28] Once the needle is placed into the joint, a small test injection of contrast can be performed; contrast should be seen readily flowing away from the needle tip. After intraarticular confirmation is made, the remainder of the iodinated contrast for CT or gadolinium-based contrast for MRI can be injected under fluoroscopic monitoring. The usual volume of contrast injected is 3 to 4 mL[1] (Figure 5-14). Fluoroscopy is continued while the wrist is moved into radial and ulnar deviation. Fluoroscopic monitoring is extremely important to identify communication between joint compartments (through torn ligaments) before overlying contrast obscures the abnormality.

When injecting the midcarpal joint, various sites can be selected, including the distalmost scaphocapitate and triquetrohamate spaces.[28] Again, site selection should be on the side opposite of the patient's symptoms. The usual injected contrast volume for this joint is 3 to 4 mL.[28]

Injection of the distal radioulnar joint requires the needle to be directed toward the head of the ulna near its radial margin. After the needle touches the ulnar head, it should be slightly directed radially to advance deeper into the joint space.[28] The typical volume of injected contrast for this joint is 1 to 2 mL.[28]

When performing the triple compartment injection, some authors advocate first injecting the midcarpal compartment; if communication is seen with the radiocarpal joint, then additional contrast will be injected. If communication is seen to both the radiocarpal and distal radioulnar joint, additional contrast will be injected to a total volume of about 7 to 9 mL.[28] If communication is not seen, then injections of the other joints should proceed from distal to proximal.

Indications

Through the use of MR/CT arthrography, a detailed evaluation of the small ligamentous structures of the wrist can be performed. These structures include the scapholunate ligament,[31] the lunotriquetral ligament,[32] and the triangular fibrocartilage complex.[31,32] In patients with a clinical diagnosis of rheumatoid arthritis, MR and CT arthrography are useful because the joints of the hands and wrists are the first to be affected and these techniques can assist in the evaluation of synovial hypertrophy and ligamentous integrity and help to confirm subtle osseous erosions.[33,34] In many cases, however, MRI without arthrography may be sufficient for this diagnosis (Table 5-4).

Findings

Normally, contrast injected into the radiocarpal compartment fills the radiocarpal joint space, the prestyloid recess, and small anterior recesses but does not fill other compartments. Contrast that fills the radioulnar joint indicates a triangular fibrocartilage (TFCC) tear, whereas filling of the midcarpal row indicates a tear of the scapholunate or lunate triquetral ligaments (Figures 5-15 to 5-17). These are often distinguished during the fluoroscopic portion of the examination. Irregularity of the joint margins, filling defects, and lymphatic filling may be seen in inflammatory arthritis.

ELBOW ARTHROGRAPHY

Historically, complex motion tomography with or without arthrography was the gold standard for the evaluation of the elbow joint surfaces.[5] Arthrography of the elbow is now used for specific indications or as a problem-solving technique. The application of newer modalities (MR or CT arthrography) has allowed not only the evaluation of the articular surfaces, but also evaluation of the

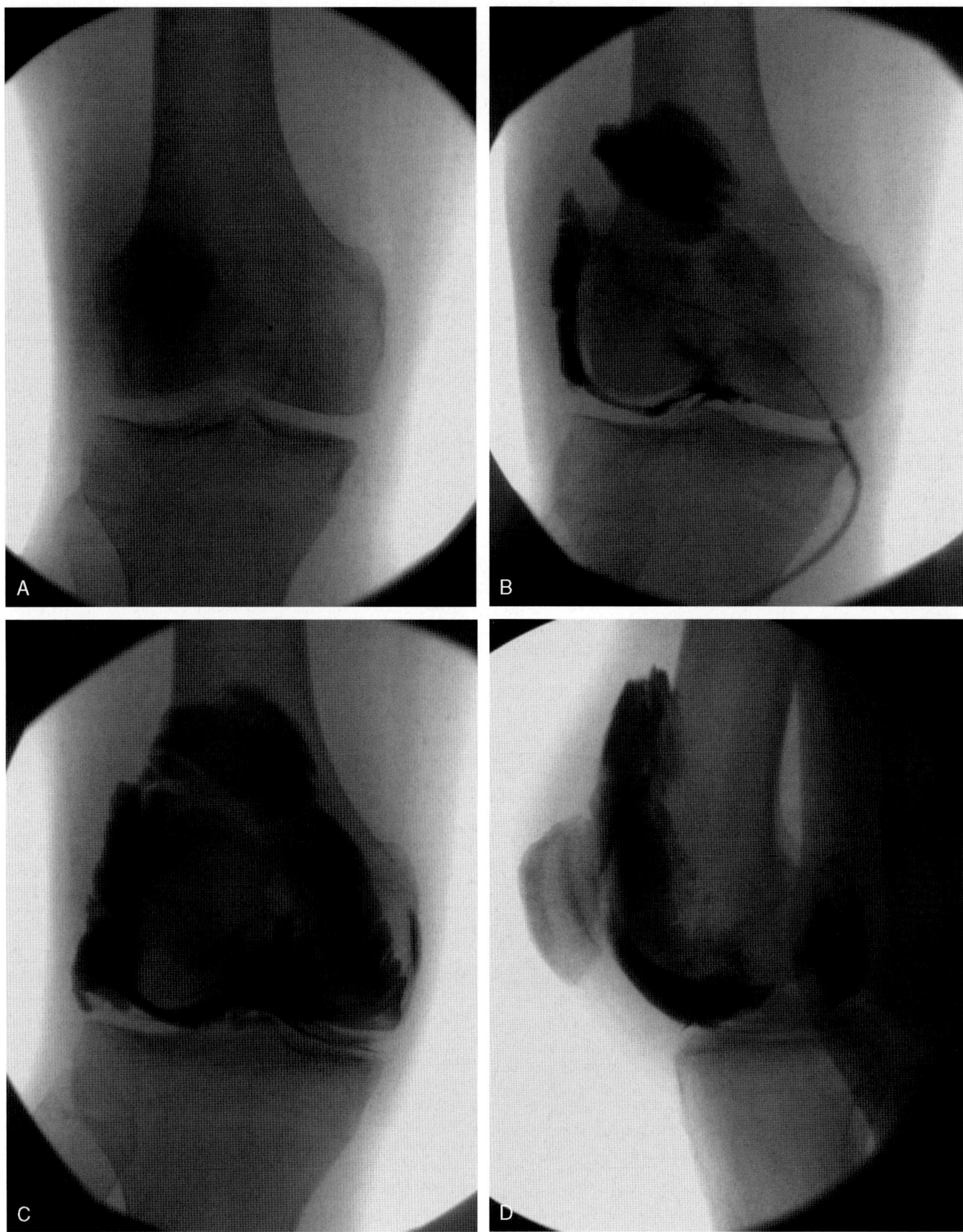

FIGURE 5-12. Arthrography of the knee. **A,** A marker was placed by palpation along the medial inferior aspect of the patella prior to placing the arthrography needle. **B,** The needle was advanced into the joint and contrast was instilled. Confirmation of placement within the joint was confirmed with a frontal view of the knee during injection. Anteroposterior **(C)** and lateral **(D)** postinjection fluoroscopic views display contrast filling the joint. The slight irregularity of the capsule suggests synovitis.

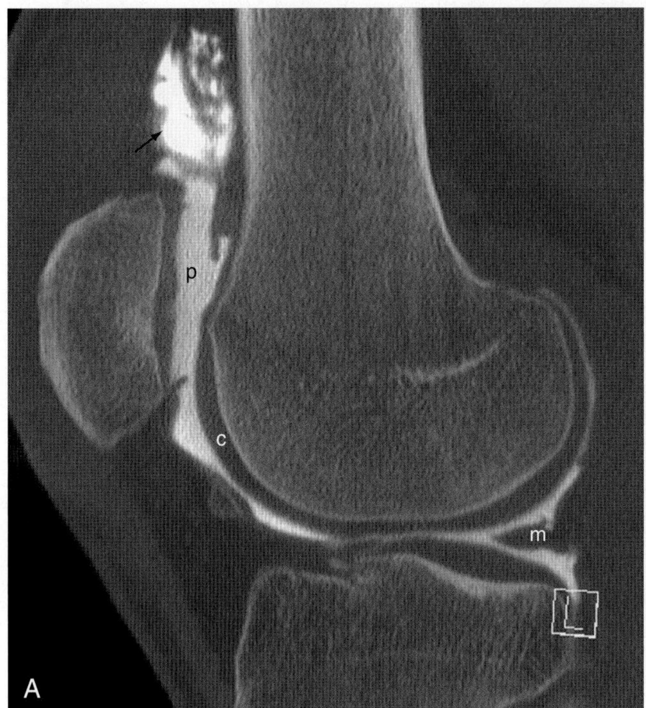

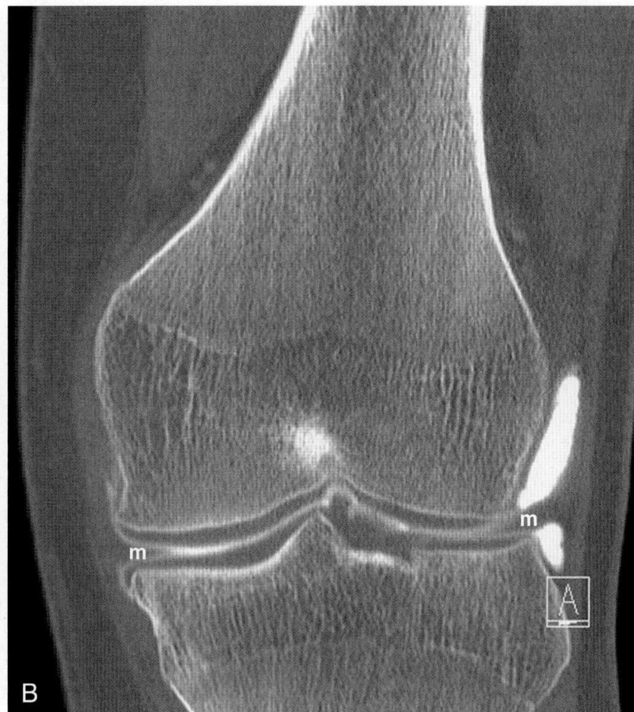

FIGURE 5-13. CT arthrography of the knee in a patient with a pacemaker (a contraindication for MRI). **A,** The lateral multiplanar reconstruction of the left knee displays contrast extending into the suprapatellar pouch *(p)*. An irregular collection *(arrow)* on the undersurface of the quadriceps tendon is consistent with contrast extravasation from faulty injection or injury. The cartilage surfaces are coated with contrast, allowing the thickness and contour of the cartilage *(c)* to be assessed. **B,** The medial and lateral menisci *(m)* appear as triangular structures clearly outlined with contrast and were normal on this examination.

collateral ligaments and the adjacent soft tissues. Currently, MR arthrography is considered to be the gold standard in the evaluation of elbow ligament tears, but CT arthrography is just as beneficial in situations in which MR is contraindicated or cannot be performed.[5]

Technique

The patient is usually positioned lying prone with the arm above the head and the elbow flexed and parallel to the fluoroscopy table. The lateral aspect of the elbow should be facing up. The skin over the elbow is prepared and draped using sterile technique. The overlying tissues are anesthetized. A 22 G needle is placed over the radiocapitellar joint and advanced under fluoroscopic guidance into the elbow joint. Any fluid present in the joint should be aspirated prior to injecting contrast. Correct placement within the joint is confirmed by injection of a small amount of radiopaque contrast material. A total volume of 8 to 12 mL of contrast should be injected[1] (Figure 5-18). Following injection of the contrast agent, the needle is withdrawn and the elbow is gently moved to distribute the contrast evenly throughout the joint. Excessive exercise should be avoided because it may lead to rupture of a distended capsule. Following this, the patient is transported to either the MRI or CT suite for completion of the examination.

Indications

MR and CT arthrography are most effective in the evaluation of the articular surfaces of the elbow. They are useful for identifying and characterizing chondral lesions as well as staging osteochondral lesions.[5,17] In the evaluation of the ligamentous structures, MR arthrography is considered to be the gold standard.[35] In any patient presenting with "clicking" or "catching," a loose body should be considered as a cause of symptoms and MR or CT arthrography would be excellent examinations for this purpose[5,36] (Table 5-5) (see Figure 5-18).

Findings

Contrast fills the elbow joint. Extension of contrast beyond its normal confines may be seen in ligamentous injury. For example, contrast between the medial collateral ligament and its insertion on the sublime tubercle of the ulna indicates a tear.

ANKLE ARTHROGRAPHY

Multiple imaging modalities exist for the assessment of ankle disorders. The modality chosen for the evaluation of the patient should be tailored to his or her specific clinical symptoms. These modalities include radiography, bone scintigraphy, ultrasound, CT, MRI, and injection procedures (CT or MR arthrography). If there is clinical concern for ligamentous or soft tissue injury, an MR examination is commonly performed. If there is not a significant effusion within the ankle joint, the evaluation of the intrinsic structures may be limited. Through the addition of intraarticular contrast, complete evaluation of the ankle cartilage and joint lining can be accomplished and any contrast extravasation indicating ligamentous injury can be identified.

Technique

When performing ankle arthrography, the patient is placed in the supine position on the fluoroscopy table with the ankle in the lateral position and the front of the ankle facing the examiner.

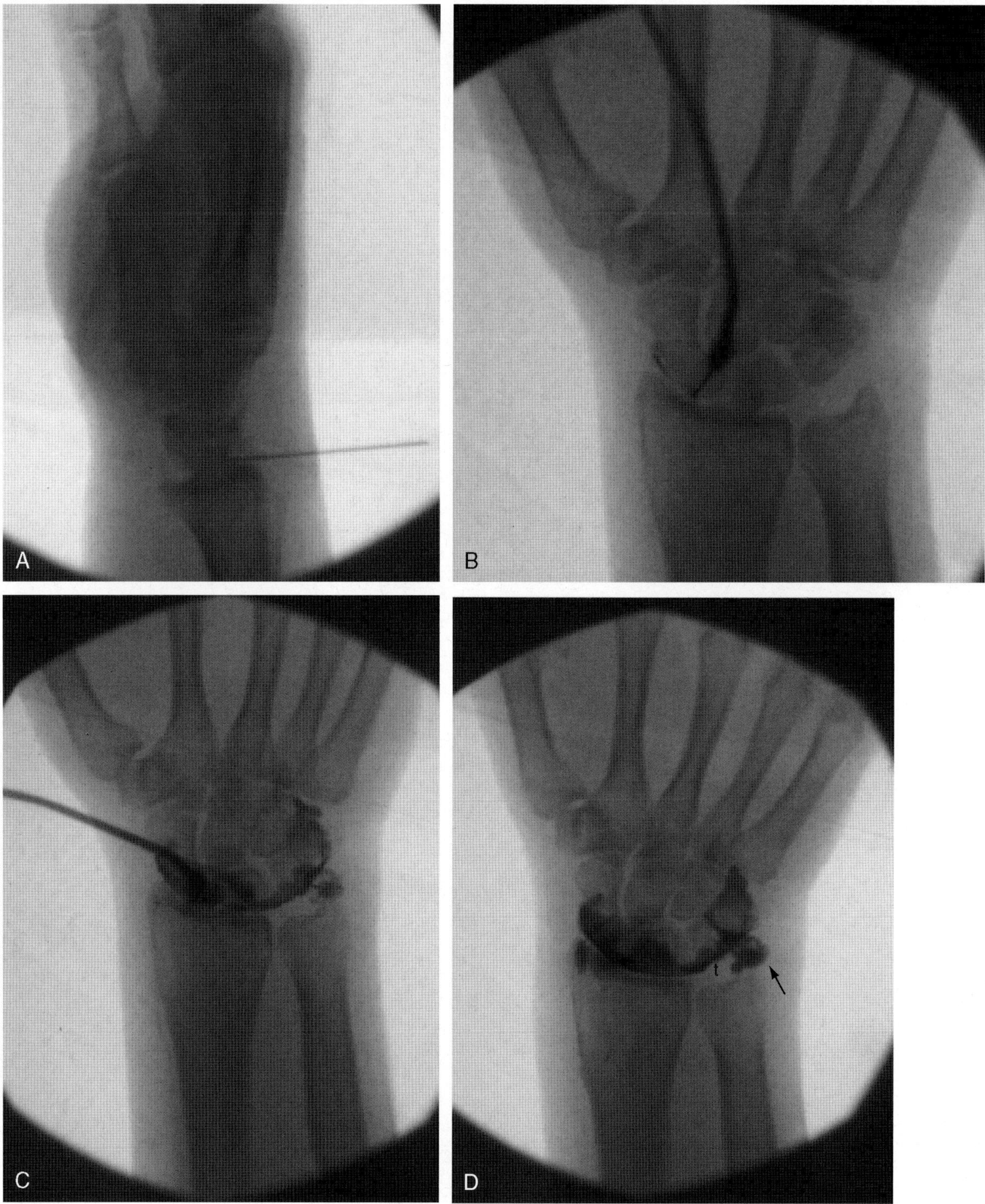

FIGURE 5-14. Normal wrist arthrogram. This 52-year-old female presented with ulnar-sided chronic wrist pain. Lateral **(A)** and frontal **(B)** fluoroscopic images during needle placement for radiocarpal contrast injection. The needle was placed at the radial aspect of the radiocarpal joint, away from the scapholunate ligament. **C,** Once placed within the joint, a small amount of contrast was instilled that flowed away from the needle tip, confirming intraarticular placement. **D,** Following injection, contrast remains contained within the radiocarpal joint with no leakage into the midcarpal joint or distal radialulnar joint to suggest ligamentous tears. The prestyloid recess *(arrow)* is noted, as is filling of the pisiform triquetral recess. The distal surface of the triangular fibrocartilage *(t)* is outlined by contrast.

TABLE 5-4. Uses of CT or MR Arthrography of the Wrist

Imaging Technique	Uses
MR arthrography	Evaluation of the triangular fibrocartilage complex (TFCC)
	Evaluation of the intrinsic ligaments including the scapholunate ligament and the lunotriquetral ligament
	Ulnar impaction syndrome
	Postoperative wrist
	Rheumatoid arthritis
CT arthrography	All of the above indications if there are contraindications for MRI
	Postoperative wrist, especially if adjacent prostheses are present

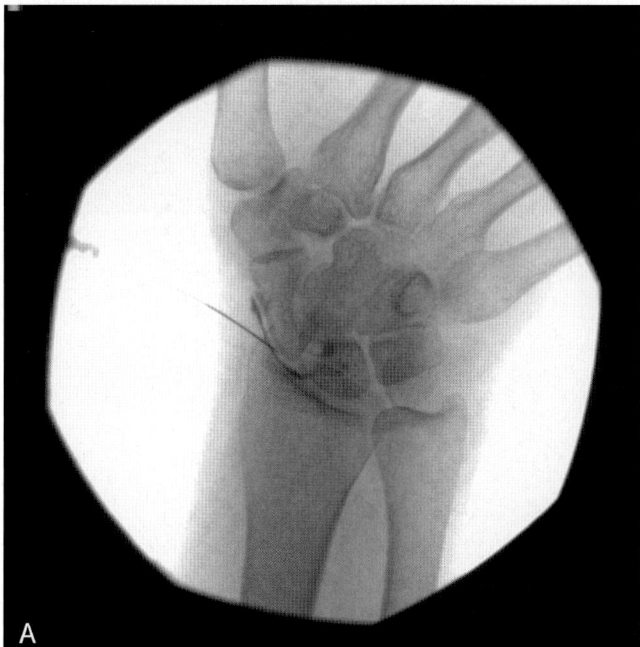

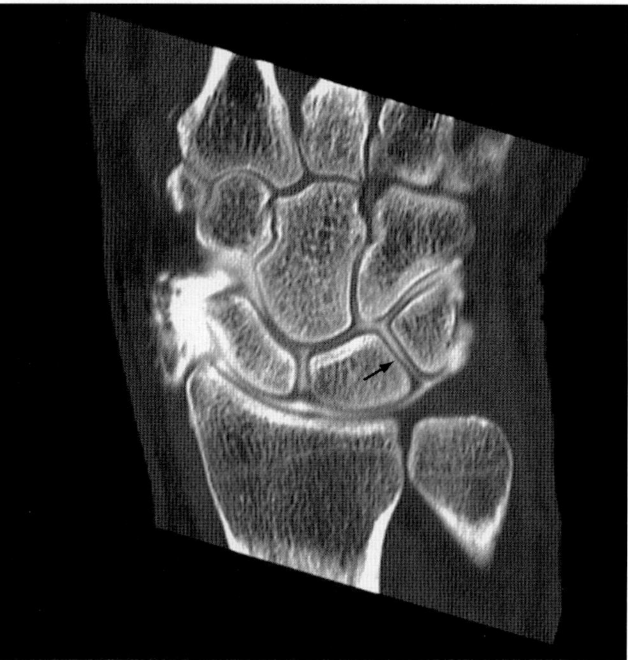

FIGURE 5-16. Lunotriquetral ligament tear in a 35-year-old male with ulnar-sided wrist pain. Coronal image from a CT arthrogram after injection of the radiocarpal joint demonstrates contrast filling the entire length of the lunotriquetral joint *(arrow)* and extending into the mid-carpal joint. These findings indicate a lunotriquetral ligament tear. There is retrograde filling of the scapholunate joint.

The position of the dorsalis pedis artery is palpated and its course is marked in order to avoid puncturing it during needle placement. After sterile preparation of the overlying skin at the site of access, these tissues are anesthetized. Then, a 22 G or 23 G needle is inserted into the tibiotalar joint medial to the extensor hallucis longus tendon and advanced under fluoroscopic guidance with a slight cranial tilt to avoid the overhanging anterior margin of the tibia.[37] Once the needle is seen projecting between the anterior

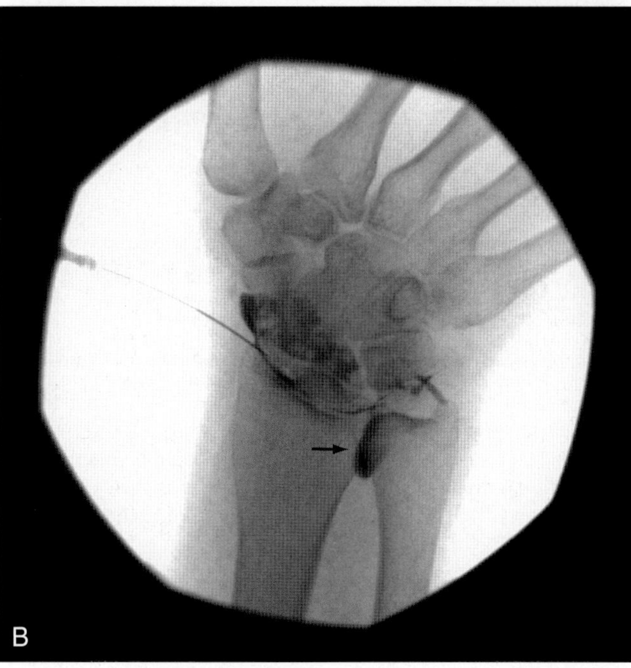

FIGURE 5-15. TFCC tear. This patient presented with ulnar wrist pain. **A,** Fluoroscopic image shows the needle was placed at the radial aspect of the radiocarpal joint with slight volar angulation to enter the joint. Once placed within the joint, a small amount of contrast was seen filling the radiocarpal joint. **B,** Subsequent fluoroscopic image shows contrast filling the distal radioulnar joint *(arrow)*, indicating a tear of the TFCC.

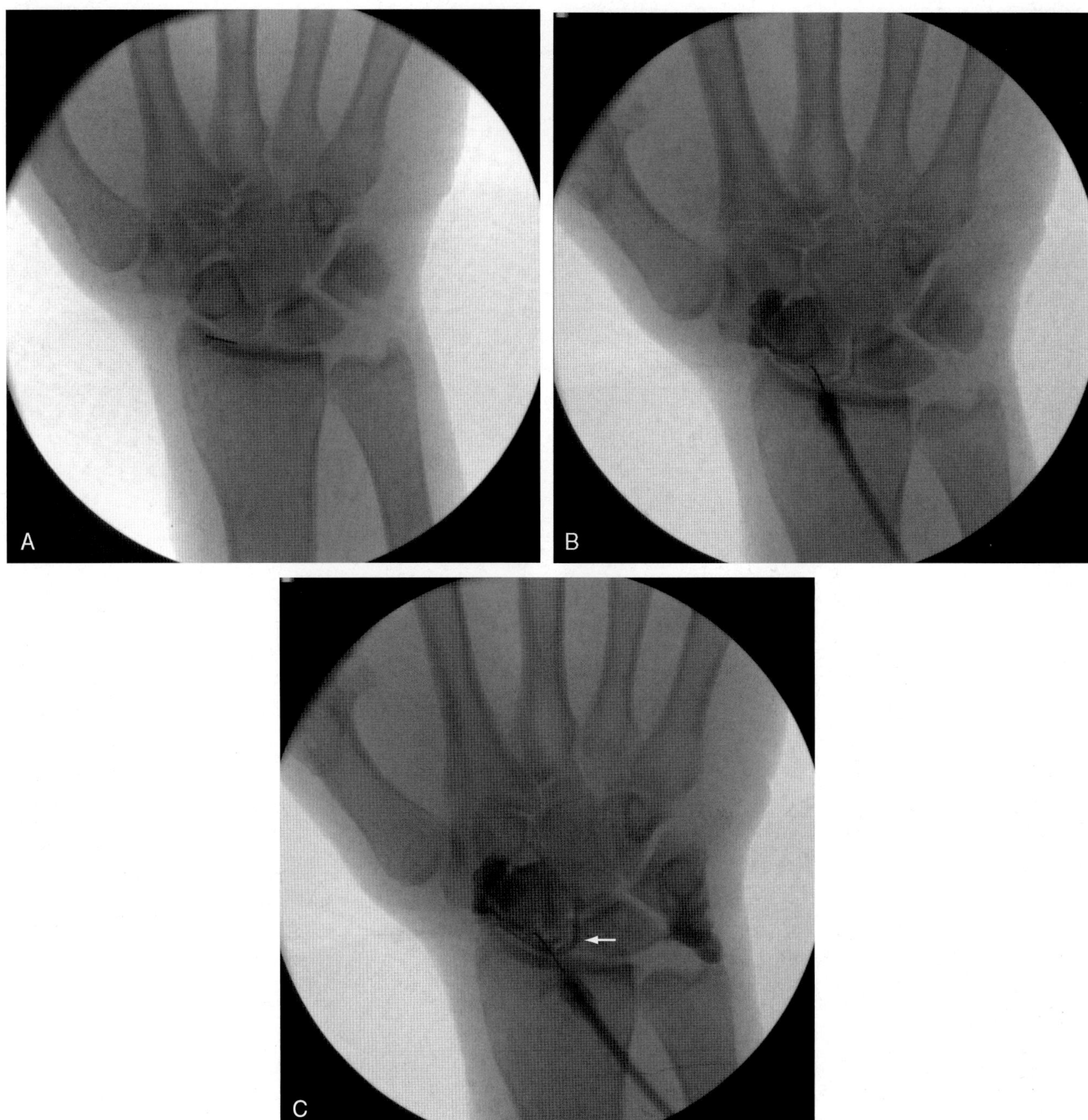

FIGURE 5-17. Arthrographic demonstration of a scapholunate ligament tear in a 44-year-old male with central dorsal-sided wrist pain after a recent fall. **A** to **C**, Three sequential fluoroscopic images were obtained after contrast injection into the radiocarpal joint. **C** demonstrates contrast flowing through the scapholunate ligament to fill the scapholunate articulation *(arrow)* and the mid-carpal joint.

margin of the tibia and the dome of the talus, an intraarticular position can be assumed (Figure 5-19). Using an alternative approach, the needle may be inserted just medial to the tibialis anterior tendon in a similar fashion. Once the needle is placed within the joint, any fluid within the joint should be aspirated. A small amount of non-ionic iodinated contrast can be injected into the joint to confirm needle placement. A total of 6 to 8 mL of contrast should be instilled into the joint.[1] Following injection, the needle is removed and the ankle can be manipulated for additional fluoroscopic images. The patient is then transferred to either the CT or MRI suite for completion of the examination.

Indications

MR and CT arthrography are excellent tools for the evaluation of the location and extent of ligamentous tears, especially the lateral

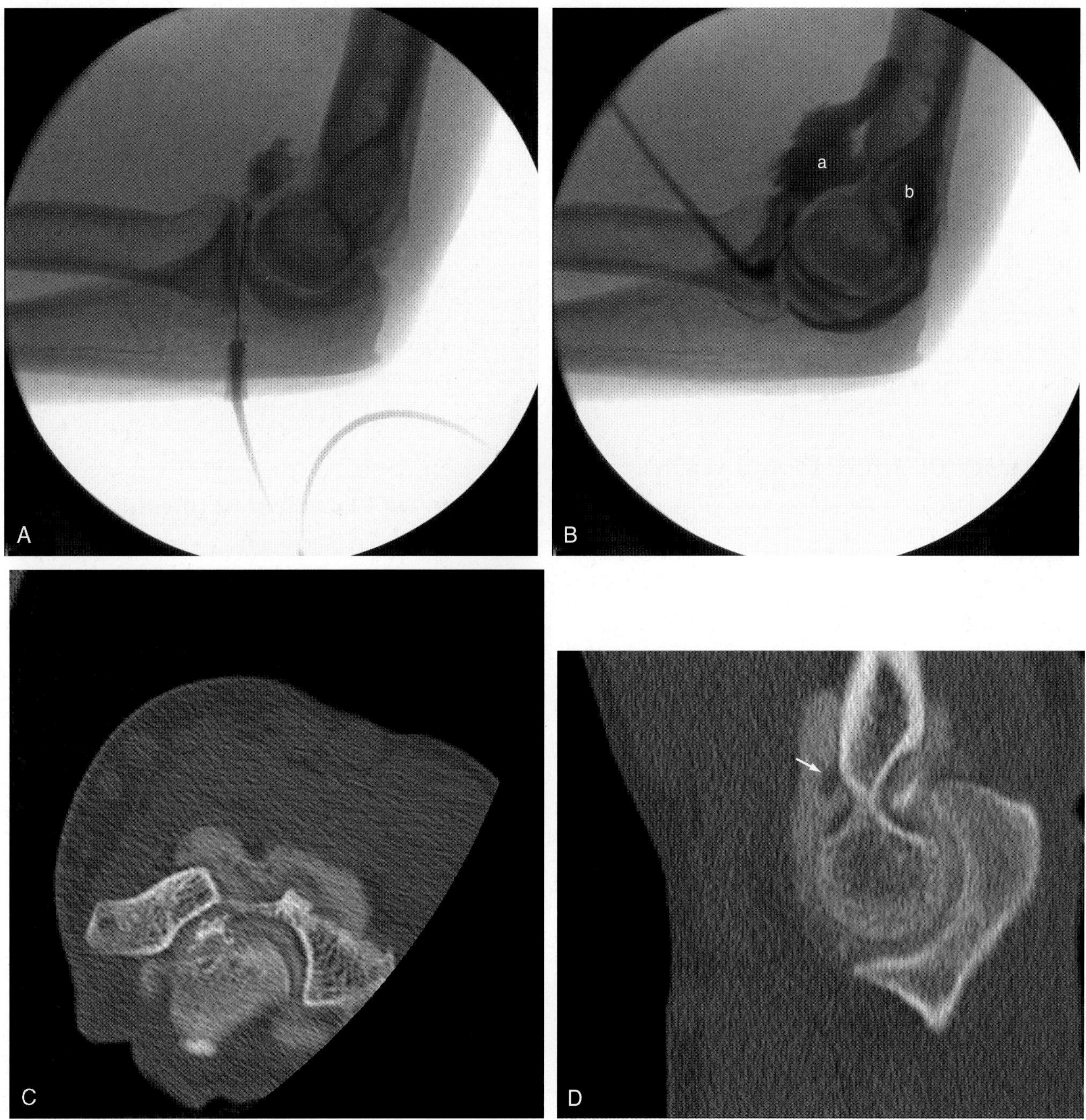

FIGURE 5-18. Elbow arthrogram in a 51-year-old male with pain on extension. **A, B,** Lateral fluoroscopic images. Using a lateral approach the elbow joint is accessed near the radial head and contrast is seen to flow away from the needle tip to fill the joint including the anterior *(a)* and posterior *(b)* recesses. Axial **(C)** and sagittal **(D)** CT images after the needle has been removed show an intraarticular body *(arrow)* surrounded by contrast in the anterior joint recess. A calcified body is also present in the posterior recess.

collateral ligamentous complex (Figure 5-20). These modalities are also good for the evaluation of various ankle impingement syndromes, especially anterolateral impingment.[38] The articular cartilage can be evaluated[39] along with identification of intraarticular bodies, communication with subchondral cysts (Figure 5-21), and determination of the stability of osteochondral lesions[28,40] (Box 5-3). In patients who have suffered previous injury, these studies can accurately detect adhesive capsulitis.[41]

Findings

The normal ankle joint shows anterior and posterior recesses. Communication with the flexor hallucis longus tendon may be normal, but filling of the peroneal tendon sheath is associated with injury to the calcaneofibular and anterior talofibular ligaments. Osteochondral lesions of the talus are frequent findings and the integrity of the overlying cartilage and the stability of the fragment can be better assessed with contrast (see Figure 5-21).

TABLE 5-5. Uses of CT or MR Arthrography of the Elbow

Imaging Technique	Uses
MR arthrography	Evaluation of the medial and lateral ligament complexes of the elbow
	Osteochondral injuries of the capitellum
	Identification of intraarticular cartilaginous bodies
CT arthrography	Osteochondral injuries to the capitellum
	Detection of chondral or osteochondral bodies in the elbow
	Any of the above indications if contraindications exist for performance of MRI

SUMMARY OF JOINT EVALUATION

MRI, with its high soft tissue contrast, is an excellent method for the noninvasive evaluation of joints. Although arthrography is an invasive procedure, it is relatively safe when performed using sterile technique and imaging guidance. There are relatively few contraindications. The intraarticular administration of contrast material, reduction of capsular redundancy, and separation of adjacent structures improves the overall evaluation of the joint. Because of both the excellent delineation of intraarticular structures and the ability to evaluate periarticular structures, MR arthrography is considered to be the gold standard in joint imaging. It has proven to be beneficial in the differentiation of full-thickness and partial-thickness rotator cuff tears, evaluation of a joint following surgery, and presurgical planning. CT arthrography is a revitalized older technique that, due to the application of modern multidetector technology, allows for high spatial resolution and serves as an effective alternative to MR arthrography, especially in patients who have undergone a failed MR arthrogram or those who have contraindications to MR arthrography. The spatial resolution is greater with CT than with MR arthrography, so small structures (e.g., articular cartilage defects) may be well seen.

INJECTION PROCEDURES

Injection of joints under image guidance is particularly useful for deeper joints (e.g., the hip, sacroiliac [SI] joints), larger patients, or difficult areas such as the midfoot where palpation may be limited (Box 5-4). Ultrasound, CT or fluoroscopy, and even MRI may be used for needle placement, but usually fluoroscopy is adequate. CT is often utilized in large patients or to inject the joints in the spine.

The accuracy of injections into various joints without imaging for needle placement was assessed in 109 patients by mixing the depot methylprednisolone with a radiographic contrast medium prior to injection.[8] Approximately 28% of knee, 33% of ankle, 25% of wrist, and 30% of shoulder injections were shown to be extraarticular. Although it seems intuitive that return of joint fluid should indicate intraarticular needle placement, even after successful aspiration of joint fluid, the needle tip may not be entirely intraarticular. Thus aspiration of synovial fluid did not predict intraarticular placement of corticosteroid injections; nearly half (14/31) of the extraarticular injections were associated with aspiration of synovial fluid.

> Even after aspiration of joint fluid, injection may not be intraarticular!

When no joint effusion is present, accurate positioning of a needle into the joint space may be difficult without imaging. Jackson et al. studied the accuracy of intraarticular needle placement into the knee when no effusion was present.[24] The lateral midpatellar approach was most effective at producing intraarticular needle placement. However, even these injections were intraarticular only 93% of the time. Imaging techniques can improve accurate intraarticular needle placement. Several studies have demonstrated the improved ability of ultrasound, for example, to localize fluid collections for aspiration as compared with clinical examination.

> Accuracy of joint aspiration can be improved by imaging.

Is Accurate Placement of Injections Necessary?

Hall and Buchbinder note that the "...clinical efficacy of corticosteroid injection may not depend on intraarticular needle placement."[42] Several studies, however, have indicated greater therapeutic benefit with accurate placement of corticosteroid injection.[43] The necessity for image-guided corticosteroid injection in most cases remains uncertain. As summarized by Hall, "while some joints such as the hip and midtarsal joints demand imaging for any accuracy of steroid placement, for most joints which have conventionally been injected by rheumatologists following an anatomical landmark approach, imaging guided injection should be reserved for those cases who have not responded to injection following anatomical landmarks."[42] Multiple uses for corticosteroid injection have been suggested (Box 5-5).

Inflammatory arthritis is the classic indication for injection, but osteoarthritis may also respond to corticosteroid injection. Ravaud et al. reported a randomized, controlled multicenter trial to evaluate the results of joint lavage and corticosteroid injection into the painful knees of patients with osteoarthritis.[46] Pain relief from intraarticular corticosteroid was maximal at week 1 and lasted for up to 4 weeks. Wise noted that response to hip injections, under fluoroscopic guidance, may last as long as 8 to 12 weeks in a majority of patients with milder osteoarthritis.[6] Resting the joint after the injection has been advised, although exact protocols differ.[47]

Contraindications to Joint Injection

Contraindications, precautions and techniques for joint injection are generally the same as for arthrography procedures. A review by Wise indicated the following potential complications of intraarticular corticosteroid injection (Box 5-6)[6]:

- Infection (1:10,000)[48]
- Soft tissue irritation
- Flare of symptoms
- Tendon tears
- Avascular necrosis
- Fistula formation

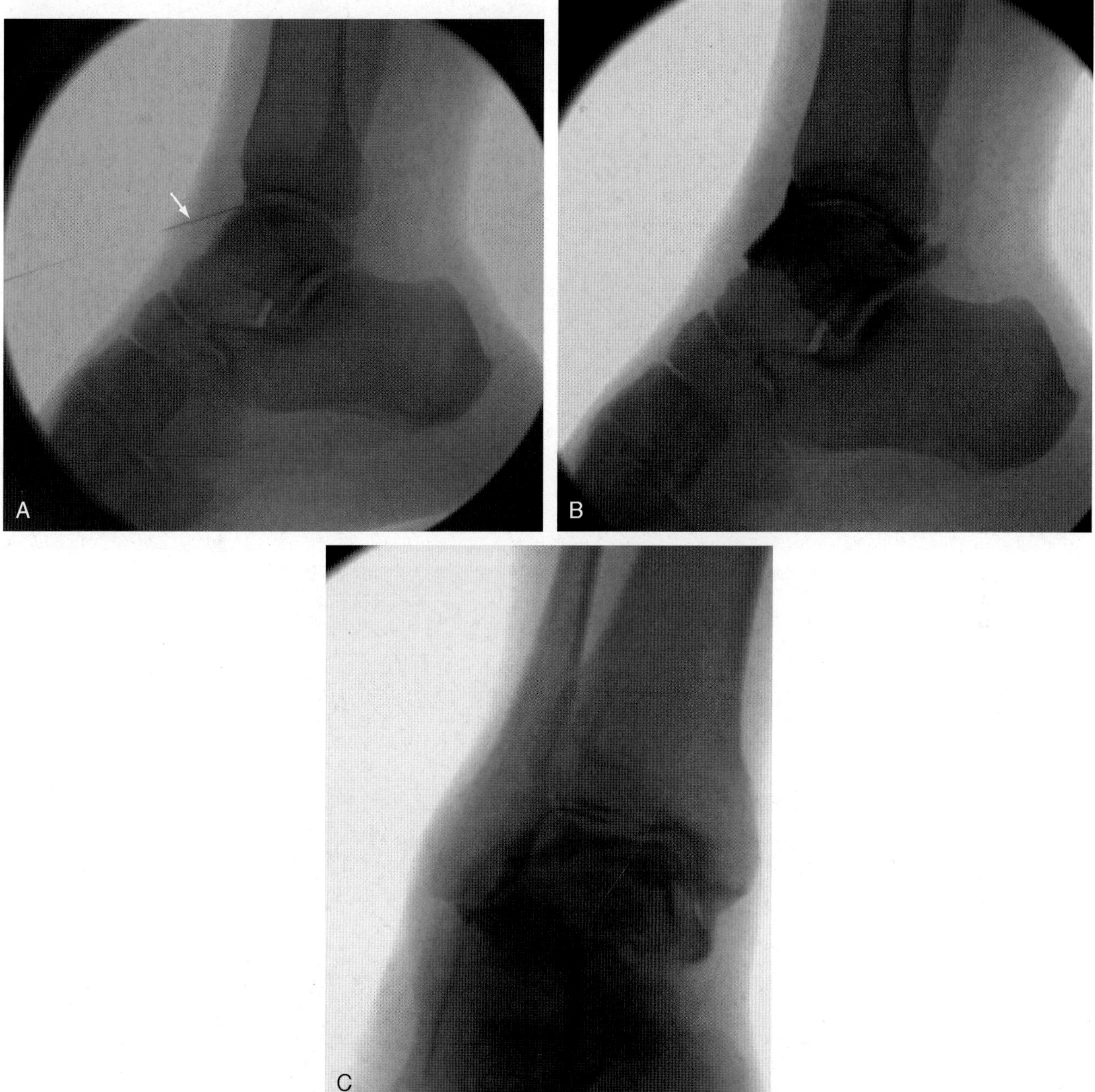

FIGURE 5-19. Normal ankle arthrography in a 44-year-old male with chronic ankle pain. **A,** Lateral fluoroscopic image shows needle positioning for arthrography. The needle *(arrow)* was advanced along the medial aspect of the flexor hallucis longus after locating the dorsalis pedis artery. A slight cranial tilt is given to the needle to advance it into the joint. Lateral **(B)** and oblique **(C)** fluoroscopic images obtained after contrast injection confirm filling of the tibiotalar joint. No extraarticular leakage of contrast or filling defects are noted. The cartilage surfaces are outlined and are smooth.

Infection introduced into the joint during injection is rare. In one series of 400,000 injections the incidence of infection was 0.005%.[49] A flare of symptoms may occur beginning a few hours after injection and last for up to 2 or 3 days. The incidence of tendon rupture is generally low but is highest in the Achilles tendon and plantar fascia, so direct tendon injection of these areas should be avoided. Systemic absorption of the locally injected corticosteroid occurs. Patients may exhibit erythema, warmth, and diaphoresis within minutes to hours after corticosteroid injection. This is most likely related to systemic absorption, but idiosyncratic reaction to preservatives may occur. Metabolic effects may occur including transiently elevated blood glucose or decreases in peripheral blood eosinophil or lymphocyte counts.[6] Avascular necrosis is uncommon.

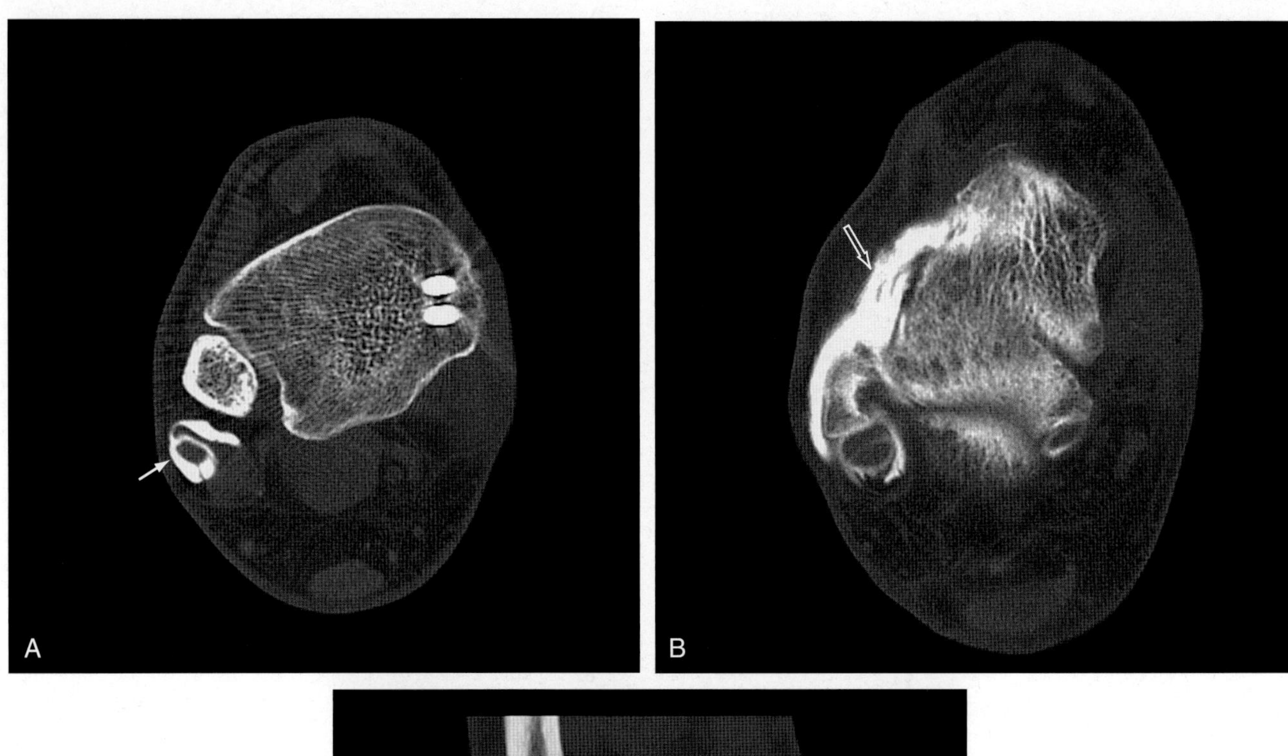

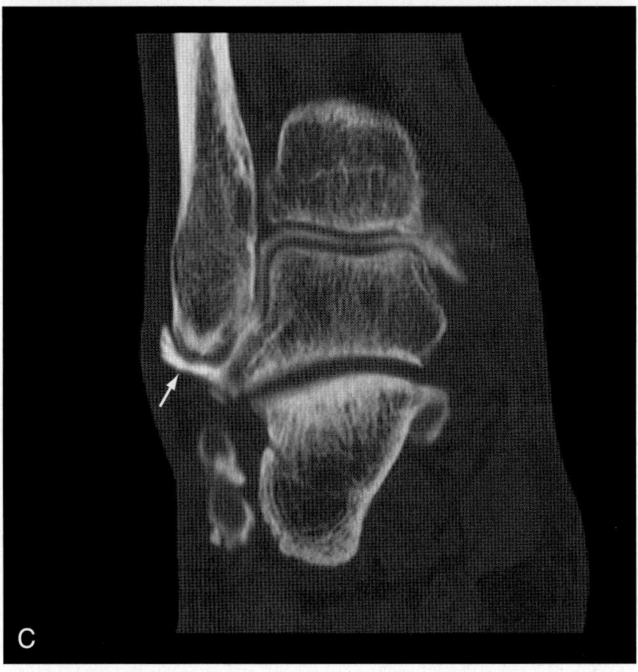

FIGURE 5-20. Ankle pain after injury. Axial CT image through the tibia **(A)**, axial CT image at the level of the talus **(B)**, and coronal reformatted CT image **(C)** are shown after an arthrogram of the tibiotalar joint. There is contrast filling the peroneal tendons *(arrows)*, indicating a tear of the calcaneofibular ligament. There is a tear of the anterior talofibular ligament causing contrast extravasation anteriorly (open arrow in **B**). Contrast is seen around the fibula, indicating an anterior calcaneofibular ligament tear (arrow in **C**).

Corticosteroid Injection

Generally, a long-acting corticosteroid preparation and/or a long-acting anesthetic are injected into the joint depending on the clinical indication. Aspiration of as much joint fluid as possible is performed prior to corticosteroid injection, as this increases the effectiveness of the injection.[6] Several corticosteroid preparations are available that differ in potency and solubility.[51] At the Brigham and Women's Department of Radiology, usually Depo-Medrol (methylprednisolone acetate injectable suspension, USP 40 mg/mL) is used. For the hip or SI joint, generally 40 to 80 mg of Depo-Medrol are injected. Forty milligrams are generally used in the shoulder. Twenty milligrams are injected into the subtalar joint. Long-acting anesthetics may also be injected (using a separate syringe) if clinically indicated. Because of potential adverse affects on cartilage, Rifat and Moeller recommend no more than three injections per location per year and note that if three injections do not provide relief, it is unlikely that more injections will.[50]

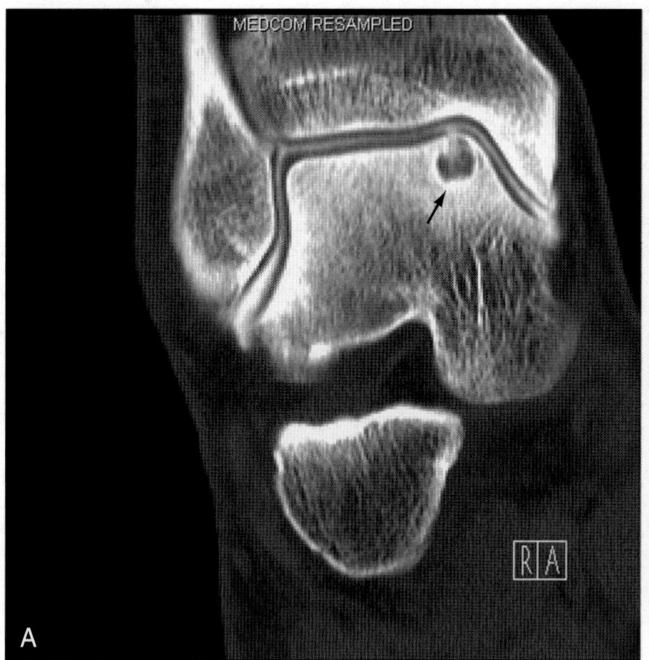

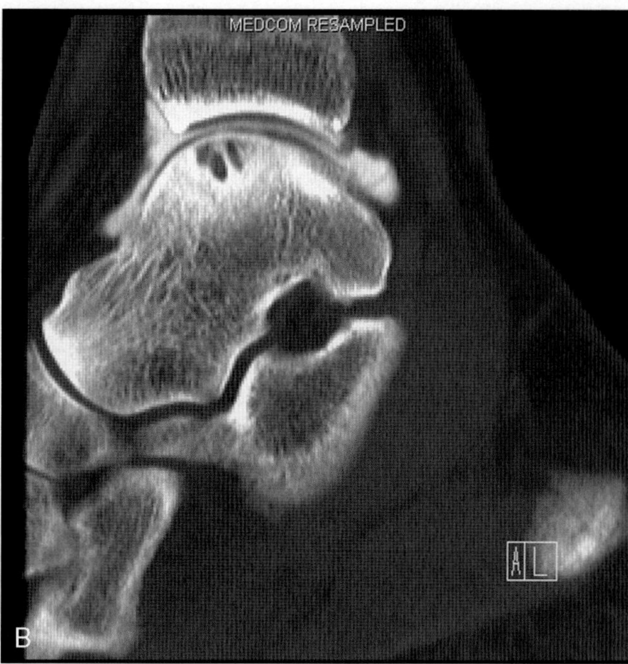

FIGURE 5-21. CT arthrography of an osteochondral injury of the talus. This 49-year-old female presented with ankle pain. Coronal **(A)** and sagittal **(B)** reformatted CT arthrographic images show a lucent lesion of the medial dome of the talus *(arrow)*. The instilled contrast is seen extending into this lesion through a defect in the adjacent articular cartilage. This confirms the bony lesion as a subchondral cyst with overlying articular cartilage damage (posttraumatic osteochondral injury).

BOX 5-3. Some Uses of Ankle Arthrography (CT and MR)

EVALUATION OF:
The lateral collateral ligament complex
Ankle impingement (anterior, anterolateral, anteromedial, and posterior impingement)
Articular cartilage
Osteochondral lesions
Adhesive capsulitis following trauma
Synovitis

BOX 5-4. Potential Sites for Image-Guided Injections

Spine
Sacroiliac joints[44]
Mid-foot joint
Subtalar joint
Hip joint
Wrist compartments

Anesthetic Injection

Anesthetic injection may be used as a diagnostic tool to isolate the source of pain or may be used in conjunction with corticosteroid administration. Long-acting anesthetic affects begin in 30 minutes and last for about 8 hours. (Rifat) We usually inject about 3 to 5 mL of bupivacaine* 0.25% in larger joints or about 2 mL in smaller joints. It is helpful to inject 1 to 2 mL of short-acting anesthetic at the same time for immediate pain relief. In the hip, pain relief is good evidence that that joint is the source of symptoms, whereas the lack of pain response is nonspecific.

*Bupivacaine HCL injection USP (2.5 mg/mL), Hospira, Inc., Lake Forest, Ill.

BOX 5-5. Potential Uses for Corticosteroid Injection[6,45]

INFLAMMATORY ARTHRITIS (1 OR 2 JOINTS)
Rheumatoid
Juvenile chronic arthritis
Ankylosing spondylitis

CRYSTAL DISEASE
Gout
Pseudogout

OSTEOARTHRITIS

BOX 5-6. Possible Complications of Intraarticular Corticosteroid Injection

Infection (1:10,000)[48]
Soft tissue irritation
Flare of symptoms
Tendon tears
Avascular necrosis
Fistula formation
Bleeding

REFERENCES

1. Helgason JW, Chandnani VP, Yu JS: MR arthrography: a review of current technique and application, *AJR Am J Roentgenol* 168:1473-1480, 1997.
2. Binkert CA, Verdun FR, Zanetti M et al: CT arthrography of the glenohumeral joint: CT fluoroscopy versus conventional CT and fluoroscopy—comparison of image guidance techniques, *Radiology* 229:153-158, 2003.
3. Dubberley JH, Faber KJ, Patterson SD et al: The detection of loose bodies in the elbow: the value of MRI and CT arthrography, *J Bone Joint Surg (Br)* 87:684-686, 2005.
4. Steinbach LS, Palmer WE, Schweitzer ME: Special focus session: MR arthrography, *Radiographics* 22:1223-1246, 2002.
5. Buckwalter KA: CT arthrography, *Clin Sports Med* 25:899-915, 2006.
6. Wise C: The rational use of steroid injections in arthritis and nonarticular musculoskeletal pain syndromes, *Bull Rheum Dis* 52:1-4, 2003.
7. Thumboo J, O'Duffy JD: A prospective study of the safety of joint and soft tissue aspirations and injections in patients taking warfarin sodium, *Arthritis Rheum* 41:736-739, 1998.
8. Jones A, Regan M, Ledingham J et al: Importance of placement of intra-articular steroid injections, *Br Med J* 307:1329-1330, 1993.
9. Schulte-Altedorneburg G, Gebhard M, Wohlgemuth WA et al: MR arthrography: pharmacology, efficacy and safety in clinical trials, *Skeletal Radiol* 32:1-12, 2003.
10. Stiles RG, Otte MT: Imaging of the shoulder, *Radiology* 188:603-613, 1993.
11. Jacobson JA, Lin J, Jamadar D et al: Aids to successful shoulder arthrography performed with a fluoroscopically guided anterior approach, *Radiographics* 23:373-379, 2003.
12. Chung CB, Dwek JR, Feng S et al: MR arthrography of the glenohumeral joint: a tailored approach, *AJR Am J Roentgenol* 177:217-219, 2001.
13. Depelteau H, Bureau NJ, Cardinal E et al: Arthrography of the shoulder: a simple fluoroscopically guided approach for targeting the rotator cuff interval, *AJR Am J Roentgenol* 182:329-332, 2004.
14. Jbara, M, Chen Q, Marten P et al: Shoulder MR arthrography: how, why, when, *Radiol Clin N Am* 43:683-692, 2005.
15. Catalano OA, Manfredi R, Vanzulli A et al: MR arthrography of the glenohumeral joint:modified posterior approach without imaging guidance, *Radiology* 242:550-554, 2007.
16. Palmer WE, Caslowitz PL: Anterior shoulder instability: diagnostic criteria determined from prospective analysis of 121 MR arthrograms, *Radiology* 197:819-825, 1995.
17. Osinski T, Malfair D, Steinbach L: Magnetic resonance arthrography, *Orthop Clin N Am* 37:299-319, 2006.
18. Schmid MR, Notzli HP, Zanetti M et al: Cartilage lesions in the hip: diagnostic effectiveness of MR arthrography, *Radiology* 226:382-386, 2003.
19. Nishii T, Tanaka H, Katsuyuki N et al: Fat-suppressed 3D spoiled gradient-echo MRI and MDCT arthrography of articular cartilage in patients with hip dysplasia, *AJR Am J Roentgenol* 185:379-385, 2005.
20. Pfirrmann CW, Mengiardi B, Dora C et al: Cam and pincer femoroacetabular impingement: characteristic MR arthrographic findings in 50 patients, *Radiology* 240:778-785, 2006.
21. Chung CB, Isaza IL, Angulo M et al: MR arthrography of the knee: how, why, when, *Radiol Clin N Am* 43:733-746, 2005.
22. Brinkert CA, Zanetti M, Hodler J: Patient's assessment of discomfort during MR arthrography of the shoulder, *Radiology* 221:775-778, 2001.
23. Faber JM: CT arthrography and postoperative musculoskeletal imaging with multichannel comuted tomography, *Semin Musculoskelet Radiol* 8:157-166, 2004.
24. Jackson DW, Evans NA, Thomas BM: Accuracy of needle placement into the intra-articular space of the knee, *J Bone Joint Surg* 84:1522-1527, 2002.
25. McCauley TR, Elfar A, Moore A et al: MR arthrography of anterior cruciate ligament reconstruction grafts, *AJR Am J Roentgenol* 181:1217-1223, 2003.
26. Kramer J, Stiglbauer R, Engel A et al: MR contrast arthrography (MRA) in osteochondrosis dissecans, *J Comput Assist Tomogr* 16:254-260, 1992.
27. Bohndorf K: Osteochondritis (osteochondrosis) dissecans: a review and new MRI classification, *Eur Radiol* 8:103-112, 1998.
28. Attarian DE, Guilak F: Observations on the growth of loose bodies in joints, *Arthroscopy* 18:930-934, 2002.
29. Berna-Serna JD, Martinez, F, Reus M et al: Wrist arthrography: a simple method, *Eur Radiol* 16:469-472, 2006.
30. Zinberg EM, Palmer AK, Coren AB et al: The triple-injection wrist arthrogram, *J Hand Surg (Am)* 13:803-809, 1988.
31. Schnitt R, Christopoulos G, Meier R et al: Direct arthroscopy: a prospective study on 125 patients, *Rofo Fortschr Geb Rontgenstr Neuen Bildgeb Verfahr* 175:911-919, 2003.
32. Kovanlikaya I, Camli D, Cakmakci H et al: Diagnostic value of MR arthrography in detection of intrinsic carpal ligament lesions: use of cine-MR arthrography as a new approach, *Eur Radiol* 7:1441-1445, 1997.
33. Scott DL, Coulton BL, Popert AJ: Long term progression of joint damage in rheumatoid arthritis, *Arthritis Rheum* 31:315-324, 1988.
34. Taouli B, Zaim S, Peterfy CG et al: Rheumatoid arthritis of the hand and wrist: comparison of three imaging techniques, *AJR Am J Roentgenol* 182:937-943, 2004.
35. Potter H, Weiland AJ, Schatz J et al: Posterolateral rotary instability of the elbow: usefulness of MR in the diagnosis, *Radiology* 204:185-189, 1997.
36. Dubberley JH, Faber KJ, Patterson SD et al: The detection of loose bodies in the elbow: the value of MRI and CT arthrography, *J Bone Joint Surg (Br)* 87:684-686, 2005.
37. Cerezal L, Abascal F, Garcia-Valtuille R et al: Ankle MR arthrography: how, why, when, *Radiol Clin N Am* 43:693-707, 2005.
38. Robinson P, White LM, Salonen D et al: Anteromedial impingement of the ankle: using MR arthrography to assess the anteromedial recess, *AJR Am J Roentgenol* 178:601-604, 2002.
39. Imhof H, Nobauer-Huhmann IM, Krestan C et al: MRI of the cartilage, *Eur Radiol* 12:2781-2793, 2002.
40. Schmid MR, Pfirrmann CW, Hodler J et al: Cartilage lesions in the ankle joint: comparison of MR arthrography and CT arthrography, *Skeletal Radiol* 32:259-265, 2003.
41. DeSmet AA, Dalinka MK, Daffner RH et al: Chronic ankle pain, American College of Radiology Appropriateness Criteria Expert Panel on Musculoskeletal Imaging, *ACR* 8:321-322, 2005.
42. Hall S, Buchbinder R: Do imaging methods that guide needle placement improve outcome? *Ann Rheum Dis* 63:1007-1008, 2004.
43. Eustace JA, Brophy DP, Gibney RP et al: Comparison of the accuracy of steroid placement with clinical outcome in patients with shoulder symptoms, *Ann Rheum Dis* 56:59-63, 1997.
44. Rosenberg JM, Quint TJ, de Rosayro AM: Computerized tomographic localization of clinically-guided sacroiliac joint injections, *Clin J Pain* 16:18-21, 2000.
45. Padeh S, Passwell JH: Intraarticular corticosteroid injection in the management of children with chronic arthritis, *Arthritis Rheum* 41:1210-1214, 1998.
46. Ravaud P, Moulinier L, Giraudeau B et al: Effects of joint lavage and steroid injection in patients with osteoarthritis of the knee: results of a multicenter, randomized, controlled trial, *Arthritis Rheum* 42:475-482, 1999.
47. Chakravarty K, Pharoah PD, Scott DG: A randomized controlled study of post-injection rest following intra-articular steroid therapy for knee synovitis, *Br J Rheumatol* 33:464-468, 1994.
48. Hunter JA, Blyth TH: A risk-benefit assessment of intra-articular corticosteroids in rheumatic disorders, *Drug Saf* 21:353-365, 1999. [Review.]
49. Hollander JL: Intrasynovial corticosteroid therapy in arthritis, *Md State Med J* 19:62-66, 1970.
50. Rifat SF, Moeller JL: Basics of joint injection. General techniques and tips for safe, effective use, *Postgrad Med* 109:157-160, 165-166, 2001.

CHAPTER 6

Dual X-Ray Absorptiometry

LEON LENCHIK, MD

KEY FACTS

- Central dual x-ray absorptiometry (DXA) scanning has become the clinical gold standard for bone mineral density assessment.
- Measurement of hip bone mineral density (BMD) by DXA is a better predictor of hip fracture than are measurements at other sites.
- Several guidelines for obtaining BMD measurements are available.
- T-scores are usually used to diagnose osteoporosis or osteopenia.
- Z-scores compare patients with age-matched controls.
- Proper positioning and analysis are critical in performing DXA scans and in following patients over time.

The use of quantitative technologies for measuring bone mineral density (BMD) is widespread. These technologies are commonly classified according to the skeletal sites that they are able to measure.[1] *Central* methods including dual x-ray absorptiometry (DXA) and quantitative computed tomography (QCT) allow measurement of the spine and proximal femur. *Peripheral* methods including peripheral dual x-ray absorptiometry (pDXA) and peripheral quantitative computed tomography (pQCT) allow measurement of the distal femur, tibia, calcaneus, forearm, or phalanges. Although it does not measure BMD, quantitative ultrasound is often included with peripheral methods.[2]

In clinical practice, central DXA is considered the gold standard for measuring BMD.[3,4] This is justified by the fact that this technique has been the most widely studied. Central DXA has been used in most epidemiologic studies aimed at determining the relationship between BMD and fracture risk.[5-10] It has also been used in most pharmaceutical trials of antiresorptive agents.[11-23] In addition, DXA has excellent reproducibility (< 0.5% coefficient of variation at the spine)[24-26] and low radiation dose (effective dose, 1 microSv).[27] Perhaps most importantly, current World Health Organization (WHO)[28] diagnostic criteria for osteoporosis and current National Osteoporosis Foundation (NOF)[29] treatment guidelines for osteoporosis are based on central DXA measurements.

DXA IMAGING PRINCIPLES

Central DXA scanners include an x-ray source (tube), x-ray collimators, and x-ray detectors. Typically the x-ray source is below the scanner table and is coupled with a C-arm to x-ray detectors found above the table. During scan acquisition, the scanner C-arm moves but does not contact the patient.

Manufacturers of densitometers use different approaches for producing and detecting dual-energy x-rays. X-ray photons are differentially attenuated by the patient based in part on their energy and on the density of the tissue through which they pass.[30] Dual-energy x-rays are needed to determine how much of the attenuation of x-ray photons is attributable to bone rather than soft tissue.[30] One approach for producing dual-energy x-rays uses K-edge filtering to divide the polyenergetic x-ray beam into high- and low-energy components (used by General Electric densitometers). These devices use energy-discriminating detectors and an external calibration phantom. The second approach uses voltage switching between high and low kVp during alternate half-cycles of the main power supply (used by Hologic Inc. densitometers). These devices use current-integrating detectors and an internal calibration drum or wheel. Different approaches for producing and detecting dual-energy x-rays explains in part why the results from densitometers made by different manufacturers are not necessarily comparable.[30]

> The densitometry results obtained by different manufacturers' scanners are not necessarily comparable.

DXA densitometers also differ according to the size and the orientation of the x-ray beam. *Pencil beam* densitometers have a collimated x-ray beam and a single detector that move in tandem. *Fan beam* densitometers have an array of x-rays and detectors. There are two types of fan beam densitometers, wide angle and narrow angle. The wide-angle fan beam is oriented transverse to the long axis of the body (used by Hologic Inc.) whereas the narrow-angle fan beam is parallel to the long axis of the body (used by General Electric). In general, fan beam densitometers have shorter scan acquisition times and higher image resolution.

BMD measurements obtained with DXA have several limitations. Perhaps the most important is that DXA provides an *areal* measurement of BMD (in g/cm^2) rather than the *volumetric* measurement (in mg/cm^3) provided by QCT.[1] Areal measurements do not take into account bone thickness and are influenced by body size and bone size.[30] In particular, young men typically have higher *areal* BMD than young women who have smaller skeletons.

Some investigators[31-37] have tried to address this issue by adjusting areal BMD for bone size either by (1) dividing *areal* BMD by height, height squared, or square root of height; (2) estimating vertebral volume from posteroanterior (PA) and lateral spine scans; or (3) calculating the volumetric bone mineral apparent density (BMAD). BMAD is calculated as follows: BMC/A$^{3/2}$ for the spine and as BMC/A^2 for the femoral neck, where *A* is the projected area. Unfortunately, in clinical practice, there is no simple way to account for this limitation because the standard scanner software does not perform any volumetric adjustment.

Another limitation of DXA is that it integrates cortical and trabecular BMD in the path of the x-ray beam.[1] In contrast, QCT allows differentiation of trabecular and cortical compartments of bone.[1]

Despite these limitations, central DXA is widely used for clinical measurement of BMD. This is appropriate because areal BMD measured by DXA has been shown to predict bone strength in biomechanical studies and to predict risk of fracture in epidemiologic studies.

Biomechanical studies[38-45] have shown: (1) material properties of trabecular bone specimens vary according to BMD and anatomic site, (2) 60% to 90% variability in elastic modulus is explained by BMD, and (3) there is high inverse association between femoral BMD and failure load. Curiously, the correlations between vertebral BMD and failure load are higher for DXA ($r = 0.80$ to 0.94) than QCT ($r = 0.30$ to 0.66). This may reflect the contributions of both the size of the bone (which influences areal BMD) as well as the cortical component of bone to biomechanical strength.[43-45]

Many cross-sectional and longitudinal studies have shown that BMD measured at various skeletal sites is highly associated with osteoporotic fractures.[5-10] In general, for each standard deviation decrease in BMD, the risk of fracture doubles.[5] DXA measurements at the hip predict hip fracture better than measurements at other skeletal sites (relative risk range 1.9 to 3.8).[5]

> In general, for each standard deviation decrease in BMD, the risk of fracture doubles.

DXA has also been used in most pharmaceutical trials for both selection of study subjects and for monitoring them over time.[11-23] All medications currently approved by the Food and Drug Administration (FDA) for the treatment of osteoporosis have shown either maintenance or increase in BMD measured by DXA.

Perhaps the main reason DXA is so widely used is because there is emerging consensus on how to use its results: to help with the diagnosis of osteoporosis, assess fracture risk, determine which patients are candidates for pharmacologic therapy, and monitor therapy.[28,29,46-54]

CLINICAL APPLICATIONS OF DXA MEASUREMENTS

Who Should Have a BMD Measurement?

The NOF[29] recommends BMD measurement in all women 65 years or older regardless of risk factors, in younger postmenopausal women with one or more risk factors (other than being Caucasian, postmenopausal, or female), and in postmenopausal women who present with fractures (Box 6-1).

Apart from the NOF, other groups including the American College of Rheumatology, American Gastroenterological Association, and American Association of Clinical Endocrinologists (AACE) have published guidelines for measurement of BMD.[49-54]

The AACE guidelines[52] are the most comprehensive and recommend BMD measurement in all women older than 65 years, in all women 40 years or older who have sustained a fracture, in women with x-ray findings suggesting osteoporosis, in women beginning or receiving long-term glucocorticoid therapy, and in adult women with symptomatic hyperparathyroidism, nutritional deficiencies, or diseases associated with bone loss (Box 6-2).

The cost of DXA is covered by Medicare and by most third-party insurance companies. Medicare recognizes the following indications: estrogen-deficient women at clinical risk for osteoporosis as determined by the physician, individuals with x-ray evidence of osteopenia or vertebral fracture, individuals receiving or planning to receive long-term glucocorticoid therapy (expected use over 3 months with > 7.5 mg prednisone or equivalent), individuals with primary hyperparathyroidism, and individuals being monitored for response on an FDA-approved osteoporosis drug therapy.

BOX 6-1. National Osteoporosis Foundation: Guidelines for BMD Measurement

- All women ≥ 65 years regardless of risk factors*
- Younger postmenopausal women with one or more risk factors (other than being white, postmenopausal, and female)
- Postmenopausal women who present with fractures (to confirm the diagnosis and determine disease severity)

*Note: Medicare covers BMD testing for the following individuals aged 65 and older:

- Estrogen-deficient women at clinical risk for osteoporosis
- Individuals with vertebral abnormalities
- Individuals receiving, or planning to receive, long-term glucocorticoid (steroid) therapy
- Individuals with primary hyperparathyroidism
- Individuals being monitored to assess the response or efficacy of an approved osteoporosis drug therapy

Retrieved September 4, 2008, from http://www.nof.org/osteoporosis/bonemass.htm.

BOX 6-2. American Association of Clinical Endocrinologists: Guidelines for Bone Densitometry

- All women > 65 years
- All women > 40 years who have had a fracture
- Women with radiographic findings suggesting osteoporosis
- Women on long-term glucocorticoid therapy
- Adult women with symptomatic hyperparathyroidism, nutritional deficiencies, or diseases associated with bone loss

Hodgson SF, Watts NB, Bilezikian JP et al: American Association of Clinical Endocrinologists 2001 Medical Guidelines for Clinical Practice for the Prevention and Management of Postmenopausal Osteoporosis, *Endocr Pract* 7:293-312, 2001.

Medicare permits individuals to repeat BMD testing every 2 years. Exceptions for more frequent testing are made when medically necessary, for example, patients on glucocorticoid therapy or patients who need baseline measurement to allow monitoring if the initial examination was performed with a different technique from the proposed monitoring technique.

What Bones Should be Measured?

Typically, BMD is measured at the lumbar spine and proximal femur.[46,47] About 20% to 30% of patients have significant spine-hip discordance, where T-scores at one site are of a different diagnostic category than the other site.[55,56] Causes of DXA-measured spine-hip discordance include differences in the age at which peak bone mass is reached and in the rate of bone loss at different skeletal sites. For example, in perimenopausal women, the rate of bone loss is greater in cancellous bone (vertebra) than cortical bone (proximal femur). Another reason for measuring both spine and hip is that the spine BMD is a better predictor of spine fractures, whereas the hip BMD is a better predictor of hip fractures.[5] This is not true in patients with severe degenerative disease of the spine. Advanced degenerative disease of the spine can falsely raise the measured BMD, making hip BMD a more accurate measure of the risk of spine fracture.

When spine or the proximal femur measurements are invalid, distal radius measurements are commonly obtained. For example, patients with spine instrumentation, fractures, severe degenerative disease, or scoliosis may benefit from a distal radius BMD measurement.[46,47] Patients with bilateral hip replacements or other instrumentation, severe hip osteoarthritis, or patients who exceed the weight limit of the table are also candidates. Finally, a forearm BMD measurement is useful in patients with hyperparathyroidism, where cortical bone loss exceeds trabecular bone loss, because the midradius region of interest contains mostly cortical bone.[46,47]

Lateral spine measurement is less influenced by degenerative changes than the PA spine. Drawbacks are the frequent overlap of the L2 vertebral body by ribs and the L4 vertebral body by the pelvis. Using lateral spine BMD for diagnosis of osteoporosis is not recommended.[46,47] Lateral scans have been adapted for lateral vertebral assessment (LVA™) or instantaneous vertebral assessment (IVA™) to detect vertebral fractures rather than measure BMD.

How Are DXA Results Expressed?

Although DXA printouts vary according to the manufacturer and software version, common features include summary of patient demographics, image of the skeletal site scanned, a plot of patient age versus BMD, and numerical results. The presentation of numerical results is usually configurable by the DXA operator. Typically, the BMD values in g/cm^2, T-scores, Z-scores, and other data (e.g., BMC, area, %BMD, vertebral height) for various regions of interest are presented. These results help clinicians to diagnose osteoporosis, assess risk of fracture, select patients for pharmacologic therapy, and monitor that therapy.

Diagnosis of Osteoporosis with DXA

In most cases, the diagnosis of osteoporosis is made according to the T-score, a standardized score that is unique to bone densitometry. T-scores are calculated by subtracting mean BMD of a young-normal reference population from the subject's measured BMD and dividing by the standard deviation of a young-normal reference population. In postmenopausal Caucasian women, the WHO criteria[28] of osteoporosis, osteopenia, and normal are widely used (Box 6-3).

T-scores rather than absolute BMD values are used to make the diagnosis of osteoporosis in part because different approaches to BMD measurement have been used. Manufacturers use different approaches for producing dual-energy x-rays and detecting them, calibrating the densitometers, and sometimes defining the regions of interest where the BMD is measured. Thus the same BMD value cannot be used for diagnosis of osteoporosis using different devices. The use of a diagnostic threshold based on a T-score enables the same diagnostic criteria to be used regardless of the DXA manufacturer.

BMD measurements are also expressed with a Z-score. The Z-score is calculated similarly to the T-score except that an age matched reference population is used. In postmenopausal women, a low Z-score may be helpful in documenting greater than usual bone loss in comparison with age-matched controls and indicate the need for additional testing (e.g., for hyperparathyroidism). Z-scores are used instead of T-scores in the evaluation of children and some premenopausal women.[47]

BOX 6-3. World Health Organization Criteria

Osteoporosis: T-score ≤ -2.5
Osteopenia: T-score between -1.0 and -2.5
Normal: T-score ≥ -1.0

When using DXA for the diagnosis of osteoporosis, the lower of the T-scores of the PA spine and hip is used.[46,47] In the spine, using the region of interest that includes L1 through L4 is preferred. Only those vertebrae affected by focal structural abnormalities (i.e., fracture, focal degenerative disease, surgery) should be excluded from analysis.

> The lower of the T-scores of the PA spine and hip is used for patient diagnosis. The lower T-score of the femoral neck and total hip regions should be used for diagnosis of the hip status.

In the hip, using the lower T-score of the total hip and femoral neck regions of interest is recommended. Ward's region should not be used to diagnose osteoporosis. Ward's region is a triangular region in the femoral neck that is created by the intersection of tensile, compressive, and intertrochanteric trabecular bundles. On DXA scans, Ward's region is a square that is variably placed (depending on the manufacturer) on the femoral neck. It has high precision error because of its small area.

Diagnostic Pitfalls

When interpreting DXA examinations it is important to check whether correct patient demographics were entered into the DXA computer. Wrong age, gender, and race may influence T-scores or Z-scores.

Disregarding improper scan acquisition or analysis is among the most common pitfalls of interpreting DXA results. It is important to evaluate the DXA image for proper patient positioning, scan analysis, and artifacts. On a properly positioned PA spine scan, the spine is aligned with the long axis of scanner table, both iliac crests are visible, and the scan extends from the middle of L5 to the middle of T12 (Figure 6-1). On a properly positioned hip scan, the femoral shaft is aligned with the long axis of the scanner table, the hip is internally rotated, and the scan includes the ischium and the greater trochanter (Figure 6-2). The lesser trochanter is a posterior structure, and its size is the best sign of the degree of rotation of the proximal femur; the lesser trochanter appears small when the hip is internally rotated. BMD values are affected by the degree of rotation of the proximal femur and the position of the femoral neck region of interest (ROI). On properly positioned forearm scan, the radius and ulna are aligned with the long axis of the scanner table, and their distal ends are visible.

The images should also show correct scan analysis: ROI size and location. On PA spine scans, the vertebral bodies should be numbered correctly (see Figure 6-1). This is especially true in patients with four or six lumbar vertebrae, where numbering should begin at the iliac crest—typically, corresponding to the L4-5 disk space. On hip scans, the femoral neck region must not include the greater trochanter or the ischium (see Figure 6-2). Femoral neck region placement is manufacturer specific; therefore it is important to follow the manufacturer's recommendations. General Electric scanners measure the midportion of the femoral neck, whereas Hologic Inc. scanners measure the base of the femoral neck.

Identification of artifacts on DXA images is especially important because they frequently affect the measured BMD (Box 6-4).[57-61] Artifacts on spine scans may be inherent to the spine or may be due to overlap of structures.

Degenerative disease of the spine may show disk space narrowing, subchondral sclerosis, osteophytosis, or facet hypertrophy (Figure 6-3). All of these changes can result in an increase in the measured BMD.[57,58] When degenerative disease of the spine is limited to several vertebrae, it should be excluded from the ROI used for diagnosis or for monitoring.[46-48]

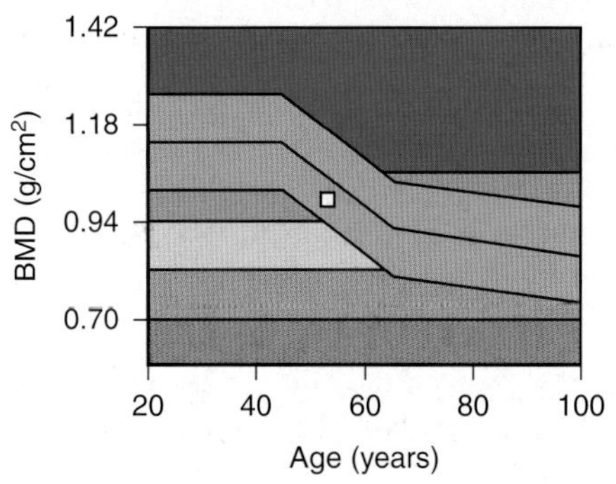

Region	BMD[1] g/cm²	Young-adult[2] %	T	Age-matched[3] %	Z
L1	0.859	76	−2.3	86	−1.1
L2	0.984	82	−1.8	92	−0.7
L3	1.040	87	−1.3	98	−0.2
L4	1.053	88	−1.2	99	−0.1
L1-L4	0.992	84	−1.6	95	−0.5

FIGURE 6-1. Properly positioned PA spine DXA. Note that the spine is positioned centrally, and the iliac crests are included. The vertebrae are correctly numbered.

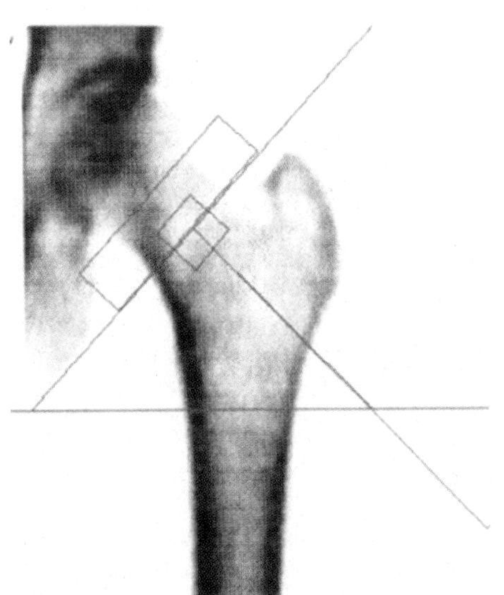

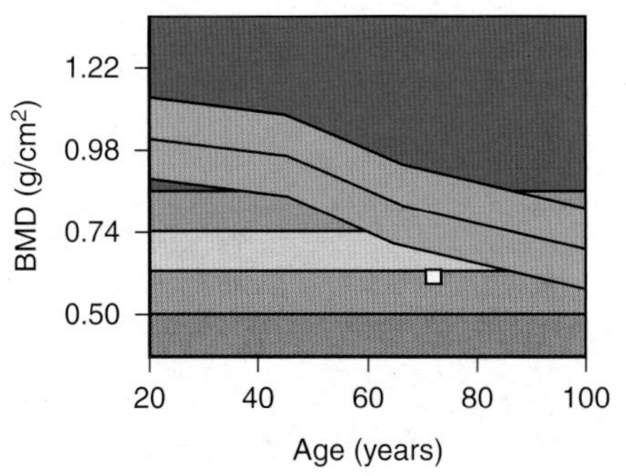

Region	BMD[1] g/cm²	Young-adult[2] %	T	Age-matched[3] %	Z
NECK	0.606	62	−3.1	77	−1.5
WARDS	0.436	48	−3.6	69	−1.5
TROCH	0.390	49	−3.6	56	−2.7
SHAFT	0.721	–	–	–	–
TOTAL	0.570	57	−3.3	68	−2.0

FIGURE 6-2. Properly positioned hip DXA. The hip is internally rotated, making the lesser trochanter inapparent. This positioning optimizes evaluation of the femoral neck. The reference lines and the rectangular femoral neck ROI are shown. The small square is the Ward's triangle ROI.

Severe degenerative disease of the hip may increase measured BMD in the femoral neck or total hip, given buttressing of the medial femoral neck that occurs in this condition. However, the trochanteric region of interest is unaffected by degenerative changes.[59]

Vertebral compression fractures typically also result in an increase in measured BMD (Figure 6-4). Vertebral fractures often appear as having decreased height compared with adjacent vertebrae. Occasionally, the PA spine DXA image will not show a known fracture. In such cases, discrepant BMD values for individual vertebrae may signal the presence of a compression fracture. Comparison with a lateral DXA image or lumbar spine x-ray is necessary to identify such fractures. Fractures must be excluded from the ROI used for scan analysis to prevent overestimation of BMD. Prior vertebroplasty will also falsely increase BMD.

Postsurgical vertebrae should also be excluded from the ROI used. Laminectomy defects usually result in a decrease in the measured BMD (Figure 6-5).

Other artifacts such as vascular calcifications, gallstones, renal stones, pancreatic calcifications (Figure 6-6), gastrointestinal (GI) contrast material (Figure 6-7), and ingested calcium tablets may result in a false increase or decrease in the measured BMD (depending on their location).

External artifacts such as buttons, zippers, bra clips, wallets, and jewelry all result in overestimation or underestimation of BMD. These should be removed before scanning. Patient motion during scan acquisition may increase or decrease measured BMD.

The same pitfalls that potentially confound the diagnosis of osteoporosis using DXA may have adverse effects on other applications of DXA results, including fracture risk assessment, selection of patients for therapy, and monitoring of therapy.

Finally, in making the diagnosis of osteoporosis using DXA, it is essential to recognize that the finding of a low BMD does not explain its etiology. In particular, low BMD in postmenopausal women does not diagnose postmenopausal osteoporosis due to estrogen deficiency, as secondary causes of osteoporosis may be causative. Also, a single low BMD result may evolve in different ways over time. For example, a single low BMD may be due to a low peak BMD in a particular patient followed by a normal rate of loss. Alternatively, a patient may have a normal peak BMD with accelerated rate of bone loss.

BOX 6-4. Artifacts That Affect BMD Measurement

ARTIFACTS THAT MAY INCREASE BMD:

- Degenerative disease
- Fracture
- Vertebroplasty
- Paget disease
- GI contrast
- Abdominal calcifications (e.g., chronic pancreatitis, cholelithiasis, urolithiasis)
- Vascular calcifications
- Patient motion

ARTIFACTS THAT MAY DECREASE BMD:

- Laminectomy
- GI contrast
- Abdominal calcifications (e.g., chronic pancreatitis, cholelithiasis, urolithiasis)
- Vascular calcifications
- Patient motion

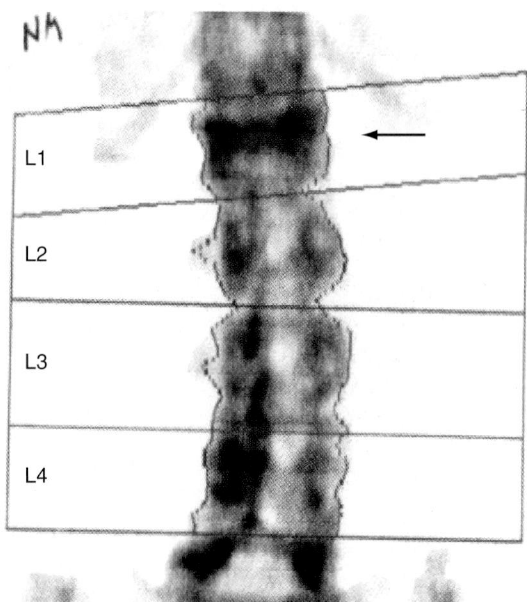

FIGURE 6-4. Vertebral fracture. PA spine DXA shows an L1 vertebral fracture *(arrow)*, which falsely increased BMD. A mild scoliosis is also noted. In this instance, hip evaluation and forearm density may be more useful.

Assessment of Fracture Risk

Epidemiologic trials[3] have shown that for each standard deviation decrease in BMD there is a 1.5- to threefold increase in risk of fracture. However, in clinical practice, it is difficult to assign numerical fracture risk to an individual patient. In particular, for younger women, non-Caucasian individuals, patients with secondary osteoporosis, and patients on therapy, the relationship between BMD and fracture risk is not known.

In all patients, non-BMD risk factors contribute substantially to overall fracture risk. Age is a powerful predictor of fracture risk: an 80 year old with a T-score of −3 has a much greater risk for fracture than a 60 year old with the same T-score. Similarly, history of previous fracture further increases fracture risk, regardless of BMD level.

In deciding an individual patient's prognosis, clinicians must be able to assess these and other non-BMD risk factors (e.g., family history, smoking, low weight). Careful history should provide clinicians with information that can be used in combination with BMD to help determine an individual's risk of fracture.

Selection of Patients for Therapy

Clinicians commonly use the results of DXA examinations to decide which patients should be offered pharmacologic therapy. Using BMD thresholds to help select patients for therapy is recommended by many organizations including the NOF,[29] which recommends pharmacologic therapy in patients with T-scores below −2. Such an approach is appropriate because evidence for fracture reduction exists mainly in subjects enrolled in pharmaceutical trials based on the presence of low BMD or the presence of a vertebral fracture.

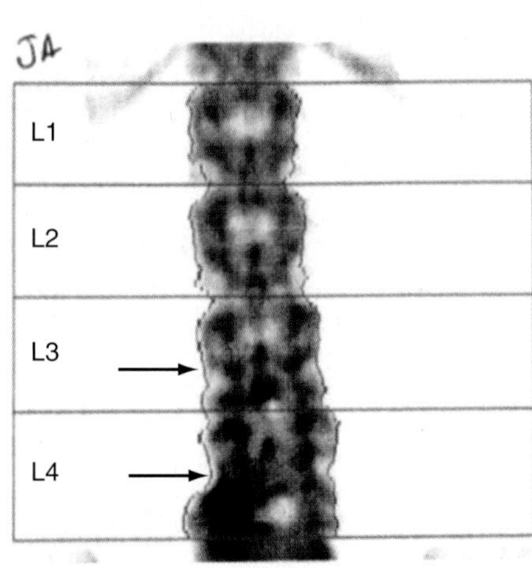

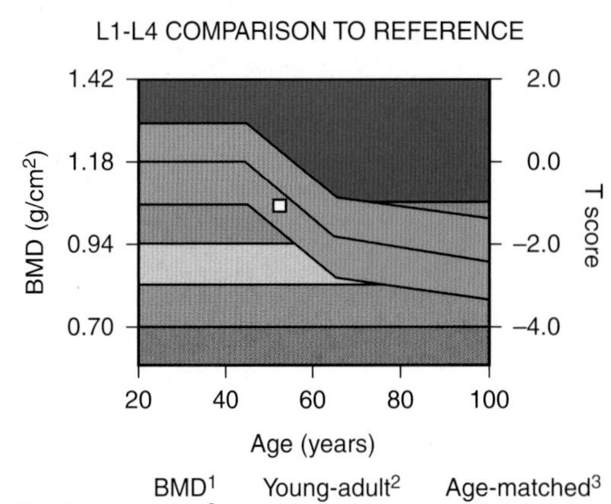

Region	BMD[1] g/cm²	Young-adult[2] %	Young-adult[2] T	Age-matched[3] %	Age-matched[3] Z
L1	0.858	76	−2.3	83	−1.5
L2	0.891	74	−2.6	80	−1.8
L3	1.080	90	−1.0	98	−0.2
L4	1.241	103	0.3	112	1.1
L1-L4	1.047	89	−1.1	96	−0.3

FIGURE 6-3. Degenerative changes. PA spine DXA shows degenerative changes involving the L3 and L4 vertebrae, which falsely increase BMD. These areas should be excluded from analysis.

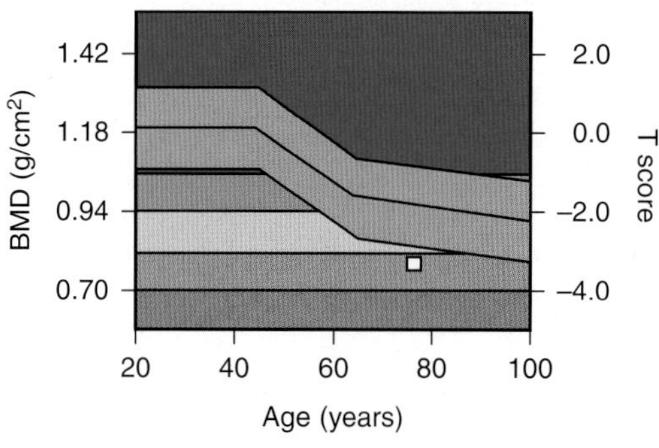

Region	BMD[1] g/cm²	Young-adult[2] %	Young-adult[2] T	Age-matched[3] %	Age-matched[3] Z
L1	0.807	71	−2.7	90	−0.8
L2	0.881	73	−2.7	91	−0.7
L3	0.852	71	−2.9	88	−1.0
L4	0.643	54	−4.6	66	−2.7
L1-L4	0.785	67	−3.3	83	−1.4

FIGURE 6-5. Laminectomy. PA spine DXA shows L4 laminectomy, which falsely decreased BMD.

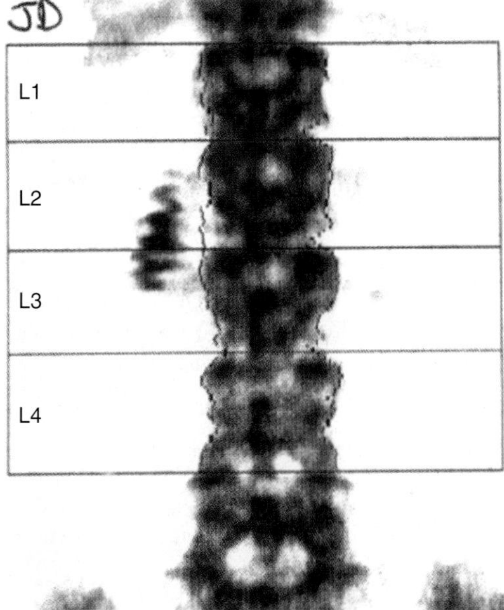

FIGURE 6-6. Pancreatic calcification. PA spine DXA shows pancreatic calcifications, which falsely increased BMD. This patient has six lumbar-type vertebrae. Designating the L4-5 level at the tip of the iliac crest would have moved the analyzed levels down by one inferiority (what is now L1 would be L2), which is the preferred method of analysis.

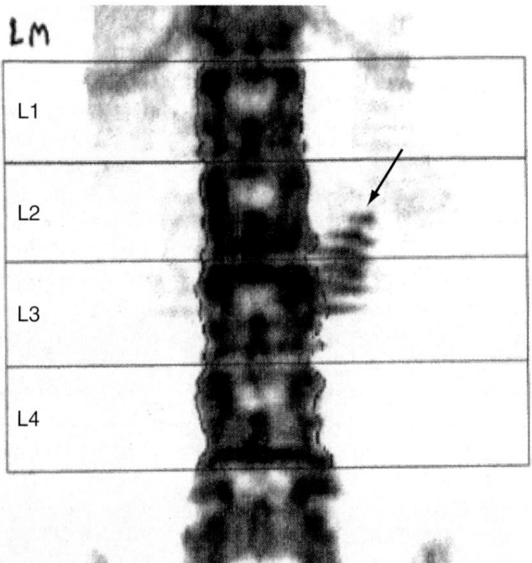

FIGURE 6-7. Artifact from retained contrast. PA spine DXA shows GI contrast, which falsely decreased BMD. Scan repeated 2 days later showed no residual contrast. T-score at L1-4 increased from −2.5 to −2.2.

The WHO is in the process of publishing 10-year risk of fracture data that will be used as thresholds for treatment instead of the current T-score–based thresholds.[62] These new thresholds will be based on femoral neck BMD, age, gender, race, family history, and other non-BMD risk factors. The revised approach should result in better targeting of pharmacologic therapy to high-risk populations.

Monitoring of Therapy

Monitoring of therapy using BMD measurements is possible as long as the devices used have low precision errors and measure skeletal sites that respond well to therapy.[48,63] Due to excellent precision and greatest responses to therapy, measurement of the spine BMD with DXA is preferable to other measurement sites.

When monitoring patients with DXA it is important that follow-up scans show consistent patient positioning and scan analysis.[48] DXA images on the two comparison studies should be inspected to make sure the ROI is the same size and position. If the measured area differs by more than 5%, the ROI should be reexamined for improper positioning, incorrect scan analysis, or artifacts (e.g., fractures, degenerative changes) that may explain the difference.

When monitoring patients, BMD values rather than T-scores should be compared because the T-scores depend on a normative database that may change with software upgrades.[48] To find out whether a change in BMD is significant, each center should determine the precision error of its equipment and then calculate the least significant change (LSC), which equals the precision error × 2.77. A change in absolute BMD greater than the LSC constitutes a significant change.

WHO Controversy

Although the WHO diagnostic criteria are appropriate for DXA measurement at certain skeletal sites (PA spine, proximal femur, and midradius), the diagnostic criteria for other skeletal sites (lateral spine, heel, phalanges) are controversial.[46,47] Also, although the WHO criteria are commonly applied to premenopausal women, men, and non-Caucasian individuals, such an approach is not universally accepted.[47,64] The peak bone mass and the change in BMD with aging and disease vary between the sexes and among ethnic groups.[65-67]

The WHO diagnostic criteria have several other important limitations. The use of any threshold for diagnosing osteoporosis may be misleading. The fact that any diagnostic threshold may be confused with a "fracture threshold" is problematic because the relationship between decreasing BMD and increasing risk of fracture is continuous rather than threshold based.[3] Because of great overlap in BMD among patients with and without fracture, it is impossible to define a threshold BMD value for a population below which everyone will experience fracture or above which no one will experience fracture. It is more appropriate to consider osteoporosis as a continuum of BMD, with the patients with the lowest BMD values having the greatest risk of fracture.

In the current health care environment in the United States, disease *risk* is not interchangeable for the *diagnosis* of a disease. Usually, a defined level of disease risk is linked with a particular diagnosis. Various threshold-based diagnostic approaches are used for hypertension, hypercholesterolemia, and type 2 diabetes, where similar continuous relationships between measured and outcome variables exist.

The T-score approach to diagnosis is also problematic because T-scores are dependent on an "appropriate" reference database. However, there is poor agreement among reference databases of different manufacturers and between reference data from various study populations.[68-70] Different manufacturers may use different inclusion and exclusion criteria when gathering normative data. Also, the same manufacturer may use different reference populations at different skeletal sites and ROIs. If the standard deviations are different, the resultant T-scores are different, even when the mean BMD values for two normative populations are the same.[69] For these reasons, the same patient measured on different devices is likely to have different T-scores.

Finally, the T-score approach to diagnosis does not adequately account for the discordance among skeletal sites and regions of interest. In fact, patterns of bone loss vary according to skeletal site and region. Using the same T-score cutoff for the same skeletal site (e.g., total hip, femoral neck, trochanter) identifies different populations of patients with different risk of fracture.[70]

The use of T-scores has been widely debated. In the next few years, T-scores will be abandoned in favor of an intervention threshold based on 10-year risk of fracture. However, the use of T-scores for the diagnosis of osteoporosis is likely to continue.

DOSE CONSIDERATIONS

Although DXA is a safe examination, clinicians should be aware that it uses radiation, which has associated risks. The radiation dose with DXA is approximately 1 to 5 mSv.[27] The dose is approximately one tenth of that of a chest x-ray.

> The radiation dose with DXA is approximately 1 to 5 mSv, approximately one tenth that of a chest x-ray.

There is a very small risk of radiation-induced carcinoma. The risk exists with any amount of ionizing radiation (no threshold dose) but increases as the dose increases. The risk of radiation induced cancer for a 30-year-old woman having one DXA examination has been estimated as 1 in 16 million.

SAFETY ISSUES

There are no major safety issues with DXA. The examinations are typically quick and comfortable for the patient. The patient lies on the scanner table during scan acquisition. Positioning aids may be used to elevate or rotate the legs. The examination time is between 5 and 30 minutes depending on the type of equipment and the number of skeletal sites that are scanned.

CONTRAINDICATIONS

DXA should not be performed if the potential risks of the examination outweigh its benefits. In particular, if the results would not influence patient management, then the DXA study should not be performed.

Relative contraindications include pregnancy (potential risk from ionizing radiation to the fetus outweighs the benefit of the examination), recent GI contrast (contrast in soft tissues invalidates the BMD result), an obese patient (DXA scanner tables have a weight limit of 250 to 450 lb), and an uncooperative patient.

SUMMARY

DXA is considered the gold standard for measuring BMD in clinical practice. Current diagnostic criteria for osteoporosis and treatment guidelines for osteoporosis are based on central DXA. Interpretation of DXA scans requires a systematic approach. Once proper patient positioning has been ensured and artifacts have been excluded, diagnosis is made using the lowest T-score of the total spine, total hip, and femoral neck. Monitoring is performed using absolute BMD compared with the least significant change, ensuring the regions of interest are comparable in size and position.

Although there are no major safety issues with DXA and the radiation dose is low, DXA examinations should only be performed if the results are likely to influence patient management.

REFERENCES

1. Genant HK, Engelke K, Fuerst T et al: Noninvasive assessment of bone mineral and structure: state of the art, *J Bone Miner Res* 11:707-730, 1996.
2. Glüer CC: Quantitative ultrasound techniques for the assessment of osteoporosis: expert agreement on current status. The International Quantitative Ultrasound Consensus Group, *J Bone Miner Res* 12:1280-1288, 1997.
3. National Institutes of Health: *Osteoporosis prevention, diagnosis and therapy. NIH consensus statement* 17:1-45, 2000.
4. American College of Radiology: *ACR practice guideline for the performance of adult dual or single x-ray absorptiometry (DXA/pDXA/SXA),* Reston, VA, 2002, ACR.
5. Marshall D, Johnell O, Wedel H: Meta-analysis of how well measures of bone mineral density predict occurrence of osteoporotic fractures, *Br Med J* 312:1254-1259, 1996.
6. Cummings SR, Black DM, Nevitt MC et al: Bone density at various sites for prediction of hip fractures, *Lancet* 341:72-75, 1993.
7. Melton LJ 3rd, Atkinson EJ, O'Fallon WM et al: Long-term fracture prediction by bone mineral assessed at different skeletal sites, *J Bone Miner Res* 8:1227-1233, 1993.
8. de Laet CE, Van Hout BA, Burger H et al: Hip fracture prediction in elderly men and women: validation in the Rotterdam study, *J Bone Miner Res* 13:1587-1593, 1998.
9. Kroger H, Huopio J, Honkanen R et al: Prediction of fracture risk using axial bone mineral density in a perimenopausal population: a prospective study, *J Bone Miner Res* 10:302-306, 1995.
10. Schott AM, Cormier C, Hans D et al: How hip and whole-body bone mineral density predict hip fracture in elderly women: the EPIDOS Prospective Study, *Osteoporos Int* 8:247-254, 1998.
11. Black DM, Cummings SR, Karpf DB et al: Randomised trial of effect of alendronate on risk of fracture in women with existing vertebral fractures, *Lancet* 348:1535-1541, 1996.
12. Liberman UA, Weiss SR, Broll J et al: Effect of oral alendronate on bone mineral density and the incidence of fractures in postmenopausal osteoporosis, *N Engl J Med* 333:1437-1443, 1995.
13. Cummings SR, Black DM, Thompson DE: Effect of alendronate reduces on risk of fracture in women with low bone density but without vertebral fractures: results from the Fracture Intervention Trial, *J Am Med Assoc* 280:2077-2082, 1998.
14. Orwoll ES, Oviatt SK, McClung MR et al: The rate of bone mineral loss in normal men and the effects of calcium and cholecalciferol supplementation, *Ann Intern Med* 112:29-34, 1990.

15. Saag KG, Emkey R, Schnitzer TJ et al: Alendronate for the prevention and treatment of glucocorticoid-induced osteoporosis, *N Engl J Med* 339:292-299, 1998.
16. Chesnut CH 3rd, Silverman S, Andriano K et al: A randomized trial of nasal spray salmon calcitonin in post-menopausal women with established osteoporosis: the prevent recurrence of osteoporotic fractures study. PROOF Study Group, *Am J Med* 109:267-276, 2000.
17. Dawson-Hughes B, Harris SS, Krall EA et al: Effect of calcium and vitamin D supplementation on bone density in men and women 65 years of age or older, *N Engl J Med* 337:670-676, 1997.
18. Delmas PD, Bjarnason NH, Mitlak BH et al: Effects of raloxifene on bone mineral density, serum cholesterol concentrations, and uterine endometrium in postmenopausal women, *N Engl J Med* 337:1641-1647, 1997.
19. Felson DT, Zhang Y, Hannan MT et al: The effect of postmenopausal estrogen therapy on bone density in elderly women, *N Engl J Med* 329:1141-1146, 1993.
20. Francis RM: The effects of testosterone on osteoporosis in men, *Clin Endocrinol* 50:411-414, 1999.
21. Reginster JY, Adami S, Lakatos P et al: Efficacy and tolerability of once-monthly oral ibandronate in postmenopausal osteoporosis: 2 year results from the MOBILE study, *Ann Rheum Dis* 65:654-661, 2006.
22. McClung MR, Geusens P, Miller PD et al: Effect of risedronate on the risk of hip fracture in elderly women. Hip Intervention Program Study Group, *N Engl J Med* 344:333-340, 2001.
23. Neer RM, Arnaud CD, Zanchetta JR et al: Effect of parathyroid hormone (1-34) on fractures and bone mineral density in postmenopausal women with osteoporosis, *N Engl J Med* 344:1434-1441, 2001.
24. Lilley J, Walters BG, Heath DA et al: In vivo and in vitro precision for bone density measured by dual-energy X-ray absorption, *Osteoporos Int* 1:141-146, 1991.
25. Haddaway MJ, Davie MW, McCall IW: Bone mineral density in healthy normal women and reproducibility of measurements in spine and hip using dual-energy X-ray absorptiometry, *Br J Radiol* 65:213-217, 1992.
26. Sievanen H, Oja P, Vuori I: Precision of dual energy x-ray absorptiometry in determining bone mineral density and content of various skeletal sites, *J Nucl Med* 33:1137-1142, 1992.
27. Lloyd T, Eggli DF, Miller KL et al: Radiation dose from DXA scanning to reproductive tissues of females, *J Clin Densitom* 1:379-383, 1998.
28. World Health Organization: *Assessment of fracture risk and its application to screening for postmenopausal osteoporosis. WHO Technical Report Series*, Geneva, 1994, WHO.
29. National Osteoporosis Foundation. *Osteoporosis: physician's guide to prevention and treatment of osteoporosis*, Washington DC, 2003, NOF.
30. Blake GM, Fogelman I: Technical principles of dual energy x-ray absorptiometry, *Semin Nucl Med* 27:210-228, 1997.
31. Nevill AM, Holder RL, Maffulli N, et al: Adjusting bone mass for differences in projected bone area and other confounding variables: an allometric perspective, *J Bone Miner Res* 17:703-708, 2002.
32. Melton LJ 3rd, Khosla S, Achenbach SJ et al: Effects of body size and skeletal site on the estimated prevalence of osteoporosis in women and men, *Osteoporos Int* 11:977-983, 2000.
33. Taaffe DR, Cauley JA, Danielson M et al: Race and sex effects on the association between muscle strength, soft tissue, and bone mineral density in healthy elders: the Health, Aging, and Body Composition Study, *J Bone Miner Res* 16:1343-1352, 2001.
34. Fieldings KT, Backrach LK, Hudes ML et al: Ethnic differences in bone mass of young women vary with method of assessment, *J Clin Densitom* 5:229-238, 2002.
35. Reid IR, Evans MC, Ames RW: Volumetric bone density of the lumbar spine is related to fat mass but not lean mass in normal postmenopausal women, *Osteoporos Int* 4:362-367, 1994.
36. Martini G, Valenti R, Giovani S et al: Age-related changes in body composition of healthy and osteoporotic women, *Maturitas* 27:25-33, 1997.
37. Nguyen TV, Howard GM, Kelly PJ et al: Bone mass, lean mass, and fat mass: same genes or same environments? *Am J Epidemiol* 147:3-16, 1998.
38. Carter DR, Hayes WC: The compressive behavior of bone as a two-phase porous structure, *J Bone Joint Surg (Am)* 59:954-962, 1977.
39. Gibson LJ: The mechanical behaviour of cancellous bone, *J Biomech* 18:317-328, 1985.
40. Hvid I, Jensen NC, Bunger C et al: Bone mineral assay: its relation to the mechanical strength of cancellous bone, *Eng Med* 14:79-83, 1985.
41. Hvid I, Hansen SL: Trabecular bone strength patterns at the proximal tibial epiphysis, *J Orthop Res* 3:464-472, 1985.
42. Linde F, Hvid I, Pongsoipetch B: Energy absorptive properties of human trabecular bone specimens during axial compression, *J Orthop Res* 7:432-439, 1989.
43. Moro M, Hecker AT, Bouxsein ML et al: Failure load of thoracic vertebrae correlates with lumbar bone mineral density measured by DXA, *Calcif Tissue Int* 56:206-209, 1995.
44. Cheng XG, Nicholson PH, Boonen S et al: Prediction of vertebral strength in vitro by spinal bone densitometry and calcaneal ultrasound, *J Bone Miner* 12:1721-1728, 1997.
45. Eriksson SA, Isberg BO, Lindgren JU: Prediction of vertebral strength by dual photon absorptiometry and quantitative computed tomography, *Calcif Tissue Int* 44:243-250, 1989.
46. Hamdy RC, Petak SM, Lenchik L: Which central dual X-ray absorptiometry skeletal sites and regions of interest should be used to determine the diagnosis of osteoporosis? *J Clin Densitom* 5(Suppl):S11-S18, 2002.
47. The International Society for Clinical Densitometry: *The ISCD's 2005 Updated Official Positions*, 2005. Retrieved March 2, 2007, from http://www.iscd.org/Visitors/positions/OfficialPositionsText.cfm.
48. Lenchik L, Kiebzak GM, Blunt BA: What is the role of serial bone mineral density measurements in patient management? *J Clin Densitom* 5(Suppl):S29-S38, 2002.
49. Kanis JA, Torgerson D, Cooper C: Comparison of the European and USA practice guidelines for Osteoporosis, *Trends Endocrinol Metab* 11:28-32, 2002.
50. Scientific Advisory Board, Osteoporosis Society of Canada: Clinical practice guidelines for the diagnosis and management of osteoporosis, *Can Med Assoc J* 155:1113-1133, 1996.
51. Consensus Statement. The prevention and management of osteoporosis. Australian National consensus conference 1996, *Med J Aust* 167:S1-S15, 1997.
52. Hodgson SF, Watts NB, Bilezikian JP et al: American Association of Clinical Endocrinologists 2001 Medical Guidelines for Clinical Practice for the Prevention and Management of Postmenopausal Osteoporosis, *Endocr Pract* 7:293-312, 2001.
53. American College of Rheumatology Ad Hoc Committee on Glucocorticoid-Induced Osteoporosis: Recommendation for the prevention and treatment of glucocorticoid-induced osteoporosis: 2001 Update, *Arthritis Rheum* 44:1496-1503, 2001.
54. American Gastroenterological Association: American Gastroenterological Association Medical Position Statement: guidelines on osteoporosis in gastrointestinal diseases, *Gastroenterology* 124:791-794, 2003.
55. Varney LF, Parker RA, Vincelette A et al: Classification of osteoporosis and osteopenia in postmenopausal women is dependent on site-specific analysis, *J Clin Densitom* 3:275-283, 1999.
56. Woodson G: Dual X-ray absorptiometry T score concordance and discordance between the hip and spine measurement sites, *J Clin Densitom* 3:319-324, 2000.
57. Yu W, Gluer CC, Fuerst T et al: Influence of degenerative joint disease on spinal bone mineral measurements in postmenopausal women, *Calcif Tissue Int* 57:169-174, 1995.
58. Drinka PJ, DeSmet AA, Bauwens SF et al: The effect of overlying calcification on lumbar bone densitometry, *Calcif Tissue Int* 50:507-510, 1992.
59. Preidler KW, White LS, Tashkin J et al: Dual-energy X-ray absorptiometric densitometry in osteoarthritis of the hip. Influence of secondary bone remodeling of the femoral neck, *Acta Radiol* 38:539-542, 1997.
60. Akesson K, Gardsell P, Sernbo I et al: Earlier wrist fracture: a confounding factor in distal forearm bone screening, *Osteoporos Int* 2:201-204, 1992.
61. Smith JA, Vento JA, Spencer RP et al: Aortic calcification contributing to bone densitometry measurement, *J Clin Densitom* 2:181-183, 1999.
62. Kanis JA, Johnell O, Oden A et al: Ten year probabilities of osteoporotic fractures according to BMD and diagnostic thresholds, *Osteoporos Int* 12 989-995, 2001.
63. Bonnick SL, Johnston CC Jr, Kleerekoper M et al: Importance of precision in bone density measurements, *J Clin Densitom* 4:105-110, 2001.
64. Binkley NC, Schmeer P, Wasnich RD et al: What are the criteria by which a densitometric diagnosis of osteoporosis can be made in males and non-Caucasians? *J Clin Densitom* 5(Suppl):S19-S27, 2002.
65. Hui SL, Zhou L, Evans R et al: Rates of growth and loss of bone mineral in the spine and femoral neck in white females, *Osteoporos Int* 9:200-205, 1999.
66. Baroncelli GI, Saggese G: Critical ages and stages of puberty in the accumulation of spinal and femoral bone mass: the validity of bone mass measurements, *Horm Res* 54(Suppl 1):2-8, 2000.
67. Yu W, Qin M, Xu L et al: Normal changes in spinal bone mineral density in a Chinese population: assessment by quantitative computed tomography and dual-energy X-ray absorptiometry, *Osteoporos Int* 9:179-187, 1999.
68. Faulkner KG, Roberts LA, McClung MR: Discrepancies in normative data between Lunar and Hologic DXA systems, *Osteoporosis Int* 6:432-436, 1996.
69. Faulkner KG, Von Stetten E, Miller PD: Discordance in patient classification using T scores, *J Clin Densitom* 2: 343-350, 1999.
70. Grampp S, Genant HK, Mathur A et al: Comparisons of noninvasive bone mineral measurements in assessing age-related loss, fracture discrimination, and diagnostic classification, *J Bone Miner Res* 12:697-711, 1997.

CHAPTER 7

Ultrasound

GANDIKOTA GIRISH, MBBS, FRCS(ED), FRCR, *and* JON A. JACOBSON, MD

KEY FACTS

- Ultrasound is now a well-established imaging modality helping early diagnosis and follow-up of rheumatologic disorders.
- Dynamic ultrasound imaging and assessment of vascularity are among the most useful contributions of ultrasound.
- **Color and power Doppler** examination demonstrate subtle intra/periarticular synovial vascularity, which correlate well with the underlying inflammatory activity.
- **High frequency transducers** (7.5-20 MHz) deliver high resolution imaging of superficial structures, a resolution greater than that of magnetic resonance imaging or computed tomography.
- Joint aspiration/injection can be performed more accurately under direct ultrasound guidance.
- **Anisotropy** should not be mistaken for tendinosis. Anisotropy occurs when the sound beam is oblique to the tendon fibers producing an artifactual hypoechoic appearance.
- Diagnostic accuracy of musculoskeletal ultrasound relies heavily on the experience of the sonographer and technology.

HISTORY OF MUSCULOSKELETAL ULTRASOUND IN RHEUMATOLOGY

Since the publication of the first B-scan image of joint in 1972 by Daniel G. McDonald and George R. Leopold[1] for differentiation of Baker's cyst from thrombophlebitis, extensive technical advancements have taken place in the field of diagnostic ultrasound, leading to much improved visualization of soft tissues and more consistent demonstration of abnormalities. Tremendous progress has been made since the first demonstration of synovitis in rheumatoid arthritis (RA) in 1978,[2] which was later followed by the first application of power **Doppler** demonstrating hyperemia in musculoskeletal disease in 1994.[3] Thousands of publications have followed the first report of quantitative ultrasound by K.T. Dussik in 1958,[4] and musculoskeletal (MSK) sonography is now considered by many as an indispensable integral part in the management of inflammatory arthritis.

IMAGING PRINCIPLES

Ultrasound is now a well-established imaging modality that assists in early diagnosis and follow-up of rheumatologic disorders in many leading centers throughout the world. Its popularity results from the distinct advantages it offers when compared with other modalities (Box 7-1). More centers can afford ultrasound machines than magnetic resonance imaging (MRI) machines. Unlike computed tomography (CT), no ionizing radiation is involved, yet ultrasound can deliver multiplanar capability in real time. Often a radiologist lacks clinical history. Ultrasound provides the opportunity to interact with the patient during the examination. This helps in targeted examination generating a focused report. Comparison with the asymptomatic contralateral side is helpful to confirm and assess the extent of subtle findings. Dynamic ultrasound imaging and assessment of vascularity are among the most useful contributions of ultrasound.

When available, MRI remains the gold standard for early diagnosis of rheumatologic disorders. However, many places do not have ready access to MRI, and even when available, it can be expensive. Widespread use of MRI for diagnosis and follow-up may not be practical in many institutions. Ultrasound has an undoubted complementary role in this situation. In the correct hands, it can act as a primary modality in the absence of MRI, both for diagnosis and follow-up. Interaction with the patient is a significant advantage—radiologists are all too aware that the diagnostic accuracy is greatly enhanced by the availability of correct history.

There are, however, many variables in ultrasound imaging. Diagnostic accuracy of MSK ultrasound relies heavily on the experience of the **sonographer** (the ultrasound technologist) and on the technology itself. Among various modalities, ultrasound is shown to have the largest interobserver and intraobserver variation in reproducibility.

> Ultrasound examinations generally are operator dependent.

A long learning curve is a significant limiting factor, as it takes the operator a long time to train and to perform at acceptable standards; more importantly, partial training may reduce the diagnostic yield and accuracy and reflects badly on the outcome of ultrasound studies.

BOX 7-1. Advantages and Disadvantages of Ultrasound Imaging

ADVANTAGES
No ionizing radiation
Real time evaluation
Blood flow assessment
Multiplanar

DISADVANTAGES
Operator dependent
Cannot identify bone marrow edema
Not all areas are accessible to study

Ultrasound has some technical limitations. The most serious technical disadvantage for rheumatologic studies is the inability to identify marrow edema, which is considered by some as pre-erosive change.

> Bone marrow edema may be a pre-erosive change; bone marrow edema cannot be demonstrated on ultrasound but can be documented on MRI examination.

Treatment initiated at this stage could produce long remission without development of erosions.

Terminology and Scanning Planes

An understanding of normal anatomy in **gray scale** is crucial to diagnosing abnormalities.

> In ultrasound imaging, the position and intensities of returning echoes are shown as a two-dimensional image.

Normal echogenicity of various soft tissues should be well understood (Table 7-1). Structures examined under ultrasound can be **hyperechoic, isoechoic, hypoechoic,** or **anechoic** or show mixed echogenicity relative to surrounding tissue. A cystic fluid collection is anechoic with posterior **through-transmission** of sound waves. Compressibility of the lesion suggests fluid content. Similarly, septated cystic collections could represent abscess, hematoma, or seroma. Correlation with history is vital for correct diagnosis.

Tendons and ligaments are generally hyperechoic and show characteristic fibrillar echotexture (Figure 7-1). A tendon affected by tendinosis is hypoechoic. Tendinosis is the preferred term to tendinitis as often there is no histologic evidence of inflammation. Synovial proliferation (synovitis) can be easily demonstrated very early by ultrasound as hypoechoic, isoechoic, or hyperechoic relative to surrounding tissues. However, synovitis is a nonspecific finding and can be seen in all types of inflammatory arthritis including infection. Depending on the location (i.e., site of interest being accessible by probe), early erosions and periosteal reaction can also be easily visualized in most occasions prior to their demonstration on radiographs. An abnormality is traditionally scanned in its longitudinal and transverse planes. Dynamic examination also provides an opportunity to scan in various planes to better define the extent of the pathology and its relation to surrounding anatomy.

Recent Advances in Technology

The role of ultrasound is developing as technology evolves. High-frequency transducers (7.5 to 20 Mhz) deliver high-resolution imaging of superficial structures, a resolution greater than that of MRI or CT. Current ultrasound equipment is already capable of resolving power of less than 0.1 mm, which is not possible by CT or MRI.[5,6] This high resolution is unfortunately at the expense of tissue penetration. Hence the depth of resolution is extremely limited with high-frequency transducers. Musculoskeletal structures being analyzed are mostly superficially located and thus extremely amenable to scanning with high-resolution probes.

> High-resolution scanning uses high-frequency transducers to evaluate superficial structures such as tendons.

Color and power Doppler examinations demonstrate subtle intraarticular/periarticular synovial vascularity, which correlates well with the underlying inflammatory activity.[7,8]

> **Color Doppler** is a technique in which colors superimposed on an image of a blood vessel indicate the speed and direction of blood flow in the vessel. Power Doppler is many times more sensitive in detecting blood flow than color Doppler.

Power Doppler has the ability to differentiate inflammatory arthritis from other types of synovial proliferation.[6] However, ultrasound in general cannot differentiate between aseptic and septic joint effusions.[9] Power Doppler has been shown to be equivalent to contrast-enhanced MRI in the assessment of inflammatory activity.[10]

Intravenous **microbubble** contrast agents significantly increase the sensitivity of detecting tissue vascularity by power Doppler examination. Their use may help quantify inflammatory activity by estimating the signal intensity changes following contrast administration.[11] Their role in rheumatology is evolving. They also have a potential but so far undefined role in drug delivery and release at the target tissue.[12]

Three-dimensional (3D) imaging (sometimes termed *four dimensional* [4D] because of real-time dynamic component) is a result of ongoing new technical advances. Its role is evolving in the general management of the rheumatology patient. Further research is needed to establish its usefulness in clinical practice. In the future there is a potential for 3D imaging of the target tissue to be performed in seconds by somebody with limited training. 3D reconstructions in the desired plane could then be recreated on the workstation similar to other cross-sectional studies.[13] Likely indications for 3D technology include early detection of erosions or enthesitis and better definition of partial tendon tears.[14]

Extended field of view technology associated with development of small and more maneuverable probes further promotes the utility of ultrasound in rheumatology practice. This technology is helpful in defining the extent of an abnormality (e.g., tendon tear, tendinosis), which is greater than the probe size, thereby providing a global perspective.

MUSCULOSKELETAL APPLICATIONS

General Indications of Ultrasound in Rheumatology

Early Diagnosis of Arthritis

Traditionally radiographs have been obtained to look for osseous changes such as erosions, but these are late features of the disease process. Ultrasound is an excellent modality to target symptomatic sites for assessment of early soft tissue changes (hyperemia, synovitis), which invariably precede osseous changes. This helps in early diagnosis and facilitates early treatment. Institution of disease modifying therapy aims to reverse these soft tissue changes, control irreversible tissue damage, and leads to better long-term remission of the disease.

Assessment and Quantification of Inflammatory Activity of Rheumatoid Arthritis

Histologically, activity of synovial proliferation directly correlates with hyperemia detected by Doppler ultrasound.[15,16] It has been shown that highly perfused active pannus leads to erosive change in the adjacent bone.[17] Advancements in Doppler technology make it a realistic possibility to assess microvascular blood flow in synovial proliferation and enthesis inflammation.[7,18,19] In the future, there is a potential for further increase in the sensitivity of Doppler imaging to detect tissue vascularity with the use of ultrasound microbubble contrast agents.[11,20]

TABLE 7-1. Ultrasound Characteristics

	Description	Examples	Illustration
Anechoic	Absence of echoes (dark) on a sonographic image	Simple fluid Cyst	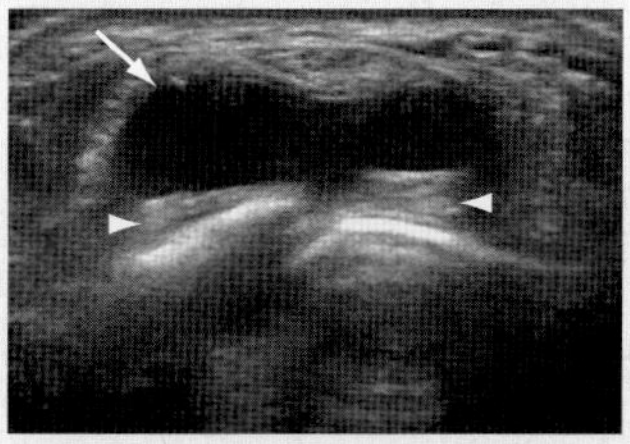 Sonographic image transverse over the dorsal aspect of the scaphoid and lunate bones shows anechoic dorsal wrist ganglion cyst *(arrow)*. Note increased through transmission *(between arrowheads)* deep to the cyst
Hypoechoic	Low-level echoes on a sonographic image	Muscle	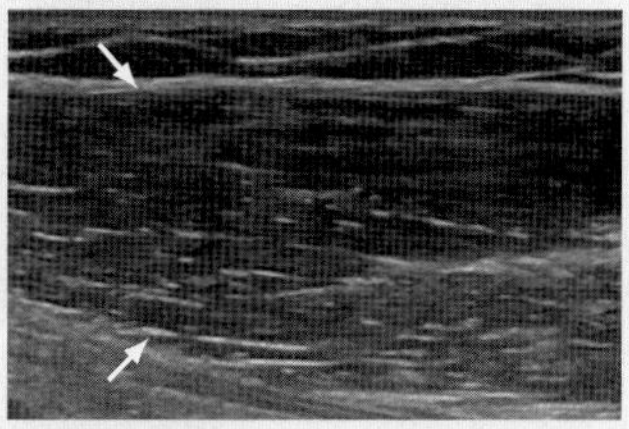 Sonographic image longitudinal to the deltoid muscle *(between arrows)* shows normal hypoechoic muscle with interspersed hyperechoic linear fibroadipose septa
Hyperechoic (Echogenic)	The presence of increased echoes (bright) on a sonographic image	Tendons	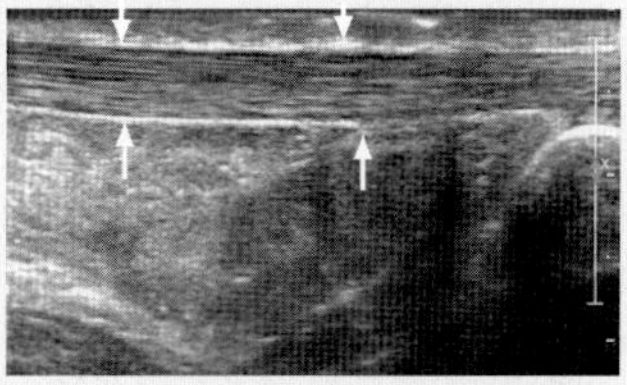 Sonographic image longitudinal to the Achilles tendon *(between arrows)* shows normal hyperechoic and fibrillar tendon echotexture
Posterior enhancement (Through transmission)	A hyperechoic region deep to a fluid-filled structure	Cysts	See Anechoic illustration above
Acoustic shadowing	Anechoic region, indicating absence of sound waves, caused by complete reflection of all waves at an interface of acoustic impedance mismatch	Gallstones Bone	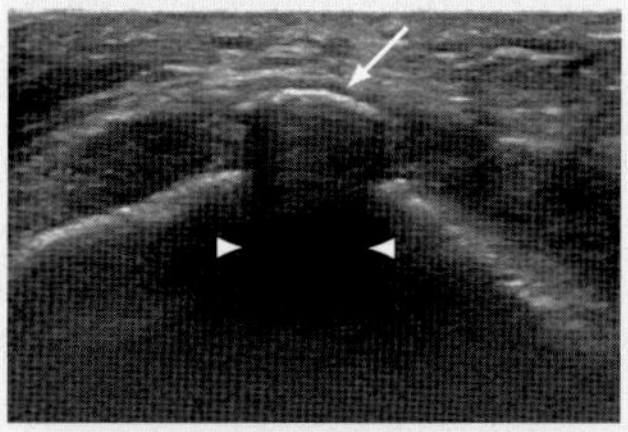 Sonographic image transverse to the superior patellar pole shows hyperechoic avulsion fracture fragment *(arrow)*. Note posterior acoustic shadowing *(between arrowheads)* deep to the bone fragment

Assessment of Response to Treatment

Early and intensive disease-modifying therapy has been advocated to delay and sometimes prevent long-term damage of RA, which includes erosions and fibrosis. The drugs used are strong and can be potentially toxic. To limit its side effects, the drug dose should be balanced with the effectiveness in response. Ultrasound is a very useful tool in monitoring drug effectiveness in response to treatment. Studies have shown that activity of disease is directly proportional to the perfusion.[21-23] Intensity of Doppler signals decreases dramatically with anti-tumor necrosis factor (TNF)-alpha,[24] corticosteroid,[25] and soluble TNF-alpha receptor–etanercept[26] treatment and hence is very useful in monitoring response. Similarly,

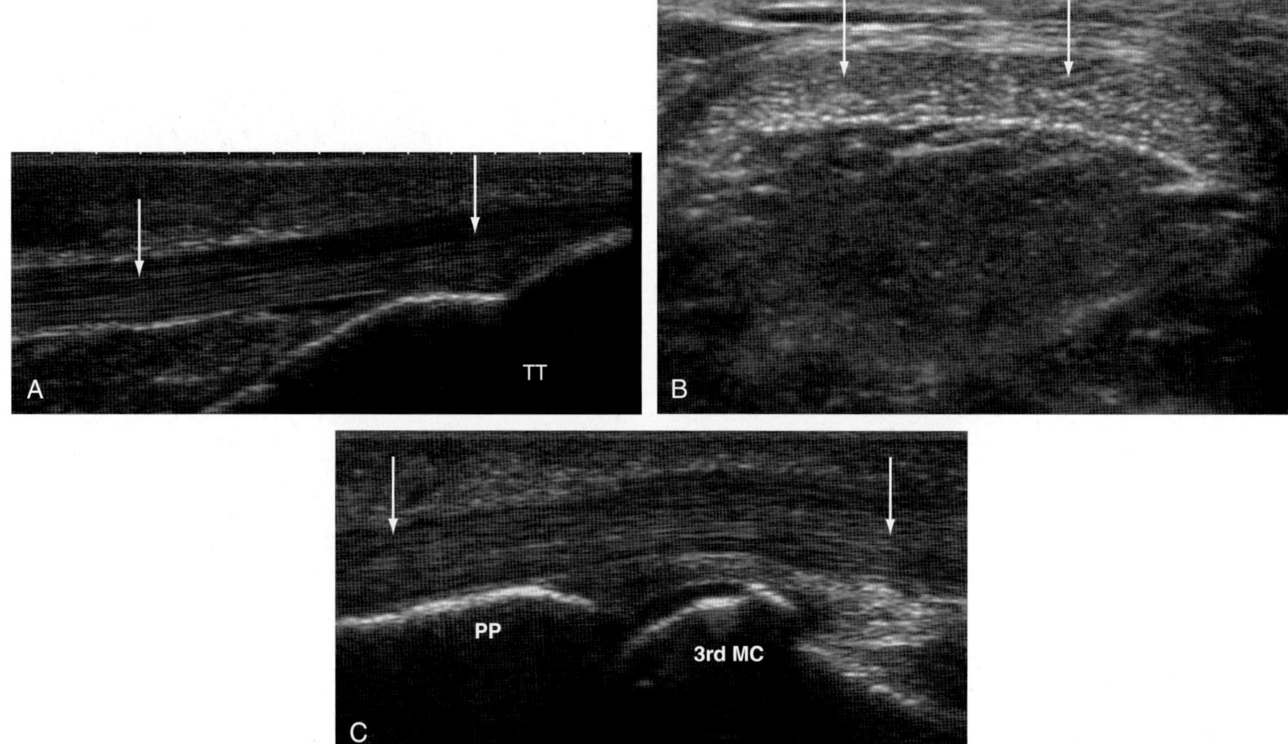

FIGURE 7-1. Normal tendon fibrillar echotexture. **A,** Longitudinal scan over the patellar tendon. *TT,* Tibial tuberosity. **B,** Transverse scan over the patellar tendon (different patient). **C,** Longitudinal scan over the flexor digitorum profundus along the volar aspect of the third finger. *MC,* Metacarpal; *PP,* proximal phalanx. *Arrows* point to the normal linear fibrillar echotexture of these tendons.

contrast-enhanced ultrasound has also shown increased sensitivity in demonstrating synovial vascularity and hence has a strong potential for monitoring therapy.[27]

Invasive Procedure Guidance: Diagnostic and Therapeutic

Ultrasound is very sensitive in detecting fluid collections in joints, tendons, and bursae.[28] It is often better and more consistent than clinical examination in diagnosing subtle joint effusions and therefore is the investigation of choice, potentially significantly affecting patient management.[29,30]

Joint aspiration can be performed under direct ultrasound guidance (generally for the deeper joints or more difficult fluid collections). Using ultrasound only for the purpose of surface marking of the skin can also be followed by aspiration as an alternative. A skin mark is generally placed at the intersection of the two planes (longitudinal and transverse) where the fluid is best visualized; the depth of fluid is maximal and easily accessible while avoiding the neurovascular structures in the needle path. Ultrasound-guided joint aspiration is often two to three times more successful than conventional joint aspiration by a clinician.[31] Intraarticular needle placement is twice as likely to be successful with than without ultrasound guidance.[32] Studies have shown that more than 30% of intended intraarticular injections miss the target when attempted without imaging guidance.[33,34] Despite a dry aspiration attempt following correct needle placement, joint lavage and aspiration can be helpful in small joints for obtaining synovial cells, often essential for the diagnosis of crystal arthropathy.[32,35]

Where possible, therapeutic soft tissue injections should be performed under image guidance, and ultrasound is generally the preferred modality. It has been shown that the desired results are more likely to be obtained by ultrasound guidance, avoiding inadvertent injection of steroids into tendons and fascia, which can result in degeneration and rupture.[36-38] Ultrasound is also very helpful in guiding soft tissue/synovial biopsies and draining abscesses.

Assessment of Long-Term Complications (e.g., Tendon Tears, Tendinosis) and Role in Follow-Up

Ultrasound is a useful modality, is readily available, and is helpful in assessing treatment response of synovitis, resolution of hematoma, abscess formation, and joint effusion. Tendon tears can be reliably assessed and separation of torn tendon ends clearly measured following dynamic examination. Ultrasound follow-up is typically more feasible than MRI and can be equally accurate.

Rheumatoid Arthritis

Ultrasound can be routinely used for early diagnosis, monitoring therapy, and guiding intervention in RA. Early rheumatologic changes such as hyperemia and synovial proliferation are nonosseous in nature and well demonstrated by ultrasound and color Doppler imaging.

> Early changes of synovial proliferation and hyperemia may be demonstrated on ultrasound before bone changes are visible on radiographs.

Early and aggressive treatment of the disease by potent disease-modifying therapy helps delay the progression of the disease and prevent irreversible changes such as erosions and fibrosis.

Joints most commonly involved in early RA and assessed by ultrasound are those of the wrists, hands, and feet. For diagnostic purposes all symptomatic joints can be assessed. Image findings include hyperemia, synovial proliferation, effusion, erosions, tenosynovitis, tendinosis, and tendon tears. All these findings are important for diagnosis but are not specific for RA. Clinical history and pattern of joint involvement are most important in providing definitive diagnosis. RA patients often present with bilaterally symmetric polyarthritis, predominantly involving small joints of the hands.

Hyperemia

Hyperemia is the earliest finding of RA that can be imaged.[39] It signifies ongoing acute inflammation or acute exacerbation of a chronic disease process. Color Doppler ultrasound can detect subtle flow and quantify the vascularity[23,26,40,41] (Figure 7-2). There is high correlation between color Doppler ultrasound and contrast-enhanced MRI for detection of hyperemia and synovitis.[10,42] As previously discussed, this is most useful in assessing the activity of the disease and monitoring response to treatment.

Synovitis

Ultrasound is sensitive in detecting early synovitis, with a limiting factor being accessibility of the joint. Assessment of synovial volume is important, as it directly relates to disease activity. Assessing synovial volume is time consuming and has mostly been performed by MRI. However, with the advent of volumetric imaging in ultrasound, this assessment may become an easier task. Pannus is described as focal mass-like proliferation of synovium of inflammatory origin, ranging from hypoechoic to hyperechoic relative to the surrounding soft tissues (Figure 7-3). Sometimes a conglomeration of focal synovial masses is seen in the late phase of RA, grouped together as extensive pannus formation. Pannus can demonstrate increased vascularity or can be avascular.

Joint Effusion

When joint effusion is seen as a solitary finding, infection should be excluded, as the appearance of fluid is not specific whether due to infection, inflammation, or crystal deposition disease.

> All joint effusion appears similar on ultrasound, with the exception of acute hemorrhage.

Hemorrhage into the joints will also have similar appearance, although acutely it will appear hyperechoic. Ultrasound is very sensitive in detecting joint effusions and is capable of visualizing 2 1 to mL of joint fluid[43,44] (Figure 7-4). In active inflammatory arthritis, effusion often coexists with synovitis.

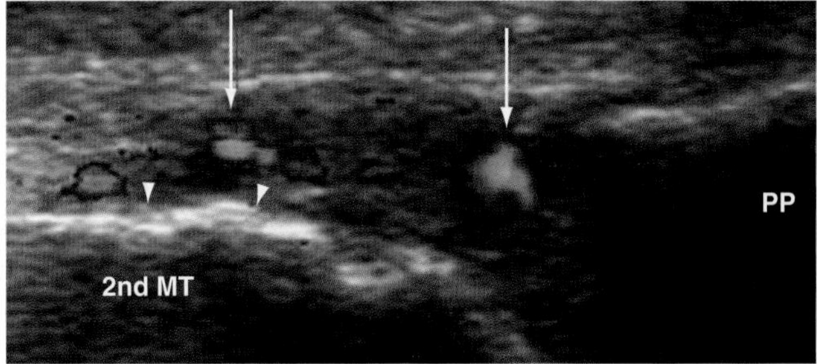

FIGURE 7-2. Hyperemia. Longitudinal scan over the second metatarsophalangeal joint. Arrows demonstrate hypervascularity in the synovial tissue. *MT*, Metatarsal; *PP*, proximal phalanx. The bony structures are outlined by a thin white linear interface *(arrowheads)*.

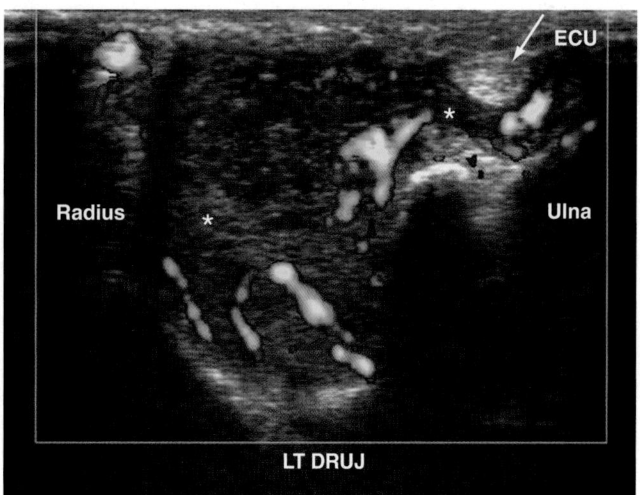

FIGURE 7-3. Extensive synovial proliferation. Transverse scan over the dorsal aspect of the distal radioulnar joint showing extensive synovial proliferation *(asterisks)* and increased vascularity, extending to involve the extensor carpi ulnaris (ECU) tendon sheath.

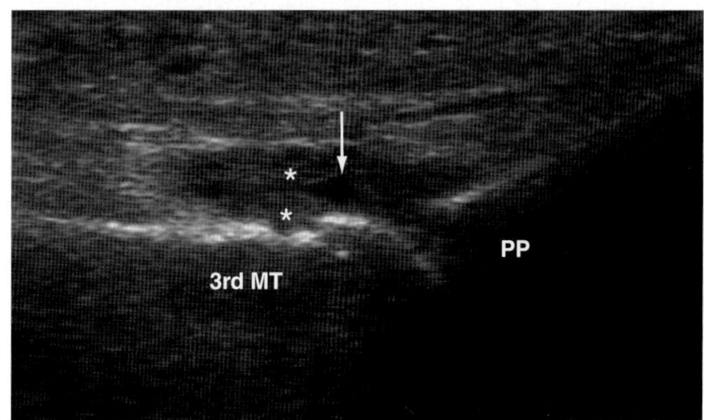

FIGURE 7-4. Early synovitis and joint effusion. Longitudinal scan over the third metatarsophalangeal joint space demonstrating early synovitis *(asterisks)* and anechoic joint effusion *(arrow)*. *MT*, Metatarsal; *PP*, proximal phalanx.

Erosions

Erosions are often associated with synovitis and are generally irreversible. Erosive change is suspected when juxtaarticular cortical irregularity is seen adjacent to synovitis (Figure 7-5). About 47% of patients may develop radiographic evidence of erosions within 1 year of diagnosis.[45] This study was published before the advent of early aggressive combination therapy with disease-modifying antirheumatic drugs (DMARDs), which seems to have significantly influenced the outcome of the disease. In 1999, McQueen et al.[46] reported detecting more carpal erosions by MRI (45%) than by radiography (15%), 4 months after onset of symptoms. Ultrasound can detect and monitor erosions[47] and is more sensitive than radiography and comparable to MRI in assessing finger joint[10,48] and metatarsophalangeal (MTP) joint[49] erosions. In fact, ultrasound is seven times more likely to demonstrate erosions compared with radiography.[50] It is also possible to assess the vascularity adjacent to an erosion, hence demonstrating synovial inflammatory activity.[21,41]

However, ultrasound has significant limitations. It cannot assess marrow edema, considered by many to be a preerosive change. Also it is limited by probe accessibility, being excellent

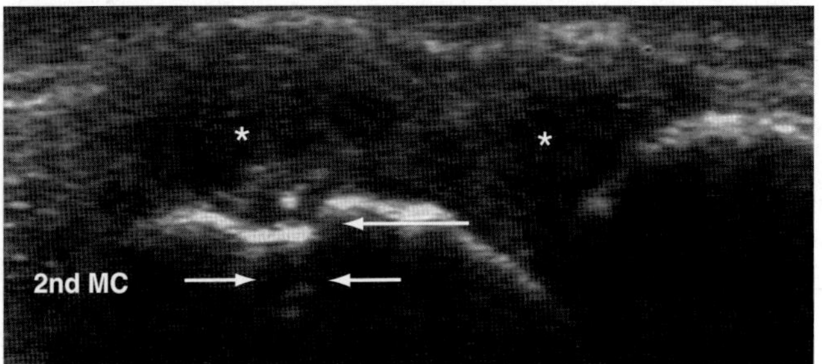

FIGURE 7-5. Erosion. Longitudinal scan over the second MCP joint. Erosion *(long white arrow)* is noted adjacent to synovitis *(asterisks)* along the dorsal aspect of the second metacarpal *(MC)* head. Two short white arrows demonstrate the reverberation artifact that may accompany early erosion.

in assessing joints such as the second and fifth metacarpophalangeal (MCP) joint and the first and fifth MTP joints but more limited in assessing others such as the carpal joints of the wrist.

> The joints of the wrist have limited accessibility to ultrasound examination. MRI would be a more appropriate choice of advanced imaging techniques to identify synovitis or early erosion.

Tenosynovitis, Tendinosis, and Tendon Tear

Ultrasound can be considered a reference standard for assessment of superficial tendons.[39] Tenosynovitis can be a coexistent early finding in RA, especially around the wrist (Figure 7-6). Comparison with an asymptomatic side may help in assessing subtle tenosynovitis; however, because RA is a systemic disease with symmetric involvement and the other asymptomatic side may demonstrate subclinical involvement, comparison may be problematic. Tendinosis and tendon tear are findings generally not seen in acute phase RA. Tendinosis generally results in a hypoechoic tendon with focal increase in volume, sometimes demonstrating increased vascularity (Figure 7-7). Tendon tear is a late complication.

Absence of extensive proliferative bone changes such as enthesitis or periosteal reaction assists in differentiating RA from seronegative arthropathies (e.g., psoriasis, Reiter's syndrome, ankylosing spondylitis). Some of the specific points of individual joint involvement in RA are described in the following section.

Wrist

The tendon sheath of the extensor carpi ulnaris is typically the early site of tenosynovitis in the wrist[39] (Figure 7-8). Early erosive changes seen in the ulnar styloid are partially related to its close proximity to the extensor carpi ulnaris.[39] Tenosynovitis of flexor tendons at the wrist as they pass beneath the flexor retinaculum can result in decrease in the volume of the carpal tunnel, causing carpal tunnel syndrome. Carpal tunnel syndrome can be satisfactorily assessed by ultrasound and later confirmed by invasive nerve conduction studies when needed (Figure 7-9).

> Carpal tunnel syndrome may be evaluated by ultrasound and confirmed by more invasive nerve conduction studies as clinically warranted.

Early synovial proliferation is often seen in the joint recesses as there is space for synovium to proliferate. Recesses are located on the ulnar and radial sides of the joints; the dorsal joint recesses of the radiocarpal and midcarpal joints are also easily accessible. The distal radioulnar joint may also be involved, leading to subluxation

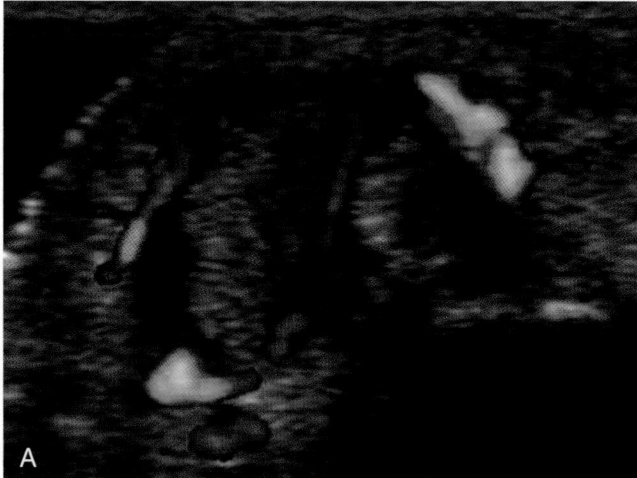

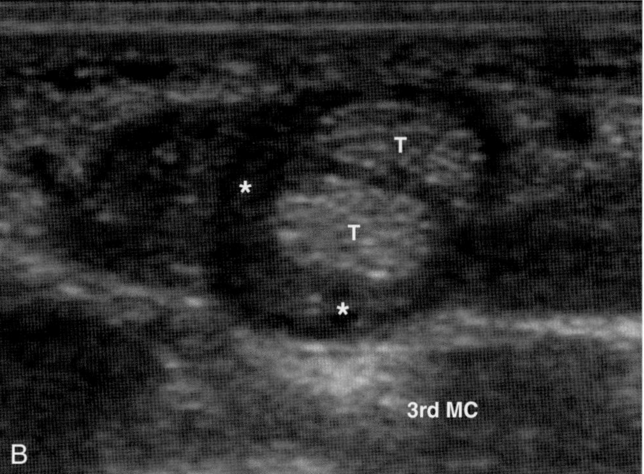

FIGURE 7-6. Tenosynovitis. **A,** Transverse scan over the first extensor compartment tendons. Hypoechogenicity and vascularity are noted in tissue surrounding the first extensor compartment tendons in keeping with tenosynovitis. **B,** Transverse scan over the volar aspect of the third metacarpophalangeal joint (3rd MC) demonstrating thickened hypoechoic rim *(asterisks)* around the flexor tendons *(T)* in keeping with tenosynovitis.

and dislocation in late stages. Intrinsic carpal ligaments (e.g., scapholunate, lunotriquetral) are involved late in the disease process, leading to tear resulting in malalignment of carpal bones. This leads to secondary osteoarthritis changes and may rarely proceed to fusion.

Hands

The second and third MCP and proximal intraphalangeal (PIP) joints typically show the earliest sonographic changes.[39] The thumb MCP joint is a common site for OA changes; hence the specificity of findings is very limited for the diagnosis of inflammatory arthritis. Synovitis and effusion can distend the MCP and interphalangeal joints (Figure 7-10). Tenosynovitis of flexor tendons of the hand may be an early finding in RA that is easily demonstrated by ultrasound. Extensor tendon subluxation may lead to ulnar deviation in the late phase of the disease.

Ankle/Foot

RA typically exhibits bilateral symmetric involvement of predominantly the MTP and PIP joints of the foot. Although all the midfoot joints can be affected, imaging changes of the midfoot are

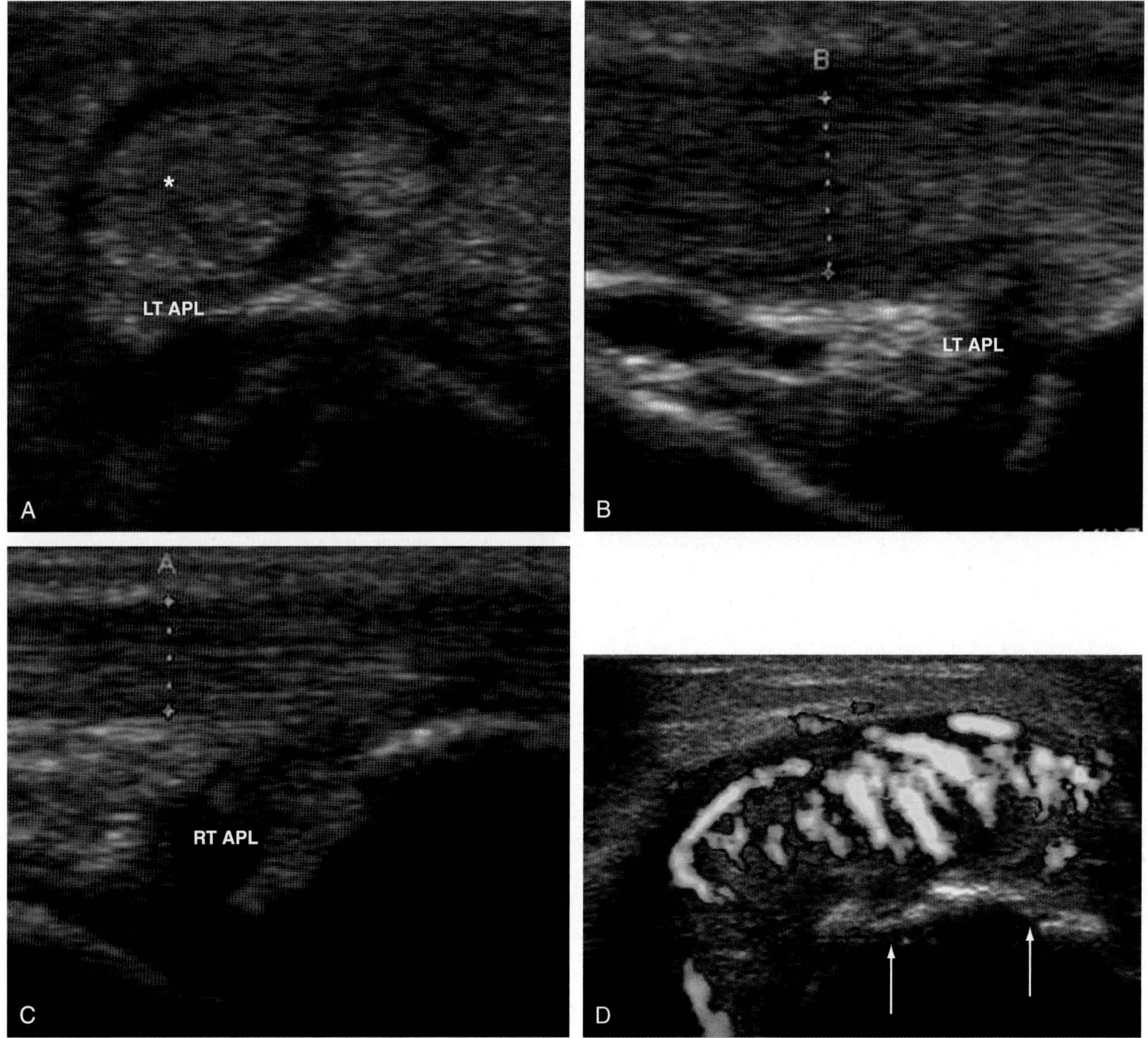

FIGURE 7-7. Tendinosis. Transverse **(A)** and longitudinal **(B)** scan over the abductor pollicis longus *(APL)* tendon of the left wrist demonstrates tendon thickening (asterisk in **A** and dashed line in **B**) and hypoechogenicity in keeping with tendinosis. **C,** Compare this with the normal, thinner, more hyperechoic APL tendon *(dashed line A)* on the asymptomatic right wrist. **D,** Transverse scan over distal triceps showing hypoechogenicity, thickening, and vascularity in keeping with tendinosis. Arrows point to the erosive change in the olecranon process.

more often seen at the talonavicular, subtalar, and tarsometatarsal joints.[51] Accessibility limits ultrasound evaluation of some of the midfoot joints; sometimes the dorsal aspect of the joint is the only accessible portion. Indications for ultrasound at this site include evaluation of soft tissue swelling as is commonly caused by ganglia. However, MTP joints, especially the first and fifth, are well suited for ultrasound assessment. Often the first changes of RA in the foot involve the fifth MTP joint, which is easily accessible to examination by ultrasound probe and hence (when expert musculoskeletal ultrasound is available) should be a part of standard investigation to detect early synovitis and/or erosions.[52] Tendinosis and tenosynovitis changes can be seen in RA involving all the ankle tendons and sinus tarsi. Rupture of the tibialis anterior tendon dorsally is an uncommon but known complication of RA.[53] Tibialis posterior involvement may lead to tendon tear and pes planus deformity.

Acromioclavicular Joint

The acromioclavicular joint can be involved early in the disease process. Synovitis is easy to detect given its superficial nature, and erosions can also be diagnosed early. The deep portion of the joint is not well visualized. Fluid distension of the acromioclavicular joint may present as a soft tissue mass, many times associated with a massive rotator cuff tear, analogous to the arthrographic geyser sign.

> The "geyser sign" is an arthrographic indicator of a rotator cuff tear. It consists of communication between contrast injected into the glenohumeral joint and the acromioclavicular joint. Normally these are separated by the intact rotator cuff. Clinically this sign correlates with the finding of a mass (fluid collection) over the acromioclavicular joint in a patient with a chronic rotator cuff tear.

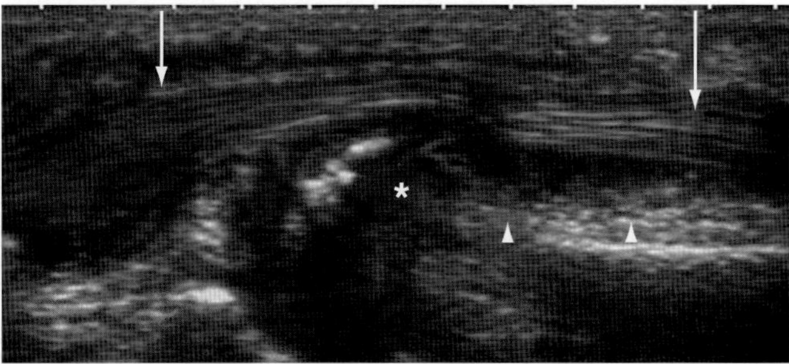

FIGURE 7-8. Longitudinal scan over the flexor carpi ulnaris tendon *(arrows)* showing hypoechoic surrounding tenosynovitis *(arrowheads)* and erosions involving the distal ulna and styloid process *(asterisk)*.

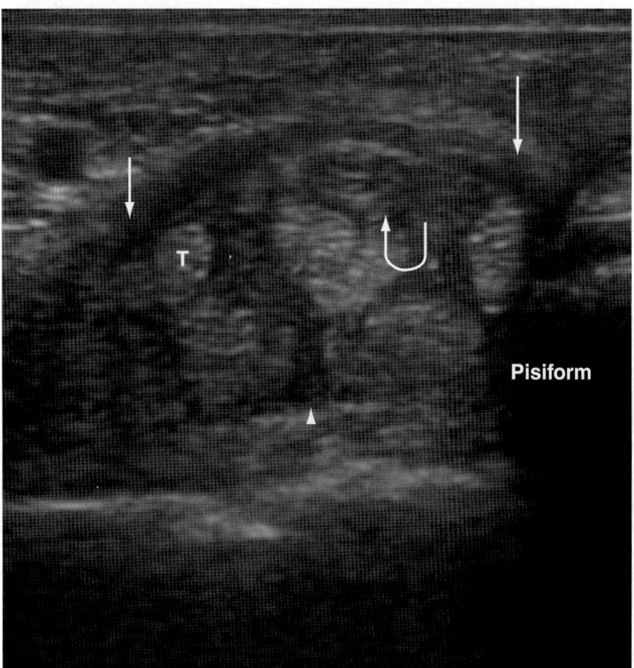

FIGURE 7-9. Flexor tenosynovitis. Transverse scan at the level of the distal crease on the volar aspect of the wrist. Tenosynovitis *(arrowhead)* of the flexor tendons is shown, which has resulted in bowing and thickening of the flexor retinaculum *(straight arrows)*. Curved arrow shows minimally flattened median nerve. This patient had carpal tunnel syndrome. The flexor tendons (one labeled *T*) appear as rounded hyperechoic structures.

Shoulder

Common sonographic findings include biceps tenosynovitis and subacromial-subdeltoid bursitis, both accurately assessed by ultrasound.[39] Biceps tenosynovitis is generally noted in the proximal bicipital groove and is usually focal (located anterior or posterior to the biceps tendon) but is sometimes diffuse, encircling the biceps tendon with fluid. It is best imaged on a transverse scan. Because glenohumeral joint fluid normally communicates with the long head of the biceps brachii tendon sheath, it is important to consider communicating joint effusion as a cause for fluid surrounding the biceps tendon. The presence of focal heterogeneous fluid or synovitis with increased flow on color Doppler imaging suggests tenosynovitis as opposed to communicating joint fluid.

The subacromial-subdeltoid bursa, as the name suggests, is located between the overlying deltoid and acromion and the underlying rotator cuff tendons, and it facilitates normal gliding movement of cuff tendons under the coracoacromial arch with various shoulder movements. Even though thickness of the bursa of more than 2 mm in transverse imaging is considered abnormal, possibly from bursitis, it is the authors' experience that a prominent bursa measuring just less than 2 mm can also be symptomatic, especially if pooling of bursal content is seen on dynamic shoulder extension movements while testing for impingement.

Early glenohumeral joint fluid is usually noted around the biceps tendon in the bicipital groove. A small joint effusion can also be localized in the posterior aspect of the joint. A distance of more than 2 mm between posterior labrum and infraspinatus tendon is indicative of effusion.[54] Often the first erosive change is seen involving the superolateral juxtaarticular surface of the humeral head—a typical ("bare area") location.

Late findings include complete tear and atrophy of rotator cuff tendons with superior migration of the humeral head (Figure 7-11). A large amount of fluid and soft tissue debris is seen in the subacromial-subdeltoid bursa, which communicates with the glenohumeral joint given the full-thickness tear of the rotator cuff tendons. Extensive cortical irregularity involving the lesser and greater tuberosities brings about loss of normal bony landmarks, sometimes making a scan difficult to interpret.

Elbow

Intraarticular synovial proliferation in the elbow joint is not uncommon. Sometimes extensive pannus formation is seen involving the entire elbow joint. Pannus echogenicity is usually mixed, becoming hyperechoic in the late stage of the disease. This may

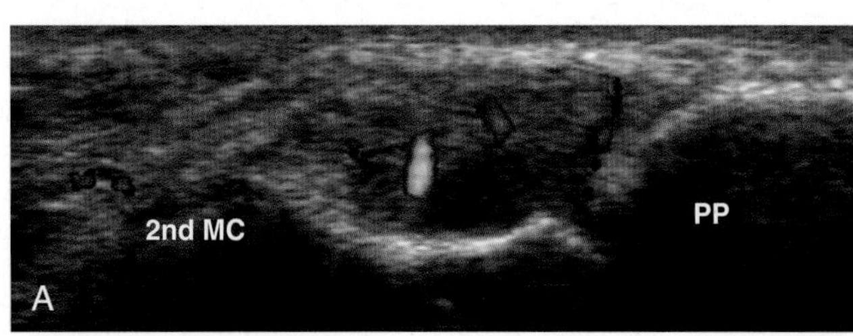

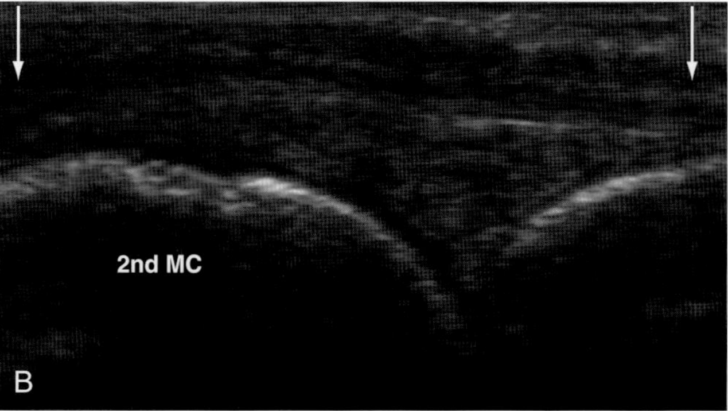

FIGURE 7-10. Joint recess. **A,** Early synovitis is demonstrated in the joint recesses located on the radial or ulnar side of the midline. Compare this with the longitudinal scan in the midline **(B)**, which fails to show synovitis. Arrows point to the extensor tendon overlying the midline of the dorsal aspect of the second metacarpophalangeal joint. Note the rounded contour of the metacarpal head in **B** in comparison with **A** *MC,* Metacarpal head.

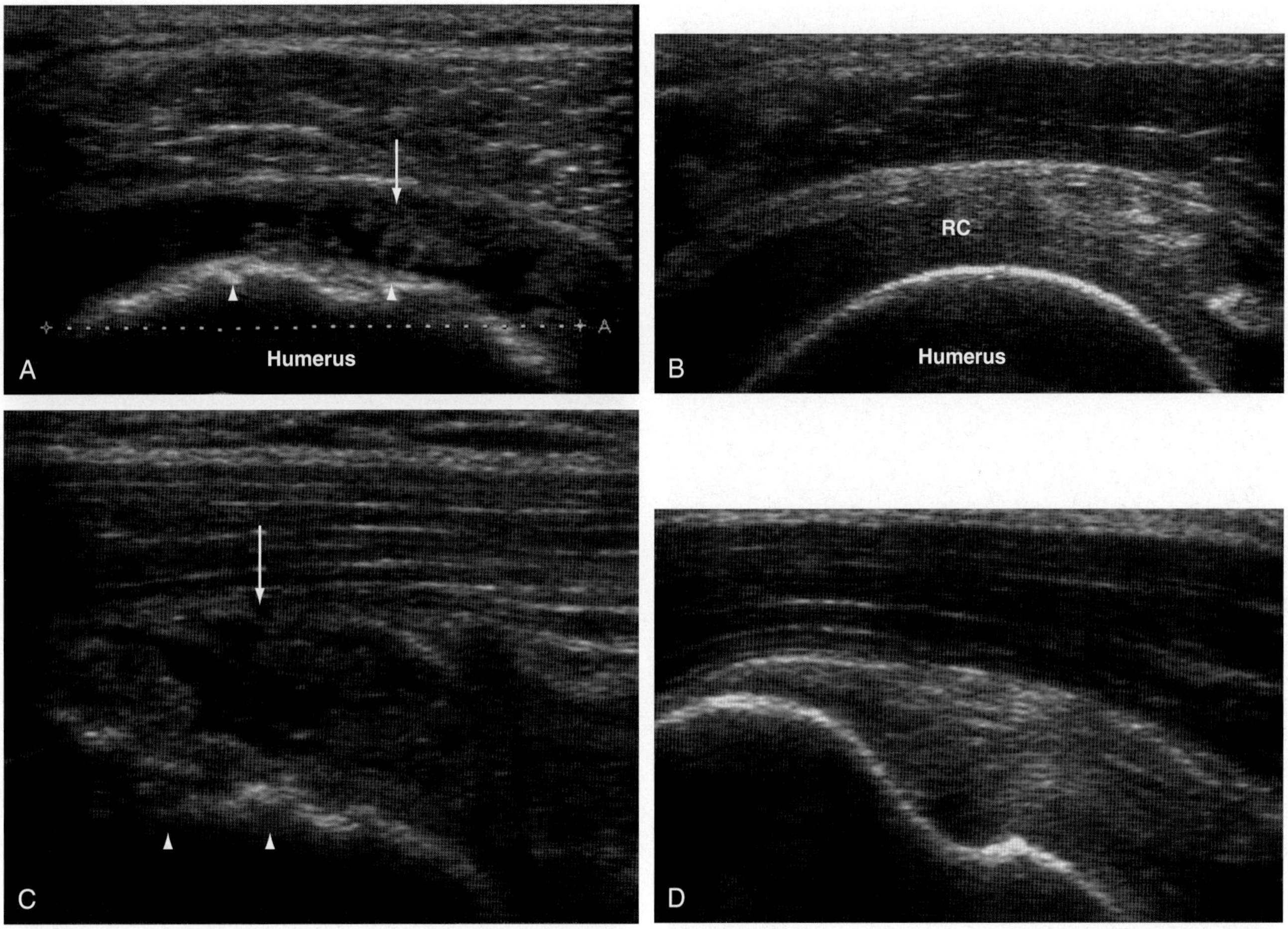

FIGURE 7-11. Complete rotator cuff tear. **A,** Transverse scan over the rotator cuff tendons shows complete rotator cuff tear. **B,** Normal transverse scan for comparison. **C,** Longitudinal scan over the supraspinatus tendon showing a full-thickness tear of the supraspinatus tendon. **D,** Normal longitudinal scan for comparison. The defect in the torn tendon is filled with fluid and residual synovitis *(arrows)*. Note also the bony erosions *(arrowheads)*.

relate to the concentration of fibrin and extravascular coagulation that is known to occur in RA.[55,56] The olecranon bursa is another common site for synovial proliferation and pannus formation late in the disease (Figure 7-12). Gout is considered in the differential diagnosis.

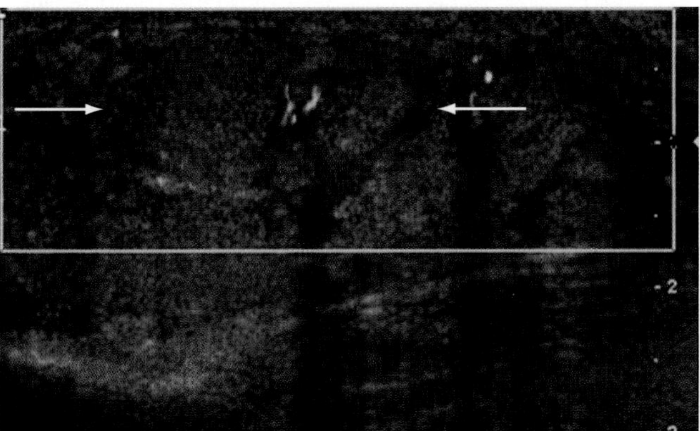

FIGURE 7-12. Olecranon bursitis. Longitudinal scan over the posterior aspect of the olecranon. Mixed echogenic mass similar to synovial proliferation *(arrows)* is demonstrated.

Knee

Ultrasound can detect subtle joint effusion, synovitis. and erosions. Ultrasound is the investigation of choice in the diagnosis of a Baker's cyst (popliteal cyst) and assessment of its intrinsic characteristics (Figure 7-13). Baker's cyst is usually seen in osteoarthritis but can also be found in any condition that causes increased joint fluid or synovitis, such as inflammatory arthritis.

> Ultrasound can identify a popliteal cyst and differentiate it from thrombophlebitis. It cannot demonstrate internal derangement of the knee, such as a meniscal tear, which may be the cause of a popliteal cyst.

Seronegative Spondyloarthritis

Types of seronegative spondyloarthritis include ankylosing spondylitis, psoriatic arthritis, and Reiter's syndrome. Ultrasound is useful in these conditions as it is more sensitive in detecting peripheral enthesitis than is clinical examination,[57,58] and enthesitis is more commonly seen in seronegative spondyloarthropathy than in RA.[18]

> *Enthesitis* refers to inflammation at ligament or tendon insertions. It is more common in seronegative spondyloarthritis than in RA.

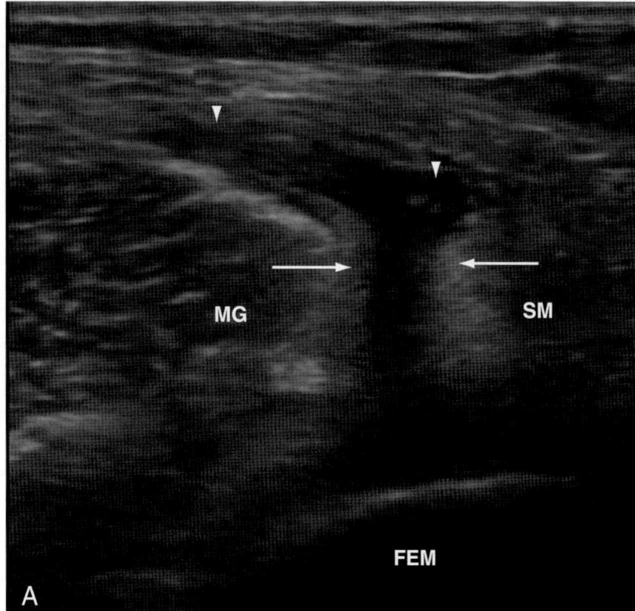

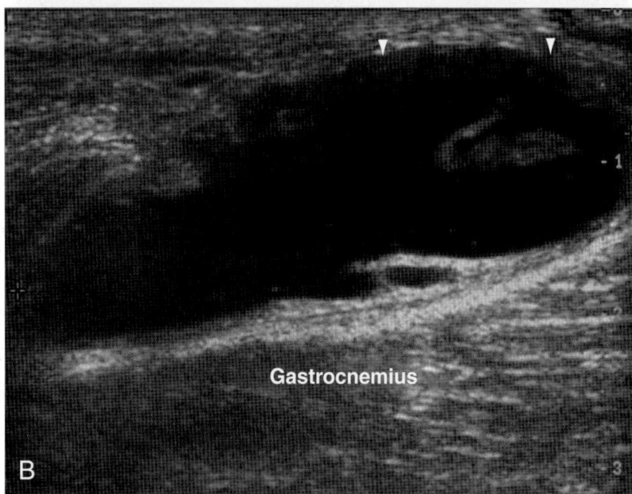

FIGURE 7-13. Baker's cyst. **A,** Transverse scan along the posteromedial aspect of the knee joint showing superficial collection *(arrowheads)* communicating with the deeper joint space via a narrow neck *(arrows)* between the medial head of the gastrocnemius *(MG)* and the semimembranosus *(SM)*. **B,** Longitudinal scan over the posterior aspect of proximal calf showing the inferior extension of the superficial fluid collection—Baker's cyst.

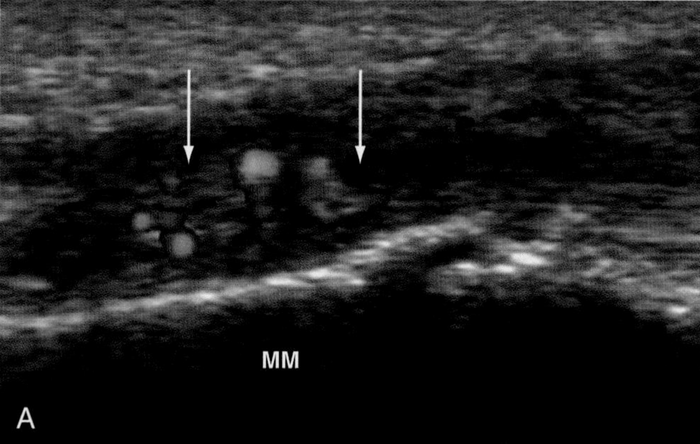

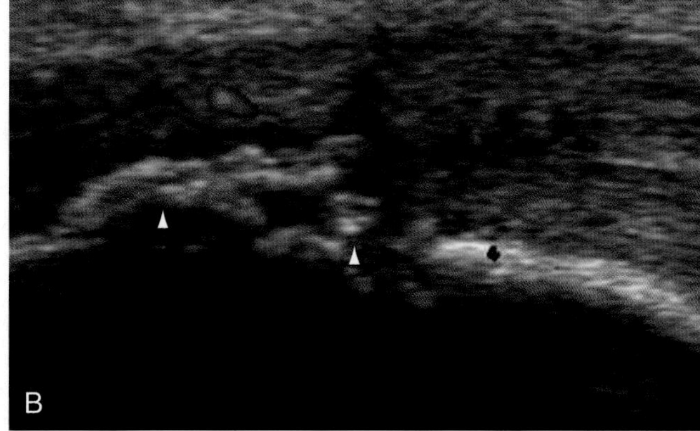

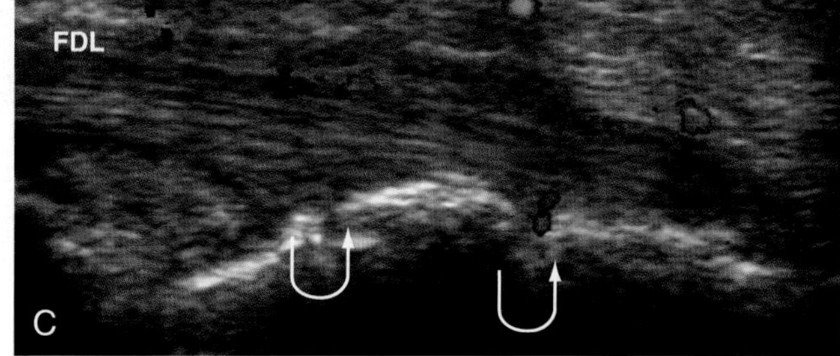

FIGURE 7-14. Seronegative arthritis. **A,** Longitudinal scan over the flexor digitorum longus (FDL) showing tenosynovitis *(straight arrows)* involving the malleolar portion of the FDL. **B,** Bone proliferation *(arrowheads)* is present adjacent to tenosynovitis. **C,** Longitudinal scan at the distal attachment of the FDL shows enthesitis changes *(curved arrows)*.

Ultrasound findings of enthesitis include a hypoechoic tendon at its attachment site, tendon thickening, tendon calcification, and enthesophyte formation.

> An enthesophyte is a bony outgrowth at the site of ligament or tendon insertions; these are seen in the spondyloarthropathies including psoriatic arthritis.

Increased vascularity may also be seen.

Different patterns of joint involvement are seen in seronegative spondyloarthritis compared with RA. Bony proliferation, irregular periosteal reaction, and bony ankylosis are more often encountered in seronegative arthropathies. Ultrasound is helpful in assessing soft tissue and bone changes at the attachment sites of tendons and ligaments, can demonstrate subtle periosteal reaction, and can suggest the presence of bone proliferation (Figure 7-14).

Unlike RA, bone erosion and ill-defined bone proliferation can occur simultaneously in psoriatic arthritis. Intraarticular sonographic changes are nonspecific and similar to those seen in other inflammatory arthritides. The pattern of joint involvement and the more prominent enthesitis are likely to help in differentiating seronegative arthritis from RA. In addition, joint involvement is often asymmetric and may be oligoarticular.

Psoriatic Arthritis

In psoriatic arthritis, the hands are more likely to be involved than the feet. In the hands, distal intraphalangeal (DIP) joints are often the first to be affected and can sometimes be associated with diffuse swelling (dactylitis).

> A diffusely swollen, "sausage" digit may be a manifestation of psoriatic arthritis.

Ultrasound is a reliable method of assessing dactylitis.[59] Common ultrasound findings of dactylitis include flexor tenosynovitis, subcutaneous edema, and tendinosis, with articular synovitis being a less prominent and less frequent early finding. Similarly, in the foot the interphalangeal joint of the first toe is most often affected.[60] Sonographic changes can also be seen in other interphalangeal joints and MTP joints of the feet. Late changes include periosteal reaction, pencil and cup deformity, gross osteolysis progressing to arthritis mutilans, and, in some cases, fusion. Sacroiliac joint involvement (seen in 25% to 75% of cases) is asymmetric and is much more common in psoriatic arthritis than in RA. Color Doppler ultrasound with microbubble contrast agent correlates well with MRI in diagnosing sacroiliitis. Ultrasound is also useful in guiding corticosteroid injections into the synovial portion of the joint.

Inflammatory changes are more frequent at tendon and ligament attachment sites when compared with intraarticular changes.[61] These changes at tendon attachments, termed *enthesitis*, are documented by ultrasound findings including enthesophyte formation, tendinosis often with increased flow,[18] erosive bone changes, and adjacent bursitis. Ultrasound can identify subtle changes of enthesitis at tendon distal attachment sites very early on in the disease process even when the psoriatic patient is clinically asymptomatic.[62] The Achilles' tendon is commonly involved, but the proximal deltoid and quadriceps tendon attachment sites may also be affected (Figure 7-15). Enthesitis of the proximal attachment site of the deltoid presents clinically as impingement syndrome and is a specific finding of psoriasis.[63] This is clinically indistinguishable from rotator cuff pathology but is easily diagnosed by ultrasound.

When the ankle joint is involved in the disease process, common ultrasound findings include ankle tendon tenosynovitis and enthesitis. Joint changes such as effusion and synovial proliferation are not frequently encountered.[57] Enthesophyte formation at the distal Achilles' tendon attachment site on the posterior calcaneus is a nonspecific finding seen in psoriatic arthritis, RA, and osteoarthritis. However, erosions at the enthesophyte attachment site are only seen in inflammatory arthritis such as psoriatic arthritis or RA. Plantar fasciitis is commonly seen in inflammatory arthritis. Focal hypoechoic thickening (4 mm or more) is noted at the proximal attachment site of the plantar fascia on the calcaneus (Figure 7-16).

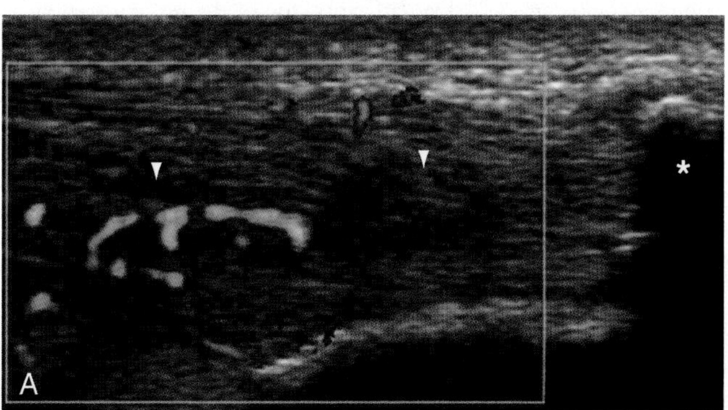

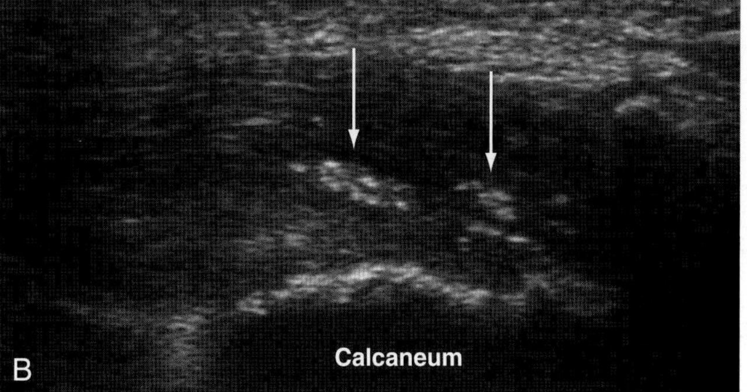

FIGURE 7-15. Achilles' tendon enthesitis. **A, B,** Longitudinal scan over the distal Achilles' tendon attachment site showing tendon thickening, hypoechogenicity *(arrowheads)*, increased vascularity, intratendinous calcification *(arrows)*, and enthesophyte formation *(asterisk)*.

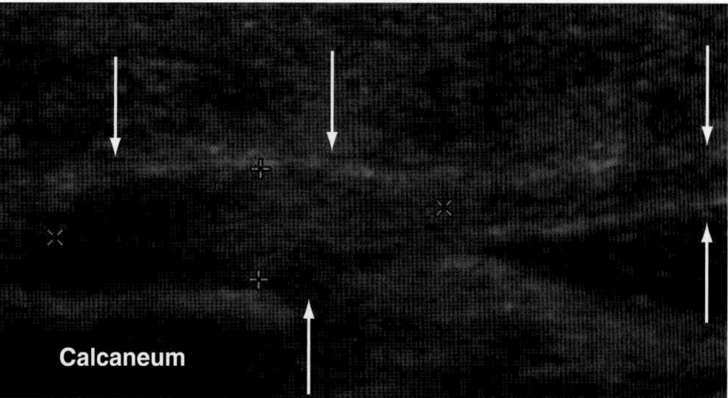

FIGURE 7-16. Plantar fascitis. Longitudinal scan over the plantar aspect of the proximal foot showing thickened plantar fascia *(arrows)* at its attachment site on the calcaneus in keeping with plantar fascitis. The crosshairs mark the area of abnormality.

Ultrasound also appears to be more sensitive than clinical examination in demonstrating psoriatic arthritis changes of the hands and wrists.[64] This challenges the traditional approach for diagnosis and is likely to become a part of the diagnostic process. Psoriatic synovitis of the knee and its response to treatment with anti–TNF-alpha can be reliably assessed by ultrasound.[65]

Crystal Deposition Disease

Crystals implicated in arthritis are calcium pyrophosphate dihydrate (CPPD), hydroxyapatite deposition disease (HADD), and sodium urate monohydrate (gout). When accessible via probe, ultrasound has demonstrated sensitivity and specificity similar to radiography in identifying CPPD crystal deposition.[66] CPPD calcifications show a sparkling appearance and cause posterior acoustic shadowing when they reach the size of 10 mm or more.[66] In contrast, CHAD crystals are generally hypoechoic in nature and cause posterior shadowing at a much smaller size (2 to 3 mm).[67] The knee, wrist, and shoulder are the commonly involved joints. Acute manifestations of crystal deposition disease mimic infection. Redness, tenderness, and swelling are clinical findings of gout or pseudogout attacks or calcific tendinitis. Hematologic laboratory values with joint aspiration and synovial fluid analysis for crystals can help differentiate these. Studies indicate a strong role of CPPD and CHAD in early cartilage degeneration in osteoarthritis.[68,69]

CPPD Crystal Deposition Disease

CPPD crystals are preferentially deposited within the joint (hyaline and fibrocartilage, synovium, and capsule). Cartilage calcification results and is termed *chondrocalcinosis* (Figure 7-17), which can be reliably demonstrated by ultrasound, when the anatomy is accessible by probe.[63] Extraarticular deposition is less common and often occurs in linear fashion. The usual extraarticular sites include the gastrocnemius, quadriceps, triceps tendons, and rotator

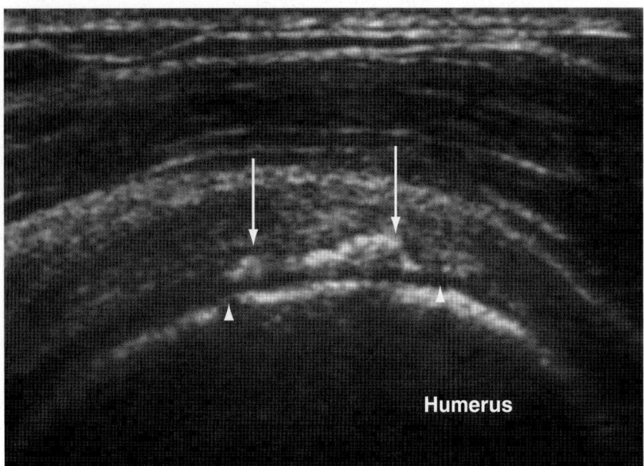

FIGURE 7-17. Calcium pyrophosphate deposition. Transverse scan over the rotator cuff tendons shows hyperechoic focal deposits *(arrows)* overlying the hyaline cartilage *(arrowheads)*. Occasionally, significant posterior acoustic shadowing may not be seen.

cuff. Globular mass-like extraarticular crystal deposition is rare and is a more common finding with hydroxyapatite and urate crystals.

Deposition Disease Hydroxyapatite (HADD)

Hydroxyapatite crystals are preferentially deposited in tendons, a common site being the rotator cuff. Crystal deposition can be asymptomatic. It can also present as acute calcific tendinitis. Some calcifications undergo resorption following an acute episode, whereas some persist and can lead to chronic calcific tendinitis causing chronic bouts of pain, signs of impingement, and focal symptoms. Sonographically acute calcific tendinitis demonstrates significant increase in vascularity, focal echogenic calcifications with shadowing, and tendinosis at the site of maximum tenderness. Chronic calcific tendinitis may not demonstrate increased vascularity but does show organized crystal deposition in the form of larger conglomerate echogenic calcification within the tendon with shadowing. Ultrasound-guided needle aspiration and breakdown of the deposits have been performed with encouraging short-term results.

Gout

Acute gouty attacks (sodium urate monohydrate crystals) are common during spring, whereas pseudogout (CPPD) is more commonly seen during fall and winter.[70] Ultrasound findings are nonspecific and show synovitis sometimes associated with characteristic erosions with an overhanging edge (Figure 7-18). The diagnosis

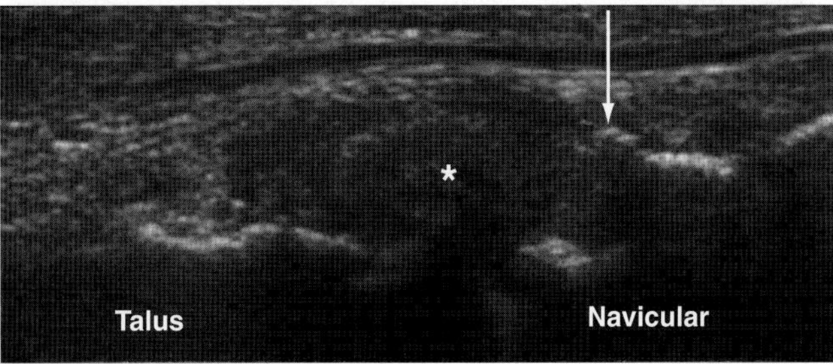

FIGURE 7-18. Gout. Longitudinal scan over dorsal aspect of the talonavicular joint showing synovitis *(asterisk)* and erosion with overhanging edge *(arrow)*.

is based on synovial fluid analysis for crystals. An attack of pseudogout can be triggered by intraarticular injections of hyaluronic acid preparations used in the symptomatic relief of osteoarthritis. Tophaceous gout is known to occur in rotator cuff tendons, the quadriceps tendon, and the mitral cardiac valve.[71-73] The usual location is the medial aspect of the first MTP joint. Olecranon bursitis is a common associated finding.

Osteoarthritis

Osteoarthritis is generally seen in weight-bearing joints, classically involving hip and knee joints and the first carpometacarpal joints of hands. It can be seen in non–weight-bearing joints following trauma or following overuse as the result of sporting activity or occupation. The hallmark of osteoarthritis is osteophytosis; other imaging findings include joint space narrowing, subchondral sclerosis, and subchondral cyst formation. Radiographs still remain the mainstay for diagnosis, as the osseous findings are characteristic. Quantifying cartilage loss using ultrasound can be performed in some large joints such as the femoral condyle of the knee. Thinning of cartilage, loss of normal echogenicity, smudging of cartilage joint space interface, and increased intensity of the cartilage bone interface have all been notable early findings.[74,75] However, sonography may be unreliable when dealing with small joints and joints with underlying cortical irregularity. Obviously the limiting factor of cartilage assessment is probe accessibility. MRI is ideal in demonstrating the entire cartilage and for global assessment, especially of large joints.

Ultrasound and Vasculitis

Ultrasound appearances of large vessel vasculitis are characteristic. Hypoechoic thickened arterial wall with surrounding edema gives rise to a "halo sign."[76] Irregular narrowing of the lumen is an associated finding. One limitation is the presence of wall calcification, which obscures the underlying abnormalities due to shadowing. Ultrasound can complement angiography by helping to assess the walls of accessible arteries. Ongoing research suggests quantification of arterial flow by ultrasound is possible, thus helping the diagnosis of Raynaud's phenomenon. Ultrasound evaluation of the thickness of the intimal layer of vasculature can help differentiate primary and secondary Raynaud's disease.[77,78] Ultrasound assessment of salivary glands in Sjögren's syndrome is helpful in diagnosis.[79,80]

Giant Cell Arteritis

The role of ultrasound in the diagnostic workup of giant cell arteritis is evolving. With the advent of color Doppler ultrasound, the sensitivity of diagnosing giant cell arteritis approaches 100%.[76,81] In the future, ultrasound has the potential to replace temporal artery biopsy for diagnosis. Skip lesions are often encountered in the disease process; hence ultrasound is helpful in guiding biopsy thereby increasing the diagnostic yield.

Scleroderma

Ultrasound appears to have a role in the diagnosis of scleroderma and assessment of its chronicity by evaluation of skin thickness over the forearm and proximal phalanx of the right second finger.[82] Studies have shown that skin thickness of the forearm is inversely proportional to the duration of the disease process. Soft tissue calcifications associated with scleroderma appear as hyperechoic foci with variable posterior acoustic shadowing.

ULTRASOUND PITFALLS

Anisotropy should not be mistaken for tendinosis; anisotropy occurs when the sound beam is oblique to the tendon fibers, producing an artifactual hypoechoic appearance. Another pitfall is that the lack of increased flow on color or power Doppler imaging does not always indicate inactive synovitis. It is hypothesized that increased synovial volume in a tight joint space with stretched capsule may demonstrate a pressure effect, inhibiting the detection of vascularity. Synovial proliferation seen in inflammatory arthritis should be differentiated from less common synovial proliferative disorders, such as pigmented villonodular synovitis and synovial chondromatosis. Intraarticular amyloidosis could have a similar appearance. Cortical contour variation representing the normal physeal plate should not be mistaken for erosion in the small joints of the hand (Table 7-2).

LIMITATIONS

The sonographer and health care provider should recognize ultrasound's long learning curve, which is almost endless given the fast pace of technical advances. To learn and constantly update basic skills is an ongoing challenge. Probably the most serious limitation is the inability of ultrasound to demonstrate marrow edema. Marrow edema is often considered a precursor to erosion, hence a vital finding of early RA, when strong therapy can force the disease process into remission. This limitation is somewhat offset by the increased sensitivity of ultrasound in detecting subclinical synovitis. Also, color and power Doppler examination helps detect hyperemia very early in the process. Synovitis is considered a precursor to marrow edema, which progresses to erosions if not treated. Ultrasound is therefore excellent at detecting the earliest changes of RA, namely hyperemia and synovial proliferation, and is thus very helpful in initiating early disease-modifying therapy. Interobserver variation can be significant because of training issues and lack of universally accepted standardized technique.[83] However, this is changing, and a standardized approach is being formulated.[84,85]

TRAINING ISSUES

Ultrasound is the most operator-dependent modality. New ultrasound machines are like the new generation of racecars: capable of delivering a winning performance, the limiting factor being the capability and skills of the team in charge. Traditionally radiologists have been the medical specialty performing musculoskeletal ultrasound. However, there is often a delay in completing such examinations or decreased interest because of busy radiology departments worldwide. There is much interest among rheumatologists to perform ultrasound scans and possibly rightly so. There are many advantages to this. The ultrasound scan can be performed without any delay as a part of the clinical examination. The scan can be focused based on the clinical needs of the patient and the results correlated with the clinical history. The major problem, however, is to master the scanning technique and image interpretation. Lack of standardized training in the past has led to some misconceptions about this modality and less than optimal results. Recently, attempts are being made to set global standards for best practice. The American College of Radiology recommends a minimum of 3 months of ultrasound training demonstrating involvement in at least 500 ultrasound scans; this figure is also supported by the American Institute of Radiology.[86]

TABLE 7-2. Ultrasound Pitfalls in Musculoskeletal System Evaluation

Pitfall	Explanation
Anisotropy	Artifactual hypoechoic appearance of a tendon due to obliquity of the ultrasound beam
Lack of flow on Doppler imaging may not indicate inactive synovitis	Hypothesized to be due to increased intraarticular pressure
Ultrasound depiction of synovitis may not indicate inflammatory arthritis	Other causes of synovitis, such as amyloidosis, could produce similar findings
Not all bone irregularities are erosions	Normal appearances, especially in the small joints of the hand, may be mistaken for erosions

SUMMARY

It is the opinion of these authors that ultrasound will be indispensable in the assessment of inflammatory arthritis. It is more readily available than MRI in most institutions around the world. There are no dose considerations, as it does not involve ionizing radiation. Hence it is a safe modality with no real contraindications. With the advancement in technology and standardization of training and scanning technique, ultrasound could become the mainstay in diagnosing arthritis and monitoring the response to treatment. It will also have a significant role in guiding intervention.

REFERENCES

1. McDonald DG, Leopold GR: Ultrasound B-scanning in the differentiation of Baker's cyst and thrombophlebitis, *Br J Radiol* 45:729-732, 1972.
2. Cooperberg PL, Tsang I, Truelove L et al: Gray scale ultrasound in the evaluation of rheumatoid arthritis of the knee, *Radiology* 126:759-763, 1978.
3. Newman JS, Adler RS, Bude RO et al: Detection of soft-tissue hyperemia: value of power Doppler sonography, *AJR Am J Roentgenol* 163:385-389, 1994.
4. Dussik KT, Fritch DJ, Kyriazidou M et al: Measurements of articular tissues with ultrasound, *Am J Phys Med* 37:160-165, 1958.
5. Grassi W, Filippucci E, Farina A et al: Sonographic imaging of tendons, *Arthritis Rheum* 43:969-976, 2000.
6. Kane D, Balint PV, Sturrock R et al: Musculoskeletal ultrasound—a state of the art review in rheumatology. Part 1: current controversies and issues in the development of musculoskeletal ultrasound in rheumatology, *Rheumatology (Oxford)* 43:823-828, 2004.
7. Kiris A, Ozgocmen S, Kocakoc E et al: Power Doppler assessment of overall disease activity in patients with rheumatoid arthritis, *J Clin Ultrasound* 34:5-11, 2006.
8. Schmidt WA: Doppler sonography in rheumatology, *Best Pract Res Clin Rheumatol* 18:827-846, 2004.
9. Strouse PJ, DiPietro MA, Teo EL et al: Power Doppler evaluation of joint effusions: investigation in a rabbit model, *Pediatr Radiol* 29:617-623, 1999.
10. Szkudlarek M, Court-Payen M, Strandberg C et al: Power Doppler ultrasonography for assessment of synovitis in the metacarpophalangeal joints of patients with rheumatoid arthritis: a comparison with dynamic magnetic resonance imaging, *Arthritis Rheum* 44:2018-2023, 2001.
11. Szkudlarek M, Court-Payen M, Strandberg C et al: Contrast-enhanced power Doppler ultrasonography of the metacarpophalangeal joints in rheumatoid arthritis, *Eur Radiol* 13:163-168, 2003.
12. Blomley MJ, Cooke JC, Unger EC et al: Microbubble contrast agents: a new era in ultrasound, *Br Med J* 322:1222-1225, 2001.
13. Downey DB, Fenster A, Williams JC: Clinical utility of three-dimensional US, *Radiographics* 20:559-571, 2000.
14. Wallny TA, Schild RL, Schulze Bertelsbeck D et al: Three-dimensional ultrasonography in the diagnosis of rotator cuff lesions, *Ultrasound Med Biol* 27:745-749, 2001.
15. Carotti M, Salaffi F, Manganelli P et al: Power Doppler sonography in the assessment of synovial tissue of the knee joint in rheumatoid arthritis: a preliminary experience, *Ann Rheum Dis* 61:877-882, 2002.
16. Schmidt WA, Volker L, Zacher J et al: Colour Doppler ultrasonography to detect pannus in knee joint synovitis, *Clin Exp Rheumatol* 18:439-444, 2000.
17. Schmidt WA: Value of sonography in diagnosis of rheumatoid arthritis, *Lancet* 357:1056-1057, 2001.

18. D'Agostino MA, Said-Nahal R, Hacquard-Bouder C et al: Assessment of peripheral enthesitis in the spondyloarthropathies by ultrasonography combined with power Doppler: a cross-sectional study, *Arthritis Rheum* 48:523-533, 2003.
19. Wakefield RJ, Brown AK, O'Connor PJ et al: Power Doppler sonography: improving disease activity assessment in inflammatory musculoskeletal disease, *Arthritis Rheum* 48:285-288, 2003.
20. Klauser A, Frauscher F, Schirmer M: Value of contrast-enhanced power Doppler ultrasonography (US) of the metacarpophalangeal joints on rheumatoid arthritis, *Eur Radiol* 14:545-546; author reply 547–548, 2004.
21. Hau M, Schultz H, Tony HP et al: Evaluation of pannus and vascularization of the metacarpophalangeal and proximal interphalangeal joints in rheumatoid arthritis by high-resolution ultrasound (multidimensional linear array), *Arthritis Rheum* 42:2303-2308, 1999.
22. Terslev L, Torp-Pedersen S, Qvistgaard E et al: Spectral Doppler and resistive index. A promising tool in ultrasonographic evaluation of inflammation in rheumatoid arthritis, *Acta Radiol* 44:645-652, 2003.
23. Qvistgaard E, Rogind H, Torp-Pedersen S et al: Quantitative ultrasonography in rheumatoid arthritis: evaluation of inflammation by Doppler technique, *Ann Rheum Dis* 60:690-693, 2001.
24. Ribbens C, Andre B, Marcelis S et al: Rheumatoid hand joint synovitis: gray-scale and power Doppler US quantifications following anti-tumor necrosis factor-alpha treatment: pilot study, *Radiology* 229:562-569, 2003.
25. Stone M, Bergin D, Whelan B et al: Power Doppler ultrasound assessment of rheumatoid hand synovitis, *J Rheumatol* 28:1979-1982, 2001.
26. Hau M, Kneitz C, Tony HP et al: High resolution ultrasound detects a decrease in pannus vascularisation of small finger joints in patients with rheumatoid arthritis receiving treatment with soluble tumour necrosis factor alpha receptor (etanercept), *Ann Rheum Dis* 61:55-58, 2002.
27. Klauser A, Demharter J, De Marchi A et al: Contrast enhanced gray-scale sonography in assessment of joint vascularity in rheumatoid arthritis: results from the IACUS study group, *Eur Radiol* 15:2404-2410, 2005.
28. Schmidt WA, Schmidt H, Schicke B et al: Standard reference values for musculoskeletal ultrasonography, *Ann Rheum Dis* 63:988-994, 2004.
29. Kane D, Balint PV, Sturrock RD: Ultrasonography is superior to clinical examination in the detection and localization of knee joint effusion in rheumatoid arthritis, *J Rheumatol* 30:966-971, 2003.
30. Karim Z, Wakefield RJ, Conaghan PG et al: The impact of ultrasonography on diagnosis and management of patients with musculoskeletal conditions, *Arthritis Rheum* 44:2932-2933, 2001.
31. Balint PV, Kane D, Hunter J et al: Ultrasound guided versus conventional joint and soft tissue fluid aspiration in rheumatology practice: a pilot study, *J Rheumatol* 29:2209-2213, 2002.
32. Raza K, Lee CY, Pilling D et al: Ultrasound guidance allows accurate needle placement and aspiration from small joints in patients with early inflammatory arthritis, *Rheumatology (Oxford)* 42:976-979, 2003.
33. Jackson DW, Evans NA, Thomas BM: Accuracy of needle placement into the intra-articular space of the knee, *J Bone Joint Surg (Am)* 841522-1527, 2002.
34. Jones A, Regan M, Ledingham J et al: Importance of placement of intra-articular steroid injections, *Br Med J* 307:1329-1330, 1993.
35. Guggi V, Calame L, Gerster JC: Contribution of digit joint aspiration to the diagnosis of rheumatic diseases, *Joint Bone Spine* 69:58-61, 2002.
36. Sofka CM, Collins AJ, Adler RS: Use of ultrasonographic guidance in interventional musculoskeletal procedures: a review from a single institution, *J Ultrasound Med* 20:21-26, 2001.
37. Ford LT, DeBender J: Tendon rupture after local steroid injection, *South Med J* 72:827-830, 1979.
38. Acevedo JI, Beskin JL: Complications of plantar fascia rupture associated with corticosteroid injection, *Foot Ankle Int* 19:91-97, 1998.
39. Campbell RS, Grainger AJ: Current concepts in imaging of tendinopathy, *Clin Radiol* 56:253-267, 2001.
40. Terslev L, Torp-Pedersen S, Qvistgaard E et al: Estimation of inflammation by Doppler ultrasound: quantitative changes after intra-articular treatment in rheumatoid arthritis, *Ann Rheum Dis* 62:1049-1053, 2003.
41. Taylor PC: VEGF and imaging of vessels in rheumatoid arthritis, *Arthritis Res* 4 (Suppl 3):S99-S107, 2002.
42. Terslev L, Torp-Pedersen S, Savnik A et al: Doppler ultrasound and magnetic resonance imaging of synovial inflammation of the hand in rheumatoid arthritis: a comparative study, *Arthritis Rheum* 48:2434-2441, 2003.
43. Jacobson JA, Andresen R, Jaovisidha S et al: Detection of ankle effusions: comparison study in cadavers using radiography, sonography, and MR imaging, *AJR Am J Roentgenol* 170:1231-1238, 1998.
44. Moss SG, Schweitzer ME, Jacobson JA et al: Hip joint fluid: detection and distribution at MR imaging and US with cadaveric correlation, *Radiology* 208:43-48, 1998.
45. Fex E, Jonsson K, Johnson U et al: Development of radiographic damage during the first 5-6 yr of rheumatoid arthritis. A prospective follow-up study of a Swedish cohort, *Br J Rheumatol* 35:1106-1115, 1996.
46. McQueen FM, Stewart N, Crabbe J et al: Magnetic resonance imaging of the wrist in early rheumatoid arthritis reveals progression of erosions despite clinical improvement, *Ann Rheum Dis* 58:156-163, 1999.
47. Grassi W, Filippucci E, Farina A et al: Ultrasonography in the evaluation of bone erosions, *Ann Rheum Dis* 60:98-103, 2001.
48. Backhaus M, Kamradt T, Sandrock D et al: Arthritis of the finger joints: a comprehensive approach comparing conventional radiography, scintigraphy, ultrasound, and contrast-enhanced magnetic resonance imaging, *Arthritis Rheum* 42:1232-1245, 1999.
49. Szkudlarek M, Narvestad E, Klarlund M et al: Ultrasonography of the metatarsophalangeal joints in rheumatoid arthritis: comparison with magnetic resonance imaging, conventional radiography, and clinical examination, *Arthritis Rheum* 50:2103-2112, 2004.
50. Wakefield RJ, Gibbon WW, Conaghan PG et al: The value of sonography in the detection of bone erosions in patients with rheumatoid arthritis: a comparison with conventional radiography, *Arthritis Rheum* 43:2762-2770, 2000.
51. Sommer OJ, Kladosek A, Weiler V et al: Rheumatoid arthritis: a practical guide to state-of-the-art imaging, image interpretation, and clinical implications, *Radiographics* 25:381-398, 2005.
52. Grassi W, Salaffi F, Filippucci E: Ultrasound in rheumatology, *Best Pract Res Clin Rheumatol* 19:467-485, 2005.
53. Kainberger F, Bitzan P, Erlacher L et al: [Rheumatic diseases of the ankle joint and tarsus], *Radiologe* 39:60-67, 1999.
54. Naredo E, Aguado P, De Miguel E et al: Painful shoulder: comparison of physical examination and ultrasonographic findings, *Ann Rheum Dis* 61:132-136, 2002.
55. Worth WD, Hermann E, Meudt R et al: [Value of arthrosonography in the evaluation of exudative and proliferative synovitis], *Z Rheumatol* 45:263-266, 1986.
56. Busso N, Morard C, Salvi R et al: Role of the tissue factor pathway in synovial inflammation, *Arthritis Rheum* 48:651-659, 2003.
57. Galluzzo E, Lischi DM, Taglione E et al: Sonographic analysis of the ankle in patients with psoriatic arthritis, *Scand J Rheumatol* 29:52-55, 2000.
58. Balint PV, Kane D, Wilson H et al: Ultrasonography of entheseal insertions in the lower limb in spondyloarthropathy, *Ann Rheum Dis* 61:905-910, 2002.
59. Kane D, Greaney T, Bresnihan B et al: Ultrasonography in the diagnosis and management of psoriatic dactylitis, *J Rheumatol* 26:1746-1751, 1999.
60. Ory PA, Gladman DD, Mease PJ: Psoriatic arthritis and imaging, *Ann Rheum Dis* 64 (Suppl 2):55-57, 2005.
61. Frediani B, Falsetti P, Storri L et al: Ultrasound and clinical evaluation of quadricipital tendon enthesitis in patients with psoriatic arthritis and rheumatoid arthritis, *Clin Rheumatol* 21:294-298, 2002.
62. De Simone C, Guerriero C, Giampetruzzi AR et al: Achilles tendinitis in psoriasis: clinical and sonographic findings, *J Am Acad Dermatol* 49:217-222, 2003.
63. Falsetti P, Frediani B, Filippou G et al: Enthesitis of proximal insertion of the deltoid in the course of seronegative spondyloarthritis. An atypical enthesitis that can mime impingement syndrome, *Scand J Rheumatol* 31:158-162, 2002.
64. Milosavljevic J, Lindqvist U, Elvin A: Ultrasound and power Doppler evaluation of the hand and wrist in patients with psoriatic arthritis, *Acta Radiol* 46:374-385, 2005.
65. Fiocco U, Ferro F, Vezzu M et al: Rheumatoid and psoriatic knee synovitis: clinical, grey scale, and power Doppler ultrasound assessment of the response to etanercept, *Ann Rheum Dis* 64:899-905, 2005.
66. Foldes K: Knee chondrocalcinosis: an ultrasonographic study of the hyalin cartilage, *Clin Imaging* 26:194-196, 2002.
67. Frediani B, Filippou G, Falsetti P et al: Diagnosis of calcium pyrophosphate dihydrate crystal deposition disease: ultrasonographic criteria proposed, *Ann Rheum Dis* 64:638-640, 2005.
68. Ryan LM, Cheung HS: The role of crystals in osteoarthritis, *Rheum Dis Clin North Am* 25:257-267, 1999.
69. McCarthy GM: Crystal-induced inflammation and cartilage degradation, *Curr Rheumatol Rep* 1:101-106, 1999.
70. Rovensky J, Mikulecky M, Masarova R: Gout and pseudogout chronobiology, *J Rheumatol* 26:1426-1427, 1999.
71. Bond JR, Sim FH, Sundaram M: Radiologic case study. Gouty tophus involving the distal quadriceps tendon, *Orthopedics* 27:18, 90-112, 2004.
72. Iacobellis G, Iacobellis G: A rare and asymptomatic case of mitral valve tophus associated with severe gouty tophaceous arthritis, *J Endocrinol Invest* 27:965-966, 2004.
73. O'Leary ST, Goldberg JA, Walsh WR: Tophaceous gout of the rotator cuff: a case report, *J Shoulder Elbow Surg* 12:200-201, 2003.
74. Grassi W, Lamanna G, Farina A et al: Sonographic imaging of normal and osteoarthritic cartilage, *Semin Arthritis Rheum* 28:398-403, 1999.
75. Hodler J, Resnick D: Current status of imaging of articular cartilage, *Skeletal Radiol* 25:703-709, 1996.
76. Schmidt WA, Gromnica-Ihle E: Incidence of temporal arteritis in patients with polymyalgia rheumatica: a prospective study using colour Doppler ultrasonography of the temporal arteries, *Rheumatology (Oxford)* 41:46-52, 2002.
77. Cheng KS, Tiwari A, Boutin A et al: Differentiation of primary and secondary Raynaud's disease by carotid arterial stiffness, *Eur J Vasc Endovasc Surg* 25:336-341, 2003.
78. Seitz WS, Kline HJ, McIlroy MB: Quantitative assessment of peripheral arterial obstruction in Raynaud's phenomenon: development of a predictive model of obstructive arterial cross-sectional area and validation with a Doppler blood flow study, *Angiology* 51:985-998, 2000.
79. Carotti M, Salaffi F, Manganelli P et al: Ultrasonography and colour doppler sonography of salivary glands in primary Sjogren's syndrome. *Clin Rheumatol* 20:213-219, 2001.
80. Makula E, Pokorny G, Kiss M et al. The place of magnetic resonance and ultrasonographic examinations of the parotid gland in the diagnosis and follow-up of primary Sjogren's syndrome, *Rheumatology (Oxford)* 39:97-104, 2000.
81. Schmidt WA, Kraft HE, Vorpahl K et al: Color duplex ultrasonography in the diagnosis of temporal arteritis, *N Engl J Med* 337:1336-1342, 1997.
82. Scheja A, Akesson A: Comparison of high frequency (20 MHz) ultrasound and palpation for the assessment of skin involvement in systemic sclerosis (scleroderma), *Clin Exp Rheumatol* 15:283-288, 1997.

83. Scheel AK, Schmidt WA, Hermann KG et al. Interobserver reliability of rheumatologists performing musculoskeletal ultrasonography: results from a EULAR "Train the trainers" course, *Ann Rheum Dis* 64:1043-1049, 2005.
84. Brown AK, O'Connor PJ, Roberts TE et al: Recommendations for musculoskeletal ultrasonography by rheumatologists: setting global standards for best practice by expert consensus, *Arthritis Rheum* 53:83-92, 2005.
85. Brown AK, Wakefield RJ, Karim Z et al: Evidence of effective and efficient teaching and learning strategies in the education of rheumatologist ultrasonographers: evaluation from the 3rd BSR musculoskeletal ultrasonography course, *Rheumatology (Oxford)* 44:1068-1069, 2005.
86. Speed CA, Bearcroft PW: Musculoskeletal sonography by rheumatologists: the challenges, *Rheumatology (Oxford)* 41:241-242, 2002.

SECTION II

IMAGING OF DEGENERATIVE AND TRAUMATIC CONDITIONS

CHAPTER 8

Osteoarthritis

BARBARA N. WEISSMAN, MD

KEY POINTS

- Osteoarthritis involves all structures of the joint.
- Osteoarthritis is the most common form of arthritis.
- There is no direct correlation between radiographic findings and symptoms.
- Radiographs are insensitive indicators of osteoarthritis.
- Magnetic resonance imaging can delineate articular cartilage changes as well as evaluate changes to the other articular structures.

DEFINITION

Osteoarthritis (OA) (also called *osteoarthrosis* or *degenerative joint disease*) is a "heterogeneous group of conditions that lead to joint symptoms and signs, which are associated with defective integrity of articular cartilage, in addition to related changes in the underlying bone at the joint margins."[1] In contrast to some definitions emphasizing that OA is a disease of hyaline articular cartilage, the disorder is now believed to involve the entire joint including cartilage, bone, ligaments, menisci, periarticular muscles, capsule, and synovium.[2]

The disorder occurs due to altered local mechanical factors in a susceptible individual. Local factors include joint malalignment, muscle weakness, injury, previous knee surgery, occupational bending and lifting, or meniscal tears.[2,3] Increasing age, female sex, possibly nutritional deficiencies, and genetic predisposition are examples of systemic predisposing factors. Obesity increases the likelihood of developing OA.

Joint involvement is asymmetric and focal, unlike the more diffuse involvement of inflammatory arthritis. Localized areas of cartilage loss can increase stress on that area, leading to further cartilage loss. Eventually, large areas of deficient cartilage or bony remodeling result in malalignment, which leads to further focal joint loading and further damage.[3]

> The changes of OA in a joint are asymmetric.

SCOPE OF THE PROBLEM

OA is the most common form of arthritis[4] and the leading cause of disability in the elderly.[5] More than 43 million individuals have degenerative joint disease in the United States.[6] Peat et al. found the prevalence of painful, disabling knee OA in people older than 55 years in the United Kingdom and the Netherlands to be 10%.[5] One quarter of these people were severely disabled. As the population ages, the disorder is likely to increase in frequency and its consequences to public health will become more profound.

PATHOLOGIC FEATURES

The pathologic features of OA have been summarized by Felson.[4] Cartilage is composed of an extensive extracellular matrix made of type II collagen and aggrecan and other molecules surrounding chondrocytes (cells that synthesize the matrix and the enzymes that break it down). Aggrecan contains highly negatively charged glycosaminoglycan (GAG) chains that are held in proximity to each other by collagen II chains interwoven in the matrix. The negatively charged glycosaminoglycan chains repel each other, providing the compressive stiffness of the cartilage.

Hyaline cartilage is the site of the initial changes in osteoarthritis.[4] In early OA, the net concentration of aggrecan falls (degradation is greater than synthesis), the negative charges are exposed, and these charges attract water into the cartilage, leading to swelling. Deterioration in the biomechanical properties of cartilage and aggrecan and collagen loss and injury lead to wearing away of cartilage, eventually exposing the subchondral bone. Subchondral bone remodeling leads to denser bone with filling in of the spaces between trabeculae, which can be seen on radiographs. Endochondral bone formation occurs at the margins of the joint, resulting in chondroosteophytes (usually called *osteophytes*). These help stabilize the joint. Synovitis occurs in 20% to 30% of cases.[4] Muscle changes also develop with decreased strength and atrophy of the fast twitch fibers that help stabilize the joint or respond to unanticipated stresses.[4]

DIAGNOSIS

The diagnosis of OA is suggested clinically when an older patient complains of pain and stiffness and there is decreased mobility and absence of systemic features.[2] The hands, knees, and hips are the most commonly affected joints. Typically pain is worse with activity and improved with rest. Rest pain may be seen, however, with severe symptomatic disease but should suggest that other disorders be considered (e.g., inflammatory arthritis).[3] Unlike inflammatory arthritis, morning stiffness lasts less than 30 minutes.[3] The diagnosis of OA is supported by typical findings on radiographs, but these are insensitive for confirming early disease.[2] Radiographs are indicated if pain is nocturnal or at rest or persists after effective treatment. Magnetic resonance imaging (MRI) can exclude other causes of pain and directly allow any cartilage damage to be assessed.

> Typically the pain of OA occurs with activity and improves with rest.

GENERAL IMAGING FEATURES

Radiography

Correlation of Radiographic Findings with Cartilage Changes

Correlation of arthroscopic findings with radiographic features has shown that significant cartilage degeneration may be present in the absence of radiologic findings.[7]

Correlation of Radiographic Findings with Symptoms

Osteophytes at the knee and cartilage space narrowing at the hip are more strongly correlated with joint pain than is a global grade of OA severity.[8] Felson et al. correlated clinical OA with a variety of definitions of radiographic OA.[9] They determined that a knee should be classified as having radiographic OA if there is either an osteophyte of grade 2 or greater severity (0 to 3 scale) or there is moderate to severe joint space narrowing ($\geq$ 2 on a 0 to 3 scale) as well as a bony feature in the affected compartment. Lanyon et al. assessed the correlation between radiographic features of OA and knee pain.[10] The presence of osteophytes at either the tibiofemoral or patellofemoral joint were more efficient at predicting pain than was assessment of cartilage space. Evaluation of the patellofemoral joint in addition to the tibiofemoral joint is important, as the patellofemoral articulation is often a source of pain.

Radiographic Scoring

Scoring systems are utilized primarily for investigational purposes such as drug trials, but review of these systems highlights the significance of various radiologic features in diagnosis generally.

- **What is assessed:** Radiographic grading of OA typically includes assessment of osteophytes and cartilage space narrowing. Other features such as sclerosis and cyst formation have lower reproducibility but are included in some grading systems.[11] Clinical and laboratory assessment may also be evaluated.
- **Reproducibility of cartilage width assessment:** Of the features of OA, cartilage space width is the most sensitive radiographic measurement for detecting change over time.[12,13] The rate of cartilage loss in patients with hip or knee OA is about 0.25 mm per year.[14] Because articular changes may be small, the reproducibility of cartilage thickness measurement is critical in following subjects over time. Reproducibility relates to several factors including uniform patient positioning on follow-up visits and measurement technique.[12]

Some Grading Systems

Kellgren and Lawrence

Kellgren and Lawrence developed a system of grading OA that remains in use today.[15] Various joints could be assessed, and a set of standardized radiographs was provided for reference.

The radiologic features that were considered in this grading system were as follows:

1. The formation of osteophytes on the joint margins or, in the case of the knee joint, on the tibial spines
2. Periarticular ossicles; these were found chiefly in relation to the distal and proximal interphalangeal joints (Figure 8-1)
3. Narrowing of the joint cartilage associated with sclerosis of subchondral bone
4. Small pseudocystic areas with sclerotic walls situated usually in the subchondral bones, particularly in the head of the femur

Grades of OA were described as follows (Table 8-1):

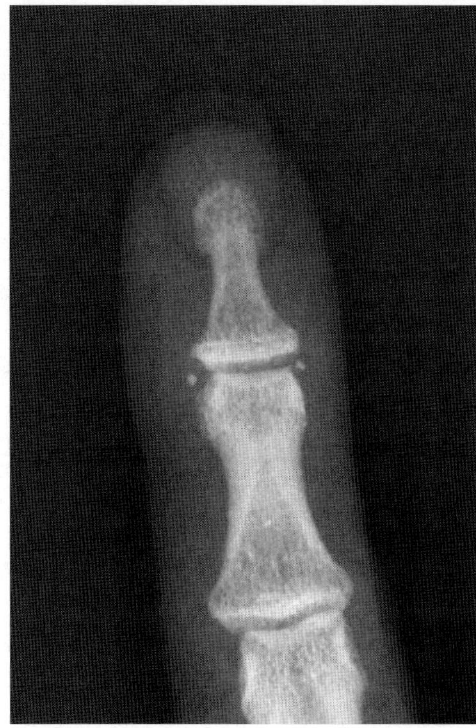

FIGURE 8-1. OA of the DIP joint. This PA radiograph of the index finger shows small periarticular ossicles, which are indicators of OA.

0: None—a definite absence of the changes of OA
1: Doubtful
2: Minimal—definitely present but of minimal severity
3: Moderate
4: Severe

Kellgren and Lawrence noted that interobserver bias could result in prevalence of disease estimates that differed by ± 31%.[16] It has subsequently been noted that this system has several additional limitations including overemphasizing the importance of osteophytes, and the failure of grading to correspond with symptoms or disability.[11] It has been suggested that grading

TABLE 8-1. Examples of Kellgren Lawrence Grades

Grade	Example
1: Doubtful	

TABLE 8-1. Examples of Kellgren Lawrence Grades—cont'd

Grade	Example
2: Minimal	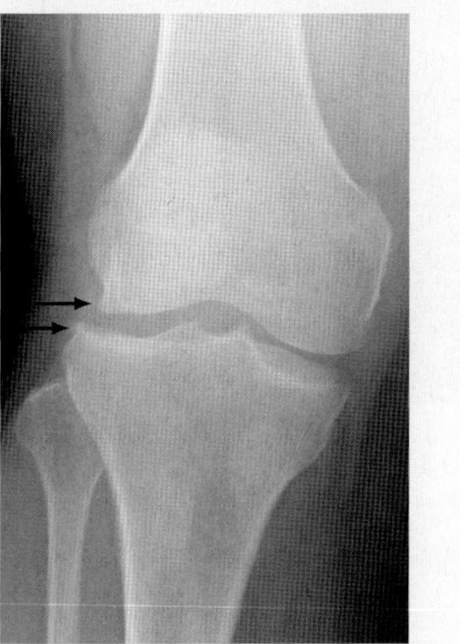
3: Moderate	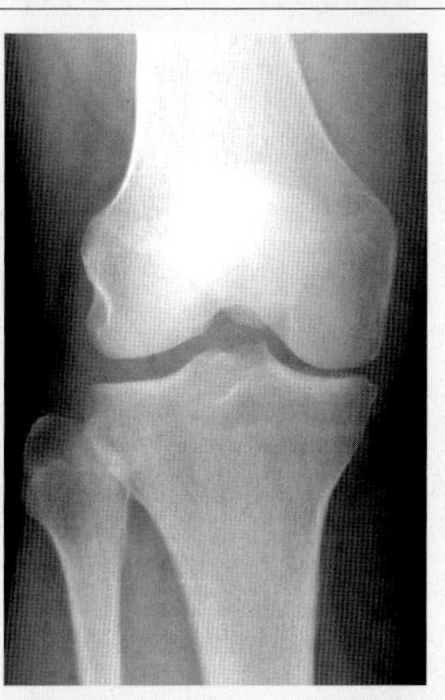
4: Severe	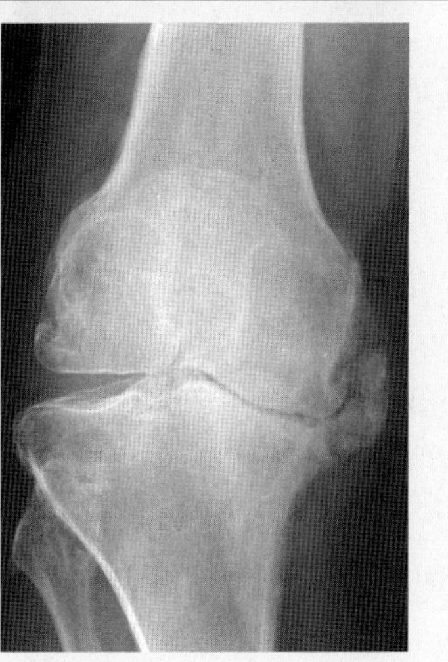

of OA may differ between joints.[17] Using the Kellgren-Lawrence scale, if no osteophytes are present, osteoarthritis can not be diagnosed even if cartilage space narrowing is present.[18] Brandt et al. also note that the Kellgren-Lawrence scale does not allow appropriate grading for patients with osteophytes and "definite" cartilage space narrowing who do not have sclerosis. These patients would be classified as having grade II (minimal) disease although cartilage loss could be prominent.

Other Scoring Systems

In 1995, an atlas (Osteoarthritis Research Society International [OARSI]) was published that illustrated the individual findings of OA in each joint or joint compartment.[8] These could be used as reference standards for clinical trials.

A line drawing atlas that may simplify scoring has also been introduced.[11] This atlas includes osteophytes and cartilage space narrowing as separate criteria. The use of line drawings (rather than radiographs) allows only one of these abnormalities to be presented on each illustration so that analysis of osteophytes, for example, is not influenced by the presence of cartilage space narrowing. Cartilage space narrowing was assessed separately for men and women. Both the femorotibial and patellofemoral joints were evaluated.

Magnetic Resonance Imaging

Virtually all the structures of a joint are involved in OA, and MRI is capable of delineating the morphology and to some degree the integrity of these tissues. Osteophytes are often more apparent on MRI than on radiographs.[19] The cortex of the osteophyte and the marrow are continuous with those of the host bone, and these features are well demonstrated on MRI (Figure 8-2). Subchondral edema, sclerosis, and cysts can be seen. Edema-like signal produces areas of intermediate to low signal on T1-weighted or intermediate-weighted images and bright signal on fluid-sensitive sequences. Subchondral fibrosis and trabecular thickening replacing normal marrow (which contains fat) result in hemispherical subchondral areas that are intermediate in signal on T1-weighted images and intermediate to low in signal on T2-weighted images.[20] Cystic changes may occur within the areas of subchondral sclerosis, producing well-defined regions that contain fluid signal.[21] Synovial hypertrophy occurs in OA to a lesser degree than in rheumatoid arthritis but may be visible on MRI.[22]

Optimal imaging of the joint and particularly of the articular cartilage is technically complex and requires very high spatial resolution (Figure 8-3). At the same time, examination times must be kept short to avoid motion artifact. Imaging parameters need to be adjusted so that articular cartilage can be differentiated both from the subjacent bone and also from the joint fluid.[23] Because MRI techniques vary, it is important to review these technical factors when evaluating published studies or assessing images of articular cartilage (see Chapter 4). MRI has been shown to provide accurate assessment of articular cartilage volume, cartilage erosion, fissuring, thinning, signal change, and thickness in cadaver knees.[24,25] The presence of changes in cartilage volume can be determined, but these advanced techniques are currently usually reserved for investigational purposes.[24,25]

MRI generally allows detection of only intermediate-to-advanced osteoarthritic change in clinical cases.[19] Correlative clinical and MRI studies have shown relationships between pain and synovitis,[26] large effusions, patellofemoral osteophytes or more than four osteophytes in the knee,[27] and enlarging bone marrow lesions.[28]

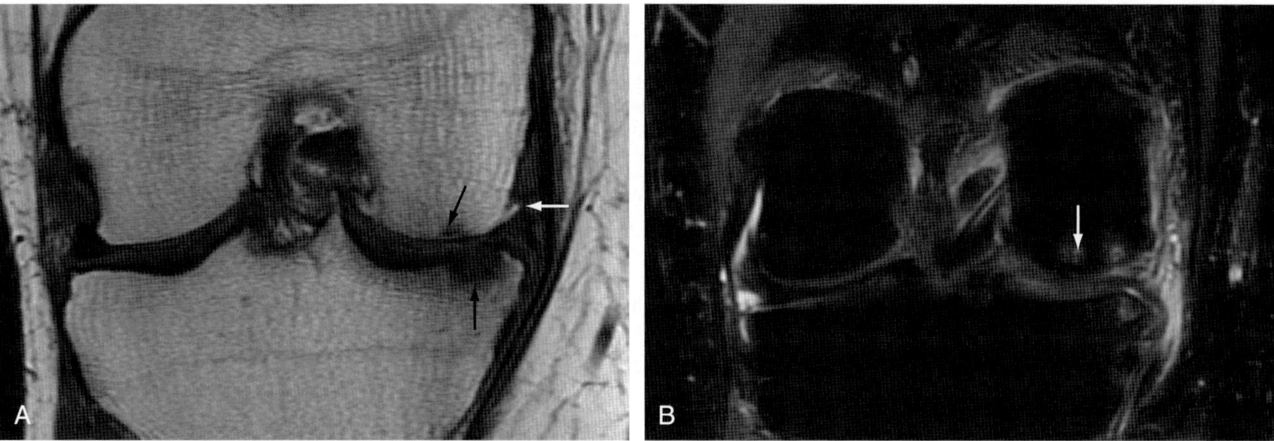

FIGURE 8-2. Changes of OA on MRI. **A,** The T1-weighted coronal image of the knee shows marginal osteophytes *(white arrow)* and sharpening of the tibial spines. The medial subchondral bone shows areas of replacement of marrow fat by intermediate signal *(black arrows)*. **B,** STIR image at another level shows high signal, termed *edema-like marrow signal,* in the abnormal areas seen in **A.** Tiny, well-defined fluid signal regions within these larger areas are consistent with subchondral cysts (one marked with *arrow*).

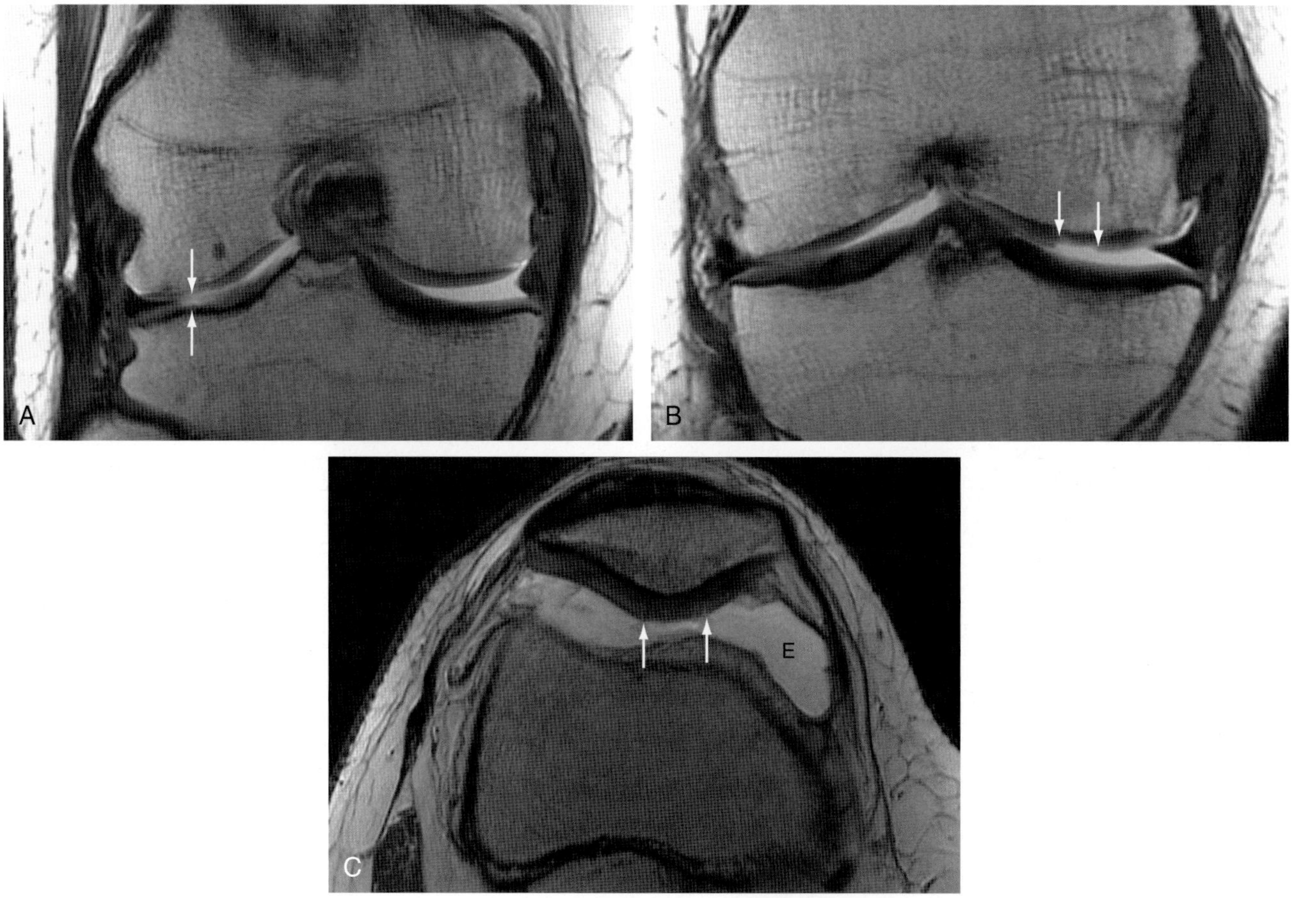

FIGURE 8-3. Evaluation of articular cartilage on MR arthrography. **A,** A coronal image of the knee obtained after the intraarticular administration of a dilute gadolinium solution demonstrates the smooth intermediate signal articular cartilage of this portion of the medial femoral condyle and tibial plateau in comparison to the irregular fissuring and thinning of the lateral cartilage surfaces *(arrows)*. The medial compartment is capacious owing to the ligament laxity medially. The medial meniscus is abnormally small consistent with a tear. **B,** Coronal image further anteriorly shows a focal 50% thinning of the medial femoral cartilage *(arrows)*. **C,** An axial view of the patellofemoral joint shows fissuring of the patellar cartilage *(arrows)*. The bright joint effusion (due to the contrast injection, *E*) is noted.

Immediate imaging after intravenous contrast may be useful to evaluate synovitis (as is often done in patients with rheumatoid arthritis) (see Chapter 20), but in OA, delayed imaging after intravenous contrast (indirect arthrography) may also be useful. Delayed imaging provides an arthrographic effect that allows the articular cartilage to be better delineated.[28a]

d-GEMERIC

Largely investigational MRI techniques include T2 relaxation mapping, T1 rho relaxation mapping, and d-GEMERIC (delayed gadolinium-enhanced MRI of cartilage) to provide molecular information about articular cartilage.[29,30] The d-GEMERIC technique utilizes MRI examination after intravenously administered gadolinium to noninvasively image the GAG concentration of articular cartilage.[31] This is possible because GAG has a negative fixed charge density and Gadolinium DTPA (Magnevist, Berlex, NJ) is a divalent anion. GAG concentration is related to the mechanical properties of cartilage and is decreased in diseased cartilage. Intraarticular contrast injection may offer improved imaging but requires a more invasive injection technique.[32]

Nomenclature for MRI

Standard nomenclature has been promulgated to facilitate communication.[33] Interpretation criteria have been proposed, such as the KOSS scoring system[34] and the WORMS score.[35]

Ultrasound

Articular cartilage is seen on ultrasound as a hypoechoic band with sharp margins.[21] Osteophytes and synovitis can also be evaluated. Not all areas can be assessed, and this technique requires operator expertise to be effective.

Positron Emission Tomography

Positron emission tomography (PET) is a functional imaging technique that enables metabolic mapping of the tissues in vivo using positron-emitting radionuclides. Fluorine 18 fluorodeoxyglucose (F-18 FDG) is the most commonly used radiopharmaceutical for PET scanning, and the degree of cellular uptake of FDG is proportional to cellular glucose metabolism. Integration with CT scanning allows precise localization of F-18 FDG–positive lesions, greatly facilitating image interpretation. Isotope uptake may also be quantified. PET scanning is usually used for evaluation of tumors, but labeled FDG is not a specific marker for cancer, and sites of infection and inflammation may also show high tracer uptake (Figure 8-4).

HANDS/WRISTS

Although OA of the hands is one of the most prevalent diseases, diagnostic criteria are not clear.[36] The American College of Rheumatology has proposed criteria for OA of the hand that provide a sensitivity of 94% and a specificity of 87%[36] (Box 8-1).

The most common areas of involvement, in decreasing order, are the distal interphalangeal (DIP) joints, the bases of the thumbs, the proximal interphalangeal (PIP) joints, and the metacarpophalangeal (MCP) joints.[38] Findings are relatively symmetric.[39] OA of other joints may accompany OA of the hand.

Clinically apparent bony nodules about the DIP joint (Heberden's nodes) and similar features about the PIP joints (Bouchard's nodes) likely (but not always) correspond to palpable osteophytes.[36,40,41]

As in other joints, the hallmarks of OA of the hand are cartilage space narrowing, subchondral sclerosis, osteophytosis, and subluxation. Erosion and ankylosis are not typically present (Figure 8-5). The significance of osteophytes without cartilage space narrowing is unclear; this finding could be an age-related change.[36]

Interphalangeal Joints

Multiple joint involvement of the distal and proximal interphalangeal rows are characteristic features of OA, with DIP joint involvement significantly more common than PIP joint involvement.[38] The highest incidence of hand OA is in the second DIP joint.[38] DIP joint involvement may occur in the absence of PIP involvement; solitary PIP changes are rare. Cartilage loss results in apposition and remodeling of the subchondral bone, producing a characteristic osseous configuration likened to the wings of a bird (the "gull wing" sign).[42] Osteophytes are marginal spike-like bony growths extending proximally from the distal phalanx at the DIP joint and proximally from the base of the middle phalanx at the PIP joint.[43,44] There is a predilection for dorsal and volar osteophyte formation, which are therefore best seen on steep oblique or lateral views of the hand. Subluxation at the joint line usually occurs in the radial and ulnar directions, producing a characteristic zigzag appearance. This may in part be due to the tendency for osteophyte formation along the dorsal and volar joint margins, inhibiting subluxation in those directions.

> Osteophytes are most common at the DIP and PIP joints and are best seen on lateral or steep oblique radiographs. Prominent MCP disease should suggest other underlying conditions.

Metacarpophalangeal Joints

MCP joint changes[45] may be seen in OA but are less prominent than the changes seen in the interphalangeal joints. Unlike the asymmetric cartilage space narrowing in large joints, cartilage space narrowing seen with osteoarthritis in the MCP joints tends to be uniform. Marginal osteophytes at the MCPs are typically smaller than those in the interphalangeal joints, and subchondral cysts are generally small.

Prominent osteoarthritic changes in the second through fifth MCP joints are classically associated with other arthropathies such as rheumatoid arthritis, calcium pyrophosphate dihydrate deposition (CPDD) syndrome, and hemochromatosis (see Secondary OA on page 127) or with certain occupations involving repetitive stress on these joints.[46]

Thumb Base

Radiographic changes of OA of the thumb base usually involve the trapeziometacarpal joint or, less often, the trapezioscaphoid joint.[47] Findings of the disorder include cartilage space narrowing, sclerosis, cystic changes, osteophytosis, bony fragmentation, and radial subluxation (Figure 8-6). If degenerative changes are seen at the trapezioscaphoid joint, 84% of these patients will have coexisting involvement of the trapeziometacarpal joint.[47] Degenerative changes seen in isolation at the trapezioscaphoid joint, however, suggest other etiologies including CPPD and rheumatoid arthritis.

Anteroposterior (AP), lateral, and oblique views of the thumb are typically used for evaluation. A basal joint stress view[48,49] provides clearer visualization of all trapezial facets and defines any subluxation of the joint.[48]

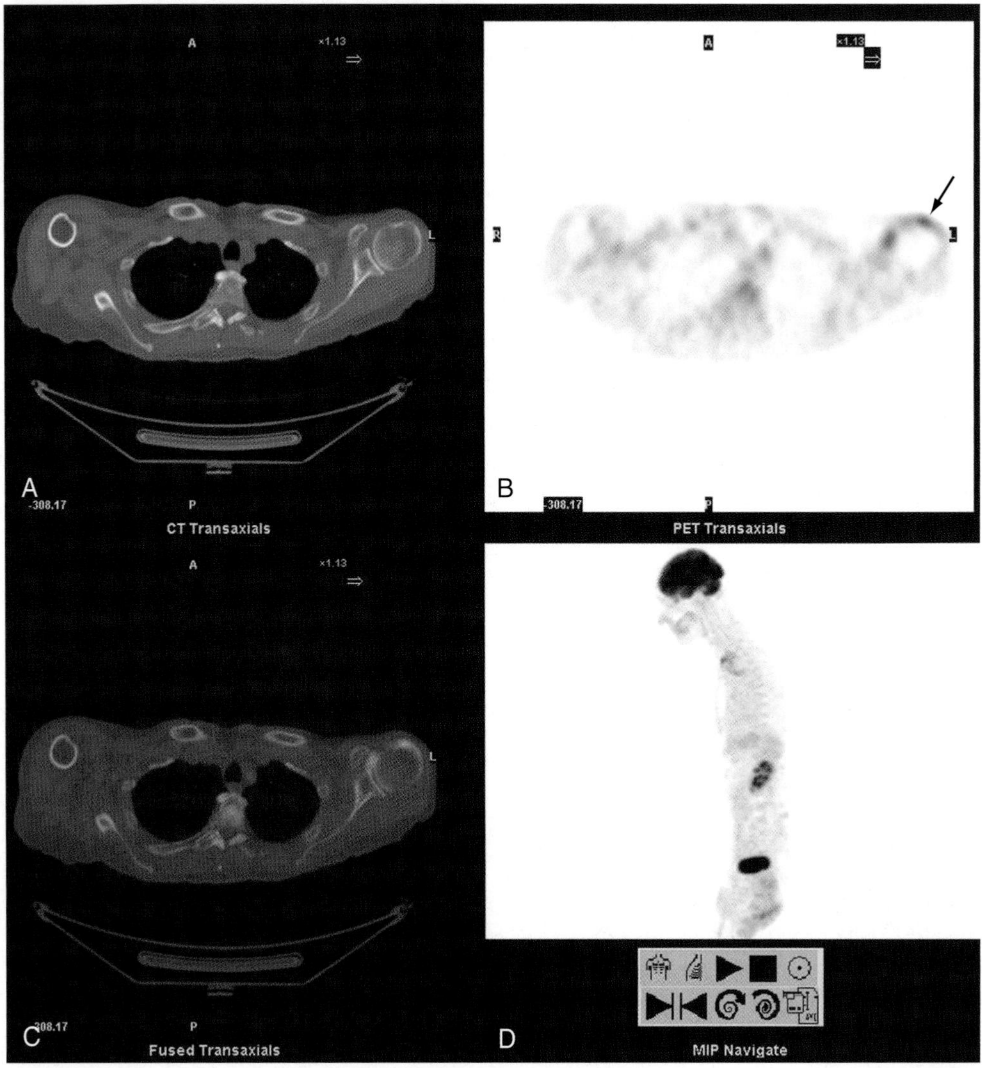

FIGURE 8-4. PET/CT scan showing nonspecific uptake around the shoulder. **A,** The axial CT scan through the shoulders shows no lytic or blastic lesions. **B,** The axial PET image shows a curvilinear area of increased activity around the shoulder *(arrow)*. **C,** The fused image confirms the activity to be localized near the greater tuberosity, consistent with degenerative changes related to the rotator cuff. A second area of increased activity is noted anteromedially that is unexplained. **D,** 3D MIP (maximum intensity projection) image. (Courtesy of Victor Gerbaudo, PhD, Brigham and Women's Hospital, Boston, MA.)

BOX 8-1. The American College of Rheumatology Criteria for OA of the Hand

Hand pain aching or stiffness for most days of the prior month plus three or four of the following four criteria:

- Hard tissue enlargement of ≥ 2 of 10 selected hand joints*
- MCP joint swelling in fewer than 3 joints
- Hard tissue enlargement of ≥ 2 DIP joints
- Deformity of at least 1 of 10 selected hand joints

*The 10 selected hand joints include bilateral second and third DIP joints, second and third PIP joints, and first carpometacarpal joints.
From Altman R, Alarcón G, Appelrouth D et al: The American College of Rheumatology criteria for the classification and reporting of osteoarthritis of the hand, *Arthritis Rheum* 33:1601–1610, 1990.

It has been postulated that chronic loading leads to progressive instability and laxity of the trapezial ligaments and trapezial tilt away from the trapezoid.[50,51] This "trapezial tilt" causes abnormal shear forces on the trapeziometacarpal joint, possibly leading to OA.[50] There is a positive correlation between increased trapezial tilt angle and the severity of trapeziometacarpal OA.[51] The trapezial tilt angle can be measured from the Robert's view, which is a true AP view of the thumb.[52]

Inflammatory (Erosive) OA

Inflammatory OA is a disorder most commonly affecting middle-aged women and characterized by acute episodes of inflammation of the interphalangeal joints of the hands.[53] The relationship of erosive osteoarthritis to OA generally is uncertain; it may be a separate entity or an aggressive form of OA.[54-57]

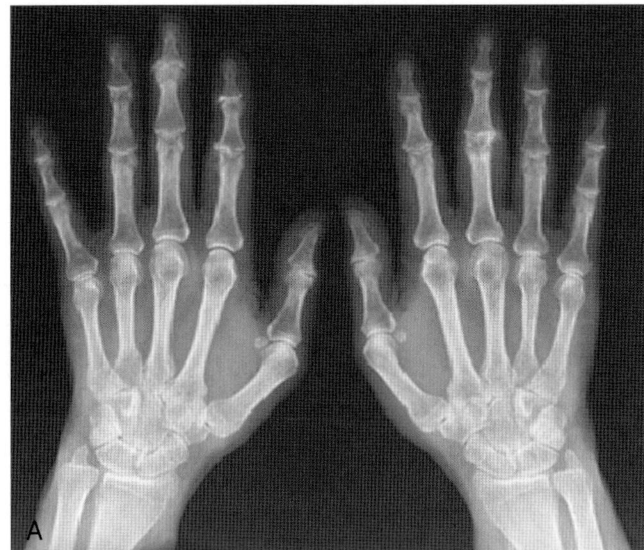

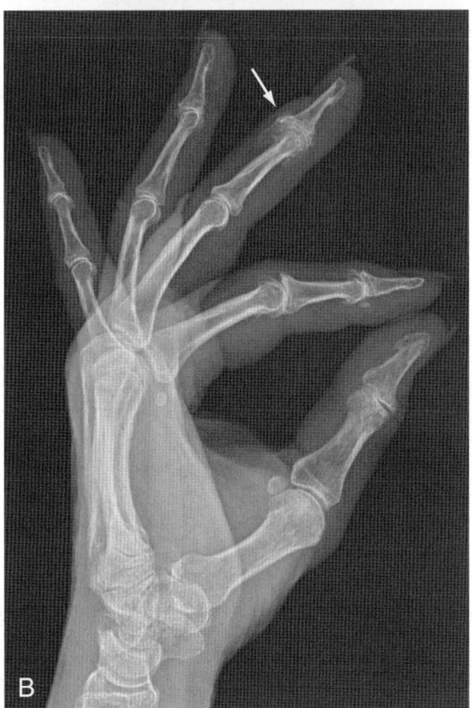

FIGURE 8-5. OA of the hands. **A,** There is asymmetric cartilage space narrowing of the DIP and many of the PIP joints. The MCP joints are normal. There is a "gull wing" appearance to the left middle finger DIP. **B,** The lateral projection of the left hand shows the osteophytes to advantage *(arrow)*, as they tend to be larger on the dorsal and palmar surfaces.

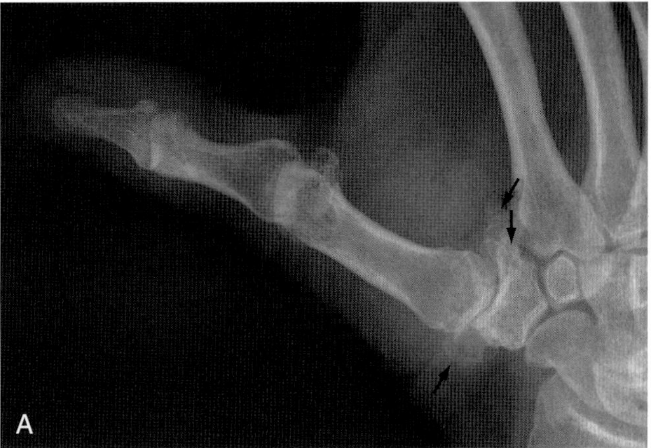

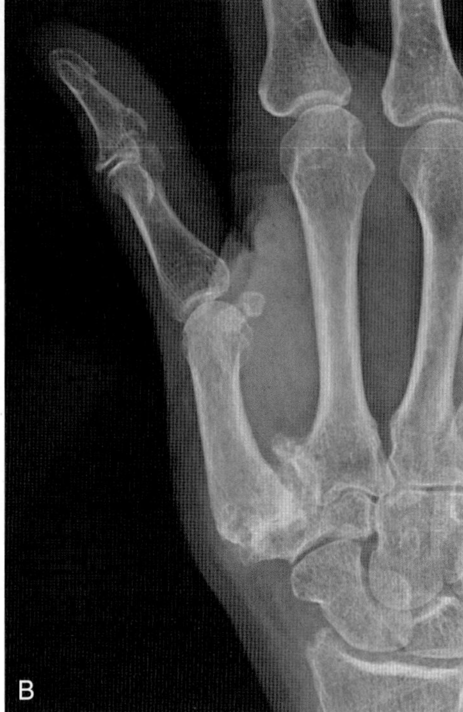

FIGURE 8-6. OA of the thumb bases. **A,** An oblique radiograph of the thumb shows severe cartilage space narrowing and osteophytic lipping *(arrow)* at the thumb carpometacarpal joint. **B,** An oblique radiograph in another patient shows severe cartilage space narrowing and hypertrophic changes at the thumb carpometacarpal. There is thenar muscle atrophy and hyperextension of the MCP joint.

Radiography

Radiographic examination shows marginal osteophytes with or without bony erosions (Figure 8-7). When erosions develop, they initially occur in the central portion of the subchondral bone, resulting in sharply marginated defects that eventually produce a "gull wing" deformity. These changes can be difficult to differentiate from psoriatic arthritis, although the presence of marginal erosion and fluffy new bone formation (a "mouse ears" appearance) is typical of psoriatic arthritis and may allow accurate diagnosis to be made.[42] Bony ankylosis across the joint may occur but is a more typical feature of psoriatic arthritis.

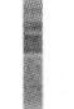

Erosive OA results in a typical pattern of central erosion and remodeling that, because of its contour, has been termed the "gull wing" deformity.

Magnetic Resonance Imaging

High-resolution MRI has shed new light on this condition. In a study of 15 patients with OA of the small joints of the hand, micro-MRI revealed erosions, synovitis, and bone marrow edema—identical to the changes seen in inflammatory arthritis—in many joints. This suggests that erosive OA may actually be part of the spectrum of OA rather than a separate entity.[58]

The MRI features of DIP joint changes of patients with OA have been compared with the changes seen in patients with

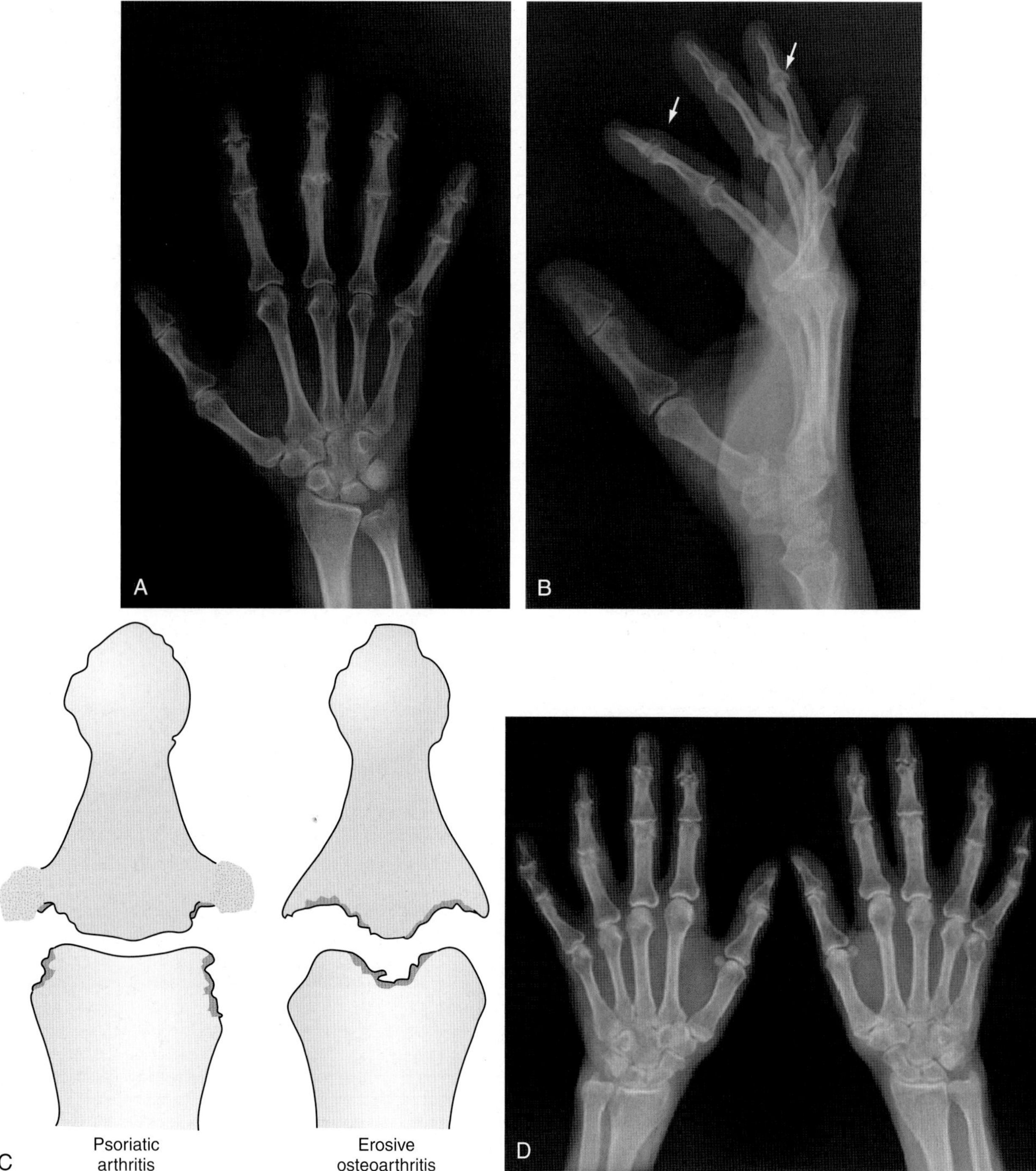

FIGURE 8-7. Erosive OA versus psoriatic arthritis. **A,** Erosive OA. PA radiograph of the hand and wrist shows swelling of the index finger DIP and the middle finger PIP. Asymmetric cartilage space narrowing is seen at several of the DIP and PIP joints with interdigitation of bony surfaces. There is erosion at the index finger DIP. **B,** The lateral radiograph of the fingers in the same patient confirms swelling and shows osteophytes *(arrows)* at the dorsal aspects of several DIP and PIP joints. **C,** Diagram of the changes of erosive OA compared with psoriatic arthritis. **D,** PA radiograph in another patient shows "gull wing" deformities and fusion of the right ring finger DIP. The latter is a more typical finding in psoriatic arthritis but may be seen in erosive OA. (**C,** Reprinted with permission from Martel W, Stuck KJ, Dworin AM et al: Erosive osteoarthritis and psoriatic arthritis: a radiologic comparison in the hand, wrist, and foot, *Am J Roentgenol* 134:125-135, 1980.)

psoriatic arthritis.[59] Generally, osteoarthritic joints showed ligamentous and entheseal changes but much less inflammation than that seen in joints with psoriatic involvement. Difficulty was found in separating ligamentous changes of patients with OA from older control subjects. Osteoarthritic joints showed diffusely thickened ligaments, some with enhancement, extensor tendon enthesitis, and thickening of the extensor tendon. Ligament and tendon changes are seen even when cartilage appeared normal. Edema-like signal was noted only in joints with complete cartilage loss. In contrast, psoriatic patients showed greater enhancement at the origins and insertions of ligaments and the extensor tendon insertions, greater extracapsular enhancement with diffuse involvement of the nail bed, and diffuse bone marrow edema. Synovitis may be a component of OA as well as of rheumatoid arthritis. Dynamic contrast enhancement has been utilized to differentiate the synovitis in these two conditions.[60]

Positron Emission Tomography

PET scanning is a potentially useful method of detecting early synovitis.[61] Usually PET scans obtained for whole body evaluation of tumors do not allow assessment of the hands and wrists,[61] but specific techniques may be used to evaluate these areas. Comparison of F18–FDG PET scanning of the hands and wrists of 14 patients with rheumatoid arthritis, 6 patients with primary OA, and 5 control patients (with fibromyalgia) has shown no increased uptake in control subjects.[61] Joints with rheumatoid arthritis and clinical synovitis showed increased uptake in most but not all sites. A smaller number of joints showed increased uptake in patients with OA, suggesting that synovitis was also present in some areas. No distinction can be made based on the presence of uptake between rheumatoid arthritis and OA.

SHOULDERS

Radiographs

Multiple radiographic projections have been developed to assess various maladies of the glenohumeral joint (Figure 8-8). A 40-degree posterior oblique, external rotation view (the Grashey projection) allows the glenohumeral cartilage space to be seen in profile and is therefore helpful for the assessment of arthritis. This projection is usually supplemented by an internal rotation AP view and by other views depending on the clinical question. Apple et al. suggest a Grashey view with the arm abducted and the patient holding a 1-lb weight to produce a loading force across the joint that approximates that of body weight.[62-64] This may demonstrate cartilage space narrowing not visible on other radiographs. The axillary projection is helpful in delineating posterior subluxation that may complicate OA of the shoulder.

> Because tumors of the lung apex may occasionally mimic shoulder symptoms, the apex of the lung is included on one radiographic view of each shoulder series at the Brigham and Women's Hospital.

Radiographic findings of OA generally occur late in the disease.[6] Marginal osteophytes develop around the anatomic neck and may be prominent medially[65] (Figure 8-9). The size of osteophytes

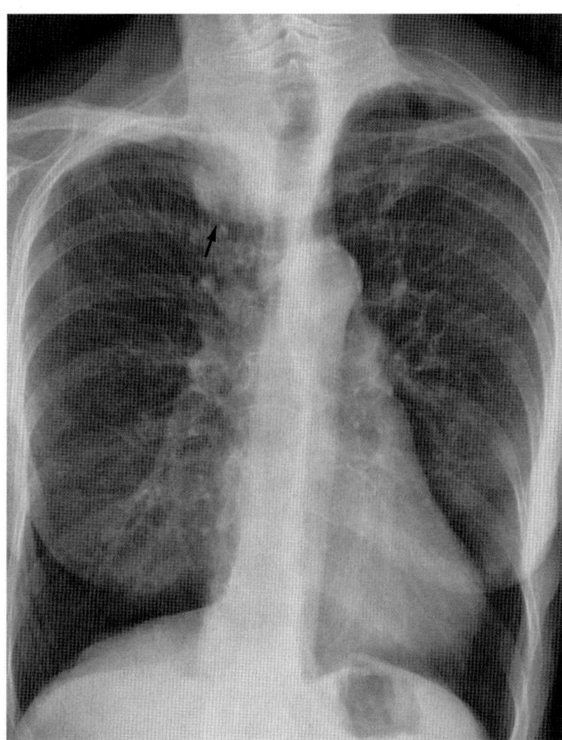

FIGURE 8-8. Pancoast tumor. This woman presented with deep shoulder pain. The PA radiograph of the chest, obtained after radiographs of the shoulder suggested an apical mass, confirmed a mass in the apex of the lung *(arrow)* with destruction of the underlying bone. Because of the possibility of such a tumor, the lung apex is included on one radiograph of the shoulder at many institutions.

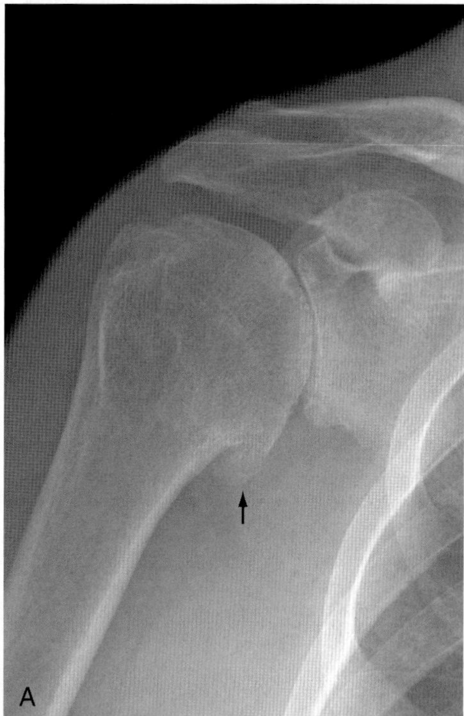

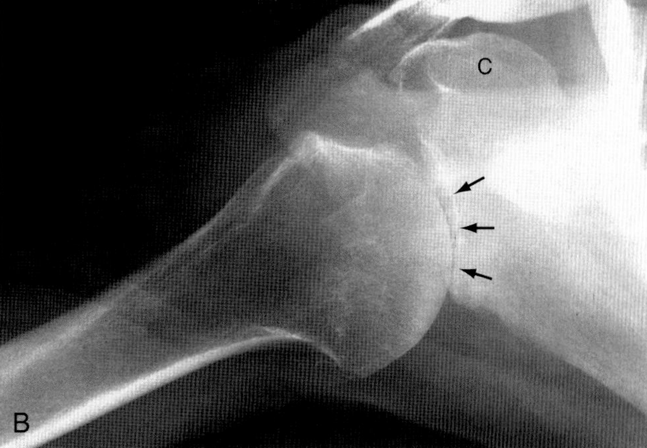

FIGURE 8-9. Shoulder OA with posterior subluxation. **A,** The posterior oblique, external rotation (Grashey) view of the shoulder shows marked narrowing of the glenohumeral joint with tiny subchondral cysts and a large humeral osteophyte (*arrow*, Grade 3). **B,** The axillary view shows posterior subluxation of the humeral head. *Arrows,* Glenoid articulation; *C,* coracoid.

from the inferior humeral head and glenoid margins on AP radiographs has been used to grade the severity of shoulder OA[66] (Table 8-2). Results of a cadaver study, however, have indicated the reliability of this system to be fair to poor.[67] Eventually, the humeral head becomes flat and enlarged and subluxes posteriorly. Corresponding posterior glenoid erosion occurs and CT may be useful in preoperative planning to assess the degree of posterior bone loss.[64,65,68] Rotator cuff tears are not a prominent feature of shoulder OA.

Positron Emission Tomography

Shoulder uptake may be seen as an incidental finding on PET scanning performed for evaluation of malignant disease. Assessment of the pattern of uptake may be helpful because circumferential diffuse uptake has been correlated with the presence of OA.[69] This is thought to be due to increased metabolic activity associated with low-grade inflammation. Patients with rotator cuff disease or frozen shoulder demonstrated more focal patterns of uptake.

Ultrasound

In experienced hands and with proper equipment, ultrasound examination of joints can be remarkably helpful.[70] In OA, ultrasound can be used to demonstrate any associated rotator cuff disruption. Intraarticular bodies can be identified and joint aspiration can be guided by ultrasound.

Magnetic Resonance Imaging

MRI can reveal findings of glenohumeral OA including osteophyte formation and subchondral marrow changes. It may be difficult to evaluate articular cartilage thickness, however. Acromioclavicular joint changes are frequently seen in asymptomatic individuals, and their presence should be correlated with clinical symptoms.[71]

HIPS

Although early articular cartilage changes may be asymptomatic, progressive disease with the formation of osteophytes and subchondral sclerosis can lead to symptoms of generalized hip pain, pain in the lateral and anterior thigh or groin, and pain with prolonged ambulation.[64] Physical examination may show an antalgic gait, decreased range of motion, pain on internal rotation, and a positive Trendelenburg sign.[64]

Radiographs

Standard radiographic projections include a supine AP view of the pelvis, an AP view of the hip, and a "frog leg" lateral view of the hip with the patient rolled toward the affected side. Supine examination of the hip is generally satisfactory because changes in cartilage space are generally minimal between supine and weight bearing.[72] The AP projections are obtained with the feet in internal rotation to correct for anteversion of the femoral neck (Figure 8-10). When the hips are internally rotated, the lesser trochanters will be partially obscured, whereas the lesser trochanters are seen in profile when there is external rotation. The "false profile" view is an oblique lateral projection of the hip obtained in the erect position. It has been shown to be more sensitive than conventional AP views for detecting early cartilage space narrowing.[16]

Normally, the acetabular roof ("sourcil") shows uniform sclerosis and does not tilt upward (upward tilt suggests dysplasia).[73] The cartilage space normally measures 3 to 8 mm in thickness superolaterally and 2 to 6 mm superomedially and is smaller in women than men.[74] In about 80% of normal subjects, the cartilage space is wider superolaterally than superomedially. Usually the cartilage spaces are bilaterally symmetric, but asymmetry has been found in almost 6% of subjects.[74] The smallest detectable difference in measuring cartilage space on serial radiographs is about 0.5 mm.[75]

> The normal hip cartilage space is uniform or slightly thinner superomedially. Superolateral thinning is likely abnormal.

CT Arthrography

Evaluation of cartilage in radiographically normal hips has shown that cartilage thickness on the acetabular and femoral sides is not identical.[76] The acetabular cartilage is thicker peripherally than centrally, and the femoral cartilage is thinner peripherally than centrally. Imagers should be aware of this normal nonuniform cartilage thickness when evaluating studies of patients suspected of having OA.

Results of a multicenter study clarified clinical and radiographic criteria for reporting OA in symptomatic patients.[77] The radiographic findings of OA in the painful hip that were present more often than in control patients include: (1) cartilage space narrowing, (2) osteophytes, (3) subchondral cysts, (4) subchondral sclerosis, (5) femoral neck buttressing, and (6) femoral head remodeling. Of these, cartilage space narrowing was the most sensitive (91%) but the least specific (60%). Medial femoral neck buttressing was the most specific (92%). Osteophytes had the best overall balance of high sensitivity (89%) and specificity (90%) in detecting hip OA. Radiographic evaluation and reporting should include each of these features.

> The imaging features of hip osteoarthritis are asymmetric cartilage space narrowing, osteophytes, subchondral cysts, subchondral sclerosis, femoral neck buttressing, and femoral head remodeling.

Osteophytes

Osteophyte formation is the most characteristic feature of osteoarthritis. Osteophytes may be described as marginal, central, and periosteal or synovial depending on their origin.[64] Marginal osteophytes occur at the periphery of the femoral head or the margins of the fovea (Figure 8-11). Central osteophytes extend from the subarticular surface and appear on radiographs as flat or button-like bony projections producing contour deformities of the femoral head. Periosteal or synovial osteophytes form as bony outgrowths from periosteum or synovial membranes. This is most apparent in the medial femoral neck, producing cortical thickening or a line of new bone formation termed *buttressing*.[64,78,79] Buttressing bone is thought to be due to altered stress loads on the femoral neck and is most commonly seen with OA and less often with osteonecrosis (Figure 8-12). Buttressing is rarely seen in patients with rheumatoid arthritis or psoriasis,[64,77,78] and the identification of this finding makes these diagnoses unlikely.

> Buttressing bone along the femoral neck is a feature of OA or osteonecrosis but not of inflammatory arthritis.

Subchondral Sclerosis

Redistribution of stress with progressive cartilage loss is thought to lead to hypervascularity and venous engorgement of the adjacent subchondral bone. Subchondral sclerosis occurs at these sites with

TABLE 8-2. Samilson and Prieto Grading of Glenohumeral OA

Grade	Description	Diagram	Example
Mild	Inferior humeral or glenoid *exostosis**, or both, measuring less than 3 mm	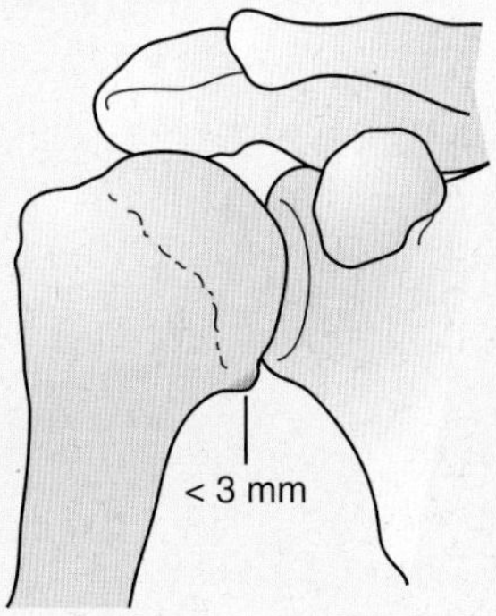 < 3 mm	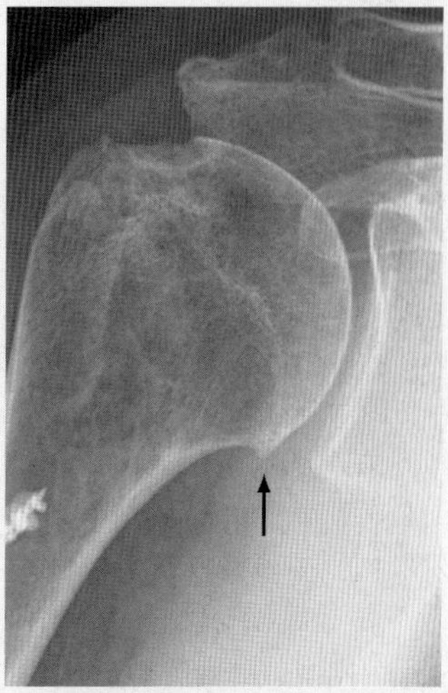
Moderate	Inferior humeral or glenoid exostosis, or both, measuring 3-7 mm and slight glenohumeral joint irregularity	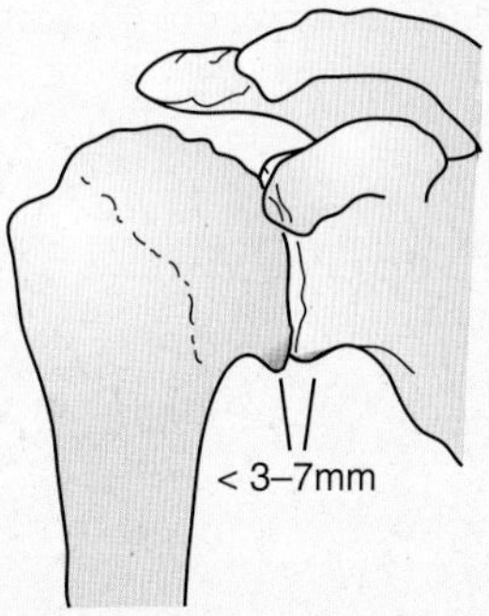 < 3–7mm	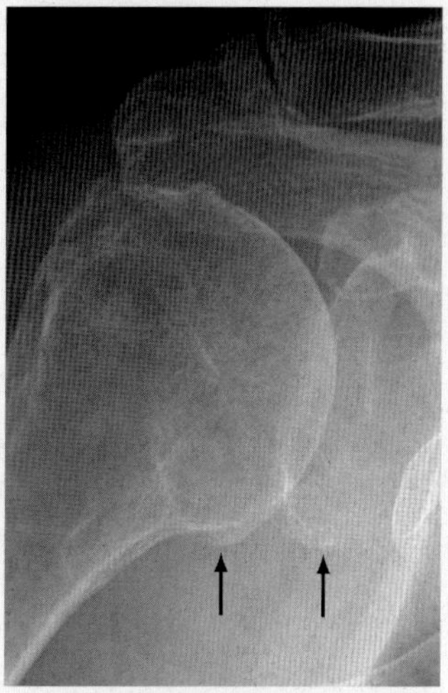
Severe	Inferior humeral or glenoid exostosis, or both, measuring more than 7 mm in height with narrowing of the glenohumeral joint and sclerosis	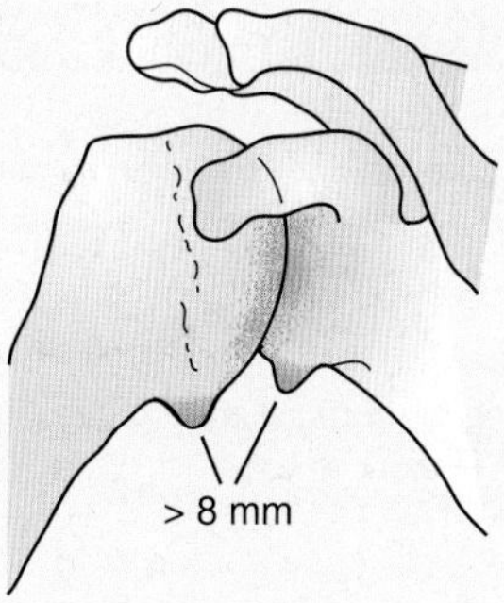 > 8 mm	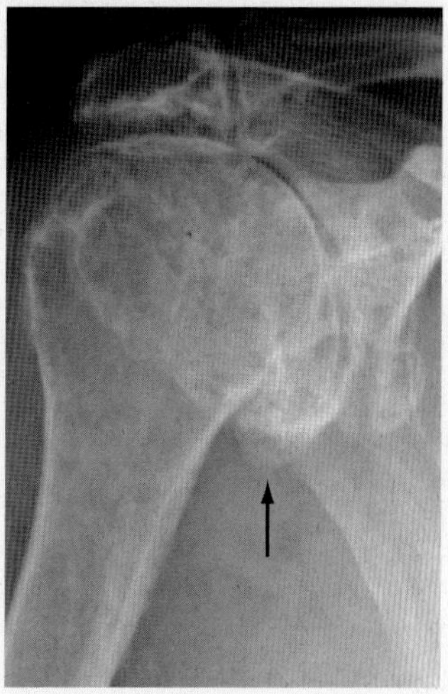

*The term exostosis was used to describe marginal osteophytes.
Diagrams redrawn from Samilson RL, Prieto V: Dislocation arthropathy of the shoulder, *J Bone Joint Surg Am* 65:456-460, 1983.

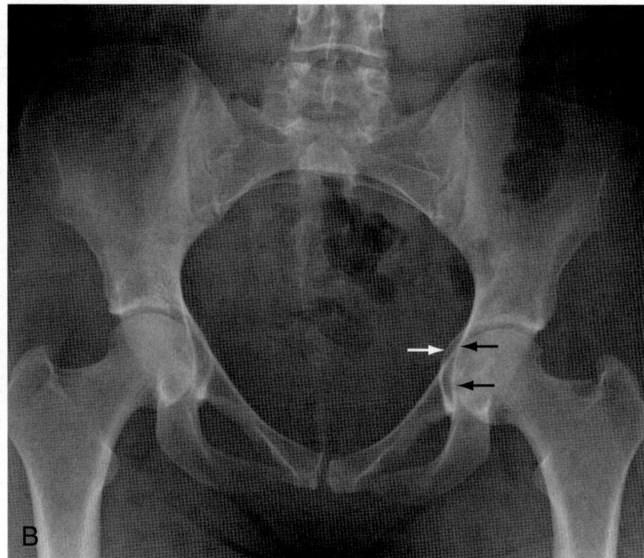

FIGURE 8-10. Normal hip appearance and protrusio deformity. **A,** Normal AP view of the pelvis shows that the lesser trochanters are partially obscured due to the internal rotation of the hips for this projection. The cartilage spaces are uniform in width and there is uniform thickness to the acetabular roofs. The anterior and posterior rims of the acetabulum are separated *(lines)* due to the normal acetabular anteversion. **B,** Protrusio deformity. The left medial acetabulum *(white arrow)* projects medial to the ilioischial line *(black arrows).*

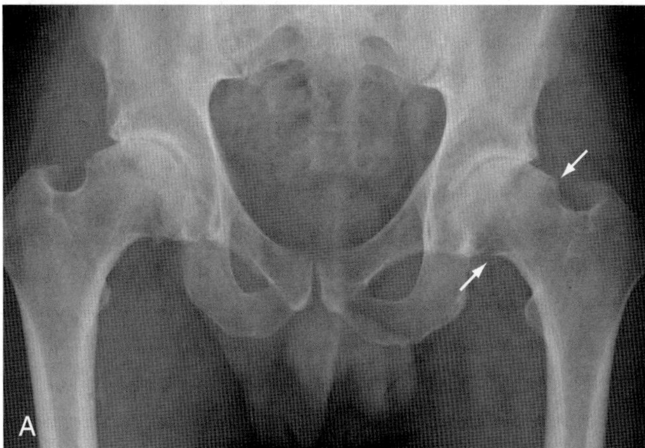

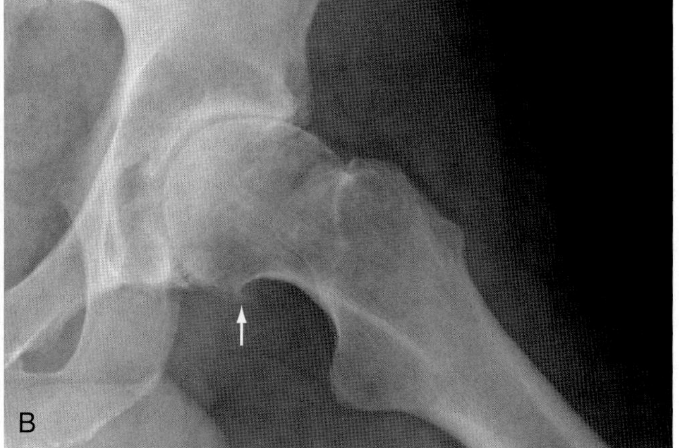

FIGURE 8-11. OA of the hip. **A,** An AP radiograph of the pelvis shows moderate to severe superolateral cartilage space narrowing bilaterally. There is osteophytic lipping *(arrows)* at the femoral head-neck junctions. **B,** The "frog leg" lateral view of the left hip shows the medial femoral head osteophyte *(arrow)* to advantage.

deposition of new bone on preexisting trabeculae and trabecular microfracture with callus formation[64] (Figure 8-13).

Subchondral Cysts

Subchondral cysts may be as large as 15 mm and are often multiple. Histologically, they can contain myxoid and adipose tissue, as well as occasional cartilage with surrounding fibrous components and are bordered by a peripheral margin of sclerotic bone.[64,80] Acetabular subchondral cysts have been termed *Eggers cysts.*[64]

Intraosseous Ganglia

Intraosseous ganglia are acetabular lesions that contain gelatinous fluid. They may be evident on radiographs if they produce a visible mass with erosion of the adjacent superolateral acetabulum or if they contain gas. The latter feature is a nearly diagnostic finding of an intraosseous ganglion and is apparently due to nitrogen tracking into the ganglion from the joint (Figure 8-14).

MRI can confirm the fluid characteristics of the mass. The signal intensity of the fluid within the ganglion may actually be greater on T1-weighted images than that of joint fluid due to the greater protein content of the ganglion[64] (see Figure 8-14).

Hip Position

As cartilage loss occurs, the femoral head position changes, "migrating" superolaterally in most cases (78%) or medially (22%)[81] (Figure 8-15). Superior migration in association with sclerosis, cysts, and osteophytes is nearly diagnostic for OA. An axial migration pattern with cartilage loss along the axis of the femoral neck is rare in primary OA, and other arthropathies such

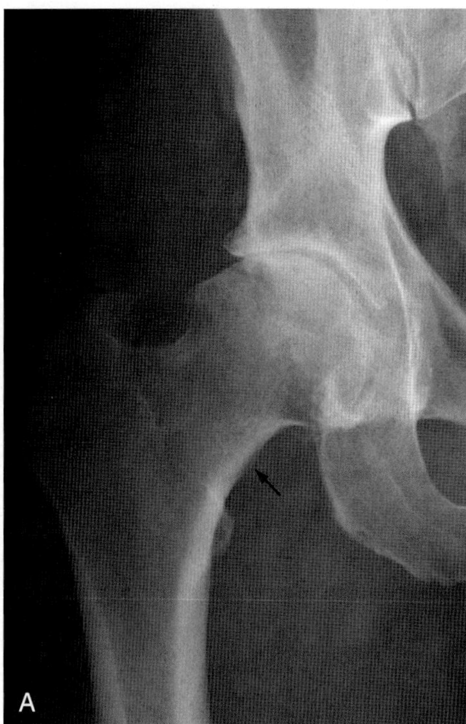

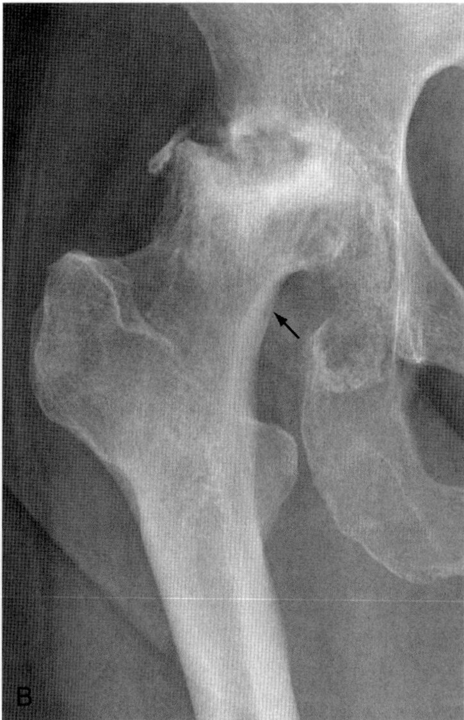

FIGURE 8-12. Buttressing bone. **A,** An AP view of the hip in a patient with OA (same patient as in Figure 8-11) shows a thin line of periosteal reaction along the femoral neck, termed *buttressing (arrow).* **B,** Avascular necrosis with buttressing new bone in a patient with sickle thalassemia. The AP radiograph of the hip shows a triangular region of collapse and sclerosis of the femoral head due to avascular osteonecrosis. There is severe secondary cartilage space narrowing (OA). Buttressing bone *(arrow)* producing cortical thickening is seen. A cortical defect from a prior core decompression is noted. Buttressing bone is typically seen in OA and osteonecrosis.

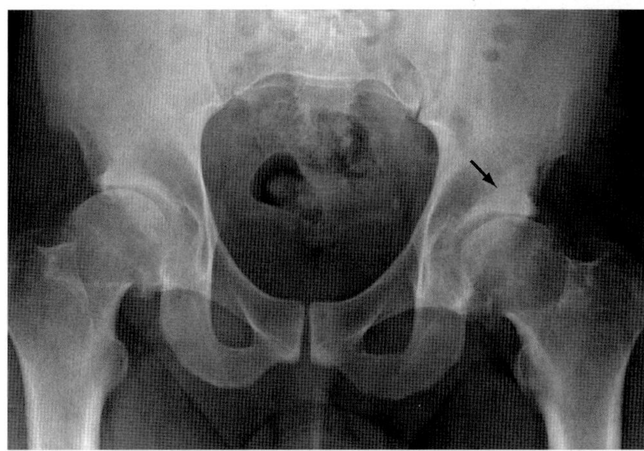

FIGURE 8-13. OA with subchondral sclerosis. The AP radiograph of the pelvis shows marked superolateral cartilage space narrowing bilaterally with prominent osteophytes at the femoral head-neck junctions. A triangular region of subchondral sclerosis *(arrow)* has developed on the patient's left, and there is thickening of the sourcil on the right side in response to changes in stress in these areas.

as rheumatoid arthritis or CPPD should be considered when this pattern is seen[64] (Figure 8-16).

The axial migration pattern is rare in primary OA, and other arthropathies such as rheumatoid arthritis should be considered first.

Diagnosis

Osteophytes from the superolateral acetabulum without other radiographic findings have been seen in the absence of OA.[77] Altman et al.[77] found that radiographic and clinical findings in patients with painful hips separated patients with hip OA from controls better than did clinical criteria alone. The parameters evaluated were: osteophytes, cartilage space narrowing, or erythrocyte sedimentation rate (ESR) < 22 mm/hr. In patients with pain, if two of these criteria were met, hip OA was diagnosed with 89% sensitivity and 91% specificity. However, using clinical criteria alone the sensitivity was 86% and the specificity 75%. A proposed classification tree of (1) hip pain and osteophytosis or (2) hip pain and cartilage space narrowing and ESR < 22 mm/hr yields 91% sensitivity and 89% specificity.

Using history, physical, laboratory, and radiographic information, OA can be diagnosed if there is hip pain and two of the following: ESR < 20 mm/hr, femoral and/or acetabular osteophytes on radiographs, or radiographic joint space narrowing.[77]

In patients with mechanical hip pain in whom radiographs are normal, MRI is usually performed. If these studies are normal or equivocal, CT or MR arthrography may be helpful.[82] Alvarez et al. identified 18 patients in whom, despite normal radiographs, helical CT arthrography demonstrated cartilage lesions.

In patients with mechanical hip pain and normal radiographs, MR or CT arthrography may show abnormalities of OA.

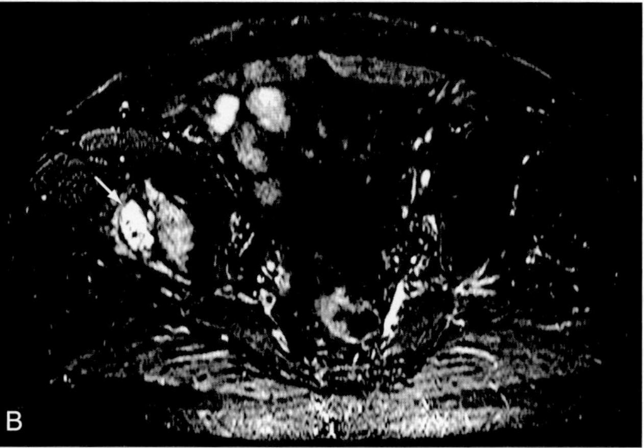

FIGURE 8-14. Intraosseous ganglion. **A,** The radiograph shows severe superolateral cartilage space narrowing. Gas is noted in the adjacent soft tissues *(arrows)*. **B,** An axial T2-weighted image shows the ganglion *(arrow)* with high signal (consistent with fluid) and central low signal (consistent with gas). (Courtesy of Dr. Leyla Alparslan.)

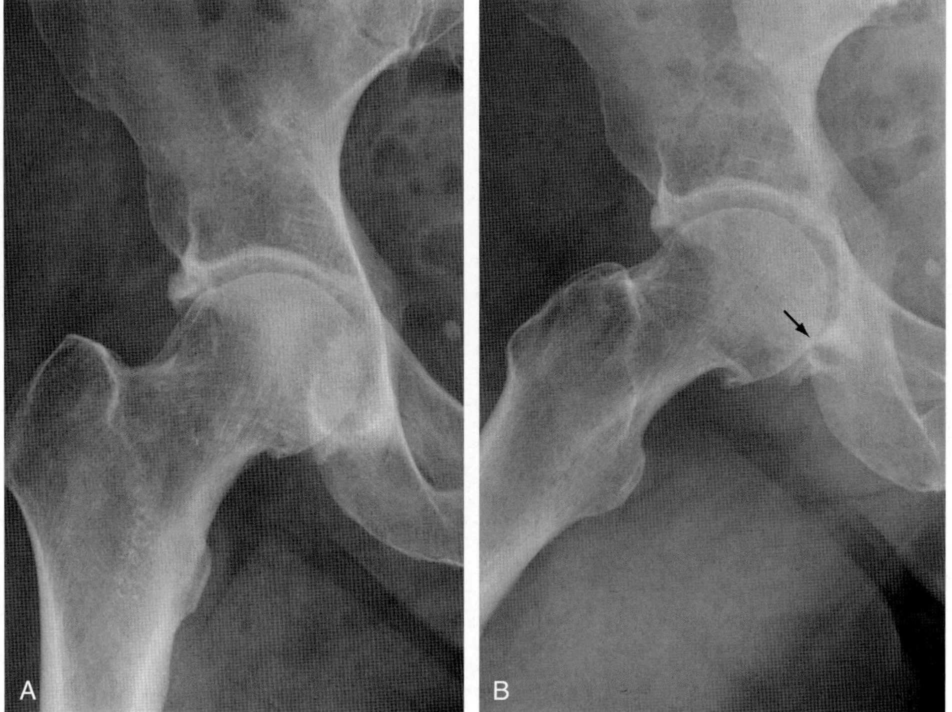

FIGURE 8-15. OA with medial cartilage space narrowing. **A,** The right hip shows medial cartilage space narrowing. There is osteophytic lipping from the acetabular margin and buttressing bone medially and probably laterally along the femoral neck. **B,** The "frog leg" lateral radiograph confirms inferomedial cartilage space narrowing and a cyst *(arrow)*.

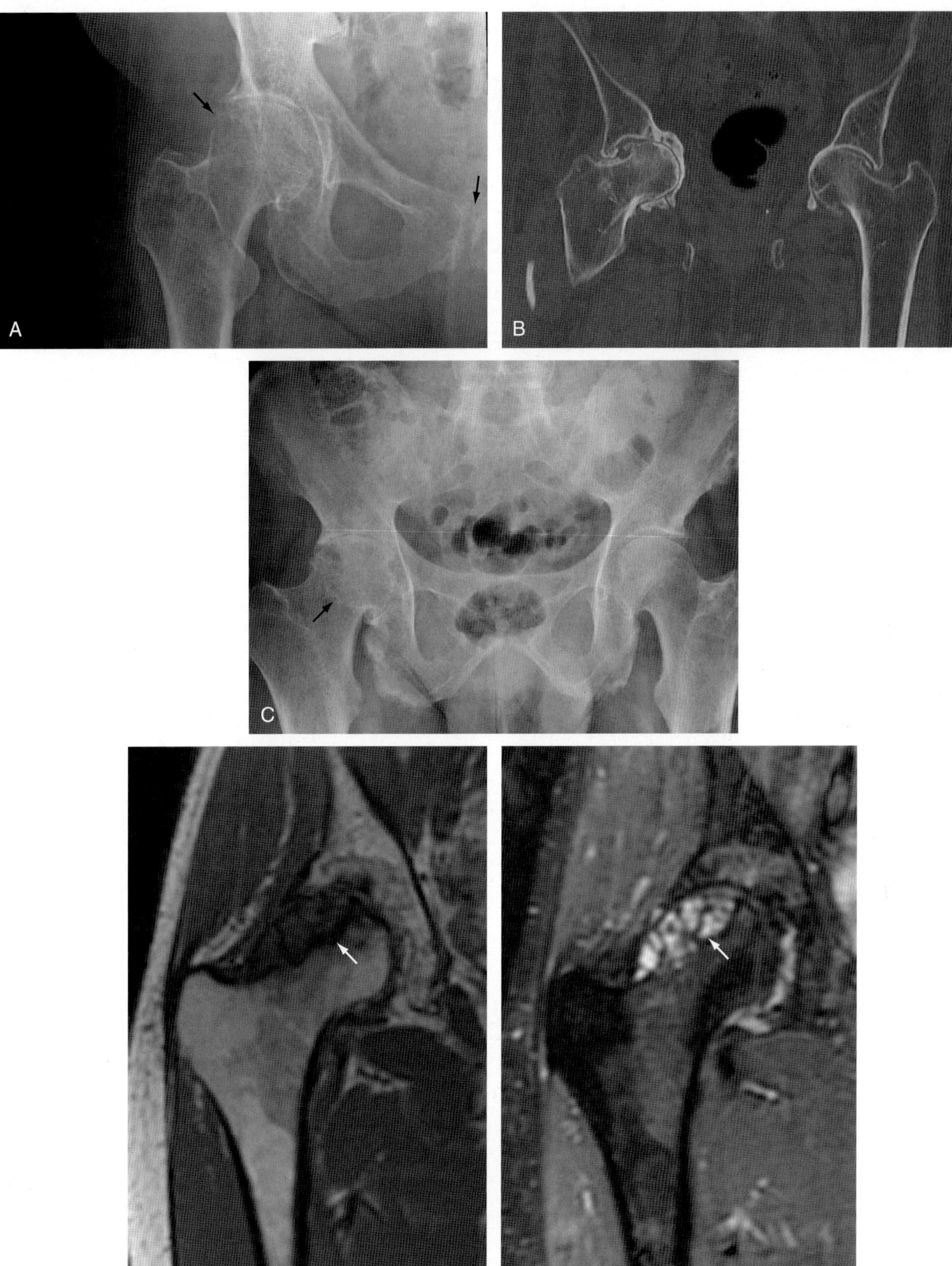

FIGURE 8-16. Secondary OA with axial cartilage loss. **A,** AP radiograph of the hip in a patient with CPPD arthropathy shows concentric cartilage space narrowing. Chondrocalcinosis is noted both in the hip articular cartilage *(arrow)* and in the pubic symphysis. The latter is a common site for identifying calcification in CPPD. **B,** Protrusio deformity in a patient with rheumatoid arthritis and secondary OA. This coronal reformatted image from a CT scan of the pelvis obtained for another purpose shows axial migration (hip displacement along the axis of the femoral necks) of the femoral heads and striking remodeling of the acetabula. There is complete cartilage loss axially. **C,** This patient shows the typical features of ankylosing spondylitis affecting the hip. There is diffuse cartilage space narrowing of the right hip with axial migration as may be seen in inflammatory arthritis, but there is a rim of osteophytes at the head neck junction *(arrows)*. Fusion of the sacroiliac joints, bony bridging in the spine, and new bone formation at the ischial entheses are also noted. There is mild osteophyte formation in the left hip medially. Coronal T1-weighted **(D)** and **(E)** coronal STIR images of a patient with hemochromatosis. There is superolateral hip cartilage space narrowing. The marked cyst-like changes in the femoral head *(arrows)* are atypical for OA.

Follow-Up

Cartilage space narrowing by 2 mm in 1 year or 4 mm after 2 years has been shown to be clinically relevant,[64] although smaller amounts of cartilage space narrowing are often present.[92] When using radiographs to assess progression of hip OA, combining cartilage space narrowing with subchondral cysts or cartilage space narrowing with subchondral sclerosis produces the best sensitivity.[13]

Image-Guided Injection of Corticosteroid

For patients unresponsive to or unable to take usual medical therapy, hip injection with corticosteroids has been proposed to decrease pain and reduce synovitis.[83] A recent placebo-controlled trial of injection of corticosteroids into the hip joint has shown the procedure to provide effective pain relief that often lasted 3 months.[83] Improvement in stiffness and physical function also occurred from baseline to 2 months. Severity of disease at the time of injection did not affect the outcome.

Technique

Because the hip joint is deep, image guidance is necessary to ensure intraarticular needle placement. Often this is fluoroscopic guidance, but ultrasound can also be used. Joint effusion is aspirated prior to injection. A small amount of iodinated contrast is injected to confirm intraarticular needle placement (Figure 8-17). Lambert et al. used a mixture of bupivacaine and 40 mg triamcinolone hexacetonide; triamcinolone was used as the corticosteroid because of its insolubility and long duration of effect. Robinson et al. compared the efficacy of 40 mg of methylprednisolone acetate (depomedrone 40 mg/cc Pfizer, New York, N.Y.) with 80 mg (each dose mixed with 3 to 4 cc 0.5% bupivacaine (Marcain, AstraZeneca, Wilmington, Del.) to make 5 mL of injectate.[84] The 80-mg dose provided a response that was maintained at 12 weeks.[84] Resting the joint for 24 hours after injection is advised.[83,85]

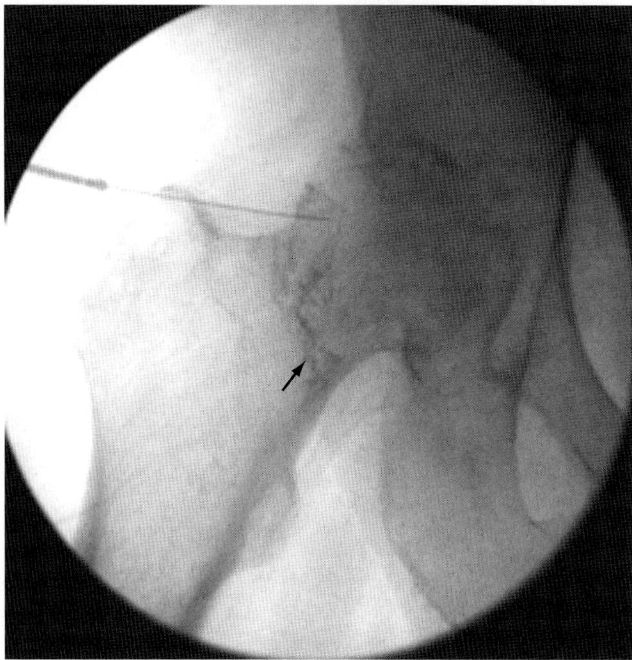

FIGURE 8-17. Injection of corticosteroid into the hip. The fluoroscopic spot film taken shortly after the start of contrast injection shows that the contrast *(arrow)* is beginning to fill the joint. If the injection were extraarticular, the contrast would collect around the needle tip.

Contraindications for corticosteroid injection include local or systemic infection, allergy to anesthetic or contrast, and possibly anticoagulation. Weight-bearing joints should not be injected more than once a month and no more than four times a year.[86] An atrophic appearance on radiographs may be associated with a poor response.

Peak effects occur by 2 to 3 weeks after injection.[87,88] Complications are uncommon and consist of postinjection flare or crystal-induced arthritis, which usually lasts less than 48 hours or infection, which is very rare.[29]

RAPID DESTRUCTIVE OSTEOARTHRITIS

Rapid destructive osteoarthritis (RDO) (also known as *Postel's osteoarthritis* or *rapidly destructive arthrosis* [RDA]) is an uncommon form of hip OA that results in striking bone and cartilage loss, often within weeks to months. The disorder usually affects elderly women, is usually unilateral,[89] and produces severe pain. The cause is not known but an insufficiency fracture of the femoral head has been found on pathologic examination.[90] Yamamoto and colleagues indicate that RDO is likely multifactorial.[64] Watanabe et al. have found mild acetabular dysplasia and posterior pelvic tilt in most cases of RDO[91] and postulate that RDO is initially triggered by mechanical factors such as insufficiency fractures caused by osteopenia, posterior pelvic tilt, and mild acetabular dysplasia and progresses to end-stage disease by inflammation due to granulation tissue.[91]

Radiographic Findings

RDO has been defined by cartilage space narrowing of at least 2 mm per year whereas, in the usually seen form of OA, cartilage space narrowing of 0 to 0.8 mm is noted yearly.[92] Rapid, marked bone loss from the femoral head and acetabulum occurs (Figure 8-18).[89] Osteophytes are small or absent, and buttressing bone is absent. Cyst-like changes and sclerosis are typical. The radiographic features may mimic osteonecrosis with secondary OA, rheumatoid arthritis, seronegative arthropathies, infection, or neuropathic arthropathy. Exclusion of septic arthritis (by joint aspiration) and of neuropathic arthropathy (by clinical features) is of critical importance preoperatively.

FEMOROACETABULAR IMPINGEMENT

Hip impingement is thought to be a potentially correctable condition that if untreated may result in OA. The source of impingement is important to identify because surgical treatment differs depending on the underlying abnormality.[93]

Two major types of femoroacetabular impingement (FAI) have been described, both of which may coexist:

1. *Cam type:* This cause of impingement is characterized by an abnormal shape of the femoral head-neck junction. This deformity leads to jamming of the femoral head-neck junction into the acetabulum during forceful flexion and internal rotation.[93] Linear contact occurs between the acetabular rim and the femoral head-neck junction, causing damage to the anterior-superior acetabular cartilage and secondary development of a labral tear or detachment.

   Causes of cam-type impingement include femoral head abnormalities (asphericity, slipped capital femoral epiphysis, absent anterior offset) or femoral neck abnormalities (retroversion, coxa vara, femoral neck malunion).
2. *Pincer type:* This condition is characterized by abnormal acetabular morphology with acetabular overcoverage. These patients have a deep acetabular socket or localized overcoverage due to

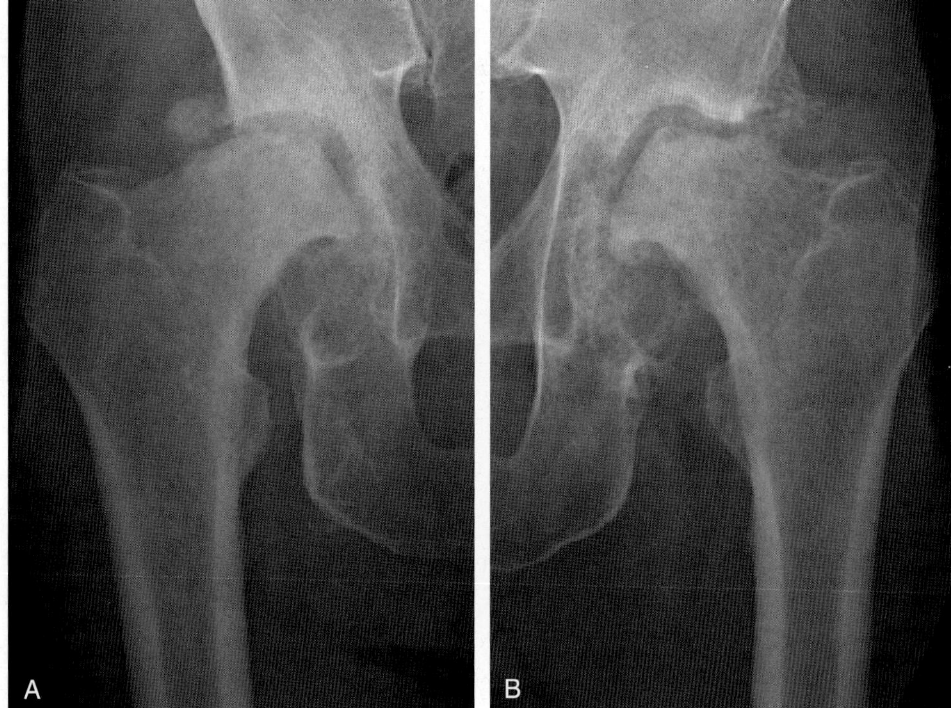

FIGURE 8-18. Rapidly progressive OA. AP view of the right hip **(A)** and AP view of the left hip **(B)** in an elderly man demonstrates severe bone loss bilaterally. Bone destruction had markedly progressed in less than 1 year. Usually this disorder is seen in elderly women and is unilateral.

acetabular retroversion.[94] Labral abnormalities occur first followed by rim ossification. Chondral injury may be present in the contrecoup region of the acetabulum (posterior-inferior). In addition, combined abnormalities may be present.

Cam impingement is usually seen in young athletic males, whereas pincer impingement is more often seen in middle-aged women.[93]

Imaging Findings

The following abnormalities have been identified in impingement.

Radiographic Findings: Cam Impingement

Deformity of the anterosuperior head/neck junction: The lack of femoral head-neck offset in the frontal plane has been called the "pistol grip" deformity and is a characteristic feature of cam impingement as described by Stulberg.[95] Several views may demonstrate the abnormal head neck junction including a cross-table lateral projection in internal rotation; AP or cross-table lateral views in external rotation may not show asphericity of the superolateral head-neck contour. The bump present anteriorly and superiorly may also be well seen on three-dimensional CT[96] (Figure 8-19).

Herniation pits (Pitt's pits): These rounded areas of radiolucency in the superolateral aspect of the femoral neck have been thought to represent incidental findings. They are reported to occur in about 5% of the population.[94] A study by Leunig et al. comparing patients with clinical and imaging features of FAI with patients with developmental dysplasia and no evidence of impingement showed these fibrocystic changes to be present in 33% of FAI hips (39/117) and in no hips with developmental dysplasia. MRI was more sensitive than radiography in detecting these lesions. The authors concluded that the high prevalence of juxtaarticular fibrocystic changes at the anterosuperior femoral neck and their spatial relation to the impingement site suggested an association and possibly a causal relationship between these findings and FAI.[94]

Os acetabuli: Normally, the os acetabuli (the epiphysis of the pubis) develops at about age 8 years and unites with the pubis at about age 18 years.[93] Separated bone fragments or os acetabuli may be observed in cam-type FAI.[97]

Large alpha angles: See below.

Radiographic Features: Pincer Impingement

Figure-eight sign, the crossover sign of acetabular retroversion: Normally the acetabulum is anteverted. Retroversion is thought to be a cause of FAI,[94,98] allowing the femoral head to abut the prominent anterior acetabular rim. This abnormality may be detected by careful radiographic analysis of the acetabular rims, especially their proximal portions near the acetabular roofs.[6]

In the normal hip, the edge of the anterior rim is projected medial to the edge of the posterior rim and the distance between the rims increases distally. The distance between the anterior and posterior margins measures at least 1.5 cm (measured along a line through the center of the femoral head, perpendicular to the anterior acetabular rim). In patients with acetabular retroversion, the posterior margin of the acetabulum is projected medial to the anterior margin proximally. More distally, the posterior rim returns to the more normal position, lateral to the anterior rim; thus the posterior and anterior rims cross over each other. This crossover or figure-eight sign confirms acetabular retroversion if patient positioning is correct (e.g., no pelvic tilt is present) (see Figure 8-19).

"Posterior wall" sign: The normal posterior margin of the acetabular rim passes through the center of the femoral head or lateral to it. The retroverted acetabular posterior rim passes medial to the center of the head.[6]

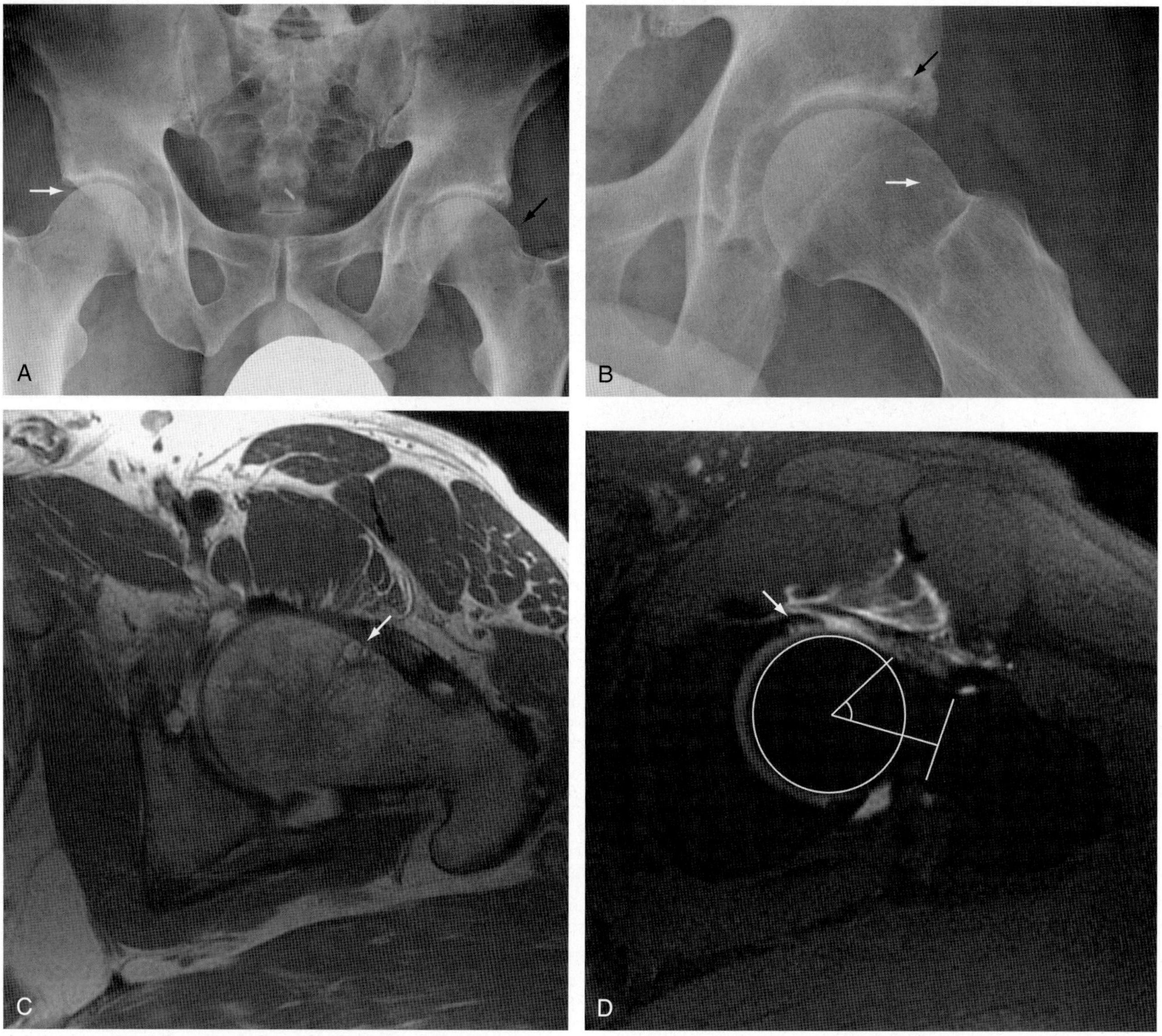

FIGURE 8-19. Hip impingement. **A,** A radiograph of the pelvis in a 45-year-old man shows an os acetabuli *(white arrow)* on the right and slight hypertrophic bone at the femoral head-neck junction *(arrow)*. The findings on the symptomatic left side are more marked with a larger bony bump at the femoral head-neck junction and cystic-like changes in the superior/lateral acetabulum. No herniation pits were definitively seen on this radiograph. **B,** The "frog leg" lateral radiograph of the left side shows the cyst-like changes of the acetabulum *(black arrow)* and a possible herniation pit *(white arrow)* anterolaterally. **C,** An oblique axial non–fat-saturated image from the MR arthrogram shows an anterior herniation pit *(arrow)* that is more often seen in patients with femoroacetabular impingement than in the general population. **D,** Oblique axial image obtained after injection of the joint with a dilute gadolinium solution shows some contrast extravasation anteriorly. A tear of the anterior labrum is seen demonstrating irregular contrast extension into the undersurface of the labrum *(arrow)*. Measurement of the alpha angle showed it to be abnormally high (65 degrees), consistent with impingement. The method of calculating this angle is shown: a line is drawn perpendicular to the femoral neck at its narrowest point. A second line is drawn perpendicular to this line bisecting the femoral neck. A "best fit" circle is drawn, outlining the femoral head. The alpha angle is formed between the femoral neck line and a line from the center of the head to the point where the femoral head protrudes anterior to the circle (after Kassarjian A, Yoon L, Belzile E: Triad of MR arthrographic findings in patients with CAM-type femoroacetabular impingement, *Radiology* 236:588-592, 2005.).

Protrusio acetabuli: An abnormally deep acetabulum may cause impingement. Apparently, this configuration is normal during development. After about 8 years of age, a deep acetabulum may be responsible for impingement. McBride et al. defined protrusio deformity as present when the medial wall of the acetabulum projects medial to the ilioischial line.[99] Other measurements have been used. For example, a medial acetabulum to ilioischial line distance of greater than 3 mm in men or 6 mm or more in women indicates this deformity (see Figure 8-10).[99a]

Acetabular rim ossification: Ossification of the acetabular rim may indicate impingement.

MRI Features: Cam Type

Abnormal alpha angle: Transverse oblique MR images are obtained. On the central slice, a circle is drawn outlining the femoral head. The alpha angle is constructed between one line drawn from the center of the circle to the point where the circle

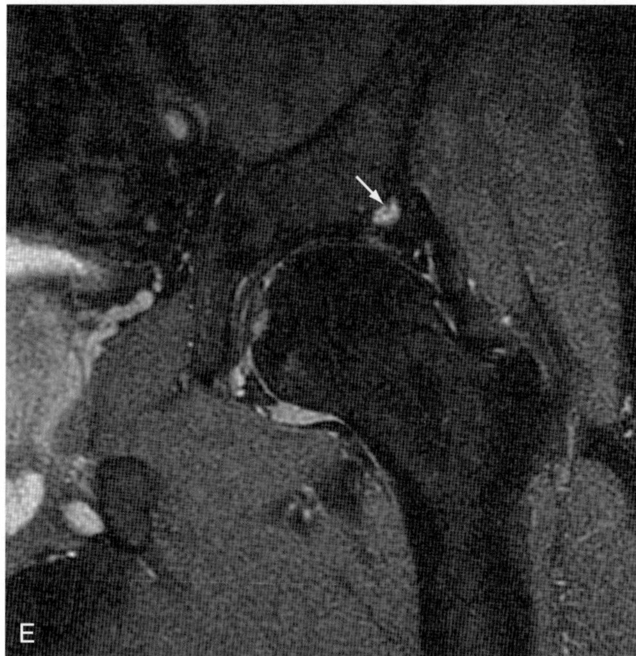

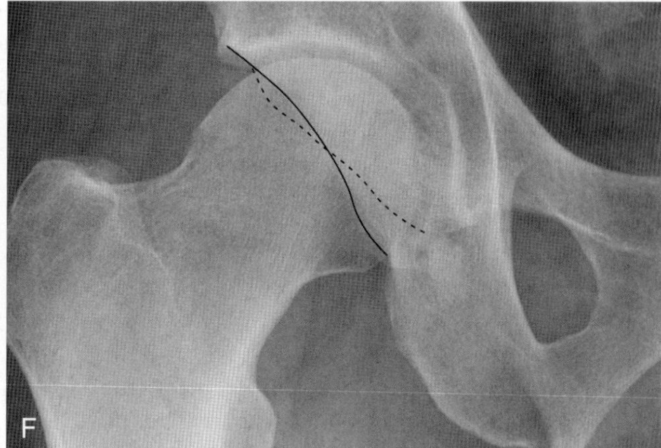

FIGURE 8-19—cont'd. E, A coronal STIR image shows the cyst-like change seen on the radiograph to contain fluid signal *(arrow)*. **F,** Pelvis radiograph shows the lines of the anterior and posterior rims of the right acetabulum (*dashed line* anterior, *solid* posterior). The crossover of these lines centrally is consistent with acetabular retroversion. (Compare with Figure 8-10A.)

and the femoral head neck junction meet and a second line is drawn from the center of the circle through the center of the femoral neck. The angle between these two lines (the alpha angle) is normally 55 degrees or less.[93] It is larger in cam-type impingement.

Cartilage damage: On MRI examination,[93] Pfirrmann et al. noted anterosuperior cartilage lesions to be significantly larger in patients with cam-type impingement than in those with pincer-type impingement. "Outside in" abrasion of anterior acetabular cartilage was noted. Other findings are avulsion/chondral flaps from inner labral edge and labral degeneration.

Osseous bump at the femoral neck: The bony bump seen on radiography is also seen on MRI.

MRI Features: Pincer Type

Posteroinferior cartilage damage: Patients with pincer-type impingement develop posteroinferior cartilage damage and labral lesions more often than do those with cam-type impingement.[93] This is thought to be due to a contrecoup mechanism.

Acetabular deformity: The abnormally deep acetabulum can be detected on MRI as well as on radiographs.

KNEES

As determined by radiographs, OA of the knee occurs in 14% to 30% of individuals older than 45 years.[100] It is more prevalent in women, increases in prevalence with age, and may be symptomatic in up to 80% of individuals with radiographically detected OA. Evaluation of both the femorotibial and patellofemoral joints is necessary to evaluate OA.[101] In patients with OA, the correlation with pain is imperfect. Articular cartilage does not have pain fibers; pain in OA is most often related to the patellofemoral joint, the bone, synovial inflammation, effusion with stretching of the joint capsule, or bursitis.[3] The finding of chondrocalcinosis is not consistently associated with symptoms.[3]

Radiographs

Joints Examined

Radiographic examination seeks to evaluate both the femorotibial and patellofemoral joints. Because the patellofemoral joint may be an important source of symptoms in OA, tangential patellar views are suggested. A number of techniques have been proposed to examine the tibiofemoral joint; these are discussed briefly below.

> The patellofemoral joint may be responsible for symptoms and should be evaluated on imaging studies of the knee.

Ideal Positioning

Ideally, the frontal projection should show the tibial spines to be centered under the femoral intercondylar notch, and the tibial plateau should be in profile. It is particularly desirable to view the medial compartment in profile because it is the site of OA in 80% of cases.[72] Mazzuca et al. considered the medial tibial plateau position to be satisfactory when its anterior and posterior margins were within 1 mm of each other.[102] Because the tibial plateau slopes downward posteriorly to a particular degree in each individual, no set angulation of the radiographic beam or knee flexion can provide this perfect view in all individuals. Fluoroscopy has been suggested to achieve ideal positioning and to obtain equivalent positioning on follow-up examinations.[103]

Structures Evaluated

Cartilage Space

The space between the femur and tibia on weight-bearing radiographs is thought to reflect the thickness of the articular cartilage (hence the term *cartilage space* used in this chapter). Cartilage space narrowing on weight-bearing radiographs therefore has traditionally been used as a marker of cartilage loss. However, in the knee, alterations in the menisci may also influence the thickness of the measured cartilage space.[2] Hunter et al. compared weight-bearing fluoroscopically positioned radiographic measurements of the medial joint space with the appearance of the articular cartilage and menisci, including meniscal degeneration and extrusion, on MRI. They found that meniscal position and meniscal degeneration as well as cartilage morphology contributed to the prediction of joint space narrowing. Other variables include weight bearing, positioning of the joint, and radiographic quality.[72]

Cartilage loss in osteoarthritis is not uniform, and there is often a disparity between compartments. Uniform cartilage space narrowing, even if osteophytes are present, should suggest secondary osteoarthritis such as occurs in rheumatoid arthritis. Eventually, cartilage loss and bone remodeling lead to malalignment of the joint, which further increases the stress on the affected compartment.

Supine versus Upright Views

Knee cartilage space thickness can change considerably between supine and upright films and even between films obtained standing on one leg or both[72] (Figure 8-20).

The normal cartilage space on a standing view measures 3 mm or more. Ahlback defined cartilage space narrowing on standing views as a cartilage space of less than 3 mm, or half or less the width of the same area in the opposite normal knee or by the presence of cartilage space narrowing on weight-bearing as compared with non–weight-bearing views.[104]

Unfortunately, comparison of the standing view with the knee extended to articular cartilage examination at surgery has shown that normal radiographs did not predict normal cartilage at surgery and abnormal radiographs did not necessarily predict a cartilage abnormality at surgery.[104]

The standing view of the legs (the mechanical axis): The standing view of the legs is an important study for the evaluation of osteoarthritic deformity or for surgical planning. The view is obtained using a long cassette to include the hips to the ankles. The patient stands with weight equally distributed on both legs and the patellae or tibial tubercles (not the feet) directed forward. In a normal individual, the mechanical axis (a line drawn from the center of the femoral head to the center of the ankle) passes just medial to the center of the knee joint (Figure 8-21). When varus knee alignment is present, the axis falls medial to this point. The distance in millimeters from the mechanical axis to the center of the knee helps quantify the deformity and is termed the *mechanical axis deviation.*

Flexed views: Knee flexion plays an important role in cartilage space evaluation because cartilage loss may occur preferentially posteriorly and these areas may be profiled on flexed views.[105] Several flexion views have been suggested[106]:

The tunnel view: As initially described, the tunnel view is obtained prone with the knee in 75 degrees of flexion.[107] The non–weight-bearing tunnel view may demonstrate cartilage loss not visible on supine or on standing views.[108]

The standing tunnel view: Several authors have indicated that flexed standing views of the knees are helpful in assessing the presence of cartilage space narrowing in OA,[105,109] but the degree of recommended flexion varies. Buckland-Wright et al. investigated the use of the posteroanterior (PA) semi-flexed standing view. This projection is a standing view but, using fluoroscopic positioning, the knee is slightly flexed (179 to 160 degrees) until the tibial plateau is parallel to the x-ray beam and the floor and perpendicular to the film.[106] The precise positioning would depend on the individual's tibial plateau slope. The foot is rotated internally or externally so that the tibial spines are centered with relation to the femoral intercondylar notch. Microfocal radiographs are obtained.

The Lyon Schuss view: This is a PA view obtained with the knees in 20 to 30 degrees of flexion. This view places the posterior femorotibial cartilage space in profile. The AP flexed radiograph is performed by having the patient flex the knee until the tibial plateau is parallel to the floor and the x-ray beam. This results in less flexion than is possible on the Lyon Schuss view, where the thighs are braced against the x-ray table.[110] Other positions have also been advocated.[111]

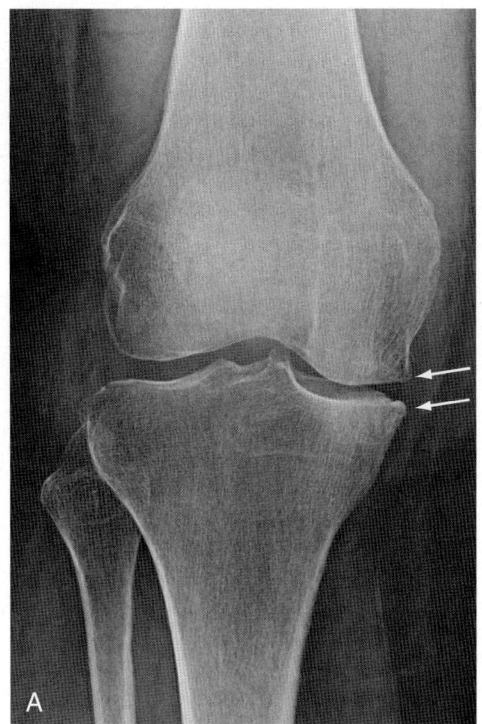

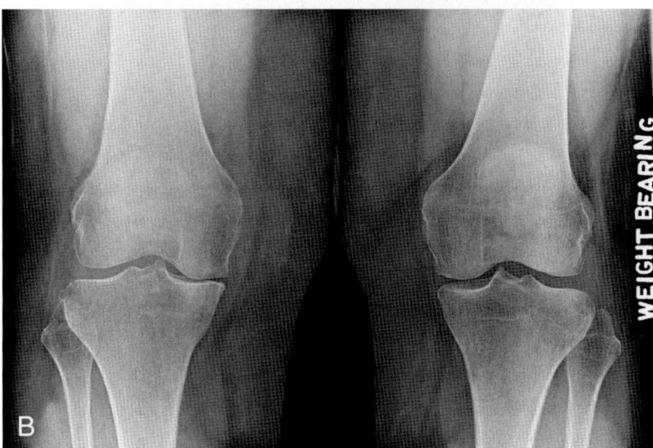

FIGURE 8-20. OA of the knee. **A,** The supine radiograph on the right knee shows marginal osteophytes from the femur and tibia *(arrows)*. The medial cartilage space appears slightly narrow. However, the subchondral sclerosis on either side of the joint *(open arrows)* is highly suggestive of severe cartilage loss. **B,** The standing AP view of both knees shows moderate to severe cartilage space narrowing on the right.

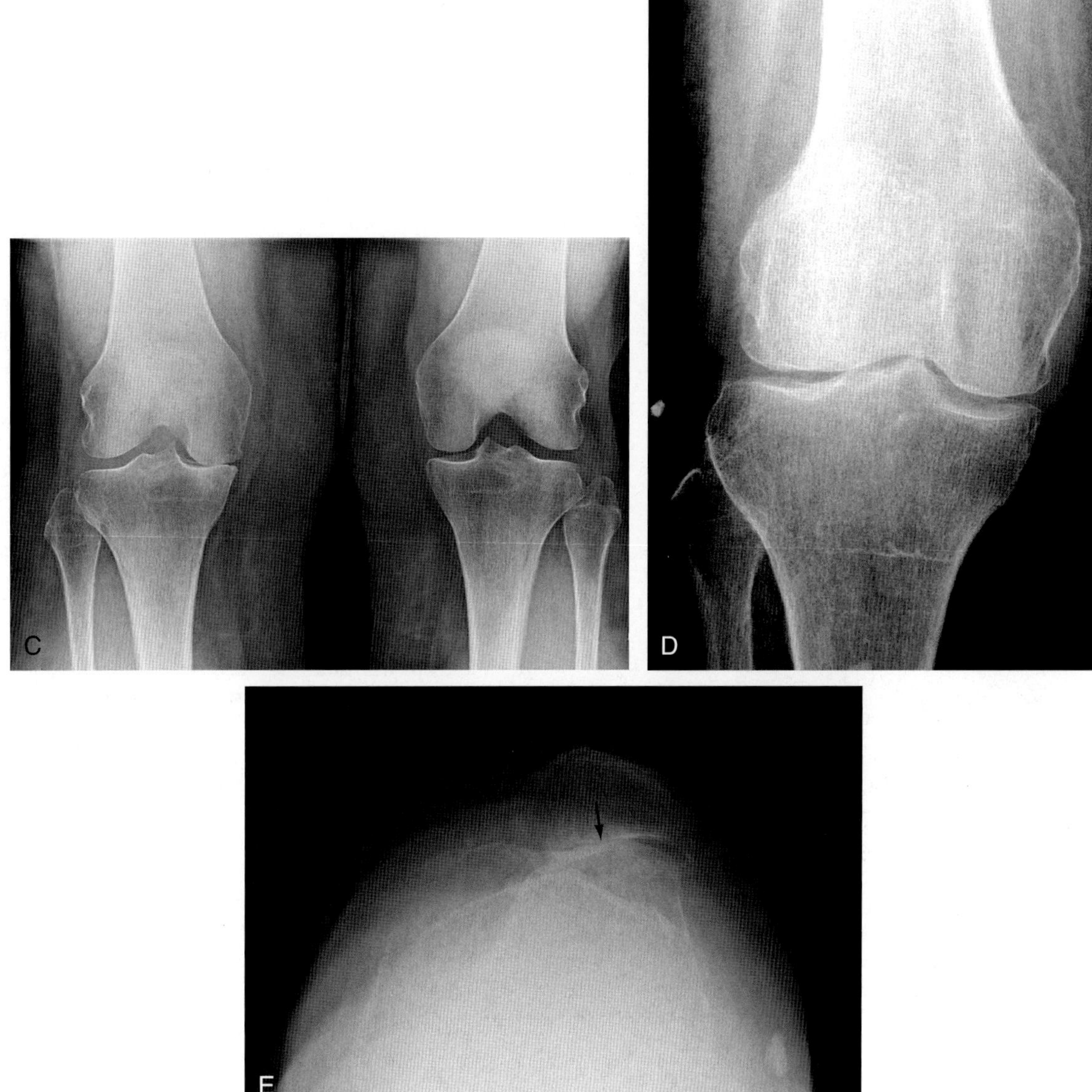

FIGURE 8-20—cont'd. **C,** The PA flexed (Rosenberg) view confirms that severe cartilage space narrowing is present. The left knee is normal. **D,** An AP radiograph in another patient shows normal femorotibial cartilage space. **E,** The tangential patellar view (same patient as **D**) shows marked patellofemoral cartilage space narrowing *(arrow)*.

The Rosenberg view: Rosenberg et al. noted that cartilage thinning was seen at arthroscopy in areas corresponding to 30 to 60 degrees of flexion and therefore they recommended the knees be flexed at 45 degrees for radiography.[109] The radiograph is obtained posteroanteriorly with weight equally distributed on each foot, the toes pointing forward, and the patellae touching the cassette. The x-ray beam is centered at the inferior pole of the patella and directed 10 degrees caudally. These authors indicate that normally the cartilage space on these radiographs measures 4 mm or more medially and 5 mm or more laterally. Using a definition of 2 mm or more of narrowing as indicating major cartilage loss, these radiographs were found to be more sensitive than standing views for the demonstration of either medial or lateral cartilage loss and also more specific (see Figure 8-20, *C*).

Following Patients Over Time

Attention to detail is critical if cartilage space narrowing over time is to be detected and followed. The degree of flexion, foot rotation, or beam inclination can change the visible cartilage space width.

Cartilage space narrowing is not a normal sequela of aging.[10] Cartilage space narrowing occurs at a mean rate of 0.26 mm per year in patients with knee OA in clinical research cohorts and at about half that rate in population-based cohorts of community elders with radiographic OA not treated by a physician.[102] Therefore sensitive and reproducible measurement techniques are necessary for evaluation. Methods have been developed to measure the minimum joint space width (JSW), the mean JSW, or the joint space area.[72] Vignon indicates that the smallest detectable difference by a single observer for minimum JSW is 0.3 mm. Variability

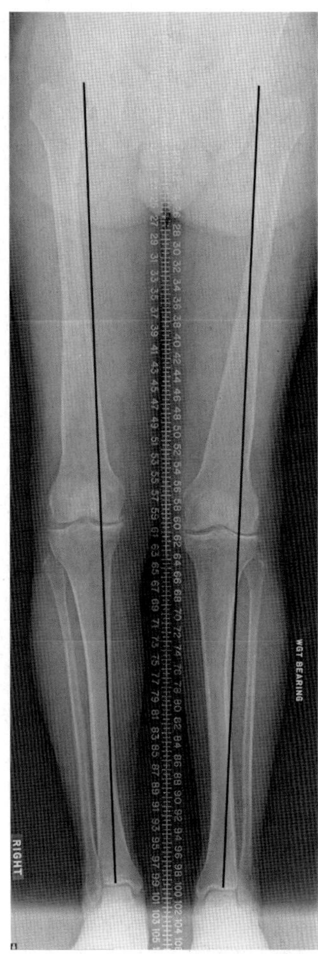

FIGURE 8-21. The mechanical axis. This AP radiograph of the legs is obtained with the patient standing. A line is drawn from the center of the femoral head to the center of the tibial plafond. Normally, this passes just medial to the center of the knee. In this case, the axis falls further medially on the right, indicating varus alignment (due to medial compartment osteoarthritis and cartilage loss), and lateral to the center of the joint on the left, indicating valgus alignment (due to lateral compartment OA).

reflects difficulty in the choice of the narrowest area and the experience of the observer.[72] More difficulty occurs in the knee than in the hip. Even with optimal positioning, the smallest detectable difference in JSW can be 0.6 mm.[72]

Bruyere et al. found a moderate association between changes in JSW and changes in cartilage volume or thickness as demonstrated by MRI in the knee joint of patients with OA.[112]

Patellofemoral Joint

Patellofemoral OA is common, may occur without tibiofemoral disease, and can cause disability[113] (see Figure 8-20). Tangential patellar ("sunrise") views are generally superior to lateral radiographs for evaluation of this joint and should be included as part of the routine examination for OA. There are numerous radiographic techniques for obtaining patellofemoral radiographs. The degree of knee flexion is an important variable because cartilage space thickness can vary with changes in flexion.

The cartilage space on the tangential patellar view can be measured from the anterior convex margin of the articular surface of the medial or lateral trochlea to the deep (anterior) subchondral cortex of the patella.[114] Boegard et al. found cartilage space of less than 5 mm usually indicates that cartilage defects are present on MRI.[114] Joint effusion can increase the patellofemoral joint space.

Osteophytes

Osteophytes are the radiographic hallmark of OA (although they alone do not define the clinical syndrome). The diagnosis of knee OA can be made with 83% sensitivity and 93% specificity if a patient with knee pain has osteophytes on radiographic examination.[1]

Osteophyte Location, Size, and Shape

Osteophytes may be described as marginal, intercondylar, on the tibial spines, or internal. The size of marginal osteophytes has been found to increase with decreasing cartilage space width.[114] In addition to local cartilage space narrowing, osteophyte size is related to varus malalignment and bone loss.[115] The shape of osteophytes has also been examined. A downward slope of a medial tibial osteophyte has been found to be associated with medial meniscal displacement (extrusion) and meniscal tear on MRI examination.[116] The authors postulate that this type of medial osteophyte may be a risk factor for developing severe OA of the knee. Enlargement of osteophytes can be accompanied by a change in their shape from horizontal to vertical.[115]

Relationship of Osteophytes to Symptoms

Knee osteophytes and the Kellgren Lawrence grading, which emphasizes osteophytes, have been shown to be predictors of knee pain.[10,100]

Relationship of Osteophytes to Cartilage Damage

The significance of the finding of "spiking" of the tibial spines has been debated. Isolated spiking of the tibial spines has been thought to be an unreliable sign of OA[117,118] whereas others indicate this to be an early sign of OA. Comparison of spiking of the tibial spines to MRI-detected cartilage defects has shown that the predictive value of the finding is related to the degree and size of the spikes.[119]

The presence of marginal osteophytes has been shown to correlate with MRI-identified cartilage defects.[120] Similarly, examination of extended-knee, weight-bearing radiographs of patients undergoing arthroscopy found osteophytes to be the most sensitive feature for the detection of OA[7]; the sensitivity of medial compartment osteophytes was 67% and the specificity 73%. Cartilage space narrowing had a lower sensitivity but a higher specificity (46% sensitivity and 95% specificity).

No relation has been found between central osteophytes and MRI-detected cartilage lesions.[118]

Malalignment

Varus alignment is more often seen in patients with OA than in those with rheumatoid arthritis (Figure 8-22).

Subchondral Sclerosis

Increased stress across a compartment may be associated with subchondral sclerosis. Sclerosis in the subchondral bone of both the tibia and femur indicates severe cartilage loss and should suggest the true severity of the disorder even when the cartilage space does not seem narrowed on the radiograph (see Figure 8-22).

Magnetic Resonance Imaging

Although there are many advantages to radiographic evaluation of OA, such as low cost and widespread availability, several limitations

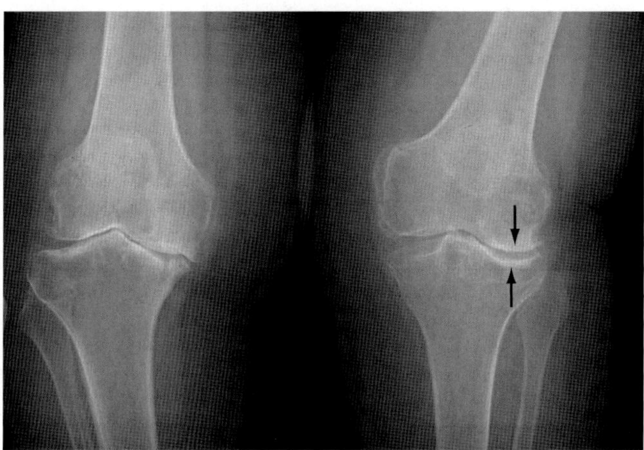

FIGURE 8-22. OA of the knees with a "windblown" appearance. This standing view of both legs shows severe cartilage space narrowing medially on the right and laterally on the left. Despite the weight-bearing nature of this examination, the degree of cartilage loss is underestimated; it appears as though some lucency (suggesting cartilage) is present in the affected compartments. The sclerosis of the subchondral bone on either side of the joint *(arrows)* and bone remodeling indicate that complete cartilage loss is present, however.

have been noted. These include the ability to evaluate only portions of the cartilage space in profile, insensitivity to bone marrow changes and osteophytes, and imperfect correlation with clinical symptoms.[121]

MRI allows evaluation of the many structures involved in OA including cartilage, synovium, and subchondral bone. Chan et al. found MRI to be more sensitive than radiography and CT for assessing the extent and severity of osteoarthritic changes and frequently showed tricompartmental disease in patients in whom radiography and CT show only bicompartmental involvement.[122] Hayes and colleagues prospectively compared radiographic severity with self-reported pain and MRI features of OA in 232 knees of more than 1000 women being followed for OA.[121] Cartilage defects and "bone marrow edema" were found even in patients with normal radiographs. MRI abnormalities were noted in the patellofemoral joint, an area not assessed with the Kellgren Lawrence system. Cartilage defects showed a statistically significant correlation with pain.

Bone Marrow Edema

Poorly defined areas of increased signal on fluid sensitive images (e.g., STIR) with corresponding decreased signal on T1-weighted images are often thought to be due to bone marrow edema (see Figure 8-2). However, histologic correlation of these changes by Zanetti and colleagues has shown that edema is actually a minor feature in these areas and was also present in normal areas.[123] The areas of increased STIR signal were shown to consist of a combination of normal marrow elements (fatty marrow, intact trabeculae, and blood vessels) as well as smaller amounts of abnormal elements (bone marrow necrosis, abnormal trabeculae, marrow fibrosis, bone marrow edema, and bleeding). Importantly, comparison of normal and abnormal regions found no difference in the prevalence of bone marrow edema. The zones did differ significantly in the presence of bone marrow necrosis, fibrosis, and abnormal trabeculae. Thus the "bone marrow edema pattern" is not due to bone marrow edema specifically and has prompted the more accurate term *edema-like MRI abnormality.*

Meniscal Tears

Medial and lateral meniscal tears are common findings in the knees of both asymptomatic (76% prevalence) and symptomatic (91% prevalence) patients with OA.[124] Meniscal tears do not correlate with severity of pain or affect functional status in these patients. Englund et al found the prevalence of a meniscal tear to be 63% among those with knee pain, aching, or stiffness on most days and 60% among those without these symptoms.[124a]

> Meniscal tears occur with high prevalence in patients with OA with or without symptoms, and the meaning of this imaging finding needs to be clinically assessed.

F18-FDG PET Scanning

F18–FDG PET scanning has been evaluated in knee osteoarthritis. Increased uptake has been noted in some osteoarthritic knees in the intercondylar notch and along the posterior cruciate ligament, around osteophytes, and in subchondral lesions and bone marrow corresponding on MRI to areas of bone marrow edema signal.

Treatment

Treatment options for knee osteoarthritis have been reviewed by Hunter and Felson.[2] Early changes are now believed to be reversible; previously the condition was thought to be inevitably progressive.[4] Unlike the hip, injection rarely requires imaging guidance.

FEET AND ANKLES

In contrast to knee OA, most cases of ankle arthritis are related to prior injury.[125] Recurrent ankle sprains or even a single ankle sprain with continued pain may lead to this condition. Cartilage space loss is asymmetric and best demonstrated on weight-bearing views.[126] A bony excrescence from the dorsal aspect of the talar neck is thought to be due to capsular traction and can be seen in athletes; it is not an indicator of OA.[127]

Osteoarthritis of the great toe metatarsophalangeal (MTP) joint can result in painful dorsiflexion. Characteristic dorsal osteophytes are seen on the lateral projection of the joint (Figure 8-23).

SECONDARY OA

Secondary OA is a response to preceding cartilage damage from trauma, arthritis, infection, metabolic conditions, or other causes.[64] Several of these underlying conditions may be suspected by careful review of radiographic findings. In particular, OA in an atypical distribution for primary OA or in young patients should suggest an underlying cause (Figure 8-24).

For example, hemochromatosis may result in an arthropathy that may resemble primary OA but is in an unusual distribution. In hemochromatosis, the MCP joints and the patellofemoral and radiocarpal joints can be affected. Subchondral cysts may be prominent. Chondrocalcinosis occurs in about 40% of cases[64] (Figure 8-25). Subtle findings (e.g., involvement of metacarpals 4 and 5 and hooklike osteophytes from the metacarpal heads) may help suggest hemochromatosis rather than idiopathic CPPD arthropathy.[128] This is important because radiographic findings may provide a clue to a previously undiagnosed condition before permanent visceral changes have occurred. A hemochromatosis-like arthropathy has also been described in diabetes mellitus without hemochromatosis,[129] long-term dialysis,[130] and manual laborers

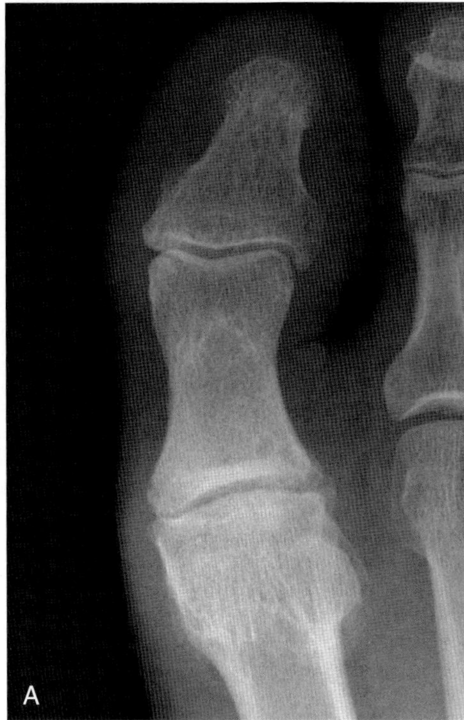

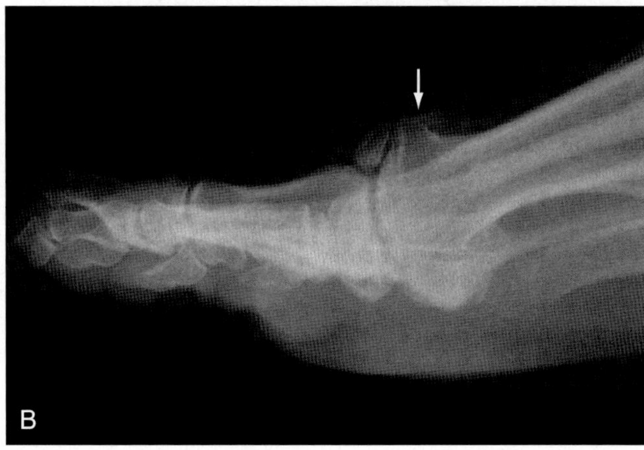

FIGURE 8-23. Hallux rigidus. **A,** PA radiograph of the great toe shows cartilage space narrowing and hypertrophic lipping. **B,** The lateral radiograph shows a prominent dorsal osteophyte *(arrow).*

("Missouri metacarpal syndrome")[46] and with OA of the elbow.[131] (See Chapter 28 for additional information.)

Acromegaly is another condition that may result in secondary OA possibly related to overgrowth of cartilage with inadequate nutrition of the thickened cartilage or its poor quality.[132] The knees, hips, and shoulders are affected most often.[132] At first, the cartilage spaces are noted to be unusually thick (MCP cartilage space greater than 3 mm in males or greater than 2 mm in females, hip cartilage spaces greater than 6 mm) (Figure 8-26). Later cartilage space narrowing occurs as secondary arthritis develops. Osteophytes may be very large.

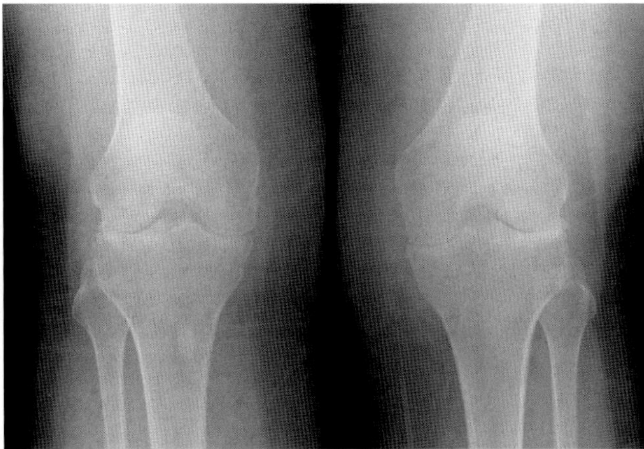

FIGURE 8-24. Secondary OA due to rheumatoid arthritis. A standing flexed view of both knees shows fairly symmetric medial and lateral cartilage space narrowing. This distribution is unusual for OA, in which one compartment is usually much more involved than the other. Both knees are affected.

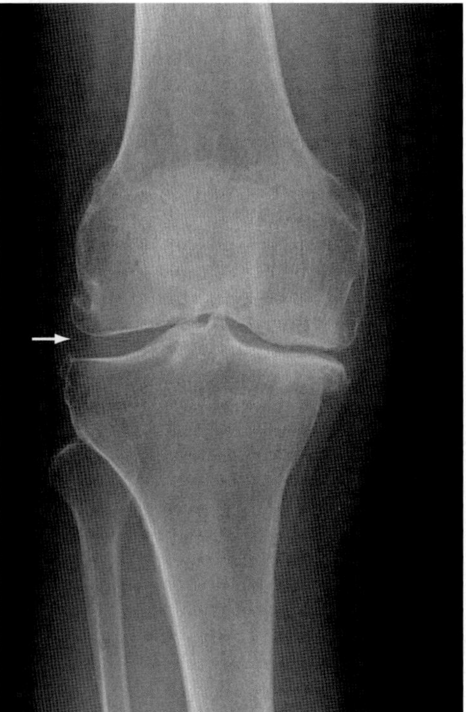

FIGURE 8-25. Hemochromatosis with OA. The frontal radiograph shows moderate medial cartilage space narrowing with sclerosis and osteophyte formation. There is chondrocalcinosis *(arrow)* of the meniscus and articular cartilage. These findings are nonspecific and could be due to OA alone. However, this patient had underlying hemochromatosis.

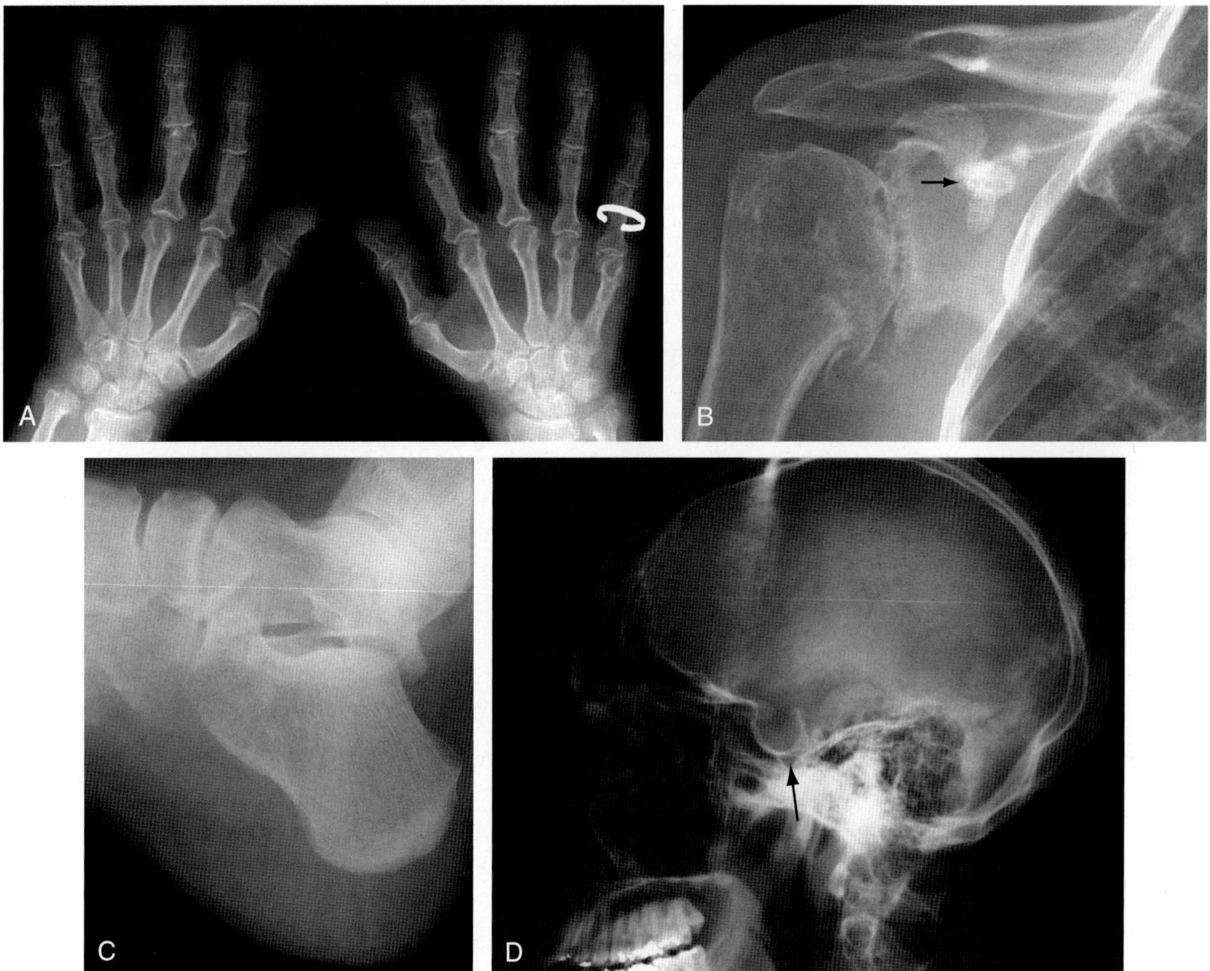

FIGURE 8-26. Acromegaly. **A,** PA radiograph of the hands shows in a patient with acromegaly shows the wide MCP cartilage spaces. The distal phalanges have a spade-like appearance. The soft tissues have enlarged as documented by the cut ring. **B,** An oblique radiograph of the shoulder in another patient with acromegaly shows severe cartilage space narrowing and large osteophytes. Several intraarticular bodies *(arrow)* are noted within the joint recesses. **C,** The lateral radiograph of the heel shows a thick fat pad. **D,** The skull shows the large sella turcica *(arrow)*, the large frontal sinuses, and the prognathic mandible.

REFERENCES

1. Altman R, Asch E, Bloch D et al: Development of criteria for the classification and reporting of osteoarthritis. Classification of osteoarthritis of the knee. Diagnostic and Therapeutic Criteria Committee of the American Rheumatism Association, *Arthritis Rheum* 29:1039-1049, 1986.
2. Hunter DJ, Felson DT: Osteoarthritis [see comment], *Br Med J* 332:639-642, 2006.
3. Felson DT: Osteoarthritis of the knee, *New Engl J Med* 354:841-844, 2006.
4. Felson DT: An update on the pathogenesis and epidemiology of osteoarthritis, *Radiol Clin North Am* 42:1-9, 2004.
5. Peat G, McCarney R, Croft P: Knee pain and osteoarthritis in older adults: a review of community burden and current use of primary health care [see comment], *Ann Rheum Dis* 60:91-97, 2001.
6. Banks KP, Beall DP, McCollum MJ et al: The accuracy of magnetic resonance imaging in the assessment of glenohumeral articular degenerative disease, *J Okla St Med Assoc* 100:52-56, 2007.
7. Kijowski R, Blankenbaker DG, Stanton PT et al: Radiographic findings of osteoarthritis versus arthroscopic findings of articular cartilage degeneration in the tibiofemoral joint, *Radiology* 239:818-824, 2006.
8. Altman R, Hochberg M, Murphy WA Jr et al: Atlas of individual radiographic features in osteoarthritis, *Osteoarthritis Cartilage* 3:3-70, 1995.
9. Felson DT, McAlindon TE, Anderson JJ et al: Defining radiographic osteoarthritis for the whole knee, *Osteoarthritis Cartilage* 5:241-250, 1997.
10. Lanyon P, O'Reilly S, Jones A et al: Radiographic assessment of symptomatic knee osteoarthritis in the community: definitions and normal joint space, *Ann Rheum Dis* 57: 595-601, 1998.
11. Nagaosa Y, Mateus M, Hassan B et al: Development of a logically devised line drawing atlas for grading of knee osteoarthritis, *Ann Rheum Dis* 59:587-595, 2000.
12. Ravaud P, Giraudeau B, Auleley GR et al: Variability in knee radiographing: implication for definition of radiological progression in medial knee osteoarthritis, *Ann Rheum Dis* 57:624-629, 1998.
13. Altman RD, Fries JF, Bloch DA et al: Radiographic assessment of progression in osteoarthritis, *Arthritis Rheum* 30:1214-1225, 1987.
14. Lequesne M, Brandt K, Bellamy N et al: Guidelines for testing slow acting drugs in osteoarthritis, *J Rheumatol* 41 (Suppl):65-71, 1994; discussion 72-73. [Erratum appears in *J Rheumatol* 21(Suppl):2395, 1994.]
15. Kellgren J, Lawrence J: Radiological assessment of osteoarthrosis, *Ann Rheum Dis* 16:494-501, 1957.
16. Lequesne MG, Laredo JD: The faux profil (oblique view) of the hip in the standing position. Contribution to the evaluation of osteoarthritis of the adult hip, *Ann Rheum Dis* 57:676-681, 1998.
17. Cooper C: Radiographic atlases for the assessment of osteoarthritis, *Osteoarthritis Cartilage* 3(Suppl A):1-2, 1995
18. Brandt KD, Fife RS, Braunstein EM et al: Radiographic grading of the severity of knee osteoarthritis: relation of the Kellgren and Lawrence grade to a grade based on joint space narrowing, and correlation with arthroscopic evidence of articular cartilage degeneration, *Arthritis Rheum* 34:1381-1386, 1991.

19. Waldschmidt JG, Braunstein EM, Buckwalter KA: Magnetic resonance imaging of osteoarthritis, *Rheum Dis Clin North Am* 25:451-465, 1999.
20. Bergman AG, Willén HK, Lindstrand AL et al: Osteoarthritis of the knee: correlation of subchondral MR signal abnormalities with histopathologic and radiographic features, *Skeletal Radiol* 23:445-448, 1994.
21. Ostergaard M, Court-Payen M, Gideon P et al: Ultrasonography in arthritis of the knee: a comparison with MR imaging, *Acta Radiol* 16:36(1)19-24, 1995.
22. Ostergaard M, Stoltenberg M, Løvgreen-Nielsen P et al: Magnetic resonance imaging-determined synovial membrane and joint effusion volumes in rheumatoid arthritis and osteoarthritis: comparison with the macroscopic and microscopic appearance of the synovium, *Arthritis Rheum* 40:1856-1867, 1997.
23. Gold GE, Burstein D, Dardzinski B et al: MRI of articular cartilage in OA: novel pulse sequences and compositional/functional markers, *Osteoarthritis Cartilage* 14(Suppl):A76-A86, 2006.
24. Eckstein F, Burstein D, Link TM: Quantitative MRI of cartilage and bone: degenerative changes in osteoarthritis, *NMR Biomed* 19:822-854, 2006.
25. Eckstein F: Quantitative magnetic resonance imaging of osteoarthritis, *Summary Future Rheumatol* 1:699-715, 2006.
26. Hill CL, Hunter DJ, Niu J et al: Synovitis detected on magnetic resonance imaging and its relation to pain and cartilage loss in knee osteoarthritis, *Ann Rheum Dis* 66:1599-1603, 2007.
27. Kornaat PR, Bloem JL, Ceulemans RY et al: Osteoarthritis of the knee: association between clinical features and MR imaging findings, *Radiology* 239:811-817, 2006.
28. Felson DT, Niu J, Guermazi A et al: Correlation of the development of knee pain with enlarging bone marrow lesions on magnetic resonance imaging, *Arthritis Rheum* 56:2986-2992, 2007.
28a. Winalski BN, Aliabadi P, Wright RJ et al: Intravenous gadolinium-DTPA enhancement of joint fluid. A less invasive alternative for MR arthrography, *Radiology* 181(P):384, 1991.
29. Gray RG, Tenenbaum J, Gottlieb NL: Local corticosteroid injection treatment in rheumatic disorders, *Semin Arthritis Rheum* 10:231-254, 1981.
30. Borthakur A, Mellon E, Niyogi S et al: Sodium and T1rho MRI for molecular and diagnostic imaging of articular cartilage, *NMR Biomed* 19:781-821, 2006.
31. Tiderius CJ, Jessel R, Kim YJ et al: Hip dGEMRIC in asymptomatic volunteers and patients with early osteoarthritis: the influence of timing after contrast injection, *Magn Reson Med* 57:803-805, 2007.
32. Boesen M, Jensen KE, Qvistgaard E et al: Delayed gadolinium-enhanced magnetic resonance imaging (dGEMRIC) of hip joint cartilage: better cartilage delineation after intra-articular than intravenous gadolinium injection, *Acta Radiol* 47:391-396, 2006.
33. Eckstein F, Ateshian G, Burgkart R et al: Proposal for a nomenclature for magnetic resonance imaging based measures of articular cartilage in osteoarthritis, *Osteoarthritis Cartilage* 14:974-983, 2006.
34. Kornaat PR, Ceulemans RY, Kroon HM et al: MRI assessment of knee osteoarthritis: Knee Osteoarthritis Scoring System (KOSS)—inter-observer and intra-observer reproducibility of a compartment-based scoring system, *Skeletal Radiol* 34:95-102, 2005.
35. Peterfy CG, Guermazi A, Zaim S et al: Whole-Organ Magnetic Resonance Imaging Score (WORMS) of the knee in osteoarthritis, *Osteoarthritis Cartilage* 12:177-190, 2004.
36. Kloppenburg M, Stamm T, Watt I et al: Research in hand osteoarthritis: time for reappraisal and demand for new strategies. An opinion paper, *Ann Rheum Dis* 66:1157-1161, 2007.
37. Altman R, Alarcón G, Appelrouth D et al: The American College of Rheumatology criteria for the classification and reporting of osteoarthritis of the hand, *Arthritis Rheum* 33:1601-1610, 1990.
38. Chaisson CE, Zhang Y, McAlindon TE et al: Radiographic hand osteoarthritis: incidence, patterns, and influence of pre-existing disease in a population based sample, *J Rheumatol* 24:1337-1343, 1997.
39. Lane NE, Bloch DA, Jones HH et al: Osteoarthritis in the hand: a comparison of handedness and hand use, *J Rheumatol* 16:637-642, 1989.
40. Alexander CJ: Heberden's and Bouchard's nodes, *Ann Rheum Dis* 58:675-678, 1999.
41. Campion G, Dieppe P, Watt I: Heberden's nodes in osteoarthritis and rheumatoid arthritis, *Br Med J Clin Res Ed* 287:1512, 1983.
42. Martel W, Stuck KJ, Dworin AM et al: Erosive osteoarthritis and psoriatic arthritis: a radiologic comparison in the hand, wrist, and foot, *AJR Am J Roentgenol* 134:125-135, 1980.
43. Brower A: *Arthritis in black and white,* ed 2, Philadelphia, 1997, Saunders.
44. Resnick D: *Diagnosis of bone and joint disorders,* ed 3, vol 3, Philadelphia, 1995, Saunders.
45. Martel W, Snarr JW, Horn JR: The metacarpophalangeal joints in interphalangeal osteoarthritis, *Radiology* 108:1-7, 1973.
46. Williams WV, Cope R, Gaunt WD et al: Metacarpophalangeal arthropathy associated with manual labor (Missouri metacarpal syndrome). Clinical radiographic, and pathologic characteristics of an unusual degeneration process, *Arthritis Rheum* 30:1362-1371, 1987.
47. North ER, Eaton RG: Degenerative joint disease of the trapezium: a comparative radiographic and anatomic study, *J Hand Surg Am* 8:160-166, 1983.
48. Eaton RG, Littler JW: Ligament reconstruction for the painful thumb carpometacarpal joint, *J Bone Joint Surg Am* 55:1655-1666, 1973.
49. Barron OA, Glickel SZ, Eaton RG: Basal joint arthritis of the thumb, *J Am Acad Orthop Surg* 8:314-323, 2000.
50. Bettinger PC, Smutz WP, Linscheid RL et al: Material properties of the trapezial and trapeziometacarpal ligaments, *J Hand Surg Am* 25:1085-1095, 2000.
51. Bettinger PC, Linscheid RL, Cooney WP 3rd et al: Trapezial tilt: a radiographic correlation with advanced trapeziometacarpal joint arthritis, *J Hand Surg Am* 26:692-697, 2001.
52. Lasserre C, Pauzat D, Derennes R: Osteoarthritis of the trapezio-metacarpal joint, *J Bone Joint Surg Br* 31:534-536, 1949.
53. Belhorn LR, Hess EV: Erosive osteoarthritis, *Semin Arthritis Rheum* 22:298-306, 1993
54. Cobby M, Cushnaghan J, Creamer P et al: Erosive osteoarthritis: is it a separate disease entity? *Clin Radiol* 42:258-263, 1990.
55. Smith D, Braunstein EM, Brandt KD et al: A radiographic comparison of erosive osteoarthritis and idiopathic nodal osteoarthritis, *J Rheumatol* 19:896-904, 1992.
56. Peter JB, Pearson CM, Marmor L: Erosive osteoarthritis of the hands, *Arthritis Rheum* 9:365-388, 1966.
57. Ehrlich GE: Osteoarthritis beginning with inflammation. Definitions and correlations, *J Am Med Assoc* 232:157-159, 1975.
58. Grainger A, Farrant JM, O'Connor PJ et al: MR imaging of erosions in interphalangeal joint osteoarthritis: is all osteoarthritis erosive? *Skeletal Radiol* 36:737-745, 2007.
59. Tan AL, Grainger AJ, Tanner SF et al : A high-resolution magnetic resonance imaging study of distal interphalangeal joint arthropathy in psoriatic arthritis and osteoarthritis: are they the same? *Arthritis Rheum* 54:1328-1333, 2006.
60. Kirkhus E, Bjørnerud A, Thoen J et al: Contrast-enhanced dynamic magnetic resonance imaging of finger joints in osteoarthritis and rheumatoid arthritis: an analysis based on pharmacokinetic modeling, *Acta Radiol* 47:845-851, 2006.
61. Elzinga EH, van der Laken CJ, Comans EF et al: 2-Deoxy-2-[F-18]fluoro-D-glucose joint uptake on positron emission tomography images: rheumatoid arthritis versus osteoarthritis. *Mol Imaging Biol* 9:357-360, 2007.
62. Apple AS, Pedowitz RA, Speer KP: The weighted abduction Grashey shoulder method, *Radiol Technol* 69:151-156, 1997.
63. Goldman AB: Some miscellaneous joint diseases, *Semin Roentgenol* 17:60-80, 1982.
64. Gupta KB, Duryea J, Weissman BN: Radiographic evaluation of osteoarthritis, *Radiol Clin North Am* 42:11-41, 2004.
65. Green A, Norris TR: Imaging techniques for glenohumeral arthritis and glenohumeral arthroplasty, *Clin Orthop Relat Res* (307):7-17, 1994.
66. Samilson RL, Prieto V: Dislocation arthropathy of the shoulder, *J Bone Joint Surg Am* 65:456-460, 1983
67. Ilg A, Bankes MJ, Emery RJ: The intra- and inter-observer reliability of the Samilson and Prieto grading system of glenohumeral arthropathy, *Knee Surg Sports Traum Arthrosc* 9:187-190, 2001.
68. Walch G, Boulahia A, Boileau P et al: Primary glenohumeral osteoarthritis: clinical and radiographic classification. The Aequalis Group, *Acta Orthop Belg* 64(Suppl 2): 46-52, 1998.
69. Wandler E, Kramer EL, Sherman O et al: Diffuse FDG shoulder uptake on PET is associated with clinical findings of osteoarthritis, *AJR Am J Roentgenol* 185:797-803, 2005.
70. Bianchi S, Martinoli C, Bianchi-Zamorani M et al: Ultrasound of the joints, *Eur Radiol* 12: 56-61, 2002.
71. Needell SD, Zlatkin MB, Sher JS et al: MR imaging of the rotator cuff: peritendinous and bone abnormalities in an asymptomatic population, *AJR Am J Roentgenol* 166:863-867, 1996.
72. Vignon E, Conrozier T, Hellio Le Graverand MP: Advances in radiographic imaging of progression of hip and knee osteoarthritis, *J Rheumatol* 32:1143-1145, 2005.
73. Weiss JJ, Good A, Schumacher HR: Four cases of "Milwaukee shoulder," with a description of clinical presentation and long-term treatment, *J Am Geriatr Soc* 33:202-205, 1985.
74. Lequesne M, Malghem J, Dion E: The normal hip joint space: variations in width, shape, and architecture on 223 pelvic radiographs, *Ann Rheum Dis* 63:1145-1151, 2004.
75. Altman RD, Bloch DA, Dougados M et al: Measurement of structural progression in osteoarthritis of the hip: the Barcelona consensus group, *Osteoarthritis Cartilage* 12:515-524, 2004.
76. Wyler A, Bousson V, Bergot C et al: Hyaline cartilage thickness in radiographically normal cadaveric hips: comparison of spiral CT arthrographic and macroscopic measurements, *Radiology* 242:441-449, 2007.
77. Altman R, Alarcon G, Appelrouth D et al: The American College of Rheumatology criteria for the classification and reporting of osteoarthritis of the hip, *Arthritis Rheum* 34:505-514, 1991. [Comment.]
78. Dixon T, Benjamin J, Lund P et al: Femoral neck buttressing: a radiographic and histologic analysis, *Skeletal Radiol* 29:587-592, 2000.
79. Moore RJ, Fazzalari NL, Manthey BA et al: The relationship between head-neck-shaft angle, calcar width, articular cartilage thickness and bone volume in arthrosis of the hip, *Br J Rheumatol* 33:432-436, 1994.
80. Milgram JW: Morphologic alterations of the subchondral bone in advanced degenerative arthritis, *Clin Orthop Relat Res* (173):293-312, 1983.
81. Resnick D: Patterns of migration of the femoral head in osteoarthritis of the hip. Roentgenographic-pathologic correlation and comparison with rheumatoid arthritis, *Am J Roentgenol Radium Ther Nucl Med* 124:62-74, 1975.
82. Alvarez C, Chicheportiche V, Lequesne M et al: Contribution of helical computed tomography to the evaluation of early hip osteoarthritis: a study in 18 patients, *Joint Bone Spine Rev Rheum* 72:578-584, 2005.
83. Lambert RG, Hutchings EJ, Grace MG et al: Steroid injection for osteoarthritis of the hip: a randomized, double-blind, placebo-controlled trial, *Arthritis Rheum* 56:2278-2287, 2007.
84. Robinson P, Keenan AM, Conaghan PG: Clinical effectiveness and dose response of image-guided intra-articular corticosteroid injection for hip osteoarthritis, *Rheumatology* 46:285-291, 2007.

85. Chakravarty K, Pharoah PD, Scott DG: A randomized controlled study of post-injection rest following intra-articular steroid therapy for knee synovitis [see comment], *Br J Rheumatol* 33:464-468, 1994.
86. Hochberg MC, Altman RD, Brandt KD et al: Guidelines for the medical management of osteoarthritis. Part I. Osteoarthritis of the hip, American College of Rheumatology, *Arthritis Rheum* 38:1535-1540, 1995. [Comment.]
87. Kullenberg B, Runesson R, Tuvhag R et al: Intraarticular corticosteroid injection: pain relief in osteoarthritis of the hip? *J Rheumatol* 31:2265-2268, 2004.
88. Qvistgaard E, Christensen R, Torp-Pedersen S et al: Intra-articular treatment of hip osteoarthritis: a randomized trial of hyaluronic acid, corticosteroid, and isotonic saline, *Osteoarthritis Cartilage* 14:163-170, 2006.
89. Rosenberg ZS, Shankman S, Steiner GC et al: Rapid destructive osteoarthritis: clinical, radiographic, and pathologic features, *Radiology* 182:213-216, 1992.
90. Yamamoto T, Bullough PG: The role of subchondral insufficiency fracture in rapid destruction of the hip joint: a preliminary report, *Arthritis Rheum* 43:2423-2427, 2000.
91. Watanabe W, Itoi E, Yamada S: Early MRI findings of rapidly destructive coxarthrosis, *Skeletal Radiol* 31:35-38, 2002.
92. Lequesne M: Les coxopathies rapidement destructrices, *Ann Radiol* 36:62-64, 1993.
93. Pfirrmann CW, Mengiardi B, Dora C et al: Cam and pincer femoroacetabular impingement: characteristic MR arthrographic findings in 50 patients, *Radiology* 240:778-785, 2006. [See comment.] [Erratum appears in *Radiology* 244:626, 2007.]
94. Leunig M, Beck M, Kalhor M et al: Fibrocystic changes at anterosuperior femoral neck: prevalence in hips with femoroacetabular impingement, *Radiology* 236: 237-246, 2005.
95. Stulberg S, Cordell L, Harris W et al: Unrecognized childhood hip disease: a major cause of idiopathic osteoarthrtis of the hip. In Editor (ed): The hip. *Proceedings of the 3rd Meeting of The Hip Society*, 1975, Mosby, St. Louis, pp 212-228.
96. Beaule PE, Zaragoza E, Motamedi K et al: Three-dimensional computed tomography of the hip in the assessment of femoroacetabular impingement, *J Orthop Res* 23: 1286-1292, 2005.
97. Kassarjian A, Yoon LS, Belzile E et al: Triad of MR arthrographic findings in patients with cam-type femoroacetabular impingement, *Radiology* 236:588-592, 2005.
98. Siebenrock KA, Schoeniger R, Ganz R: Anterior femoro-acetabular impingement due to acetabular retroversion. Treatment with periacetabular osteotomy, *J Bone Joint Surg Am* 85:278-286, 2003.
99. McBride MT, Muldoon MP, Santore RF et al: Protrusio acetabuli: diagnosis and treatment, *J Am Acad Orthop Surg* 9:79-88, 2001.
99a. Armbuster TG, Guerra J, Resnick D et al: The adult hip: anatomic study 1. The bony landmarks, *Radiology* 128:1, 1978.
100. Spector TD, Hart DJ, Byrne J et al: Definition of osteoarthritis of the knee for epidemiological studies, *Ann Rheum Dis* 52:790-794, 1993.
101. Davies AP, Vince AS, Shepstone L et al: The radiologic prevalence of patellofemoral osteoarthritis, *Clin Orthop Relat Res* (402):206-212, 2002.
102. Mazzuca SA, Brandt KD, Dieppe PA et al: Effect of alignment of the medial tibial plateau and x-ray beam on apparent progression of osteoarthritis in the standing anteroposterior knee radiograph, *Arthritis Rheum* 44:1786-1794, 2001.
103. Buckland-Wright JC: Quantitative radiography of osteoarthritis, *Ann Rheum Dis* 53:268-275, 1994.
104. Ahlback S: Osteoarthrosis of the knee. A radiographic investigation, *Acta Radiol Diag* 8(Suppl):277-282, 1968.
105. Messieh SS, Fowler PJ, Munro T: Anteroposterior radiographs of the osteoarthritic knee, *J Bone Joint Surg Br* 72:639-640, 1990.
106. Buckland-Wright JC, Macfarlane DG, Jasani MK et al: Quantitative microfocal radiographic assessment of osteoarthritis of the knee from weight bearing tunnel and semiflexed standing views, *J Rheumatol* 21:1734-1741, 1994.
107. Holmblad EM: Postero-anterior x-ray view of knee in flexion, *J Am Med Assoc* 109:1196-1197, 1937.
108. Resnick D, Vint V: The "Tunnel" view in assessment of cartilage loss in osteoarthritis of the knee, *Radiology* 137:547-548, 1980.
109. Rosenberg TD, Paulos LE, Parker RD et al: The forty-five-degree posteroanterior flexion weight-bearing radiograph of the knee, *J Bone Joint Surg Am* 70: 1479-1483, 1988.
110. Merle-Vincent F, Vignon E, Brandt K et al: Superiority of the Lyon schuss view over the standing anteroposterior view for detecting joint space narrowing, especially in the lateral tibiofemoral compartment, in early knee osteoarthritis, *Ann Rheum Dis* 66:747-753, 2007.
111. Buckland-Wright JC, Wolfe F, Ward RJ et al: Substantial superiority of semiflexed (MTP) views in knee osteoarthritis: a comparative radiographic study, without fluoroscopy, of standing extended, semiflexed (MTP), and schuss views, *J Rheumatol* 26:2664-2674, 1989.
112. Bruyere O, Genant H, Kothari M et al: Longitudinal study of magnetic resonance imaging and standard x-rays to assess disease progression in osteoarthritis, *Osteoarthritis Cartilage* 15:98-103, 2007.
113. McAlindon TE, Snow S, Cooper C et al: Radiographic patterns of osteoarthritis of the knee joint in the community: the importance of the patellofemoral joint, *Ann Rheum Dis* 51:844-849, 1992.
114. Boegard T, Rudling O, Petersson IF et al: Joint-space width in the axial view of the patello-femoral joint. Definitions and comparison with MR imaging, *Acta Radiol* 39:24-31, 1998.
115. Nagaosa Y, Lanyon P, Doherty M: Characterisation of size and direction of osteophyte in knee osteoarthritis: a radiographic study, *Ann Rheum Dis* 61:319-324, 2002.
116. Nakamura M, Sumen Y, Sakaridani K et al: Relationship between the shape of tibial spurs on x-ray and meniscal changes on MRI in early osteoarthritis of the knee, *Magn Res Imaging* 24:1143-1148, 2006.
117. Donnelly S, Hart DJ, Doyle DV et al: Spiking of the tibial tubercles—a radiological feature of osteoarthritis? *Ann Rheum Dis* 55:105-108, 1996.
118. Boegard T, Rudling O, Petersson IF et al: Correlation between radiographically diagnosed osteophytes and magnetic resonance detected cartilage defects in the patellofemoral joint, *Ann Rheum Dis* 57:395-400, 1998.
119. Unlu Z, Tarhan S, Goktan C et al: The correlation between magnetic resonance detected cartilage defects and spiking of tibial tubercles in osteoarthritis of the knee joint, *Acta Med Okayama* 60:207-214, 2006.
120. Boegard T, Rudling O, Petersson IF et al: Correlation between radiographically diagnosed osteophytes and magnetic resonance detected cartilage defects in the tibiofemoral joint, *Ann Rheum Dis* 57:401-407, 1998.
121. Hayes CW, Jamadar DA, Welch GW et al: Osteoarthritis of the knee: comparison of MR imaging findings with radiographic severity measurements and pain in middle-aged women, *Radiology* 237:998-1007, 2005.
122. Chan WP, Lang P, Stevens MP et al: Osteoarthritis of the knee: comparison of radiography, CT, and MR imaging to assess extent and severity, *AJR Am J Roentgenol* 157:799-806, 1991.
123. Zanetti M, Bruder E, Romero J et al: Bone marrow edema pattern in osteoarthritic knees: correlation between MR imaging and histologic findings, *Radiology* 215: 835-840, 2000.
124. Bhattacharyya T, Gale D, Dewire P et al: The clinical importance of meniscal tears demonstrated by magnetic resonance imaging in osteoarthritis of the knee, *J Bone Joint Surg Am* 85:4-9, 2003. [See comment.]
124a. Englund M, Guermazzi A, Gale D: Incidental meniscal findings on knee MRI in middle-aged and elderly persons, *N Engl J Med* 359:1108-1115, 2008.
125. Saltzman CL, Salamon ML, Blanchard GM et al: Epidemiology of ankle arthritis: report of a consecutive series of 639 patients from a tertiary orthopaedic center, *Iowa Orthop J* 25:44-46, 2005.
126. Harrington KD: Degenerative arthritis of the ankle secondary to long-standing lateral ligament instability, *J Bone Joint Surg Am* 61:354-361, 1979.
127. Keats TE, Harrison RB: Hypertrophy of the talar beak, *Skeletal Radiol* 4:37-39, 1979.
128. Adamson TC 3rd, Resnik CS, Guerra J Jr et al: Hand and wrist arthropathies of hemochromatosis and calcium pyrophosphate deposition disease: distinct radiographic features, *Radiology* 147:377-381, 1983.
129. McCarthy GM, Rosenthal AK, Carrera GF: Hemochromatosis-like arthropathy in diabetes mellitus without hemochromatosis, *J Rheumatol* 23:1453-1456, 1996.
130. Braunstein EM, Menerey K, Martel W et al: Radiologic features of a pyrophosphate-like arthropathy associated with long-term dialysis, *Skeletal Radiol* 16:437-441, 1987.
131. Doherty M, Preston B: Primary osteoarthritis of the elbow, *Ann Rheum Dis* 48: 743-747, 1989.
132. Detenbeck LC, Tressler HA, O'Duffy JD et al: Peripheral joint manifestations of acromegaly, *Clin Orthop Relat Res* 91:119-127, 1973.

CHAPTER 9

Degenerative Disorders of the Spine

TARAK H. PATEL, MD, *and* JOHN A. CARRINO, MD, MPH

KEY FACTS

- Specific terminology, available on the Internet, has been developed based on anatomy and pathology to describe lumbar spine disorders.
- Bony excrescences from the vertebrae have subtle features and accompanying findings that may allow identification of the underlying cause. Characteristic syndesmophytes of ankylosing spondylitis extend from the margin of one disk to the margin of the next and are symmetric, whereas osteophytes begin in a horizontal direction.
- Magnetic resonance imaging (MRI) findings must be correlated with clinical findings.
- Intervertebral disk herniation is a localized displacement (less than 180 degrees of the circumference) of disk material beyond the normal margin of the intervertebral disk space. The types of disk herniation are a protrusion, extrusion, and free fragment (sequestration).
- Differences in the anatomy and stresses placed upon the thoracic and cervical areas provide challenges to diagnostic MRI.

This chapter reviews the more common imaging findings of spine degenerative disease and associated conditions. Radiographs are often a useful first imaging step for evaluation of low back pain. The manifestations of disk degeneration from an imaging perspective, especially focusing on magnetic resonance imaging (MRI) findings, including the significance of marrow changes and high-intensity zones are highlighted. The imaging of cervical and thoracic degenerative disease is also discussed.

IMAGING FINDINGS OF DEGENERATIVE DISK DISEASE

The intervertebral disk is a composite structure consisting of three distinct components: the anulus fibrosus, the nucleus pulposus, and the cartilaginous endplates. They are cartilaginous joints (intervertebral symphyses). The anulus fibrosis is the limiting capsule of the nucleus pulposus. It is attached superiorly and inferiorly to the vertebral body ring apophysis by Sharpey fibers and is confluent with the anterior and posterior longitudinal ligaments. The anulus fibrosis is made predominantly of type 1 collagen and, because of the absence of free protons and a dense lamellar structure, is normally hypointense on all MRI pulse sequences. The nucleus pulposus portion of the disk is mainly made up of glycosaminoglycans (GAG) and has approximately 85% to 90% water content under normal conditions. Its signal intensity is intermediate on T1-weighted images and hyperintense on T2-weighted images, reflecting the high water binding of the GAGs. The bilocular appearance of the adult nucleus pulposus results from the development of a central horizontal band of fibrous tissue and is considered a sign of normal maturation. The intervertebral disk height reflects the status of the nucleus pulposus and in the lumbar spine typically increases gradually as one goes from cephalad to caudad, with the exception of the lumbosacral junction, which may be narrower than the remainder of the lumbar intervertebral disks. The end plates are covered by hyaline cartilage that serves as the biomechanical and metabolic interface between vertebral body and nucleus pulposus. The intervertebral disk configuration is different among the cervical, thoracic, and lumbar segments (Figure 9-1, *A* to *C*). In the lumbar spine, the anulus fibrosis tends to be thicker ventrally than dorsally.

> In the normal lumbar spine, without segmentation anomalies, the widest intervertebral disk is at L4-5.

Disk degeneration begins early in life with the cervical spine preceding the lumbar spine (second to third decades versus fourth to fifth decades) and the thoracic spine being intermediate; the etiologies may be related to normal aging, genetic predisposition, or environmental factors. Component changes can occur in the nucleus pulposus, anulus fibrosus, cartilaginous end plates, and subjacent marrow. The nucleus pulposus typically shows desiccation, fibrosis, or a vacuum phenomenon (gas) while the anulus fibrosus undergoes mucinous degeneration. Fissuring may occur from radial tearing in the vertical or transverse direction leading to rupture of Sharpey fibers near the ring apophysis. The cartilaginous end plates may demonstrate marginal osteophytes and subarticular marrow signal alteration.

There is some confusion over the terminology of degenerative joint disease in general. Osteoarthritis or osteoarthrosis is a process of synovial joints. Therefore, in the spine, these terms are appropriately applied to the zygoapophyseal (Z-joint, facet), atlantoaxial, costovertebral, and sacroiliac joints. In the author's practice, *degenerative disk disease* (DDD) is a term applied specifically to clinical findings accompanying intervertebral disk degeneration.

> *Osteoarthritis* refers to degenerative changes in synovial joints, whereas *degenerative disk disease* refers to degenerative changes of the intervertebral disk. Spondylosis deformans (often shortened to *spondylosis*) is a degenerative process of the spine involving essentially the anulus fibrosus and characterized by anterior and lateral marginal osteophytes arising from the vertebral body apophyses, while the intervertebral disk height is normal or only slightly decreased.

The widely endorsed nomenclature for lumbar intervertebral disks is supported by many subspecialty groups and should be the basis for describing disk-related pathology among different types

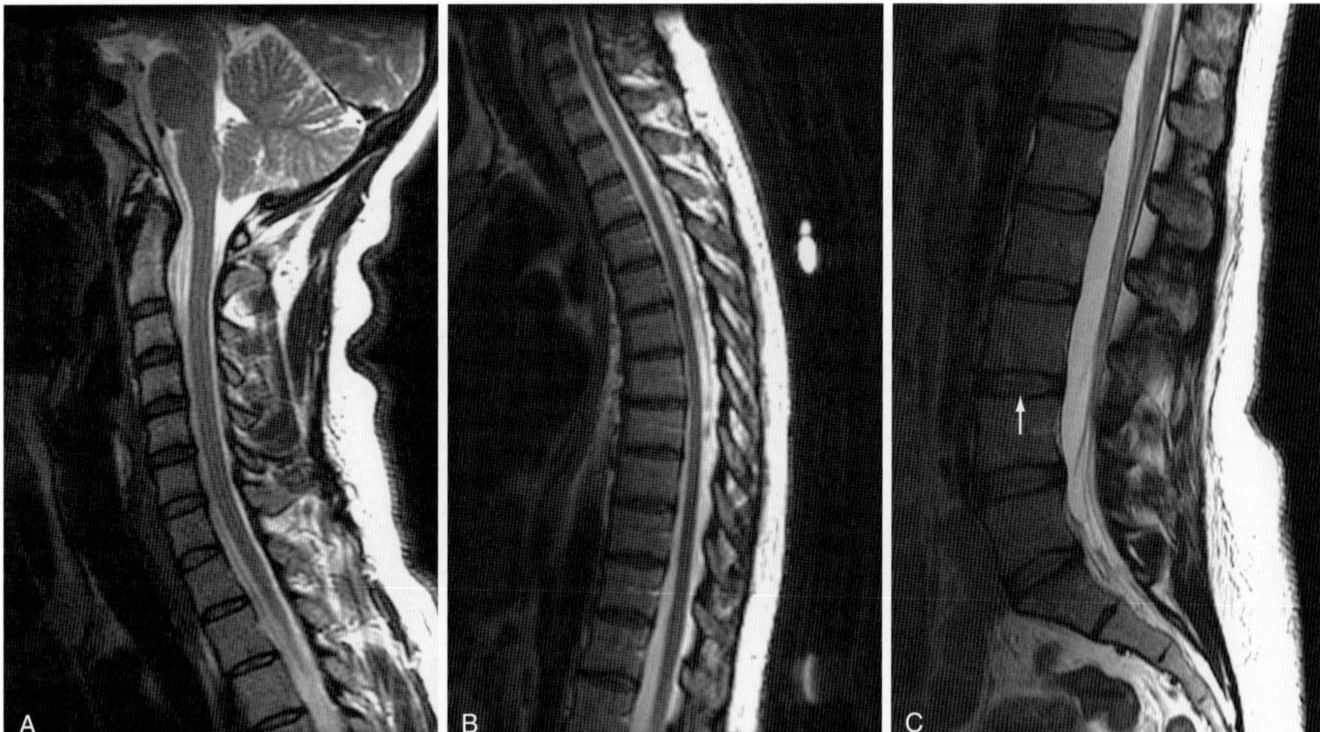

FIGURE 9-1. Normal MRI of the intervertebral disk. **A,** Sagittal T2-weighted image without fat suppression shows the cervical disks are relatively hypointense, reflecting early desiccation. **B,** Sagittal T2-weighted image without fat suppression shows the thoracic intervertebral disk heights are relatively narrow compared with other segments of the spine. **C,** Sagittal T2-weighted image without fat suppression shows that lumbar disks are relatively hyperintense (can be near fluid signal), reflecting normal water content of the nucleus pulposus; thin horizontal intervertebral clefts are often present *(arrow)*.

of providers.[1] It is important to recognize that the definitions of diagnoses should not define or imply external etiologic events such as trauma and should not imply relationship to symptoms. The definitions may, however, imply need for specific treatment. The terminology used in this chapter is supported by the "Nomenclature and Classification of Lumbar Disk Pathology" document available online.[2]

The disk derives its structural properties largely through its ability to attract and retain water. *Internal disk disruption* (IDD) is a term that was coined in the 1970s to describe pathologic changes of the internal structure of the disk. Decreased tissue cellularity and altered matrix architecture characterize intervertebral disk degeneration. The physiochemical change of diminished water binding capacity in the GAGs is heralded on MRI by loss of T2 signal and has been called the "desiccated disk." Thus some refer to this condition as "dark disk disease" or "black disk disease."

Disk degeneration is accompanied by decreased water binding in the nucleus pulposus and therefore low signal on T2-weighted images, known as "dark disk disease."

Osteophytosis is a hallmark of degenerative disk disease and should be differentiated from paravertebral calcification/ossification, syndesmophytes, and longitudinal ligament calcification/ossification. Marginal osteophytes tend to be horizontal and parallel to the disk margin, as though they are creating additional articular surface.

Osteophytes tend to project horizontally from the bone margins.

However, osteophytes can be bridging (i.e., from one level to the next). Anterior and lateral marginal osteophytes have been found in 100% of skeletons of individuals older than 40 years and are believed to be a consequence of normal aging, whereas posterior osteophytes have been found in only a minority of skeletons of individuals older than 80 years and thus are not inevitable consequences of aging.[3] The *claw osteophyte of McNabb* is defined as the bony outgrowth arising very close to the disk margin from the vertebral body apophysis, directed with a sweeping configuration, toward the corresponding part of the vertebral body opposite the disk. These are findings of spondylosis deformans. Small horizontal bony projections are more likely to be associated with instability. Paravertebral calcification/ossification tends to come off the midportion of the vertebral body and can be seen in HLA B27 seronegative spondyloarthropathies such as psoriasis and reactive arthritis (formerly known as Reiter disease). There is often a paucity of DDD, which can be helpful in the differential diagnosis. Syndesmophytes are calcifications along the outer margin of the anulus fibrosus and have a thin vertical orientation from one disk margin to the next. These are hallmarks of ankylosing spondylitis and occur in young men with only minimal disk disease. Calcification may also occur in the anterior longitudinal ligament or posterior longitudinal ligament. Ossification of the posterior longitudinal ligament (OPLL) is a degenerative-related condition typically seen in the cervical spine (Figure 9-2, *A*) and not often seen in the lumbar spine.

Ossification of the posterior longitudinal ligament may cause cervical spinal cord compression.

Anterior longitudinal ligament mineralization is predominantly seen in the thoracolumbar spine (Figure 9-2, *B*). This is believed to be a senescent condition usually with only minimal

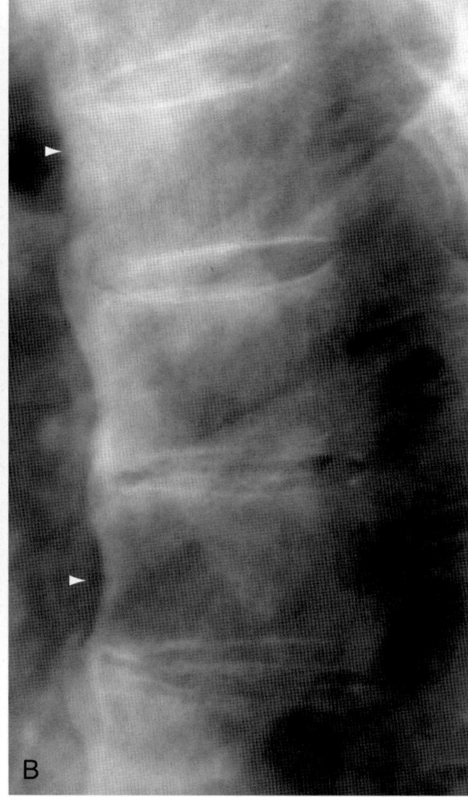

FIGURE 9-2. Paravertebral ossification (diffuse idiopathic skeletal hyperostosis [DISH]). This patient has difficulty swallowing. **A,** Cervical spine: Lateral radiograph shows contiguous ossification of the anterior longitudinal ligament from C4-7 *(white arrow)*. There is also associated ossification of the posterior longitudinal ligament *(black arrow)*. Note also the displacement of the upper pharynx by ossification at C1 and C2. This can interfere with swallowing. **B,** Thoracic spine: Lateral radiograph shows contiguous ossification of the anterior longitudinal ligament over at least four spinal segments *(arrowheads)*. This is the most classic appearance of DISH.

disk height loss; when it involves greater than four contiguous segments, it is referred to as *diffuse idiopathic skeletal hyperostosis* (DISH).

> DISH is characterized by flowing ossification along four or more contiguous vertebrae with normal disk spaces and sacroiliac joints.

Schmorl nodes are intervertebral disk herniations and may be considered a transosseous disk extrusion. Herniation of the nucleus pulposus occurs through the cartilaginous end plate into the vertebral marrow space. They often have a characteristic round or lobulated appearance. They may be enhanced after contrast administration, with ring-like enhancement being most common. They are often incidental and likely to be developmental or posttraumatic[4] rather than purely degenerative or adaptive. The distribution is most frequent around the thoracolumbar junction. There is imaging evidence of a significant genetic association between the COL9A3 tryptophan allele (Trp3 allele), Scheuermann's disease, and intervertebral disk degeneration among symptomatic patients.[5]

Intradiscal calcification is most often incidental and can be seen in the pediatric population but is also frequently seen with DDD or simply as senescent change.[6] However, when associated with predominantly nucleus pulposus disease (i.e., loss of disk height, present at virtually every lumbar segment), this is pathognomonic for alkaptonuria (ochronosis). Ochronosis is a hereditary disorder of amino acid metabolism leading to the accumulation of a dark pigment (organized polymer of homogentisic acid) in connective tissues. The imaging manifestations are marked height loss, vacuum cleft formation, and sclerosis. Osteophytosis is minimal, as this is primarily a nucleus pulposus disease. The radiographic hallmark is dystrophic calcification universally present in all disks.

Disk contour changes are part of the degenerative or maturation process and are broadly characterized as bulges and herniations. The following is a summary of the accepted nomenclature for abnormal disk contours as applied primarily to the lumbar spine. MRI is well suited to reveal the severity of disease and to characterize contour abnormalities in regard to size, morphology, and location. Mass effect on the spinal cord and nerve roots can also be demonstrated. However, the MRI findings need to be correlated with the clinical syndrome. Hence, the following are pathoanatomic descriptors that do not imply a specific pathoetiology or syndrome.

The posterior disk margin tends to be concave in the upper lumbosacral spine (Figure 9-3, *A*) and is straight or slightly convex at L4-5 and L5-S1. The posterior margin typically projects no more than 1 mm beyond the end plate.

> Normally, the posterior disk margin tends to be concave in the upper lumbosacral spine and straight or slightly convex at L4-5 and L5-S1. The posterior margin of the disk projects no more than 1 mm beyond the end plate.

An anular bulge is described as a generalized displacement (greater than 180 degrees or 50% of the circumference of the disk) of disk margin beyond the normal margin of the intervertebral

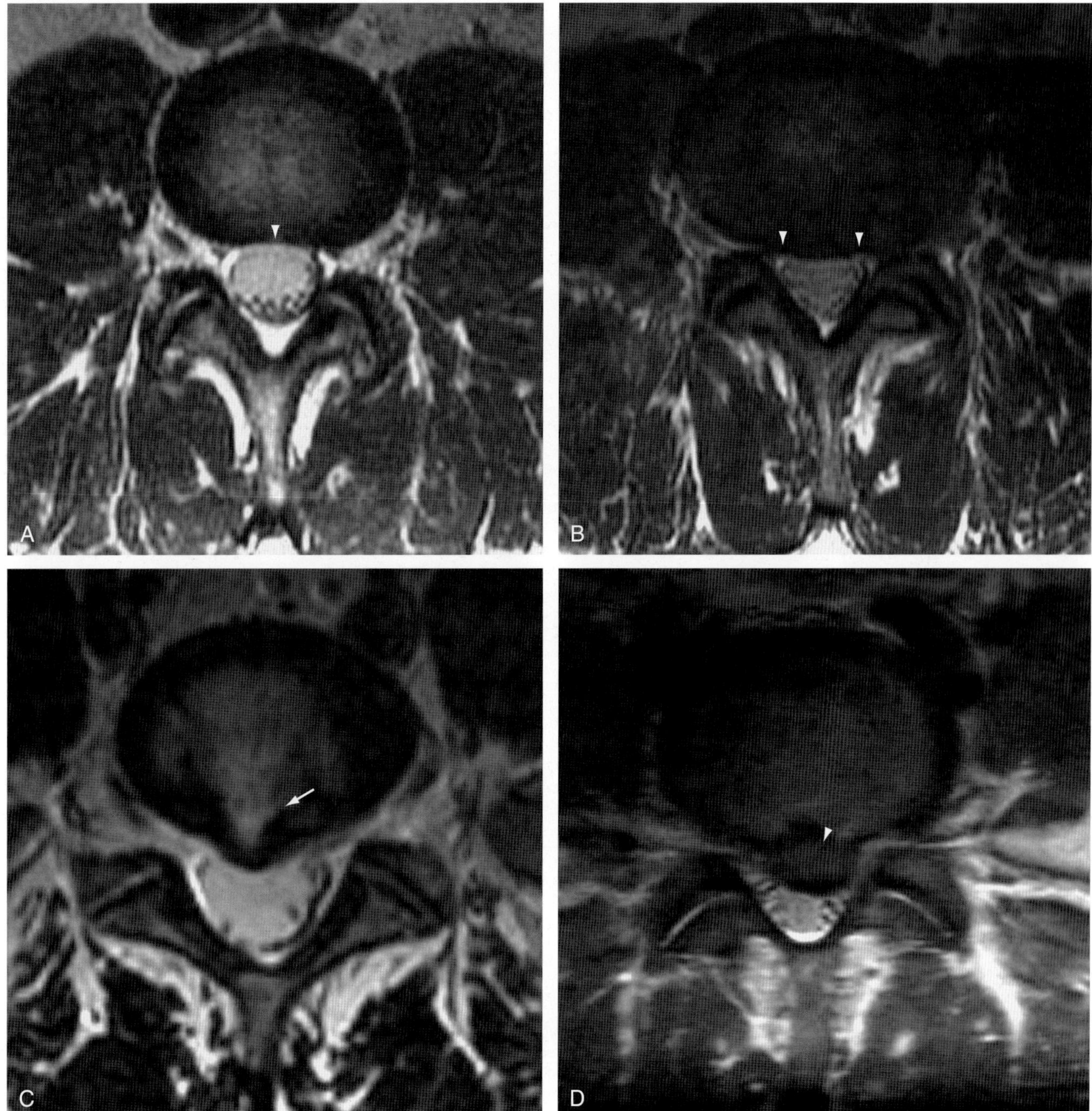

FIGURE 9-3. Lumbar spine disk contour abnormalities. **A,** Normal: Axial T2-weighted image shows a concave posterior margin *(arrowhead)*. **B,** Bulge: Axial T2-weighted image shows a generalized displacement of greater than 180 degrees of the disk margin beyond the normal margin of the intervertebral disk space manifested by a convex posterior margin *(arrowheads)*. **C,** Herniation, protrusion type: Axial T2-weighted image shows a focal contour abnormality with the base against the parent disk margin broader than the component displaced into the canal. Extension of nucleus pulposus through a defect of the inner anulus is identified *(arrow)*. **D,** Herniation, extrusion type *(arrowhead)*: Axial T2-weighted image shows a focal contour abnormality with the base against the parent disk margin narrower than the component displaced into the canal (either anteroposterior or craniocaudal dimension). This was confirmed on sagittal images. Substantial mass effect is present, causing moderate central canal and severe left foraminal zone stenosis.

disk (Figure 9-3, *B*). The normal margin is defined by the vertebral body ring apophysis exclusive of osteophytes. Bulges can be the result of disk degeneration with a grossly intact anulus. Disk margins tend to be smooth, symmetric, or eccentric (asymmetric) and nonfocal and may have a level-specific appearance in the lumbar spine.

A bulging disk is a disk in which the contour of the outer anulus extends, or appears to extend, in the horizontal (axial) plane beyond the edges of the disk space, over greater than 50% (180 degrees) of the circumference of the disk and usually less than 3 mm beyond the edges of the vertebral body apophyses.

Intervertebral disk herniation is a localized displacement (less than 180 degrees of the circumference) of disk material beyond the normal margin of the intervertebral disk space (Figure 9-3, *C*). This material may consist of nucleus pulposus, cartilage, fragmented apophyseal bone, or fragmented anular tissue. It is often the result of disk degeneration with some degree of focal anular disruption. The types of disk herniation are a protrusion, extrusion, and free fragment (sequestration). *Protrusion* refers to a herniated disk in which the greatest distance, in any plane, between the edges of the disk material beyond the disk space is less than the distance between the edges of the base in the same plane. In disk protrusion the base against the parent disk margin is broader than any other diameter of the herniation; extension of the nucleus pulposus may occur through a partial defect in the anulus but is contained by some intact outer anular fibers and the posterior longitudinal ligament.

> Disk protrusion is a type of herniation in which the base against the parent disk margin is broader than any other diameter of the herniation; extension of the nucleus pulposus may occur through a partial defect in the anulus but is contained by some intact outer anular fibers and the posterior longitudinal ligament.

Extrusion refers to a herniated disk in which, in at least one plane, any one distance between the edges of the disk material beyond the disk space is greater than the distance between the edges of the base in the same plane, or when no continuity exists between the disk material beyond the disk space and that within the disk space (Figure 9-3, *D*). An extrusion is characterized by the following: the base against the parent disk margin tends to be narrower than any other diameter of the herniation, with extension of the nucleus pulposus through a complete focal defect in the anulus fibrosus. Extruded disks in which all continuity with the disk of origin is lost may be further characterized as sequestrated. Disk material displaced away from the site of extrusion may be characterized as migrated whether sequestered or not; it may stay subligamentous, contained by the posterior longitudinal ligament, or may migrate widely. A chronic disk herniation may also show calcification, ossification, or gas (a vacuum phenomenon) (Table 9-1).

> A disk extrusion is characterized by having the base against the parent disk margin narrower than any other diameter of the herniation, with extension of the nucleus pulposus through a complete focal defect in the anulus fibrosus.

A staging system has been proposed for lumbar DDD,[7] but most providers will report findings using the designations of minimal, moderate, and severe. The following scheme is used to define the degree of canal compromise produced by disk displacement or spinal

TABLE 9-1. Terminology

Term[2]	Definition	Diagram
Disk bulge	A disk in which the contour of the outer anulus extends, or appears to extend, in the horizontal (axial) plane beyond the edges of the disk space, over greater than 50% (180 degrees) of the circumference of the disk and usually less than 3 mm beyond the edges of the vertebral body apophyses	90° 90° 90° 90° "Symmetrical bulging disk" / "Asymmetrical bulging disk"
Herniated disk: protrusion	A herniated disk in which the greatest distance, in any plane, between the edges of the disk material beyond the disk space is less than the distance between the edges of the base in the same plane	Protrusion
Herniated disk: extrusion	A herniated disk in which, in at least one plane, any one distance between the edges of the disk material beyond the disk space is greater than the distance between the edges of the base in the same plane, or when no continuity exists between the disk material beyond the disk space and that within the disk space	Extrusion

TABLE 9-1. Terminology—cont'd

Term[2]	Definition	Diagram
Herniated disk: extrusion, sequestrated disk	An extruded disk in which a portion of the disk tissue is displaced beyond the outer anulus and maintains no connection by disk tissue with the disk of origin.	

Figures redrawn from Fardon DF, Milette PC: Nomenclature and classification of lumbar disk pathology. Recommendations of the combined task forces of the North American Spine Society, American Society of Spine Radiology, and American Society of Neuroradiology, *Spine* 26:E93-E113, 2001.

stenosis based on the goals of being practical, objective, reasonably precise, and clinically relevant. Measurements are typically taken from an axial section at the site of the most severe compromise. Canal compromise of less than one third of the canal at that section is "minimal"; that between one third and two thirds is "moderate" (Figure 9-4, *A*); and that more than two thirds is "severe" (Figure 9-4, *B*). This scheme may also be applied to defining the degree of foraminal (neural canal) narrowing.

> Canal compromise of less than one third of the canal is minimal; that between one third and two thirds is moderate; and that more than two thirds is severe.

Endplate-Related Marrow Signal Alteration: "Modic Change"

Modic et al.[8] initially described vertebral marrow end plate findings in association with DDD; this spectrum of findings is popularly referred to as "Modic changes." Type 1 is "fluid-like" and shows T1 hypointensity and T2 hyperintensity (i.e., follows fluid signal). Type 1 Modic changes show bone marrow edema (Figure 9-5, *A* and *B*), have mild enhancement that may involve the disk, and are identified in 4% of patients scanned. On contrast-enhanced MRI, the enhancement is proportional to reactive granulation tissue present at the peripherally herniated nucleus pulposus, anular tear, or degenerated end plate. Type 2 Modic

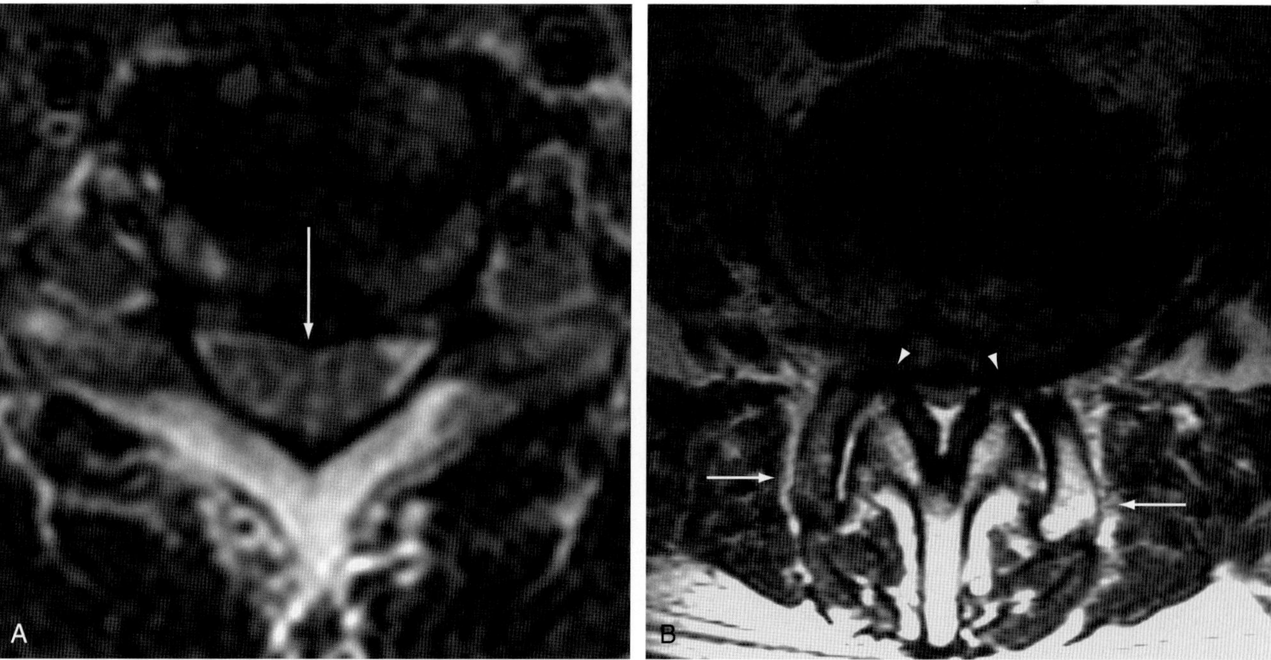

FIGURE 9-4. Spinal stenosis. **A,** Cervical spine moderate stenosis: Axial T2-weighted image shows prominent disk osteophyte complex contacting the spinal cord *(arrow)*, causing mild flattening with a paucity of surrounding cerebrospinal fluid. **B,** Lumbar spine severe stenosis: Axial T2-weighted image shows hypertrophic facet joint osteoarthritis *(arrows)* and moderate disk bulge *(arrowheads)*. This combination is causing severe central spinal stenosis with effacement of cerebrospinal fluid from around the traversing nerves.

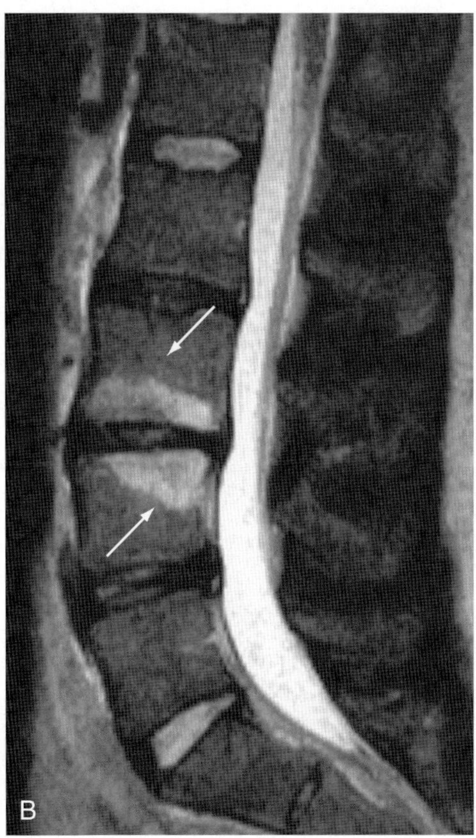

FIGURE 9-5. Vertebral marrow endplate signal alteration (Modic changes): Type 1. Sagittal T1-weighted **(A)** and sagittal T2-weighted **(B)** MR images show disk height loss and desiccation at multiple levels. At the L3-4 level, this is associated with rounded areas of signal alteration that abut the end plate and follow fluid-like signal with T1 hypointensity and T2 hyperintensity *(arrows)*.

changes are "fat-like" and follow fat signal intensity on all pulse sequences (Figure 9-6, *A* and *B*). Therefore type 2 changes show T1 and T2 hyperintensity without fat suppression or T2 hypointensity with fat suppression. Type 2 Modic changes are identified in 16% of patients scanned for lumbar disease. Type 3 Modic changes are "sclerosis-like" and show hypointensity on all pulse sequences (Figure 9-7, *A* and *B*). Type 3 changes can also be identified on radiography as a rounded area of sclerotic opacity abutting the end plate, known as *discogenic vertebral sclerosis.* The characteristic feature of Modic changes is that they are related to the endplate. They can be round or hemispheric, but this is not a requirement. The disk shows degeneration, meaning that there is at least some degree of desiccation of the nucleus pulposus. The differential diagnosis may include infection. One way to distinguish this is that infection should have intradiscal fluid-like signal and end plate erosions. Modic findings are typically believed to span a spectrum from type 1 to type 3; however, mixed end plate findings are often present and are generally associated with more severe spondylosis. Also, moderate and severe Modic type 1 and type 2 end plate abnormalities are useful in predicting discography positive pain response in patients with symptomatic low back pain.[9] Others have found that Modic changes are a relatively specific but insensitive sign of a painful lumbar disk in patients with discogenic low back pain.[10]

HIGH-INTENSITY ZONE

High-intensity zone (HIZ) is the imaging term used to describe an area of hyperintense signal in the region of the anulus fibrosus on T2-weighted MR images (Figure 9-8, *A* and *B*). A posterior location tends to be more common than an anterior one. In the patient population undergoing MRI for lumbar back pain, this finding may be noted in approximately 25%. The presence of an HIZ correlates with an anular tear and an approximately 85% chance that there will be concordant pain reproduction at discography.[11,12] Others have also concluded that the lumbar disk HIZ in patients with low back pain is likely to represent painful internal disk disruption.[13]

> The presence of an HIZ correlates with an anular tear and about an 85% chance that there will be concordant pain reproduction at discography. However, asymptomatic patients may also have this finding.

However, studies comparing symptomatic to asymptomatic people undergoing both MRI and discography have revealed that, as in other disk-related MRI findings, asymptomatic HIZs may also be encountered. The presence of an HIZ does not reliably indicate the presence of symptomatic internal disk disruption; it is a marker of pathoanatomy and not a specific painful syndrome. Although a higher percentage of HIZs exists in symptomatic patients, the prevalence in asymptomatic individuals with degenerative disk disease (25%) is too high for meaningful clinical use. However, a similar percentage of asymptomatic and symptomatic individual disks with an HIZ were shown to be painful at discography.[14] Therefore merely the presence of an HIZ does not define a group of patients with particular clinical features.[15]

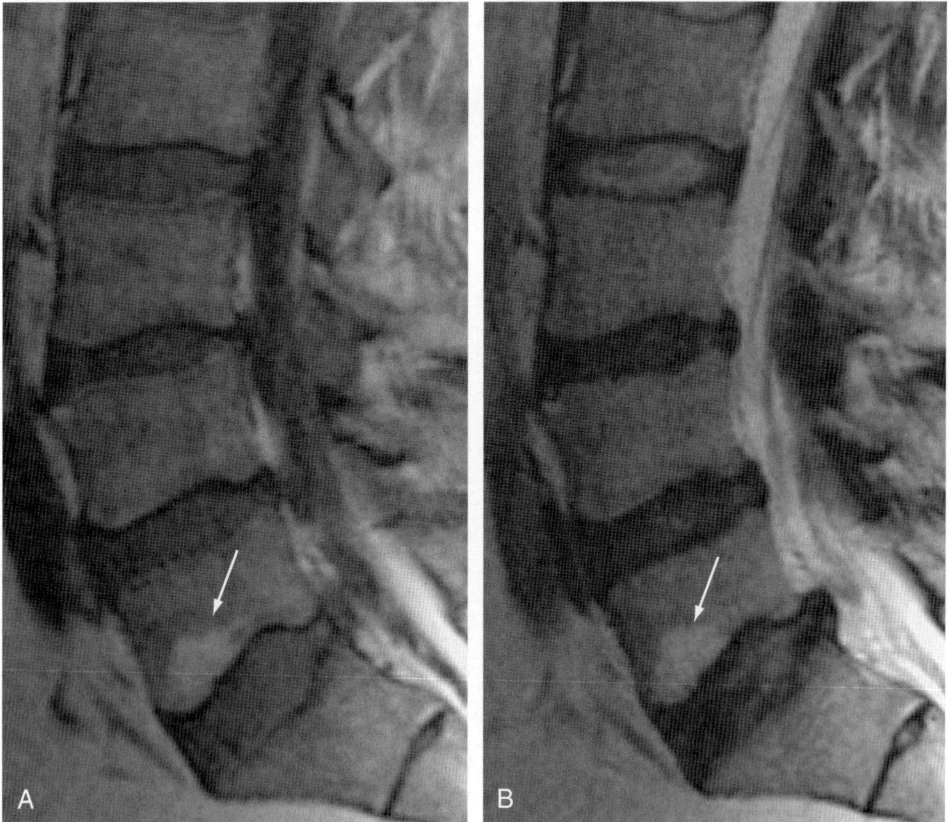

FIGURE 9-6. Vertebral marrow end plate signal alteration (Modic changes): Type 2. Sagittal T1-weighted MR image **(A)** and sagittal T2-weighted MR image without fat suppression **(B)** show disk desiccation at multiple levels. At the L5-S1 level, this is associated with a rounded area of signal abnormality in the anteroinferior aspect of L5 abutting the end plate *(arrows)*. This follows fat signal on all pulse sequences and is hyperintense on T1-weighted and T2-weighted images without fat suppression (on the fat suppression image the signal would suppress similar to fat elsewhere).

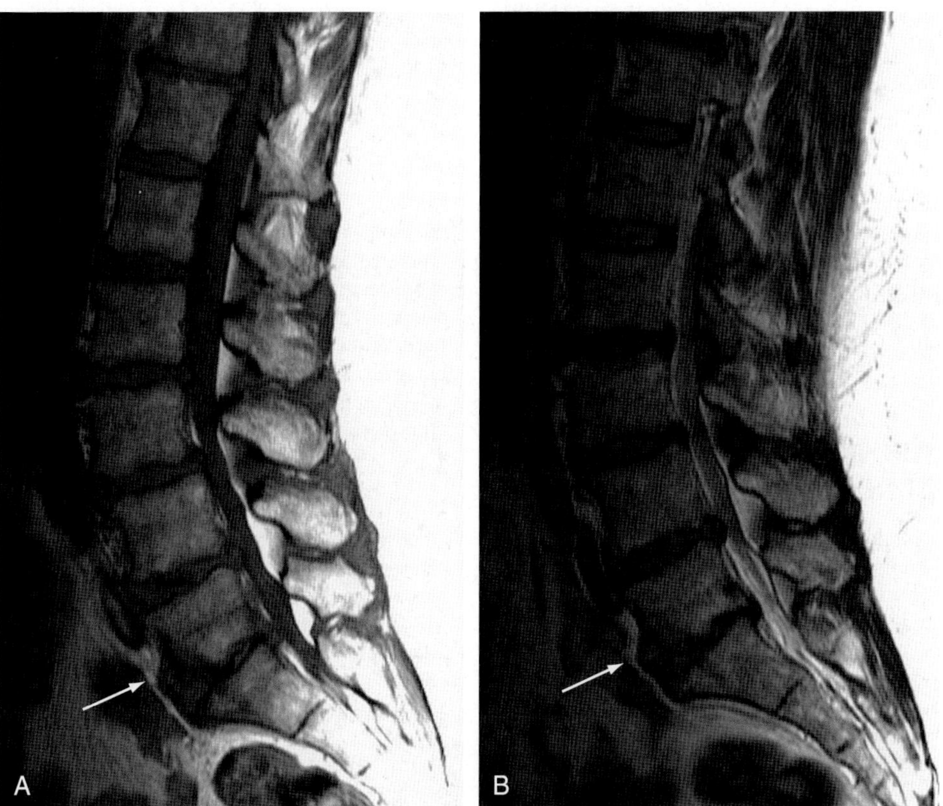

FIGURE 9-7. Vertebral marrow end plate signal alteration (Modic changes): Type 3. Sagittal T1-weighted MR image **(A)** and sagittal T2-weighted MR image without fat suppression **(B)** show degenerative disk disease at the lumbosacral junction. The anteroinferior aspect of L5 *(arrow)* shows a well-defined area of T1 and T2 hypointensity abutting the end plate.

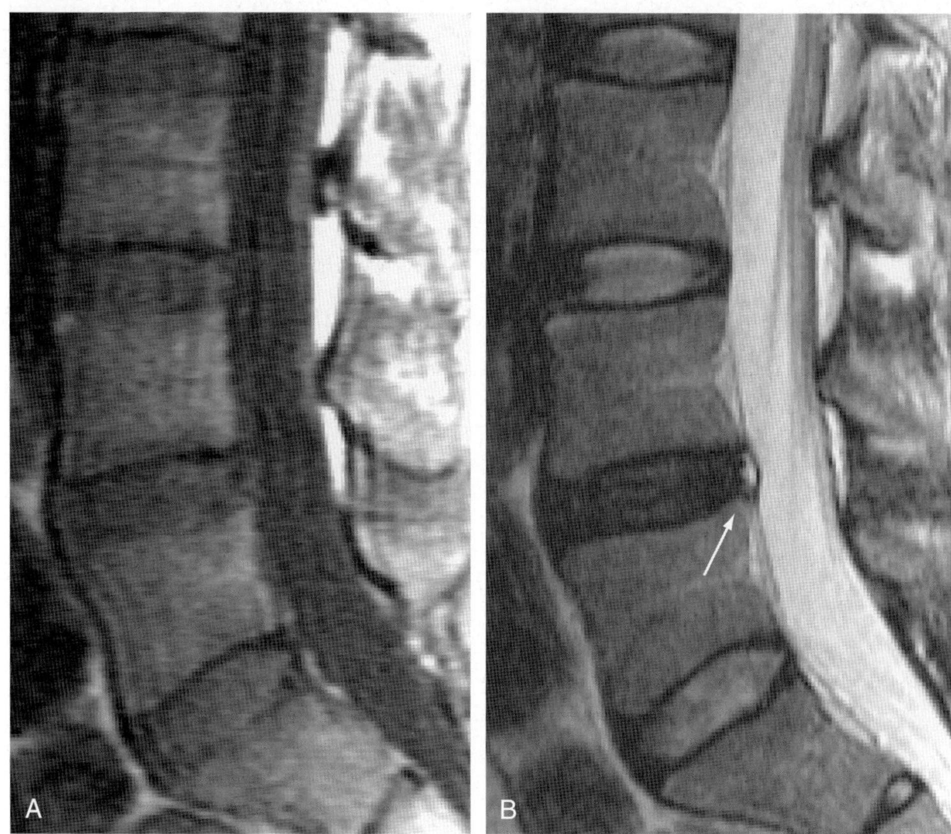

FIGURE 9-8. High-intensity zone: anular fissure (tear). **A,** Sagittal T1-weighted image shows no abnormality. **B,** Sagittal T2-weighted image shows a small focus of hyperintensity *(arrow)* within the posterior anulus fibrosis, which reflects an anular fissure (tear).

The nature of the HIZ finding remains unknown, but it probably represents an area of secondary inflammation as a result of an anular tear. As has been well demonstrated, HIZs correlate with peripheral anular tears demonstrated at discography (painful or not). The focal T2 hyperintense areas may indicate fragmentation of the outer collagenous anulus fibrosis. The preferred term for such lesions is *fissures* rather than *tears*, because of the traumatic etiology connotation, but *tear* is so entrenched in medical practice that it is likely to persist. An HIZ may be enhanced after contrast administration, reflecting the fibrovascular ingrowth into the region of the anular tear. In addition, nerve tissue has also been seen by histology in this lesion and is the purported mechanism by which peripheral anular tears generate pain.[16] Given the current data, the prognostic or therapeutic significance of this finding has not yet been elucidated.

ROLE OF COMPUTED TOMOGRAPHY AND MR MYELOGRAPHY

For computed tomography (CT) imaging, soft tissue contrast is best between highly compact/dense structures (e.g., tendons, ligaments, anulus fibrosus), water-containing structures (e.g., muscle, thecal sac), fat (epidural or fascial), and gas. Thus CT is a reasonable modality for detection of disk herniations causing thecal sac or nerve compression (Figure 9-9, *A*). This is an improvement over projectional radiography, which requires approximately a 10% change of full scale to detect contrast differences. One mechanism to improve contrast resolution is to administer a contrast agent through one of several routes. The most commonly employed routes for spine imaging are intravenous, intrathecal, and intradiscal.

MRI is not only limited in specificity but in some instances also inaccurately depicts the pathoanatomic state. CT myelography (in which CT is performed after iodinated contrast is instilled in the thecal sac) continues to be requested extensively. It is as accurate as MRI and can be more specific because of its ability to distinguish bone (osteophytes) from soft tissue (Figure 9-9, *B*). The advantages of MRI include providing excellent visualization of regions proximal and distal to severe stenosis or a block. It often avoids the need for contrast, although contrast improves conspicuity. The main reasons cited for using CT myelography in conjunction with or in lieu of MRI are: improved visualization of the extent of disk herniations, demonstration of focal neural compression by small herniations, and clarification of abnormalities of the facets, including synovial cysts. However, an opportunity for refinement of the indications for CT myelography remains, particularly given the large variability of utilization.

MR myelography can also be obtained without contrast injection by using heavily T2-weighted images with fat suppression. MR myelography yields images that resemble conventional myelography and may be used to help confirm abnormalities seen on conventional MRI in selected cases; however, there are a large number of false-positive and false-negative findings.[17] Although MR myelography does not significantly improve the diagnostic accuracy of MRI, it does allow a better overall view of the dural sac and root sleeves, making it easier to diagnose spinal stenosis and disk herniation in a minority of cases.[18] The development of better 3D pulse sequences with isotropic voxels combined with improved signal and spatial resolution available on higher field strength systems (e.g., 3 Tesla) may make MRI competitive with the spatial resolution and anatomic detail that surgeons seem to favor in CT myelography.

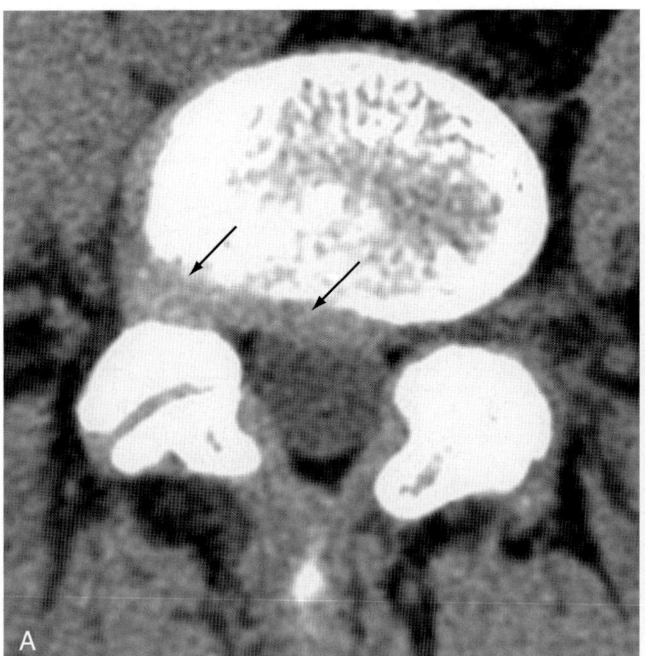

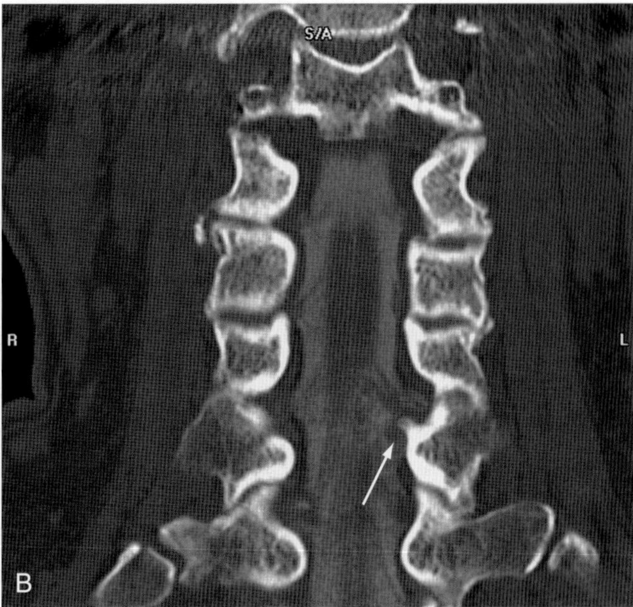

FIGURE 9-9. CT imaging. **A,** Axial CT image shows a focal disk contour abnormality *(arrows),* obliterating the right neural foramen representing an intervertebral disk herniation. **B,** Multislice CT myelography in a patient after anterior cervical fusion: Coronal oblique multiplanar reformation (MPR) shows an osseous ridge compressing the nerve roots *(arrow).* MPRs are created in planes that correct for any patient rotation to generate more useful sections based on true anatomic landmarks.

DDD IN THE CERVICAL AND THORACIC SPINE

Degenerative changes of the cervical and thoracic spine are less common than these changes in the lumbar spine. Although the radiographic findings reflect similar pathologic events, the cervical and thoracic spine segments are anatomically unique compared with the lumbar spine and with each other.

The cervical spine is the most biomechanically challenged segment of the spine. Recent anatomic reevaluation has determined that the annulus fibrosis of the cervical spine is a crescentic anterior interosseous ligament rather than a completely circumferential "O-ring" that surrounds the nucleus pulposus, as in the lumbar spine. It tapers laterally where the uncinate processes exist and is deficient in the posterolateral aspects. Posteriorly there is a thin layer of vertically oriented intervertebral fibers reinforced by the posterior longitudinal ligament (PLL). This anatomic structure is not present in the human fetus, child, or adolescent and is believed to represent a normal phenomenon of maturation. When bipeds turn their heads, a rotational component is involved, which in quadrupeds is mostly achieved with lateral side bending. Therefore uncovertebral joints are unique to vertebrate species that maintain an erect posture, and this biomechanical condition causes uncovertebral hypertrophy as a normal aging (presumably degenerative) phenomenon. In the cervical spine, intradural connections between adjacent nerves may account for the greater than expected overlap of dermatomal pain patterns in this region. Because of these considerations, chronic cervical spine pain of an axial nature is difficult to evaluate and treat. Because of this unique anatomy in the cervical spine, radicular pain is more often from osseous proliferation of the uncovertebral joints causing neural foraminal stenosis (Figure 9-10, *A* and *B*) rather than an intervertebral disk herniation (Figure 9-10, *C*).

The thoracic spine is stabilized by the ribs and has less range of motion than the other segments of the spinal column. Thoracic pain is relatively uncommon. However, it is important from a management perspective because dorsal back pain can be as disabling as cervical and lumbar pain. Although histologic studies of the thoracic disks are currently being reevaluated, it has been revealed that branches of the rami communicantes may provide innervation circumferentially. MRI reveals that a substantial number (up to 27%) of asymptomatic degenerative or protruded disks also exist in the thoracic spine.[17] However, anatomic changes on imaging studies do not necessarily equate with pain generation, and in one investigation approximately one fourth of the disks injected provoked a pain response that did not match MRI findings or morphology findings at discography.[18] One case series on thoracic discography[19] concluded that useful information is obtained for treatment planning. In this study, in addition to painful segments, control disks were also injected, which did not provoke pain. The challenge with thoracic spine MRI is the number of segments necessitating a large field of view for the sagittal images and artifacts generated from cardiac, respiratory, and cerebrospinal fluid motion. Similar to the lumbar spine, axial images along the disk plane are best at characterizing contour abnormalities (Figure 9-11, *A* and *B*).

CONCLUSION

Spine imaging can provide exquisite information regarding pathoanatomy with respect to DDD but often does not define a specific painful clinical syndrome for a patient. The more common imaging findings of disk degeneration and associated conditions have been described in this chapter. However, abnormal imaging findings of the disks may be degenerative, adaptive, genetic, or a combination of environmental and undetermined factors. Many findings may simply represent senescent changes that are the natural consequence of stress applied during

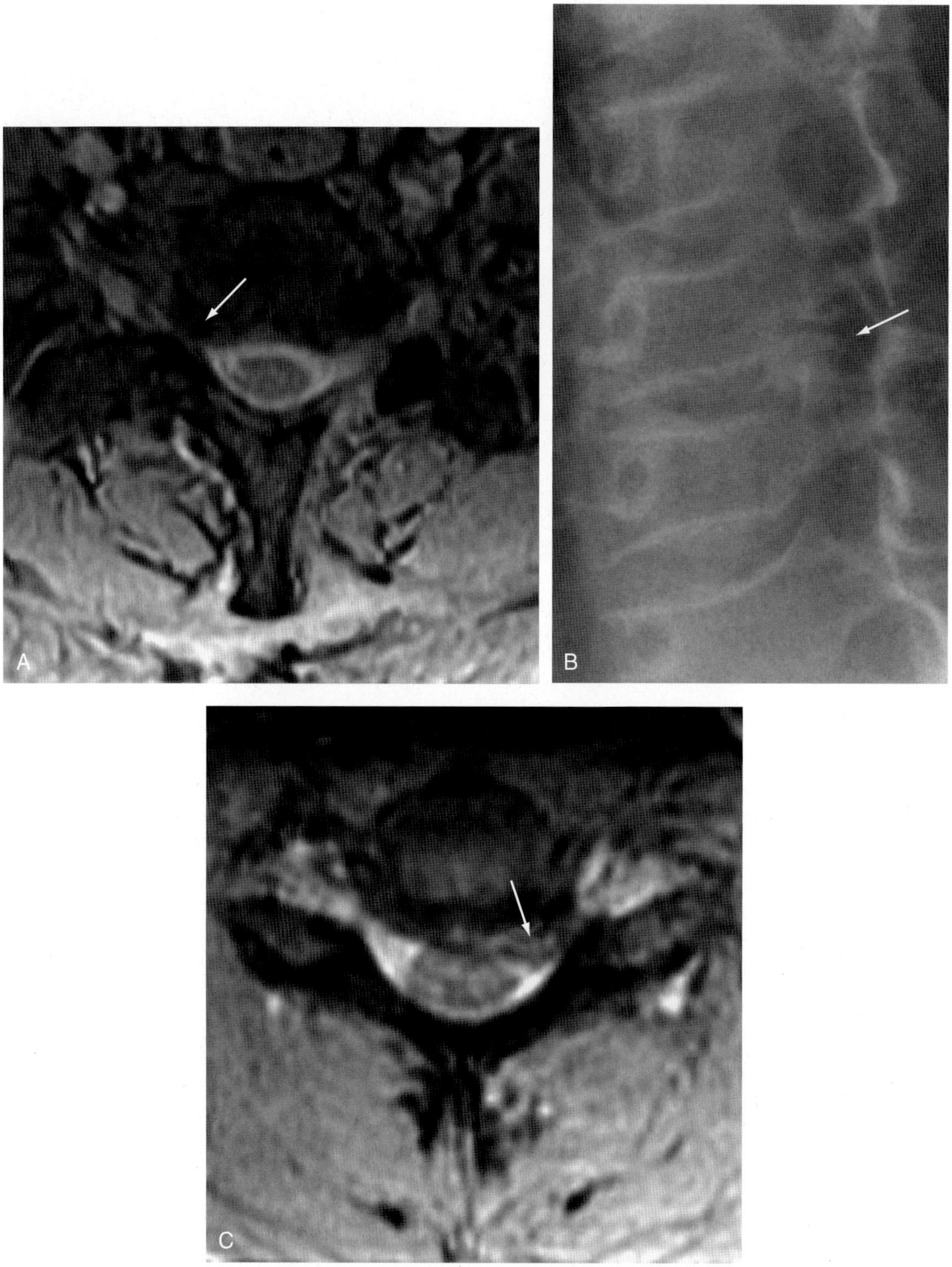

FIGURE 9-10. Cervical spine foraminal lesions. **A,** Axial T2*-weighted image showing neural foraminal stenosis from a hypointense disk-osteophyte complex related to uncovertebral hypertrophy *(arrow)*. **B,** Oblique radiograph shows osseous proliferation of the posterolateral aspect of the intervertebral disk (uncovertebral hypertrophy, *arrow*) causing neural foraminal stenosis correlating to the MRI findings shown in **A**. **C,** Axial T2*-weighted image shows an intervertebral disk herniation with extruded nucleus pulposus *(arrow)*.

the course of a lifetime. The imaging appearance of spine degenerative disease has a similar incidence between symptomatic and nonsymptomatic populations. Therefore the appropriate utilization of imaging modalities within a defined clinical context is paramount. For some patients with complicated or recalcitrant symptoms, the most useful application of advanced imaging techniques may be in the exclusion of more serious causes of axial low back pain such as infection, neoplasm, or fracture rather than the inclusion of any specific degenerative findings.

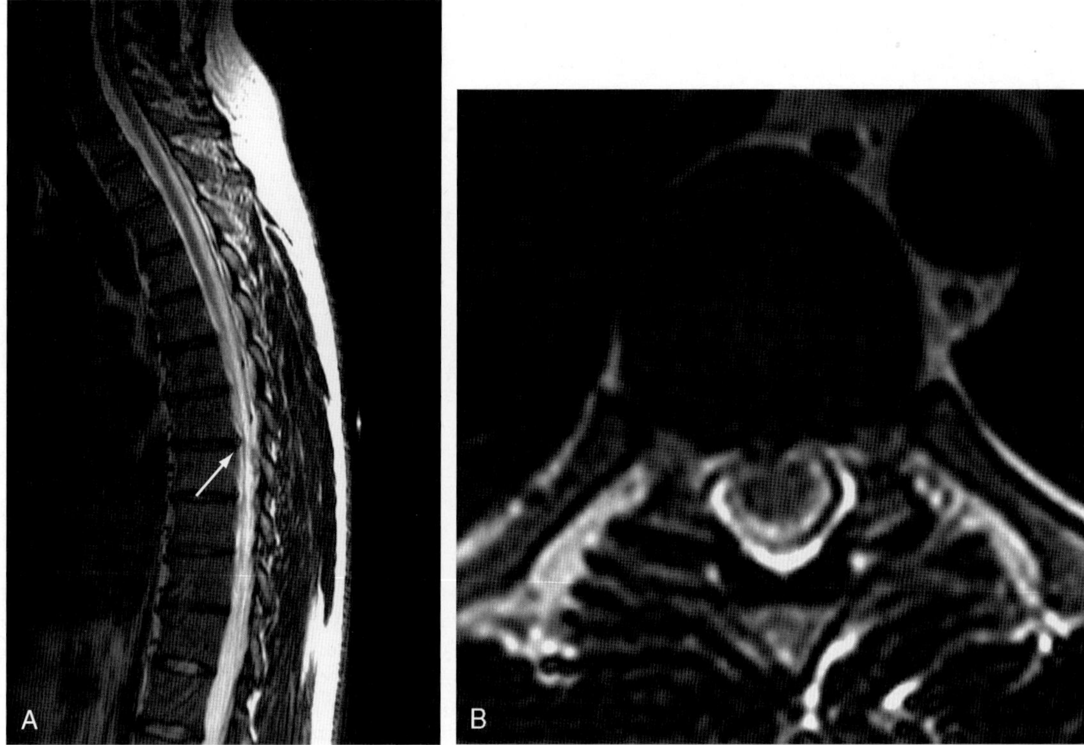

FIGURE 9-11. Thoracic spine disk herniation. **A,** Sagittal T2-weighted image with fat suppression shows an intervertebral disk contour abnormality *(arrow)*. **B,** Axial T2-weighted image without fat suppression characterizes the contour abnormality as an extruded disk herniation.

REFERENCES

1. Fardon DF, Milette PC: Nomenclature and classification of lumbar disc pathology. Recommendations of the Combined Task Forces of the North American Spine Society, American Society of Spine Radiology, and American Society of Neuroradiology, *Spine* 26:E93-E113, 2001.
2. Retrieved September 15, 2006 from http://www.asnr.org/spine_nomenclature.
3. Nathan H: Osteophytes of the vertebral column. An anatomical study of their development according to age, race, and sex, with consideration as to their etiology and significance, *J Bone Joint Surg* 44:243-268, 1962.
4. Pfirrmann C, Resnick D: Schmorl nodes of the thoracic and lumbar spine: radiographic-pathologic study of prevalence, characterization, and correlation with degenerative changes of 1,650 spine levels in 100 cadavers, *Radiology* 219:368-374, 2001.
5. Karppinen J, Paakko E, Paassilta P et al: Radiologic phenotypes in lumbar MR imaging for a gene defect in the COL9A3 gene of type IX collagen, *Radiology* 227:143-148, 2003.
6. Cheng XG, Brys P, Nijs J et al: Radiological prevalence of lumbar intervertebral disc calcification in the elderly: an autopsy study, *Skeletal Radiol* 25:231-235, 1996.
7. Pfirrmann CW, Metzdorf A, Zanetti M et al: Magnetic resonance classification of lumbar intervertebral disc degeneration, *Spine* 26:1873-1878, 2001.
8. Modic MT, Steinberg PM, Ross JS et al: Degenerative disk disease: assessment of changes in vertebral body marrow with MR imaging, *Radiology* 166:193-199, 1998.
9. Weishaupt D, Zanetti M, Hodler J et al: Painful lumbar disk derangement: relevance of endplate abnormalities at MR imaging, *Radiology* 218:420-427, 2001.
10. Braithwaite I, White J, Saifuddin A et al: Vertebral end-plate (Modic) changes on lumbar spine MRI: correlation with pain reproduction at lumbar discography, *Eur Spine J* 7:363-368, 1998.
11. Aprill CN, Bogduk N: High-intensity zone: a diagnostic sign of painful lumbar disc on magnetic resonance imaging, *Br J Radiol* 65:361-369, 1992.
12. Schellhas KP, Pollei SR, Gundry CR et al: Lumbar disc high-intensity zone. Correlation of magnetic resonance imaging and discography, *Spine* 21:79-86, 1996.
13. Lam KS, Carlin D, Mulholland RC: Lumbar disc high-intensity zone: the value and significance of provocative discography in the determination of the discogenic pain source, *Eur Spine J* 9:36-41, 2000.
14. Carragee EJ, Paragioudakis SJ, Khurana S: 2000 Volvo Award winner in clinical studies: lumbar high-intensity zone and discography in subjects without low back problems, *Spine* 25:2987-2992, 2000.
15. Rankine JJ, Gill KP, Hutchinson CE et al: The clinical significance of the high-intensity zone on lumbar spine magnetic resonance imaging, *Spine* 24:1913-1919, 1999.
16. Ross JS, Modic MT, Masaryk TJ: Tears of the anulus fibrosus: assessment with Gd-DTPA-enhanced MR imaging, *AJR Am J Roentgenol* 154:159-162, 1990.
17. Thornton MJ, Lee MJ, Pender S et al: Evaluation of the role of magnetic resonance myelography in lumbar spine imaging, *Eur Radiol* 9:924-929, 1999.
18. Pui MH, Husen YA: Value of magnetic resonance myelography in the diagnosis of disc herniation and spinal stenosis, *Australas Radiol* 44:281-284, 2000.
19. Jensen MC, Brant-Zawadzki MN, Obuchowski N: Magnetic resonance imaging of the lumbar spine in people without back pain, *N Engl J Med* 331:69-73, 1994.

CHAPTER 10

Imaging of Diabetes Mellitus and Neuropathic Arthropathy: The Diabetic Foot

MARK E. SCHWEITZER, MD, *and* MELISSA BIRNBAUM, MD

KEY FACTS

- Pedal complications are very common in the diabetic population due to neurologic and vascular disease and cause significant morbidity.
- Neuropathic arthropathy results from a combination of sensory, motor, and autonomic dysfunction.
- The Schon classification is based on the location of Charcot joints and their severity.
- Neuropathy, ligamentous injury, tendinopathy, and muscle atrophy lead to foot deformity and abnormal biomechanics resulting in callus formation. Progressive breakdown of the callus leads to focal ulceration and superimposed infection.
- The most accurate way of determining the presence of osteomyelitis is to find the ulcer and sinus tract and closely assess the adjacent bones, either clinically or more accurately by imaging.
- It is often difficult to distinguish neuropathic arthropathy from osteomyelitis. Neuroarthropathy commonly occurs in the midfoot, whereas osteomyelitis is seen predominantly in the metatarsal heads and hindfoot. Nuclear scintigraphy is frequently used to differentiate the two.

Diabetes has become a health care problem of increasing concern in the United States as the number of people affected has risen tremendously over the past 2 decades. From 1980 through 2003, the number of Americans with diabetes has nearly tripled and will continue to rise to near epidemic proportions.[1] Approximately 15 million persons in the United States alone have been estimated to have diabetes, and this number is predicted to rise to 22 million by 2025.[2]

The diabetic foot has had a significant impact both on society and on individual patients. An estimated 15% to 20% of all individuals with diabetes in the United States will be hospitalized at some point for a foot-related complication.[3] Health-economic consequences are enormous, with costs of healing an infected ulcer without amputation totaling $17,500.[4] However, amputation is often a necessary treatment in the diabetic patient, with approximately 50,000 lower extremity amputations performed each year in the United States at a cost of over $1 billion.[5] Diabetes is the most common cause of nontraumatic amputation, with a rate 15 times higher among the diabetic population compared with the nondiabetic population.[6] The incidence of complication involving the contralateral foot is also increased within 2 years after surgery, which reflects the weight-bearing shift onto the intact extremity. The overall quality of life following amputation is reduced in the diabetic patient as well.[7]

Early care and management of the diabetic foot is extremely important and can improve quality of life. Effective interventions include optimizing glycemic control, intensive podiatric care, debridement of calluses, orthotics, and in some cases surgical revascularization, including bypass grafts and peripheral angioplasty. These interventions may contribute to a decreased risk of foot ulcerations and therefore favorable consequences to the individual and society.

The foot is susceptible to multiple complications that are largely due to the cumulative effects of neurologic and vascular disease. Diabetic patients show evidence of peripheral vascular disease, both macrovascular and microvascular, which lead to chronic ischemia, decreased ability to fight infection, and poor wound healing. Diabetic patients also exhibit peripheral neuropathy, motor and sensory as well as autonomic, which contribute to the pedal disorder. The decreased sensation of the diabetic foot allows unrecognized microtrauma with incomplete healing, the formation of calluses, and consequent tissue breakdown and ulceration. Superimposed infection may occur as a result of bacterial colonization via direct implantation and contiguous spread. Furthermore, repetitive trauma to the foot and ischemia result in neuropathic osteoarthropathy, or joint deformity.

Imaging is essential in the evaluation of the sequelae of the diabetic foot. It is key for identifying vascular disease and soft tissue, articular, and bony complications. Radiographs and computed tomography (CT) are useful for osseous anatomic information. Bone and leukocyte scintigraphy are often used to distinguish infection, although localization is sometimes imprecise. Magnetic resonance imaging (MRI) has become the primary imaging tool for evaluation of the diabetic foot, demonstrating both osseous and soft tissue infection in addition to improved anatomic depiction.

PATHOGENESIS

A combination of metabolic dysfunction, neuropathy, immunopathy, and peripheral vascular disease contribute to the development of the diabetic foot. On the microvascular level, diabetic patients show thickening of the capillary basement membrane and accumulation of advanced glycation end products on the membrane, impairing transfer of molecules and contributing to an abnormal hyperemic response. Vasomotor changes and formation of arteriovenous shunting lead to decreased perfusion to bone, muscle, skin, and subcutaneous tissue, which is thought to play a role in the onset of both ischemic changes and the neuropathic foot.

Macrovascular disease affects the diabetic population and occurs in the form of atherosclerosis. This complication is believed to arise from metabolic mechanisms increased by hyperglycemia, including nonenzymatic glycation, diacylglycerol-protein kinase C activation, sorbitol-polyol pathway, and redox alterations.[8] These abnormal pathways promote accelerated atherosclerosis, particularly in the lower extremity. An additional contributor to atherosclerosis is the cell mediator, nitric oxide, which interferes with cell adhesion to vasculature and leads to smooth muscle proliferation and increased negative vascular tone.

Neuropathy primarily originates from the direct effects of hyperglycemia. The "sorbitol theory" explains the mechanism by which excess glucose enters an alternative pathway and is converted to sorbitol. The by-product of this pathway is that the redox potential of the cell is lowered, thus impairing fatty acid metabolism, reducing axonal transport. A second mechanism for the development of neuropathy is nonenzymatic glycosylation. This activity occurs in several tissues including the nerve, vascular basement membrane, and connective tissue. Exposure of these tissues, including nerve myelin, to hyperglycemia leads to covalent bonding of advanced glycation end products, which disrupt protein function.[9]

Sensory neuropathy, seen as distal sensory loss and numbness, results in failure to recognize foot trauma. Motor neuropathy and ischemia lead to atrophy of the intrinsic muscles, promoting foot deformity. This structural change leads to loss of the plantar arch, increased pressure points in several areas, and ulcer formation. Autonomic neuropathy causes impaired thermoregulation of the microvasculature and anhidrosis. As a result, diabetic patients often have dry scaly skin with cracks and fissures, which provides an entrance for infection. Autonomic dysfunction may manifest as a failure of the parasympathetic system with a loss of regulation of heart rate or sympathetic failure with dysregulated neurogenic control of blood flow.[10]

Furthermore, hyperglycemia and metabolic derangements impair the immune system, causing increased susceptibility to infection. Hyperglycemia impairs neutrophil function and diminishes aspects of host defense such as chemotaxis and phagocytosis. Impaired leukocyte function leads to poor granuloma formation and impaired wound healing. Studies have shown that up to 50% of diabetics have an inadequate leukocyte response to severe foot infection.[11] The pedal manifestations of these derangements include osteomyelitis and septic arthritis (Table 10-1).

TABLE 10-1. Multiple Factors Causing Diabetic Foot Disorders

Photogenesis	Mechanism	Effects
Vascular disease	Small vessel disease	Decreased perfusion, neuropathy
	Large vessel disease	Decreased perfusion
Nerve disease	Motor	Muscular atrophy, deformity, pressure points
	Sensory	Numbness, failure to recognize trauma
	Autonomic	Dry skin, portal for infection
Immunologic abnormalities		Increased susceptibility to infection

VASCULAR DISEASE

Peripheral vascular disease is very common in the diabetic patient and is four times more likely to develop in such a patient than in the general population.[12] It is characterized by both atherosclerotic occlusive disease of the lower extremities and arteriosclerotic disease, which is more diffuse, premature, and accelerated in the diabetic patient.[13] Plaques develop circumferentially along the vessel, and calcification occurs within the tunica media.[9] Perfusion is compromised, resulting in chronic ischemia of the lower extremity.

Atherosclerosis is found most commonly at the aortic bifurcation, at the tibial trifurcation, and in the superficial femoral artery at the adductor hiatus. Peripheral vascular disease tends to spare the internal iliac, profunda femoris, and peroneal arteries. Patterns of atherosclerosis have been classified based on vessel involvement. Type 1 disease involves the aorta and common iliac arteries. Type 2 disease involves the aorta, common iliac, and external iliac arteries. Type 3 disease extends from the aorta and iliac to the femoral, popliteal, and tibial arteries. Diabetic patients often have patterns of type 2 and 3. In addition to the major vessels, the distal arterioles and capillaries of the diabetic patient are affected as well and to a greater degree than in nondiabetic individuals.[14,15] Atherosclerotic narrowing of the vessels in the upper extremity is fairly uncommon but may be seen in some cases.

Radiographically, proximal arterial disease is seen as calcification of the vessel wall and angiographically as stenosis.

> Calcification of the vessels distal to the Lisfranc joint in patients younger than 50 years is fairly specific for diabetes.

Conventional angiography, CT angiography, and MR angiography have all played a role in the diagnosis of peripheral vascular disease of the diabetic patient.[16] In each of these imaging techniques, arterial stenosis is seen as a localized narrowing of the vessel, abrupt cutoff of blood flow, or nonvisualization of a vessel branch.[17] With chronic disease, collateralization of vessels may develop in the attempt to increase perfusion to the extremity (Figure 10-1). Although these imaging modalities are accurate in the diagnosis of macrovascular disease and are useful to assess the role of bypass grafts or angioplasty with stents to treat proximal disease, they are not effective in diagnosing the more important microvascular disease.[18] Revascularization techniques may improve blood flow to distal vessels, but disease of the periphery still exists and is more difficult to manage.

Current theory suggests that the microvascular disease may not be anatomic, but rather part of the autonomic dysfunction. Dysfunctional sympathetic control of the neurovascular system leads to capillary hypertension, impaired vasoconstriction, arteriovenous shunting of blood, and consequently decreased perfusion. Injury to the foot is less likely to heal in the face of disease of distal vessels as a result of baseline ischemia and decreased vascular reserve.[19] Callus formation and gradual breakdown in these ischemic areas promotes the development of ulceration and infection.

MRI of peripheral vascular disease is promising. This imaging can be anatomic and show proximal major vessels. However, distal imaging and the assessment of tissue perfusion are more important. One method of assessing tissue perfusion is a comparison between precontrast and postcontrast imaging sequences after administration of intravenous gadolinium. Ischemia and tissue devitalization can be detected as a focal or regional lack of soft tissue contrast enhancement.[20]

> Lack of tissue enhancement after intravenous gadolinium can indicate tissue ischemia and devitalization.

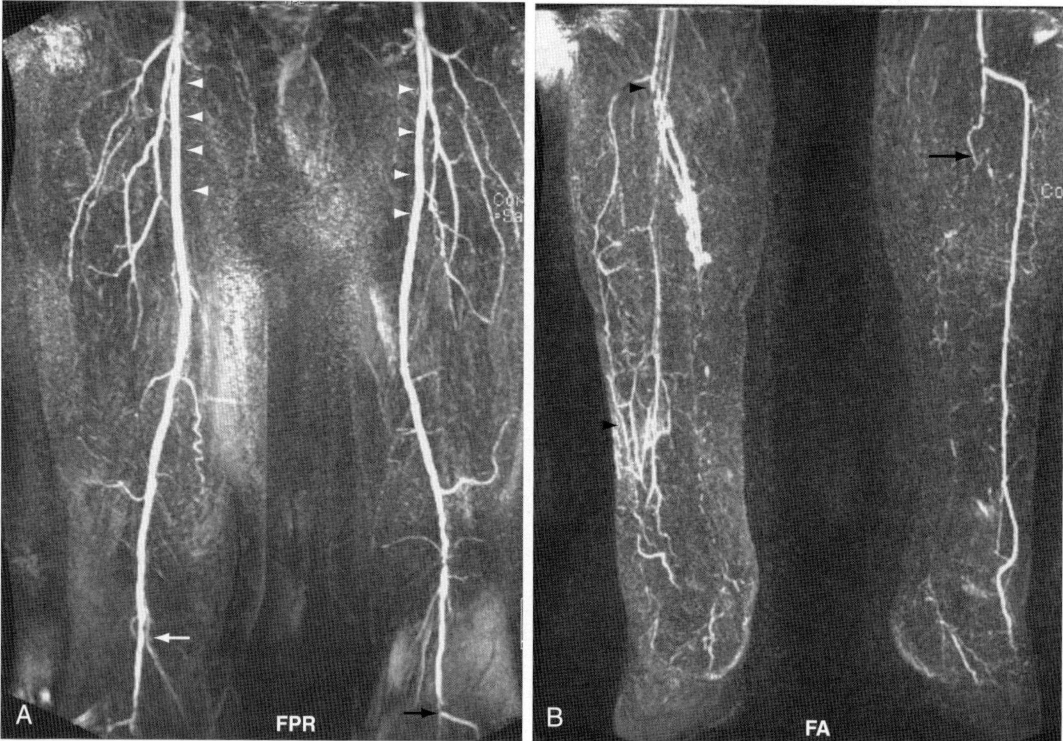

FIGURE 10-1. MR angiogram of the lower extremities. **A,** The common femoral, superficial femoral, and profunda femoris arteries are patent. Mild atherosclerotic plaque is noted diffusely through the superficial femoral arteries *(white arrowheads)* producing irregularities in the vessel contours. Focal narrowing is also seen in the right popliteal artery at the level of the knee joint, resulting in a high-grade stenosis *(white arrow)*. High-grade stenosis of the left popliteal is present just above the knee *(black arrow)*. **B,** The right anterior tibial artery is occluded in the proximal calf with collateral formation that continues to the foot *(black arrowheads)*. The posterior tibial artery is occluded proximally. The left anterior tibial artery is patent to the dorsalis pedis artery. The left tibioperoneal trunk is occluded proximally *(black arrow)*.

Surrounding soft tissue may show increased enhancement representative of hypervascular, reactive tissue. T1-weighted and T2-weighted images show nonspecific alterations in signal, and therefore contrast enhancement is necessary to recognize devitalization. Ischemic tissue that has not yet devitalized may show subtle MRI changes, such as mildly decreased enhancement in comparison with surrounding tissue (Figure 10-2). Arterial spin labeling is an alternative method, not requiring the use of contrast, to obtain similar information.

With the loss of adequate blood supply, gangrene may ensue. Gangrene can be classified as wet or dry, meaning superinfected or not, respectively. Gangrenous tissue shows localized soft tissue loss, mostly in the distal digits. This is often easy to identify on radiographs but is sometimes more difficult to see on MRI.

Soft tissue air may be seen as low-density (dark) structures on radiographs or CT or as signal voids in areas of devitalization on MRI. Gas may be a sign of overlying infection; however, it does not always imply gas gangrene, as it may be seen when an overlying skin ulceration allows air to enter the underlying soft tissues.

> Not all gas within soft tissues in diabetic patients indicates infection. Gas may be introduced into the soft tissues through an ulcer without infection being present.

It is important to note that underlying infections such as osteomyelitis and abscess may not enhance within the necrotic area; in these cases, T1-weighted and T2-weighted images should be used to diagnose infection.[20] Furthermore, even using these signs, false-negative studies may occur.

Finally, in areas of chronic foot ischemia accompanying diabetes, bone infarction is not rare. Bone infarcts are demonstrated by longitudinally oriented regions of signal abnormality in the fatty medullary cavity. They have well-defined margins and a serpiginous configuration.[21,22] Surrounding marrow, if noninfected, is typically normal. It is not uncommon to see multiple bones infarcted in a region of chronic, even fairly mild ischemia.

NEUROPATHY

Neuropathic osteoarthropathy is a complication of diabetes that is sometimes overlooked clinically or is misdiagnosed.[23] This deforming, destructive arthritis is suggested to result from sensory, motor, and autonomic dysfunction.[24] First, the diabetic patient experiences diminished sensation of the distal extremities, classically referred to as having a "stocking and glove" distribution. This sensory neuropathy leads to multiple episodes of minor trauma to the foot with the patient unaware of the injury or the inadequate healing. Immunopathy and chronic baseline ischemia further contribute to the delayed wound healing. Second, motor neuropathy leads to intrinsic foot muscular atrophy and some minimal calf muscle atrophy.[21] This results in shifted weight bearing of the lower extremity and exacerbates the articular injury. Third, autonomic dysfunction occurs involving both sympathetic and parasympathetic systems, leading to soft tissue change and accelerated

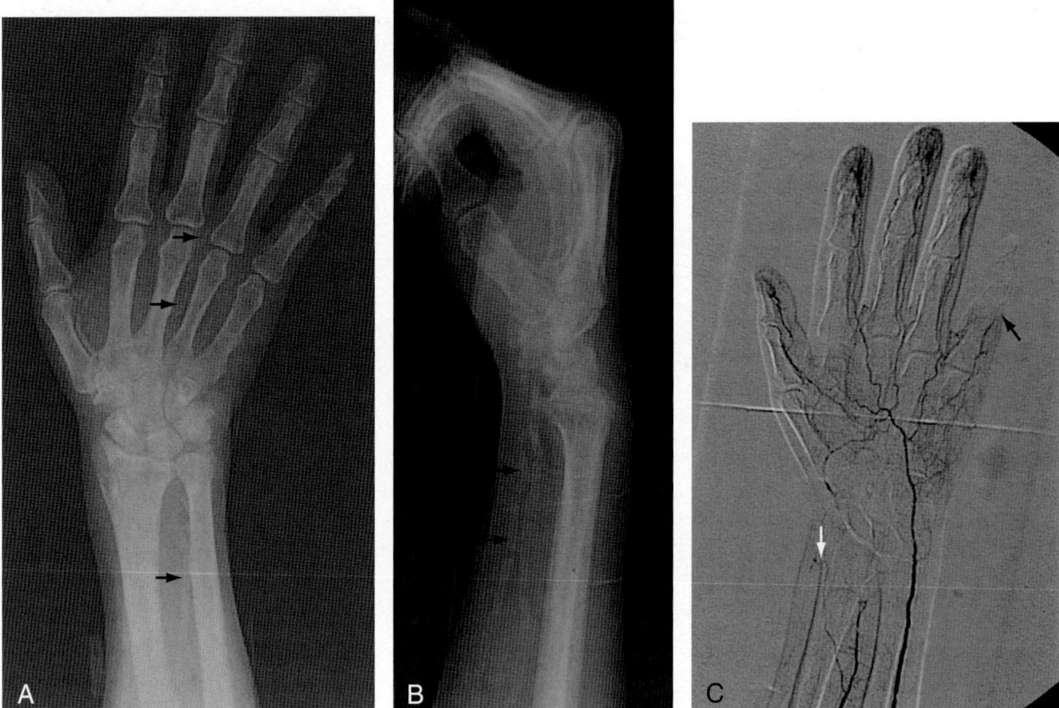

FIGURE 10-2. Upper extremity peripheral vascular disease. Posteroanterior **(A)** and lateral **(B)** radiographs of a patient with diabetes show extensive vascular calcification *(black arrows)* that extends into the digits. Marked atrophy of the soft tissues around the middle and distal phalanges of the fifth finger is seen. **C,** Arteriogram of the hand shows ulnar artery patency with only a single arch filling. There is occlusion of the right radial artery *(white arrow)*. There is also complete obstruction of the right fifth digital artery *(black arrow)*. The digital vessels supplying the other digits are intact.

ulceration.[9] Neuropathic osteoarthropathy or Charcot's arthropathy is the product of this multifaceted pathologic interplay.

Charcot's neuroarthropathy has been further explained by two main theories. The first is a neurotraumatic mechanism in which the joints are insensitive to pain and proprioception and therefore undergo destruction from repetitive microtrauma. The second theory suggests that joint destruction is secondary to a neurally stimulated vascular reflex causing periarticular bone resorption and ligamentous insufficiency.[25]

Ligamentous injury is a significant contributor to neuropathic arthritis. Tendon injury occurs as well, at an increased incidence, particularly in the posterior tibialis tendon, promoting deformity.[26] Tendon and—more significantly—ligamentous injury, in addition to muscular atrophy, joint injuries, and microtrauma, cause a severe foot deformity with arch collapse leading to deformities such as the "rocker bottom" foot.[27] These effects on the peripheral nervous system of the diabetic patient gradually lead to alteration in the distribution of plantar pressure, progressive ulceration, and finally superimposed infection.

Multiple classification systems have characterized diabetic neuroarthropathy into several patterns. Schon classified Charcot joints based on the location and degree of involvement (Table 10-2). There are four patterns of involvement, each divided into three subtypes. The first pattern is Lisfranc, the second is the naviculocuneiform, the third is the perinavicular, and the fourth is the transversal tarsal pattern. The staging system allows for the prediction of disease progression and sites where future ulceration may occur as well as assessing risk for infection. Thus neuropathic arthropathy can occur at multiple locations including the Lisfranc joint, the hindfoot and ankle, the talonavicular joint, and the metatarsophalangeal joints.[28]

Neuroarthropathy can be identified in the acute or chronic stage. In the acute form, there is edema, erythema, tenderness, and associated warmth that may mimic cellulitis. As the disease progresses, joint fragmentation and/or destruction occur, as well as subluxation, bony proliferation, and sclerosis. The diabetic foot then exhibits a chronic deformity.

Radiography is often the first imaging modality used in the diagnosis of the neuroarthropathic foot (Table 10-3).

Imaging findings in the acute phase of the Charcot foot may be absent at the time of presentation.[29] If radiographic change is evident, it may be minimal soft tissue swelling and slight resorption of bone around the affected joint. There also may be an offset of the arch or slight subluxation. Findings on radiography in the chronic phase of the neuropathic foot are more prominent and include deformity, dislocation, destruction, and debris.[30] The arthropathy appears on radiographs as a mixed pattern of both bone destruction and production, as opposed to a predominant proliferative or erosive pattern as seen in the rest of the body.

Hypertrophic neuroarthropathy is manifested by sclerosis of the marginal bone, preservation of bone density, and large osteophytes. Osteophytes that form are ill defined and grow large in the late stage of the arthropathy. Periosteal new bone formation is also characteristic. This can extend up to the mid metatarsals and mimic infection.

Hypertrophic neuroarthropathy is characterized by the "D's" including *d*ebris, *d*estruction, *d*islocation, and no *d*emineralization (Table 10-3).

Atrophic neuroarthropathy shows joint erosion, destruction, and disorganization. The fragmentation of articular surfaces causes

TABLE 10-2. The Schon Classification System

Type	Pattern
I	**Lisfranc**
IA	Breakdown along medial side of Lisfranc joints, primarily the first, second, and third metatarsocuneiform joints; hallux valgus possible; no rocker bottom.
IB	Medial rocker from excessive abduction of foot. Minimal fullness under the fourth and fifth metatarsocuboid joint but no plantar lateral rocker bottom.
IC	Extension plantarly of medial rocker toward the lateral side of midfoot under the fourth and fifth metatarsocuboid joint. Central rocker often ulcerates, with risk for infection.
II	**Naviculocuneiform**
IIA	Instability of naviculocuneiform joint, lowers medial arch, leads to fullness under fourth and fifth metatarsocuboid joints.
IIB	Medial arch lowers further, but deformity is occurring more proximally in medial foot, therefore no medial rocker. Later rocker develops under the fourth and fifth metatarsocuboid joints.
IIC	Extension of lateral rocker to central and medial plantar region of foot. Prominence can ulcerate, with risk for infection.
III	**Perinavicular**
IIIA	Avascular necrosis of navicular or displaced fracture of navicular. Minimal lowering of medial arch, fullness under fourth and fifth metatarsocuboid joint from decrease in lateral arch height.
IIIB	Fragmentation of navicular, dorsal subluxation on the talus, shortening of medial column. Lateral rocker develops under fourth and fifth metatarsocuboid joint.
IIIC	Rocker bottom shifts more proximally under cuboid toward midfoot. Talus is plantar flexed and navicular is dorsally located on neck of talus. Dorsal translation of medial column may be complete, with cuneiform metatarsals dorsally on neck of talus. Ulceration and infection likely.
IV	**Transverse tarsal pattern**
IVA	Lateral subluxation of navicular on talus with abduction of foot and valgus of calcaneus. Dorsal translation of cuboid relative to calcaneus. Central-lateral fullness over calcaneocuboid joint.
IVB	Progressive adduction of foot on head of talus, decreased height of medial arch. Plantar central rocker under calcaneocuboid joint.
IVC	Destruction of calcaneocuboid articulation or dorsal translation of cuboid relative to calcaneus. Extreme abduction of navicular on talus and complete dislocation may occur. Central proximal rocker because posterior calcaneal tuberosity is non–weight bearing. All weight on distal end of calcaneus and cuboid. Medial rocker under navicular and central rocker under calcaneus. Osteomyelitis of distal calcaneus or talus is often seen because it is uncovered by navicular.

With permission from Schon LC, Easley ME, Weinfeld SB: Charcot neuroarthropathy of the foot and ankle, *Clin Orthop Relat Res* 349:116-131, 1998.

TABLE 10-3. Radiographic Findings in Diabetic Neuroarthropathy

Classification	Findings
Acute	Swelling
	Slight subluxation
	Slight bone resorption
Chronic	"The D's":
	*D*eformity
	*D*islocation
	*D*estruction
	*D*ebris
	No *D*emineralization
Hypertrophic	Sclerosis of juxtaarticular bone
	Generally normal bone density
	Large osteophytes
	Periosteal bone proliferation
Atrophic	Erosion, bone loss
	Destruction
	Dislocation
	Fracture

bony debris and intraarticular bodies to form, and parts of the tarsal bones may dissolve. Fractures of neighboring bones are often found in neuropathic arthropathy. They are usually spontaneous or occur with minimal trauma and tend to be horizontal fractures, as opposed to those caused by trauma, which are spiral or oblique. The most common finding on radiography is the Lisfranc fracture dislocation with destruction and fragmentation of the tarsometatarsal joints (Figure 10-3). Calcaneal fractures, talar collapse and angulation, and less commonly distal fibular fractures occur as well.

The patterns of radiographic changes in the neuropathic foot are found at the tarsometatarsal joints, the metatarsophalangeal and interphalangeal joints, and the anterior medial column of the foot, with talus, talonavicular, and naviculocuneiform destruction.[31] In the forefoot, osteolysis of the distal ends of the metatarsals combined with a broadening of bases of the proximal phalanges produce "pencil and cup" deformities. Flattening or fragmenting of the metatarsals may occur as well. Dorsiflexion of the toes accompanied by plantar subluxation of the metatarsal heads leads to ulceration under the heads of the metatarsals or at the dorsal aspects of the distal interphalangeal (DIP) joints. The midfoot and hindfoot experience continuous trauma and exhibit a rapidly destructive process with fragmentation, subluxation, and dislocation (Figure 10-4).

The Charcot process has been well characterized by the presence of bone destruction, joint destruction, and subluxation or dislocation and fragmentation, as well as periosteal reaction.[31] These changes are characteristically found in the midfoot of the diabetic patient. In a group of neuropathic patients with foot ulcers, there was a 16% prevalence of hypertrophic Charcot changes.[32]

A three-phase bone scan has been a useful tool in demonstrating neuropathic disease. Sensitivity of bone scintigraphy is high for neuropathic arthropathy at 85% to 100%; however, specificity is low at 0% to 54%.[33] The latter is a particular problem, as the usual clinical question is whether infection is present. Neuropathic arthropathy has been divided into five scintigraphic stages according to uptake (Table 10-4). Stage zero has swelling and pain clinically. Radiographs are normal while the bone scan shows increased radiouptake in all three phases. In stage one, radiographs show erosion and periarticular cysts, and the bone scan shows increased uptake in phases I and II with diffuse uptake in phase III. Stage two and three show joint subluxation on radiographs, and the bone scan shows increased uptake in all three phases. Stage four

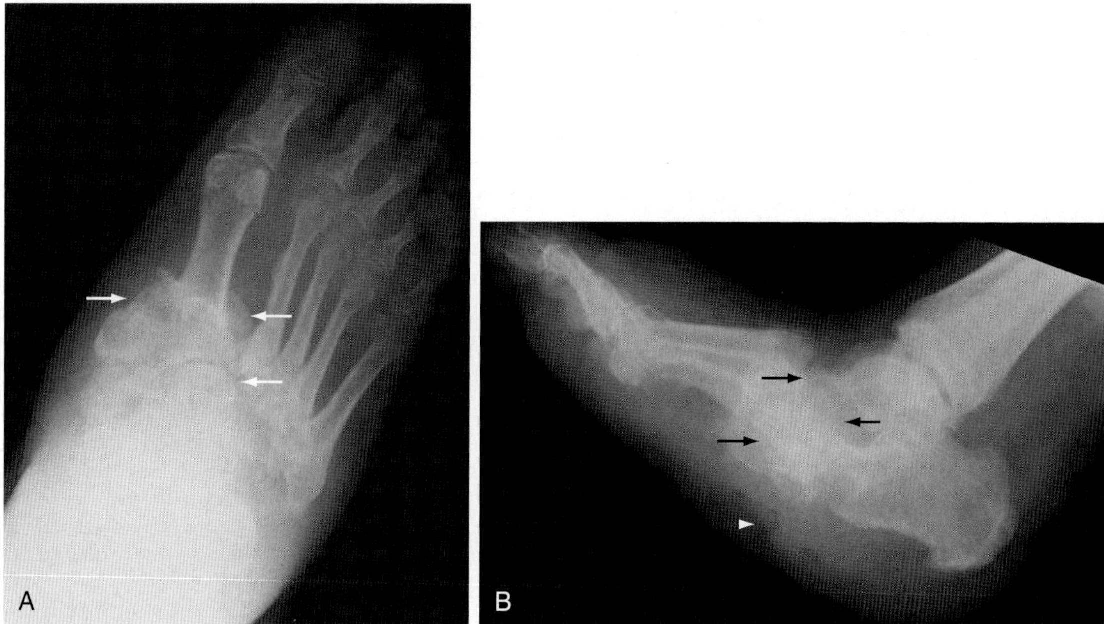

FIGURE 10-3. Neuropathic foot with Lisfranc joint deformity. **A,** An anteroposterior view of the foot shows diffuse soft tissue swelling. There is destruction, offset, and new bone formation at the Lisfranc (tarsometatarsal) joints *(white arrows)*. This is consistent with Schon stage 1B. **B,** Lateral view of the foot demonstrates severe deformity of the midfoot involving the cuboid, navicular, and cuneiform bones with collapse *(black arrows)*. An ulcer containing gas is seen in the plantar soft tissues *(arrowhead)*, in the usual location following midfoot collapse. This is Schon stage IIIB.

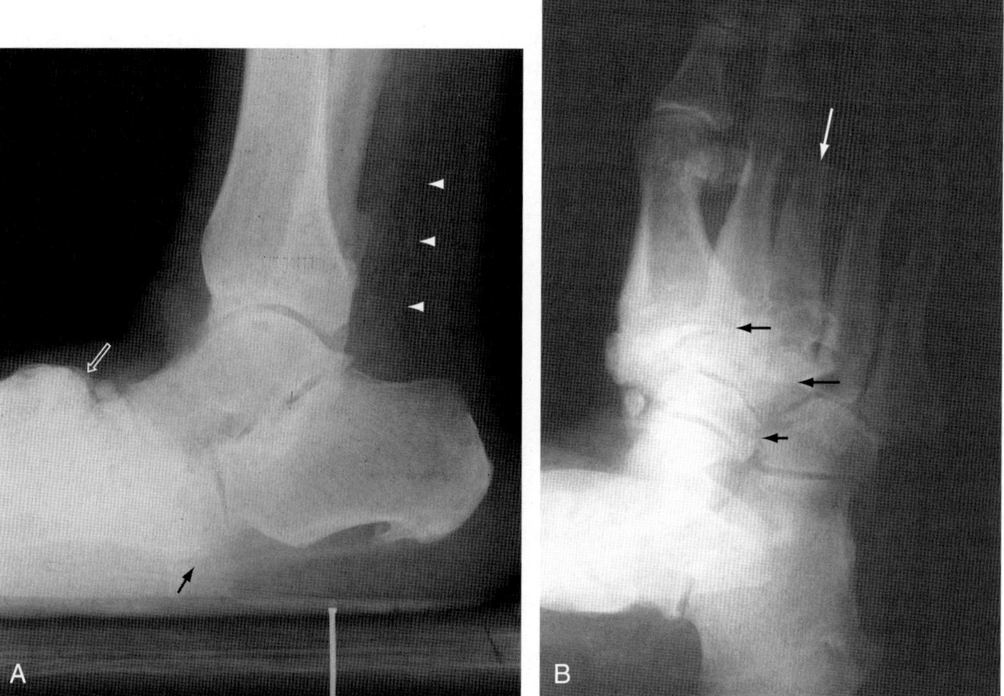

FIGURE 10-4. Neuropathic disease of the foot. **A,** A lateral radiograph shows collapse of the plantar arch and midfoot rocker bottom deformity *(arrow)*. There is dorsal subluxation of the metatarsals *(open arrow)*. Diffuse soft tissue swelling and vascular calcifications *(arrowheads)* are evident. This represents Schon pattern type IIB. **B,** There is fragmentation of the cuneiforms and bony sclerosis of the metatarsals, cuneiforms, and navicular *(black arrows)*. Prior amputations of the third digit through the distal metatarsal *(white arrow)*, as well as amputations of the fourth and fifth digit distal phalanges were related to prior infections.

TABLE 10-4. Staging of Neuropathic Joints by Scintigraphy

Stage	Radiographic Appearance	Scintigraphic Appearance
Stage 0	Normal	Increased uptake in phases I–III of bone scan
Stage 1	Erosion and cystic changes	Increased uptake phases I, II Diffuse uptake phase III
Stage 2	Subluxation	Increased uptake phases I, II, III
Stage 3	Dislocation	Increased uptake phases I, II, III
Stage 4 (rare, fusion, stable patient)	Bone fusion	Increased uptake phase III Normal phases I, II

From Aliabadi P, Nikpoor N, Alparslan L: Imaging of neuropathic arthropathy, *Semin Musculoskel Radiol* 7:217-225, 2003.

is a clinically stable patient with the rare fusion of joint spaces and increased uptake on the delayed phase; phases 1 and 2 are normal.[34] Therefore in the early stage of neuropathic joints, uptake is seen on the early and late phase of the bone scan due to bone turnover and increased vascularity at the articular surface. In the late stage of disease, uptake is seen on the delayed images only.[35]

The use of bone scanning may be limited related to vascular disease in the diabetic patient where decreased perfusion may affect distribution and hence uptake of the radiotracer. Also, the amount of hyperemia in the acute stage of neuropathy is variable and therefore scintigraphy may not be accurate. Combined bone and radiolabeled white blood cell scans may be used for the detection of infection in the neuropathic foot. This combination has been found to be more specific in diagnosing osteomyelitis of the Charcot foot than MRI or radiography.[36]

The combination of bone scanning and white blood cell scans may be helpful in diagnosing osteomyelitis of the Charcot foot and may be more helpful than MRI.

MRI is somewhat nonspecific in the diagnosis of neuropathic arthropathy. The acute hyperemic stage is characterized by soft tissue edema and osseous edema with no bone destruction (Box 10-1). Joint effusions are also common and show rim enhancement with contrast. Bone marrow edema and enhancement centered at the subchondral bone reflect the articular pattern of disease.[37] Periarticular edema also occurs, and enhancement may be seen. Subcutaneous fat is preserved in this setting, which helps to differentiate this edema from cellulitis. Chronic neuropathic arthropathy shows dislocation or subluxation of the joints with bony proliferation at the joint margins.[38] Fragmentation, debris, and deformity are prominent. Soft tissue edema is frequently seen in the diabetic foot, largely due to decreased venous drainage (Figures 10-5 to 10-7).

Acute neuropathic arthropathy may be superimposed on chronic changes. In this situation, acute episodes are usually intermittent and there is foot deformity in addition to soft tissue and bone marrow edema, suggesting acute injury or instability.

The management for the Charcot foot is immobilization and proper foot protection in a total contact cast at the time of acute presentation. Reconstructive surgery to realign the joints is typically reserved for patients with chronic ulcerations from deformity, unstable joints that are unbraceable, and recurrent infected ulcers associated with a bony prominence, although this has been unsuccessful in severe midfoot collapse.[39] The goals of surgery are to remove any bony prominences and perform an arthrodesis (fusion) of the affected joints. Percutaneous lengthening of the Achilles' tendon has also significantly reduced plantar pressures in diabetic feet.[40]

CALLUS

An exceedingly common complication in the foot of the diabetic patient is callus formation and progressive ulceration. A combination of abnormal biomechanics and friction against footwear lead

BOX 10-1. MRI Features of Diabetic Feet

ACUTE HYPEREMIA
Soft tissue and bone marrow edema
Joint effusions
May have contrast enhancement of periarticular bone
Adjacent fat is preserved (unlike infection)

CHRONIC NEUROPATHIC FOOT
Dislocation or subluxation
Debris
Deformity
Soft tissue edema

CALLUS
Subcutaneous mass-like density with low signal on T1-weighted and T2-weighted images

ULCERATION
Skin defect
Granulation tissue at the ulcer base shows low T1 and high T2 signal and contrast enhancement

CELLULITIS
Thickened skin
Reticulated subcutaneous tissue
Edema signal in the subcutaneous tissues (low signal on T1-weighted, bright signal on T2-weighted) similar to nonspecific edema but with poorly defined septal enhancement in patients with cellulitis
Gas (low signal foci on all sequences) in an area of absent enhancement raises the possibility of infection in devitalized tissue

SINUS TRACTS
May be difficult to see
May emanate from an ulcer
Postcontrast fat-suppressed images allow the hyperemic bright walls of the tracts to be delineated

ABSCESS
Focal fluid collection (intermediate to low signal on T1-weighted and high signal on T2-weighted images with thick low signal wall)
Wall enhancement after contrast
Adjacent soft tissues are edematous

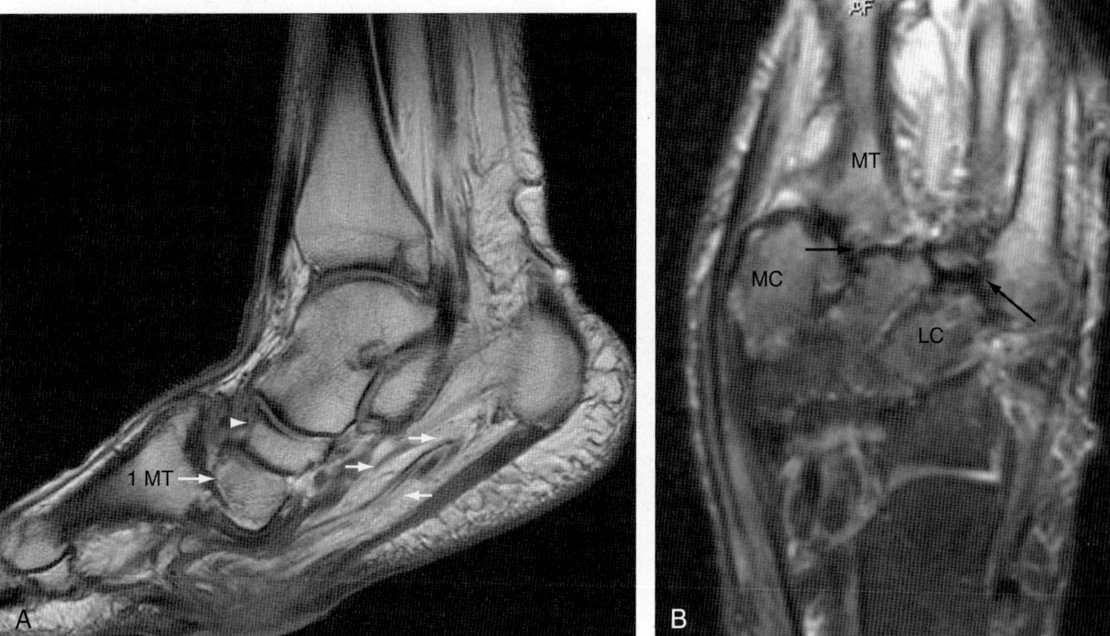

FIGURE 10-5. MR images of chronic neuropathy. **A,** Sagittal T1-weighted image of the midfoot shows plantar subluxation of the medial cuneiform *(white arrow)* with relation to the first metatarsal (1MT) with fracture and destruction of the cuneiform and navicular *(white arrowhead)* (Schon classification 3). Note the fatty replacement of the intrinsic muscles *(small arrows)*. An unusually distal rocker bottom deformity is present with ulceration of the medial plantar soft tissues. **B,** Axial STIR image of the forefoot demonstrates deformity and subluxation of the Lisfranc joint *(black arrows)*. Note the relative absence of marrow edema and joint effusions in this chronic neuroarthropathy. *LC,* Lateral cuneiform; *MC,* medial cuneiform; *MT,* second metatarsal.

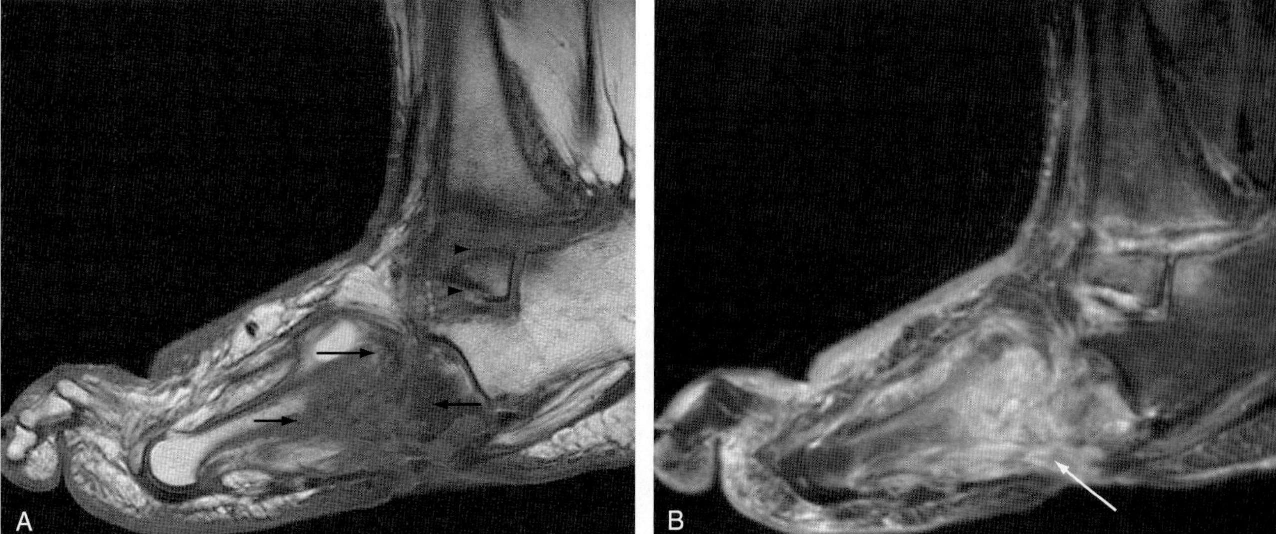

FIGURE 10-6. Charcot arthropathy. **A,** Sagittal T1-weighted MR image shows a diffuse Charcot arthropathy involving the hindfoot, midfoot, and Lisfranc joint with marrow edema replacing the normally bright marrow fat. There is dissolution and fracture of the talus, leaving a small remnant *(arrowheads)*. Rocker bottom deformity is noted with an adjacent ulcer *(black arrows)*. This represents Schon type IV. Although the low marrow signal of the cuboid is similar to that of the rest of the tarsus, because it is located adjacent to an ulcer, it is consistent with chronic osteomyelitis. **B,** Sagittal T2-weighted MR image demonstrates high signal abnormality in the metatarsal and cuboid compatible with osteomyelitis. Note the relative lack of edema of the residual (noninfected) talus fragment. The *white arrow* indicates the area of ulceration and edema.

to the formation of skin callus. The basis for this change in biomechanics is the deformity of the diabetic foot, which is multifactorial and related to ligamentous disorders, as well as tendinopathy, muscular atrophy, and sensory neuropathy. The diabetic foot shows dry skin with cracking due to a lack of perspiration from autonomic dysfunction of the peripheral nerves. This lack of moisture contributes to the formation of a skin callus that may be complicated by superimposing initially superficial polymicrobial infection.

Skin callus in the diabetic foot occurs at pressure points. Sites most commonly involved are positioned under the metatarsal heads, usually the first or second, or laterally at the fifth metatarsal

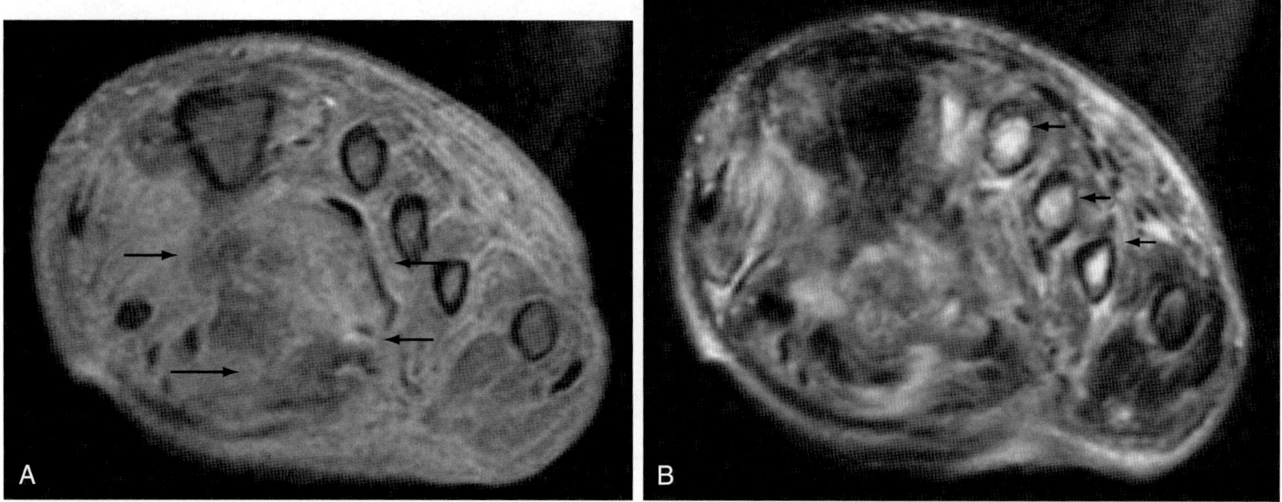

FIGURE 10-7. Bone marrow edema in the acute neuropathic foot. **A,** T1-weighted fat-suppressed coronal MR image after intravenous gadolinium. Note the relative lack of enhancement of the plantar soft tissue consistent with ischemia and devitalization *(arrows)*. **B,** Coronal T2-weighted image shows extensive marrow edema in the second through fourth metatarsals *(arrows)*. Marrow edema and periosteal reaction can extend significantly up the metatarsal shaft from neuropathic disease. This is common in acute neuroarthropathy and does not necessarily represent osteomyelitis.

head. In neuropathic feet with toe deformity, there are prominent calluses under the first and second metatarsal bones, at the fifth metatarsophalangeal (MTP) joint, and on the plantar surface of the posterior calcaneus.[41] In addition, callus often forms dorsally next to the proximal interphalangeal joint or the distal interphalangeal joint. In the case of hallux valgus, frequently found in neuropathic foot patients, callus is located medial to the first metatarsal. In the neuropathic case where midfoot deformity and a rocker-bottom foot are common, callus formation is most prominent under the cuboid.

Another common finding of the diabetic foot, the claw toe deformity, results in skin callus under the forefoot and over the dorsal toes. Without the modifying forces of the intrinsic foot muscles to flex the MTP joints and extend interphalangeal joints, the opposite occurs. There is extension of the MTP joints and flexion of the intraphalangeal joints. This clawing results in sites of increased pressure. Callus, followed by ulceration, occurs under the tip of the toe where it hits the floor or over the dorsum of the proximal intraphalangeal joint where it strikes the shoe.

MRI of skin callus shows low signal intensity on T1-weighted and T2-weighted images. The callus is a prominent focal area within the subcutaneous fat, often almost mass-like. Following use of contrast, the callus may enhance often prominently, mimicking a soft tissue infection. Careful attention to location of focal enhancement and lack of additional soft tissue change excludes the development of an ulcer (Figure 10-8).

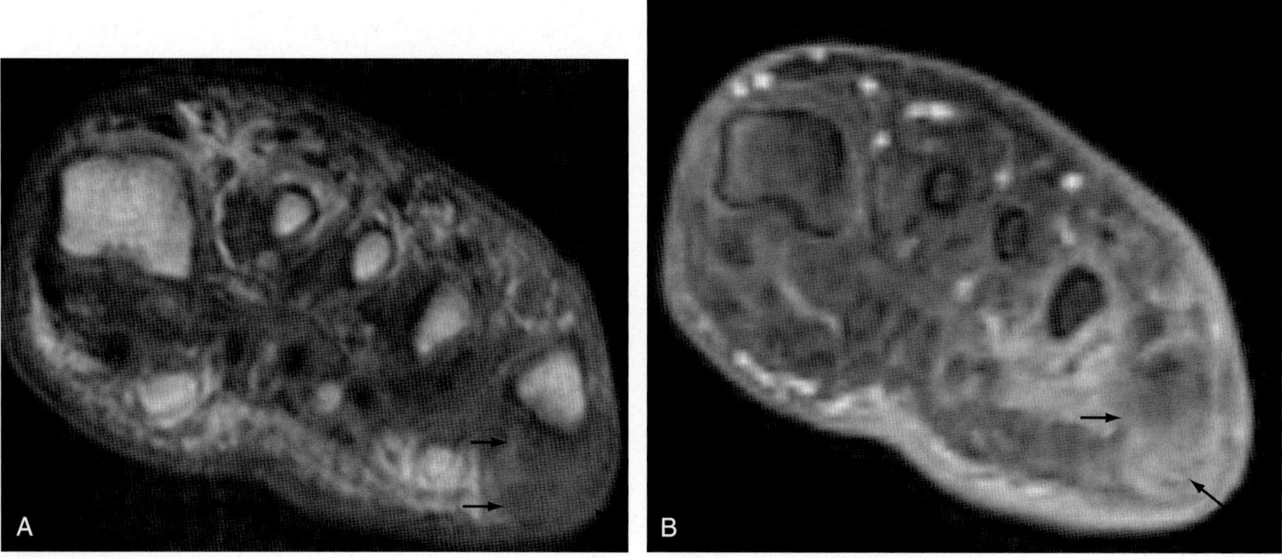

FIGURE 10-8. Skin callus. **A,** Coronal T1-weighted MR image shows a mass-like area of low signal tissue in the plantar soft tissue *(arrows)* adjacent to the fifth metatarsal head. **B,** Coronal T1-weighted (fat saturated) image post intravenous gadolinium shows significant enhancement of the callus *(arrows)*. Note the lack of enhancement of the rest of the foot, consistent with devitalization. The plantar skin and subcutaneous fat is enhancing from superimposed cellulitis.

Ulceration

Weight-bearing shifts, dry skin, neuropathy, and friction with poorly fitted shoes lead to a gradual breakdown of the callus. The product of this breakdown is ulceration. Minor trauma to the diabetic foot can lead to ulcer formation, because trauma can go unrecognized with the sensory and motor neuropathy of the diabetic foot. The trauma may be as insignificant as toenail cutting or more substantial such as stepping on an object. In addition, peripheral arterial disease and immune suppression increase the patient's susceptibility to infection.

On MRI, ulceration is shown as a skin defect overlying subcutaneous tissues. Flatter ulcers may be easily missed unless care is taken to assess the integrity of the skin at common sites of ulceration. Larger ulcers often have a significant ischemic component and are more frequently seen dorsally above the toes and in the shin. Granulation tissue lining the ulcer should be low signal intensity on T1-weighted images and high signal intensity on T2-weighted images. Following contrast administration, intense enhancement of the ulcer base is shown,[42] and tract-like enhancement of the rim is seen.

Suppression of the immune system in diabetes mellitus facilitates inoculation of organisms through the ulcer. Infection of diabetic ulcers tends to be polymicrobial and require broad-spectrum antibiotics for treatment and immediate wound care including sharp debridement of devitalized tissue and callus with sterile dressings.[43] In the case of inadequate treatment, progression of ulcers to cellulitis, sinus tracts, abscess formation, and osseous infection often results. Deep ulcerations are particularly significant, as they lead to sinus tracts and have a strong association with osteomyelitis and, therefore if marrow signal abnormality is present contiguous with a skin defect on imaging, osteomyelitis should be suspected (Figure 10-9).

SOFT TISSUE INFECTION

Soft tissue infections such as cellulitis, sinus tracts, abscesses, and foreign body granulomas most often arise from inadequately treated and infected ulcers. Bacteria spread first to the subcutaneous fat. Clinical manifestations of cellulitis are an edematous, erythematous, warm lower extremity. Because diffuse soft tissue edema is a common presentation in imaging the diabetic patient and is not necessarily indicative of inflammation or infection, it is important to differentiate systemic causes of edema from cellulitis. In diabetes mellitus, peripheral vascular disease results in chronic ischemia and loss of autonomic regulation of the microvasculature. As a result, venous drainage is significantly decreased, causing an increase of fluid in the soft tissue.[44] Fluid also accumulates in muscular tissue as a result of muscle atrophy and ischemia. On MRI, T1-weighted images show thickened skin and reticulated subcutaneous fat, and T2-weighted images may show increased signal in both areas. Administration of contrast is somewhat useful in distinguishing between "benign" edema and cellulitis. Cellulitis will show ill-defined septal enhancement, as opposed to edema from diabetic vascular insufficiency, which does not show significant enhancement.

Gas may be seen in devitalized tissue, although rarely. Because devitalized tissue does not enhance, the presence of gas in an area of nonenhancement may be a sign of underlying infection.[17] On MRI, gas can be seen as several small, often subtle, foci of signal void that bloom on gradient echo images (Figure 10-10).

> Gas is seen on MRI as small, round low signal areas that become more prominent on gradient echo images.

Sinus Tracts

Sinus tracts are commonly associated with osteomyelitis and adjacent skin ulceration.[42] Sinus tracts also may show reverse flow and form the route through which pus attempts to drain out to the skin. Then tracts are demonstrated on MR images as discrete thin lines of fluid signal extending through the tissue. The tracts may be difficult to see directly as they blend with adjacent tissue edema. In addition, some of the sinus tracts are collapsed and not actively draining fluid, and therefore fluid signal will not always be evident within them. Fat-suppressed T1-weighted images after contrast administration are helpful in viewing the tracts due to the linear enhancement of the hyperemic margins. The tracts are seen as tram track linear enhancement extending from the ulcer.

> Tram track linear enhancement may indicate a tract or fistula that is otherwise difficult to see.

Abscesses

Soft tissue abscesses are frequently seen in the diabetic population and have been estimated to be present in 10% to 50% of cases of osteomyelitis.[45] More likely the number is lower, as a recent study demonstrated that abscesses occur in 18% of patients suspected to have osteomyelitis. The majority of abscesses are located in the forefoot; however, they occur with nearly 50% frequency in the midfoot and hindfoot.[46] Abscesses are typically more common in musculoskeletal infections of the child than the adult; however, diabetic patients are a notable exception to this rule.

MRI is useful in evaluating the presence and location of abscess formation. It allows for excellent soft tissue contrast and provides the capability to visualize infection in several planes. MR images demonstrate low to intermediate signal on T1-weighted images and focal fluid signal on T2-weighted images with thick rim enhancement following intravenous contrast. Often there is adjacent soft tissue edema and inflammation. The abscesses can be located intermuscularly or intramuscularly and vary in size from large to fairly small. Other abscesses show multiloculation and association with sinus tracts. Because most abscesses in diabetic patients are fairly small, it may be difficult to differentiate microabscesses from undulating sinus tracts imaged transversely (Figure 10-11).

Foreign Bodies

It is not uncommon for a foreign body to be found residing in the soft tissue of the diabetic foot. An object may be imbedded deep within the pedal tissue, often associated with a sensory neuropathy that creates an inability to recognize injury. No ulceration or adjacent abscesses need be present. Oftentimes, the patient is unable to recall any such trauma to the foot, and therefore discovery of the foreign body may be unsuspected clinically. MRI shows signs of inflammatory reaction in the soft tissue and granuloma formation. T1-weighted images usually show a low signal, and T2-weighted images show a high signal from the foreign body. Contrast administration typically shows enhancement. A T1-weighted gadolinium-enhanced fat-suppressed image can demonstrate surrounding soft tissue enhancement, which is consistent with a granulomatous response. There may be no change seen on MRI, and radiographs, CT, or ultrasound may be a necessary supplement to identify the object. The foreign body is often subtle and difficult to detect unless carefully searched for on gradient echo images. They are usually seen plantarly, often under the metatarsal heads, less commonly at the tips of the toes (Figure 10-12).

> Ultrasound or MRI may be useful for defining nonradiopaque foreign bodies.

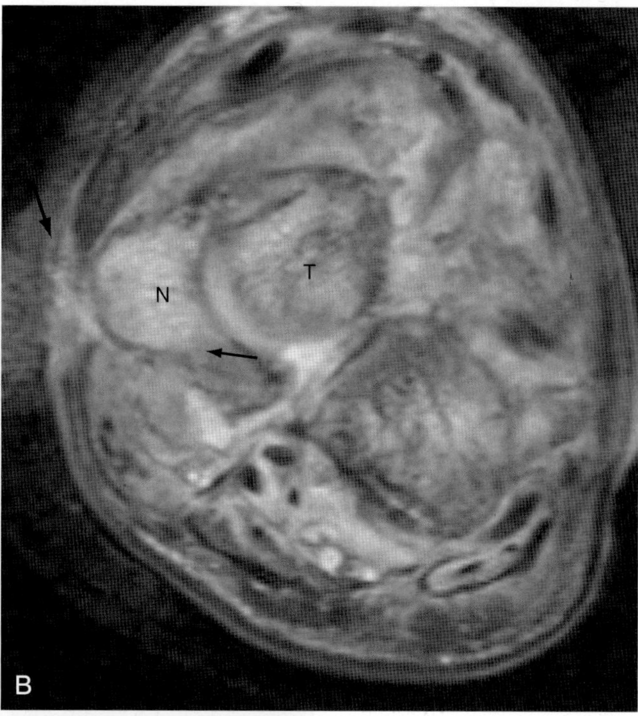

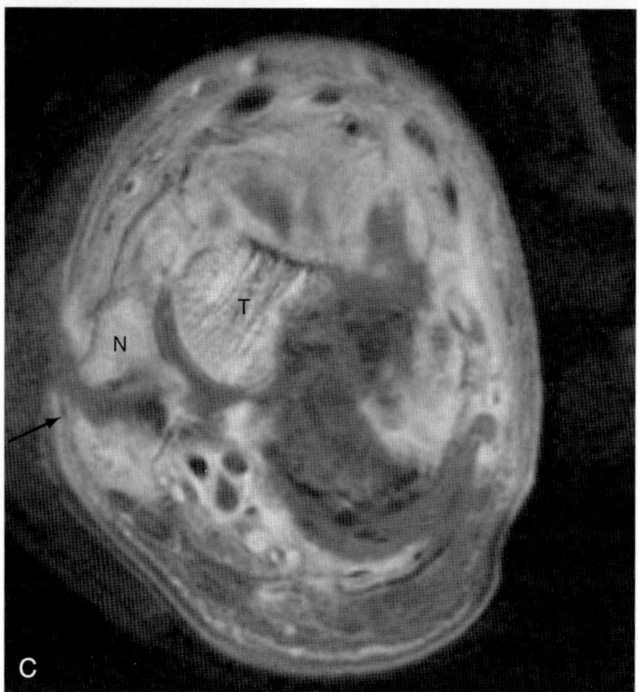

FIGURE 10-9. Ulcer with sinus tract and navicular osteomyelitis. **A,** Coronal T1-weighted MR image pre-contrast of the midfoot shows a focal soft tissue ulcer at medial aspect of foot with a tract extending to the navicular *(arrow).* There is low signal at the base of the ulcer and decreased T1 signal in the adjacent bone marrow. **B,** Coronal T1-weighted post-contrast fat-saturated image shows enhancement (high signal) of granulation tissue at the base of the ulcer. Also seen is abnormal high signal in the adjacent navicular bone compatible with osteomyelitis. (*Large arrow,* Ulcer; *small arrow,* base of ulcer with granulation tissue). **C,** A more posterior coronal T1-weighted gadolinium-enhanced MR image shows tram track linear enhancement (sinus tract) extending from the ulcer base *(arrow). N,* Navicular bone; *T,* talus.

Fascial Compartments

The foot is composed of three fascial compartments. The first compartment, the medial, extends to the base of the first metatarsal. The second is the lateral compartment, which extends to the base of the fifth metatarsal. The central compartment extends proximally into the midfoot and hindfoot and becomes contiguous with the calf muscles.[41] These divisions are partial barriers to infection, and infection spreads proximally instead of between compartments. It must be recognized that the fascial barriers of the foot are not perfect and therefore spread may occur between neighboring compartments.[47]

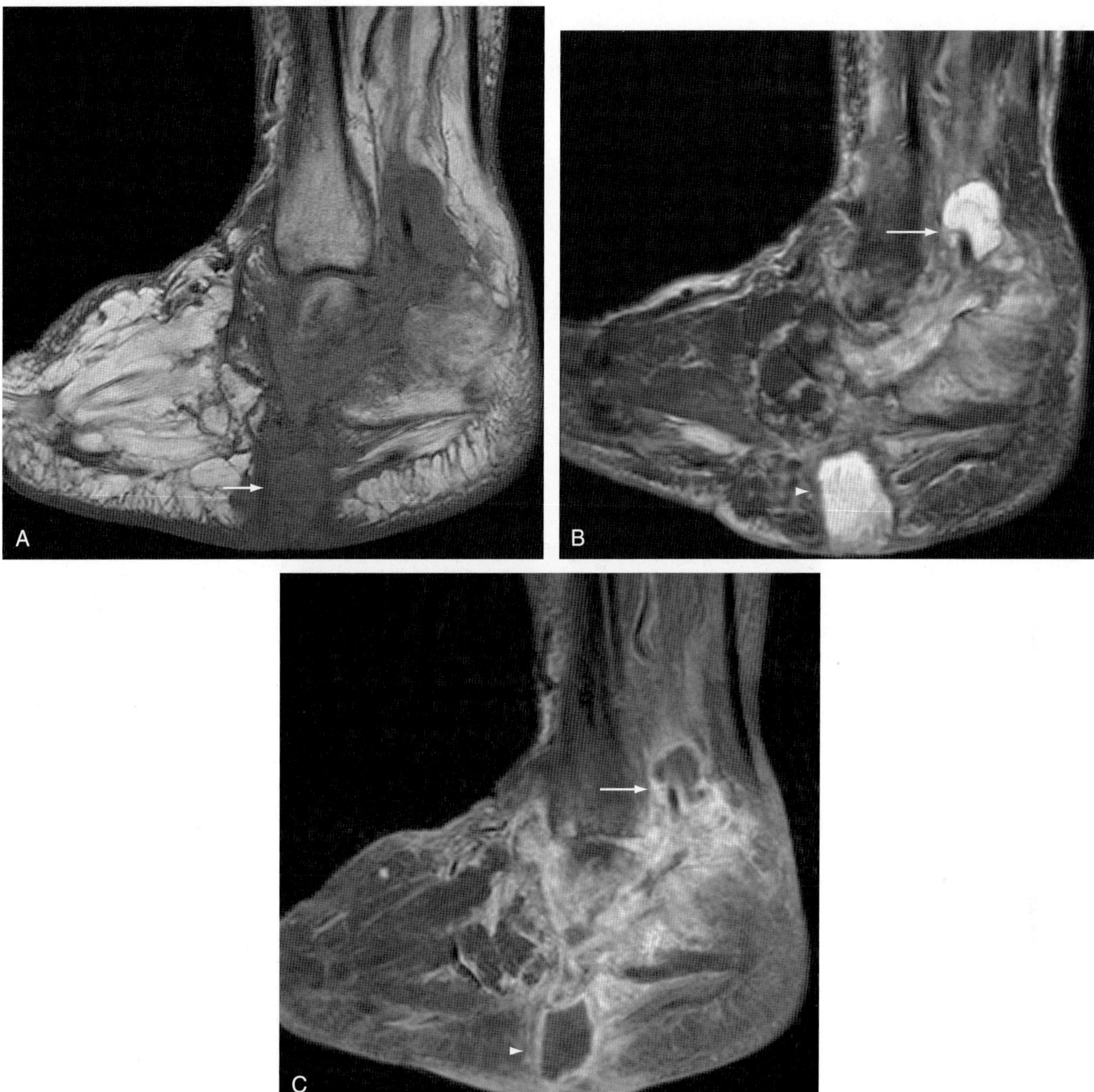

FIGURE 10-10. Soft tissue abscess and tenosynovitis. **A,** Sagittal T1-weighted MR image demonstrates severe neuropathic changes with rocker bottom deformity. There is destruction of the talus, calcaneus, and cuboid. This represents Schon stage IVC. There is low signal intensity in the plantar tissues of the midfoot *(arrow)* due to an ulcer. **B,** Sagittal T2-weighted MR image shows a focal fluid signal intensity collection deep to the ulcer in the plantar soft tissue *(arrowhead)* and at the level of the ankle joint. There is also a large amount of high signal fluid in the flexor hallucis tendon sheath *(arrow)*. **C,** Sagittal fat-suppressed T1-weighted image post-intravenous gadolinium demonstrates a rim-enhancing fluid collection *(arrowhead)* representing an abscess extending from the ulcer. Infectious tenosynovitis is also present with rim enhancement of the fluid in the distended flexor hallucis tendon sheath *(arrow)*.

OSTEOMYELITIS

Osteomyelitis is a challenging disease to diagnose, and imaging studies play a central role in the evaluation of the patient suspected of having bone marrow infection. Osteomyelitis may arise from hematogenous spread of bacteria, contiguous spread from soft tissue infection, or direct inoculation following trauma or surgery. Although hematogenous spread is the most common cause of osteomyelitis in most parts of the body, contiguous spread and direct inoculation are more common in the foot and ankle. Furthermore, the diabetic foot is commonly ulcerated, a predisposing risk factor for subsequent infection of soft tissue and adjacent bone.

Clinical manifestations of osteomyelitis vary with duration and location, but typical presentation includes bone pain, tenderness, lower extremity warmth, and swelling. Osteomyelitis is more difficult to clinically diagnose in the diabetic patient with peripheral vascular disease, ulcers, or superficial infection, and infection is probably somewhat more chronic. The most accurate way of

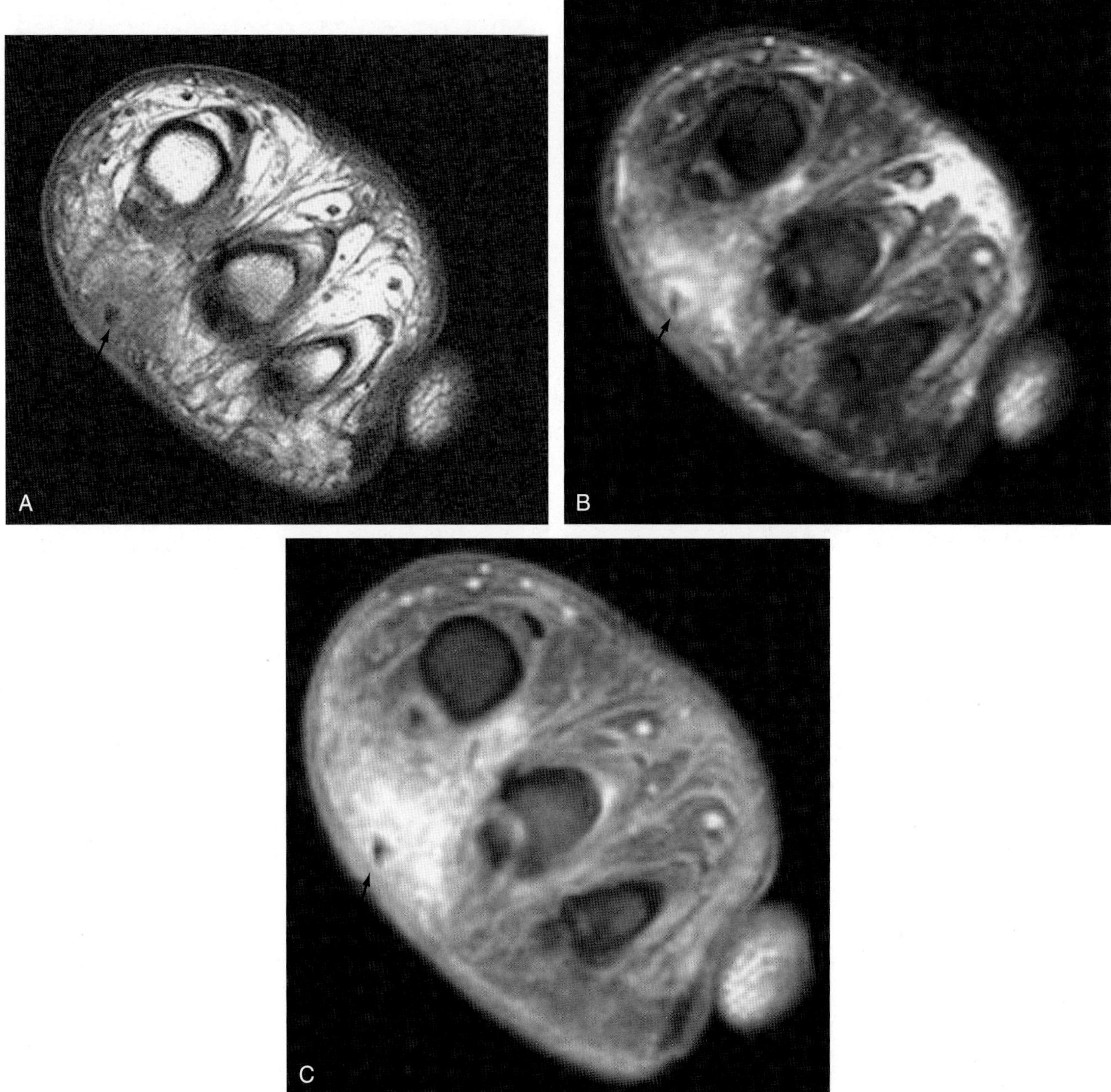

FIGURE 10-11. Foreign body. **A,** A coronal T1-weighted MR image shows a small, well-defined area of low signal intensity in the plantar soft tissues at the base of the first toe proximal phalanx, consistent with a foreign body *(arrow)*. **B,** Coronal T2-weighted MR image shows high signal soft tissue edema and granuloma formation surrounding the low signal body *(arrow)*. **C,** Coronal T1-weighted MR image post-intravenous gadolinium administration demonstrates focal soft tissue and non–mass-like enhancement surrounding the foreign body *(arrow)*. This represents granulomatous inflammatory change, not an abscess.

determining the presence of osteomyelitis is to find the ulcer and sinus tract and closely assess the adjacent bones, either clinically or more accurately by imaging.[21]

If osteomyelitis is suspected, the initial imaging study should be radiography. In the early stage of infection, the radiograph is often normal or shows soft tissue swelling only. Moreover, radiographic changes can be delayed up to 2 weeks and are relatively insensitive[48,49] for diagnosis because a 30% to 50% loss of bone density must occur before it is seen on a radiograph. Therefore the primary role of radiography is in advanced disease and for diagnosis of concomitant neuroarthropathy.

When visible on radiographs, osteomyelitis shows evidence of local rarefaction of bone, periosteal reaction, decreased bone density, and gradual bone destruction (Box 10-2). Periostitis is rare in the bones of the foot except for the metatarsals. However, periostitis is also frequently seen in neuropathic feet.

CT scan is infrequently used in patients with suspected osteomyelitis, but it can accurately display cortical bony detail and detect

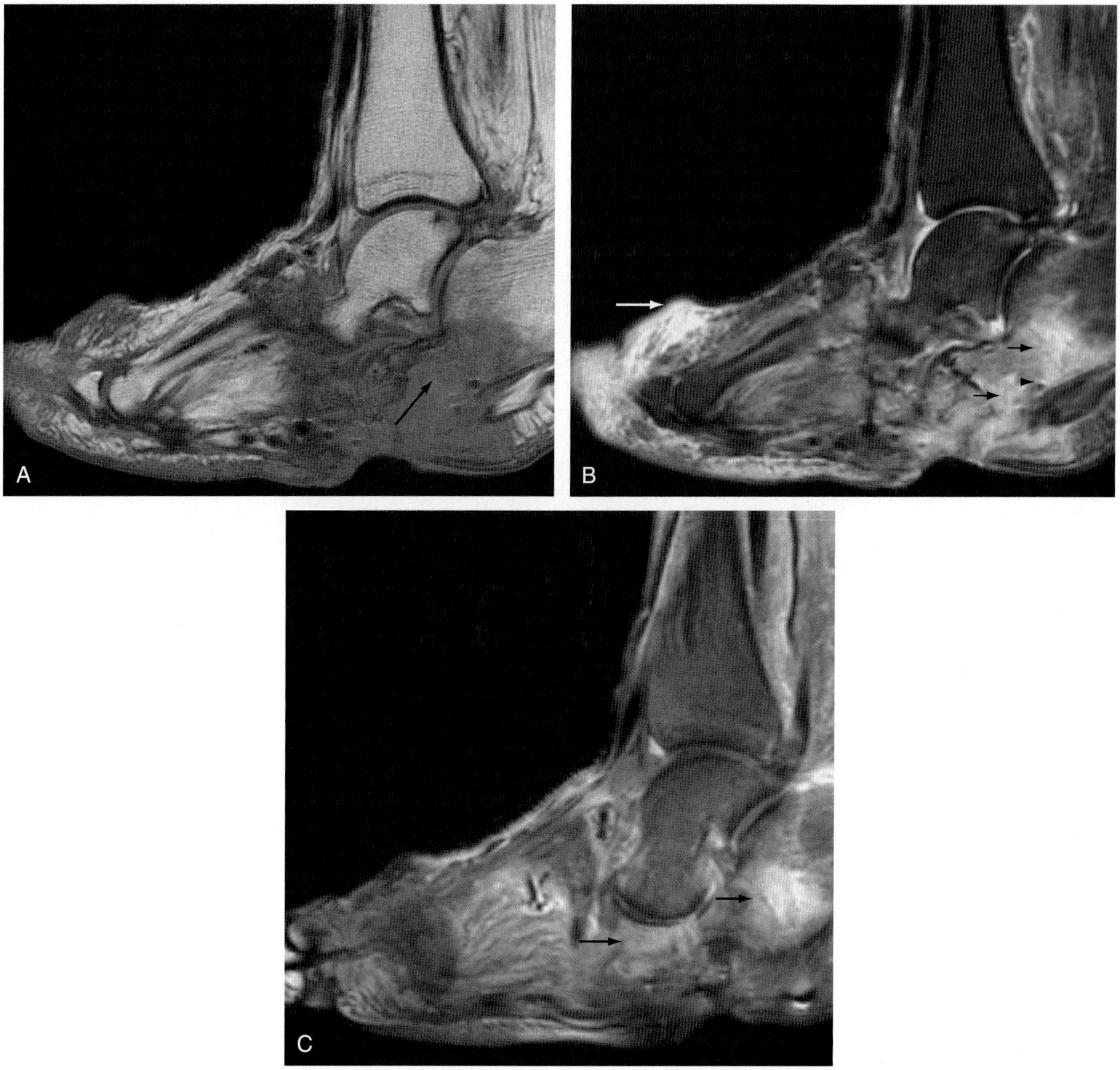

FIGURE 10-12. Osteomyelitis of the calcaneus with associated ulcer and sinus tract. **A,** Sagittal T1-weighted MR image shows decreased signal in the anterior portion of the calcaneus *(arrow)* associated with an adjacent ulcer and tract. **B,** Sagittal T2-weighted fat saturated MR image shows significant bone marrow edema in the calcaneus *(black arrows)*. The tissue around the sinus tract enhances, making the low signal tract *(arrowhead)* visible. High signal of the soft tissues of the toe is consistent with cellulitis *(white arrow)*. **C,** A sagittal T1-weighted post-gadolinium image again shows enhancement of the cuboid and calcaneus, as well as edematous tissue *(black arrows)*. Nonenhancing debris can be seen as well. Note also the chronic neuropathic findings including collapse of the medial column with a plantar flexed talus and fragmented cuneiforms and cuboid bones. Also seen is muscle atrophy and mild dorsal foot edema.

cortical destruction, intraosseous gas, periosteal reaction, and soft tissue extension.[50] In the era of multislice CT, detailed anatomic information required for surgical planning may best be obtained by CT.

> CT is useful in confirming a sequestrum, which is evidence of chronic active osteomyelitis.

Scintigraphy is commonly used to assess pedal infections. Three-phase bone scan is very sensitive in the detection of osteomyelitis; however, it proves somewhat limited localization of the anatomic site of infection, causing potential difficulty in surgical planning. 99m-Tc bound to phosphorus accumulates in areas of increased osteoblast activity or reactive new bone formation. Regional radiotracer uptake is seen on the early phase and localized uptake is seen on the later phase in areas of infection. If no uptake is seen on the bone scan, osteomyelitis can be excluded with confidence except in the diabetic patient due to the likely presence of peripheral vascular disease, a possible barrier for the tracer. The bone scan has a low specificity due to other disease entities that may result in hyperemia and increased bone turnover, including neuropathic osteoarthropathy, fractures, and osteoarthritis, which can cause a false-positive result.

BOX 10-2. Imaging Features of Osteomyelitis

RADIOGRAPHS
Delay of 7-10 days in seeing abnormalities
Periosteal reaction
Bone erosion or rarefaction

CT
Can detect cortical destruction, intraosseous gas, periosteal reaction, soft tissue extension, sequestra

THREE-PHASE BONE SCAN
Very sensitive but not specific
May be falsely normal if vascular disease limits tracer distribution
Limited for localization

INDIUM-111 LABELED LEUKOCYTE SCINTIGRAPHY
88% sensitivity
85% specificity for infection
Increased specificity when combined with sulfur colloid scan

MRI
> 90% sensitivity and specificity
Bone marrow edema (low signal on T1-weighted images and high signal on T2-weighted and STIR images) and marrow enhancement after intravenous gadolinium
T1-weighted images and contrast image findings are more specific

Indium-111 labeled leukocyte scintigraphy has been used to detect infection in the diabetic foot. Radiolabeled leukocytes have a high specificity in the imaging of osteomyelitis.[51] The scan reflects the distribution of white blood cells in the body, and activity outside the normal distribution is evidence for infection. A review of the results of various studies determined overall sensitivity and specificity to be 88% and 85%, respectively.[52] However, labeled leukocyte accumulation in active marrow of the neuroarthropathic foot has led to many false-positive results for the diagnosis of osteomyelitis. Theories for leukocyte uptake in the noninfected diabetic foot include inflammation, thus the migration of polymorphonuclear cells to involved areas, multiple fractures in the Charcot foot stimulating a reparative process, and increased cytokine activity in arthropathy leading to stimulated marrow. Abnormal marrow activity in the Charcot foot decreases the specificity of the indium scan. Therefore combined indium-111 labeled leukocyte scan and 99mTc-sulfur colloid marrow scan are proposed as a highly accurate method to differentiate between active marrow and infection of the neuropathic foot.[53]

> The combination of the Indium-111 scan and the 99mTc labeled sulfur colloid marrow scan increases the specificity for differentiating neuropathic arthropathy from infection.

The marrow scan uses 99mTc labeled sulfur colloid as the radioactive tracer, which is normally only taken up by the bone marrow, spleen, and liver. Comparison of the combined scintigraphy will allow congruent images on marrow and leukocyte scans to exclude an infectious process, whereas incongruent results will favor the diagnosis osteomyelitis. This is superior to both the bone scan and combined leukocyte/bone scintigraphy.

MRI for osteomyelitis has increased in use over the past decade and has recently been the focus of many studies. Sensitivity and specificity have been documented at greater than 90%.[54] Disease processes such as neuropathic osteoarthropathy, inflammatory disease, fracture, infarction, and prior surgery may lower the specificity of MRI. On MRI, osteomyelitis shows a low marrow signal on T1-weighted images and a high marrow signal on T2-weighted images and inversion recovery images. Following contrast administration, marrow enhancement is usually present in osteomyelitis.

> Osteomyelitis shows low marrow signal on T1-weighted images and high marrow signal on T2-weighted and inversion recovery images. Following contrast administration, marrow enhancement is usually present in osteomyelitis.

Osseous involvement is better determined on T1-weighted images and postcontrast sequences due to higher specificity.[42,54] T2-weighted sequences and STIR sequences are more sensitive but can lead to an overdiagnosis of osteomyelitis.

> The best way to identify osteomyelitis is to follow an ulcer and sinus track down to the bone; if there is adjacent abnormal marrow signal on T1-weighted images, then osteomyelitis should be suspected.

More than 90% of cases of osteomyelitis of the foot and ankle are a result of contiguous spread.[55] The pattern and distribution of the marrow signal are important when considering osteomyelitis in order to differentiate it from other entities. Identification of a fracture line or adjacent arthritis may help to exclude osteomyelitis (Figure 10-13).

Bone infection has been frequently located in the first and fifth metatarsal bones and at the distal phalanx of the first toe, in close association with the common location of diabetic ulcerations. With hindfoot involvement, the calcaneus and lateral malleolus are most commonly involved, and the midfoot is less frequently involved, occurring in association with a rocker bottom deformity, especially with involvement of the cuboid.[54,56] With the use of MRI, the extent of infection can be anatomically delineated in accurate detail, leading to improved surgical planning for the patient.

SEPTIC ARTHRITIS

Septic arthritis is both a sequela of the systemic disease and a complication of the diabetic foot. In the latter, it is typically the result of contiguous spread from adjacent soft tissue infection. Diabetics have also shown an increased incidence of septic arthritis in larger joints such as the knee and hip. A delay in the diagnosis of septic arthritis may lead to osteomyelitis, osteonecrosis, and consequent severe secondary osteoarthritis.[57] Therefore it is important clinically to inspect all joints of the diabetic foot for signs of erythema, swelling, warmth, and tenderness in order to exclude infection. Adequate drainage of the infected synovial fluid, appropriate antibiotics, repetitive joint aspiration, and immobilization of the joint are essential in treatment. If necessary, early surgical intervention can achieve successful outcomes in most cases.[60]

Protective mechanisms exist at the level of the joint space. Normal synovial cells have phagocytic capabilities to engulf microorganisms, and the synovial fluid contains bactericidal activity.

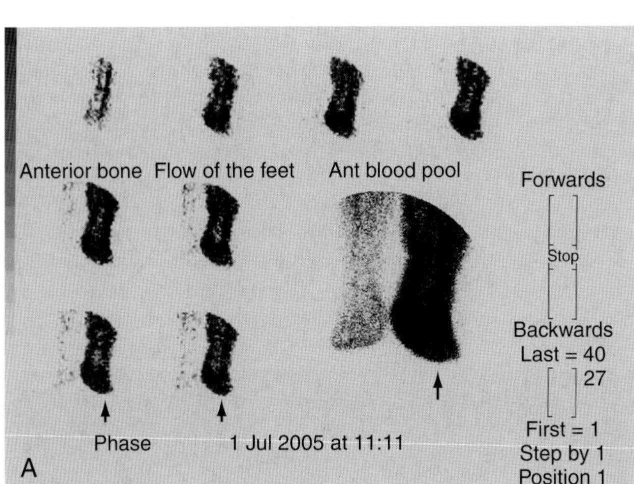

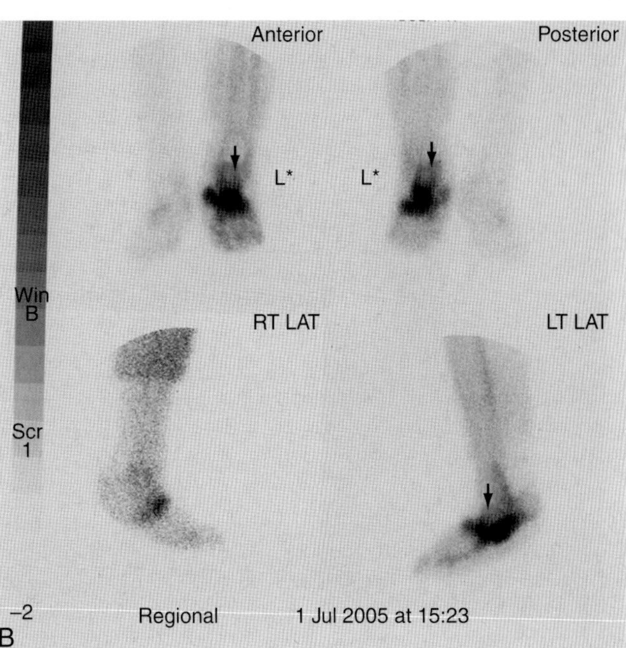

FIGURE 10-13. Bone scan findings in osteomyelitis with soft tissue infection and inflammation. **A,** Blood pool phase of both feet and ankles. There is markedly increased blood flow to the left foot relative to the right side and significantly increased soft tissue activity in the left leg, ankle, and foot *(arrows)*. **B,** Delayed image shows a focal area of increased radiotracer activity in the left midfoot and hindfoot *(arrows)*. This corresponds to the site of the patient's known ulcer and osseous structures deep to the ulcer.

Diabetic patients have impaired defense mechanisms (decreased phagocytosis and chemotaxis) as a result of the immunopathy related to metabolic dysfunction. This increases the susceptibility of the diabetic foot to infection by direct inoculation, spread from adjacent periarticular tissue, or even hematogenous infections.

Septic arthritis commonly occurs in the diabetic foot because pedal ulcers are usually located near joints.[54] The joints commonly involved in this infectious process are the interphalangeal and MTP joints, particularly the first and fifth.[54,58] Hindfoot infection involves the subtalar joint, whereas septic arthritis of the midfoot is rare but occasionally may be seen in the neuropathic foot. Not uncommonly, malleolar ulcers spread to the ankle joint.

Radiographic findings of septic arthritis are difficult to visualize in early stages of infection (Box 10-3). Subtle changes such as soft tissue swelling and joint effusions should be present. Advanced stages of disease typically show larger joint effusions with cartilage loss, bone erosions, and destruction. Juxtaarticular osteomyelitis may also be seen on radiographs when late in the process (Figure 10-14).

> The early diagnosis of septic arthritis depends on joint aspiration.

MRI has been useful in the diagnosis of septic arthritis. One third of patients with advanced pedal infection show evidence of joint infection on MRI.[54] On MR images, septic joints show

BOX 10-3. Imaging Features of Septic Arthritis

RADIOGRAPHS
Early: Nonspecific joint effusion
Diffuse swelling
Later: Cartilage space narrowing
Subchondral bone erosion

MRI
Articular cartilage loss
Marrow edema—if present on T1-weighted images, then osteomyelitis is likely
Bone erosion
Joint effusion
Synovial enhancement and thickening
Perisynovial edema
Capsular distension and fluid outpouchings

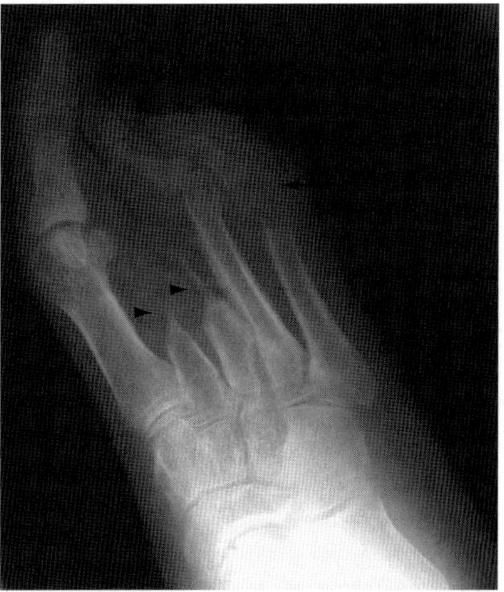

FIGURE 10-14. Septic arthritis. Anteroposterior radiograph shows advanced stage septic arthritis of the fifth MTP joint. Bone erosion is present *(arrow)*. Amputation of the second and third toes through the mid metatarsals can be seen related to prior osteomyelitis *(arrowheads)*.

cartilaginous destruction, marrow edema, and bone erosions. Bone erosions have been found to be twice as frequent in septic joints when compared with noninfected inflamed joints.[59]

However, joint effusions are often present, and in some joints physiologic fluid can mimic an effusion. This is especially true in the first MTP joint. Distension of the joint recesses is the best sign of an effusion.[41] It has been shown that one third of patients will lack an effusion, typically in the small joints where increased fluid may not be evident.[59]

Joint effusion is expected but not essential for the diagnosis of septic arthritis.

With contrast administration, synovial enhancement and thickening is seen. A recent study demonstrated synovial enhancement in 98% of cases of septic arthritis.[58] Other findings on MRI include perisynovial edema, capsular distension, and fluid outpouching. Adjacent bone may show reactive edema, with increased signal on T2-weighted images only. This should be differentiated from osteomyelitis by looking at the T1-weighted image.

If the edema is low in signal intensity on T1-weighted images, then osteomyelitis is present.[59]

An MRI triad of bone erosions, marrow edema, and cartilage destruction is highly suggestive of septic arthritis. Unfortunately there is no single MRI finding that is considered pathognomonic for a septic joint; most changes on MRI are nonspecific and may also be seen in noninfectious types of inflammatory arthropathy[60] (Figure 10-15).

An MRI triad of bone erosions, marrow edema, and cartilage destruction is highly suggestive of septic arthritis in the appropriate clinical situation.

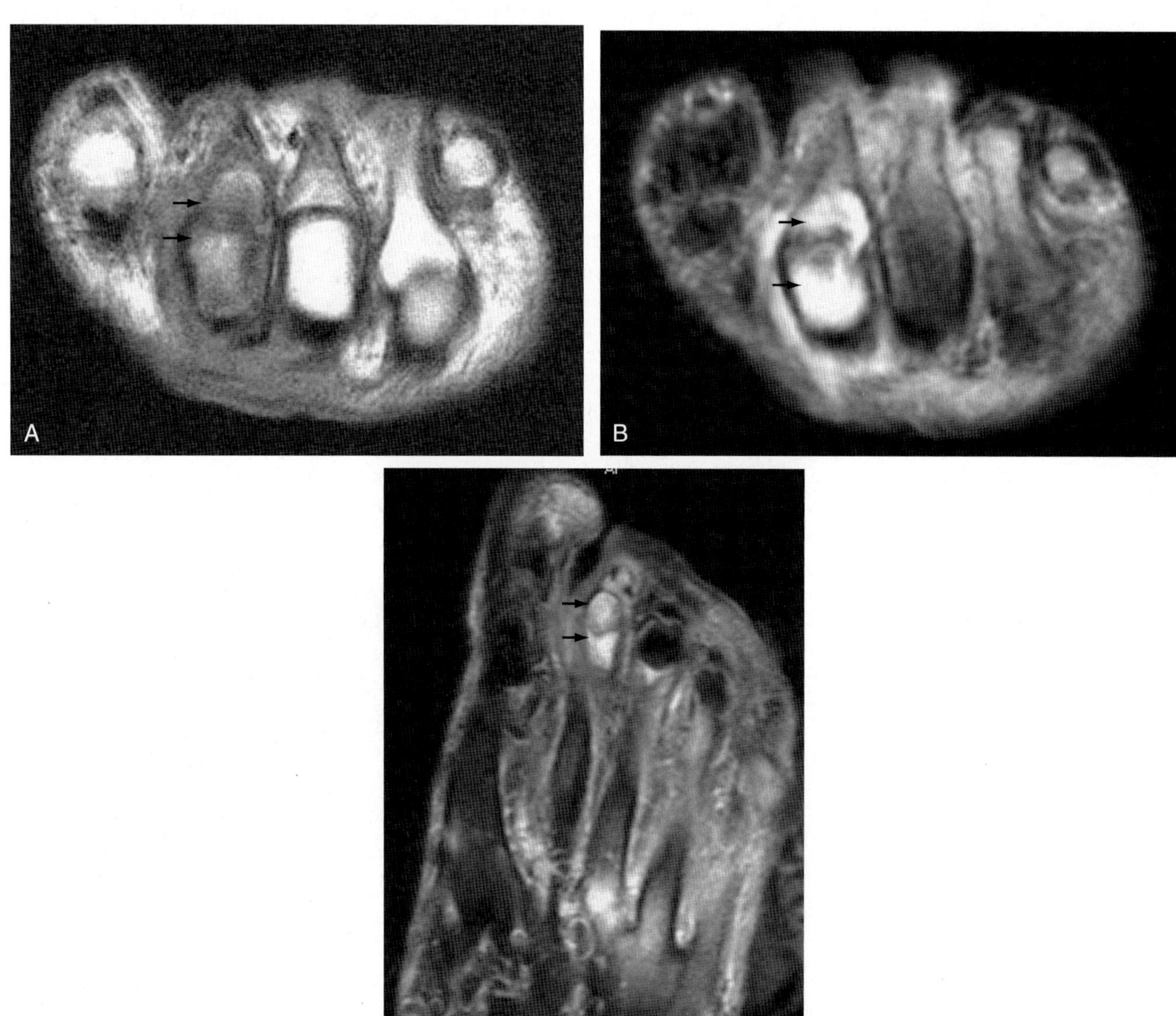

FIGURE 10-15. MR images of septic arthritis of the MTP joint. **A,** Coronal T1-weighted MR image shows decreased signal intensity of the second toe proximal phalanx and metatarsal head, consistent with osteomyelitis *(arrows)*. **B,** Coronal T2-weighted image shows increased signal intensity of the second toe proximal phalanx and metatarsal head *(arrows)*. **C,** Axial T2-weighted MR image of the forefoot shows increased fluid at the second metatarsophalangeal joint and bone marrow edema in the proximal phalanx and metatarsal head of the second digit *(arrows)*. There is adjacent soft tissue edema at this level with high signal consistent with tissue inflammation. Changes are consistent with septic arthritis and osteomyelitis.

Radionuclide scans are of limited use in diagnosing septic arthritis. Ga-67 and Tc99m scans can nonspecifically localize areas of inflammation; however, the scans are unable to demonstrate joint detail precisely. Therefore it may be difficult to differentiate among bone, joint, and soft tissue inflammation. Bone scans will show increased periarticular activity on the dynamic and blood pool phases of the scan that can persist on delayed images. Indium111 leukocyte scintigraphy has been helpful in imaging acute septic arthritis and is shown to be positive in 60% of patients with septic arthritis.[61] The problem is that many false-positive results occur in patients with synovitis secondary to inflammatory arthritis. As a result, leukocyte scans are typically used to rule out concomitant osteomyelitis, not to diagnose septic arthritis.

TENOSYNOVITIS

Tendons located in areas of soft tissue infection and adjacent to ulceration are more likely to become involved in infection through contiguous spread; however, tendons and their sheaths are not a common route for further spread. Infection of the flexor hallucis longus can occur in a patient who has septic arthritis of the ankle and subtalar joints because there is a normal communication between the flexor sheath and the joint.

The most commonly infected tendons are the peroneals because ulceration is prominent at the lateral malleolus. The flexor tendons may also be affected. In addition, the Achilles' tendon, often silent clinically, frequently becomes infected as a result of posterior calcaneal osteomyelitis.

MRI demonstrates fluid within the tendon sheath in infected tendons. Enhancement of a tendon sheath should raise concern for infective tenosynovitis. The thick rim of enhancement after contrast administration represents the inflamed, hypertrophic synovium. It is important to note that tendon sheaths rarely provide a route for the spread of proximal infection. Tenosynovitis occurs in approximately one half of the patients who require surgery and has altered surgical management in many of these patients.[62]

> Enhancement of a tendon sheath should raise concern for infective tenosynovitis.

DIABETIC MUSCLE INFARCTION

Diabetic muscle infarction is a rare complication of diabetes mellitus that has become more frequently recognized in the past few years and should be considered in the differential diagnosis of a diabetic patient with severe muscular pain. It is typically seen in patients who have a long history of diabetes and have many of the late complications including retinopathy, nephropathy, neuropathy, and peripheral vascular disease.[63] A patient typically presents with acute severe pain, tenderness, and swelling in one or more muscles of the thigh in the absence of trauma.

> Diabetic muscle infarction should be suspected in patients with long-standing insulin-dependent diabetes with systemic complications and acute severe pain, tenderness, and swelling in one or more muscles of the thigh and no history of trauma.

The onset of pain may be sudden or gradual. Infarction has been reported to occur in the thigh muscles, most commonly the quadriceps followed by the thigh adductors and the hamstrings, as well as the calf muscles and may be seen bilaterally in up to one third of patients. The pain is present during rest and worsens with movement. The pathogenesis of diabetic muscle infarction is not completely clear; however, several hypotheses have been proposed. Hypoxia-reperfusion injury may play a role in the infarction process. It has been suggested that muscle necrosis is brought on initially by a small thrombotic event causing muscle ischemia. A potent inflammatory response follows with hyperemia and reperfusion with generation of reactive oxygen species leading to greater muscle damage. Muscle edema from the inflammatory response causes a compartment syndrome, resulting in further muscle damage.[64]

The differential diagnosis for muscle infarction is rather large and includes deep vein thrombosis, muscle hematoma, muscle tear, pyomyositis, abscess, and soft tissue sarcoma; thus misdiagnosis is common. Imaging has become extremely useful in determining the correct diagnosis in a diabetic patient with muscle pain.

Radiography may show evidence of vascular mineralization and gross soft tissue swelling. CT also allows only limited evaluation of the soft tissue. Ultrasonography can better localize the region of soft tissue involvement and show focal muscle edema, demonstrating decreased echogenicity in comparison with normal muscle. Bone scanning may show focal increased uptake during the vascular phase in the soft tissue of the involved area but has also been found to be normal.[65]

Currently MRI is the most accurate method for delineating the infarcted muscle groups (Box 10-4). T2-weighted MR images and STIR sequences demonstrate edematous, enlarged muscles with increased signal abnormality of the involved area (Figure 10-16). There may be signs of subcutaneous edema and subfascial edema on T2-weighted images. The signal on T1-weighted images may be normal.

> If there is increased muscle signal on enhanced images localized to one muscle compartment, it is important to consider compartment syndrome as an emergent complication that should be managed immediately.

Treatment for diabetic muscle infarction includes analgesic therapy and physiotherapy. Symptoms typically resolve without need for surgery. Biopsy is usually contraindicated. Recurrence of symptoms is not uncommon and may be seen in the affected or contralateral limb.

> Biopsy is usually contraindicated in patients with diabetic muscle infarction.

NEUROPATHIC ARTHROPATHY VERSUS OSTEOMYELITIS

Neuropathic arthropathy in the diabetic foot is often difficult to differentiate from osteomyelitis. Neuropathic arthropathy, a progressive, degenerative process of the foot and ankle, presents with similar symptoms to osteomyelitis including erythema, tenderness, and edema. MRI may show similar subchondral bone marrow signal abnormalities, and soft tissue changes with periosteal reaction are seen in both disorders.

BOX 10-4. MRI Features of Diabetic Muscle Infarction

- Edematous enlarged muscles (bright on T2-weighted and STIR images)
- Subcutaneous and subfascial edema may be present
- Muscle enhancement in one compartment may indicate compartment syndrome

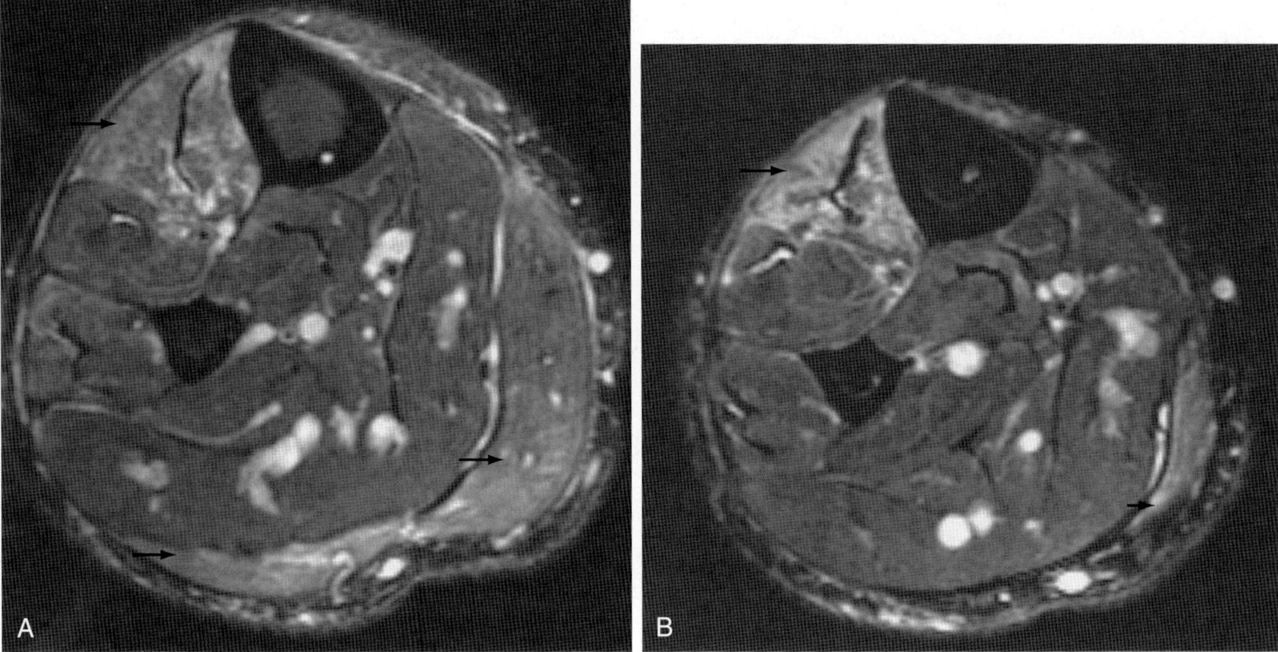

FIGURE 10-16. Diabetic muscle infarction. **A, B,** Axial T2-weighted MR images of the left leg show patchy muscle edema in several muscle groups of the calf including the anterior tibialis and medial and lateral gastrocnemius *(arrows)*. This appearance and distribution is characteristic for diabetic muscle infarction in the appropriate clinical setting.

The best rules to use in order to make a distinction between a neuropathic joint and osteomyelitis are location, adjacent soft tissue ulceration, and pattern of edema and enhancement. Neuropathic arthropathy commonly occurs in the midfoot, whereas osteomyelitis is seen predominantly in the metatarsal heads, interphalangeal joints, and hindfoot.

Neuropathic arthropathy commonly occurs in the midfoot, whereas osteomyelitis is seen predominantly in the metatarsal heads, interphalangeal joints, and hindfoot. If osteomyelitis is present in the midfoot, it typically results from adjacent ulceration of a deformed foot. Infection in the foot occurs from contiguous spread; thus osteomyelitis is likely to result from an adjacent skin ulceration, sinus tract, or soft tissue infection. Without these features, the diagnosis of infection is unlikely. Neuropathic arthropathy tends to involve multiple joints in an area, whereas osteomyelitis appears to be more focal and spreads centripetally.

The acute stage of neuroarthropathy may be difficult to differentiate from osteomyelitis. This is because bone marrow edema and joint effusions are prominent findings of both conditions. With chronic progression of the neuropathic foot, deformity is a significant aspect and may aid in the differentiation of neuroarthropathy from infection.

Occasionally, but not frequently, osteomyelitis may be superimposed on neuropathic disease. The "ghost sign" has been used to establish whether or not infection is present.

If the T1-weighted images show bones that appear to be dissolved but become more regular morphologically on the postcontrast T1-weighted images and on T2-weighted images, infection should be suspected.

Nuclear scintigraphy is a frequently used tool in the diagnosis of infection versus diabetic neuropathy. Indium-labeled leukocyte scans demonstrate areas of infection; however, they are not reliable alone because the uninfected neuropathic joint also demonstrates uptake of labeled leukocytes. Inflammation, bone remodeling, and hematopoietically active marrow explain why white cell uptake occurs in the neuropathic joint, making it difficult to differentiate from infection. Combined leukocyte and marrow scans are a more accurate way to determine whether leukocyte uptake results from infection or from increased marrow activity of a neuropathic joint. The combined scintigraphy has been reported to have high sensitivity and specificity (100% and 94%, respectively).[52] This study is superior to the bone scan and the combined bone and leukocyte study.[33]

Combined leukocyte and marrow scans are a more accurate way to determine whether leukocyte uptake results from infection or increased marrow activity due to a neuropathic joint.

Positron emission tomography (PET) has more recently been studied as an accurate method in the evaluation of infection in patients with diabetic neuroarthropathy and superimposed osteomyelitis. One study demonstrated that PET imaging using 18F-FDG is able to localize the precise anatomic site of increased uptake and accurately identify osteomyelitis of the diabetic foot.[66] Another study showed that PET (ring or hybrid) could be used to distinguish between Charcot's neuroarthropathy and osteomyelitis.[67]

CONCLUSION

Diabetes is a prevalent disease in the United States and continues to increase in numbers. Pedal foot problems cause significant morbidity for the diabetic patient and, if not treated in the early stage, major complications can develop. Peripheral vascular disease, neuropathy, and immunopathy contribute to a cascade of events resulting in ischemia, muscle atrophy, deformity, ulceration, and infection. Imaging has been critical in the management of the diabetic foot and in the prevention of the devastating consequences of amputation. Radiographs, nuclear scintigraphy, and MRI have paved the way for accurate diagnoses, allowing for successful treatment and early intervention. Imaging has created a reliable way to delineate the extent of infection as well as thoroughly describe the extent of joint deformity, influencing surgical planning. Radiology is an evolving field, with continual improvement and exploration of new ways to diagnose disease and assess the diabetic foot. In the future, PET scans, dynamic imaging, and nuclear scintigraphy may play a larger role in this disease.

REFERENCES

1. Centers for Disease Control and Prevention, National Center for Health Statistics, Division of Health Interview Statistics, data from the National Health Interview Survey. U.S. Bureau of the Census, census of the population and population estimates.
2. Barriers to chronic disease care in the United States of America: The case of diabetes and its consequences. Yale University Schools of Public Health and Medicine and the Institute for Alternative Futures, 2005.
3. Smith DM, Weinberger M, Katz BP: A controlled trial to increase office visits and reduce hospitalizations of diabetic patients, *J Gen Intern Med* 2:232-238, 1987.
4. Tennvall GF, Apelqvist J: Health economic consequences of diabetic foot lesions, *Clin Infect Dis* 39:132-139, 2004.
5. Apelqvist J, Ragnarson-Tennvall G, Persson U et al: Diabetic foot ulcers in a multidisciplinary setting. An economic analysis of primary healing and healing with amputation, *J Intern Med* 235:463-471, 1994.
6. Mayfield JA, Rieber GE, Sanders LJ et al: Preventative foot care in people with diabetes, *Diabetes Care* 21:2161-2177, 1998.
7. Pell JP, Donnan PT, Fowkes FG et al: Quality of life following lower limb amputation for peripheral arterial disease, *Eur J Vasc Surg* 7:448-451, 1993.
8. Faries PL, Teodorescu VJ, Morrissey NJ et al: The role of surgical revascularization in the management of diabetic foot wounds, *Am J Surg* 187:34-37, 2004.
9. Guyton GP, Saltzman CL: The diabetic foot: basic mechanisms of disease, *J Bone Joint Surg* 83:1084-1096, 2001.
10. Low PA, Zimmerman BR, Dyck PJ: Comparison of distal sympathetic and vagal function in diabetic neuropathy, *Muscle Nerve* 9:592-596, 1986.
11. Eneroth M, Apelqvist J, Stenstrom A: Clinical characteristics and outcome in 223 diabetic patients with deep foot infections, *Foot Ankle Int* 18:716-722, 1997.
12. Dyet JF, Nicholson AA, Ettles DF: Vascular imaging and intervention in peripheral arteries in the diabetic patient, *Diabetes Metab Res Rev* 16:16-22, 2000.
13. American Diabetes Association: Peripheral arterial disease in people with diabetes, *Diabetes Care* 26:333-341, 2003.
14. Arora S, LoGerfo FW: Lower extremity macrovascular disease in diabetics, *J Am Podiatr Med Assoc* 87:327-331, 1997.
15. Tooke JE: Microvascular function in human diabetes: a physiological perspective, *Diabetes* 12:721-726, 1995.
16. Alson MD, Lang EV, Kaufman JA: Pedal arterial imaging, *J Vasc Interven Radiol* 6:589-594, 1997.
17. Morrison WB, Ledermann HP: Work-up of the diabetic foot, *Radiol Clin North Am* 40:1171-1192, 2002.
18. Carpenter JP, Golden MA, Barker CF et al: The fate of bypass grafts to angiographically occult runoff vessels detected by magnetic resonance angiography, *J Vasc Surg* 23:483-489, 1996.
19. Stadelmann WK, Digenis AG, Tobin GF: Impediments to wound healing, *Am J Surg* 17:39-47, 1998.
20. Ledermann HP, Schweitzer ME, Morrison WB: Non-enhancing tissue on MR imaging of pedal infection: characterization of necrotic tissue and associated limitations for diagnosis of osteomyelitis and abscess, *AJR Am J Roentgenol* 178:215-222, 2002.
21. Schweitzer ME, Morrison WB: MR imaging of the diabetic foot, *Radiol Clin North Am* 42:61-71, 2004.
22. Munk PL, Helms CA, Holt RG: Immature bone infarcts: findings on plain radiographs and MR scans, *AJR Am J Roentgenol* 152:547-549, 1989.
23. Shah MK, Hugghins SY: Charcot's joint: an overlooked diagnosis, *J La State Med Soc* 154:246-250, 2002.
24. Younger DS, Bronfin L: Overview of diabetic neuropathy, *Semin Neurol* 16:107-113, 1996.
25. Brower AC, Allman RM: Pathogenesis of the neurotropic joint: neurotraumatic vs neurovascular, *Radiology* 139:349-354, 1981.
26. Schweitzer ME, Karasick D: MR imaging of disorders of the posterior tibialis tendon, *AJR Am J Roentgenol* 15:627-635, 2000.
27. Schon LC, Easley ME, Weinfeld SB: Charcot neuroarthropathy of the foot and ankle, *Clin Orthopaed Rel Res* 349:116-131, 1998.
28. Armstrong DG, Todd WF, Lavery LA et al: The natural history of acute Charcot's arthropathy in a diabetic foot specialty clinic, *Diabetic Med* 87:357-363, 1997.
29. Caputo GM, Ulbrecht J, Cavanagh PR: The charcot foot in diabetes: six key points, *Am Fam Physician* 57:2705, 1998.
30. Gil HC, Morrison WB: MR imaging of diabetic foot infection, *Semin Musculoskel Radiol* 8:189-198, 2004.
31. Cofield RH, Morrison MJ, Beabout JW: Diabetic neuroarthropathy in the foot: patient characteristics and patterns of radiographic change, *Foot Ankle* 4:15-22, 1983.
32. Cavanagh PR, Young MJ, Adams JE et al: Radiographic abnormalities in the feet of patients with diabetic neuropathy, *Diabetes Care* 17:201-209, 1994.
33. Palestro CJ, Mehta HH, Patel M et al: Marrow versus infection in the Charcot joint: indium-111 leukocyte and technetium-99m sulfur colloid scintigraphy, *J Nucl Med* 39:346-350, 1998.
34. Aliabadi P, Nikpoor N, Alparslan L: Imaging of neuropathic arthropathy, *Semin Musculoskel Radiol* 7:217-225, 2003.
35. Crim JR, Seeger LL: Imaging evaluation of osteomyelitis, *Crit Rev Diagn Imaging* 35:201-256, 1994.
36. Lipman BT, Collier BD, Carrera G et al: Detection of osteomyelitis in the neuropathic foot: nuclear medicine, MRI, and conventional radiography, *Clin Nucl Med* 23:77-82, 1998.
37. Yu JS: Diabetic foot and neuroarthropathy: magnetic imaging evaluation, *Top Magnet Res Imaging* 9:295-310, 1998.
38. Clouse ME, Gramm HF, Legg M et al: Diabetic osteoarthropathy. Clinical and roentgenographic observations in 90 cases, *AJR Am J Roentgenol Radium Therm Nucl Med* 121:22-34, 1974.
39. Early JS, Hansen ST: Surgical reconstruction of the diabetic foot: a salvage approach for midfoot collapse, *Foot Ankle Int* 17:325-330, 1996.
40. Armstrong DG, Stacpoole-Shea S, Nguyen H et al: Lengthening of the Achilles tendon in diabetic patients who are at high risk for ulceration of the foot, *J Bone Joint Surg* 81:535-538, 1999.
41. Chatha DS, Cunningham PM, Schweitzer ME: MR imaging of the diabetic foot: diagnostic challenges, *Radiol Clin North Am* 43(4):747-759, 2005.
42. Morrison WB, Schweitzer ME, Batte WG et al: Osteomyelitis of the foot: relative importance of primary and secondary MR imaging signs, *Radiology* 207:625-632, 1998.
43. Joshi N, Caputo GM, Weitekamp MR et al: Primary care: infections in patients with diabetes mellitus, *N Engl J Med* 341:1906-1912, 1999.
44. Hill SL, Holtzman GI, Buse R: The effects of peripheral vascular disease with osteomyelitis in the diabetic foot, *Am J Surg* 177:282-286, 1999.
45. Beltran J, Campanini DS, Knight C et al: The diabetic foot: magnetic resonance imaging evaluation, *Skelet Radiol* 19:37-41, 1990.
46. Ledermann HP, Morrison WB, Schweitzer ME: Pedal abscesses in patients suspected of having pedal osteomyelitis: analysis with MR imaging, *Radiology* 224:649-655, 2002.
47. Ledermann HP, Morrison WB, Schweitzer ME: Is soft tissue infection in pedal infection contained by fascial planes? MR analysis of compartmental involvement in 115 feet, *Am J Radiol* 178:605-612, 2002.
48. Erdman WA, Tamburro F, Jayson HT et al: Osteomyelitis: characteristics and pitfalls of diagnosis with MR imaging, *Radiology* 180:533-539, 1991.
49. Yuh, WT, Corson JD, Baraniewski HM et al: Osteomyelitis of the foot in diabetic patients: evaluation with plain film, 99mTc-MDP bone scintigraphy, and MR imaging, *AJR Am J Roentgenol* 152:795-800, 1989.
50. Gold RH, Tong D, Crim JR et al: Imaging the diabetic foot, *Skelet Radiol* 24:563-571, 1995.
51. Newman LG, Waller J, Palestro CJ et al: Unsuspected osteomyelitis in diabetic foot ulcers: diagnosis and monitoring by leukocyte scanning with indium in 111 oxyquinoline, *J Am Med Assoc* 266:1246-1251, 1991.
52. Schauwecker DS: The scintigraphic diagnosis of osteomyelitis, *AJR Am J Roentgenol* 158:9-18, 1991.
53. Palestro CJ, Rounmanas P, Swyer AJ et al: Diagnosis of musculoskeletal infection using combined In-111 labeled leukocyte and Tc-99m SC marrow imaging, *Clin Nucl Med* 17:269-273, 1991.
54. Ledermann HP, Morrison WB, Schweitzer ME: MR image analysis of pedal osteomyelitis: distribution, patterns of spread, and frequency of associated ulceration and septic arthritis, *Radiology* 223:747-755, 2002.
55. Lipsky BA, Pecoraro RE, Wheat LJ: The diabetic foot: soft tissue and bone infection, *Infect Dis Clin North Am* 4:409-432, 1990.
56. Bamberger DM, Daus GP, Gerding DN: Osteomyelitis in the feet of diabetic patients: long-term results, prognostic factors, and the role of antimicrobial and surgical therapy, *Am J Med* 83:653-660, 1987.
57. Mitchell M, Howard B, Haller J et al: Septic arthritis, *Radiol Clin North Am* 26:1295-1313, 1995.
58. Karchevsky M, Schweitzer ME, Morrison WB et al: MRI findings of septic arthritis and associated osteomyelitis in adults, *Am J Roentgenol* 182:119-122, 2004.
59. Graif M, Schweitzer ME, Deely D et al: The septic versus nonseptic inflamed joint: MRI characteristics, *Skelet Radiol* 28:616-620, 1999.
60. Gottlieb T, Atkins BL, Shaw DR: Soft tissue bone and joint infections, *Med J Austr* 176:609-615, 2002.
61. Shirtliff ME, Mader JT: Imaging in osteomyelitis and septic arthritis, *Curr Treat Options Infect Dis* 5:323-335, 2003.
62. Ledermann HP, Morrison WB, Schweitzer ME et al: Tendon involvement in pedal infection: MR analysis of frequency, distribution and spread of infection, *Am J Radiol* 179:939-947, 2002.
63. Grigoriadis E, Fam AG, Starok M et al: Skeletal muscle infarction in diabetes mellitus, *J Rheumatol* 27:1063-1068, 2000.
64. Silberstein L, Britton KE, Marsh FP et al: An unexpected cause of muscle pain in diabetes, *Ann Rheum Dis* 60:310-312, 2001.
65. Aboulafia AJ, Monson DK, Kennon RE: Clinical and radiologic aspects of idiopathic diabetic muscle infarction: rational approach to diagnosis and treatment, *J Bone Joint Surg* 81:323-326, 1999.
66. Keider Z, Militianu D, Melamed E: The diabetic foot: initial experience with 18F-FDG PET/CT, *J Nucl Med* 46:444-449, 2005.
67. Hopfner S, Krolak C, Kessler S et al: Preoperative imaging of Charcot neuroarthropathy in diabetic patients; comparison of ring PET, hybrid PET, and magnetic resonance imaging, *Foot Ankle Int* 25:890-895, 2004.

CHAPTER 11

Stress Injuries to Bone

RICHARD H. DAFFNER, MD, FACR

KEY FACTS

- Characteristics of fatigue fractures include: (1) the activity is new or different for the individual; (2) it is strenuous; and (3) the activity is repeated with a frequency that ultimately produces symptoms.
- Insufficiency fractures result from normal or physiologic muscular activity on a bone that is deficient in mineral or in elastic resistance.

Stress injuries of bone comprise a constellation of abnormalities that have as their common denominator overuse of the involved bones. This category of diseases includes stress fractures, the most common of the group; toddler's fractures; and "shin splints." Classically, stress fractures may be divided into two broad categories: fatigue fractures and insufficiency fractures.[1] *Fatigue fractures* are the result of overuse of bones of normal mineralization; *insufficiency fractures* result from normal activity on bones that are either deficient in mineral (the most common) or have abnormal mineralization (e.g., Paget's disease).

> *Fatigue fractures* result from overuse on bones of normal mineralization; *insufficiency fractures* result from normal activity on bones that are either deficient in mineral or have abnormal mineralization.

Toddler's fractures are a variant of stress fractures because they occur in infants learning how to walk, at an age when their bones are not sufficiently mineralized to take the loading that is placed upon them. *Shin splints* is a generic term for any kind of pretibial pain that may result from overactivity. The actual injuries suffered by patients so afflicted may range from muscle or fascial tears to ligament strain, or stress fracture.

Stress injuries are common and are specific in both their location, as well as in regard to the activity that produced them.[1-5] Although stress injuries are common, the diagnosis is often delayed because trauma is frequently not considered as the etiology for these lesions. The wide interest in physical fitness over the past 2 decades, however, has resulted in greater attention being paid to stress injuries.[6-8] Furthermore, insufficiency fractures are receiving greater attention, particularly as they frequently occur in patients with known malignancy.[9-11]

This chapter describes the pertinent aspects of stress injury to bone, focusing on those entities commonly encountered and the role that diagnostic imaging plays in establishing the diagnosis. Particular attention will be placed upon the use of magnetic resonance imaging (MRI), which has not only a high sensitivity for finding an abnormality but also has a fairly high specificity. Furthermore, the chapter will also discuss the occurrence of stress fractures in female athletes and in children. Finally, the chapter will discuss insufficiency fractures in the osteoporotic and elderly populations to provide a greater degree of awareness of this entity to readers.

PATHOPHYSIOLOGY

Overuse of the limbs is the cause of stress injuries. A fatigue fracture results from repetitive and prolonged muscular action on a bone that has not yet adapted itself to that action.

> A fatigue fracture results from repetitive and prolonged muscular action on a bone that has not yet adapted itself to that action.

One of the interesting phenomena in medical science is that many concepts often evolve in a circular fashion. Initially, stress fractures were believed to be due to direct impact on bone. In the early 1970s, Devas demonstrated that stress fractures were the result of muscular action on bone instead of direct impact.[12] This concept was widely accepted, and it was only recently that new evidence emerged from sports medicine research that both weight loading and direct impact play a role in the development of certain stress fractures of the lower limbs. Longitudinal stress fractures of the tibia are a prime example.[7] What is certain, however, is the fact that any individual with a fatigue fracture has engaged in vigorous activity that is either totally new to him or her or is one to which he or she has not yet become conditioned. By definition, fatigue fractures result from the application of abnormal muscular stress or torque to a bone with normal elastic resistance. There is a common triad with most fatigue fractures: (1) the activity is new or different for the individual; (2) it is strenuous; and (3) the activity is repeated with a frequency that ultimately produces symptoms.[1,2] Insufficiency fractures, on the other hand, result from normal or physiologic muscular activity applied to a bone that is deficient in mineral or in elastic resistance. The term *pathologic fracture* is not used to describe these injuries because it implies that a preexisting tumor or infection has weakened the bone.

> A pathologic fracture occurs due to weakening of the bone by tumor or infection.

Bone is a dynamic tissue in which the mineral content is quite "fluid." As a result, bones respond to the muscular load that is placed upon them. With greater muscular activity, the bones become stronger as additional mineral is deposited. Conversely,

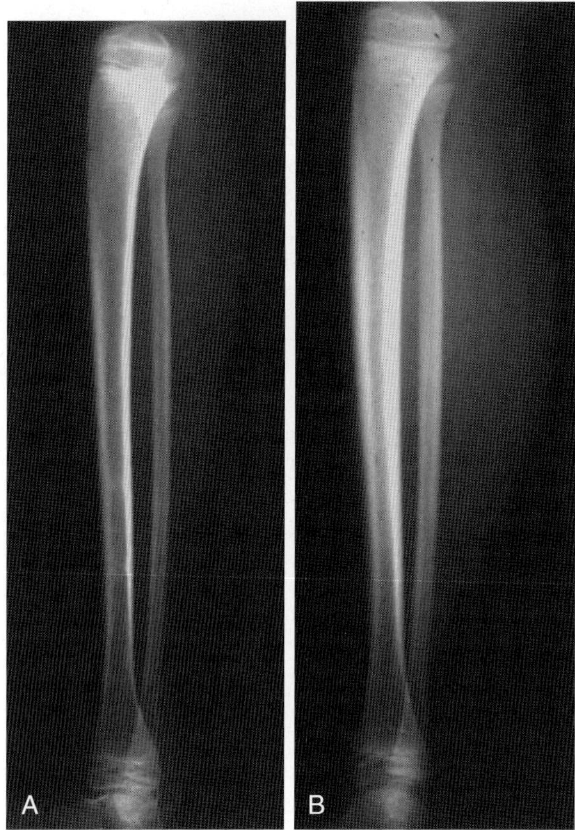

FIGURE 11-1. Response of bone and muscles to use. Child with cerebral palsy affecting the right side of the body. **A,** The right leg shows the bones to be gracile and osteopenic. The muscles are smaller than on the normal left side. **B,** The left leg shows normal bone thickness and muscle development.

in the absence of significant muscular activity, bones rapidly lose their mineral content (develop osteopenia) and become weaker (Figures 11-1 and 11-2).

In an ideal world, increased muscle activity would produce an increase in the strength of the muscles involved as well as the bones at an equal rate. Unfortunately, the muscles tone up much faster than the bones, and this results in a mechanical imbalance. Every novice recreational runner has experienced positive cardiovascular effects within a few days of beginning training. As a result, muscle tone and strength have increased to the point at which the individual feels capable of extending the distances run. Unfortunately, there has not been an equal increase in the skeletal strength to match that of the muscle tone. As a result, extending the running distance produces overuse on bones not yet ready to accept the added stress loading. Furthermore, fatigue of opposing muscle groups, which frequently prevent one group of muscles from overexerting their effect on the involved bone, may produce a further imbalance and accelerate bone failure.

From a purely architectural standpoint, bone behaves as do other structural materials such as metal, wood, ceramics, or plastic. When these materials are placed under stress, they behave according to Wolff's law[13] (Figure 11-3). According to Wolff's law, as the amount of loading on bone (or any other structural material) increases, there is progressive deformity up to the critical point. Any deformity up to this point occurs within what is referred to as the *elastic range,* meaning that relaxation or removal of the loading force will result in a return of the bone to its original configuration. Once the critical point is exceeded, further loading takes the bone into the *plastic range* of deformity. It is at this stage that permanent deformity occurs as the result of microfractures, a fact that has been verified experimentally.[13,14] Within the plastic range, relaxation or removal of the loading force will not result in the original configuration being restored because the microfractures have occurred. Furthermore, as the number of microfractures increases, small cortical cracks occur and progress as the stress loading increases. Generally, the crack propagates through subcortical infractions. Ultimately, the fatigue point is exceeded, and structural failure with complete or catastrophic fractures results.[15] Additional factors that contribute to the abnormal muscle pull can produce overload on stressed bones. The first is poor posture, producing a change in the center of gravity for which the body must compensate. This results in an increase in the effect of direct muscle pull on bone and also leads to fatigue of the opposing muscle groups. Second, environmental conditions may also result in increased stress on the bones. Typically, in runners, changes in terrain, running surface, or equipment (different shoes) may all result in a change or an increase in muscle pull on the bones of the lower limbs. Running uphill or downhill, instead of on a level surface, increases the forces by as much as 14 times.[16] A change from a grass surface to a hard surface may result in an unconscious protective curling of the feet to cushion the footfall. A similar occurrence may occur as the result of improperly fitted running shoes. Finally, we now recognize the effects of direct impact on the production of stress fractures, particularly longitudinal stress fractures of the tibia.[5,7]

Table 11-1 lists the location of fatigue fractures and the activities that typically produce them.

Insufficiency fractures, as previously mentioned, are the result of normal activity in patients with abnormal bone mineral content or elasticity. In some instances, the individual may have engaged in a new activity that ordinarily would not be associated with excessive stress on the bones. Although the majority of these injuries occur in elderly women with postmenopausal osteoporosis, insufficiency fractures may occur in patients suffering from osteoporosis of any cause, including corticosteroid use, rheumatoid arthritis, diabetes mellitus, and renal disease. Box 11-1 lists the common locations of insufficiency fractures. Box 11-2 lists the conditions likely to predispose a patient to insufficiency fractures.

Stress fractures are more likely to occur in nonosteoporotic bones at the sites of previous surgery. Screw holes and excision sites produce stress risers in bone.[17] Patients who have undergone muscle or tendon transfers will have the pull vectors of those muscles or tendons altered, which can increase the stress on the underlying bones. A common example of this is a stress fracture of the second or third metatarsal as the result of bunion surgery.[18,19]

Recent advances in sports medicine have produced a greater awareness of injuries to the female athlete. There have been a number of reports of an increase in the incidence of stress fractures in female athletes that have been attributed to a variety of factors.

Female athletes may be particularly prone to stress fractures.

These factors include genetics, ethnicity (Caucasian), low body weight, lack of weight-bearing exercise, mechanical factors, hormonal disorders such as oligomenorrhea or amenorrhea, eating disorders, and inadequate calcium intake.[4,20]

Finally, there are disturbing reports of an increasing incidence of stress fractures occurring in the pediatric population. This may be due to a trend of increasing pressure by parents and coaches on talented young people as well as the tendency toward beginning training at an earlier age.[21-23] The areas of risk for stress fractures in children include not only the same areas of the lower limbs as in adults from similar activities, but also the distal

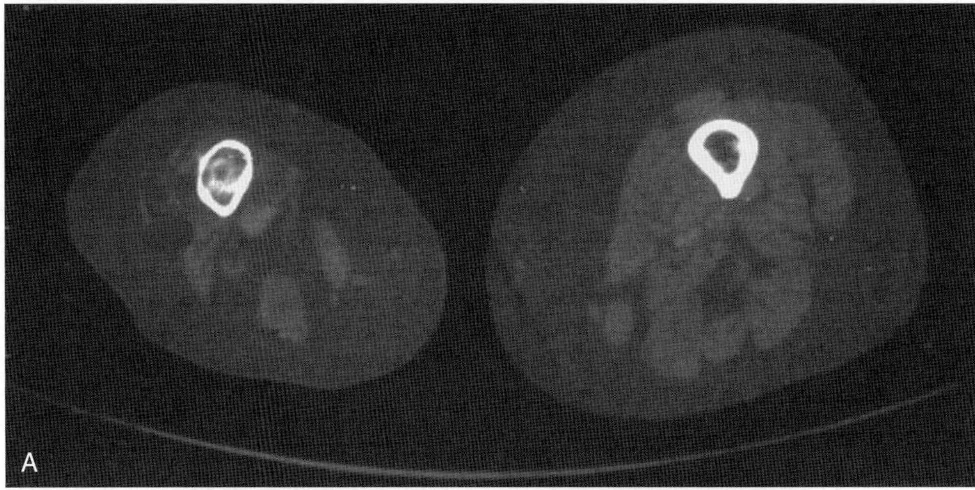

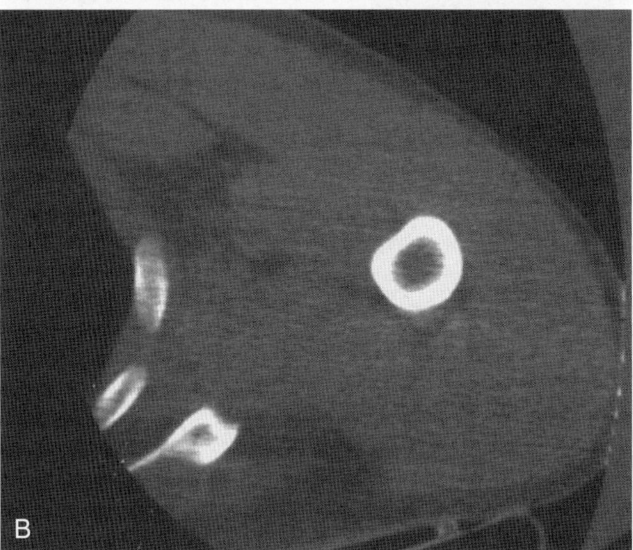

FIGURE 11-2. Response of bone and muscles to use. **A,** CT of the lower femurs in an elderly patient with an infected total knee implant on the right. Note the bone and muscle atrophy on the affected side compared with the normal side. **B,** CT of the upper throwing arm of a professional baseball pitcher. Note the thickness of the bony cortex as well as the hypertrophy of the muscles. Compare with **A.**

humerus and elbow in throwing sports, the wrists in gymnasts, the pars interarticularis in gymnasts and dancers, and the ribs in those who row or play golf or basketball.

CLINICAL FEATURES

The typical history of a fatigue fracture is that of a patient who experiences pain during a particular activity. The pain is typically relieved by rest as well as by analgesics and is made worse by continuing the activity. In contrast, all other pathologic lesions typically have pain with activity as well as at rest. Interestingly, the symptoms are often worse at night.

> Pain associated with tumor occurs with activity and at rest, whereas pain due to fatigue fracture is usually relieved with rest.

The fact that the lesion is relieved by analgesics should not be used for diagnostic purposes. In most instances, the activity is either new or different for the individual. These characteristic features must be actively sought when obtaining the patient's history. For example, a recreational runner who decides to increase his or her distance from 2 to 5 miles may suffer a fatigue fracture. Conditioned professional athletes also may suffer stress fractures if they have broken training, returned from an injury, or decided to increase the amount of effort expended when they perform their particular athletic feat.

As mentioned previously, the clinical history is paramount in making a diagnosis of stress fracture. The patient must be questioned closely with particular attention paid to the sequence of events that led up to the onset of pain in the affected limb. Clinicians should make no assumptions, particularly of nonathletic-appearing patients. Recreational walking is a low-impact activity with excellent aerobic cardiovascular effects. This activity is now popular among many middle-aged and elderly individuals and has resulted in an increasing number of insufficiency fractures.

It is important for clinicians and radiologists to recognize stress fractures, so the patient may be instructed to abstain from those activities that produced the injuries. Sustained activity on a bone (particularly in the leg) with a stress fracture may result in a complete fracture of that bone, in distraction of the bone fragments, in

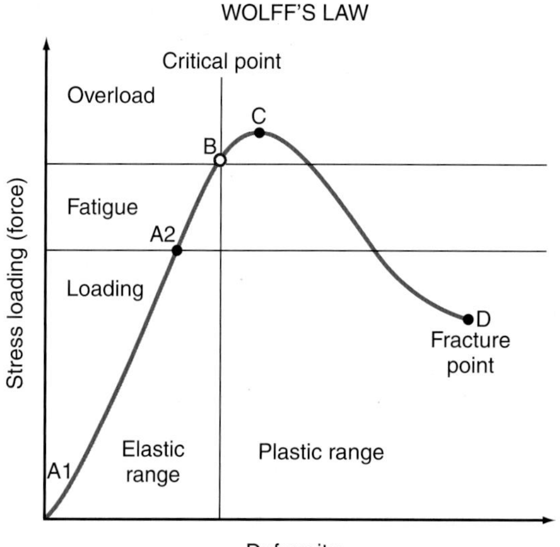

FIGURE 11-3. Wolff's law showing the response of architectural structures to stress. As a stressing force is applied to any rigid material, measurable deformity occurs. The deformity is in the elastic range until the critical point *(B)* is reached and a release of the stress results in the original architectural configuration being restored. Once the critical point is exceeded, microfractures occur, ultimately leading to catastrophic failure. If the stress is released, permanent deformity (plastic deformity) will remain because of the microfractures. The degree of deformity depends on the number of microfractures.

the fracture of another bone in the same limb, or in a fracture of the same bone in the opposite limb, due to the individual shifting weight to the opposite side.

Regarding insufficiency fractures, two subsets of patients deserve special mention. Patients with rheumatoid arthritis have an increased risk of insufficiency fractures attributed to the osteopenia that accompanies the disease, disuse atrophy of the affected bones, and the use of corticosteroids.[24,25] In addition, patients with rheumatoid arthritis who have recently undergone total joint replacement may suffer stress fractures when they begin ambulation. The second group comprises patients with a history of pelvic malignancy who have undergone radiation therapy. These patients frequently have a higher incidence of sacral and pelvic insufficiency fractures.[10,11,26]

Patients with pelvic malignancy treated with irradiation have a higher incidence of pelvic and sacral insufficiency fractures. Clinical history and imaging studies can usually differentiate these fractures from metastatic lesions.

IMAGING

The types of imaging studies performed for patients with suspected stress fractures run the entire gamut including radiography, computed tomography (CT), nuclear imaging, and MRI. Ultrasound does not have a place in the diagnostic armamentarium for these conditions. Radiography is most often the initial imaging study performed. Unfortunately, it is not the most sensitive tool that we have for establishing a diagnosis in the early stages. Figure 11-4 shows the gamut of imaging and the points in time at which they are likely to yield positive results. The radiographic appearance depends on the time sequence between the onset of injury and the radiographic examination, as well as whether or not the patient continued participation in the activity. Mulligan described the earliest radiographic change as a "graying" or indistinctness of the cortex that he believed most likely represented localized bone or periosteal edema.[27] Occasionally, in the early phase, the fracture in the shaft of a long bone may appear as a lucency through the cortex without any evidence of periosteal reaction or callus (Figure 11-5). In cancellous bone, such as the calcaneus, the first manifestation may be a linear area of sclerosis that is frequently oriented perpendicular

TABLE 11-1. Location of Fatigue Fracture by Activity

Location	Activity
Lower limb	
Sesamoids under metatarsals	Prolonged standing, running
Metatarsals	Marching, ballet, postoperative bunionectomy, skating
Navicular	Marching, running, basketball
Calcaneus	Jumping, parachuting, prolonged standing, recent immobilization
Tibia: proximal shaft	Walking, running
Tibia: mid and distal shaft	Running, leaping (basketball), ballet, aerobic dance
Fibula: distal shaft	Running, aerobics
Fibula: proximal shaft	Jumping, parachuting
Patella	Hurdling, gymnastics, basketball, aerobics
Femur: shaft	Ballet, running
Femur: neck	Ballet, marching, running, gymnastics
Trunk	
Sacrum	Running, aerobics
Pelvis: obturator ring	Stooping, bowling, gymnastics
Lumbar vertebra (pars interarticularis)	Ballet, running, gymnastics, heavy lifting, scrubbing floors
Lower cervical, upper thoracic spinous process	Clay shoveling
Ribs	Carrying heavy pack, ice hockey, golf, coughing
Upper limb	
Clavicle	Postoperative radical neck, typing
Coracoid of scapula	Trap shooting, golf
Humerus: distal	Throwing a ball
Ulna: coronoid	Pitching a ball
Ulna: shaft	Pitching a ball, pitchfork work, propelling a wheelchair
Hook of hamate	Holding golf clubs, tennis racquet, baseball bat

BOX 11-1. Location of Insufficiency Fractures

Sacrum
Pubic arches
Acetabulum
Femoral neck
Tibia
Calcaneus

BOX 11-2. Conditions Predisposing to Insufficiency Stress Fractures

Osteoporosis of any cause
Rheumatoid arthritis
Postirradiation
Osteomalacia/rickets
Hyperparathyroidism
Diabetes mellitus
Fibrous dysplasia
Paget disease
Pyrophosphate arthropathy
Healing tibial fracture
Scurvy
Surgery
Osteogenesis imperfecta
Osteopetrosis

to the trabeculae (Figure 11-6). Once healing begins, solid or thick lamellar periosteal reaction occurs on both the endosteal as well as the periosteal surface, confined to a small area of the cortex (Figure 11-7). This fusiform area of reactive bone is typically smaller than that encountered in an osteoid osteoma. In addition, stress fractures typically involve only one of the cortical surfaces as opposed to the entire circumference of the bone, as in the case of sclerosing osteomyelitis. As periosteal reaction thickens, any fracture line that may have been present disappears.

Insufficiency fractures of the sacrum and pelvis are not typically diagnosed by radiographs at their early stages. On occasion, a stress fracture of the sacrum may be seen on a radiograph as it heals (Figure 11-8).

The choice of an imaging modality beyond radiography will depend on the clinician's "need to know." The elite athletes and other individuals whose livelihood depends on the use of injured limbs should undergo either radionuclide imaging or MRI if initial radiography is inconclusive or normal.

Radionuclide Imaging

The radionuclide bone scan has been a mainstay for diagnosing patients with suspected stress fractures, particularly those patients with normal radiographs.[28-30] The purpose of this study is to differentiate between an actual bony lesion and nonskeletal lesions. This is particularly important for the competitive athlete or for the individual in whom cessation of a particular activity would be detrimental to his or her livelihood. In these individuals, the finding of increased tracer activity within the suspected bone is highly suggestive of stress fracture. As shown in Figure 11-4, the radionuclide image becomes positive early in the course of the stress fracture by showing slightly increased tracer activity. In the later stages of the injury, there are well-marginated areas of increased activity (Figure 11-9). Radionuclide scanning is also useful in patients with insufficiency fractures of the sacrum and pelvis (Figure 11-10). The usual indication for this study being performed is the suspicion of metastatic disease (when the clinician does not consider stress fracture as the primary diagnosis). In the sacrum, one pattern is highly suggestive of stress fractures; patients with bilateral sacral stress fractures frequently will demonstrate an H-shaped radionuclide distribution called the "Honda sign" (Figure 11-11).

> Bilateral sacral insufficiency fractures will produce H-shaped uptake on bone scan, referred to as the "Honda sign."

Furthermore, in unilateral fractures, increased tracer activity is frequently found in a linear vertical pattern (see Figure 11-10, *A*, and Figure 11-11, *A*) rather than in a globular pattern such as occurs in a malignancy. The finding of either of these uptake patterns should prompt follow-up with a CT scan to confirm the diagnosis (see Figure 11-10, *B*, and Figure 11-11, *C*).[31]

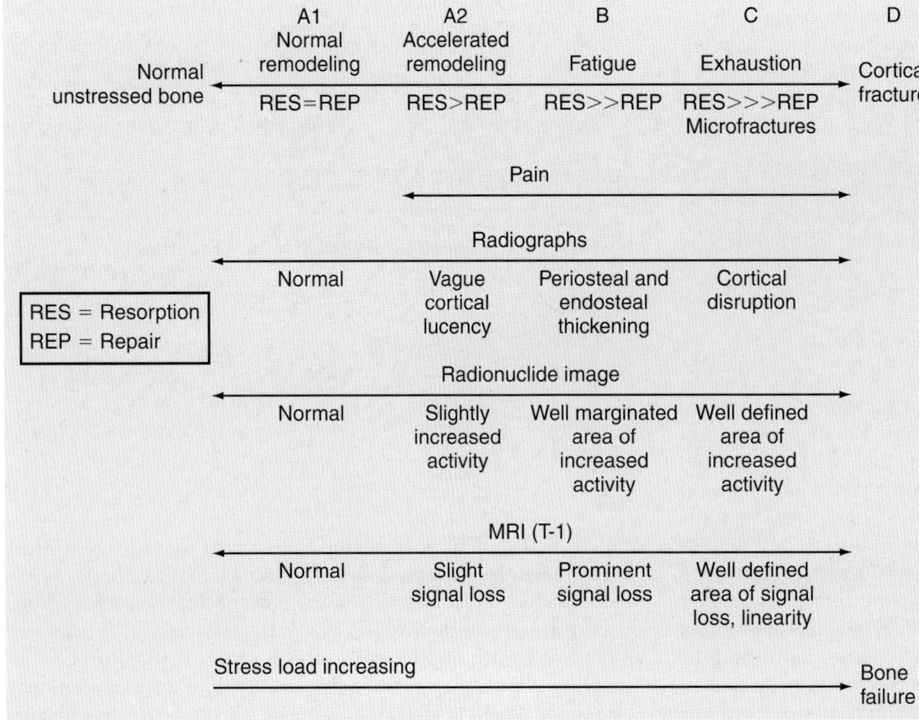

FIGURE 11-4. Graph showing the relationship of bone stress, clinical symptoms, and imaging findings to timing of the stress. The letters correspond to the points on the Wolff's law graph shown in Figure 11-3.

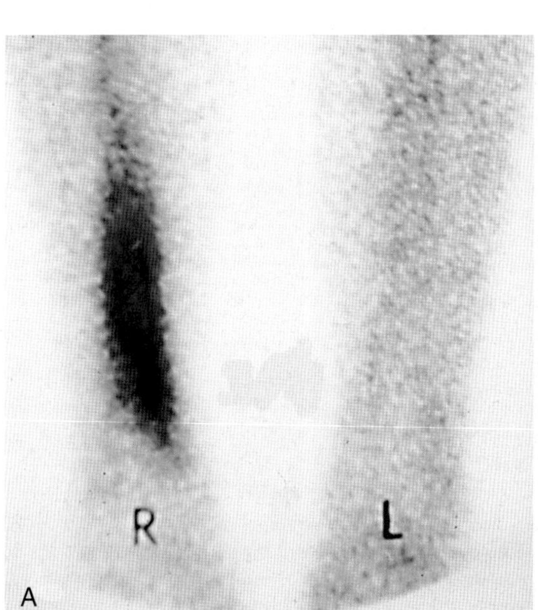

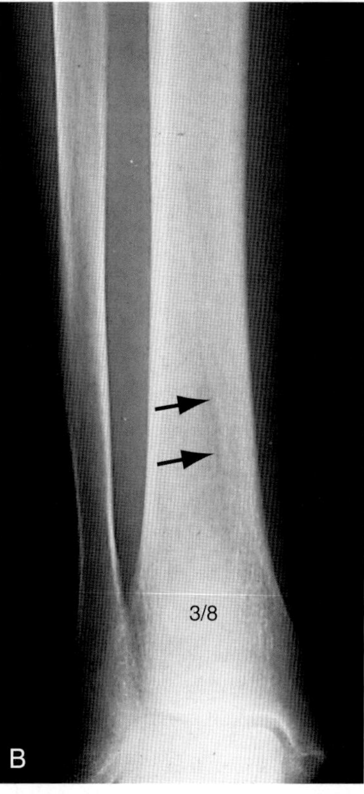

FIGURE 11-5. Longitudinal stress fracture of the tibia. **A,** Radionuclide bone scan shows an area of intense increase in tracer activity in the right tibia. **B,** Radiograph shows the vertical stress fracture *(arrows)*.

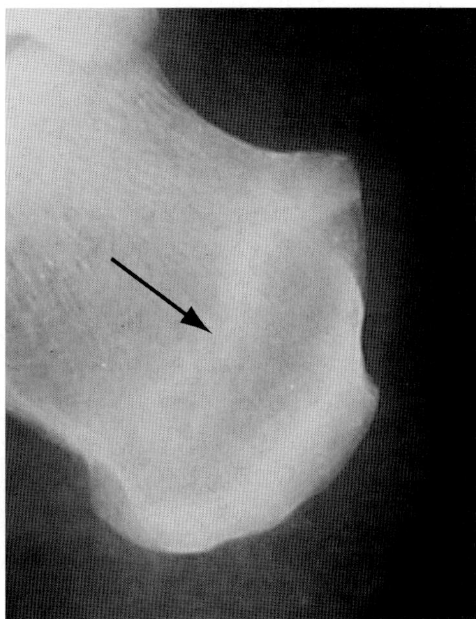

FIGURE 11-6. Calcaneal stress fracture. The fracture presents as a zone of condensation *(arrow)* oriented perpendicularly to the long axis of the calcaneus.

Although radionuclide images may be nonspecific in the early stage, a pattern considered fairly specific for stress fractures is uptake that is both *linear* as well as *vertical.* As mentioned previously, tumors and infections frequently have globular increases in tracer activity.

Computed Tomography

CT should not be used as a primary investigative tool for most patients with suspected stress fractures. With the exception of sacral and longitudinal tibial stress fractures, the findings are often inconclusive in demonstrating areas of periosteal and endosteal new bone as well as fracture lines. CT is best used for follow-up, particularly in the sacrum (see Figure 11-8, *B,* and Figure 11-11, *B*) to confirm a diagnosis suspected by another imaging study.

Magnetic Resonance Imaging

MRI is now used extensively to confirm or exclude the diagnosis in patients with suspected stress fractures.[31-38] MRI examination is frequently performed when a diagnosis other than stress fracture is entertained and in some patients with a history of previous malignancy in whom insufficiency fractures of the sacrum or pelvis may occur. In this group of patients, the MRI findings may be sufficiently characteristic to allow a confident diagnosis of insufficiency fractures to be made and preclude biopsy or additional testing.[31]

Stress injuries may also affect tendons, ligaments, muscles, and the neurovascular structures as well as the bones. A prime example of this is "shin splints." Because MR imaging is so sensitive, it can depict all of the structures that may be involved with the injury.

It is often not necessary to do an extensive MRI evaluation. Patients with suspected stress injuries can be studied with a limited series that combines a fast spin echo (FSE) T1-weighted sequence with short tau inversion recovery (STIR) images in two planes. Such screening studies provide rapid and potentially inexpensive "tailored" diagnostic examinations that are frequently

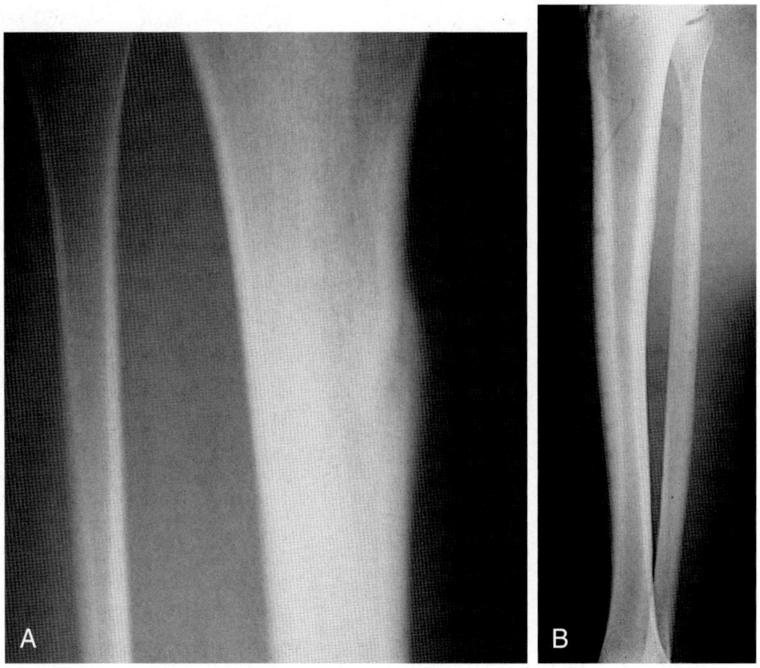

FIGURE 11-7. Healing stress fractures. **A,** Tibial stress fracture in a runner. Detailed view shows the lucent fracture line with solid overlying periosteal reaction. **B,** Anterior tibial striations (stress fractures) in a basketball player with "shin splints." Note the multiple faint horizontal lucencies perpendicular to the cortex along the anterior shaft of the tibia. The other leg showed similar findings. Note the thickening of the anterior cortex as well.

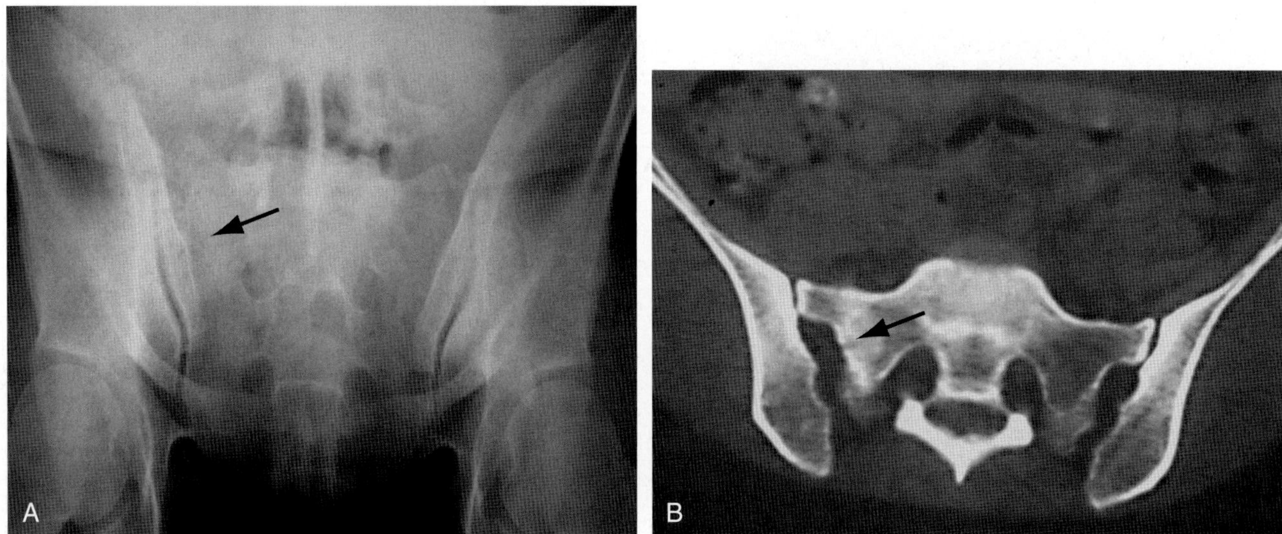

FIGURE 11-8. Healing stress fracture of the sacrum. **A,** Pelvic outlet view shows a vertical area of linear sclerosis in the body of the sacrum on the right *(arrow)*. These are infrequently visible on radiographs. **B,** CT image shows the healing fracture *(arrow)* to advantage. CT is the gold standard for imaging sacral stress fractures.

very specific as to the diagnosis (Figure 11-12). On T1-weighted sequences, stress fractures appear as areas of low signal. These areas show increased signal intensity on T2-weighted images (Figure 11-13). Following intravenous enhancement with a gadolinium compound, the area of abnormality will show increased signal (Figure 11-14). With STIR imaging, there is an intense increase in signal activity reflecting the edema of the affected bone (Figure 11-15). Frequently, the fracture line itself will be demonstrated (Figures 11-16 and 11-17).[10,31-38] When follow-up studies are performed, the bone marrow edema typically resolves within 6 months of the initial diagnosis. If this abnormal marrow signal intensity persists, it most likely represents a recurrent injury.

Although the MRI manifestations of stress injuries are not site-specific, the location of the abnormalities may suggest the diagnosis. As mentioned previously, stress fractures tend to occur in

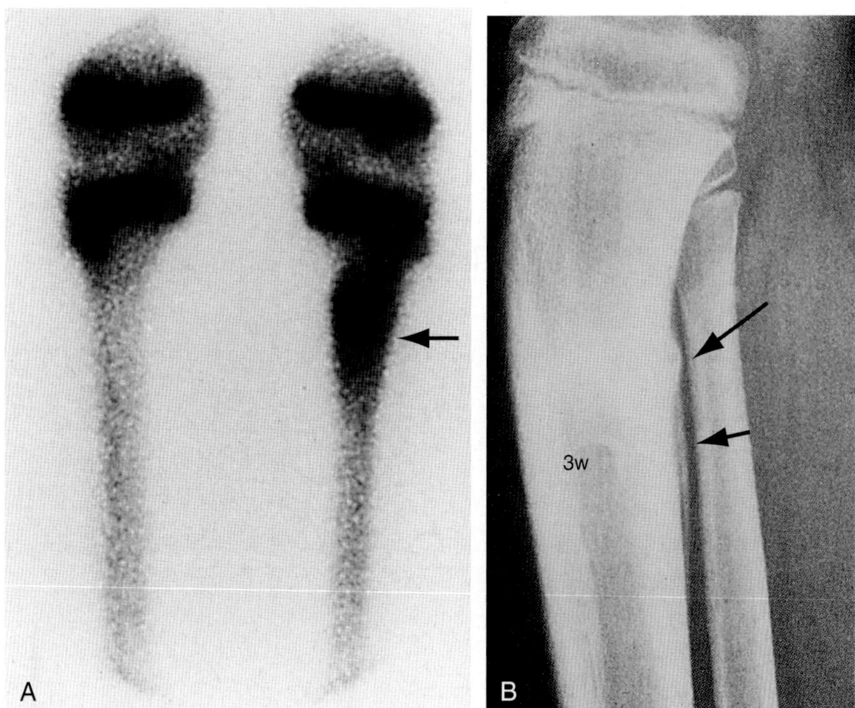

FIGURE 11-9. Use of radionuclide bone scan to identify a stress fracture in a 12-year-old runner. Radiograph was normal. **A,** Bone scan performed 10 days after the initial radiograph shows an intense area of increased tracer activity *(arrow)* in the left proximal tibia. Note the marked uptake of isotope in the normal femoral and tibial epiphyses. **B,** Radiograph taken 3 weeks after onset of symptoms shows the healing stress fracture *(large arrow)* as well as solid laminar periosteal reaction *(small arrow)*.

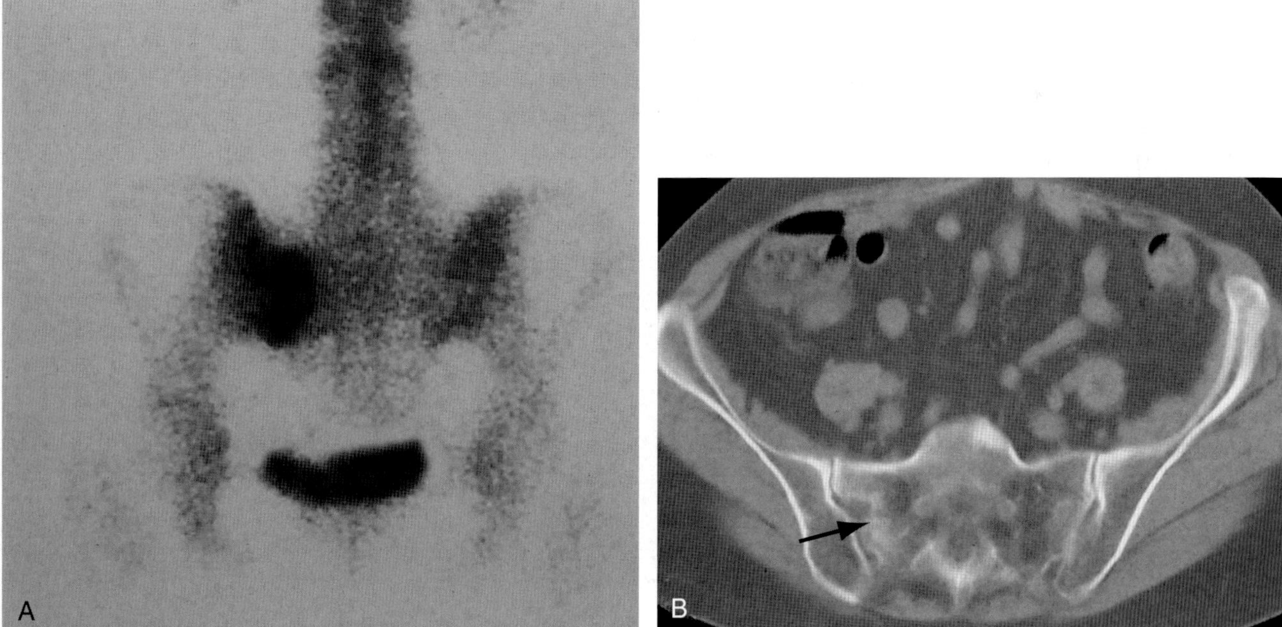

FIGURE 11-10. Insufficiency fracture of the sacrum. **A,** Radionuclide bone scan shows unilateral increase in tracer activity on the right. **B,** CT image shows the healing stress fracture *(arrow)*.

specific locations. Regarding pelvic stress fractures, fatigue fractures occur in the femoral neck, the pubis, and the sacrum. Insufficiency fractures most commonly involve the ischiopubic rami, the sacrum, the supraacetabular region, and the femoral head and neck.

Fatigue fractures occur in the femoral neck, the pubis, and the sacrum. Insufficiency fractures most commonly involve the ischiopubic rami, the sacrum, the supra-acetabular region, and the femoral head and neck.

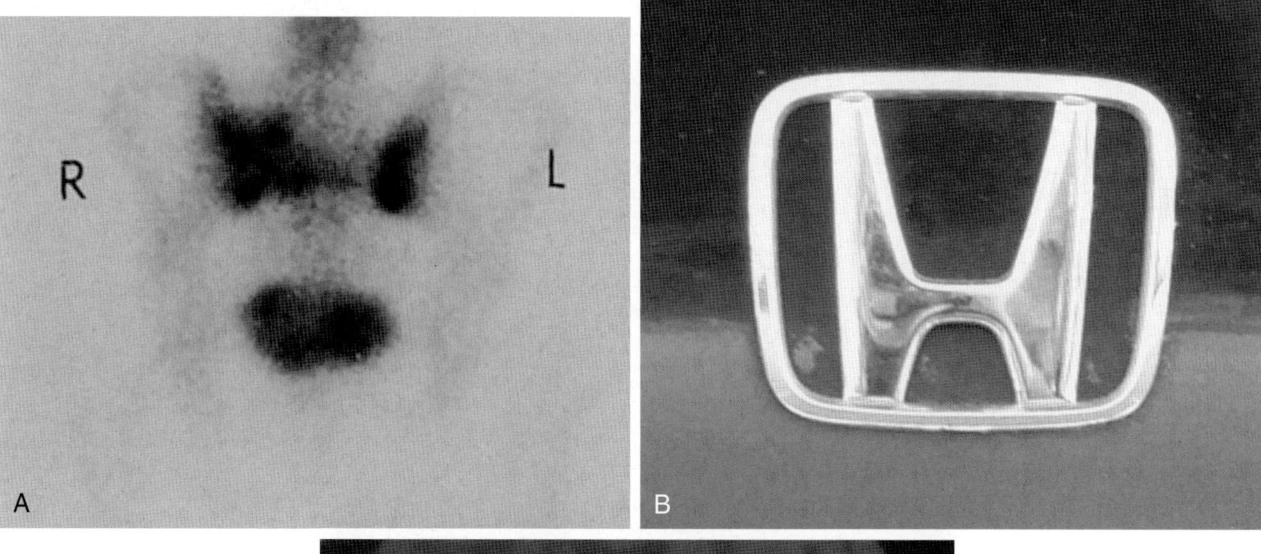

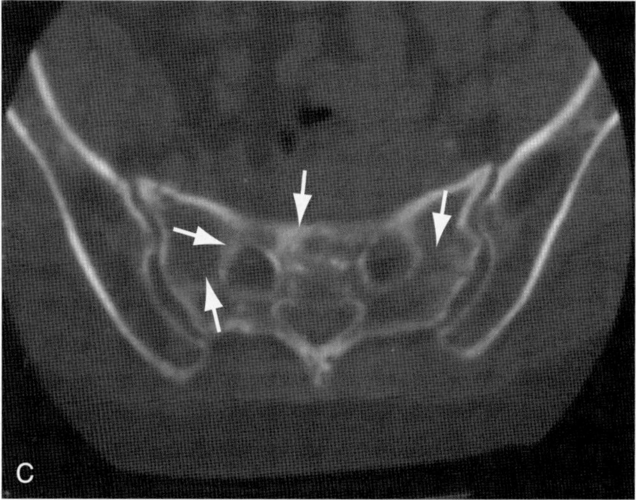

FIGURE 11-11. Insufficiency fractures of the sacrum. **A,** Radionuclide bone scan shows bilateral vertically oriented areas of increased tracer activity with a small central connecting area ("Honda sign"). **B,** Honda logo. Note the resemblance to the findings in **A. C,** CT image shows bilateral and central areas of sclerosis *(arrows)* and anterior discontinuity on the right representing the healing stress fractures.

Although MRI findings are typically nonspecific, they may be encountered in a variety of conditions that cause hyperemia. However, the presence of linearity and vertical orientation, particularly in the sacrum, should alert the radiologist to the correct diagnosis. Metastases typically produce globular areas of abnormal signal similar to that seen in radionuclide bone scans. Radiation fibrosis typically produces a diffuse pattern of signal abnormality conforming to the shape of the portal.

One should be able to establish the diagnosis of a stress fracture clinically when a specific activity is associated with the onset of symptoms in an area where stress fractures typically occur. Unfortunately, patients frequently cannot recall an inciting activity. Nonetheless, radiologists and clinicians should seek clues in the history pointing to the presence of an underlying stress fracture when a lesion occurs in a location common for these entities. If there is any possibility that a bone lesion may represent a healing stress fracture, *biopsy should be avoided* because a specimen through any recent fracture often contains immature bone cells that represent the healing process, and these may be misinterpreted on pathologic examination as representing an osteosarcoma. When any stress fracture is suspected, patients should be radiographically reexamined in 1 to 2 weeks. If the area is difficult to examine on radiographs, CT with multiplanar reconstruction is indicated. If the individual has stopped the activity that produced the injury, there should be evidence of healing within that period of time and these imaging modalities should allow the proper diagnosis to be made. In the absence of findings of sepsis, a delay of several weeks will not prove to be detrimental. Thus "tincture of time" should be applied when stress fractures are suspected and biopsies should be avoided until there is clear-cut radiographic evidence that no healing has occurred.

Sacral insufficiency fractures may take months to heal.

DIFFERENTIAL DIAGNOSIS

The differential diagnosis of stress fractures includes four entities: osteoid osteoma, chronic sclerosing osteomyelitis, osteomalacia, and metastases. Classically, osteosarcoma and Ewing's tumor have been included in the differential diagnosis; however, these two entities should never be seriously confused with stress fractures because their radiographic features are fairly typical of a neoplasm.

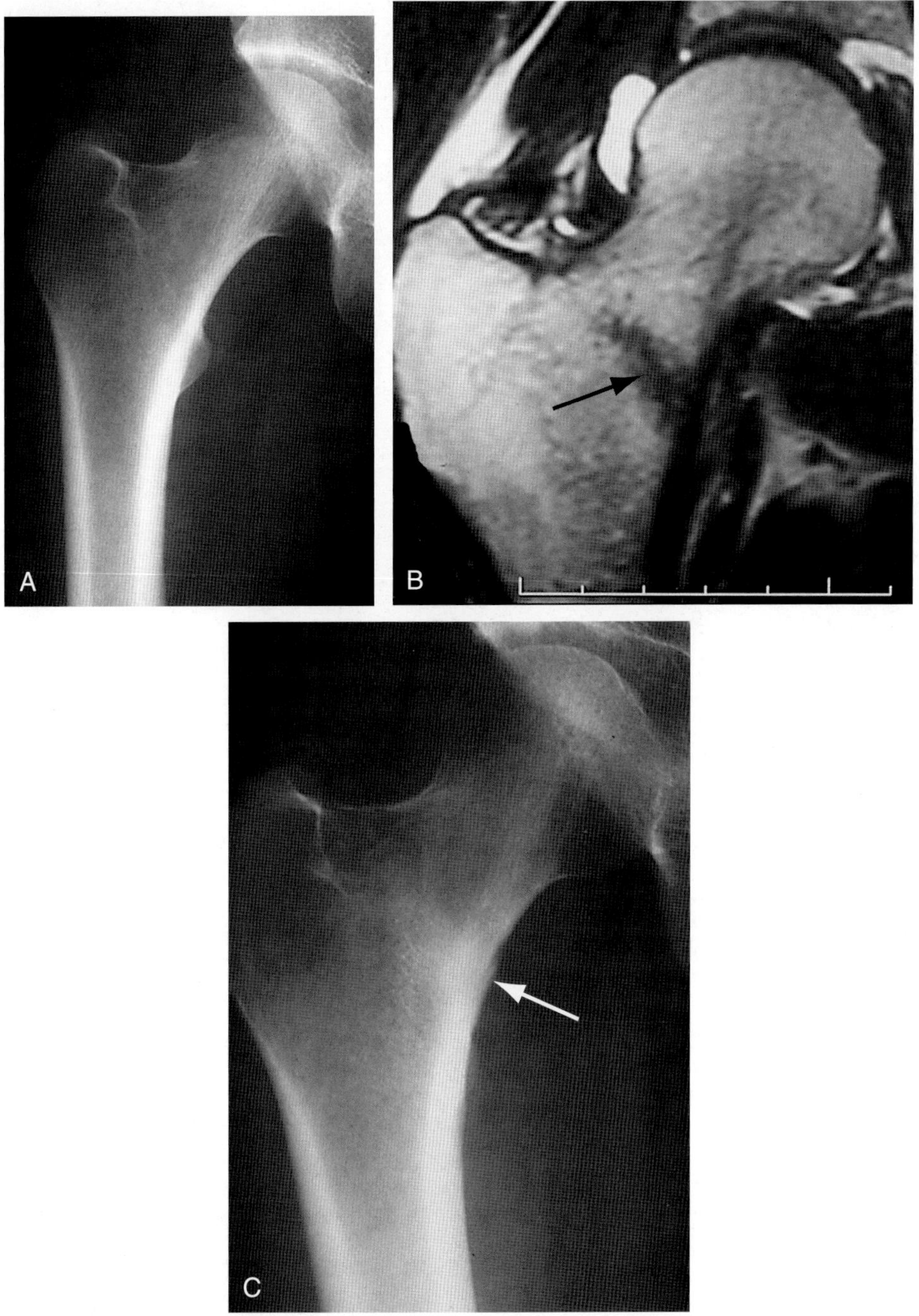

FIGURE 11-12. Use of MRI to diagnose an occult stress fracture in a 21-year-old professional soccer player with hip pain. **A,** Initial radiograph 2 days after onset of symptoms is normal. **B,** T1-weighted coronal MR image taken 1 day later shows a linear area of low signal in the inferior femoral neck *(arrow)*. **C,** Follow-up radiograph 6 weeks after onset of symptoms shows the healing stress fracture of the femoral neck *(arrow)*.

Osteoid osteoma is a benign neoplasm characteristically manifested clinically by night pain relieved by antiinflammatory medication. Pain may or may not be associated with activity. In contradistinction, stress fractures typically produce pain that is made worse by activity and is relieved by rest. Radiographically, the typical osteoid osteoma has a dense sclerotic area or reaction surrounding a lucent nidus (Figure 11-18). CT may be needed to identify this nidus. Osteoid osteomas are generally eccentric, whereas stress fractures often involve both sides of the shaft of the affected bone. With an osteoid osteoma, there is an intense sclerotic reaction that is fusiform and long. Periosteal reaction is typically seen after a stress fracture.

Sclerosing osteomyelitis is characterized by a dense sclerotic bone reaction that may contain a central lucency. The lesion is centered within the medullary cavity, typical of infections in general. The lesion usually involves the entire circumference of the bone and is much more widespread than is a stress fracture (Figure 11-19). The thin linear sclerotic appearance of a trabecular stress fracture should be sufficiently characteristic to allow differentiation between the two lesions. Sclerosing osteomyelitis will show

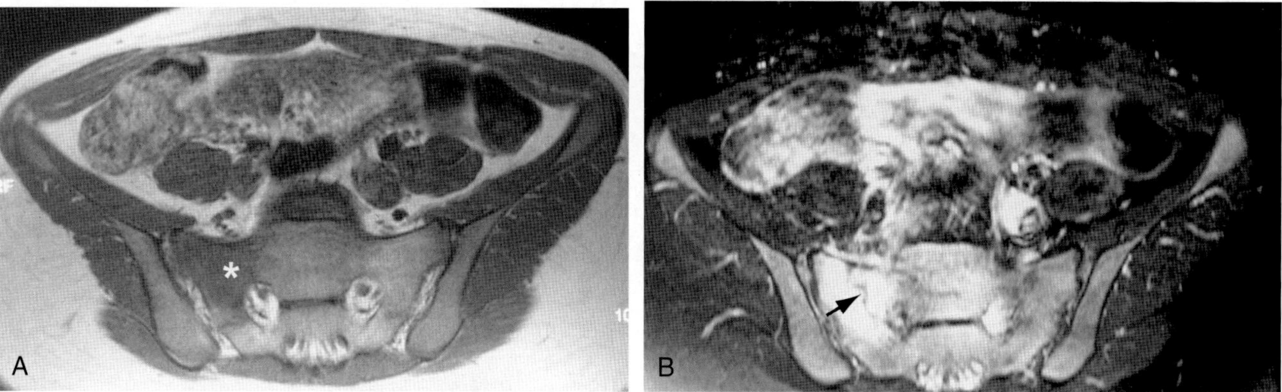

FIGURE 11-13. MR signal changes in sacral insufficiency fracture. This is the same patient as in Figure 11-10. **A,** T1-weighted image shows low signal in affected area *(asterisk)* replacing the normal bright fat. **B,** T2-weighted image shows the increased signal in the affected area owing to the edema with a low signal central fracture line *(arrow)*.

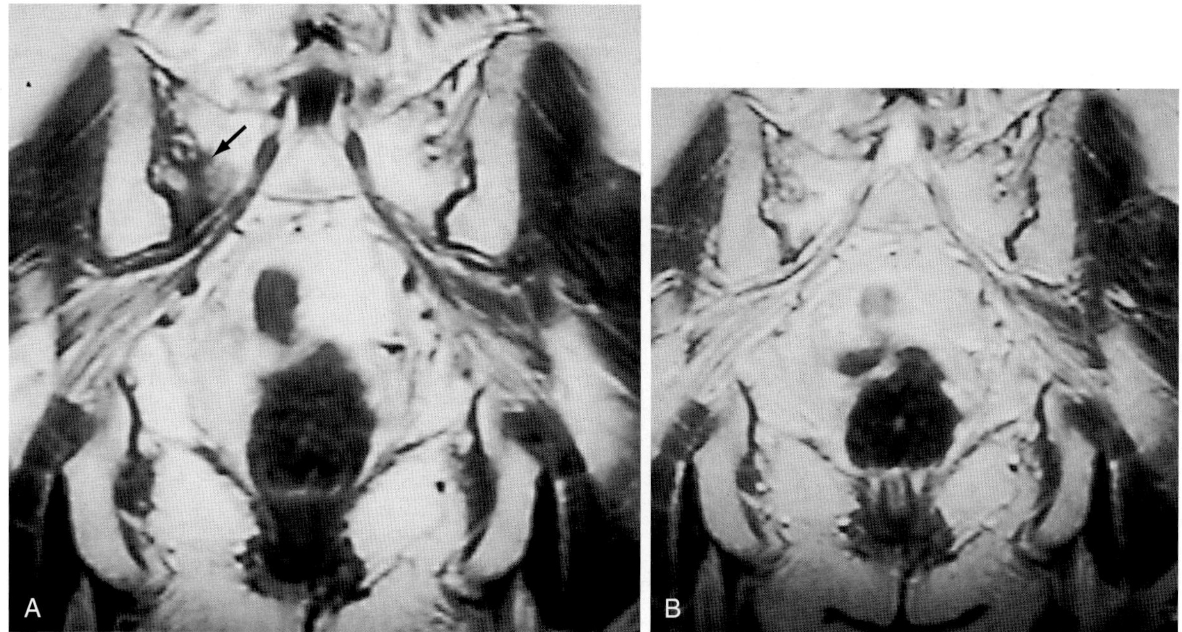

FIGURE 11-14. MR signal in sacral insufficiency fracture after gadolinium enhancement. **A,** T1-weighted coronal image shows a linear area of low signal representing the fracture and surrounding edema *(arrow)*. **B,** T1-weighted image following gadolinium administration shows an increase in signal in the affected area. The intense enhancement obscures the fracture.

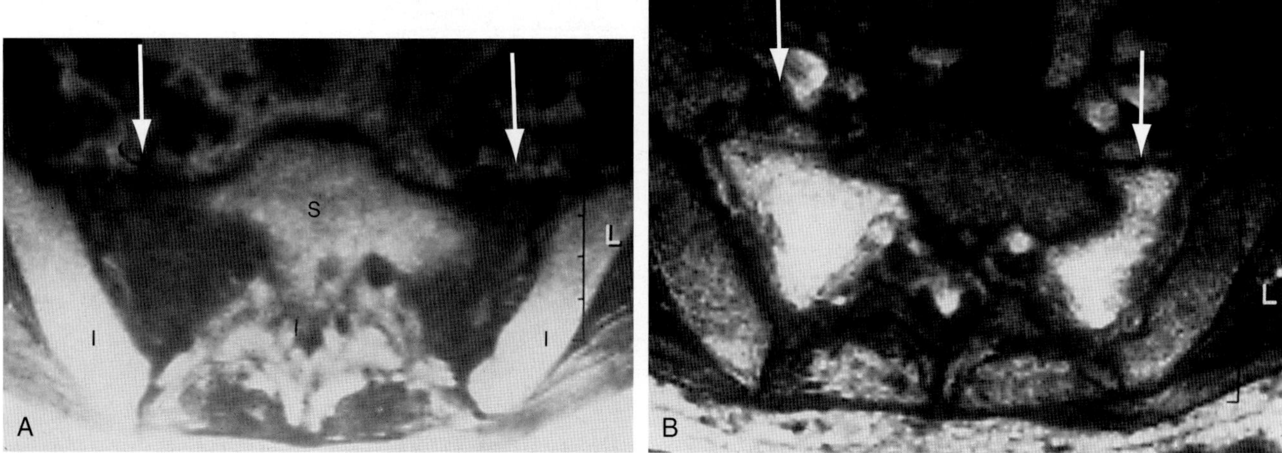

FIGURE 11-15. MR signal changes in a sacral insufficiency fracture using STIR sequence. This is the same patient as in Figure 11-11. **A,** T1-weighted axial image shows bilateral areas of low signal in the sacral ala. **B,** STIR sequence image shows intense signal increase in affected areas. *I,* Ilium; *S,* sacrum.

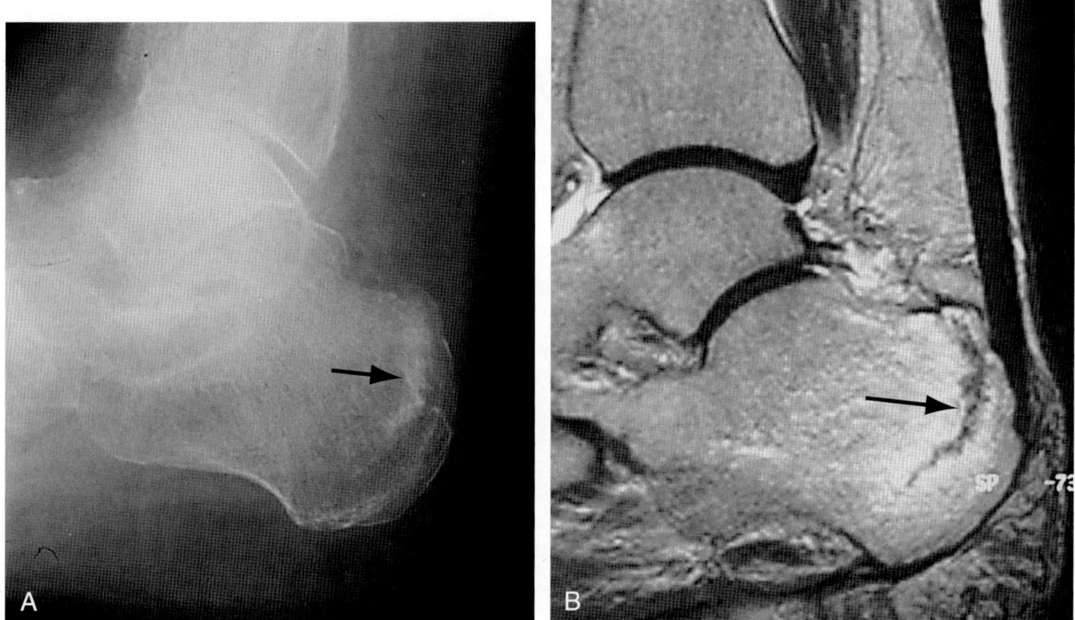

FIGURE 11-16. Healing calcaneal insufficiency fracture. **A,** Radiograph shows the linear area of condensing bone repair *(arrow)*, establishing the diagnosis of a fracture. **B,** T2-weighted sagittal image shows the fracture line *(arrow)* surrounded by a zone of edema. There is no added diagnostic value from this MRI study.

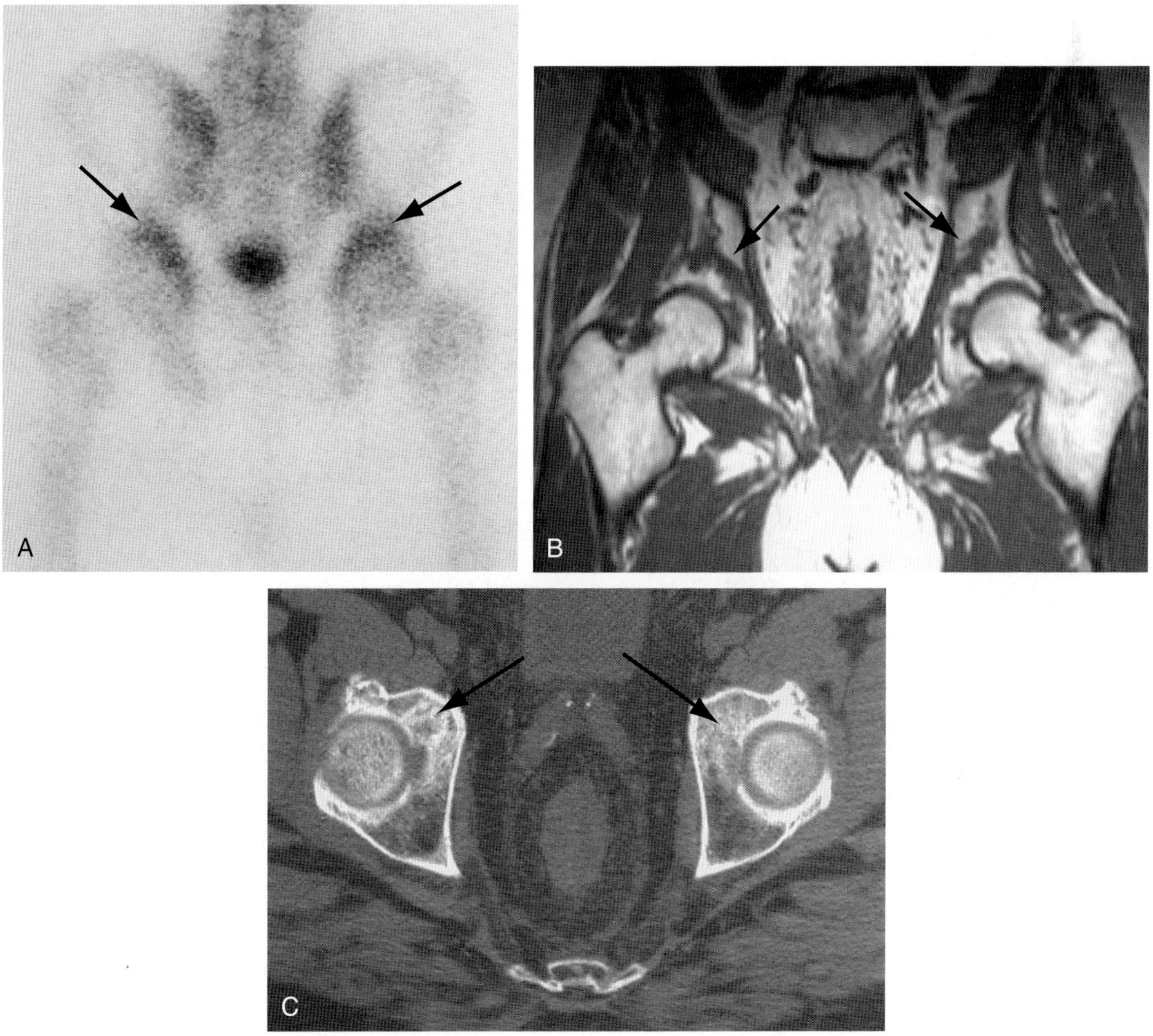

FIGURE 11-17. Bilateral acetabular insufficiency fractures demonstrated by MRI. The radiograph was normal. **A,** Radionuclide bone scan shows areas of bilateral increased tracer activity in the acetabula *(arrows)*. **B,** T1-weighted coronal MR image shows the fracture lines in both acetabula *(arrows)*. **C,** Axial CT image shows the sclerotic fracture lines *(arrows)*.

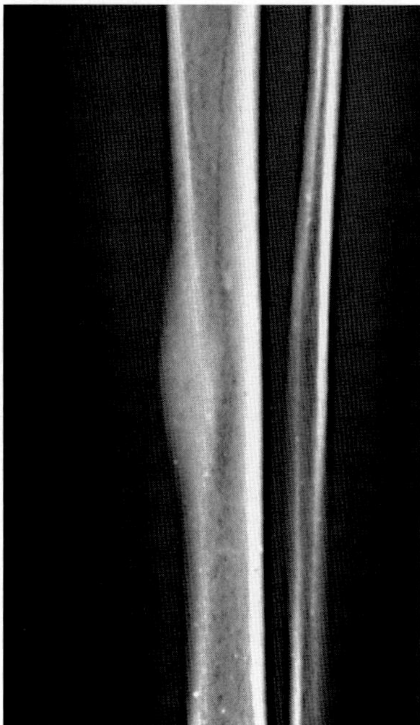

FIGURE 11-18. Osteoid osteoma of the mid-tibia. There is fusiform hyperostosis involving the endosteal as well as the periosteal surfaces of the bone. Stress fractures do not have this pattern.

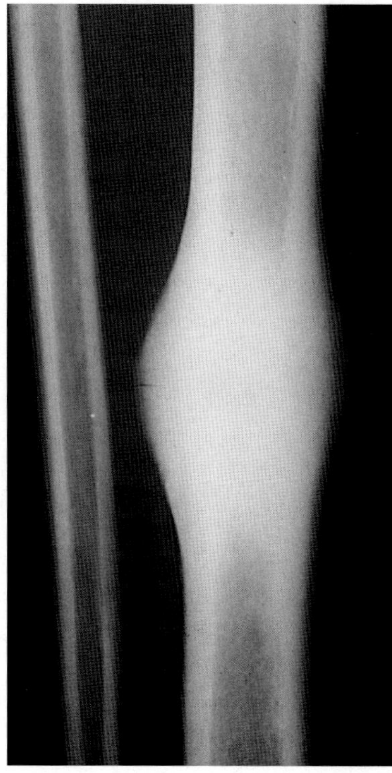

FIGURE 11-19. Sclerosing osteomyelitis. There is fusiform hyperostosis involving both sides of the tibia. The epicenter of the lesion is in the medullary cavity. Stress fractures do not have this appearance.

little or no change on serial radiographs, whereas the course of stress fracture rapidly evolves over several weeks.

Looser zones or osteoid seams are insufficiency fractures that occur in patients with osteomalacia. They occur more commonly in adults than in children. Looser zones typically occur as lucencies

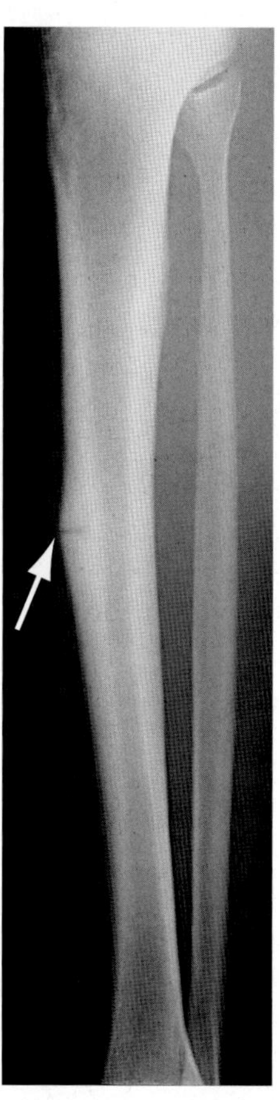

FIGURE 11-20. Anterior tibial stress fracture in a basketball player. The fracture *(arrow)* is perpendicular to the long axis of the bone. There is normal bone density. Looser zones have similar appearances, with the added features of decreased bone density, blurred trabeculae, some poorly defined callus, and often stigmata of renal osteodystrophy (hyperparathyroidism, rugger jersey spine, soft tissue calcification).

perpendicular to the cortex of the bone. They may be differentiated from a stress fracture (Figure 11-20) by the fact that they are associated with typical findings of osteomalacia such as decreased bone density, blurring of the trabeculae, and occasionally bowing of the long bones. Because nearly all of these affected patients have chronic renal disease, other manifestations such as hyperparathyroidism or "rugger jersey spine" may be encountered. From a historical standpoint, Milkman described what he thought was a new disease in 1934 when he published a case of osteomalacia with "multiple spontaneous idiopathic symmetrical fractures." What he really described were insufficiency fractures.[39]

Stress fractures may also be confused with metastases or pathologic fractures.[40] Although insufficiency fractures in the sacrum and pelvis have been described in the recent radiologic literature,[10,31,34,41] there still is a general lack of appreciation for them on the part of clinicians and radiologists. These fractures may be confused with other lesions if there is bony resorption at the fracture ends (Figure 11-21). The typical patient is one with a known pelvic malignancy who developed sudden onset of low back, hip, or groin pain. Trivial stresses such as walking may produce them. However, because of the vertical and linear orientation of these fractures in the sacrum, the imaging findings may be highly suggestive of the correct diagnosis (see Figure 11-13). CT is confirmatory and shows, in addition to the fracture line, sclerosis indicating

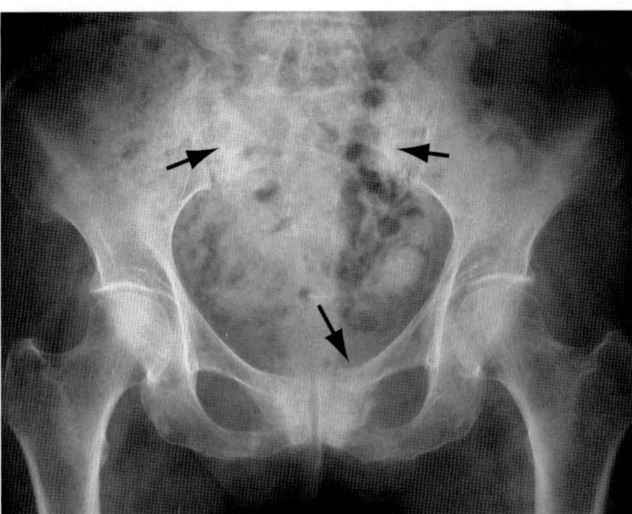

FIGURE 11-21. Insufficiency fractures in a patient with previous pelvic malignancy. The sacral fractures show sclerosis *(short arrows)*. The left pubic fracture has bizarre bone reaction *(long arrow)* suggesting malignancy. A follow-up radiograph 1 week later showed further healing of the pubic fracture without evidence of bone destruction to indicate malignancy.

healing. Radiographs are of little help because the faint callus is obscured by overlying bowel gas and content.

Pathologic fractures occur due to weakening of the bone by an underlying lesion. Therefore, on MRI, the underlying marrow lesion is usually well defined and there is frequently adjacent soft tissue extension. Stress fractures, on the other hand, show marrow edema that is poorly defined. There is associated edema in the adjacent soft tissues. There is no evidence of marrow or soft tissue invasion.[40]

Osteosarcoma and occasionally Ewing's tumor are often listed in the differential diagnosis for stress fractures. However, their appearance is sufficiently characteristic that they should not be confused with stress fractures. Osteosarcomas are typically located in the metaphysis of the involved bone and have a "moth-eaten" lytic pattern of destruction, sclerosis due to accompanying tumor bone and an aggressive, often spiculated, and irregular periosteal reaction. The lytic destructive appearance of Ewing's tumor, particularly in the diaphysis of a long bone, is usually sufficiently characteristic of an aggressive lesion to not be confused with a benign stress fracture. Both of these lesions show MRI findings that are typical of malignant bone sarcomas such as extensive marrow infiltration, cortical breakthrough, and extension into the adjacent soft tissues. Stress fractures have none of these features.

REFERENCES

1. Daffner RH, Pavlov H: Stress fractures: current concepts, *AJR Am J Roentgenol* 159:245-252, 1992.
2. Anderson MW, Greenspan A: Stress fractures, *Radiology* 199:1-12, 1996.
3. Bennell KL, Brukner PD: Epidemiology and site specificity of stress fractures, *Clin Sports Med* 16:179-196, 1997.
4. Reeder MT, Dick BH, Atkins JK et al: Stress fractures: current concepts of diagnosis and treatment, *Sports Med* 22:198-212, 1996.
5. Umans H, Pavlov H: Stress fractures of the lower extremities, *Semin Roentgenol* 29:176-193, 1994.
6. Matheson GO, Clement DB, McKenzie DC et al: Stress fractures in athletes: a study of 320 cases, *Am J Sports Med* 15:46-58, 1987.
7. Keating JF, Beggs I, Thorpe GW: Three cases of longitudinal stress fracture of the tibia, *Acta Orthop Scand* 66:41-42, 1995.
8. Kiss ZS, Khan KM, Fuller PJ: Stress fractures of the tarsal navicular bone: CT findings in 55 cases, *AJR Am J Roentgenol* 160:111-115, 1993.
9. DeSmet AA, Neff JR: Pubic and sacral insufficiency fractures: clinical course and radiologic findings, *AJR Am J Roentgenol* 145:601-606, 1985.
10. Blomlie V, Lien HH, Iversen T et al: Radiation-induced insufficiency fractures of the sacrum: evaluation with MR imaging, *Radiology* 188:241-244, 1993.
11. Mumber MP, Greven KM, Haygood TM: Pelvic insufficiency fractures associated with radiation atrophy: clinical recognition and diagnostic evaluation, *Skeletal Radiol* 26:94-99, 1997.
12. Devas MB: Stress fractures, London, 1975, Churchill Livingstone.
13. Chamay A, Tschants P: Mechanical influence in bone remodeling: experimental research on Wolff's law, *J Biomech* 5:173-180, 1972.
14. Carter DR, Caler WE: Cycle-dependent and time-dependent bone fracture with repeated loading, *J Biomech Eng* 105:166-170, 1983.
15. Wright TM, Hayes WC: The fracture mechanics of fatigue crack propagation in compact bone, *J Biomed Mater Res* 7:637-648, 1976.
16. Daffner RH, Martinez S, Gehweiler JA Jr et al: Stress fractures of the proximal tibia in runners, *Radiology* 142:63-65, 1982.
17. Brooks DB, Burstein AH, Frankel VH: The biomechanics of torsional fractures: the stress concentration of a drill hole, *J Bone Joint Surg (Am)* 52:507-514, 1970.
18. Danon G, Pokrassa M: An unusual complication of the Keller bunionectomy: spontaneous stress fractures of all lesser metatarsals, *J Foot Surg* 28:335-339, 1989.
19. Crotty JG, Berlin SJ, Donick II: Stress fracture of the first metatarsal after Keller bunionectomy, *J Foot Surg* 28:516-520, 1989.
20. Nattiv A, Armsey TD Jr: Stress injury to bone in the female athlete, *Clin Sports Med* 16:197-224, 1997.
21. Coady CM, Micheli LJ: Stress fractures in the pediatric athlete, *Clin Sports Med* 16:225-238, 1997.
22. Grier D, Wardell S, Sarwark J et al: Fatigue fractures of the sacrum in children: two case reports and a review of the literature, *Skeletal Radiol* 22:515-518, 1993.
23. Haasbeek JF, Green NE: Adolescent stress fractures of the sacrum: two case reports, *J Pediatr Orthop* 14:336-338, 1994.
24. Miller B, Markheim HR, Towbin MN: Multiple stress fractures in rheumatoid arthritis, *J Bone Joint Surg (Am)* 49:1408-1414, 1967.
25. Schneider R, Kaye JJ: Insufficiency and stress fractures of the long bones occurring in patients with rheumatoid arthritis, *Radiology* 116:595-600, 1975.
26. Abe H, Nakamura S, Takahashi S et al: Radiation-induced insufficiency fractures of the pelvis: evaluation with 99mTc-methylene diphosphonate scintigraphy, *AJR Am J Roentgenol* 158:599-602, 1992.
27. Mulligan ME: The "gray cortex": an early sign of stress fracture, *Skeletal Radiol* 24:201-203, 1995.
28. Geslien GE, Thrall JH, Espinosa JL et al: Early detection of stress fractures using 99mTc-polyphosphate, *Radiology* 121:683-687, 1976.
29. Wilcox JR, Moniot AL, Green JP: Bone scanning in the evaluation of exercise related stress injuries, *Radiology* 123:699-703, 1977.
30. Roub LW, Gumerman LW, Hanley EN Jr: Bone stress: a radionuclide imaging perspective, *Radiology* 132:431-438, 1979.
31. Daffner RH, Fedyshin PJ: Insufficiency fractures of the sacrum, *Emerg Radiol* 8:59-64, 2001.
32. Brahme SK, Cervilla V, Vint V et al: Magnetic resonance appearance of sacral insufficiency fractures, *Skeletal Radiol* 19:489-493, 1990.
33. Blomlie V, Rofstad EK, Talle K et al: Incidence of radiation-induced insufficiency fractures of the female pelvis: evaluation with MR imaging, *AJR Am J Roentgenol* 167:1205-1210, 1996.
34. Grangier C, Garcia J, Howarth NR et al: Role of MRI in the diagnosis of insufficiency fractures of the sacrum and acetabular roof, *Skeletal Radiol* 26:517-524, 1997.
35. Hosono M, Kobayashi H, Fujimoto R et al: MR appearance of parasymphyseal insufficiency fractures of the os pubis, *Skeletal Radiol* 26:525-528, 1998.
36. Tyrell PNM, Davies AM: Magnetic resonance imaging appearances of fatigue fractures of the long bones of the lower limb, *Br J Radiol* 67:332-338, 1994.
37. Umans HR, Kaye JJ: Longitudinal stress fractures of the tibia: diagnosis by magnetic resonance imaging, *Skeletal Radiol* 25:319-324, 1996.
38. Otte MT, Helms CA, Fritz RC: MR imaging of supra-acetabular insufficiency fractures, *Skeletal Radiol* 26:279-283, 1997.
39. Milkman LA: Multiple spontaneous idiopathic symmetrical fractures, *AJR Am J Roentgenol* 32:622-634, 1934.
40. Fayad LM, Kawamoto S, Kamel IR et al: Distinction of long bone stress fractures from pathologic fractures on cross-sectional imaging: how successful are we? *AJR Am J Roentgenol* 185:915-924, 2005.
41. Moreno A, Clemente J, Concepción C et al. Pelvic insufficiency fractures in patients with pelvic irradiation, *Int J Radiat Oncol Biol Phys* 44:61-66, 1999.

CHAPTER 12

Traumatic Muscle Injuries

TARA LAWRIMORE, MD, FRCPC, *and* WILLIAM PALMER, MD

KEY FACTS

- Muscle is a dynamic tissue that can be subject to direct and indirect traumatic injuries.
- Type 1 muscle fibers contain more numerous mitochondria, enabling longer, sustained contractions that are more resistant to fatigue (e.g., soleus). Type 2 fibers elicit faster, shorter, more powerful contractions, which are optimal for short energy bursts and tend to hypertrophy with training (e.g., hamstring muscles).
- In skeletally immature individuals, the apophyseal growth plate represents the weakest point along the myotendinous unit.
- Delayed-onset muscle soreness is a symptom of exercise-induced, indirect muscle damage that typically begins gradually, approximately 8 to 12 hours postexercise.
- Myotendinous strain injuries are among the most common activity-related indirect traumatic muscle injuries. Acute injury occurs at the myotendinous junction and is classified as first degree (stretch injury), second degree (partial tear), or third degree (complete rupture).
- Direct traumatic muscle injuries include contusions and lacerations.
- Tendinopathy denotes a continuum of disorders of the tendon including degeneration (tendinosis), partial tear, and complete rupture, which develop over an extended period of time.
- Complications of traumatic muscle injuries include hematoma formation, myonecrosis, and myositis ossificans.
- Calcification in myositis ossificans may take at least 6 to 8 weeks to be seen, making follow-up radiographs or computed tomography useful. Because calcification is difficult to see on magnetic resonance imaging, the appearance of myositis ossificans may be confused with other lesions including tumors.

The late 20th and early 21st century societies have seen an increase in consumer health consciousness and physical fitness as individuals are in constant pursuit of longer and healthier lives. It is generally widely accepted, and evidence continues to show that physical activity is associated with overall good mental and biologic health.[1] A regular exercise regimen is associated with reduced risk of death and morbidity from a number of major diseases including cardiovascular, which has ranked as the number one cause of mortality in society for a number of years.[2,3] Coincident with a rise in the so-called baby boomer and elderly generations, an increasing number of individuals are engaging in exercise and participating in sports, activities that have traditionally been associated more with the adolescent, young adult, amateur, or professional athlete. Although health benefits are seen with moderate, well-balanced activity programs, enthusiastic and sometimes overzealous "weekend warriors" challenge themselves and the limits of their anatomy to the breaking point, literally. Pain and disability result as a consequence of traumatic injury, which is often muscular in nature.

This chapter focuses on the spectrum of traumatic muscle injuries. A large percentage of traumatic muscle injuries are frequently clearly associated with precipitating activity, as in the setting of the acute muscle strains. More direct forms of traumatic muscle injuries include lacerations and contusions. Although imaging plays a limited role in diagnosis in the acute setting when a clear temporal relationship between an activity or direct injury correlates with the onset of pain and loss of function, it may assist in grading the extent and severity of injury. Imaging may assist in treatment planning, performance prognosis, and evaluation of delayed complications such as myositis ossificans. In clinical circumstances where confounding history or delayed presentation hinders the practitioner's diagnosis, imaging may play a crucial role in patient assessment. For instance, a number of neoplastic or inflammatory conditions can frequently masquerade as muscle injury. For these reasons, patients are often referred for imaging evaluation.

In order to recognize the appearance of traumatic muscle injuries, one must have an understanding of the normal anatomic structure and organization of muscle, and this chapter will begin with an overview of muscle morphology and risk factors for muscle injury. Imaging techniques will be discussed briefly, with an emphasis on magnetic resonance (MR) technology as the imaging modality of choice. The remainder of the chapter will then address specific traumatic muscle injuries. Common acute injuries to skeletal muscle include strains and contusions. The importance of myotendinous strain will be emphasized, given that this represents the most frequently encountered form of traumatic muscle injury in clinical practice.[4]

ANATOMIC CONSIDERATIONS AND RISK FACTORS

Muscle is a biologic tissue whose structure is uniquely tailored for force generation and movement. Based on percentage mass, muscle is the single largest tissue in the body, comprising up to 50% of the total body weight in some individuals.[5] The basic structural unit of muscle is the myofiber, which consists of a multinucleated cell that is the smallest complete contractile system. In the maturation of muscle fibers, a unique characteristic metabolic profile may develop, dividing structural muscle units into type 1 and type 2 fibers. Every muscle is composed on a combination of both types of fibers in varying percentages that helps to define its metabolism. Type 1 fibers contain more numerous mitochondria, enabling longer, sustained contractions that are more resistant to fatigue. A good example of muscle dominant in type 1 fibers would include a postural muscle such as the soleus. Type 2 fibers elicit faster, shorter, more powerful contractions, which are optimal for short energy bursts and tend to hypertrophy with training, as in the hamstring muscles.

Numerous myofibers are bundled into fascicles, which in turn are grouped into the entities we recognize as individually named muscles. Highly compartmentalized skeletal muscles are architecturally arranged in a manner to establish their functional properties, which in the majority of instances is to produce joint motion.[6] Compartmentalized muscle is generally bounded by fascia, a tough connective tissue investment. In addition to maintaining the structural integrity of muscle, fascia plays an important role in the pathogenesis of muscle disorders such as muscle herniation and compartment syndrome and influences the patterns of spread of neoplastic and infectious processes.[7]

Muscles function to produce movement by acting across joints. Most muscles cross one joint, but a number of muscles span two joints. Methods of generating force across joints include concentric and eccentric muscle contractions. Concentric contraction occurs when the load acting on the muscle is less than the maximum tetanic tension generated by that muscle, resulting in active muscle shortening, as one might witness with biceps curls. Eccentric contraction occurs when the force on a muscle increases beyond the maximum force that muscle is capable of generating, resulting in active muscle lengthening.

With respect to activity-related traumatic injuries, and with myotendinous strain injuries predominating, the most commonly affected muscles tend to involve those that cross two joints. As a result, these muscles are generally activated as they are being stretched, resulting in a propensity for eccentric contractions.[8,9] These muscles also tend to possess a greater proportion of type 2, fast twitch fibers. Muscles most susceptible to injury during rapid acceleration and speed activities based on these biomechanical and anatomic considerations include the hamstrings (i.e., semimembranosus), gastrocnemius, and rectus femoris.[10]

> Muscles that cross two joints, such as the hamstrings, are most susceptible to myotendinous strain injuries.

A multitude of other risk factors are known to play a role in traumatic and, more specifically, activity-related muscle injury. A history of muscle strain injury represents one of the most recognized risk factors for future insult to that muscle.[11] Inadequate or overzealous rehabilitation resulting in early return to activity before complete healing is another recognized risk factor for injury.[12] Poor conditioning, insufficient muscle strength, abrupt higher performance activity level, and increasing age are among some of the other known clinical risk factors.[13-15]

Risk factors for activity-related muscle injury include a history of muscle strain, return to activity before complete healing, poor conditioning, insufficient muscle strength, abrupt increase in activity level, and increasing age.

Another feature to be considered in muscle injuries is the viscoelasticity properties of skeletal muscle. A simplified explanation of this concept is that repetitive stretching of a muscle reduces the load on the muscle-tendon unit at any given length, thereby increasing its viscoelasticity profile. Viscoelasticity is also temperature dependent. These principles provide a simplified explanation for the way warm-up combined with stretching prior to exercise seems to be beneficial in improving the viscoelasticity profile of muscle that, in turn, is protective against strain injuries.[16,17]

Finally, in discussing the pathophysiology of traumatic muscle injuries, the importance of the myotendinous unit should be understood. The myotendinous unit consists of the muscle, the myotendinal (muscle-tendon) junction, the tendon, and the osseous attachment sites of the tendon. The myotendinous unit transmits the forces generated by muscles to their points of attachment to bone via the tendons of origin and insertion. When muscle injury occurs, the severity and location of injury along the entire myotendinous unit is influenced by a multitude of factors, including age; the rate, magnitude, and duration of stress loading; and the presence of underlying disorders such as tendinopathy.[18] Normal tendons without underlying disease are much stronger than either their osseous attachment sites or the myotendinal junction.[19]

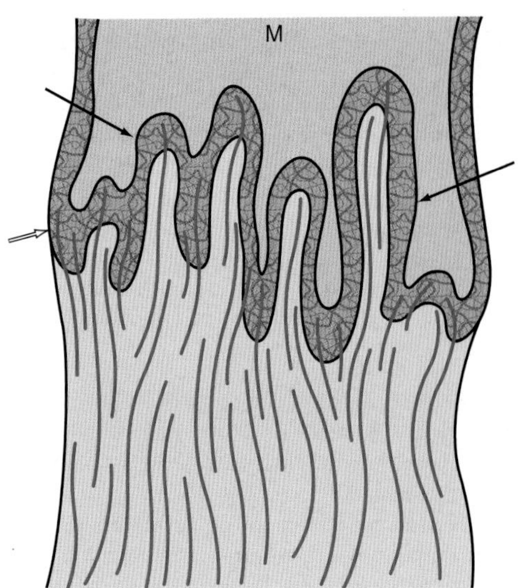

FIGURE 12-1. Schematic drawing demonstrating the ultrastructure of the myotendinal junction. Each muscle cell *(M)* has a thick basement membrane *(open arrow)* covering multiple finger-like processes *(black arrows)*. Collagen fibrils from the tendon insert deeply between the processes and penetrate the basement membrane. This ultrastructure allows for an increased contact area between myocytes and tendon, resulting in dissipation of forces during muscle contraction and protection of the myotendinal junction from strain injury.

The myotendinal junction contains interdigitating tendinous fibers amongst finger-like processes of skeletal muscle linked by a thick basement membrane[20] (Figure 12-1). Despite its complex ultrastructure, the myotendinal junction represents the relative weak point of the normal myotendinous unit. The myotendinal junction possesses poor intrinsic viscoelastic properties and lower capacity for energy absorption when compared with muscle, tendon, or its osseous attachments, thereby placing it at great risk for acute strain injury.[18]

> The myotendinous junction is the area most vulnerable to acute strain injury.

IMAGING CONSIDERATIONS IN THE DIAGNOSIS OF TRAUMATIC MUSCLE INJURIES

Acute traumatic muscle injuries are mostly self-limited and generally do not require imaging for diagnosis or management.[21] The diagnosis begins with a careful history, taking close note of the relationship of onset of symptoms with the occurrence of trauma. Physical examination is confirmatory when there is evidence of swelling or ecchymosis and functional muscle testing reveals a loss or limitation of function supporting the clinical history. However, there are certain clinical circumstances where imaging might provide important information to the evaluating clinician (Box 12-1). For example, in high-performance or professional athletes, imaging may help to determine whether a conservative treatment regimen or surgical repair is indicated. Imaging in these instances helps to grade the severity and localize the extent of injury.[22,23] The additional information garnered through imaging helps in assessing the

BOX 12-1. Some Indications for Imaging Muscle Injury

In a high-performance athlete to determine whether conservative or surgical treatment is appropriate
Determining the presence of underlying tendinopathy
Muscle pain or mass of uncertain cause
Detecting complications of muscle injury (hematoma, herniation, myositis ossificans)

individual's risk of possible re-injury if an insufficient treatment regimen is prescribed.[24] Another situation whereby imaging plays an important role is in determining the presence of underlying tendinopathy as a potential risk factor for future injury.[25] Muscle pain or a soft tissue mass of uncertain etiology in the setting of confounding history or without a specific inciting traumatic incident would also be important to assess with imaging, as specific findings may direct the radiologist to suggest an unsuspected muscle injury (rather than a tumor) as a source.[26] Finally, potential complications of muscle injuries, such as hematoma, herniation, and myositis ossificans, can also be evaluated by imaging.[27]

The imaging of traumatic muscle injuries, as in all facets of musculoskeletal imaging, has evolved over the past several decades. Radiography can be helpful in the acute setting if associated bony injury is also suspected. This technique can be useful in the assessment of apophyseal avulsion injuries that frequently occur in children and adolescents. Chronic sequelae of muscle injury may also be seen and diagnosed using radiographs, as in the case of myositis ossificans. Bone scintigraphy can be more sensitive than radiography in detecting early stages of myositis ossificans.[28] However, radiography and bone scintigraphy are limited by their inability to fully characterize soft tissue abnormalities.

Computed tomography (CT) is an important adjunctive procedure in the evaluation and diagnosis of musculoskeletal trauma. It is generally widely available, easy and fast to perform, and capable of providing multiplanar and three-dimensional image reconstructions. CT is superior to radiography in the imaging of complex osseous trauma and does add some further characterization of soft tissues that is far superior to that of radiography. The disadvantages of CT include its use of ionizing radiation and its improved but less than ideal soft tissue representation that is limited in terms of detail and specific lesion characterization when compared with other modalities available, such as ultrasound and magnetic resonance imaging (MRI).[29] However, CT offers its greatest advantage in being able to demonstrates soft tissue calcifications that are frequently overlooked by MRI.

Ultrasound is a very versatile imaging tool that is highly adaptable to clinical practice and assessment of muscle. Traumatic muscle injuries such as complete tendon ruptures or intramuscular hematomas from direct or indirect injuries can be assessed. Generally, ultrasound evaluation of muscle is ideally performed with high-frequency (5 to 10 MHz) linear array transducers. Deeper-seated muscle abnormalities may require the use of a low frequency (2 to 4 MHz) curvilinear probe. The field of view (FOV) can be a limitation for ultrasound in the imaging of relatively larger muscles groups; the introduction of extended FOV imaging helps to improve the accuracy and representation of spatial relationships within muscles.[30,31] However, with the advent of MRI, exquisite anatomic detail and characterization of soft tissues with a large FOV to incorporate imaging of an entire limb segment has made this modality one of the best suited for evaluation of traumatic muscle injuries, which are frequently soft tissue in nature. MRI is highly sensitive to hemorrhage and edema that may result from muscle injury, also making it the imaging method of choice for muscles, tendons, and ligaments.[32]

TECHNICAL CONSIDERATIONS AND PRINCIPLES OF MRI IN TRAUMATIC MUSCLE INJURIES

Standard MRI Protocol

The goal of imaging is to identify, localize, and characterize abnormalities, which are predominantly soft tissue in nature with respect to traumatic muscle injuries. There are general imaging principles that may be applied with respect to designing a protocol suitable for imaging of muscle. First, a capsule may be placed over the patient's point of maximal symptoms to help localize the abnormality. Longitudinal (long axis) and orthogonal transverse (short axis) planes should be included in all imaging studies. The longitudinal plane is used to identify an abnormality and determine its length. The orientation of the longitudinal plane varies according to the location of the suspected lesion relative to bone. For lesions anterior or posterior in location, sagittal imaging is favored, whereas coronal imaging is preferred for lesions at the medial or lateral aspects of the limb. The transverse plane aids in additional lesion localization and establishing its anatomic relationship to adjacent structures, such as the myotendinous junction and neurovascular bundle. The FOV should be large enough to allow visualization of the full length of the lesion in question. In the thigh or lower leg, the FOV may be expanded as such to include the asymptomatic side for comparison. This aids in the detection of subtle, asymmetric abnormalities in the symptomatic leg and also allows for assessment of subtle changes in overall muscle bulk that can help to determine the chronicity of the injury.

Once protocol imaging planes are established, pulse sequences are prescribed to characterize tissue according to its T1 and T2 relaxation properties. A combination of pulse sequences may be used, and at least one should employ a fat-suppression technique. For example, when evaluating a suspected muscle abnormality in the thigh, a combination of T1-weighted and inversion recovery (IR) fast spin echo (FSE) sequences can demonstrate most lesions. Fat-suppressed T2-weighted images may also be used to supplement IR pulse sequences. The T1-weighted sequences optimize depiction of fat and normal anatomic planes. Inconspicuous areas of edema, hemorrhage, and intramuscular lesions that cannot be detected on T1-weighted sequences are often better evaluated on IR images. Because of its outstanding sensitivity to edema and subtle abnormalities, the IR or fat-suppressed T2-weighted images are best suited for detecting most pathologic changes. Transverse imaging may employ a combination of T2-weighted and high-resolution fat-suppressed proton density sequences.

Specialized Adjuncts to Routine MRI

Supplemental sequences can be added to a routine protocol as additional tools for further injury or lesion characterization. Gradient-echo images with T2* weighting accentuate certain paramagnetic effects. The most useful application of this technique is increased conspicuity of the blood product hemosiderin, whose paramagnetic properties result in an accentuated "blooming" effect.

> Hemosiderin is low in signal on all pulse sequences but is particularly prominent on gradient echo sequences.

These distinctive findings can help to identify and demonstrate myotendinous abnormalities related to remote strain.

Intravenous administration of gadolinium-based contrast material is not routinely necessary as an aid to the diagnosis of muscle injury. In certain circumstances, it can assist in distinguishing between solid and necrotic lesions or may assist in assessing for enhancing components indicating potentially hemorrhagic neoplasm that could masquerade as an intramuscular hematoma. Areas of myonecrosis (muscle infarction), a potential complication of a traumatic muscle injury, could also be detected as areas that do not enhance after intravenous contrast administration.

TRAUMATIC MUSCLE INJURIES: SPECIFIC CONDITIONS

An extensive array and wide spectrum of injuries may be associated with trauma to skeletal muscle. A practical approach to muscle trauma is to categorize injuries in terms of mechanism as direct or indirect (Box 12-2). In direct injuries, as implied, a force is contiguously applied to muscle resulting in immediate trauma to the underlying tissue as may occur with laceration, contusion, or pressure necrosis. Indirect injuries occur through a more complex mechanism of action and dissipation of forces than may be seen with myotendinous strain injuries during forceful eccentric muscle contractions. The remainder of the chapter will focus on various imaging features of the most common traumatic muscle injuries and the potential complications that may arise as a result of such injuries.

Indirect Muscle Injury

Exercise and Delayed-Onset Muscle Soreness

Muscle pain, tenderness, and swelling that develop approximately 24 hours following an unfamiliar or unaccustomed exercise or activity is a common experience for both the elite athlete and the deconditioned "couch potato." The symptoms, which can range from mild tenderness to functionally limiting pain, are usually referred to as *delayed-onset muscle soreness* (DOMS).[33,34] There is no specific instant at which an injury occurs, nor is there generally one particular moment of trauma or acute onset of pain recalled by the patient. Rather, DOMS is a symptom of exercise-induced, indirect muscle damage that typically begins gradually, approximately 8 to 12 hours postexercise. Activities that consist of predominantly eccentric muscle action have the potential to cause this condition. Soreness continues to increase, especially when the affected muscle contracts, stretches, or is palpated, culminating in maximal symptoms at about 2 to 3 days after the activity. Symptoms then slowly dissipate by approximately 1 week. Although the precise mechanism remains uncertain, it is generally thought that DOMS is caused by reversible ultrastructural damage and inflammation mediated through a variety of physiologic factors and is usually self-limited.[35]

BOX 12-2. Traumatic Muscle Injuries: Specific Conditions

DIRECT	INDIRECT
Contusion	Exercise (DOMS)
Laceration	Avulsion: apophyseal or tendinous
Pressure necrosis	Myotendinous strain

DOMS can be commonly seen in muscle groups such as the quadriceps following downhill running or walking activities or the lower back muscles with stressful physical labor.[36] The MRI appearance of DOMS shows diffuse muscle swelling and intramuscular edematous changes as high signal intensity on T2-weighted or IR sequences[37] (Figure 12-2). An important practical fact to keep in mind is that exercise may also cause immediate, transient increases in signal intensity on MRI that may persist up to half an hour after the activity. This effect, which could be confused for pathologic edema or DOMS, is secondary to an increase in extracellular water that accompanies exercise.[38] Fortunately, most individuals are not usually imaged immediately following a workout on the elliptical machine.

The clinical diagnosis of DOMS is usually not a difficult one, but the diagnostician should be aware of this entity because muscle signal abnormalities on MRI may remain despite resolution of symptoms.[34] In addition, not infrequently, the T2 hyperintense muscle edema pattern can appear similar to findings seen in mild grade 1 myotendinous strain injuries. However, the lack of acute onset of symptoms with DOMS allows for easy clinical differentiation from myotendinous strain injuries.

Injuries of the Myotendinous Unit

Building upon the fundamentals of an understanding of myotendinous anatomic structures and considerations discussed earlier in the chapter, a pathophysiologic approach to the interpretation of imaging of myotendinal unit injuries may be applied. When an eccentric stretching force is applied to skeletal muscle, exceeding the capacity of the system, injury occurs somewhere along the myotendinal unit. A number of risk factors can influence the point at which an injury is likely to occur, and several of these have been alluded to previously in the chapter. For example, age is one

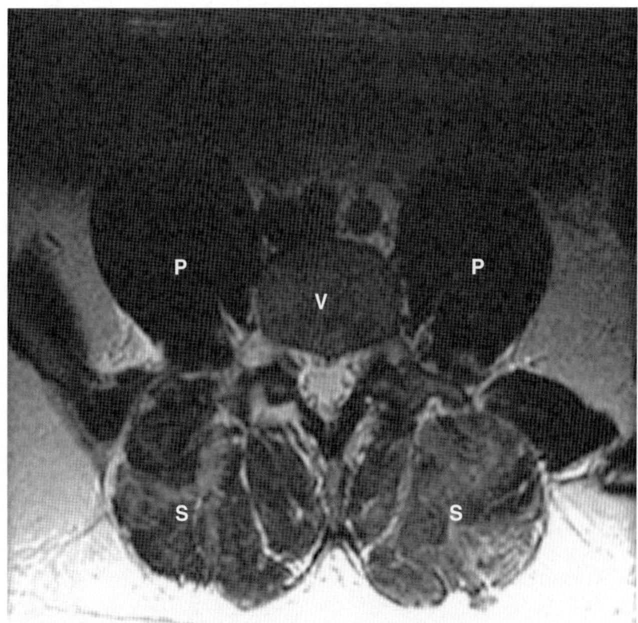

FIGURE 12-2. DOMS in a 57-year-old man 2 days after heavy lifting activities helping his son move into a college dormitory. Axial T2-weighted MR image shows feathery pattern of symmetrically increased signal intensity within the paraspinal musculature *(S)*. Although the imaging appearance of intramuscular edema is nonspecific and DOMS is a diagnosis of exclusion, the temporal relationship of a delayed onset of symptoms following unaccustomed physical activity suggests the diagnosis. *p*, Psoas muscle; *V*, vertebral body.

important factor to consider. In children and adolescents, the unfused apophysis serves as an attachment site for tendons to the central skeleton. When the apophyseal growth plate is open, it represents the weakest point along the bone-tendon-muscle interface. Therefore apophyseal avulsions are more likely to occur than other myotendinal injuries.

> In children, the unfused apophysis is more vulnerable to injury than the musculotendinous junction, explaining the higher incidence of avulsion injuries in this age group. In adults, the tendon is more vulnerable and an avulsion fracture should suggest an underlying bone abnormality such as metastasis.

As the apophysis fuses in young adults, biomechanical failure tends to involve the myotendinous junction at the muscle-tendon interface, which represents the weakest link and site of injury with forceful, eccentric, muscle contractions. In contrast, as the tendon itself becomes diseased, as may be seen in older adults or as a result of overuse or impingement syndromes, failure tends to occur at the level of the degenerated tendon or at its weakened attachment site to bone. It is thus important for radiologists and clinicians to be aware of how these factors influence the pattern and site of injury that occurs along the myotendinal chain of muscle, tendon, and bone.

Apophyseal Avulsion Injuries

Age is an important factor in determining the weakest point along the myotendinous unit. In skeletally immature individuals, the apophyseal growth plate represents the weakest point along the myotendinous unit and is frequently the site of injury. As the force generated by muscle exceeds the attachment of the apophysis to the skeleton, an apophyseal avulsion injury results.

The most frequent sites of apophyseal avulsion injuries occur around the pelvis (Box 12-3). Avulsion of the ischial apophysis by the hamstrings is common in dancers and runners. Other common sites associated with sprinting and kicking sports include the anterosuperior and anteroinferior iliac spines. Patients typically present with loss of function and localized tenderness at the avulsive injury site.[39]

Familiarity with the anatomy of the major tendinous attachments sites to bone is indispensable in arriving at the correct diagnosis.[40,41] In the acute phase, radiography is often diagnostic (Figure 12-3). A displaced apophyseal fracture fragment is usually evident unless the apophysis is not yet ossified or is only minimally displaced. In this instance, MRI may be beneficial. The findings on MRI are along a spectrum depending on the timing and severity of the injury. In minimally displaced avulsive injuries, localized edema with increased T2 hyperintense fluid signal cleft at the apophyseal junction might be the only indication of an injury (Figure 12-4). As the degree of displacement increases, abnormal signal in the muscle and surrounding soft tissues from hematoma

BOX 12-3. Common Sites of Avulsion Injuries: Pelvis

SITE OF TENDON-BONE ATTACHMENT	MUSCLE
Anterior superior iliac spine	Sartorius
Anterior inferior iliac spine	Rectus femoris
Ischial tuberosity	Hamstrings (semimembranosus, semitendinosis, biceps femoris)
Lesser trochanter of femur	Iliopsoas
Greater trochanter of femur	Gluteus medius

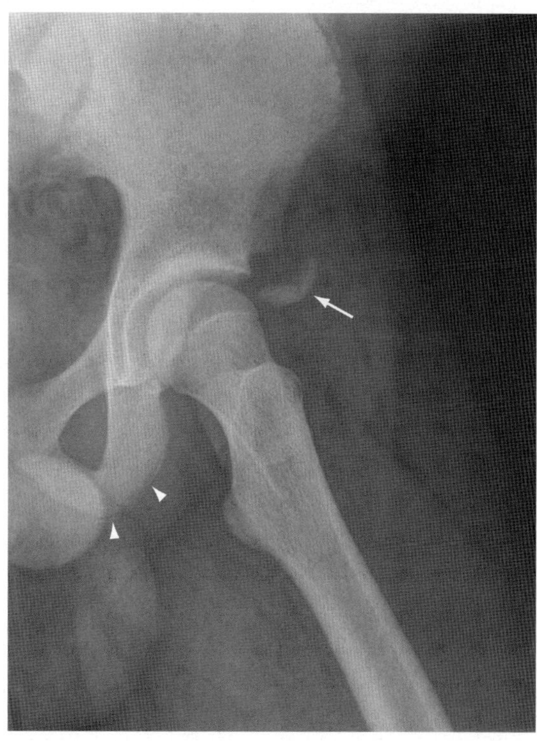

FIGURE 12-3. Acute apophyseal avulsion injury. Frog-leg lateral radiograph of the left hip in an adolescent male demonstrates an avulsed ossified apophyseal fragment *(arrow)* from the anterior inferior iliac spine at the rectus femoris origin. Note the normal ischial apophysis *(arrowheads)*.

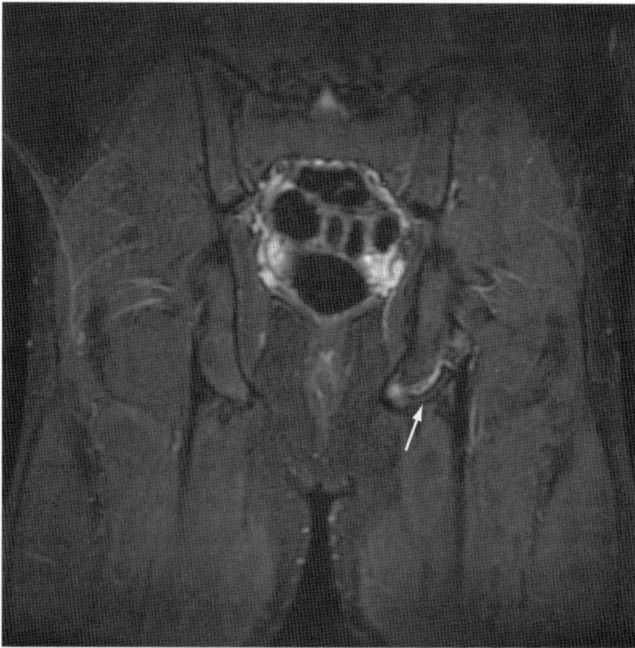

FIGURE 12-4. Nondisplaced apophyseal avulsion injury in a 16-year-old male. Coronal STIR image demonstrates a T2 hyperintense fluid cleft *(above the arrow)* separating the ischium from the apophyseal origin of the common hamstring tendon, consistent with a nondisplaced apophyseal avulsion injury.

and inflammation can be quite striking. Displaced bone fragments can also sometimes be difficult to identify by MRI alone.

Radiographs are important adjuncts to MRI because bone fragments and calcium deposits may be difficult to see on MRI.

In the subacute to chronic setting, osteolysis at the fracture (avulsion site) and callus formation can result in a mixed lytic and sclerotic appearance. If not significantly displaced from bone, the observer might mistake this appearance for an aggressive lesion, such as a bone neoplasm (i.e., osteosarcoma), or infection.[42] Radionuclide evaluation with a Tc99m MDP bone scan may also show localized increased uptake of radiopharmaceutical at the site of avulsive injury, which is nonspecific and should always be interpreted with concurrent radiographs[43] (Figure 12-5).

Myotendinous Strain Injuries

Myotendinous strain is a common form of indirect traumatic muscle injury occurring in sport and exercise-related settings. An acute strain occurs at the myotendinal junction because this represents the weakest point of the normal myotendinous unit, based on its poor intrinsic viscoelastic properties and lower energy absorption, as characterized earlier in our discussion regarding anatomic considerations of muscle injuries. Therefore, as an eccentric contraction and force exceeds the loading capacity of a long, fusiform muscle such as the hamstring, acute injury occurs at the myotendinous junction. It should be noted that ultrasonography, with proper technique and expertise, can be extremely useful for the assessment of myotendinous strain and is relatively inexpensive and widely available. However, MRI is also now widely available and accessible to most patients. Due to its superior soft tissue characterization and multiplanar capability, MRI is an ideal modality to localize, characterize, and grade the severity of myotendinous injury and will be highlighted in this section.

The severity of the strain injury depends on a number of factors, including the rate, magnitude, and duration of the loading force. Clinical grades of muscle strain injuries can range from a minor strain, where there is minimal loss of function, to a severe strain, in which there is complete loss of function. The MRI grade of myotendinous strain injuries parallels the clinical grade and is classified as a first-degree (stretch injury), second-degree (partial tear), or third-degree (complete rupture) injury[44] (Table 12-1).

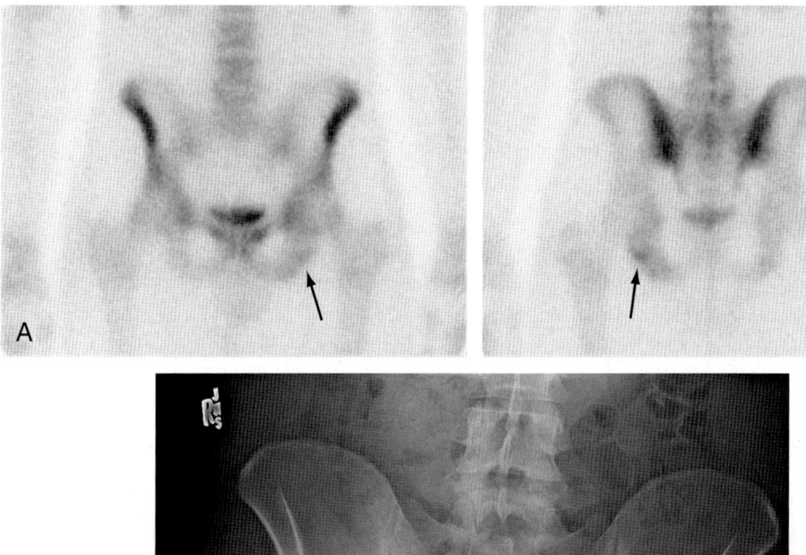

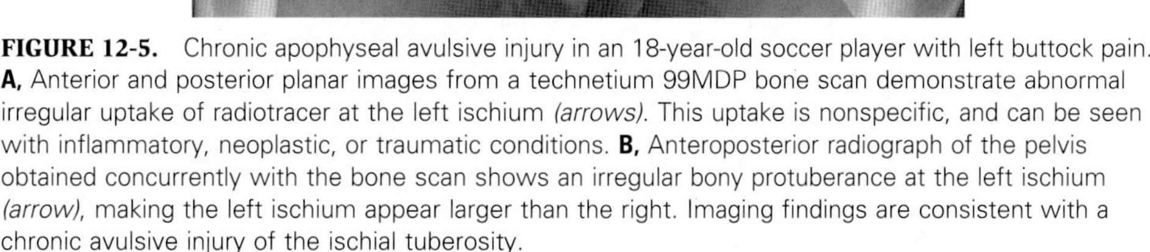

FIGURE 12-5. Chronic apophyseal avulsive injury in an 18-year-old soccer player with left buttock pain. **A,** Anterior and posterior planar images from a technetium 99MDP bone scan demonstrate abnormal irregular uptake of radiotracer at the left ischium *(arrows)*. This uptake is nonspecific, and can be seen with inflammatory, neoplastic, or traumatic conditions. **B,** Anteroposterior radiograph of the pelvis obtained concurrently with the bone scan shows an irregular bony protuberance at the left ischium *(arrow)*, making the left ischium appear larger than the right. Imaging findings are consistent with a chronic avulsive injury of the ischial tuberosity.

TABLE 12-1. Grading of Myotendinous Strain Injuries

Grade	Injury	Degree of Fiber Disruption
Grade 1 strain	Stretch	Microscopic
Grade 2	Partial tear	Macroscopic
Mild Moderate Severe		Less than one third Between one third and two thirds Greater than two thirds
Grade 3	Complete tear	Rupture

First-Degree Strain

In a first-degree strain, which represents a mild stretch injury characterized by microscopic fiber disruption, T2-weighted and short tau inversion recovery (STIR) images through the involved muscle demonstrate high signal intensity edema and hemorrhage in the acute setting, centered at and surrounding the myotendinous junction (Figure 12-6). A feathery pattern of edema may also be seen as fluid and blood dissipates along the muscle fascicles.[45] The tendon is intact, and T1-weighted sequences are usually normal in appearance. Patients with first-degree strains generally heal following conservative treatment and rest without any functional impairment. Imaging abnormalities also resolve completely.

The location of the edema at the myotendinous junction is a characteristic feature of muscle strain injury and helps differentiate it from other abnormalities such as tumors.

Second-Degree Strain

As the severity of injury increases, partial, macroscopic tearing of the myotendinous junction occurs and characterizes a second-degree strain. Depending on the severity of the injury and extent of fiber disruption, functional impairment may ensue and patients may continue to have long-term pain and weakness. The severity of the tear can be subclassified as low grade (mild) if less than one third of the fibers are disrupted and high grade (severe) if greater than two thirds are torn, with injuries in between one third to two thirds torn falling in the moderate category.[46]

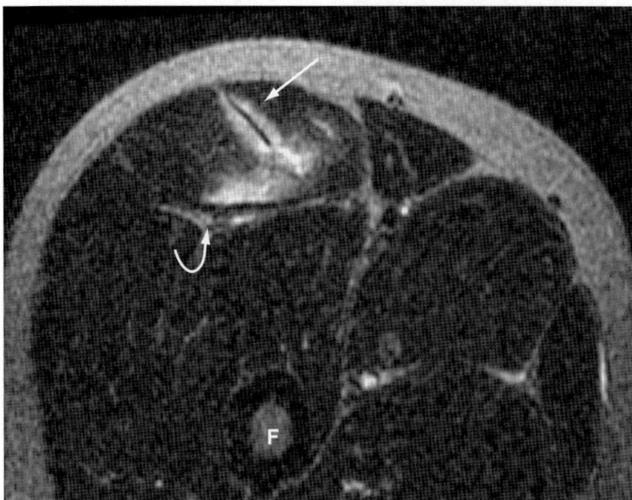

FIGURE 12-6. Grade 1 rectus femoris strain involving the proximal *(straight arrow)* and distal *(curved arrow)* myotendinous junctions in a 21-year-old hurdler. Axial gradient echo image through the thigh shows high signal intensity edema and hemorrhage surrounding the proximal, centrally positioned and distal, more deeply positioned myotendinous junctions. The location of the edema (bright signal) around the tendon (linear dark signal) is typical for a strain injury. *F,* Femur.

The MRI appearance will vary depending on the severity and acuity of the injury. In the acute setting, MRI will continue to demonstrate high signal intensity edema and hemorrhage on T2-weighted and STIR sequences, but findings in a second-degree strain will be more extensive than those seen in a first-degree strain. Edema and hemorrhage is also more prominent along the fascial planes, and irregular thinning and mild laxity of tendon fibers may be visible. There is usually no significant retraction of tendon or bunching of muscle however because tearing is incomplete and the myotendinous junction remains partially intact. A hematoma at the myotendinous junction is a defining, pathognomonic finding in second-degree strains[5,44] (Figure 12-7). The appearance of the hematoma by MRI on T1-weighted and T2-weighted sequences varies depending on its composition according to its age. In the setting of old second-degree strains, hemosiderin or fibrosis may result in low signal intensity on T2-weighted sequences.

Treatment of second-degree myotendinous strains, in most instances, consists of a conservative regimen that reestablishes normal strength and range of motion without significant functional limitation. Treatment options include rest, activity modification, physical therapy, therapeutic ultrasound, and nonsteroidal antiinflammatory medications. Typically, most strains resolve clinically within several weeks. However, individuals suffering from second-degree strains and persistent pain following conservative treatment may be susceptible to recurrent myotendinous injury if the original injury is not given sufficient time to heal.[47] Therefore MRI can be helpful not only in grading the severity of injury, but also in assisting management by evaluating the status of recovery.[48] Persistent signal alterations by MRI in a strained muscle might indicate an ongoing vulnerable period and increased risk of reinjury despite improvement in clinical signs and symptoms.[49,50]

Third-Degree Strain

Continued tearing of the myotendinous junction to complete rupture characterizes the most severe injury, the third-degree strain. Patients present acutely with significant symptoms, including loss of function of the respective muscle, combined with physical examination findings that help to support the suspected diagnosis, obviating the need for imaging. There are two possible indications for imaging in this setting. First, if confounding factors such as patient guarding, swelling and variable weakness owing to recruitment of synchronal muscles confuses the clinical picture and examination, imaging can be helpful in arriving at the correct diagnosis. Second, should a surgical repair be contemplated in a patient with a confident clinical diagnosis of a myotendinous strain, MRI may provide the orthopedic surgeon with information regarding the location of injury and condition of the underlying tendon. Given the severe nature of the injury in the grade 3 strain, MR images demonstrate extensive hemorrhage and distortion of the normal anatomic structures, including the myotendinous junction. There may be visible separation of tendon margins and secondary bunching of muscle secondary to retraction and interposed hematoma formation in the gap created by the tear (Figure 12-8). Untreated, there is generally no reestablishment of normal muscle function, and long-term sequelae of muscular atrophy or scarring and fibrosis results.[51]

Tendon Degeneration

Tendinopathy denotes a continuum of disorders of the tendon including degeneration (tendinosis), partial tear, and complete

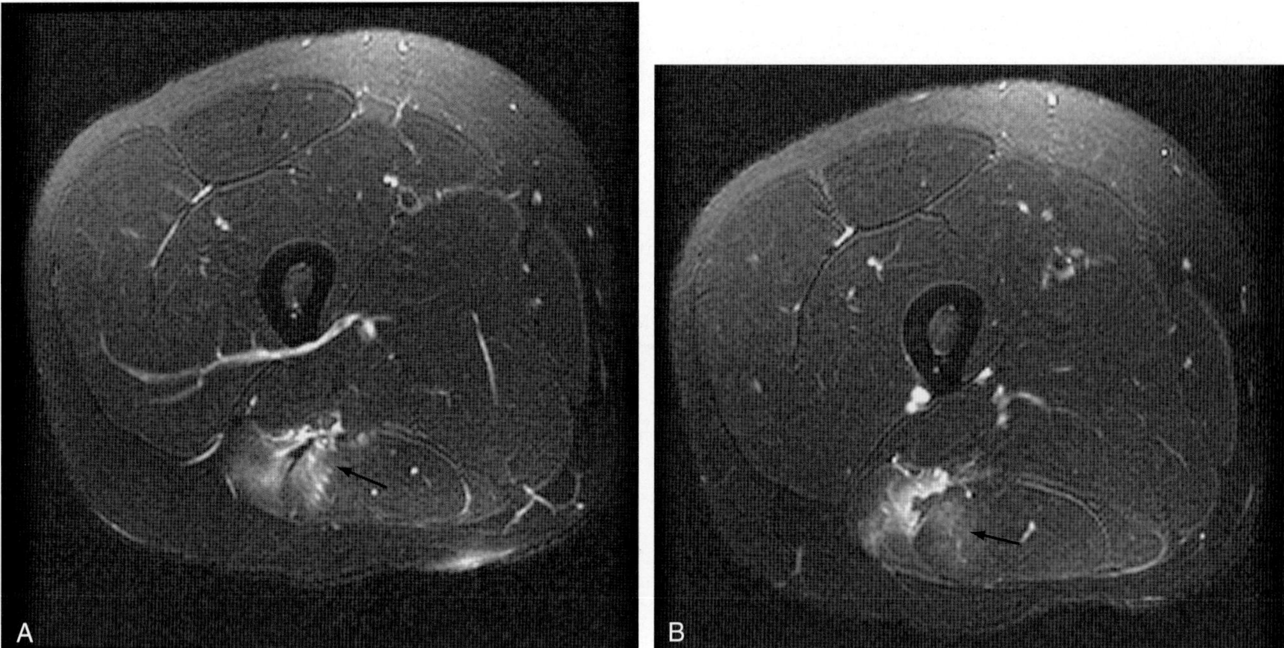

FIGURE 12-7. Grade 2 biceps femoris strain injury in a 17-year-old man with acute onset of posterior thigh pain during a football game. **A,** Axial fat-suppressed T2-weighted image shows edema and hemorrhage (bright signal) adjacent to the myotendinous junction (low signal tendon) of the biceps femoris muscle *(arrow)*. **B,** Axial fat-suppressed T2-weighted image more caudal to **A** shows partial disruption and irregularity of the myotendinous junction *(arrow)* with hemorrhage.

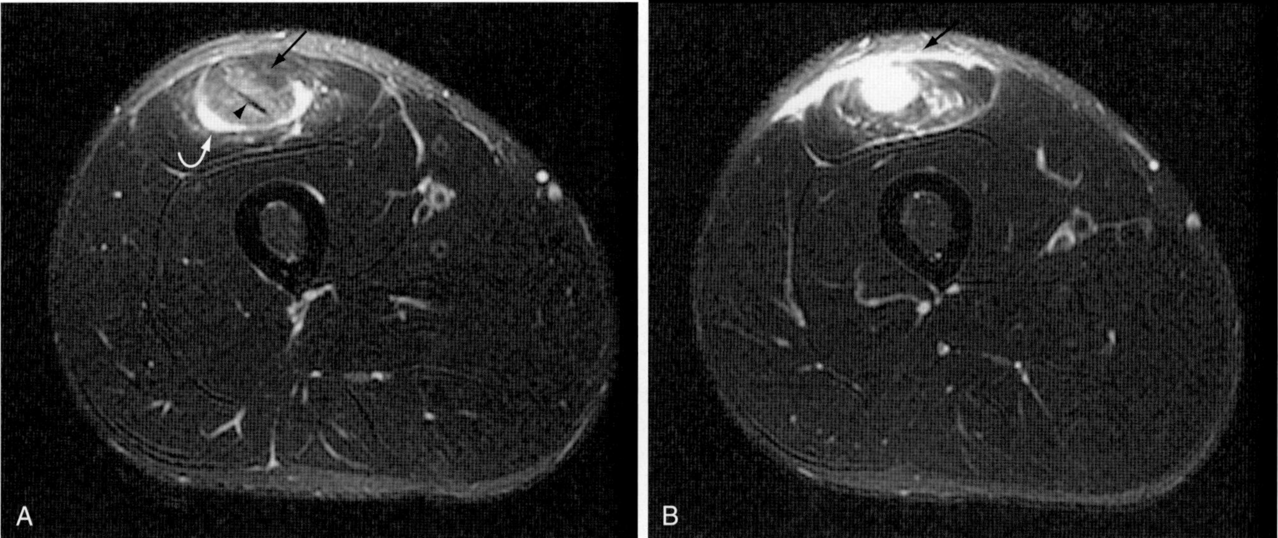

FIGURE 12-8. Grade 3 rectus femoris strain in an 18-year-old soccer player with acute onset of anterior thigh pain. **A,** Axial fat-suppressed T2-weighted image shows increased signal intensity at the proximal myotendinal junction of the rectus femoris muscle *(arrow)*. A hyperintense semilunar fluid cleft is seen posteriorly *(curved arrow)*. The intact low signal tendon *(arrowhead)* is clearly seen. **B,** On a more caudal image than **A,** the proximal myotendinal junction shows complete disruption (absent low signal tendon), with fluid and hematoma formation *(arrow)* in the cleft created by the disrupted, retracted myotendinous junction. There is also surrounding muscle and perifascial edema and hemorrhage.

rupture that tends to develop over an extended period of time. When the site of degeneration and abnormality occurs at the osseous attachment site of tendons, it is termed *enthesopathy.* There are a multitude of conditions that can predispose to development of tendinopathy and enthesopathy. Systemic disorders such as diabetes, rheumatoid arthritis, seronegative spondyloarthropathy, and hyperparathyroidism may cause tendon disease (Box 12-4). More common causes include overuse and mechanical impingement syndromes and long-term corticosteroid therapy. Chronically, the conditions cause tendon degeneration and predispose to injuries.

As the degree of tendon degeneration progresses, the tendon itself can replace the myotendinous junction as the site most susceptible to injury in the bone-tendon-muscle unit. Frequently, the tensile force from eccentric muscle contraction that is required to injure and potentially rupture a degenerated tendon is much less

BOX 12-4. Causes of Tendon Degeneration

Diabetes
Rheumatoid arthritis
Seronegative spondyloarthropathy
Hyperparathyroidism
Gout
Chronic injury
Impingement
Corticosteroids
Ciprofloxacin

than would be compulsory for a myotendinous strain. As a result, injury occurs in the form of partial tear or complete rupture of the weakened tendon or its undermined attachment to bone. MRI is helpful in characterizing not only the site of injury in the myotendinous unit, but also in assessing the integrity and health of the underlying tendon (Figure 12-9).

Direct Muscle Injury

Muscle Contusions

A contusion injury results after direct trauma to a muscle, in which there is injury to the underlying tissue, typically by a blunt object, without disruption of the overlying skin. Clinically, patients present with varying degrees of swelling and pain that may result in weakness and diminished range of motion acutely.[52] Blunt trauma and the resulting muscle contusion presumably represent variable degrees of muscle damage combined with hematoma formation and reactive hyperemia in the adjacent tissues. Depending on the severity of injury, contusive injuries are not necessarily superficial and can be quite deeply located in the soft tissues, as is frequently the case in the thigh.

On MRI of muscular contusions, edema and hemorrhage within muscle are seen as high signal on T2-weighted and IR FSE sequences. The pattern of increased signal change may adopt very geographic or more diffuse, ill-defined margins. There may be an accompanying increase in the girth of the muscle, but typically no fiber discontinuity or laxity is appreciated. The abnormal area of signal intensity may be hyperintense as a result of subacute blood products, although signal characteristics of blood will vary depending on the age of the contusion injury. If the contusion injury is severe enough, possible complications include myonecrosis (Figure 12-10). Frequently, the imaging appearance may overlap and mimic those of grade 1 or mild to moderate grade 2 strains. However, the lack of localization at the myotendinous junction helps to distinguish muscular contusion from strain injuries on imaging.[53]

Muscle Laceration

Muscle laceration is another form of direct muscle injury but, unlike contusion, laceration results from a penetrating injury. These types of injuries are infrequently evaluated with imaging in the acute setting unless a neurovascular or associated parenchymal injury is suspected. MRI findings include discontinuity of normal muscle, edema, and hemorrhage, often in a linear configuration along the trajectory of the penetrating injury that causes laceration of the soft tissues (Figure 12-11). Frequently, soft tissue gas is present secondary to the penetrating nature of the injury, which is easily visible on CT but can be frequently overlooked on MRI. In the chronic setting, the sequelae of prior lacerating injuries may be visible by imaging, such as muscular fatty atrophy, fibrosis, or herniation.

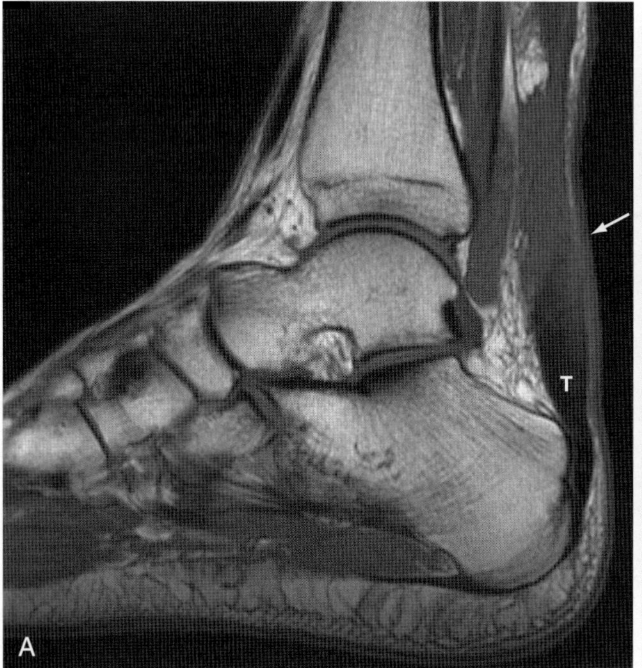

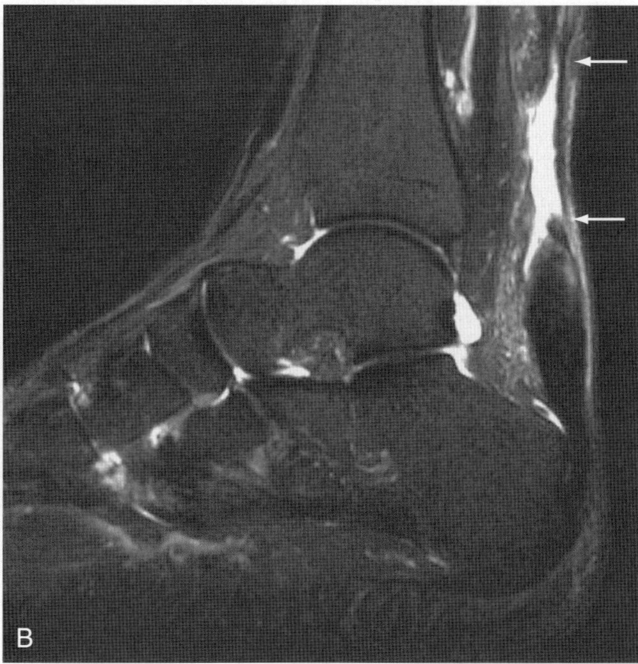

FIGURE 12-9. A 38-year-old man who presented with acute rupture of the Achilles' tendon following a hiking trip. The patient had a long-standing history of insulin-dependent diabetes resulting in chronic tendinopathy, leading to rupture after minimal trauma. **A,** Sagittal T1-weighted MR image shows that the normally low signal Achilles' tendon is disrupted *(arrow)* approximately 5 cm from its osseous attachment site at the calcaneus and is retracted proximally. There is thickening of the distal Achilles' tendon *(T)*. **B,** Sagittal fat-suppressed T2-weighted MR image shows hyperintense fluid and hemorrhage in the cleft between the ruptured and retracted tendon margins *(arrows)*.

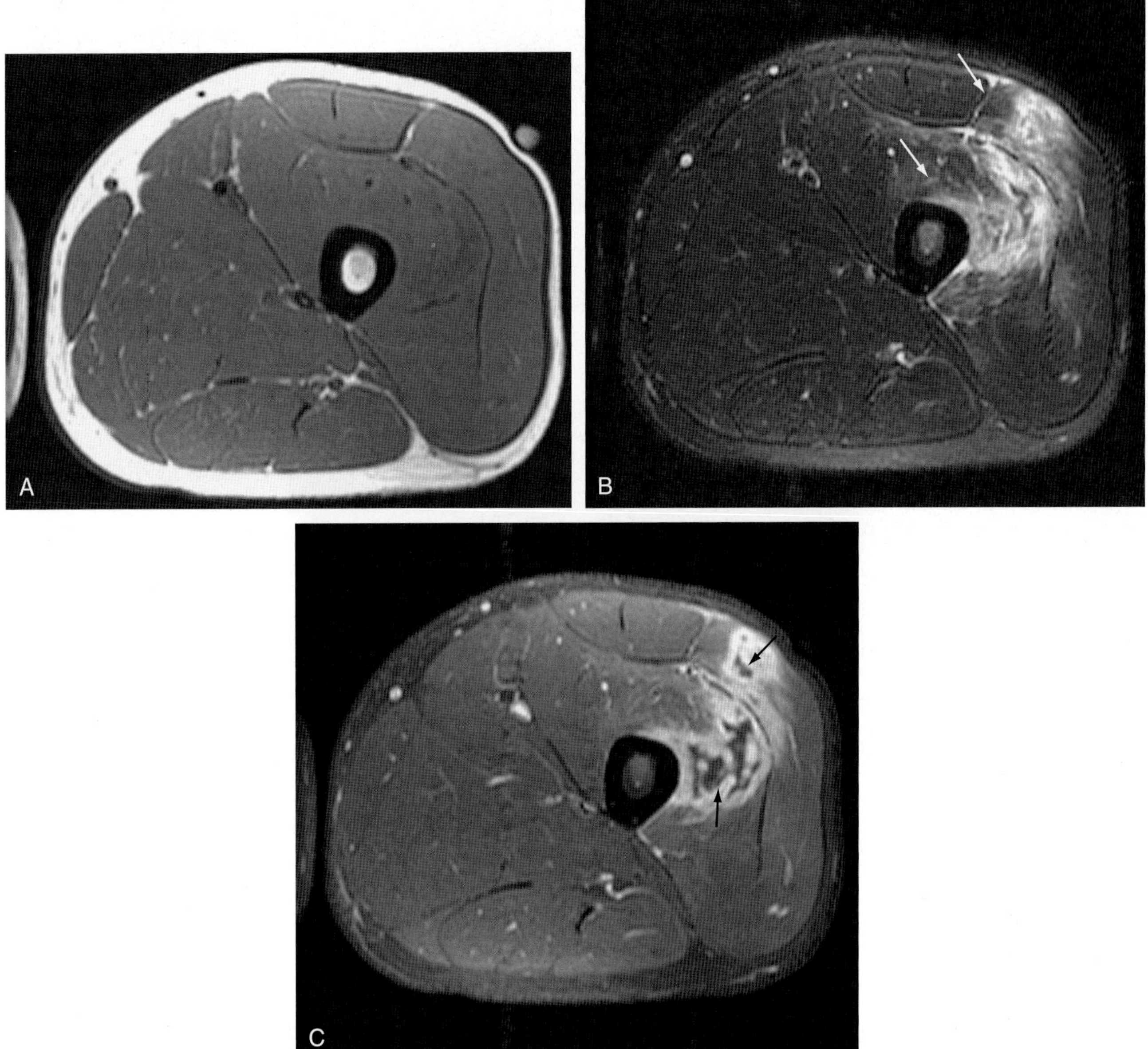

FIGURE 12-10. Myonecrosis secondary to direct pressure to the thigh from the surgical table during a spine operation with the patient in a prone position. **A,** Axial T1-weighted image through the thigh shows that the vastus intermedius appears thickened with subtle hypointense signal. The fat planes in the vastus intermedius and lateralis are effaced. A vitamin E skin marker has been placed at the site of pain. **B,** Axial fat-suppressed T2-weighted image demonstrates high signal intensity edema and hemorrhage diffusely extending in a continuous fashion superficially from the vastus lateralis through the vastus intermedius up to the underlying femur margin along the direction of compressive force *(arrows)*. **C,** Axial fat-suppressed T1-weighted image following gadolinium administration shows low signal intensity nonenhancing regions *(arrows)* corresponding to infarcted muscle.

Muscle Herniation

Muscle herniation consists of protrusion of muscle through a focal defect or breach of the fascia. There are two main causes of muscle herniations. The first and more common of the two mechanisms occurs in the setting of muscle hypertrophy as a result of exercise. As the muscle hypertrophies, intracompartmental pressures increase, resulting in secondary distension of inherently weak fenestrations in the fascia through which blood vessels and nerves traverse.[54] As these fascial openings widen under increasing tension, muscle can subsequently herniate through.[55] Second, and less common, a rent or tear of the fascia may occur as a result of blunt or penetrating trauma. Clinically, patients sometimes complain of a mass that may become more prominent with active muscle engagement during exercise.

> Muscle herniation may produce a mass that may become larger with activity. It is most frequent in the anterior compartment of the leg.

Although frequently asymptomatic, pain and localized tenderness may also accompany small herniations with activity. Rarely with large herniations, cosmetic complaints or nerve entrapments may occur.[56] The most common location for muscle herniations

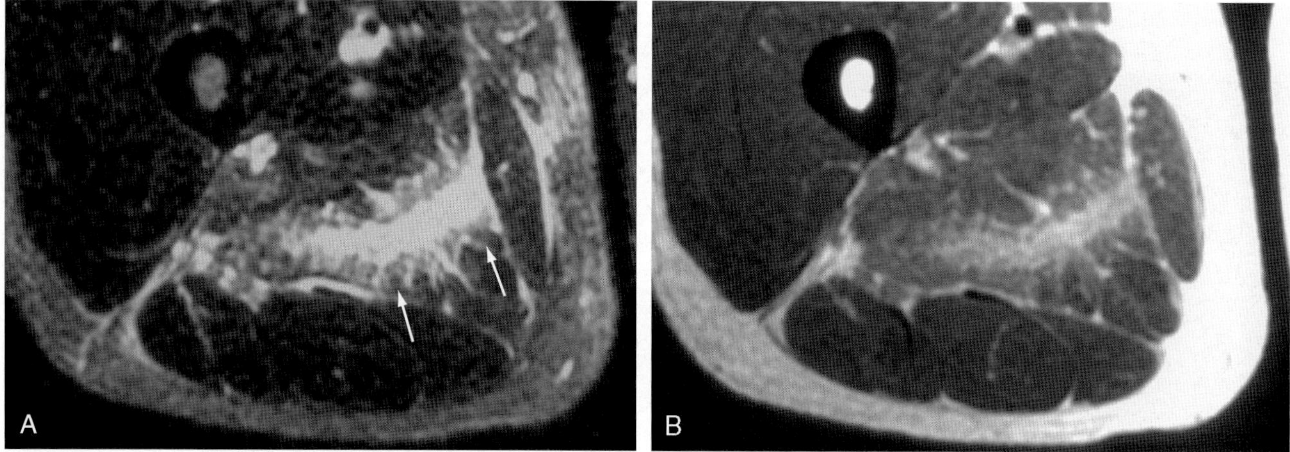

FIGURE 12-11. Laceration of the posterior thigh in a 32-year-old man following a gunshot injury. **A,** Axial fat-suppressed T2-weighted image through the thigh reveals a linear defect that demonstrates elevated signal intensity *(arrows)* in the posterior musculature consistent with hemorrhage in a muscle laceration. **B,** Axial proton density weighted MR image shows high signal blood products in the wound.

is in the lower extremity, with the tibialis anterior muscle most commonly affected.[57] The treatment of asymptomatic muscle hernias is usually conservative, with more aggressive management options such as fascial repairs or fasciotomies reserved for severely symptomatic herniations.[58,59]

Owing to its better delineation and characterization of soft tissue detail, MRI is far superior to CT in the evaluation of suspected muscle herniations. Frequently, an irregular peripheral contour sometimes associated with an outward bulging of muscle is identified at the time of imaging. The identification of a discrete fascial defect is inconsistent, and in certain situations, dynamic MRI during muscle contraction and relaxation employing very fast gradient echo MRI may accentuate definition of the muscle herniation.[60] Similarly, dynamic ultrasound can be extremely useful in the identification of fascial defects in the muscle aponeurosis. With the ability to have the patient contract and relax during real-time evaluation, ultrasound may more visually depict subtle contour abnormalities associated with small hernias[61] (Figure 12-12).

Dynamic imaging during muscle contraction and relaxation may be necessary to identify a muscle herniation.

SEQUELAE OF TRAUMATIC MUSCLE INJURIES

Hematoma and Pseudotumor

Hematomas, which are localized collections of blood, can be seen following any traumatic muscle injury but are most commonly seen associated with muscle strains and contusions.[62] A well-defined, sharply marginated mass is typical of an intramuscular hematoma. The MRI appearance on T1-weighted and T2-weighted sequences is affected by many factors, including the age of the hematoma, tissue clearance, and the relative concentration of protein and methemoglobin (Table 12-2).[63] Acutely, hematomas imaged within 48 hours are usually isointense on T1-weighted images. In general, imaging occurs

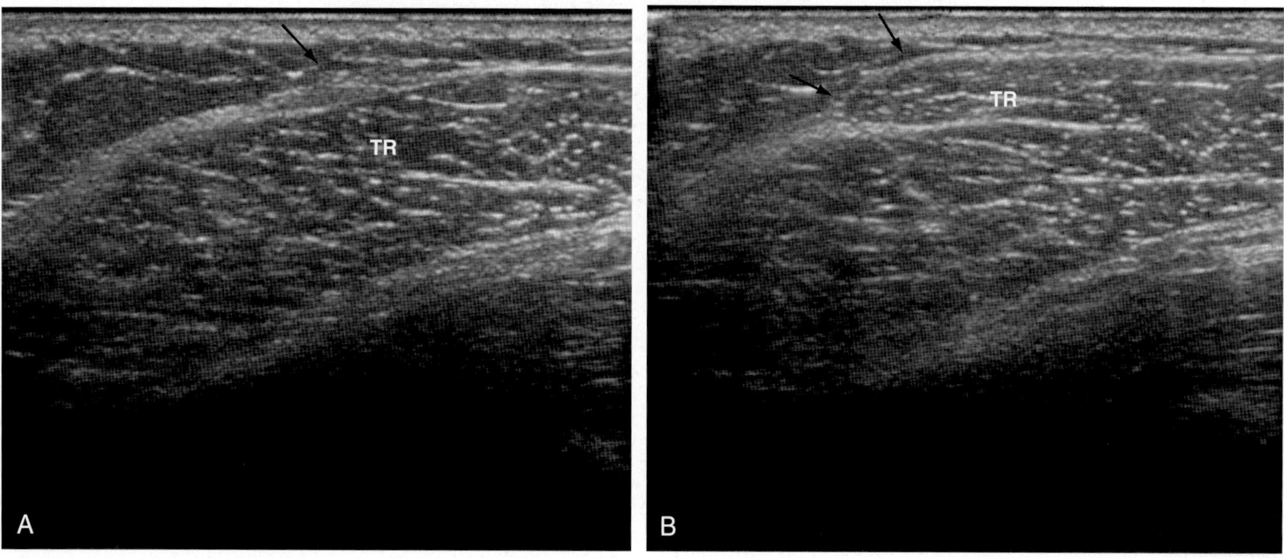

FIGURE 12-12. Muscle herniation in a 42-year-old woman with shoulder pain. **A,** Longitudinal ultrasound image of the trapezius muscle *(TR)* at rest shows a subtle contour deformity of the fascia overlying the muscle *(arrow)*. **B,** Voluntary contraction of the muscle while imaging clearly depicts and accentuates the hernia *(arrows)*.

TABLE 12-2. MRI Appearance of Hematomas

Chronicity	Appearance
< 48 hours	T1 isointense, T2 hyperintense
Subacute	T1 hyperintense, T2 hyperintense
Chronic	Hypointense (hemosiderin) rim

during the subacute phase following an injury as methemoglobin products accumulate and result in characteristic signal intensities on T1-weighted and T2-weighted images. As the hematoma evolves, a bull's-eye configuration results from the sequential laying down of breakdown products and hemosiderin accumulates, creating a dark signal intensity rim around the hematoma.

On MR images, hematoma following myotendinous strain may be intramuscular or intermuscular in location but is anatomically localized to the myotendinous junction. Spontaneous intramuscular hematoma may occur in the setting of patients receiving anticoagulation therapy. Imaging features can help to discriminate between these two occurrences (Figure 12-13). In the case of spontaneous intramuscular hematoma, the myotendinous junction remains intact and the muscle surrounding the hematoma is normal in appearance or demonstrates only minimal inflammatory reaction. This is in contrast to myotendinous disruption, and the feathery T2-weighted signal changes in the muscle adjacent to a strain-related hematoma.[27]

Contusion injuries are more commonly intramuscular in location, directly related to the site of blunt trauma, and may vary in size depending on factors such as the severity of the injury and blunt force applied. In severe contusion injuries, the degree of muscle damage that occurs as it is crushed against underlying bone may result in myonecrosis (see Figure 12-10). Imaging will show prominent reactive edema and inflammatory changes, and hematoma formation is also extremely common. Although these MRI characteristics mimic those seen in strain injuries, the lack of localization of findings relative to the myotendinous junction helps to arrive at the correct diagnosis. In cases of myonecrosis resulting as a consequence of very severe contusive injuries, with time the necrotic muscle may heal in a variety of ways. Cavitation with liquefaction of the dead muscle may result in a fluid-like cavity frequently outlined by a peripheral margin of fibrosis, hemosiderin, or calcification that may appear as low signal on T1-weighted and T2-weighted sequences, mimicking a chronic hematoma.[27]

It is not uncommon in clinical practice to have patients referred for imaging evaluation of a soft tissue mass with an equivocal or remote history of trauma. Although traumatic muscular injuries are in the differential consideration, the experienced clinician recognizes that occult neoplastic, and occasionally malignant, lesions may cause symptoms initially attributed incorrectly to minor or enigmatic trauma. For these reasons, patients may be referred for imaging.

> Neoplasms, even malignancies, may first be recognized or may erroneously be attributed to a traumatic event.

Intramuscular neoplasms rarely demonstrate any relationship to the myotendinous junction, and any association to it anatomically is coincidental. Lesions arising near the myotendinous junction will displace the tendon, rather than encompass or disrupt it (Figure 12-14). Frequently, neoplasms may demonstrate MRI characteristics that may have a similar appearance to an intramuscular hematoma. For example, fat within hemangiomas, lipomas, or sarcomas could be confused for subacute blood products but may be more irregularly contoured or distributed in a manner not typical for hematoma. Fat-suppressed images will show diminished signal in fat-containing lesions, whereas high signal from a hematoma would remain unchanged.

Caution should also be exercised when interpreting complex hematomas because neoplasms may undergo hemorrhagic necrosis and could be mistaken for complex blood collections. Administration of contrast can be helpful in excluding a neoplasm if there is complete lack of enhancement, but potential diagnostic pitfalls

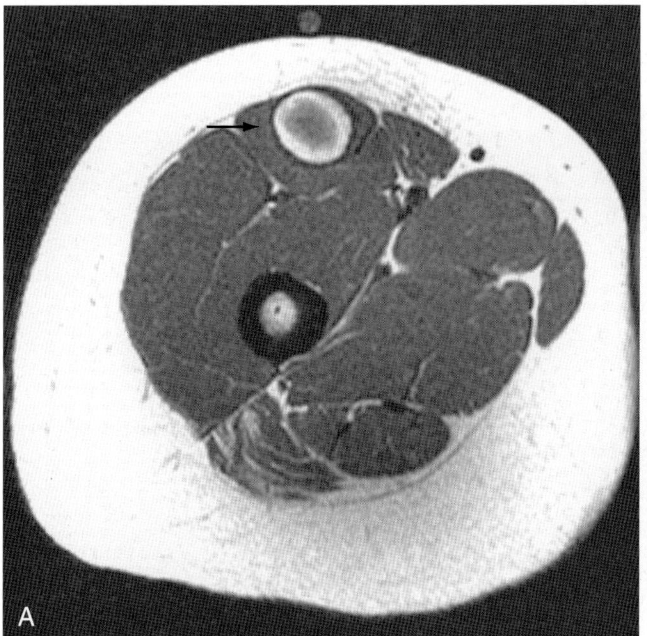

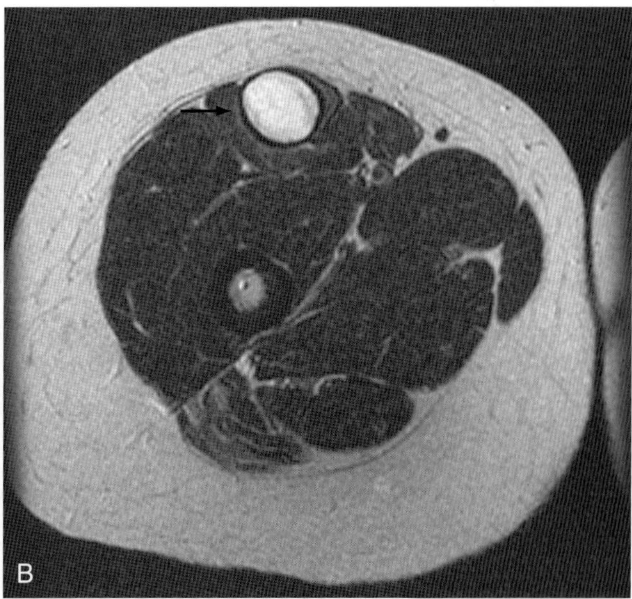

FIGURE 12-13. Spontaneous rectus femoris hematoma in a 57-year-old man receiving anticoagulation therapy with supratherapeutic levels of Coumadin. **A,** Axial T1-weighted MR image shows a hematoma *(arrow)* in the rectus femoris muscle characterized by peripheral increased signal intensity outlined by a sharply circumscribed low signal rim. **B,** Axial T2-weighted MR image reveals no edema surrounding the well-circumscribed hematoma *(arrow)*. The very low signal rim, due to hemosiderin deposition, outlines the peripheral margins of the hematoma. *(Continued)*

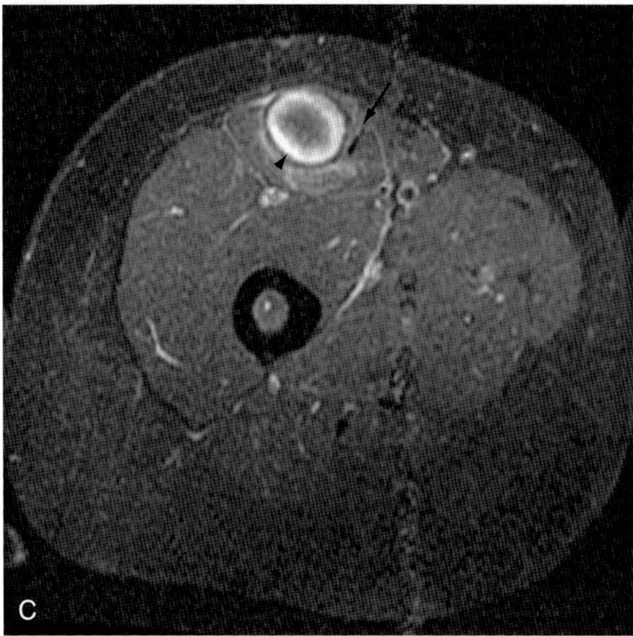

FIGURE 12-13—cont'd. C, Axial gadolinium-enhanced fat-suppressed T1-weighted MR image demonstrates that the low signal central proximal tendon of the rectus femoris *(arrow)* is separate from the laterally positioned hematoma. The peripheral high signal intensity *(arrowhead)* is unchanged compared with **A** and therefore represents methemoglobin from blood breakdown, rather than contrast enhancement.

exist when fibrovascular tissue and inflammation from an evolving hematoma are present, which may make it difficult to exclude an underlying neoplasm. When the diagnosis of a hematoma is probable but in doubt, a follow-up MR examination should be suggested to assess the presumed evolution of the hematoma and confirm the suspected etiology.

Because the clinical and imaging characteristics of hematoma and neoplasm may be similar, follow-up examination or biopsy may be necessary to differentiate these conditions.

Myositis Ossificans

Myositis ossificans is an aberrant reparative process that represents the formation of benign heterotopic ossification in skeletal muscle. The use of the word *myositis* is somewhat misleading, because it is not usually a primary inflammatory pathophysiologic process of muscle. There are a number of predisposing factors and possible causes, most commonly traumatic injury such as muscle contusion, in addition to surgery, burns, neurologic insults, and chronic immobilization.[64] Clinically, myositis ossificans may present as a painful, palpable soft tissue mass that may be confused for neoplastic or inflammatory conditions, especially if there is a vague or remote history of trauma confounding the clinical picture. Myositis ossificans most commonly affects large muscles of the lower extremity but can occur in any muscle[65] (Figure 12-15).

Clinically, myositis ossificans may present as a painful soft tissue mass that could be confused with tumor or inflammatory lesions.

Myositis ossificans undergoes phases of evolution and as such has a variable appearance by imaging depending on the stage at which it is investigated. In the acute to subacute stages, imaging is disturbingly nonspecific, especially by MRI. Frequently, a soft tissue abnormality of muscle with mass effect is identified with variable inflammatory features that frequently enhance following contrast administration, simulating neoplasm and creating diagnostic confusion.[66] Radiography and CT may only show nonspecific soft tissue swelling. During the subacute phase, which generally follows 2 to 6 weeks after the onset of imaging, radiography and CT scans may begin to demonstrate faint areas of mineralization. However, these subacute stages of myositis ossificans, consisting of a mass with foci of mineralization, can frequently be confused with soft tissue

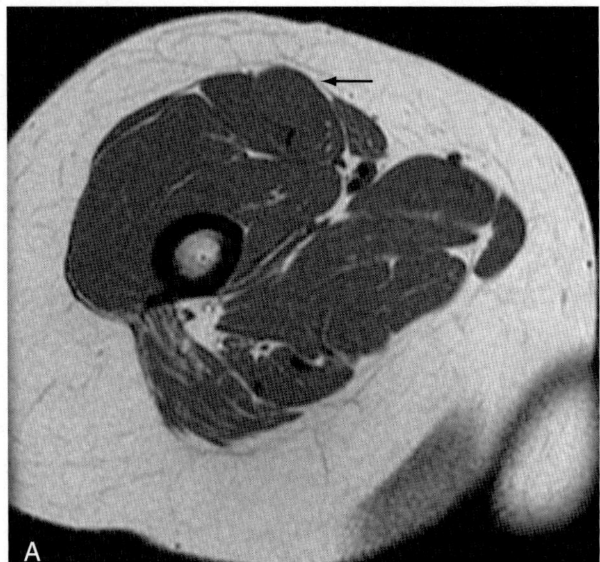

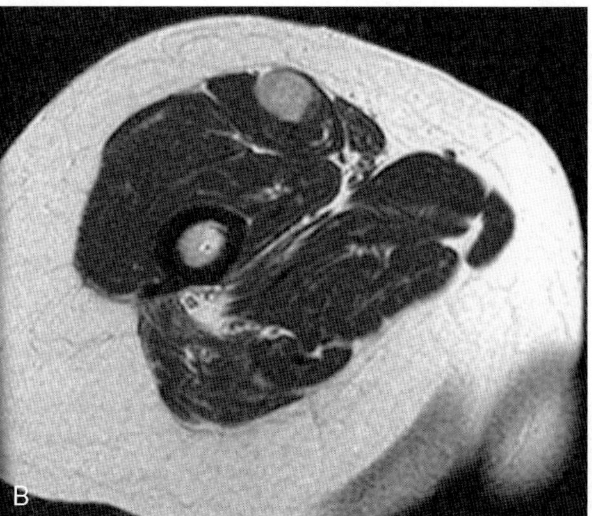

FIGURE 12-14. Fibroma of the rectus femoris in a 43-year-old female. **A,** Axial T1-weighted image through the thigh shows a subtle contour abnormality of the rectus femoris muscle anteriorly *(arrow)* owing to a mass that is isointense to muscle on this sequence. **B,** On the axial T2-weighted image at the same level, the sharply marginated intramuscular mass that is mildly hyperintense becomes apparent. The lesion is located at the level of the central tendon of the rectus femoris but is anterior to and displaces but does not disrupt the myotendinal junction.

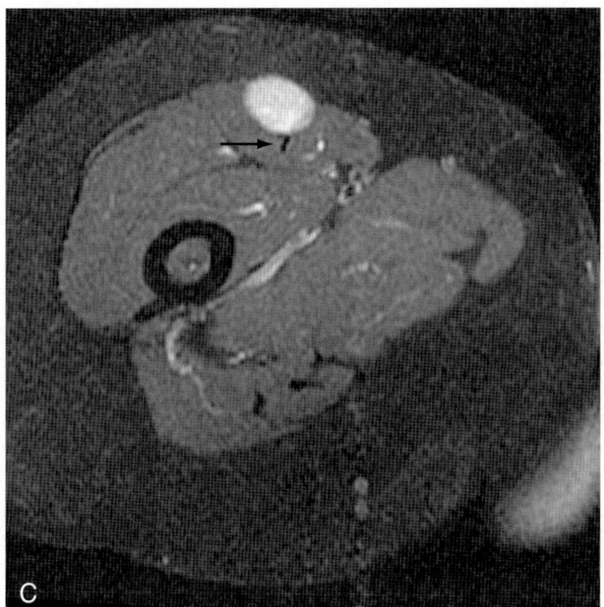

FIGURE 12-14—cont'd. C, Axial contrast-enhanced T1-weighted fat-suppressed MR image shows diffuse enhancement, consistent with a solid neoplasm. Note the mass effect exerted posteriorly on the central tendon *(arrow)*. The relationship of this fibroma to the myotendinal junction is entirely coincidental and differs from the typical myotendinal location of muscle strains.

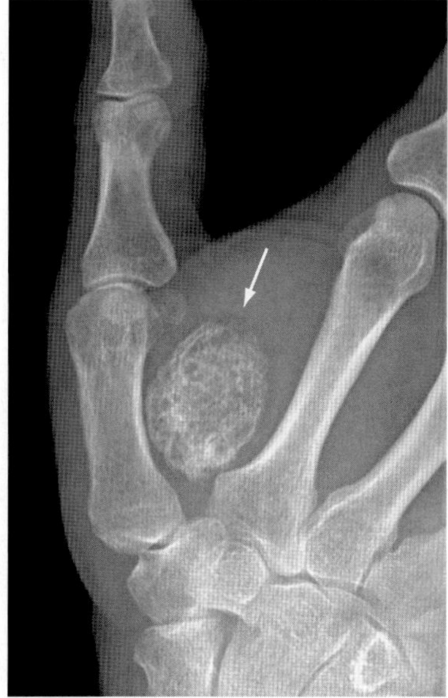

FIGURE 12-15. Myositis ossificans in a 34-year-old female with a painful, palpable mass. Posteroanterior radiograph of the hand demonstrates a round, well-organized, mineralized mass *(arrow)* with a peripheral rim of compact bone, consistent with myositis ossificans.

sarcomas. It is only in the chronic stages that imaging findings allow for a confident differentiation of myositis ossificans from neoplasm. The case in Figure 12-16 highlights the value of obtaining radiographs to supplement MRI examination. These findings include a well-defined, sharply marginated ossific mass containing mature peripheral cortical (compact) bone with central trabecular (lamellar) bone.[27] Conventional radiography and CT can take up to 6 to 8 weeks or longer following symptom onset to confirm the characteristic bone formation of myositis ossificans. On MRI, even long-standing, stable heterotopic ossification can be mistaken for other abnormalities because of poor depiction of calcification.

Typically, tumors associated with bone formation show the ossification to be most dense centrally, whereas the characteristic calcification/ossification of myositis ossificans occurs peripherally.

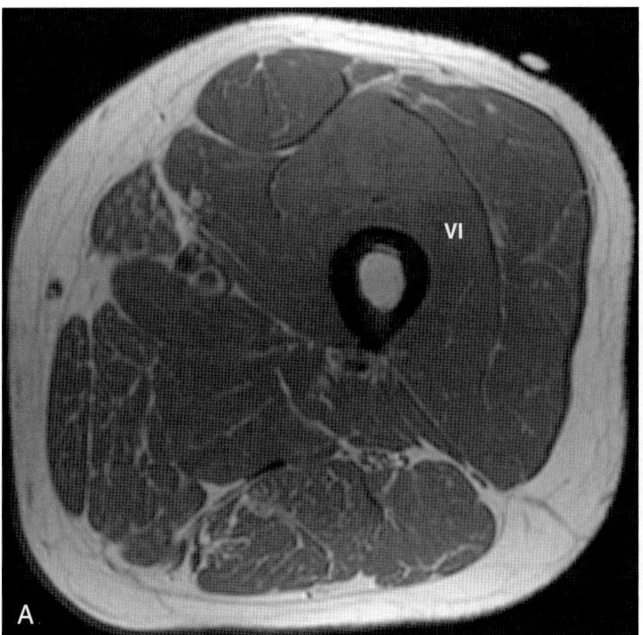

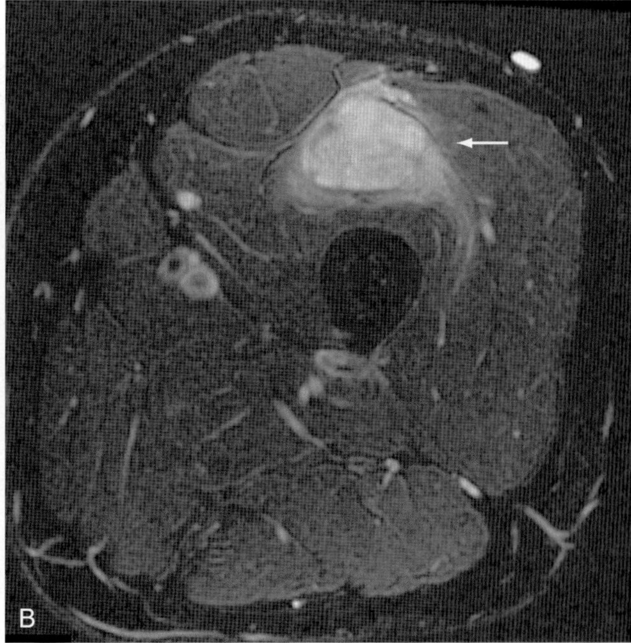

FIGURE 12-16. Myositis ossificans in a 36-year-old male with a painful, palpable mass in the thigh. There was no history of recent trauma. **A,** Axial T1-weighted image through the thigh shows a soft tissue contour abnormality of the vastus intermedius *(VI)*. **B,** Axial T2-weighted fat-suppressed sequence shows heterogeneously increased signal intensity with surrounding edema and inflammation *(arrow)*.

(Continued)

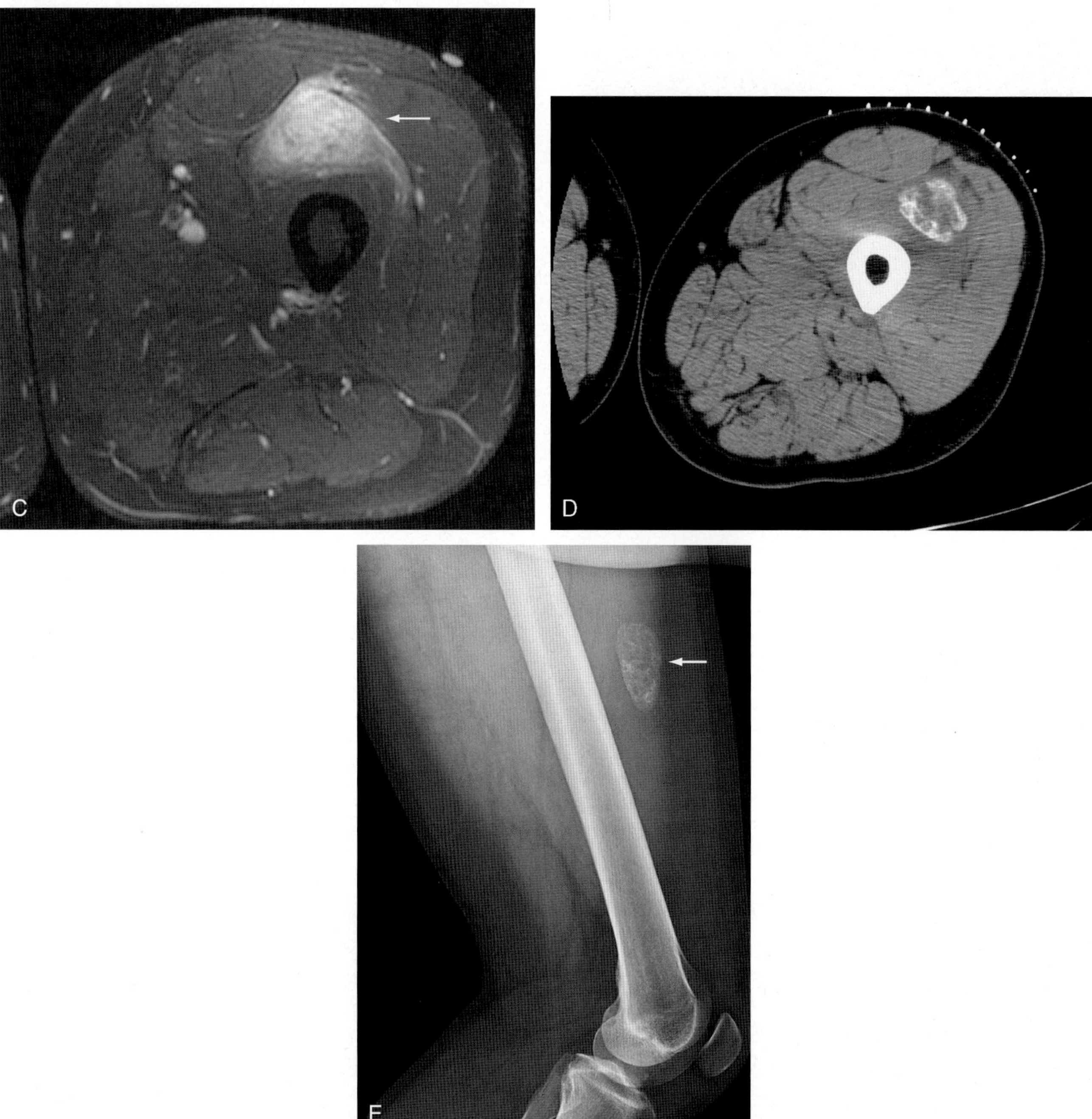

FIGURE 12-16—cont'd. **C,** Axial contrast-enhanced T1-weighted fat-suppressed image shows diffuse enhancement suspicious for neoplasm *(arrow);* the patient was scheduled for CT-guided biopsy. **D,** Preliminary CT image obtained at the time of biopsy shows calcification in a pattern characteristic of myositis ossificans. The biopsy was cancelled. **E,** Follow-up lateral radiograph of the thigh obtained 1 month later shows a well-circumscribed mineralized mass *(arrow)* with peripheral rim of bone, consistent with myositis ossificans.

REFERENCES

1. Lee IM, Paffenbarger RS Jr: Associations of light, moderate and vigorous intensity physical activity with longevity: the Harvard Alumni Health Study, *Am J Epidemiol* 151:293-299, 2000.
2. Noda H, Iso H, Date C et al: Walking and sports participation and mortality from coronary heart disease and stroke, *J Am Coll Cardiol* 46:1761-1767, 2005.
3. Hu G, Sarti C, Jousilahti P et al: Leisure time, occupational and commuting physical activity and the risk of stroke, *Stroke* 36:1994-1999, 2005.
4. Peterson L, Renstrom P: *Sports injuries: their prevention and treatment*, Chicago, 1986, Yearbook Medical, pp 25-36.
5. El-Khoury GY, Brandser EA, Kathol MH et al: Imaging of muscle injuries, *Skeletal Radiol* 25:3-11, 1996.
6. Armbrustmacher VW: Skeletal muscle. In Rubin E, Farber JL (eds): *Pathology*, Philadelphia, 1994, Lippincott, pp 1349-1370.
7. Anderson MW, Temple HT, Dussault RG et al: Compartmental anatomy: relevance to staging and biopsy of musculoskeletal tumors, *AJR Am J Roentgenol* 173:1663-1671, 1999.
8. Krejci V, Koch P: *Muscle and tendon injuries in athletes*, Chicago, 1979, Yearbook Medical, pp 74-79.
9. Zarins B, Ciullo JV: Acute muscle and tendon injuries in athletes, *Clin Sports Med* 2:167-182, 1983.
10. Garrett WE Jr: Muscle strain injuries, *Am J Sports Med* 24(Suppl):S2-S8, 1996.
11. Croisier JL: Factors associated with recurrent hamstring injuries, *Sports Med* 34:681-695, 2004.
12. Hoskins W, Pollard H: The management of hamstring injury—Part 1: issues in diagnosis, *Man Ther* 10:96-107, 2005.
13. Verrall GM, Slavotinek JP, Barnes PG et al: Clinical risk factors for hamstring muscle strain injury: a prospective study with correlation of injury by magnetic resonance imaging, *Br J Sports Med* 35:435-439, 2001.
14. Orchard JW: Intrinsic and extrinsic risk factors for muscle strains in Australian football, *Am J Sports Med* 29:300-303, 2001.
15. Verrall GM, Slavotinek JP, Barnes PG: The effect of sports specific training on reducing the incidence of hamstring injuries in professional Australian Rules football players, *Br J Sports Med* 39:363-368, 2005.
16. Kirdendall DT, Garrett EW Jr: Clinical perspective regarding eccentric muscle injury, *Clin Orthop Relat Res* 403(Suppl):S81-S89, 2002.
17. Witvrouw E, Danneels L, Asselman P et al: Muscle flexibility as a risk factor for developing muscle injuries in male professional soccer players. A prospective study, *Am J Sports Med* 31:41-46, 2003.
18. Palmer WE, Kuong SJ, Elmadbouh HM: MR imaging of myotendinous strain, *AJR Am J Roentgenol* 173:703-709, 1999.
19. Noonan TJ, Garrett WE Jr: Injuries at the myotendinous junction, *Clin Sports Med* 11:783-806, 1992.
20. Jozsa LG, Kannus P: *Human tendons: anatomy, physiology, and pathology*, Champaign, Ill, 1997, Human Kinetics, pp 105-108.
21. Pleacher MD, Glazer JL: Lower extremity soft tissue conditions, *Curr Sports Med Rep* 5:255-261, 2005.
22. Connell DA, Schneider-Kolsky ME, Hoving JL et al: Longitudinal study comparing sonographic and MRI assessment of acute and healing hamstring injuries, *AJR Am J Roentgenol* 183:974-984, 2004.
23. Pomeranz SJ, Heidt RS Jr: MR imaging in the prognostication of hamstring injury, *Radiology* 189:897-900, 1993.
24. Orchard J, Best TM: The management of muscle strain injuries: an early return versus the risk of recurrence, *Clin J Sport Med* 12:3-5, 2002.
25. Schweitzer ME, Karasick D: MR imaging of disorders of the Achilles tendon, *AJR Am J Roentgenol* 175:613-625, 2000.
26. Fleckenstein JL, Weatherall PT, Parkey RW et al: Sports-related muscle injuries: evaluation with MR imaging, *Radiology* 172:793-798, 1989.
27. Palmer W: Myotendinous unit: MR imaging diagnosis and pitfalls. In Buckwalter KA, Kransdorf MJ (eds): *Musculoskeletal imaging: exploring new limits*, Oak Brook, Ill, 2003, Radiological Society of North America, pp 25-35.
28. Sud AM, Wison MW, Mountz JM: Unusual clinical presentation and scintigraphic pattern in myositis ossificans, *Clin Nucl Med* 17:198-199, 1992.
29. Brandser EA, El-Khoury GY, Kathol MH et al: Hamstring injuries: radiographic, conventional tomographic, CT, and MR imaging characteristics, *Radiology* 197:257-262, 1995.
30. Campbell RSD, Wood J: Ultrasound of muscle, *Imaging* 14:229-240, 2002.
31. Peetrons P: Ultrasound of muscles, *Eur Radiol* 12:35-43, 2002.
32. De Smet AA, Fisher DR, Heiner JP et al: Magnetic resonance imaging of muscle tears, *Skeletal Radiol* 19:283-286, 1990.
33. Armstrong RB: Mechanisms of exercise-induced delayed onset muscular soreness: a brief review, *Med Sci Sports Exerc* 16:529-538, 1984.
34. Gulick DT, Kimura IF: Delayed-onset muscle soreness: what is it and how do we treat it? *J Sport Rehabil* 5:234-243, 1996.
35. Zainuddin Z, Newton M, Sacco P et al: Effects of massage on delayed-onset muscle soreness, swelling and recovery of muscle function, *J Athl Train* 40:174-180, 2005.
36. Cheung K, Hume P, Maxwell L: Delayed onset muscle soreness: treatment strategies and performance factors, *Sports Med* 33:145-164, 2003.
37. Evans GF, Haller RG, Wyrick PS et al: Submaximal delayed-onset muscle soreness: correlations between MR imaging findings and clinical measures, *Radiol* 208:815-820, 1998.
38. Fleckenstein JL, Canby RC, Parkey RW et al: Acute effects of exercise on MR imaging of skeletal muscle in normal volunteers, *AJR Am J Roentgenol* 151:213-237, 1988.
39. Fernbach SK, Wilkinson RH: Avulsion injuries of the pelvis and proximal femur, *AJR Am J Roentgenol* 137:581-584, 1981.
40. Tehranzadeh J: The spectrum of avulsion and avulsion-like injuries of the musculoskeletal system, *Radiographics* 7:945-973, 1987.
41. Brandser EA, El-Khoury GY, Kathol MH et al: Hamstring injuries: radiographic, conventional tomographic, CT and MR imaging characteristics, *Radiol* 197:257-262, 1995.
42. Barnes ST, Hinds RB: Pseudotumor of the ischium, *J Bone Joint Surg* 54:645-647, 1972.
43. Annett P, Bruce W, Sweetland K et al: Scintigraphy of an avulsion injury of the rectus femoris muscle, *Clin Nucl Med* 26:781-782, 2001.
44. Palmer WE, Kuong SJ, Elmadbouh HM: MR imaging of myotendinous strain, *AJR Am J Roentgenol* 173:703-709, 1999.
45. De Smet AA, Best TM: MR imaging of the distribution and location of acute hamstring injuries in athletes, *AJR Am J Roentgenol* 174:393-399, 2000.
46. Connell DA, Potter HG, Sherman MF et al: Injuries of the pectoralis major muscle: evaluation with MR imaging, *Radiology* 210:785-791, 1999.
47. Taylor DC, Dalton JD Jr, Seaber AV et al: Experimental muscle strain injury: early functional and structural deficits and the increased risk for reinjury, *Am J Sports Med* 21:190-194, 1993.
48. Orchard J, Best TM, Verrall GM: Return to play following muscle strains, *Clin J Sport Med* 6:436-441, 2005.
49. Fleckenstein JL, Weatherall PT, Parker RW et al: Sports-related muscle injuries: evaluation with MR imaging, *Radiology* 172:793-798, 1989.
50. Greco A, McNamara MT, Escher RM et al: Spin-echo and STIR MR imaging of sports-related muscle injuries at 1.5 T, *J Comput Assist Tomogr* 15:994-999, 1991.
51. Blasier RB, Morawa LG: Complete rupture of the hamstring origin from a water skiing injury, *Am J Sports Med* 18:435-437, 1990.
52. Diaz JA, Fischer DA, Rettig AC et al: Severe quadriceps muscle contusions in athletes. A report of three cases, *Am J Sports Med* 31:289-293, 2003.
53. Kneeland JP: MR imaging of muscle and tendon injury, *Eur J Radiol* 25:198-208, 1997.
54. Braunstein JT, Crues JV 3rd: Magnetic resonance imaging of hereditary hernias of the peroneus longus muscle, *Skeletal Radiol* 24:601-604, 1995.
55. Blankenbaker DG, De Smet AA: MR imaging of muscle injuries, *Applied Radiol* 33:14-26, 2004.
56. Alhadeff J, Lee CK: Gastrocnemius muscle herniation at the knee causing peroneal nerve compression resembling sciatica, *Spine* 20:612-614, 1995.
57. Zeiss J, Ebraheim NA, Woldenberg LS: Magnetic resonance imaging in the diagnosis of anterior tibialis muscle herniation, *Clin Orthop* 244:249-253, 1988.
58. Siliprandi L, Martini G, Chiarelli A et al: Surgical repair of an anterior tibialis muscle hernia with Mersilene mesh, *Plast Reconstr Surg* 53:154-157, 1993.
59. Miniaci A, Rorabeck CH: Tibialis anterior muscle hernia: a rationale for treatment, *Can J Surg* 30:79-80, 1987.
60. Mellado JM, Perez del Palomar L: Muscle hernias of the lower leg: MRI findings, *Skeletal Radiol* 28:465-469, 1999.
61. Peetrons P: Ultrasound of muscles, *Eur Radiol* 12:35-43, 2002.
62. Shellock FG, Mink J, Deutsch AL: MR imaging of muscle injuries, *Appl Radiol* 2:11-16, 1994.
63. Steinback LS, Fleckenstein JL, Mink JH: MR imaging of muscle injuries, *Semin Muscllulokelet Radiol* 1:127-41, 1997.
64. Vanden Bossche L, Vanderstraeten G: Heterotopic ossification: a review, *J Rehabil Med* 37:129-136, 2005.
65. Jayasekera N, Joshy S, Newman-Sander A: Myositis ossificans traumatica of the thenar region, *J Hand Surg* 30:507-508, 2005.
66. Shirkhoda A, Armin AR, Bis KG et al: MR imaging of myositis ossificans: variable patterns at different stages, *J Magn Reson Imaging* 5:287-292, 1995.

CHAPTER 13

Imaging of Tendons and Bursae

MARY G. HOCHMAN, MD, ARUN J. RAMAPPA, MD,
JOEL S. NEWMAN, MD, *and* STEPHEN W. FARRAHER, MD

KEY FACTS

- *Tendinopathy* refers to the full spectrum of tendon pathology, including tendon degeneration and tear, tenosynovitis, and calcific tendinitis. *Tendinosis* refers to tendon degeneration. The term *tendinitis* is currently considered less accurate, because inflammatory cells are rarely present in common tendon conditions.
- Radiographs are an important first step in the evaluation of tendon or bursal pathology and serve as an adjunct to further workup with magnetic resonance imaging (MRI), ultrasound, or computed tomography (CT). Although only a few tendons can be directly visualized on radiographs, important information regarding secondary signs of tendon pathology or alternative explanations for symptoms can be demonstrated.
- MRI and, in experienced hands, ultrasound are the current modalities of choice for direct visualization of tendon and bursal pathology. Ultrasound of tendons and bursae requires appropriate high-frequency transducers for optimal technique. Depending on the specific tendon site, the two modalities have respective strengths and weaknesses and may play complementary roles. Accuracy for diagnosis of tendon pathology in experienced hands is often strikingly similar between the two modalities, despite the great difference in technologies. Ultrasound is particularly well-suited for guiding interventions, compared with MRI.
- On MRI, the normal tendon is low in signal on all conventional sequences. Tendinosis appears as high signal on proton density weighted and T1-weighted sequences, but low signal on T2-weighted or fat-saturated T2-weighted sequences. Tendon tears appear as fluid-like high signal on all sequences. When tendons cross at 55 degrees to the main magnetic field, high signal due to magic angle artifact can mimic tendinosis.
- CT effectively depicts tendon course and caliber and certain forms of tendon pathology, such as tenosynovitis. It is particularly helpful to demonstrate calcification or ossification within a tendon, to demonstrate the relationship between tendon and surrounding bony structures, and when a patient has a contraindication to MRI. CT is used less commonly to image tendons than MRI or ultrasound, because it is less sensitive for depiction of tendon degeneration and some tendon tears. Bursae are rarely visible on CT unless distended with fluid.
- Shoulder arthrography can be used to diagnose full-thickness tears of the rotator cuff. MR arthrograms can be used to diagnose partial articular surface tears, as well as complete tears, and provide additional information related to the size and location of tear, quality of the tendon and shape of the coracoacromial arch, and presence of tendon retraction and muscle atrophy. CT shoulder arthrograms can also be used to detect rotator cuff tears but involve additional radiation exposure and are not commonly performed unless MRI is contraindicated.
- Tenograms and bursograms are rarely performed for diagnostic purposes but may be performed as part of an aspiration procedure or a therapeutic injection.
- Nuclear medicine studies, which are based on administration of radioactive pharmaceuticals, may show incidental evidence of peritendinous inflammation and enthesitis, but they are not a primary modality for tendon imaging. However, because the degree of tracer activity on positron emission tomography (PET) scans is related to the level of glucose metabolism, a possible future role for PET scanning in assessment of the degree or peritendinous or bursal inflammation and response to therapy has been suggested.

Tendons connect muscle to bone, transmitting force from muscle contraction to effect motion of joints and limbs. Tendon abnormalities are common—the result of degeneration and overuse, instantaneous trauma, and local and systemic disease processes. Tendon abnormalities can result in considerable morbidity and disability. Although history and physical examination remain the mainstay for evaluating tendon dysfunction, imaging examinations provide important supplementary information for the diagnosis and characterization of tendon pathology.

A tendon is composed of longitudinally oriented collagen fibrils that are bundled into fibers ranging in size from 5 to 30 mm (Figure 13-1). The collagen fibers are organized into successively larger bundles—microfibrils, fibrils, and fascicles—to form a tendon. These successively larger bundles are enveloped and bound together by an endotenon, a network of collagen connective tissue that permits longitudinal motion of fascicles and conducts blood vessels, lymphatics, and nerves. The endotenon invests every fiber.[1] The entire tendon, including the endotenon, is enveloped by a collagenous epitenon covering. As a tendon emerges from muscle, it is enveloped by a thin adventitial layer, termed a *paratenon*, formed from the fascial covering of the muscle. The paratenon is composed of collagen fibrils running parallel to the long axis of the tendon. A paratenon typically surrounds tendons that move in a straight line and helps to facilitate sliding motion of the tendon within the surrounding tissue. Together, the epitenon and paratenon comprise the peritenon.[2] In some tendons, the paratenon is replaced by a tenosynovium, a synovial sheath composed of two layers lined by synovial cells. The tenosynovium provides lubrication and promotes gliding of the tendon. The synovial sheath also facilitates a cellular response to tendon injury.[1] The Achilles' tendon is an example of a tendon with a paratenon, whereas the flexor tendons of the hand are surrounded by a tenosynovium.

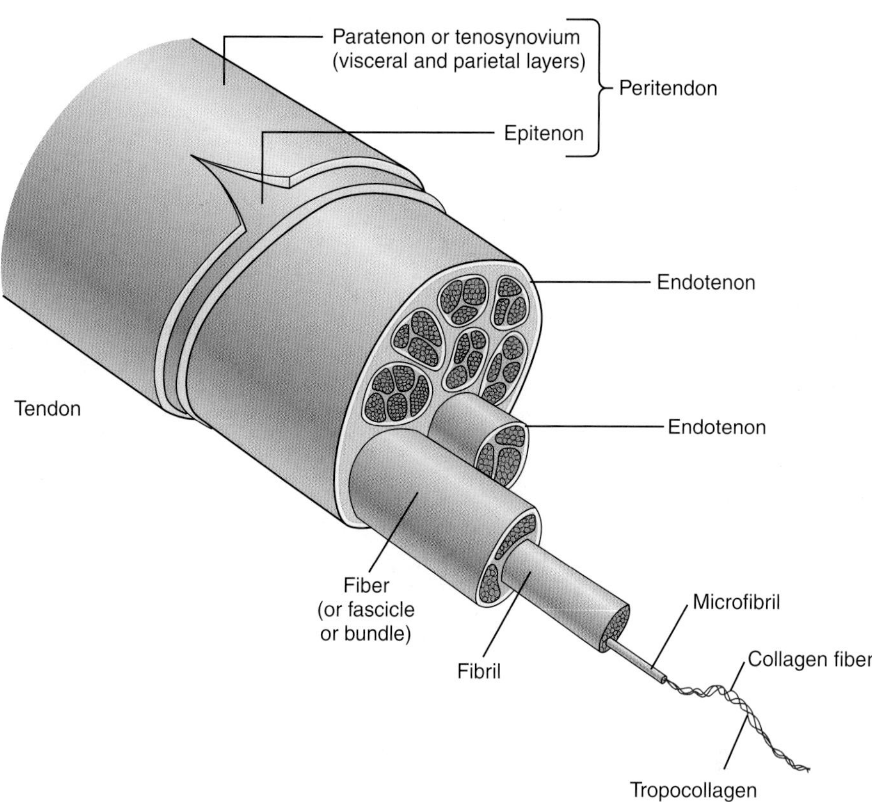

FIGURE 13-1. Normal tendon anatomy. A tendon is composed of longitudinally oriented collagen fibrils that are bundled into fibers ranging in size from 5 to 30 mm. The collagen fibers are organized into successively larger bundles—microfibrils, fibrils and fascicles—to form a tendon. These successively larger bundles are enveloped and bound together by an endotenon. The entire tendon, including the endotenon, is enveloped by a collagenous epitenon covering. As a tendon emerges from muscle, it is enveloped by the paratenon, formed from the fascial covering of muscle. Together, the epitenon and paratenon comprise the peritenon. In some tendons, the paratenon is replaced by a tenosynovium, a synovial sheath composed of two layers (visceral and parietal) lined by synovial cells. (Illustration by Steven Moskowitz.)

The normal adult tendon is composed predominantly of type I collagen, with less than 5% other types of collagen (types III, IV, V, and VI) and 2% elastin, in an extracellular matrix composed of ground substance and water. Collagen provides tensile strength, whereas elastin provides compliance and elasticity. The degree of cross-linking within and between longitudinally arrayed collagen molecules is the key to the tensile strength and resistance to degradation of collagen.[2,3] Ground substance consists of proteoglycans, glycosaminoglycans (GAGs), structural glycoproteins, plasma proteins, and various small molecules. The water-binding capacity of ground substance helps account for the viscoelastic properties of tendon. Cellular elements are relatively sparse, composed of specialized forms of fibroblasts, known as *tenocytes* and *tenoblasts.*[2,4]

The force of muscle contraction is transmitted from tendon to bone at the osteotendinous junction. At a direct insertion site, the tendon attaches to bone via transition through four distinct histologic zones: tendon, unmineralized fibrocartilage, mineralized fibrocartilage, and bone. At an indirect insertion site, the tendon attaches to the periosteum via collagenous fibers known as *Sharpey fibers.*[4,5]

Tendons develop independently in the mesenchyme; their connection with muscle occurs secondarily. At the myotendinous junction, collagen fibers from tendons insert into clefts formed by muscle cells. This structure greatly increases the contact surface between the tendon and muscle, reducing the force per unit area during muscle contraction.[6] The musculotendinous junction represents a weak link—it is less able to withstand loads than a normal tendon is. As a result, the myotendinous junction is a common site of failure (i.e., strain, tear) due to injury, when the tendon is normal and the individual is skeletally mature.[7]

The blood supply to the tendon has several sources: the perimysium of muscle, the periosteal attachments, and the surrounding tissues. Some tendons are surrounded by a paratenon and receive vessels along their borders. Other tendons are contained within tendon sheaths and receive their blood supply via discrete conduits called *mesotenons* or *vinculae.*[2] This latter arrangement results in areas of relative avascularity along the length of the tendon, which are nourished only by diffusion of synovial fluid.[8] These areas of relative avascularity are considered prone to injury.

To perform their role in transmitting muscle force to bone, tendons must be capable of resisting high tensile force with limited elongation.[2] Tendon strength correlates with total collagen content, density of stable (pyridinoline) cross-links, collagen organization, and fibril diameter and correlates inversely with type III (reparative) collagen and the proteoglycan-collagen ratio.[6] Large variations in ultimate tensile strength and maximum strain are seen with differences in type and age of tendons.[2,7] When mechanical load is excessive, it may produce inflammation and fiber damage, delayed and reduced collagen maturation, and inhibited collagen cross-linking.[4] Age-related changes in tendon biochemistry, which can be seen as early as the third decade of life, may result in a less compliant tendon with decreased tensile strength and may predispose the tendon to overuse injury and tear.[4,9-11] Older tendons also demonstrate decreased healing capacity.[4] Accumulation of degenerative histologic changes within the tendon, such as hypoxic or mucoid changes, may also predispose to injury.[4,12]

Tendon injuries may be acute, chronic, or acute-on-chronic. Acute injury includes direct injury, such as contusion or laceration, and indirect injury, such as acute tensile overload. Acute tensile overload usually causes either injury to the myotendinous junction (because the healthy tendon can withstand higher tensile loads than the muscle)[6] or an avulsion fracture. Myotendinous strain usually occurs in the setting of rapid, forceful, eccentric muscle contraction (i.e., the muscle lengthens while it is simultaneously contracting). Muscles that cross two joints, such as the rectus femoris, hamstring, and gastrocnemius muscles, are thought to be predisposed to acute myotendinous strain, because they can develop tension on the basis of passive joint positioning alone.[13] When it occurs in the setting of chronic tendon degeneration, acute tensile overload can also result in intrasubstance tendon tears. For example, many eccentric Achilles' tendon ruptures occur due to acute injury superimposed on chronic tendon degeneration.

Chronic repetitive microtrauma can lead to overuse injury to the tendon,[14] a much more common form of injury than myotendinous strain. When the tendon is strained repeatedly to 4% to 8% of its original length, the adaptive and reparative ability of the tendon can be exceeded.[4,6] This can result in microscopic and/or macroscopic injury to collagen fibrils, noncollagenous matrix, and the microvasculature.

Tendinopathy is a term used to describe the combination of tendon pain, swelling, and impaired performance.[13] It is a clinical descriptor and is used independent of underlying histopathology. The term *tendinosis* refers to intrasubstance tendon degeneration. Tendinosis, which can be asymptomatic,[4] is characterized by histopathologic alterations to cells, collagen fibers, and noncollagenous matrix components.[13] Both degenerative and reparative processes are observed. As microfailure of tendon fibers occurs, fibers may fail to heal effectively, perhaps due to decreased vascular supply or other factors. Histopathologic degenerative changes include angiofibroblastic hyperplasia (proliferation of fibroblasts and new capillaries), mucoid degeneration, hypoxic degeneration, hyaline degeneration, fatty degeneration, fibrinoid degeneration, chondroid metaplasia, calcification, and vascular changes.[1,2,4,15] These histopathologic changes result in a decreased tensile strength of the tendon.[6] Loss of functional tendon fibers leads to increased load on the remaining tendon, which, in turn, increases risk for progressive failure.[7] Of note, inflammation within the tendon is not a feature in tendinosis,[13,15,16] so the term "tendinitis" is considered by many to be a misnomer.

Continued tendon overload and chronic peritendinitis may result in tendon degeneration, although a causal relationship has not been conclusively established.[4,17] Asymptomatic microscopic tendinosis has been documented in approximately one third of persons older than age 35.[18] The source of pain in chronic tendon disorders is not clearly understood; certain biochemical compounds may irritate the pain receptors.[19]

Distinct pathology can occur at the osteotendinous junction. In the skeletally immature child, tensile overload can lead to pathologic changes at the apophysis, with small avulsions from the apophyseal ossification center and resultant apophysitis.[4,13] This process occurs most commonly at the tibial tuberosity (Osgood-Schlatter's disease) and calcaneus (Sever's disease). In adults, insertional tendinopathy can occur at the osteotendinous junction, with collagen fragmentation and disorganization and thickening of the fibrocartilage zone. Such changes are not infrequently seen at the Achilles' tendon insertion site onto the calcaneus and at the rotator cuff insertion site onto the greater tuberosity.

Calcific tendinitis refers to a process that is distinct from tendinosis and degenerative tendon calcification.[20] Calcific tendinitis is a common, self-limited process of unknown etiology, in which calcium hydroxyapatite forms in a tendon and then is ultimately spontaneously resorbed, with healing of the tendon.[21] It occurs commonly in the rotator cuff tendons but has also been reported in other tendons, including the pectoralis major, deltoid, flexor carpi ulnaris, gluteus maximus and medius, and adductor magnus.[22] Calcium hydroxyapatite deposition is often asymptomatic, but resorption can be associated with significant pain.[23]

> Calcific tendinitis is due to the deposition of calcium hydroxyapatite within a tendon; it may be the cause of symptoms or an incidental finding on radiographs.

A bursa is a synovial-lined structure that lies between a tendon and a nearby bony prominence or other compressive structure.[13,24] The bursa facilitates gliding motion of the tendon through the surrounding soft tissue. Some bursae develop in utero and many are present at birth.[24] Some bursae remain isolated, whereas others develop a secondary communication with a joint.[24] Bursal anatomy can be variable, even at established anatomic sites. In addition, synovial-lined adventitial bursae may develop at any point in life, in response to local friction.

OSTEOARTICULAR IMAGING FEATURES OF TENDONS AND BURSAE

Radiographs

Although radiographs are of limited utility in imaging of tendons and bursae, they represent an important first step in the evaluation of symptoms, helping to detect associated ossification or bony pathology, exclude other causes of symptoms, and evaluate for potential complications. Tendons are visible on radiographs when they are surrounded by fat and lie tangential to the x-ray beam, as is the case with the Achilles' and patellar tendons (Figure 13-2, *A*, and Figure 13-3, *A*). In these instances, they may be assessed for their thickness, uniform diameter, and the preservation of surrounding fat. With edema or fibrosis in the fat surrounding the tendon, however, the tendon contours will be effaced. Tendinosis or intrasubstance tearing may cause focal or diffuse thickening of the usual tendon contour (Figure 13-2, *B*), but, in general, these intrasubstance changes will not be visible radiographically. Gross disruption of the tendon may be evident as a result of marked changes in the normal contour of the tendon, often with tendon waviness (Figure 13-2, *C*, and Figure 13-3, *B*), but partial tears or nondistracted complete tears may not be apparent. When the tendon envelops a bony sesamoid or ossicle, retraction of the bony structure can provide radiographic evidence of tendon tear. This is seen most commonly with tears of the quadriceps or patellar tendons when they cause retraction of the patella but also is observed, less commonly, as a sign of tear in the posterior tibial or peroneal tendons of the hindfoot. Avulsion fractures at tendon insertion sites provide a similar radiographic sign of functional tendon disruption, which is seen, among other sites, at the flexor tendon insertion onto the middle phalanx of the hand ("volar plate fracture"), the triceps tendon insertion site onto the olecranon, and the Achilles' tendon insertion onto the calcaneus (Figure 13-4). Occasionally, the absence of a tendon may become apparent because of loss of its usual mass effect. Such is the case in chronic rotator cuff tear, when the rotator cuff outlet space is effaced and the humeral head abuts the undersurface of the acromion. Acromial humeral narrowing of $\leq$ 7 mm has a high correlation with rotator cuff tear [25] (Figure 13-5).

> Narrowing of the space between the humeral head and the acromion to 7 mm or less usually indicates a chronic rotator cuff tear.

Tendon laxity or rupture may also be inferred from abnormal bone alignment in certain locations, such as flexion of the distal interphalangeal joint of the finger ("mallet finger") indicating rupture of the extensor tendon (Figure 13-6, *A*) or pes planus on a standing view of the foot due to insufficiency of the posterior tibial tendon (Figure 13-6, *B*).

Radiographs may demonstrate calcifications within the tendon associated with insertional tendinopathy (e.g., at insertion of the Achilles' tendon or rotator cuff) (see Figure 13-2, *D*), heterotopic ossification associated with osteochondroses at a tendon-bone interface (e.g., Sindig-Larsen-Johanssen and Osgood-Schlatter

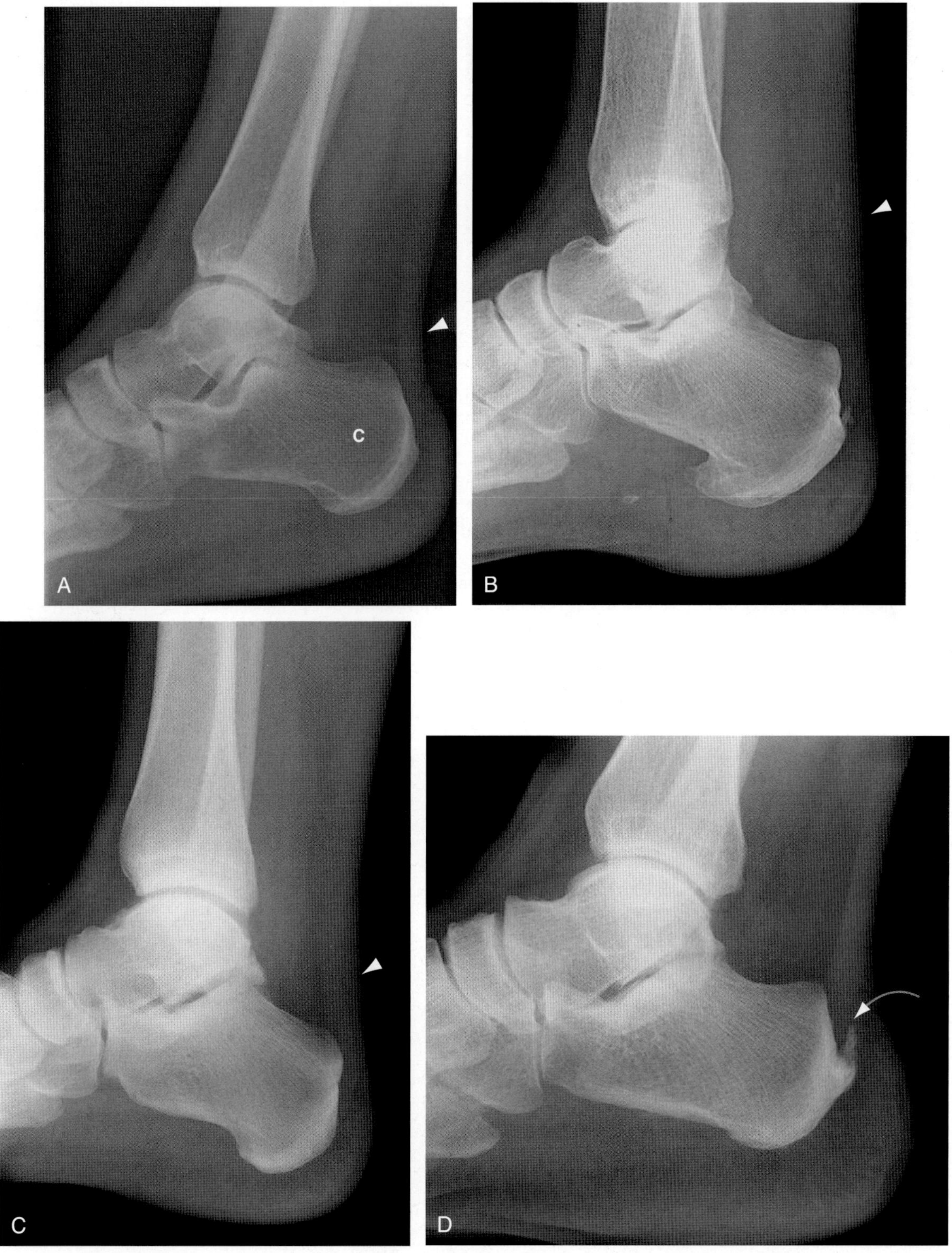

FIGURE 13-2. Radiography of the Achilles' tendon. **A,** The normal Achilles' tendon is visible on radiographs *(arrowhead)* when surrounded by fat and tangential to the x-ray beam. It demonstrates uniform thickness and a well-defined interface with the surrounding fat. *c,* Calcaneus. **B,** Achilles' tendinosis appears as a thickened tendon. Metaplastic ossification *(arrowhead)* can be a feature of tendinosis. **C,** The Achilles' tendon is completely ruptured, with diffuse thickening *(arrowhead)*, but the tear itself is not evident radiographically. Tendon tear and tendinosis can be difficult to distinguish. In other cases, a torn tendon may lose its distinct structure. **D,** Insertional tendinosis. The distal tendon is thickened at its site of insertion onto the calcaneus and an insertional enthesophyte has formed *(curved arrow)*.

changes at the proximal and distal edges of the patellar tendon, respectively) (Figure 13-7), or metaplastic ossification within a degenerated tendon. Radiographs may also reveal bony findings that are associated with tendon pathology, such as an accessory navicular bone associated with a predisposition to posterior tibial tendon tears, nonaggressive periosteal new bone formation along the distal radius laterally occurring secondary to degeneration of the first extensor compartment tendons (DeQuervain's tenosynovitis),[26] similar periostitis along the distal tibia medially associated with posterior tibia tendon degeneration (Figure 13-6, *C*),

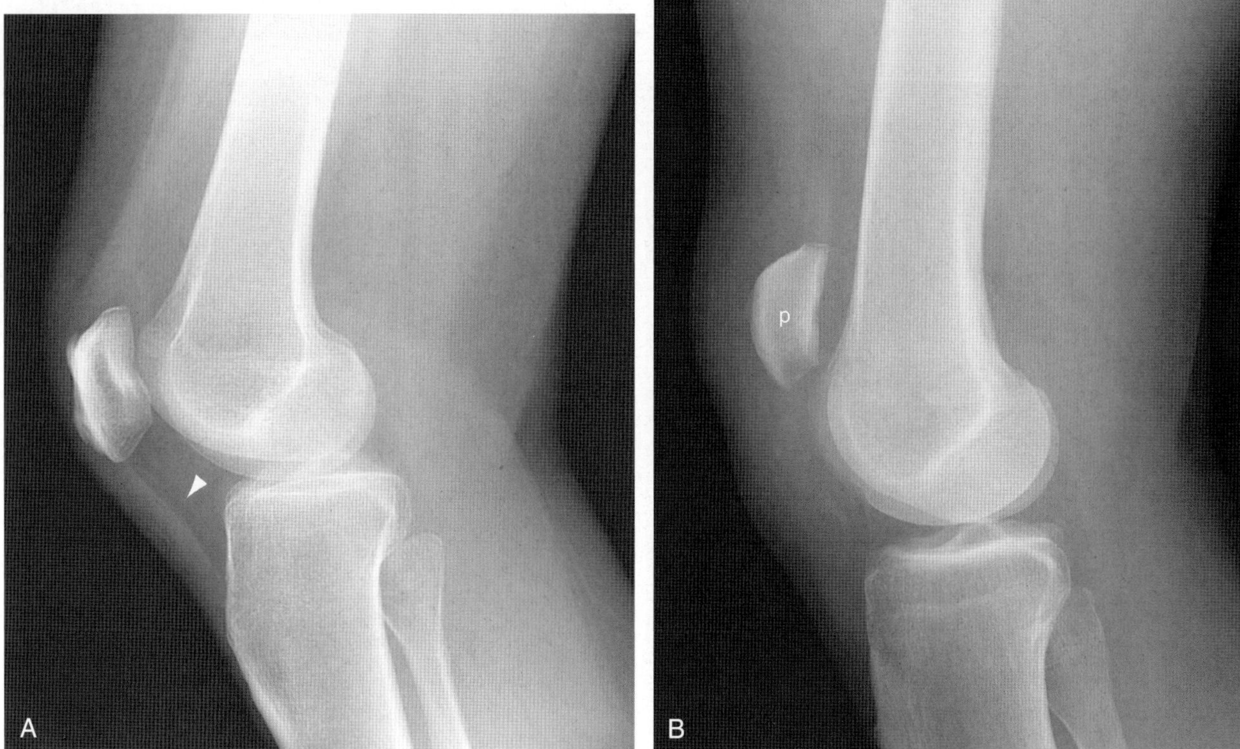

FIGURE 13-3. Radiography of the patellar tendon. **A,** The normal patellar tendon is visible on radiographs *(arrowhead)* when surrounded by fat and tangential to the x-ray beam. Like the normal Achilles' tendon, the normal patellar tendon demonstrates uniform thickness and a well-defined interface with the surrounding fat. **B,** When the patellar tendon is completely ruptured, its interface with surrounding fat become indistinct and it is no longer visible. The patella *(p)* may be retracted proximally ("patella alta"), as it is in this case.

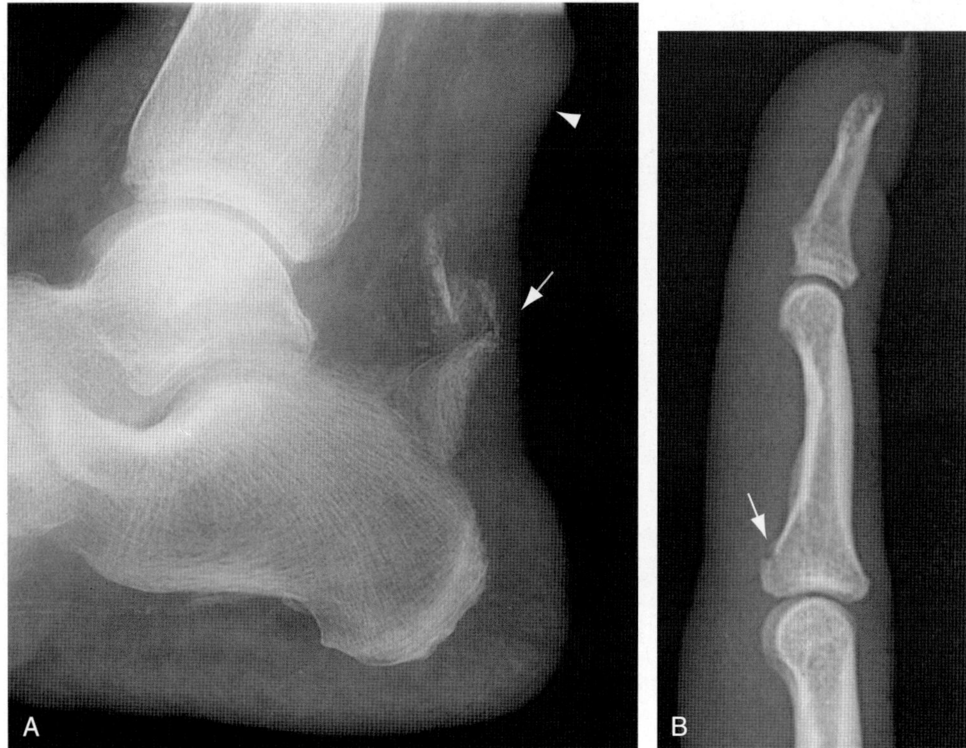

FIGURE 13-4. Tendon avulsion with fracture at avulsion site. **A,** Achilles' tendon avulsion. The Achilles' tendon has avulsed its insertion site at the posterosuperior calcaneus. The tendon contour is thickened and irregular *(arrowhead)* and the avulsed fragment of bone is retracted proximally *(arrow)*. **B,** Flexor digitorum tendon avulsion. The flexor digitorum tendon has avulsed from its insertion site onto the middle phalanx, creating a small "volar plate" avulsion fracture *(arrow)*. This is a common injury, often caused by hyperextension of the digit, that requires urgent treatment to ensure restoration of normal flexor tendon function.

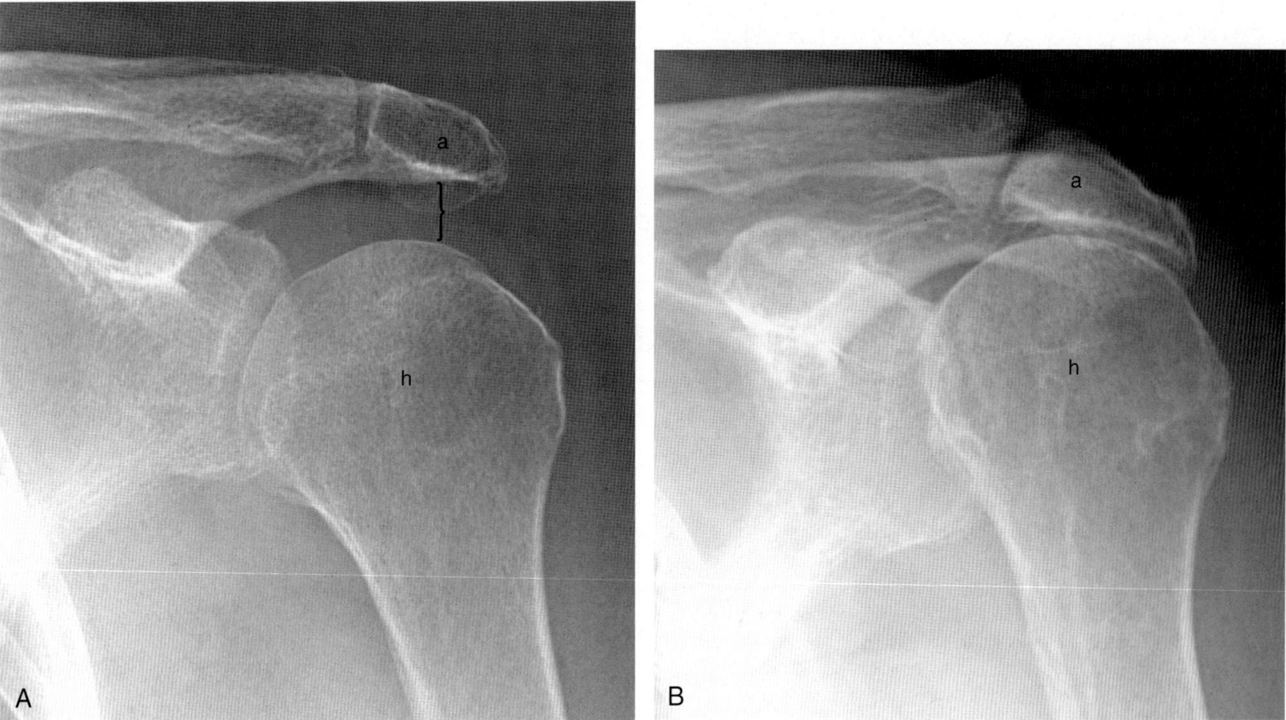

FIGURE 13-5. Chronic rotator cuff tear. **A,** The relatively radiolucent soft tissues of the rotator cuff tendons, particularly the supraspinatus, fill the space between the acromion and the humeral head *(bracket)*. **B,** In a chronic rotator cuff tear, the acromiohumeral distance becomes narrowed. Remodeling of the undersurface of the acromion by the humeral head is indicative of chronicity. *a,* Acromion; *h,* humeral head.

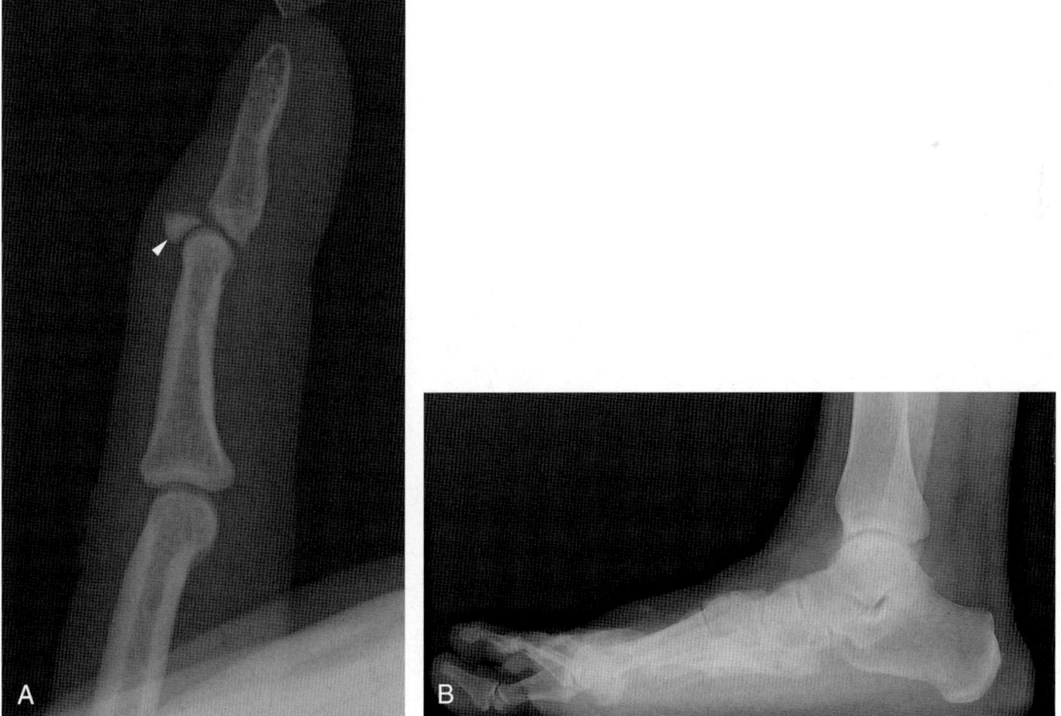

FIGURE 13-6. Abnormal bone alignment as a sign of tendon failure. **A,** Mallet finger. A lateral view of the digit shows an avulsion fracture at the site of insertion of the extensor digitorum tendon onto the distal phalanx. The avulsed fracture fragment is seen dorsally *(arrowhead)*. Because the action of the flexor tendon on the distal phalanx is no longer opposed by the extensor tendon, there is abnormal alignment of the phalanges: the distal phalanx has subluxed slightly in a volar direction with respect to the middle phalanx, creating the "mallet finger" deformity. **B,** A standing lateral view of the foot demonstrates pes planus (i.e., loss of the usual longitudinal arch). The presence of pes planus is associated with posterior tibial tendon tendinopathy, as the posterior tibial tendon plays an important role in helping to maintain the longitudinal arch.

(Continued)

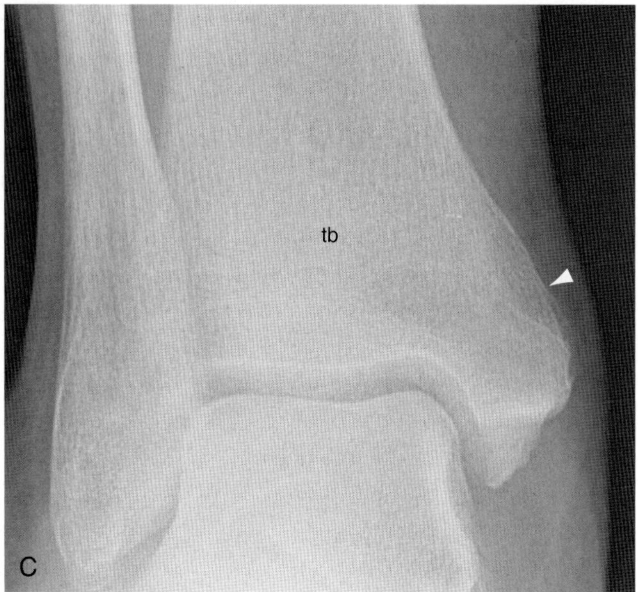

FIGURE 13-6—cont'd. C, Mature periosteal new bone formation or spurring along the distal tibia medially *(arrowhead)* has been described as a sign of posterior tibial tendon tendinopathy. A similar finding along the distal radius laterally has been reported as a sign of DeQuervain's tenosynovitis. *tb,* Tibia.

or irregularity along the greater tuberosity of the proximal humerus, which can be seen with rotator cuff pathology.[27] Of note, radiographs are instrumental in demonstrating and diagnosing calcium hydroxyapatite deposits associated with calcific tendinitis, a finding that is often overlooked or misinterpreted on magnetic resonance imaging (MRI) scans and can be the key to explaining a patient's symptoms (Figure 13-8).

Calcification may be less apparent on MRI than on radiographs.

Bursae are generally not visible radiographically. However, when a bursa abuts or is surrounded by fat and is tangential to the x-ray beam, it may become visible when distended. Distended pre-patellar, olecranon, and retrocalcaneal bursae may be visible on radiographs (Figure 13-9). There may be edema in the surrounding fat. Bony osteolysis or reactive sclerosis may be visualized. The presence or absence of infection within a bursa cannot be determined on the basis of imaging. Calcification outlining the bursa suggests the presence of hydroxyapatite and associated calcific bursitis. Multiple loose bodies within the bursa may have migrated from a communicating osteoarthritic joint or may indicate a rare occurrence of intrabursal synovial osteochondromatosis.[27a]

Computed Tomography

Tendons, particularly tendon course and caliber, are well depicted by computed tomography (CT). However, CT images have less intrinsic soft tissue contrast than MRI or ultrasound and thus are less effective in depicting the full range of tendon pathology. As a result, CT is not considered the first-line cross-sectional modality for tendon imaging. Nonetheless, CT can provide considerable useful information regarding tendons and tendon pathology and may be of particular utility when questions involve soft tissue calcification or ossification or the relation between a tendon and bone or bone fragments or when MRI or ultrasound is not feasible.

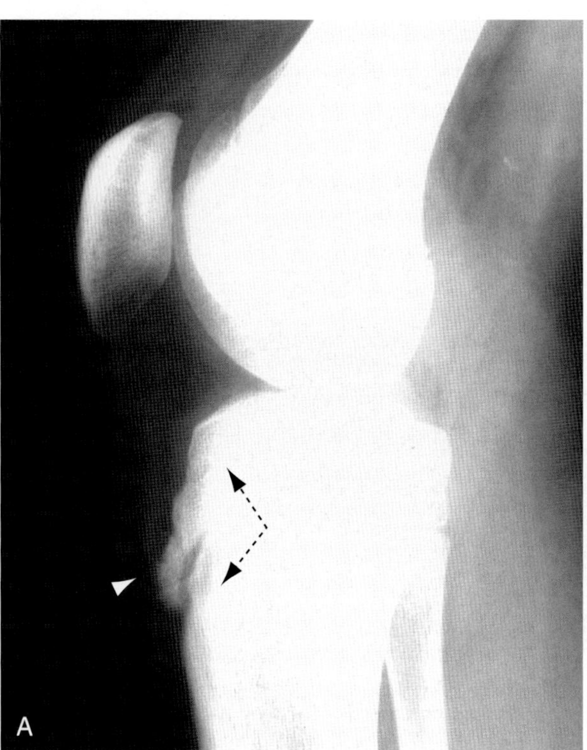

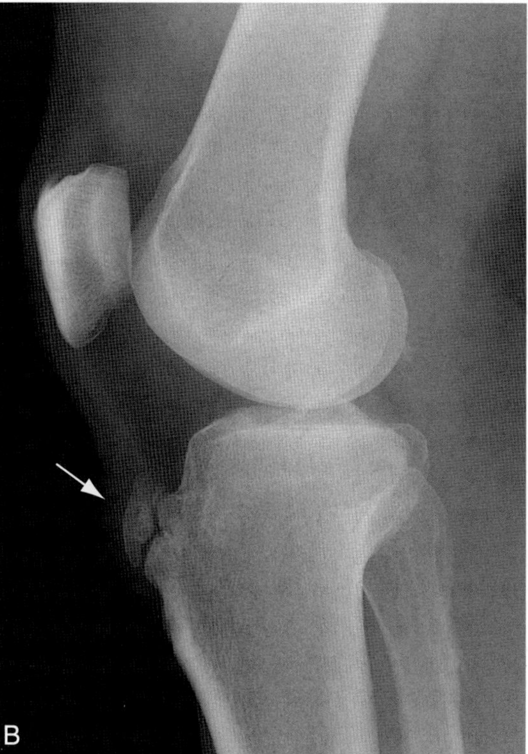

FIGURE 13-7. Osgood-Schlatter's apophysitis. Lateral views of the knee. **A,** The physes are unfused *(dotted arrow)* in this adolescent male, with tenderness over the tibial tubercle *(arrowhead).* Swelling and calcification are faintly visible in the soft tissues immediately adjacent to the tibial tubercle, in the region of the distal patellar tendon. **B,** Ossification is seen in the distal patellar tendon *(arrow),* representing residua from childhood Osgood-Schlatter's disease in an asymptomatic adult.

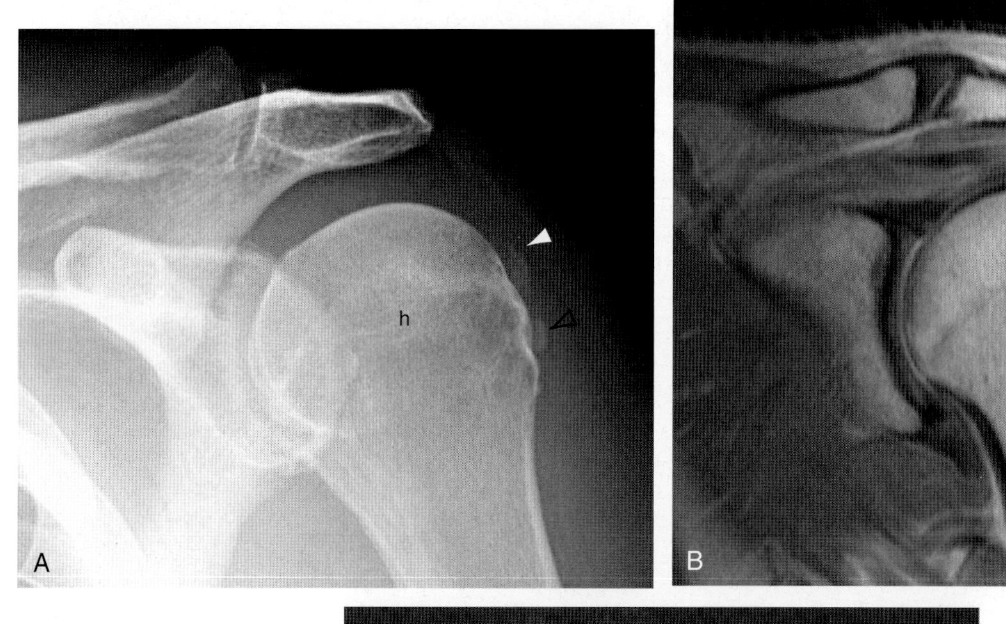

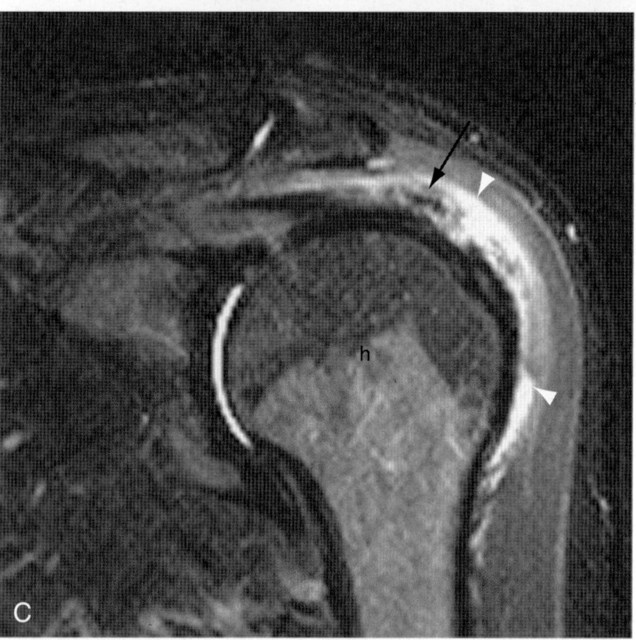

FIGURE 13-8. Calcific tendinitis. **A,** Two foci of hydroxyapatite are seen superimposed over the tendons of the rotator cuff. The more proximal focus is more amorphous *(solid arrowhead)* and the more distal focus is more discrete *(open arrowhead)*. **B,** Proton density weighted MR image and **(C)** fat-saturated T2-weighted MR image. On MRI, the focus of calcific tendinitis is seen as a region of low signal along the course of the supraspinatus tendon *(arrow)*, but this finding is easily overlooked without a correlative radiograph. There is extensive edema and fluid surrounding the focus of calcific tendinitis, seen as bright signal on **C** *(arrowheads)*. In some cases, this may be accompanied by bone marrow edema. This high T2 signal can be mistaken for infection or other causes of inflammation, if knowledge of the radiographic finding is not available. *h,* Humeral head.

CT allows for very rapid, high-resolution imaging over a large field of view and is highly reproducible and operator independent. New generation multidetector scanners provide techniques that help minimize artifact from orthopedic hardware. Exposure to ionizing radiation remains a concern, particularly with repeat exams, but radiation exposure to extremities is generally better tolerated than radiation to the torso.

Tendons are more electron dense than muscle or fat on CT and therefore appear "bright" compared to muscle and fat. Density on CT is measured by Hounsfield units (HU) and tendons measure 75 to 115 HU, considerably more electron dense than muscle (55 to 60 HU) or fat (< 0 HU) and considerably less dense than bone (930 to 953 HU).[28-30] On CT, normal tendons are seen as high-density structures, typically round, ovoid or flat, and smooth bordered and have a characteristic normal diameter (Figure 13-10, *A*). The tendon course can typically be traced from its musculotendinous origin to its insertion site. Tenosynovitis may be evident as well-demarcated lower-density material surrounding tendon along its course (Figure 13-10, *B*). Simple fluid measures < 20 HU, whereas hemorrhagic or proteinaceous fluid will show higher HU values. Tendon enlargement or attenuation can be detected. Chronic partial rupture or degeneration is seen as increased tendon diameter associated with

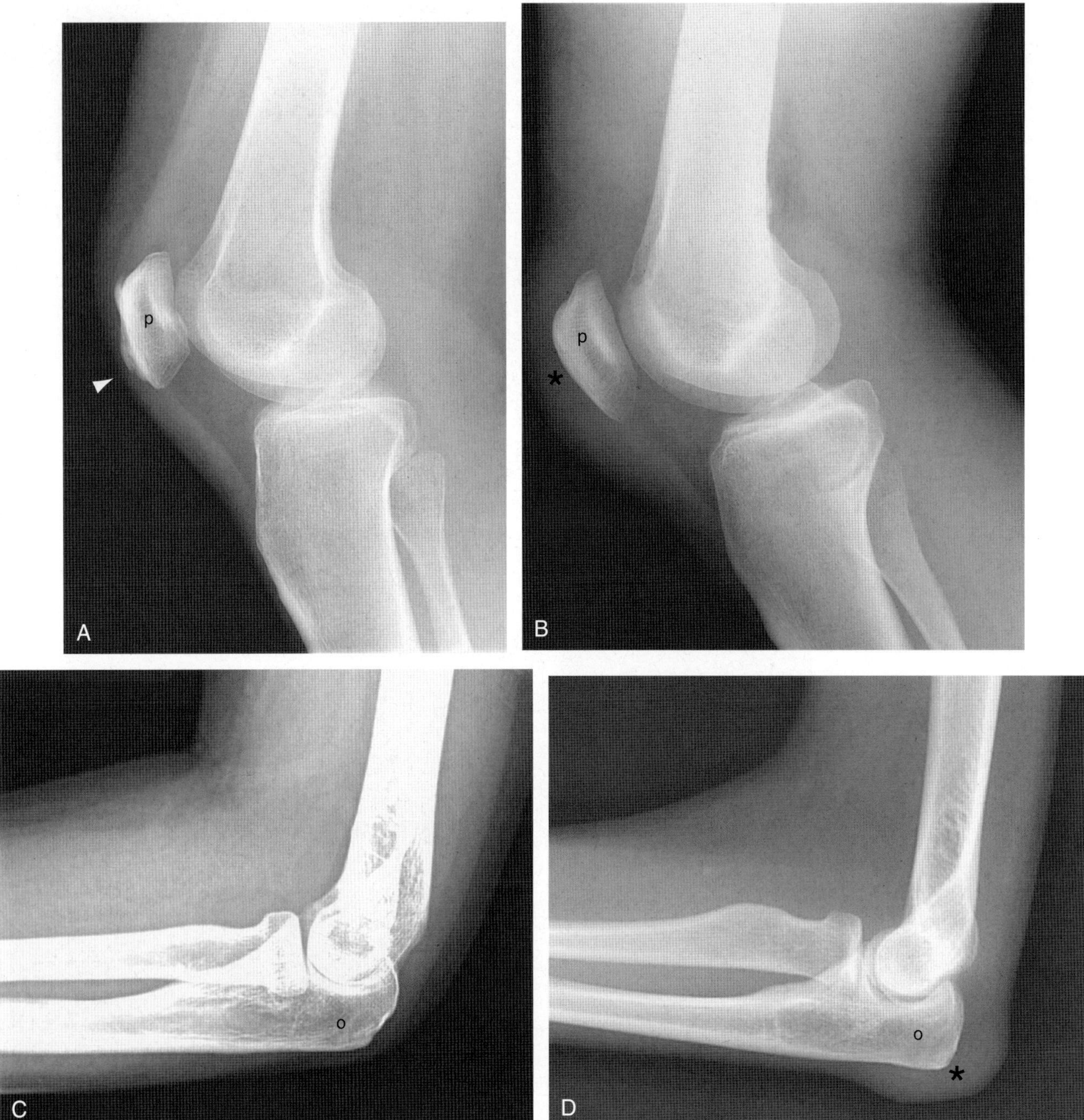

FIGURE 13-9. Bursitis on radiographs. **A,** Normal prepatellar bursa *(arrowhead)*. **B,** Prepatellar soft tissues are thickened and abnormally dense *(asterisk)*, consistent with prepatellar bursitis. The differential diagnosis includes interstitial edema in the prepatellar fat. **C,** Normal olecranon bursa. **D,** Olecranon bursitis in the setting of gout *(asterisk)*. *o*, olecranon; *p*, patella.

(Continued)

diffuse or heterogeneous decreased tendon density (30 to 50 HU) (Figure 13-10, *C*).[28,31,32] More severe tendon rupture may be visible as focal attenuation of the tendon.[31,32] Changes in tendon attenuation can be identified, including internal low density indicative of tendon degeneration and/or intrasubstance tear and high density associated with tendon calcification or ossification (Figure 13-10, *D* to *F*). However, early tendon degeneration may not be detectable on CT. A complete tendon tear, with tendon retraction, may be evident by CT, but the presence of edema or fibrosis may obscure the tendon rupture. Rosenberg et al. studied 28 cases of suspected posterior tibial tendon tear using CT, categorizing the tendons as normal or as Type I (intact, enlarged, heterogeneous); Type II (attenuated), or Type III (complete transverse rupture with gap) tears,[32] compared with surgery. Overall accuracy in detecting tendon tears was 82%. In 4 of 28 cases, CT identified the tendon rupture but underestimated the extent of tear, and, in one case CT failed to detect a type I tear. In general, CT is less effective than MRI or ultrasound in demonstrating intrasubstance tendon degeneration, longitudinal splits, partial tears,[31,32] and tenosynovial fluid[31] and less effective than MRI in demonstrating tendon contours in the setting of surrounding edema or fibrosis.[31] However, tendon subluxation is readily identified on CT,[28,33] as are bony abnormalities that might predispose to subluxation, such as a shallow retromalleolar

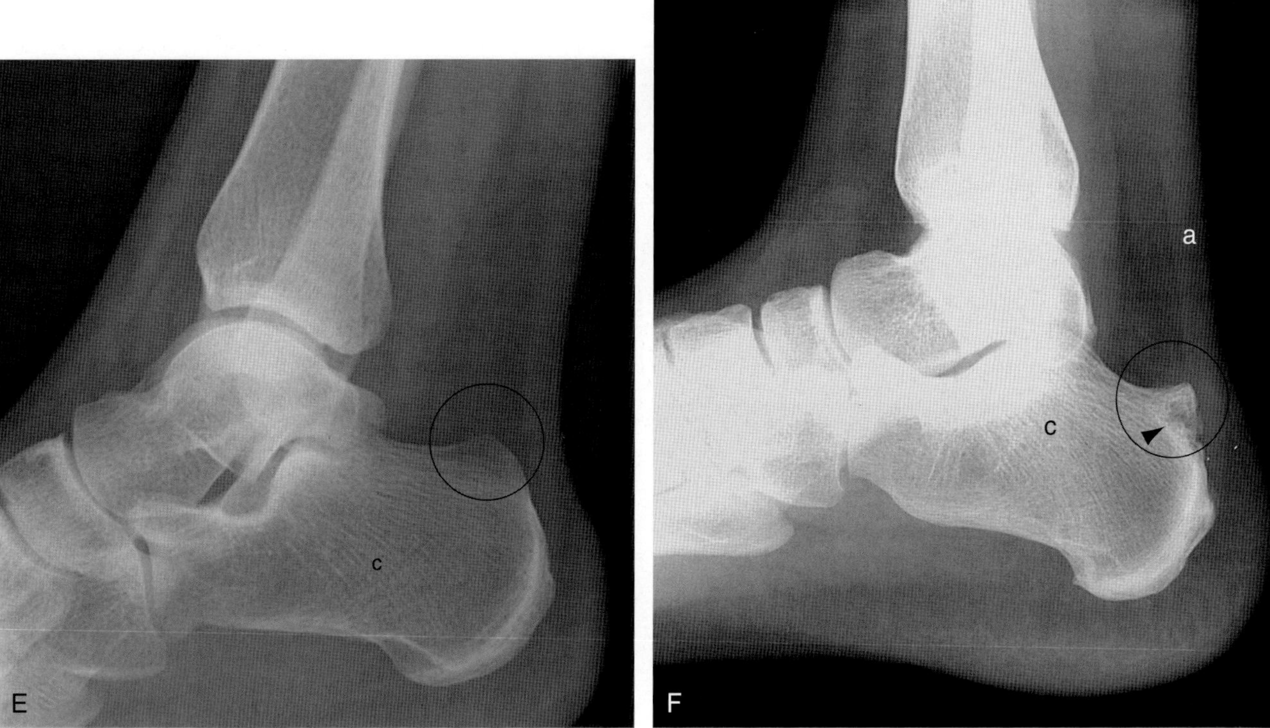

FIGURE 13-9—cont'd. **E,** Normal retrocalcaneal bursa. Tissue interposed between the posterosuperior calcaneus and distal Achilles' tendon is of normal fat density *(circle)*. **F,** Retrocalcaneal bursitis in patient with rheumatoid arthritis. The retrocalcaneal fat is obscured by fluid in the retrocalcaneal bursa. Due to the bursitis, an erosion has developed in the calcaneus *(arrowhead)*. *a,* Achilles' tendon; *c,* calcaneus.

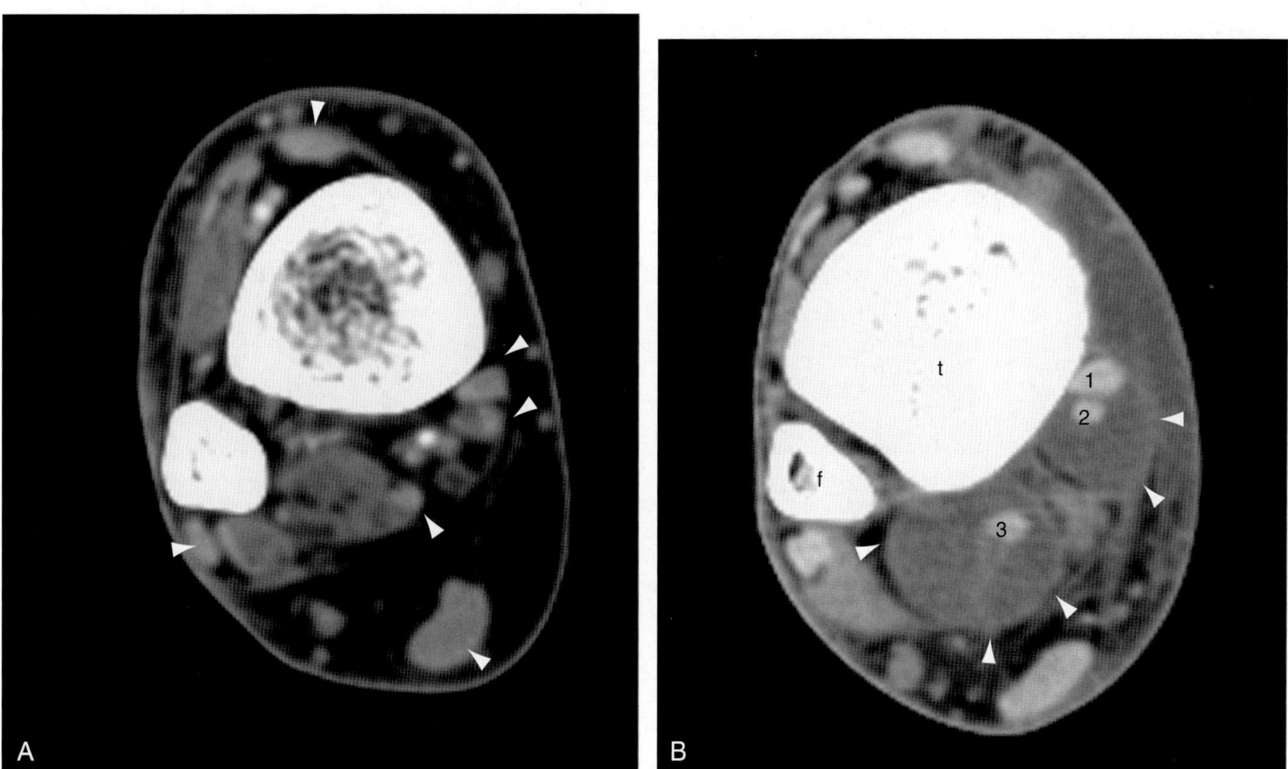

FIGURE 13-10. **A,** Normal tendons are easily visualized on CT as high-density structures with well-defined borders *(arrowheads)*. **B,** Axial image through the ankle showing tenosynovitis of the posterior tibial *(1)*, flexor digitorum *(2)*, and flexor hallucis *(3)* tendons *(arrowheads)*. Tenosynovitis is seen as material enveloping the tendon and contained within the tendon sheath. Simple fluid is lower density; complex material may shower high attenuation and may be more similar in density to the normal tendon. *f,* femur; *t,* tibia.

(Continued)

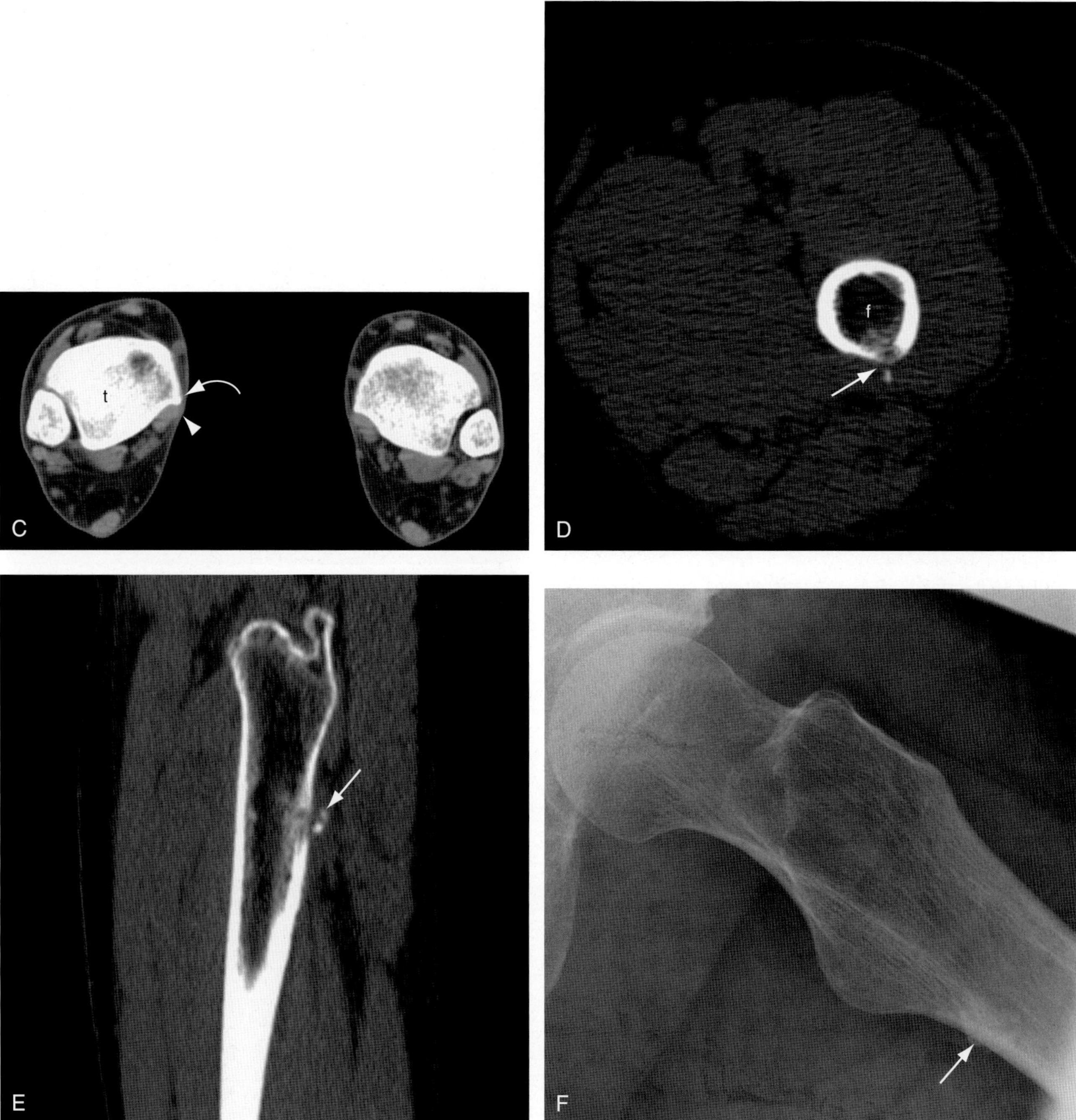

FIGURE 13-10—cont'd. **C,** Posterior tibial tendon tendinosis, seen as tendon enlargement, worse on the right side *(arrowhead).* Note the medial tibial spurring *(curved arrow).* **D,** Axial image through the thigh shows calcific tendinitis involving the gluteus maximus tendon insertion site onto the proximal posterior femur *(arrow).* As in this case, it can be associated with cortical erosion. **E,** Sagittal reformatted image through the same area helps to better demonstrate the relationship of the calcification *(arrow)* to the gluteus maximus tendon insertion site. **F,** The calcification *(arrow)* and its anatomic significance is much better demonstrated on the CT images, than on the corresponding radiograph; an experienced practitioner may recognize the significance of the finding if it is visualized on the radiograph, but an inexperienced practitioner may not. *f,* Femur; *t,* tibia.

groove in the distal fibula.[34] CT also readily demonstrates tendon entrapment by fracture fragments[33] (Figure 13-11), bone spurs that might contribute to tendon pathology, and bony periostitis that is associated with tendon degeneration in the distal radius or tibia (Figure 13-10, *C*).

CT can demonstrate tendon tears but is less effective than MRI or ultrasound in demonstrating subtle abnormalities.

CT images are acquired axially, but, using newer generations of multidetector and volume CT scanners, the axial sections acquired are so thin that the resultant voxels are near-isotropic and can be reconstructed along any plane of interest (multiplanar reconstruction) while retaining high spatial resolution (see Figure 13-11). This is of particular utility for tendons that may follow an oblique or curved course. Images acquired in routine protocols can also be post-processed as three-dimensional (3D) volume rendered

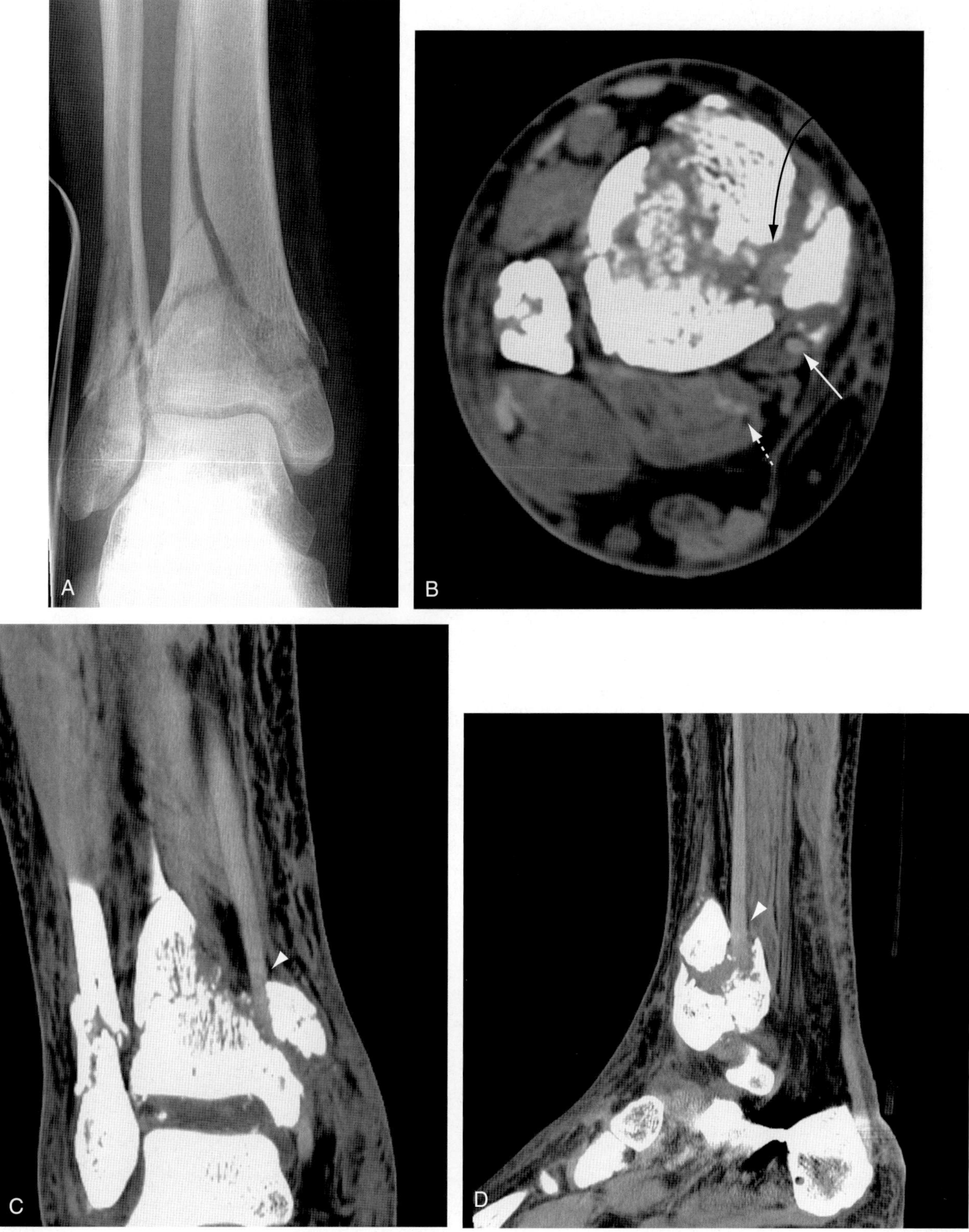

FIGURE 13-11. Tendon entrapment by fracture fragments. **A,** AP radiograph demonstrating a comminuted fracture of the distal tibia. Findings related to specific soft tissue structures are limited. **B,** On axial images acquired through the fracture site, an ovoid high-density structure consistent with the posterior tibial tendon *(PTT)* is seen entrapped by fracture fragments *(curved arrow).* The flexor digitorum *(solid arrow)* and flexor hallucis *(dashed arrow)* tendons appear normal and lie in their anatomic positions. **(C)** Coronal and **(D)** sagittal reformatted images, generated from post-processing the acquired axial images, depict the abnormal course of the PTT as it becomes entrapped by the fracture fragments *(arrowheads).*

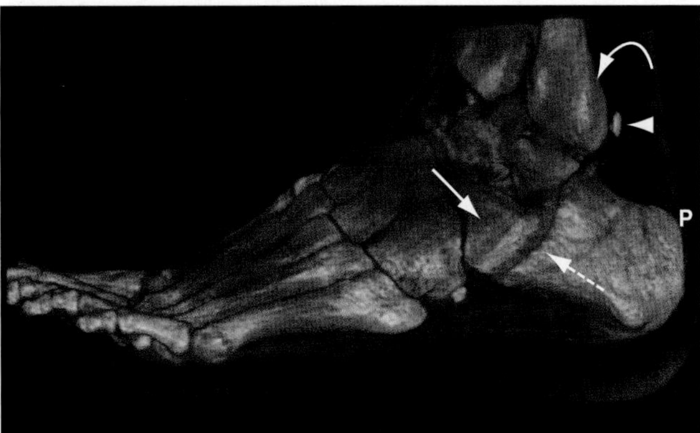

FIGURE 13-12. 3D volume rendered CT image of tendons. Multidetector CT scans can produce 3D or volumetric data sets that can be post-processed to produce volume-rendered 3D images of both bone and soft tissue anatomy. Routine axial images can be manipulated in this way to depict tendons and their relation to the bony surfaces. In conjunction with standard imaging, this technique may aid in preoperative planning. Here, the peroneal tendons (peroneus brevis, *solid arrow*; peroneus longus, *dotted arrow*) are subluxed anteriorly with respect to their usual position in the groove *(curved arrow)* along the posterior surface of the fibula, due to disruption of the superior peroneal retinaculum. A small bony fragment *(arrowhead)* represents an avulsion fracture at the insertion site of the superior peroneal retinaculum onto the distal fibula,

reformatted images, which help depict tendons in relation to their bony landmarks and have shown early promise for helping in the preoperative planning of tendon rupture repair[35] (Figure 13-12). Unlike MRI, the CT images can be obtained rapidly over a lengthy field of view. However, limitations regarding sensitivity for detection of tendon tear remain. In addition, to date, distal tendons in the hand, particularly on the extensor side, are not well demonstrated with this technique.[35]

Normal bursae are generally not visible on CT. A distended bursa is visible as a discrete fluid or soft tissue density structure, in a characteristic location (Figure 13-13). Simple fluid within the bursa measures shows low density, similar to water. Hemorrhage or proteinaceous fluid or pus measures greater than 20 HU. Thickened synovium yields variable density measurements, typically more than simple fluid. Following administration of intravenous (IV) contrast, several different enhancement patterns may be seen: (1) a non-inflamed fluid-filled bursa will demonstrate a thin rim of peripheral enhancement; (2) an inflamed fluid-filled bursa will demonstrate a somewhat thickened rim of enhancement; or (3) a bursa containing thickened synovium will show variable internal enhancement corresponding to the volume and distribution of hypertrophic synovial tissue present. Rare instances of intrabursal masses, such as pigmented villonodular synovitis or other soft tissue masses, may also demonstrate internal enhancement within the bursa. When there is edema, inflammation, or fibrosis in the tissue surrounding the bursa, bursal borders may be obscured. As with other modalities, the presence or absence of infection within a bursa cannot be determined on the basis of imaging. Calcification within the bursa may be due to calcific bursitis, synovial osteochondromatosis, or (in bursae that communicate with a joint) loose bodies. The CT imaging features of iliopsoas bursitis[36] (Figure 13-13, *A*), greater trochanteric bursitis,[37] anserine bursitis,[38] radiobicipital bursitis,[39] and adventitial bursitis of the scapulothoracic articulation[40] have been described. Spence et al. noted that CT was less sensitive for detection of septae within bursae than ultrasound and less sensitive than MRI for detection of rice bodies.[39]

> Although a distended bursa may be detected on CT, the presence or absence of infection within a bursa cannot be determined by imaging.

Magnetic Resonance Imaging

MRI is an extremely effective method for imaging of tendons and bursae. Tendons and bursae throughout the body, both superficial and deep, can be imaged in their entirety. Unlike ultrasound, the technique is not operator dependent and interpretation skills are more broadly disseminated. Although MRI protocols vary from institution to institution, most protocols are well suited to the depiction of tendon and bursae and their attendant pathology.

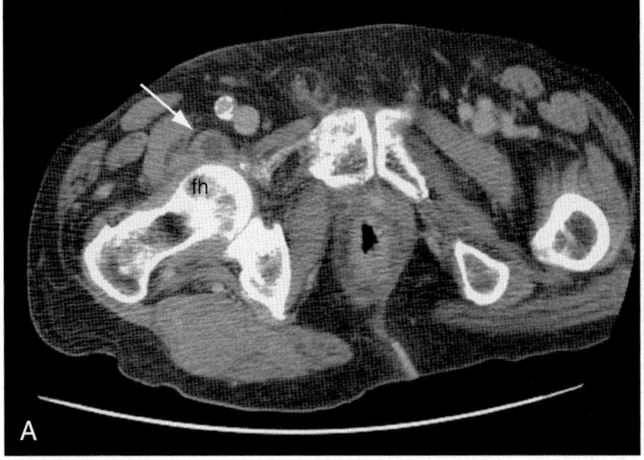

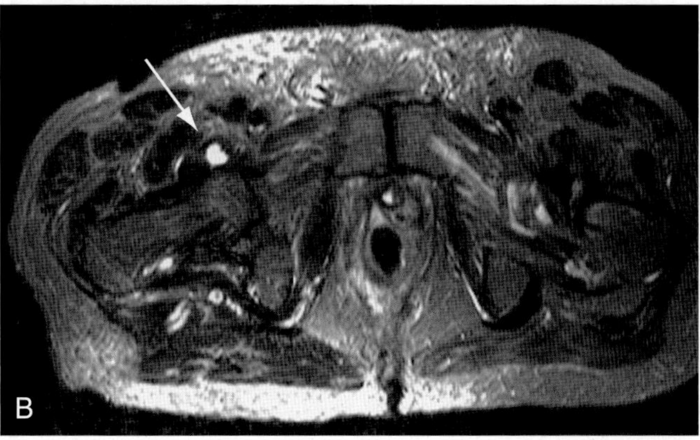

FIGURE 13-13. Iliopsoas bursitis. **A,** Axial CT images through the low pelvis and right hip joint shows a rounded fluid density structure immediately anterior to the femoral head *(arrow)*, without an associated hip joint effusion, consistent with iliopsoas bursitis. The iliopsoas bursa can communicate with the hip joint and may become distended when there is a joint effusion. Here, the disproportionate amount of fluid in the iliopsoas bursa, compared with the hip joint, is highly suggestive of bursitis. **B,** Axial T2-weighted MR image at the same level in the same patient demonstrates analogous findings, with high T2 fluid or hyperemic synovium within the iliopsoas bursa *(arrow)*. *fh,* Femoral head.

Tendinosis, partial and complete tears, tear size and associated muscle atrophy, tenosynovitis and paratenonitis, tendon subluxation/dislocation, insertional tendinopathy, and injury to the musculotendinous junction can be depicted. Bursal distension with fluid or synovitis can be demonstrated. Because soft tissue calcification and small bony fragments are not well depicted on MRI, correlative radiographs are an important adjunct to an MRI exam.

Radiographs can provide information that is helpful for MRI interpretation.

MRI is often performed at field strengths of 1.5T, but imaging is also performed on lower field strength magnets, on newer 3T magnets, and on dedicated extremity machines ranging in field strength from 0.2T to 1T. In general, high field strengths can be used to produce images of higher spatial resolution and/or shorter duration. 3T magnets are new to the market, and their clinical accuracy is only beginning to be evaluated.[41,42] High-resolution imaging is dependent on the use of a local receiver coil, a specialized antennae designed to lie in close proximity to the tissue of interest in order to increase sensitivity for detection of signal. Use of a local coil allows for higher signal-to-noise ratio (SNR), which can be used to produce images with higher spatial resolution. In all instances, the anatomic area of interest must lie in the craniocaudad center of the magnet. In newer short-bore magnets, most patients' knees and ankles can be imaged with the head outside the magnet. The wrist and elbow are optimally imaged with the patient lying prone and the arm extended overhead, but these joints can also be imaged with the patient supine and the arm down at the side. Dedicated extremity magnets allow the patient to sit outside the bore of the magnet while extending the limb of interest into the bore of the magnet and permit imaging from elbow to hand and from knee to foot.[43] Because these are lower-field magnets, they trade-off lower spatial resolution against longer duration of exam.[44] Depending on specifics of hardware and technique, subtle pathology and smaller structures may not be optimally visualized on these lower-field magnets.

The typical musculoskeletal MR examination lasts from 25 to 45 minutes. It consists of several individual sequences, each lasting 2 to7 minutes. Different sequences are designed to highlight different tissue characteristics. Typical sequences include proton density weighted or T1-weighted sequences to highlight anatomic structures and T2-weighted sequences or fat-saturated proton density weighted or T2-weighted sequences to highlight edema and fluid (as indicators of pathology). Sequences are obtained in multiple planes, typically axial, oblique coronal, and oblique sagittal planes, with planes optimized to depict the anatomy for the joint or limb of interest. The axial plane is often, but not always, the most useful for examining tendons. In some instances, an oblique axial plane may be used to help display a tendon in true cross section. Because the ankle tendons follow a curvilinear course when the ankle is at 90 degrees, the ankle may be imaged in plantar flexion in order to achieve true axial images through these tendons. For evaluation of the rotator cuff, each of the three planes—oblique coronal, oblique sagittal, and axial—may provide useful unique information. The use of an oblique sagittal image plane angled perpendicular to the curve of the tendons over the humeral head has also been described but yielded only minor improvements in diagnostic accuracy in that study.[45] It is important to obtain thin section images with high spatial resolution and sufficient SNR in order to optimize the ability to detect small tendon abnormalities; small tendon tears or small foci of degeneration may not be visible on images obtained with insufficient resolution or SNR. Gadolinium contrast is not usually employed for MR evaluation of tendons. However, under certain circumstances, IV gadolinium contrast may be administered. Gadolinium contrast can help to distinguish cystic from solid structures and can help to better delineate tissues planes. In particular, gadolinium contrast can be used to distinguish fluid in a tendon sheath or bursa from hyperemic thickened synovium.[46] Hyperemic synovium will enhance within the first few minutes after contrast administration; fluid will not. Contrast enhancement can be quantitated over time, providing indirect information about the degree of vascularity and the volume of interstitial space.[47,48] MR arthrography can be performed by instilling dilute gadolinium contrast directly into a joint and is used to detect labral tears, articular cartilage defects, and—in some joints—partial and complete tendon tears[49] (Figure 13-14). When intraarticular gadolinium is used, fat-saturated T1-weighted images are employed to highlight the bright signal from gadolinium contrast. For certain exams, special positioning can aid in evaluating the tendon. For example, in the shoulder, external rotation provides optimal separation of the supraspinatus and infraspinatus tendons. In the ankle, imaging the Achilles' tendon with the foot in plantar flexion can aid in assessing the potential for successful apposition of tendon tear edges when casted. When peroneal tendon subluxation is suspected, axial images of tendon can be obtained in both plantar and dorsiflexion. Although techniques for kinematic MRI of the joints have been described,[50] they usually employ specialized frames that restrict the motion to a single plane and are not in common clinical use.

The **normal tendon** is characterized by low signal intensity on all sequences (Figure 13-15) (Table 13-1). Normal collagen microfibrils bind water tightly and, because there is a paucity of mobile protons, the signal from tendons is low.[51,52] In pathologic states, the mobile water content of the tendon increases and higher signal areas appear within the tendon.[52] However, high signal can be seen within the normal tendon on short echotime (TE) sequences, when the tendon lies at an angle of 55 degrees to the main magnetic field, due to magic angle artifact. (Magic angle artifact is seen in anisotropic structures such as tendons when they are oriented at 55 degrees to the main magnetic field, due to an effect governing molecular relaxation; this effect is dependent on the value of Cos θ, a value that approaches 0 at 55 degrees.) When present, magic angle artifact is seen in all imaging planes (Figure 13-16). If the tendon position is adjusted within the magnet away from the 55-degree angle, the artifactual signal will be eliminated.[53] When the main magnetic field extends along the bore of the magnet, as is the case with most contemporary 1.5T magnets, magic angle artifact can be seen in the rotator cuff tendon. It can also be seen in the peroneal and other tendons when the ankle is imaged with the toes pointing upward, but it is eliminated when the ankle is imaged in plantar flexion. (When the main magnetic field runs perpendicular to the bore of the magnet, as is the case in a smaller subset of magnets, the sites of magic angle artifact within tendons will be shifted.) Tendon appearance varies due to differences in intrinsic tendon morphology, such as when the patellar tendon is uniformly low signal, whereas the quadriceps tendon is seen as a laminated structure with alternating low and high signal layers. Fusiform, unipennate, bipennate, multipennate, bicipital, and triangular musculotendinous morphologies can be distinguished.

High signal, simulating an abnormality, can be seen within a normal tendon on short TE sequences, when the tendon lies at an angle of about 55 degrees to the main magnetic field. This is termed "magic angle artifact."

Tendon degeneration can result in focal or diffuse tendon enlargement. In general, tendon degeneration appears as an area of high signal on proton density signal on proton density weighted or T1-weighted images and low to intermediate (but not as bright as fluid) on T2-weighted images (Figure 13-17). The use of fat saturation on T2-weighted images can accentuate the high signal seen within the tendon and, as a result, may make it more difficult to distinguish advanced degeneration from a partial tear.[54-57] Different

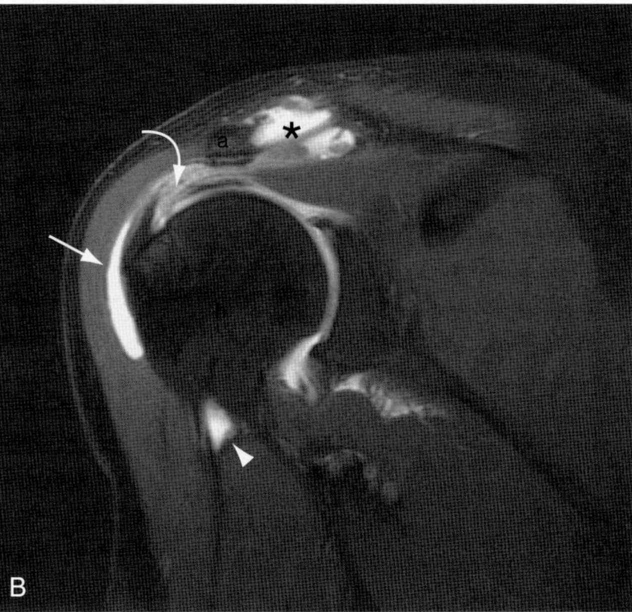

FIGURE 13-14. MR arthrogram with tendon tears. **A,** As a preliminary step in performing an MR arthrogram, contrast is instilled into the joint under x-ray fluoroscopic guidance. Here, a spot image from the fluoroscopy procedure shows that contrast that was injected into the glenohumeral joint has extravasated into the subacromial-subdeltoid bursa *(arrow)*. This indicates the presence of rotator cuff tear, although it does not provide detailed information regarding the location or size of the tear. Faint contrast within the joint outlines the humeral head cartilage *(arrowhead)* and fills the axillary recess *(ax)* of the glenohumeral joint. **B,** Coronal fat-saturated T1-weighted image through the shoulder. Gadolinium contrast, instilled under fluoroscopic guidance, appears bright or high signal. Contrast is seen not only within the joint, but also extending through a tear in the supraspinatus tendon *(curved arrow)*, into the subdeltoid bursa *(straight arrow)*. Contrast has also broken through into the acromioclavicular joint *(asterisk)*. Contrast surrounding the biceps tendon *(arrowhead)* is a normal finding, as the biceps tendon sheath communicates with the glenohumeral joint. *a,* Acromion; *h,* humeral head.

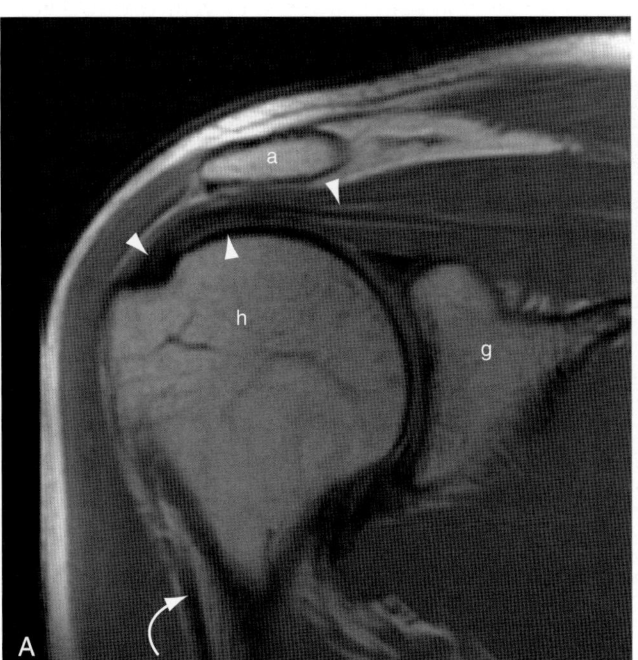

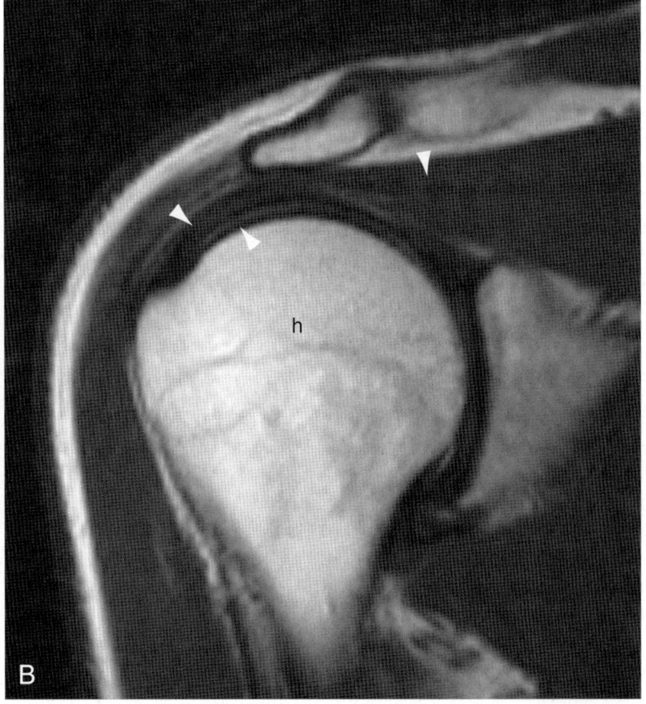

FIGURE 13-15. MRI of normal tendon. **A,** Coronal proton density weighted image through the shoulder. The tendon itself is very dark or low signal, in contrast to muscle, which is intermediate signal, and fat, which is bright. The supraspinatus tendon *(arrowheads)* is a smooth, thin, linear low signal structure that inserts on the greater tuberosity. Normal biceps tendon also appears dark *(curved arrow)*. **B,** Coronal T2-weighted image though the shoulder. Again, the normal tendon appears as a dark or low signal structure *(arrowheads)*. *a,* Acromion; *g,* glenoid; *h,* humeral head.

TABLE 13-1. Tendinopathy: Signal on MR Images

	Proton Density Weighted/T1-Weighted	T2-Weighted/Fat-Saturated T2- Weighted
Normal tendon	Low signal (dark)*	Low signal (dark)
Tendinosis	High signal (bright)	Low or intermediate signal (dark)
Tendon tear	High signal (bright)	High signal (bright)
Tenosynovitis	Low signal (dark) surrounding the tendon	High signal (bright) surrounding the tendon
Magic angle artifact	High signal (bright)	Low signal (dark)

*Signal on proton density weighted and T1-weighted images is similar but not exactly the same. Simple fluid will be lower signal on T1-weighted than on proton density weighted images, for example.

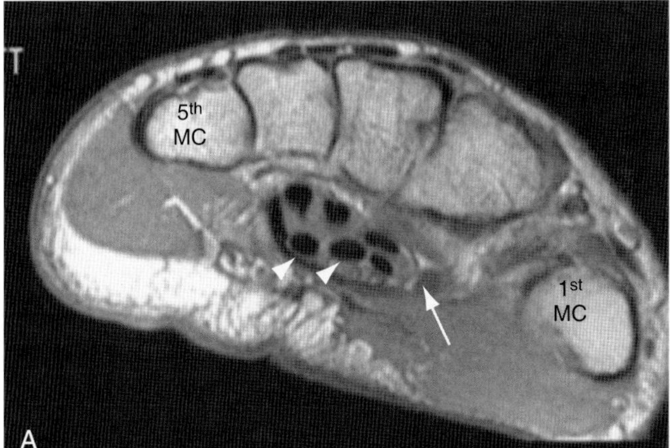

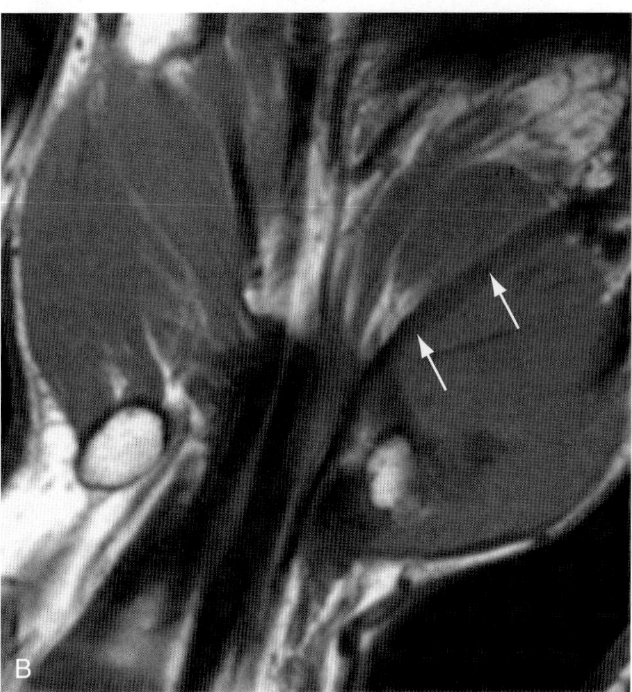

FIGURE 13-16. Magic angle artifact. When the tendon crosses at 55 degrees to the main magnetic field, artifactual high signal can be seen within the tendon on some sequences. It will appear in images obtained at any orientation but will disappear if the tendon position within the magnet is altered. **A,** Axial proton density weighted image through the wrist shows abnormally elevated signal within the flexor pollicis longus tendon *(arrow).* Deep and superficial flexor tendons, passing through the carpal tunnel, show normal low signal intensity *(arrowheads).* In this instance, the high signal represents magic angle artifact and should not be mistaken for tendinosis. **B,** Coronal T1-weighted image through the wrist and hand shows how the flexor pollicis tendon *(arrows),* unlike the flexor tendons to digits 2 through 5, follows a curved course that causes it to cross at 55 degrees to the main magnet field. *MC,* Metacarpal.

forms of tendon degeneration can result in different MRI appearances: fibromatous or hypoxic tendinopathy tends to cause tendon enlargement with maintenance of normal low signal; mucoid degeneration causes tiny foci of high T2 signal, which can coalesce to form interstitial tears; lipoid tendinopathy is not well characterized on MRI but may account for diffuse tendon thickening and very subtle internal signal; and calcific or osseous tendinopathy may have low signal related to calcification or, alternatively, signal intensity similar to bone and bone marrow.[15,58,59] As noted above, magic angle artifact can mimic tendon degeneration with high signal on proton density weighted or T1-weighted images and low signal on T2-weighted images and should be considered in the differential when the tendon is crossing at 55 degrees to the main magnet field. Ossification within the tendon can also mimic tendon degeneration with intermediate to high signal on short TE sequences and intermediate signal on T2-weighted images. For that reason, radiographs should be reviewed for ossification, either within the substance of the tendon or at its insertion site, and correlated with MR images.

> Tendon degeneration and tears appear as an area of high signal on proton density weighted or T1-weighted images; on T2 weighted images, however, degeneration shows low to intermediate signal intensity, whereas tendon tears show high (fluid) signal.

On MRI, **tendon tears** appear as high signal on both short TE (proton density weighted and T1-weighted) and long TE (T2-weighted) sequences (Figure 13-18). Signal on T2-weighted sequences must be as high as simple fluid to constitute a tear. Tendon tears may be partial or complete. **Partial tears** may be contained within the substance of the tendon (intrasubstance tear) or may extend to the tendon surface (Figure 13-19). Fraying of the tendon surface represents a form of partial tear. In the rotator cuff, partial tears may involve either the articular or bursal surface. In unusual cases, an intratendinous or intramuscular ganglion cyst may develop, providing a secondary sign of a partial tendon tear

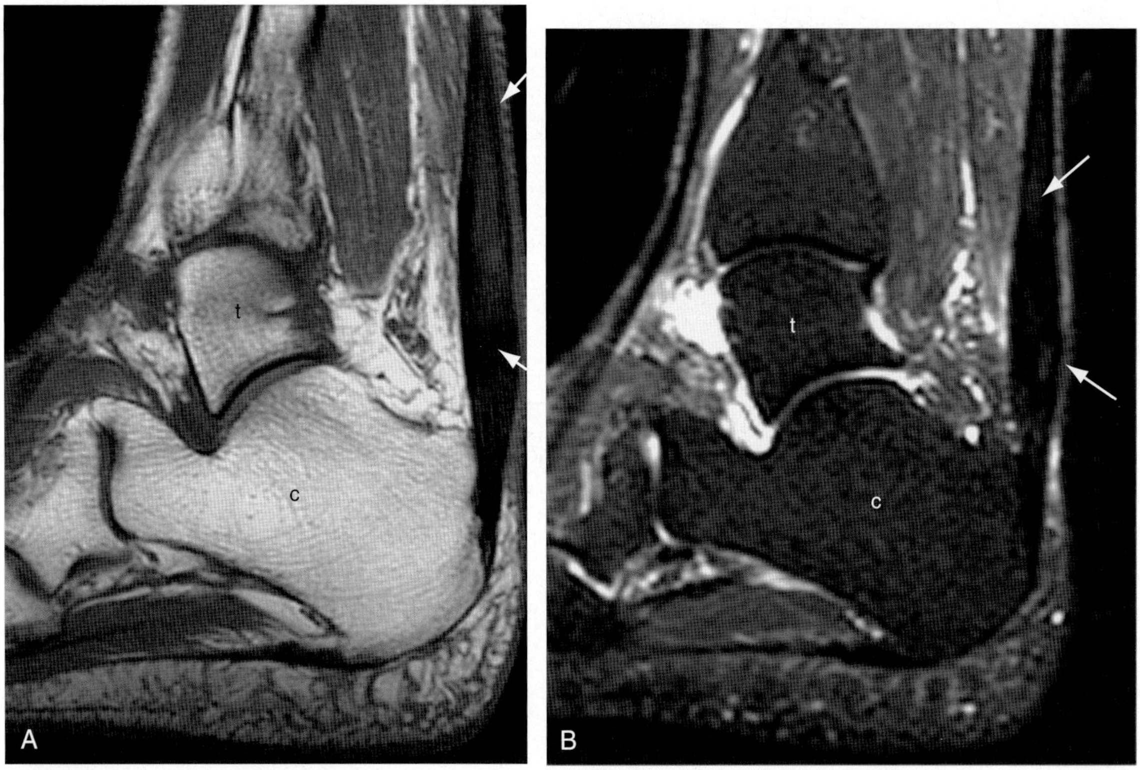

FIGURE 13-17. Tendinosis. **A,** Sagittal T1-weighted image through the ankle shows that the Achilles' tendon is thickened and contains abnormally high T1 signal *(arrows)*. Similar findings would be expected on a proton density weighted image. **B,** Most of the areas that are abnormal on the T1-weighted image show normal low signal on the fat-saturated T2-weighted image. Similar findings would be expected on a T2-weighted image. Punctate intrasubstance high signal could represent a focus of more severe degeneration or could represent a small intrasubstance tear. The high signal seen immediately anterior and posterior to the tendon is indicative of paratenonitis. *c,* Calcaneus; *t,* talus.

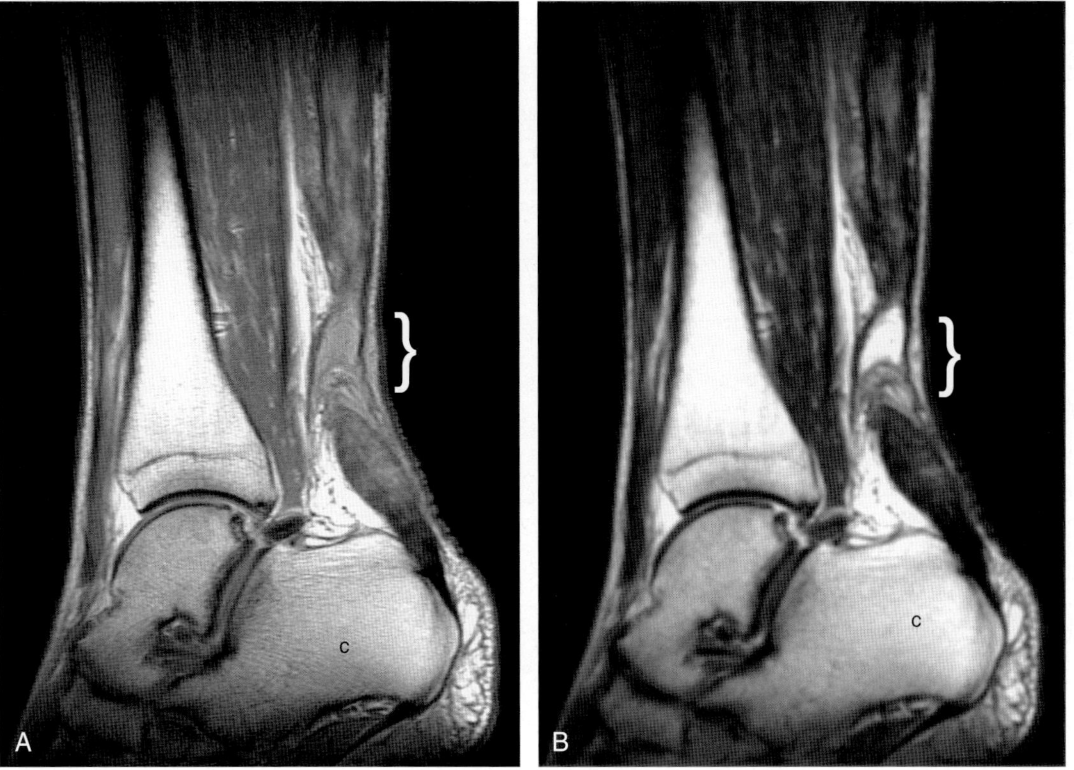

FIGURE 13-18. Tendon tears. **(A)** Sagittal proton density weighted, **(B)** T2-weighted, and

(Continued)

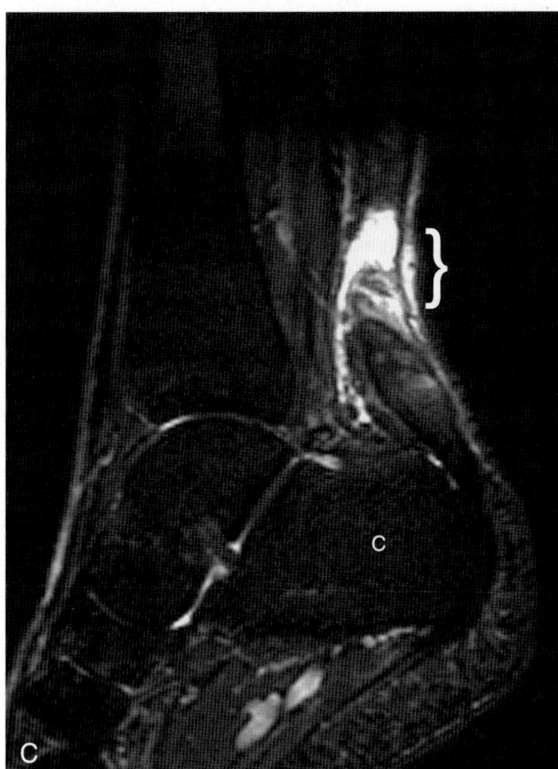

FIGURE 13-18—cont'd. **(C)** fat-saturated T2-weighted images through the ankle show a complete tear through the Achilles' tendon *(brackets)*. The site of the complete tear is higher signal intensity than the proton density weighted images, suggesting hemorrhage and high signal on T2-weighted images due to fluid. *c,* Calcaneus.

(Figure 13-19, *C*). The tear serves as a "one-way valve" allowing fluid to accumulate within the substance of the muscle, usually tracking within the tendon toward the musculotendinous junction. The ganglion cyst appears as a well-circumscribed, lobulated high T2 mass with variable signal on proton density weighted and T1-weighted images, which extends along the long axis of the tendon and muscle.[60-62] *Longitudinal splits* refer to tendon tears that extend along the longitudinal axis of the tendon and may be partial or complete. A surfacing longitudinal tear may or may not demonstrate high T2 signal (Figure 13-20). **Complete tendon tears** are seen as a transverse gap traversing the length of the tendon, with high T2 signal extending across the complete thickness of the tendon (see Figure 13-18). The torn tendon is often wavy and retracted. The tendon edges may be frayed and edematous, with a swollen appearance and high T2 signal. The surrounding tendon may show evidence of tendinosis and/or additional tears. When the tendon tear is acute, there is usually high signal in the surrounding soft tissues on both T1-weighted and T2-weighted images. High signal on T1-weighted images corresponds to hemorrhage, whereas high signal on T2-weighted images corresponds to edema or fluid. In the supraspinatus tendon, it is not unusual to have a complete tear through one portion of the tendon, while the remainder of the tendon is intact (e.g., a complete tear involving the anterior fibers of the distal supraspinatus tendon, with intact middle and posterior supraspinatus tendon fibers).

A "complete" rotator cuff tear involves the entire thickness of the tendon(s) from the bursal to the articular surface but not necessarily the entire width of the tendon(s) from anterior to posterior.

MRI allows for accurate characterization of the precise site and size of tendon gap. In a study of 16 patients with shoulder pain who underwent arthroscopy, Teefy and Rubin et al. found that

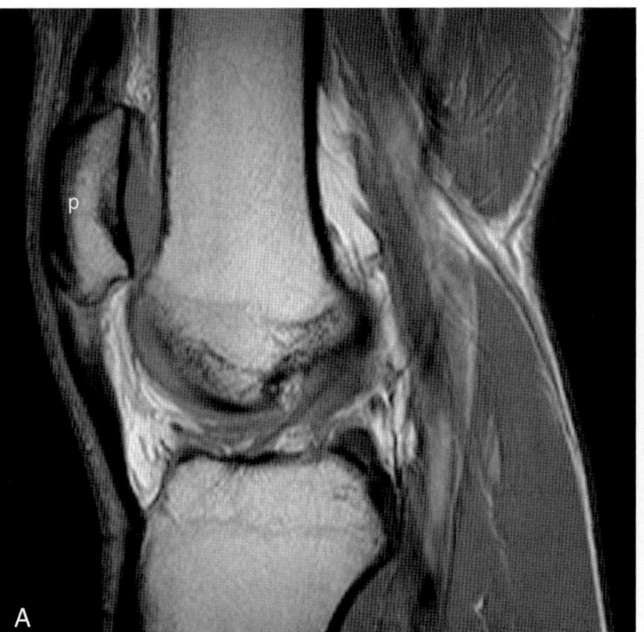

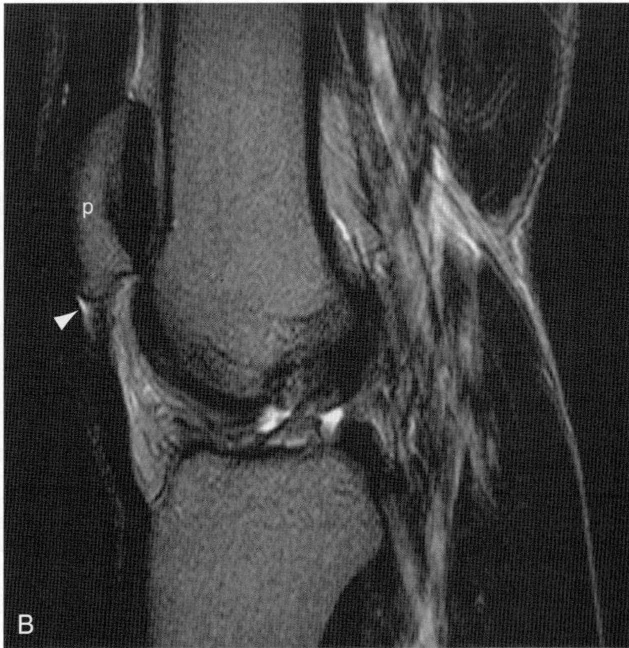

FIGURE 13-19. Partial tears. Sagittal **(A)** proton density weighted and **(B)** T2-weighted images through the patellar tendon show a partial intrasubstance tear *(arrowhead)* superimposed on a larger area of tendon degeneration. Although both degeneration and tear are high signal on the proton density weighted image, the tear is very high signal on the T2-weighted images, whereas the area of degeneration becomes dark on T2-weighted images.

(Continued)

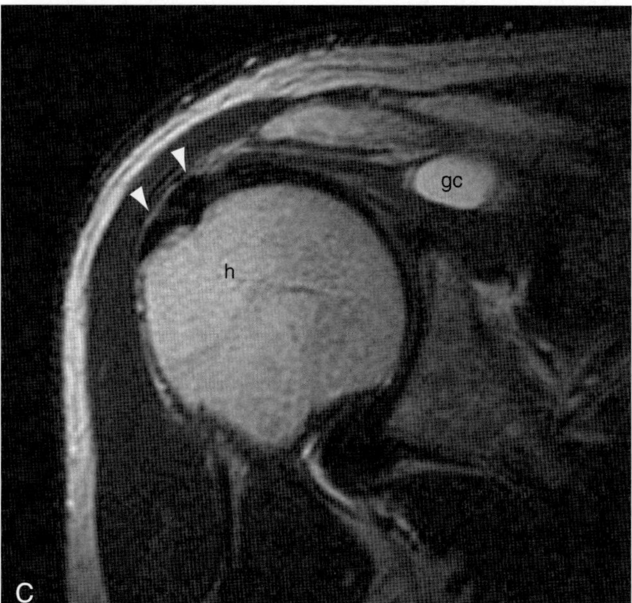

FIGURE 13-19—cont'd. **C,** Coronal T2-weighted image through the shoulder. A fluid filled ganglion cyst *(gc)* is seen within the substance of the supraspinatus muscle, adjacent to the musculotendinous junction, implying the presence of partial tendon tear. No distinct high T2 signal tendon tear is visualized, but there is slight irregularity along the bursal surface of the tendon *(arrowheads)* that may represent the site of the partial tear. *h,* Humeral head; *p,* patella.

MRI correctly identified 100% of complete rotator cuff tears and 63% of partial tears, with an overall accuracy of 87%. MRI correctly predicted the length (63%) and width (80%) of complete tears and the length (75%) and width (75%) of partial tears.[63] However, the apparent size of the tear can be influenced by the position of the joint or limb. For example, the size of an Achilles' tendon tear will be greater when ankle is imaged with the foot in neutral position or dorsiflexion than when the foot is plantar flexed. As patients may be treated with casting in plantar flexion, it may be helpful to image with the foot in plantar flexion; unless the tendon edges are apposed in plantar flexion, the tendon is unlikely to heal with casting alone.[64]**Chronic tears** may be appreciated as nonvisualization of the tendon, typically without surrounding edema or hemorrhage. The chronically torn tendon may be atrophic and/or retracted (Figure 13-21). Fibrosis may develop in or around the site of tendon tear and may limit retraction and obscure portions of the tear.[65] Changes in the muscle associated with the torn tendon may be evident. Early changes of muscle atrophy may be seen as high signal edema on T2-weighted and fat-saturated T2-weighted images. Eventually, muscle mass will decrease and fatty infiltration of the muscle may be seen[66] (see Figure 13-21). Prognosis for tendon repair is less favorable in the setting of muscle atrophy.[67,68] It should be noted that similar changes can be seen due to post-denervation change or other forms of muscle injury. Description of tear size, background tendinosis, and muscle edema or atrophy is important information for surgical planning available from MRI scans.[69]

Paratenonitis refers to inflammation of the paratenon or fascial covering of a tendon (see Figure 13-17). The Achilles' and patellar

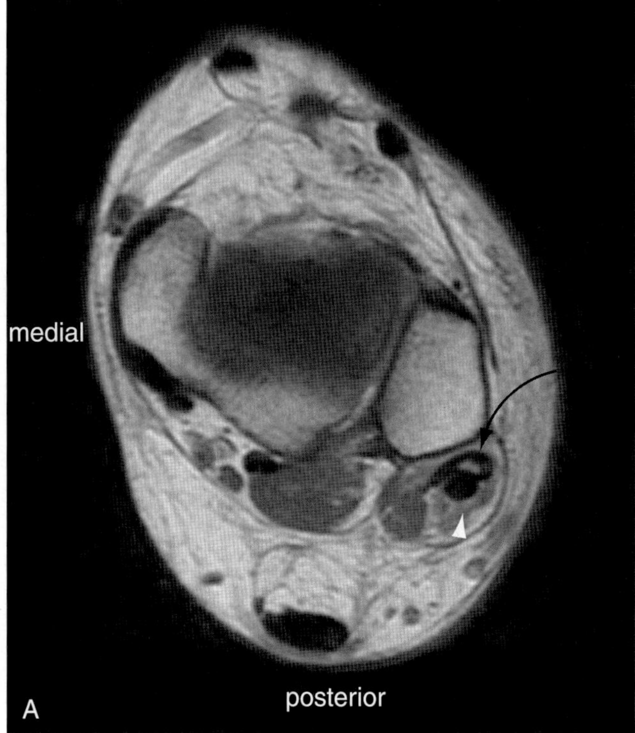

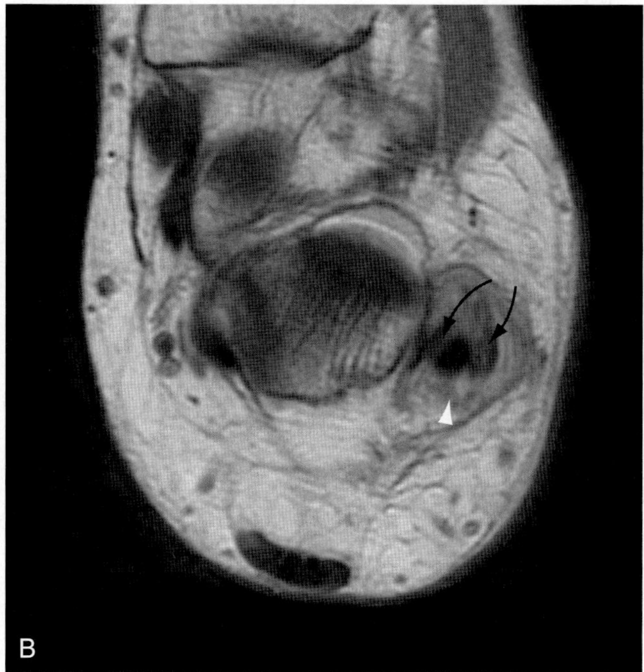

FIGURE 13-20. Longitudinal split tear. Axial T1-weighted images through the ankle. Proximally, the peroneus brevis *(curved arrow)* and peroneus longus *(dark oval structure above arrowhead)* tendons are normal in appearance. More distally, there is a longitudinal split tear of the peroneus brevis tendon, resulting in two separate tendon fragments *(curved arrows)*. The peroneus longus *(arrowhead)* remains intact.

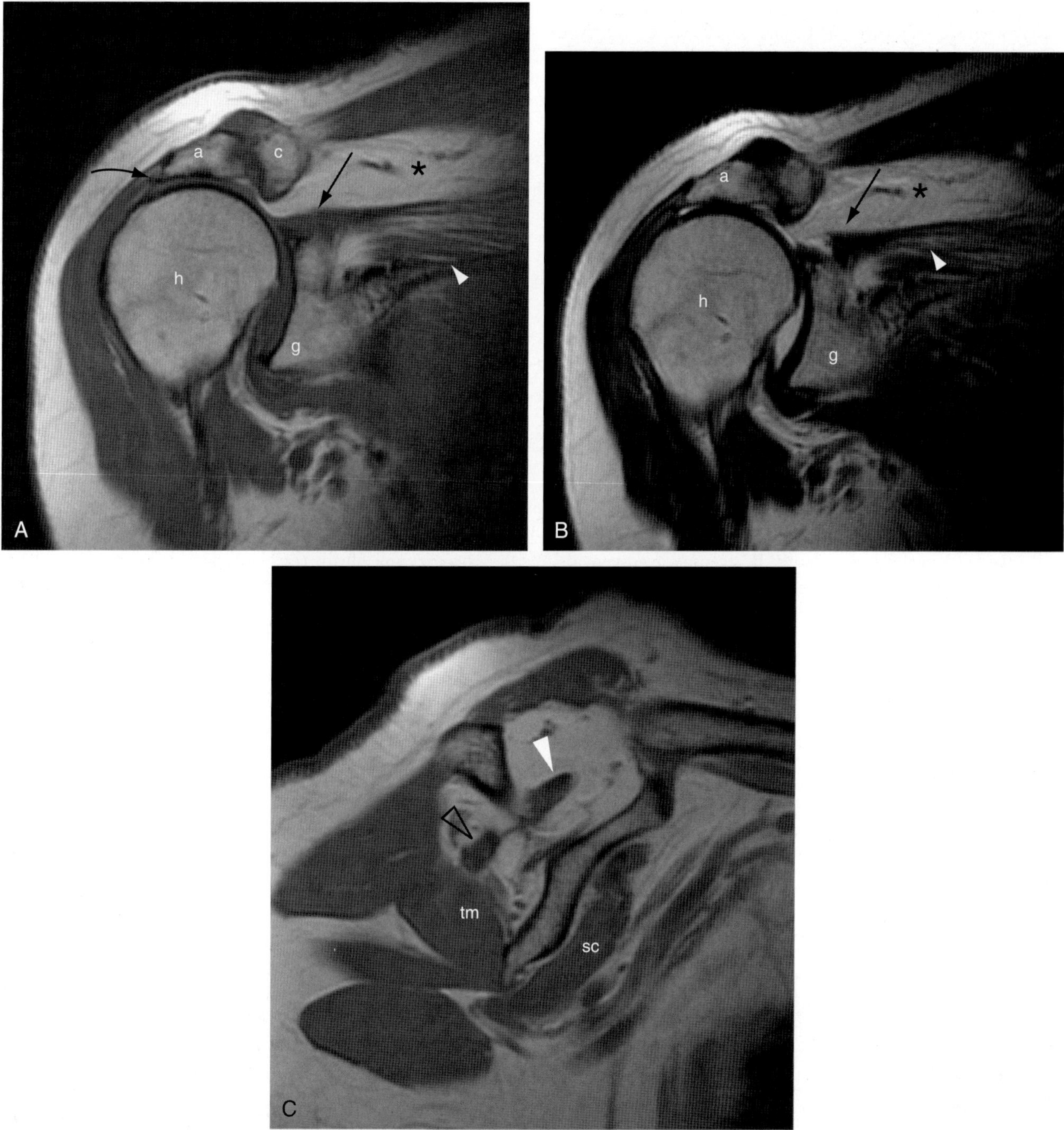

FIGURE 13-21. Chronic tendon tear. Coronal **(A)** proton density weighted and **(B)** T2-weighted images through the shoulder in an individual with a complete tendon tear. There is marked acromiohumeral narrowing, with no tendon visualized in the acromiohumeral interval *(curved arrow)*. The torn edge of the supraspinatus tendon is retracted medially *(arrow)*. Fatty stranding is seen as high signal stranding between muscle fibers on both sequences *(arrowhead)*, as well as overall muscle atrophy, with high signal fat seen in the space usually occupied by the muscle belly *(asterisk)*. **C,** Sagittal proton density weighted image through the rotator cuff in the same patient shows marked atrophy of the supraspinatus and infraspinatus muscles. Both the supraspinatus tendon *(white arrowhead)* and infraspinatus tendon *(open arrowhead)* are surrounded by fat instead of muscle. *a,* Acromion; *c,* clavicle; *g,* glenoid; *h,* humerus; *sc,* subscapularis muscle; *tm,* teres minor muscle.

tendons, for example, are enveloped by a paratenon rather than a synovial sheath.[13] In the Achilles' tendon, the normal paratenon is a thin, homogeneous layer visible along the posterior, medial, and lateral aspects of the Achilles' tendon, best seen on the axial images; it is clearly distinct proximally but becomes less distinct distally as it inserts onto the periosteum of the calcaneus.[70] It is slightly higher in signal intensity than the normal Achilles tendon on T1-weighted and short tau inversion recovery (STIR) images.[70] In some cases, the normal paratenon may be of high signal intensity in the middle third (longitudinally) and may have more prominent high STIR signal.[70] In paratenonitis (also referred to as *paratendonitis*[15] and *paratendinitis* or *peritendinitis*[71]), there is generalized inflammation in the pre-Achilles fat and in the soft tissues surrounding the tendon.[71,72] This is seen as strand-like signal in the fat surrounding the tendon: low signal on T1- and proton density weighted sequences and high signal on T2-weighted sequences. The paratenon, seen as a curvilinear line visible posterior to the Achilles' tendon, may become thickened.[73] Areas of high T2 signal seen in the acute setting may progress to low signal scarring in the chronic setting. The underlying tendon may be normal or abnormal. **Tenosynovitis** (i.e., fluid and/or synovial thickening within the tendosynovial lining of the tendon) is seen as high T2 signal within a distended tendon sheath, surrounding a normal or abnormal tendon (Figure 13-22). The normal synovial sheath may not be appreciable on MRI images or may appear as a thin structure outlining the tendon that is low signal on all sequences. In some tendons, such as the flexor hallucis longus tendon, a small amount of tenosynovial fluid may be a normal finding. High T2 signal within the tendon sheath may represent either simple fluid or thickened hyperemic synovium—these two entities can only be distinguished by administration of gadolinium contrast. When IV gadolinium is administered, thickened synovium will enhance very rapidly, whereas tenosynovial fluid will not. Synovitis may also be visible on nonenhanced T2-weighted images as small low signal "fronds" extending out at right angles from the inner surface of the synovial sheath. With fluid in the tendon sheath, the mesotenon may be visible as a thin low T2 signal, linear, tether-like strand extending from the surface of the tendon to the low signal synovial sheath. In stenosing tenosynovitis, two distinct appearances have been described: (1) the high T2 fluid column surrounding the tendon may develop scattered areas of narrowing—this pattern has been described in the flexor hallucis longus tendon[71]; or (2) in addition to tenosynovial fluid and internal debris, the fat immediately surrounding the tendons (peritenonous fat) becomes low signal, with blurring of the usual smooth borders of the tendon, and may show edema on fat-saturated T2-weighted images. This second pattern has been seen in the first extensor compartment tendons of the wrist, in the setting of DeQuervain's tenosynovitis.[74,75] Septic tenosynovitis may be indistinguishable from tenosynovitis related to noninfectious inflammatory or traumatic causes and therefore requires a high clinical vigilance to diagnose. In a classic presentation, there will be a disproportionate amount of complex fluid surrounding a tendon or tendons, but the volume or signal intensity of the fluid is not diagnostic. The tenosynovial fluid is often complex and demonstrates a thick rim of contrast enhancement, corresponding to inflamed proliferative synovium.[76] There may be edema in the surrounding bones and soft tissues. MRI provides an overview to help localize the infection and assess its extent. Direct sampling is required to confirm the diagnosis and characterize the organism, and, if performed percutaneously, ultrasound guidance is most feasible.[77,78] Loose bodies may be seen as nonspecific low signal debris within the synovial sheath on T2-weighted images or may have a characteristic ossific appearance with a thick low signal cortex peripherally and marrow signal within. Multiple ossific bodies of relatively similar sizes suggest the diagnosis of synovial osteochondromatosis. Signal intensity is variable, reflecting variation in the histologic composition of the "bodies."[79] In this case, radiographs may help to clarify the diagnosis. In inflammatory arthritides as well as chronic low-grade infectious synovitis, small fibrinous structures known as "rice bodies" may accumulate within the tendon sheath, together with marked synovial thickening—when present, they appear as small linear or ovoid intermediate to low signal structures on T1-weighted and T2-weighted images. Rice bodies are not calcified and do not demonstrate blooming.[39]

Tendon subluxation or dislocation is seen as displacement of the tendon from its normal location (Figure 13-23) and can be seen, for example, with the long head biceps tendon at the shoulder,[1,80] the extensor carpi ulnaris (ECU) tendon at the distal ulna,[81] and the peroneal tendons in the ankle.[82] There may or may not be associated tendon pathology.

Myotendinous strain or tear usually occurs in the setting of rapid, forceful, eccentric muscle contraction (i.e., the muscle lengthens while it is simultaneously contracting). These injuries tend to occur in muscles that cross two joints, such as the rectus femoris, hamstring, and gastrocnemius muscles.

MRI can demonstrate the severity of muscle injury.

In first-degree or mild strain, there is microscopic injury to muscle or tendon with fewer than 5% of fibers disrupted. There is negligible loss of strength or range of motion. On MRI, edema and hemorrhage can be seen at the musculotendinous junction.[83,84] Because the musculotendinous junction is actually composed of

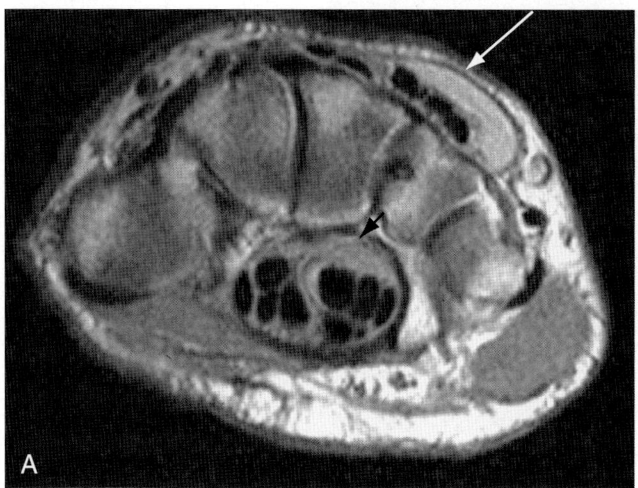

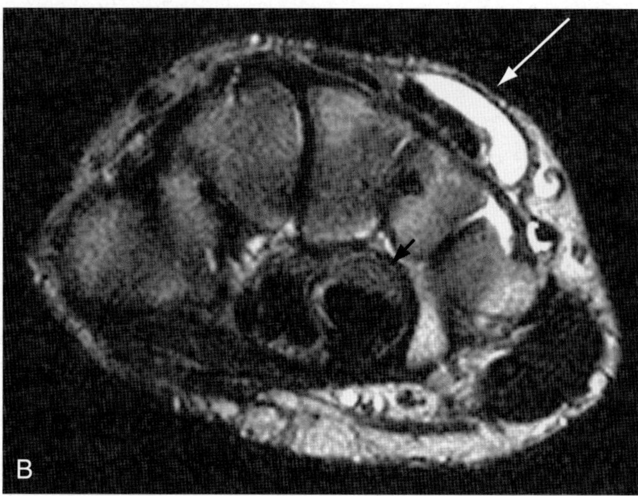

FIGURE 13-22. Tenosynovitis. Axial **(A)** proton density weighted and **(B)** T2-weighted images through the wrist. Hyperemic synovium surrounds the extensor carpi radialis and brevis tendons *(long arrows)* and appears slightly brighter than muscle on proton density weighted images and bright like fluid on T2-weighted images. Examination after intravenous contrast confirmed enhancement due to synovitis. There is also thickened synovium surrounding some flexor tendons within the carpal tunnel *(short arrows)*. In this case, it is also slightly brighter than muscle on proton density weighted images but is low signal and darker than fluid on T2-weighted images. This low signal is consistent with fibrotic—rather than hyperemic—tenosynovitis.

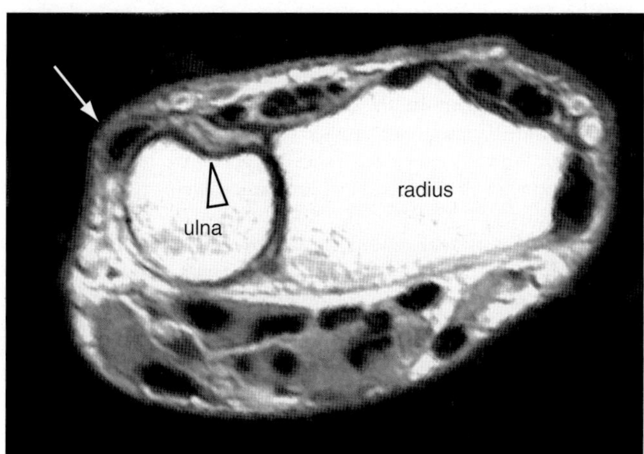

FIGURE 13-23. Tendon dislocation. Axial image through the wrist shows that the extensor carpi ulnaris tendon *(arrow)* has dislocated out of the distal ulnar sulcus *(arrowhead)*. Whether this is a permanent or transient finding cannot be determined from static MR images. The tendon appears otherwise normal.

innumerable sites distributed over a large area within the muscle, these findings can be distributed widely throughout the muscle. High T2 signal may track between muscle fascicles, causing a characteristic feathery appearance, and a rim of T2 hyperintense fluid may track along fascial planes and surround nearby muscles[83,84] (Figure 13-24). The overall architecture of the muscle remains intact. Pain and imaging findings resolve after a brief period of rest and conservative treatment.[85] In second-degree or moderate strain, there is a macroscopic partial thickness tear, although some fibers remain intact. Second-degree strain may be further categorized as low, moderate, or high grade, based on whether disruption involves less than one third, one third to two thirds, or greater than two thirds of the muscle, with corresponding loss of strength. The MRI appearance will vary with severity and acuity.[83] Edema, hemorrhage, and perifascial fluid will be present. A focal hematoma at the musculotendinous junction is a characteristic finding.[84,86] Late findings include low signal fibrosis and hemosiderin at the injury site. Persistent altered signal intensity may be associated with a window of vulnerability to reinjury.[83,87] In third-degree or severe strain, there is complete disruption of fibers, often with retraction and focal palpable defect and apparent "soft tissue mass," with loss

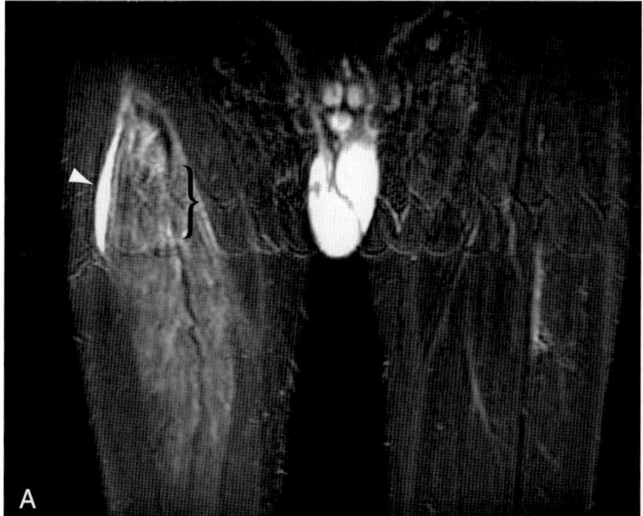

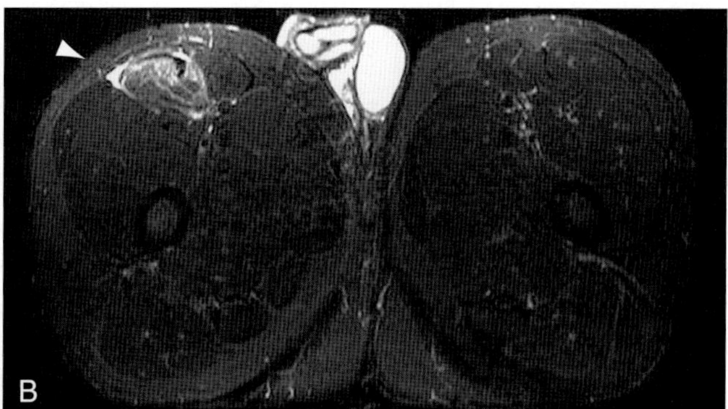

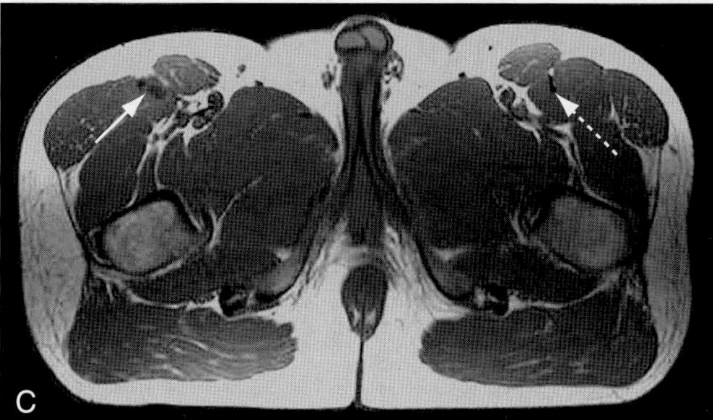

FIGURE 13-24. Myotendinous strain. **(A)** Coronal fat-saturated T2-weighted, **(B)** axial fat-saturated T2-weighted, and **(C)** axial T1-weighted images through the thigh show a grade I to II myotendinous strain involving the rectus femoris tendon and muscle. The T2-weighted images show high signal fluid and edema extending throughout the muscle, reflecting the wide dispersion of microscopic musculotendinous junction sites throughout the muscle. The tendon is torn and wavy *(bracket)* and fluid is collecting along the fascia surrounding the muscle *(arrowhead)*. On the axial T1-weighted image, a retracted portion of the tendon is abnormally thickened and indistinct *(arrow)*, and there is subtle high signal in the rectus muscle due to hemorrhage, both appreciated when compared with the contralateral side *(dashed arrow)*.

of strength in the involved muscle group. Clinical assessment in this setting can be difficult. MRI reveals complete discontinuity of fibers, with evidence of fiber laxity[84] (Figure 13-24, *A*). A hematoma may be present at the site of fiber discontinuity. Muscle atrophy begins within the first day and may be irreversible by 4 months.[83] Hematomas associated with muscle injury tend to show high T1 and T2 signal consistent with methemoglobin, with a characteristic high T1 rim, but the appearance depends on acuity and local biochemical microenvironment.[83] Following a moderate or severe strain, intramuscular or intermuscular hematomas often resorb spontaneously over 6 to 8 weeks.[88] The hematoma itself is a nonspecific finding, and an underlying malignant mass cannot be excluded on the basis of imaging appearance alone. Indeed, the hematoma can demonstrate contrast enhancement due to fibrovascular tissue related to healing, which can be confused with evidence of tumor. Residual high T2 signal at the site of injury may represent serous fluid trapped in an intramuscular pseudocyst.[89] However, intramuscular myxomas can be predominantly cystic and can mimic a postinjury seroma. For these reasons, the appearance must be correlated with the clinical presentation and other imaging findings. In some instances, a follow-up MRI to document resolution of the hematoma or stability or resolution of the seroma may be indicated.

Insertional tendinopathy refers to degenerative changes at the osteotendinous junction. It can occur at any tendon insertion site, but the most common sites are at the rotator cuff insertion, humeral epicondyle, patellar tendon origin from the inferior patella ("jumper's knee"), and Achilles' tendon insertion site onto the calcaneus[13] (Figure 13-25). Insertional tendinopathy may be associated with microtrauma due to overuse or with enthesopathic diseases such as rheumatoid arthritis or other spondyloarthropathies.[90,91] Acute forms of insertional tendinopathy are characterized by inflammatory signs without tissue degeneration; chronic forms are characterized by tendinosis.[13] Diagnosis is usually based on clinical presentation. MRI shows associated changes in the tendon and surrounding structures, which can help differentiate insertional tendinopathy from other causes of pain in the region, and—by demonstrating the extent of the changes—can provide data relevant to prognosis and treatment. However, several studies suggest that ultrasound may be more sensitive for detection of the earliest changes of insertional tendinopathy.[92,93]

Chronic insertional tendinosis has been best described in the distal Achilles' tendon.[13,94] In this location, the Achilles endotendon is continuous with the periosteum of the calcaneus, but the tendon itself inserts directly into bone, at a site free of periosteum, via collagen fibers known as *Sharpey fibers*.[13] Achilles insertional tendinopathy often presents as an overuse syndrome, most commonly seen in mid-distance and long-distance running, dancing, soccer, and tennis, and can be associated with training errors. Hyperpronation and forefoot varus are commonly associated. Patients present with pain, tenderness, and swelling over the osteotendinous junction. There may be loss of passive dorsiflexion.[90] On MRI, the distal tendon may show high proton density and high T1-weighted intratendinous signal consistent with tendinosis, high T2 signal consistent with small intrasubstance tears and, in later stages, may become thickened.[15,95] (Figure 13-25, *B, C*). The signal abnormalities may be vague or ill-defined[15] or may take the form of flame-shaped or comet tail–shaped areas, extending to the calcaneal periosteum.[96] There may be intratendinous fibrosis, calcification and/or ossification, or insertional enthesophytes, which typically occur within degenerated portions of tendon.[97]

Radiographs are more sensitive than MRI for detecting intratendinous calcification and ossification, which may appear as nonspecific signal abnormality on MRI.

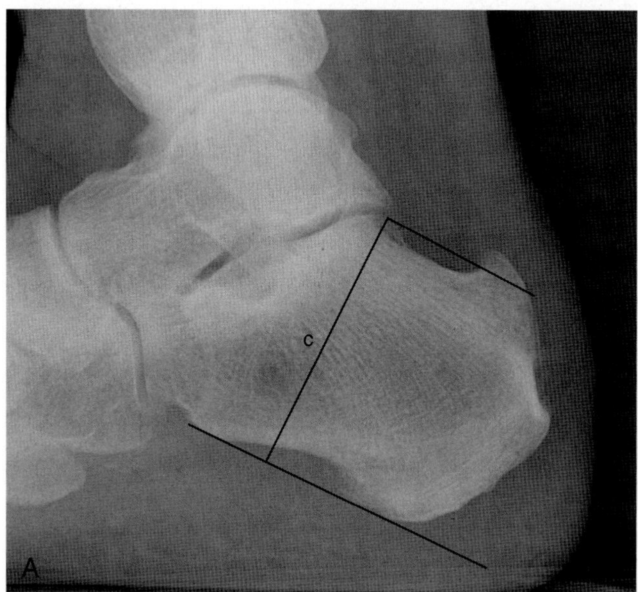

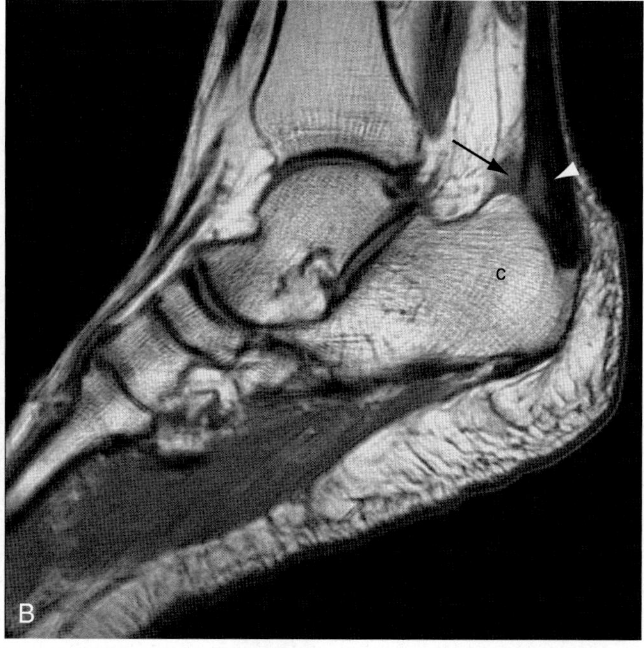

FIGURE 13-25. Insertional tendinopathy of the Achilles' tendon. **A,** Lateral radiograph of the heel. Parallel pitch lines are drawn over the calcaneus to assess for Haglund's deformity (i.e., prominence of the posterosuperior corner of the calcaneus). If present, Haglund's deformity can contribute to retrocalcaneal bursitis and insertional Achilles' tendinitis. Thickening of the distal Achilles' tendon and an enthesophyte at the Achilles' insertion site onto the calcaneus are, however, consistent with insertional tendinopathy. **B,** Sagittal T1-weighted image through the ankle shows that the distal Achilles' tendon is thickened. In addition, there is fluid in the retrocalcaneal bursa *(arrow)* and a partial tear along the anterior surface of the distal Achilles' tendon *(arrowhead)*. *c,* Calcaneus.

(Continued)

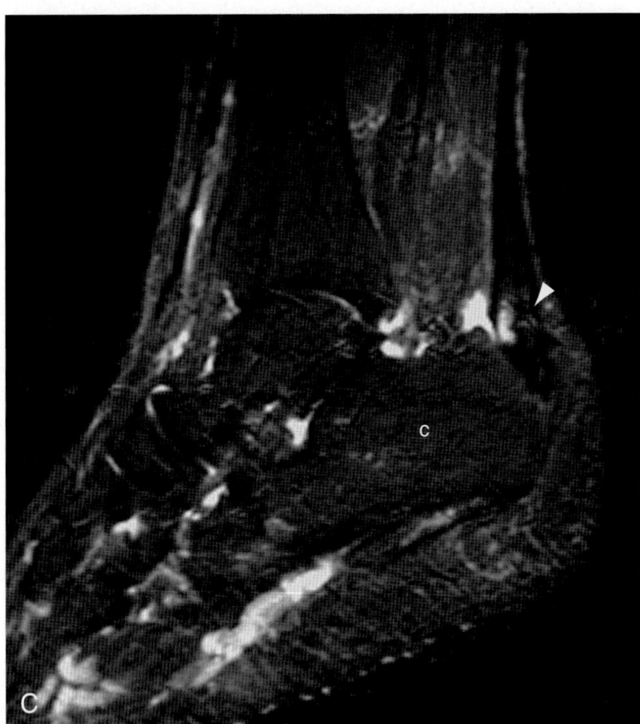

FIGURE 13-25—cont'd. C, Sagittal fat-saturated T2-weighted image through the ankle highlights the high signal fluid in the retocalnaneal bursa and in the partial tear *(arrowhead)* of the tendon. *c,* Calcaneus.

Marrow edema may be present in the adjoining portion of the calcaneus,[96] particularly in the setting of retrocalcaneal bursitis. Imaging reveals the severity of tissue alterations and can therefore be used as an indicator of prognosis.[90,98] Nicholson et al. used MRI to stratify patients with insertional tendinopathy and found that individuals who demonstrated confluent areas of intrasubstance signal change (types II and III) were unlikely to respond to nonoperative treatment.[99] There is a high association of insertional tendinopathy with retrocalcaneal bursitis, and up to 60% of patients also have Haglund deformity (i.e., prominence of the posterosuperior calcaneus).[73,90,95,100-103] Prominence of the posterosuperior calcaneus can cause inflammation in the retrocalcaneal bursa and impingement on the distal Achilles' tendon, both of which contribute to the development of tendinosis.[104] By the same token, however, insertional tendinopathy, retrocalcaneal bursitis, and Haglund's deformity can occur independently, as independent causes of heel pain.

> Prominence of the posterior superior calcaneus (Haglund's deformity) may result in chronic pressure against a shoe and inflammation of the retro-calcaneal bursa, the distal Achilles' tendon, and the superficial retro-Achilles' bursa.

The retrocalcaneal bursa is a disk-shaped cap lying between the posterosuperior corner of the calcaneus and the distal Achilles' tendon.[105] Anteriorly, the wall of the retrocalcaneal bursa is composed of fibrocartilage overlying the calcaneus; posteriorly, the wall of the bursa is indistinguishable from the epitenon of the Achilles' tendon. A small amount of high T2 signal fluid may be apparent in the normal bursa on MRI. However, fluid that distends the bursa greater than 2 mm anteroposterior, 14 mm craniocaudad, and 6 mm transverse is indicative of retrocalcaneal bursitis[106] (Figure 13-25, *C*). Plantar flexion facilitates detection of small amounts of bursal fluid.[106] The presence of a prominent posterosuperior calcaneal tuberosity, the so-called Haglund's deformity, can be evaluated by drawing parallel pitch lines on lateral radiographs or sagittal MR images[107] (Figure 13-25, *A*). Because MRI allows direct visualization of changes in the distal Achilles' tendon, calcaneal morphology, and fluid in the retrocalcaneal and retro-Achilles' bursae, it can aid in diagnosis and pretreatment planning.[15] Fluid in the retro-Achilles' bursa, which lies posterior (superficial) to the distal Achilles' tendon, is usually a phenomenon that is completely distinct from insertional tendinopathy or Haglund's syndrome. Rather, it usually occurs due to irritation of superficial soft tissue by the heel counter of a shoe and does not affect the Achilles' tendon.[73] This can also be distinguished as a separate entity on MRI.

> "Pump bumps" are due to irritation of the retro-Achilles' bursa from shoe pressure.

MRI of the **postoperative tendon** is challenging, because routine postoperative changes often mimic tendon pathology. In general, accuracy is higher for detection of complete tears than for partial tendon tears. Baseline postoperative MRI examinations, when available, can provide a useful basis for comparison. In addition to imaging the postoperative tendon itself, MRI provides for assessment of surrounding structures and associated postoperative complications. Correlative radiographs aid in the evaluation of the postoperative tendon, by providing for evaluation of hardware failure, heterotopic ossification, and bone quality and alignment.

Although most studies evaluating MRI of the postoperative tendon have focused on the rotator cuff and Achilles' tendon, many of the same principles are more broadly applied. The appearance of the normal postoperative rotator cuff depends on the surgery performed. General findings include distortion of fat planes, fibrosis, and metallic susceptibility artifact (Figure 13-26). Metallic susceptibility artifact may be visible even when no metal is seen on radiographs, due to microscopic particles introduced by the routine passage of surgical instrumentation.

> Postoperative metal susceptibility artifact may be present on MRI even when no metal is visible on radiographs.

In patients' status post acromioplasty, which is commonly performed at the time of rotator cuff repair, the acromion may appear small, absent, or sclerotic (Figure 13-26, *B*), with loss of the normal fat signal in the subacromial-subdeltoid peribursal fat plane due to scarring. In addition, fluid may be present in the subacromial-subdeltoid bursa and can mimic bursitis[108-110] (Figure 13-26, *A*). The coracoacromial ligament may be resected and absent; occasionally the acromioclavicular joint and distal clavicle may also be resected. In tendon-to-bone repair, a small surgical trough may be visible at the site of tendon fixation. Granulation tissue around suture material in the cuff or bone trough may cause intermediate to high proton density or T2 signal that can mimic the respective appearance of tendon degeneration or tear[109,111] (Figure 13-26, *A, B*). In a study of asymptomatic patients status post rotator cuff repair, Spielmann et al. found that only 10% had normal low signal intensity tendons. Fifty-three percent showed slightly increased signal intensity (consistent with tendinosis) and 37% had high T2 signal within the tendon (suggestive of partial or complete rotator cuff tears).[112] Small or moderate glenohumeral joint effusions and bone marrow edema were present in these asymptomatic postoperative patients, even several years out from surgery[110,112] (Figure 13-26, *A*). Zanetti et al. examined 14 asymptomatic and 32 symptomatic patients at 27 to 53 months status post open tendon-to-bone rotator cuff repair.[110] Findings consistent with full-thickness tendon tears (high T2 signal) were seen in 21% of asymptomatic patients. Tears tended to be smaller in the asymptomatic patients, with a mean width of 8 mm in the asymptomatic group versus 32 mm in the symptomatic group.

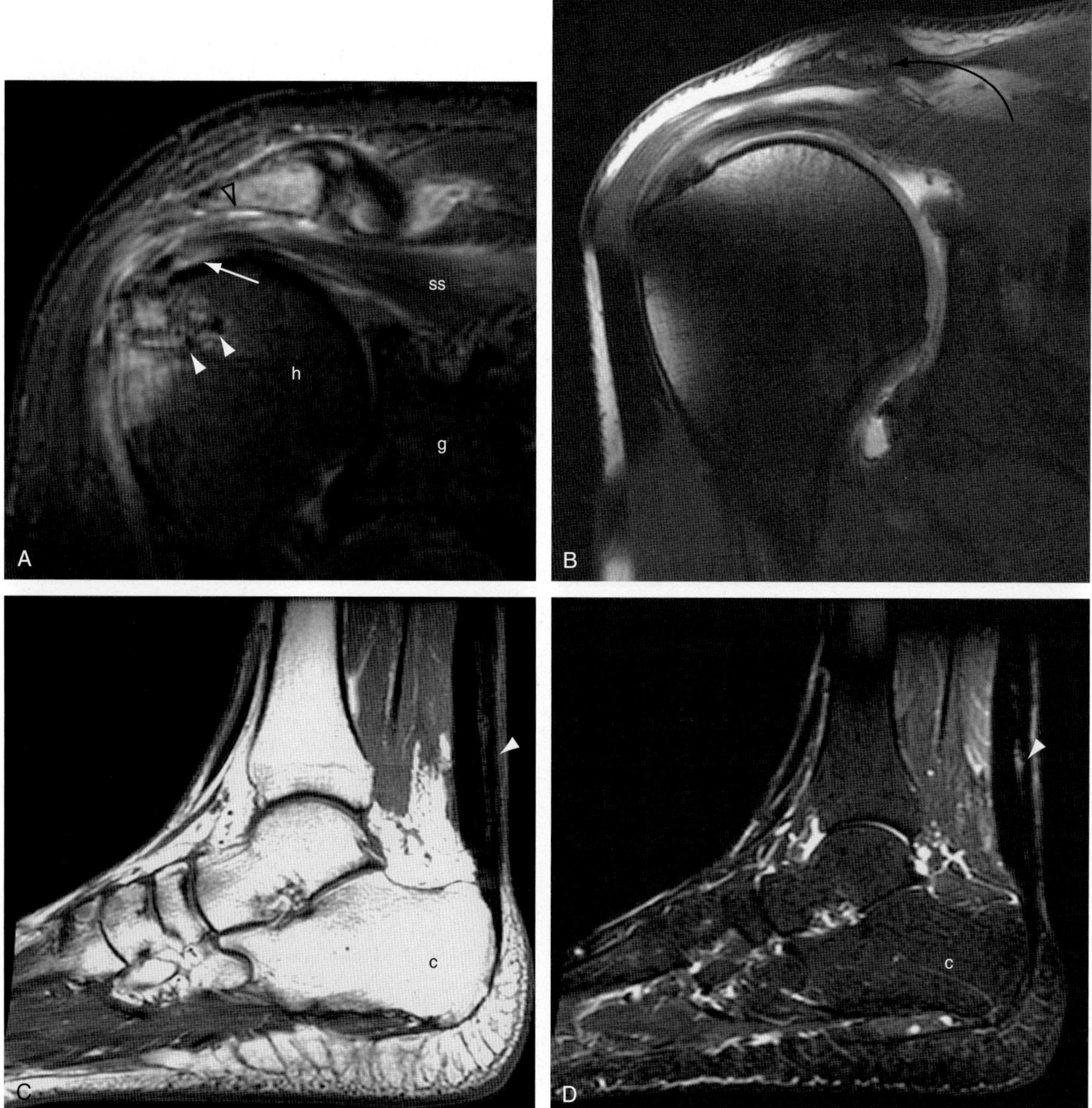

FIGURE 13-26. Postoperative tendon. **A,** Coronal fat-saturated T2-weighted image through the shoulder following rotator cuff repair. The supraspinatus tendon inserts onto the greater tuberosity, but is thinned and irregular *(arrow)*; the muscle *(ss)* is somewhat atrophied. Two anchors *(arrowheads)* extend into the humeral head, securing the tendon. There is surrounding high signal marrow edema. There is edema and a small amount of fluid in the subacromial bursa *(open arrowhead)*. *g,* Glenoid; *h,* humeral head. **B,** Coronal fat-saturated T1-weighted image through the shoulder after instillation of bright, high signal gadolinium into the glenohumeral joint. There is also contrast in the subacromial-subdeltoid bursa. Although this indicates a tear in a native rotator cuff, it can be a normal postoperative finding, as in this case. Subcutaneous fat appears artifactually bright due to inhomogeneous fat saturation. The acromion *(curved arrow)* is small and sclerotic, due to acromioplasty performed at the time of surgery. **(C)** Sagittal T1- and **(D)** sagittal fat-saturated T2-weighted images through the ankle status post Achilles' tendon repair. The tendon is thickened due to postoperative fibrosis. Linear high signal within the tendon is compatible with granulation tissue, an expected postoperative finding. In a preoperative tendon, similar high signal could be seen due to tendinosis. *c,* Calcaneus.

High signal intensity on T2-weighted images (suggesting a tear) may be seen in asymptomatic patients after rotator cuff repair. Symptomatic lesions tend to be larger.

Additional asymptomatic postoperative findings include slight superior migration of the humeral head[113] and, when open repair with re-attachment of the deltoid muscle has been performed, thinning of the deltoid muscle near its acromial attachment.[113] This normal postoperative thinning should be distinguished from the rare, but very serious, complication of deltoid detachment or dehiscence, which manifests as fluid traversing the deltoid at its acromial attachment site and which leads to deltoid atrophy and retraction, with concomitant loss of strength. The postoperative appearance of severe rotator cuff tear repairs may demonstrate transfer of the latissimus dorsi, pectoralis minor, or pectoralis major tendon. Visualization of arthrographic contrast within the subacromial-subdeltoid bursa is not a reliable sign of cuff tear in the postoperative patient (Figure 13-26, *B*). Few cuff repairs are "water tight": contrast can easily flow through a rotator cuff repair, even when it is clinically intact.[108,114,115] Moreover, even when a tear is present, contrast may fail to extravasate through the tear and into the bursa, due to adhesions and granulation tissue.[108]

The criteria for rotator cuff tears remain the same in the postoperative patient as they are in the preoperative individual, notwithstanding their considerable overlap with normal postoperative findings. Diagnosis of complete tendon tear in the postoperative setting is based on the presence of high T2 fluid-like signal traversing the full thickness of the tendon or on nonvisualization of the tendon. Atrophy or retraction of the muscle can be a useful secondary sign.[113] Partial tears are seen as high T2 signal defects along the bursal or articular surface of the tendon or, nonsurfacing, within the substance of the tendon. Owen et al. found that nonarthrographic MRI had a sensitivity of 86%, specificity of 92%, and accuracy of 90% for detection of residual or recurrent full-thickness tears. Owen et al. failed to identify five partial tears that were identified at follow-up surgery—although the tendon signal was elevated, the signal was not as high as fluid and therefore not interpreted as a tear.[108] Magee et al. found a sensitivity of 100% and specificity of 97% in identifying either a full-thickness or partial-thickness tear, as opposed to an intact tendon.[116] However, the positive predictive value for partial tears was only 65%, compared with 84% for full-thickness tears.[116] Magee et al. noted that sensitivity for detection of partial tears was higher in their study than in that of Owen et al.; they attributed the difference to their use of a fat-saturated T2-weighted sequence, which was more sensitive for detection of fluid than T2-weighted images that lacked fat saturation. There are limited data on the use of MR arthrography to evaluate the postoperative rotator cuff. [117] As noted above, contrast flowing from the glenohumeral joint, through the repaired cuff, into the subacromial-subdeltoid bursa is not considered a reliable sign of failed repair.[108,114,115] In one retrospective study of 48 patients who had undergone postoperative MR arthrography followed by surgery, 85% to 90% (two independent readers) of full-thickness supraspinatus tears and 42% to 52% of partial-thickness supraspinatus tears were detected, based on direct visualization of contrast-filled defects within the tendon.[118] It should be noted that fat saturation, which usually plays an important role in MR arthrographic images, may be ineffective and may actually obscure findings in the postoperative shoulder, due to metallic susceptibility artifact and resultant inhomogeneous fat saturation. The magnitude of this effect is an empiric phenomenon that varies from case to case.

In addition to imaging the postoperative tendon itself, MRI provides for assessment of surrounding structures and associated postoperative complications. Potential causes of persistent postoperative pain include not only new or recurrent rotator cuff tear, but also residual coracoacromial impingement; adhesions; deltoid weakness secondary to detachment or denervation; suprascapular nerve palsy due to postoperative fibrosis, perisuture reaction, or paralabral ganglion cyst; osteonecrosis of the humeral head; biceps tendinopathy or dislocation; reactive synovitis; and infection.[109] Gusmer cautions that large amounts of fluid in the subacromial space should raise concern for infection, perisutural inflammation, or synovitis secondary to bioabsorbable surgical tacks or loose bodies.[113]

The postoperative appearance of the Achilles' tendon has also been described. Tears of the Achilles' tendon may be treated with direct end-to-end anastomosis, tendon flaps, or synthetic graft, with a wide variety of specific techniques.[104,119] Dillon et al. examined patients at 3 and 6 months following both conservative and surgical Achilles' tendon repair and found intrasubstance fluid-signal foci, mimicking tears, within the healing tendons [Figure 13-26, *C, D*). Signal intensity tended to decrease as the tendon healed over a period of months to 1 year.[73,120,121] The tendon remained thickened, mimicking tendinosis, even after signal normalized.[73,120] The authors cautioned against overreading these normal early postoperative changes as evidence of poor healing, retear, or failed surgical repair.[71,73] Karjalainen et al. similarly found high proton density and high T2 signal within 19 of 21 postoperative tendons they examined. In their group, large lesions were associated with poor clinical outcomes.[122] It should be noted that focal high signal within the tendon can be caused by suture granuloma and can mimic abcess.[123] Liem et al. studied patients who underwent repair of Achilles' tendon rupture using a graft composed of polymer of lactic acid [PLA]. In these individuals, the tendon appeared fusiform and thickened, with intrasubstance intermediate T1 streaking and intermediate T2 intrasubstance signal. These areas decreased in signal over time, a change that was attributed to a collagenous response surrounding the implant.[124] Recurrent Achilles' tendon tears are seen in 0% to 5% of surgical repairs and as high as 39% with conservative repairs.[2]

Calcium hydroxyapatite deposits within a tendon can be very difficult to detect by MRI. The deposit is generally low signal and can be difficult to distinguish from the low signal tendon, unless it causes focal enlargement of the tendon. As a result, it is helpful to review the MRI in conjunction with a correlative radiograph. If gradient echo sequences are employed, the hydroxyapatite signal void may become more prominent ("blooming") on the gradient echo images, a feature which would suggest the presence of calcification. In its acute phase, calcific tendinitis can be accompanied by surrounding soft tissue and marrow edema, sometimes quite extensive. If the tendon calcification is not recognized, this soft tissue edema can be readily mistaken for infection or other inflammatory or posttraumatic processes. In some cases of calcific tendinitis, there is frank bony erosion[22] as well as marrow edema,[125] which may also prompt concern for an aggressive process such as infection or tumor. These potential pitfalls highlight the necessity of reviewing a contemporaneous radiograph for the characteristic appearance of calcium hydroxyapatite, in order to accurately interpret the MRI findings (see Figure 13-8, *B, C*).

MRI is well-suited to imaging of **soft tissue masses** associated with tendons. In general, MRI has limited ability to characterize a mass but provides important information for preoperative planning, including the size and extent of the mass, its relationship to surrounding structures, and its degree of vascularity. Several kinds of masses are characteristically associated with tendons and the MRI appearance, while not definitive, can be suggestive. Giant cell tumor of the tendon sheath is a benign entity that typically presents as a round or ovoid low T2 signal mass adherent to the surface of the tendon. The presence of hemosiderin (due to the friable nature of this vascular mass) causes low T2 signal and can cause "blooming" (accentuation of low signal) on T2*-weighted gradient echo sequences. Giant cell tumors typically demonstrate prominent homogeneous or heterogeneous gadolinium enhancement[126] (Figure 13-27). Ganglion cysts can occasionally arise from the surface of a tendon. Ganglion cysts are typically seen as lobulated well-circumscribed masses that are homogeneously high signal on T2-weighted images, with a very thin rim of enhancement and occasional thin septations. They need not demonstrate communication with the tendon sheath or joint.[126] Xanthomas, which are usually found in the setting of familial hypercholesterolemia, can occur in any tendon but are often seen often in the Achilles' tendon. Xanthomas give rise to heterogeneous intrasubstance signal and stippling within

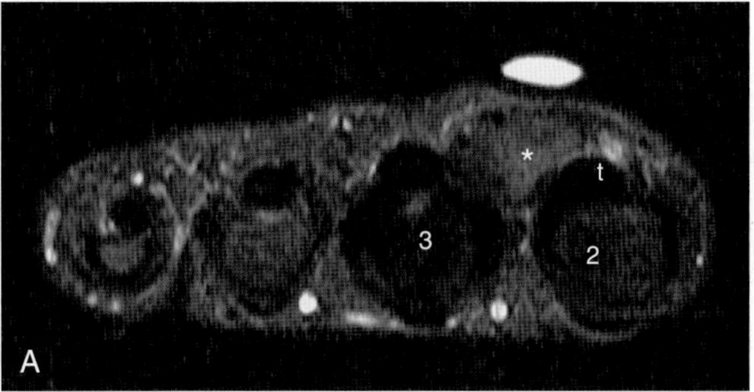

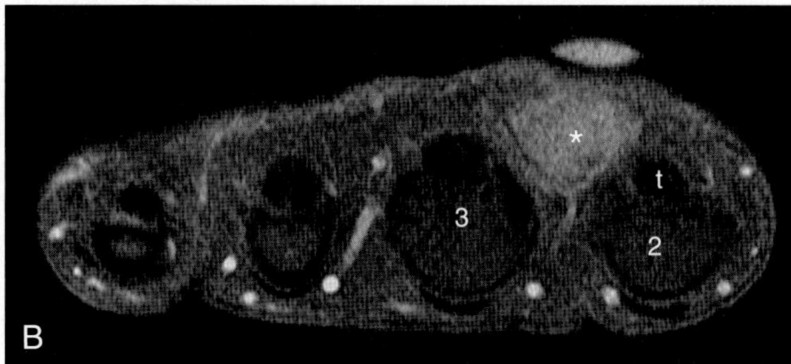

FIGURE 13-27. Giant cell tumor of the tendon sheath. **A,** Axial fat-saturated T2-weighted image through the hand. The giant cell tumor of the tendon sheath is seen as a low signal ovoid mass *(asterisk)* lying along the volar aspect of the interspace between the second *(2)* and third *(3)* digits. The mass abuts the flexor tendon of the second digit *(t)* and actually arises from it. The bright ovoid structure on the skin surface is a marker placed over the palpable abnormality. **B,** Axial post-contrast fat-saturated T1-weighted image through the same level in the hand. The giant cell tumor is a vascular mass *(asterisk)* that enhances with contrast and appears bright.

the tendon with fusiform enlargement. Although the differential diagnosis includes Achilles' tendinosis, xanthoma should be considered when the abnormality is bilateral and, in particular, when there is evidence of lipoid degeneration.[73,127] It is important to keep in mind that the benign or malignant nature of mass cannot be definitely determined from MRI and that additional evaluation or appropriate follow-up will be required.

> The benign or malignant nature of a mass cannot be definitely determined from MRI, and additional evaluation or appropriate follow-up will often be required.

MR-guided interventions are not a common part of the workup or treatment of tendon or bursal pathology. The use of MR guidance for procedures related to MR arthrography of the shoulder and aspiration of the perilabral cyst in the shoulder has been reported by sites with special interest in these techniques.[128-130]

MRI is very sensitive for depiction of **bursal** fluid (Figure 13-28; see also Figure 13-13, *B*). In most cases, a fluid-filled bursa will appear as a discrete, well-circumscribed structure. Certain bursae, however, may be poorly defined and difficult to distinguish from surrounding interstitial edema. A small amount of fluid may be visible in some bursae as a normal finding.[106,131] For example, in the retrocalcaneal bursa, up to 2 mm (anteroposterior [AP] dimension) of fluid is considered normal.[106] Fat-saturated high T2-weighted images are extremely sensitive to small amounts of edema and often demonstrate edema in the region of the greater

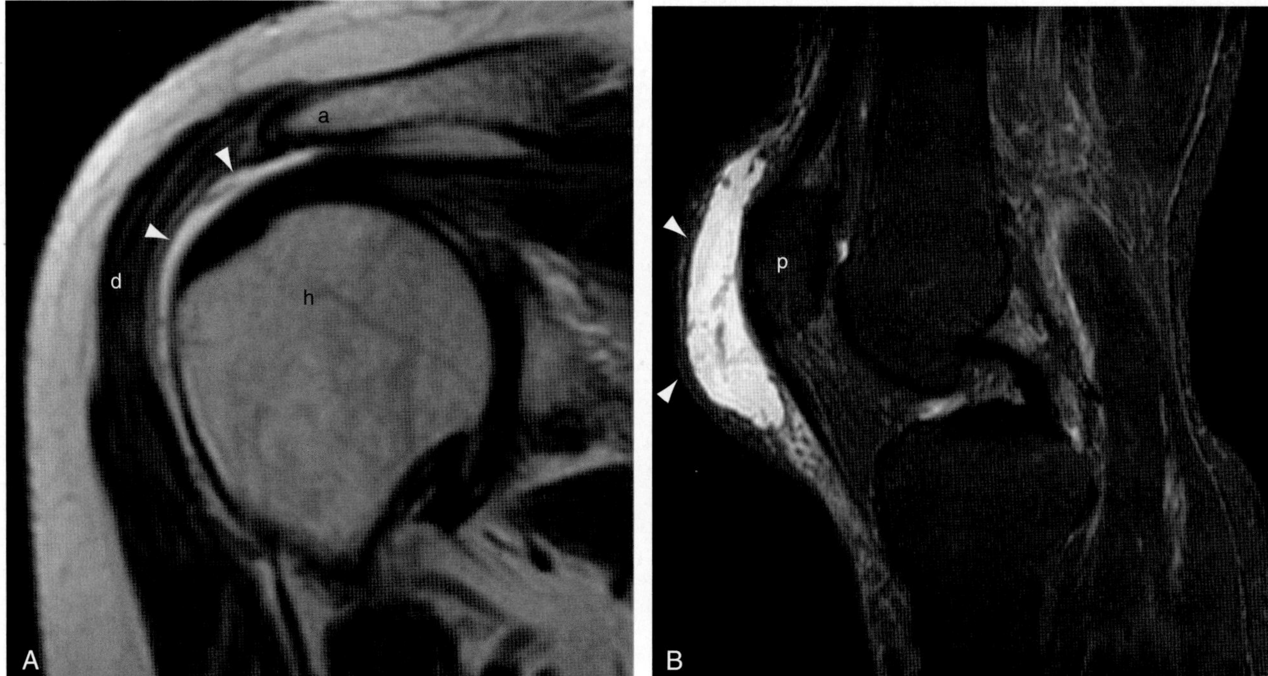

FIGURE 13-28. Bursitis. **A,** Coronal T2-weighted image through the shoulder shows high signal fluid in the subacromial-subdeltoid bursa *(arrowheads)* in the presence of an intact rotator cuff, consistent with subacromial-subdeltoid bursitis. *a,* Acromion; *d,* deltoid; *h,* humeral head. **B,** Sagittal fat-saturated T2-weighted image through the knee shows a high signal lenticular structure *(arrowheads)* anterior to the patella *(p)*, consistent with prepatellar bursitis.

(Continued)

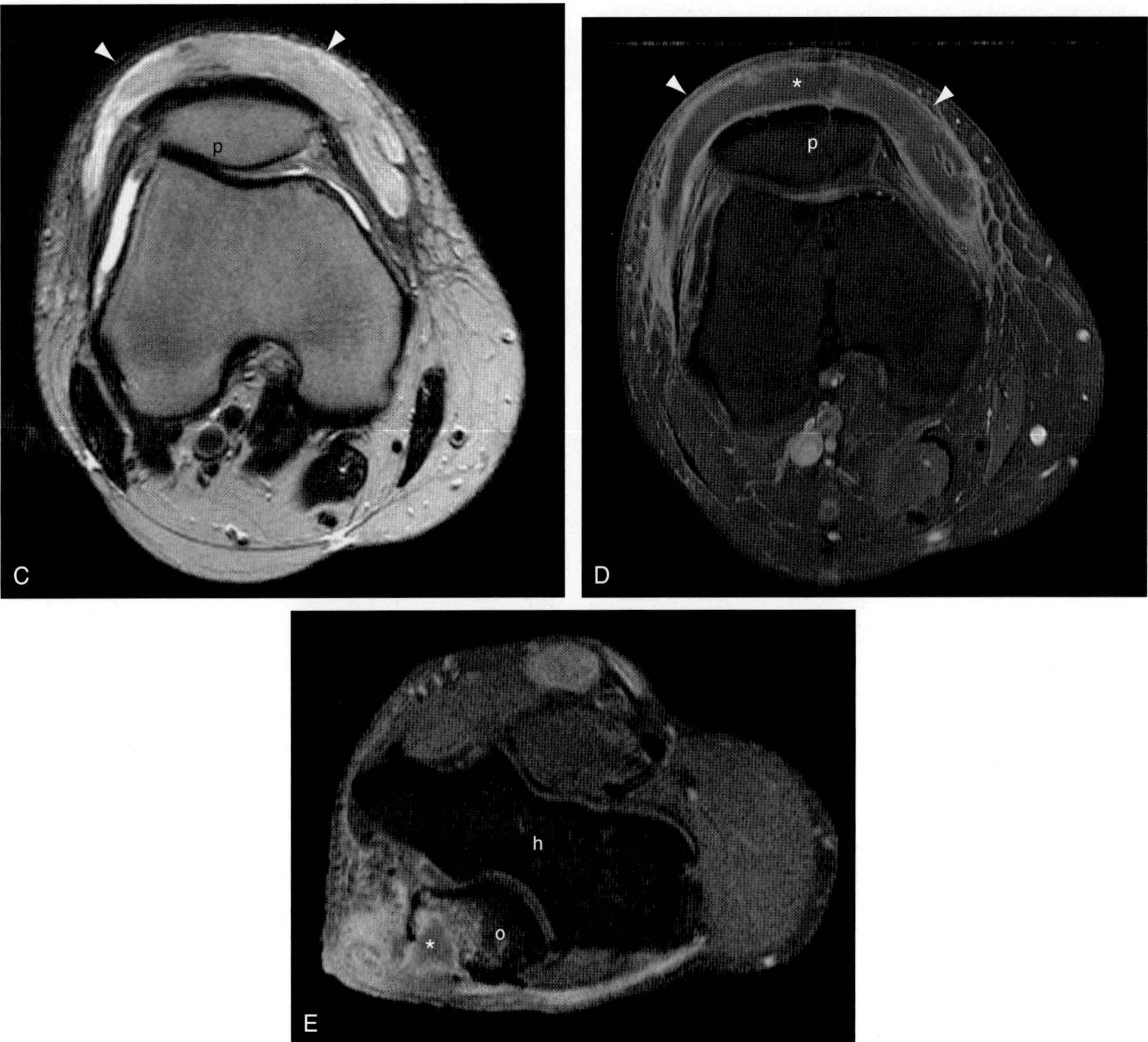

FIGURE 13-28—cont'd. **C,** Axial T2-weighted image through the knee shows a distended prepatellar bursa *(arrowheads)*, filled with material that is high in signal on T2-weighted images. High T2 signal could represent either fluid, thickened hyperemic synovium, or both. **D,** Axial fat-saturated T1-weighted image through the same level in the knee, following intravenous administration of gadolinium contrast. The gadolinium contrast appears bright. Thickened synovium will appear bright with contrast, whereas fluid will appear dark. This demonstrates that the prepatellar bursa is composed predominantly of nonenhancing, low signal fluid *(asterisk)*, whereas the walls of the bursa are enhancing *(arrowheads)* due to slightly thickened synovium and/or mild surrounding inflammatory change. **E,** Axial post-contrast fat-saturated T1-weighted image through the elbow showing high signal enhancement surrounding darker fluid within an infected olecranon bursa. Fluid from the bursa *(asterisk)* has eroded into the olecranon. There is enhancement of the adjacent bone marrow. *h,* Humerus; *o,* olecranon.

trochanteric bursa and the subacromial/subdeltoid bursa; the significance of this finding is uncertain. In some cases it may be a normal finding. Abnormal distension of a bursa is consistent with bursitis and may be due to acute or chronic trauma or to inflammatory or infectious processes. Both simple fluid and hyperemic synovium are isointense to muscle on T1-weighted images and hyperintense on T2-weighted images and are not easily distinguishable in the absence of IV gadolinium contrast. Proteinaceous or hemorrhagic fluid is often hyperintense to muscle on T1-weighted images and of variable signal intensity on T2-weighted images.[132] A fluid level may present; simpler fluid will be lower signal on T1-weighted images and higher signal on T2-weighted images, compared with fluid bound to proteinaceous material. Hemorrhage may also cause fibrinous low signal T2-weighted stranding. Fronds of fibrotic (low T2) synovium, septations, synechiae, and loose bodies may be present. Loose bodies may be low signal on T2-weighted images; if ossified, the loose bodies will be similar in signal to intramedullary fat centrally and surrounded by low signal cortical rim. Bursal calcification and calcified or ossified loose bodies may not be readily apparent on MRI and require correlation with radiographs for reliable detection. Following administration of IV gadolinium, the bursal synovium will enhance and, depending on the degree of synovial hypertrophy, variable amounts of internal enhancement will be seen (Figure 13-28, *D* to *F*). Edema (high T2 signal) and/or hemorrhage (high T1 signal) may be present in the surrounding soft tissue. If so, the borders of a well-circumscribed bursa may be less distinct. Bursal distension should be distinguished from focal interstitial edema; background tissue texture should not be visible within the distended bursa. Although an infected bursa will tend to have higher T1 signal, may be less well defined and may show more internal enhancement and surrounding edema than a noninfected bursa; the presence or absence of infection within a bursa cannot be determined on the basis of MRI.[133] If there is clinical suspicion for septic bursitis, then aspiration must be performed. In rare circumstances, bursae can become involved with processes that affect synovium elsewhere, including synovial osteochondromatosis, pigmented villonodular synovitis, and lipoma arborescens. In synovial osteochondromatosis, MRI demonstrates rounded or somewhat faceted bodies within the bursa that tend to have a thick low signal cortical rim and an intramedullary cavity that follows the signal intensity of normal bone marrow on all sequences. Pigmented villonodular synovitis may be focal or diffuse. The most characteristic appearance is a low T2 signal mass, with low signal that is even more pronounced on a T2*-weighted (long echo time) gradient echo image, but, in the absence of sufficient hemosiderin, the MRI appearance may be nonspecific. In lipoma arborescens, the submucosal layer deep to the synovium accumulates fat and high T1 signal mass protrudes into the bursa.[134] Adventitial bursae may be seen at sites of increased friction, including over osteochondromas[135] and in amputation stumps[136] (Figure 13-29).

Scintigraphy

At present, nuclear medicine studies do not play a significant role in the assessment of tendons or bursae. Nuclear medicine bone scans, performed with technetium-99m methylene diphosphonate, may show increased uptake of the radionuclide agent within bone that abuts abnormal or inflamed tendons or bursae (Figure 13-30, *A*) and, in case reports, can demonstrate response to treatment.[137] Inflamed synovium in a tendon or bursa may be directly demonstrated on the blood pool phase of a triple phase bone scan due to hypervascularity.[138] Positron emission tomography (PET) scans, which show activity related to the metabolism of ^{18}F-2-flourodeoxyglucose (F18-FDG) and are currently used primarily for evaluation of tumor and tumor metastases in certain cancers, also show increased tracer uptake in areas of inflammation associated with peritendinous or bursal inflammation.[139] PET-CT scans (i.e., PET scans obtained with a correlative CT scan) can further localize an area of increased activity to a specific anatomic structure, such as a tendon or bursa, on a CT scan (Figure 13-30, *B*). Because the degree of tracer activity reflects the level of glucose metabolism, the potential use of PET scanning to assess activity of inflammatory disease and its response to therapy has been suggested.[140] In early studies of patients with rheumatoid arthritis, FDG uptake was observed not only about joints, but also in the synovium of tendons and bursae and demonstrated decreased activity in response to treatment.[141]

Arthrography, Tenography, and Bursography

Shoulder **arthrography** can aid in evaluation of rotator cuff tendons. Traditional shoulder arthrography is performed using x-ray fluoroscopy to follow the passage of radiopaque contrast instilled into the glenohumeral joint. Although techniques may vary, the most common technique involves placement of a 22G needle into

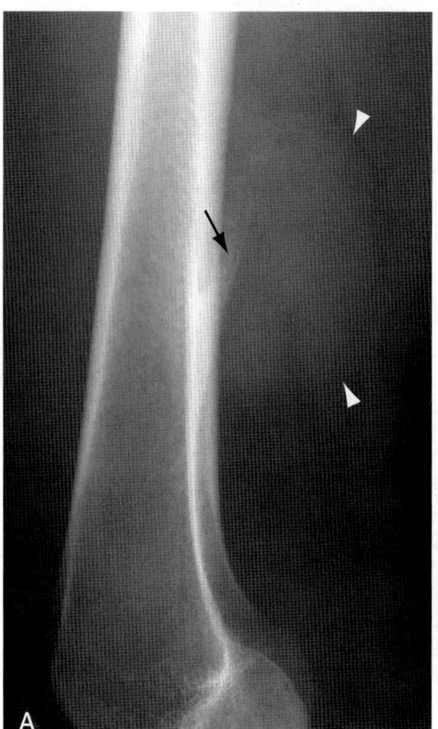

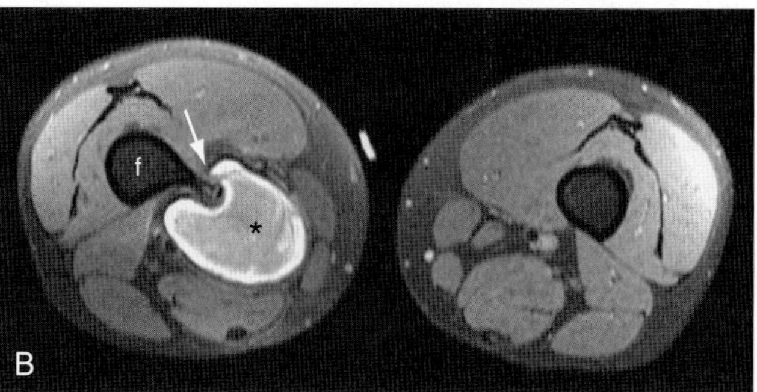

FIGURE 13-29. Adventitial bursitis. **A,** Lateral radiograph of the femur shows a pedunculated osteochondroma projecting off the posterior aspect of the distal femur *(arrow)*. The fluid distended bursa is large and dense enough to be visible radiographically *(arrowheads)*. Poor visualization of the distal tip of the osteochondroma is due to technical factors: higher kilovoltage needed to penetrate soft tissues of the thigh "burns through" the thin ossified tip. **B,** Axial fat-saturated T1-weighted images through the both thighs show the osteochondroma *(arrow)* projecting off the femur *(f)* into the surrounding soft tissues. The distended adventitial bursa *(asterisk)* can be seen forming around it. Linear signal through the extreme tip of the osteochondroma raises the question of a fracture through it.

(Continued)

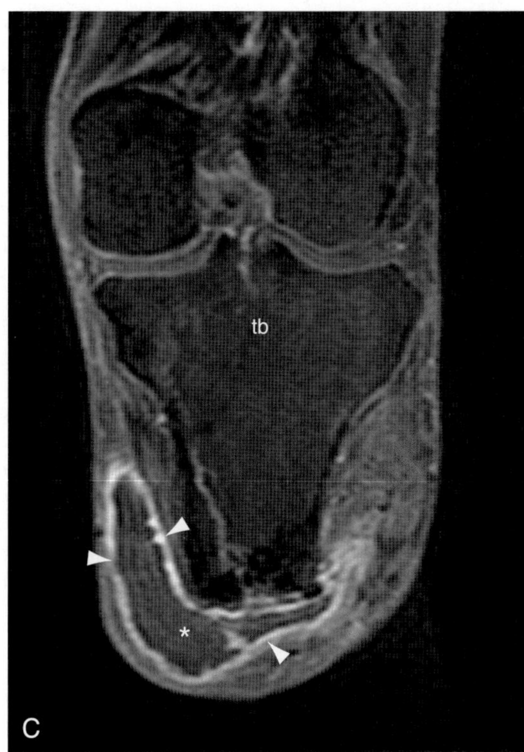

FIGURE 13-29—cont'd. **C,** Coronal post-contrast fat-saturated T1-weighted image through the knee and upper calf in an individual status post below-the-knee amputation. An adventitial bursa has formed at the lower edge of the tibial stump *(asterisk)* and shows a thin rim of high signal contrast enhancement *(arrowheads). tb,* tibia.

the glenohumeral joint under fluoroscopic guidance and instillation of 8 to 12 mL of contrast material into the joint. The appearance of contrast in the subacromial-subdeltoid bursa implies the presence of a rotator cuff tear (see Figure 13-14, *A*).

> A full-thickness ("complete") rotator cuff tear is indicated on arthrography by the passage of contrast injected into the glenohumeral joint through the tear and into the subacromial-subdeltoid bursa.

A partial articular surface tear may be visible as focal surface irregularity along the articular surface of the cuff. Arthrography is very accurate for diagnosis of complete tears of the rotator cuff. Mink et al. found overall accuracy of greater than 99% for detection of complete rotator cuff tears with double contrast arthrography in 152 surgically confirmed cases. They also found a strong correlation for the quantitative and qualitative assessment of tear size.[142,143] Sensitivity for diagnosis of partial articular surface tears is more limited.[144] Arthrography cannot effectively diagnose bursal-sided tears and does not provide as much information about background tendon degeneration, muscle atrophy, or other potential sources of shoulder pain as MRI or ultrasound. Techniques for performing arthrography under ultrasound guidance have also been described.[145]

At present, the fluoroscopic procedure is usually followed by cross-sectional imaging of the fluid-distended joint using MRI or CT.[49,146,147] If MR arthrography is performed, then single contrast technique is employed (no air in the joint), and, once the joint is localized, the remaining 10 mL or so of fluid instilled into the joint is composed of dilute gadolinium. The advantage of MRI is that it allows detailed depiction of the site and size of the tear and of the quality of the tendon edges, tendon substance, and other abnormalities about the shoulder. With the advent of

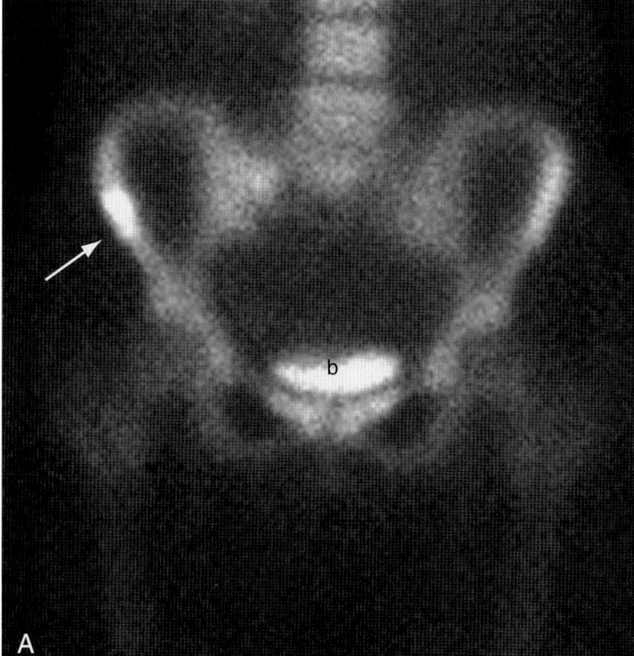

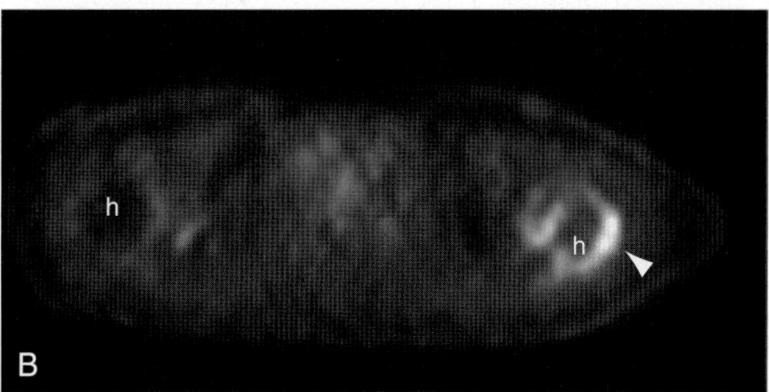

FIGURE 13-30. Radionuclide studies. **A,** AP view of the pelvis from a technetium-99m pertechnetate bone scan. An area of increased activity is seen at the anterior superior iliac spine *(arrow)*. This reflects reactive bony hyperostosis forming at the origin of the sartorius tendon, either due to chronic repetitive trauma or inflammatory change. High signal is also seen in the bladder, due to accumulation of excreted radionuclide. **B,** Axial image through the shoulder girdle from an FDG-PET scan. High signal, indicating areas of increased metabolism, is seen in the left subacromial-subdeltoid bursa *(arrowhead)*, reflecting the presence of a benign aseptic bursitis. *B,* Bladder; *h,* humeral head.

multidetector CT scanners, there is renewed interest in the use of CT arthrography to evaluate the glenohumeral joint and labrum, but the use of CT arthrography for evaluation of rotator cuff tendons remains limited. Recent studies suggest a high sensitivity and specificity for detection of rotator cuff tears and excellent quantification of tear size compared with arthroscopy.[147] However, CT arthrography of the rotator cuff would seem to provide little added value as compared with the combination of fluoroscopy (presence/absence of tear) and MR arthrography (location and size of tear and condition of tendon) for assessment of the rotator cuff, raising the question of whether the additional radiation exposure is justified. CT arthrography may be performed in individuals who have contraindications to MRI. In that case, the CT arthrogram is performed as a double contrast procedure with only a small amount of positive contrast and the remaining volume composed of air injected into the joint. As with a conventional arthrogram, contrast or air seen in the subacromial/subdeltoid bursa indicates the presence of a complete tear, and irregularity along the articular surface of the rotator cuff indicates the presence of an articular surface tear.

Conventional arthrography or CT arthrography can be used to diagnose a rotator cuff tear in patients with contraindications to MRI.

Tenography, once a mainstay of imaging for diagnosis of tendon pathology, is no longer commonly practiced, having been supplanted by MRI and ultrasound. Tenography refers to imaging of tendons via the percutaneous instillation of radiographic contrast material into the tenosynovial space surrounding the tendon, under fluoroscopic guidance and imaging[148,149] (Figure 13-31). It has been used to evaluate the integrity of the tendon, tendon sheath, adjoining capsule, and (calcaneofibular) ligaments and to assess inflammatory conditions involving the tendon sheaths of the ankle, foot, and wrist.[150-154] On tenography, the normal tendon appears as a longitudinal defect in the contrast column surrounding it. Tendon rupture can be seen as contrast extending into or through the expected contrast defect or as a mass-like defect within the tendon sheath. Tendon avulsion may appear as interruption of the contrast column itself. When synovial proliferation is present, the contrast column about the tendon may be narrowed and irregular with nodularity and multiple outpouchings or sacculations. Stenosing tenosynovitis is seen as areas of abnormal constriction of the contrast column. Constrictions at the site of retinacula represent normal findings (e.g., flexor retinaculum about the posterior tibial tendon at the level of the tibial plafond and superior and inferior peroneal retinacula about the peroneal tendons at levels proximal and distal to the sustentaculum tali), which should not be mistaken for pathologic constriction. Loose bodies within the tendon sheath are seen as rounded filing defects within the contrast column. Tenography provides for dynamic imaging of a tendon and, as such, has proven useful in the diagnosis of snapping iliopsoas tendon.[155] Advocates suggest that tenography helps confirm the tendon as the site of symptoms and helps identify patients who will benefit from surgery.[156] However, diagnostic tenography provides limited specificity: poor filling of the tendon sheath may be caused by sheath fibrosis, tendon enlargement, extrinsic compression, or tumor. Moreover, tenography does not allow for assessment of tendinosis or for quantification of a tendon tear.

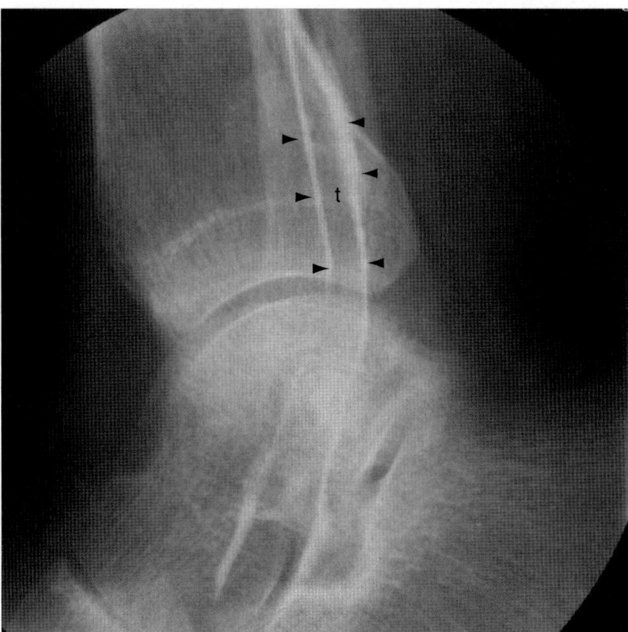

FIGURE 13-31. Tenography. Sagittal image through the ankle in a patient with a normal posterior tibial tendon. Contrast instilled under fluoroscopic guidance enters and distends the tendon sheath and is seen as a column of white material following the course of the tendon sheath *(arrowheads)*. The tendon itself appears as a tubular filling defect *(t)* within the contrast-distended tendon sheath. Because the normal tendon is continuous and uniform in width, areas of tendon thickening, thinning, or interruption can be identified. (Image courtesy of Arthur Newberg, MD.)

In a limited number of practices, tenograms are still performed in conjunction with therapeutic injections. Although originally performed under fluoroscopic guidance, therapeutic tenography can also be performed under ultrasound guidance.[145] The tendon sheath is distended with contrast to aid in lysing adhesions, and anesthetic and corticosteroids are injected. In follow-up evaluation of 111 patients who underwent therapeutic tenography for symptoms refractory to conservative treatment, 48% (31/65) of patients treated for posterior tibial tendon symptoms and 46% (18/39) of patients treated for peroneal symptoms reported complete or near-complete resolution of symptoms. However, tonographic appearance did not correlate with response to symptoms.[156] Potential complications of tenography are rare but include infection and tendon rupture and, when steroids are administered, discoloration of overlying skin. In order to avoid tendon rupture, practitioners recommend preprocedure imaging to assess for partial or complete tendon tears—in these instances (and when a mass suggestive of rupture is encountered at tenography), steroid injection is unlikely to be beneficial and risks potential interference with collagen healing.[156] Practitioners also recommend that the patient refrains from sports or strenuous activities for up to 6 weeks following the tonogram and suggest the use of short leg cast or walking boot after posterior tibial tendon injections to avoid tendon rupture and subsequent development of pes planus.[156]

Bursography refers to percutaneous instillation of contrast into a bursa under fluoroscopic guidance and, like tenography, is also now rarely performed.[148,154,157] Injection of contrast into the subacromial-subdeltoid bursa has been performed to detect irregularity of the superficial surface of the supraspinatus tendon and thereby diagnose a partial bursal surface tendon tear.[154] Injection of dilute gadolinium contrast into the bursa to aid in MRI visualization of partial bursal surface tears has been described, but many of these tears can be visualized on routine MRI examinations, and the technique is not commonly performed. Injection of contrast into the retrocalcaneal bursa in order to detect tears of the distal Achilles' tendon has been performed.[154] Although findings at bursography were found to correlate well with findings at surgery, this technique has largely been abandoned.[158]

Some practitioners may perform bursography in conjunction with either aspiration of a bursa for diagnosis of suspected infection or therapeutic injections for symptomatic bursal inflammation. Common sites include the subacromial-subdeltoid, olecranon, greater trochanteric, and prepatellar bursae. These bursal interventions may also be performed under ultrasound guidance.[145]

Ultrasound

In experienced hands, ultrasound is an effective method for imaging tendons and bursae. Normal and abnormal tendons and bursae can be demonstrated with high spatial resolution and high accuracy. Results are highly dependent on the quality of the equipment, the sonographer, and the interpreting physician. The examination allows for direct interaction with the patient and, as a result, facilitates detailed assessment of the specific site of symptoms. Ultrasound images are generated in real-time, which allows for dynamic evaluation—tendons can be imaged through a range of motion to aid in detecting subluxation and impingement, and tissue motion in response to compression by the ultrasound transducer can be assessed to aid in detecting tendon tears and distinguishing fluid from synovitis. Ultrasound also permits real-time guidance for interventional procedures, such as aspiration or injection of bursae, tendon sheaths, peritendinous tissues, and symptomatic foci of calcific tendinitis, while helping to avoid injection into the tendon. Examination of deep structures with ultrasound is limited using the high-frequency transducers that are optimal for imaging of superficial tendons, but use of 5-MHz transducers and extended field of view imaging with appropriately focused positioning is helpful in the evaluation of deep tendons.[159] Although imaging of the postoperative tendon may be difficult due to postoperative changes in the tissues, orthopedic hardware does not generally interfere with ultrasound examination of tendons or bursae. Ultrasound examination is generally well tolerated by patients and can be performed in individuals who are claustrophobic or have pacemakers or other electronic implants. However, serial ultrasound evaluation of a particular structure or process over time can be more challenging than with MRI.

Advantages of ultrasound include real time imaging during range of motion, patient interaction to correlate imaging and clinical findings, and the absence of ionizing radiation.

Ultrasound imaging is based on insonating tissues with sound waves.[160]

Insonate means "to expose to ultrasound waves."

The amplitude of reflected sound is translated into a gray scale to create an image: areas of high reflectivity appear bright on images and are considered highly echogenic or hyperechoic, areas of low reflectivity appear less bright and are considered hypoechoic, and areas that do not scatter or reflect sound waves appear dark or anechoic. The quality of ultrasound images, visibility of certain structures, and even the ultrasound appearance of tissues are highly dependent on the ultrasound equipment employed.[161] Although evaluation of tendons was limited with older generations of equipment, development of broadband high-frequency ultrasound transducers has allowed for high-resolution imaging of musculoskeletal structures such as tendons and bursae. High-quality musculoskeletal imaging is now performed with small-footprint linear transducers in the 7.5- to 15-MHz range. High frequencies are important in order to achieve high (axial) spatial resolution but have limited penetration into deep tissues. Although lower frequency transducers allow for deeper penetration, they provide only limited spatial resolution. Visualization of characteristic tissue texture and subtle pathology in tendons is dependent on having sufficiently high transducer frequency.[159,162] Linear array transducers are preferred for tendon imaging, because the alternative curved or sector-design transducers have divergent beam geometry that accentuates artifacts in tendons due to anisotropy.

Anisotropy refers to a property that varies with direction of measurement through a structure.

Ultrasound examination is based on positioning the patient and obtaining standardized views that are tailored to the joint or limb in question. In all instances, tendons and bursae should be imaged in both longitudinal and axial planes. Good technique with standard views must be employed to minimize artifacts that can interfere with the examination, such as anisotropy. Anisotropy results in areas of low echogenicity within a tendon and can mimic tendinosis or tendon tear. In order to avoid artifacts due to anisotropy, the ultrasound beam must be directed perpendicular to the surface of the tendon. Even when the transducer is tilted as little as 5 to 10 degrees, anisotropy artifacts can occur.[52,162] This artifact can occur in all tendons but creates a particular challenge in imaging tendons that follow a curvilinear path, such as tendons of the rotator cuff and ankle.

Power Doppler imaging is a very useful technique for imaging of tendons and bursae. It is sensitive to slow blood flow and small vessels and is used to detect areas of increased vascularity that are associated with inflammation within or around a tendon or bursa. Because artifactual power Doppler signal can arise from any strongly reflective tissue (tendon, ligament, fascia, bone), care should be taken not to mistake this artifactual signal for evidence of tendinitis.[162] Methods for reproducible quantitation of perfusion using power Doppler imaging are currently being developed.

Tendons that can be examined with ultrasound include the rotator cuff and long head of the biceps tendons at the shoulder; brachii distal biceps and triceps tendons and common flexor and extensor tendons at the elbow; flexor and extensor tendons of the wrist and hand; iliopsoas, gluteus, adductor, and hamstring tendons at the hip; quadriceps and patellar tendons at the knee; and Achilles' and other major tendons of the ankle and foot.

The **normal tendon** appears as a band of fine, dense, parallel linear echoes in a fibrillar pattern on longitudinal scans and as a flat, rounded or ovoid structure composed of multiple small closely packed echogenic foci on transverse scans (Figure 13-32, *A, B*). Echoes visible within the tendon are thought to correspond to the interface between the tendon bundles and the surrounding endotenon.[159,163] The tendon surface is bounded by a hyperechoic rim corresponding to either the paratenon or the synovial sheath.[52] Occasionally a small amount of anechoic physiologic fluid may be visible within the sheath as a thin hypoechoic line interposed between the echogenic rim and the tendon surface.[159] Although often well demarcated, the tendon outline may be less distinctly visible when it is surrounded by echogenic fat. Under normal conditions, no flow is detected within a tendon on power Doppler imaging. Retinculae restraining tendons may be visible on high-resolution imaging and are seen as linear hyperechoic structures.

Tendinosis, or tendon degeneration, is seen as focal or diffuse cross-sectional enlargement of the tendon[160] and focal or diffuse decreased echogenicity within the tendon[164] (Figure 13-33).

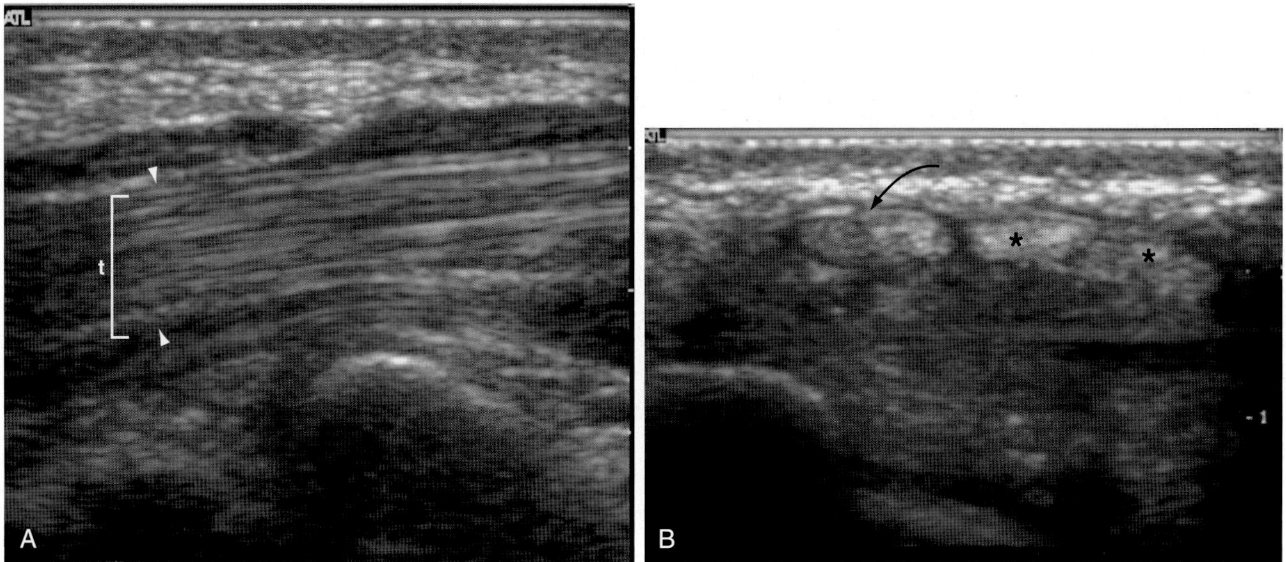

FIGURE 13-32. Normal tendon. **A,** Longitudinal view through adjoining flexor tendons in the wrist (*t,* with *bracket*) demonstrates the typical fibrillar echotexture of a tendon, consisting of a band of fine, dense, parallel echogenic lines. Echoes visible within the tendon are thought to correspond to the interface between the tendon bundles and the surrounding endotenon. The surface of the tendon is bounded by an echogenic outline *(arrowheads).* **B,** Transverse view through a normal extensor tendon in the hand *(curved arrow).* In cross section, the normal tendon appears as a flat, rounded or ovoid structure composed of multiple small closely packed echogenic foci. Additional tendons are seen nearby *(asterisks).*

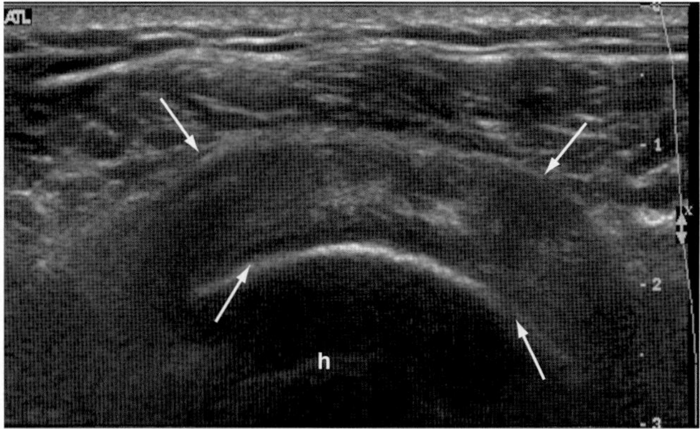

FIGURE 13-33. Tendon degeneration. The degenerated supraspinatus tendon *(arrows)* is abnormally thickened with loss of the normal fibrillar pattern and heterogeneous echotexture. The echogenic surface of the tendon is uninterrupted. *h,* Humeral head.

> Tendinosis, or tendon degeneration, is seen as focal or diffuse cross-sectional enlargement of the tendon and focal or diffuse decreased echogenicity within the tendon.

Hypoechoic foci within the tendon reflect the presence of various forms of histologic degeneration, including hypoxic and mucoid degeneration. Small anechoic cystic foci, focal echogenic dystrophic calcification or ossification, or tiny echogenic calcific foci may also be visible. Peritendinous fluid may be present.[165] When the paratenon is abnormal, it can be difficult to visualize the paratenon as a structure distinct from the degenerated tendon on gray-scale images. In this setting, power Doppler imaging may demonstrate flow within the paratenon and may help to distinguish the paratenon from the tendon.[166] However, power Doppler signal can be seen within the tendon due to angiofibroblastic changes in symptomatic tendinosis.[27,167,168] In fact, some authors have suggested that the presence of hyperemia on power Doppler imaging may help localize areas of tendon that will respond to therapeutic injection. Although ultrasound has been shown to have a high positive predictive value for tendinosis, a false-negative exam can occur in symptomatic individuals.[161,169] It has been suggested that these individuals may have a better outcome than those with positive ultrasonographic findings.[170] False-positive exams may also occur with findings of abnormal hypoechoic foci in asymptomatic tendons. Some observers believe that these false-positive findings are associated with an increased likelihood of future tendon symptoms.[170]

Ultrasound is useful in detecting **tendon tears,** determining the location and size of the gap, and, in some anatomic sites, locating retracted tendon edges. Criteria for diagnosis of tear vary from anatomic site to site, but, in general, a **complete tendon tear** is seen as a discrete, well-marginated, hypoechoic full-thickness cleft across the tendon with focal loss of the normal fibrillar echotexture (Figure 13-34, *A*).

> A complete tendon tear shows a discrete, well-marginated, hypoechoic full-thickness cleft across the tendon with focal loss of the normal fibrillar echotexture.

Additional criteria include detachment and retraction of a tendon from a bony insertion site, with or without a small hyperechoic focus of avulsed bone, and nonvisualization of the tendon. Tendon edges may be seen as a poorly reflective echogenic lines.[170] Focal or diffuse thinning of the tendon may be evident. Even with a complete tendon tear, the paratenon may remain intact. Some signs of tendon tear may be site specific. For example, in the rotator cuff, signs of tear include widening of the gap between the biceps and supraspinatus tendons, alteration in the appearance of the nearby subacromial-subdeltoid bursa as it sags down into the tear, exposure of a bare area of bone and cartilage, and focal increased reflectivity of humeral head cartilage and bone due to fluid in the tear (Figure 13-34, *B*). Fluid within a tendon tear can serve to accentuate the tear, but echogenic hematoma and

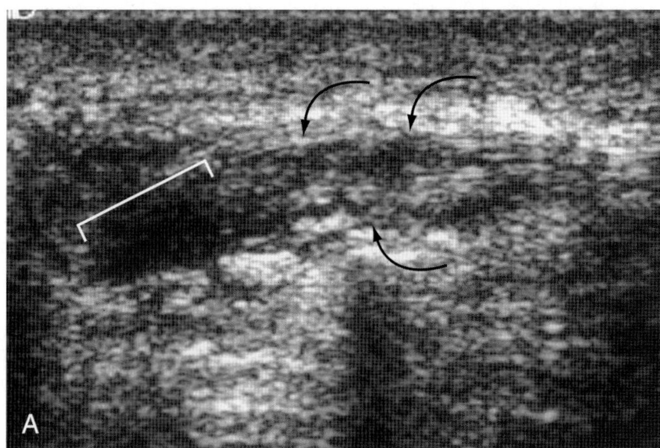

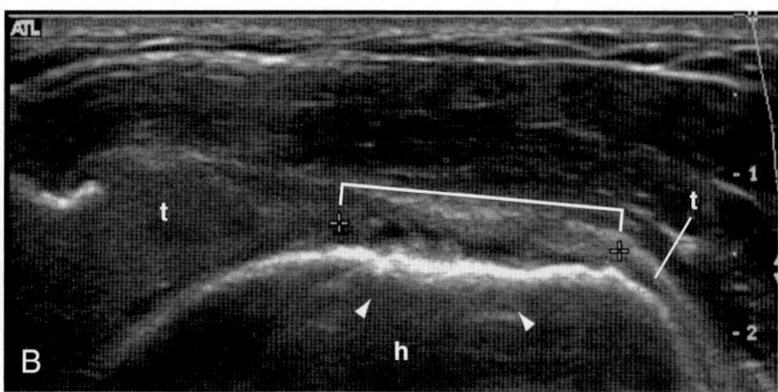

FIGURE 13-34. Tendon tear. **A,** Complete tear through the posterior tibial tendon. Longitudinal image shows a hypoechoic fluid-filled gap in the tendon *(bracket)* and irregular fibers at the torn tendon edge *(curved arrows)*. **B,** Tear through the supraspinatus tendon of the rotator cuff. The tear is seen as an anechoic fluid-filled gap extending through the echogenic tendon *(bracket)*. The frayed, swollen ends of the supraspinatus tendon *(cross hairs)* are seen at either edge of the tendon tear. Loss of the normal fibrillar pattern within the tendon fragments *(t)* indicates underlying tendon degeneration and/or edema. The irregularity of the cortical surface of the humeral head, seen here as an irregular, highly echogenic white line *(above arrowheads)*, is often seen in the setting of cuff arthropathy.

debris may also help to obscure an acute tear. **Chronic tears** may be obscured by scar, granulation tissue, or calcification. Gentle compression with the ultrasound transducer can help to highlight the tendon tear by displacing fluid and by revealing discontinuous motion of the tendon edges[170] (Figure 13-35). Secondary signs may be useful in making the diagnosis of tendon tear. For example, in a study by Hollister et al., the presence of fluid in both the glenohumeral joint and subacromial bursa had a 95% positive predictive value for rotator cuff tear and was present in only 1.7% of asymptomatic shoulders.[171] The accuracy of ultrasound for detection of tendon tears varies from anatomic site to site, but, in general, ultrasound demonstrates high sensitivity for detection of complete tendon tears[159,172] and has shown accuracy similar to MRI for the diagnosis of some types of tendon tears.[63] For example, in a study by Teefey et al., ultrasound correctly identified all 65 full-thickness rotator cuff tears (sensitivity of 100%) found at arthroscopy, with 17 true-negative and 3 false-positive exams (specificity 85%) and an overall accuracy of 96%. However, ultrasound is less sensitive for detection of partial tears than for detection of complete tears.[161,173,174] In the study by Teefey, only 10 of 15 partial-thickness tears diagnosed on arthroscopy were detected by ultrasound.[174]

FIGURE 13-35. Chronic tear with compression. Under pressure from the transducer, fluid fills a gap *(bracket)* formed by a rotator cuff tear. The resultant acoustic window allows for visualization of the surface of the hyaline cartilage as a thin echogenic line above the humeral cortex *(arrowheads)*. *h,* Humeral head; *t,* rotator cuff tendon.

Quantification of tear size is important for determining surgical technique and for evaluating prognosis. In many instances, ultrasound provides for accurate measurement of the dimensions of a complete tendon tear. In some cases, accurate assessment of tear size is not possible due to the presence of hemorrhage, debris, or fibrosis within or around the tear. Measurement of the tear may sometimes be precluded by retraction of the tendon beyond the ultrasound-visible acoustic window, as in the case of a massive rotator cuff tear. Measurements may also be influenced by differences in positioning at ultrasound exam versus surgery.[161] In two prospective studies of patients with suspected rotator cuff tears, ultrasound and MRI were comparable in accuracy for quantification of tear size,[63,175,176] but ultrasound was less accurate for quantifying tendon retraction greater than 30 mm. Use of a "curved line" measurement technique for large tears helped to avoid underestimation of tear size.[176] The use of ultrasound to identify muscle atrophy in the setting of a chronic tendon tear has been described, but ultrasound does not appear to be as sensitive as MRI for detection of mild fatty infiltration.[177] Atrophic changes in muscle (seen as increased echogenicity) may develop in the subacute and chronic phases following a tendon tear, but, at present, no reliable method for quantitation of echogenicity by ultrasound is available. Comparison to the normal contralateral side may be useful in assessing relative muscle mass, but it is important to recognize that measurements must be made on truly comparable views and that side-to-side differences can be seen due to normal variation. Loss of muscle mass may also be difficult to quantify at specific sites, such as the rotator cuff, where the muscle is partially obscured by bone.

A drawback to using ultrasonography for the assessment of the rotator cuff is some limitation in quantifying fatty infiltration and atrophy of the affected muscles; these are important parameters for treatment planning.

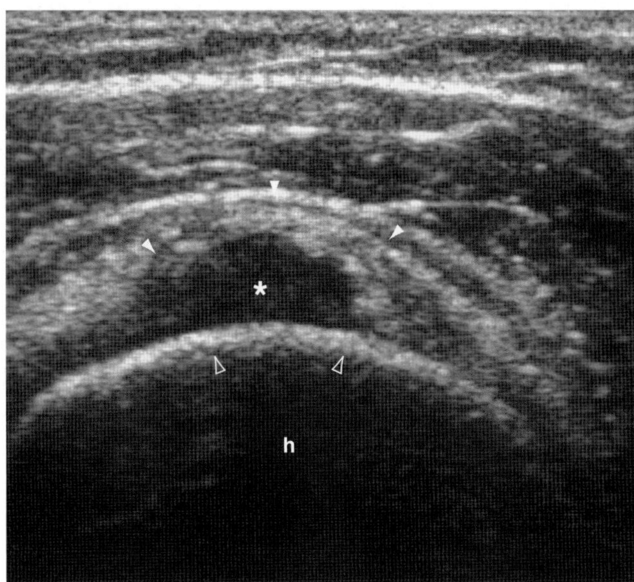

FIGURE 13-36. Partial tear through the supraspinatus tendon. Transverse image through the shoulder shows a partial articular surface tear *(asterisk)*. The superficial or bursal portion of the supraspinatus tendon remains intact *(arrowheads)*. The cortex of the humerus *(h)* appears as a highly echogenic curved white line *(open arrowheads)*.

Partial tears can be quite difficult to distinguish from severe tendinosis on ultrasound exam.[159,174,178] A partial tear appears as a hypoechoic focus along the bursal or articular surface of the tendon or as a nonsurfacing focus within the substance of the tendon that is seen on two planes or as a mixed hypoechoic/hyperechoic focus[159] (Figure 13-36). Careful graded compression of a tear site and dynamic assessment in flexion and extension may aid in differentiating partial tear from tendinosis.[161] Identification of power Doppler flow within the tendon supports a diagnosis of tendinosis rather than partial tear.[179] Presence of fluid within the tendon sheath may help to outline partial tears, but arthrosonography is not commonly used to diagnose tears. Improvements in ultrasound technology may lead to improved diagnostic accuracy in the detection of partial tears. Some authors argue that detection of partial tears on ultrasound examination is of doubtful clinical significance, in that severe partial tears may be functionally indistinguishable from complete tears, whereas small partial tears may respond to treatment for tendinosis. In practice, treatment of partial tears varies depending on the patient population and other clinical considerations. Whether ultrasound or MRI is more sensitive for detection of partial tears is controversial[160,161] and, no doubt, depends upon local expertise. In a recent large comparative study of rotator cuff tears by Teefey et al., ultrasound and magnetic resonance imaging had comparable accuracies for identifying and measuring the size of partial-thickness tears.[63] Ultrasound and MRI correctly identified 13 of 19 and 12 of 19 partial-thickness rotator cuff tears and correctly predicted the width of 54% and 75% of partial-thickness tears, respectively.[63]

In **acute paratenonitis**, the tendon may appear swollen and its edges may be blurred, either focally or along the entire tendon.[179] There may be increased power Doppler signal in the inflamed paratenon and peritendinous soft tissues.[180] Comparison with the contralateral side may help to assess the degree of abnormality. In **chronic paratenonitis**, the tendon contour may be irregular and bumpy. Tiny echogenic foci may be visible, with or without shadowing, due to tiny intratendon calcifications.[181] Paratenonitis may or may not be associated with changes in the underlying tendon. **Tenosynovitis** may involve tendons of the biceps, wrist, hand, iliopsoas, ankle, or foot. Tenosynovitis appears as a sheath of simple or complex material surrounding the tendon (Figure 13-37, *A, B*). A small amount of simple fluid surrounding the tendon can be a normal finding in some locations, such as the long head of the biceps tendon in the shoulder or the flexor hallucis tendon in the ankle. Simple fluid should be anechoic. Complex echogenic material surrounding the tendon may indicate the presence of either pus or thickened synovium.[179,182] Complex fluid will demonstrate swirling debris with transducer percussion, whereas thickened synovium will not. Pus and thickened synovium can be distinguished using power Doppler imaging (Figure 13-37, *C, D*). Pus may show hypervascularity surrounding the fluid collection, but the purulent fluid itself should not show signal on power Doppler imaging. Thickened synovium—whether due to overuse or inflammatory arthritis—should demonstrate hypervascularity within the distended tendon sheath on power Doppler imaging.[180,183]

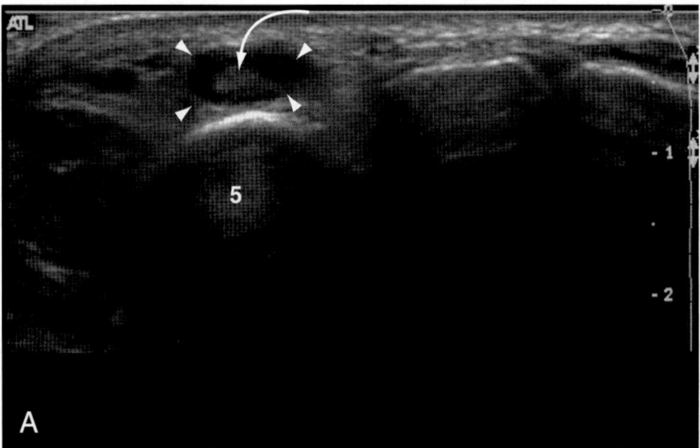

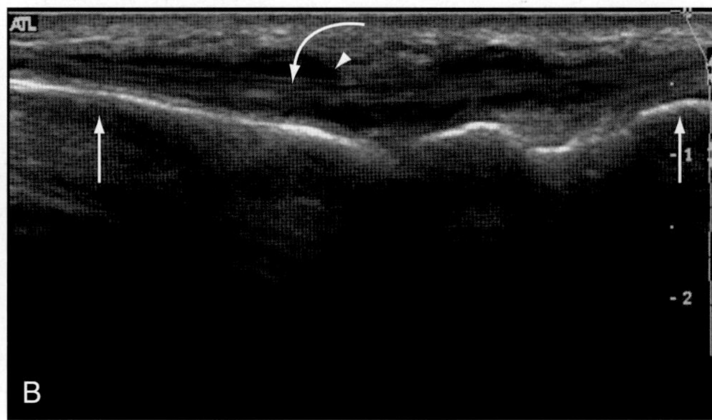

FIGURE 13-37. Tenosynovitis. **(A)** Transverse and **(B)** longitudinal images through the extensor digiti minimi tendon of the hand. The tendon *(curved arrow)*, with its echogenic fibrillar pattern, is surrounding by hypoechoic material representing fluid within the tenosynovial sheath *(arrowheads)*. On the longitudinal image, the tenosynovial sheath appears sacculated, with an undulating contour, reflecting the presence of stenosing tenosynovitis. The thin, highly echogenic white line deep to the tendon and its surrounding tenosynovitis represents the cortex of the bone *(arrows)*. The remainder of the bone is shadowed, due to the highly reflective quality of the cortical surface.

(Continued)

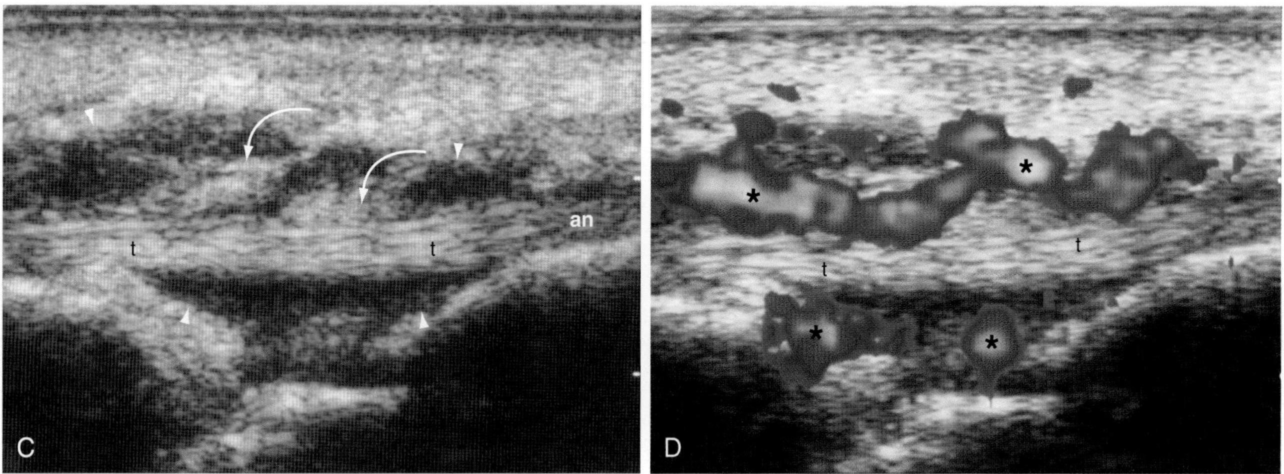

FIGURE 13-37—cont'd. **C, D,** Infectious tenosynovitis. **C,** Longitudinal image through the biceps tendon in a diabetic patient. The tendon itself *(t)* appears relatively normal, with relatively uniform thickness and preservation of the fibrillar echotexture. However, there is heterogeneous material surrounding the tendon, consisting predominantly of anechoic material *(arrowheads)* but also containing areas of increased echogenicity *(curved arrows)*. This is compatible with a complex tenosynovitis and could represent hemorrhage, pus, inflammatory material, or other proteinaceous or solid material within the tenosynovial sheath. Note the area of artifactually decreased echogenicity within the tendon due to anisotropy, as the tendon angles in relation to the transducer *(an)*. **D,** Power Doppler imaging applied in the same area as **C** shows considerable increased vascularity within the tenosynovial sheath *(asterisks)*, indicating either an infectious or a noninfectious inflammatory tenosynovitis. Aspiration confirmed the presence of an infectious tenosynovitis. Note that the tendon itself does not demonstrate increased vascularity on power Doppler imaging.

> Thickened hypermic synovium from overuse or inflammatory arthritis demonstrates hypervascularity within the distended tendon sheath on power Doppler imaging.

Marked hypoechoic thickening of the synovium with little or no fluid may be a sign of chronic tenosynovitis.[179] In stenosing tenosynovitis, the thickened tendon can be seen passing through thickened synovium at points of entrapment on dynamic ultrasound.[27] Ultrasound may be used to monitor effect of treatment on tenosynovitis by tracking change in the volume of fluid and thickened synovium and change in the degree of hypervascularity indicated by power Doppler signal.[179] Like paratenoninitis, tenosynovitis may or may not be associated with changes in the underlying tendon.

Dynamic ultrasound examination can be extremely useful in assessment of **tendon subluxation or dislocation** (Figure 13-38, *A, B*). For example, imaging the proximal humerus in external rotation can help to demonstrate instability of the long head of the biceps tendon at the bicipital groove[184]; imaging of the distal forearm in supination/pronation can help to demonstrate extensor

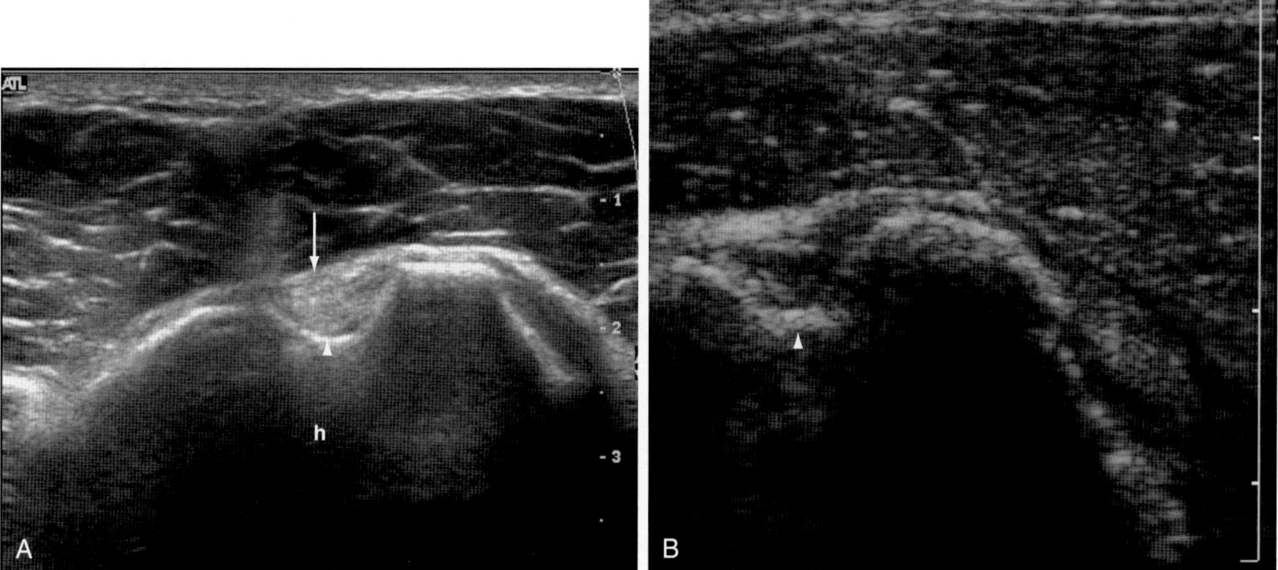

FIGURE 13-38. Tendon subluxation. **A,** Axial image through the humeral head *(h)* demonstrates the echogenic biceps tendon *(arrow)* seated in the intertubercular groove *(arrowhead)*. **B,** Axial image through similar level in another patient shows an empty intertubercular groove *(arrowhead)*. The biceps tendon has subluxed medially due to a tear in the subscapularis tendon.

carpi ulnaris instability along the distal ulnar sulcus; and imaging the ankle in plantar and dorsiflexion and eversion can help to demonstrate instability involving the peroneal tendons at the distal fibula.

The **musculotendinous junction** represents a common site of injury when excessive force is applied to a muscle. The injury can involve not only at the macroscopic musculotendinous junction, but also the microscopic musculotendinous junctions that ramify more extensively through the muscle. In grade I injuries, the muscle and musculotendinous junction may appear normal or there may be a small (< 5% total muscle volume) focus of fiber disruption, with hematoma and perifascial fluid.[185,186] Grade II injuries are partial tears that involve > 5% of muscle volume and demonstrate a hematoma that evolves over time.[185] The hematoma is initially echogenic but becomes relatively hypoechoic after 24 hours and subsequently develops echogenic granulation tissue along its periphery. Perifascial fluid is also present. Dynamic assessment helps to demonstrate the "bell clapper" sign, separation of the frayed ends of the muscle tear with either muscle contraction or transducer pressure. Grade III injuries show a complete tear of the muscle with hematoma and perifascial fluid.[185] The torn musculotendinous junction may appear rounded rather than pointed.[159,187] Dynamic imaging shows a "bell clapper" appearance across the entire width of the muscle with frayed edges and bunching of the muscle. Fluid and hemorrhage tracking along nearby nerves may be better resolved by ultrasound than by MRI.[185]

Based on observations at the Achilles' **tendon insertion** site onto the calcaneus, the normal tendon insertion site appears as a relatively well-defined hypoechoic zone in the distal tendon, triangular in shape when viewed in the longitudinal plane. The appearance is similar to that of cartilage. It is not known whether the hypoechogenicity of the tendon enthesis is related to the presence of cartilage or to anisotropy of curved fibers in the tendon attachment.[160] Insertional tendinopathy is seen as thickening of the tendon[188,189] and hyperechoic signal and shadowing due to calcification or ossification within the tendon (Figure 13-39).

Ultrasound imaging is readily performed in the setting of orthopedic hardware in the **postoperative tendon**[179] (Figure 13-40). Although metal causes considerable acoustic shadowing (it appears hyperechoic due to a strongly specular reflective surface and causes prominent ring-down artifact deep to the metal), it is usually possible to obtain an effective acoustic "window" even when metal is present.

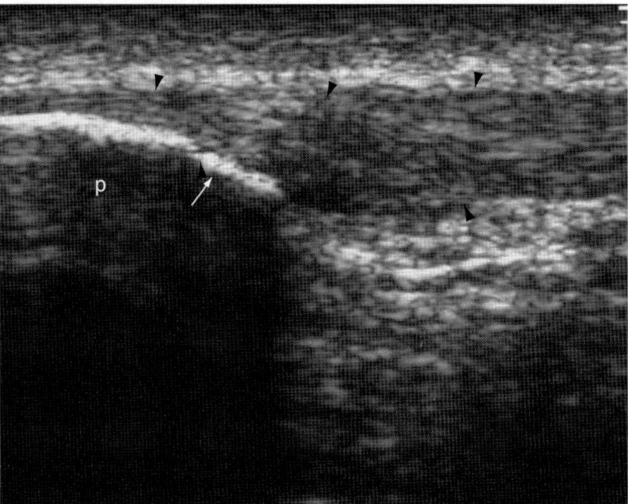

FIGURE 13-39. Insertional tendinopathy. Sagittal image through the proximal patellar tendon *(arrowheads)* shows heterogeneous signal in the tendon, adjacent to the inferior patellar *(p)* pole, with areas of hyperechogenicity and shadowing calcification *(arrow)*.

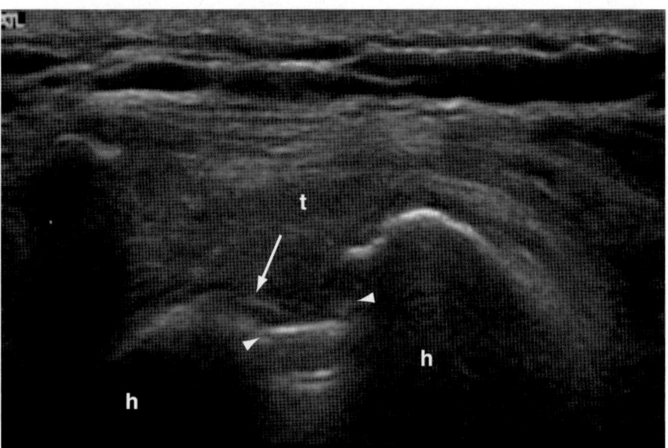

FIGURE 13-40. Postoperative tendon. Sagittal image through the humeral head *(h)* shows a supraspinatus tendon repair. The repaired tendon inserts into a trough *(arrowheads)* in the humeral head. A portion of a suture anchor is visible as a small echogenic structure *(arrow)*. The normal fibrillar echotexture of the supraspinatus tendon *(t)* is less pronounced due to postoperative changes.

> Ultrasound is an effective way of examining tendons adjacent to metallic hardware.

In fact, ultrasound can be used to assess tendon injury from nearby metallic hardware.[52,190] Even under normal circumstances, the postoperative tendon may not demonstrate a normal ultrasound appearance, which can make it difficult to detect tendinosis or residual or recurrent tear. The postoperative tendon often remains enlarged and heterogeneous, with blurred margins, for months or years.[179] Scarring may be present and may be difficult to distinguish from intact tendon. If hyperechoic foci are seen, they may be related to either calcification or suture material. Dynamic assessment of the tissues may be useful to assess for coordinated versus abnormal motion of the residual soft tissue and may help to detect occult tears. In the postoperative setting, increased Doppler activity may be related to normal hypervascularity associated with healing (rather than inflammatory change), but hypervascularity associated with healing should decrease over time.[52]

Calcific tendinitis, caused by deposition of calcium hydroxyapatite within the tendon, is well seen by ultrasound[52] (Figure 13-41, *A, B*). Ultrasound can detect calcium hydroxyapatite deposits when they are still radiographically occult.[161] Early and later phases of calcific tendinitis may be differentiated by ultrasound (Figure 13-41, *A, B*). The acute hydroxyapatite deposit appears as a globular echogenic mass, fluid-like and deformable, without acoustic shadowing and is amenable to aspiration. The chronic hydroxyapatite deposit appears as a more discrete mass with a highly echogenic superficial surface (specular reflector) and with prominent acoustic shadowing, at which point it is unlikely to be easily aspirated.[27,184] Chiou et al. observed increased Doppler signal associated with calcific tendinitis during the painful resorptive phase.[191]

> Calcific tendinitis can be demonstrated by ultrasound before it is seen on radiographs, and its appearance can indicate whether aspiration is possible.

Ultrasound can depict **soft tissue masses** associated with the tendon (Figure 13-42). As with MRI, ultrasound helps with

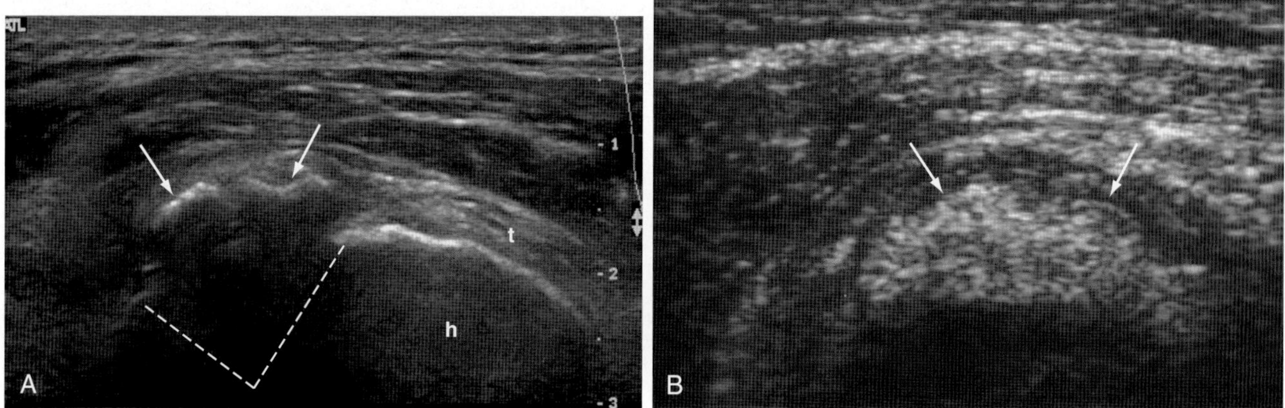

FIGURE 13-41. Calcific tendinitis. **A,** Sagittal image through the rotator cuff *(t)* shows a large focus of hydroxyapatite in the infraspinatus tendon *(arrows)*, consistent with calcific tendinitis. The superficial surface of the calcific deposit is highly echogenic and appears as a thin white curvilinear line. Because it is highly reflective to the ultrasound waves, the hydroxyapatite deposit causes severe shadowing, with areas of decreased echogenicity deep to the surface of the calcific deposit (bounded by *dashed lines*). The presence of shadowing is consistent with chronic or late-stage calcific tendinitis. **B,** Acute form of calcific tendinitis. The stage of calcific tendinitis can be distinguished based on the ultrasound appearance of the deposit. The acute form of hydroxyapatite is a more amorphous echogenic structure *(arrows)*. It contains more fluid and creates less shadowing than late-stage calcifications. *h,* Humeral head.

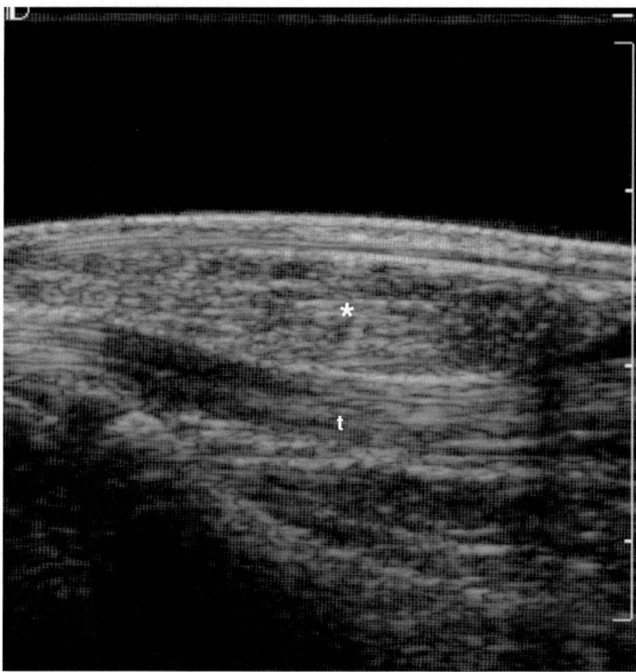

FIGURE 13-42. Ultrasound of soft tissue mass—lipoma. Ultrasound demonstrates this lipoma as an ovoid homogeneous, echogenic mass *(asterisk)*, displacing the underlying flexor tendon *(t)*. Lipomas vary in their echogenicity.

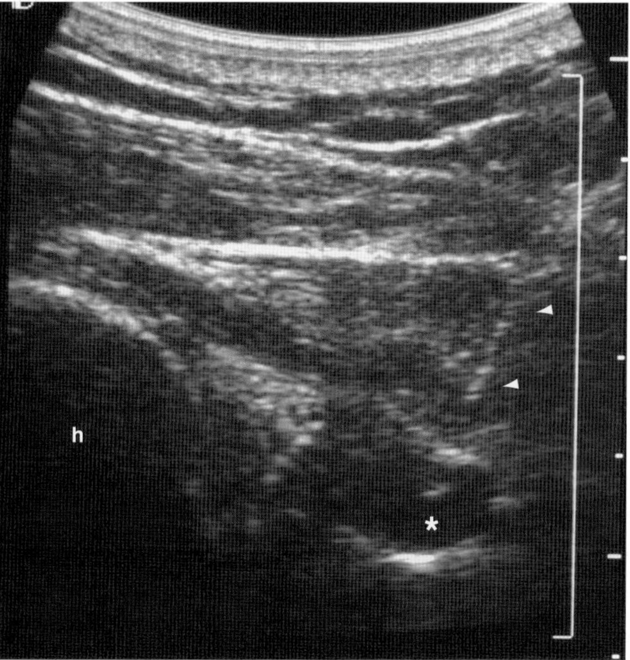

FIGURE 13-43. Ultrasound-guided aspiration of a paralabral cyst. A painful paralabral cyst in the shoulder *(asterisk)* was aspirated under ultrasound guidance and treated successfully with injection of corticosteroids. The needle is visible as an echogenic line *(arrowheads)*. *h,* Humeral head.

preoperative planning and, in some cases, may provide features supportive of a diagnosis, but it cannot definitively characterize a mass. The ultrasound appearance of giant cell tumors of the tendon sheath is nonspecific: a relatively well-circumscribed hypoechoic soft tissue mass abutting the surface of the tendon, with internal power Doppler signal.[179] Peritendinous ganglion cysts may be anechoic or somewhat echogenic, depending on their fluid content, and should have a thin echogenic rim and enhanced though-transmission, without evidence of intrasubstance perfusion on power Doppler imaging.[192] Soft tissue xanthomas, such as those that develop in familial hypercholesterolemia, appear as hypoechoic intratendinous masses and can be detected on ultrasound even before the tendon becomes clinically enlarged.[193]

Ultrasound permits real-time **guidance for interventional procedures**, such as aspiration or injection of bursae, tendon sheaths, peritendinous tissues, and symptomatic foci of calcific tendinitis (Figure 13-43). The needle and relevant anatomy, including arteries and veins, are well visualized on real-time images. Procedures are performed using a standard imaging transducer, fitted with a sterile cover, with or without an attachable needle guide. Although 21G needles are often used, larger-gauge needles can be used, when needed, to aspirate more viscous material or to perform core biopsy. Procedures involving the subacromial-subdeltoid,[145] olecranon, trochanteric, gluteal and iliopsoas,[145] prepatellar, and retrocalcaneal bursae, as well as the common extensor tendon,[145] adductor tendon,[145] posterior tibial[194] and peroneal tendons,[145] and the paratenon of the Achilles' tendon[145] have been described. Ultrasound guidance for aspiration and therapeutic injection of symptomatic calcific tendinitis has also been described.[145] Use of ultrasound guidance for steroid injection can be helpful in preventing direct injection into the tendon, a practice that has been associated with weakening and possible rupture of the tendon.[145,195] Instillation of local anesthetic or sterile fluid can be used to distend the tendon sheath and help further delineate the tendon borders. Instillation of fluid also produces an "arthrosonographic" effect that can highlight subtle tendon tears, although it is rarely used as a diagnostic technique.[196,197]

Normal **bursae** are often not visible on ultrasound examination.[179] When a small amount of physiologic fluid is present, the bursa will appear as a hypoechoic or anechoic cleft, with a thin hyperechoic rim.[159] Bursal shape varies from site to site. Bursal distension greater than 2 mm is considered abnormal.[198] However, the amount of physiologic fluid in bursae varies from site to site, and comparison with the contralateral side of the body may aid in detection of abnormal amounts of bursal fluid. Bursitis occurs most commonly in the subacromial-subdeltoid, olecranon, prepatellar, and retrocalcaneal bursae.

Simple fluid within the bursa should be anechoic and should demonstrate enhanced through-transmission (Figure 13-44, *A*). When hemorrhage or proteinaceous fluid is present, the bursal fluid will be echogenic. Synovial thickening varies in appearance from hyperechoic to near- anechoic within the bursa and may—but not always—demonstrate perfusion on power Doppler imaging[199] (Figure 13-44, *B*). The diagnosis of either acute or chronic bursitis is based on detection of a distended bursa seen in a characteristic location with increased vascularity (i.e., power Doppler signal) in the bursal wall.

> Bursitis is seen on ultrasound as a distended bursa with increased vascularity in the wall on power Doppler examination.

Bursal margins are often blurred, and the echogenic bursa may be difficult to distinguish from surrounding echogenic fat.[170] There may be evidence of synovial proliferation, fibrosis and adhesions, or loose bodies. Echogenic material may indicate the presence of hemorrhage, inflammation, or infection. In chronic bursitis, bursal fluid is generally complex, with echogenic debris, and calcification may be present.[179,200] Inflammatory bursitis can be followed for response to treatment based on the quantity of bursal fluid and thickness of the synovium[179,201] as well as the evolution of the activity seen on power Doppler imaging. The presence or absence of infection in the bursa cannot be determined by imaging. Ultrasound can be used to guide aspiration and/or injection into the bursa.

> Infection in a bursa (as in a joint) cannot be diagnosed by ultrasonography, and aspiration is necessary if this diagnosis is considered a possibility clinically.

CONCLUSIONS

Although history and physical examination play a central role in evaluating tendon dysfunction and bursal abnormalities, imaging examinations provide important supplementary information for the diagnosis and characterization of tendon and bursal pathology. MRI and, in experienced hands, ultrasound are the current modalities of choice for direct visualization of tendon and bursal pathology. Normal tendons and bursae and an extensive spectrum of tendon and bursal pathology can be depicted by both modalities. Depending on the specific tendon site, the two modalities have respective strengths and weaknesses and may play complementary roles. Accuracy for diagnosis of tendon and bursal pathology in experienced hands is often strikingly similar between the two modalities, despite the great difference in technologies. Ultrasound is particularly well suited for guiding interventions, compared with MRI. CT is not considered a primary modality for imaging of tendon and bursae but can be especially helpful in demonstrating calcification or ossification within a tendon or bursa or in demonstrating the relationship between tendon and surrounding bony

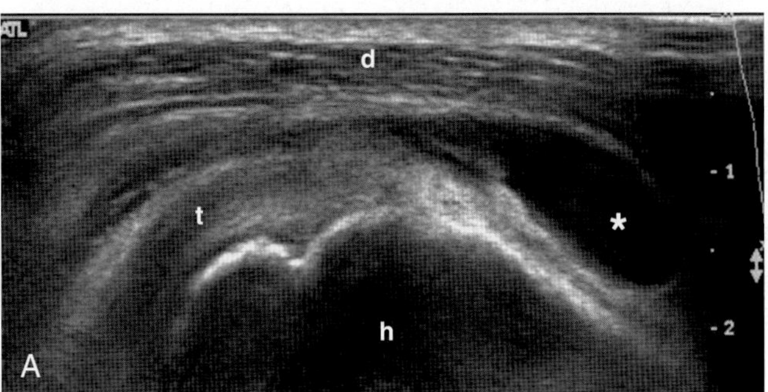

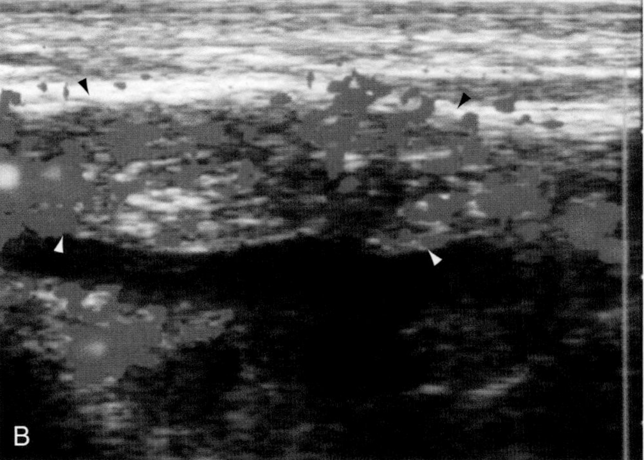

FIGURE 13-44. Bursitis. **A,** Axial image through the shoulder shows simple fluid in the subacromial-subdeltoid bursa *(asterisk)* consistent with bursitis (assuming no rotator cuff tear). Simple fluid is readily appreciated as homogeneously anechoic material within the bursa, without areas of wall thickening or internal echogenicity. Enhanced through-transmission—seen here as an area of increased echogenicity immediately deep to the bursal fluid—is an important corollary sign for simple fluid. *d,* Deltoid muscle; *h,* humerus; *t,* subscapularis tendon. **B,** Image through the region of the subdeltoid bursa, obtained with power Doppler imaging. In this case, the bursa is distended with heterogeneous echogenic material *(arrowheads)*, indicating complex fluid and/or synovial proliferation within the bursa. Power Doppler demonstrates increased vascularity within the bursa and in the surrounding soft tissues surrounding the bursa, consistent with either infectious or noninfectious inflammatory bursitis. Aspiration confirmed a diagnosis of septic subdeltoid bursitis.

structures. Radiographs serve as an important adjunct to these cross-sectional modalities, particularly in the case of MRI, where calcification and ossification can be easily overlooked.

ALGORITHM AND RECOMMENDATIONS

Radiographs are useful as a screening exam for suspected tendon or bursal pathology to identify associated findings such as calcification, ossification, spurs, erosions, and exostoses and to exclude other, confounding, sources of pathology. In general, MRI and ultrasound are the preferred techniques for direct visualization of tendon and bursal pathology. Ultrasound of tendons and bursae requires appropriate equipment and a high level of technical expertise. Power Doppler ultrasound technique can be especially helpful in delineating hyperemic changes and in differentiating thickened synovium from fluid or pus. Most tendon tears are detected by direct visualization under MRI or ultrasound. Routine fluoroscopic arthrography can be used to detect rotator cuff tears but is not as accurate in detecting or sizing some kinds of tears as direct visualization with MRI or ultrasound. MR arthrography, usually performed as a fluoroscopic procedure for contrast injection, followed by an MRI exam, is somewhat more sensitive for detection of tears, particularly partial tears, than MRI alone but does require a needle injection. When contraindications to MRI exist, CT arthrography may be performed instead. Ultrasound is the preferred technique for imaging guidance of interventional procedures related to the tendons and bursae. Tenography under fluoroscopic guidance may still be used for tendon-related aspirations or injections but represents a specialized skill. CT is generally not as effective for direct visualization of tendon or bursal pathology as MRI or ultrasound due to more limited intrinsic soft tissue image contrast, but CT can be of added value to show calcification or ossification in relation to the tendon or bursa and to detect tendon entrapment in the setting of fractures. Moreover, CT is a commonly performed study, such that tendon and bursal pathology is a common incidental finding. Newer 3D volume rendered CT techniques can depict tendons and their relation to bones and may help pre-operative planning (Table 13-2).

TABLE 13-2. Work-up of Suspected Tendon Abnormality

Tendon symptoms, without acute trauma	Screening radiograph, followed by MRI or ultrasound to assess for tendon degeneration or tear	Radiographs may show calcification, ossification, reactive osteolysis or sclerosis, erosions, periostitis, exostoses, retraction of ossicle, avulsion fracture, or other bony pathology
Suspected acute tendon tear or avulsion	Screening radiograph, followed by MRI or ultrasound	
Rotator cuff tendon tear	Screening radiograph, followed by MRI or ultrasound	Consider MR arthrography for highest MR accuracy, particularly in patients < 45 years
Suspected inflammatory tenosynovitis	Screening radiograph, followed by MRI or ultrasound	
Suspected septic tenosynovitis	Emergent situation; screening radiograph, followed by MRI or ultrasound	Conclusive diagnosis requires aspiration of infected material; ultrasound or tenography for image-guided aspiration
Paratenonitis	Screening radiograph, followed by MRI or ultrasound	
Tendon subluxation or dislocation	Screening radiograph, followed by ultrasound or MRI	Ultrasound facilitates dynamic assessment; MRI may fail to detect subluxation if tendon is not displaced at the time of imaging
Tendon entrapment by fracture fragments	CT	Multiplanar reformation may be helpful
Musculotendinous strain or tear	Screening radiograph, followed by MRI or ultrasound	May require large field of view
Insertional tendinopathy	Screening radiograph, followed by ultrasound or MRI; ultrasound may be more sensitive	
Postoperative tendon	Screening radiograph, followed by ultrasound or MRI; ultrasound preferred at site of joint replacement	Metal can cause artifacts on both MRI and ultrasound; preferred modality will depend on empiric factors
Calcific tendinitis	Screening radiograph, followed by ultrasound or MRI; calcium itself also well-demonstrated by CT	Calcification can be easily overlooked on MRI – correlative radiograph is necessary to prevent erroneous MRI diagnosis
Tendon masses	Screening radiograph, followed by MRI or ultrasound	IV contrast is usually used for MRI; power Doppler is helpful for ultrasound
Interventions	Ultrasound usually preferred – faster, more accessible	
Bursitis	Screening radiograph, followed by MRI or ultrasound	IV contrast (MRI) and power Doppler (u/s) help distinguish hyperemic synovium from fluid or pus
Septic bursitis	Screening radiograph, followed by ultrasound or MRI	Conclusive diagnosis requires aspiration of infected material; ultrasound preferred for image-guided aspiration
Adventitial bursa	Screening radiograph, followed by MRI or ultrasound	Radiograph important to assess for underlying bony irritant; IV contrast or power Doppler may be useful (see bursitis)

REFERENCES

1. Sharma P, Maffulli N: Tendon injury and tendinopathy: healing and repair, *J Bone Joint Surg Am* 87:187-202, 2005.
2. DeLee J, Drez D Jr, Miller MD (eds): *DeLee & Drez's orthopaedic sports medicine: principles and practice*, ed 2, vol 1, Philadelphia, 2003, Saunders.
3. Brodsky B, Ramshaw JA: The collagen triple-helix structure, *Matrix Biol* 15:545-554, 1997.
4. Coleman S, Rodeo SA: Tendons and ligaments around the knee: the biology of injury and repair. In Callaghan JJ, Rubah HE, Simonian PT et al (eds): *The adult knee*, Philadelphia, 2003, Lippicott, Williams and Wilkins, pp 213-224.
5. Rodeo SA, Arnoczky SP, Torzilli PA et al: Tendon-healing in a bone tunnel. A biomechanical and histological study in the dog, *J Bone Joint Surg Am* 75:1795-1803, 1993.
6. Butler DL, Grood ES, Noyes FR et al: Biomechanics of ligaments and tendons, *Exerc Sport Sci Rev* 6:125-181, 1978.
7. Towers JD, Russ EV, Golla SK: Biomechanics of tendons and tendon failure, *Semin Musculoskelet Radiol* 7:59-65, 2003.
8. Carr AJ, Norris SH: The blood supply of the calcaneal tendon, *J Bone Joint Surg Br* 71:100-101, 1989.
9. Vailas AC, Pedrini VA, Pedrini-Mille A et al: Patellar tendon matrix changes associated with aging and voluntary exercise, *J Appl Physiol* 58:1572-1576, 1985.
10. Kannus P, Paavola M, Jozsa L: Aging and degeneration of tendons. In Maffulli N, Renstrom P, Leadbetter W (eds): *Tendon injuries: basic science and clinical medicine*, London, 2005, Springer-Verlag, pp 25-31.
11. Bosco C, Komi PV: Influence of aging on the mechanical behavior of leg extensor muscles, *Eur J Appl Physiol Occup Physiol* 45:209-219, 1980.
12. Elliott DH: Structure and function of mammalian tendon, *Biol Rev Camb Philos Soc* 40:392-421, 1965.
13. Jozsa L, Kannus P: *Human tendons: anatomy, physiology and pathology*, Champaign, Ill, 1997, Human Kinetics.
14. Leadbetter WB: Cell-matrix response in tendon injury, *Clin Sports Med* 11:533-578, 1992.
15. Schweitzer ME, Karasick D: MR imaging of disorders of the Achilles tendon, *AJR Am J Roentgenol* 175:613-625, 2000.
16. Kader D, Maffulli N, Leadbetter WB et al: Achilles tendinopathy. In Maffulli N, Renstrom P, Leadbetter W (eds): *Tendon injuries: basic science and clinical medicine*, London, 2005, Springer-Verlag, pp 201-208.
17. Backman C, Boquist L, Friden J et al: Chronic Achilles paratenonitis with tendinosis: an experimental model in the rabbit, *J Orthop Res* 8:541-547, 1990.
18. Shadwick RE: Elastic energy storage in tendons: mechanical differences related to function and age, *J Appl Physiol* 68:1033-1040, 1990.
19. Maffulli N, Renstrom, P, Leadbetter W (eds): *Tendon injuries: basic science and clinical medicine*, London, 2005, Springer-Verlag.
20. Gartner J, Simons B: Analysis of calcific deposits in calcifying tendinitis, *Clin Orthop Relat Res* (254):111-120, 1990.
21. Uhthoff HK, Loehr JW: Calcific tendinopathy of the rotator cuff: pathogenesis, diagnosis, and management, *J Am Acad Orthop Surg* 5:183-191, 1997.
22. Chan R, Kim DH, Millett PJ et al: Calcifying tendinitis of the rotator cuff with cortical bone erosion, *Skeletal Radiol* 33:596-599, 2004.
23. McKendry RJ, Uhthoff HK, Sarkar K et al: Calcifying tendinitis of the shoulder: prognostic value of clinical, histologic, and radiologic features in 57 surgically treated cases, *J Rheumatol* 9:75-80, 1982.
24. Hollinshead W: *Anatomy for surgeons*, ed 3, Philadelphia, 1982, Harper and Row.
25. Saupe N, Pfirrmann CW, Schmid MR et al: Association between rotator cuff abnormalities and reduced acromiohumeral distance, *AJR Am J Roentgenol* 187:376-382, 2006.
26. Chien AJ JJ, Martel W: Radial styloid periosteal bone apposition as an indicator of de Quervain tenosynovitis, *RSNA 86th Scientific Assembly and Annual Meeting* 2000.
27. Hughes T: Imaging of tendon ailments. In Maffulli N, Renstrom P, Leadbetter W (eds): *Tendon injuries: basic science and clinical medicine*, London, 2005, Springer-Verlag, pp 49-60.
27a. Hashimoto N, Okada K: Synovial osteochondromatosis of the retrocalcaneal bursa. A case report, *J Bone Joint Surg Am* 78(11):1741-1745, 1996.
28. Rosenberg ZS, Feldman F, Singson RD et al: Ankle tendons: evaluation with CT, *Radiology* 166:221-226, 1988.
29. Rosenberg ZS, Cheung Y, Jahss MH: Computed tomography scan and magnetic resonance imaging of ankle tendons: an overview, *Foot Ankle* 8:297-307, 1988.
30. Pelc JS, Beaulieu CF: Volume rendering of tendon-bone relationships using unenhanced CT, *AJR Am J Roentgenol* 176:973-977, 2001.
31. Rosenberg ZS, Cheung Y, Jahss MH et al: Rupture of posterior tibial tendon: CT and MR imaging with surgical correlation, *Radiology* 169:229-235, 1988.
32. Rosenberg ZS, Jahss MH, Noto AM et al: Rupture of the posterior tibial tendon: CT and surgical findings, *Radiology* 167:489-493, 1988.
33. Rosenberg ZS, Feldman F, Singson RD et al: Peroneal tendon injury associated with calcaneal fractures: CT findings, *AJR Am J Roentgenol* 149:125-129, 1987.
34. Szczukowski M Jr, St Pierre RK, Fleming LL, et al: Computerized tomography in the evaluation of peroneal tendon dislocation. A report of two cases, *Am J Sports Med* 11:444-447, 1983.
35. Choplin RH, Buckwalter KA, Rydberg J et al: CT with 3D rendering of the tendons of the foot and ankle: technique, normal anatomy, and disease, *Radiographics* 24:343-356, 2004.
36. Pritchard RS, Shah HR, Nelson CL et al: MR and CT appearance of iliopsoas bursal distention secondary to diseased hips, *J Comput Assist Tomogr* 14:797-800, 1990.
37. Varma DG, Parihar A, Richli WR: CT appearance of the distended trochanteric bursa, *J Comput Assist Tomogr* 17:141-143, 1993.
38. Hall FM, Joffe N: CT imaging of the anserine bursa, *AJR Am J Roentgenol* 150:1107-1108, 1988.
39. Spence LD, Adams J, Gibbons D et al: Rice body formation in bicipito-radial bursitis: ultrasound, CT, and MRI findings, *Skeletal Radiol* 27:30-32, 1998.
40. Shackcloth MJ, Page RD: Scapular osteochondroma with reactive bursitis presenting as a chest wall tumour, *Eur J Cardiothorac Surg* 18:495-496, 2000.
41. Magee T, Williams D: 3.0-T MRI of the supraspinatus tendon, *AJR Am J Roentgenol* 187:881-886, 2006.
42. Kuo R, Panchal M, Tanenbaum L et al: 3.0 Tesla imaging of the musculoskeletal system, *J Magn Res Imaging* 25:245-261, 2007.
43. Schirmer C, Scheel AK, Althoff CE et al: Diagnostic quality and scoring of synovitis, tenosynovitis and erosions in low-field MRI of patients with rheumatoid arthritis: a comparison with conventional MRI, *Ann Rheum Dis* 66:522-529, 2007.
44. Ghazinoor S, Crues JV 3rd, Crowley C: Low-field musculoskeletal MRI, *J Magn Res Imaging* 25:234-244, 2007.
45. Tuite MJ, Asinger D, Orwin JF: Angled oblique sagittal MR imaging of rotator cuff tears: comparison with standard oblique sagittal images, *Skeletal Radiol* 30:262-269, 2001.
46. Tehranzadeh J, Ashikyan O, Anavim A et al: Enhanced MR imaging of tenosynovitis of hand and wrist in inflammatory arthritis, *Skeletal Radiol* 35:814-822, 2006.
47. Cimmino MA, Innocenti S, Livrone F et al: Dynamic gadolinium-enhanced magnetic resonance imaging of the wrist in patients with rheumatoid arthritis can discriminate active from inactive disease, *Arthritis Rheum* 48:1207-1213, 2003.
48. Furman-Haran E, Margalit R, Grobgeld D et al: Dynamic contrast-enhanced magnetic resonance imaging reveals stress-induced angiogenesis in MCF7 human breast tumors. *Proc Natl Acad Sci U S A* 93:6247-6251, 1996.
49. Palmer WE: Magnetic resonance arthrography of the shoulder. In Zlatkin MB (ed): *MRI of the shoulder*, ed 2, Philadelphia, 2003, Lippicott, Williams and Wilkins, pp 279-299.
50. Shellock FG: Functional assessment of the joints using kinematic magnetic resonance imaging, *Semin Musculoskelet Radiol* 7:249-276, 2003.
51. Koblik PD, Freeman DM: Short echo time magnetic resonance imaging of tendon, *Invest Radiol* 28:1095-1100, 1993.
52. Adler RS, Finzel KC: The complementary roles of MR imaging and ultrasound of tendons, *Radiol Clin North Am* 43:771-807, 2005.
53. Fullerton GD, Cameron IL, Ord VA: Orientation of tendons in the magnetic field and its effect on T2 relaxation times, *Radiology* 155:433-435, 1985.
54. Tsao LY, Mirowitz SA: MR imaging of the shoulder. Imaging techniques, diagnostic pitfalls, and normal variants, *Magn Res Imaging Clin North Am* 5:683-704, 1997.
55. Quinn SF, Sheley RC, Demlow T et al: Rotator cuff tendon tears: evaluation with fat-suppressed MR imaging with arthroscopic correlation in 100 patients, *Radiology* 195:497-500, 1995.
56. Reinus WR, Shady KL, Mirowitz SA et al: MR diagnosis of rotator cuff tears of the shoulder: value of using T2-weighted fat-saturated images, *AJR Am J Roentgenol* 164:1451-1455, 1995.
57. Singson RD, Hoang T, Dan S et al: MR evaluation of rotator cuff pathology using T2-weighted fast spin-echo technique with and without fat suppression, *AJR Am J Roentgenol* 166:1061-1065, 1996.
58. Jozsa L, Balint BJ, Reffy A et al: Hypoxic alterations of tenocytes in degenerative tendinopathy, *Arch Orthop Trauma Surg* 99:243-246, 1982.
59. Kannus P, Jozsa L: Histopathological changes preceding spontaneous rupture of a tendon. A controlled study of 891 patients, *J Bone Joint Surg Am* 73:1507-1525, 1991.
60. Sanders TG, Tirman PF, Feller JF et al: Association of intramuscular cysts of the rotator cuff with tears of the rotator cuff: magnetic resonance imaging findings and clinical significance, *Arthroscopy* 16:230-235, 2000.
61. Kassarjian A, Torriani M, Ouellette H et al: Intramuscular rotator cuff cysts: association with tendon tears on MRI and arthroscopy, *AJR Am J Roentgenol* 185:160-165, 2005.
62. Costa CR, Morrison WB, Carrino JA et al: MRI of an intratendinous ganglion cyst of the peroneus brevis tendon, *AJR Am J Roentgenol* 181:890-891, 2003.
63. Teefey SA, Rubin DA, Middleton WD et al: Detection and quantification of rotator cuff tears. Comparison of ultrasonographic, magnetic resonance imaging, and arthroscopic findings in seventy-one consecutive cases, *J Bone Joint Surg Am* 86:708-716, 2004.
64. Keene JS, Lash EG, Fisher DR et al: Magnetic resonance imaging of Achilles tendon ruptures, *Am J Sports Med* 17:333-337, 1989.
65. Marcus DS, Reicher MA, Kellerhouse LE: Achilles tendon injuries: the role of MR imaging, *J Comput Assist Tomogr* 13:480-486, 1989.
66. Fleckenstein JL, Watumull D, Conner KE et al: Denervated human skeletal muscle: MR imaging evaluation, *Radiology* 187:213-218, 1993.
67. Thomazeau H, Boukobza E, Morcet N et al: Prediction of rotator cuff repair results by magnetic resonance imaging, *Clin Orthop Relat Res* (344):275-283, 1997.
68. Gladstone JN, Bishop JY, Lo IK et al: Fatty infiltration and atrophy of the rotator cuff do not improve after rotator cuff repair and correlate with poor functional outcome, *Am J Sports Med* 35:719-728, 2007.
69. Morag Y, Jacobson JA, Miller B et al: MR imaging of rotator cuff injury: what the clinician needs to know, *Radiographics* 26:1045-1065, 2006.
70. Soila K, Karjalainen PT, Aronen HJ et al: High-resolution MR imaging of the asymptomatic Achilles tendon: new observations. AJR Am J Roentgenol 173(2):323-8,1999.
71. Stoller D, Ferkel, RD, Li AE, Mann, RA, Lindauer, KR: The ankle and foot. In Stoller D (ed): *Magnetic resonance imaging in orthopedics and sports medicine*, ed 3, Baltimore, 2007, Lippincott, Williams and Wilkins, pp 733-1050.

72. Rosenberg ZS, Beltran J, Bencardino JT: MR imaging of the ankle and foot, *Radiographics* 20:S153-S179, 2000.
73. Bencardino JT, Rosenberg ZS, Serrano LF: MR imaging of tendon abnormalities of the foot and ankle, *Magn Reson Imaging Clin North Am* 9:475-492, 2001.
74. Stoller D, Li AE, Lichtman DM et al: The wrist and hand. In Stoller D (ed): *Magnetic resonance imaging in orthopedics and sports medicine*, ed 3, Baltimore, 2007, Lippincott, Williams and Wilkins, pp 1627-1846.
75. Glajchen N, Schweitzer M: MRI features in de Quervain's tenosynovitis of the wrist, *Skeletal Radiol* 25:63-65, 1996.
76. Morrison WB, Ledermann HP, Schweitzer ME: MR imaging of inflammatory conditions of the ankle and foot, *Magn Reson Imaging Clin North Am* 9:615-637, 2001.
77. Berquist T: Infection. In Berquist T (ed): *Radiology of the foot and ankle*, ed 2, Philadelphia, 2000, Lippincott, Williams and Wilkins, pp 357-404.
78. Boutin RD, Brossmann J, Sartoris DJ et al: Update on imaging of orthopedic infections, *Orthop Clin North Am* 29:41-66, 1998.
79. Sugimoto K, Iwai M, Kawate K et al: Tenosynovial osteochondromatosis of the tarsal tunnel, *Skeletal Radiol* 32:99-102, 2003.
80. Klug JD, Moore SL: MR imaging of the biceps muscle-tendon complex, *Magn Reson Imaging Clin North Am* 5:755-765, 1997.
81. Egi T, Inui K, Koike T et al: Volar dislocation of the extensor carpi ulnaris tendon on magnetic resonance imaging is associated with extensor digitorum communis tendon rupture in rheumatoid wrists, *J Hand Surg Am* 31:1454-1460, 2006.
82. Shellock FG, Feske W, Frey C et al: Peroneal tendons: use of kinematic MR imaging of the ankle to determine subluxation, *J Magn Reson Imaging* 7:451-454, 1997.
83. Boutin RD, Fritz RC, Steinbach LS: Imaging of sports-related muscle injuries, *MRI Clin North Am* 11:341-371, 2003.
84. Bencardino JT, Rosenberg ZS, Brown RR et al: Traumatic musculotendinous injuries of the knee: diagnosis with MR imaging, *Radiographics* 20:S103-S120, 2000.
85. De Smet AA, Best TM: MR imaging of the distribution and location of acute hamstring injuries in athletes, *AJR Am J Roentgenol* 174:393-399, 2000.
86. Palmer WE, Kuong SJ, Elmadbouh HM: MR imaging of myotendinous strain, *AJR Am J Roentgenol* 173:703-709, 1999.
87. Fleckenstein JL, Weatherall PT, Parkey RW et al: Sports-related muscle injuries: evaluation with MR imaging, *Radiology* 172:793-798, 1989.
88. El-Khoury GY, Brandser EA, Kathol MH et al: Imaging of muscle injuries, *Skeletal Radiol* 25:3-11, 1996.
89. Hasselman CT, Best TM, Hughes CT et al: An explanation for various rectus femoris strain injuries using previously undescribed muscle architecture, *Am J Sports Med* 23:493-499, 1995.
90. Renstrom P, Hach T: Insertional tendinopathy in sports. In Maffulli N, Renstrom P, Leadbetter W (eds): *Tendon injuries: basic science and clinical medicine*, London, 2005, Springer-Verlag, pp 70-85.
91. Olivieri I, Barozzi L, Padula A et al: Clinical manifestations of seronegative spondylarthropathies, *Eur J Radiol* 27(Suppl 1):S3-S6, 1998.
92. Kamel M, Eid H, Mansour R: Ultrasound detection of knee patellar enthesitis: a comparison with magnetic resonance imaging, *Ann Rheum Dis* 63:213-214, 2004.
93. De Simone C, Di Gregorio F, Maggi F: Comparison between ultrasound and magnetic resonance imaging of achilles tendon enthesopathy in patients with psoriasis, *J Rheumatol* 31:1465, 2004.
94. Kamel M, Eid H, Mansour R: Ultrasound detection of heel enthesitis: a comparison with magnetic resonance imaging, *J Rheumatol* 30:774-778, 2003.
95. Karjalainen PT, Soila K, Aronen HJ et al: MR imaging of overuse injuries of the Achilles tendon, *AJR Am J Roentgenol* 175:251-260, 2000.
96. Zoga AC, Schweitzer ME: Imaging sports injuries of the foot and ankle, *Magn Reson Imaging Clin North Am* 11:295-310, 2003.
97. Fiamengo SA, Warren RF, Marshall JL et al: Posterior heel pain associated with a calcaneal step and Achilles tendon calcification, *Clin Orthop Relat Res* 167:203-211, 1982.
98. Astrom M, Gentz CF, Nilsson P et al: Imaging in chronic achilles tendinopathy: a comparison of ultrasonography, magnetic resonance imaging and surgical findings in 27 histologically verified cases, *Skeletal Radiol* 25:615-620, 1996.
99. Nicholson CW, Berlet GC, Lee TH: Prediction of the success of nonoperative treatment of insertional Achilles tendinosis based on MRI, *Foot Ankle Int* 28:472-477, 2007.
100. Myerson MS, McGarvey W: Disorders of the Achilles tendon insertion and Achilles tendinitis, *Instr Course Lect* 48:211-218, 1999.
101. Schepsis AA, Jones H, Haas AL: Achilles tendon disorders in athletes, *Am J Sports Med* 30:287-305, 2002.
102. Stephens MM: Haglund's deformity and retrocalcaneal bursitis, *Orthop Clin North Am* 25:41-46, 1994.
103. Bencardino J, Rosenberg ZS, Delfaut E: MR imaging in sports injuries of the foot and ankle, *Magn Reson Imaging Clin North Am* 7:131-149, 1999.
104. Wapner KL, Bordelon RL: Heel pain. In DeLee J, Drez D Jr, Miller MD (eds): *DeLee & Drez's orthopaedic sports medicine: principles and practice*, ed 2, vol 2, Philadelphia, 2003, Saunders, pp 2446-2473.
105. Canoso JJ, Liu N, Traill MR et al: Physiology of the retrocalcaneal bursa, *Ann Rheum Dis* 47:910-912, 1988.
106. Bottger BA, Schweitzer ME, El-Noueam KI et al: MR imaging of the normal and abnormal retrocalcaneal bursae, *AJR Am J Roentgenol* 170:1239-1241, 1998.
107. Pavlov H, Heneghan MA, Hersh A et al: The Haglund syndrome: initial and differential diagnosis, *Radiology* 144:83-88, 1982.
108. Owen RS, Iannotti JP, Kneeland JB et al: Shoulder after surgery: MR imaging with surgical validation, *Radiology* 186:443-447, 1993.
109. Feller J, Howey TD, Plaga BR: MR imaging of the postoperative shoulder. In Steinbach LS, Tirman PFJ, Feller, JF (ed): *Shoulder magnetic resonance imaging*, Philadelphia, 1998, Lippincott-Raven, pp 187-219.
110. Zanetti M, Jost B, Hodler J et al: MR imaging after rotator cuff repair: full-thickness defects and bursitis-like subacromial abnormalities in asymptomatic subjects, *Skeletal Radiol* 29:314-319, 2000.
111. Berquist T, Peterson JJ: Shoulder and arm. In Berquist T (ed): *MRI of the musculoskeletal system*, ed 5, Philadelphia, 2006, Lippincott, Williams and Wilkins, pp 557-656.
112. Spielmann AL, Forster BB, Kokan P et al: Shoulder after rotator cuff repair: MR imaging findings in asymptomatic individuals—initial experience, *Radiology* 213:705-708, 1999.
113. Gusmer PB, Potter HG, Donovan WD et al: MR imaging of the shoulder after rotator cuff repair, *AJR Am J Roentgenol* 168:559-563, 1997.
114. Calvert PT, Packer NP, Stoker DJ et al: Arthrography of the shoulder after operative repair of the torn rotator cuff, *J Bone Joint Surg Br* 68:147-150, 1986.
115. Wu J, Covey A, Katz LD: MRI of the postoperative shoulder, *Clin Sports Med* 25:445-464, 2006.
116. Magee TH, Gaenslen ES, Seitz R et al: MR imaging of the shoulder after surgery, *AJR Am J Roentgenol* 168:925-928, 1997.
117. Mohana-Borges AV, Chung CB, Resnick D: MR imaging and MR arthrography of the postoperative shoulder: spectrum of normal and abnormal findings, *Radiographics* 24:69-85, 2004.
118. Duc SR, Mengiardi B, Pfirrmann CW et al: Diagnostic performance of MR arthrography after rotator cuff repair, *AJR Am J Roentgenol* 186:237-241, 2006.
119. Kader D, Mosconi M, Benazzo F et al: Achilles tendon rupture. In Maffulli N, Renstrom P, Leadbetter W (eds): *Tendon injuries: basic science and clinical medicine*, London, 2005, Springer-Verlag, pp 187-200.
120. Dillon E, Pope CF, Barber V et al: Achilles tendon healing: 12 month follow-up with MR imaging, *Radiology* 177(P):306, 1990. [Abstract.]
121. Panageas E, Greenberg S, Franklin PD et al: Magnetic resonance imaging of pathologic conditions of the Achilles tendon, *Orthop Rev* 19:975-980, 1990.
122. Karjalainen PT, Aronen HJ, Pihlajamaki HK et al: Magnetic resonance imaging during healing of surgically repaired Achilles tendon ruptures, *Am J Sports Med* 25:164-171, 1997.
123. Bergin D, Morrison WB: Postoperative imaging of the ankle and foot, *Radiol Clin North Am* 44:391-406, 2006.
124. Liem MD, Zegel HG, Balduini FC et al: Repair of Achilles tendon ruptures with a polylactic acid implant: assessment with MR imaging, *AJR Am J Roentgenol* 156:769-773, 1991.
125. Flemming DJ, Murphey MD, Shekitka KM et al: Osseous involvement in calcific tendinitis: a retrospective review of 50 cases, *AJR Am J Roentgenol* 181:965-972, 2003.
126. Maldjian C, Rosenberg ZS: MR imaging features of tumors of the ankle and foot, *Magn Reson Imaging Clin North Am* 9:639-657, 2001.
127. Dussault RG, Kaplan PA, Roederer G: MR imaging of Achilles tendon in patients with familial hyperlipidemia: comparison with plain films, physical examination, and patients with traumatic tendon lesions, *AJR Am J Roentgenol* 164:403-407, 1995.
128. Genant JW, Vandevenne JE, Bergman AG et al: Interventional musculoskeletal procedures performed by using MR imaging guidance with a vertically open MR unit: assessment of techniques and applicability, *Radiology* 223:127-136, 2002.
129. Lewin JS, Petersilge CA, Hatem SF et al: Interactive MR imaging-guided biopsy and aspiration with a modified clinical C-arm system, *AJR Am J Roentgenol* 170:1593-1601, 1998.
130. Carrino JA, Blanco R: Magnetic resonance—guided musculoskeletal interventional radiology, *Semin Musculoskelet Radiol* 10:159-174, 2006.
131. White EA, Schweitzer ME, Haims AH: Range of normal and abnormal subacromial/subdeltoid bursa fluid, *J Comput Assist Tomogr* 30:316-320, 2006.
132. Donahue F, Turkel D, Mnaymneh W et al: Hemorrhagic prepatellar bursitis, *Skeletal Radiol* 25:298-301, 1996.
133. Floemer F, Morrison WB, Bongartz G et al: MRI characteristics of olecranon bursitis, *AJR Am J Roentgenol* 183:29-34, 2004.
134. Doyle AJ, Miller MV, French JG: Lipoma arborescens in the bicipital bursa of the elbow: MRI findings in two cases, *Skeletal Radiol* 31:656-660, 2002.
135. Griffiths HJ, Thompson RC Jr, Galloway HR et al: Bursitis in association with solitary osteochondromas presenting as mass lesions, *Skeletal Radiol* 20:513-516, 1991.
136. Foisneau-Lottin A, Martinet N, Henrot P et al: Bursitis, adventitious bursa, localized soft-tissue inflammation, and bone marrow edema in tibial stumps: the contribution of magnetic resonance imaging to the diagnosis and management of mechanical stress complications, *Arch Phys Med Rehabil* 84:770-777, 2003.
137. Aburano T, Yokoyama K, Taki J et al: Tc-99m MDP bone imaging in inflammatory enthesopathy, *Clin Nucl Med* 15:105-106, 1990.
138. Yon JW Jr, Spicer KM, Gordon L: Synovial visualization during Tc-99m MDP bone scanning in septic arthritis of the knee, *Clin Nucl Med* 8:249-251, 1983.
139. Nuutila P, Kalliokoski K: Use of positron emission tomography in the assessment of skeletal muscle and tendon metabolism and perfusion, *Scand J Med Sci Sports* 10:346-350, 2000.
140. Palmer WE, Rosenthal DI, Schoenberg OI et al: Quantification of inflammation in the wrist with gadolinium-enhanced MR imaging and PET with 2-[F-18]-fluoro-2-deoxy-D-glucose, *Radiology* 196:647-655, 1995.
141. Goerres GW, Forster A, Uebelhart D et al: F-18 FDG whole-body PET for the assessment of disease activity in patients with rheumatoid arthritis, *Clin Nucl Med* 31:386-390, 2006.

142. Mink JH, Harris E, Rappaport M: Rotator cuff tears: evaluation using double-contrast shoulder arthrography, *Radiology* 157:621-623, 1985.
143. Goldman AB, Ghelman B: The double-contrast shoulder arthrogram. A review of 158 studies, *Radiology* 127:655-663, 1978.
144. Levey D, Berry M, Sartoris, DJ: Technical aspects: flouroscopy and contrast arthrography. In Sartoris D (ed): *Principles of shoulder imaging,* New York, 1995, McGraw-Hill, pp 13-31.
145. McNally E: Musculoskeletal interventional ultrasound. In McNally EG (ed): *Practical musculoskeletal ultrasound,* Philadelphia, 2005, Elsevier, pp 283-308.
146. Wilson AJ, Totty WG, Murphy WA et al: Shoulder joint: arthrographic CT and long-term follow-up, with surgical correlation, *Radiology* 173:329-333, 1989.
147. Charousset C, Bellaiche L, Duranthon LD et al: Accuracy of CT arthrography in the assessment of tears of the rotator cuff, *J Bone Joint Surg Br* 87:824-828, 2005.
148. Greenspan A: *Orthopedic radiology: a practical approach, ed 2, Philadelphia, 1996, Lippincott-Raven.*
149. Schreibman KL: Ankle tenography: what, how, and why, *Semin Roentgenol* 39:95-113, 2004.
150. Palmer DG: Tendon sheaths and bursae involved by rheumatoid disease at the foot and ankle, *Australas Radiol* 14:419-428, 1970.
151. Resnick D, Goergen TG: Peroneal tenography in previous calcaneal fractures, *Radiology* 115:211-213, 1975.
152. Teng MM, Destouet JM, Gilula LA et al: Ankle tenography: a key to unexplained symptomatology. Part I: Normal tenographic anatomy, *Radiology* 151:575-580, 1984.
153. Gilula LA, Oloff L, Caputi R et al: Ankle tenography: a key to unexplained symptomatology. Part II: Diagnosis of chronic tendon disabilities, *Radiology* 151:581-587, 1984.
154. Baker KS, Gilula LA: The current role of tenography and bursography, *AJR Am J Roentgenol* 154:129-133, 1990.
155. Harper MC, Schaberg JE, Allen WC: Primary iliopsoas bursography in the diagnosis of disorders of the hip, *Clin Orthop Relat Res* 221:238-241, 1987.
156. Jaffee NW, Gilula LA, Wissman RD et al: Diagnostic and therapeutic ankle tenography: outcomes and complications, *AJR Am J Roentgenol* 176:365-371, 2001.
157. Tehranzadeh J, Mossop EP, Golshan-Momeni M: Therapeutic arthrography and bursography, *Orthop Clin North Am* 37:393-408, 2006.
158. Allenmark C: Partial Achilles tendon tears, *Clin Sports Med* 11:759-769, 1992.
159. Bianchi S, Martinoli C, Abdelwahab IF: Ultrasound of tendon tears. Part 1: general considerations and upper extremity, *Skeletal Radiol* 34:500-512, 2005.
160. van Holsbeeck M, Introcaso JH: *Musculoskeletal ultrasound,* St Louis, 2001, Mosby.
161. McNally E: Ultrasound of the rotator cuff. In McNally EG (ed): *Practical musculoskeletal ultrasound,* Philadelphia, 2005, Elsevier, pp 43-58.
162. Read JW: Musculoskeletal ultrasound: basic principles, *Semin Musculoskelet Radiol* 2:203-210, 1998.
163. Martinoli C, Derchi LE, Pastorino C et al: Analysis of echotexture of tendons with US, *Radiology* 186:839-843, 1993.
164. Sell S, Schulz R, Balentsiefen M et al: Lesions of the Achilles tendon. A sonographic, biomechanical and histological study, *Arch Orthop Trauma Surg* 115:28-32, 1996.
165. Weinberg EP, Adams MJ, Hollenberg GM: Color Doppler sonography of patellar tendinosis, *AJR Am J Roentgenol* 171:743-744, 1998.
166. Richards PJ, Dheer AK, McCall IM: Achilles tendon (TA) size and power Doppler ultrasound (PD) changes compared to MRI: a preliminary observational study, *Clin Radiol* 56:843-850, 2001.
167. Zanetti M, Metzdorf A, Kundert HP et al: Achilles tendons: clinical relevance of neovascularization diagnosed with power Doppler US, *Radiology* 227:556-560, 2003.
168. Astrom M, Westlin N: Blood flow in chronic Achilles tendinopathy, *Clin Orthop Relat Res* 308:166-172, 1994.
169. Khan KM, Forster BB, Robinson J et al: Are ultrasound and magnetic resonance imaging of value in assessment of Achilles tendon disorders? A two year prospective study, *Br J Sports Med* 37:149-153, 2003.
170. McNally E: Ultrasound of the foot and ankle. In McNally EG (ed): *Practical musculoskeletal ultrasound,* Philadelphia, 2005, Elsevier, pp 167-190.
171. Hollister MS, Mack LA, Patten RM et al: Association of sonographically detected subacromial/subdeltoid bursal effusion and intraarticular fluid with rotator cuff tear, *AJR Am J Roentgenol* 165:605-608, 1995.
172. Crass JR, Craig EV, Feinberg SB: Clinical significance of sonographic findings in the abnormal but intact rotator cuff: a preliminary report, *J Clin Ultrasound* 16:625-634, 1988.
173. van Holsbeeck MT, Kolowich PA, Eyler WR et al: US depiction of partial-thickness tear of the rotator cuff, *Radiology* 197:443-446, 1995.
174. Teefey SA, Hasan SA, Middleton WD et al: Ultrasonography of the rotator cuff. A comparison of ultrasonographic and arthroscopic findings in one hundred consecutive cases, *J Bone Joint Surg Am* 82:498-504, 2000.
175. Bryant L, Shnier R, Bryant C et al: A comparison of clinical estimation, ultrasonography, magnetic resonance imaging, and arthroscopy in determining the size of rotator cuff tears, *J Shoulder Elbow Surg* 11:219-224, 2002.
176. Kluger R, Mayrhofer R, Kroner A et al: Sonographic versus magnetic resonance arthrographic evaluation of full-thickness rotator cuff tears in millimeters, *J Shoulder Elbow Surg* 12:110-1116, 2003.
177. Strobel K, Hodler J, Meyer DC et al: Fatty atrophy of supraspinatus and infraspinatus muscles: accuracy of US, *Radiology* 237:584-589, 2005.
178. Falchook FS, Zlatkin MB, Erbacher GE et al: Rupture of the distal biceps tendon: evaluation with MR imaging, *Radiology* 190:659-663, 1994.
179. Fornage BD: The case for ultrasound of muscles and tendons, *Semin Musculoskelet Radiol* 4:375-391, 2000.
180. Breidahl WH, Stafford Johnson DB, Newman JS et al: Power Doppler sonography in tenosynovitis: significance of the peritendinous hypoechoic rim, *J Ultrasound Med* 17:103-107, 1998.
181. Fornage BD, Rifkin MD, Touche DH et al: Sonography of the patellar tendon: preliminary observations, *AJR Am J Roentgenol* 143:179-182, 1984.
182. Jeffrey RB Jr, Laing FC, Schechter WP et al: Acute suppurative tenosynovitis of the hand: diagnosis with US, *Radiology* 162:741-742, 1987.
183. Newman JS, Adler RS, Bude RO et al: Detection of soft-tissue hyperemia: value of power Doppler sonography, *AJR Am J Roentgenol* 163:385-389, 1994.
184. Farin PU, Jaroma H: Acute traumatic tears of the rotator cuff: value of sonography, *Radiology* 197:269-273, 1995.
185. Robinson P: Ultrasound of muscle injury. In McNally EG (ed): *Practical musculoskeletal ultrasound,* Philadelphia, 2005, Elsevier, pp 223-244.
186. Takebayashi S, Takasawa H, Banzai Y et al: Sonographic findings in muscle strain injury: clinical and MR imaging correlation, *J Ultrasound Med* 14:899-905, 1995.
187. Bianchi S, Martinoli C, Abdelwahab IF et al: Sonographic evaluation of tears of the gastrocnemius medial head ("tennis leg"), *J Ultrasound Med* 17:157-162, 1998.
188. Merkel KH, Hess H, Kunz M: Insertion tendopathy in athletes. A light microscopic, histochemical and electron microscopic examination, *Pathol Res Pract* 173:303-309, 1982.
189. Genc H, Cakit BD, Tuncbilek I et al: Ultrasonographic evaluation of tendons and enthesal sites in rheumatoid arthritis: comparison with ankylosing spondylitis and healthy subjects, *Clin Rheumatol* 24:272-277, 2005.
190. Westhoff B, Wild A, Werner A et al: The value of ultrasound after shoulder arthroplasty, *Skeletal Radiol* 31:695-701, 2002.
191. Chiou HJ, Chou YH, Wu JJ et al: Evaluation of calcific tendonitis of the rotator cuff: role of color Doppler ultrasonography, *J Ultrasound Med* 21:289-295; quiz 96–97, 2002.
192. Cardinal E, Buckwalter KA, Braunstein EM et al: Occult dorsal carpal ganglion: comparison of US and MR imaging, *Radiology* 193:259-262, 1994.
193. McNally E: *Practical musculoskeletal ultrasound,* Philadelphia, 2005, Elsevier.
194. Brophy DP, Cunnane G, Fitzgerald O et al: Technical report: ultrasound guidance for injection of soft tissue lesions around the heel in chronic inflammatory arthritis, *Clin Radiol* 50:120-122, 1995.
195. Unverferth LJ, Olix ML: The effect of local steroid injections on tendon, *J Sports Med* 1:31-37, 1973.
196. Adler RS, Sofka CM: Percutaneous ultrasound-guided injections in the musculoskeletal system, *Ultrasound Q* 19:3-12, 2003.
197. Zingas C, Failla JM, Van Holsbeeck M: Injection accuracy and clinical relief of de Quervain's tendinitis, *J Hand Surg Am* 23:89-96, 1998.
198. Fornage BD: *Musculoskeletal ultrasound,* New York, 1995, Churchill Livingstone.
199. Newman JS, Laing TJ, McCarthy CJ et al: Power Doppler sonography of synovitis: assessment of therapeutic response—preliminary observations, *Radiology* 198: 582-584, 1996.
200. Friedman L, Chhem, RK: Ultrasound of knee pathology. In McNally EG (ed): *Practical musculoskeletal ultrasound,* Philadelphia, 2005, Elsevier, pp 143-166.
201. van Holsbeeck M, van Holsbeeck K, Gevers G et al: Staging and follow-up of rheumatoid arthritis of the knee. Comparison of sonography, thermography, and clinical assessment, *J Ultrasound Med* 7:561-566, 1988.

CHAPTER 14

Entrapment Syndromes

MARY G. HOCHMAN, MD*

KEY FACTS

- Peripheral nerves are vulnerable to compression at sites of fibrous and fibroosseous tunnels.
- Early diagnosis is important because early nerve injuries may be reversible, whereas late injuries are not.
- Nerve compression can be caused by many different factors: (1) space occupying lesions (e.g., ganglion cysts, soft tissue tumors, bony spurs, bursitis, hematoma, callus, mass effect from inflammation of surrounding structures); (2) edema and tenosynovitis caused by overuse or inflammatory arthritis or edema and thickening of connective tissue caused by hormonal changes; (3) edema and fibrosis caused by mechanical friction about the nerve; and (4) dynamic compression of the nerve caused by normal or near-normal anatomic structures during certain movements.
- Initial diagnosis is based on presenting symptoms and physical exam. Electrodiagnostic testing helps to confirm the diagnosis and localize the site of injury. In difficult cases, imaging can help to define the site and etiology of nerve compression or to establish an alternative cause for the symptoms.
- Radiographs are the first step in the workup of nerve compression. They are useful for demonstrating osseous causes of nerve compression but are of limited utility in demonstrating the nerve and surrounding soft tissues. Specialized radiographic views and computed tomography scans can help to delineate bony anatomy of the carpal, cubital, and tarsal tunnels.
- Magnetic resonance imaging (MRI) and, in experienced hands, ultrasound are used to visualize nerves and surrounding soft tissue structures directly. On T1-weighted MR images, the normal nerve (seen in cross-section) is a smooth, rounded, or oval low signal structure, surrounded by bright T1 fat. In the median and sciatic nerves, individual fascicles are visible on MR images. When seen on ultrasound, normal nerves demonstrate a fascicular pattern of internal echoes. Both MRI and ultrasound can also be used to assess for post-denervation muscle edema and atrophy. As with electromyography, the distribution of muscle changes on MRI and ultrasound can be used to determine the site of nerve injury.

Peripheral nerves are vulnerable to compression at sites of fibrous and fibroosseous tunnels. Depending on the nature of the insult and the types of fibers that constitute the nerve at that site, nerve injury may result in sensory and/or motor symptoms. Early diagnosis of nerve compression is important because early nerve injuries may be reversible, whereas late injuries are not. Initial treatment may consist of conservative therapy, but early surgical intervention (release) may also be indicated in order to help prevent permanent nerve injury.

Initial diagnosis of nerve injury is based on presenting symptoms and physical exam. Electrodiagnostic testing is used to confirm the diagnosis and help localize the site of injury. Definitive diagnosis based on the clinical and neurophysiologic exam may be difficult when findings are nonspecific or inconsistent, when multiple nerves or multiple sites of compression are involved, or when another condition mimics the symptoms of nerve compression or coexists with the nerve compression. In these cases, imaging can play a role in helping to define the site and the etiology of nerve compression or in helping to identify an alternative etiology for the symptoms. Radiographs and computed tomography (CT) scan can help to identify bony lesions that can cause nerve impingement. Magnetic resonance imaging (MRI) and ultrasound provide direct visualization of the nerve and any surrounding abnormalities.

This chapter reviews compression neuropathies of the upper and lower extremities (Box 14-1) and describes the role of imaging modalities in their diagnostic evaluation.

NERVES AND NERVE INJURY

A peripheral nerve is composed of many nerve fibers bound together (Figure 14-1). Depending on its function, the peripheral nerve contains varying combinations of motor, sensory, and autonomic fibers. Motor (efferent) fibers deliver impulses from the central nervous system (CNS) to skeletal muscles for voluntary activity. Sensory (afferent) fibers transmit impulses from skin receptors to the CNS. Autonomic fibers (efferent) control certain smooth muscle, glandular, and trophic functions.

The nerve may be injured by direct trauma (crush or transection), traction, mechanical or functional compression, or repetitive local friction. When nerve conduction is interrupted, nerve function is impaired. When motor nerves are affected, weakness, paralysis, and muscle atrophy can occur. When sensory nerves are affected, subjective sensations of pain and paresthesia (e.g., numbness, tingling, crawling sensation) and objective findings of analgesia and anesthesia can occur. When autonomic nerves (to the skin) are affected, dryness, cyanosis, hair loss, brittle nails, ulceration, and slow wound healing can develop. Injury to a nerve may take the form of neurapraxia, axonotmesis, or neurotmesis.[1] Although early nerve compression results in neurapraxic injury, severe or chronic compression can progress to axonotmesis or neurotmesis. Different grades of injury can coexist in the same nerve. Neurapraxia, the least severe category

*The author wishes to thank Dr. Elizabeth Raynor, Dr. Robert Kane, Dr. Stephen Farraher, Clotell Forde, and Ronald Kukla for their assistance in preparation of this chapter and to thank Steven Moskowitz for his assistance in preparation of the diagrams presented here.

BOX 14-1. Nerve Compression Syndromes in the Upper and Lower Extremities

SHOULDER
Suprascapular notch (suprascapular nerve and its supraspinatus and infraspinatus nerve branches)
Quadrilateral space (axillary nerve)

ELBOW/FOREARM
Radial tunnel (radial nerve, PION)
Cubital tunnel (ulnar nerve)
Pronator teres syndrome (median nerve)
Kiloh-Nevin's syndrome (AION)

WRIST
Carpal tunnel (median nerve)
Ulnar tunnel or Guyon's canal (ulnar nerve)

PELVIS/HIP
Piriformis syndrome (sciatic nerve)

KNEE
Tibial nerve compression in popliteal fossa (tibial nerve)
Peroneal or fibular tunnel (common peroneal nerve and its superficial, deep, and recurrent nerve branches)

ANKLE
Tarsal tunnel syndrome (posterior tibial nerve and its medial and lateral plantar nerve branches)
Sinus tarsi syndrome (terminal branch of the deep peroneal nerve)

FOOT
Morton's neuroma at metatarsal heads (plantar digital nerve)

of injury, involves focal damage to the myelin sheath, without axonal disruption. The mildest form of neurapraxia results from transient ischemia rather than actual loss of myelin; an example is the symptoms that develop from crossing one's legs. Uncomplicated neurapraxia usually resolves spontaneously and relatively quickly (sometimes hours to days and usually within 3 months) as the myelin regenerates. Axonotmesis, a more severe level of injury, results when the axon is interrupted, but the Schwann cell basal lamina and endoneurium remain intact. When focal axonal disruption occurs, the axon distal to the site of injury also degenerates after several days (Wallerian degeneration). Because the supporting structure surrounding the axon is not destroyed, the axon can regenerate along intact pathways, at a rate of approximately 1 mm/day. Prognosis for recovery from axonotmesis is good, but recovery can take weeks to months, depending on the rate of regeneration and the distance between the site of injury and the target organ. Neurotmesis is the most severe level of injury, characterized by complete axonal disruption and discontinuity of some or all of the surrounding connective tissue. Neurotmesis may occur due to mechanical disruption or due to severe scarring. Wallerian degeneration of the distal axon occurs, but because the lattice surrounding the axon is also disrupted, regeneration cannot occur. This severe degree of injury requires surgical repair and nerve reconstruction in order for function to be restored.

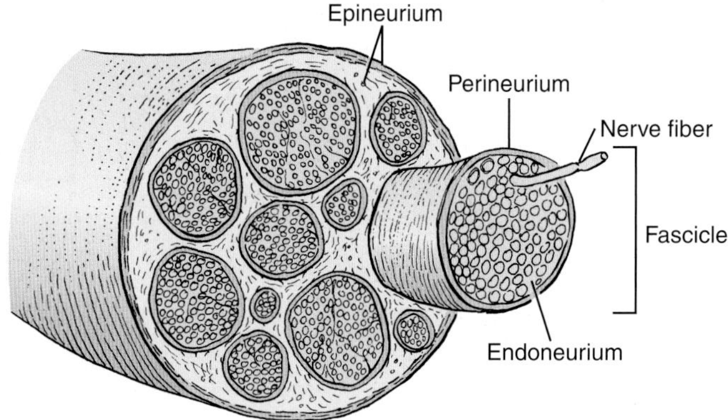

FIGURE 14-1. The peripheral nerve. Each nerve cell consists of a cell body; multiple dendrites, which receive impulses from adjacent cells; and a single long axon. The nerve axon conducts nerve impulses to several terminal buttons. The axon is enveloped by a myelin sheath formed by the cell membrane of the Schwann cell. A specialized connective tissue called the *endoneurium* surrounds the axon and Schwann cell, creating an endoneural tube. Multiple nerve fibers with their surrounding endoneurium are packed together into a nerve fascicle, which is enveloped by a thin sheath of perineurium. Multiple fascicles and their surrounding interfascicular epineurium, in turn, are packed together into a nerve trunk, which is surrounded by an external epineurium. The epineurium of the nerve trunk is surrounded by loose areolar tissue, the mesoneurium, which supplies a framework for the blood vessels that penetrate the nerve and facilitates motion of the nerve without undue traction on the blood supply. (Modified with permission from Hochman MG, Zilberfarb MG: Nerves in a pinch: imaging of nerve compression syndromes, *Radiol Clin North Am Arthritis Imaging* 42:221-245, 2004.)

COMPRESSION-ENTRAPMENT NEUROPATHY

Compression neuropathy refers to nerve damage resulting from pressure on a nerve. Some authors distinguish entrapment neuropathy as a subset of compression neuropathy involving pressure on a nerve from an anatomic or pathoanatomic structure (e.g., flexor retinaculum in carpal tunnel syndrome).[2] Almost any peripheral nerve in the body can be compressed, but nerve compression tends to occur at certain sites where the area around the nerve is more constrained, most often within known fibrous or fibroosseous tunnels. Compression injury can be acute, chronic, or intermittent.

> Damage to a nerve from pressure is termed *compression neuropathy*; entrapment neuropathy is a subset of this, caused by pressure due to anatomic structures or anatomic variations.

There are numerous causes of compression entrapment neuropathies; the relative incidence varies with location. A nerve may be predisposed to compression due to congenital narrowing of its osseous tunnel or abnormal thickening of its soft tissue roof. Fractures or joint instability can cause abnormalities of bony alignment that can narrow the fibroosseous canal and can result in nerve compression. Compression neuropathies can be caused by space-occupying lesions, such as ganglion cysts, soft tissue tumors, bony spurs, bursitis, hematoma, or callus, impinging on the nerve. Inflammation of structures surrounding the nerve can also produce mass effect. Edema and tenosynovitis due to overuse or inflammatory arthritis or edema and thickening of connective tissue caused by hormonal changes can result in nerve compression. Mechanical friction about the nerve can lead to local edema and fibrosis and can contribute to nerve compression as well. Dynamic compression of the nerve can occur when normal anatomic structures—fibrous, muscular, or tendinous bands overlying the nerve—result in compression during certain motions. This dynamic compression can occur in the setting of only minimal anatomic variation and can be especially problematic when associated with chronic repetitive activities. When two sites of compression occur in tandem along a single nerve, "double crush" syndrome may occur.[3] The presence of the proximal lesion lowers the threshold for development of symptoms from the distal lesion. The classic example of double crush syndrome is nerve impingement in the cervical spine predisposing to development of carpal tunnel syndrome. A similar phenomenon is seen in patients with an underlying polyneuropathy and can be seen in a number of systemic diseases such as diabetes mellitus, rheumatoid arthritis, hyperthyroidism, alcoholism, malnutrition, renal failure, and hematologic disorders.

> The presence of proximal compression on a nerve or of a polyneuropathy, such as that due to diabetes mellitus, lowers the threshold for a more distal second compressive lesion to become manifest.

The effect of compression on the nerve is mediated by ischemia and edema.[4] Compression of the vasa nervorum can result in ischemia, disruption of the blood-nerve barrier, and venous congestion. This, in turn, leads to epineurial and endoneurial edema and increased pressure within the endoneurium. In early stages, symptoms may be intermittent, with interval recovery of intraneural circulation and resolution of intraneural edema. As the disease progresses, prolonged edema of the epineurium may result in fibrosis, further constricting the nerve. Long-standing compression causes damage to the myelin sheath and ultimately results in axonal interruption and distal degeneration, with permanent loss of nerve function and atrophy of the denervated muscles.[5]

Signs and symptoms of compression neuropathy can be nonspecific.[6] Patients may present with paresthesias and sharp burning pain in the distribution of the affected nerve; the symptoms are often worse with motion and worse at night. There may be muscle weakness, with or without associated cutaneous sensory loss. Compression of motor nerves can cause deep, diffuse, poorly localized pain. In advanced cases, muscle atrophy will be seen. Trophic changes due to autonomic nerve dysfunction may be present. The pattern of sensory and muscle involvement reflects the site of nerve compression. However, it may difficult to distinguish between two different sites of compression if their respective fields overlap.

Treatment of nerve compression depends on location, etiology, chronicity, and extent of existing damage. Initial treatment is generally conservative. When conservative measures fail, however, early surgical decompression is indicated in order to minimize permanent nerve injury.[2,6] Conservative measures include eliminating aggravating activities, immobilization, heat, antiinflammatory medications, orthotics, and physical therapy. In some instances, local injection of corticosteroids can help alleviate symptoms and thereby also help confirm the diagnosis. Surgical treatment may include decompression of the nerve as well as nerve transposition, tenosynovectomy, arthrodesis, or osteotomy. Thorough decompression at every site of compression is a major goal and is important to prevent postsurgical recurrence of symptoms.

ELECTRODIAGNOSTIC EXAMINATION

Electrodiagnostic examination can help to confirm a diagnosis of peripheral nerve compression, localize a lesion, determine its pathophysiology, and grade its severity. The electrodiagnostic examination consists of nerve conduction studies, which can be performed on both motor and sensory nerves, and electromyography (EMG).[1] Nerve conduction studies (NCS) can be performed using surface electrodes; EMG is performed using needle electrodes placed within the muscle being tested. NCS measures the velocity of nerve impulse conduction. Findings at EMG are dependent on the presence of axonal injury. Muscles studied at EMG examination are chosen specifically to localize the site of nerve injury.[1]

Electrodiagnostic studies play an important role in the evaluation of nerve compression. Early nerve compression affects myelin and is associated with slowing of nerve conduction; compression injury can progress to involve axonal destruction, which results in correlative EMG changes. However, sensitivity and specificity of electrodiagnostic exam can be limited.[6] Normal conduction time does not exclude the presence of compression. NCS can appear normal if slowing is mild or if a few fast-conducting fibers remain intact. Conduction can be slowed not only due to nerve compression, but also due to segmental demyelination from other forms of neuropathy. The sensitivity and specificity of the exam depends on the specific location and the clinical setting. It is not uncommon for results of NCS/EMG studies to be abnormal but not clearly localizing. Imaging studies can supplement electrodiagnostic exams by helping to localize and characterize a lesion at the site of suspected nerve compression or by demonstrating changes in the muscles innervated by that nerve.

OSTEOARTICULAR IMAGING FEATURES OF NERVES AND NERVE COMPRESSION

Radiographs and CT

Radiographs are an important first step in the workup of nerve compression. Radiographs best demonstrate osseous causes of nerve compression such as fracture, dislocation, callus, osteophyte, and exostosis. When necessary, specialized views have been developed to demonstrate the bony contour of certain fibroosseous tunnels. These targeted views are often now supplanted or supplemented by CT scans, which can better delineate bony contours and their relationship to nerve structures. Although CT has been used in the past for direct imaging of nerves, intrinsic soft tissue contrast on CT images is limited. Currently, MRI and, to a more limited extent, ultrasound are the methods of choice for direct imaging of nerves.

Magnetic Resonance Imaging

MR images have a high intrinsic soft tissue contrast that provides for direct depiction of normal and abnormal nerves, helps identify and characterize structures surrounding the nerve that might cause compression, and can also demonstrate post-denervation changes in muscles supplied by the affected nerve.[7-9] The precise technique for imaging nerve entrapment depends on the specific site involved. In general, techniques are based on routine imaging protocols. For imaging about the shoulder, knee, ankle, or foot, standard shoulder and extremity coils can be employed. For imaging about the wrist, elbow, forearm, or forefoot, paired surface coils or a small flexible coil can be used. In order to image small structures, high-resolution techniques, based on relatively small fields of view and high image matrices, are optimal. Images obtained in the axial plane are important for identifying the nerve and detecting extrinsic compression. T1-weighted conventional spin echo or fast spin echo sequences depict the anatomy of the nerve and surrounding structures. Proton density weighted images are similar to T1-weighted images in that respect. T2-weighted conventional spin echo or fast spin echo images help to demonstrate edema within the nerve and to characterize surrounding masses. In order to detect subtle amounts of edema within the nerve or the surrounding soft tissues, fat-saturated T2-weighted images (of which short tau inversion recovery [STIR] images are one form) are employed. Intravenous gadolinium contrast may be used to determine whether a mass is cystic or solid and to help delineate vascular anatomy. Gadolinium is used commonly for many types of MRI examinations and is generally well tolerated, even in individuals with renal failure. (It should be noted that recent experience in a small group of patients primarily using a particular formulation of gadolinium contrast agent had introduced the possibility of development of nephrogenic systemic fibrosis as a potential complication of contrast administration in patients with diminished renal function. Additional data on this issue are currently being gathered.[10])

On T1-weighted images, fat is of high signal intensity and appears bright; muscles are lower in signal intensity and appear relatively dark. A normal nerve seen in cross-section on T1-weighted images is a smooth, round, or ovoid structure that is isointense to muscle and surrounded by high T1 signal perineural fat.[11-14] On T2-weighted images, fluid is of high signal intensity or bright, and muscles appear relatively dark. Fat signal varies depending on technique and is generally higher in signal than muscle but not as bright as fluid. On T2-weighted images, the normal nerve is isointense or slightly hyperintense to muscle. In larger nerves, such as the sciatic and median nerves, the nerve in cross section demonstrates a fascicular pattern, with punctuate high signal intensity foci surrounded by lower signal intensity on both T1-weighted and T2-weighted images.[15,16] Normal fascicles are uniform in size and shape. When the nerve is damaged, endoneural free water increases and the nerve becomes considerably hyperintense to muscle on T2-weighted images.[16-18] The nerve may become enlarged, and nerve fascicles may become distorted. *MR neurography* refers to high-resolution MR sequences specifically tailored for depiction of the nerves.[19-21]

On MRI, normal nerves are smooth, round or oval in cross section, and of intermediate signal intensity. Larger nerves may show separate bundles (fascicles). Damaged nerves typically are larger and higher in signal on T2-weighted images.

Signal from arterial and venous flow proximal and distal to the nerve segment of interest are suppressed using saturation bands. The significance of gadolinium enhancement of the nerve is controversial.[22] Although some investigators associate nerve enhancement with nerve inflammation,[23,24] others have reported poor correlation between enhancement and nerve pathology.[25]

MRI can also be useful in assessing changes in muscles innervated by a compressed nerve. Muscle edema is an early postdenervation change that is seen as high signal intensity on T2-weighted and fat-saturated images.[26,27] Eventually, muscle atrophy and fatty infiltration develop, producing a muscle that is smaller than normal in size with areas of high intramuscular signal on T1-weighted images.[26] As with EMG, the distribution of muscle denervation can help to localize the level of nerve injury.[28]

MRI depicts the fibroosseous canal surrounding a nerve. The bony canal may appear diminished in size. The fibrous portion may be thickened. Spurs and osteophytes can be seen on MRI but may be quite difficult to appreciate. Additional imaging with radiographs or CT can be helpful if subtle bony spurring or soft tissue calcification is suspected. MRI is particularly effective at depicting soft tissues structures surrounding or compressing a nerve. As a result, the site and etiology of nerve compression can often be conclusively established. A ganglion cyst appears as rounded, well-circumscribed, multilobulated structure adjacent to the joint, which is isointense to high signal (bright) on T1-weighted images and high signal on T2-weighted images. The ganglion cyst does not enhance internally, although a thin enhancing rim is usually visible.[29] Lipomas are high signal intensity (bright) on T1-weighted images.[29] A neurofibroma is typically seen as a cylindric mass that is not encapsulated. It often demonstrates a characteristic target appearance on T2-weighted images, with central low signal and peripheral high signal, and enhances centrally. A schwannoma is low to intermediate signal on T1-weighted images and markedly hyperintense on T2-weighted images. It may be heterogeneous on T2-weighted images and can show hemorrhagic or necrotic foci on contrast-enhanced images. It may also have a target-like appearance, similar to neurofibromas. In many schwannomas, the nerve can be identified on one side of the mass.[29] Imaging features are not reliable for distinguishing between benign and malignant nerve sheath tumors. Heterogeneity and infiltrating margins are suggestive of malignancy but not specific for it.[29]

Ultrasonography

Although MRI is considered the modality of choice for imaging peripheral nerves, ultrasound, in the hands of an experienced practitioner, can provide a useful alternative.[30,31] The quality of ultrasound images depends heavily on the skill of the individual performing the ultrasound. It requires a relatively high level of expertise for successful nerve imaging. Ultrasound has the advantage of being noninvasive and low cost. It also facilitates imaging of the nerve over long segments and permits both static and dynamic assessment of the nerve. In the upper extremity, the radial nerve within the upper arm, the anterior osseous nerve within the forearm, the median nerve within the carpal tunnel, and the ulnar nerve within the cubital tunnel and within Guyon's canal can be examined.[32-34] In the lower extremity, the common peroneal nerve at the fibular neck, the posterior tibial and plantar nerves within the tarsal tunnel, and the interdigital nerves within the intermetatarsal spaces can be examined.[32,33,35] Experience with ultrasound of the median nerve for evaluation of carpal tunnel syndrome is growing. Experience with ultrasound imaging of other peripheral nerves is more limited, but clinical utility of the technique is well documented.

Successful nerve imaging with ultrasound depends on optimized technique.[32,33,36] Linear array transducers are preferred over sector transducers because of their wider near-field view. Sophisticated near-field focusing can eliminate the need for a stand-off pad. Recommendations regarding transducer frequency vary somewhat. In general, higher frequencies help to provide high spatial resolution and are desirable for identifying small structures and subtle differences in internal echotexture. However, lower frequencies are preferred when increased penetration is required in order to visualize deeper structures (e.g., the sciatic nerve). At our institution, we employ a compact linear array 7- to 15-MHz broadband transducer. The appearance of the nerve can be expected to vary with the resolution of the images, with the characteristic fascicular pattern becoming more apparent on higher-resolution images.[37] Use of the lowest gain setting helps minimize spurious echogenicity. *Echogenicity* refers to the intensity of echoes generated by a structure imaged using ultrasound. Highly echogenic structures appear bright on ultrasound images; hypoechoic structures contain somewhat lower levels of echoes and are less bright; anechoic structures are devoid of internal echoes and appear uniformly dark. The nerve is examined systematically in both longitudinal and transverse planes to help distinguish it from other linear echogenic structures such as tendons and aponeuroses. The transducer must be maintained perpendicular to the structures of interest to avoid artifactual decrease in echogenicity related to anisotropy, a phenomenon observed in both nerves and tendons. Real-time examination during active or passive flexion and extension helps to distinguish the nerve from surrounding tendons and muscles, because the nerve remains relatively immobile.[38] Comparison to the contralateral side helps to highlight abnormal size, echogenicity, and course of the nerve. Color Doppler imaging and power Doppler imaging, two techniques for demonstrating the presence of blood flow, can be helpful in identifying vascular landmarks and in assessing the vascularity of surrounding structures. The use of ultrasound to guide carpal tunnel release and also guide aspiration of cysts in the suprascapular notch and periacetabular region has been reported.[39,40]

Certain nerves and portions of nerves can be imaged directly with ultrasound. Nerve size and shape, echotexture, and course can be demonstrated. Normal peripheral nerves are seen as markedly echogenic linear structures with multiple hypoechoic parallel but discontinuous linear areas separated by hyperechoic bands, surrounded by an echogenic envelope, when viewed on longitudinal scans.[32,33,36,37] They are seen as oval to round structures with punctuate internal echoes, in a honeycomb-like pattern, when viewed on transverse scans. The hypoechoic foci seen interspersed between hyperechoic bands at higher frequencies correspond to neural fascicles.[37] The normal range of values for the cross-sectional area of a nerve differs from nerve to nerve and also depends on the specific site along the length of the nerve. Inflammation of the nerve appears as either diffuse or segmental thickening, with decreased internal echogenicity and loss of the usual parallel linear echotexture.

Ultrasound examination can be used to assess causes of nerve entrapment. Tendons have an appearance similar to the nerves but are somewhat more echogenic, with a fibrillar echotexture.[38] The normal tendon sheath appears as a very thin hypoechoic line around the tendon. In tenosynovitis, the tendon is surrounded by fluid, which may be anechoic or may contain internal echoes. A ganglion cyst appears as a round or oval anechoic lesion with thin regular margins and is often multilobulated.[38] When inflamed, the ganglion cyst may demonstrate thicker walls, less well-defined margins, and internal echoes. A small anechoic "duct" may be seen extending between the ganglion cyst and a nearby joint. Anomalous muscles have ultrasound characteristics typical of all muscles. Scar tissue is typically seen as an area of increased echogenicity, reflecting the presence of fibrosis. Schwannomas and neurofibromas generally appear as hypoechoic masses with increased vascularity on color Doppler.[36,38] Schwannomas tend to be round or oval, well defined, and eccentric to the nerve axis, with internal cystic areas and enhanced through-transmission. Neurofibromas tend to be lobulated and elongated along the nerve axis. The junction between the hypoechoic tumor and the normal echogenic nerve proximal and/or distal to it may be visible. However, the benign or malignant etiology of the tumor cannot be accurately determined by ultrasound.[32] A traumatic neuroma appears as a focal rounded hypoechoic or hyperechoic mass, which may be encapsulated by a fibrous sheath or adhesed to surrounding structures.[36,38,41] When there is edema in muscles surrounding a nerve, it may be seen as diffuse enlargement of the muscle, with preservation of internal architecture. Decreased internal echogenicity may or may not be appreciated. When subtle, these abnormalities may be highlighted by comparison to the contralateral limb. The use of ultrasound to demonstrate post-denervation changes in muscle has been described.[34,42] Affected muscle may demonstrate decreased bulk and increased reflectivity (due to fatty replacement). Tendon rupture, a possible alternative etiology for muscle atrophy, can be excluded by ultrasound.

SPECIFIC SYNDROMES

Suprascapular Nerve Syndrome

Suprascapular nerve syndrome occurs due to compression of the suprascapular nerve either proximally within the suprascapular notch (incisura scapulae) or more distally within the spinoglenoid notch[6,43] (Figure 14-2). The suprascapular nerve (C5, 6) is a mixed motor and sensory nerve arising directly from the brachial plexus. The nerve passes deep to the trapezius muscle, parallel to the omohyoid muscle and then courses anteroposteriorly through the suprascapular notch. On the posterior side of the scapula, the nerve runs underneath the supraspinatus muscle, dividing into the supraspinatus nerve, which supplies motor branches to the supraspinatus muscle and sensory branches to the acromioclavicular and glenohumeral joints and the infraspinatus nerve. The infraspinatus nerve continues through the spinoglenoid notch into the infraspinatus fossa, where it supplies motor branches to the infraspinatus muscle and sensory fibers to the shoulder joint and scapula. The suprascapular notch is bridged by the superior transverse scapular ligament. In about 50% of people, the spinoglenoid notch is bridged by the spinoglenoid ligament.[6,43] Compression of the nerve within the suprascapular notch will affect both the supraspinatus and infraspinatus muscles; compression in the spinoglenoid notch will affect only the infraspinatus muscle. The suprascapular

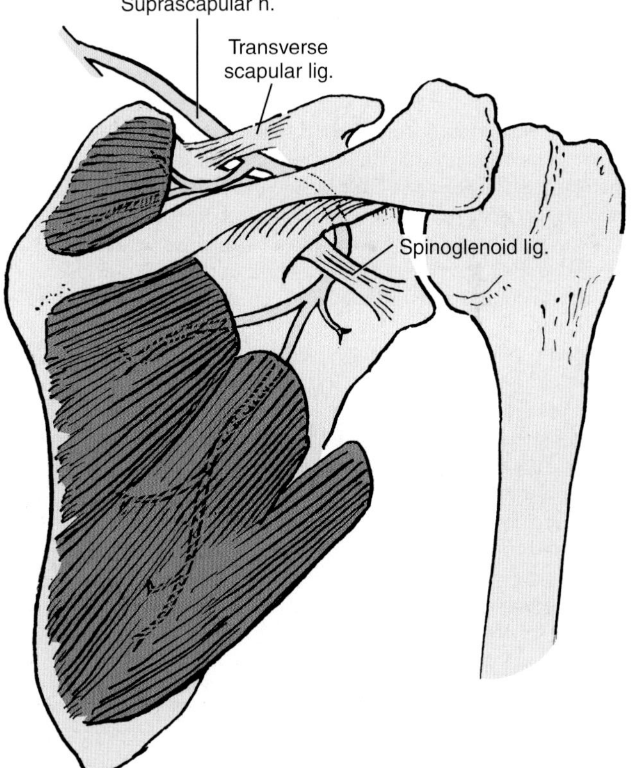

FIGURE 14-2. The suprascapular nerve, posterior view. The suprascapular nerve passes from anterior to posterior through the suprascapular notch, deep to the transverse scapular ligament, then branches into the supraspinatus and infraspinatus nerves. The infraspinatus nerve continues through the spinoglenoid notch, where it is bridged by the spinoglenoid ligament in approximately 50% of individuals. (Modified with permission from Hochman MG, Zilberfarb MG: Nerves in a pinch: imaging of nerve compression syndromes, *Radiol Clin North Am Arthritis Imaging* 42:221-245, 2004.)

artery and vein travel outside the fibroosseous tunnel, passing over the superior transverse ligament.

> Compression of the suprascapular nerve at the suprascapular notch leads to atrophy of both the supraspinatus and infraspinatus muscles, whereas compression at the spinoglenoid notch leads only to infraspinatus atrophy.

Suprascapular nerve syndrome can result from compression by ganglion cysts, lipomas and tumors, anomalous or varicose veins, or traction injuries and secondary inflammation and fibrosis.[6,43] Severe forward flexion of the shoulder, especially when the scapula is fixed, can tether the nerve in the suprascapular notch; this has been described as a mechanism of injury in pitchers. Stretching of the nerve can occur in activities with repetitive overhead motions involving the scapula, such as painting, tennis, volleyball, weightlifting, and gymnastics. Traction injuries of the nerve can occur acutely due to trauma and may also occur during rotator cuff surgery. Some individuals have a developmentally small or narrowed notch that predisposes them to entrapment. Patients with suprascapular nerve syndrome present with shoulder pain, which can mimic rotator cuff symptoms. After time, they may develop weakness and atrophy of the supraspinatus and/or infraspinatus muscles, which then limits their abduction and external rotation.

The suprascapular nerve is well visualized on routine shoulder MR images.[43] The suprascapular notch is best seen on oblique coronal images oriented along the scapula. The spinoglenoid notch is best seen on axial images. The overlying ligaments are not typically visible. The area around the nerve should be carefully assessed for a mass. Lipomas (high signal or bright on T1-weighted images) and fibrosis (low signal or dark on T2-weighted images) can be relatively subtle. If a paralabral cyst or ganglion cyst is present, it will appear as well-circumscribed, rounded, or lobulated high T2 signal mass. These cysts often arise secondary to a glenoid labral tear, although the tear itself may or may not be apparent[44] (Figure 14-3). However, not all cysts will cause nerve compression. Veins in the region of the notch appear as tubular high T2 structures with a characteristic branching pattern. Prominent veins in the region of the notch are not uncommon, but anomalous and varicose veins have been implicated in nerve compression.[45] Post-denervation edema and muscle atrophy may be seen. Muscle atrophy is often easiest to identify on oblique sagittal images. Post-denervation changes should be differentiated from other causes of shoulder girdle muscle atrophy including tendon tears and Parsonage-Turner syndrome.[46,47]

The use of ultrasound to identify ganglion cysts within the suprascapular notch has been described.[34,39] Perilabral cysts can be treated temporarily via imaging-guided percutaneous aspiration and injection of corticosteroids. However, in the setting of a labral tear, a cyst will tend to reaccumulate unless the labral tear itself is repaired.[39]

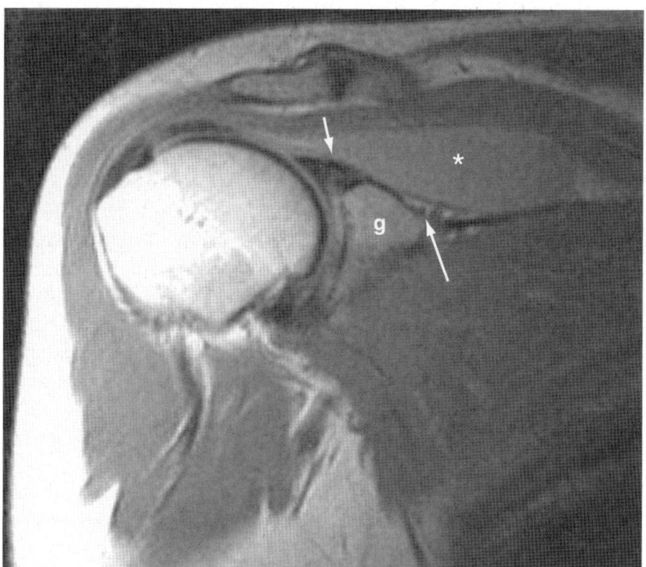

FIGURE 14-3. Paralabral cyst compressing the suprascapular nerve. Coronal proton density weighted (PD-weighted) image of the shoulder demonstrates a large paralabral cyst *(asterisk)* compressing the suprascapular nerve *(long arrow)* as it passes through the suprascapular notch. Linear high signal at the base of the superior labrum *(short arrow)* represents a portion of the labral tear that gave rise to the cyst. *g,* Glenoid. (Reprinted with permission from Hochman MG, Zilberfarb MG: Nerves in a pinch: imaging of nerve compression syndromes, *Radiol Clin North Am Arthritis Imaging* 42:221-245, 2004.)

Quadrilateral Space Syndrome (Axillary Nerve)

Quadrilateral space syndrome (also known as *lateral axillary hiatus syndrome*) occurs due to compression of the axillary nerve or one of its branches within the quadrilateral space.[48] The quadrilateral space is demarcated by the long head of the triceps brachii muscle medially, the teres minor muscle superiorly, the teres major muscle inferiorly, and the proximal humerus laterally. The axillary nerve (C5, 6) originates from the brachial plexus, passes anterior to the subscapularis muscle, and then runs dorsally, together with the posterior humeral circumflex artery, through the quadrilateral space, continuing around the posterior aspect of the humeral surgical neck.[49] The axillary nerve innervates the teres minor and deltoid muscles and the posterolateral cutaneous region of the shoulder and upper arm. The original description of the quadrilateral space syndrome referred to dynamic compression of the nerve due to extreme abduction.[48] The nerve may also be stretched or contused by trauma, including recurrent glenohumeral dislocation, or be damaged or compressed by fractures of the proximal humerus or scapula, hematomas, axillary masses including paralabral cysts, hypertrophy of the teres minor muscle, or fibrous bands. Patients with quadrilateral space syndrome present with shoulder pain and paresthesia and may describe symptoms resembling intermittent claudication. When there is chronic injury to the nerve, it results in atrophy of the teres minor and, less commonly, the deltoid muscles. Symptoms of quadrilateral space syndrome may be mistaken for rotator cuff disease, cervical spine disease, or thoracic outlet syndrome.

MRI is the method of choice for imaging the axillary nerve and for detection of any surrounding soft tissue masses[50] (Figure 14-4). The quadrilateral space is best demonstrated on oblique coronal views. The nerve and vessels are well demonstrated on routine oblique coronal, oblique sagittal, and axial images of the shoulder. Under normal circumstances, the nerve shows no kinking or focal enlargement, the surrounding fat is intact, and no mass is present. In the subacute or chronic setting, edema and atrophy of the teres minor and, more rarely, the deltoid muscle, may be seen.[51,52] Fatty atrophy of the teres minor is best identified on the oblique sagittal images.

> Quadrilateral space syndrome causes selective atrophy of the teres minor muscle and sometimes the deltoid muscle on MRI.

Radiography or CT can depict callus or bone tumors that may compress the axillary nerve. On conventional angiography and MR angiography, the diagnosis of dynamic compression of the nerve is supported by demonstration of a normal, patent posterior

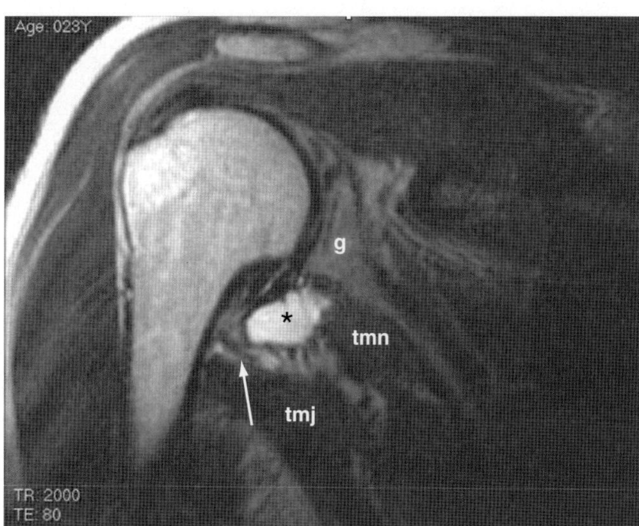

FIGURE 14-4. Paralabral cyst compressing the axillary nerve. Coronal T2-weighted image through the posterior aspect of the shoulder shows a cyst *(asterisk)* arising from a tear in the inferior glenoid labrum, compressing the axillary nerve *(long arrow)* as it passes through the quadrilateral space. The axillary nerve and posterior circumflex humeral vessels are displaced by the cyst. Only short segments of the nerve are visible on the image, seen as short linear structures at the inferior periphery of the cyst. *g,* Glenoid; *tmj,* teres major muscle; *tmn,* teres minor muscle. (Reprinted with permission from Hochman MG, Zilberfarb MG: Nerves in a pinch: imaging of nerve compression syndromes, *Radiol Clin North Am Arthritis Imaging* 42:221-245, 2004.)

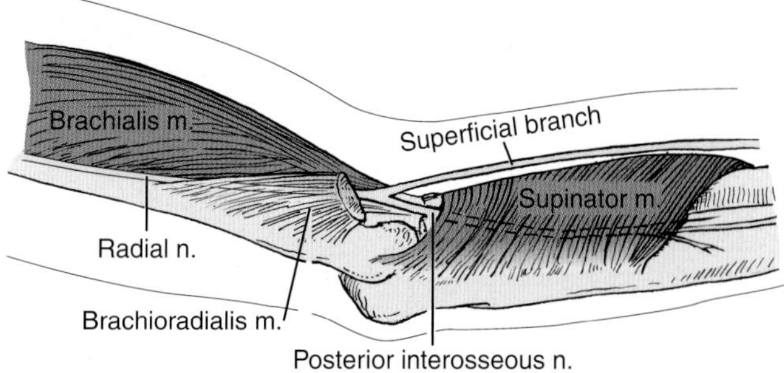

FIGURE 14-5. Radial nerve, lateral view. The radial tunnel is bounded posteriorly by the capitellum, anteromedially by the brachialis muscle, and anterolaterally by the brachioradialis (proximal) and extensor carpi radialis brevis (distal) muscles. The radial nerve can be compressed at several sites within the tunnel. Immediately distal to the elbow, the nerve divides into a superficial branch and a deep branch. The superficial branch of the radial nerve runs outside the supinator muscle. The deep branch, termed the *posterior interosseous nerve,* passes between the two heads of the supinator muscle and can be compressed by the arcade of Frohse, a fibrous band at the origin of the supinator muscle. (Modified with permission from Hochman MG, Zilberfarb MG: Nerves in a pinch: imaging of nerve compression syndromes, *Radiol Clin North Am Arthritis Imaging* 42:221-245, 2004.)

circumflex humeral artery that subsequently occludes with extreme abduction.[53] The differential diagnosis for post-denervation changes in the teres minor and deltoid muscles includes Parsonage-Turner syndrome (acute brachial neuritis), an atraumatic self-limited condition, that causes severe shoulder pain radiating down the arm, followed by loss of motor function in the affected muscles and that lasts days to weeks. In Parsonage-Turner syndrome, the long thoracic and suprascapular nerves as well as the axillary nerve may be involved.[46,47]

Radial Tunnel Syndrome and Posterior Interosseous Nerve Syndrome (Radial Nerve and Its Branches)

The *radial tunnel* refers to a space about the elbow approximately 5 cm long, extending from the capitellum to the distal edge of the supinator muscle.[6,54] It is bounded posteriorly by the capitellum, anteromedially by the brachialis muscle, and anterolaterally by the brachioradialis (proximal) and extensor carpi radialis brevis (distal) muscles (Figure 14-5). There are several potential sites of nerve compression within the radial tunnel[6,54-56]: (1) fibrous bands that can tether the radial nerve or its branches to the elbow joint at varying locations; (2) the tendinous edge of the extensor carpi radialis brevis muscle; (3) the radial recurrent artery and its vascular branches (known as the *leash of Henry*); (4) a fibrous band at the origin of the supinator muscle (known as the *arcade of Frohse*); and (5) a fibrous band at the distal end of the supinator muscle.

Within the radial tunnel, the radial nerve divides into the superficial branch of the radial nerve (SBRN) and the posterior interosseous nerve (PION).[54] This division occurs distal to the lateral epicondyle of the elbow and proximal to the supinator muscle. The SBRN runs superficial to the supinator muscle and continues along the superficial aspect of the lateral forearm, providing sensation to the dorsoradial hand. The PION runs deeper in a plane between the deep and superficial heads of the supinator muscle. There the PION can be compressed by the arcade of Frohse, a fibrous band at the origin of the supinator muscle. The PION continues into the forearm, traveling deep, along the extensor surface of the interosseous membrane. The posterior interosseous nerve supplies motor innervation to the extensor-supinator muscles.

The terms *radial tunnel syndrome* and *posterior interosseous nerve syndrome* describe two distinct clinical syndromes that arise due to compression of the radial nerve or its branches in the region of the radial tunnel.[54] Although these two syndromes can have similar causes, they may be distinguished by their differing clinical presentations. Radial tunnel syndrome presents predominantly with pain and occasional sensory disturbances but without significant weakness. Posterior interosseous nerve syndrome presents predominantly with motor weakness, but without significant sensory loss. The two syndromes can occasionally coincide, complicating the clinical diagnosis.

Patients with radial tunnel syndrome present with chronic aching pain over the lateral aspect of the elbow and proximal forearm. Symptoms can mimic lateral epicondylitis, and as a result, radial tunnel syndrome should be considered when suspected lateral epicondylitis fails to respond to treatment. The tenderness associated with radial tunnel syndrome typically occurs 6 to 7 cm distal to the lateral epicondyle. The differential also includes chronic extensor compartment syndrome and cervical radiculopathy. Some patients experience "double crush" phenomenon involving the cervical spine and radial tunnel. Patients with PION syndrome experience pain on the lateral side of the elbow, followed soon after by motor weakness. There is paresis or paralysis affecting extension of the metacarpophalangeal joints of the thumb and fingers, with inability to abduct the thumb. The wrist tends to deviate radially because of extensor carpi ulnaris paralysis.

Nerve entrapment leading to either syndrome may result from direct compression of the nerve by the structures of the radial tunnel detailed earlier. In this setting, activities that involve repetitive pronation and supination can lead to dynamic compression of the nerve; this phenomenon has been reported in violinists, music conductors, and swimmers.[54] The radial nerve can also experience mechanical compression due to ganglion cysts, lipomas, vascular malformations, synovitis,[57] bicipitoradial bursitis, swelling due to trauma, and radial head dislocation.

Radiographs can demonstrate fracture, dislocation, or bony abnormality contributing to radial nerve compression about the elbow. MRI can depict the nerves and surrounding musculature,[13] as well as surrounding masses contributing to nerve compression, such as ganglion cysts, bicipitoradial bursitis, or synovial hemangioma (Figure 14-6).[58,59] The use of high-resolution ultrasound to depict PION impingement was described in a group of four patients with forearm weakness and pain. In that study, ultrasound successfully demonstrated enlargement of the deep branch of the radial nerve on the affected side in all four patients, a finding that was confirmed by electroneurographic testing and surgical testing.[60] In this study by Bodner et al., the mean nerve diameter was 4.2 mm (transverse) by 3.3 mm (anteroposterior) in the symptomatic group, compared with 2.13 mm (transverse) by 1.3 mm (anteroposterior) in volunteers.

Cubital Tunnel Syndrome (Ulnar Nerve)

Cubital tunnel syndrome is the second most common entrapment neuropathy, after carpal tunnel syndrome.[61] Within the cubital tunnel, the ulnar nerve (C8, T1) may be compressed at two separate, but nearby and related, locations[6,61,62] (Figure 14-7). The first site is within the sulcus on the posterior surface of the medial humeral epicondyle (the sulci nervi ulnaris). The arcuate ligament

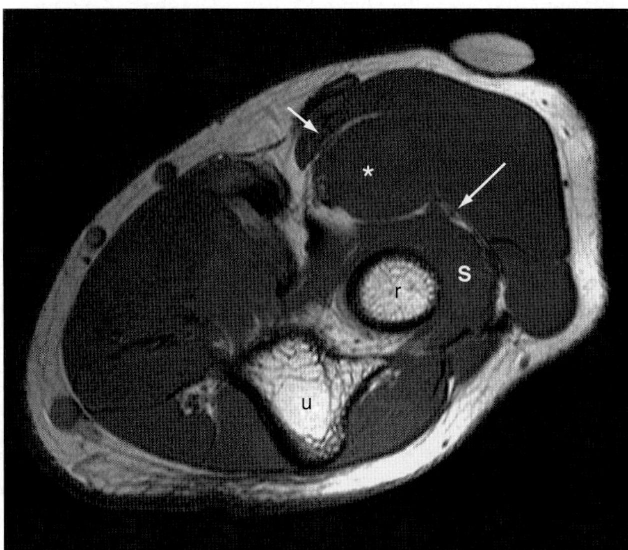

FIGURE 14-6. Schwannoma in the radial tunnel. Axial PD-weighted image in the proximal forearm. There is a rounded well-circumscribed mass (*asterisk* on center), isointense to muscle on T1-weighted images and heterogeneously high on T2-weighted images, which displaces and compresses the superficial branch of the radial nerve *(short arrow)* and the PION *(long arrow)* in the radial tunnel. The supinator muscle, through which the PION passes, wraps around the radius. The superficial branch of the radial nerve *(short arrow)* passes superficial to the supinator muscle. A marker at the location of the palpable mass indents the skin. *r,* Radius; *u,* ulna; *S,* supinator muscle. (Reprinted with permission from Hochman MG, Zilberfarb MG: Nerves in a pinch: imaging of nerve compression syndromes, *Radiol Clin North Am Arthritis Imaging* 42:221-245, 2004.)

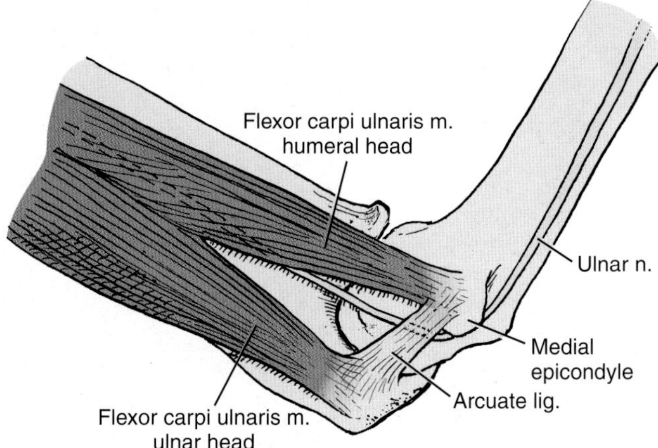

FIGURE 14-7. Cubital tunnel, lateral view. The ulnar nerve passes through a groove along the posterior surface of the medial humeral epicondyle, which is covered by the arcuate ligament of Osborne. The nerve continues deep to the two heads of the flexor carpi ulnaris muscle, where it may also be compressed. (Modified with permission from Hochman MG, Zilberfarb MG: Nerves in a pinch: imaging of nerve compression syndromes, *Radiol Clin North Am Arthritis Imaging* 42:221-245, 2004.)

of Osborne (or cubital tunnel retinaculum) spans the sulcus between the medial epicondyle and the olecranon, creating a fibroosseous tunnel. The second site lies approximately 1 cm distal to the sulcus, where the nerve runs and between the two heads (ulnar and humeral) of the flexor carpi ulnaris muscle and the medial surface of the humerus. The two heads of the flexor carpi ulnaris originate from and are connected by the arcuate ligament of Osborne.

Symptoms of cubital tunnel syndrome may be caused by acute or chronic bony deformity, ganglion cysts, and other soft tissue tumors, synovitis, and nerve enlargement.[62,63] Chronic repetitive microtrauma associated with elbow flexion/extension can cause edema and perineural scarring, resulting in nerve compression.[61] Although subluxation of the nerve with flexion can occur and may predispose to friction neuritis, it is seen in 10% to 16% of asymptomatic normals and its actual role in giving rise to cubital tunnel syndrome is unclear.[61] Recurrent traction on the ulnar nerve can lead to symptoms and can be seen in baseball pitchers,[64] boxers, jackhammer operators, and assembly line workers. Dynamic compression of the nerve can occur because of marked decrease in the volume of the cubital tunnel in flexion.[6,65] With flexion, the aponeurotic roof of the cubital tunnel is stretched and the medial collateral ligament bulges into the tunnel, reducing volume of the canal up to 50% of baseline and generating increased pressures within the canal. In some people, the ligament overlying the tunnel may be replaced by an accessory muscle—the anconeus epitrochlearis muscle—that can contribute to nerve compression. Because of its superficial location at the elbow, the ulnar nerve is also susceptible to external compression in this location. Causes of external compression include leaning on the elbow for long periods of time, application of a tourniquet, or positioning during surgery.

Patients with cubital tunnel syndrome present with paresthesias in the fifth and medial fourth fingers and can progress to muscle weakness and atrophy, with clawing of the fourth and fifth fingers.[6] Symptoms can develop acutely in the setting of trauma. Physical exam may reveal tenderness over the medial epicondyle and a palpable enlarged ulnar nerve. Tinel's sign may be elicited over the cubital tunnel. Symptoms of cubital tunnel syndrome may be confused with symptoms due to C8 radiculopathy, superior sulcus tumors, or thoracic outlet syndrome. Medial epicondylitis is also associated with localized tenderness to palpation along the medial elbow but can be distinguished because it is not accompanied by paresis or sensory changes.

Anteroposterior (AP) and lateral radiographs of the elbow can demonstrate bony changes about the cubital tunnel. The cubital tunnel view, taken with the humerus externally rotated and the elbow fully flexed and resting on the plate, depicts the cubital tunnel itself[66] but is no longer commonly obtained. CT scans are used more routinely now for imaging the bony contours of the cubital tunnel.

The ulnar nerve is well seen on routine axial MR images of the elbow[11-13,67] (Figure 14-8). In cross section, the nerve appears as a round or oval structure that is isointense to muscle and that is surrounded by normal fat. Enlargement of the nerve and abnormal elevated T2 signal within the nerve at the level of the cubital tunnel suggests cubital tunnel syndrome[67] (Figure 14-9). These findings should be interpreted in conjunction with clinical history, however, as other causes of neuropathy can create this appearance.[67] The arcuate ligament is visible on MRI and can be assessed for thickening. The recurrent ulnar artery also lines within the cubital tunnel, posterior to the nerve. Ganglion cysts, soft tissue masses, olecranon bursitis, or the normal variant anconeus epitrochlearis muscle can be diagnosed. The nerve may lie outside the canal due to subluxation or postoperative transposition. If ulnar subluxation is suspected but is not apparent on the conventional MR images, additional images with the elbow flexed can be obtained using a flexible or local surface coil.[11]

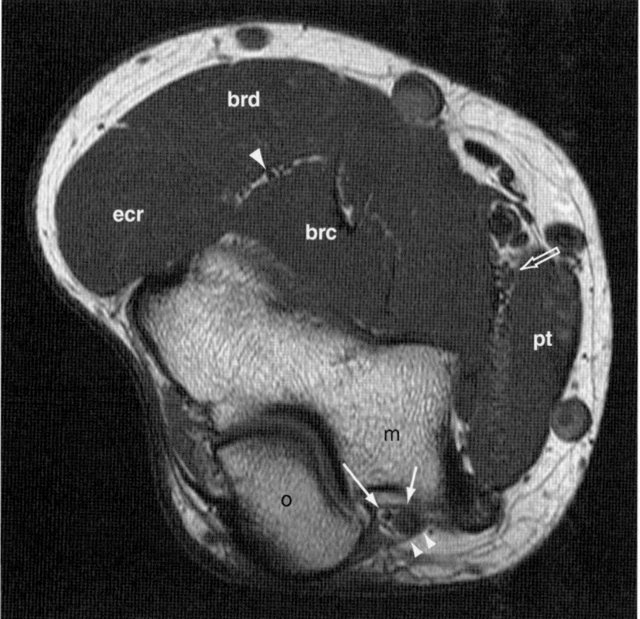

FIGURE 14-8. Normal ulnar nerve in the cubital tunnel. Axial PD-weighted image through the elbow. The ulnar nerve *(short arrow)* sits in a groove immediately behind the medial epicondyle. The recurrent ulnar artery *(long arrow)* lies posterior or lateral to the nerve. The tunnel is enclosed by the arcuate ligament of Osborne *(arrowheads)*, which extends from the medial epicondyle to the olecranon. Note also the normal radial nerve *(large arrowhead)* and median nerve *(open arrow)*. *brc,* Brachialis muscle; *brd,* brachioradialis muscle; *ecr,* extensor carpi radialis longus muscle; *m,* medial epicondyle; *o,* olecranon; *pt,* pronator teres. (Reprinted with permission from Hochman MG, Zilberfarb MG: Nerves in a pinch: imaging of nerve compression syndromes, *Radiol Clin North Am Arthritis Imaging* 42:221-245, 2004.)

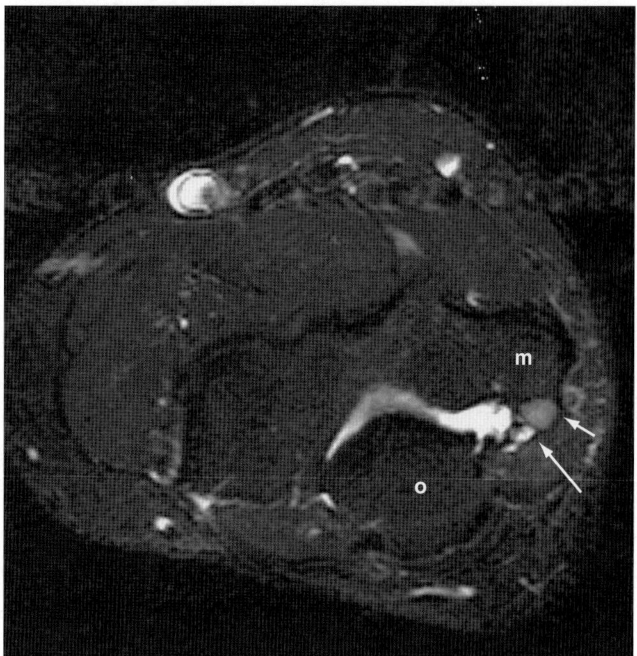

FIGURE 14-9. Enlarged ulnar nerve in cubital tunnel syndrome. Axial STIR fat-saturated T2-weighted MR image through the elbow. The ulnar nerve *(short arrow)* is enlarged and of relatively high signal intensity compared to muscle. An ulnar vessel *(long arrow)* lies immediately posterior to the nerve. *m,* Medial epicondyle; *o,* olecranon. (Reprinted with permission from Hochman MG, Zilberfarb MG: Nerves in a pinch: imaging of nerve compression syndromes, *Radiol Clin North Am Arthritis Imaging* 42:221-245, 2004.)

The literature related to ultrasound of the cubital tunnel is limited but supports the potential utility of ultrasound for clinical imaging.[32-34,68,69] On ultrasound examination, the nerve appears as an ovoid structure located (1) between the medial head of the triceps and the biceps, proximal to the elbow; (2) posterior to the medial epicondyle, at the level of the elbow; and (3) between the flexor carpi ulnaris and flexor digitorum profundus muscles, distal to the elbow. Color Doppler imaging can be used to distinguish the recurrent ulnar artery, which also lies within the tunnel. Chiou et al.[68] examined 10 controls and 14 patients with pain over the medial elbow. In their control group, mean dimensions for the ulnar nerve at the level of the medial epicondyle were 0.198 cm (short axis), 0.401 cm (long axis), and 0.068 cm^2 (area). They suggest that cubital tunnel syndrome should be considered if the area of ulnar nerve at level of epicondyle is greater than 0.075 cm^2, depending on the clinical context. Because it provides real-time imaging and easily accommodates changes in patient position, ultrasound can be used to demonstrate ulnar nerve subluxation in relation to the cubital tunnel.[70,71]

Pronator Syndrome (Median Nerve)

Pronator syndrome refers to compression of the median nerve in the vicinity of the elbow.[72] The median nerve may be compressed at one of four sites (proximal to distal): (1) the supracondylar process of the humerus; (2) a fascial extension of the biceps tendon, known as the *lacertus fibrosis*; (3) the fibrous arch of the flexor digitorum superficialis (FDS) muscle; and (4) the pronator teres muscle (Figure 14-10). However, the pronator teres muscle is the most common site of compression, whereas compression by a supracondylar process is quite uncommon. The supracondylar process is a

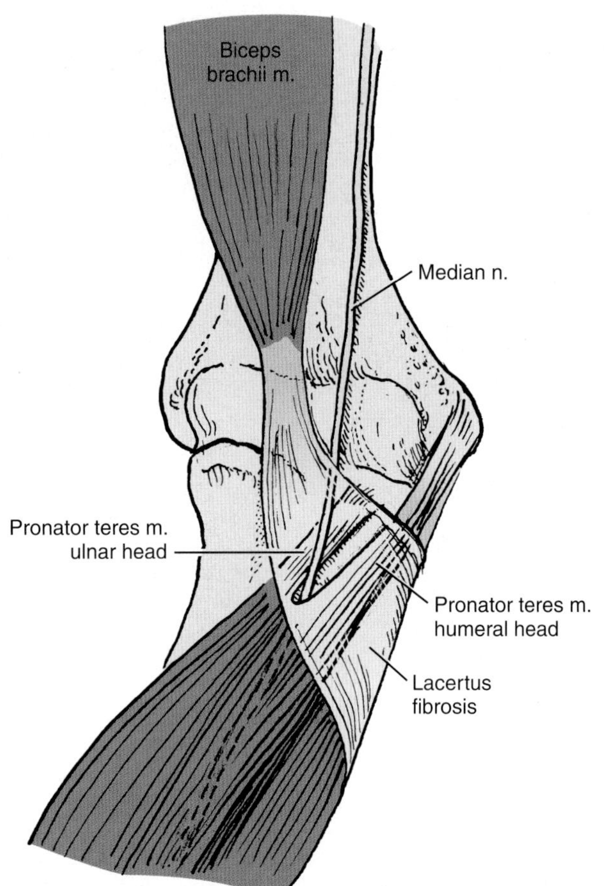

FIGURE 14-10. Median nerve, anterior view. In the region of the elbow, the median nerve passes between the two heads of the pronator teres muscle. It travels deep to the lacertus fibrosis or biceps aponeurosis. It may also be compressed when it passes under the fibrous origin of the flexor digitorum superficialis muscle, which arises from the medial epicondyle. (Modified with permission from Hochman MG, Zilberfarb MG: Nerves in a pinch: imaging of nerve compression syndromes, *Radiol Clin North Am Arthritis Imaging* 42:221-245, 2004.)

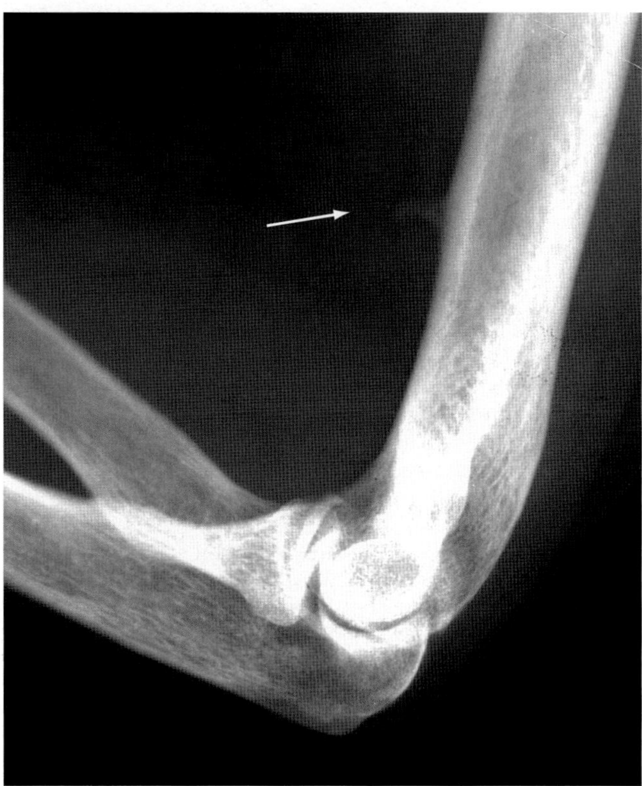

FIGURE 14-11. Supracondylar process. Lateral view of the elbow shows a bony projection, the supracondylar process, arising from the volar surface of the distal humerus *(arrow)*. Unlike an osteochondroma, the supracondylar process points toward the joint. The ligament of Struthers is not visible on radiographs but courses from the supracondylar process to the medial humeral epicondyle, creating a fibroosseous tunnel that can compress the median nerve.

rare anatomic variant found in fewer than 3% of humans. It consists of a bony exostosis arising from the ventral surface of the distal humerus, 5 to 7 cm proximal to the elbow[73] (Figure 14-11). It may be, but is not always, bilateral. The bony spur points toward the elbow joint and is often connected to the medial humeral epicondyle by a band of connective tissue known as the *ligament of Struthers*. When the ligament of Struthers is present, it creates a fibroosseous tunnel with the humerus through which the median nerve passes. In some cases, the median nerve is accompanied in the tunnel by the brachial artery, and in these cases, arterial claudication may also occur. Compression may occur due to trauma or due to dynamic compression. The lacertus fibrosis, also known as the *bicipital aponeurosis*, represents a fascial extension from the biceps tendon that overlies the pronator-flexor muscles and inserts on the antebrachial fascia. When thickened, the lacertus fibrosis can compress the pronator muscle and the median nerve. The median nerve passes between the superficial (humeral) and deep (ulnar) heads of the pronator teres muscle 2.5 to 4 cm distal to the medial epicondyle. When the elbow is extended and pronated, the two heads of the pronator teres muscle are brought closer together, which can result in dynamic compression of the nerve. The fibrous arch origin of the FDS muscle, located 2 cm distal to the deep head of the pronator teres along the proximal edge of the FDS, represents the most distal potential site for median nerve compression in the pronator teres syndrome.

Static compression of the median nerve can occur due to trauma, various masses, ulnar head abnormalities, and prolonged external compression ("honeymoon paralysis").

> "Honeymoon paralysis" is the reversible ischemic neuropathy that occurs due to compression of the arm by pressure from the head of another. It is now more broadly applied to other forms of compression of the median nerve.

Dynamic compression results from pronation and supination of the forearm. Symptoms are exacerbated when the pronator muscle becomes hypertrophied due to repetitive action (e.g., window washers and professional cleaners, hammering, prolonged driving, weight training) or the motion involves finger flexion (which tightens the fibrous arch of the FDS muscles). Patients with pronator teres syndrome present with pain in the forearm and with paresthesias and motor weakness along the distribution of the median nerve. Symptoms are aggravated by resisted pronation of the forearm. A characteristic finding on physical exam is decreased ability to oppose the thumb and to flex the thumb, index, and middle fingers. There may be pain and a positive Tinel's sign over the two heads of the pronator teres muscle. The symptoms can be confused with carpal tunnel syndrome and can lead to unsuccessful carpal tunnel release surgery.

There is relatively limited literature on imaging of pronator teres syndrome. Radiographs can demonstrate a bony supracondylar process or can reveal posttraumatic changes about the elbow.

On axial MR images, the normal median nerve is seen as a small rounded or linear low signal intensity structure lying between the pronator teres and brachialis muscles.[11,12] MRI case reports have described compression of the median nerve by a lipoma,[13] by the ligament of Struthers,[74] and by an anomalous third head of the biceps muscle.[75] MR images obtained with the elbow in pronation may demonstrate compression of the nerve by a hypertrophied pronator teres muscle.[11] Reported experience with ultrasound in the region is limited.

Kiloh-Nevin Syndrome (Anterior Interosseous Nerve)

The anterior interosseous nerve (AION) branches from the median nerve in the proximal forearm, immediately distal to the pronator teres muscle, and extends distally along the volar surface of the interosseous membrane, innervating all the deep ventral muscles of the forearm. Compression of the AION can occur anywhere along the nerve but is most common near its origin.[6] Common causes of compression include posttraumatic changes, vascular anomalies, tendinosis of the ulnar head of the pronator teres, fibrous bands, anomalous muscles, soft tissue tumors, or an enlarged bicipital bursa. More distally, compression can occur from casts or bandages about the forearm.[76]

Patients with compression of the anterior interosseous nerve present with forearm discomfort similar to that in the pronator teres syndrome, but without any sensory deficit. Motor weakness and paralysis in the flexor pollicis longus, flexor digitorum profundus, and pronator quadratus muscles results in a characteristic pinch deformity and inability to make a fist.[6] Because the AION runs adjacent to the median nerve in the proximal forearm, both nerves may be compressed simultaneously. Only portions of the AION are visible by MRI or ultrasound. However, both modalities have been used to demonstrate post-denervation changes in the muscles supplied by the AION, helping to confirm the diagnosis in a small number of cases.[28,42]

Carpal Tunnel Syndrome (Median Nerve)

Carpal tunnel syndrome (CTS) is the most common entrapment neuropathy of the upper extremity. It occurs due to compression of the median nerve at the carpal tunnel of the wrist. The carpal tunnel is formed by the transverse carpal ligament (also known as the *flexor retinaculum*) and the volar surface of the carpal bones. The tunnel contains the deep and superficial flexor tendons of the fingers, the flexor pollicis longus tendon, and the median nerve.

> The carpal tunnel contains the deep and superficial flexor tendons for the fingers, the flexor pollicis longus tendon, and the median nerve.

The transverse carpal ligament extends from the pisiform and hook of hamate bones medially to the scaphoid tuberosity and tubercle of trapezium laterally. On its radial side, the transverse carpal ligament splits into two layers to envelop the flexor carpi radialis tendon. The median nerve lies immediately deep to the transverse carpal ligament and courses superficial and parallel to the second and third flexor tendons and medial to the flexor pollicis longus tendon. The median nerve divides into two main trunks, usually at the distal edge of the transverse carpal ligament. However, the anatomy of the median nerve is quite variable.[6,77] In one variant, the motor branch of the nerve follows a course superficial to or through the transverse carpal ligament; this variant is at higher risk for injury during surgical section of the ligament in the treatment of CTS. Imaging diagnosis of this variant has not yet been reported. In another variant, the median nerve is bifid; that is, the nerve divides or is duplicated within the carpal tunnel. The bifid nerve may be separated by a persistent median artery or by an accessory muscle. The two components of the nerve may rejoin distally. The bifid median nerve may be associated with CTS. Occasionally, one of the branches of the bifid median nerve lies in a distinct compartment, which then requires targeted surgical decompression. Lanz identified seven duplicated median nerves in a series of 246 cases of carpal tunnel release. It is important to alert the surgeon to the presence of a bifid median nerve and/or persistent median artery preoperatively.

CTS is caused either by conditions that increase the volume of tunnel contents or by conditions that decrease the size of the tunnel; both phenomena result in an ischemic neuropathy.[6,77] The most common cause of CTS is tenosynovitis due to overuse and is often seen in keyboard operators. Other causes include tenosynovitis due to inflammatory arthritis; swelling related to thyroid disease, dialysis, or pregnancy; amyloid deposition; space-occupying lesions such as a ganglion cyst, lipoma, nerve sheath, or other tumors, gouty tophi, posttraumatic fibrosis, excess fat within the tunnel, persistent median artery; or anomalous musculature. CTS can also result from fractures or ligamentous instability. Patients with proximal nerve compression (e.g., cervical stenosis) or peripheral neuropathy (e.g., from alcoholism, chronic renal failure, or diabetes) have increased susceptibility to CTS on the basis of the "double crush" phenomenon.[3]

Symptoms of carpal CTS include pain and paresthesias in the distribution of the median nerve (thumb through radial side of the ring finger), often awakening the patient at night. In advanced cases, atrophy of the thenar eminence occurs, with eventual loss of abduction and opposition of the thumb. Physical exam may demonstrate a positive Tinel's sign (pain in the distribution of the median nerve elicited by percussion over the transverse carpal ligament) or a positive Phalen's sign (reproduction of paresthesias with maximal flexion of the wrist for 60 seconds). CTS may be bilateral in up to 50% of cases.

> CTS may produce pain and paresthesias of the thumb through radial side of the ring finger, thenar atrophy, loss of abduction and opposition of the thumb, and positive Tinel's and Phalen's signs.

The most common differential diagnosis is cervical radiculopathy. Additional differential considerations include neurogenic thoracic outlet syndrome and brachial plexus lesions, DeQuervain's tenosynovitis, and vitamin B[12] deficiency. History and clinical findings usually suggest the diagnosis, and NCS may be used for confirmation.

Plain radiographs of the wrist are of limited utility in CTS but can demonstrate causes of median nerve compression related to carpal malalignment or instability, bony spurring, or soft tissue calcification. A specialized carpal tunnel view can be obtained with the hand placed palm down on the x-ray cassette, in maximal dorsiflexion, and the beam projected parallel to the fourth metacarpal bone, at 25 to 30 degrees to a line perpendicular to the film.[66] CT scan provides detailed three-dimensional measurements of carpal tunnel bony anatomy but, compared with MRI and ultrasound, assessment of soft tissues on CT is quite limited.

Although MRI is rarely used for routine diagnosis of CTS, it can play a role when a mass lesion is suspected or when a patient experiences persistent symptoms following carpal tunnel release. The carpal tunnel is best demonstrated on axial proton density weighted or T1- and T2-weighted images[15] (Figure 14-12, *A*, *B*). In axial section, the normal median nerve is a round or ovoid

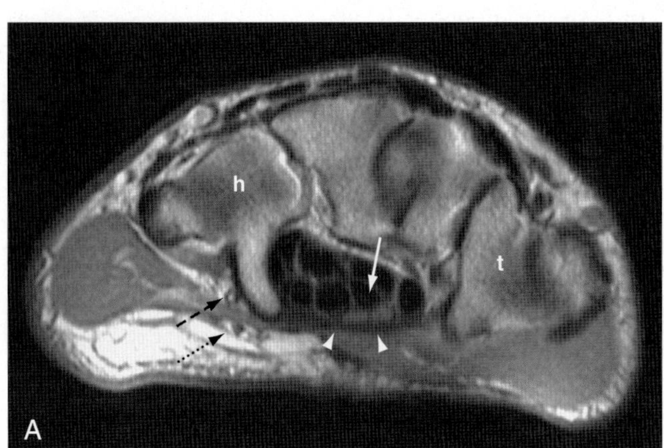

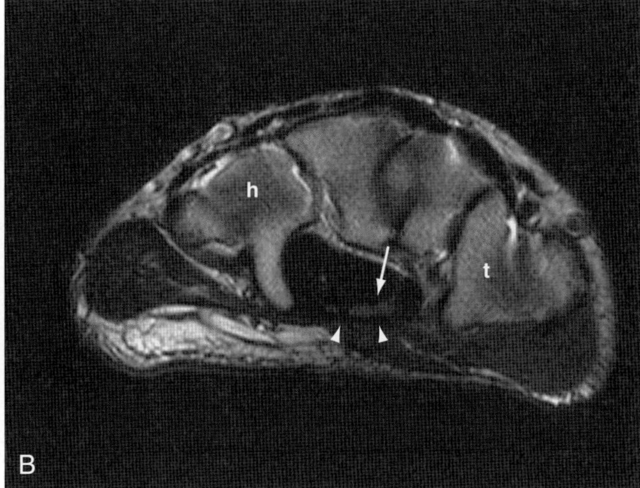

FIGURE 14-12. Normal median nerve in the carpal tunnel. Axial proton density weighted **(A)** and T2-weighted **(B)** MR images through the carpal tunnel. The median nerve *(solid arrow)* is seen as a flat ovoid structure immediately deep to the transverse carpal ligament *(arrowheads)*. Small rounded nerve fascicles, uniform in size, can be seen within the nerve. The deep and superficial flexor tendons are low signal and closely packed. The nerve is flat and of intermediate signal intensity on T2-weighted images. The ulnar nerve has divided into superficial *(dotted arrow)* and deep *(dashed arrow)* branches. *h,* Hamate; *t,* trapezium. (Reprinted with permission from Hochman MG, Zilberfarb MG: Nerves in a pinch: imaging of nerve compression syndromes, *Radiol Clin North Am Arthritis Imaging* 42:221-245, 2004.)

structure of intermediate T1 and T2 signal intensity. On high-resolution images, nerve fascicles can be visualized. The normal median nerve is flat at the level of the pisiform bone. It usually lies superficial in the carpal tunnel, immediately deep to the flexor retinaculum, but occasionally follows a deeper course. As noted, the median nerve may divide into radial and ulnar branches proximal to or within the tunnel. The normal flexor retinaculum is a thin, uniform, low signal band with mild volar bowing. The flexor tendons are ovoid low signal structures that, in the absence of synovial thickening, are closely spaced. A small amount of fat may be present within the carpal tunnel.

MRI findings of CTS include an enlarged median nerve (level of pisiform), a flattened median nerve (level of hamate), palmar bowing of the flexor retinaculum (level of hamate), and very high signal intensity within the median nerve on T2-weighted images[15,78,79] (Figure 14-13) (Box 14-2). Mesgarzadeh et al. described quantitative criteria for these characteristics.[78] However, these findings are nonspecific[80,81] and have been observed in asymptomatic individuals.[82] Signal within the median nerve can be misleading. When T2-weighted images are obtained with fat saturation, they are particularly sensitive to small amounts of edema, such that high signal within the nerve can be a normal finding. Also, when symptoms are chronic, the nerve may no longer demonstrate elevated signal on T2-weighted images. The use of contrast-enhanced MRI to demonstrate and distinguish nerve edema and ischemia has been described in a small group of patients.[24] In some cases, MRI can help to identify a cause of symptoms by demonstrating tenosynovitis, masses, or alignment abnormalities[81] (Figure 14-14).

In postoperative patients, MRI should show interruption of the flexor retinaculum, with volar migration of the carpal tunnel contents. If these findings are not demonstrated, it suggests either that the retinacular release is incomplete or that fibrotic scarring has developed.[83] Persistent proximal enlargement and distal flattening of the nerve may also be a sign of incomplete release. However, abnormally increased T2 signal within the postoperative median nerve does not necessarily indicate incomplete release. Evaluation of the postoperative patient should also include assessment for hematoma, persistent tenosynovitis or mass lesion, postoperative neuroma or perineural fibrosis, and, where indicated, the possibility of a more proximal lesion.

In the past few years, experience with ultrasound of CTS has grown and some consensus regarding diagnostic criteria is emerging.[33] On transverse scans, the normal median nerve is ovoid with a heterogeneous hypoechoic fascicular pattern and a thin echogenic rim (Figure 14-15, *A, B*). It flattens progressively as it courses distally. The nerve lies superficial to the flexor tendons,

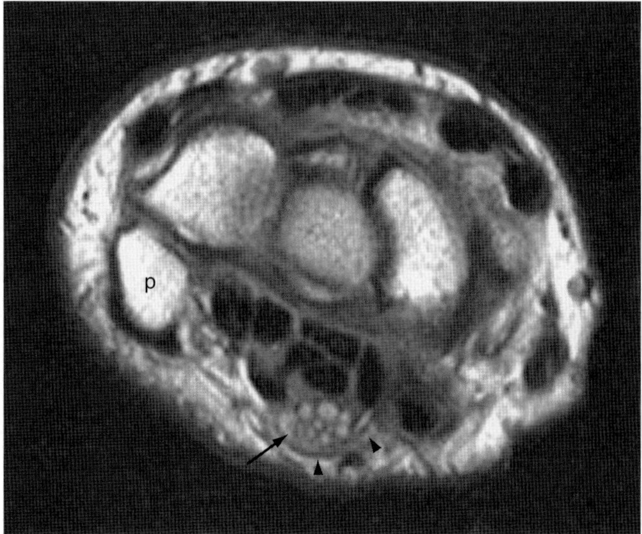

FIGURE 14-13. Median nerve enlargement in CTS. Axial proton density weighted MR image at the level of the pisiform *(p)*. The median nerve *(arrow)* is enlarged, and individual round fascicles of varying sizes are clearly evident. Note the bowed flexor retinaculum *(arrowheads)*, also known as the *transverse carpal ligament.* (Reprinted with permission from Hochman MG, Zilberfarb MG: Nerves in a pinch: imaging of nerve compression syndromes, *Radiol Clin North Am Arthritis Imaging* 42:221-245, 2004.)

BOX 14-2. MRI Findings That May Be Seen in CTS

Enlarged median nerve at the level of the pisiform
Flattened median nerve at the level of the hamate
Bowing of the flexor retinaculum at the level of the hamate
High signal intensity in the median nerve
Tenosynovitis or other causes of CTS
Edema of the thenar muscles

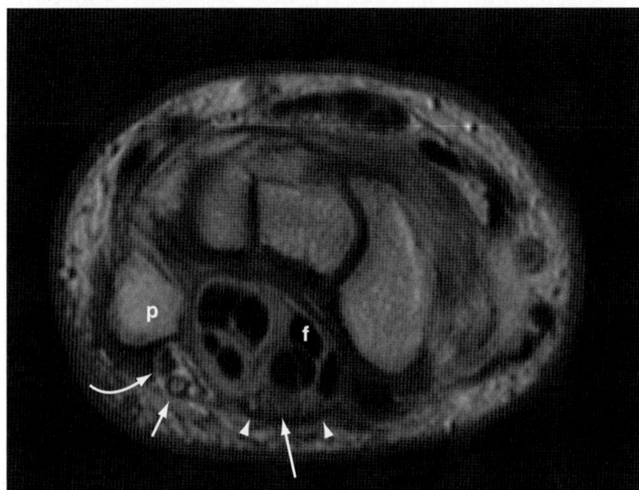

FIGURE 14-14. CTS owing to tenosynovitis. Axial proton density weighted MR images through the carpal tunnel. The low signal flexor tendons (one is labeled *f*) are surrounded by intermediate signal material, reflecting thickened tenosynovium. Resultant increased volume within the tunnel causes median nerve compression. The median nerve *(long arrow)* is prominent. The ulnar nerve *(curved arrow)* and ulnar artery *(short arrow)* are seen within Guyon's canal. The volar carpal ligament is a thin low-signal structure overlying the artery and nerve *(arrowheads)*. *p,* Pisiform bone. (Reprinted with permission from Hochman MG, Zilberfarb MG: Nerves in a pinch: imaging of nerve compression syndromes, *Radiol Clin North Am Arthritis Imaging* 42:221-245, 2004.)

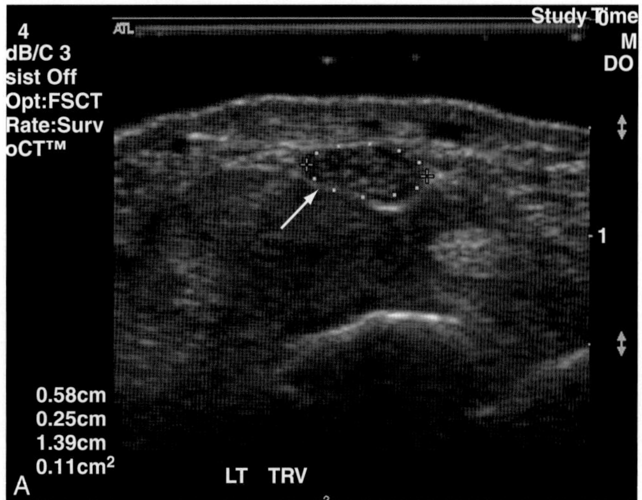

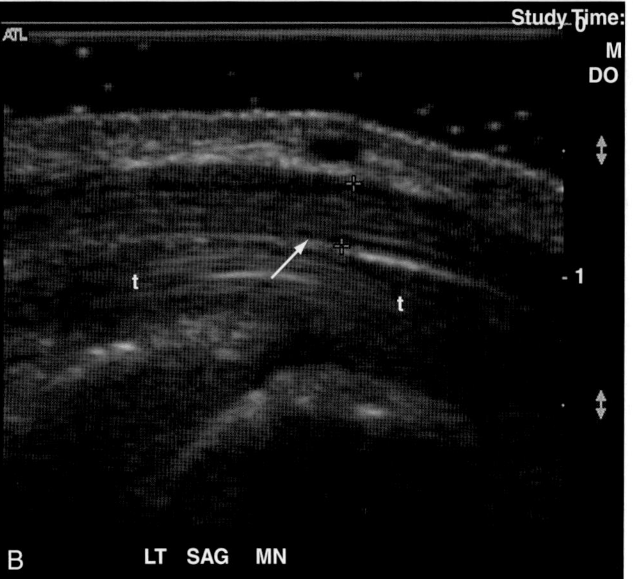

FIGURE 14-15. Normal median nerve on ultrasound. **(A)** Transverse and **(B)** sagittal images through the median nerve at the level of the carpal tunnel. **A,** On the transverse image, the nerve is a flattened ovoid structure *(arrow)* with punctate hyperechoic foci internally, reflecting its fascicular structure. The hyperechoic border of the nerve is thought to correspond to the perineurium. **B,** On the sagittal image, the nerve is an elongated structure, uniform in thickness, with a fascicular echotexture composed of internal hyperechoic (white) lines *(arrow)*. The intervening parallel hypoechoic lines within the nerve are discontinuous, unlike the hypoechoic lines within tendons. *t,* Tendon. (Reprinted with permission from Hochman MG, Zilberfarb MG: Nerves in a pinch: imaging of nerve compression syndromes, *Radiol Clin North Am Arthritis Imaging* 42:221-245, 2004.)

which have a fibrillar (rather than fascicular) pattern. The nerve usually lies directly over the superficial flexor tendon of the second digit, which is easily identified by flexing the index finger. Changes with flexion/extension of the fingers can also be used to distinguish the nerve from the tendons: On sagittal scans, the median nerve remains stable, whereas tendons glide. The normal flexor retinaculum is seen as a hyperechoic band, bridging the carpal bones superficial to the nerve and tendons. The ulnar artery, which lies outside the tunnel at its medial edge, can be distinguished by pulsation and Doppler signal. The size, shape, echogenicity, and relationship of the median nerve to the tendons and retinaculum are assessed. Continuity of the median nerve and any focal constriction or swelling is determined on sagittal/longitudinal images. The quality of the tendons and the presence of any surrounding fluid can be evaluated. The presence of any masses or anatomic variants is also evaluated.

Ultrasound criteria for median nerve compression include the classic triad of nerve swelling at the proximal tunnel (pisiform), nerve flattening in the distal tunnel (hamate), and palmar bowing of the flexor retinaculum[84-86] (Figure 14-16, *A, B*). According to Duncan et al., however, this classic triad was present in only 7% of 68 symptomatic wrists.[87] In their study, Duncan et al. determined that the best criterion for diagnosis of CTS was a median nerve cross-sectional area greater than 0.9 cm^2 at the level of the pisiform and suggested that this, in combination with median nerve width greater than 4.9 mm in the proximal tunnel, may be even more specific.[87] Wong et al. examined 35 patients with CTS and 35 asymptomatic controls and, applying receive operating characteristic curve (ROC) analysis, identified a median nerve

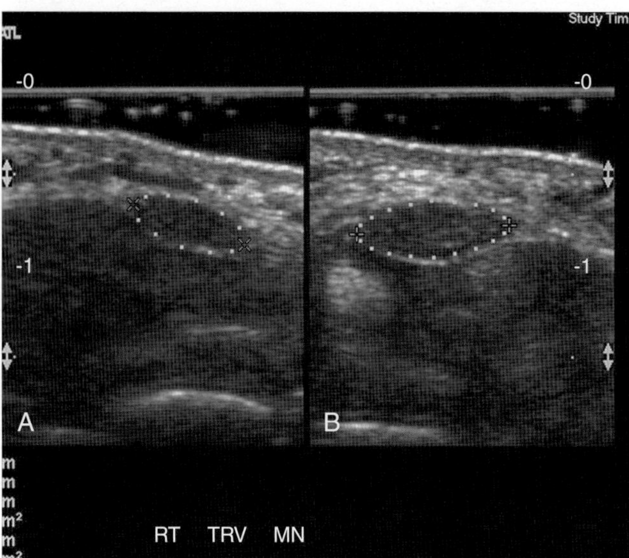

FIGURE 14-16. Abnormal median nerve in CTS. Transverse ultrasound images through the median nerve *(dotted circumference)* at the level of the distal radius **(A)** and carpal tunnel **(B)**. The distal segment of the nerve is enlarged. Although visible, the fascicular echotexture is less evident owing to edema within the nerve. (Reprinted with permission from Hochman MG, Zilberfarb MG: Nerves in a pinch: imaging of nerve compression syndromes, *Radiol Clin North Am Arthritis Imaging* 42:221-245, 2004.)

cross-sectional area cutoff > 0.098 cm^2 at the proximal tunnel for the diagnosis of CTS, with a sensitivity of 89% and a specificity of 83%.[88] Similarly, El Meidany et al. found an upper limit of normal cutoff of 10.0 mm^2 for the mean cross-sectional area of the median nerve, based on a study of 78 patients with symptoms of CTS, 78 asymptomatic controls, and comparison with electrophysiologic testing.[89] However, Wong et al. questioned the sensitivity of this criterion for detection of subtle disease. Lee found that, of several criteria, median nerve swelling at the level of the pisiform correlated best with EMG results and found that swelling ($\geq$ 15 mm^2) provided 88% sensitivity, 96% specificity, 97% positive predictive value (PPV), and 86% negative predictive value (NPV) for diagnosis of CTS.[90,91] In 172 wrists compared with NCS, Mallouhi et al. found that nerve swelling ($\geq$ 0.11 cm^2) was the most accurate (accuracy 91%) criterion on gray scale ultrasound for identifying median nerve involvement; however, the most accurate criterion overall in the Mallouhi study was intraneural hypervascularity (accuracy 95%) visualized on color Doppler sonography.[92] It should be noted that the mean cross-sectional diameter of the median nerve in some patients who have rheumatoid arthritis but no signs or symptoms of CTS may exceed the value of 10 mm^2 often cited in the literature as the upper limit of normal.[93] Ultrasound can be used to evaluate the carpal tunnel following surgery[84] but may be limited by overlying surgical scar. In this setting, persistent flattening of the median nerve is associated with persistent or recurrent compression.[94] There are few direct comparisons of ultrasound and MRI. Buchberger et al. compared CTS in 20 symptomatic wrists with both ultrasound and MR and found that measurements of cross-sectional area and flattening of the median nerve did not significantly differ between the two modalities.[95] However, bowing of the flexor retinaculum, mild compression of the median nerve, tendon sheath thickening, and ganglion cysts were better demonstrated with MRI. It is worth noting, however, that ultrasound technology has become significantly more sophisticated since this study was conducted in 1992. A small study compared newer ultrasound and MRI techniques in 15 patients with CTS, who underwent NCS to confirm the diagnosis, and 19 asymptomatic patients and found a sensitivity of 100% for both modalities.[96]

Ulnar Tunnel Syndrome (Ulnar Nerve)

Ulnar tunnel syndrome occurs due to compression of the distal ulnar nerve within Guyon's canal, a 4-cm-long fibroosseous tunnel along the ulnar aspect of the volar wrist.[62] Guyon's canal is formed dorsally by the flexor retinaculum, volarly by the palmar carpal ligament, and medially by the pisiform and hamate bones.[6,97] In the distal portion of Guyon's canal, the ulnar nerve bifurcates into a superficial sensory branch that runs with the artery and a deeper motor branch that supplies the hypothenar muscles and then crosses the palm to innervate multiple intrinsic hand muscles, including muscles of the thenar eminence. The fibrous arch of the flexor digiti minimi muscle divides the distal tunnel into two separate longitudinal channels: one containing the superficial ulnar nerve and artery, and the other containing the deep branch of the ulnar nerve.[98]

Patients with nerve compression in Guyon's canal present with pain and tingling in an ulnar nerve distribution (hypothenar region and ulnar side of fourth and fifth digits) and/or weakness of the hypothenar and other supplied intrinsic muscles. Compression proximal to the origin of the deep motor branch causes a mixed sensory and motor disturbance. Compression distal to the origin of the deep motor branch causes either a pure motor or, less commonly, a pure sensory deficit. The differential diagnosis includes compression of the ulnar nerve in the cubital tunnel, which is actually much more common.

Ulnar tunnel syndrome can be caused by fractures of the hook of the hamate or by a mass lesion within the tunnel.[99] Nerve compression can be caused by anomalous accessory muscles, which are quite common within Guyon's canal. Anomalous muscles have been reported in 22.4% of cadaveric specimens and are often present bilaterally.[98] Many of the anomalous muscles within the canal arise from the antebrachial fascia immediately proximal to the canal and insert with the abductor digit minimi muscle. The deep motor branch of the ulnar nerve can be compressed as it passes under a fibrous arch that is formed from the flexor digiti minimi and abductor digiti minimi muscles and that connects the pisiform bone to the hamate. External compression can also cause symptoms, such as bicycle handlebars, canes, crutches, or other sources of repetitive trauma. Ulnar neuropathy following carpal tunnel release has also been described.[100]

Bony anatomy about the ulnar tunnel can be surveyed using specialized radiographic views, such as the semisupinated oblique view and the lateral view with the hand in radial deviation with the thumb abducted or, alternatively, by using CT.[101] MRI using axial T1-weighted (or proton density weighted) and T2-weighted images effectively depicts Guyon's canal and provides effective direct visualization of the ulnar nerve[97] (see Figures 14-12 and 14-14). The normal nerve is a small, low signal structure that is surrounded by fat. The nerve lies medial (ulnar) to the ulnar artery. On high-resolution images, the bifurcation into superficial and deep motor branches, as well as the more distal branches of the superficial nerve, can be visualized. Only a short segment of the deep motor nerve is visible before it merges with the hypothenar muscles. A thin band representing the fibrous arch of the flexor digiti minimi brevis muscle can be seen separating the superficial from the deep canal and attaching to the hook of the hamate. Examination of the canal may reveal mass lesions, edema, fibrosis, or surrounding bony abnormalities (Figure 14-17). On ultrasound, the ulnar nerve is consistently demonstrated at the level of the pisiform as a thin round structure medial (ulnar) to the artery.[32] Ganglion and pisotriquetral cysts, anomalous muscles, and other masses can be demonstrated.

Piriformis Syndrome (Sciatic Nerve)

Piriformis syndrome is caused by compression of the sciatic nerve (L4-S3) in the pelvis, by the piriformis muscle.[6,102] Although degenerative spine disease and lumbar disk herniation are the most common causes of pain along the distribution of the sciatic nerve, a small subset of patients who present with sciatic, leg, or buttock pain are thought to have symptoms due to piriformis syndrome.[103]

> Compression of the sciatic nerve may occur due to pressure from the piriformis muscle associated with an intramuscular course of the nerve, muscle hypertrophy, traumatic changes, or alignment abnormalities.

The piriformis muscle arises from the anterior surface of the sacrum and the gluteal surface of the ilium and crosses the greater sciatic foramen to insert onto the superior border of the greater trochanter. In most instances, the sciatic nerve passes along the anterior surface of the piriformis muscle and exits the pelvis below the piriformis muscle, passing posteriorly along its inferior border (Figure 14-18, *A*). In some cases, however, a portion of the sciatic nerve passes directly through the piriformis muscle, predisposing the nerve to compression (Figure 14-18, *B*).[6]

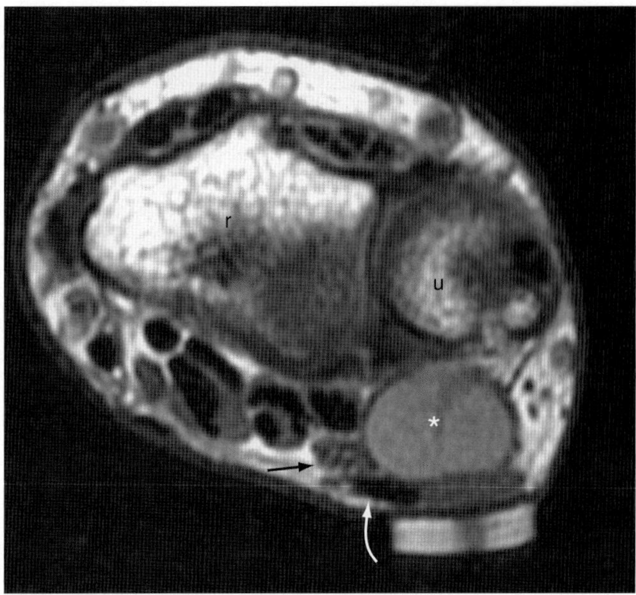

FIGURE 14-17. Ganglion cyst compressing ulnar nerve near Guyon's canal. Axial proton density weighted images through the wrist show a rounded mass representing a ganglion cyst *(asterisk)* abutting and displacing the ulnar nerve *(arrow)*, immediately proximal to Guyon's canal. The ganglion cyst lies deep to the flexor carpi ulnaris tendon *(curved arrow)*. A marker on the skin overlies the palpable abnormality. *r*, Radius; *u*, ulna.

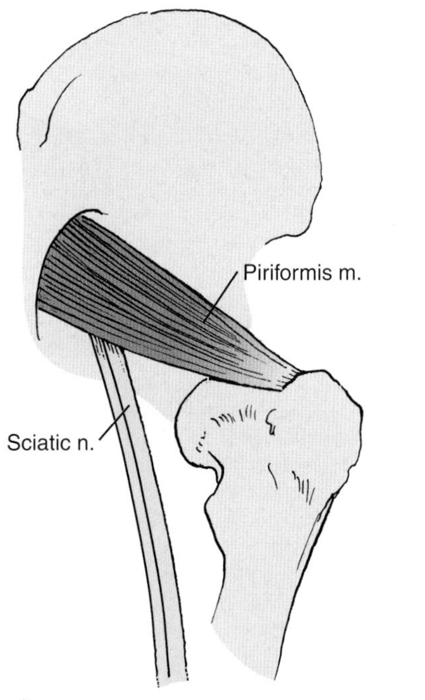

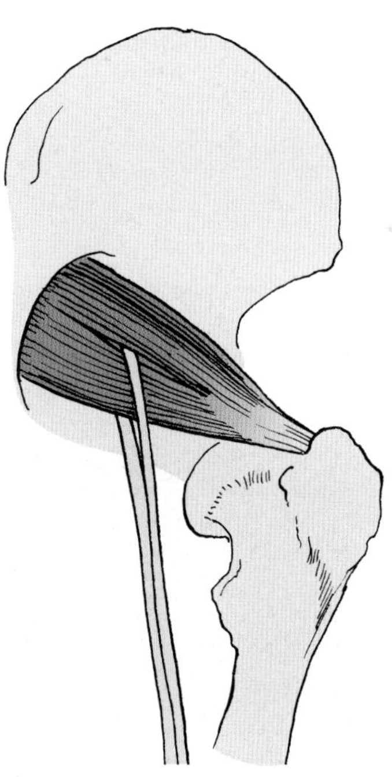

FIGURE 14-18. Piriformis muscle and sciatic nerve, posterior views. The piriformis muscle arises from the anterior surface of the sacrum and the gluteal surface of the ilium and crosses the greater sciatic foramen to insert onto the superior border of the greater trochanter. **A,** In most instances, the sciatic nerve passes along the anterior surface of the piriformis muscle and exits the pelvis below the piriformis muscle, passing posteriorly along its inferior border. **B,** In some individuals, a portion of the sciatic nerve passes through the piriformis muscle. Other anatomic variants have been described. (Modified with permission from Hochman MG, Zilberfarb MG: Nerves in a pinch: imaging of nerve compression syndromes, *Radiol Clin North Am Arthritis Imaging* 42:221-245, 2004.)

Other proposed causes of piriformis syndrome include hypertrophy of the piriformis muscle, alignment abnormalities,[104] and posttraumatic changes (hematoma, fibrosis, myositis ossificans, fracture).[6,102] The differential diagnosis for the symptoms of piriformis syndrome includes compression of the sciatic nerve due to lumbar disk disease, as well as other causes of sciatic nerve compression, such as hip joint dislocation, fracture fragments, heterotopic ossification,[105] or an acetabular cyst[106]; injury during joint reduction[107]; wear debris from total hip replacement[108]; and compression by gluteal varicosities.[109]

MRI can demonstrate local anatomy and exclude the presence of lumbar disk disease and pelvic masses.[103,104] The piriformis muscle is well displayed on routine axial, coronal, and sagittal T1-weighted and T2-weighted sequences of the pelvis. Muscle size, symmetry, and signal intensity and the presence or absence of edema, hemorrhage, or atrophy is depicted (Figure 14-19). The relationship of the sciatic nerve to the muscle can be traced, although the use of MRI to delineate specific anatomic variants has not been described. In a similar fashion, the morphology of the piriformis muscle and surrounding structures can be evaluated by CT scan, although subtle muscle edema would only be detected by MRI. A small study referring to the use of ultrasound to identify swelling and atrophy of the piriformis muscle and to guide therapeutic steroid injection of the muscle has been reported, but formal criteria for diagnosis of the syndrome were not provided.[110]

Tibial Nerve Compression in the Popliteal Fossa

The tibial nerve (L4-S3) is not part of the conventional popliteal artery entrapment syndrome. Occasionally, however, the tibial nerve may be compressed in the popliteal fossa. Nerve compression by popliteal cysts and by hemorrhage associated with popliteal muscle rupture has been reported[111,112] (Figure 14-20, *A, B*). Mastaglia described six surgically proven cases of tibial nerve entrapment by the tendinous arch of the origin of the soleus muscle.[113] The tibial nerve is well depicted on axial T1-weighted and T2-weighted MRI scans. Although dedicated images of the symptomatic leg provide high spatial resolution to better visualize the nerve, imaging both legs can highlight asymmetry of surrounding soft tissues.

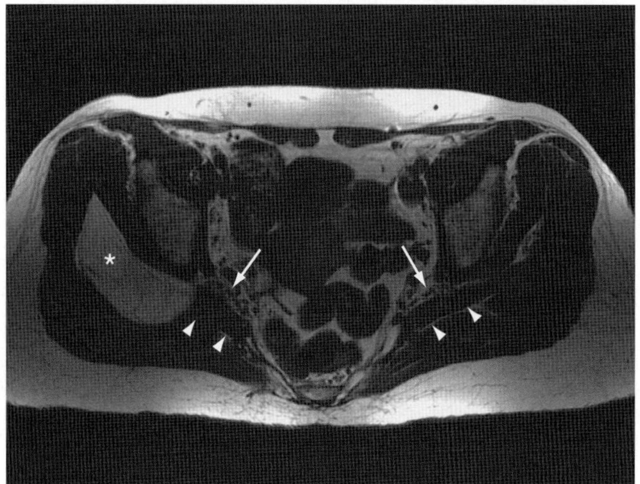

FIGURE 14-19. Piriformis syndrome caused by lipoma. Axial T1-weighted MR image through the pelvis. The right piriformis muscle *(arrowheads)* is compressed and displaced by a large lipoma *(asterisk)*, with resultant compression of the right sciatic nerve *(arrow)* as it exits the pelvis inferior to the muscle. Note the normal left piriformis muscle *(arrowheads)* and the left sciatic nerve *(arrow)*. (Reprinted with permission from Hochman MG, Zilberfarb MG: Nerves in a pinch: imaging of nerve compression syndromes, *Radiol Clin North Am Arthritis Imaging* 42:221-245, 2004.)

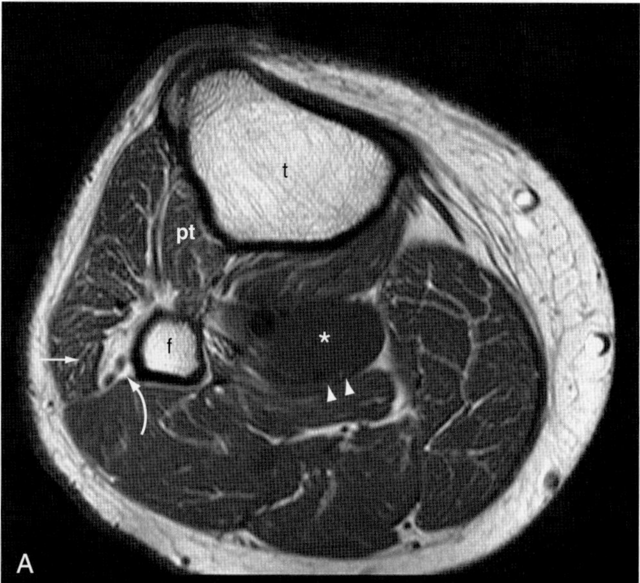

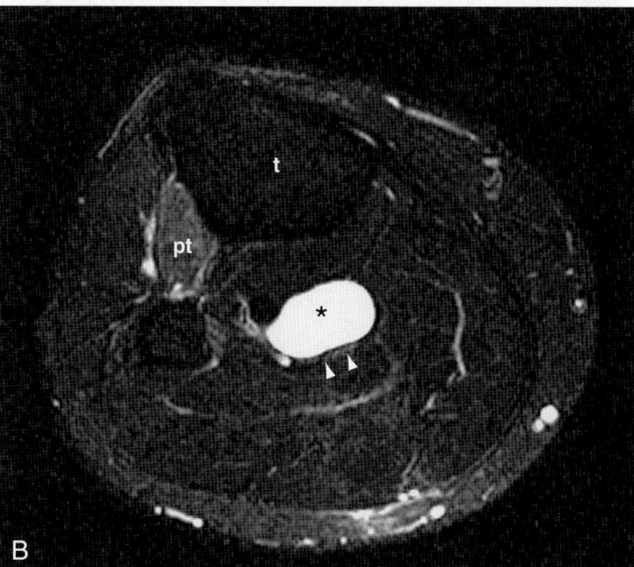

FIGURE 14-20. Tibial nerve compression by a ganglion cyst. Axial **(A)** T1-weighted and **(B)** STIR fat-saturated T2-weighted MR images through the upper calf show a ganglion cyst *(asterisk)* that arose from the proximal tibiofibular joint and is compressing the tibial nerve *(arrowheads)*. There is diffuse high signal within the posterior tibialis muscle *(pt)* on the STIR images, reflecting post-denervation edema, but it has not progressed to muscle atrophy. The popliteal artery is seen as a rounded signal void anterior to the cyst. On the T1-weighted image **(A)**, the peroneal tunnel is also visible. The deep and superficial branches of the peroneal nerve *(curved arrow)* lie between the tendon of the peroneus longus muscle *(arrow)* and the fibular neck. *f*, Fibula; *t*, tibia. (Reprinted with permission from Hochman MG, Zilberfarb MG: Nerves in a pinch: imaging of nerve compression syndromes, *Radiol Clin North Am Arthritis Imaging* 42:221-245, 2004.)

Peroneal Tunnel at the Fibular Neck (Common Peroneal Nerve and Its Branches)

The common peroneal nerve (L4-S2) usually branches from the sciatic nerve in the proximal popliteal fossa.[2] It courses anterolaterally and winds around the fibular head. As it comes along the anterior surface of the fibula, the nerve enters the peroneal or (fibular) tunnel. Within the tunnel, the nerve runs deep to the tendinous origin of the peroneus longus muscle and rests against the surface of the fibular neck (Figure 14-21). As the common peroneal nerve enters the tunnel, it divides into deep, superficial, and recurrent peroneal nerves. Plantar flexion or inversion of the foot tenses the peroneus longus muscle and compresses the nerve against the fibular neck.

Patients with nerve compression in the peroneal tunnel experience pain and tenderness along the tunnel and pain along the dermatome of the common peroneal nerve.[2,6] Symptoms can be similar to those of tibial stress fracture, deep medial tibial syndrome (shin splits), or compartment syndrome. However, peroneal nerve compression symptoms are exacerbated by forced inversion of the foot. Eventually, the patient develops sensory loss over the anterolateral leg and dorsum of the foot and weakness of dorsiflexion and inversion, with foot drop and slapping gait.

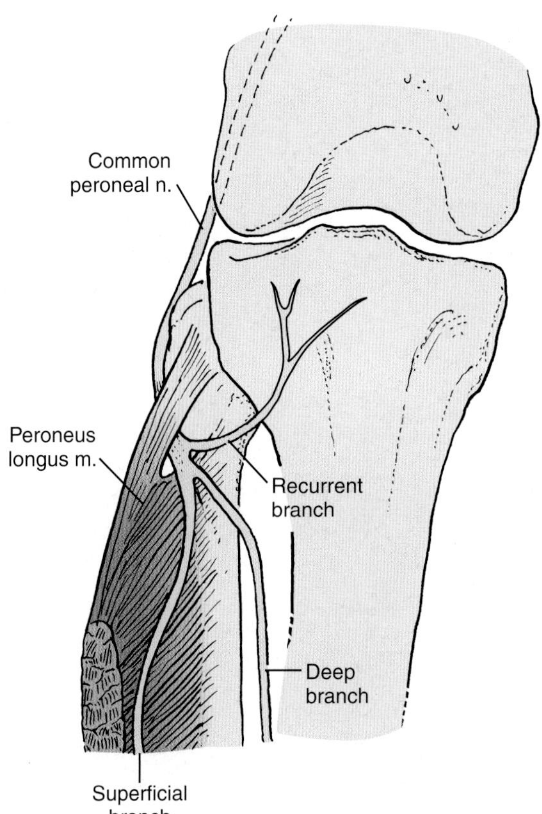

FIGURE 14-21. Peroneal tunnel, anterior view. The common peroneal nerve winds from posterior to anterior around the fibular head. As it comes along the anterior surface of the fibula, it passes through the two heads of the peroneus longus muscle and then divides into the superficial, deep, and recurrent peroneal nerves. Here the nerve can be compressed against the fibula by the tendon of the peroneus longus. (Modified with permission from Hochman MG, Zilberfarb MG: Nerves in a pinch: imaging of nerve compression syndromes, *Radiol Clin North Am Arthritis Imaging* 42:221-245, 2004.)

Peroneal nerve compression can occur with activities that involve repetitive inversion or pronation of the foot, such as running, and in occupations that involve repetitive use of a pedal. Symptoms may also result from prolonged crossing of the legs, prolonged squatting, or repetitive flexion-extension of the knee. Nerve compression can also result from fractures and hemorrhage about the fibular head, bony exostoses, altered anatomy due to knee arthroplasty, and tight-fitting casts or boots. Synovial, ganglion, and meniscal cysts; muscle herniation; and soft tissue tumors can also compress the nerve within the tunnel. When symptoms develop following a minor insult, the question of a concomitant neuropathy or lumbar spine disease ("double crush" syndrome) should be raised.

Radiographs are often unremarkable but may show bony anomalies along the expected course of the peroneal nerve. MRI directly demonstrates the anatomy of the proximal fibula, peroneus longus muscle and tendon, and fibular tunnel[14] (see Figure 14-20, *A, B*). The course of the common peroneal nerve and its branches can be followed and the presence of bony abnormalities or cystic or solid masses can be evaluated. Muscle edema and atrophy related to post-denervation changes can also be assessed. Ultrasound can be used to demonstrate the common peroneal nerve from the lateral portion of the popliteal fossa down to the fibular neck.[32] The posterior margin of the biceps femoris tendon and the echogenic cortex of the fibular head are used as landmarks.

Tarsal Tunnel Syndrome (Posterior Tibial and Plantar Nerves)

Tarsal tunnel syndrome refers to pain resulting from compression of the posterior tibial nerve and its branches as they pass through the tarsal tunnel. The tunnel is formed by the medial surfaces of the distal tibia, talus and calcaneus, the sustentaculum tali, and the flexor retinaculum. It extends from the medial malleolus proximally to the abductor hallucis muscle (inclusive) distally (Figure 14-22). The tarsal tunnel contains the posterior tibial, flexor digitorum, and flexor hallucis tendons, as well as the tibial neurovascular bundle and its branches.[6,114] The tibial nerve divides posteroinferior to the medial malleolus: the medial plantar branch runs in the upper compartment of the tunnel; the lateral branch runs in the lower compartment. The upper and lower compartments of the tarsal tunnel are delineated by the transverse interfascicular septum, which arises from the flexor retinaculum. The medial calcaneal nerve, which provides sensory innervation to the skin over the heel, originates proximal to the tarsal tunnel in approximately 35% of cases and, in those instances, is not involved in tarsal tunnel syndrome.[115]

Tarsal tunnel syndrome may be caused by bony impingement, including changes related to tarsal coalition and trauma, or by space-occupying lesions such as ganglion cysts, neurilemomas and other tumors, tenosynovitis, accessory or hypertrophic muscles, or varicosities. Tarsal tunnel syndrome can occur bilaterally in the setting of systemic diseases such as rheumatoid arthritis, tophaceous gout, diabetes, and myxedema. Certain sports activities that involve a heavy load on the ankle, such as sprinting and jumping, can trigger tarsal tunnel syndrome, particularly in the setting of anatomic or alignment abnormalities.[116] Symptoms associated with tarsal tunnel syndrome are variable and can be nonspecific, with poorly localized burning pain and paresthesias along the medial aspect of the heel and plantar aspect of the foot and toes. The clinical differential is extensive and can include plantar

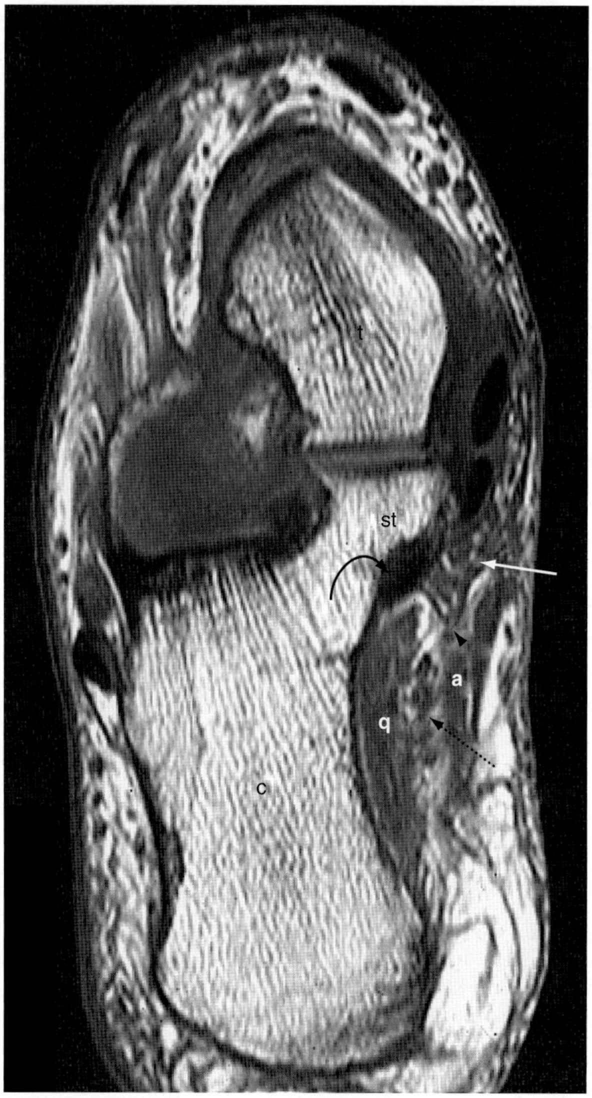

FIGURE 14-22. Anatomy of the tarsal tunnel. Coronal T1-weighted MR image through the hindfoot/midfoot. The medial *(solid arrow)* and lateral *(dotted arrow)* plantar neurovascular bundles pass between the abductor hallucis *(a)* and quadratus plantae *(q)* muscles and the surrounding bony structures. The medial and lateral branches travel in distinct compartments, separated by the transverse interfascicular septum *(arrowhead)*. Flexor hallucis longus tendon is noted coursing along the undersurface of the sustentaculum tali *(curved arrow)*. *c,* Calcaneus; *st,* sustentaculum tali; *t,* talus. (Reprinted with permission from Hochman MG, Zilberfarb MG: Nerves in a pinch: imaging of nerve compression syndromes, *Radiol Clin North Am Arthritis Imaging* 42:221-245, 2004.)

fasciitis, calcaneal bursitis, tendopathy and tenosynovitis, S1 radiculopathy, peripheral vascular disease, peripheral neuropathy, and reflex sympathetic dystrophy. Some authors describe the proximal tarsal tunnel as a distinct entity, referring to entrapment of the tibial nerve in the retromalleolar region, and distinguish it from distal tarsal tunnel syndrome involving the branches of the tibial nerve.[117,118]

Symptoms of tarsal tunnel syndrome include poorly localized burning pain and paresthesias along the medial aspect of the heel and plantar aspect of the foot and toes.

Radiographs of the foot may reveal bony deformity, spurring, or evidence of tarsal coalition. The tarsal tunnel itself can be directly visualized on specialized axial radiographs of the hindfoot, which are obtained with the patient supine, heel resting on the cassette, ankle at 90 degrees (aided by pulling on the foot with gauze), with the central ray of the x-ray beam directed at the base of the third metatarsal and angled 40 degrees toward the head.[66] Bony abnormalities can be demonstrated in greater detail using CT.[119] MRI depicts detailed anatomy of the tarsal tunnel and is the method of choice for detecting space-occupying lesions within the tunnel[120] (Figure 14-23). Pfeiffer and Cracchiolo found that surgical decompression yielded more favorable results in patients in whom a space-occupying lesion was identified prospectively.[121] MRI can also play an important role in excluding other causes of hindfoot/midfoot pain. The tarsal tunnel is generally well demonstrated on routine T1- and T2-weighted MR images of the hindfoot and midfoot. It is best seen on true axial (perpendicular to the long axis of the tibia) and thin-section sagittal images but is also well demonstrated on true coronal images. Ultrasound can demonstrate the anatomy of the tarsal tunnel, including the course of the tibial nerve and its branches and can identify and help characterize space-occupying lesions.[32,33,35]

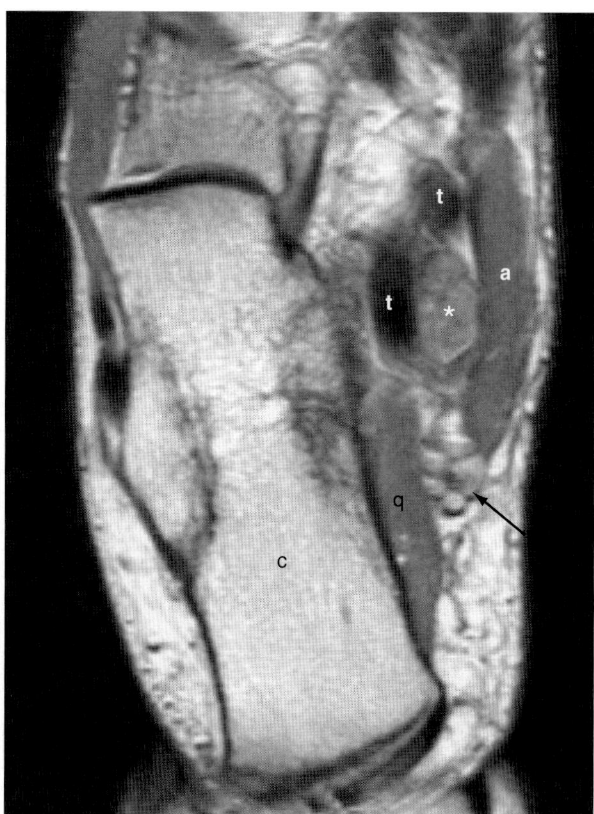

FIGURE 14-23. Ganglion cyst causing nerve compression in tarsal tunnel. Axial proton density weighted MR image through the tarsal tunnel. A lobulated ovoid ganglion *(asterisk)* causes mass effect within the tunnel, compressing the neurovascular bundle *(arrow)*. The tendons *(t)* are also splayed. *a,* Abductor hallucis muscle; *c,* calcaneus; *q,* quadratus plantae muscle. (Reprinted with permission from Hochman MG, Zilberfarb MG: Nerves in a pinch: imaging of nerve compression syndromes, *Radiol Clin North Am Arthritis Imaging* 42:221-245, 2004.)

Sinus Tarsi and Sinus Tarsi Syndrome (Nerve of Tarsal Canal)

The sinus tarsi or tarsal canal lies immediately anterior to the posterior subtalar facet, at the level of the subtalar joint, interposed between the talus and calcaneus. It is a cone-shaped space, wider laterally and narrower medially, and it runs at an angle of approximately 45 degrees to the longitudinal axis of the calcaneus. The sinus tarsi is filled with fat and contains a neurovascular bundle and several ligaments and the medial and intermediate roots of the inferior extensor retinaculum.[122] Synovial recesses from the posterior subtalar joint may extend into the sinus tarsi.[123] The sinus tarsi is innervated by a branch of the deep peroneal nerve or, less commonly, by a medial branch of the sural nerve.[124] The nerve endings within the sinus tarsi contribute to proprioception about the ankle. The two ligaments of the sinus tarsi—the cervical ligament and interosseous talocalcaneal ligament—help to stabilize the subtalar joint. The artery of the tarsal canal constitutes a branch of the posterior tibial artery.

> Sinus tarsi syndrome is characterized by pain along the lateral aspect of the foot and a subjective sensation of hindfoot instability.[122]

It is typically a chronic process. Approximately 70% of cases develop from secondary effects of trauma, commonly an ankle inversion injury.[123,125] The remaining 30% of cases are due to inflammatory arthritides (e.g., rheumatoid arthritis or ankylosing spondylitis, gout), or due to foot deformity (e.g., tarsal coalition, pes cavus, pes planus). Inflammatory changes within the tarsal canal can result in nerve compression and attendant pain. The sinus tarsi ligaments may be torn, either due to trauma or inflammation.

Diagnosis of sinus tarsi syndrome can be difficult, as chronic heel pain is a common finding with an extensive differential diagnosis. Patients with sinus tarsi syndrome report pain along the lateral aspect of the foot that is worse with standing, walking, or supination/abduction motions and improves with rest or immobilization. Pain is exacerbated by pressure applied over the sinus tarsi. However, physical exam is not definitive for the diagnosis of sinus tarsi syndrome. Radiographs may demonstrate findings supportive of the diagnosis but are not in themselves diagnostic of the entity. Radiographs, including AP, oblique, and standing lateral views of the foot, may demonstrate associated alignment abnormalities of the foot such as pes cavus or pes planus or evidence of tarsal coalition or misplaced hindfoot fusion hardware. Radiographs may also show evidence of prior inversion injury (e.g., swelling, malleolar or other fractures, ossicles about the ankle, talar dome osteochondritis dissecans (OCD), subtalar osteoarthritis) or, alternatively, may reveal erosions suggestive of inflammatory arthritis. If there has been injury to the lateral collateral ligaments of the tibiotalar joint, stress radiographs (radiographs performed with stress applied to the tibiotalar joint) may show evidence of lateral talar tilt, but this is an indirect finding of lateral inversion injury and is not diagnostic for sinus tarsi ligament injury. Subtalar arthrography (instillation of radiopaque contrast into the subtalar joint under fluoroscopic guidance) may demonstrate lack of filling of the anterior microrecesses of the subtalar joint, which has been described as a sign of sinus tarsi syndrome.[126] In Taillard's study, 15 of 21 (71%) of cases of chronic sinus tarsi syndrome had abnormal findings at arthrography. Arthrography may be performed in conjunction with image-guided injection of anesthetic and corticosteroid into the joint, and a presumptive diagnosis of sinus tarsi syndrome may be made if symptoms resolve in response to the injection.[123,127] In fact, prior to the use of MRI, this was the primary technique for diagnosing sinus tarsi syndrome. It should be noted, however, that arthrography of the subtalar joint is a specialized skill that is not universally available.

MRI effectively demonstrates the normal anatomy and pathology of the sinus tarsi.[122,128] The normal sinus tarsi is filled with fat, which is high signal on T1-weighted images, intermediate on T2-weighted images, and low signal on fat-saturated T2-weighted images (Figure 14-24, *A*). The normal sinus tarsi ligaments are seen as linear low signal structures extending between the talus and calcaneus, surrounded by higher signal fat. On MR images, the cervical ligament is visualized in 66% to 88% of normal individuals (coronal and sagittal planes, respectively) and the interosseous talocalcaneal ligament is visualized in 56% to 62% (coronal and sagittal planes, respectively).[128] Fluid-filled synovial recesses extending from the subtalar joint are seen in approximately 50% of normals.[122]

In MRI of sinus tarsi syndrome, there is loss of the normal signal of the fat in the sinus. Low signal on T1-weighted and high signal on T2-weighted images in the sinus tarsi fat indicate inflammation and synovitis (Figure 14-24, *B, C*). Low signal on T1-weighted and low signal on T2-weighted images indicate fibrosis. Small fluid collections may be present, related to small synovial cysts or distended synovial microrecesses. (The arthrographic sign of nonvisualization of subtalar recesses is not accepted as a sign of sinus tarsi syndrome on MRI, perhaps due to the differences in subtalar pressure between routine imaging and subtalar injection.) The ligaments of the sinus tarsi may demonstrate heterogeneously high signal on T1-weighted or T2-weighted images, reflecting hemorrhage and edema. Nonvisualization of the ligaments may be due to obscuration by changes in the fat or due to ligament rupture. If acutely torn, the ligament may appear interrupted or wavy. If chronically torn, the ligament may be attenuated or thickened. A high incidence of associated injuries of the lateral collateral ligaments, particularly the calcaneofibular ligament, and of the posterior tibial tendon has been described.[122] MRI may also play a role in identifying and characterizing abnormal masses within the sinus tarsi as potential causes of sinus tarsi syndrome.[123]

> MRI features of sinus tarsi syndrome include edema or fibrosis of the sinus tarsi, abnormal ligaments in the sinus tarsi, associated (but nonspecific) lateral collateral ligament injuries and posterior tibial tendon tears, and any underlying masses.

In general, ultrasound evaluation of the sinus tarsi is limited by shadowing from surrounding osseous structures, and the routine use of ultrasound for the diagnosis of sinus tarsi syndrome has not been reported. However, ultrasound has been used to guide injections into the subtalar joint and region of the sinus tarsi.[129]

Sinus tarsi syndrome may respond to conservative therapy including local injection, immobilization, and physical therapy but, in some cases, may require surgical or arthroscopic synovectomy and ligamentoplasty for more definitive treatment. In the appropriate clinical setting, correction of severe flatfoot deformity may be indicated.[123,127,130]

Morton Neuroma (Plantar Digital Nerve)

Morton neuroma refers to mass-like enlargement of the plantar digital nerve, which characteristically occurs at the level of the metatarsal heads between the deep and superficial layers of the intermetatarsal. The mass, known as a *Morton neuroma*, is

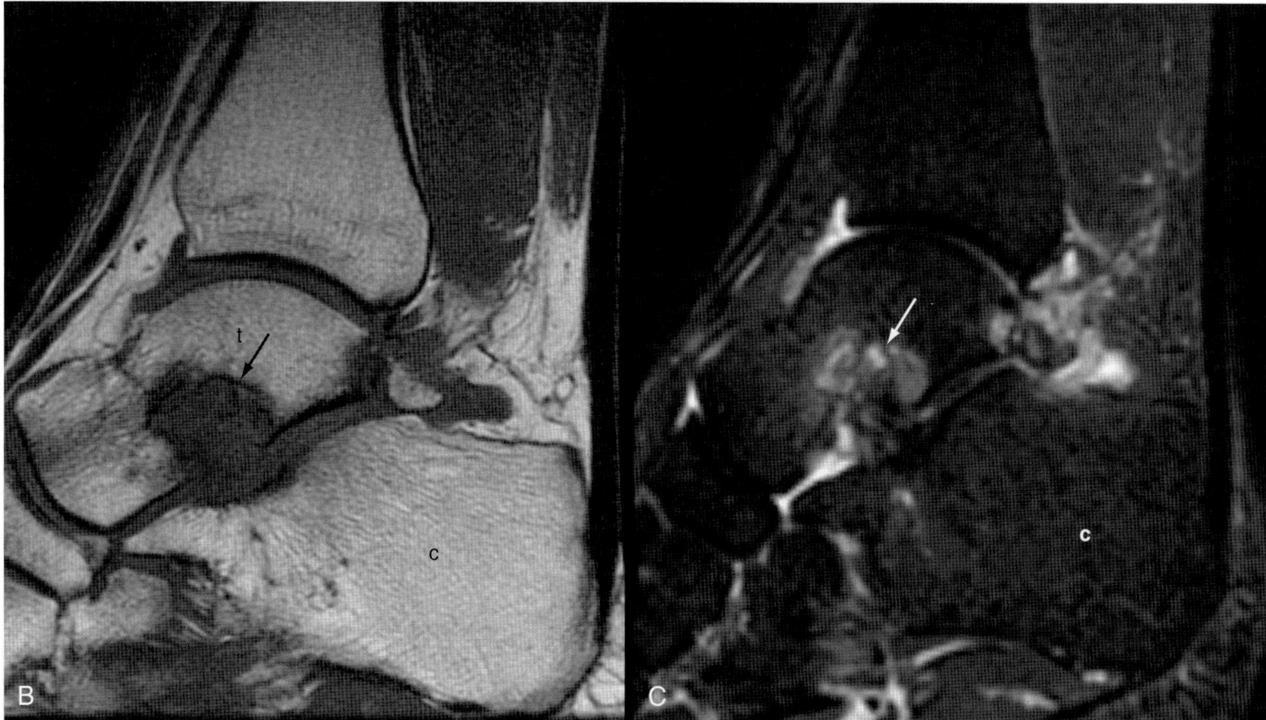

FIGURE 14-24. Sinus tarsi syndrome. **A,** Sagittal T1-weighted image showing a normal sinus tarsi *(arrows)* containing normal high signal fat. The cervical ligament is seen as a linear low signal structure extending between the talus and calcaneus *(curved arrow)*. Punctate low signal in the posterior sinus tarsi fat most likely represents a small nerve fiber. A small amount of low signal fluid extending into the sinus tarsi from the posterior subtalar joint is a normal finding *(arrowhead)*. **B,** Sagittal T1-weighted image showing evidence of sinus tarsi syndrome, with effacement of the sinus tarsi fat *(arrow)*. Cortex along the undersurface of the talus has been eroded by proliferating synovium. **C,** Sagittal fat-saturated T2-weighted image showing edema and fluid in the sinus tarsi and marrow edema associated with erosions in the adjoining talus. *c,* Calcaneus; *t,* talus.

not a true neoplastic neuroma; it is formed from nerve degeneration, endoneurial edema, epineurial and endoneural vascular hyalinization, and perineural fibrosis. It is thought to develop due to nerve entrapment and repetitive trauma.

In most cases, the diagnosis of Morton neuroma is a clinical diagnosis, based on history and physical examination.[6,131] Patients present with sharp burning or throbbing pain centered in the ball of the foot and radiating into the toes, often worse with crouching or wearing high heels. Morton neuroma is more common in middle-aged women, possibly due to chronic trauma associated with high-heeled shoes. It occurs most commonly in the third intermetatarsal space but can also be found in the second or fourth intermetatarsal spaces. Physical exam reveals focal tenderness between metatarsal heads, with or without a palpable mass. Imaging can be helpful when symptoms are atypical or coexisting neurologic conditions are present. Imaging studies may also play a role in surgical planning when multiple neuromas are suspected or when evaluating a postoperative patient with recurrent symptoms.

Radiographs of the foot, best obtained standing, can reveal splaying of the metatarsal heads when a large interdigital mass is present. They help exclude other causes of forefoot pain, such as fracture, exostosis, or foreign body. Radiographs may also demonstrate metatarsal alignment abnormalities that can account for the symptoms or that may contribute to the development of Morton neuroma.

MRI can be used for imaging of Morton neuroma, with reported accuracy of approximately 90%, PPV of 100%, and NPV of 60%.[132] Although imaging of the foot is typically performed with the patient supine, Weishaupt et al. demonstrated improved visibility for Morton neuroma when performing MRI with the patient prone compared with supine or weight-bearing positions.[133] Morton neuroma is best seen in the true coronal (transverse to the long axis of the foot) or true axial plane and is usually best appreciated on the T1-weighted images. It appears as a teardrop–shaped soft tissue mass lying between the metatarsal heads, extending into the plantar subcutaneous fat[134] (Box 14-3). Signal characteristics are nonspecific, isointense to muscle on T1-weighted images, and variable on T2-weighted images. The mass may be low signal on T2-weighted images due to fibrosis (Figure 14-25, *A, B*). There is often high T2 signal fluid adjacent to the mass in an intermetatarsal bursa. The bursa is oriented vertically and tends to be centered more dorsal than the neuroma, at the level of the metatarsal heads. Fluid in the bursa is considered physiologic when it measures less than 3 mm in width.[134] Gadolinium enhancement in Morton neuroma is variable and the utility of contrast enhancement in its evaluation is controversial.[132,135] The differential diagnosis for an intermetatarsal mass includes bursitis, inflammatory or pigmented villonodular synovitis, foreign body granuloma, and true neoplastic neuroma. MR images should also be assessed for other potential causes of forefoot pain, such as stress fracture, Freiberg's infraction, metatarsophalangeal joint dislocation, and osteomyelitis.

MRI can have a significant impact on clinical decision-making with regard to Morton neuroma.[136] It is important to realize, however, that findings suggestive of Morton neuroma are commonly detected in asymptomatic individuals.[134,137] Bencardino diagnosed Morton neuroma in 33% (19/57) of patients with no clinical evidence of the condition.[137] Zanetti et al. compared neuromas detected in 70 asymptomatic volunteers with those identified in 16 symptomatic surgically proven cases and suggested that the MRI diagnosis of Morton neuroma may be clinically relevant only when the mass is 5 mm or greater in transverse diameter and when it correlates with clinical findings.[134]

A small (< 5 mm) Morton neuroma can be an asymptomatic incidental finding.

BOX 14-3. MRI Features of Morton Neuroma

- Mass between the metatarsal heads extending into the plantar subcutaneous fat
- Mass is isointense to muscle on T1-weighted images and variable on T2-weighted images
- Variable gadolinium contrast enhancement
- High T2 signal fluid in an intermetatarsal bursa may coexist with a neuroma

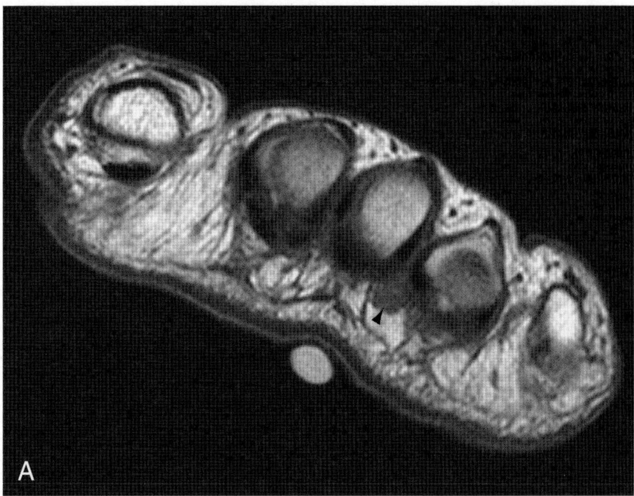

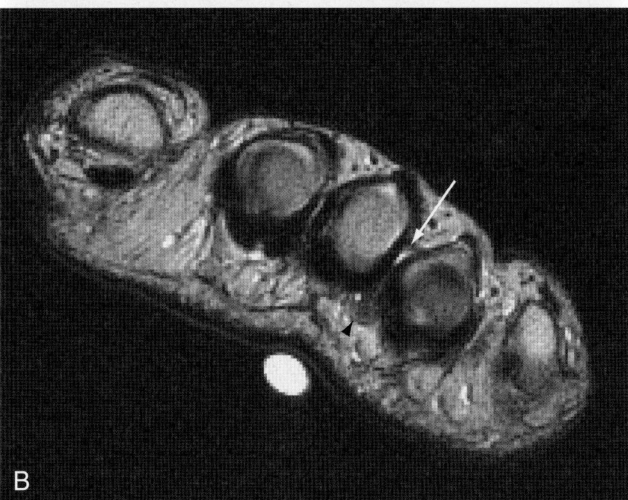

FIGURE 14-25. Morton neuroma of the plantar digital nerve. **(A)** T1-weighted and **(B)** T2-weighted MR images through the forefoot, perpendicular to the long axis of the foot. **A,** There is an ovoid mass centered in the third intermetatarsal space *(arrowhead)* and extending toward the plantar surface, replacing the normal high T1 signal fat there. Some abnormal signal is also present in the second intermetatarsal space. **B,** The T2-weighted image shows corresponding low signal within the plantar aspect of the third intermetatarsal space, representing the neuroma *(arrowhead)*. A tiny amount of high T2 signal in the dorsal portion of the intermetatarsal space *(arrow)* represents fluid within the intermetatarsal bursa.

Ultrasound is also an effective technique for imaging Morton neuroma, with reported sensitivities of 95% to 98%.[41,138,139] Sharp et al. examined 29 cases with both ultrasound and MRI examinations, prior to neurectomy for Morton neuroma, and found similar accuracies between the two modalities.[140] On ultrasound examination for Morton neuroma, the patient is scanned on the plantar and dorsal aspect of the foot, over the symptomatic interspace. Pressure applied to the foot on the surface opposite the transducer helps splay the metatarsals and improve visualization. Morton neuroma often appears as a hypoechoic intermetatarsal mass on ultrasound images, but it can be heterogeneous with hyperechoic and anechoic foci.[141] Enhanced through-transmission (hyperechoic appearance of tissues deep to the lesion, relative to surrounding tissues) may be seen. Scanning in the sagittal plane may help demonstrate continuity of the mass with a portion of the plantar digital nerve. Small neuromas may be beyond the

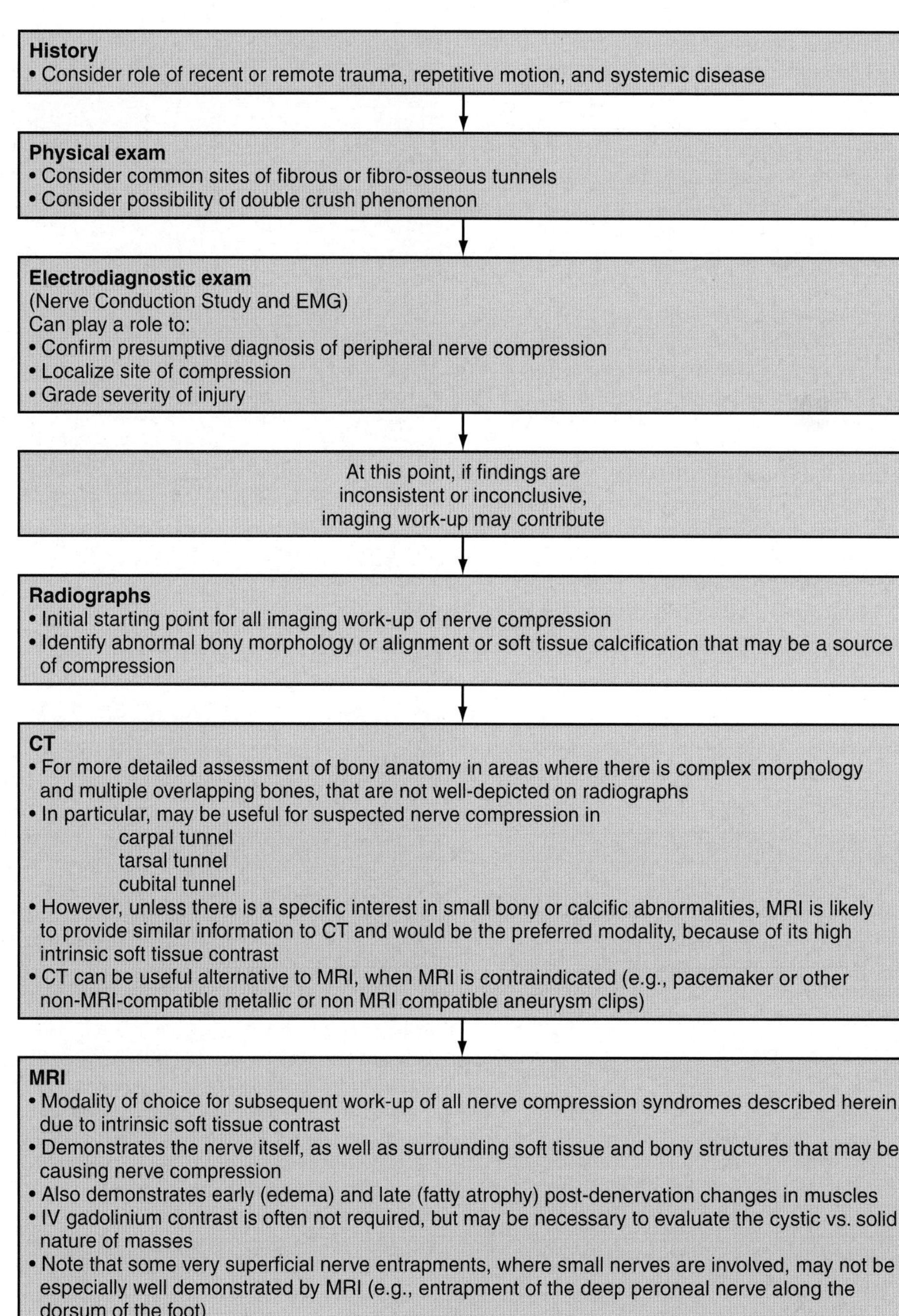

FIGURE 14-26. Recommended work-up of suspected peripheral nerve compression.

resolution limits of ultrasound, although most symptomatic neuromas tend to be larger than 5 mm.[139] As with MRI, the differential diagnosis includes fluid in the intermetatarsal bursa and other masses.

CONCLUSION

Nerve compression is a common entity that can result in considerable morbidity. There are numerous causes of nerve compression, including trauma, space-occupying lesions, inflammatory changes, and dynamic compression with motion. Early diagnosis is important in order to institute prompt treatment and minimize potential injury. Although the appropriate diagnosis is often determined by clinical exam, the diagnosis may be more difficult when the presentation is atypical or when anatomic and technical limitations complicate the clinical picture. In these instances, imaging can play an important role in helping to define the site and the etiology of nerve compression or in establishing an alternative diagnosis. Bony abnormalities contributing to nerve compression are best assessed by radiographs or CT. MRI and ultrasound provide direct visualization of the nerve and surrounding abnormalities. For both modalities, the use of high-resolution techniques is important (Figure 14-26).

REFERENCES

1. Hilburn JW: General principles and use of electrodiagnostic studies in carpal and cubital tunnel syndromes. With special, attention to pitfalls and interpretation, *Hand Clin* 12:205-221, 1996.
2. Campbell WW: Diagnosis and management of common compression and entrapment neuropathies, *Neurol Clin* 15:549-567, 1997.
3. Simpson RL, Fern SA: Multiple compression neuropathies and the double-crush syndrome, *Orthop Clin North Am* 27:381-388, 1996.
4. Yoshizawa H: Presidential address: pathomechanism of myelopathy and radiculopathy from the viewpoint of blood flow and cerebrospinal fluid flow including a short historical review, *Spine* 27:1255-1263, 2002.
5. Delfiner JS: Dynamics and pathophysiology of nerve compression in the upper extremity, *Orthop Clin North Am* 27:219-226, 1996.
6. Pecina M, Krmpotic-Nemanic J, Markiewitz A: *Tunnel syndromes: peripheral nerve compression syndromes,* ed 3, New York, 2001, CRC Press.
7. Kim S, Choi JY, Huh YM et al: Role of magnetic resonance imaging in entrapment and compressive neuropathy—what, where, and how to see the peripheral nerves on the musculoskeletal magnetic resonance image: part 1. Overview and lower extremity, *Eur Radiol* 17:139-149, 2007.
8. Kim S, Choi JY, Huh YM et al: Role of magnetic resonance imaging in entrapment and compressive neuropathy—what, where, and how to see the peripheral nerves on the musculoskeletal magnetic resonance image: part 2. Upper extremity, *Eur Radiol* 17:509-522, 2007.
9. Andreisek G, Crook DW, Burg D et al: Peripheral neuropathies of the median, radial, and ulnar nerves: MR imaging features, *Radiographics* 26:1267-1287, 2006.
10. Sadowski EA, Bennett LK, Chan MR et al: Nephrogenic systemic fibrosis: risk factors and incidence estimation, *Radiology* 243:148-157, 2007.
11. Kim YS, Yeh LR, Trudell D et al: MR imaging of the major nerves about the elbow: cadaveric study examining the effect of flexion and extension of the elbow and pronation and supination of the forearm, *Skeletal Radiol* 27:419-426, 1998.
12. Beltran J, Rosenberg ZS: Diagnosis of compressive and entrapment neuropathies of the upper extremity: value of MR imaging, *AJR Am J Roentgenol* 163:525-531, 1994.
13. Rosenberg ZS, Beltran J, Cheung YY et al: The elbow: MR features of nerve disorders, *Radiology* 88:235-240, 1993.
14. Loredo R, Hodler J, Pedowitz R et al: MRI of the common peroneal nerve: normal anatomy and evaluation of masses associated with nerve entrapment, *J Comput Assist Tomogr* 22:925-931, 1998.
15. Mesgarzadeh M, Schneck CD, Bonakdarpour A: Carpal tunnel: MR imaging. Part I. Normal anatomy, *Radiology* 171:743-748, 1989.
16. Hormann M, Traxler H, Ba-Ssalamah A et al: Correlative high-resolution MR-anatomic study of sciatic, ulnar, and proper palmar digital nerve, *Magn Reson Imaging* 21:879-885, 2003.
17. Aagaard BD, Maravilla KR, Kliot M: MR neurography. MR imaging of peripheral nerves, *Magn Reson Imaging Clin N Am* 6:179-194, 1998.
18. Aagaard BD, Lazar DA, Lankerovich L et al: High-resolution magnetic resonance imaging is a noninvasive method of observing injury and recovery in the peripheral nervous system, *Neurosurgery* 53:199-203, 2003; discussion 204.
19. Filler AG, Maravilla KR, Tsuruda JS: MR neurography and muscle MR imaging for image diagnosis of disorders affecting the peripheral nerves and musculature, *Neurol Clin* 22:643-682, vi-vii, 2004.
20. Filler AG, Howe FA, Hayes CE et al: Magnetic resonance neurography, *Lancet* 341:659-661, 1993.
21. Freund W, Brinkmann A, Wagner F et al: MR neurography with multiplanar reconstruction of 3D MRI datasets: an anatomical study and clinical applications, *Neuroradiology* 249:335-341, 2007.
22. Bendszus M, Wessig C, Solymosi L et al: MRI of peripheral nerve degeneration and regeneration: correlation with electrophysiology and histology, *Exp Neurol* 188: 171-177, 2004.
23. Jinkins JR: MR of enhancing nerve roots in the unoperated lumbosacral spine, *AJNR Am J Neuroradiol* 14:193-202, 1993.
24. Sugimoto H, Miyaji N, Ohsawa T: Carpal tunnel syndrome: evaluation of median nerve circulation with dynamic contrast-enhanced MR imaging, *Radiology* 190: 459-466, 1994.
25. Lane JI, Koeller KK, Atkinson JL: Contrast-enhanced radicular veins on MR of the lumbar spine in an asymptomatic study group, *AJNR Am J Neuroradiol* 16: 269-273, 1995.
26. Bendszus M, Koltzenburg M, Wessig C et al: Sequential MR imaging of denervated muscle: experimental study, *AJNR Am J Neuroradiol* 23:1427-1431, 2002.
27. Fleckenstein JL: Muscle water shifts, volume changes, and proton T2 relaxation times after exercise, *J Appl Physiol* 74:2047-2048, 1993.
28. Grainger AJ, Campbell RS, Stothard J: Anterior interosseous nerve syndrome: appearance at MR imaging in three cases, *Radiology* 208:381-384, 1998.
29. Kransdorf MJ: Musculoskeletal neoplasms. In Berquist TH (ed): *MRI of the musculoskeletal system,* Philadelphia, 2001, Lippincott, Williams and Wilkins, pp 842-955.
30. Chiou HJ, Chou YH, Chiou SY et al: Peripheral nerve lesions: role of high-resolution US, *Radiographics* 23:e15, 2003.
31. Stuart RM, Koh ES, Breidahl WH: Sonography of peripheral nerve pathology, *AJR Am J Roentgenol* 182:123-139, 2004.
32. Martinoli C, Bianchi S, Gandolfo N et al: US of nerve entrapments in osteofibrous tunnels of the upper and lower limbs, *Radiographics* 20:S199-S213, 2000; discussion S7.
33. Martinoli C, Bianchi S, Dahmane M et al: Ultrasound of tendons and nerves, *Eur Radiol* 12:44-55, 2002.
34. Martinoli C, Bianchi S, Pugliese F, et al. Sonography of entrapment neuropathies in the upper limb (wrist excluded). *J Clin Ultrasound* 32(9):438-50, 2004.
35. Peer S, Kovacs P, Harpf C et al: High-resolution sonography of lower extremity peripheral nerves: anatomic correlation and spectrum of disease, *J Ultrasound Med* 21:315-322, 2002.
36. Gruber H, Glodny B, Bendix N et al: High-resolution ultrasound of peripheral neurogenic tumors, *Eur Radiol* 17(11):2880-2888, 2007.
37. Silvestri E, Martinoli C, Derchi LE et al: Echotexture of peripheral nerves: correlation between US and histologic findings and criteria to differentiate tendons, *Radiology* 197:291-296, 1995.
38. Fornage BD: Musculoskeletal ultrasound, New York, 1995, Churchill Livingstone.
39. Chiou HJ, Chou YH, Wu JJ et al: Alternative and effective treatment of shoulder ganglion cyst: ultrasonographically guided aspiration, *J Ultrasound Med* 18:531-535, 1999.
40. Yukata K, Arai K, Yoshizumi Y et al: Obturator neuropathy caused by an acetabular labral cyst: MRI findings, *AJR Am J Roentgenol* 184(3 Suppl):S112-S114, 2005.
41. Pollak RA, Bellacosa RA, Dornbluth NC et al: Sonographic analysis of Morton neuroma, *J Foot Surg* 31:534-537, 1992.
42. Hide IG, Grainger AJ, Naisby GP et al: Sonographic findings in the anterior interosseous nerve syndrome, *J Clin Ultrasound* 27:459-464, 1999.
43. Fritz RC, Helms CA, Steinbach LS et al: Suprascapular nerve entrapment: evaluation with MR imaging, *Radiology* 182:437-444, 1992.
44. Tirman PF, Feller JF, Janzen DL et al: Association of glenoid labral cysts with labral tears and glenohumeral instability: radiologic findings and clinical significance, *Radiology* 190:653-658, 1994.
45. Carroll KW, Helms CA, Otte MT et al: Enlarged spinoglenoid notch veins causing suprascapular nerve compression, *Skeletal Radiol* 32:72-77, 2003.
46. Gaskin CM, Helms CA: Parsonage-Turner syndrome: MR imaging findings and clinical information of 27 patients, *Radiology* 240:501-507, 2006.
47. Scalf RE, Wenger DE, Frick MA et al: MRI findings of 26 patients with Parsonage Turner syndrome, *AJR Am J Roentgenol* 189:W39-W44, 2007.
48. Cahill BR, Palmer RE: Quadrilateral space syndrome, *J Hand Surg (Am)* 8:65-69, 1983.
49. Ball CM, Steger T, Galatz LM et al: The posterior branch of the axillary nerve: an anatomic study, *J Bone Joint Surg (Am)* 85:1497-1501, 2003.
50. Linker CS, Helms CA, Fritz RC: Quadrilateral space syndrome: findings at MR imaging, *Radiology* 188:675-676, 1993.
51. Cothran RL Jr, Helms C: Quadrilateral space syndrome: incidence of imaging findings in a population referred for MRI of the shoulder, *AJR Am J Roentgenol* 184:989-992, 2005.
52. Sofka CM, Lin J, Feinberg J et al: Teres minor denervation on routine magnetic resonance imaging of the shoulder, *Skeletal Radiol* 33:514-518, 2004.
53. Mochizuki T, Isoda H, Masui T et al: Occlusion of the posterior humeral circumflex artery: detection with MR angiography in healthy volunteers and in a patient with quadrilateral space syndrome, *AJR Am J Roentgenol* 163:625-627, 1994.
54. Kleinert JM, Mehta S: Radial nerve entrapment, *Orthop Clin North Am* 27:305-315, 1996.
55. Konjengbam M, Elangbam J: Radial nerve in the radial tunnel: anatomic sites of entrapment neuropathy, *Clin Anat* 17:21-25, 2004.
56. Ritts GD, Wood MB, Linscheid RL: Radial tunnel syndrome. A ten-year surgical experience, *Clin Orthop Relat Res* (219):201-205, 1987.
57. Fernandez AM, Tiku ML: Posterior interosseous nerve entrapment in rheumatoid arthritis, *Semin Arthritis Rheum* 24:57-60, 1994.

58. Ferdinand BD, Rosenberg ZS, Schweitzer ME et al: MR imaging features of radial tunnel syndrome: initial experience, *Radiology* 240:161-168, 2006.
59. Chien AJ, Jamadar DA, Jacobson JA et al: Sonography and MR imaging of posterior interosseous nerve syndrome with surgical correlation, *AJR Am J Roentgenol* 181: 219-221, 2003.
60. Bodner G, Harpf C, Meirer R et al: Ultrasonographic appearance of supinator syndrome, *J Ultrasound Med* 21:1289-1293, 2002.
61. Folberg CR, Weiss AP, Akelman E: Cubital tunnel syndrome. Part I: Presentation and diagnosis, *Orthopaed Rev* 23:136-144, 1994.
62. Posner MA: Compressive neuropathies of the ulnar nerve at the elbow and wrist. *Instr Course Lect* 49:305-317, 2000.
63. Kato H, Hirayama T, Minami A et al: Cubital tunnel syndrome associated with medial elbow Ganglia and osteoarthritis of the elbow, *J Bone Joint Surg (Am)* 84:1413-1419, 2002.
64. Aoki M, Takasaki H, Muraki T et al: Strain on the ulnar nerve at the elbow and wrist during throwing motion, *J Bone Joint Surg (Am)* 87:2508-2514, 2005.
65. Gelberman RH, Yamaguchi K, Hollstien SB et al: Changes in interstitial pressure and cross-sectional area of the cubital tunnel and of the ulnar nerve with flexion of the elbow. An experimental study in human cadavera, *J Bone Joint Surg (Am)* 80: 492-501, 1998.
66. Frank ED LB, Smith BJ, eds: *Merrill's atlas of radiographic positions and radiologic procedures*, ed 6, St. Louis, 1986, C.V. Mosby Co.
67. Britz GW, Haynor DR, Kuntz C et al: Ulnar nerve entrapment at the elbow: correlation of magnetic resonance imaging, clinical, electrodiagnostic, and intraoperative findings, *Neurosurgery* 38:458-465, 1996; discussion 65.
68. Chiou HJ, Chou YH, Cheng SP et al: Cubital tunnel syndrome: diagnosis by high-resolution ultrasonography, *J Ultrasound Med* 17:643-648, 1998.
69. Wiesler ER, Chloros GD, Cartwright MS et al: Ultrasound in the diagnosis of ulnar neuropathy at the cubital tunnel, *J Hand Surg (Am)* 31:1088-1093, 2006.
70. Jacobson JA, Jebson PJ, Jeffers AW et al: Ulnar nerve dislocation and snapping triceps syndrome: diagnosis with dynamic sonography—report of three cases, *Radiology* 220:601-605, 2001.
71. Grechenig W, Mayr J, Peicha G et al: Subluxation of the ulnar nerve in the elbow region—ultrasonographic evaluation, *Acta Radiol* 44:662-664, 2003.
72. Rehak DC: Pronator syndrome, *Clin Sports Med* 20:531-540, 2001.
73. Newman A: The supracondylar process and its fracture, *Am J Roentgenol Radium Ther Nucl Med* 105:844-849, 1969.
74. Pecina M, Boric I, Anticevic D: Intraoperatively proven anomalous Struthers' ligament diagnosed by MRI, *Skeletal Radiol* 31:532-535, 2002.
75. Ozan H, Atasever A, Sinav A et al: An unusual insertion of accessory biceps brachii muscle, *Kaibogaku Zasshi* 72:515-519, 1997.
76. Nagano A: Spontaneous anterior interosseous nerve palsy, *J Bone Joint Surg (Br)* 85:313-318, 2003.
77. Kulick RG: Carpal tunnel syndrome, *Orthop Clin North Am* 27:345-354, 1996.
78. Mesgarzadeh M, Schneck CD, Bonakdarpour A et al: Carpal tunnel: MR imaging. Part II. Carpal tunnel syndrome, *Radiology* 171:749-754, 1989.
79. Mesgarzadeh M, Triolo J, Schneck CD: Carpal tunnel syndrome. MR imaging diagnosis, *Magn Reson Imaging Clin North Am* 3:249-264, 1995.
80. Jarvik JG, Yuen E, Haynor DR et al: MR nerve imaging in a prospective cohort of patients with suspected carpal tunnel syndrome, *Neurology* 58:1597-1602, 2002.
81. Jarvik JG, Yuen E, Kliot M: Diagnosis of carpal tunnel syndrome: electrodiagnostic and MR imaging evaluation, *Neuroimaging Clin North Am* 14:93-102, viii, 2004.
82. Radack DM, Schweitzer ME, Taras J: Carpal tunnel syndrome: are the MR findings a result of population selection bias? *AJR Am J Roentgenol* 169:1649-1653, 1997.
83. Murphy RX Jr, Chernofsky MA, Osborne MA et al: Magnetic resonance imaging in the evaluation of persistent carpal tunnel syndrome, *J Hand Surg (Am)* 18:113-120, 1993.
84. Chen P, Maklad N, Redwine M et al: Dynamic high-resolution sonography of the carpal tunnel, *AJR Am J Roentgenol* 168:533-537, 1997.
85. Lew HL, Chen CP, Wang TG et al: Introduction to musculoskeletal diagnostic ultrasound: examination of the upper limb, *Am J Phys Med Rehabil* 86:310-321, 2007.
86. Buchberger W, Schon G, Strasser K et al: High-resolution ultrasonography of the carpal tunnel, *J Ultrasound Med* 10:531-537, 1991.
87. Duncan I, Sullivan P, Lomas F: Sonography in the diagnosis of carpal tunnel syndrome, *AJR Am J Roentgenol* 173:681-684, 1999.
88. Wong SM, Griffith JF, Hui AC et al: Discriminatory sonographic criteria for the diagnosis of carpal tunnel syndrome, *Arthritis Rheum* 46:1914-1921, 2002.
89. El Miedany YM, Aty SA, Ashour S: Ultrasonography versus nerve conduction study in patients with carpal tunnel syndrome: substantive or complementary tests? *Rheumatology (Oxford)* 43:887-895, 2004.
90. Lee D, van Holsbeeck MT, Janevski PK et al: Diagnosis of carpal tunnel syndrome. Ultrasound versus electromyography, *Radiol Clin North Am* 37:859-872, x, 1999.
91. Lee CH, Kim TK, Yoon ES et al: Correlation of high-resolution ultrasonographic findings with the clinical symptoms and electrodiagnostic data in carpal tunnel syndrome, *Ann Plast Surg* 54:20-23, 2005.
92. Mallouhi A, Pulzl P, Trieb T et al: Predictors of carpal tunnel syndrome: accuracy of gray-scale and color Doppler sonography, *AJR Am J Roentgenol* 186:1240-1245, 2006.
93. Hammer HB, Haavardsholm EA, Kvien TK: Ultrasonographic measurement of the cross-sectional area of the median nerve in patients with rheumatoid arthritis without symptoms or signs of carpal tunnel syndrome, *Ann Rheum Dis* 66(6):825-827, 2006.
94. Buchberger W: Radiologic imaging of the carpal tunnel, *Eur J Radiol* 25:112-117, 1997.
95. Buchberger W, Judmaier W, Birbamer G et al: Carpal tunnel syndrome: diagnosis with high-resolution sonography, *AJR Am J Roentgenol* 159:793-798, 1992.
96. Keberle M, Jenett M, Kenn W et al. Technical advances in ultrasound and MR imaging of carpal tunnel syndrome, *Eur Radiol* 10:1043-1050, 2000.
97. Zeiss J, Jakab E, Khimji T et al: The ulnar tunnel at the wrist (Guyon's canal): normal MR anatomy and variants, *AJR Am J Roentgenol* 158:1081-1085, 1992.
98. Dodds GA 3rd, Hale D, Jackson WT: Incidence of anatomic variants in Guyon's canal, *J Hand Surg (Am)* 15:352-355, 1990.
99. Bui-Mansfield LT, Williamson M, Wheeler DT et al: Guyon's canal lipoma causing ulnar neuropathy, *AJR Am J Roentgenol* 178:1458, 2002.
100. Pingree MJ, Bosch EP, Liu P et al: Delayed ulnar neuropathy at the wrist following open carpal tunnel release, *Muscle Nerve* 31:394-397, 2005.
101. Blum AG, Zabel JP, Kohlmann R et al: Pathologic conditions of the hypothenar eminence: evaluation with multidetector CT and MR imaging, *Radiographics* 26:1021-1044, 2006.
102. Rodrigue T, Hardy RW: Diagnosis and treatment of piriformis syndrome, *Neurosurg Clin North Am* 12:311-319, 2001.
103. Jankiewicz JJ, Hennrikus WL, Houkom JA: The appearance of the piriformis muscle syndrome in computed tomography and magnetic resonance imaging. A case report and review of the literature, *Clin Orthop Relat Res* (262):205-209, 1991.
104. Rossi P, Cardinali P, Serrao M et al: Magnetic resonance imaging findings in piriformis syndrome: a case report, *Arch Phys Med Rehabil* 82:519-521, 2001.
105. Laborde A, Hermier M, Cotton F: Clinical vignette. Sciatic nerve entrapment secondary to heterotopic ossification: imaging findings and potential effect of selective cox-2 inhibitors, *Rheumatology (Oxford)* 44:110, 2005.
106. Sherman PM, Matchette MW, Sanders TG et al: Acetabular paralabral cyst: an uncommon cause of sciatica, *Skeletal Radiol* 32:90-94, 2003.
107. Leversedge FJ, Gelberman RH, Clohisy JC: Entrapment of the sciatic nerve by the femoral neck following closed reduction of a hip prosthesis: a case report, *J Bone Joint Surg (Am)* 84:1210-1213, 2002.
108. Crawford JR, Van Rensburg L, Marx C: Compression of the sciatic nerve by wear debris following total hip replacement: a report of three cases, *J Bone Joint Surg (Br)* 85:1178-1180, 2003.
109. Bendszus M, Rieckmann P, Perez J et al: Painful vascular compression syndrome of the sciatic nerve caused by gluteal varicosities, *Neurology* 61:985-987, 2003.
110. Broadhurst NA, Simmons DN, Bond MJ: Piriformis syndrome: correlation of muscle morphology with symptoms and signs, *Arch Phys Med Rehabil* 85:2036-2039, 2004.
111. Sansone V, Sosio C, da Gama Malcher M et al: Two cases of tibial nerve compression caused by uncommon popliteal cysts, *Arthroscopy* 18:E8, 2002.
112. Logigian EL, Berger AR, Shahani BT: Injury to the tibial and peroneal nerves due to hemorrhage in the popliteal fossa. Two case reports, *J Bone Joint Surg (Am)* 71: 768-770, 1989.
113. Mastaglia FL: Tibial nerve entrapment in the popliteal fossa, *Muscle Nerve* 23: 1883-1886, 2000.
114. Finkel JE: Tarsal tunnel syndrome, *Magn Reson Imaging Clin North Am* 2:67-78, 1994.
115. Havel PE, Ebraheim NA, Clark SE et al: Tibial nerve branching in the tarsal tunnel, *Foot Ankle* 9:117-119, 1988.
116. Kinoshita M, Okuda R, Yasuda T et al: Tarsal tunnel syndrome in athletes, *Am J Sports Med* 34:1307-1312, 2006.
117. Heimkes B, Posel P, Stotz S et al: The proximal and distal tarsal tunnel syndromes. An anatomical study, *Int Orthop* 11:193-196, 1987.
118. Franson J, Baravarian B: Tarsal tunnel syndrome: a compression neuropathy involving four distinct tunnels, *Clin Podiatr Med Surg* 23:597-609, 2006.
119. Takakura Y, Kumai T, Takaoka T et al: Tarsal tunnel syndrome caused by coalition associated with a ganglion, *J Bone Joint Surg (Br)* 80:130-133, 1998.
120. Erickson SJ, Quinn SF, Kneeland JB et al: MR imaging of the tarsal tunnel and related spaces: normal and abnormal findings with anatomic correlation, *AJR Am J Roentgenol* 155:323-328, 1990.
121. Pfeiffer WH, Cracchiolo A 3rd: Clinical results after tarsal tunnel decompression, *J Bone Joint Surg (Am)* 76:1222-1230, 1994.
122. Klein MA, Spreitzer AM: MR imaging of the tarsal sinus and canal: normal anatomy, pathologic findings, and features of the sinus tarsi syndrome, *Radiology* 186:233-240, 1993.
123. Beltran J: Sinus tarsi syndrome, *Magn Reson Imaging Clin North Am* 2:59-65, 1994.
124. Dellon AL, Barrett SL: Sinus tarsi denervation: clinical results, *J Am Podiatr Med Assoc* 95:108-113, 2005.
125. Rosenberg Z, Beltran J, Bencardino JT: MR imaging of the ankle and foot. *Radiographics* 20:S153-179, 2000.
126. Taillard W, Meyer JM, Garcia J et al: The sinus tarsi syndrome, *Int Orthop* 5: 117-130, 1981.
127. Berquist T: Soft tissue trauma and overuse syndromes. In T. Berquist (ed): *Radiology of the foot and ankle*, ed 2, Philadelphia, 2000, Lippincott, Williams and Wilkins, pp 59, 105-170.
128. Beltran J, Munchow AM, Khabiri H et al: Ligaments of the lateral aspect of the ankle and sinus tarsi: an MR imaging study, *Radiology* 177:455-458, 1990.
129. Sofka CM, Adler RS: Ultrasound-guided interventions in the foot and ankle, *Semin Musculoskelet Radiol* 6:163-168, 2002.
130. Kuwada GT: Long-term retrospective analysis of the treatment of sinus tarsi syndrome, *J Foot Ankle Surg* 33:28-29, 1994.
131. Zanetti M, Weishaupt D: MR imaging of the forefoot: Morton neuroma and differential diagnoses, *Semin Musculoskelet Radiol* 9:175-186, 2005.
132. Zanetti M, Ledermann T, Zollinger H et al: Efficacy of MR imaging in patients suspected of having Morton's neuroma, *AJR Am J Roentgenol* 168:529-532, 1997.

133. Weishaupt D, Treiber K, Kundert HP et al: Morton neuroma: MR imaging in prone, supine, and upright weight-bearing body positions, *Radiology* 226:849-856, 2003.
134. Zanetti M, Strehle JK, Zollinger H et al: Morton neuroma and fluid in the intermetatarsal bursae on MR images of 70 asymptomatic volunteers, *Radiology* 203: 516-520, 1997.
135. Berquist T, McLeod RA: Bone and soft tissue tumors and tumor-like conditions. In Berquist TH (ed): *Radiology of the foot and ankle*, ed 2, Philadelphia, 2000, Lippincott, Williams and Wilkins, pp 315-356.
136. Zanetti M, Strehle JK, Kundert HP et al: Morton neuroma: effect of MR imaging findings on diagnostic thinking and therapeutic decisions, *Radiology* 213:583-588, 1999.
137. Bencardino J, Rosenberg ZS, Beltran J et al: Morton's neuroma: is it always symptomatic? *AJR Am J Roentgenol* 175:649-653, 2000.
138. Shapiro PP, Shapiro SL: Sonographic evaluation of interdigital neuromas, *Foot Ankle Int* 16:604-606, 1995.
139. Redd RA, Peters VJ, Emery SF et al: Morton neuroma: sonographic evaluation, *Radiology* 171:415-417, 1989.
140. Sharp RJ, Wade CM, Hennessy MS et al: The role of MRI and ultrasound imaging in Morton's neuroma and the effect of size of lesion on symptoms, *J Bone Joint Surg (Br)* 85:999-1005, 2003.
141. Quinn TJ, Jacobson JA, Craig JG et al: Sonography of Morton's neuromas, *AJR Am J Roentgenol* 174:1723-1728, 2000.

CHAPTER 15

Imaging Findings of Drug-Related Musculoskeletal Disorders

LEYLA H. ALPARSLAN, MD, *and* BARBARA N. WEISSMAN, MD

KEY FACTS

- Osteoporosis, osteomalacia, osteosclerosis, hyperostosis, and osteonecrosis may be related to drug effects.
- Methotrexate osteopathy is characterized by bone pain, osteoporosis, and insufficiency fractures.
- Antiepileptic drugs may cause rickets, osteomalacia, osteoporosis, and increased risk for fracture, and phenytoin can cause calvarial thickening.
- Retinoids may produce birth defects, hyperostosis, ligament calcification, or ligament ossification.
- Fluorosis results in characteristic skeletal changes, including osteosclerosis and calcification or ossification of tendons and ligaments.
- Fluoroquinolones may produce tendinopathy or tendon tears, especially in patients with other predisposing conditions.
- Demyelinating lesions in the central nervous system may occur in patients receiving antitumor necrosis factor alpha drugs.
- Infection may complicate immunosuppressive or anti-TNF alpha drugs.

In this chapter, musculoskeletal and teratogenic side effects of certain drugs and chemical substances are reviewed. Some of the medications taken for the treatment of arthritis and skin and epileptic diseases, as well as corticosteroids, anticoagulants, and antineoplastic drugs, can profoundly affect the skeleton. Osteoporosis, osteomalacia, osteosclerosis, and hyperostosis may result.

TERATOGENIC DRUGS

A teratogen is an agent that can disturb the development of the embryo or fetus, resulting in spontaneous abortion, congenital malformations, intrauterine growth retardation, mental retardation, carcinogenesis, or mutagenesis.[1,2] Known teratogens include radiation, maternal infections, chemicals, and drugs. Among possible teratogens, drugs account for approximately 1% of all congenital malformations of known etiology.[3,4] All teratogenic drugs generally produce a specific pattern or single malformation during a sensitive period of gestation with a dose-dependent effect.[5]

> Teratogenic drugs generally produce a specific pattern of abnormalities or a single malformation during a sensitive period of gestation with a dose-dependent effect.

The American Food and Drug Administration (FDA) instituted a rating system for drugs marketed after 1980 based on their safety during pregnancy. Five pharmaceutical categories have been elaborated: A, B, C, D, and X. Drugs under Category A are the safest drugs in which no fetal risks have been demonstrated during controlled human studies, while those under Category X present proven teratogenicity that clearly outweighs their benefits. Category D drugs have demonstrated risks to the human fetus, but in serious diseases or life-threatening situations their benefits outweigh these risks.[6]

Retinoids

The term *retinoids* includes all compounds, synthetic and natural, that possess vitamin A activity. Isotretinoin, etretinate, and acitretin are potent teratogens. The birth defects characteristically induced by oral retinoids known as retinoic acid embryopathy include abnormalities involving central nervous system, cardiovascular system, craniofacial structures, thymus, and skeletal system. Retinoid effects on neural crest cells during the fourth week after fertilization may be responsible for many of the observed malformations.[7]

The most common reported craniofacial and skeletal malformations include microcephaly, cleft plate, micrognathia, abnormalities of the external ears (anotia, microtia, rudimentary ears), and abnormal or absent auditory canals. Affected children may also have a depressed midface, large occiput, and narrow frontal bone.[8] Limb reduction and duplication have also been reported.[9] The clinical expression of retinoic acid embryopathy may vary with type of the retinoid; etretinate is more likely to induce acral skeletal malformations and less likely to induce cardiac malformations.[10] Cardiac malformations include atrial and ventricular septal defects, overriding aorta, interrupted or hypoplastic arch, and subclavian arteries. Central nervous system abnormalities range from retinal or optic nerve abnormalities to hydrocephalus and cognitive and behavioral changes[11-14] (Table 15-1).

Anticonvulsants

The overall risk of congenital anomalies among the infants of epileptic mothers treated with antiepileptic drugs during pregnancy is 2 to 3 times higher than the "baseline" risk of every pregnancy, which has been estimated to be between 3% and 5%.[15-19]

The risk of fetal malformation is increased up to 15% with polytherapy.[20-22] The combination of valproic acid, carbamazepine, and phenytoin or phenobarbital seems to have the highest risk.

The diphenylhydantoin syndrome occurs in 5% to 10% of babies born to a mother under therapy with the drug.[23] The

TABLE 15-1. Drugs with Teratogenic Effects to Musculoskeletal System at Therapeutic Doses

DRUGS (FDA Category)	Maternal Condition	Musculoskeletal Anomalies	Other Anomalies
Thalidomide (X)	Insomnia, oropharyngeal and esophageal ulcers associated with AIDS, immunopathologic disease, multiple myeloma, graft-versus-host disease, leprosy	Limb reduction	Cardiac defects, renal and gastrointestinal anomalies, deafness, mental retardation, autism
Retinoids (X)	Dermatologic disease	Facial dysmorphia	CNS, ear and cardiac malformations
Coumarin derivatives dicumarol, warfarin	Thromboembolic disorders	Stippled epiphyses	CNS anomalies, intracranial hemorrhage
Anticonvulsants (D) carbamazepine, clonazepam, ethosuximide, phenobarbital, phenytoin, primidone, trimethadione, valproic acid	Epilepsy	Digital hypoplasia, facial dysmorphia	CNS (neural tube defects), cardiac and genitourinary anomalies
Folic acid antagonists (D) methotrexate	Cancer, rheumatic diseases	Large fontanelles, abnormal head shape, craniosynostosis, skeletal defects	

Modified from Polifka JE, Friedman JM, Hall J: Medical genetics: 1. Clinical teratology in the age of genomics, *CMAJ* 167(3): 265-273, 2002.

syndrome includes prenatal onset of growth deficiency, large anterior fontanelle, metopic ridging, ocular hypertelorism and depressed nasal bridge, cleft lip with or without cleft palate, distal phalangeal hypoplasia, digitalized thumb and nail hypoplasia, and cardiac and genitourinary anomalies.[14,24] Valproic acid has been associated with neural tube defects.[25]

Warfarin

The oral anticoagulant warfarin has been recognized as a human teratogen for many years. Warfarin embryopathy is seen in approximately 10% of fetuses with first-trimester exposure to coumarin.[26,27] This distinct pattern of anomalies includes nasal hypoplasia, depressed nasal bridge, and "stippling" of epiphyses of spine, proximal femora, and tarsal and carpal bones, which are visible radiographically.[28,29] X-linked recessive chondrodysplasia punctata (CDPX) and warfarin embryopathy share the same phenotype.[28,30] A different pattern of anomalies with CNS defects is seen with second-trimester and third-trimester exposure to coumarin, possibly secondary to fetal hemorrhage.[31]

Folic Acid Antagonists

Aminopterin and its methyl derivative, methotrexate, are folic acid analogs with antagonistic effects. Methotrexate is currently used in high doses as an antineoplastic agent and in low doses for a variety of rheumatic conditions. These agents have been used to induce abortion in early pregnancy, but their use later in gestation results in prenatal growth deficiency, abnormal skull ossification, ocular hypertelorism, supraorbital ridge hypoplasia, malformed ears, and micrognathia. The skeletal abnormalities may also include talipes equinovarus, short extremities, syndactyly, absent digits, and multiple anomalous ribs.[5,32,33]

Thalidomide

Thalidomide was recognized as a human teratogen in the early 1960s when an unusually large number of infants with severe limb defects and other anomalies were noted in Europe in association with the maternal use of thalidomide.[1-6] It was used as a sleeping pill and to treat morning sickness during pregnancy. It is estimated that more than 10,000 pregnancies were exposed before the drug was withdrawn from the market worldwide.[5]

The risk of teratogenicity is highest between the 34th and 50th days of the pregnancy. Characteristically, thalidomide exposure produces reduction deformities of the limbs, such as dysplasia of the thumbs and radial hemimelia, phocomelia, or complete four limb amelia. Other defects of thalidomide embryopathy include hypoplasia or aplasia of the external ear canal, congenital heart defects, gastrointestinal atresia, and renal malformations.[34-37]

Originally not approved for use in the United States, in 1998 the FDA approved the use of thalidomide for treatment of erythema nodosum leprosum. Currently, its other potential uses in the treatment of AIDs, autoimmune disorders, and multiple myeloma have been suggested,[37] leading once again to concern about thalidomide-induced birth defects.[5,38]

DRUGS ASSOCIATED WITH OSTEOPOROSIS AND OSTEOMALACIA

Corticosteroids

Possible effects of local injection of corticosteroids are discussed in the chapter on joint injections (see Chapter 5).

Corticosteroid-induced osteoporosis is multifactorial and dose dependent.[39] In a metaanalysis by van Staa et al,[40] cumulative dose has been noted to be strongly correlated with loss of bone mineral density and daily dose to be strongly correlated with the risk of fracture. The risk of fracture was found to increase rapidly after the start of oral corticosteroid therapy (within 3 to 6 months) and decrease after stopping therapy. In another study by van Staa et al, a dose dependence of fracture risk was observed; with a standardized daily dose of less than 2.5 mg prednisolone, hip fracture risk was 0.99 (0.82-1.20) relative to control, rising to 1.77 (1.55-2.02) at daily doses of 2.5 to 7.5 mg, and 2.27 (1.94-2.66) at doses of 7.5 mg or greater.

Manelli and Giustina[41,42] note corticosteroid treatment to be associated with increased bone resorption, inhibition of bone formation, decreased intestinal calcium absorption, changes in vitamin D metabolism, and marked hypercalciuria, with variable changes in plasma PTH levels and inhibition of the gonadotropic and somatotropic axis.

Comparison of iliac crest samples from subjects with idiopathic osteoporosis to those with corticosteroid-induced osteoporosis has shown differences in bone microstructure. Aaron et al.[43] showed that loss of trabecular bone volume is common to both groups, but there is a difference in the distribution of the remaining bony tissue and indices of remodeling. A decrease in trabecular number accompanied by a relative increase in resorption characterized primary osteoporosis, whereas a decline in trabecular width associated with depressed formation was the predominant feature in the secondary disease. Investigational micro MRI and CT studies have been used in vivo to better understand the microarchitectural changes in trabecula in osteoporosis including corticosteroid induced osteoporosis.[44,45]

Imaging of osteoporosis is discussed in Chapter 31. Radiographic features of corticosteroid-induced osteoporosis are usually indistinguishable from those of osteoporosis. Insufficiency fractures may result, involving thoracic and lumbar vertebrae, the sacrum, the long bones, and the calcaneus. Generally in patients with acute low back pain (less than 6 weeks in duration) symptoms are self-limited and not considered an indication for imaging. However, osteoporosis or a history of prolonged corticosteroid use are "red flags" that should prompt imaging.[46] Radiographs are the first study suggested. Sclerosis along the compressed vertebral margins is a finding that may be prominent following corticosteroid-related compression fracture (Barbara Weissman, personal communication) (Figure 15-1).

In patients with painful osteoporotic compression fractures treated with vertebroplasty, subsequent fracture has been reported to be more likely to occur in corticosteroid-treated patients than in those with primary osteoporosis. Hiwatashi and Westesson[47] found the incidence of subsequent vertebral compression fractures after vertebroplasty in patients on long-term corticosteroid therapy to be 69% (11/16), compared with 23% (9/39) in those who were not on corticosteroid therapy.[47]

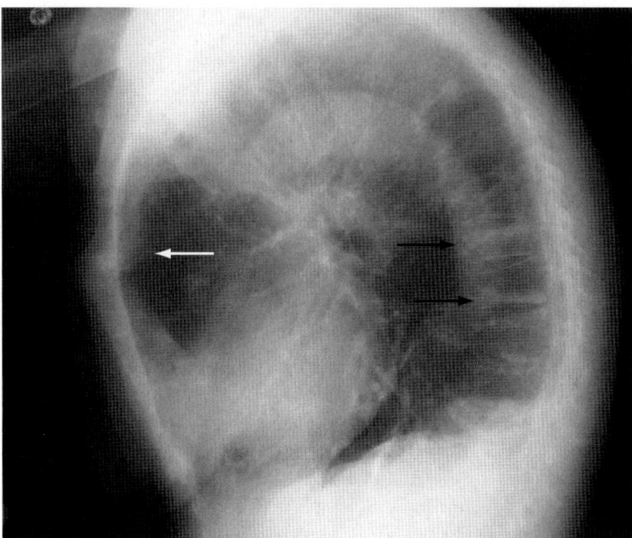

FIGURE 15-1. Osteoporotic compression fractures in a patient on long-term corticosteroids. Lateral radiograph of the chest shows a diffuse kyphosis and generally decreased bone density. There are multiple vertebral compression fractures, several of which show endplate sclerosis (*black arrows*). A displaced sternal fracture (*white arrow*) is noted. Sternal fractures may be a cause of chest pain in patients with osteoporosis and kyphotic deformity.

> Patients on corticosteroids undergoing vertebroplasty appear more likely to develop subsequent vertebral fractures than are patients with primary osteoporosis.

Methotrexate

Methotrexate (MTX) is a folate antagonist commonly used for the treatment of various childhood malignancies and in low doses to control rheumatoid arthritis and psoriasis. Its hematologic, hepatic, and pulmonary toxicities are well recognized. The use of high-dose MTX therapy in pediatric oncology, especially during treatment of acute lymphatic leukemia and osteosarcoma, has been associated with an osteopathy, which is characterized by severe bone pain, osteoporosis, and insufficiency fractures.[48-52] The radiographic changes of MTX osteopathy resemble those of scurvy with severe osteopenia, dense zones of provisional calcification, multiple transverse metaphyseal bands, and metaphyseal fractures involving multiple bones, more frequently in lower extremities (Figure 15-2). The bone pain usually improves within three to four weeks after discontinuing the drug, although the radiographic changes take about four months to resolve.[48,51] Delayed healing of fractures has also been reported, with bone union not occurring until the MTX has been discontinued.[52]

> Methotrexate osteopathy can produce changes on radiographs that resemble those of scurvy with severe osteopenia, dense zones of provisional calcification, multiple transverse metaphyseal bands, and metaphyseal fractures.

Detrimental effects of MTX on the skeleton in patients with rheumatic diseases is more controversial because most patients using MTX have other risk factors for fractures. There have been sporadic case reports of fragility fractures seen in adult patients on low-dose MTX for rheumatoid or psoriatic arthritis.[53-56] Uehara et al[57] have shown in vitro that methotrexate impairs bone formation dose dependently by inhibiting the differentiation of osteoblast precursors. The proliferation and further maturation of cells of the osteoblast lineage are not affected by treatment with MTX. Recent studies have shown no definite adverse effect of long-term, low dose MTX therapy on bone mineral density (BMD) or bone turn over.[58-63]

Antiepileptic Drugs

The antiepileptic drugs (AED) can adversely affect the bones in patients of all ages. Chronic AED therapy can cause rickets, osteomalacia, and osteoporosis with increased risk for fracture.

Several theories have been proposed to explain the link between AEDs and metabolic bone changes. These theories include increased catabolism of vitamin D, impairment of calcium absorption, alteration of bone resorption and formation, abnormal PTH release or cellular responsiveness to PTH, and abnormalities in calcitonin or vitamin K.[64] Antiepileptic drugs (phenytoin, phenobarbital, and carbamazepine) that lead to induction of the cytochrome P-450 enzyme system have been most commonly associated with bone abnormalities.[55,56] Valproate, a newer AED that inhibits the cytochrome P-450 enzyme system, also appears to affect bone adversely. The AEDs that induce cytochrome P-450 enzymes may cause increased conversion of vitamin D to inactive metabolites in the liver, reducing levels of vitamin D.[67] Reduced levels of

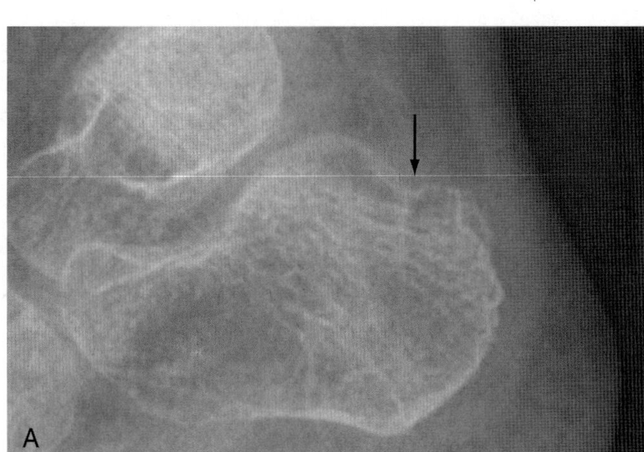

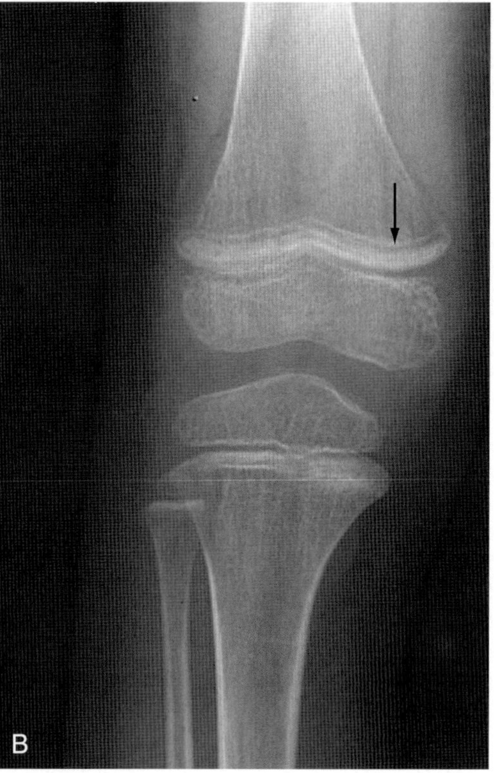

FIGURE 15-2. Methotrexate osteopathy. **A,** Lateral radiograph of a 6-year-old child with acute lymphoblastic leukemia on methotrexate shows diffuse osteopenia. There is deformity of the calcaneus at the site of an insufficiency fracture *(arrow)*. **B,** The AP radiograph of the knee shows osteopenia and dense metaphyseal bands *(arrow)*.

biologically active vitamin D lead to decreased absorption of calcium from the gut, resulting in hypocalcemia and an increase in circulating parathormone.

Early reports described a high incidence of rickets and osteomalacia in patients treated with AEDs.[68,69] However, these reports primarily involved institutionalized patients in whom low dietary calcium and vitamin D intake and reduced exercise level and sunlight exposure probably influenced outcomes. Radiologic evidence of osteomalacia and rickets is rarely found in ambulatory patients[70,71]; when present, radiographic changes are indistinguishable from those of rickets or osteomalacia resulting from other causes.[72] Radiologic findings of rickets appear as widening of growth plate, indistinctness of zones of provisional calcification, widening and cupping of the metaphysis, and deformities of bones. Osteomalacic changes of the bone are seen on radiographs as a decrease in radiographic bone density, coarsened trabecular pattern, and looser zones. Radiologic findings of secondary hyperparathyroidism may accompany these findings.[73]

> Rickets/osteomalacia or osteoporosis can be a side effect of antiepileptic drug treatment.

Children with convulsions and tuberous sclerosis appear to be particularly vulnerable to developing AED-induced rickets.[74] The diuretic acetazolamide (Diamox), which is a carbonic anhydrase inhibitor, produces a renal tubular acidosis with increased excretion of calcium and phosphorus and can accentuate AED-induced rickets or osteomalacia.[75,76]

Long-term treatment with AEDs is a recognized factor that can contribute to the development of osteoporosis. Several studies using dual x-ray absorptiometry (DXA) in patients receiving AEDs have shown significantly reduced BMD, both in adults and children.[77-82] AED use has been reported to increase the fracture risk, independent from the increased fracture rate described in epileptic patients[83,84] (Figure 15-3).

In addition, phenytoin (Dilantin) has been associated with calvarial thickening and enlargement of the heel pad, similar to the changes occurring in acromegaly.[85,86]

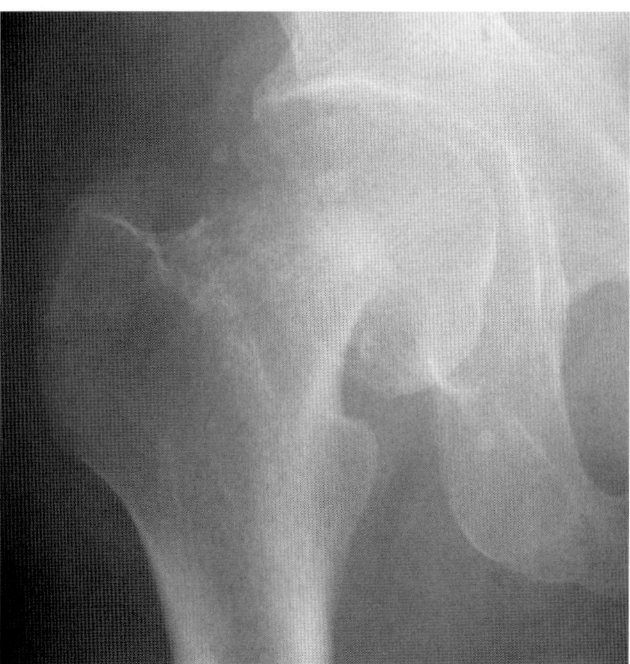

FIGURE 15-3. Dilantin bone changes. This 30-year-old man was on chronic Dilantin therapy. AP view of the hip shows a displaced subcapital femoral fracture.

Deferoxamine

Deferoxamine is an iron-chelating agent used to remove excess iron during the treatment of patients with transfusion-dependent anemias such as beta-thalassemia major. Iron overload caused by hypertransfusion may result in toxicity and dysfunction of the heart, liver, and endocrine organs. Parenteral chelation therapy with deferoxamine prolongs the life expectancy in these patients; however, deferoxamine therapy also has its own risks, causing sensorineural ototoxicity, ocular toxicity, growth retardation, and bone dysplasia. These undesirable effects of deferoxamine can be largely avoided if optimal dose and timing of the therapy is adjusted.

In 1988, de Virgiliis et al.[87] described radiologic abnormalities similar to those of rickets in the metaphyses of long bones in 70% of thalassemic patients undergoing chelation therapy. Growth retardation and metaphyseal abnormalities were noted to occur frequently in patients in whom chelation was started before the age of 3 years. The mechanism by which deferoxamine affects bone is not entirely understood. Chelation of zinc[87] and the antiproliferative effect of deferoxamine may be the underlying pathophysiologic mechanisms.[88,89]

The radiologic changes seen in metaphyses of long bones are most commonly detected in the distal ends of the ulna, radius, femur, and proximal tibia.[90-92] These include peripheral deficiency of bone at the metaphysis, asymmetric widening of the growth plate, irregular metaphyseal sclerosis, and lucencies with sclerotic margins.

> Radiographic findings following deferoxamine treatment include peripheral deficiency of bone at the metaphysis, asymmetric widening of growth plate, irregular metaphyseal sclerosis, and lucencies with sclerotic margins that are most prominent at the wrists and knees.

The thoracic and lumbar vertebrae may show flattening with loss of height. Olivieri et al.[93] demonstrated significant decline in height percentile in patients who started on deferoxamine prior to age 2 years.

MRI findings of deferoxamine-induced bone dysplasia in the distal femur and patella in thalassemic patients have been described by Chan and his colleagues.[92] They detected blurring of the physeal-metaphyseal junction, hyperintense areas in the distal metaphysis, and physeal widening. Physeal widening and distal metaphyseal hyperintensities were all more pronounced peripherally. Linear or irregular low-signal–intensity foci somewhat similar to the MR appearance of immature bone infarcts were also described in the metaphyses and epiphyses.

Vitamin D

Vitamin D intoxication in children is usually accidental but may develop during the treatment of rickets. Clinical manifestations include anorexia, weakness, hypotonia, constipation, and lethargy. The level of serum calcium becomes elevated. Metaphyseal bands of sclerosis, reflecting heavy calcification of the proliferating cartilage, can be seen in the tubular bones (Figure 15-4).

In adults, hypervitaminosis D can be seen in patients with rheumatoid arthritis, gout, or Paget's disease who are treated with excessive doses of vitamin D. It can lead to generalized osteoporosis and metastatic soft tissue calcification in the periarticular soft tissues, tendon sheaths, joint capsules, and synovial bursae.[94]

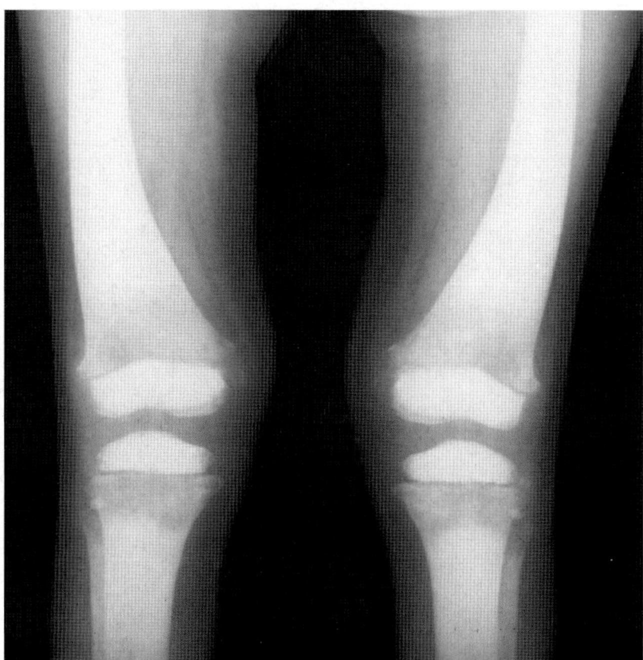

FIGURE 15-4. Vitamin D intoxication. This patient was treated for rickets. The AP view of the legs shows residual bowing of the femurs. There are areas of sclerosis in the diaphyses and epiphyses.

Other Drugs Associated with Osteoporosis and Osteomalacia

Heparin

Heparin when administered in large doses (greater than 15,000 units/day) can induce osteoporosis. Typical radiographic findings are osteopenia and multiple rib and vertebral compression fractures.

Gonadotrophin-Releasing Hormone

Gonadotrophin-releasing hormone (Gn-RH) and its analogues as androgen deprivation therapy are prescribed in patients with locally advanced or metastatic prostate cancer. Treatment with GnRH increases bone turnover,[95] decreases BMD,[95-97] and increases fracture risk.[98]

Aromatase Inhibitors

The aromatase inhibitors (AI) anastrozole, letrozole, and exemestane are used for the adjuvant treatment of estrogen-receptor–positive early and advanced breast cancer in postmenopausal patients.

Aromatase inhibitor therapy increases the risk of osteoporosis and associated bone fractures.[99]

Ifosfamide

Ifosfamide is a derivative of cyclophosphamide, commonly used in the treatment of sarcomas and other solid tumors. One potential toxicity of its use is renal tubular damage, which can lead to skeletal abnormalities, rickets in children, and osteomalacia in adults. Hypophosphatemic rickets occurs in 5% to 18% of children treated with ifosfamide and may be the first manifestation of the underlying renal damage.[100-103]

Bisphosphonates

Growth Changes

The effects of bisphosphonate therapy in growing skeleton have been described by van Persijn van Meerten et al. in 9 pediatric patients. They observed radiographic findings of band-like metaphyseal sclerosis, bone-within-bone appearance, and metaphyseal undertubulation, presumably due to inhibition of osteoclastic activity and relative increase in bone formation. It has been reported that metaphyseal sclerosis is reversible after discontinuation of medication before closure of the growth plates and in patients receiving continued medication after closure of the growth plates.[104]

Two complications of bisphosphonate treatment have received recent attention.

(1) Osteonecrosis of the mandible: Bisphosphonates are used in the treatment of postmenopausal osteoporosis, Paget's disease, steroid induced osteoporosis, multiple myeloma, and other conditions. Osteonecrosis of the mandible is a rare condition that may occur in patients taking nitrogen-containing bisphosphonates (e.g., alendronate, risedronate, pamidronate, zoledronic acid, and ibandronate[105]). Conditions that predispose to the development of this complication include cancer and anticancer treatment, intravenous administration of bisphosphonates, dental extractions and surgery involving the mandible or maxilla, duration of treatment, glucocorticoids, comorbidities such as malignancy, smoking and alcohol, and pre-existing dental or periodontal disease.[106] The incidence of osteonecrosis in patients taking oral preparations is estimated at between 1 in 10,000 and < 1 in 100,00 patient treatment years.[106] In patients with cancer receiving high doses of intravenous bisphosphonates, the incidence is higher, ranging from 1 to 10 per 100 patients.[106]

> Osteonecrosis of the mandible is a rare condition that may occur in patients taking nitrogen-containing bisphosphonates and may lead to painful areas of exposed bone that are susceptible to infection.

The mandible is affected more often than the maxilla. Areas of exposed bone are susceptible to infection and are slow to heal or do not heal. Pain is the predominant manifestation, but loose teeth or a draining fistula may occur.[105] There is no curative treatment.[105] Several articles have reviewed the features of this condition and provide recommendations for clinical management before and after bisphosphonate therapy.[105-109]

Radiographs remain the initial imaging modality although they are not early detectors of the condition.[106] Sclerosis, with mottling and bone fragmentation and sequestration and persistent extraction sockets may be seen.[110] CT can better define areas of sclerosis or bone destruction (lysis) due to secondary infection.[106] Periosteal reaction may be visible.[110] Contrast enhanced MRI may be most useful, as the area of ischemia will not enhance.[106] Unenhanced MRI is less valuable but may show loss of normal marrow signal on T1-weighted images and cortical fragmentation.[110] FDG-PET scanning has shown increased standardized uptake value (SUV-max) in areas of osteonecrosis.[110]

(2) Atypical fractures of the femoral shaft: Subtrochanteric or proximal diaphyseal femoral fractures have been seen after minimal trauma (such as a fall from a standing height or less) in postmenopausal woman treated with alendronate.[111] The pattern of these fractures on radiographs was described as "unique".[111] Thus 10 of the 15 patients demonstrated a simple transverse or oblique fracture with beaking of the cortex and diffuse cortical thickening of the proximal femoral shaft. Interestingly, cortical thickening was also seen in the contralateral femur. Kwek et al. noted that these fractures most likely represent completion of a prior stress fracture.[112] Most patients have had prodromal thigh pain, vague discomfort, or weakness. These authors therefore suggest that patients on bisphosphonates who have thigh pain should have radiographs of the femur and that any patient with a complete fracture should undergo radiographic examination of the opposite femur to detect stress changes or incomplete fractures. MRI, CT, or bone scanning may be useful in this assessment as well. The cause of these fractures remains incompletely understood.[113]

> Subtrochanteric or proximal femoral shaft fractures may occur with minimal trauma in patients taking bisphosphonates.

Other Effects

Disodium etidronate is a bisphosphonate used in low doses for treatment of Paget's disease.[114,115] The major complication of etidronate treatment is the inhibition of normal skeletal mineralization, leading to a clinical and histologic picture of "focal" osteomalacia.[116] Spontaneous fractures of uninvolved bones of patients with Paget's disease during treatment with disodium etidronate have been described.[117]

DRUGS ASSOCIATED WITH OSTEOSCLEROSIS AND PROLIFERATIVE CHANGES

Vitamin A

Vitamin A provided by the diet is found in two forms: (1) preformed vitamin A, found naturally only in animal products; and (2) carotenoid vitamin A precursors (provitamin A), found primarily in foods of plant origin. Hypercarotenemia has not been shown to have any adverse systemic effects. On the other hand, excessive intake of preformed vitamin A is toxic.[118] The clinical presentation and radiologic findings of vitamin A toxicity are related to the acute or chronic nature of vitamin abuse and the patient's age.

Acute hypervitaminosis A may occur after ingestion of 500,000 IU (100 times the recommended dietary allowance [RDA]) or more in adults (proportionately smaller doses in children) over a short period of time.[118] The most common symptoms of acute vitamin A toxicity include nausea, vomiting, headache, and irritability. In children, bulging of fontanelles and widening of the sutures due to acute transient hydrocephalus can be seen and usually resolve within 36 to 48 hours on cessation of overdosing.[94]

Chronic hypervitaminosis A in humans has been reported after recurrent intakes of retinol in amounts > 10 times the RDA in adults.[119-121] Chronic hypervitaminosis A is more common than acute hypervitaminosis and often goes unrecognized. Bone pain, eczema, hair loss, anorexia, pseudotumor cerebri, liver disease, and psychiatric complaints have been described with chronic hypervitaminosis A. Children are particularly sensitive to vitamin A, with daily intakes of 1500 IU/kg body weight reportedly leading to toxicity.[118,120,122,123] Skeletal changes observed in children exposed to high doses of chronic vitamin A are cortical thickening of the tubular bones, typically in the ulnae and metatarsal bones, cupping and splaying of metaphyses, and irregularity and narrowing of the growth plates and premature fusion of epiphyseal ossification centers[124,125] (Figure 15-5). The irreversible damage to epiphyseal cartilage can result in short stature, leg length discrepancy, and flexion contractures.

> Bone changes of chronic hypervitaminosis A in children include cupping and splaying of metaphyses, irregularity and narrowing of the growth plates, premature fusion of epiphyseal ossification centers, and cortical thickening of the tubular bones.

Bone changes in vitamin A poisoning are rare in adults, but proliferative enthesopathies involving both long bones and the flaval ligaments of the spine have been noted.[75]

In recent years, studies conducted in Scandinavia and the United States found associations between preformed vitamin A intake and hip fracture or osteoporosis.[126-129] These studies suggest that intakes as low as twice the current RDA can increase the risk for osteoporosis; however, further research is needed to clarify whether subclinical toxicity of vitamin A exists or if other synergistic nutritional or nonnutritional factors enhance bone fragility.

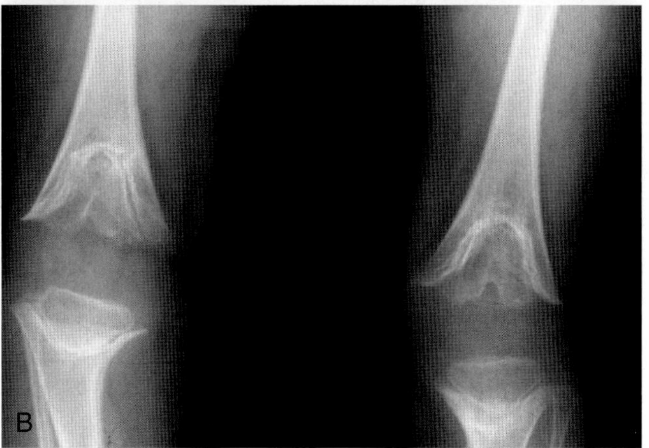

FIGURE 15-5. Vitamin A intoxication in two patients. **A,** 7-year-old boy complained of leg and arm pain. He had 2 weeks of headache, fever, lethargy, mild vomiting, and tenderness of both forearms. Symptoms improved over several days, and he was thought to have a viral syndrome. Dryness of the lips and scattered eczematoid eruptions were present. Because of the bone pain and fever, the diagnosis of leukemia was considered. A radiograph of the arm shows well-organized new bone formation along the shaft of the ulna *(arrow)*, and similar findings were noted at other sites. The radiologic findings prompted further questioning and testing that revealed Vitamin A intoxication. **B,** The history was unreliable in this patient, but it seemed that this 22-month-old girl had had received excessive doses of vitamin A. There is central fusion of the epiphyses of the distal femurs and proximal tibias. (Courtesy of Dr. Jeanne Chow, Children's Hospital, Boston, Mass.)

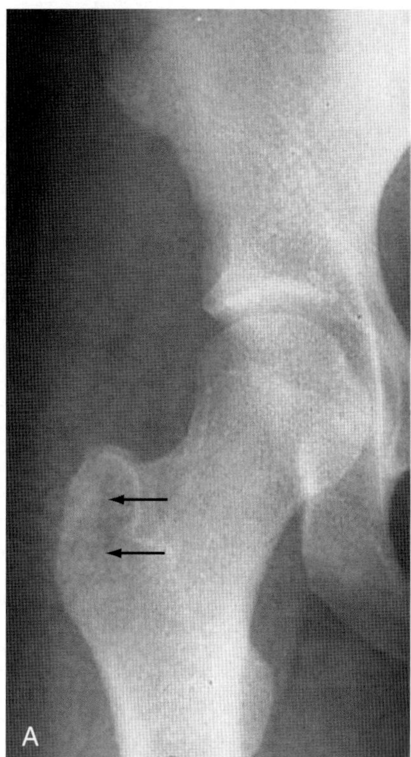

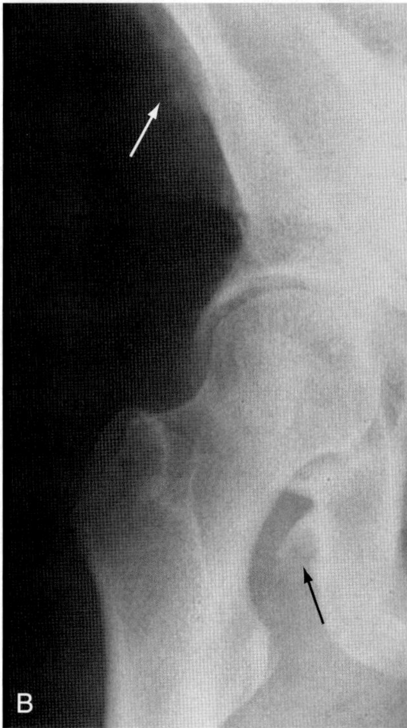

FIGURE 15-6. New bone formation following retinoic acid therapy. **A,** Radiograph of the hip in a patient with epidermolytic hyperkeratosis. The skin changes are visible as multiple irregular opacities *(arrows)* on the radiograph. **B,** 85 months following initiation of retinoid therapy, the skin changes have improved. Bony excrescences are now noted at sites of tendon attachment *(arrows)*. (Figure **A** courtesy of Dr. Jack P Lawson, Yale-New Haven Medical Center, New Haven, Conn.) (Figure **B** with permission from Lawson JP, McGuire J: The spectrum of skeletal changes associated with long-term administration of 13-cis-retinoic acid, *Skel Radiol* 16:91-97, 1987.)

Retinoids

The term *retinoids* includes all compounds, synthetic and natural, that possess vitamin A activity.

Today three generations of retinoids have been developed. Isotretinoin is a first generation drug that was confirmed to be highly effective against nodular cystic acne and gained approval from the Food and Drug Administration (FDA) in 1982 for treatment of that condition.[130] The second generation retinoids, etretinate and acitretin, also known as aromatic retinoids, are most effective in treating psoriasis and keratinizing disorders. The third generation retinoids include tazarotene and adapalene, which are FDA-approved topical agents for psoriasis and acne, respectively.

Musculoskeletal Side Effects

The main adverse skeletal effect of oral retinoids is skeletal hyperostosis, manifested as vertebral osteophytes, bony bridges, and ossification of the anterior longitudinal ligament and extraspinal ossifications of tendons and ligaments[75,131-133] (Figures 15-6 to 15-8). These findings are reminiscent of those seen in diffuse idiopathic skeletal sclerosis (DISH). Spinal alterations predominate in the cervical region. Etretinate and acitretin may selectively target the peripheral entheses most notably at the calcaneus, pelvis,

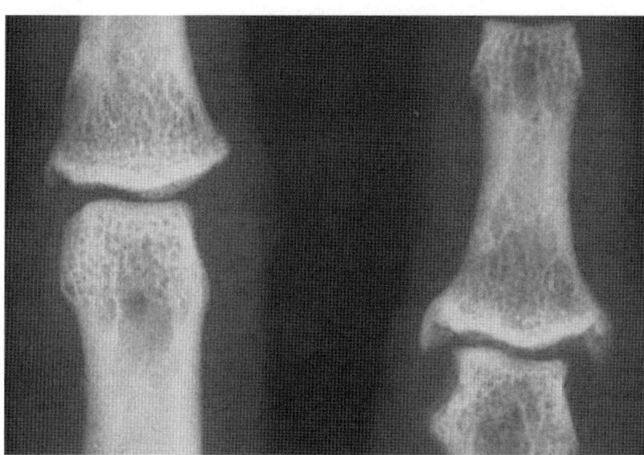

FIGURE 15-7. Retinoic acid. Hypertrophic bone is noted at the proximal interphalangeal joints. (Courtesy of Dr. Jack P Lawson, Yale-New Haven Medical Center, New Haven, Conn.)

and knee.[134,135] A few cases of ossification of the interosseous membrane at the forearm have been described in patients on etretinate.[136] The extent of radiologic ossification increases with the type, dosage, and duration of the retinoid therapy.[137] The average time for development of radiologic abnormalities is usually 24 to 36 months with etretinate and 10 months with isotretinoin.[134] Hyperostoses are irreversible, but they are generally asymptomatic.[138]

> Retinoids may result in new bone formation at entheses, hyperostosis with vertebral osteophytes, bony bridges, and ossification of the anterior longitudinal ligament and less often, the posterior longitudinal ligament.

Premature epiphyseal closure resulting in growth retardation is a recognized manifestation of chronic vitamin A toxicity and has been rarely described in children receiving oral retinoid therapy[139-141] (Figure 15-9). Other skeletal changes that have been reported include ossification of posterior longitudinal ligament, reduced bone density, periosteal thickening, nasal osteophytosis, and slender bones (Table 15-2).[75,142,143]

Myalgia, and less commonly arthralgia, have been reported in patients taking oral retinoids. Muscle symptoms can be associated with an elevated creatine phosphokinase (CPK) level that is reversible.[14]

Fluorine

Fluorine is an element widely found in various concentrations in soil, rock, and water. Both organic and inorganic compounds containing fluorine are called fluorides. Fluorine may not function as an essential trace element for human health, but it is beneficial to bone and tooth integrity and has a positive effect on prevention of dental caries.[139]

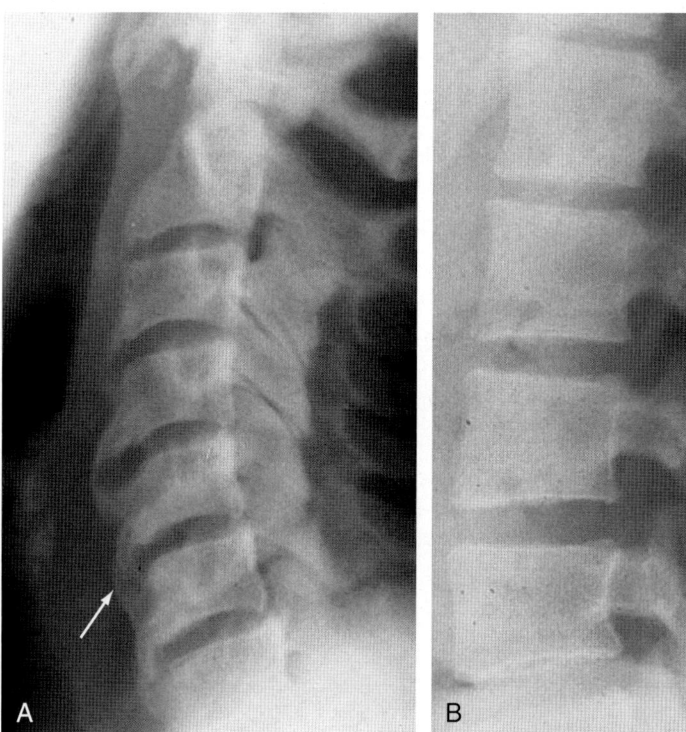

FIGURE 15-8. Spine changes following treatment with retinoic acid. **A,** Lateral radiograph of the cervical spine of the same patient as in Figure 15-6 shows bony bridging of vertebral bodies *(arrow)*. The findings are similar to those of DISH (diffuse idiopathic skeletal hyperostosis). **B,** Lateral radiograph of the lumbar spine before and (**C**) lateral radiograph of the lumbar spine after treatment with retinoic acid shows that ankylosis of the apophyseal joints has occurred producing an appearance similar to ankylosing spondylitis *(arrow)*.

(Continued)

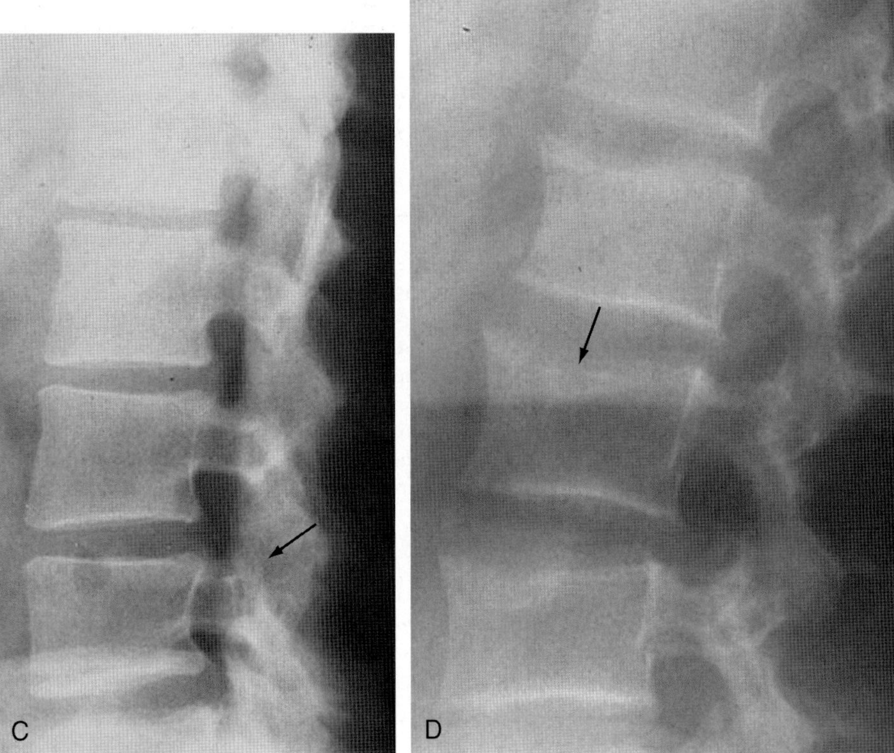

FIGURE 15-8—cont'd. D, In another patient, osteopenia has developed with end plate compressions *(arrow)*.(Courtesy of Dr. Jack P Lawson, Yale-New Haven Medical Center, New Haven, Conn.) (Figure 15-8A from Lawson JP, McGuire J: The spectrum of skeletal changes associated with long-term administration of 13-cis-retinoic acid, *Skel Radiol* 16:91-97, 1987. Figure 4A, by permission.)

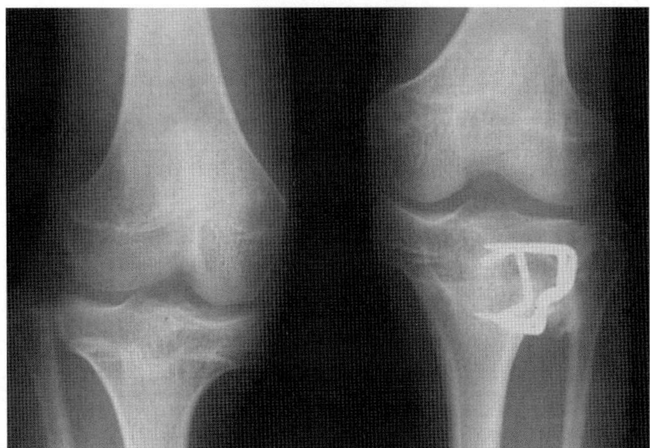

FIGURE 15-9. Retinoic acid. There is premature fusion of femoral and tibial epiphyses with resulting shortening. Note the relatively long fibulae. (Courtesy of Dr. Jack P Lawson, Yale-New Haven Medical Center, New Haven, Conn.)

TABLE 15-2. Skeletal Abnormalities Associated with Retinoid Therapy

Axial Skeleton	Appendicular Skeleton
Hyperostosis vertebral osteophytes	Tendon and ligament calcification
Ossification of the anterior longitudinal ligament	**Other less frequent findings**
Less frequently ossification of posterior longitudinal ligament	Premature epiphyseal closure
	Osteopenia
	Periosteal thickening
	Slender long bones

Chronic exposure to high quantities of fluorine, either by ingestion or inhalation, leads to a condition known as fluorosis. Fluorosis affects the teeth and skeleton and secondarily the nervous system. The most common cause of fluorosis is consumption of drinking water containing fluoride concentrations higher than 4 ppm. Endemic fluorosis due to fluoride-rich water has been recorded in tropical areas of India, China, and South Africa. Endemic fluorosis attributed to indoor coal combustion has also been reported from China.[140,141] Other recognized sources of fluorine toxicity include industrial exposure during arc welding, cryolite mining, or manufacture of aluminum, steel, or glass, fluoride therapy for osteoporosis, and drinking "brick tea" in excess.[142,143] The severity of the disease is related to the dose, period of ingestion, age, sex, meteorologic factors, and the nutritional status and physical strains to which the patients are subjected.[144]

Clinical manifestations of fluorosis include joint pain and restriction of motion, backache, rigidity of the spine, and functional dyspnea due to restriction of respiratory movements.

Palpable bony excrescences can be detected at the ulna and anterior tibia. In advanced cases, crippling deformities of the spine and extremities result in locomotor and neurologic disability.

In endemic regions, it is estimated that about 10% of those with skeletal fluorosis develop neurologic complications.[145,146] The neurologic symptoms are usually in the form of radiculomyelopathy due to mechanical compression of the spinal cord and nerve roots by osteophytes and ossification of posterior longitudinal and flaval ligaments.[147]

In children, exposure before the age of 8 years causes dental fluorosis, which is characterized by discoloration and mottled enamel of permanent teeth.[148,149]

Radiologic Findings

The primary effect of the fluoride ion is to stimulate new bone formation, which is mainly woven in character and imperfectly mineralized. Accelerated bone resorption may occur simultaneously. These pathologic changes of the bones are reflected on radiographs as a combination of osteosclerosis, osteomalacia, and osteoporosis of varying degrees.

> Osteosclerosis, osteomalacia, or rickets, and osteoporosis, ligament and tendon ossification, growth lines, and periosteal reaction may be evident on radiographs of individuals with skeletal fluorosis.

Osteosclerosis

Sclerotic changes are most marked in spine, pelvis, and ribs. In early fluorosis, the cancellous bone shows accentuation of trabeculae (Figures 15-10 and 15-11). In more advanced disease, increasing trabecular condensation eventually creates dense and chalky appearance of the bones. The skull and tubular bones are relatively spared by this sclerotic process.[150,151]

Osteopenia

Osteosclerosis of pelvis and spine is usually combined with osteoporosis of the long bones. Findings of osteomalacia may be present with decreased bone density, blurring of trabeculae, and bone deformities. In younger children, a rickets-like pattern may be detected with widened physeal plates and a lack of mineralization of the provisional zone of calcification.[152] The deformities commonly encountered are bending of tubular bones, coxa valga, genu valgum and varum, and kyphosis.[153] Protrusio acetabuli and multiple Looser zones can be seen in the pelvis.[151]

Characteristic findings of secondary hyperparathyroidism have been described.[154] Findings included subperiosteal resorption in the phalanges, loss of the lamina dura, coarse and cystic trabeculae, metaphyseal erosions, and thinning of the cortex, particularly in the pelvis, knees, and hands.

Growth Lines

Wang et al.[151] of reported growth lines in 70% of patients with skeletal fluorosis. The lines were manifested as transverse, dense linear shadows, mainly in the metaphysis adjacent to the provisional zone of calcification. Concentric growth lines were detected in flat or irregular bones, such as the pelvis and vertebral bodies, giving the appearance of bone-within-bone, a manifestation of altered bone growth in childhood.

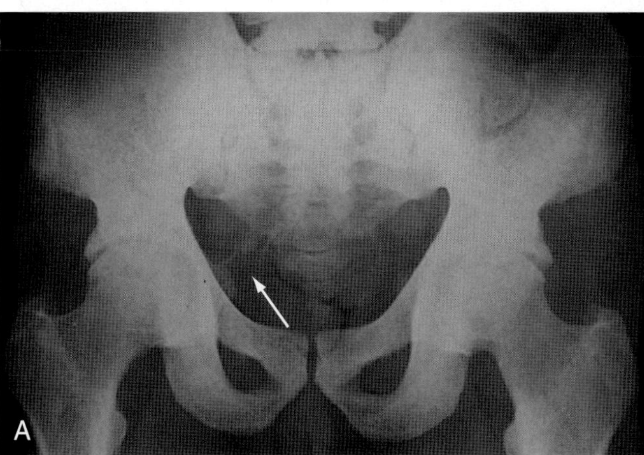

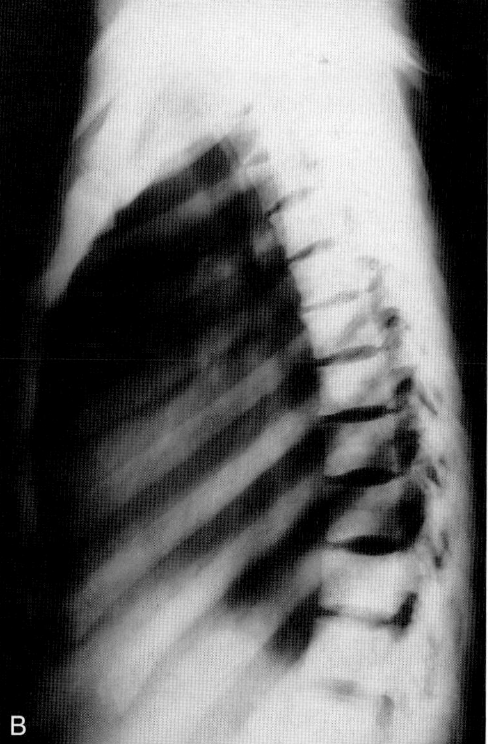

FIGURE 15-10. Fluorosis. **A,** There is diffuse sclerosis with a coarse trabecular pattern and ossification of the sacro-spinous ligament *(arrow)*. **B,** The vertebrae and ribs (of a different patient) are diffusely dense. (**A** Courtesy of Dr. UM Rao Malla, Visakhapatnam, India. **B** Courtesy of Dr. John Carrino, The Johns Hopkins Hospital, Baltimore, MD.)

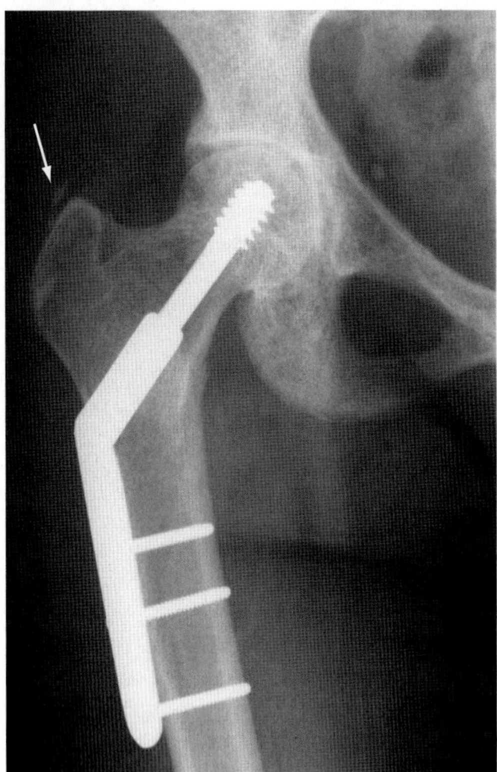

FIGURE 15-11. Fluoride changes after treatment of osteoporosis. This woman with osteoporosis suffered a femoral neck fracture. After internal fixation of the fracture she received fluoride therapy that increased the density of the bones. Note the tendon calcification *(arrow)*.

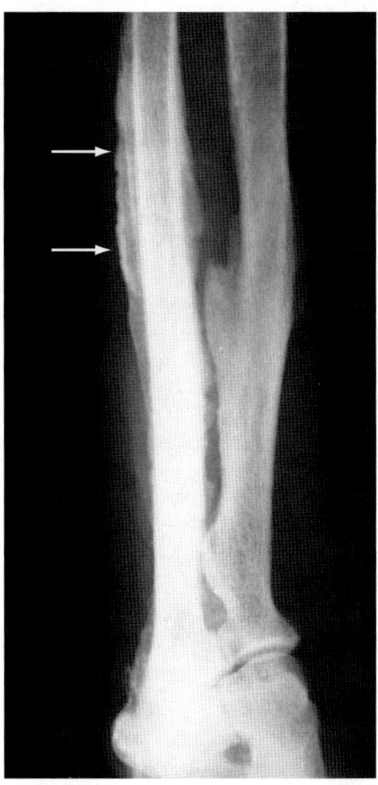

FIGURE 15-12. Radiograph of the forearm shows marked interosseous ligament calcification and periosteal reaction *(arrows)*. (Courtesy of Dr. John Carrino, Johns Hopkins Hospital, Baltimore, MD.)

Periosteal Reaction and Ligamentous Calcification

Periosteal bone formation and calcification occurs at ligamentous and tendinous insertions in both the axial and appendicular skeleton, mimicking the enthesopathy of ankylosing spondylitis and diffuse idiopathic skeletal hyperostosis (Figure 15-12). Bony excrescences develop especially in the iliac crests, ischial tuberosities, ulna, and anterior tibia. In some cases, excessive undulating periosteal new bone formation may surround the tubular bones.[155] The interosseous membranes between tibia and fibula and between radius and ulna are ossified in variable degree in most of the cases. In severe cases, the radius and the ulna can be fused by completely ossified interosseous membranes (see Figure 15-12).

Calcifications of intraspinal ligaments along with vertebral osteophytes can lead to encroachment of the spinal canal and neural foramina. Ossification of the ligamentum flavum (OLF) due to fluorosis is a rare cause of spinal stenosis in the thoracic spine. OLF can be readily demonstrated by MRI as a triangular protrusion, with a low signal intensity resembling cortical bone along the posterior aspect of the spinal canal.[156] It can be associated with ossification of posterior longitudinal ligament.

Prostaglandin

Prostaglandin E1 intravenous infusion is used in infants with cyanotic congenital heart diseases to maintain ductal patency and prolong life until palliative or corrective surgery is feasible.[157] Cortical hyperostoses, pseudowidening of the cranial sutures, soft-tissue swelling, and gastric outlet obstruction have been associated with long-term prostaglandin E1 infusion.[158-160] In the normal circulation, prostaglandins are cleared by the pulmonary bed and do not reach the systemic circulation. In neonates requiring the drug, the arterial shunt allows prostaglandin to bypass the lungs and reach the systemic circulation, leading to adverse affects.

Prostaglandin-induced periosteal reaction, also known as cortical hyperostosis, usually develops after 40 days or more of therapy but may be demonstrated as early as 9 days.[161,162] Periostitis involves long bones of the extremities, ribs, clavicles, and scapula. Unlike Caffey's disease, it rarely involves the mandible and is frequently symmetrical[163,164] (Figure 15-13). It is associated with soft-tissue swelling of the extremities. After cessation of prostaglandin administration, periosteal reaction completely incorporates into the underlying bone and undergoes remodeling over a period of 6 months to 1 year.[165,166]

> Periosteal reaction involving the long bones of the extremities, ribs, clavicles, and scapula may occur as a consequence of prostaglandin treatment in infants. In contrast to Caffey's disease, it rarely involves the mandible and is usually symmetrical.

The differential diagnosis of generalized cortical thickening in infants includes congenital syphilis, infantile cortical hyperostosis (Caffey's disease), prostaglandin-induced periosteal reaction, Interleukin-11,[167] scurvy, and hypervitaminosis A.

Musculoskeletal Side Effects of Quinolones

Fluoroquinolone antibiotics have been implicated in causing arthralgias, arthritis, tendinopathy, and tendon ruptures. In 1972, Bailey noted an association between quinolone antibiotic

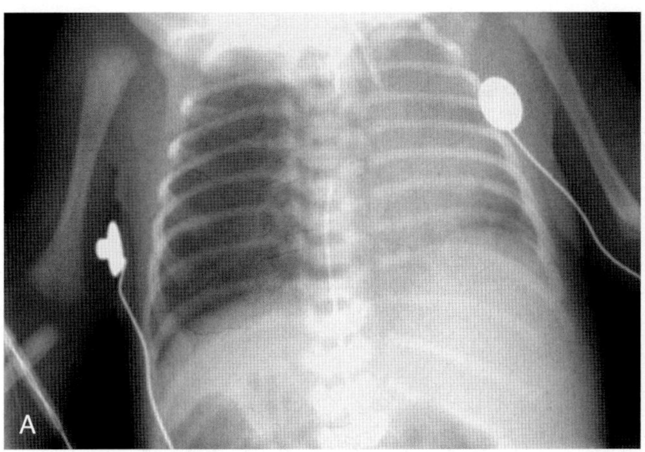

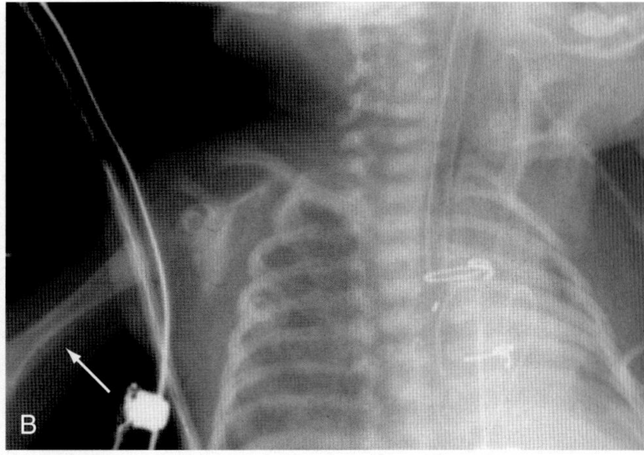

FIGURE 15-13. Prostaglandin therapy. 1700-gram girl born at 32 weeks of gestation. Cardiac catheterization revealed the tetralogy of Fallot. The patient was placed on prostaglandins to maintain patency of the ductus arteriosus to allow blood flow to the lungs. **A,** At one day of age the bones are normal. **B,** Radiograph at 1 month shows new bone formation along the humerus *(arrow)* and clavicle. No periosteal reaction is seen along the mandible such as may be seen in Caffey disease. (Courtesy of Dr. Jeanne Chow, Children's Hospital, Boston, Mass.)

and a rheumatic syndrome. He reported a patient who developed severe arthralgia while receiving nalidixic acid; the symptoms resolved upon withdrawal of the medication.[168]

Animal studies have demonstrated that fluoroquinolones are toxic to chondrocytes. Fluoroquinolone-induced joint/cartilage damage observed in juvenile animal studies is dose-specific and species-specific.[169] Macroscopically the lesions associated with fluoroquinolone use in animals include noninflammatory effusions, blisters in cartilage, and erosions of articular cartilage.[170]

Fluoroquinolones have the potential to cause arthralgia in children. A review of ciprofloxacin use in 1795 children demonstrated reversible arthralgia occurring in 1.5% of the patients.[171] Pradhan et al.[172] evaluated 58 children for quinolone related articular adverse effects. None of the children developed clinical symptoms of joint toxicity. These children also underwent MRI before and after 10 to 15 days of therapy. Blinded observers detected no difference between scans, supporting the premise that joint toxicity was absent. Long-term follow-up (22 months after treatment) also demonstrated no significant difference from the pretreatment exam.

Population data on fluoroquinolone-related chondrocyte toxicity among adults is presently lacking.[173] On the other hand, there is a definite but small increased risk of developing tendinopathy and subsequent tendon rupture in patients receiving fluoroquinolone.[174,175] Fluoroquinolone-induced tendinopathy appears more commonly in tendons under high stress; the Achilles' tendon being the most commonly affected tendon. The other reported affected tendons are the quadriceps, rectus femoris, biceps brachii, and supraspinatus tendons.[174,176,177] The median duration of fluoroquinolone treatment before the onset of tendon injury was reported as being 8 days, although symptoms can be seen as early as 2 hours after the first dose and as late as 6 months after treatment.[178]

Fluoroquinolones may be associated with tendinopathy and tendon rupture.

The exact mechanism of fluoroquinolone-induced tendinopathy is unknown, but it is thought to include matrix-degrading proteolytic activity and ischemic processes leading to an imbalance in the cell-to-matrix ratio of the fibroblasts.[179] The sudden onset of some tendinopathies also suggests a direct cytotoxic effect on the tendons.[180,181]

Both MRI and ultrasound are effective in detecting the changes of Achilles' tendinopathy. Ultrasound is inexpensive and readily available, whereas MRI offers more easily reproducible overall imaging.[176,182]

MARROW CHANGES ASSOCIATED WITH DRUG TREATMENT

Hyperplastic marrow associated with granulocyte colony stimulating factor (G-CSF) may produce focal lesions mimicking tumor on PET-CT and MRI.[183]

ANTITUMOR NECROSIS FACTOR ALPHA

Antitumor necrosis factor (TNF) agents are used to manage patients with inflammatory conditions including rheumatoid arthritis.[184] Infliximab (a chimeric monoclonal antibody against TNF-alpha), Adalimumab, and etanercept (tumour necrosis factor alpha receptor fusion protein[185]) are such agents.[184] These agents can suppress autoimmune disease but can also induce or exacerbate it.[185] Anti-TNF alpha therapy for rheumatoid arthritis has been associated with monophasic CNS demyelination, worsening of known multiple sclerosis (MS), and new onset MS.[186] MRI shows findings of demyelinization (areas of increased signal in white matter on T2-weighted images) that may enhance (Figure 15-14). Clinically, paresthesias or optic neuritis are the most usual clinical manifestations. Complete or partial resolution usually occurs after the drug is withdrawn.

Lupus-like manifestations may also be seen after treatment with anti-TNF agents.[187] Pleural or pericardial effusions, exacerbation of arthritis, skin rashes, positive ANAs, or anti-double stranded DNA antibodies have occurred after infliximab.[187] The findings regress when treatment is withdrawn.

Granulomatous infections have been reported following treatment with infliximab or etanercept.[188,189] Tuberculosis was the most frequently reported disease and was likely due to reinfection of latent disease. Candidiasis, coccidioidomycosis, histoplasmosis, listeriosis, nocardiosis, and infections due to nontuberculous mycobacteria were reported with significantly greater frequency among infliximab-treated patients (Figures 15-15 and 15-16).

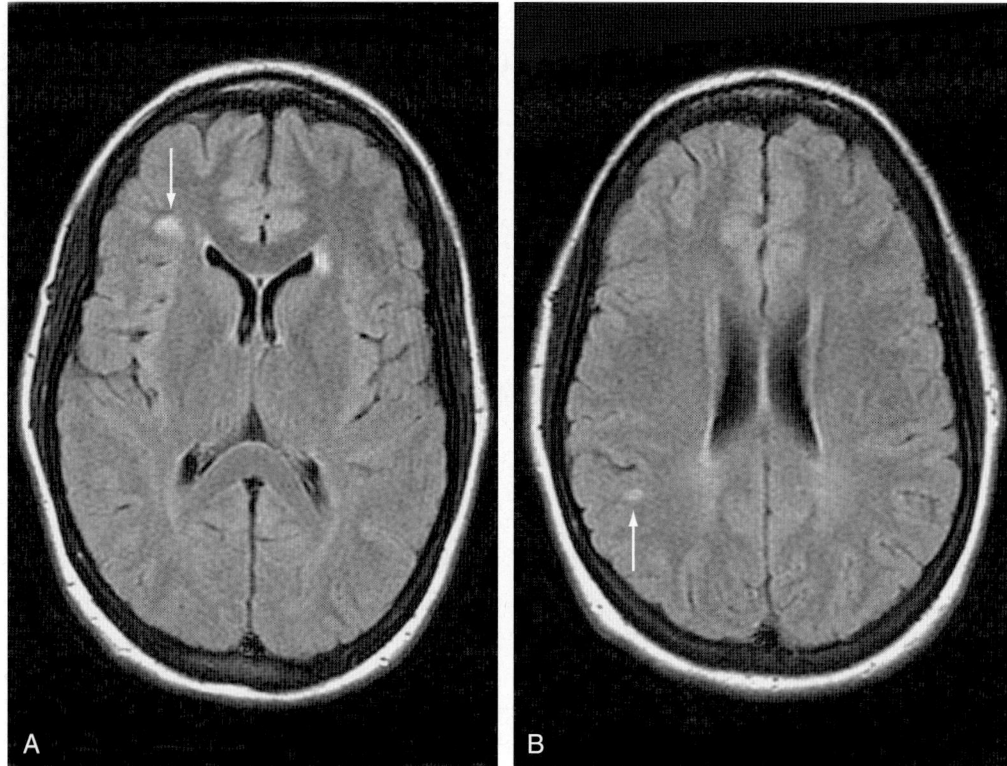

FIGURE 15-14. Demyelinating syndrome following treatment with anti-TNF alpha. A 33-year-old woman with long-standing rheumatoid arthritis on etanercept treatment, presenting with neurologic symptoms including body numbness and L'Hermitte sign (electric shock like sensation). **(A)** and **(B)** Axial brain images from a fluid-attenuated inversion recovery sequence reveal multifocal white matter lesions *(arrows)*. (David S. Titelbaum, Alexandra Degenhardt, and R. Philip Kinkel: Anti-tumor necrosis factor alpha-associated multiple sclerosis, *AJNR Am J Neuroradiol* 26:1548–1550, June/July 2005, with permission.)

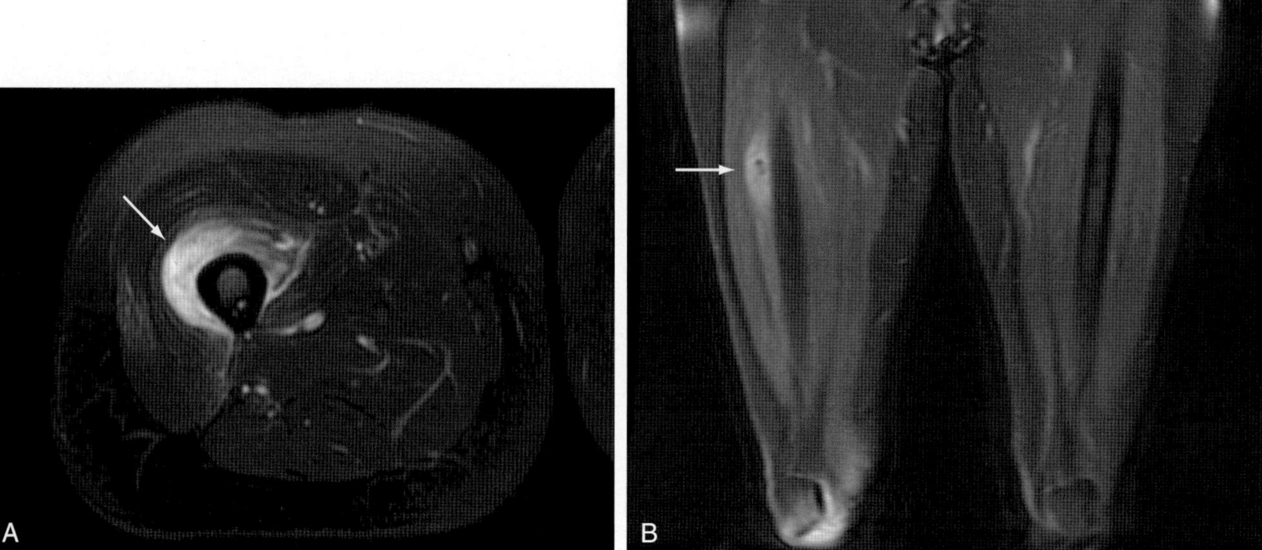

FIGURE 15-15. Presumed abscess in a 60-year-old woman with rheumatoid arthritis and acute pain and swelling over the right upper thigh. She had been receiving Remicade (infliximab) infusions. There was no history of injury. **A,** Axial STIR image shows marked edema of the vastus intermedius muscle *(arrow)*. There was no increased signal on T1-weighted images to suggest subacute blood. **B,** Coronal fat saturated T1-weighted image following intravenous contrast shows marked enhancement *(arrow)* of the area with an unenhancing center consistent with necrosis. No drainage was performed.

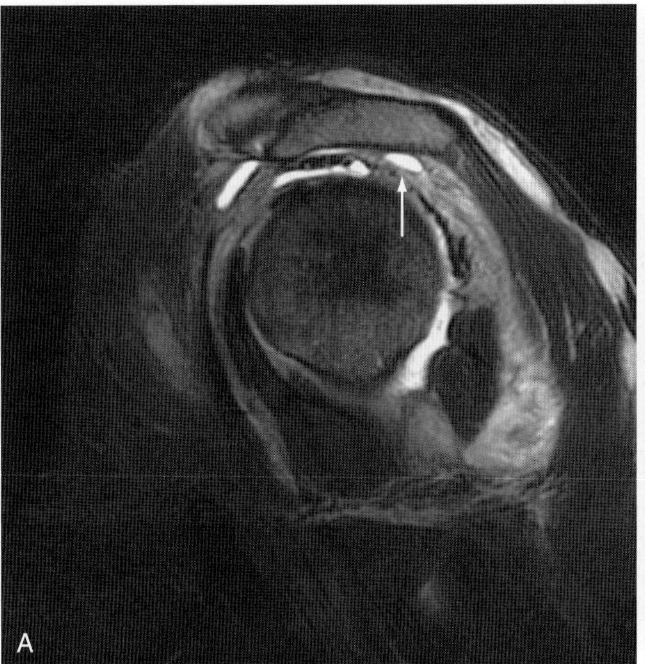

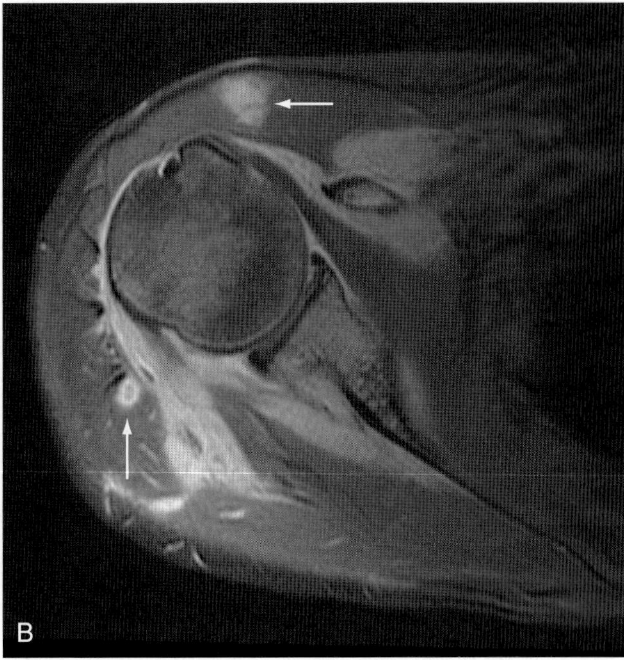

FIGURE 15-16. Disseminated Mycobacterium Kansasii infection with MRI findings consistent with infection. The patient has been on prednisone, methotrexate, and Rituxan (targets specific B-cells) for treatment of polymyositis when she developed disseminated infection with M. Kansasii. **A,** Sagittal STIR image through the right shoulder shows diffuse edema of the supraspinatus, infraspinatus and teres minor muscles. Small fluid collections *(arrow)* are noted. **B,** Axial image following intravenous contrast shows several enhancing nodular foci *(arrows)* within the deltoid muscle, as well as more diffuse enhancement of involved muscles. (Courtesy of Michael Weinblatt, MD, Brigham & Women's Hospital, Boston, MA.)

REFERENCES

1. Speight T, Holford N: *Avery's Drug Treatment.* 4th edition, Auckland, New Zealand, 1997, Adis International Limited, pp. 684-698.
2. Briggs G, Freeman RK, Yaffe SJ: *Drugs in Pregnancy and Lactation: a Reference Guide to Fetal and Neonatal Risk,* 8th edition, Baltimore, Lippincott Williams & Wilkins.
3. Koren G: *Maternal-fetal toxicology: a clinician's guide,* 2nd edition, New York, 1994, Marcel Dekker, Inc.
4. De Santis M, Straface G, Carducci B: Risk of drug-induced congenital defects, *European Journal of Obstetrics & Gynecology and Reproductive Biology* 117(1):10-19, 2004.
5. Seaver L: Adverse environmental exposures in pregnancy: teratology in adolescent in adolescent medicine practice, *Adolesc Med* 13:262-292, 2002.
6. Food and Drug Administration: Federal Register, 44:37434-37467, 1980.
7. Brecher AR, Orlow SJ: Oral retinoid therapy for dermatologic conditions in children and adolescents, *J Am Acad Dermatol* 49(2):171-186, 2003.
8. Willhite CC, Hill RR, Irving DW: Isotretinoin-induced craniofacial malformations in humans and hamsters, *J Craniofac Genet Dev Biol Suppl* 2:193-209, 1986.
9. Rizzo R, Lammer EJ, Parano E et al: Limb reduction defects in humans associated with prenatal isotretinoin exposure, *Teratology* 44(6):599-604, 1991.
10. Rosa FW, Wilk AL, Kelsey FO: Teratogen update: vitamin A congeners, *Teratology* 33(3):355-364, 1986.
11. Lammer EJ, Chen DT, Hoar RM et al: Retinoic acid embryopathy, *N Engl J Med* 313(14):837-841, 1985.
12. Adams J, Lammer EJ: Neurobehavioral teratology of isotretinoin, *Reprod Toxicol* 7(2):175-177, 1993.
13. Coberly S, Lammer E, Alashari M: Retinoic acid embryopathy case report and review of literature, *Pediatr Pathol Lab Med* 16(5):823-836, 1996.
14. Hanson JW: Teratogen update: fetal hydantoin effects, *Teratology* 33(3):349-353, 1986.
15. Brent RL: Utilization of developmental basic science principles in the evaluation of reproductive risks from pre- and postconception environmental radiation exposures, *Teratology* 59(4):182-204, 1999.
16. Kaneko S, Battino D, Andermann E et al: Congenital malformations due to antiepileptic drugs, *Epilepsy Res* 33(2-3):145-158, 1999.
17. Holmes LB, Harvey EA, Coull BA et al: The teratogenicity of anticonvulsant drugs, *N Engl J Med* 344(15):1132-1138, 2001.
18. Samren EB, van Duijn CM, Christiaens GC et al: Antiepileptic drug regimens and major congenital abnormalities in the offspring, *Ann Neurol* 46(5):739-746, 1999.
19. Polifka JE, Friedman JM: Medical genetics: 1. Clinical teratology in the age of genomics. [See comment], *CMAJ* 167(3):265-273, 2002.
20. Annegers JF, Hauser WA, Elveback LR et al: Congenital malformations and seizure disorders in the offspring of parents with epilepsy, *Int J Epidemiol* 7(3):241-247, 1978.
21. Koch S, Losche G, Jager-Roman E et al: Major and minor birth malformations and antiepileptic drugs, *Neurology* 42(4 Suppl 5):83-88, 1992.
22. Nakane Y, Okuma T, Takahashi R et al: Multi-institutional study on the teratogenicity and fetal toxicity of antiepileptic drugs: a report of a collaborative study group in Japan, *Epilepsia* 21(6):663-680, 1980.
23. Torbjorn T, Battino D: Teratogenic effects of antiepileptic drugs, *Seizure* 17:166-171, 2008.
24. Loughnan PM, Gold H, Vance JC: Phenytoin teratogenicity in man, *Lancet* 1(7794):70-72, 1973.
25. Omtzigt JG, Los FJ, Grobbee DE et al: The risk of spina bifida aperta after first-trimester exposure to valproate in a prenatal cohort, *Neurology* 42(4 Suppl 5):119-125, 1992.
26. Holzgreve W, Carey JC, Hall BD: Warfarin-induced fetal abnormalities, *Lancet* 2(7991):914-915, 1976.
27. Pauli R, Haun J: Intrauterine effects of coumarin derivatives, *Dev Brain Dysfunc* 6:229-247, 1993.
28. Franco B, Meroni G, Parenti G et al: A cluster of sulfatase genes on Xp22.3: mutations in chondrodysplasia punctata (CDPX) and implications for warfarin embryopathy, *Cell* 81(1):15-25, 1995.
29. Hall JG, Pauli RM, Wilson KM: Maternal and fetal sequelae of anticoagulation during pregnancy, *Am J Med* 68(1):122-140, 1980.
30. Savarirayan R: Common phenotype and etiology in warfarin embryopathy and X-linked chondrodysplasia punctata (CDPX), *Pediatr Radiol* 29(5):322, 1999.
31. Shaul WL, Hall JG: Multiple congenital anomalies associated with oral anticoagulants, *Am J Obstet Gynecol* 127(2):191-198, 1977.
32. Buckley LM, Bullaboy CA, Leichtman L et al: Multiple congenital anomalies associated with weekly low-dose methotrexate treatment of the mother, *Arthritis Rheum* 40(5):971-973, 1997.
33. Milunsky A, Graef JW, Gaynor MF, Jr.: Methotrexate-induced congenital malformations, *J Pediatr* 72(6):790-795, 1968.
34. McBride W: Thalidomide and congenital abnormalities, *Lancet* 2:1358, 1961.
35. Lenz W: Thalidomide and congenital abnormalities, *Lancet* 1:271, 1962.
36. Smithells RW: Thalidomide and malformations in Liverpool, *Lancet* 1(7242): 1270-1273, 1962.
37. Stirling D, Sherman M, Strauss S: Thalidomide. A surprising recovery, *J Am Pharm Assoc NS*37(3):306-313, 1997.
38. Castilla EE, Ashton-Prolla P, Barreda-Mejia E et al: Thalidomide, a current teratogen in South America, *Teratology* 54(6):273-277, 1996.
39. Vergne P, Bertin P, Bonnet C et al: Drug-induced rheumatic disorders: incidence, prevention and management, *Drug Saf* 23(4):279-293, 2000.
40. van Staa T, Leufkens HGM: The pathogenesis, epidemiology and management of glucocorticoid-induced osteoporosis, *Calcif Tissue Int* 79(3):129-137, 2006.
41. Manelli F, Giustina A: Glucocorticoid-induced osteoporosis, *Trends Endocrinol Metab* 11(3):79-85, 2000.

42. Saag KG: Glucocorticoid-induced osteoporosis, *Endocrinol Metab Clin North Am* 32(1):135-157, 2003.
43. Aaron JE, Francis RM, Peacock M et al: Contrasting microanatomy of idiopathic and corticosteroid-induced osteoporosis, *Clin Orthop Relat Res* (243):294-305, 1989.
44. Ladinsky GA, Vasilic B, Popescu AM et al: Trabecular structure quantified with the MRI-based virtual bone biopsy in postmenopausal women contributes to vertebral deformity burden independent of areal vertebral BMD, *J Bone Miner Res* 23(1): 64-74, 2008.
45. Cortet B, Dubois P, Boutry N et al: Computed tomography image analysis of the calcaneus in male osteoporosis, *Osteoporos Int* 13(1):33-41, 2002.
46. Bradley WG, Jr.: Special focus--outsourcing after hours radiology: another point of view—use of a nighthawk service in an academic radiology department. [See comment], *J Am Coll Radiol* 4(10):675-677, 2007.
47. Hiwatashi A, Westesson PL: Patients with osteoporosis on steroid medication tend to sustain subsequent fractures, *AJNR* 28(6):1055-1057, 2007.
48. Ragab AH, Frech RS, Vietti TJ: Osteoporotic fractures secondary to methotrexate therapy of acute leukemia in remission, *Cancer* 25(3):580-585, 1970.
49. Schwartz AM, Leonidas JC: Methotrexate osteopathy, *Skeletal Radiol* 11(1):13-16, 1984.
50. Eclund K, Laor T, Goorin A et al: Methotrexate Osteopathy in patients with osteosarcoma, *Radiology* 202:543-547, 1997.
51. O'Regan S, Melhorn DK, Newman AJ: Methotrexate-induced bone pain in childhood leukemia, *Am J Dis Child* 126(4):489-490, 1973.
52. Stanisavljevic S, Babcock AL: Fractures in children treated with methotrexate for leukemia, *Clin Orthop Relat Res* (125):139-144, 1977.
53. Wijnands M, Burgers A: Stress fracture in long term methotrexate treatment for psoriatic arthritis, *Ann Rheum Dis* 60(8):736-739, 2001.
54. Bologna C, Jorgensen C, Sany J: Possible role of methotrexate in the distal tibiae fractures in a patient with rheumatoid arthritis, *Clin Exp Rheumatol* 14(3):343-344, 1996.
55. Preston SJ, Terence D, Scott A et al: Methotrexate osteopathy in rheumatic disease, *Ann Rheum Dis* 52(8):582-585, 1983.
56. Rudler M, Pouchot J, Paycha F et al: Low dose methotrexate osteopathy in a patient with polyarticular juvenile idiopathic arthritis. [See comment], *Ann Rheum Dis* 62 (6):588-589, 2003.
57. Uehara R, Suzuki Y, Ichikawa Y: Methotrexate (MTX) inhibits osteoblastic differentiation in vitro: possible mechanism of MTX osteopathy, *J Rheumatol* 28(2):251-256, 2001.
58. Patel S, Patel G, Johnson D et al: Effect of low dose weekly methotrexate on bone mineral density and bone turnover, *Ann Rheum Dis* 62(2):186-187, 2003.
59. Cranney AB, McKendry RJ, Wells GA et al: The effect of low dose methotrexate on bone density, *J Rheumatol* 28(11):2395-2399, 2001.
60. Carbone LD, Kaely G, McKown KM et al: Effects of long-term administration of methotrexate on bone mineral density in rheumatoid arthritis, *Calcif Tissue Int* 64(2):100-101, 1999.
61. Minaur NJ, Kounali D, Vedi S et al: Methotrexate in the treatment of rheumatoid arthritis. II. In vivo effects on bone mineral density, *Rheumatology* 41(7):741-749, 2002.
62. Minaur NJ, Jeferiss C, Bhalla AK et al: Methotrexate in the treatment of rheumatoid arthritis. I. In vitro effects on cells of the osteoblast lineage, *Rheumatology* 41(7): 735-740, 2002.
63. O'Dell JR: Methotrexate use in rheumatoid arthritis, *Rheum Dis Clin North Am* 23(4):779-796, 1997.
64. Pack AM, Gidal B, Vazquez B: Bone disease associated with antiepileptic drugs, *Cleve Clin J Med* 71 Suppl 2:S42-48, 2004.
65. Gough H, Goggin T, Bissessar A et al: A comparative study of the relative influence of different anticonvulsant drugs, UV exposure and diet on vitamin D and calcium metabolism in out-patients with epilepsy, *Q J Med* 59(230):569-577, 1986.
66. Beerhorst K, Huvers FC, Renier WO: Severe early onset osteopenia and osteoporosis caused by antiepileptic drugs, *Neth J Med* 63(6):222-226, 2005.
67. Perucca E: Clinical implications of hepatic microsomal enzyme induction by antiepileptic drugs, *Pharmacol Ther* 33(1):139-144, 1987.
68. Richens A, Rowe DJ: Disturbance of calcium metabolism by anticonvulsant drugs, *Br Med J* 4(5727):73-76, 1970.
69. Dent CE, Richens A, Rowe DJ et al: Osteomalacia with long-term anticonvulsant therapy in epilepsy, *Br Med J* 4(5727):69-72, 1970.
70. Crosley CJ, Chee C, Berman PH: Rickets associated with long-term anticonvulsant therapy in a pediatric outpatient population, *Pediatrics* 56(1):52-57, 1975.
71. Livingston S, Berman W, Pauli LL: Anticonvulsant drugs and vitamin D metabolism, *JAMA* 224(12):1634-1635, 1973.
72. Pitt J: Rickets and osteomalacia, in Resnick D. (ed): *Diagnosis of bone and joint disorders*, 4th edition, Philadelphia, 2002, WB Saunders Company, pp 1901-1945.
73. Campbell JE, Tam CS, Sheppard RH: "Brown tumor" of hyperparathyroidism induced with anticonvulsant medication. *J Can Assoc Radiol* 28(1):73-76, 1977.
74. Addy P: Rickets associated with anticonvulsant therapy in children with tuberous sclerosis, *Arch Dis Child* 51:972-974, 1997.
75. Lawson JP, McGuire J: The spectrum of skeletal changes associated with long-term administration of 13-cis-retinoic acid, *Skeletal Radiol* 16(2):91-97, 1987.
76. Mallette LE: Acetazolamide-accelerated anticonvulsant osteomalacia, *Arch Intern Med* 137(8):1013-1017, 1977.
77. Farhat G, Yamout B, Mikat MA et al: Effect of antiepileptic drugs on bone density in ambulatory patients. [See comment], *Neurology* 58(9):1348-1353, 2002.
78. Andress DL, Ozuna J, Tirschwell D et al: Antiepileptic drug-induced bone loss in young male patients who have seizures, *Arch Neurol* 59(5):781-786, 2002.
79. Valimaki MJ, Tiihonen M, Laitinen K et al: Bone mineral density measured by dual-energy x-ray absorptiometry and novel markers of bone formation and resorption in patients on antiepileptic drugs, *J Bone Miner Res* 9(5):631-637, 1994.
80. Sato Y, Kondo I, Ishida S et al: Decreased bone mass and increased bone turnover with valproate therapy in adults with epilepsy, *Neurology* 57(3):445-449, 2001.
81. Pack AM, Olarte LS, Morrell MJ et al: Bone mineral density in an outpatient population receiving enzyme-inducing antiepileptic drugs, *Epilepsy Behav* 4(2):169-174, 2003.
82. Sheth RD, Binkley N, Hermann BP: Progressive bone deficit in epilepsy. [See comment], *Neurology* 70(3):170-176, 2008.
83. Vestergaard P, Tigaran S, Rejnmark L et al: Fracture risk is increased in epilepsy, *Acta Neurol Scand* 99(5):269-275, 1999.
84. Espallargues M, Sampietro-Colom L, Estrada MD et al: Identifying bone-mass-related risk factors for fracture to guide bone densitometry measurements: a systematic review of the literature, *Osteoporos Int* 12(10):811-822, 2001.
85. Kattan KR: Calvarial thickening after Dilantin medication, *Am J Roentgenol Radium Ther Nucl Med* 110(1):102-105, 1970.
86. Kattan KR: Thickening of the heel-pad associated with long-term Dilantin therapy. *Am J Roentgenol Radium Ther Nucl Med* 124(1):52-56, 1975.
87. De Virgiliis S, Longia M, Frau F et al: Deferoxamine-induced growth retardation in patients with thalassemia major, *J Pediatr* 113(4):661-669, 1988.
88. Lederman HM, Cohen A, Lee JW et al: Deferoxamine: a reversible S-phase inhibitor of human lymphocyte proliferation, *Blood* 64(3):748-753, 1984.
89. Estrov Z, Tawa A, Wang XH et al: In vitro and in vivo effects of deferoxamine in neonatal acute leukemia, *Blood* 69(3):757-761, 1987.
90. Brill PW, Winchester RP, Giardina PJ et al: Deferoxamine-induced bone dysplasia in patients with thalassemia major. *Am J Roentgenol* 156(3):561-565, 1991.
91. Orzincolo C, Scutellari PN, Castaldi G: Growth plate injury of the long bones in treated beta-thalassemia, *Skeletal Radiol* 21(1):39-44, 1992.
92. Chan YL, Li CK, Pang LM et al: Desferrioxamine-induced long bone changes in thalassanemic patients—radiographic features, prevalence and relations with growth, *Clin Radiol* 55(8):610-614, 2000.
93. Olivieri NF, Koren G, Harris J et al: Growth failure and bony changes induced by deferoxamine, *Am J Pediatr Hematol Onco* 14(1):48-56, 1992.
94. Resnick D: Hypervitaminosis and hypovitaminosis, in Resnick D (ed): *Diagnosis of Bone and Joint Disorders*, 4th Edition, Philadelphia, 2002, WB Saunders Company pp. 3456-3464.
95. Smith MR, McGovern FJ, Zeitman AL et al: Pamidronate to prevent bone loss during androgen-deprivation therapy for prostate cancer. [See comment], *N Engl J Med* 345(13): 948-955, 2001.
96. Maillefert JF, Sibilia J, Michel F et al: Bone mineral density in men treated with synthetic gonadotropin-releasing hormone agonists for prostatic carcinoma, *J Urol* 161 (4):1219-1222, 1999.
97. Diamond T, Campbell J, Bryant C et al: The effect of combined androgen blockade on bone turnover and bone mineral densities in men treated for prostate carcinoma: longitudinal evaluation and response to intermittent cyclic etidronate therapy. *Cancer*, 1998. 83(8): p. 1561-1566.
98. Shahinian VB, Kuo YF, Freeman JL et al: Risk of fracture after androgen deprivation for prostate cancer, *N Engl J Med* 352(2):154-164, 2005.
99. Weng MY, Lane NE: Medication-induced osteoporosis, *Curr Osteoporos Rep* 5(4):139-145, 2007.
100. Burk CD, Restaino I, Kaplan BS et al: Ifosfamide-induced renal tubular dysfunction and rickets in children with Wilms tumor. [See comment], *J Pediatr* 117(2 Pt 1):331-335, 1990.
101. Suarez A, McDowell H, Niaudet P et al: Long-term follow-up of ifosfamide renal toxicity in children treated for malignant mesenchymal tumors: an International Society of Pediatric Oncology report, *J Clin Oncol* 9(12):2177-2182, 1991.
102. Skinner R et al: Risk factors for ifosfamide nephrotoxicity in children. [See comment], *Lancet* 348(9027):578-580, 1996.
103. Church DN, Hassan AB, Harpers J et al: Osteomalacia as a late Metabolic Complication of Ifosfamide Chemotherapy in Young Adults: Illustrative Cases and Review of the Literature, *Sarcoma* :91586, 2007.
104. van Persijn van Meerten EL, Kroon HM, Papapoulos SE: Epi- and metaphyseal changes in children caused by administration of bisphosphonates, *Radiology* 184(1):249-254, 1992.
105. Shenker NG, Jawad AS: Bisphosphonates and osteonecrosis of the jaw, *Rheumatology* 46(7):1049-1051, 2007.
106. Khosla S, Burr D, Cauley J et al: Bisphosphonate-associated osteonecrosis of the jaw: report of a task force of the American Society for Bone and Mineral Research, *J Bone Miner Res* 22(10):1479-1491, 2007.
107. Ruggiero SL, Mehrotra B, Rosenberg TJ et al: Osteonecrosis of the jaws associated with the use of bisphosphonates: a review of 63 cases, *J Oral Maxillofac Surg* 62(5):527-534, 2004.
108. Marx RE, Sawatari Y, Fortin M et al: Bisphosphonate-induced exposed bone (osteonecrosis/osteopetrosis) of the jaws: risk factors, recognition, prevention, and treatment. [See comment], *J Oral Maxillofac Surg* 63(11):1567-1575, 2005.
109. Woo SB, Hellstein JW, Kalmar JR: Narrative [corrected] review: bisphosphonates and osteonecrosis of the jaws. [See comment][erratum appears in *Ann Intern Med* 1;145(3):235, 2006]. *Ann Intern Med* 144(10):753-761, 2006.
110. Raje N, Woo SB, Hande K et al: Clinical, radiographic, and biochemical characterization of multiple myeloma patients with osteonecrosis of the jaw, *Clin Cancer Res* 14(8):2387-2395, 2008.
111. Lenart BA, Lorich DG, Lane JM: Atypical fractures of the femoral diaphysis in postmenopausal women taking alendronate, *N Engl J Med* 358(12):1304-1306, 2008.
112. Kwek EB, Koh JS, Howe TS: More on atypical fractures of the femoral diaphysis. [comment], *N Engl J Med* 359(3):316-318, 2008.
113. Lee P, Seibel MJ: More on atypical fractures of the femoral diaphysis. [See comment], *N Engl J Med* 359(3):317-318, 2008.

114. Smith R, Russell RG, Bishop M: Diphosphonates and Page's disease of bone, *Lancet* 1(7706):945-947, 1971.
115. Jowsey J, Riggs BL, Kelly PJ et al: The treatment of osteoporosis with disodium ethane-1, 1-diphosphonate, *J Lab Clin Med* 78(4):574-584, 1971.
116. Boyce BF, Smith L, Fogelman I et al: Focal osteomalacia due to low-dose diphosphonate therapy in Paget's disease, *Lancet* 1(8381):821-824, 1984.
117. MacGowan JR, Pringle J, Morris VH et al: Gross vertebral collapse associated with long-term disodium etidronate treatment for pelvic Paget's disease, *Skeletal Radiol* 29(5):279-282, 2000.
118. Bendich A, Langeth L: Safety of Vitamin A, *Am J Clin Nutr* 49:358-371, 1989.
119. Biesalski HK, Seelert K: Vitamin A deficiency. New knowledge on diagnosis, consequences and therapy, *Z Ernahrungswiss* 28(1):3-16, 1989.
120. Hathcock JN et al: Evaluation of vitamin A toxicity, *Am J Clin Nutr* 52(2):183-202, 1990.
121. Olson J: Vitamin A: In: Rucker RB. Suttie JW, McCormick DB, Machlin LJ, editors: *Handbook of Vitamins*, 2001, New York, Marcel Dekker Inc, pp. 1-50.
122. Coghlan D, Cranswick NE: Complementary medicine and vitamin A toxicity in children, *Med J Aus* 175(4):223-224, 2001.
123. Penniston KL, Tanumihardjo SA: The acute and chronic toxic effects of vitamin A. [See comment], *Am J Clin Nutr* 83(2):191-201, 2006.
124. Siverman A, Ellis CN, Vorhees J: Hypervitaminosis A syndrome: paradigm of retinoid side effect, *J Am Acad Derm* 16:1027-1039, 1987.
125. Pease CN: Focal retardation and arrestment of growth of bones due to vitamin A intoxication, *JAMA* 182:980-985, 1962.
126. Lim LS, Harnack LJ, Lazovich D et al: Vitamin A intake and the risk of hip fracture in postmenopausal women: the Iowa Women's Health Study, *Osteoporos Int* 15(7): 552-559, 2004.
127. Michaelsson K, Lithell H, Vessby B et al: Serum retinol levels and the risk of fracture. [See comment], *N Engl J Med* 348(4):287-294, 2003.
128. Promislow JH, Goodman-Gruen D, Slymen DJ et al: Retinol intake and bone mineral density in the elderly: the Rancho Bernardo Study. [See comment], *J Bone Miner Res* 17(8):1349-1358, 2002.
129. Feskanich D, Singh V, Willett WC et al: Vitamin A intake and hip fractures among postmenopausal women. [See comment], *JAMA* 287(1):47-54, 2002.
130. Peck GL, Yoder F, Strauss J et al: Prolonged remissions of cystic and conglobate acne with 13-cis-retinoic acid. [See comment], *N Engl J Med* 300(7):329-333, 1979.
131. Yoder FW: Isotretinoin: a word of caution, *JAMA* 249(3):50-51, 1983.
132. Pennes DR, Ellis CN, Madison KC et al: Early skeletal hyperostoses secondary to 13-cis-retinoic acid, *AmJ Roentgenol* 142(5):979-983, 1984.
133. Archer CB, Griffiths WA, MacDonald L: Spinal hyperostosis and etretinate, *Lancet* 1(8535):41, 1987.
134. Vincent V, Zabraniecki L, Loustau O et al: Acitretin-induced enthesitis in a patient with psoriatic arthritis, *J Rheum* 72(7):646-649, 2004.
135. DiGiovanna JJ, Helfgott RK, Gerber LH et al: Extraspinal tendon and ligament calcification associated with long-term therapy with etretinate, *N Engl J Med* 315 (19):1177-1182, 1986.
136. Krause E, Zabarino P, Guilhou JJ et al: Ossification symptomatique de la membrane interosseuse antibrachiale induite par les retinoides. A propos d'une observation. *Rev Rhum Mal Osteoartic* 56(8-9):601-603, 1989.
137. White SI, MacKie RM: Bone changes associated with oral retinoid therapy, *Pharmacol Ther* 40(1):137-144, 1989.
138. Hanson N, Neachman S: Safety issues in isotretinoin therapy, *Sem in Cutan Med & Surg* 20:166-183, 2001.
139. Halkier-Sorensen L, Laurberg G, Andresen J: Bone changes in children on long-term treatment with etretinate, *J Am Acad Dermatol* 16(5 Pt 1):999-1006, 1987.
140. Milstone LM, McGuire J, Ablow RC: Premature epiphyseal closure in a child receiving oral 13-cis-retinoic acid, *J Am Acad Dermatol* 7(5):663-666, 1982.
141. Prendiville J, Bingham EA, Burrows D: Premature epiphyseal closure--a complication of etretinate therapy in children, *J Am Acad Dermatol* 15(6):1259-1262, 1986.
142. Pennes DR, Martel W, Ellis CN: Retinoid-induced ossification of the posterior longitudinal ligament, *Skeletal Radiol* 14(3):191-193, 1985.
143. Novick NL, Lawson W, Schwartz IS: Bilateral nasal bone osteophytosis associated with short-term oral isotretinoin therapy for cystic acne vulgaris, *Am J Med* 77(4):736-739, 1984.
144. Krishnamachari KA: Skeletal fluorosis in humans: a review of recent progress in the understanding of the disease, *Prog Food Nutr Sci* 10(3-4):279-314, 1986.
145. Haimanot RT, Fekadu A, Bushra B: Endemic fluorosis in the Ethiopian Rift Valley, *Trop Geogr Med*, 39(3):209-217, 1987.
146. Singh A, Jolly SS: Skeletal fluorosis and its neurological complications, *Lancet* 28:197-200, 1961.
147. Maloo J, Radhakrishnan A, Thacker AK et al: Fluorotic radiculomyelopathy in a Libyan male, *Clin Neurol Neurosurg* 92:63-65, 1990.
148. Browne D, Whelton D, O'Mullane D: Fluoride metabolism and fluorosis, *J Dent* 33(3):177-186, 2005.
149. Jolly SS, Singh BM, Mathur OC: Endemic fluorosis in Punjab (India), *Am J Med* 47(4):553-563, 1969.
150. Mithal A, Triuvedl N, Gupta S: Radiological spectrum of endemic fluorosis: relationship with calcium intake, *Skeletal Radiol* 22(4):257-261, 1993.
151. Wang Y, Yin Y, Gilula LA et al: Endemic fluorosis of the skeleton: radiographic features in 127 patients, *Am J Roentgenol* 162(1):93-98, 1994.
152. Christie DP: The spectrum of radiographic bone changes in children with fluorosis, *Radiology* 136(1):85-90, 1980.
153. Krishnamachari KA, Krishnaswamy K: Genu valgum and osteoporosis in an area of endemic fluorosis, *Lancet* 2(7834):877-879, 1973.
154. Teotia SP, Teotia M: Secondary hyperparathyroidism in patients with endemic skeletal fluorosis, *Br Med J* 1(5854):637-640, 1973.
155. Soriano M, Manchon F: Radiological aspects of a new type of bone fluorosis, periostitis deformans, *Radiology* 87(6):1089-1094, 1966.
156. Wang W, Kong L, Zhao H et al: Thoracic ossification of ligamentum flavum caused by skeletal fluorosis. *Eur Spine J* 16(8):1119-1128, 2007.
157. Donahoo JS, Roland JM, Kan J et al: Prostaglandin E1 as an adjunct to emergency cardiac operation in neonates, *J Thorac Cardiovasc Surg* 81(2):227-231, 1981.
158. Peled N, Dagan O, Babyn P et al: Gastric-outlet obstruction induced by prostaglandin therapy in neonates. [See comment], *N Engl J Med* 327(8):505-510, 1992.
159. Joshi A, Berdon WE, Brudnicki A et al: Gastric thumbprinting: diffuse gastric wall mucosal and submucosal thickening in infants with ductal-dependent cyanotic congenital heart disease maintained on long-term prostaglandin therapy, *Pediatr Radiol* 32(6):405-408, 2002.
160. Estes K, Nowicki M, Bishop P: Cortical hyperostosis secondary to prostaglandin E1 therapy, *J Pediatr* 151(4):441, 2007.
161. Kaufman MB, El-Chaar GM: Bone and tissue changes following prostaglandin therapy in neonates, *Ann Pharmacother* 30(3):269-274, 1996.
162. Nadroo AM, Shringari S, Garg M et al: Prostaglandin induced cortical hyperostosis in neonates with cyanotic heart disease, *J Perinat Med* 28(6):447-452, 2000.
163. Poznanski AK, Fernbach SK, Berry TE: Bone changes from prostaglandin therapy, *Skeletal Radiol* 14(1):20-25, 1985.
164. Matzinger M, Briggs HJ, Udjus DJ et al: Plain film and CT observations in prostaglandin-induced bone changes, *Pediatr Radiol* 22(4):264-266, 1992.
165. Drvaric DM, Parks WJ, Wyly JB et al: Prostaglandin-induced hyperostosis. A case report, *Clin Orthop Relat Res* (246):300-304, 1989.
166. Ueda K, Saito A, Nakano H et al: Cortical hyperostosis following long-term administration of prostaglandin E1 in infants with cyanotic congenital heart disease, *J Pediatr* 97(5): 834-836, 1980.
167. Milman E, Berdon WE, Garvin JH et al: Periostitis secondary to interleukin-11 (Oprelvekin, Neumega). Treatment for thrombocytopenia in pediatric patients, *Pediatr Radiol* 33(7):450-452, 2003.
168. Bailey RR, Natale R, Linton AL: Nalidixic acid arthralgia, *Can Med Assoc J* 107(7):604 passim, 1972.
169. Grady R: Safety profile of quinolone antibiotics in the pediatric population, *Pediatr Infect Dis J* 22(12):1128-1132, 2003.
170. Amacher D, Schomaker SJ, Gootz TD et al: Proteoglycan and procollagen synthesis in rat embryo limb bud cultures treated with quinolone antibacterials, *Altern Methods Toxicol* 7:307-312, 1989.
171. Hampell B, Hulmann R, Schmidt H: Ciprofloxacin in pediatrics: worldwide clinical experience based on compassionate use: safety report, *Ped Infec Dis J* 16:127-129, 1997.
172. Pradhan K, Arora NK, Jena A et al: Safety of ciprofloxacin therapy in children: magnetic resonance images, body fluid levels of fluoride and linear growth, *Acta Paediatr* 84(5):555-560, 1995.
173. Stahlmann R, Lode H: Fluoroquinolones in the elderly: safety considerations, *Drugs Aging* 20(4):289-302, 2003.
174. Mor A, Pillinger MH, Wortmann RL et al: Drug-induced arthritic and connective tissue disorders, *Semin Arthritis Rheum* (in print), 2007.
175. van der Linden P, van Puijenbroek EP, Feenstra J et al: Tendon disorders attributed to fluoroquinolones: a study on 42 spontaneous reports in the period 1988 to 1998, *Arthritis Rheum June* 45(3): 235-239, 2001.
176. Yu C, Giuffre B: Achilles tendinopathy after treatment with fluoroquinolone, *Australas Radiol* 49:407-410, 2005.
177. Karistinos A, Paulos LE: "Ciprofloxacin-induced" bilateral rectus femoris tendon rupture, *Clin J Sport Med* 17(5):406-407, 2007.
178. Khaliq Y, Zhanel GG: Fluoroquinolone-associated tendinopathy: a critical review of the literature, *Clin Infect Dis* 36(11):1404-1410, 2003.
179. Magra M, Maffulli N: Matrix metalloproteases: a role in overuse tendinopathies, *Br J Sports Med* 39(11):789-791, 2005.
180. Williams RJ, III, Attia E, Wichiewicz TL et al: The effect of ciprofloxacin on tendon, paratenon, and capsular fibroblast metabolism. [See comment], *Am J Sports Med* 28(3):364-369, 2000.
181. Sendzik J, Shakibaei M, Shafer-Korting M et al: Fluoroquinolones cause changes in extracellular matrix, signalling proteins, metalloproteinases and caspase-3 in cultured human tendon cells, *Toxicology* 212(1):24-36, 2005.
182. Jacobson JA: Ultrasound in sports medicine, *Radiol Clin North Am* 40(2):363-386, 2002.
183. Kouba M, Maaloufova J, Campr V et al: G-CSF stimulated islands of haematopoiesis mimicking disseminated malignancy on PET-CT and MRI scans in a patient with hypoplastic marrow disorder, *Br J Haematol* 130(6):807, 2005.
184. Haraoui B, Keystone EC, Thorne JC et al: Clinical outcomes of patients with rheumatoid arthritis after switching from infliximab to etanercept, *J Rheumatol* 31(12):2356-2359, 2004.
185. Watts R: Musculoskeletal and systemic reactions to biological therapeutic agents, *Curr Opin Rheumatol* 12:49-52, 2000.
186. Titelbaum DS, Degenhardt A, Kinkel RP: Anti-tumor necrosis factor alpha-associated multiple sclerosis, *Am J Neuroradiol* 26(6):1548-1550, 2005.
187. Haraoui B, Keystone E: Musculoskeletal manifestations and autoimmune diseases related to new biologic agents, *Curr Opin Rheumatol* 18(1):96-100, 2006.
188. Wallis RS, Broder M, Wong J et al: Granulomatous infections due to tumor necrosis factor blockade: correction, *Clin Infect Dis* 39(8):1254-1255, 2004.
189. Wallis RS, Broder MS, Wong JY et al: Granulomatous infectious diseases associated with tumor necrosis factor antagonists. [See comment], *Clin Infect Dis* 38(9):1261-1265, 2004.

CHAPTER 16

Infarction and Osteonecrosis

MURRAY K. DALINKA, MD, *and* JOHN D. MACKENZIE, MD

KEY FACTS

- The terms *osteonecrosis* (ON) and *avascular necrosis* (AVN) are usually used interchangeably. The term *infarct* usually refers to identical changes occurring in the marrow cavity rather than in the subchondral bone.
- One theory indicates that bone marrow edema may lead to increased intramedullary pressure and osteonecrosis.
- The "crescent sign" on radiographs is a subchondral fracture resulting from bone resorption. It is characteristic of ON but is not an early finding.
- Magnetic resonance imaging (MRI) is the most sensitive and specific test for the diagnosis of ON (or infarct), but false-negative cases have been reported.
- The margin of an osteonecrotic segment is well defined. A low signal rim with an inner high signal band on T2-weighted sequences, "the double line sign," is a characteristic MRI feature of ON.
- If there is a clinical question of ON, radiographs should be done including a "frog leg" lateral view. If these are negative on one or both sides and treatment is considered, MRI without contrast is indicated. If MRI and radiographs are normal and clinical suspicion of early ON remains, contrast-enhanced MRI examination or bone scan could be done.
- Bone marrow edema may be seen in patients with ON, transient osteoporosis, or insufficiency fracture. The differentiation between these conditions may be difficult on imaging studies early in their course. Clinical correlation and follow-up studies may be necessary.
- Spontaneous osteonecrosis of the knee (SONK) affects older women, is abrupt in onset, and usually affects the medial femoral condyle. It may be due to a subchondral insufficiency fracture.

OSTEONECROSIS

Avascular necrosis (AVN) is also known as *ischemic necrosis, osteonecrosis,* or *aseptic necrosis.* All these terms refer to bone death resulting from insufficient blood supply to the subchondral bone. The term *infarction* is usually applied to the identical changes occurring in the marrow cavity rather than in the subchondral bone.

Osteonecrosis may be posttraumatic occurring secondary to femoral neck fractures, hip dislocations, or the forcible reduction of the hip in patients with developmental dysplasia. In these cases, the trauma interrupts the medial and lateral femoral circumflex arteries, causing osteonecrosis. This chapter reviews nontraumatic osteonecrosis.

> Osteonecrosis is the underlying reason for 5% to 12% of total hip replacements.[1]

Causes

Osteonecrosis (AVN) has been described to result from a host of different abnormalities with the common end point being mechanical failure followed by collapse of the articular surface. In one large series, 90% of cases occurred in patients who were alcohol abusers or were on corticosteroids.[1]

> The minimum dose of corticosteroids necessary to result in osteonecrosis is thought to be equivalent to 4000 mg for a period of 3 months, although this complication has been reported with even low-dose, short courses of treatment.[2]

Other etiologies of osteonecrosis include hemoglobinopathies, in particular sickle cell and Sickle-C disease, marrow packing disorders (Gaucher's disease), and barotrauma (Box 16-1). In approximately 5% of patients with osteonecrosis, the cause is not apparent (idiopathic), but in many of these patients the cause is unrecognized alcohol abuse. There is an increased risk of osteonecrosis with as little as 400 mL of alcohol per week, which is the equivalent of approximately 20 beers.[3]

The pathophysiology of osteonecrosis is unknown and multiple theories have been proposed. Ficat[4] and others[5,6] believe that bone is a fixed compartment and increased intraosseous pressure resulting from ischemia and marrow edema resulting in osteonecrosis. The increased pressure may be secondary to venous abnormalities, which can be seen in sickle cell disease secondary to sickling in the intraosseous veins, and venous obstruction could be caused by nitrogen bubbles in dysbaric osteonecrosis.[5] Extravascular obstruction can occur secondary to marrow packing in Gaucher's disease. This compartment theory forms the basis for core decompression as treatment,[6,7] in which a cylindric core is removed from the femoral head and neck to decrease intraosseous pressure. Jones[8] believes that osteonecrosis is multifactorial and that abnormal fat metabolism with stasis, hypercoagulability, and endothelial damage by free fatty acids lead to fatty emboli and osteonecrosis in patients who abuse alcohol or are on corticosteroids.

Pathologic Findings

Sweet and Madewell[9] divided the histologic appearance of osteonecrosis into four characteristic zones: a central area of cell death surrounded by an area of ischemia, an area of hyperemia, and an area of normal bone (Figure 16-1). The "reactive zone" or interface is made up of the areas of hyperemia and ischemia. Histologically, the findings of ischemic necrosis are identical to those seen in bone infarction; the difference is based upon the location of the ischemia; when ischemia occurs in the subchondral bone it is referred to as *osteonecrosis* or *AVN,* and when it occurs in the shaft

BOX 16-1. Causes of Osteonecrosis

Trauma
Vasculitis
Corticosteroids
Sickle cell disease, Sickle C
Barotrauma (nitrogen emboli)
Gaucher's disease
Alcoholism (multifactorial)

or metadiaphyseal region, the lesions are termed *"bone infarcts"* (Figure 16-2).

Radiologic and histologic correlation reveals that initially normal findings are followed by bone resorption with a fibrous margin. Bone deposition at the margin or peripheral area of repair causes a sclerotic rim, giving the appearance of a "cyst like" lesion. Increased bone resorption results in macrofractures and eventually a visible crescent sign due to a subchondral fracture. This is followed by macrofracture with femoral head collapse and secondary osteoarthritis.

Standard radiography is insensitive for the early diagnosis of AVN and magnetic resonance imaging (MRI) is considered the most sensitive imaging study for diagnosis.[10,11] MRI is occasionally negative, however. Koo and colleagues[12] reported 28 hips (in 22 patients suspected clinically of having AVN) that had normal MRI examinations but had osteonecrosis diagnosed by angiography, scintigraphy, and intraosseous pressure measurements with biopsy. These patients were observed for 1 to 2 years. Eleven of the angiographically positive hips remained negative on MRI as did 14 of the 15 angiographically negative hips. None of the lesions that became positive on MRI showed characteristic findings of osteonecrosis. Five symptomatic patients underwent core decompression with relief of pain. The same authors stated that "the clinical implications of failure to detect early-stage osteonecrosis using MR imaging are uncertain, and it is still unknown whether these high-risk femoral heads will progress to a further stage." Sakamota and associates[13] performed serial MRI examinations in 48 patients receiving high doses of corticosteroids for autoimmune related conditions. The findings of osteonecrosis were seen in 31 hips in 17 patients and there was no correlation with pulse corticosteroid therapy or the cumulative dose of prednisolone between 4 and 12 weeks. All the initial findings of AVN were detected between 2.5 and 6 months after initiation of corticosteroid treatment. No additional lesions were detected in the remaining hips with a mean follow-up of 2 years and 6 months.

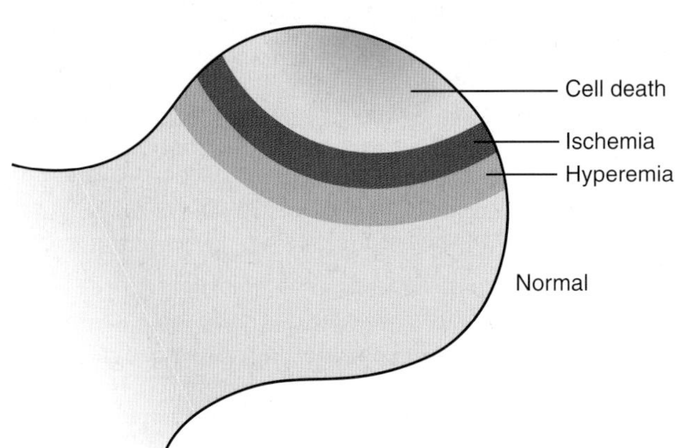

FIGURE 16-1. Gross representation of histologic zones of AVN.

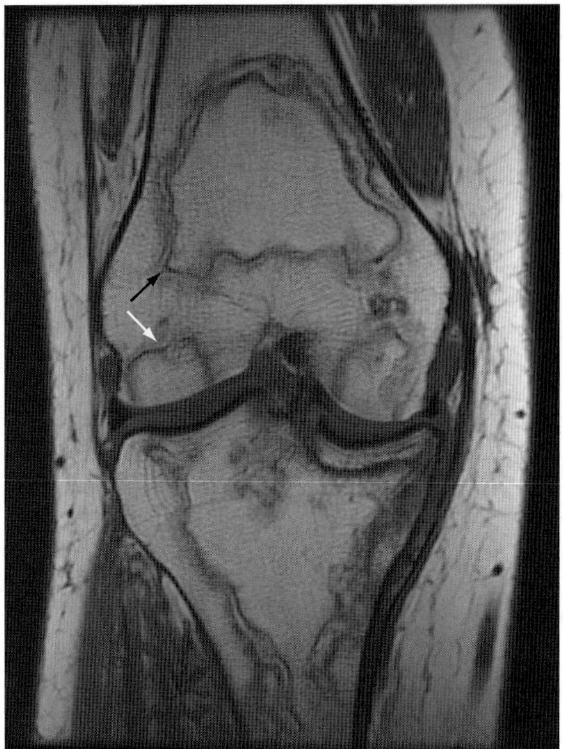

FIGURE 16-2. Bone infarcts *(black arrow)* and ischemic necrosis *(white arrow)* of the knee in a patient with systemic lupus erythematosus. Note that the findings are the same but the location is the basis for distinction. A subchondral fracture is present in the medial tibia.

In that series, the lesions regressed or disappeared in 14 hips and most patients remained asymptomatic during follow-up except for three hips with large lesions that progressed to collapse.

> Patients with osteonecrosis may be aymptomatic.[13]

Staging

Emphasis has been placed on developing a staging system for osteonecrosis as a basis for determining comparative prognosis and treatment. The early and sometimes still utilized classification was a clinical radiographic classification devised by Ficat and Arlet[14] (Table 16-1). Stage 0 was preclinical, stage 1 was painful and preradiologic, and stage 2 was radiographically positive with sclerosis, "cyst formation," and osteopenia but prior to collapse of the femoral head. Stage 3 indicated femoral head collapse, and in stage 4 there was degenerative joint disease. Interobserver and intraobserver variation is high with this classification, suggesting that this system is of limited utility.[15,16]

The International Classification is now the most commonly used classification for osteonecrosis.[1] It also consists of five stages. Stage 0 is biopsy positive but imaging negative. This is uncommon, as biopsies are rarely performed in patients with negative MRIs and/or bone scans. Stage 1 disease has a positive bone scan or MRI and negative radiographs. Stage 2 disease has radiographic findings with an intact humeral head In stage 3 disease a crescent sign or subchondral fracture is present, and in stage 4 the femoral head has a flattened articular surface and degenerative joint disease. Steinberg and colleagues[17] have added quantification to the classification of AVN as the extent of

TABLE 16-1. Staging of AVN (Osteonecrosis) Based on Radiographs

Classification	Description	Example
Ficat and Arlet		normal; abnormal MRI
Stage 0	Preclinical	
Stage 1	Pain; normal radiographs	
Stage 2	Abnormal radiographs; no subchondral collapse	
Stage 3	Subchondral collapse	
Stage 4	Degenerative joint disease	
International Classification		cystic changes; crescent
Stage 0	Imaging negative, biopsy positive	
Stage 1	Normal radiographs; abnormal MRI or bone scan	
Stage 2	Abnormal radiographs; intact femoral head	
Stage 3	Crescent sign	
Stage 4	Flattening of the femoral head; degenerative joint disease	
Steinberg classification*		flattening; osteoarthritis
Stage 0	Normal or nondiagnostic radiograph, bone scan, or MRI	
Stage 1	Normal radiograph; abnormal bone scan or MRI	
Stage 2	Cystic or sclerotic changes on radiograph	
Stage 3	Crescent sign	
Stage 4	Flattening of the femoral head	
Stage 5	Cartilage space narrowing with or without acetabular involvement	
Stage 6	Advanced degenerative changes	

*A modifier is placed after stages to indicate the extent of involvement of the femoral head and acetabulum: mild = A; moderate = B; severe = C.

involvement and location have a strong prognostic value and stages 1 to 3 can be subdivided dependent upon the location and extent of involvement.

Osteonecrosis most frequently affects the hip, although the shoulders, knees (see Figure 16-2), and small joints of the hands and feet may be involved. The hip is almost invariably involved when osteonecrosis is present in other joints and will be used as illustrative of the findings of this condition generally. In 50% to 80% of patients, both hips are involved although typically the findings are asymmetric (Figure 16-3).

> Most patients with AVN have bilateral, asymmetric involvement of the hips.

The increased incidence of bilateral disease has become more evident since the advent of MRI.

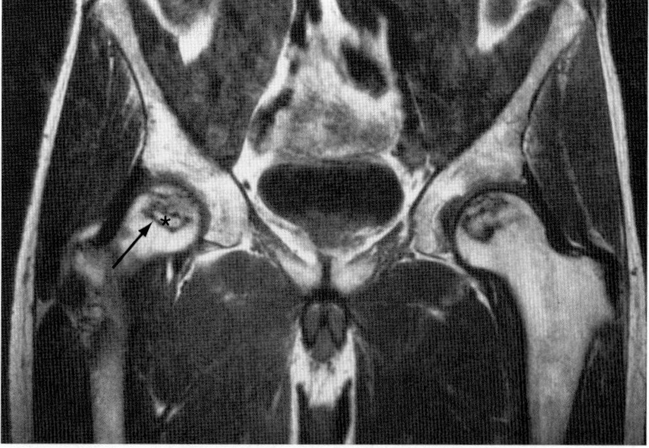

FIGURE 16-3. Osteonecrosis. Patient with bilateral AVN of the hips with low signal margin *(arrow)* surrounding central area of fat *(asterisk)*. This is a common finding in osteonecrosis, which may be x-ray negative or asymptomatic.

Imaging Features

In a multicenter study of 277 hips in 224 patients, Sugano and colleagues[18] identified five highly specific criteria for the diagnosis of AVN: (1) collapse of the femoral head with an intact acetabulum and joint space, (2) a femoral head lesion with a sclerotic margin in an otherwise normal femur, (3) "cold and hot" appearance on bone scan, (4) low signal margin to the lesion on T1-weighted MR images, and (5) positive biopsy. The authors stated that the sensitivity and specificity of diagnosis was 99% when any combination of two of these criteria was met. Glickstein and colleagues[19] found that MRI was 97% sensitive and 98% specific in differentiating AVN from normal hips and 91% sensitive in differentiating AVN from other disorders.

MRI findings often precede clinical symptoms. The MRI appearance in early AVN, prior to collapse, typically consists of a lesion with a low signal margin in the anterior femoral head

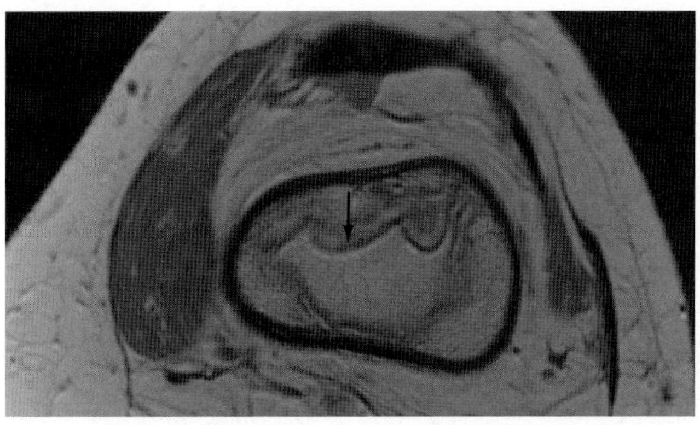

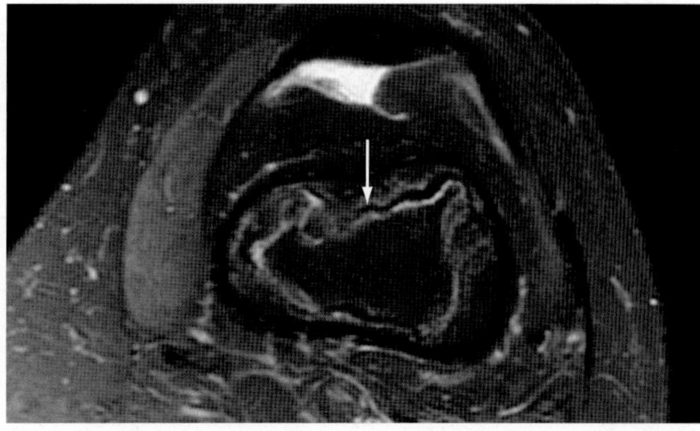

FIGURE 16-4. "Double line" sign. **A,** The axial proton density image of the femur (same patient as Figure 16-2) shows a serpentine low-signal line *(arrow)*. **B,** The corresponding T2-weighted image shows the double-line sign with a low-signal rim and an inner high-signal rim *(arrow)*.

with a central area containing the signal characteristics of fat (see Figure 16-3). Mitchell and colleagues[20] described the "double line" sign in which T2-weighted images exhibited an area of high signal within the low signal margin of the lesion. This "reactive zone" likely represents a combination of granulation tissue and chemical shift artifact and is characteristic of ischemic necrosis of the hip[20-22] (Figure 16-4). With fat suppression, this reactive zone may appear as a high signal margin surrounding the lesion (Figure 16-5). In the late stages of osteonecrosis, there is often low signal within the central area, typically representing fibrosis.[20] The area central to the low signal margin may change over the course of the disease but geographic progression of the lesion is extremely rare on histopathologic examination.[23] The lesions of AVN are typically bilateral and asymmetric. When symptomatic, prior to collapse, there is often edema on the symptomatic side.[24,25] This edema involves the entire femoral head and neck

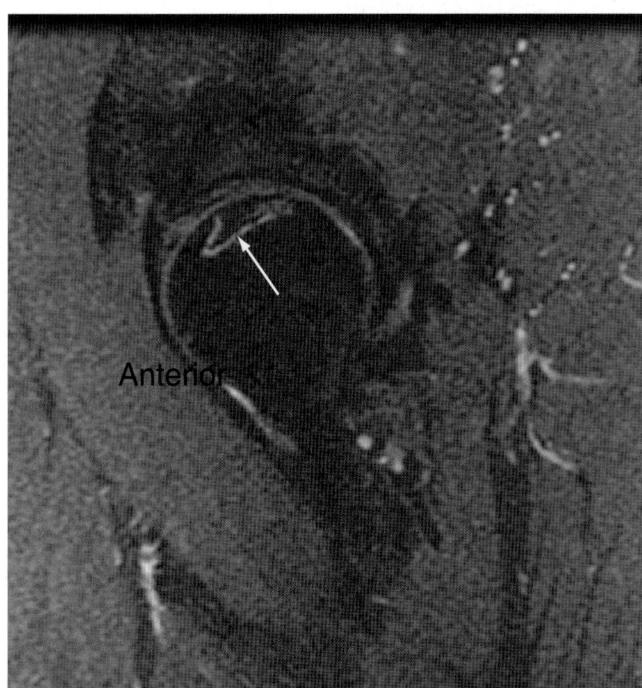

FIGURE 16-5. "Double line" sign. T2-weighted fat-suppressed sagittal image shows a high signal line *(arrow)* surrounding the area of AVN.

and is frequently associated with a joint effusion.[25] The presence of edema correlates with late collapse of the femoral head in patients with corticosteroid-induced osteonecrosis.[26] Following core decompression, the pain and edema resolve, but typically the associated lesion of osteonecrosis remains (Figure 16-6).

> The chances of collapse are highly dependent upon the size of the lesion and the percentage of the weight-bearing surface involved; larger lesions are more likely to result in collapse.[27,28]

Yamamoto and colleagues,[23] in a histopathologic study of 606 consecutive hips removed for osteonecrosis, concluded that an increase in size of the osteonecrotic lesion was extremely uncommon (seen in only 2 of 606 cases) and that osteonecrosis was therefore likely to be secondary to a single event. Shimizu and colleagues[28] followed 50 patients with osteonecrosis of the hip over an average of 45 months. They did not observe a change in the size of the lesions, and they believed that prognosis was determined by the size and location of the original lesion. Defects in the contour of the femoral head occur with collapse and are best seen on sagittal images (Figure 16-7). Stevens and colleagues[29] believe that CT is best for subchondral fractures, although we rarely perform CT in patients with osteonecrosis.

Osteonecrosis may occur in the upper extremity, where it typically involves the humeral head. Other areas of upper extremity osteonecrosis such as Kienbock's disease (lunate osteonecrosis) and osteonecrosis of the capitellum are typically posttraumatic and are not included in this chapter.

Mont and colleagues,[30] in a review of 1056 patients with atraumatic osteonecrosis of any joint, detected AVN in 127 shoulders in 73 patients (7% of cases with AVN). Bilateral shoulder involvement was present in 74% of these cases (54/73). Standard radiography and MRI were utilized for diagnosis and staging. At least one other joint was involved in 96% of the cases, with three or more joints involved in more than 25% of cases. Hip involvement was present in 81% of the patients (59/73), and the knee was involved in 41% (30/73).

Differential Considerations on Imaging Studies

Radiographic examination when abnormal is usually diagnostic, although other epiphyseal lesions such as chondroblastoma (in children), eosinophilic granuloma, or indolent infection such as

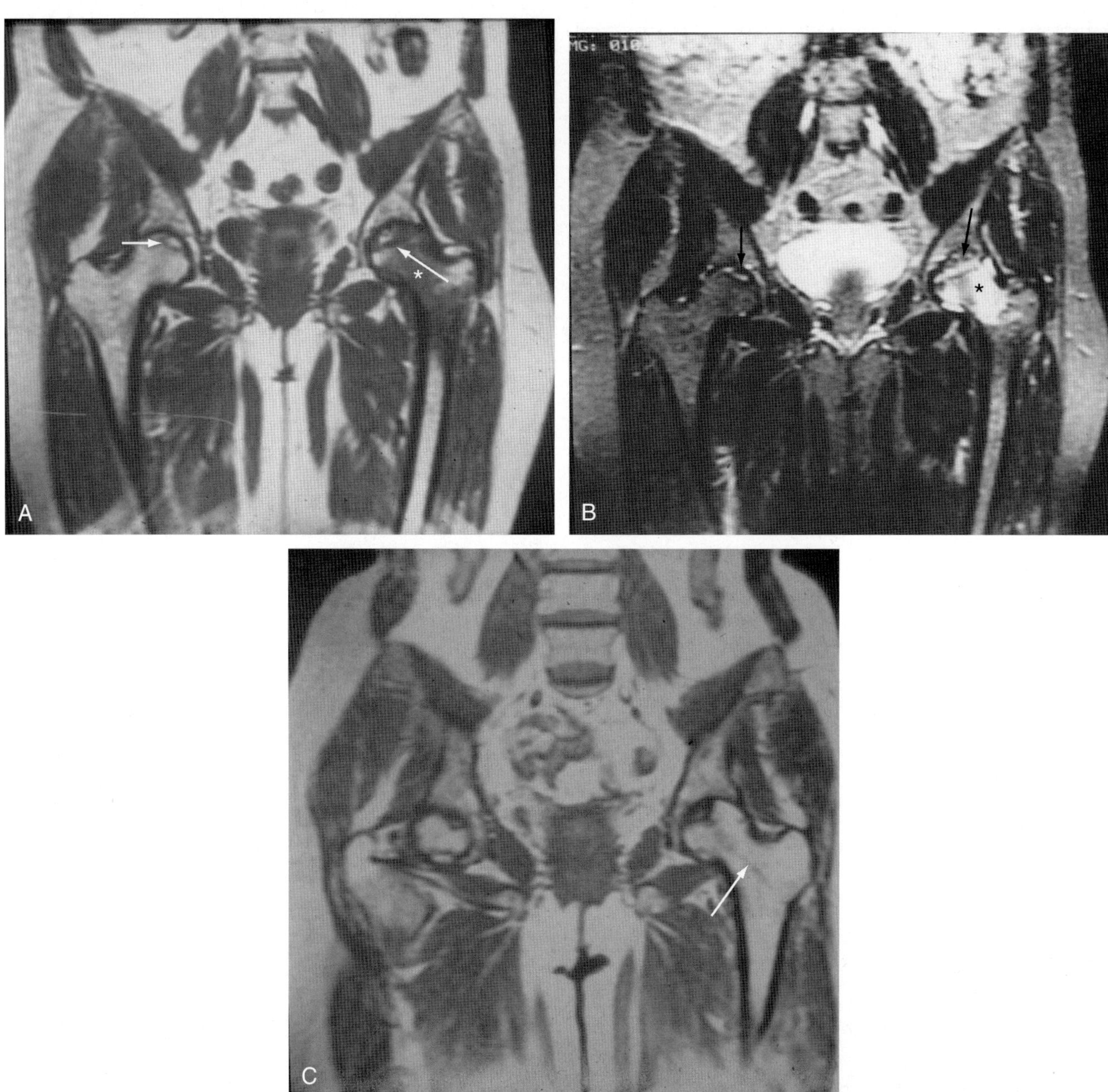

FIGURE 16-6. Osteonecrosis treated with core decompression. **A,** T1-weighted image shows triangular areas of subchondral bone delineated by low signal lines indicating bilateral AVN *(arrows).* On the left there is low signal replacing the normal fatty marrow, consistent with marrow edema *(white asterisk)* of the femoral head and neck. **B,** T2-weighted image shows the bright signal marrow edema *(black asterisk)* and the "double line" sign *(arrows)* indicating osteonecrosis within the femoral heads. **C,** T1-weighted image following core decompression. The *arrow* points to the core tract. The edema has resolved, but bilateral osteonecrosis is still present.

cystic tuberculosis may produce lytic epiphyseal lesions that might cause confusion (Box 16-2). The finding of a crescent sign is diagnostic of AVN and not present in these other conditions.

MRI findings may also cause diagnostic difficulties.

> The major entities confused with AVN on MRI are transient marrow edema (transient osteoporosis) and subchondral insufficiency fractures.

Transient Osteoporosis

Transient osteoporosis is a disorder of unknown etiology, primarily affecting the hip in middle-aged males or females in the third trimester of pregnancy.[31] The patients typically present with unilateral, severe hip pain and limitation of motion, and the radiographs typically reveal osteoporosis. This entity is generally reversible, with return to normal appearances in 9 to 12 months. On occasion, similar symptoms later develop in the opposite hip or other joints, particularly in the lower extremity. Involvement of other joints is usually sequential and typically occurs 1 to 2 years following resolution of the initial lesion (Figure 16-8). This condition has been termed *transient migratory osteoporosis.*[32]

On MRI examination, patients with transient osteoporosis exhibit unilateral bone marrow edema involving the femoral head and neck, which resolves spontaneously over time. Many patients with an identical clinical story present with normal radiographs and an identical marrow edema pattern on MRI, which, because of the absence of osteoporosis, is called *transient marrow edema*

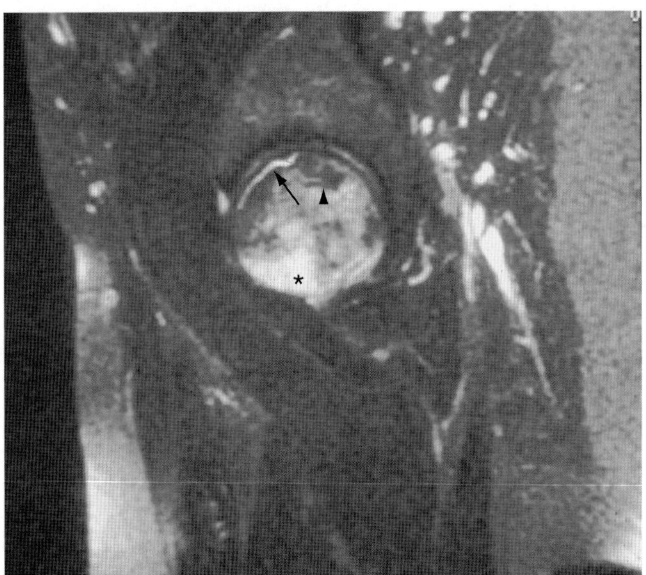

FIGURE 16-7. Subchondral crescent. Sagittal T2-weighted image demonstrates bright marrow edema *(asterisk)* and a high signal crescent sign *(arrow)* in the femoral head. The "double line" sign is also visible *(arrowhead)*. There is slight irregularity of the subchondral bone superficial to the crescent sign, indicating subchondral collapse.

syndrome.[33] It is believed that with the advent of MRI the diagnosis is made at an earlier stage, prior to the onset of osteoporosis. Patients with or without osteoporosis are typically treated in the same conservative fashion and taken off weight bearing. The patients may become asymptomatic with reversal of the marrow edema in as little as 6 weeks[34] (Figure 16-9). It is likely that prior to MRI patients with a less severe form of this disorder presented with unexplained hip pain that resolved spontaneously without ever developing osteoporosis. Some patients, in whom the diagnosis is

BOX 16-2. Epiphyseal "Cystic" Lesions on Radiographs

Cystic changes related to osteoarthritis or other arthritides (e.g., rheumatoid, PVNS)
Avascular necrosis (osteonecrosis)
Chondroblastoma (children)
Giant cell tumor (adults)
Eosinophilic granuloma
Infection (e.g., cystic tuberculosis)

not made, may develop hip fractures, particularly those presenting in the third trimester of pregnancy in which the fracture may not be detected until after delivery.[35]

Clinically, patients with transient osteoporosis have no predisposing factors for AVN and the MRI reveals edema but without an underlying lesion and a normal opposite hip. The marrow edema is reversible, and the appearance of the involved hip returns to normal. Some patients develop a similar pattern in the opposite hip or other joints years after resolution.

Plenk et al.[36] performed functional exploration of bone in 32 hips with marrow edema and suspected osteonecrosis, 80% of the patients had documented risk factors. Bone marrow pressures, intraosseous venography, and core biopsies were performed. Intramedullary pressure was increased in all cases and the intraosseous venograms were reported as abnormal in all cases. These authors believed that the bone marrow edema was likely caused by venous stasis leading to increased intramedullary pressure as is also seen in AVN. There was appositional new bone formation, which can be seen with trichrome stains but could be easily overlooked with hematoxylin and eosin preparations in decalcified bone sections. There was no osteoporosis or structural bone loss, but there was increased osteoid volume and significant undermineralization, which may explain the osteopenic appearance on radiographs.

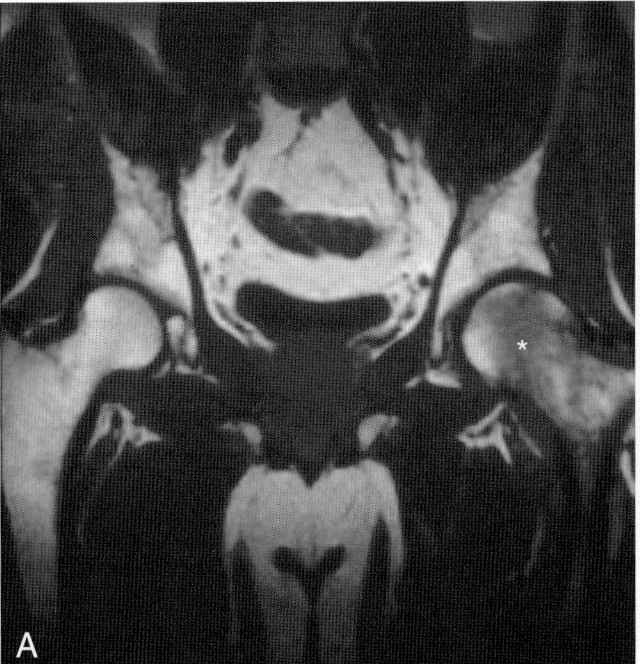

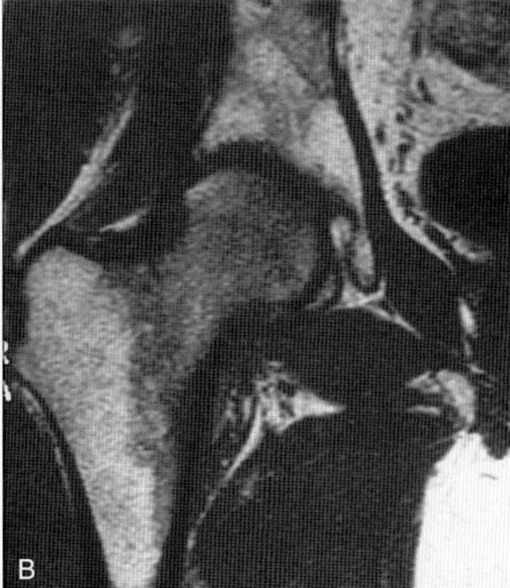

FIGURE 16-8. Transient osteoporosis. **A,** Low-field T1-weighted image of a patient with transient marrow edema involving the left femoral head and neck shows low signal edema replacing the normal marrow fat *(asterisk)*. There is no osteonecrotic lesion seen in the subchondral region. **B** and **C,** T1-weighted and T2-weighted coronal images of the same patient 5 years later with findings of marrow edema on the right.

(Continued)

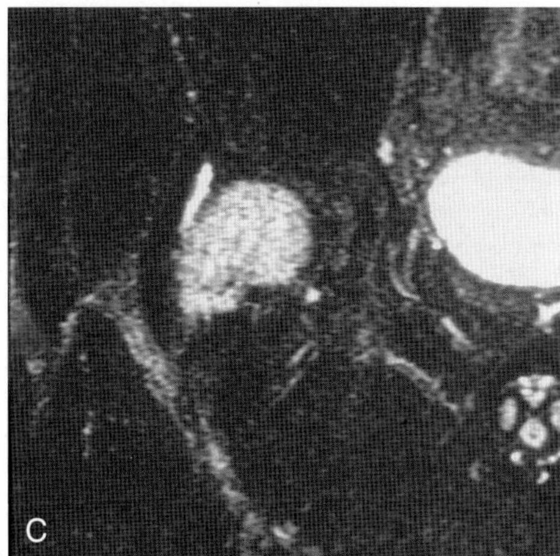

FIGURE 16-8—cont'd.

The undermineralization may cause reduction in the mechanical properties of bone, predisposing these patients to fracture. The histology of this disorder differs from AVN in that no osteonecrosis is present in the marrow or trabeculae. The live trabecula and increased active bone formation were thought to be responsible for repair and the reversible nature of the syndrome. Edema and fibrosis may be present surrounding the marrow. There may be focal areas of thin trabecula, active osteoblasts, and osteoid seams, which may resemble osteonecrosis. The authors concluded that the changes of bone marrow edema were likely the initial event in ischemic necrosis, which was reversible prior to the formation of a reactive interface that indicated the onset of irreversible disease.[36] Note that these were patients with suspected AVN, 80% of whom had documented risk factors.

Turner and associates[37] described six painful hips in 5 patients with diffuse marrow edema without a focal lesion that went on to develop osteonecrosis; they proposed a relationship between the two entities.

Spontaneous Osteonecrosis

Spontaneous osteonecrosis of the knee (SONK) was described by Ahlback in 1968[38] in patients with a sudden onset of intense medial knee pain with normal radiographs and a positive bone scan (Box 16-3). This entity most commonly involves the medial femoral condyle but has also been reported in the lateral femoral condyle or proximal tibia. Most commonly SONK is seen in middle-aged or elderly females who are often overweight. Pain is severe, acute in onset, and unilateral. These cases have no risk factors for osteonecrosis. Medial meniscal tears are often present. A subchondral insufficiency fracture may be the underlying cause.

> Spontaneous osteonecrosis of the knee usually occurs in elderly women, is acute in onset, involves the medial femoral condyle, and may be associated with a meniscal tear and insufficiency fracture.

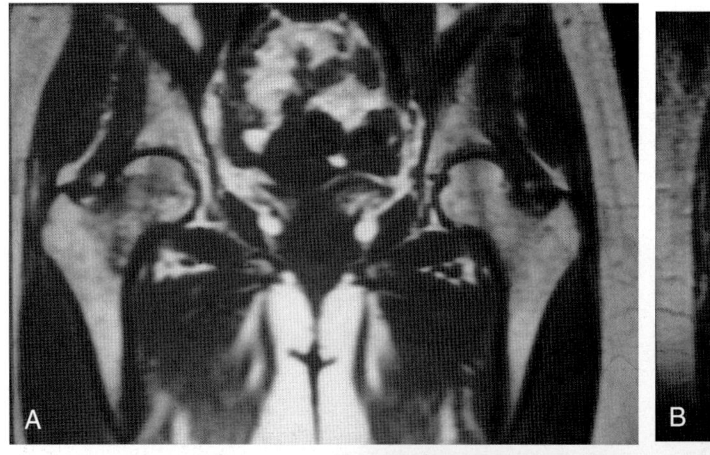

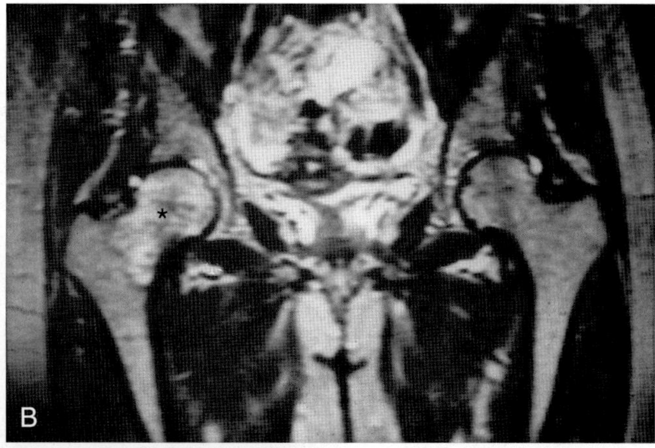

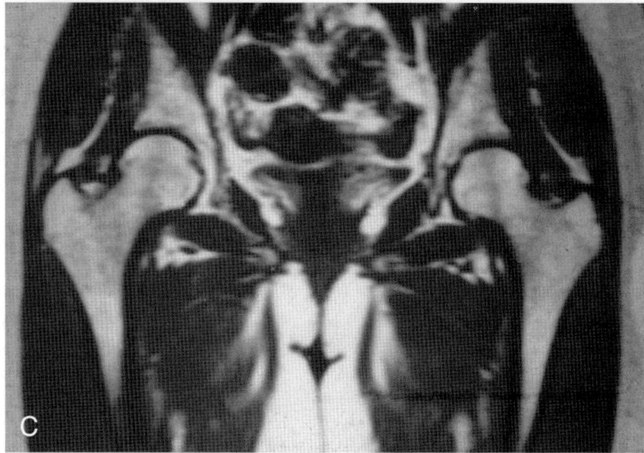

FIGURE 16-9. Transient marrow edema. **A** and **B,** Marrow edema is present in the right hip in a 55-year-old patient with hip pain and radiographs reported as normal. Note the decreased signal of the femoral head and neck on T1 images **(A)**, which increases in signal on T2 weighting **(B)**, consistent with edema *(asterisk)*. **C,** The same patient returned nearly to normal after 6 weeks of non–weight bearing.

BOX 16-3. Features of Spontaneous Osteonecrosis

Acute onset of knee pain, especially in elderly women
Most often affects the medial femoral condyle
Meniscal tears often present
May be due to insufficiency fracture
Radiographs normal initially; subchondral lucent zone and flattening of the subchondral bone are typical later
MRI shows an area of subchondral edema; a low signal line may be present just beneath the subchondral bone, suggesting an insufficiency fracture
Extensive MRI abnormalities may presage articular collapse

Ahlback's patients later developed abnormalities of the medial femoral condyle, typically flattening or subchondral lucency in the condyle.[38] Later papers described patients with an identical symptom complex, normal radiographs, and a positive bone scan in whom there was spontaneous resolution of the symptoms with the return of the bone scan to normal and without subsequent collapse of the femoral condyle.[39] On MRI it may be possible to differentiate between the patients in whom the marrow signal will return to normal and those who will go on to develop collapse.[40] The patients in whom a subchondral low signal area on T2-weighted images was more than 4 mm thick or greater than 14 mm long typically go on to collapse, as do those patients with defects in the contour of the epiphysis or deep low signal linear areas within the condyle (Figure 16-10). Work by Yamamoto and Bullough[41] strongly suggests that the inciting event in this entity is an insufficiency fracture with subsequent osteonecrosis (see Figure 16-10).

Subchondral Insufficiency Fractures

Box 16-4 describes features of subchondral insufficiency fractures.

Rafii and colleagues[42] reported 3 patients with insufficiency fractures of the femoral head that simulated AVN on MRI. In all 3 cases there was considerable bone marrow edema. These patients were all osteopenic and older than 63 years, and none had risk factors for AVN. All lesions resolved. Vande Berg and associates[43] reported similar insufficiency fractures in patients with chronic renal disease who also went on to complete resolution. The same group[44] studied patients with bone marrow edema without a reactive interface to suggest AVN. They utilized a small field of view and surface coils to obtain high-resolution MR images. In the 24 patients without subchondral changes the lesions were all transient and completely resolved. In 48 patients with this diffuse marrow pattern and focal subchondral marrow changes, 15 were irreversible (Figure 16-11). Characteristic findings of AVN developed in 9 patients and small residual subchondral changes remained in 6 patients. Irreversible lesions were at least 4 mm thick and 12.5 mm long, similar to the cases of knee marrow edema that went on to collapse in another paper from the same group.

The authors and others[45] believe that many cases reported with marrow edema that "progressed to osteonecrosis" are likely examples of subchondral insufficiency fracture with collapse. The clinical picture in these cases of insufficiency fracture is very different from classic osteonecrosis. The patients are often older, overweight, and osteopenic, and the opposite-side hip is normal. Risk factors for osteonecrosis are often absent.

BOX 16-4. Subchondral Insufficiency Fractures of the Hip

Affect older osteopenic women
Present with hip pain
MRI demonstrates marrow edema with a low signal subchondral fracture line on T1-weighted images

> Patients with insufficiency fractures as opposed to osteonecrosis typically do not have risk factors for osteonecrosis, are older and osteopenic, have acute onset of symptoms, and have a normal opposite joint.

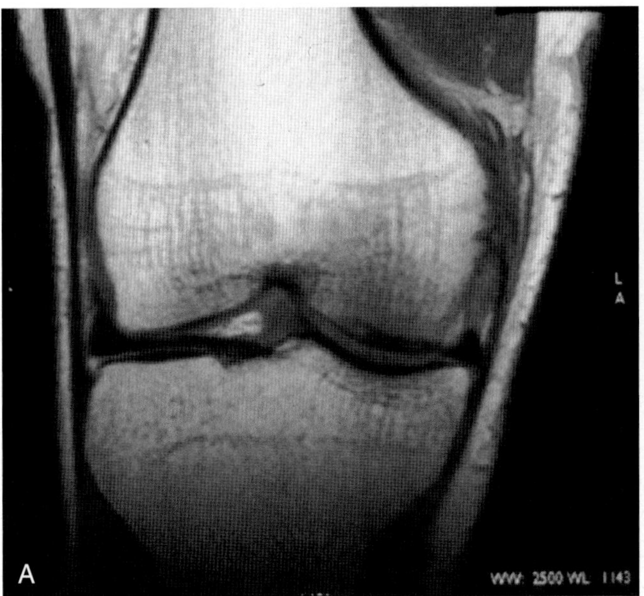

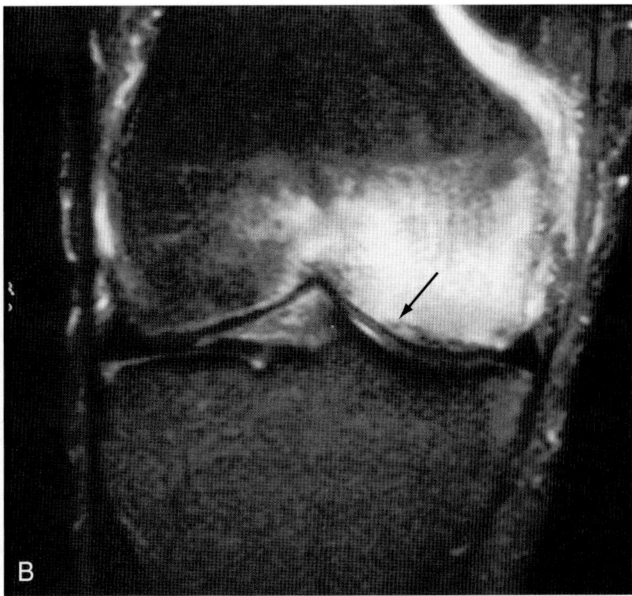

FIGURE 16-10. Spontaneous osteonecrosis of the knee with insufficiency fracture. **A,** T1-weighted and **B,** STIR images of the knee show extensive edema of the medial femoral condyle. The low signal line in the medial condyle, represents a presumed insufficiency fracture.

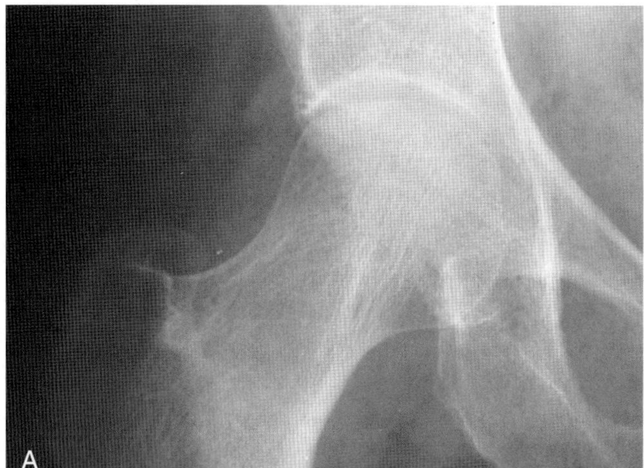

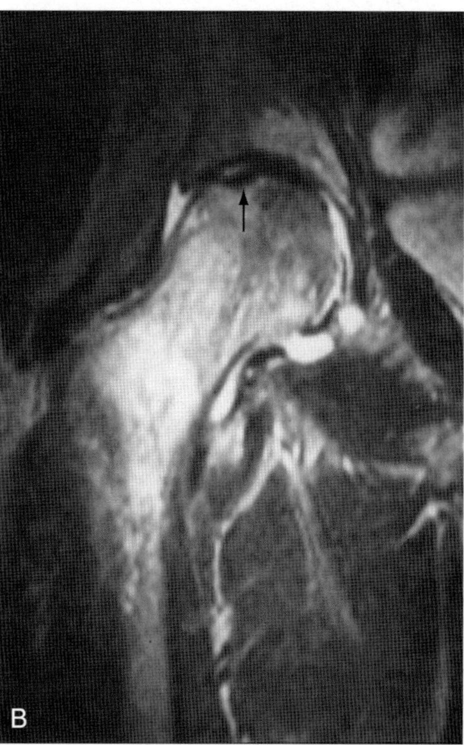

FIGURE 16-11. Insufficiency fracture in a 75-year-old osteopenic patient with hip pain. **A,** Radiograph shows decrease in trabecula due to osteoporosis. **B,** MRI reveals edema of the femoral head and neck and subchondral irregularity *(arrow)*, indicating an insufficiency fracture simulating osteonecrosis.

Summary

This chapter is a review of osteonecrosis and abnormalities that may be confused with or possibly overlap osteonecrosis. Emphasis has been placed on the imaging appearance of these entities and how they differ clinically and radiologically.

Nontraumatic AVN is usually bilateral and frequently asymmetric. The vast majority of patients with this entity have risk factors that predispose them to osteonecrosis. These include corticosteroid treatment, alcoholism, sickle cell disease, barotraumas, and marrow packing disorders. Patients with AVN of the hips not infrequently have similar findings in other joints, particularly the shoulders and knees.

On MRI the lesions of AVN are surrounded by a well-defined border with a low signal margin; the signal within the lesion may vary but the lesion almost never increases in size. The lesion may be surrounded by edema in the femoral head and this typically is associated with pain and is thought to be a predictor of late collapse. The edema is the major reason that AVN is confused with transient marrow edema and subchondral insufficiency fractures.

Patients with transient marrow edema typically have no risk factors, and the disorder is unilateral on presentation. Involvement of other joints may occur, but the involvement is sequential rather than concomitant. The major imaging factor that differentiates transient marrow edema from osteonecrosis is the absence of a low signal lesion within the area of edema and its spontaneous disappearance and return to normal. Although "reversible" AVN has been described, it has never been described with surrounding edema. Although some cases have been reported to progress from edema to osteonecrosis, the authors believe that this is truly uncommon and these cases likely had unrecognized subchondral insufficiency fractures.

REFERENCES

1. Mont MA, Hungerford DS: Non-traumatic avascular necrosis of the femoral head, *J Bone Joint Surg Am* 77:459-474, 1995.
2. McKee MD, Waddell JR, Kudo PA et al: Osteonecrosis of the femoral head in men following short-course corticosteroid therapy: a report of 15 cases, *Can Med Assoc J* 164:205, 2001.
3. Ono K, Sugioka Y: Epidemiology and risk factors in avascular necrosis of the femoral head. In Schoutens A, Arlet J, Gardeniers JWM et al (eds): *Bone circulation and vascularization in normal and pathological conditions*, New York, 1993, Plenum Press, pp 241-248.
4. Ficat RP: Idiopathic bone necrosis of the femoral head: early diagnosis and treatment, *J Bone Joint Surg Br* 67:3-10, 1985.
5. Hungerford DS, Lennox DW: The importance of increased intraosseous pressure in the development of osteonecrosis of the femoral head: implications for treatment, *Orthop Clin North Am* 16:635-654, 1985.
6. Hungerford DS: Core decompression for the treatment of avascular necrosis of the femoral head, *Semin Arthrop* 2:182-188, 1991.
7. Fairbank AC, Bhatia D, Jinnah RH et al: Long-term results of core decompression for ischaemic necrosis of the femoral head, *J Bone Joint Surg Br* 77:42-48, 1995.
8. Jones JP Jr: Etiology and pathogenesis of osteonecrosis, *Semin Arthrop* 2:160-168, 1991.
9. Sweet DE, Madewell JE: Osteonecrosis pathogenesis. In Resnick DK (ed): *Diagnosis of bone and joint disorders*, ed 3, Philadelphia, 1994, Saunders, pp 3445-3494.
10. Mitchell MD, Kundel HL, Steinberg ME et al: Avascular necrosis of the hip: comparison of MR, CT, and scintigraphy, *AJR Am J Roentgenol* 67:71, 1986.
11. Owen RS, Dalinka MK: Imaging modalities for early diagnosis of osteonecrosis of the hip, *Semin Arthroplasty* 2:169-174, 1991.
12. Koo KH, Kim R, Cho SH et al: Angiography, scintigraphy, intraosseous pressure, and histologic findings in high-risk osteonecrotic femoral heads with negative magnetic resonance images, *Clin. Orthop* 308:127-138, 1994.
13. Sakamoto M, Shimizu K, Iida S et al: Osteonecrosis of the femoral head, *J Bone Joint Surg Br* 79:213-219, 1997.
14. Ficat RP, Arlet J: Functional investigation of bone under normal conditions. In Hungerford DS (ed): *Ischemia and necrosis of bone*, Baltimore, 1980, Williams and Wilkins, pp 29-52.
15. Kay RM, Lieberman JR, Dorey FJ et al: Inter-and intraobserver variation in staging patients with proven avascular necrosis of the hip, *Clin Orthop* 307:124-129, 1994.
16. Smith SW, Meyer RA, Connor PM et al: Interobserver reliability and intraobserver reproducibility of the modified Ficat Classification System of Osteonecrosis of the Femoral Head, *J Bone Joint Surg Am* 70:1702-1706, 1996.

17. Steinberg ME, Hayken GD, Steinberg DR: A quantitative system for staging for staging avascular necrosis. *J Bone Joint Surg Br* 77:34-41, 1995.
18. Sugano N, Kubo T, Takaoka K et al: Diagnostic criteria for non-traumatic osteonecrosis of the femoral head, *J Bone Joint Surg Br* 81:590-595, 1999.
19. Glickstein MF, Burk DL, Schiebler ML et al: Avascular necrosis versus other diseases of the hip: sensitivity of MR imaging, *Radiology* 169:213-215, 1988.
20. Mitchell DG, Rao VM, Dalinka MK et al: Femoral head avascular necrosis: correlation of MR imaging, radiographic staging, radionuclide imaging, and clinical findings, *Radiology* 162:709-715, 1987.
21. Coleman BG, Kressel KY, Dalinka MK et al: Radiographically negative avascular necrosis: detection with MR imaging, *Radiology* 168:525-528, 1988.
22. Duda SH, Laniado M, Schick F et al: The double-line sign of osteonecrosis: evaluation on chemical shift MR images, *Euro J Rad* 16:233-238, 1993.
23. Yamamoto T, DiCarlo EF, Bullough PG: The prevalence and clinicopathological appearance of extension of osteonecrosis in the femoral head, *J Bone Joint Surg Br* 81:328-332, 1999.
24. Koo KH, Ahn IO, Kim R et al: Bone marrow edema and associated pain in early stage osteonecrosis of the femoral head: prospective study with serial MR images, *Radiology* 213:715-722, 1999.
25. Huang GS, Chan WP, Chang YC et al: MR imaging of bone marrow edema and joint effusion in patients with osteonecrosis of the femoral head: relationship to pain, *AJR Am J Roentgenol* 181:545-549, 2003.
26. Iida S, Harada Y, Shimizu K et al: Correlation between bone marrow edema and collapse of the femoral head in steroid-induced osteonecrosis, *AJR Am J Roentgenol* 174:735-743, 2000.
27. Sugano N, Takaoka K, Ohzono K et al: Prognostication of nontraumatic avascular necrosis of the femoral head, *Clin Orthop* 303:155-164, 1994.
28. Shimizu K, Moriya H, Sakamoto M et al: Prediction of collapse with magnetic resonance imaging of avascular necrosis of the femoral head, *J Bone Joint Surg Am* 76:215-222, 1994.
29. Stevens K, Tao C, Lee SU et al: Subchondral fracture in osteonecrosis of the femoral head: comparison of radiography, CT, and MR imaging, *AJR Am J Roentgenol* 180:363-368, 2003.
30. Mont MA, Payman RK, Laporte DM et al: Atraumatic osteonecrosis of the humeral head, *J Rheumat* 27:1766-1772, 2000.
31. Rosen RA: Transitory demineralization of the femoral head, *Radiology* 94:509-512, 1970.
32. Duncan H, Frame B, Frost HM et al: Migratory osteolysis of the lower extremities, *Ann Intern Med* 66:1165-1173, 1967.
33. Wilson AJ, Murphy WA, Hardy DC et al: Transient osteoporosis: transient bone marrow edema? *Radiology* 167:757-760, 1988.
34. Watson RM, Roach NA, Dalinka MK: Avascular necrosis and bone marrow edema syndrome, *Radiol Clin North Am* 42:207-219, 2004.
35. Fingeroth RJ: Successful operative treatment of a displaced subcapital fracture of the hip in transient osteoporosis of pregnancy, *J Bone Joint Surg Am* 77:127-130, 1995.
36. Plenk HJr, Hofmann S, Eschberger J et al: Histomorphology and bone morphometry of the bone marrow edema syndrome of the hip, *Clin Orthop* 334:73-84, 1997.
37. Turner DA, Templeton AC, Selzer PM et al: Femoral capital osteonecrosis: MR finding of diffuse marrow abnormalities without focal lesions, *Radiology* 171:135-140, 1989.
38. Ahlback S, Bauer GCH, Bohne WH: Spontaneous osteonecrosis of the knee, *Arthritis Rheum* 11:705-733, 1968.
39. Lotke PA, Ecker ML, Alavi A: Painful knees in older patients: radionuclide diagnosis of possible osteonecrosis with spontaneous resolution, *J Bone Joint Surg Am* 59:617-621, 1977.
40. Lecouvet FE, Vande Berg BC, Maldague BE et al: Early irreversible osteonecrosis versus transient lesions of the femoral condyles: prognostic value of subchondral bone and marrow changes on MR imaging, *AJR Am J Roentgenol* 170:71-77, 1998.
41. Yamamoto T, Bullough PG: Spontaneous osteonecrosis of the knee: the result of subchondral insufficiency fracture, *J Bone Joint Surg Am* 82:858-866, 2000.
42. Rafii M, Mitnick H, Klug J et al: Insufficiency fracture of the femoral head: MR imaging in the three patients, *AJR Am J Roentgenol* 168:159-163, 1997.
43. Vande Berg B, Malghem J, Goffin EJ et al: Transient epiphyseal lesions in renal transplant recipients: presumed insufficiency stress fractures, *Radiology* 191:403-407, 1994.
44. Vande Berg BC, Malghem JJ, Lecouvet FE et al: Idiopathic bone marrow edema lesions of the femoral head: predictive value of MR imaging findings, *Radiology* 212:527-535, 1999.
45. Yamamoto T, Schneider R, Bullough PG: Subchondral insufficiency fracture of the femoral head: histopathologic correlation with MRI, *Skeletal Radiol* 30:247-254, 2001.

CHAPTER 17

Imaging Arthropathies Associated with Malignant Disorders

BARBARA N. WEISSMAN, MD

KEY POINTS

- Secondary hypertrophic osteoarthropathy (HOA) is most often due to malignancies, especially non-small cell lung cancer.
- HOA may be due to nonpulmonary conditions.
- Bone scan findings of HOA can usually be distinguished from those of metastatic disease.
- Amyloid arthropathy, which may occur in patients with multiple myeloma, has a distinctive appearance on magnetic resonance imaging.

HYPERTROPHIC OSTEOARTHROPATHY

Definition and Terminology

Hypertrophic osteoarthropathy (HOA) (also called *hypertrophic pulmonary osteoarthropathy* or *Pierre-Marie-Bamberger syndrome*)[1,2] is a syndrome consisting of clubbing of the fingers and toes; pain and swelling of the distal ends of the limbs; symmetric periosteal reaction, especially of the tubular bones; synovitis; and arthralgia.[3] The disorder has two forms, primary and secondary.[4] The primary form, pachydermoperiostosis or Touraine-Solente-Gole syndrome, is inherited as an autosomal dominant trait with variable expression.[5] The acquired condition is termed *secondary hypertrophic osteoarthropathy* or *pachydermoperiostosis acquisita.* The designation "hypertrophic pulmonary osteoarthropathy" has been replaced by *hypertrophic osteoarthropathy* because nonpulmonary etiologies of the condition have been increasingly recognized.

Etiology

The incidence of HOA is rare in certain countries such as Japan but more common in others.[4] In the United States the incidence has been reported as 0.8%.[6] Up to 90% of cases of HOA are associated with malignancy, usually non-small cell lung cancer.[4] Some of the causes of the secondary form are listed in Box 17-1.

HOA is associated with increased blood flow and arteriovenous shunting.[4] Armstrong et al. have summarized the theories explaining the underlying cause(s) of HPOA.[4] A neurogenic cause was first postulated in response to the observation that resolution of HOA could occur with interruption of the vagus nerve even if the tumor remained.[7] The entire spectrum of manifestations of the condition (e.g., facial skin thickening), however, were not adequately explained, and a humoral cause was postulated, such as growth hormone or hepatocyte growth factor.[4] These factors could either be produced by tumor cells and delivered to the periphery, or there could be a failure to remove or deactivate them in the lungs due to arteriovenous shunting.[4,8] A unifying theory suggests that unfragmented megakaryocytes bypass the pulmonary circulation due to conditions such as cyanotic heart disease and stimulate the endothelium to produce platelet-derived growth factors (PDGF) and vascular endothelial growth factor (VEGF). These lead to angiogenesis, endothelial hyperplasia, clubbing, and HOA. It is postulated that if the cause of HOA is carcinoma-derived growth factor, tumor resection will lead to improvement, whereas if shunting is prominent (fewer cases), tumor resection will not ameliorate the symptoms.[4]

The cause of HPOA in chronic cholestatic liver disease is uncertain, but resolution can occur with improvement in liver disease or after liver transplantation.[9]

Clinical Features

Clubbing of the fingers and toes is the most frequent manifestation of HOA.[4] Periosteal reaction of the long bones is common. Skin thickening may develop that is so prominent that ridges and furrows resembling the gyri of the brain are seen on the scalp and forehead.[5] These features may be confused with acromegaly. Synovitis with noninflammatory fluid is a recognized manifestation, but inflammatory arthritis has also been documented. Armstrong et al. reported two patients with inflammatory synovitis who presented with several months of swelling of the wrists and ankles, elbow and shoulder, and clubbing of the fingers and toes.[4] Both patients were found to have periosteal reaction, elevated sedimentation rates, and lung tumors (small cell in one and non-small cell in the other).

> Clubbing, symmetric periosteal reaction, and arthritis are typical manifestations of HOA.

An interesting presentation is seen in patients with infected vascular grafts where the findings of HOA are localized to the areas distal to the vascular prosthesis.[11]

Imaging Findings

The clinical manifestations should lead to imaging evaluation. An underlying pulmonary lesion can be detected using standard radiography and computed tomography (CT). Care must be taken because pulmonary infections and benign lesions and malignancies may result in HOA and even in uptake on fluorodeoxyglucose positron emission tomography (FDG-PET) scanning.[13] Therefore tissue diagnosis is necessary.

BOX 17-1. Some Causes of HOA

Pulmonary
- Bronchial carcinoma
- Secondary lung carcinoma
- Mesothelioma
- Solitary fibrous tumor of the lung
- Pulmonary fibrosis
- Empyema
- Cystic fibrosis
- Chronic infections
- Arteriovenous fistulae

Cardiac
- Congenital cyanotic heart disease
- Infective endocarditis

Mediastinal

Esophageal carcinoma

Thymoma

Achalasia

Liver
- Cirrhosis
- Liver carcinoma
- Biliary atresia
- Cholestatic liver disease

Intestinal
- Gastrointestinal carcinoma
- Inflammatory bowel disease
- Chronic infections
- Laxative abuse
- Polyposis
- Whipple disease
- Lymphoma

Miscellaneous
- Graves' disease
- Thalassemia
- Childhood tumors (e.g., nasopharyngeal, lymphoma)
- POEMS (polyneuropathy, organomegaly, endocrinopathy, monoclonal gammopathy, skin changes)
- Syphilis

Localized
- Aneurysms
- Infective arteritis
- Vascular prosthesis infection
- Patent ductus arteriosus
- Hemiplegia
- Chronic venous stasis
- Takayasu arteritis

*From Alonso-Bartolome P, Martínez-Taboada VM, Pina T et al: Hypertrophic osteoarthropathy secondary to vascular prosthesis infection: report of 3 cases and review of the literature, *Medicine* 85:183-191, 2006; Armstrong RD, Crisp AJ, Grahame R et al: Hypertrophic osteoarthropathy and purgative abuse, *Br Med J Clin Res Ed* 282:1836, 1981; Katsicas M, Ciocca M, Rosanova M et al: Hypertrophic osteoarthropathy in two children with cholestatic hepatic disease, *Acta Paediatr* 94:1152-1155, 2005; and Kuloğlu Z, Kansu A, Ekici F et al: Hypertrophic osteoarthropathy in a child with biliary atresia, *Scand J Gastroenterol* 39:698-701, 2004.

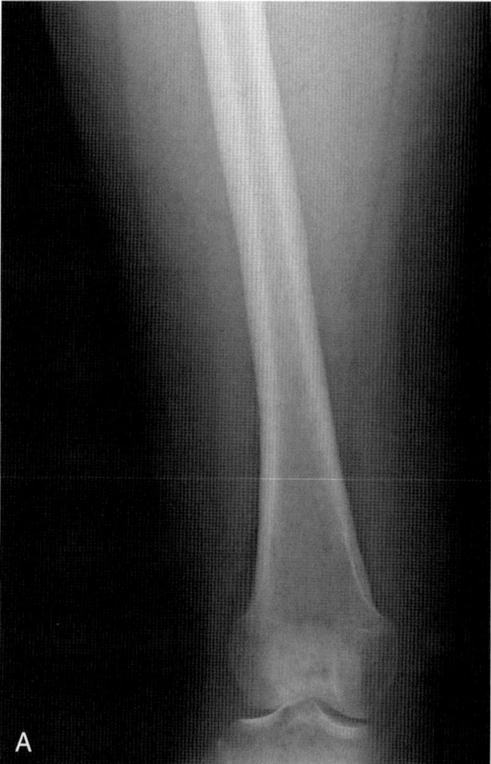

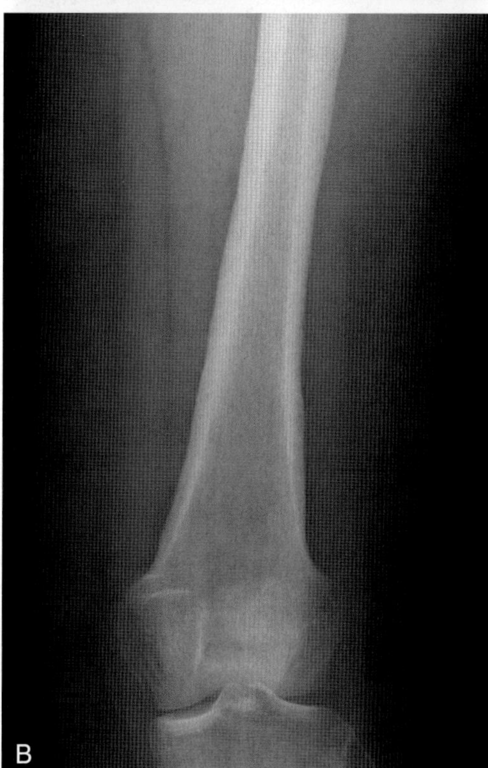

FIGURE 17-1. HOA in a patient with cyanotic congenital heart disease. **(A)** Anteroposterior radiograph of the right femur and **(B)** anteroposterior radiograph of the left femur show periosteal reaction bilaterally, producing an undulating contour to the bones.

Radiographs

The disorder is characterized on radiographs by the presence of periostitis that usually involves the diaphyses of long tubular bones (Figures 17-1 and 17-2). Although periosteal reaction can be seen on radiographs, these are less sensitive than bone scan or magnetic resonance imaging (MRI) for early diagnosis. Periosteal reaction is seen first along the proximal and distal shafts and metaphyses of long tubular bones as a single layer.[14] As the condition progresses, the periosteal reaction becomes more marked, extends to the epiphysis, and becomes laminated or multilayered. Eventually it can involve all of the tubular bones, causing increased cortical

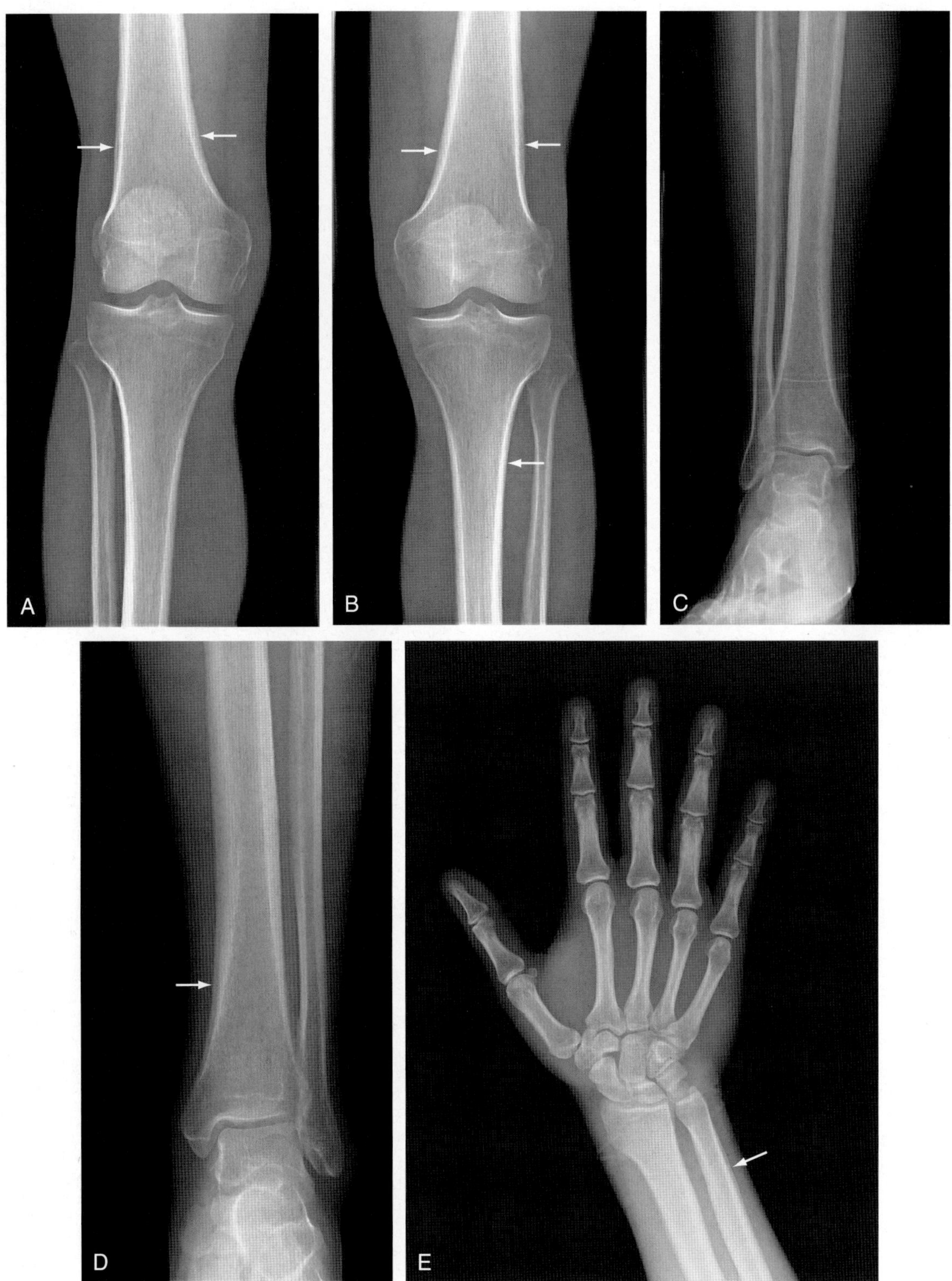

FIGURE 17-2. HOA in a patient with cystic fibrosis. **A,** Right knee. **B,** Left knee. **C,** Right ankle. **D,** Left ankle. **E,** Posteroanterior view, right hand and wrist.

(Continued)

thickness and an irregular surface. The interosseous membranes can ossify.[14]

The periosteal reaction becomes thicker and more extensive with longer disease duration.[14] Comparison by Pineda et al. of patients with cyanotic heart disease to those with lung cancer showed that those with congenital cyanotic heart disease (CCHD) or primary HOA demonstrated periosteal new bone formation along the diaphyses, metaphyses, and epiphyses whereas epiphyseal involvement was not seen in patients with HOA secondary to lung carcinoma. Also, the configuration of

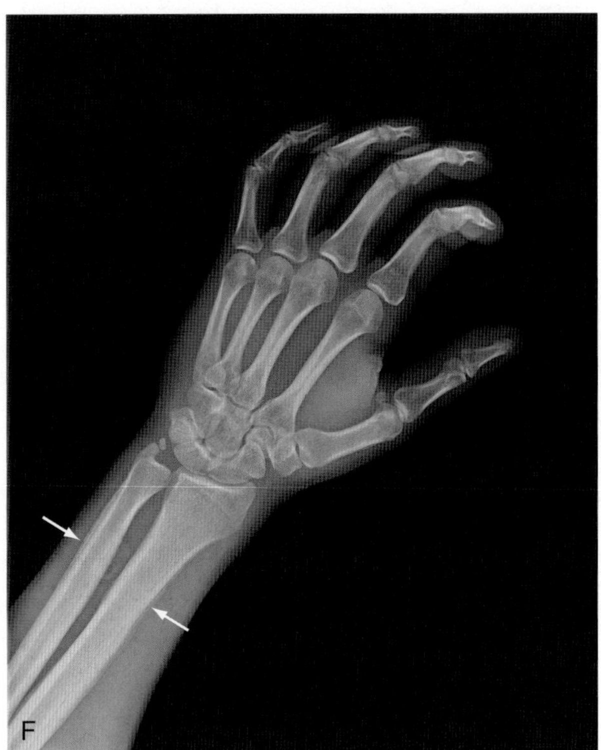

FIGURE 17-2—cont'd. F, Oblique view, left hand and wrist. Note the periosteal reaction at each of these sites *(arrows).* The oblique view of the hand and wrist shows clubbing of the nails.

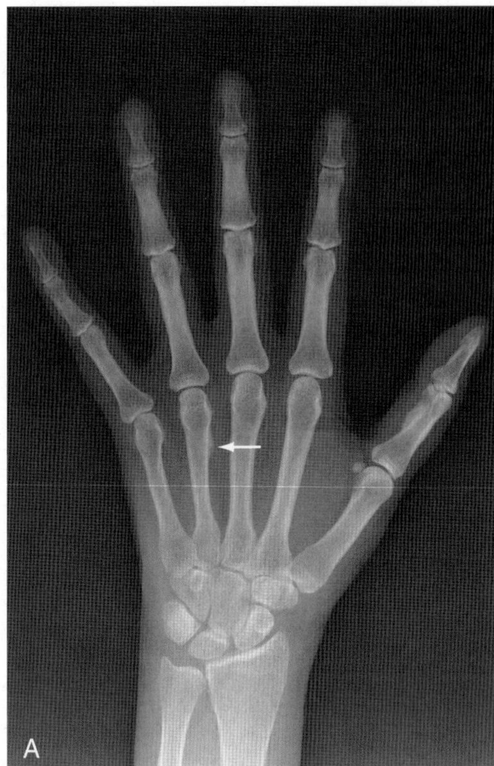

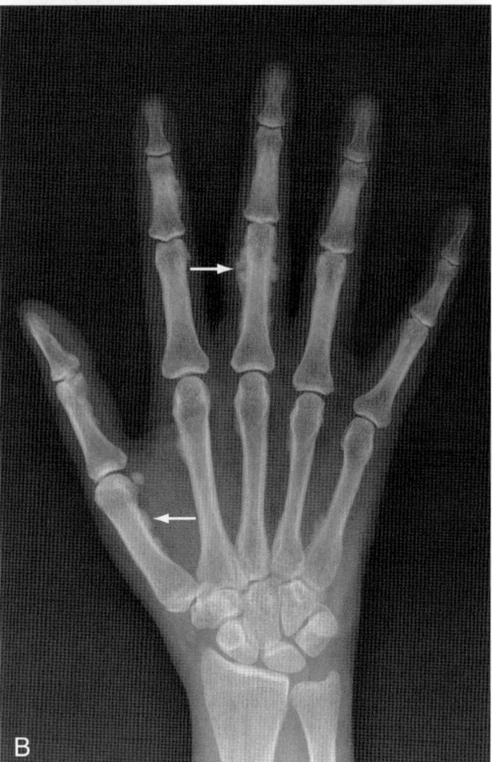

FIGURE 17-3. Hypertrophic osteoarthropathy. This patient with cystic fibrosis underwent a lung transplant. The posteroanterior view of the **(A)** left and **(B)** right hands shows irregular periosteal reaction *(arrows)* thought to be due to HOA.

the periosteal reaction seems to be related to disease duration. Thus, in the same study, periosteal reaction in primary HOA and in CCHD was usually multilayered and an irregular pattern was seen in one third of those patients (Figure 17-3). In the patients with lung cancer–related HOA, the most frequent appearance was a single layer of periosteal new bone and no irregular periostitis was seen.[14]

Acroosteolysis has been described in the fingers of patients with primary pachydermoperiostosis and with HOA.[15] Correlation with other signs is necessary to exclude other causes of this abnormality.

Scintigraphy

Bone scan findings in HOA are characterized by symmetrical increased uptake along the cortices of long bones (the "parallel track" or "double stripe" sign) consistent with periosteal new bone formation.[16] The regions covered by periosteum are usually involved, but extension to the epiphyses can be present and can be seen on radiographs. Ali noted the involvement to be "regular" in 85% of cases and symmetric in 83%.[16] It was more active in the lower as compared with the upper extremities in 98% of cases, with activity greater in the long bones distal to the knees and elbows (Figure 17-4). Either the tibias or the fibulas were involved in all cases.[16] In another publication, Love noted the uptake pattern to be most commonly nonuniform, irregular cortical uptake involving the long bones. Unexpectedly, involvement was seen by Ali et al. in the metatarsals, metacarpals, calcanei, and distal phalanges (attributed to the improved imaging technology of the time) and in the scapulas (67%), clavicles (33%), skull (42%), and mandible. Involvement of the pelvis occurred in only one case, and spine and sacral involvement were not seen.

> Involvement of the pelvis and spine is not a feature of HOA and should suggest metastatic disease.

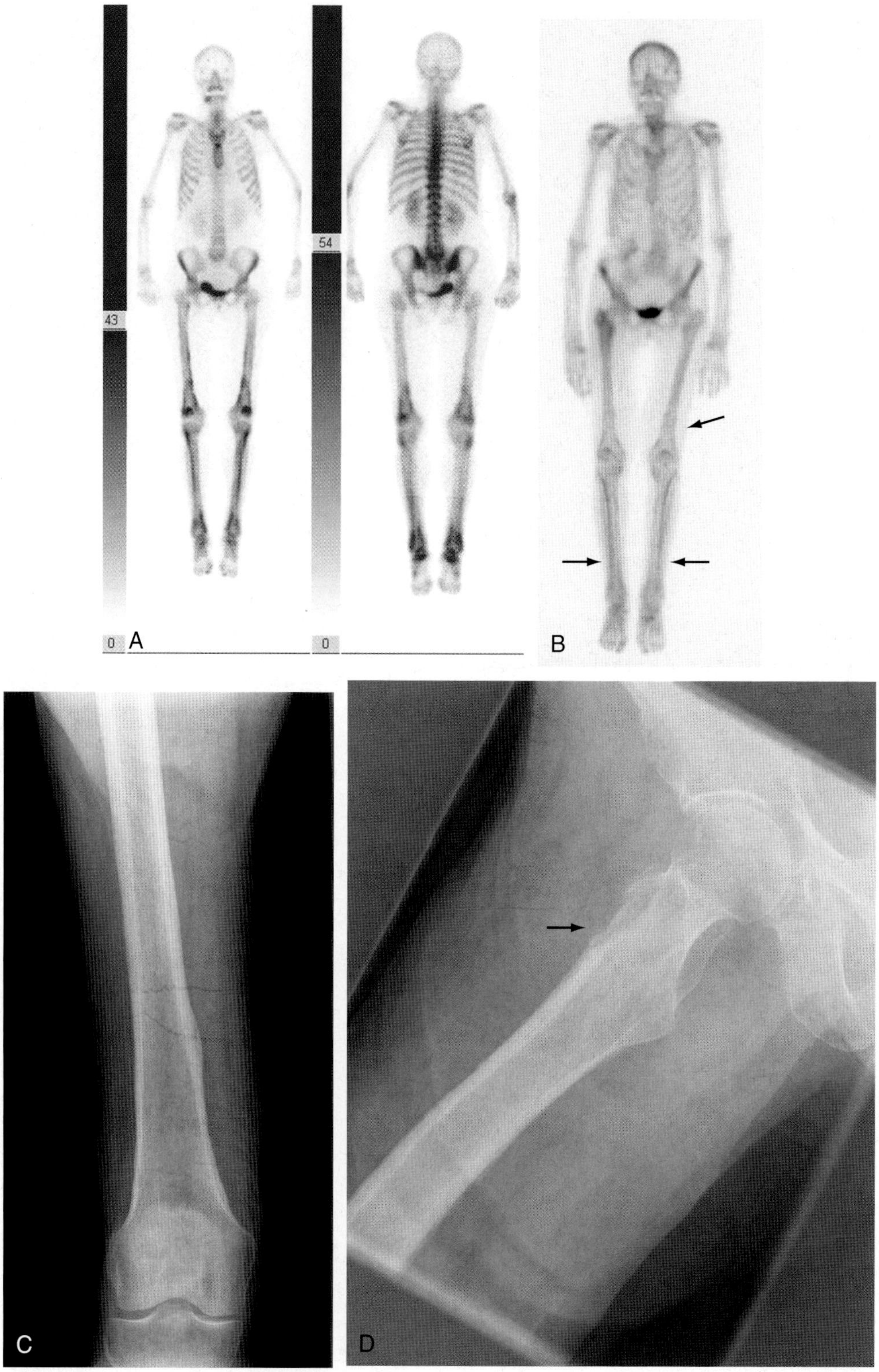

FIGURE 17-4. Bone scan in HOA. **A,** The anterior *(left)* and posterior *(right)* images from a bone scan show increased uptake along the femurs and tibias consistent with HOA in this patient with lung carcinoma. **B,** Bone scan of another patient shows increased uptake along the shafts of the femurs and tibias *(arrows)*. There is also a focal area of increased uptake in the right proximal femur. **C,** Radiograph of the distal femur shows periosteal reaction consistent with HOA. **D,** "Frog leg" lateral radiograph of the right hip shows a destructive lesion of the greater trochanter *(arrow)* consistent with a metastatic lesion from the patient's known non-small cell lung cancer. (**A,** Courtesy of Victor Gerbaudo, PhD, Brigham and Women's Hospital, Boston; **B** to **D,** courtesy of Niall Philip Sheehy, MBBCh, BAO, Brigham and Women's Hospital, Boston.)

Increased radionuclide uptake is also present around joints affected with synovitis and in the fingertips due to clubbing or to acroosteolysis.[17]

Magnetic Resonance Imaging

MRI findings mirror the bone scan findings with symmetric increased signal around the diaphyses and metaphyses of the femur, tibia, and fibula on short tau inversion recovery (STIR) images, indicating periosteal reaction.[3] This may precede radiographic identification of periosteal new bone formation.

Fluorodeoxyglucose Positron Emission Tomography (FOG-PET)

Increased FDG accumulation is seen in the associated primary pulmonary tumor (or infection), and faint uptake has been noted along the femurs in a patient with HOA associated with non-small cell lung cancer.[18]

The imaging findings of HOA may precede the diagnosis of the underlying condition (or its recurrence or the development of metastases) even by many months.[19] Symptoms may improve or resolve after removal of the tumor or treatment of the underlying condition, and imaging findings can similarly regress or disappear after treatment.[16]

Differential Diagnosis of Imaging Features

Other conditions may result in periosteal reaction, but the constellation of imaging and clinical findings usually allows the proper diagnosis to be made. The pattern of symmetric juxtacortical uptake in HOA can be readily distinguished from the more central and medullary uptake seen in metastatic disease in most cases. Involvement of the spine, pelvis, or ribs is rare in HOA and frequent in metastatic disease.[16] Periosteal reaction in the hands may be seen in psoriatic arthritis or juvenile rheumatoid arthritis, in association with human immunodeficiency virus, and in thyroid acropachy.[20] The scintigraphic features, when confined to the lower extremities, however, should be diagnosed with caution because a similar distribution of uptake may be seen with chronic venous stasis or lower limb edema.[16,21]

ARTICULAR INVOLVEMENT IN MULTIPLE MYELOMA

Multiple myeloma is a malignant proliferation of plasma cells that produces a monoclonal paraprotein.[22] Articular involvement in multiple myeloma is occasionally a presenting manifestation of the disease. Arthritis associated with multiple myeloma may take the form of an oligoarthritis or a rheumatoid-like polyarthritis.[22] Possible mechanisms for arthritis in multiple myeloma are summarized by Molloy et al. as (1) infection, (2) gout, (3) local synovial precipitation of paraproteins or immunoglobulin crystals inciting an inflammatory response, (4) deposition of amyloid or immunoglobulins resulting in carpal tunnel syndrome, or (5) direct invasion of the synovium.[22] Sumrall et al. reported infection of multiple joints as the initial manifestation of multiple myeloma[23] (Figure 17-5). Rarely, multiple myeloma may present as an acute interstitial nephritis and rheumatoid-like polyarthritis.[24]

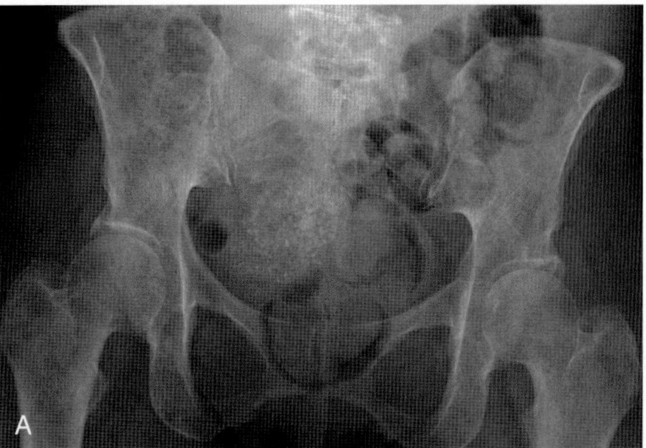

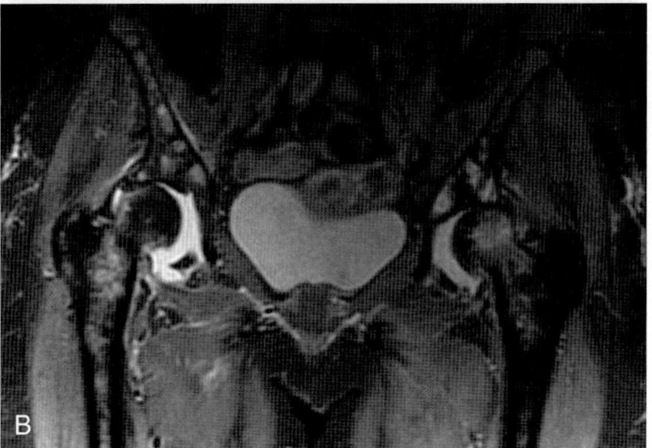

FIGURE 17-5. Joint disease in multiple myeloma. **A,** Radiograph of the pelvis shows barely visible lucent lesions, most prominent in the proximal right femur. **B,** Follow-up STIR image from an MRI scan of the pelvis approximately 2 years later shows the multiple high signal bone lesions. There is now severe cartilage loss in each hip, large hip joint effusions, and adjacent marrow edema. The specific cause of the changes is not known.

Amyloidosis may complicate multiple myeloma. Fautrel et al. found proven peripheral amyloid arthropathy in 11 of 311 patients with multiple myeloma on retrospective review.[25] The arthropathy occurred within 6 months after the diagnosis of multiple myeloma in most cases. Shoulder arthropathy and a rheumatoid-like polyarthritis were the most frequent types of articular involvement.

Radiographs may show erosive changes.[26] A characteristic (but not entirely specific) appearance of amyloid is seen on MRI examination. The involved joint is distended with intraarticular masses that are low in signal on both T1-weighted and STIR images[27] (Figure 17-6).

MISCELLANEOUS DISORDERS

Imaging may be useful in detecting tumors associated with paraneoplastic syndromes.[28] Palmar fasciitis and polyarthritis have been associated with ovarian and nonovarian carcinomas.[29] MRI can confirm the clinical findings, and imaging can identify the associated malignancy (Figure 17-7).

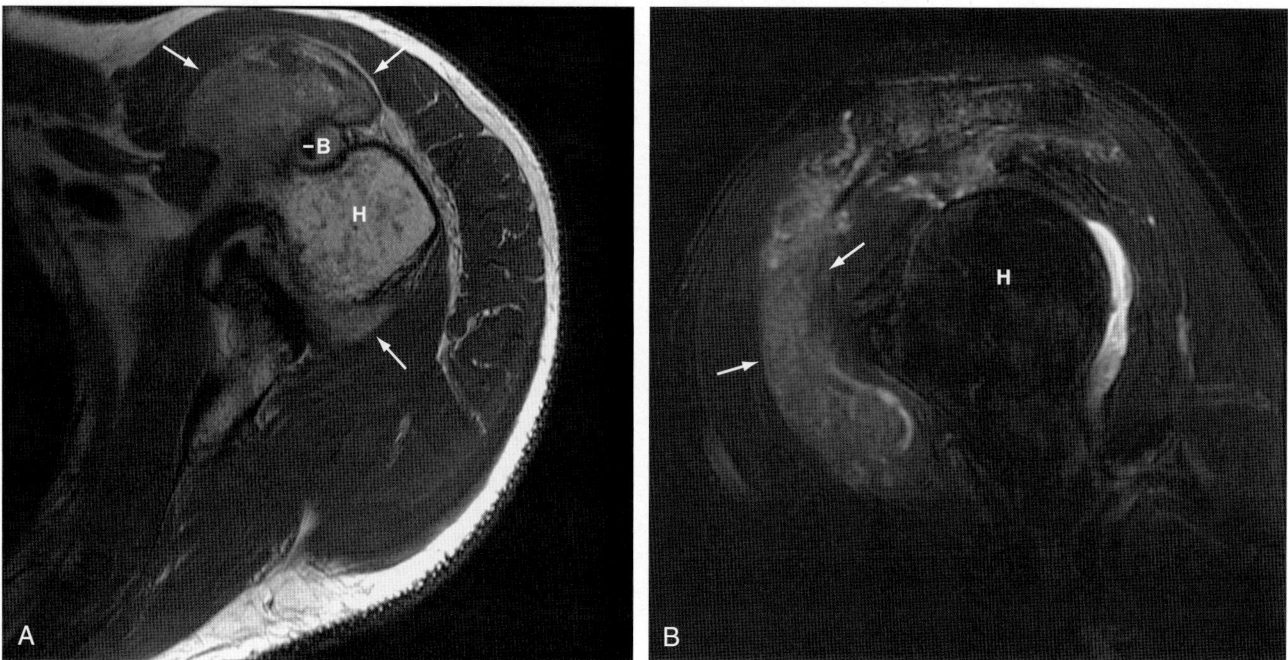

FIGURE 17-6. Amyloid arthropathy in a patient with multiple myeloma presenting with a palpable mass anterior to the shoulder. **A,** Axial proton density image from an MRI scan shows marked distension of the subscapularis recess *(two arrows)* and of the joint *(single arrow)* by intermediate signal material. *B,* Biceps tendon; *H,* humerus. **B,** The sagittal STIR image shows the large distended anterior recess to be filled with intermediate to low signal material consistent with amyloid *(arrows)*. This was proven at biopsy but was characteristic from the imaging appearance given the clinical information. *H,* Humerus.

Metastatic lesions may invade joints (Figure 17-8). Leukemia may present with rheumatologic complaints, and initial radiographs may alert the clinician to the diagnosis. Jones et al.[30] compared clinical and laboratory findings of patients presenting to a rheumatology clinic who were subsequently found to have juvenile rheumatoid arthritis or acute lymphocytic leukemia. The frequency of abnormal radiographic findings was similar between the two groups. The findings of radiolucent bands, sclerosis, lytic lesions, and periosteal elevation were seen only in children with acute lymphocytic leukemia, however. Osteopenia and joint effusions were seen in both groups[31,32] (Figure 17-9).

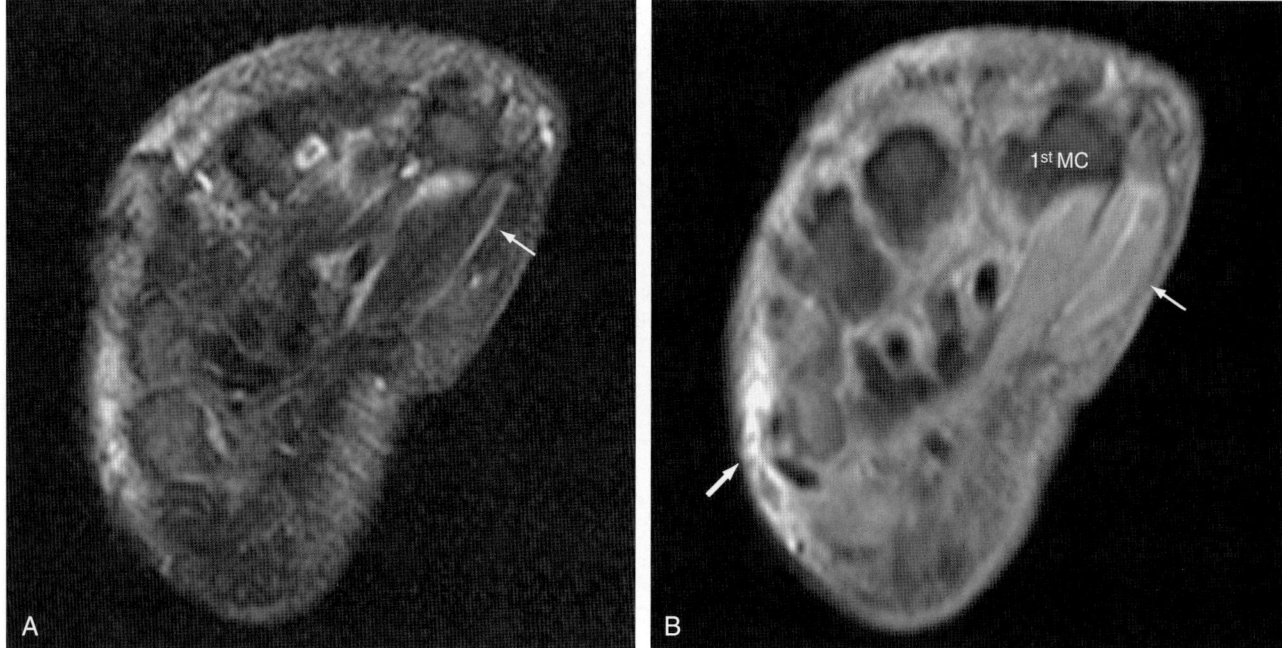

FIGURE 17-7. Palmar fasciitis in a patient later proven to have ovarian carcinoma. **A,** The axial STIR MR image of the hand shows edema along the dorsum of the hand and along the fascia of the thenar eminence *(arrow)*. **B,** After intravenous contrast, there is enhancement in these same regions. *1st MC,* first metacarpal.

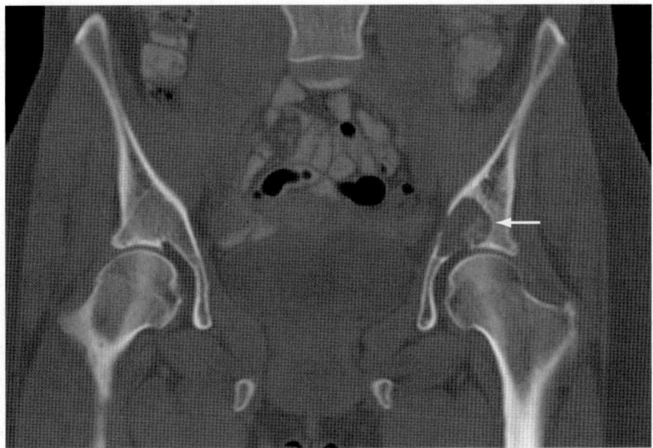

FIGURE 17-8. Metastatic breast carcinoma. Coronal reformatted image from a CT scan shows a lytic lesion *(arrow)* that destroys the medial acetabulum and the acetabular roof.

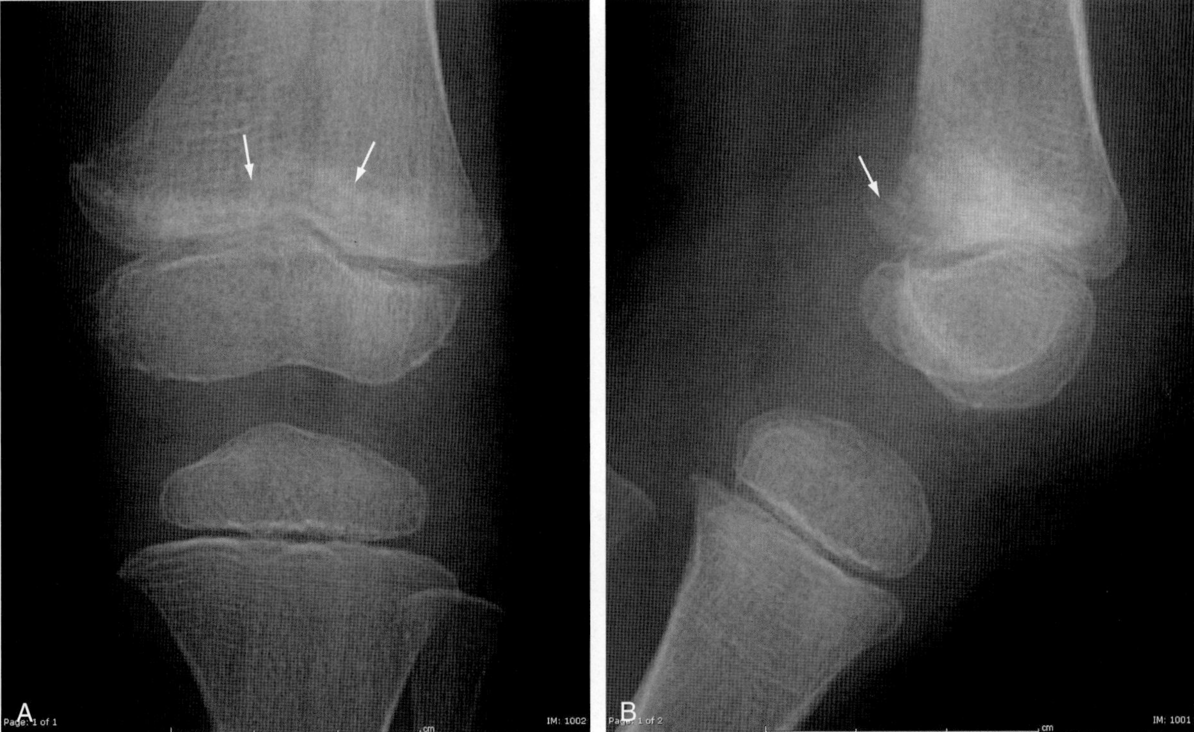

FIGURE 17-9. Acute lymphocytic leukemia in a 4-year-old child. **A,** Anteroposterior radiograph of the knee shows a metaphyseal lucent band *(arrows)*. **B,** Lateral radiograph shows the cortical defect posteriorly *(arrow)* due to the metaphyseal lucency. The diagnosis was suggested on the basis of the radiographic appearance.

(Continued)

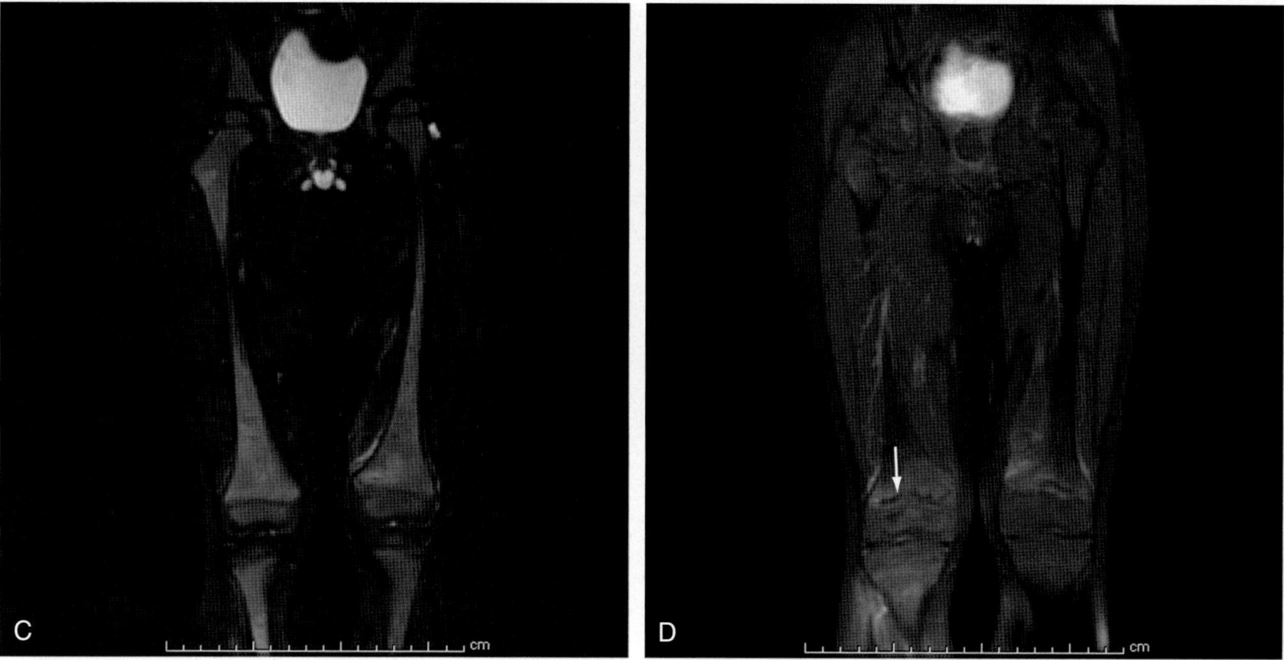

FIGURE 17-9—cont'd. **C,** Coronal STIR image shows the abnormal bone marrow to be diffusely increased in signal. The low signal metaphyseal band is faintly visible. **D,** After intravenous contrast there is enhancement along the metaphyseal bands bilaterally *(arrow)*. (Courtesy of Dr. Michele Walters, Brigham & Women's Hospital and Children's Hospital, Boston.)

REFERENCES

1. Von Bamberger E: Veranderungen der Rohrrenknochen bei Bronchiektasie, *Wien Klin Wochenschr* 2:226, 1889.
2. Marie P: De l'osteo-arthropathie hypertrophiante pneumique, *Rev Med Paris* 10:1, 1890.
3. Sainani NI, Lawande MA, Parikh VP et al: MRI diagnosis of hypertrophic osteoarthropathy from a remote childhood malignancy, *Skeletal Radiol* 36(Suppl 1):S63-S66, 2007.
4. Armstrong DJ, McCausland EM, Wright GD: Hypertrophic pulmonary osteoarthropathy (HPOA) (Pierre Marie-Bamberger syndrome): two cases presenting as acute inflammatory arthritis. Description and review of the literature, *Rheumatol Int* 27:399-402, 2007.
5. Cannavo SP, Guarneri C, Borgia F et al: Pierre Marie-Bamberger syndrome (secondary hypertrophic osteoarthropathy), *Int J Dermatol* 44:41-42, 2005.
6. Segal AM, Mackenzie AH: Hypertrophic osteoarthropathy: a 10-year retrospective analysis, *Semin Arthritis Rheumat* 12:220-232, 1982.
7. Rutherford RB, Rhodes BA, Wagner HN Jr: The distribution of extremity blood flow before and after vagectomy in a patient with hypertrophic pulmonary osteoarthropathy, *Dis Chest* 56:19-23, 1969.
8. Spicknall KE, Zirwas MJ, English JC 3rd: Clubbing: an update on diagnosis, differential diagnosis, pathophysiology, and clinical relevance, *J Am Acad Dermatol* 52:1020-1028, 2005.
9. Katsicas M, Ciocca M, Rosanova M et al: Hypertrophic osteoarthropathy in two children with holestatic hepatic disease, *Acta Paediatr* 94:1152-1155, 2005.
10. Armstrong RD, Crisp AJ, Grahame R et al: Hypertrophic osteoarthropathy and purgative abuse, *Br Med J Clin Res Ed* 282:1836, 1981.
11. Alonso-Bartolome P, Martínez-Taboada VM, Pina T et al: Hypertrophic osteoarthropathy secondary to vascular prosthesis infection: report of 3 cases and review of the literature, *Medicine* 85:183-191, 2006.
12. Kuloğlu Z, Kansu A, Ekici F et al: Hypertrophic osteoarthropathy in a child with biliary atresia, *Scand J Gastroenterol* 39:698-701, 2004.
13. McNaughton DA, Nguyen BD: AJR teaching file: cavitated mass with hypertrophic osteoarthropathy, *AJR Am J Roentgenol* 188(3 Suppl):S7-S9, 2007.
14. Pineda CJ, Martinez-Lavin M, Goobar JE et al: Periostitis in hypertrophic osteoarthropathy: relationship to disease duration, *AJR Am J Roentgenol* 148:773-778, 1987.
15. Joseph B, Chacko V: Acro-osteolysis associated with hypertrophic pulmonary osteoarthropathy and pachydermoperiostosis, *Radiology* 154:343-344, 1985.
16. Ali A, Tetalman MR, Fordham EW et al: Distribution of hypertrophic pulmonary osteoarthropathy, *AJR Am J Roentgenol* 134:771-780, 1980.
17. Rosenthall L, Kirsh J: Observations of radionuclide imaging in hypertrophic pulmonary osteoarthropathy, *Radiology* 120:359-362, 1976.
18. Strobel K, Schaffer NG, Hasarik TF et al: Pulmonary hypertrophic osteoarthropathy in a patient with nonsmall cell lung cancer: diagnosis with FDG PET/CT, *Clin Nucl Med* 31:624-626, 2006.
19. Staalman CR, Umans U: Hypertrophic osteoarthropathy in childhood malignancy, *Med Pediatr Oncol* 21:676-679, 1993.
20. Restrepo CS, Lemos DF, Gordillo H et al: Imaging findings in musculoskeletal complications of AIDS, *Radiographics* 24:1029-1049, 2004.
21. Gensburg RS, Kawashima A, Sandler CM: Scintigraphic demonstration of lower extremity periostitis secondary to venous insufficiency, *J Nucl Med* 29:1279-1282, 1988.
22. Molloy C, Peck RA, Bonny SJ et al: An unusual presentation of multiple myeloma: a case report, *J Med Case Reports* 10:84, 2007.
23. Sumrall A, Muzny C, Bell J et al: Pneumococcal septic arthritis as the initial presentation of multiple myeloma, *Int J Lab Hem* 30:82-83, 2008.
24. Ardalan MR, Shoja MM: Multiple myeloma presented as acute interstitial nephritis and rheumatoid arthritis-like polyarthritis, *Am J Hematol* 82:309-313, 2007.
25. Fautrel B, Fermand JP, Sibilia J et al: Amyloid arthropathy in the course of multiple myeloma, *J Rheumatol* 29:1473-1481, 2002.
26. Bukhari M, Freemont AJ, Noble J et al: Erosive amyloidosis of the wrist and knee associated with oligoclonal bands, *Br J Rheumatol* 36:494-497, 1997.
27. Prokaeva T, Spencer B, Kaut M et al: Soft tissue, joint, and bone manifestations of AL amyloidosis: clinical presentation, molecular features, and survival, *Arthritis Rheum* 56:3858-3868, 2007.
28. Crotty E, Patz EF Jr: FDG-PET imaging in patients with paraneoplastic syndromes and suspected small cell lung cancer, *J Thorac Imaging* 16:89-93, 2001.
29. Shiel WC Jr, Prete PE, Jason M et al: Palmar fasciitis and arthritis with ovarian and non-ovarian carcinomas. New syndrome, *Am J Med* 79:640-644, 1985.
30. Jones OY, Spencer CH, Bowyer SL et al: A multicenter case-control study on predictive factors distinguishing childhood leukemia from juvenile rheumatoid arthritis, *Pediatrics*, 117:e840-e844, 2006.
31. Spilberg I, Meyer GJ: The arthritis of leukemia, *Arthritis Rheum* 15:630-635, 1972.
32. Rogalsky RJ, Black GB, Reed MH: Orthopaedic manifestations of leukemia in children, *J Bone Joint Surg Am* 68:494-501, 1986.

CHAPTER 18

Juxtaarticular Cysts and Fluid Collections: Imaging and Intervention

JOEL S. NEWMAN, MD

KEY FACTS

- Cysts and ganglia demonstrate similar imaging characteristics but may be distinguished in some instances by their location.
- Cysts and ganglia may cause nerve compression. This occurs most often in the shoulder due to paralabral cysts (suprascapular nerve) or in the knee due to tibiofibular ganglia (peroneal nerve).
- Symptomatic improvement may follow drainage and injection of corticosteroids into cysts.
- Not all lesions that appear well defined and homogeneously bright on T2-weighted images are cysts. Intravenous gadolinium can differentiate solid tumors from cystic masses; vascular masses will enhance centrally, whereas cystic collections will enhance only peripherally or not at all. Ultrasound may also differentiate solid masses from cysts.

Juxtaarticular cysts and fluid collections may develop as an extension of intracapsular pathology or may present in the absence of intrinsic joint disease. Cysts may form adjacent to large and small joints both in the appendicular and axial skeleton. Commonly encountered cystic lesions include synovial cysts and ganglia. Bursal distension with fluid is common around joints; adventitial bursae may form in response to repeated localized frictional injury, particularly in the foot. Meniscal cysts develop secondary to meniscal tears, and paralabral cysts are formed in the setting of labral tears at the shoulder or hip.[1]

Assigning the appropriate nomenclature to juxtaarticular cysts is often difficult and results in considerable confusion. A large majority of the cysts detailed below develop secondary to a process occurring within the joint capsule. Some represent distension of preexisting anatomic connections to the joint; others a de novo outpouching from the capsule. Elucidating the etiology of the cyst is far more important than assigning the correct name; in fact, these lesions share very similar imaging characteristics.

Synovial cysts are commonly encountered about joints, large and small. These synovial cell–lined cysts represent outpouching or herniation of the synovial membrane through the joint capsule. Synovial cysts may develop secondary to a variety to intracapsular processes including inflammatory arthropathy (Figure 18-1), degenerative joint disease (DJD), or, rarely, crystal arthropathies.[2-4]

> Synovial cysts are diverticula or herniations of the synovial membrane through the joint capsule, often in response to increased intraarticular pressure. These cysts are lined by synovium.

Soft tissue ganglion cysts may arise from joints or tendon sheaths. Ganglia are considered to represent degenerative lesions.[5] Given their similar imaging appearances to synovial cysts, differentiation of the two entities may be difficult, if not impossible. Some contend that unlike synovial cysts, ganglion cysts lack a synovial cell lining.[6] Histologically, ganglia are unilocular or multilocular and are filled with a mucinous substance.[5] On cytologic examination, histiocytes may be present.[7,8] As will be detailed subsequently, many ganglia are filled with fluid more viscous than typical joint fluid; this may simply reflect desiccation of synovial fluid that no longer freely communicates with its source.

> Ganglia are cyst-like structures filled with a mucinous fluid and lacking a synovial lining. They are difficult to differentiate on imaging studies from synovial cysts.

Bursae are synovium-lined sacs that may lie in apposition to bony prominences or between tendons and ligaments. Adventitial bursae may develop in the subcutaneous tissues adjacent to sites of repetitive frictional trauma. Some bursae may communicate with adjacent joints, including the iliopsoas bursa at the hip and semimembranosus-gastrocnemius bursa at the knee. In this regard, their behavior is analogous to synovial cysts, becoming distended secondary to a variety of intraarticular conditions.[9,10]

> Bursae are synovium-lined sacs that are present at sites of friction such as adjacent to bony prominences. When bursae communicate with joints (e.g., the Baker's cyst in the knee) they behave as synovial cysts and distend in response to intraarticular increases in pressure.

Juxtaarticular cysts may be asymptomatic, although many present with localized swelling, the perception of deep pain or fullness by the patient, or as a mass confirmed on physical examination. In rare cases, nerve compression by a cyst may result in pain, motor weakness, or muscle atrophy. Some cysts, encountered in the appropriate clinical setting, may be amenable to aspiration in the clinician's office. In most cases, however, initial imaging is warranted to define the anatomy, elucidate any related intracapsular

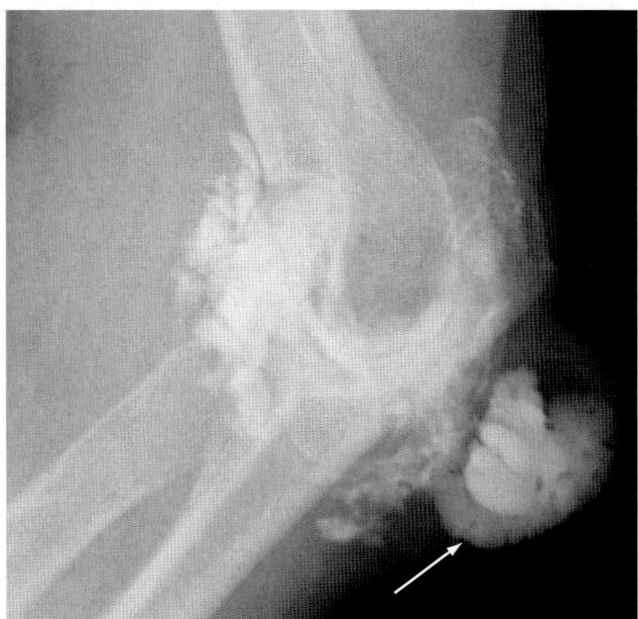

FIGURE 18-1. Rheumatoid arthritis with synovial cyst. Lateral elbow radiograph taken following contrast injection into the joint shows a markedly irregular joint capsule with filling defects due to hyperplastic synovium. A synovial cyst posterior to the olecranon *(arrow)* fills with contrast.

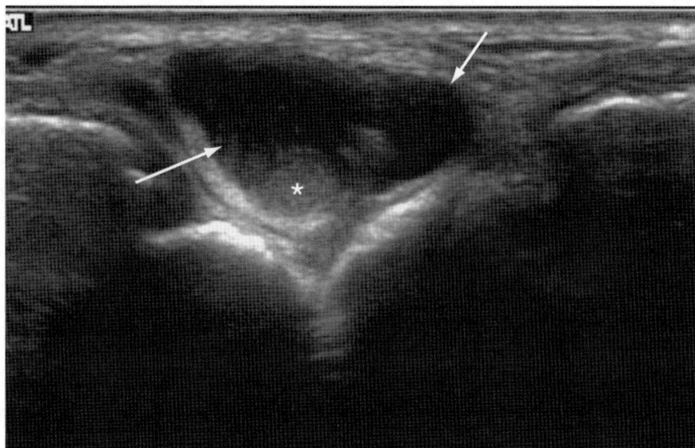

FIGURE 18-2. Dorsal wrist ganglion—sonography. Sagittal image of the dorsum of the wrist shows an ovoid, predominantly anechoic mass *(arrows)* situated superficial to the radiocarpal joint. There is debris within the dependent portion of the ganglion cyst *(asterisk)*.

pathology, and confirm that the palpable finding is indeed a cyst and not a solid or partially solid mass. If clinically indicated, aspiration, with or without corticosteroid injection, may be readily performed by the radiologist under imaging guidance.

IMAGING

Suspected cystic lesions around joints in the appendicular skeleton are initially evaluated with radiography followed by sonography or magnetic resonance imaging (MRI) to document the cystic nature of the mass. Deeper lesions and those in the axial skeleton may be difficult to image with ultrasound, necessitating MRI. Radiographs should be performed initially at all painful joints, even if a discrete mass is palpable, in order to evaluate for underlying arthropathies, osseous lesions, and soft tissue calcification. A cyst may be visible as a water-density soft tissue mass on radiographs, although a solid mass may be indistinguishable in its appearance. By virtue of its more limited contrast resolution, computed tomography (CT) is recommended for the evaluation of juxtaarticular cysts only in limited situations. This includes deeper lesions adjoining joint prostheses and other implants where MRI is limited by virtue of metal artifact. CT does remain a useful modality, however, for image-guided aspiration of some lesions.

On sonography, cystic lesions have a variable appearance, similar to other fluid collections, ranging from anechoic, to largely anechoic with low level echoes, to hypoechoic.[11] Some chronic synovial cysts, for example, may have considerable avascular, solid debris along the cyst walls or layering dependently within the cyst cavity (Figure 18-2). Increased through-transmission may be evident in many cases. Color or power Doppler sonography may be useful in confirming the avascular nature of the cyst, despite a heterogeneous appearance on gray-scale imaging.[12] Synovial cysts that have developed in continuity to articulations with severe DJD may contain chondral and/or osteochondral bodies, the latter resulting in "shadowing." Septations may be observed in many cysts.

On MRI, juxtaarticular cysts have a relatively typical appearance, being of similar signal intensity to fluid on all sequences.[1] On T1-weighted scans, cyst fluid is of moderately low signal intensity. On T2-weighted scans, cyst fluid exhibits high signal intensity. If cysts are filled with highly proteinaceous fluid, or, in the setting of subacute hemorrhage within a cyst, modestly elevated signal on T1-weighted scans may be identified. In synovium-lined cysts with acute or chronic inflammation, wall thickening may be observed. Innumerable, small filling defects within cyst fluid may reflect fronds of hyperplastic synovium. Ossified bodies in the cyst cavity exhibit very low signal intensity (signal void) but centrally may contain high signal on T1-weighted images, indicating bone marrow elements.

Although the majority of juxtaarticular cysts are readily diagnosed on MRI by virtue of their anatomic location and imaging appearances, some cysts may exhibit atypical characteristics mimicking a solid mass, particularly a homogeneous-appearing neoplasm, such as a myxoma[13] (Figure 18-3). In equivocal cases, such as these, T1-weighted MRI should be performed before and after intravenous (IV) gadolinium administration. The avascular cyst contents will fail to exhibit contrast enhancement (Figure 18-4); with solid masses, enhancement is generally visualized (Figure 18-5). Rim enhancement of cysts, however, is not uncommon.

> Cyst vs. solid: Masses that exhibit homogeneous fluid signal on MRI (intermediate signal on T1-weighted images and high signal on T2-weighted images) are not necessarily cysts. Tumors with high water content, such as myxomas, can exhibit similar imaging findings. In cases in which location or appearance suggest the possibility of a solid mass, IV contrast should be administered. The central part of the mass will enhance if it is a tumor but not if it is a fluid collection. Ultrasound can also distinguish cystic from solid lesions.

Knee

Cystic lesions about the knee are common and are readily detected at the time of MRI examination performed after acute knee injury or in the setting of chronic knee pain. Popliteal cysts, meniscal cysts, bursal collections, and ganglia may be encountered. Clinical manifestations are variable based on location and the presence or absence of intracapsular pathology.

Popliteal cysts are synovial cysts that extend posterior and medial to the knee, situated between the semimembranosus tendon and the proximal medial head of gastrocnemius muscle and

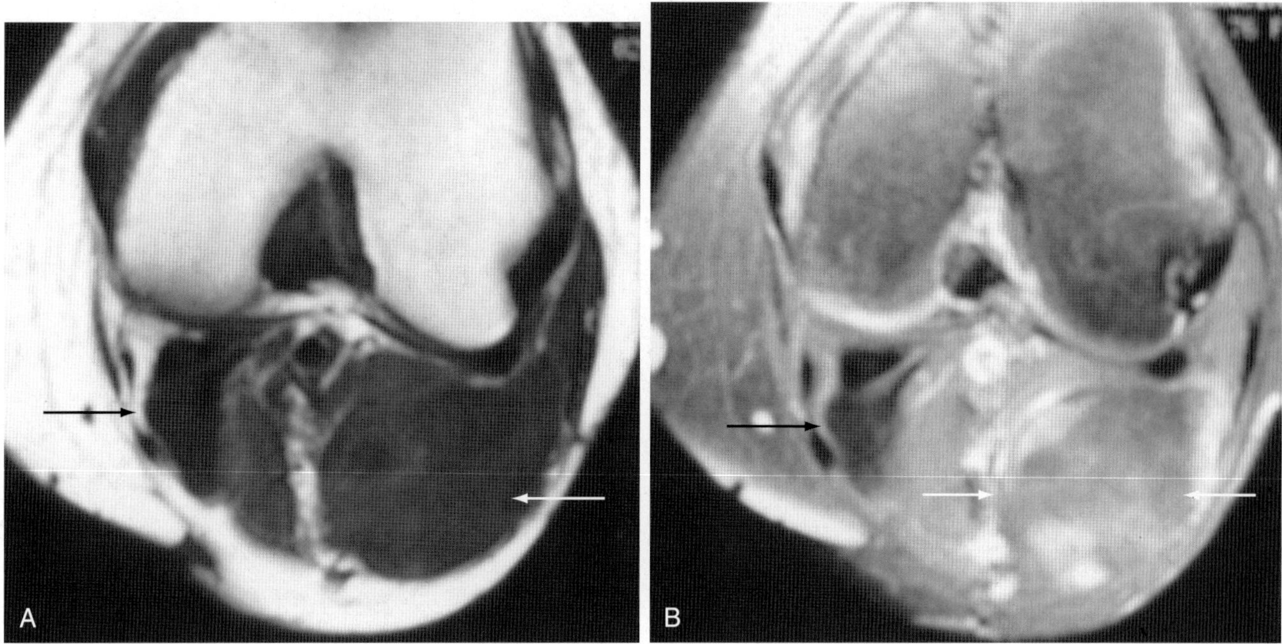

FIGURE 18-3. Myxoid liposarcoma: popliteal fossa. **A,** Axial T1-weighted image of the knee shows a slightly heterogeneous mass along the posterolateral knee *(white arrow)*. A small popliteal cyst *(black arrow)* is also present. **B,** Axial T1-weighted fat-suppressed image following gadolinium administration shows mild, patchy enhancement of the mass *(white arrows)*, which was shown to represent a myxoid liposarcoma at biopsy. Note the lack of enhancement of the central fluid contents of the popliteal cyst *(black arrow)*.

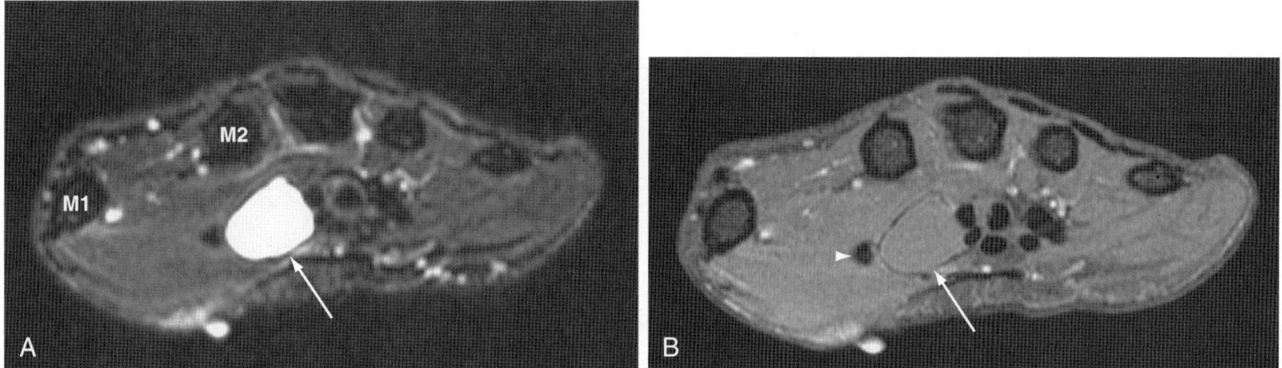

FIGURE 18-4. Palmar ganglion—MRI. **A,** Axial inversion recovery scan shows a homogeneous, hyperintense mass *(arrow)* along the palmar aspect of the wrist, between the thumb and index finger flexor tendons. The thumb *(M1)* and index *(M2)* metacarpals are noted. **B,** Axial T1-weighted fat-suppressed MR image following IV gadolinium administration shows no enhancement within the ganglion cyst *(arrow)*. The flexor pollicis longus tendon is indicated by an *arrowhead*.

tendon. This potential space is referred to as the *semimembranosus-gastrocnemius bursa;* the nomenclature itself may be a source of confusion.[14] In most cases, there is a potential communication between joint and bursa, allowing decompression of joint fluid into the bursa (Figure 18-6). When large, these cysts dissect caudad and occasionally cephalad. Patients with popliteal cysts may report a sensation of fullness posterior to the knee. Large cysts may be palpable or even manifest visible swelling or mass on physical examination.

Popliteal cysts typically form in the setting of increased intracapsular pressure, with the joint effusion decompressing posteriorly. These cysts frequently accompany both DJD and inflammatory arthropathies and can be seen with meniscal tears.[4,15] Intracapsular chondroosseous bodies may extend into the cyst in the setting of DJD or with primary synovial osteochondromatosis.

On radiographs, large popliteal cysts may be visible as a soft tissue density mass in the popliteal fossa; osseous bodies within the cyst may be visualized. In the patient with posterior knee pain and fullness, sonography is a rapid means of diagnosing a popliteal cyst and excluding other conditions such as popliteal deep venous thrombosis. These cysts are typically ovoid in shape and longest in the longitudinal axis (Figure 18-7). When imaged transversely, a comma shape may be observed due to the narrow neck extending anteriorly between the semimembranosus tendon and the medial head of the gastrocnemius (Figure 18-8). The cyst contents are variable, from anechoic to complex,[11] with occasional wall thickening and septation. Ultrasound is more sensitive than physical examination for the detection of popliteal cysts.[16] On MRI in the transverse plane, the typical comma shape may also be observed with signal intensities reflecting its largely fluid content.

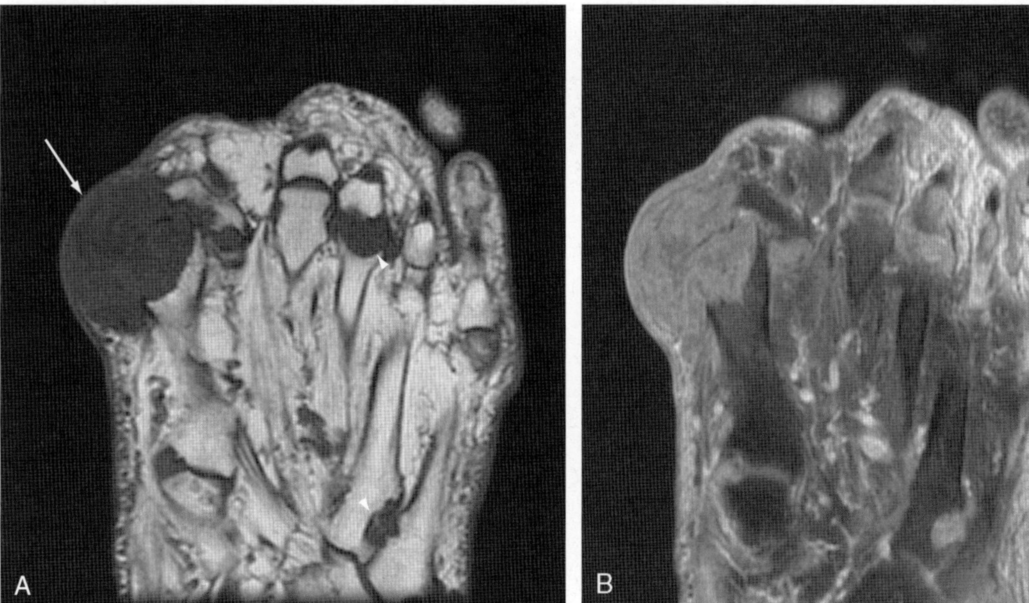

FIGURE 18-5. Chronic tophaceous gout—MRI. **A,** An oblique axial T1-weighted MR image of the forefoot shows a large soft tissue mass *(arrow)* eroding the distal great toe metatarsal, compatible with a tophus. Note the sharply marginated erosion of bone along the tophus. Additional tophi with erosive changes are indicated by *arrowheads.* **B,** Following IV gadolinium administration, a fat-suppressed T1-weighted MR image shows enhancement of the tophi.

Popliteal cyst rupture presents as sudden severe calf pain and swelling as the cyst fluid typically dissects caudad and superficial to the medial head of the gastrocnemius muscle. MRI and/or ultrasound examination of the popliteal fossa and calf are generally indicated to exclude other conditions with a similar presentation, including gastrocnemius or soleus musculotendinous strain, plantaris rupture (Figure 18-9), or deep venous thrombosis.[17,18]

Acute pain and swelling may indicate popliteal cyst rupture, especially in patients with rheumatoid arthritis. Ultrasound is usually the easiest method to document cyst rupture and exclude deep venous thrombosis. MRI is most useful in documenting an underlying cause for the cyst (e.g., meniscal tear) or other conditions such as muscle strains that may simulate cyst rupture.

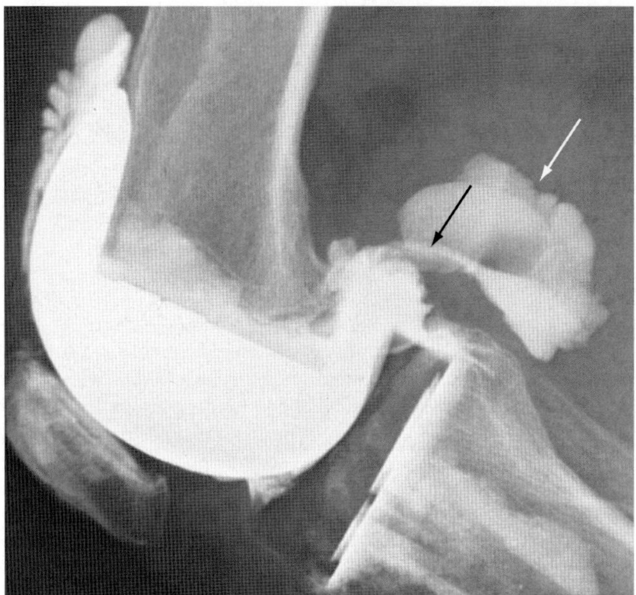

FIGURE 18-6. Popliteal cyst. Lateral post-arthrogram radiograph of the knee in a patient with a total knee arthroplasty shows contrast filling a popliteal cyst *(white arrow).* The thin connection to the joint is visible *(black arrow)* and may act as a one-way valve with fluid entering but not exiting the cyst.

Another commonly encountered cyst about the knee is the meniscal cyst. By definition, these cysts develop secondary to meniscal tears and reflect joint fluid being forced out through a meniscal tear via a one-way or ball-valve mechanism. These cysts originate along the margin of the meniscal tear (Figure 18-10), although they may dissect some distance from the tear.

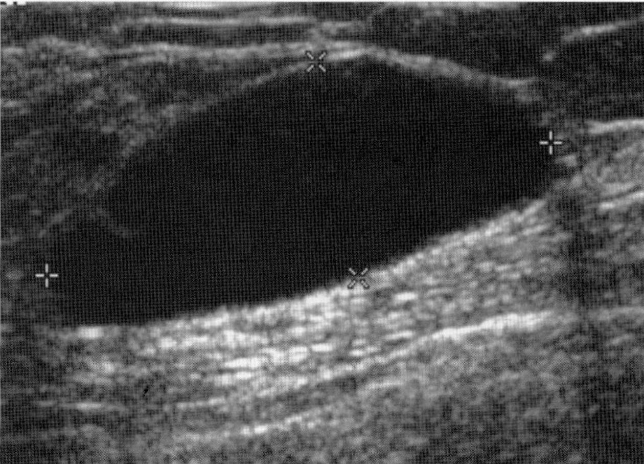

FIGURE 18-7. Popliteal cyst—sonography. Sagittal image of the popliteal fossa shows an ovoid, anechoic mass *(between cursors)* with increased through-transmission, compatible with a popliteal cyst.

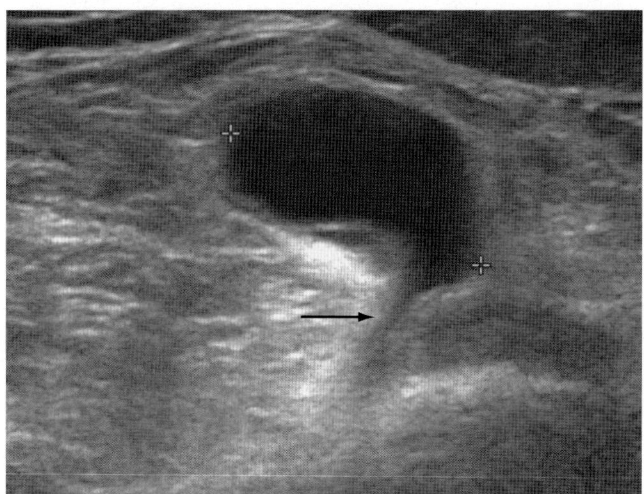

FIGURE 18-8. Popliteal cyst—sonography. Transverse image of a popliteal cyst *(between cursors)* showing the typical appearance of the cyst neck *(arrow)* extending between the semimembranosus tendon and the medial head of gastrocnemius to communicate with the knee joint capsule.

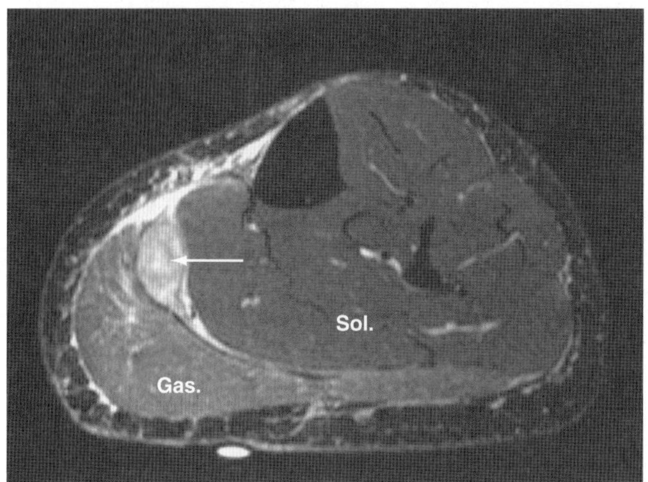

FIGURE 18-9. Plantaris rupture—MRI. Axial fat-suppressed proton density MR image of the calf in a patient with sudden calf pain and swelling following an athletic injury. Hematoma *(arrow)* interposed between the medial head of the gastrocnemius *(Gas.)* and the soleus *(Sol.)* is a typical finding in plantaris rupture.

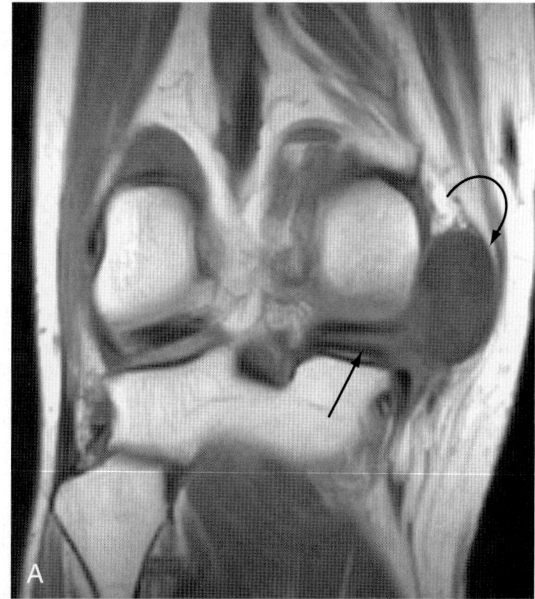

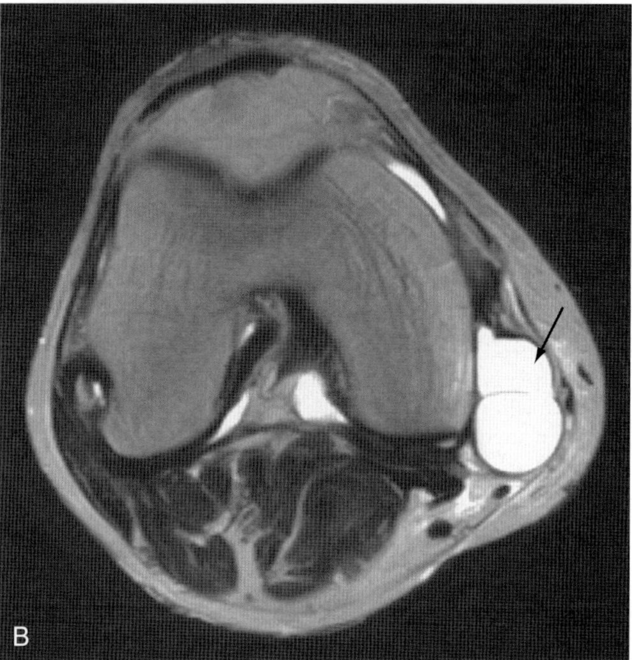

FIGURE 18-10. Meniscal cyst—MRI. **A,** Coronal T1-weighted MR image of the knee shows a heterogeneous mass *(curved arrow)* along the posteromedial aspect of the knee, in contiguity with the posterior horn of the medial meniscus. The horizontal high signal cleft traversing the meniscus represents the meniscal tear *(straight arrow)*. **B,** Axial T2-weighted MR image shows the typical high signal of the cyst contents *(arrow)*. A linear septation is seen.

Meniscal cysts have been described in association with both medial and lateral meniscal tears. MRI is a highly sensitive means for the detection of meniscal cysts[19]; in fact, these cysts have been detected in asymptomatic knees using MRI.[1]

Multiple bursae lie along the medial aspect of the knee. Bursal distension may result in medial joint line pain, simulating a meniscal tear and/or medial femorotibial DJD. The pes anserine bursa is located adjacent to the confluence of the semitendinosus, gracilis, and sartorius tendons as they course along the anterior aspect of the medial proximal tibia.

> The pes anserinus (goose's foot) bursa lies along the anteromedial tibia, deep to the sartorius, gracilis, and semitendinosus tendons and superficial to the medial collateral ligament.

This bursa is centered distal to the medial joint line. The clinical presentation of painful pes anserine bursitis may mimic that associated with a meniscal tear.[20]

> Pes anserinus bursitis is a cause of pain over the anteromedial tibia and is usually seen in overweight women, older patients with osteoarthritis, and young athletes (especially runners). Tenderness is present 2 to 5 cm below the anteromedial joint margin. Pain occurs especially with stair climbing.[20a]

The semimembranosus bursa is more posterior in location and slightly more proximal. Bursal distension results in a C-shaped collection draped over the semimembranosus tendon.[21] Fluid may be observed in the semimembranosus bursa along with distension of the semimembranosus-gastrocnemius bursa (popliteal cyst). The medial collateral ligament (MCL) bursa is a potential space deep to the superficial MCL fibers. An MCL bursal collection will typically have a crescent shape, conforming to the undersurface of the MCL and spanning the joint line.[22]

Anterior to the knee and adjacent to the extensor mechanism are the prepatellar and superficial infrapatellar bursae. Prepatellar bursitis is generally the result of friction on the prepatellar soft tissues, such as may be seen in the setting of repetitive kneeling.[23] Fluid collects superficial to the patella and may result in considerable swelling. Hematomas may collect in the prepatellar bursa following direct trauma. Small amounts of fluid are frequently identified incidentally on MRI or sonography within the deep infrapatellar bursa, which lies just deep to the distal patellar tendon.[1]

An important site of cyst formation about the knee is along the inner margin of the tibiofibular joint. These collections, referred to as *tibiofibular joint ganglia*, are variable in size. Due to the close proximity of tibiofibular joint ganglia to the peroneal nerve, some cysts may result in nerve irritation.[24]

Intraarticular ganglia at the knee have been described. These often lie adjacent to the anterior cruciate ligament (ACL) or posterior cruciate ligament (PCL) and are variable in size. Ganglia have been reported to occur in Hoffa's fat pad.[25,26] These lesions have also been reported in association with mucoid degeneration of the ACL.[27] Some intraarticular ganglia may be associated with pain.

Shoulder

Cystic lesions at the shoulder may lie in proximity to the glenohumeral joint or to the acromioclavicular (AC) joint. Synovial cysts are commonly encountered in rheumatoid arthritis. Fluid may collect in the subacromial-subdeltoid bursa in the setting of direct trauma, impingement, or with a full-thickness rotator cuff tear when joint and bursa are in direct communication. The paralabral cyst forms secondary to glenoid labral tear, dissecting along the scapular neck. As detailed below, some paralabral cysts may become symptomatic.

Although the osseous and articular manifestations of rheumatoid arthritis at the shoulder are beyond the scope of this chapter, there are a number of soft tissue abnormalities to consider. Synovial cysts may extend from the glenohumeral joint capsule. These may become quite large, presenting as a soft tissue mass.[28] On MRI, these cysts will show typical high signal intensity of fluid. In addition, the cyst contents will appear complex, with multiple, small filling defects representing hyperplastic synovial fronds, or "rice bodies." Glenohumeral joint arthrography will show communication between joint and synovial cysts; it is therefore not surprising that the appearance of the cyst contents would parallel those of joint fluid. In addition to synovial cysts, distension of the subacromial/subdeltoid bursa may be seen with rheumatoid arthritis; this can be massive.[29]

Massive distension of the subacromial bursa may be present in rheumatoid arthritis, tuberculosis, and amyloidosis, the latter described as the "shoulder pad sign."[30]

Of all cystic lesions at the shoulder, imaging plays the greatest role in the diagnosis and management of paralabral cysts. These cystic lesions form in response to glenoid labral tears, commonly posterior and/or superior in location.[31,32] The mechanism of formation is probably analogous to meniscal cysts at the knee: a ball-valve mechanism forcing synovial fluid from the joint through the labral rent. Although cysts may be encountered anteriorly, they are far more common posterior and superior in location. Tiny paralabral cysts are of no clinical significance; when large, these cysts may exert mass effect resulting in nerve compression.

MRI has revolutionized the diagnosis of paralabral cysts and offers not only precise anatomic localization but also the ability to define the sequelae of nerve compression. By virtue of their location, these cysts may not be optimally visualized at glenohumeral arthroscopy,[33] and paralabral cysts remain an important consideration in the differential diagnosis of shoulder pain, particularly in the setting of a normal rotator cuff. Prior to the widespread use of shoulder MRI, these cysts often went undiagnosed.

Most paralabral cysts dissect into the spinoglenoid notch (Figure 18-11); some extend to the supraspinous region. Less commonly, the cysts may be entirely supraspinous in location. Within the spinoglenoid notch, paralabral cysts may compromise the suprascapular nerve motor branch to the infraspinatus. More superiorly, in the supraspinous region, the motor branch to the supraspinatus may be compromised as well. Although the suprascapular nerve is primarily a motor nerve, it must be emphasized that, due to sensory branches, some patients experience deep pain with paralabral cysts.[34,35]

The diagnosis of nerve compromise, or denervation, can be confirmed with electromyography (EMG)[33] or diagnosed at the time of MR examination. In acute denervation, muscle edema is visualized. Depending on the location of suprascapular nerve compromise, this edema will involve the infraspinatus or infraspinatus and supraspinatus. Muscle edema may be subtle and is always best confirmed on proton density or T2-weighted scans with fat saturation or on inversion recovery scans. Long-standing denervation may result in muscle atrophy. On MRI, muscle atrophy manifests as progressively decreasing muscle bulk with increasing fatty infiltration.[36]

> Paralabral cysts may cause compression of the suprascapular nerve; when this occurs in the suprascapular notch, both the branch to the supraspinatus and infraspinatus muscles are affected; when it occurs at the spinoglenoid notch, only the infraspinatus muscle is affected. The resulting denervation will thus cause predictable patterns of muscle atrophy.

Traditionally, the treatment of symptomatic paralabral cysts required open surgery[33] as access via arthroscopy may be difficult. Minimally invasive percutaneous therapy will be discussed later in this chapter.

Hip

Paralabral cysts are common about the hip, occurring in the setting of acetabular labral tears. Labral tears have a variety of etiologies including traumatic, degenerative, and dysplastic.[37] Recent investigations have focused on a predisposition for acetabular labral tears in patients with developmental dysplasia of the hip (DDH) and those with femoroacetabular impingement (FAI). FAI reflects abnormal femoral and/or acetabular morphology predisposing to impaction of the femoral head/neck on the acetabular rim during specific motions. Although labral tears and accelerated DJD have been described with both conditions, paralabral cysts appear to be more common with labral tears associated with DDH.[38,39]

The diagnosis of paralabral cysts at the hip is often made incidentally at the time of pelvic or hip MRI performed for a variety of indications. Evaluation of the acetabular labrum and joint capsule is best accomplished with MR arthrography, where the joint capsule is distended with a dilute solution of gadolinium in sterile saline prior to MRI. In our experience with more than 2500 hip MR arthrograms performed at our institution, actual communication between the joint and cyst via the labral tear is observed only occasionally (Figure 18-12). It is likely that these cysts become sequestered with progressively increasing viscosity of the contents, similar to what is often observed with paralabral cysts at the shoulder.

Distension of the iliopsoas bursa is commonly observed, as the bursa may communicate with the hip joint capsule[40,41]

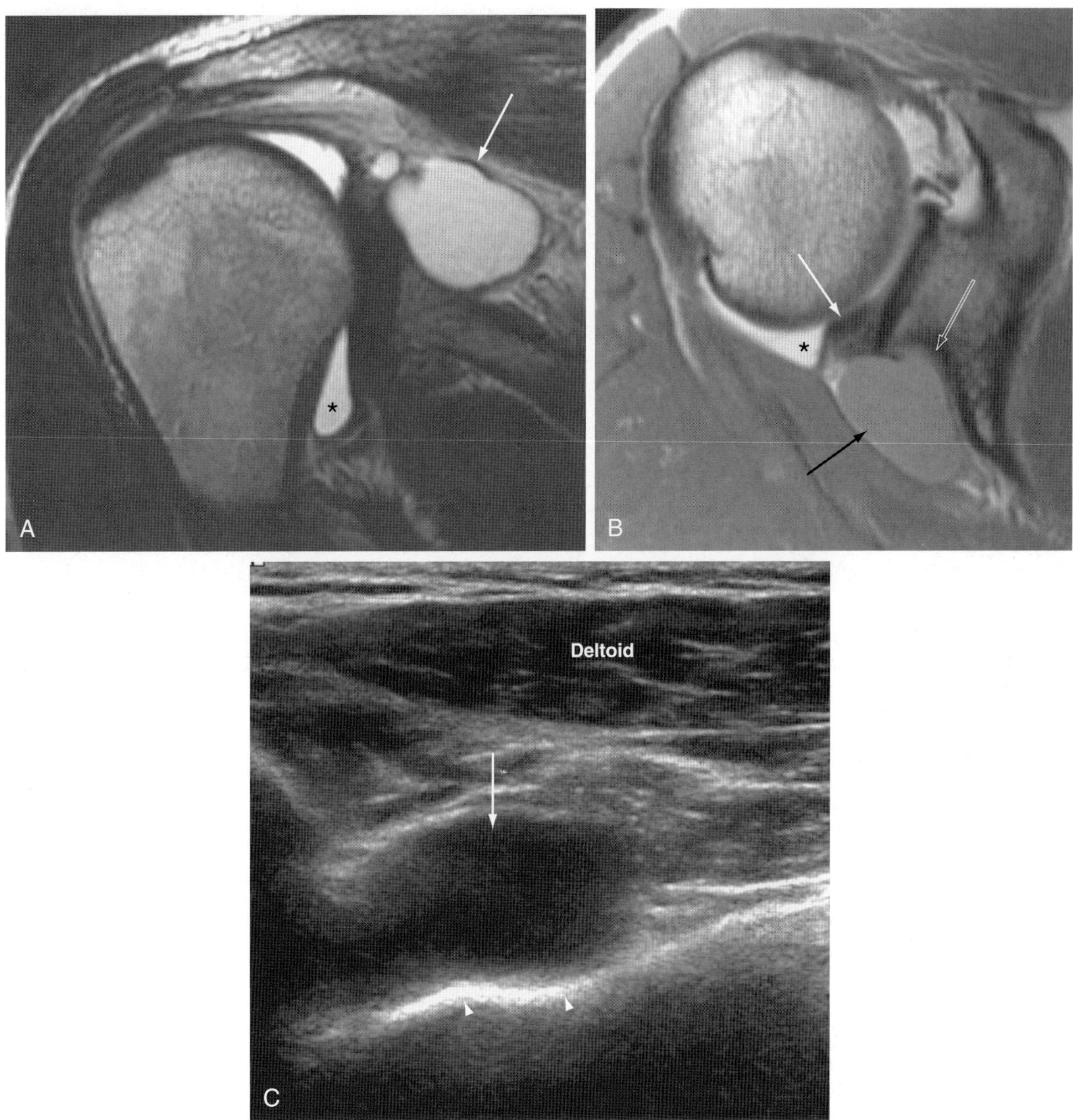

FIGURE 18-11. Glenoid paralabral cyst—MR arthrography and sonography. **A,** Oblique coronal T2-weighted MR image and (**B**) axial proton density MR image show a large, fluid-appearing mass (*white arrow* in **A**; *black arrow* in **B**) in the spinoglenoid notch *(open arrow)* in a patient with a posterosuperior labral tear. The degenerated labrum is indicated by a *white arrow* in **B**. Fluid in joint capsule represents a dilute gadolinium mixture injected at the time of arthrography *(asterisk)*. **C,** Ultrasound shows a hypoechoic mass representing the paralabral cyst *(arrow)*. The scapular cortex is indicated by *arrowheads*.

(Figure 18-13). Although the distended bursa may be present distally, at the level of the hip, intrapelvic bursal distension may also be observed and discovered incidentally at the time of pelvic CT or MRI. When large, these distended bursae may present with localized groin pain and swelling. Imaging-guided aspiration and injection of the distended iliopsoas bursa may be readily performed. Another commonly symptomatic bursa at the hip is the trochanteric bursa, situated along the greater trochanter.

Distal Appendicular Skeleton

Cystic lesions are not encountered as frequently at the elbow as at other articulations. Ganglion cysts are not typical, although there are two important bursae at the elbow that may become distended—the olecranon and bicipitoradial bursae.

Olecranon bursitis is common and may be seen in the setting of trauma with hemorrhage, as well as with rheumatoid arthritis and crystal arthropathies. Septic arthritis may result from the innoculation of the bursal space during trauma.[42] Patients with olecranon bursitis present with dorsal swelling along the proximal ulna. Sonography reveals a pancake-shaped collection superficial to the ulna. The bursal fluid may appear complex with hypoechoic particulate material. On MRI, olecranon bursitis exhibits typical high signal on T2-weighted images. There is considerable overlap in the appearance of septic and nonseptic olecranon bursitis on MRI[43]; aspiration and microbiologic analysis may be required for differentiation. In all cases of inflammatory collections about the elbow, it is important to exclude concomitant elbow joint effusion, a finding that may imply intracapsular infection.

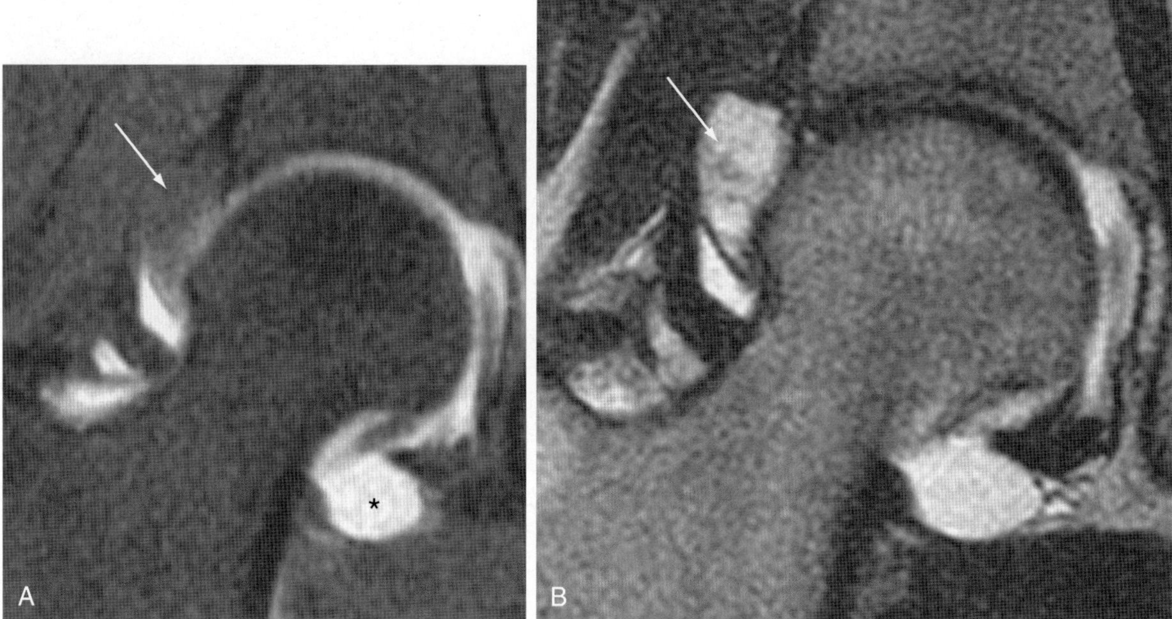

FIGURE 18-12. Paralabral cyst of the hip—MR arthrography. **A,** Coronal fat-suppressed T1-weighted image and **(B)** coronal T2-weighted MR image show a paralabral cyst (*arrows*) adjacent to the superolateral acetabulum. The cyst does not fill with injected dilute gadolinium (high signal, *asterisk*) as the cyst remains of low signal intensity on the T1-weighted image.

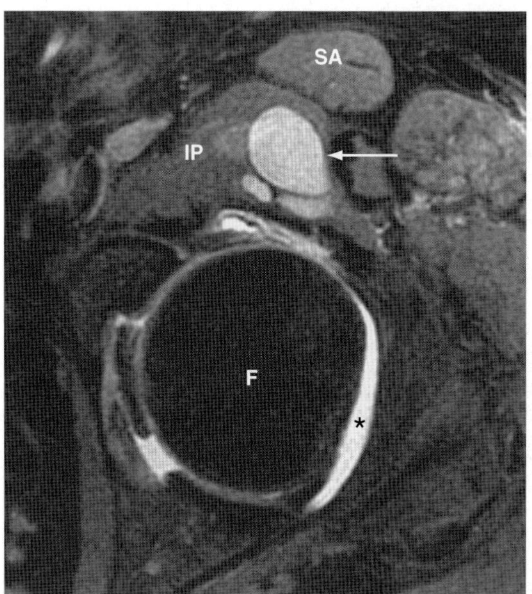

FIGURE 18-13. Distended iliopsoas bursa—MR arthrography. Axial fat-suppressed proton density image shows fluid distending the iliopsoas bursa *(arrow)*. Injection of the hip joint at the time of arthrography may demonstrate communication with the iliopsoas bursa. *F*, Femoral head; *IP*, iliopsoas muscle; *SA*, sartorius muscle. *Asterisk* indicates injected contrast.

Differentiation of septic versus aseptic bursitis cannot be reliably done by imaging alone; fluid sampling is required if there is a clinical question of infection. The presence of an elbow joint effusion in addition to bursitis raises the possibility of elbow joint infection, although a reactive effusion may also occur.

Fluid collections along the olecranon should be differentiated from a common solid mass, the rheumatoid nodule. On MRI, these soft tissue masses typically exhibit isointense signal intensity to muscle on T1-weighted images with intermediate to high signal intensity on T2-weighted images. Enhancement is variable on post-contrast images.[44] As patients with rheumatoid arthritis may experience both olecranon bursitis and rheumatoid nodules, imaging may be required to differentiate between the two entities.

The bicipitoradial bursa is situated along the distal biceps tendon at the elbow and serves to reduce friction between the biceps tendon and the radial tuberosity. When distended, this bursa typically manifests as a C-shaped collection about the distal biceps. A distended bicipitoradial bursa may be seen in the setting of repetitive trauma and inflammatory arthropathy and may accompany biceps tendon injury or tear[45] (Figure 18-14).

Ganglion cysts are common in the soft tissues about the wrist and hand. These cysts may present with localized soft tissue swelling or mass, particularly in the fingers. A large number of carpal ganglion cysts are not palpable due to their small size or deep location. Occult carpal ganglia are frequently diagnosed on MRI or ultrasound and are an important cause of wrist pain.[46,47] Many ganglia arise from the radiocarpal joint; a narrow neck leading down to the joint may be visualized on imaging. Wrist ganglia may be dorsal or volar. When dorsal, these collections are typically deep to the extensor tendons. Volar cysts are frequently observed along the radial aspect of the joint adjacent to the flexor carpi radialis tendon (Figure 18-15). Transmitted pulsation from the radial artery may simulate a pseudoaneurysm on physical exam (Figure 18-16). Doppler ultrasound readily depicts the radial artery and its relationship to the ganglion, which is important if surgical excision is contemplated.

There is a subset of wrist ganglia that arise along the dorsal aspect of the scapholunate interosseous ligament. These ganglia appear to result from scapholunate ligament tears and may be analogous to meniscal or paralabral cysts in their pathophysiology. Similarly, ganglia have been described in association with injury

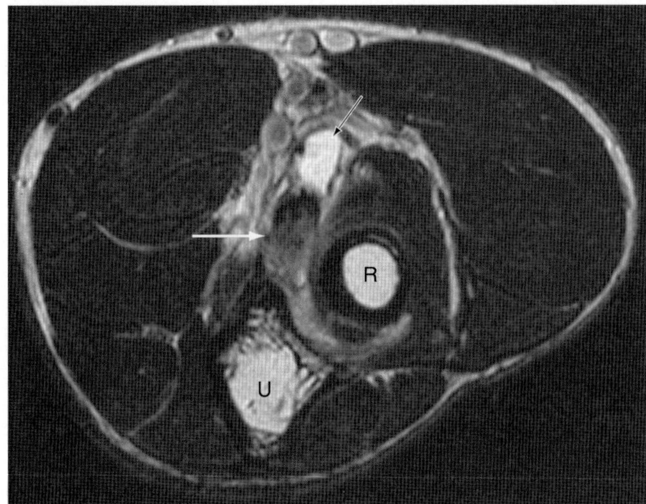

FIGURE 18-14. Bicipitoradial bursitis—MRI. Axial FSE T2-weighted MR image shows a fluid collection *(black arrow)* anterior to the distal biceps tendon *(white arrow)* indicating a distended bicipitoradial bursa. Note the swollen, amorphous biceps tendon in this patient with injury resulting in a partial tendon tear. *R,* Radius; *U,* ulna.

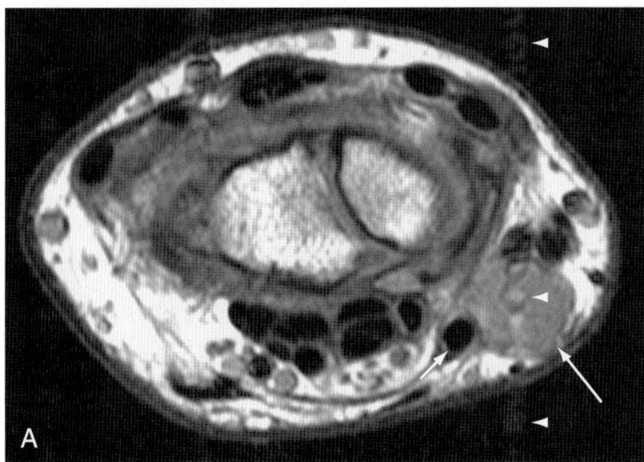

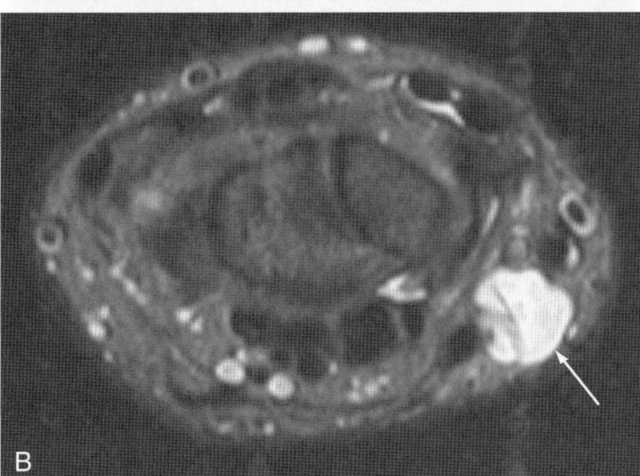

FIGURE 18-15. Radial-side volar wrist ganglion—MRI. **A,** Axial T1-weighted and **(B)** inversion recovery MR images show a homogeneous mass *(arrows)* along the volar aspect of the wrist just lateral to the flexor carpi radialis tendon (*short arrow* in **A**). Note the ring-like pulsation artifact *(arrowheads)* within the ganglion and in a line extending past the wrist in **A** from the adjacent radial artery, which is deep to the cyst.

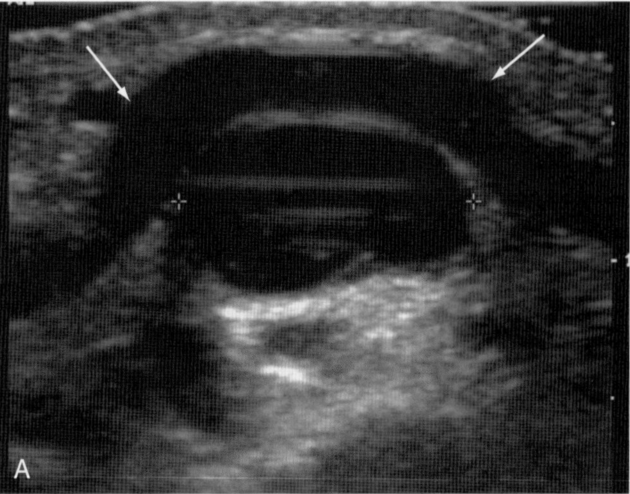

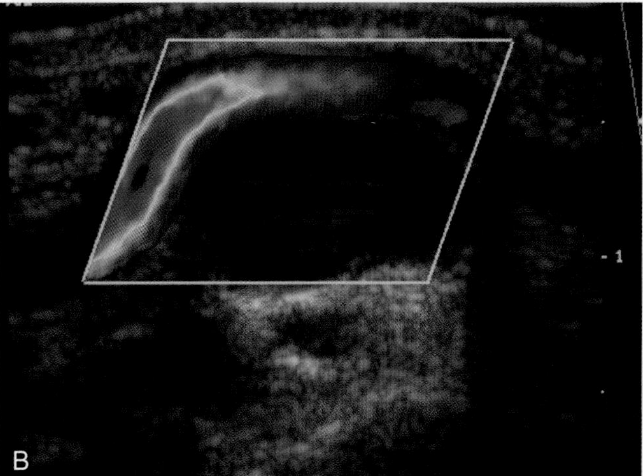

FIGURE 18-16. Ganglion deep to radial artery at the wrist simulating a pseudoaneurysm—sonography. **A,** Gray-scale and **(B)** color Doppler images show the radial artery (*white arrows* in **A**; color filled in **B**) draped over a ganglion (between cursors in **A**). The patient presented with a pulsatile wrist mass.

to the triangular fibrocartilage complex (TFCC). Ganglion cysts at the wrist have also been observed to arise from the triscaphe (scaphoid–trapezium–trapezoid joint)[48] (Figure 18-17).

> The origin of ganglia is most important if surgical excision is planned, as removal of the tract is important to avoid recurrence.

In the fingers, ganglion cysts arising from tendon sheaths are encountered.[49] The differential diagnosis for soft tissue masses in the fingers also includes mucous cysts,[50] neurogenic tumors such as schwannomas and neurofibromas, localized giant cell tumors of tendon sheath, and glomus tumors. The differentiation of cystic from solid is important and may be accomplished with MRI performed after IV gadolinium administration. Cystic lesions such as ganglia will be centrally nonenhancing. Neurogenic tumors typically show robust enhancement.[51] Giant cell tumor of tendon sheath may exhibit predominantly low signal on all MR sequences by virtue of its hemosiderin content[52] (Figure 18-18). Glomus tumors are typically distal in location, in close proximity to the nail bed.[53]

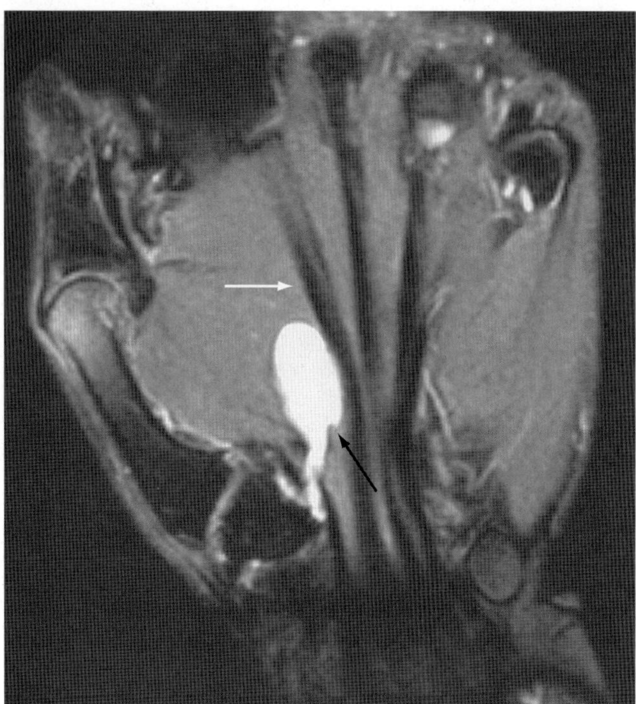

FIGURE 18-17. Ganglion arising from the scaphoid-trapezium-trapezoid (triscaphe) joint of the wrist—MRI. Coronal fat-suppressed proton density image of the palm shows a ganglion *(black arrow)* originating via a thin channel from the triscaphe joint and extending to abut the index finger flexor tendons *(white arrow)*.

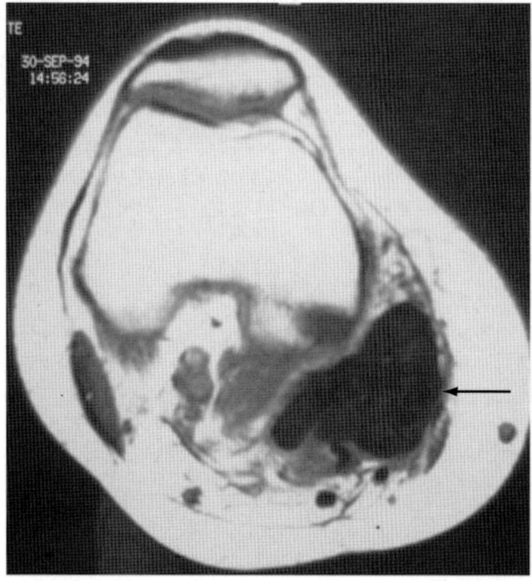

FIGURE 18-18. Pigmented villonodular synovitis (PVNS) presenting as posterior knee mass. Axial T1-weighted MR image shows a very low signal intensity mass along the posteromedial knee *(arrow)*, proven at excision to represent focal PVNS. The hemosiderin-laden tissue in this condition is responsible for the very low signal intensity on MRI.

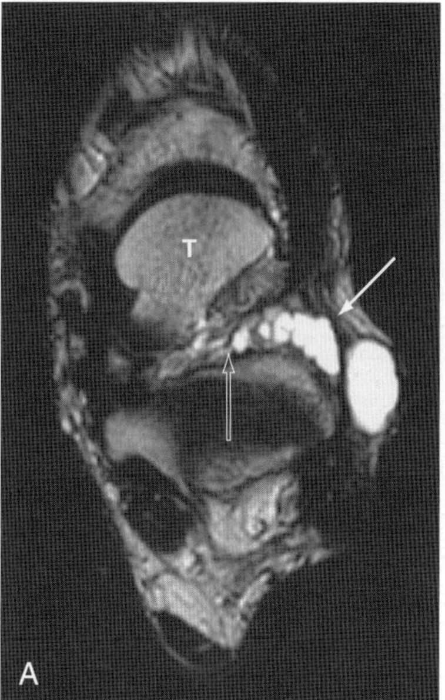

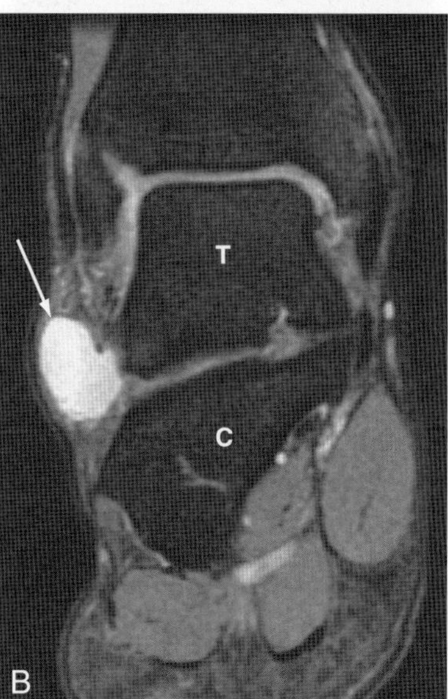

FIGURE 18-19. Ganglion—sinus tarsi—MRI. **A,** Axial T2 weighted and **(B)** coronal proton density with fat-suppression MR images show a multiseptated, fluid-appearing mass *(arrows)* originating in the sinus tarsi, dissecting to the superficial, lateral hindfoot. This mass was excised surgically. *C,* Calcaneus; *T,* talus; *open arrow,* sinus tarsi.

Cystic lesions about the foot and ankle are common and include ganglia (Figure 18-19) and fluid-filled bursae. Adventitial bursae typically develop along the plantar surface of the foot, at sites of repetitive frictional trauma, such as beneath the metatarsal heads[54] (Figure 18-20). The retrocalcaneal bursa is located anterior to the Achilles' tendon at the calcaneal insertion and may become distended with fluid from repeated trauma.[55,56] The intermetatarsal bursa lies in the web space between the toes. This relatively small, slit-like fluid collection is readily detected on MRI. Intermetatarsal bursal distension may accompany interdigital or Morton's neuromas, or it may be seen in asymptomatic individuals.[57,58] Focal, "cyst-like" distension of tendon sheaths may be observed, particularly about the ankle.

A number of solid masses at the foot and ankle must be distinguished from cysts (Figure 18-21). This can be accomplished with sonography or via MRI. Intravenous gadolinium may be necessary to confirm the solid nature of some masses. Fibromas are common along the plantar aponeurosis of the foot and have a relatively typical MRI appearance, exhibiting low signal on both T1-weighted and T2-weighted scans[59] (Figure 18-22). Interdigital or Morton's

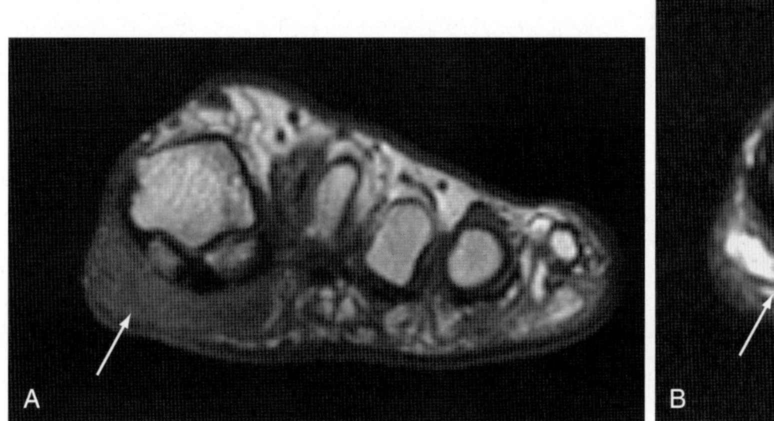

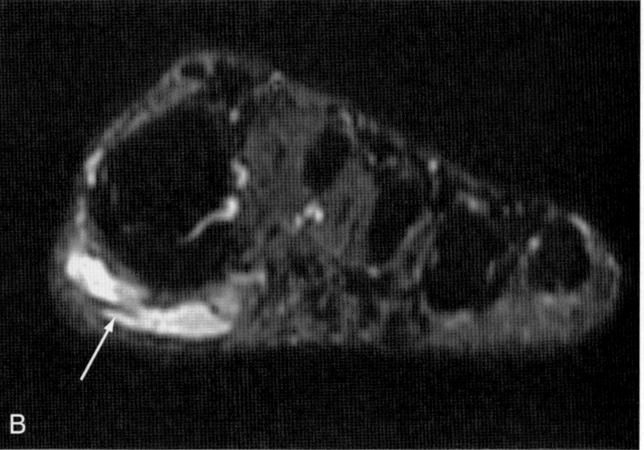

FIGURE 18-20. Adventitial bursa—forefoot—MRI. **A,** Coronal T1-weighted and **(B)** inversion recovery MR images show a homogeneous, fluid-intensity mass plantar to the sesamoids of the great toe in keeping with an adventitial bursa.

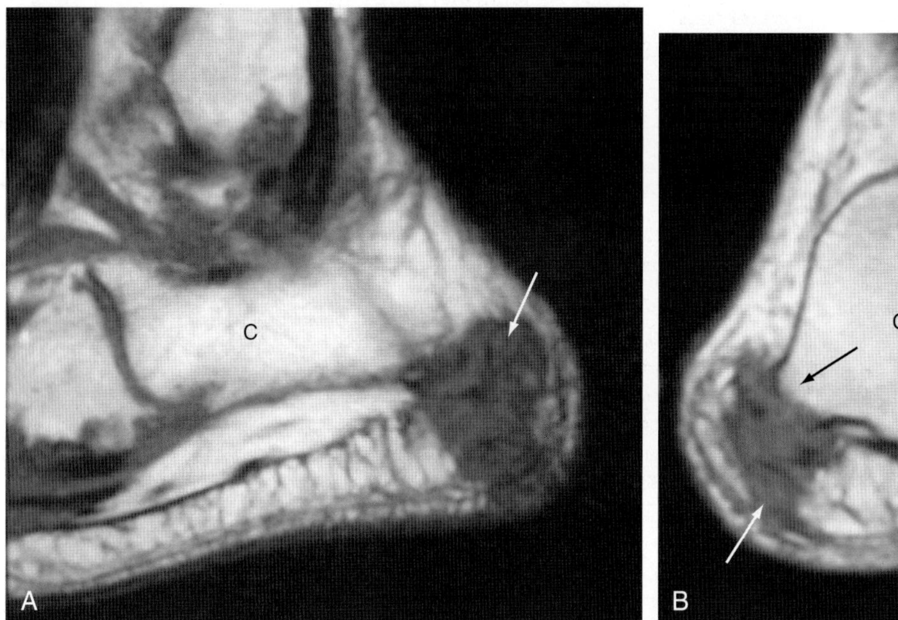

FIGURE 18-21. Rheumatoid nodule—plantar hindfoot. **A,** Sagittal and **(B)** coronal T1-weighted MR images show a heterogeneous low signal intensity mass along the plantar surface of the heel *(white arrows).* Subtle cortical erosion in **B** is indicated by the *black arrow. C,* Calcaneus.

neuromas represent perineural fibrosis of the plantar digital nerve and occur most commonly between the third and fourth or second and third metatarsals. These exhibit similar MR features as other fibrous lesions. Enhancement following gadolinium administration may be observed[58] (Box 18-1).

Spine

Facet joint synovial cysts are diagnosed with greater frequency with the increasing use of CT and MRI for the evaluation back pain.[60] These cysts are associated with facet joint osteoarthritis, spondylolisthesis, and facet instability[61,62] and are encountered in the lumbar and cervical spine (Figure 18-23). Facet synovial cysts in the thoracic spine are quite rare.[63]

Ganglion cysts are felt to arise from spinal ligaments, frequently the ligamentum flavum in the lumbar spine, or rarely, in the cervical spine.[64,65] These lesions are often in close proximity to the facet joints, making differentiation from synovial cysts difficult on imaging studies alone.[66]

IMAGING-GUIDED INTERVENTIONS

As detailed in this chapter, many juxtaarticular cysts are symptomatic. Compression of adjacent neurovascular structures may occur in some cases. In others, persistent mass effect from the cyst results in localized pain, a sensation of fullness or swelling. In patients with long-standing symptoms, direct intervention may be warranted. Although some cysts respond to treatment of an underlying condition within the joint, many will not respond in this approach. Some chronic cysts are treated with surgical excision with inherent risks of morbidity and lengthy recovery. Palpable cysts may be aspirated in the clinician's office. Improvements in imaging-guided intervention now allow aspiration of cysts that are not palpable or deep to the skin surface or those in close proximity to vessels and nerves.

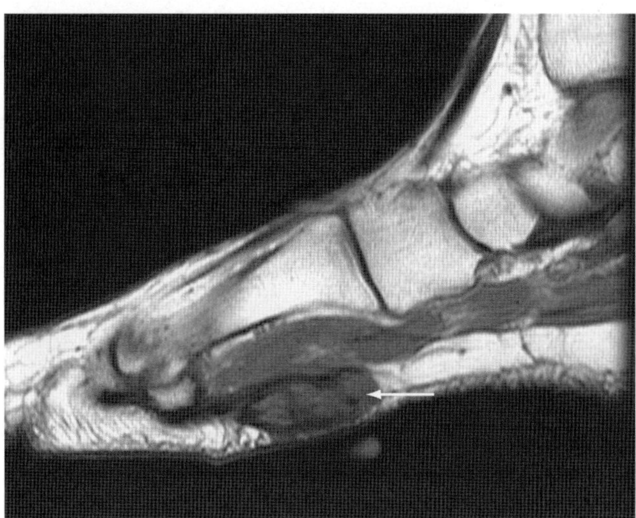

FIGURE 18-22. Plantar fibroma—MRI. T1-weighted sagittal MR image shows an ovoid, heterogeneous, low signal intensity, superficial plantar mass *(arrow)* representing a plantar fibroma.

BOX 18-1. Morton's Neuroma

Perineural fibrosis of a plantar digital nerve
Most often occurs between second and third or between third and fourth metatarsal heads
Women most often affected; high heels or narrow shoes exacerbate condition
Pain in the ball of the foot may radiate to the toes
MRI: low signal masses, may enhance after contrast, prone position at scanning may make them visible
Ultrasound: mass in typical location

Aspiration of cysts does not, in and of itself, prevent recurrence. Despite this, many patients experience long-term or even permanent symptomatic relief from aspiration. If cysts recur, they may be reaspirated, with surgical management a last resort, reserved for recalcitrant cases.

In our practice, all juxtaarticular cysts that are aspirated are also injected with a corticosteroid and a long-acting anesthetic. A potential role for corticosteroids in preventing cyst recurrence is not proven,[67] yet the combination of corticosteroid and anesthetic injection would offer potentially increased long-term pain relief over aspiration alone. We typically inject methylprednisolone, 40 to 80 mg along with up to 4 mL of bupivacaine 0.5%, the total volume of anesthetic and corticosteroid injected not to exceed total aspirated cyst volume. It is important to instruct the patient regarding possible recurrence of pain once the anesthetic wears off, given the expected 2- to 3-day delay before onset of any therapeutic benefit from the corticosteroid.

> The therapeutic effect of cyst aspiration and corticosteroid injection may not be evident for 2 to 3 days.

Cysts may be aspirated and injected using ultrasound, CT, or even MR guidance. Fluid collections near bony landmarks may even be aspirated and injected under fluoroscopy alone. Sonography is preferred in most cases of cyst aspiration, by virtue of the lack of ionizing radiation, real-time imaging guidance during the entire procedure, and easy characterization of the fluid contents of the cyst. CT and particularly CT fluoroscopy are helpful for localizing and aspirating deep fluid collections and those partially obscured by osseous structures. If clinically indicated, aspirated fluid may be submitted for laboratory analysis, including cultures, cell count, and crystal analysis.

One of the most compelling indications for imaging-guided aspiration is the paralabral cyst at the shoulder. As detailed earlier, these cysts may compress the suprascapular nerve resulting in muscle weakness. Cyst contents are often very viscous (Figures 18-24 and 18-25). Recent studies have documented successful cyst decompression via arthroscopy,[68,69] obviating a more invasive open surgical procedure with longer recovery and increased morbidity.

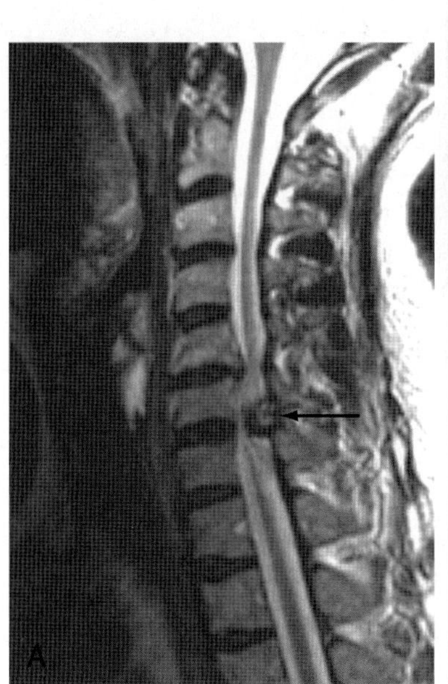

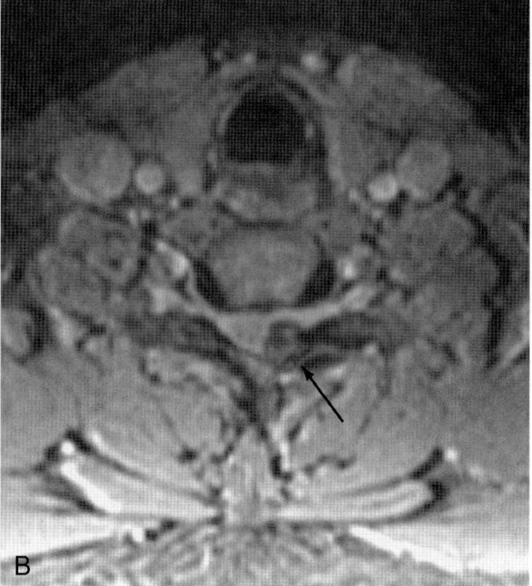

FIGURE 18-23. Facet synovial cyst—cervical spine—MRI. **A,** Sagittal T2-weighted and **(B)** axial gradient-echo MR images show a mass (*arrows*) arising from the posterior spinal elements with compromise of the spinal canal. A synovial cyst was excised at surgery.

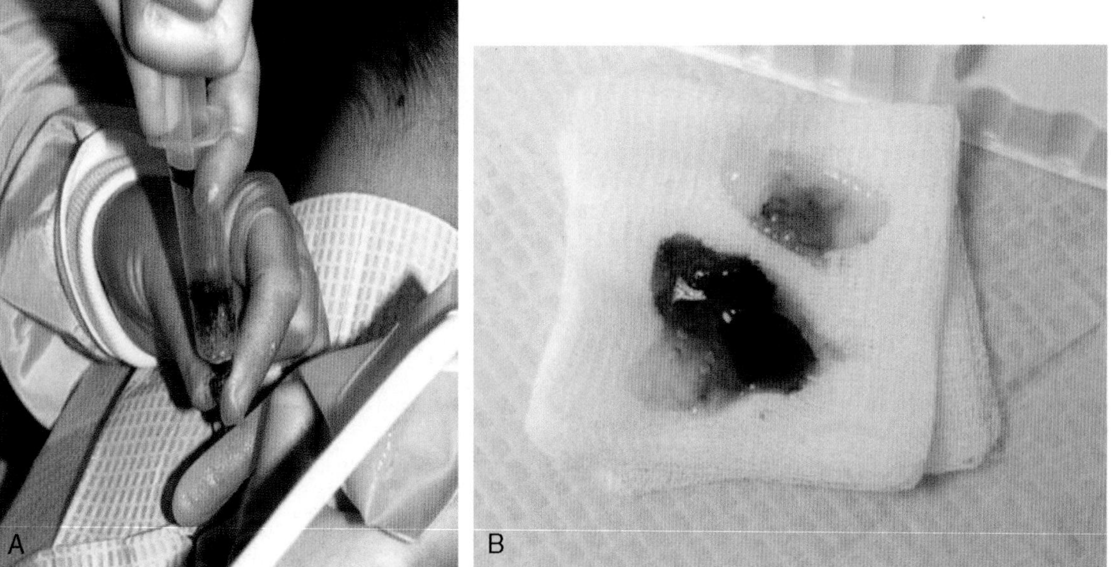

FIGURE 18-24. Supraspinous paralabral cyst—aspiration under ultrasound guidance. **A,** Cyst aspiration technique. An assistant holding an ultrasound transducer (probe) covered with a sterile glove is visible to the right of the needle. **B,** Viscous cyst contents following aspiration.

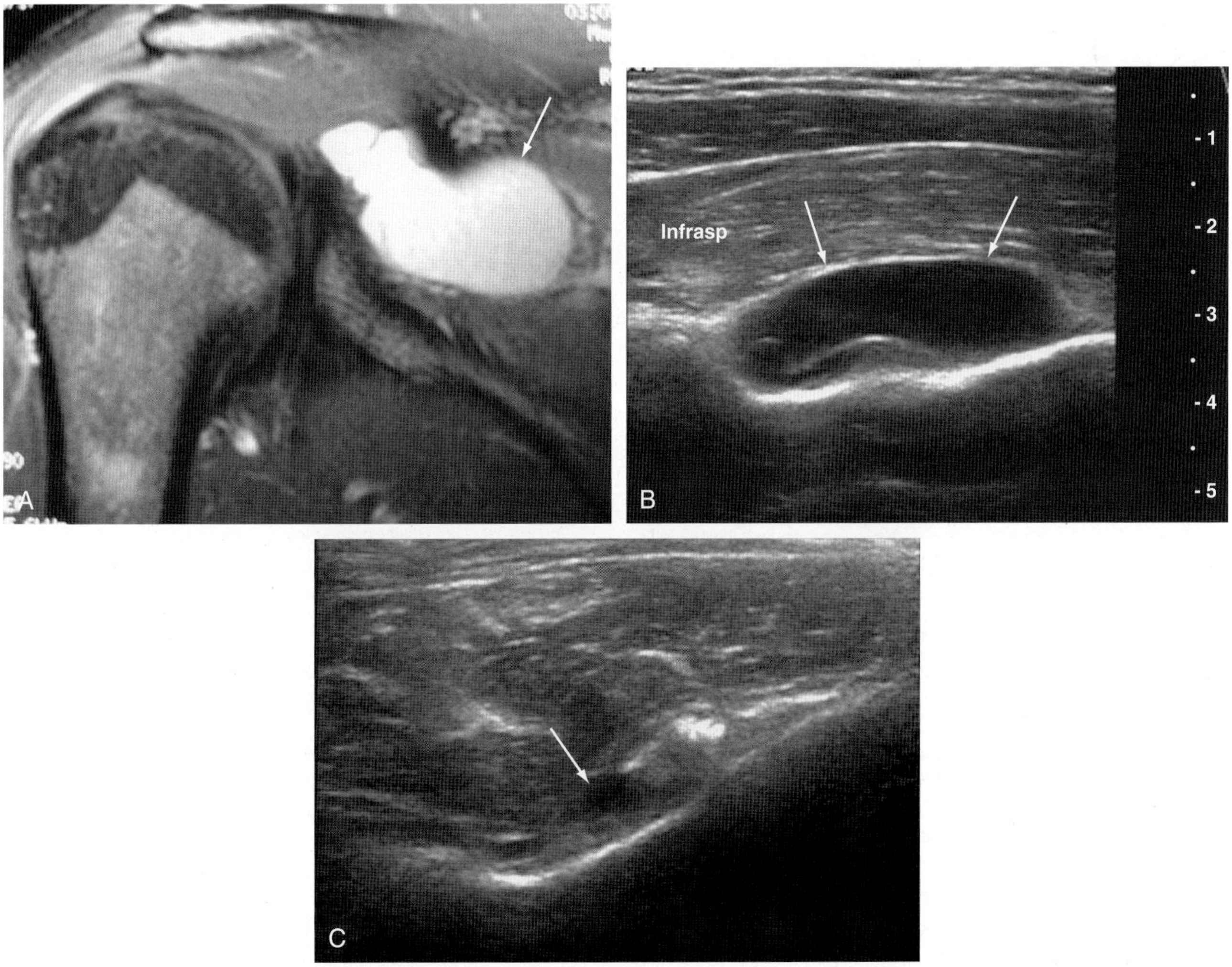

FIGURE 18-25. Female bodybuilder with shoulder pain and large spinoglenoid paralabral cyst—ultrasound-guided aspiration. **A,** Coronal fat-suppressed proton density MR image shows a large paralabral cyst *(arrow)*. **B,** Ultrasound image shows the spinoglenoid notch cyst *(arrows)* deep to the infraspinatus *(Infrasp)* muscle. **C,** Following aspiration and injection of corticosteroids and long-acting anesthetic, the residual cyst components *(arrow)* are visible.

Nevertheless, surgical treatment may be reserved for cysts that continue to recur despite less invasive interventions.

Piatt and colleagues described 5 recurrences in 11 patients in whom paralabral cysts were treated with aspiration alone, without corticosteroid injection.[70] In our practice, some patients do experience partial cyst recurrence or less than complete aspiration due to high fluid viscosity; despite this, many of these patients report long-term pain relief and improvements in rotator cuff strength following the procedure. This may reflect the benefits of the corticosteroid injection into the cyst cavity, although this remains unproven. Moreover, recurrent cysts resulting in symptoms may be reaspirated under imaging guidance.

Breidahl and Adler reported on their experiences with ultrasound-guided aspiration and injection of ganglia, the majority at the wrist. All ganglia were injected with a mixture of corticosteroid and long-acting anesthetic. Nine of ten patients experienced either complete resolution of the ganglion or symptomatic relief with reduction in size of the ganglion.[71]

SUMMARY

Juxtaarticular cysts are common and frequently result from underlying intracapsular pathologies. Cross-sectional imaging, particularly ultrasound and MRI, have facilitated accurate diagnosis and precise anatomic localization of these cysts and fluid collections. Although it may be difficult to differentiate between the various types of "cysts," be they ganglia, synovial cysts, or distended bursae, therapeutic management will be predicated upon patient symptoms and anatomic considerations rather than nomenclature. Image-guided aspiration with corticosteroid and anesthetic injection is a minimally invasive approach to treating these conditions.

REFERENCES

1. Tschirch F, Schmid M, Pfirrmann C et al: Prevalence and size of meniscal cysts, ganglionic cysts, synovial cysts of the popliteal space, fluid-dilled bursae, and other fluid collections in asymptomatic knees on MR imaging, *AJR Am J Roentgenol* 180:1431-1436, 2003.
2. Palmer DG: Synovial cysts in rheumatoid disease, *Ann Intern Med* 70:61-68, 1969.
3. Gadgil AA, Eisenstein SM, Darby A et al: Bilateral symptomatic synovial cysts of the lumbar spine caused by calcium pyrophosphate deposition disease: a case report, *Spine* 27:E428-E431, 2002.
4. Stone KR, Stoller D, De Carli A et al: The frequency of Baker's cysts associated with meniscal tears, *Am J Sports Med* 24:670-671, 1996.
5. Dodd LG, Major NM: Fine-needle aspiration of articular and periarticular lesions, *Cancer Cytopathol* 96:157-165, 2002.
6. Malghem J, Vandeberg BC, Lebon C et al: Ganglion cysts of the knee: articular communication revealed by delayed radiography and CT after arthrography, *AJR Am J Roentgenol* 170:1579-1583, 1998.
7. Dodd LG, Layfield LJ: Fine-needle aspiration of ganglion cysts, *Diagn Cytopathol* 15:377-381, 1996.
8. Oertel YC, Beckner ME, Engler WF: Cytologic diagnosis and ultrastructure of fine-needle aspirates of ganglion cysts, *Arch Pathol Lab Med* 110:938-942, 1986.
9. Robinson P, White LM, Agur A et al: Obturator externus bursa: anatomic origin and MR imaging features of pathologic involvement, *Radiology* 228:230-234, 2003.
10. Dunn T, Heller CA, McCarthy SW et al: Anatomical study of the "trochanteric bursa", *Clin Anat* 16:233-240, 2003.
11. Ward EE, Jacobson J, Fessell DP et al: Sonographic detection of Baker's cysts: comparison with MR imaging, *AJR Am J Roentgenol* 176:373-380, 2001.
12. Newman JS, Adler RS: Power Doppler sonography: applications in musculoskeletal imaging, *Semin Musculoskelet Radiol* 2:331-340, 1998.
13. Murphey MD, McRae GA, Fanburg-Smith JC et al: Imaging of soft-tissue myxoma with emphasis on CT and MR and comparison of radiologic and pathologic findings, *Radiology* 225:215-224, 2002.
14. Handy JR: Popliteal cysts in adults: a review, *Semin Arthritis Rheum* 31:108-118, 2001.
15. Curl WW: Popliteal cysts: historical background and current knowledge, *J Am Acad Orthop Surg* 4:129-133, 1996.
16. Kane D, Balint PV, Sturrock RD: Ultrasonography is superior to clinical examination in the detection and localization of knee joint effusion in rheumatoid arthritis, *J Rheumatol* 20:966-971, 2003.
17. Helms CA, Fritz RC, Garvin GJ: Plantaris muscle injury: evaluation with MR imaging, *Radiology* 195:201-203, 1995.
18. Parellada AJ, Morrison WB, Reiter SB et al: Unsuspected lower extremity deep venous thrombosis simulating musculoskeletal pathology, *Skeletal Radiol* 2006; 35:659-664.
19. Campbell SE, Sanders TG, Morrison WB: MR imaging of meniscal cysts: incidence, location, and clinical significance, *AJR Am J Roentgenol* 177:409-413, 2001.
20. Rennie WJ, Saifuddin A: Pes anserine bursitis: incidence in symptomatic knees and clinical presentation, *Skeletal Radiol* 34:395-398, 2005.
20a. Glencross PM, Little JP: Pes Anserinus Bursitis. http://www.emedicine.com/pmr/topic104.htm (accessed November 6, 2006).
21. Rothstein CP, Laorr A, Helms CA et al: Semimembranosus-tibial collateral ligament bursitis: MR imaging findings, *AJR Am J Roentgenol* 166:875-877, 1996.
22. DeMaeseneer M, Shahabpour M, Van Roy F et al: MR imaging of the medial collateral ligament bursa: findings in patients and anatomic data derived from cadavers, *AJR Am J Roentgenol* 177:911-917, 2001.
23. Myllymaki T, Tikkakoski T, Typpo T et al: Carpet-layer's knee. An ultrasonographic study, *Acta Radiol* 34:496-499, 1993.
24. Iverson DJ: MRI detection of cysts causing common peroneal neuropathy, *Neurology* 65:1829-1831, 2005.
25. Bui-Mansfield LT, Youngberg RA: Intraarticular ganglia of the knee: prevalence, presentation, etiology and management, *AJR Am J Roentgenol* 168:123-127, 1997.
26. Recht MP, Applegate G, Kaplan P et al: The MR appearance of cruciate ganglion cysts: report of 16 cases, *Skeletal Radiol* 23:597-600, 1994.
27. Bergin D, Morrison WB, Carrino JA et al: Anterior cruciate ligament ganglia and mucoid degeneration: coexistence and clinical correlation, *AJR Am J Roentgenol* 182:1283-1287, 2004.
28. Bussiere JL, Zmantar C, Cauhape P et al: [Giant synovial cyst of the shoulder. apropos of a case], *Rev Rheum Mal Osteoartic* 59:145-148, 1992.
29. Kay-Geert AH, Backhaus M, Schneider U et al: Rheumatoid arthritis of the shoulder joint: comparison of conventional radiography, ultrasound and dynamic contrast-enhanced magnetic resonance imaging, *Arthritis Rheum* 48:3338-3349, 2003.
30. Carlos de Moura GG, de Souza SP: The "shoulder pad" sign. Images in clinical medicine, *N Engl J Med* 351:e23, 2004.
31. Tung GA, Entzian D, Stern JB et al: MR imaging and MR arthrography of paraglenoid labral cysts, *AJR Am J Roentgenol* 174:1707-1715, 2000.
32. Tirman PF, Feller JF, Jnazen DL et al: Association of glenoid labral cysts with labral tears and glenohumeral instability: radiologic findings and clinical significance, *Radiology* 190:653-658, 1994.
33. Westerheide KJ, Karzel RP: Ganglion cysts of the shoulder: technique of arthroscopic decompression and fixation of associated type II superior labral anterior to posterior lesions, *Orthop Clin North Am* 34:521-528, 2003.
34. Romeo AA, Rotenberg DD, Bach BR: Suprascapular neuropathy, *J Am Acad Orthop Surg* 7:358-367, 1999.
35. Cummins CA, Messer TM, Nuber GW: Current concepts review: suprascapular nerve entrapment, *J Bone Joint Surg Am* 82: 415-424, 2000.
36. Boutin RD, Fritz RC, Steinbach LSL: Imaging of sports-related muscle injuries, *Radiol Clin North Am* 40:333-362, 2002.
37. Boutin RD, Newman JS: MR imaging of sports-related hip disorders, *Magn Reson Imaging Clin N Am* 11:1-27, 2003.
38. Ganz R, Parvizi J, Beck M et al: Femoroacetabular impingement: a cause for osteoarthritis of the hip, *Clin Orthop* 417:112-120, 2003.
39. Beck M, Kalhor M, Leunig M et al: Hip morphology influences the pattern of damage to articular cartilage: femoroacetabular impingement as a cause of early osteoarthritis of the hip, *J Bone Joint Surg Br* 87:1012-1018, 2005.
40. Steinbach LS, Schneider R, Goldman AB et al: Bursae and abscess cavities communicating with the hip: diagnosis using arthrography and CT, *Radiology* 156:303-307, 1985.
41. Kozlov DB, Sonin AH: Iliopsoas bursitis: diagnosis by MRI, *J Comput Assist Tomogr* 22:625-628, 1998.
42. McAfee JH, Smith DL: Olecranon and prepatellar bursitis: diagnosis and treatment, *West J Med* 149:607-610, 1998.
43. Floemer F, Morrison WB, Bongartz G et al: MRI characteristics of olecranon bursitis, *AJR Am J Roentgenol* 183:29-34, 2004.
44. Theodorou DJ, Theodorou SJ, Farooki S et al: Disorders of the plantar aponeurosis: a spectrum of MR imaging findings, *AJR Am J Roentgenol* 176:97-104, 2001.
45. Skaf AY, Boutin RD, Dantas RWM et al: Bicipitoradial bursitis: MR imaging findings in eight patients and anatomic data from contrast material opacification of bursa followed by routine radiography and MR imaging in cadavers, *Radiology* 212:111-116, 1999.
46. Lee D: Sonography of the wrist and hand, *Semin Musculoskelet Radiol* 2:237-244, 1998.
47. Anderson SE, Steinbach LS, Stauffer E et al: MRI for differentiating ganglion and synovitis in the chronic painful wrist, *AJR Am J Roentgenol* 186:812-818, 2006.
48. El-Noueam KI, Schweitzer ME, Blasbalg R: Is a subset of wrist ganglia the sequela of internal derangements of the wrist joint? MR imaging findings, *Radiology* 212:537-540, 1998.
49. Abe Y, Watson HK, Renaud S: Flexor tendon sheath ganglion: analysis of 128 cases, *Hand Surg* 9:1-4, 2004.
50. Drape JL, Idy-Peretti I, Goettman S et al: MR imaging of digital mucoid cysts, *Radiology* 200:521-536, 1996.
51. Lacour-Petit MC, Lozeron P, Ducreux D: MRI of peripheral nerve lesions of the lower limbs, *Neuroradiology* 45:166-170, 2003.
52. Jelinek JS, Kransdorf MJ, Shmookler BM et al: Giant cell tumor of the tendon sheath: MR findings in nine cases, *AJR Am J Roentgenol* 162:919-922, 1994.
53. Ozdemir O, Coskunol E, Ozalp T et al: Glomus tumor of the finger: a report of 60 cases, *Acta Orthop Traumatol Turc* 37:244-248, 2003.

54. Ashman CJ, Klecker RJ, Yu JS: Forefoot pain involving the metatarsal region: differential diagnosis with MR imaging, *Radiographics* 21:1425-1440, 2001.
55. Aronow MS: Posterior heel pain (retrocalcaneal bursitis, insertional and noninsertional Achilles tendinopathy), *Clin Podiatr Med Surg North Am* 22:19-43, 2005.
56. Bottger BA, Schweitzer ME, El-Noueam KI et al: MR imaging of the normal and abnormal retrocalcaneal bursae, *AJR Am J Roentgenol* 170:1239-1241, 1998.
57. Zanetti M, Weishaupt D: MR imaging of the forefoot: Morton neuroma and differential diagnoses, *Semin Musculoskelet Radiol* 9:175-186, 2005.
58. Murphey MD, Smith WS, Smith SE et al: Imaging of musculoskeletal neurogenic tumors: radiologic-pathologic correlation, *Radiographics* 19:1253-1280, 1999.
59. Wetzel LH, Levine E: Soft-tissue tumors of the foot: value of MR imaging for specific diagnosis, *AJR Am J Roentgenol* 155:1025-1030, 1990.
60. Liu SS, Williams KD, Drayer BP et al: Synovial cysts of the lumbosacral spine: diagnosis by MR imaging, *AJR Am J Roentgenol* 154:163-166, 1990.
61. Doyle AJ, Merrilees M: Synovial cysts of the lumbar facet joints in a symptomatic population: prevalence on magnetic resonance imaging, *Spine* 15:874-878, 2004.
62. Tillich M, Trummer M, Lindbichler F et al: Symptomatic intraspinal synovial cysts of the lumbar spine: correlation of MR and surgical findings, *Neuroradiology* 43:1070-1075, 2001.
63. Cohen-Gadol AA, White JB, Lynch JJ et al: Synovial cysts of the thoracic spine, *J Neurosurg Spine* 1:52-57, 2004.
64. Sze CI, Kindt G, Huffer WB et al: Synovial excrescences and cysts of the spine: clinicopathologic features and contributions to spinal stenosis, *Clin Neuropathol* 23:80-90, 2004.
65. Yamamoto A, Nishiura I, Handa H et al: Ganglion cyst of the ligamentum flavum of the cervical spine causing myelopathy: report of two cases, *Surg Neurol* 56:390-395, 2001.
66. Shima Y, Rothman SL, Yasura K et al: Degenerative intraspinal cyst of the cervical spine: case report and literature review, *Spine* 27:E18-E22, 2002.
67. Acebes JC, Sanchez-Pernaute O, Diaz-Oca A et al: Ultrasonographic assessment of Baker's cysts after intraarticular corticosteroid injection in knee osteoarthritis, *J Clin Ultrasound* 34:113-117, 2006.
68. Abboud JA, Silverberg D, Glaser DL et al: Arthroscopy effectively treats ganglion cysts of the shoulder, *Clin Orthop Relat Res* 444:129-133, 2006.
69. Chen AL, Ong BC, Rose DJ: Arthroscopic management of spinoglenoid cysts associated with SLAP lesions and suprascapular neuropathy, *Arthroscopy* 19:E15-E21, 2003.
70. Piatt BE, Hawkins RJ, Fritz RC et al: Clinical evaluation and treatment of spinoglenoid notch ganglion cysts, *J Shoulder Elbow Surg* 11:600-604, 2002.
71. Breidahl WH, Adler RS: Ultrasound-guided injection of ganglia with corticosteroids, *Skeletal Radiol* 25:635-638, 1996.

CHAPTER 19

Imaging of Infection

AMY ROSEN LECOMTE, MD, MOHAMAD OSSIANI, MD, *and* PIRAN ALIABADI, MD

KEY FACTS

- Infections of the bones and joints result from one of three mechanisms of spread: (1) hematogenous, (2) contiguous, or (3) direct implantation.
- Radiographic hallmarks of osteomyelitis are cortical and medullary destructive osteolysis with soft tissue swelling in the acute phase and reactive sclerosis and periosteal reaction in the subacute to chronic phase; sequestrum and involucrum formation with sinus tracts differentiate chronic active from background chronic inactive osteomyelitis.
- Pediatric osteomyelitis occurs most commonly in the metaphysis of a long bone, usually around the knee, and is often multifocal. Adult osteomyelitis occurs most commonly in the diaphysis of a long bone.
- *Staphylococcus aureus* is the most common organism regardless of age.
- Brodie's abscess, or focal subacute osteomyelitis, is a walled-off infection with no sequestrum. It has a four-layered target appearance on contrast-enhanced magnetic resonance imaging (MRI). It can be differentiated from an osteoid osteoma with confidence when a sinus tract is identified to the growth plate. Bone abscess should be considered for any destructive metaphyseal lesion extending into the epiphysis.
- MRI hallmarks of spine infection are disk space narrowing, vertebral end plate destruction/loss of sharp disk outline, and paraspinal mass.
- Radiographic hallmarks of septic arthritis are periarticular osteoporosis, joint effusion, and soft tissue swelling in the early phase, with cartilage destruction and subchondral plate destruction in the later phase.
- Tuberculous arthritis is characterized by the Phemister triad of periarticular osteoporosis, peripheral erosions, and absence of joint space narrowing. Although similar in appearance to rheumatoid arthritis, when involvement is monoarticular and erosions are poorly defined, tuberculosis should be considered.
- Immunocompromised patients are prone to aggressive soft tissue infection. Diabetic patients are prone to foot infection.
- Technetium-99m three-phase bone scan, although nonspecific, is useful to differentiate soft tissue infection from joint or bone infection, especially in children. To improve specificity for infection, bone scan may be combined with gallium 67 citrate or indium 111 labeled white blood cell scanning.
- Percutaneous aspiration or biopsy should be used to confirm infection and obtain an organism for treatment planning.

Imaging studies are important adjuncts to clinical history, tissue cultures, and laboratory tests in patients with suspected musculoskeletal infection. Once the diagnosis is considered, appropriate imaging studies should always include radiographs, with ultrasound, magnetic resonance imaging (MRI), computed tomography (CT), or radionuclide scans selectively used to help confirm diagnosis, determine extent of involvement, and facilitate pathologic diagnosis through biopsy or aspiration.

In this chapter we will divide musculoskeletal infections first by their anatomic involvement—the bones, joints, or soft tissues with special attention to infection in the spine and foot. Then we will consider the interplay of acuity of infection, route of infectious spread, organisms involved, and host age and immune status. The imaging features that characterize each type of infection will be explored by modality, identifying the benefits and drawbacks of each technique.

ADULT OSTEOMYELITIS

Infection involving the bone is termed *osteomyelitis.* Bone is at risk for such infection when its integrity is compromised by trauma, a large inoculum, or foreign body. The ensuing infection may then resolve or become chronic. Rather than being an inevitable stepwise progression from one entity to the next, multiple factors come into play to determine whether acute osteomyelitis will progress, including host factors (immunocompromised status, comorbidities) and treatment instituted (whether sufficiently early and appropriate). These are important for long-term prognosis, as the sequelae of these infections become graver with progression of disease. In the appropriate clinical context, when osteomyelitis is suspected, imaging is a valuable adjunct to laboratory findings for early confirmation, which in turn will facilitate the early treatment necessary to improve outcome. Complications of delayed treatment include pathologic fracture, growth disturbance, and, infrequently, malignancy in a chronically draining sinus tract.

There are three clinical manifestations of osteomyelitis based on acuity of infection (Table 19-1):

1. *Acute:* Begins with marrow edema, cellular infiltration, hyperemia, and possibly microabscess.
2. *Subacute:* Increased pressure spreads infection from the marrow to the cortex via haversian and Volkmann's canals, extending subperiosteally, eventually through the periosteum and into the soft tissues or joint. Local hyperemia and inflammation cause osteolysis and surrounding soft tissue degradation. Cortical compromise can lead to fracture, slipped epiphysis, premature growth plate closure, and chronic infection. Subacute infection may present with fever, pain, and periosteal elevation. Brodie's abscess, or focal subacute osteomyelitis, often presents with long-standing dull pain without fever.
3. *Chronic:* Defined by symptoms persistent for more than 1 month before therapy or following inadequate treatment of acute osteomyelitis; chronic osteomyelitis is characterized clinically by drainage at the site of infection and low-grade fever.

TABLE 19-1. Stages of Osteomyelitis

Stage	Time Course	Pathologic Features	Example
Acute	7-10 days	Bone marrow edema,* cellular infiltration	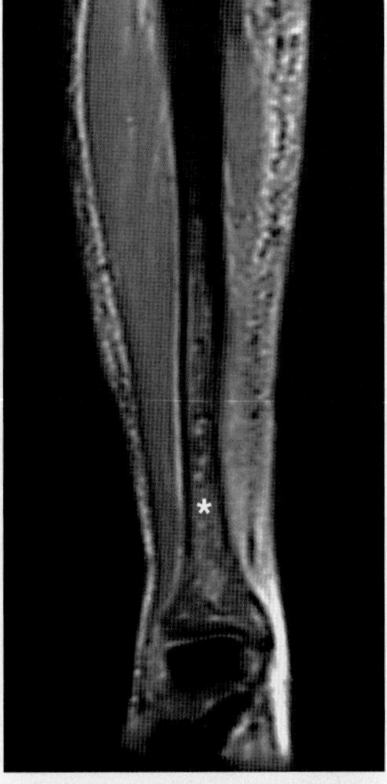
Subacute	2 weeks-month	Spread of infection through the cortex Focal subacute: Brodie's abscess; walled-off infection *(arrow)*	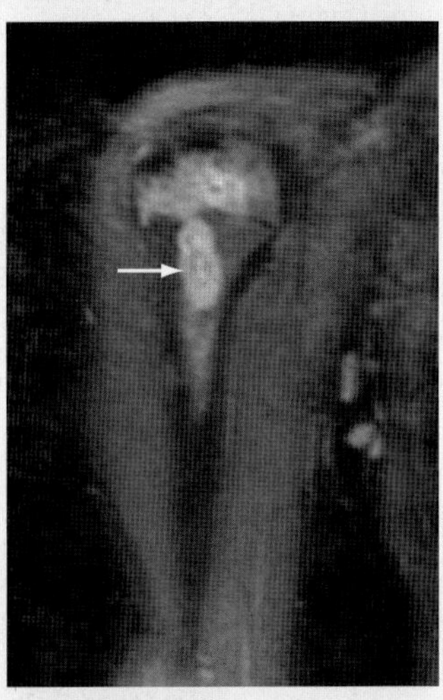
Chronic	> 1 month	Sequestrum of necrotic bone *(arrow)*	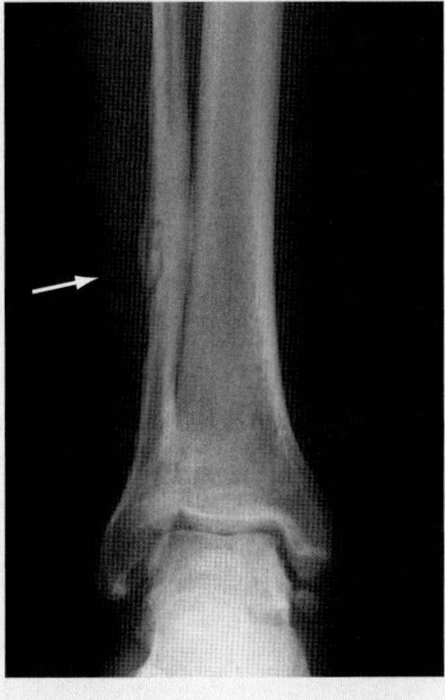

TABLE 19-2. Methods of Osteomyelitis Spread

Method of Spread	Cause	Usual Organisms
Hematogenous	Bloodborne infection	*S. aureus*
Contiguous	From adjacent ulcer	Multiple organisms
Direct implantation	Posttraumatic or postoperative	Multiple organisms

The hallmark in adults is a necrotic sequestrum, the result of ischemic necrosis caused by increased intramedullary intraosseous pressure.

> A sequestrum is the hallmark of chronic active osteomyelitis and consists of a fragment of devitalized bone.

The sequestrum may be surrounded by granulation tissue or living reactive new bone (i.e., involucrum), often within the thickened cortex. The sequestrum may be extruded to the skin surface through the involucrum via a cloaca (sinus tract).[1]

Osteomyelitis can spread by three routes (Table 19-2):

1. *Hematogenous:* Hematogenous infection is most commonly caused by *Staphylococcus aureus.* In adults, acute hematogenous osteomyelitis usually begins in the diaphyses; infection can spread throughout the medullary canal to include the epiphysis and joint. The periosteum is tightly attached in adults, resulting in less periosteal elevation than is seen in children.[2] Cortical breakthrough usually leads to soft tissue abscess, and sinus tracts develop from sequestrations to the skin; in children, who have the periosteum more loosely adherent to bone, subperiosteal abscess rather than soft tissue abscess results. Intramedullary abscess most commonly occurs as a single lesion near the metaphysis of the distal tibia.
2. *Contiguous:* This type of spread occurs most commonly in adults, particularly in the diabetic foot, from adjacent soft tissue or decubitus ulcers.
3. *Direct implantation, posttraumatic or postoperative:* Organisms are introduced through acute inoculation into bone at the time of trauma or spread from adjacent soft tissue infection. This category includes infections from interventions. As opposed to hematogenous spread, infections due to direct implantation are usually caused by multiple organisms including *S. aureus* and coagulase-negative staphylococci 75% of the time, as well as gram-negative bacilli and anaerobic organisms.[1]

Imaging Features

Radiographs

Acute Osteomyelitis

Within 1 to 2 days postinfection there is soft tissue swelling with loss of fascial planes.

> Swelling in osteomyelitis obliterates fascial planes, whereas tumors usually displace facial planes.

Focal osteopenia may be noted.

By 7 to 10 days there is destructive bony lysis, but radiographs can be normal for 10 to 21 days postinfection, as 30% to 50% loss of medullary bone is required to see changes on radiographs.

> Radiographs are insensitive for early osteomyelitis because bone changes may be inapparent for several weeks after infection.

Bone changes in early osteomyelitis therefore lag about 2 weeks behind the infection itself, and following treatment, radiographic improvement generally lags behind clinical improvement.

Following treatment, radiographic improvement generally lags behind clinical improvement.

The sensitivity of radiographs ranges from 43% to 75% and the specificity from 75% to 83% for evidence of osteomyelitis.[2,3] Early radiographs are useful, however, for evaluating alternate diagnoses such as neoplasm, injury, or osteoarthritis.

By 2 to 6 weeks, radiographs generally show destruction of cortical and medullary bone, periosteal reaction, and new bone formation (Figure 19-1, *A*).

Subacute osteomyelitis

Subacute osteomyelitis can occur in the setting of inadequate treatment or when the underlying bone is abnormal. The cortex becomes more lucent as infection spreads into cortical haversian and Volkmann's canals. Although uncommon in adults, subperiosteal abscess is evidenced by periostitis with subperiosteal new bone and involucrum formation. Periosteal disruption with adjacent soft tissue abscess is evidenced by soft tissue swelling and mass-like opacity obliterating fat planes, with bony disruption commonly leading to pathologic fracture in adults.

Focal subacute osteomyelitis (Brodie's abscess)

Radiographs of a patient with a Brodie's abscess show a sharply defined radiolucent lesion with a sclerotic margin that fades peripherally such that the outer border appears fuzzy. These lesions can also appear on imaging studies as elongated serpiginous lucencies. There is no associated sequestrum. Brodie's abscess occurs most frequently at the metaphysis of long tubular bones, often the tibia or femur (Table 19-1).

Brodie's abscess is a focus of subacute osteomyelitis that is usually in the metaphysis of a long bone.

Chronic osteomyelitis

By 6 to 8 weeks, signs of chronic active osteomyelitis appear after inadequate treatment or treatment in immunocompromised patients. A sequestrum (necrotic bone) is formed as the blood supply to the metaphyseal and periosteal vessels is disrupted by infectious thrombi. The sequestrum is surrounded by an involucrum (periosteal new bone), which forms when pus penetrates the cortex, stimulating periosteal new bone formation. Sinus tracts form in the soft tissues relatively frequently in adults, which may extrude sequestra that then migrate to the skin surface[4] (Figure 19-1, *B*). The cortex is thickened with the bone having an expanded appearance.[5] Garre's sclerosing osteomyelitis is a type of chronic osteomyelitis characterized by marked cortical thickening or periosteal reaction producing a very dense appearance on radiographs.[6]

Sequestration is a hallmark of chronic active osteomyelitis, and adequate treatment requires surgical removal of this necrotic bone nidus (Figure 19-2).

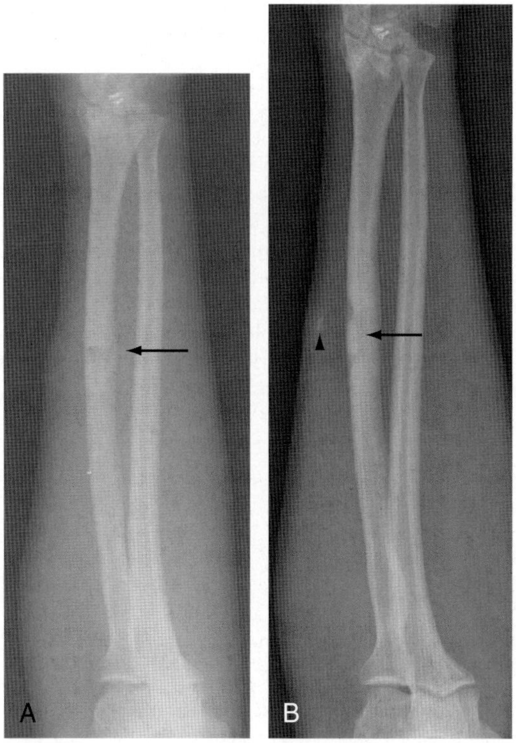

FIGURE 19-1. Pin tract infection. 33-year-old man with external fixator placed status post delayed treatment of wrist fracture. **A,** Posteroanterior radiograph of the forearm after hardware removal demonstrates periosteal reaction and indistinctness of the margins of the pin tract *(arrow)* within the midradial diaphysis, consistent with acute osteomyelitis. **B,** Posteroanterior radiograph 5 years later demonstrates sequestrum formation *(arrow)* with soft tissue calcification within sinus tract *(arrowhead)*, findings consistent with chronic active osteomyelitis.

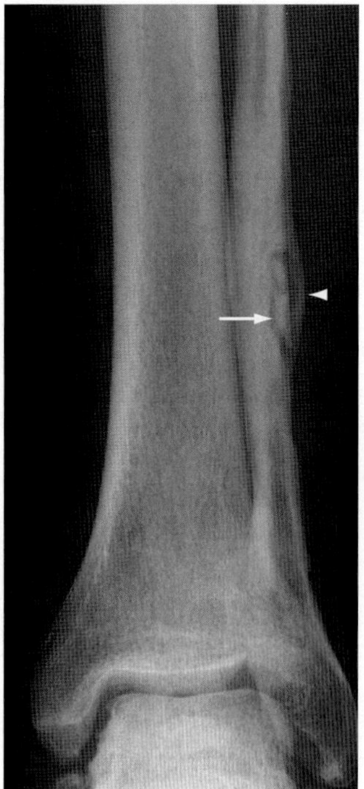

FIGURE 19-2. Chronic osteomyelitis with sequestrum. 27-year-old man status post motor vehicle accident with a closed fibular fracture, status post removal of internal fixation, with a draining sinus tract. Anteroposterior radiograph demonstrates sequestrum formation *(arrow)* with involucrum *(arrowhead)* representing chronic osteomyelitis. Pathologic examination was consistent with *S. aureus* chronic osteomyelitis with a draining fistula.

TABLE 19-3. Radiographic Features of Chronic Active Osteomyelitis

Finding	Example	Finding	Example
Destruction of medullary bone with mottled lucencies *(arrow)*	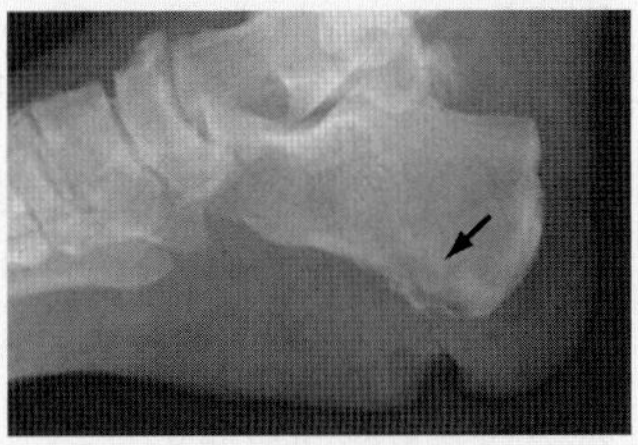	Cortical thickening and reactive sclerosis	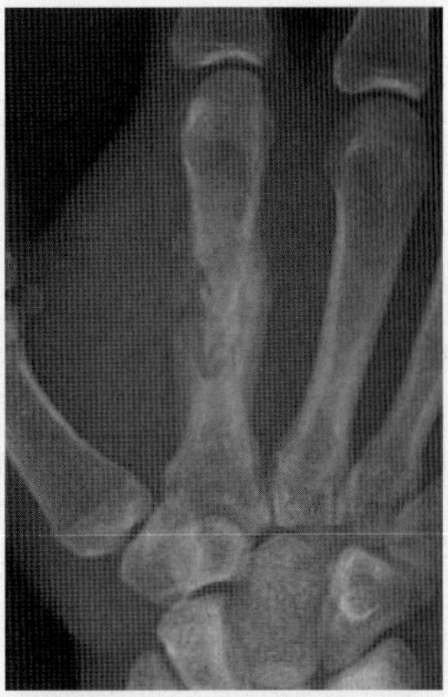
Periosteal new bone formation or reaction	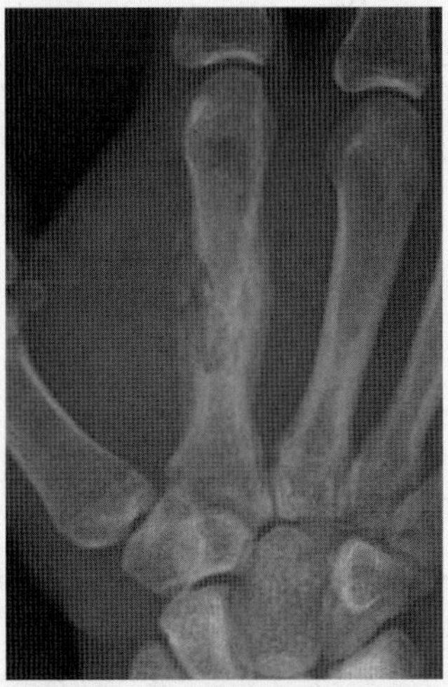	Sinus tract *(arrow)*	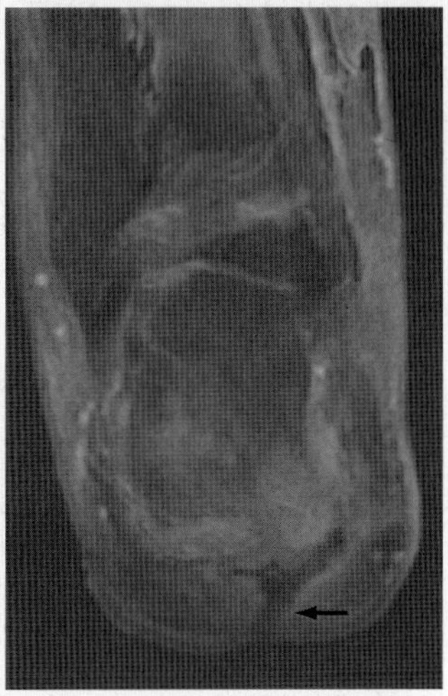
Sequestration *(arrow)*	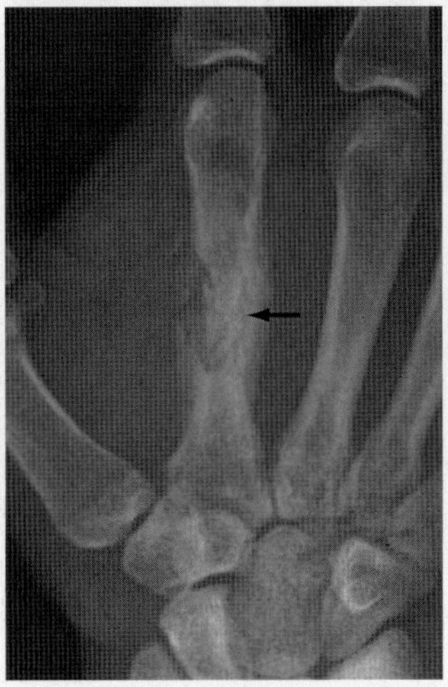		

The presence of a sequestrum, which can best be documented by CT, indicates chronic active osteomyelitis. It requires surgical removal.

Sensitivity of radiographs for identifying sequestration in chronic active osteomyelitis has been reported at 9% to 33%.[7]

Classic radiographic features of chronic active osteomyelitis thus include the following (Table 19-3):

- Destruction of medullary bone with mottled lucencies (Figure 19-3, *A, B*)
- Periosteal new bone formation (Figure 19-4, *A*)
- Cortical thickening and reactive sclerosis (Figure 19-5, *A*)
- Sequestration (Table 19-3)
- Soft tissue calcification suggesting a sinus tract[4]

Computed Tomography (CT)

Acute osteomyelitis

In early osteomyelitis, CT can be a useful adjunct to radiographs, as it can be more sensitive for detection of cortical destruction and new bone formation, periosteal reaction and soft tissue involvement, as well as medullary increased attenuation, and medullary cavity constriction. Intraosseous gas is an uncommon but pathognomonic manifestation of osteomyelitis.

In acute osteomyelitis, MRI is preferred to CT. In chronic osteomyelitis, CT is helpful in documenting a sequestrum and will complement MRI findings.

Drawbacks to CT include lower specificity of findings such as increased medullary density, which can be seen in hemorrhage, neoplasm, stress fracture, and postradiation change. Scatter metallic artifact can degrade the images and therefore be a limiting factor.

Serial CT is specifically considered the optimal imaging technique to distinguish cranial osteomyelitis from soft tissue infection. It is useful for monitoring of the response to therapy in elderly diabetic patients who may present with a rare but potentially lethal *Pseudomonas* infection of necrotizing external otitis.[8]

Chronic osteomyelitis

To differentiate chronic active osteomyelitis from a background of chronic inactive osteomyelitis requires careful evaluation for irregular foci of destructive osteolysis, fluffy periostitis (Figure 19-3, *C*), soft tissue swelling, sequestra, and sinus tracts, which are all signs of an active infection.[4] CT is particularly useful to visualize small sequestra in areas of bony sclerosis, periosteal reaction, cortical erosion, foreign bodies, and subtle sinus tracts in bone. CT can be better than MRI to identify marrow calcification and cortical destruction. Tumeh et al. found CT 100% sensitive for sequestra, but the examination can be falsely positive due to bone remodeling and sclerosis from old healed infections.[5]

Nonspecific CT findings of inflammation include medullary hyperattenuation, which can be seen with a differential diagnosis of hemorrhage, neoplasm, fracture, and radiation. Increased specificity is seen with cortical bone destruction, new bone formation, decrease in size of the medullary space, sequestration, and intraosseous gas

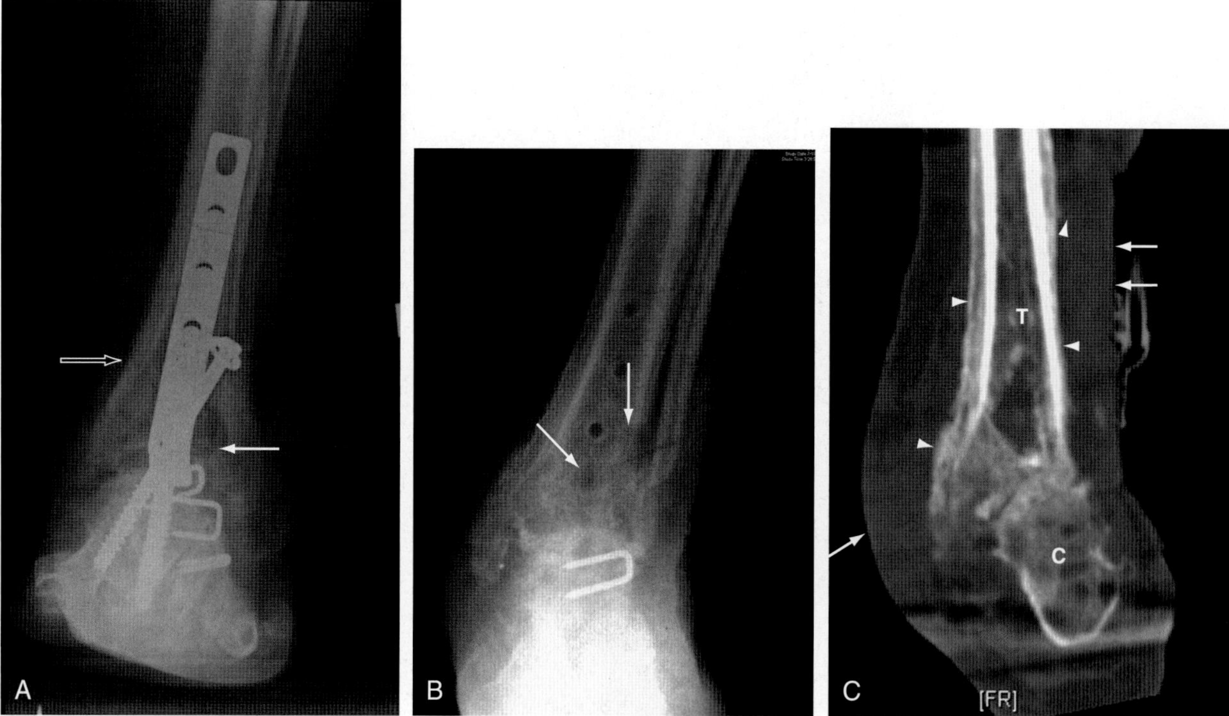

FIGURE 19-3. Osteomyelitis. This 44-year-old woman with Charcot-Marie-Tooth polyneuropathy was status post tibiotalar, talonavicular, and calcaneocuboid fusion. Internal fixation hardware was replaced with external fixator due to nonunion. MRSA positive wound infection with tibial osteomyelitis then complicated external fixation necessitating its removal. **(A)** AP radiograph before and **(B)** after removal of most of the fixation hardware demonstrate prominent lucency centered at the lateral aspect of the tibiotalar joint *(arrows)*, and prominent periosteal reaction of the distal tibia *(open arrow)*. The distal fibula has been resected in **B. C,** Coronal reformatted CT demonstrates periosteal reaction *(arrowheads)* and lucency along the distal tibia with adjacent soft tissue swelling *(arrows)* consistent with osteomyelitis. Subcutaneous swelling is indicated by replacement of the subcutaneous fat tissue by fluid density. *C,* Calcaneus; *T,* tibia.

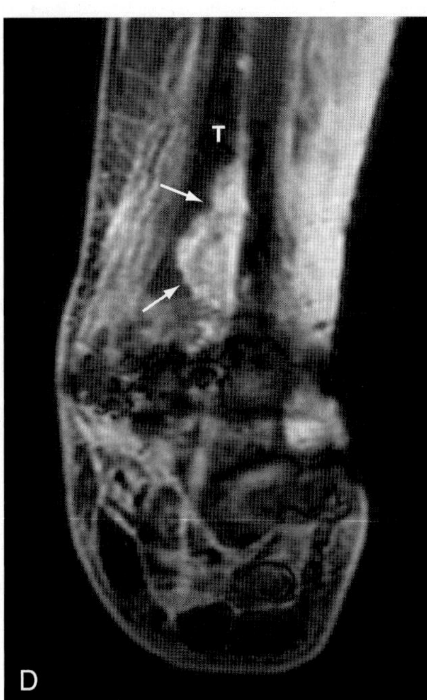

FIGURE 19-3—cont'd. **D,** Coronal T1-weighted fat-suppressed MRI after intravenous gadolinium demonstrates contrast enhancement within the distal tibia *(arrows)* consistent with osteomyelitis, with marked enhancement in the lateral soft tissues.

(Figure 19-4, *B, C*). Localization of the sequestrum is important, as this needs to be surgically removed to adequately treat the infection or else it will continue to serve as a nidus of active osteomyelitis.

Magnetic Resonance Imaging

Acute osteomyelitis

MRI is the most useful modality for early diagnosis and determination of extent of infection, offering better marrow and soft tissue evaluation than CT and greater anatomic detail than nuclear medicine examination.

> MRI is the method of choice for imaging acute osteomyelitis. Intravenous contrast is indicated when evaluating possible osteomyelitis. Radiographs should also be obtained in most cases prior to MRI to exclude other diagnoses and for correlation with MRI findings.

On T1-weighted spin echo imaging, fatty bone marrow normally shows bright signal, cortical bone shows dark signal, and cartilage shows intermediate signal. Marrow replacement by higher-water-content material may be due to a wide variety of conditions such as neuropathic osteoarthropathy, tumor, infarct, ischemia, fracture, or infection. In all of these conditions, the marrow fat will be replaced and the marrow will appear darker on T1-weighted images and brighter on T2-weighted images. A greater degree of T2 signal intensity does, however, seem to correlate with a greater likelihood of osteomyelitis.[8] Often the pattern of the marrow changes or other findings will help identify the presence of infection. These supporting

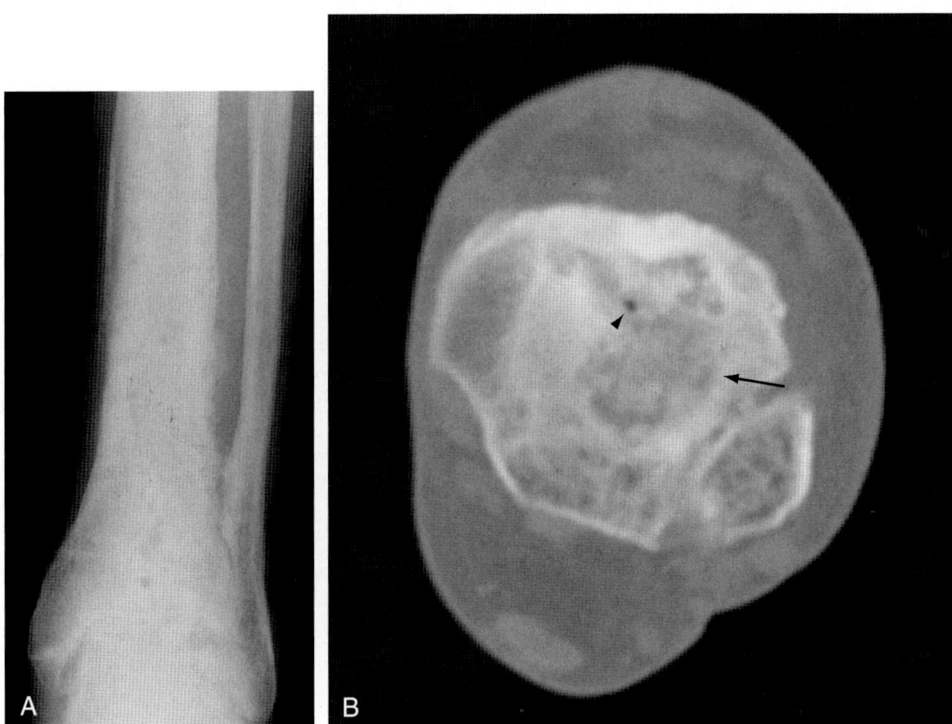

FIGURE 19-4. Osteomyelitis with intraosseous gas and positive bone scan. 51-year-old man status post removal of fixation hardware for distal tibial and fibular fractures. **A,** Radiograph demonstrates cortical thickening with well-organized periosteal reaction along the distal tibial fracture site. **B,** CT demonstrates destructive lesion *(arrow)* in the intramedullary tibial plafond with intraosseous gas *(arrowhead)*, consistent with active osteomyelitis. The wound culture grew *Streptococcus.*

(Continued)

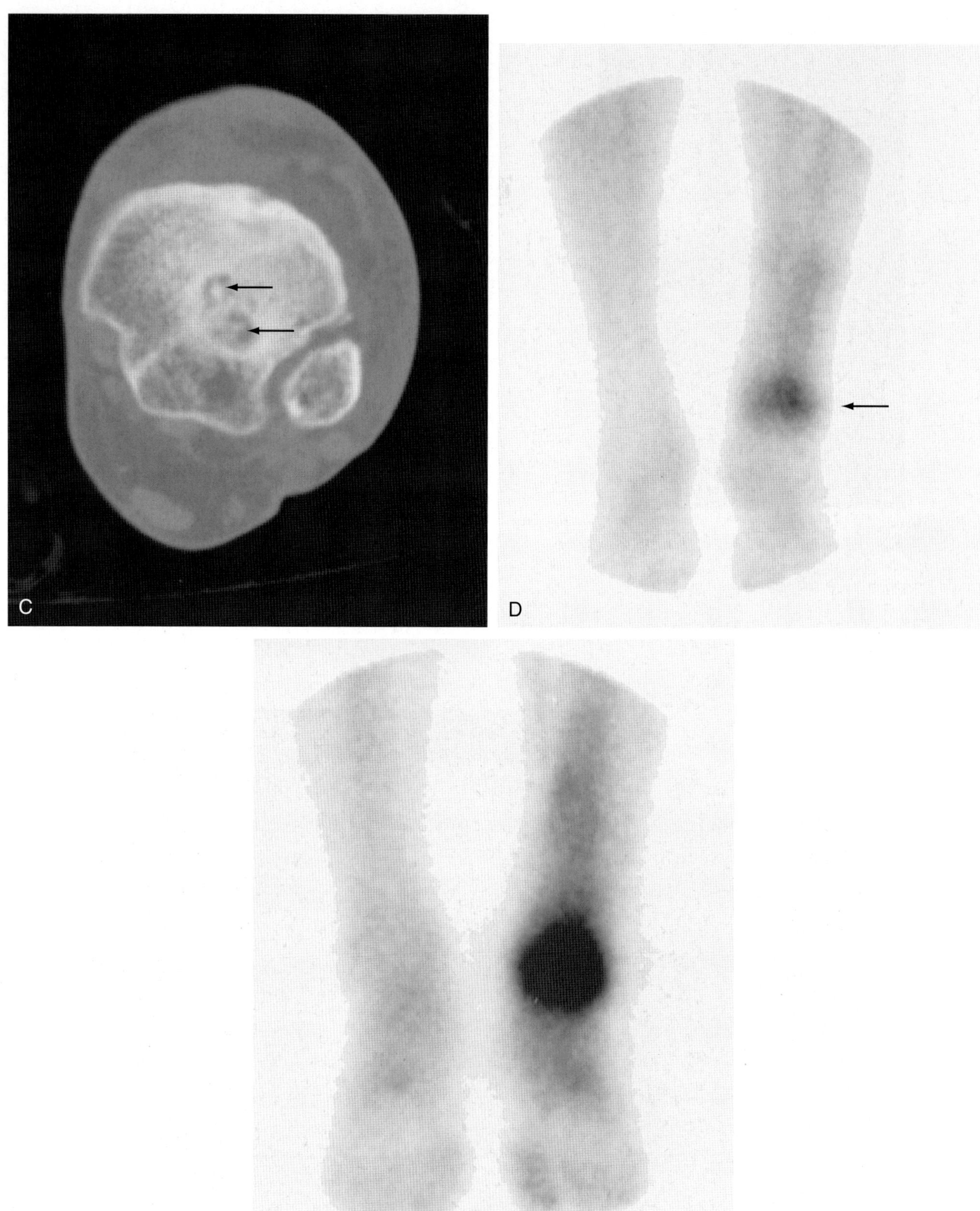

FIGURE 19-4—cont'd. **C,** CT scan shows small dense fragments, sequestra *(arrows)*. **D,** Bone scan demonstrates increased uptake on the initial blood pool image *(arrow)*. **E,** Delayed bone scan image shows increased uptake at the site of osteomyelitis.

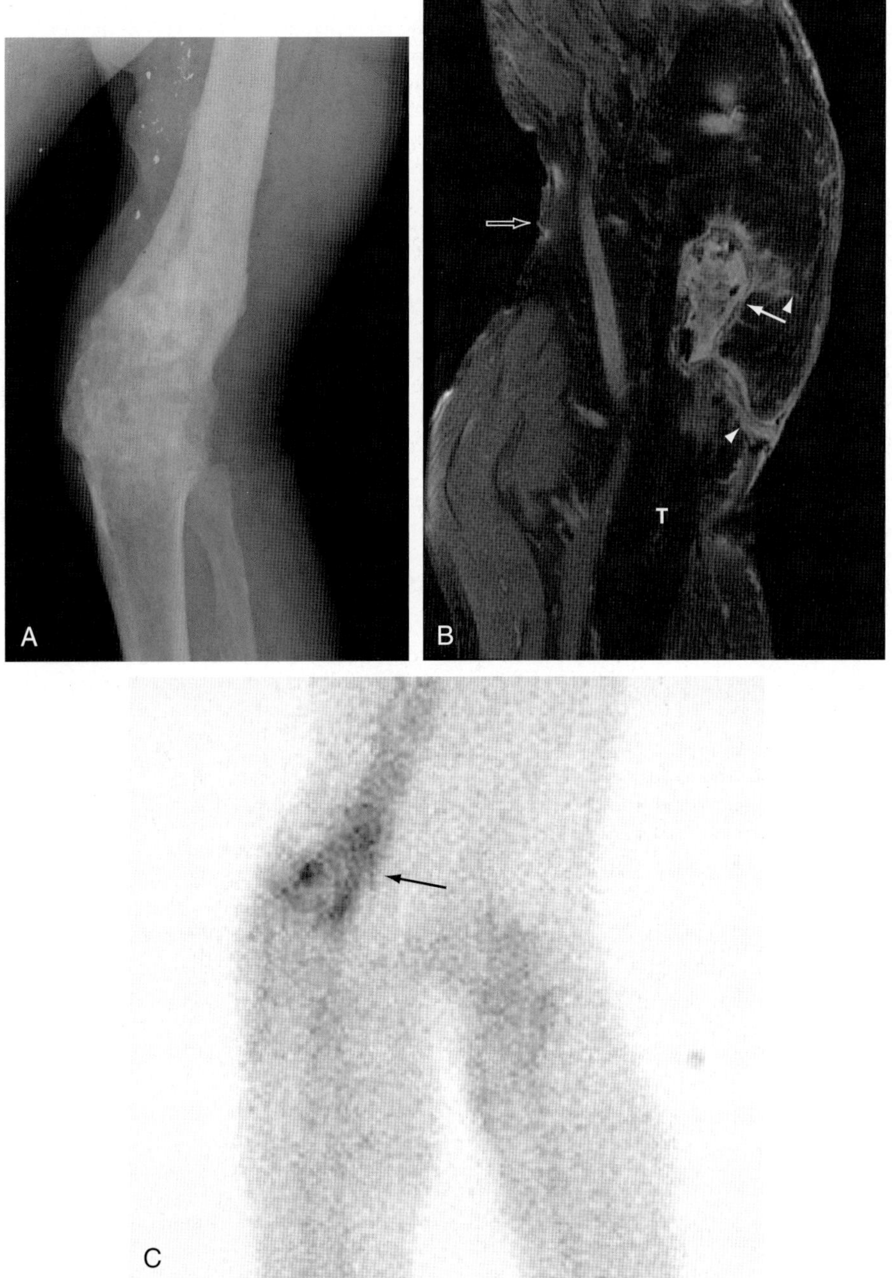

FIGURE 19-5. Chronic osteomyelitis. 84-year-old man with World War II–era gunshot wound to the knee, with a 60-year history of intermittent drainage from the distal femur. **A,** Oblique radiograph demonstrates knee fusion with cortical thickening and periosteal reaction of the distal femur. Multiple metal fragments are noted in the anterior soft tissues. **B,** T1-weighted MRI after intravenous gadolinium demonstrates a fluid signal area in the distal femoral metadiaphysis with a peripheral rim sign *(arrow)* and two sinus tracts *(arrowheads)* to the skin, consistent with the patient's penicillin-sensitive *S. aureus*–positive chronic active osteomyelitis. The internal low signal areas are consistent with foreign material. Note the site of soft tissue scarring *(open arrow)* that was evident on the radiograph. **C,** Bone scan showing mild delayed uptake in the distal femoral metadiaphysis *(arrow)*.

secondary MRI signs for osteomyelitis include: soft tissue ulcer, cellulitis, soft tissue abscess, sinus tract, and cortical interruption. MRI examination may be limited to various degrees by artifact from metallic prostheses, and the ability of the patient to tolerate the examination due to their hemodynamic status or claustrophobia.

Modic et al. also report that some culture positive cases of osteomyelitis show low signal on T1-weighted and T2-weighted imaging, with similar signal characteristics to fibrous dysplasia, bone infarction, and benign sclerosis.[9] In the presence of metallic prostheses, the degree of artifact limits the utility of MRI, making indium-labeled white blood cell (WBC) scanning generally more sensitive and specific in this scenario, as well as in the immediate postoperative or posttraumatic period.

When metallic prostheses are present, indium-labeled WBC scanning may be more helpful than MRI because of the artifacts associated with prostheses on MRI examination.

MRI is more useful than nuclear imaging for differentiating soft tissue infection with periostitis from osteomyelitis.[9]

MRI is the most useful modality to identify or exclude osteomyelitis when soft tissue infection and periosteal reaction are present.

The sensitivity of MRI (using fat-suppression technique) for osteomyelitis is variable, generally ranging from 82% to 100%, with specificity ranging from 75% to 100%,[2] which is greater than radiographs or CT and comparable to radionuclide studies.[6] However, sensitivity has been reported as low as 60% and specificity as low as 50%.[8] Short tau inversion recovery (STIR) sequences are highly sensitive but less specific than spin echo sequences, with negative predictive value of STIR for acute osteomyelitis reportedly near 100% but with limited spatial resolution that cannot reliably differentiate abscess from edema.[8]

A normal STIR sequence on MRI essentially rules out osteomyelitis.

Pitfalls of MRI for diagnosing osteomyelitis include evaluation for marrow abnormalities in anemic patients and in other marrow replacement abnormalities, with diagnosis particularly difficult in small and flat bones.

Focal subacute osteomyelitis

T1-weighted post-gadolinium images of Brodie's abscess characteristically show a "target" lesion with four layers, the central abscess being low signal, surrounded by enhancing intermediate signal granulation tissue lining the inner wall ("double line" sign) of the abscess, surrounded by a sharp low signal "rim sign" of fibrosis, and, most peripherally, higher signal endosteal reaction/hyperemia.[2]

Brodie's abscess typically shows a target lesion with four layers on T1-weighted MRI.

Chronic osteomyelitis

In chronic osteomyelitis, tissue planes become more sharply demarcated. Intraosseous edema also becomes more sharply demarcated with a peripheral "rim sign" of low T1 and T2 signal due to devascularized fibrosis. This gain is reportedly seen in 93% of patients with posttraumatic chronic osteomyelitis.[5] T2 bright sinus tracts may be present (Figure 19-5, *B*).

In the difficult clinical quandary of diagnosing reactivation of osteomyelitis in a site of chronic posttraumatic osteomyelitis, MRI has a reported sensitivity of 100%, specificity of 60%, and accuracy of 79%, with negative predictive value of 100%.[6] Sequestra, cloacae, and soft tissue and subperiosteal abscesses should suggest an active component.

A negative MRI is highly reliable in ruling out active osteomyelitis in a patient with chronic posttraumatic osteomyelitis.

Higher signal at T1-weighted images signal can suggest healed infection with fatty marrow replacement rather than active infection. Sequestra tend to be low signal on all sequences and nonenhancing when derived from cortical bone but higher signal intensity when derived from cancellous bone. Soft tissue abscesses are well-demarcated T2 bright foci. Gadolinium administration allows for high sensitivity but cannot reliably differentiate infection (see Figure 19-3, *D*) from adjacent joint inflammation, trauma, osteoarthritis, diabetic osteoarthropathy, neoplasm, or radiation (Figure 19-6, *A* and *B*). Lack of enhancement, on the other hand, offers good support against infection. Gadolinium can help differentiate chronic from acute processes, with infarcted sequestra showing no enhancement, and can help differentiate abscesses from tumor, as abscesses do not enhance.

Complications of longstanding chronic osteomyelitis include squamous cell carcinoma development within a sinus tract in 0.23% to 1.6% of such patients.[6] This can be identified by the presence of new lytic bone lesions on radiographs or by a soft tissue mass on MRI.

MRI can aid in surgical planning to determine extent of disease, involvement of critical structures, and the presence of devitalized tissue.[6]

Scintigraphy

Nuclear medicine provides physiologic information regarding inflammation, but with lower anatomic resolution than MRI. Three radionuclide classes are most commonly used: (1) technetium-99m (Tc-99m) MDP bone scan, (2) gallium-67 (Ga-67) citrate, and (3) indium-111 (In-111) labeled or Tc-99m hexamethylpropyleneamine oxime (HMPAO) labeled WBCs. The accuracy of the bone scan is increased by combining it with gallium-labeled or indium-labeled WBC scanning. A number of additional radiopharmaceuticals, however, are being evaluated for improved accuracy. This topic is explored in greater depth in the nuclear medicine section, Chapter 2.

Acute osteomyelitis

Three-phase bone scan is a routine technique used to distinguish cellulitis from osteomyelitis; the former shows increased uptake on the first two phases of the bone scan but not on delayed imaging, and the latter shows increased uptake on all phases within 1 to 3 days of symptom development. Bone scan has high sensitivity but low specificity in diagnosing osteomyelitis, with a sensitivity ranging from 69% to 100% and specificity ranging from 38% to 82%.[2] The relatively low specificity can be attributed to numerous diagnoses resulting in increased bone turnover, including infection, neoplasm, and trauma, that show a similar appearance by this technique. In postoperative, posttraumatic, or neuropathic patients, infection may therefore be difficult to differentiate from the underlying disease.[2] Bone scan does offer the opportunity to detect multiple sites of infection simultaneously. Three-phase whole-body bone imaging, developed by Yang et al. in 1988, has also been used to differentiate between cellulitis and sites of active and inactive osteomyelitis.[10]

Bone scan followed by Ga-67 scan, which tends to be more specific, shows increased uptake with inflammation and decreased uptake in response to therapy. In-111 labeled WBC imaging has both a high sensitivity and specificity for diagnosing acute osteomyelitis, especially in the extremities, with a reported sensitivity of 83%, specificity of 94%, and accuracy of 88% for osteomyelitis.[4]

Three phase bone scan can distinguish cellulotis from osteomyelitis.

Chronic osteomyelitis

Any form of osteomyelitis can progress to a chronic form involving necrotic bone. Three-phase bone scan remains useful to distinguish

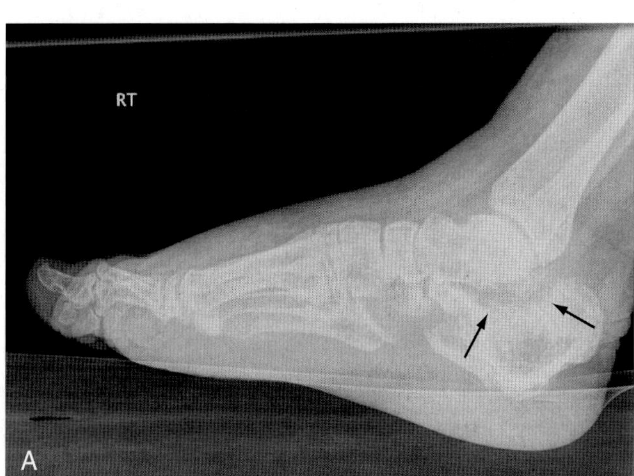

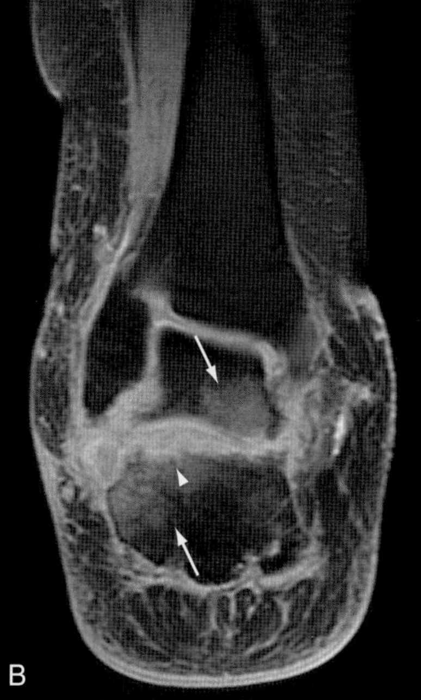

FIGURE 19-6. Limitations of imaging in excluding active infection. 75-year-old man with foot pain following remote calcaneal fracture. **A,** Lateral radiograph of the foot demonstrates lysis and widening along the subtalar joint *(arrows)*, suspicious for osteomyelitis in the clinical setting of prior calcaneal fracture. A similar appearance could be seen in a neuropathic joint. **B,** Post-contrast fat-suppressed T1-weighted coronal MR image demonstrates deformity of the calcaneus and posterior subtalar joint, with adjacent abnormal fluid signal and enhancement in the talus and calcaneus *(arrows)* as well as erosions *(arrowhead)* suspicious for osteomyelitis. There is a complex subtalar joint effusion. Bone biopsy showed chronic changes with destruction of subchondral bone and new bone formation, but no active osteomyelitis or infectious organisms were found.

cellulitis from osteomyelitis (see Figure 19-4, *D*, Figure 19-4, *E*, and Figure 19-5, *B*). Combined bone scan and leukocyte scan is limited in the setting of low-grade chronic infections (see Figure 19-5, *C*), in closely adherent soft tissue infection, in the central skeleton where there is a predominance of hematopoietic marrow, and posttraumatic or postsurgical cases that have ectopic hematopoietic marrow. Combined bone scan and gallium scan are the current radionuclide gold standard for vertebral infection. To diagnose chronic active osteomyelitis, Tc-99m sulfur colloid marrow imaging combined with In-111–labeled WBC imaging has been advocated.[4] Tumeh et al. found scintigraphy to be a helpful adjunct imaging technique in excluding the presence of active disease when the CT is falsely positive for sequestra, hence avoiding surgery.[7]

Positron Emission Tomography

As an alternative to combined nuclear medicine scanning, 18-F-fluoro-D-deoxyglucose positron emission tomography, or FDG-PET, has shown particularly promising results in evaluating patients with chronic osteomyelitis. These images are not compromised by metallic implants and can differentiate between scar tissue and active inflammation. It is of particular utility for its greater accuracy in the axial skeleton, where alternate nuclear imaging techniques are compromised. It may become useful for more specific follow-up of therapeutic response to antibiotics, as it quantitatively images activated inflammatory cells rather than the hyperemia that is imaged with bone scan, CT, and MRI.[11] Stumpe et al. evaluated 45 whole- or partial-body FDG-PET examinations to detect soft tissue and bone infections. Sensitivity of PET was found to be 96% for soft tissue infections and 100% for bone infections. Specificity for this group ranged from 70% to 99%.[12]

PET scanning may be a method for accurately identifying and following acute infection.

Ultrasonography

Ultrasound is easily accessible, inexpensive, without ionizing radiation, and allows dynamic real time examination to guide biopsy, aspiration, or drainage. The utility in evaluation of osteomyelitis is in the evaluation for subperiosteal fluid collections, which are diagnostic in the appropriate clinical setting. Changes highly suspicious for osteomyelitis include abscess or fluid collections next to the cortex. Ultrasound evaluation is not hampered by metallic prostheses, as is the case with cross-sectional modalities.

ADULT SPINAL INFECTION

Infection in the spine can involve several anatomic areas and is usually spread by the hematogenous route but can also be spread by contiguous infection or direct implantation.[4] Areas involved can include the vertebral body, the disk, the paravertebral soft tissues, or the epidural space.

Infection beginning in the anterior inferior body suggests spread from the anterior spinal artery. Segmental vertebral arteries usually bifurcate to supply two adjacent vertebrae, and infection usually involves these vertebrae and their intervening disk.

Typically, infection involves two adjacent vertebrae and the intervening intervertebral disk. This is distinct from tumor involvement that usually spares the disk.

Of hematogenous vertebral osteomyelitis, approximately 50% of cases involve lumbar vertebrae, 30% involve thoracic vertebrae, and 20% involve cervical vertebrae. Forty percent of adult vertebral osteomyelitis is reportedly associated with retrograde urinary tract infection (UTI) spread through Batson's venous plexus. Other causes are IV drug use, endocarditis, diabetes, and sickle cell disease. In IV drug use, the incidence of cervical vertebral involvement increases (27%) and thoracic vertebral involvement decreases (4.5%).[1]

Vertebral osteomyelitis may quickly spread to adjacent vertebrae and cause discitis, epidural and subdural abscesses, meningitis, paravertebral, retropharyngeal, mediastinal, subphrenic, or retroperitoneal abscesses.

The most common organism involved is *S. aureus* in normal patients (accounts for 90% of spine infections), or aerobic gram-negative rods including *Pseudomonas aeruginosa* and *Serratia marcescens* in IV drug users and patients with urinary tract infections.[1] Granulomatous infection is also seen including tuberculosis (TB), brucellosis, or coccidioidomycosis.

Imaging Features

Radiographs

Disk space narrowing and vertebral endplate irregularity are seen with pyogenic spondylodiscitis, which can progress to vertebral collapse (Figure 19-7, *A*).

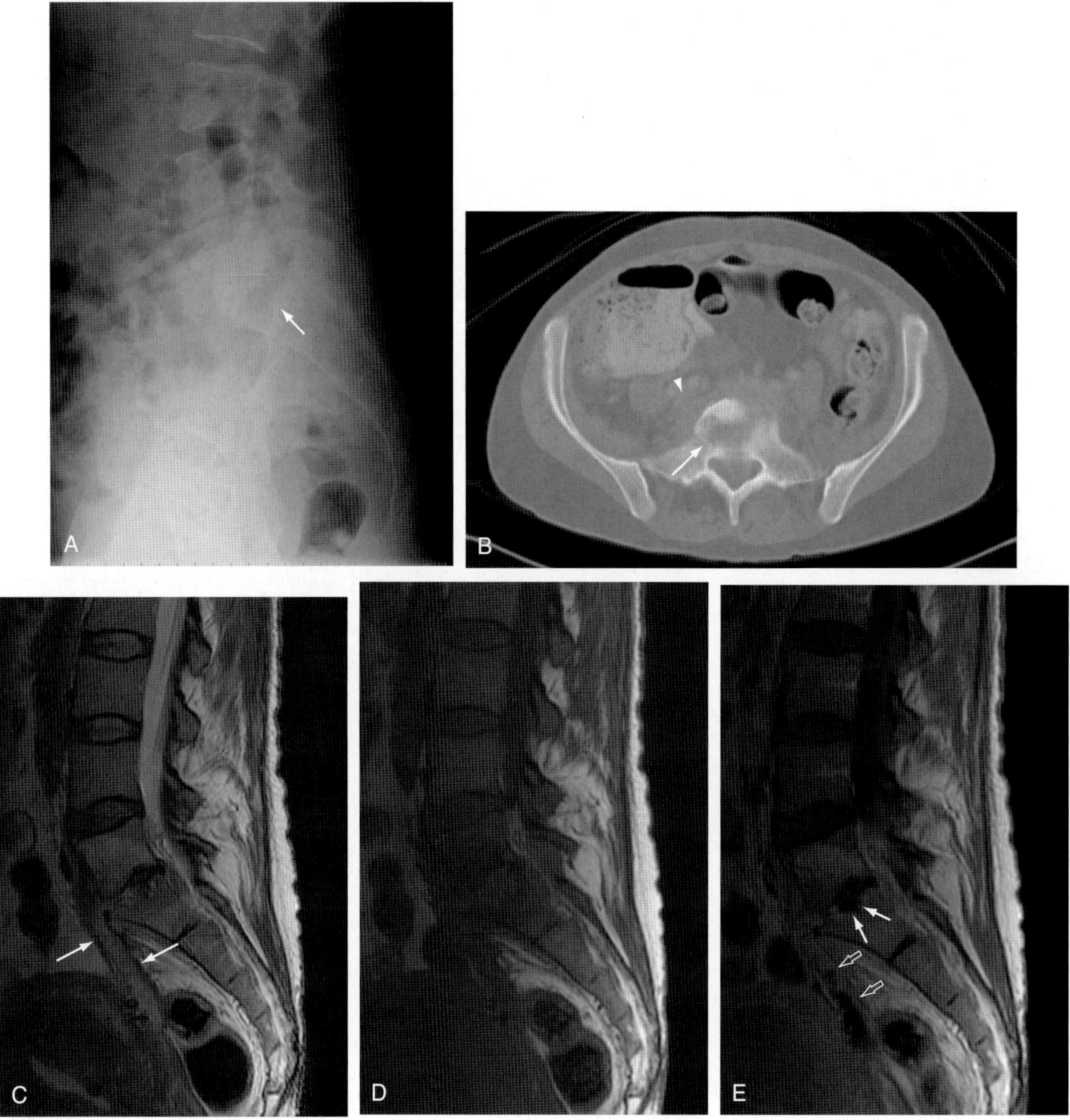

FIGURE 19-7. Spinal osteomyelitis/discitis. This 53-year-old woman developed back pain following colpopexy mesh placement for uterine prolapse, which was complicated by an infected hematoma. The patient developed L5/S1 discitis/osteomyelitis with an epidural abscess as well as fistula formation to the pelvis. **A,** Radiograph demonstrates disk space narrowing and bone erosion adjacent to the L5/S1 disk *(arrow)*. **B,** CT demonstrates circumferential soft tissue *(arrowhead)* anterior to the L5/S1 disk space, with end plate irregularity *(arrow)*. **C,** T2-weighted sagittal MR image demonstrates disk space narrowing with T2 bright edema signal within the disk space and adjacent end plates as well as in the paravertebral musculature. A T2 bright fistula *(arrows)* extends from the rectouterine space. **(D)** T1-weighted pre-gadolinium MRI sequence **(E)** T1-weighted post-gadolinium MRI sequence demonstrate enhancing L5-S1 disk space and adjacent end plates *(arrows)*, with enhancement along the fistulous tract to the pelvis *(open arrows)* and within the paravertebral musculature.

(Continued)

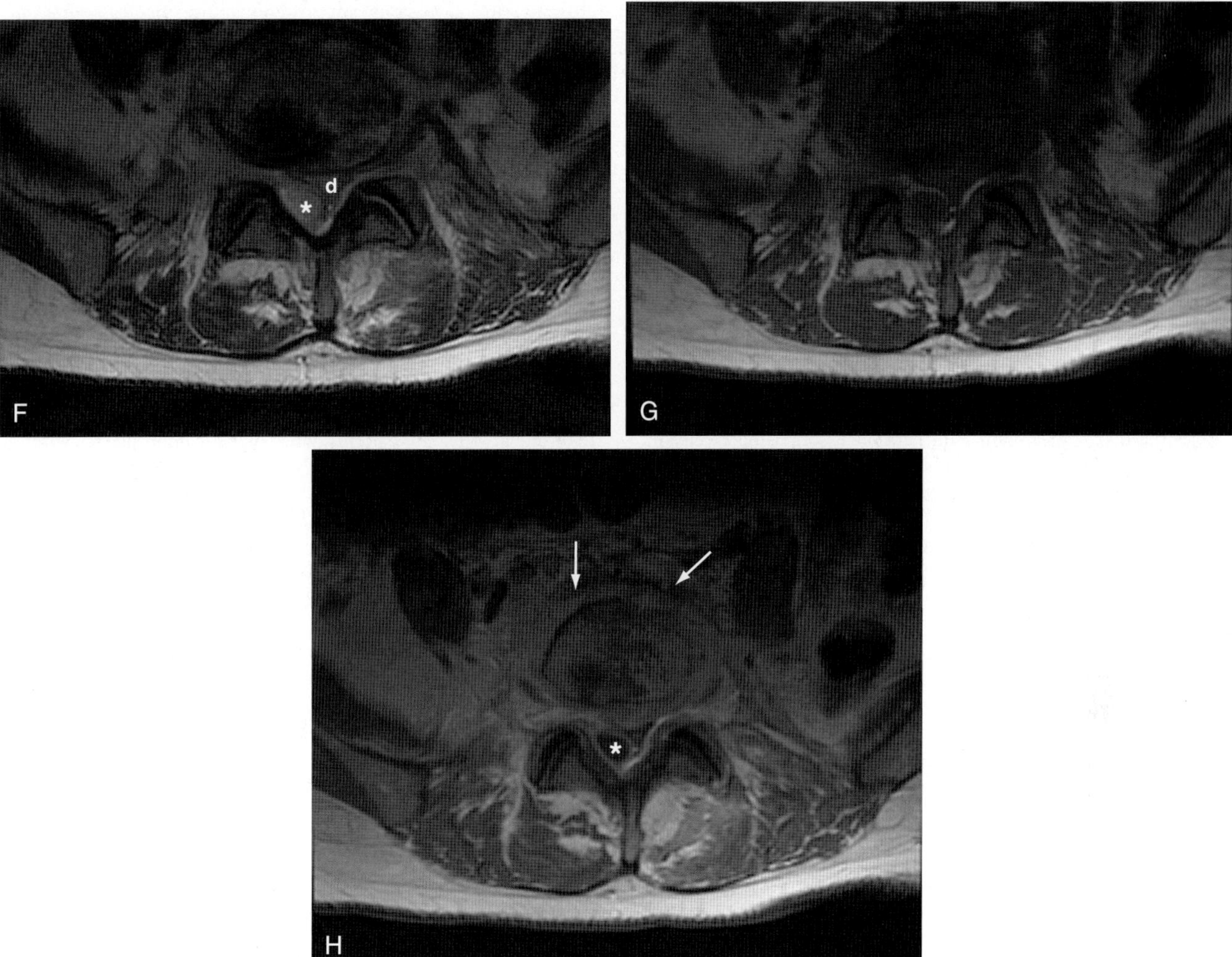

FIGURE 19-7—cont'd. **F,** T2-weighted axial MR image best demonstrates T2 bright fluid collections within the epidural space *(asterisk)*. *d,* Dural sac with cauda equina. **(G)** T1-weighted MR image pre-gadolinium and **(H)** T1-weighted MR axial image post-gadolinium demonstrate peripheral enhancement of the right posterior epidural abscess *(asterisk)*. The enhancement of the left paraspinal muscles and the anterior soft tissue swelling *(arrows)* is well seen. **F,** T2-weighted axial MR image best demonstrates T2 bright fluid collections within the epidural space *(asterisk)*. *d,* Dural sac with cauda equina. **(G)** T1-weighted MR image pre-gadolinium and **(H)** T1-weighted MR axial image post-gadolinium demonstrate peripheral enhancement of the right posterior epidural abscess *(asterisk)*. The enhancement of the left paraspinal muscles and the anterior soft tissue swelling *(arrows)* are well seen.

Tuberculous spondylitis, or Pott's disease, can involve the vertebrae or disk, and the lower thoracic and upper lumbar vertebrae are affected 25% to 50% of the time. Brucellosis, in comparison, often involves the lower lumbar spine and maintains vertebral bodies intact with the disk spaces decreased, posterior elements not affected, and epidural and paraspinal spaces less affected than with TB. In disseminated coccidioidomycosis, the granulomatous infection of the southwestern United States, the spine can be involved 10% to 50% of the time with multiple foci throughout the vertebrae but with disk spaces preserved.[5]

Computed Tomography

Vertebral osteomyelitis can be evaluated with contrast enhanced CT, which will show end plate erosions, paravertebral masses, and hyperemic disk enhancement (Figure 19-7, *B*). If the soft tissue mass extends around most of the vertebral body, infection rather than tumor is likely.

Magnetic Resonance Imaging

MRI has proven to be the modality of choice to evaluate spine infection, as it shows vertebral infection with a sensitivity of 96% and specificity of 93%[2] and allows delineation of epidural and paraspinal abscesses.

> MRI with gadolinium is the modality of choice for evaluating possible spine infection.

In the spine, vertebral osteomyelitis is characterized by disk height loss, confluent low T1 signal in the vertebrae and disks with blurring of the end plate margins, and high T2 signal and enhancement within the vertebrae and usually within the disk (Figure 19-7, *C-E*). On T2-weighted imaging, normally the disk is high signal bisected by a thin dark line, or cleft, which is thought to be fibrous tissue and is seen normally by age 30. Changes within the disk with infection include obliteration or irregularity of this cleft.[9] Epidural abscesses are well-defined, usually T1 isointense, T2 hyperintense foci, but can show signal heterogeneity and partial or diffuse enhancement with gadolinium (Figure 19-7, *F-H*).

MRI can be more useful than radiography or nuclear scintigraphy in differentiating degenerative or neoplastic involvement from infectious involvement. Degenerative disks are distinct from the vertebral end plates on T1-weighted imaging and show low T2 signal, as opposed to high T2 signal in infection or neoplasm. Neoplasm does not show abnormality crossing the disk space on both the T1-weighted and T2-weighted imaging as occurs with active osteomyelitis that has progressed to disk involvement.

In tuberculous spondylitis, findings include disk space narrowing and destruction of the adjacent endplates, often with a paraspinal psoas abscess. Complications include most commonly spinal stenosis with paraplegia, but vertebral collapse with kyphosis and gibbus formation can also occur, with MRI being useful to evaluate any cord compromise.[4] When coccidioidomycosis involves the spine, it rarely involves the disk, can present with paraspinal soft tissue extension, and does not tend to cause the gibbus deformity seen with TB.[4]

Following treatment, MRI signal can remain abnormal for 6 weeks to 1 year. The long duration of healing change is likely related to fibrous scar tissue and new bone formation.[9]

Scintigraphy

Gallium scanning is useful for diagnosis of vertebral osteomyelitis[13] and can be more accurate than MRI in evaluating for isolated epidural abscess, as the signal can be obscured on MRI by the adjacent similar cerebrospinal fluid signal.[9] In the presence of antibiotics, gallium scans may return to normal, which can be an indicator of clinical response.

DIABETIC FOOT

Diabetic patients are prone to ulceration by the combination of angiopathy/ischemia and peripheral neuropathy. Ulceration can progress to infection and osteomyelitis more frequently in diabetic than in nondiabetic patients. Imaging can aid in early diagnosis of osteomyelitis, which can in turn decrease the likelihood of amputation.

Osteomyelitis occurs most frequently at sites of pressure—the first and fifth metatarsal heads, the phalanges, and the calcaneus—but can also involve the talus, distal fibula, and tibia. These are usually multiorganism infections including *S. aureus*, coagulase-negative *Staphylococcus, Streptococcus, Enterococcus*, gram-negative bacilli, and anaerobes.

Imaging Features

Radiographs

Degenerative or inflammatory arthritis and neuropathic joints can have a similar radiographic appearance. Radiographs are less sensitive but comparably specific compared with bone scan in identifying osteomyelitis in the diabetic foot. Changes of osteomyelitis may be atypical in the diabetic, as ischemia inhibits bone resorption, periosteal reaction, and new bone formation. The bony sclerosis, pathologic fractures, and subluxations seen with chronic infection can mimic the findings of neuroarthropathy. Differentiating osteomyelitis from alternate diagnoses such as sterile nonunion can be difficult, and judging the extent of involvement by osteomyelitis can be problematic. Radiographs are nonetheless a good starting point, being inexpensive and available and providing minimal ionizing radiation.

The earliest findings of infection on radiographs are soft tissue swelling obliterating tissue planes, focal osteoporosis, and medullary bone resorption. When present, osteoporosis and ill-defined erosions are suspicious for osteomyelitis, whereas with pure neuroarthropathy, bone density tends to be preserved or hypertrophic in the midfoot and hindfoot (but still atrophic in the forefoot).[14]

With contiguous spread, periosteal reaction is present (Figure 19-8, *A*) except in the toes, which show cortical resorption and adjacent soft tissue swelling. The differential diagnosis of periosteal reaction is trauma or chronic venous stasis.[8]

Magnetic Resonance Imaging

MRI has been reported to have the highest accuracy of imaging modalities for the evaluation of osteomyelitis in diabetic feet. A sensitivity of 82% and specificity of 80% in diabetic patients, compared with a sensitivity of 89% and specificity of 94% in nondiabetic patients, has been noted. Contiguous osteomyelitis is reported at 15% in patients with diabetic foot ulcers, with one third of these patients with advanced pedal osteomyelitis showing septic arthritis by MRI (Figure 19-8, *B*).[6]

MRI does allow differentiation of bone from soft tissue infection with marrow edema seen in cases of osteomyelitis; however, the presence of marrow edema (bright marrow signal T2-weighted and low signal on T1-weighted images) is nonspecific and can be found with fracture, tumor, osteonecrosis, and postsurgical changes. The utility of MRI to differentiate infection from reactive bone marrow is being continuously explored. Ledermann et al. evaluated contrast-enhanced MRI in 161 cases of suspected pedal osteomyelitis that went to surgery. These authors found almost all true osteomyelitis to be contiguous with ulcers, the first and fifth metatarsophalangeal joints at the areas of highest pressure to usually be affected, one fifth of cases to be in the hindfoot, and rare occurrence in the midfoot.[15]

> By MRI, neuroarthropathy generally results in low marrow signal on T1-weighted and T2-weighted imaging, whereas osteomyelitis demonstrates high signal on T2-weighted imaging.

Collins et al. sought to differentiate osteomyelitis from reactive bone marrow when they focused on the T1-weighted imaging characteristics of 80 patients with osteomyelitis by MRI who went to surgery. They suggest that osteomyelitis can be excluded if low marrow signal on T1-weighted images is not in a geographic, medullary distribution with a confluent pattern. T2 signal approaching fluid and cortical irregularity were both supportive of osteomyelitis. An ill-defined, reticulated pattern of low signal on T1-weighted images was strongly suggestive of reactive marrow regardless of the T2 and post-gadolinium signal.[16] Ledermann et al reviewed 110 contrast-enhanced MRI foot studies, the majority in diabetic patients, looking for areas of nonenhancement to determine the added value of contrast administration. Contrast helped to diagnose necrotic tissue, which showed a sharp area of nonenhancement, usually in diabetic patients because of their poor peripheral perfusion. This is important for treatment, as debridement of the necrotic area is necessary to avoid progression to gangrene.[17]

Osteomyelitis may therefore be more likely when MRI shows greater marrow signal abnormality and adjacent soft tissue ulcers beneath the weight-bearing metatarsal heads or calcaneus. Evaluation of the foot for osteomyelitis and neuropathic arthropathy is limited by inhomogeneous fat suppression, which may be improved by chemical shift MRI.

> MRI appearance of acute, rapidly progressive neuroarthropathy may be indistinguishable from osteomyelitis.[6]

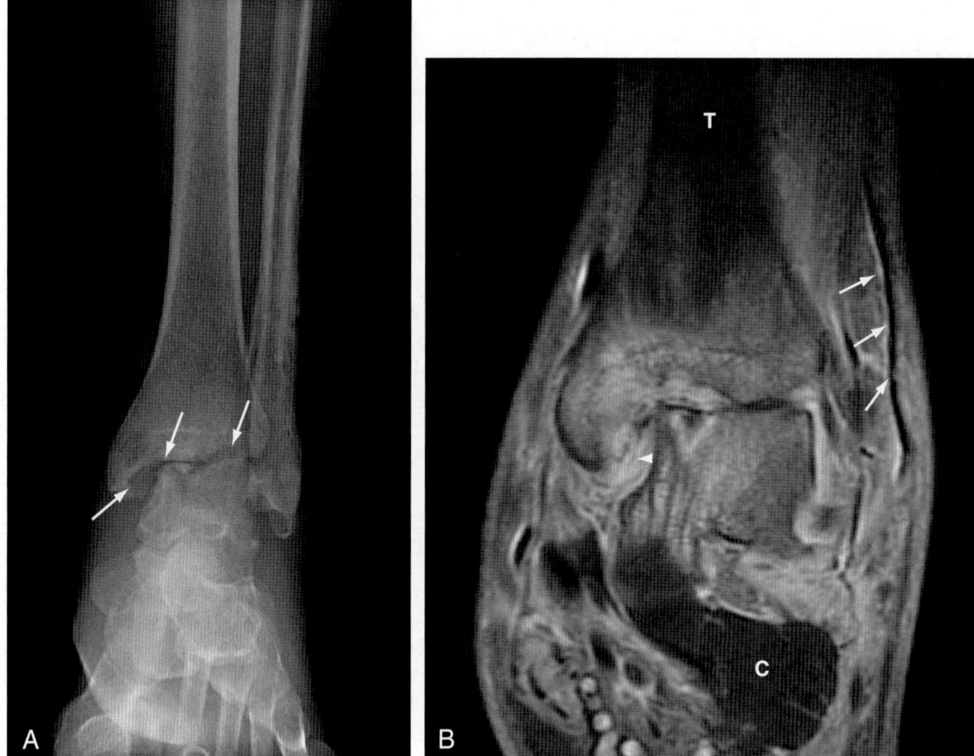

FIGURE 19-8. Tibial *Pseudomonas* osteomyelitis and ankle septic arthritis. This 71-year-old diabetic man had a recurrent lateral ankle soft tissue ulcer growing *Pseudomonas aeruginosa* and *Pseudomonas acinetobacter*. **A,** Anteroposterior radiograph demonstrates cortical irregularity and periosteal reaction in the distal fibular shaft and metaphysis, as well as bony erosions involving the distal tibia *(arrows)* and talus. The tibiotalar cartilage space is markedly narrowed. There is moderate soft tissue swelling. **B,** T1-weighted fat-suppressed MR image after intravenous gadolinium demonstrates bony enhancement in the distal tibia, fibula, and talus, with numerous osseous erosions *(arrowhead)* and bony destruction along the distal tibia and talar dome. For comparison, note the normal dark marrow of the unaffected calcaneus *(C)* and proximal tibia *(T)*. Contrast-enhanced fluid *(white)* and unenhanced fluid *(dark)* track superiorly within the fibular periosteum consistent with subperiosteal abscess *(arrows)*. Enhancing soft tissue edema surrounds the ankle.

Scintigraphy

In the diabetic foot, radiographs and bone scan have similar specificity for the diagnosis of osteomyelitis, but often bone scan in combination with In-111–labeled WBC imaging can differentiate osteomyelitis from soft tissue infection.[4,13] Accuracy of nuclear imaging in the foot is lower than elsewhere.

NONPYOGENIC OSTEOMYELITIS

The most common nonpyogenic infectious organisms seen involving bone are TB, syphilis, and fungal infections.[4]

TB Infection

Usually via hematogenous spread from the lung or genitourinary tract, skeletal TB is seen in 3% of patients with TB and accounts for 30% of extrapulmonary TB infections. Ten percent to 15% of cases involve osteomyelitis without arthritis. In children, osteoarticular TB most commonly affects the metaphyses of long bones, whereas in adults the joints are usually involved.

Imaging Features

TB may present with the typical changes of osteomyelitis, but with little or no reactive sclerosis or periosteal reaction. TB can cause fusiform enlargement of the diaphysis of a short tubular bone in the hand or foot (spina ventosa), destruction in the mid-diaphysis of such bones (tuberculous dactylitis), or multifocal lytic lesions of bones (cystic tuberculosis).[4]

Syphilitic Infection

The chronic systemic infection of congenital syphilis passed from mother to fetus can present as osteochondritis, periostitis, or osteitis. The tibia is the most common site of involvement, which is often symmetric and multifocal.

Imaging Features of Syphilitic Osteomyelitis

Congenital syphilitic lesions show the characteristic "Wimberger sign" of destruction of the metaphysis at the junction with the physis. The "saber shin" deformity is the appearance of chronic anterior tibial deformity. In the acquired form of the disease, syphilis can present as chronic osteitis or as syphilitic abscesses, known as *gummas*, that do not contain sequestra.[4]

Fungal Infections

The most common fungal infections of bone are coccidioidomycosis, blastomycosis, actinomycosis, and nocardiosis. These tend to involve bony prominences or the ribs or vertebrae. Bone infection can occur in 10% to 50% of patients with disseminated coccidioidomycosis.[4]

Imaging Features

These indolent fungal infections can resemble TB radiographically and tend to form an abscess and draining sinus. Coccidioidomycosis is characterized by punched-out, well-marginated lytic lesions involving the long and flat bones, as permeative bony destruction without significant periosteal reaction, or as monoarticular septic arthritis (indistinguishable from TB septic arthritis), almost always in conjunction with osteomyelitis. Coccidioidomycosis lesions appear bubbly, lytic, and expansile by CT and are T1 dark and T2 bright by MRI.[4]

PEDIATRIC OSTEOMYELITIS

Osteomyelitis occurs in boys more frequently than girls, equally in neonates. Spread in children and infants is usually hematogenous to the metaphyses of long bones. Involvement is most common at the knee, followed by the distal humerus and radius and proximal femur and humerus, metaphyseal equivalent sites of flat bones (at growth centers and periarticular sites along the pubic symphysis and sacroiliac joints), and spine.

> Apophyses are growth centers at bony prominences that do not contribute to the length of the bone. Areas deep to apophyses are metaphyseal equivalent areas and are subject to the same diseases as other metaphyses such as infection.

Although *S. aureus* remains the most common organism regardless of age, the appearance of hematogenous osteomyelitis varies with age based on differences in vascular distribution: in infants younger than 1 year, capillaries cross the growth plate, increasing the likelihood of epiphyseal involvement and a septic joint (Table 19-4). The periosteum is loosely attached, resulting in decompression of the medullary space via elevation of the periosteum. In childhood, from age 1 to physeal closure, the transphyseal arteries recede and the metaphyses and epiphyses have separate blood supplies. The avascular growth plate blocks spread of infection to the epiphysis and joint space unless, such as in the case of the elbow, shoulder, and hip joint, the metaphysis is intracapsular, increasing the susceptibility to a septic joint. Hematogenous infection otherwise tends to reside in the metaphysis or metaphyseal equivalent areas (i.e., femoral trochanters, calcaneal apophyses). The periosteum is again loosely attached, resulting in pus perforating through the cortex and elevating the periosteum with a greater frequency of subperiosteal abscess, as well as a tendency towards greater sequestrum formation due to the less adherent blood supply than adults. Multifocal osteomyelitis can be seen in 7% of children and 22% of neonates with osteomyelitis. The incidence of osteomyelitis is increased in patients with sickle cell disease. Pediatric osteomyelitis in sickle cell disease tends to occur in the diaphysis of the humerus, femur, and tibia rather than the metaphysis; occurs multifocally; and is associated with more severe sequelae.[2]

TABLE 19-4. Variations in Osteomyelitis by Age

Age or Comorbidity	Findings
< 1 year	Increased incidence of epiphyseal and joint involvement. Prominent periosteal elevation
> 1 to physeal closure	Metaphyses or metaphyseal equivalent areas involved. Only joints that are intraarticular are involved (shoulder, elbow, hip)
With sickle cell	Diaphyses, multifocal

Complications of limb osteomyelitis include septic joint in a reported 33% of cases, pathologic fracture, and growth disturbance. Osteochondroma has been reported following posttraumatic osteomyelitis involving the growth plate.[3]

Infectious organisms involved are most commonly *S. aureus*, which represents 80% to 90% of pediatric osteomyelitis, with group B beta-hemolytic streptococcus less commonly seen.[18] Neisseria meningitidis with septic emboli involving the growth plates is seen in Waterhouse-Friderichsen's syndrome. *S aureus*, group B streptococcus, and *Candida albicans* are associated with instrumentation. *S. aureus* and salmonella are most common in sickle cell patients. Chicken pox is classically complicated by osteomyelitis. Pseudomonas is associated with penetrating wounds, most often affecting the plantar calcaneus as opposed to hematogenous spread to the posterior calcaneus. Congenital syphilis involves the metaphysis in newborns. Immunization has drastically reduced *Haemophilus influenzae* as an offending organism. With chronic inactive osteomyelitis, usually no bacteria are found on biopsy.

Neonatal osteomyelitis is usually due to hematogenous spread but can be from a contiguous source or posttraumatic/postsurgical cause. It is described in babies less than 2 months old, often with a history of prematurity or line sepsis. The infection tends to involve the hips more frequently than the shoulder, knee, elbow, ankle, or small bones of the hand. Infection can often be multifocal and involve the adjacent joint.[2] External fixator devices are particularly at risk, given the presence of associated open skin wounds. Heel puncture technique can put infants at risk for calcaneal osteomyelitis.

Chronic recurrent multifocal osteomyelitis is seen most frequently in the age range of 19 months to 27 years and presents as multifocal metaphyseal lesions of the tibia, femur, clavicle, and spine that tend to occur symmetrically (Box 19-1).

The etiology is unclear and the condition may be viral or mycoplasmal. It may be part of the SAPHO syndrome (*s*ynovitis, *a*cne, *p*ustulosis, *h*yperostosis, and *o*steitis), which is characterized by osteocondensation and osteolysis. Multifocal osteomyelitis is a diagnosis of exclusion to be differentiated from pyogenic osteomyelitis and eosinophilic granuloma.

Sequelae, which are uncommon, include growth disturbance and kyphosis. Lesions become increasingly sclerotic, which is seen as a sign of healing, and can resolve in approximately 2 years.[2]

Imaging Features

To improve prognosis, multiple imaging techniques must be considered to aid in diagnosis and determination of the extent of infection.

Radiographs

Acute osteomyelitis

Radiographs are always the initial imaging modality of choice, and changes can be seen by 48 hours after onset of symptoms. In

BOX 19-1. Features of Multifocal Osteomyelitis

Children and young adults
May be associated with SAPHO syndrome
Multifocal metaphyseal lesions
Diagnosis of exclusion
Healing manifested by sclerosis

children, comparative images of the opposite side may be helpful to identify subtle abnormalities. Radiographic findings range from normal to soft tissue swelling early, with metaphyseal bone destruction and periosteal reaction beginning 10 to 15 days postinfection.

> Soft tissue swelling is an early finding of osteomyelitis; metaphyseal bone destruction and periosteal reaction occur 10 days to 2 weeks after onset.

Intraosseous infection expands to subperiosteal abscess and eventually soft tissue abscess. Early radiographs are predominantly useful to exclude alternate diagnoses. Differential diagnosis of acute osteomyelitis in children includes histiocytosis, leukemia, trauma, and Ewing's sarcoma.[3]

Subacute osteomyelitis

The differential diagnosis of Brodie's abscess in children includes osteoid osteoma, eosinophilic granuloma, tuberculosis, enchondroma, osteosarcoma, Ewing's sarcoma, and chondroblastoma. A serpentine sinus tract can often be seen extending to the growth plate, which helps to differentiate Brodie's abscess from osteoid osteoma.[3]

> A serpentine lucency in the metaphysis extending to the growth plate is a characteristic sign of osteomyelitis.

Chronic osteomyelitis

Chronic osteomyelitis shows mottled radiolucency and bony sclerosis/cortical thickening and a dense sequestrum, involucrum, or sinus tract formation when active. The differential diagnosis for chronic osteomyelitis in children includes bone neoplasms.

Chronic recurrent multifocal osteomyelitis

Radiographs show multifocal lytic or mixed lytic and sclerotic metaphyseal lesions with or without a sclerotic rim, sometimes with periosteal reaction, and usually without sequestrum formation.

Computed Tomography

With a lower sensitivity than MRI for the diagnosis of osteomyelitis, the specific utility of contrast-enhanced CT is to identify cortical erosion, small foreign bodies, periosteal reaction, and intraosseous gas, with contrast helping to identify soft tissue abscess by its rim enhancement. CT is particularly useful in surgical planning and identifying sequestra, involucra, and cloaca. CT can help to differentiate sequestra from calcified osteoid osteoma nidus, as the inner surface of the radiolucent nidus is said to be smooth with osteoid osteoma and irregular with osteomyelitis. The calcified nidus in osteoid osteoma is said to be located centrally but is eccentric in sequestra. CT is helpful for characterization of cortical osteitis, seen as an oblong radiolucent area and periosteal reaction, with differential diagnosis including osteoid osteoma, stress fracture, chronic tendinosis, and cortical bone metastases.[3] CT evaluation is limited in the setting of metallic prostheses due to beam-hardening artifact. It is a useful modality to guide biopsy for tissue diagnosis.

Magnetic Resonance Imaging

Children pose a unique difficulty in differentiating normal hematopoietic marrow from marrow edema, pus, and inflammatory cells, which generally show higher signal on T2-weighted and STIR sequences. MRI can distinguish between acute osteomyelitis, which shows diffuse changes with a wide zone of transition between the infected area and the normal bone and poor soft tissue plane demarcation, and chronic osteomyelitis, which shows a more narrow zone of transition in the bone and cortical thickening, with infarcted fibrotic areas of marrow sequestration that show low T1 and T2 signal and do not enhance (Box 19-2). Gadolinium aids in identifying active bone and soft tissue inflammation without necrosis by enhancement, with abscess showing nonenhancement centrally but enhancement peripherally.[2,18] Sinus tracts appear as linear or curvilinear T2 bright signal that may or may not be enhancing. MRI is particularly useful for detailing bony and soft tissue changes in the spine, pelvis, and appendicular skeleton; for surgical planning; or for cases that extend into the physis or show poor response to treatment.

> MRI usually requires sedation in children younger than 6 years.

Although periosteal reaction and erosions can mimic neoplasms, MRI can be useful to differentiate acute osteomyelitis from eosinophilic granuloma (EG) or Ewing's sarcoma. Acute osteomyelitis shows soft tissue swelling and obliteration of the fascial planes, whereas with EG or Ewing's sarcoma, a soft tissue mass that preserves fascial planes is seen.[4] In differentiating chronic recurrent multifocal osteomyelitis from pyogenic osteomyelitis, MRI can demonstrate findings supportive of the latter, such as abscess, sequestra, or sinus tracts.

Scintigraphy

Three-phase bone scan is most commonly used initially to diagnose uncomplicated acute or subacute osteomyelitis in children, with the main utility being its ability to identify multiple sites of infection, as is common in children. It is the modality of choice prior to MRI in children, as it usually does not require sedation and can evaluate the whole body simultaneously when it is difficult to localize symptoms. Normal physeal cartilage activity in children can pose a pitfall in diagnosis. Combined bone marrow or bone scan imaging and gallium scanning can be used to differentiate osteomyelitis from bone infarct in sickle cell patients.[8]

Ultrasound

Ultrasound is particularly useful in children, following radiographs and scintigraphy, as it is quick to perform, easily available, well tolerated and lacks ionizing radiation. However, it does allow for only a narrow anatomic field of examination at any given time. Ultrasound changes can be seen as early as 1 to 2 days following symptom onset.[19]

BOX 19-2. MRI Features of Osteomyelitis in Children

Acute osteomyelitis
- Gradual transition from lesion to marrow
- Soft tissue planes obliterated by edema
- Marrow enhancement

Chronic osteomyelitis
- Well-demarcated marrow lesion
- Cortical thickening
- Nonenhancing, low signal (on T1-weighted and T2-weighted images), infarcted marrow
- Abscesses and sinus tracts

The sonographic features of osteomyelitis include soft tissue swelling that is maximal near the bone, the "sandwich sign" of periosteal thickening with hypoechoic areas deep and superficial to it, and a hypoechoic or anechoic zone elevating periosteum by greater than 2 mm.[3]

A subperiosteal abscess is the most important finding that can be seen by ultrasound, as this confirms the clinical diagnosis of osteomyelitis. This can be used to help differentiate infarct from osteomyelitis in sickle cell disease.[3] Later in osteomyelitis, ultrasound can identify cortical bony defects. Ultrasound is a useful technique for guiding aspiration or drainage for pathologic confirmation and then for following response to therapy.

PEDIATRIC SPINAL INFECTION

> In children as opposed to adults, infection can involve the disk alone.

In addition to vessels in the connective tissue surrounding the disk annulus, children have vascular anastomoses between the vertebral endplate and the disk annulus as well as to the metaphysis through vessels along the periphery of the disk, allowing infection to cross from the metaphysis of one vertebral body across the disk space to the next vertebral body (Box 19-3). Discitis most commonly occurs in children aged 6 months to 4 years and 10 to 14 years. Girls are affected twice as often as boys, and usually the lumbar spine is involved. Whether discitis is an infectious or inflammatory process is controversial. Although *S. aureus* is again the most common etiologic organism, cultures are positive only 50% to 60% of the time.[1] Spinal infections can also include mycobacterial and brucella spondylodiscitis.[19a]

Imaging Features

Radiographs

Early paravertebral soft tissue swelling can be seen, followed by disk space narrowing after 1 week to 10 days. Erosion and destruction of vertebral end plates and new bone formation occur after several weeks of infection. Vertebral height loss typically involving the anterior portion of the vertebrae and paraspinal abscess are seen later in the course of infection.

Computed Tomography

CT demonstrates end plate erosion, paravertebral masses, and an enhancing disk.

> As in adults, contrast is necessary when scanning for possible vertebral osteomyelitis or discitis.

Magnetic Resonance Imaging

Fluid signal within the disk is normally higher in children than adults, decreasing the sensitivity for increased T2 signal changes seen with diskitis.[9] In chronic recurrent multifocal osteomyelitis, involvement of the intervertebral disk space is uncommon. TB can show large paraspinal and intraspinal abscesses that may track the length of the psoas muscle. Vertebral destruction and epidural abscess can cause cord compression. Following treatment, disk space narrowing remains and can lead to vertebral fusion.[2]

BOX 19-3. Discitis in Children

- Disk may be affected without bone involvement due to disk vascularity
- 6 months-4 years and 10-14 years old affected
- Girls twice as often as boys
- *S. aureus* most common but cultures may be negative

Scintigraphy

Bone scan shows increased uptake in the disk and adjacent vertebrae on all three phases with high specificity; sensitivity is improved with the addition of gallium scanning.[2]

SEPTIC ARTHRITIS

When infection involves the joint, including synovium and articular cartilage, it is termed *septic arthritis.* Septic arthritis comprises about 23% of musculoskeletal infections.[20-23] Infection can spread to the joint by three routes: (1) hematogenous, (2) contiguous, or (3) direct implantation. In adults, spread is most commonly via hematogenous seeding of the synovium from bacteremia or contiguous spread from adjacent bone or soft tissue. Alternatively, direct inoculation can occur in any joint during procedures or penetrating trauma.[20,24-26] In children, when metaphyses are intraarticular, such as in the hip, osteomyelitis can spread contiguously to produce septic arthritis. In children, more than 90% of cases are monoarticular, usually involving the hip, knee, shoulder, elbow, or ankle.[4]

Pyogenic septic arthritis can be classified as gonococcal or nongonococcal. Nongonococcal infection is usually acute, the offending organism most commonly *S. aureus*[21,23,25,27,28] less frequently group A streptococcus or *S. pneumoniae.* Group B streptococcus can be seen in neonates. Septic arthritis constitutes a medical emergency because pus in the joint can increase pressure to the point of epiphyseal ischemia.

> Septic arthritis is a medical emergency.

After 24 to 48 hours, if left untreated, permanent loss of joint function has been seen in 10% to 73% of patients.[1] Long-term sequelae of undiagnosed and untreated septic arthritis include dislocation, femoral head destruction, degenerative arthritis, and growth deformity. A mortality rate of 5% to 20% occurs from the associated transient or chronic bacteremia associated with seeding the joint.[2]

Neisseria gonorrhoeae can be seen in sexually active adolescents. Gonococcal arthritis follows a much more indolent course than pyogenic infection with a low morbidity and good prognosis. Chronic infections usually from mycobacteria or fungi also follow a chronic indolent course.[1]

Sterile/reactive arthritis can occur as an inflammatory reaction to distant infection and can be seen preceding hepatitis or postgastrointestinal infections with salmonella or *Shigella.*[1] Other organisms are seen, particularly in patients at risk for hematogenous spread to unusual locations by IV drug use, such as *Pseudomonas aeruginosa, Enterobacter cloacae, Klebsiella pneumoniae, C. albicans,* and *Serratia marcescens.*[2]

Imaging Features

Conventional Radiographs

Radiographs show juxtaarticular osteoporosis, peripheral erosions, sclerotic reaction, and joint space narrowing with cortical destruction as well as joint effusion and soft tissue swelling. Indistinctness of the cortex is consistent with nonspecific inflammation secondary to infection, synovitis, or chondrolysis. Early signs of septic arthritis are swelling of soft tissues and signs of joint effusion such as fat pad displacement and joint space widening. Later signs are diffuse joint space narrowing from cartilage destruction, changes of osteomyelitis (Figure 19-9, *A*), osteoarthritis, joint fusion, periarticular calcifications, or subchondral bone loss with ensuing reactive sclerosis. Sensitivity of 73% and specificity of 79% for joint effusion have been reported for radiographs.[2]

> When there is a question of septic arthritis, radiographs are useful in excluding other diagnoses or documenting signs of osteomyelitis or effusion. Joint aspiration is mandatory.

Computed Tomography

CT can demonstrate large joint effusions, soft tissue swelling, and periarticular abscess and offer supportive evidence for septic arthritis, by detecting adjacent osteomyelitis (Figure 19-9, *B*). CT offers good cortical bony detail but may not be helpful in early septic arthritis when changes may not be evident. CT can also be useful for guiding bone biopsy and aspiration or selecting an appropriate surgical approach.

Magnetic Resonance Imaging

MRI is recommended in diagnosing septic arthritis,[1] as gadolinium-enhanced MRI with fat suppression has been reported to offer excellent sensitivity (up to 100%) for detection of septic arthritis with joint effusion and enhancing hypertrophic synovium, with specificity of 77%.[2]

Transient synovitis can produce similar MRI and radiographic findings. Differentiating septic arthritis from transient synovitis has been attempted by MRI, with additional findings indicating septic arthritis such as increased signal in the juxtaarticular bone marrow on T2-weighted images (Figure 19-9, *C*) and gadolinium-enhanced T1-weighted imaging (Figure 19-9, *D*).[2,20,24-26,29]

High T2 signal within the joint capsule is consistent with a joint effusion but cannot alone determine whether this fluid is infected. Graif et al. evaluated the gadolinium-enhanced MRI of 30 patients suspected of having septic arthritis to determine among five groups of MRI signs those most useful in differentiating septic from nonseptic joints. They found a great deal of overlap, but bone erosions, particularly in the presence of marrow edema on either side of the joint, were found to be a significant indicator highly suggestive of septic arthritis. Additional supportive evidence for septic arthritis included synovial thickening, synovial edema, soft tissue edema, and bone marrow enhancement. They found that lack of joint effusion could not be used to exclude septic arthritis or negate the need for aspiration, and the signal characteristics of joint fluid did not necessarily indicate presence of infection.[30]

> Joint effusions of infected or noninfected joints appear identical on MRI. The absence of joint effusion does not indicate the absence of septic arthritis.

Intraarticular effusion and articular cartilage destruction with loss of intermediate signal intensity can be seen with or without subchondral bone destruction. Percutaneous aspiration or image-guided biopsy confirms the diagnosis and obtains an organism for treatment.

Ultrasound

Ultrasound is appealing as it is devoid of known risks, is relatively inexpensive, allows real-time imaging, and enables aspiration and drainage for pathologic diagnosis and treatment of collections as small as 1 to 2 mL. The characteristic septic effusion is non–echo-free. Echo-free effusions may be more suggestive of transient synovitis or fresh hemorrhagic effusion than infection, but this should be determined by aspiration.[2]

Arthrography

Arthrography (imaging of a joint following injection of radiopaque contrast) confirms intraarticular needle placement for joint aspiration and defines fistulae. In patients with prostheses, arthrography can demonstrate loosening of the prosthesis and abscess formation as well as provide fluid for culture.

SOFT TISSUE INFECTIONS

Soft tissue infection is most commonly due to direct introduction of organisms and is often a complication of diabetes. Imaging can help to differentiate superficial cellulitis (usually secondary to gram-positive cocci) from soft tissue abscess, pyomyositis, or necrotizing fasciitis.

Cellulitis

Cellulitis is an infectious process affecting the skin and subcutaneous tissue.[20,24,31-33] The causative agent is usually gram-positive cocci that are part of the skin flora. The diagnosis of cellulitis is clinical but diagnostic imaging helps in defining the extent of the infection. CT and MRI have been used in differentiating superficial cellulitis and cellulitis associated with deep soft tissue infection.[20,24,25,34]

Imaging Features

Conventional radiographs

Radiography offers limited resolution of fascial layers and, therefore, although it shows soft tissue swelling, it is of limited value. Gas caused by gas-forming organisms can be easily recognized on radiographs and usually indicates gangrene caused by anaerobes.

Gas in the soft tissues can be a sign of infection but can also be seen in diabetic patients as a consequence of skin ulceration even when no infection is present.

Computed tomography

In superficial cellulitis, CT and MRI reveal enhancement and inflammatory changes involving the subcutaneous fat, but no extension beyond the superficial fascia is seen. Other abnormal findings include skin thickening, septation of subcutaneous fat and thickening of the superficial fascia, loss of distinction of tissue planes, and heterogeneous enhancement, all confined to the subcutaneous tissues, with sparing of the fascial planes and muscles. CT demonstrates inflammation and edema as areas of increased density with increased attenuation in the range of 90 to 120 HU.[20,34]

Magnetic resonance imaging

MRI is more sensitive and shows subcutaneous infection as areas of ill-defined, mildly enhancing decreased signal on T1-weighted images and striated bright signal on T2-weighted images[20,24,35,36] interspersed within subcutaneous fat without focal fluid collections.

Ultrasound

Ultrasound shows subcutaneous tissue with increased echogenicity, thickening, and loss of distinction of tissue planes with hypoechoic fluid between fat lobules.

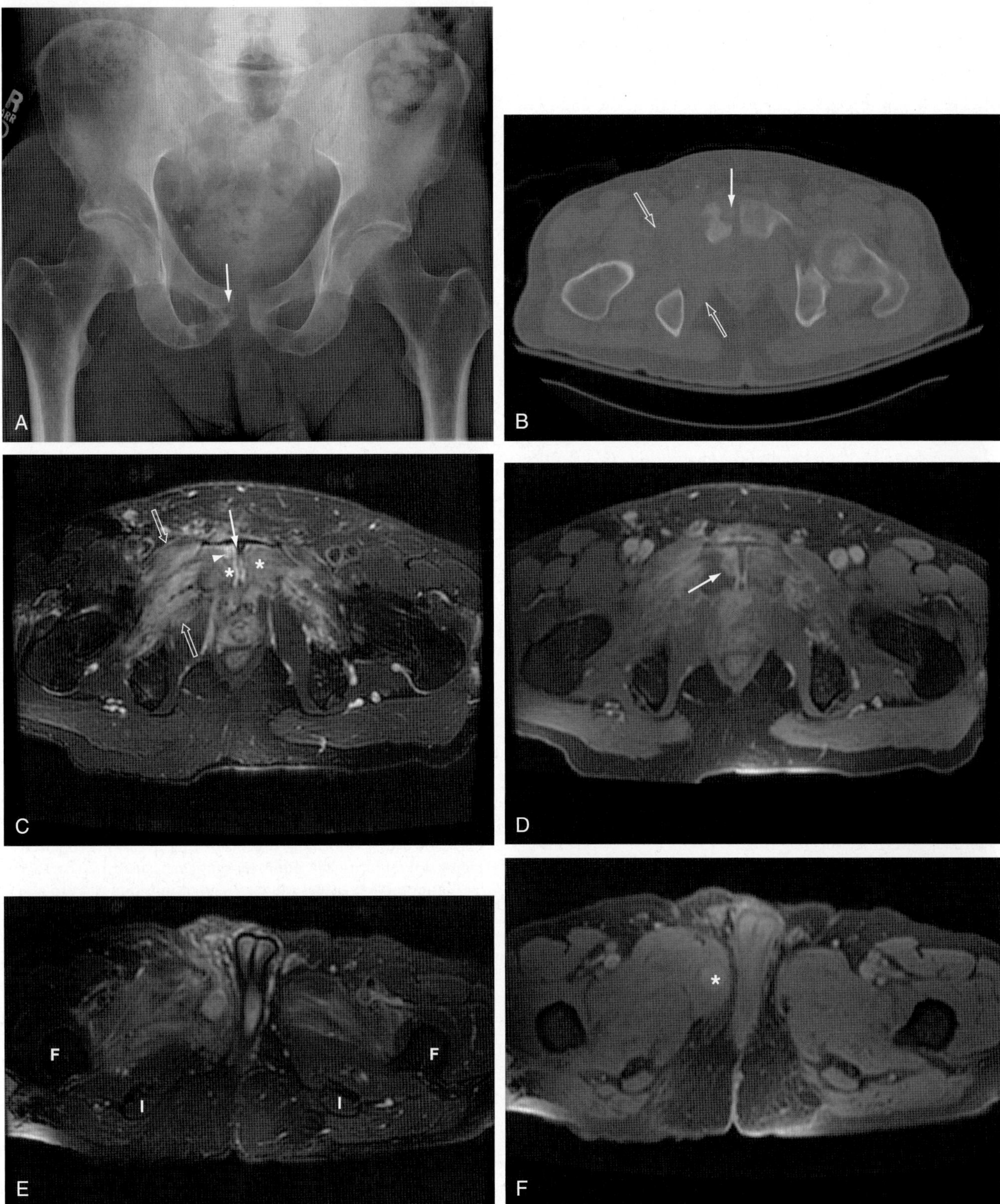

FIGURE 19-9. *S. aureus* osteomyelitis and septic arthritis of the pubic symphysis, and soft tissue abscess. This 49-year-old diabetic man developed osteomyelitis following spontaneous pubic ramus fracture. **A,** Anteroposterior radiograph demonstrates erosion and destruction *(arrow)* of the pubic symphysis and right pubic bone, consistent with osteomyelitis and septic arthritis. **B,** CT scan demonstrates lysis of the right *(arrow)* greater than the left pubic bone adjacent to a widened pubic symphysis. There is surrounding soft tissue swelling with obliteration of the intermuscular fat planes, particularly on the right *(open arrows)*. Note that the CT image better demonstrates bone contours in comparison to the MR image or radiograph. The bones are better seen than the soft tissues on this image displayed with "bone windows." **C,** Fast spin echo (FSE) fat-suppressed T2-weighted MR image demonstrates T2 bright edema signal in the pubic bones *(asterisks)* abutting the pubic symphysis, with fluid in the pubic symphysis *(arrow)*. A focal erosion in the right pubis contains fluid signal *(arrowhead)*. Normal bone marrow is low signal *(black)* on this sequence. Normal muscles are gray (intermediate signal) but the muscles in the area of infection are white (bright) *(open arrows)*, indicating fluid (edema with or without infection). **D,** Fat-suppressed T1-weighted MR image post gadolinium demonstrates corresponding area of enhancement in the right pubic bone abutting the pubic symphysis *(arrow)*, with peripheral enhancement of fluid in the pubic symphysis shown to represent osteomyelitis/septic arthritis pathologically. **E,** MRI demonstrates well-defined T2 bright fluid signal in the right adductor longus muscle. *F,* Femur; *I,* ischium. **F,** Fat-suppressed T1-weighted MR image post gadolinium demonstrates corresponding area of enhancement consistent with right adductor longus muscle soft tissue abscess *(asterisk)*.

Soft Tissue Abscesses

Bacterial infection in soft tissues develops into abscess in immunologically compromised patients.

Imaging Features

Conventional radiographs

Radiographs show soft tissue swelling and may show gas collections.

Computed tomography

CT shows a somewhat high attenuation (greater than 20 HU) fluid collection that can contain air, surrounded by a thick enhancing rim after contrast (Figure 19-10, *A*).

Magnetic resonance imaging

Abscess is seen as a well-defined, thick, enhancing low T2 signal fibrous capsule surrounding a high T2, low T1 signal round or elongated loculated fluid collection (Figure 19-9, *E, F*).[25,26,29,37,38] Sinus tracts to the skin may be present (Figure 19-10, *B*). Necrotic debris may show central low T2 signal. Infected tenosynovitis appears identical to noninfected tenosynovitis with T1 dark, T2 bright fluid signal within tendon sheaths (Figure 19-11, *A-C*).[4]

Ultrasound

Ultrasound of an abscess shows a focal collection of mixed echogenicity surrounded by hyperechoic wall.

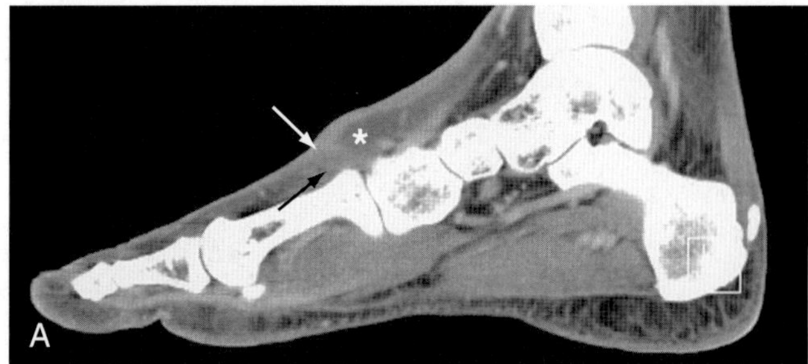

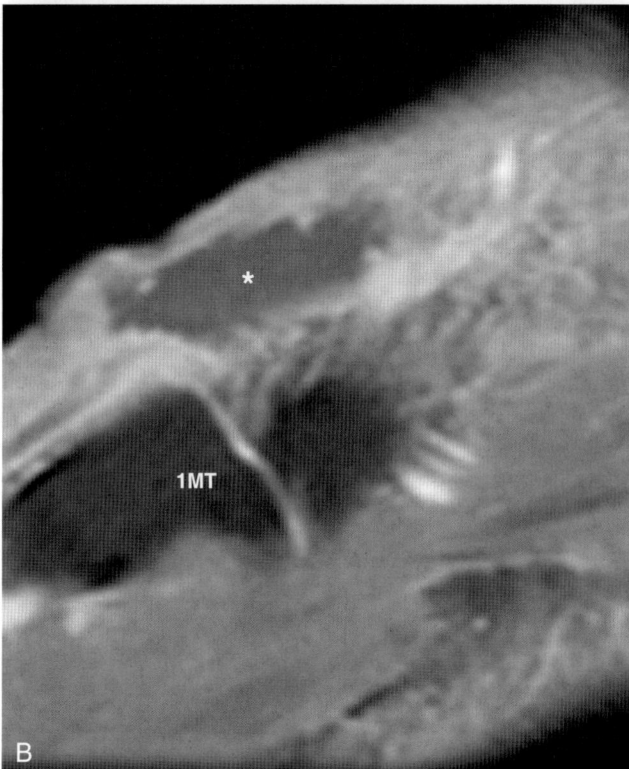

FIGURE 19-10. Abscess. 48-year-old man status post spider bite on the dorsum of the foot, with *S. aureus*–positive soft tissue abscess and sinus tract to the skin. **A,** CT after intravenous contrast demonstrates well-defined low attenuation collection *(asterisk)* in continuity with the skin surface. The wall of the abscess has enhanced after contrast administration *(arrows)*. **B,** Fat-suppressed T1-weighted gadolinium-enhanced MR image demonstrates peripherally enhancing low T1 signal collection *(asterisk)* in continuity with the skin surface at the site of the spider bite. The normal low signal base of the first metatarsal *(1MT)* and the adjacent bright joint are noted.

Necrotizing Fasciitis

Necrotizing fasciitis is caused commonly by trauma in immune-suppressed patients.[33,39,40] It is a rare entity with rapid progression. The hallmark of this disease is extensive skin necrosis with extension of infection along fascial planes. The condition can lead to septic shock, hypovolemia, and delirium. This is a surgical emergency, as the delay in diagnosis of necrosis represents one of the most important predictors of mortality.[24,33] Treatment within 4 days of onset lowers the mortality rate from 73% to 12%. Patients with necrotizing fasciitis should be followed for late development of necrosis.[24,33,35,40]

Imaging Features

> The detection of necrotizing fasciitis is an emergency.

Computed tomography

CT and MRI show the extent and depth of inflammation and any involvement of the osseous structures. CT shows gas and low attenuation along the fascial planes early on, with deeper fluid collections as the infection progresses.

Magnetic resonance imaging

MRI can differentiate severe cellulitis from fasciitis.[33,40] The defining characteristic is deep fascial involvement.

> Involvement of the deep fascia and muscle, differentiate necrotizing fasciitis from superficial cellulitis.

Although both entities can have similar imaging findings of fascial thickening with linear areas of T2 bright, T1 intermediate to low signal with variable enhancement along the superficial fascial planes, the imaging findings of necrotizing fasciitis include involvement of the deeper fascia and muscle.

Pyomyositis

Pyomyositis is a bacterial infection of striated muscle, considered to only occur in damaged muscle or in immunosuppressed patients, as in patients with prior trauma, diabetes mellitus, chronic steroid use, connective tissue disorders, malignancy, and malnutrition, as well as concurrent infection with human

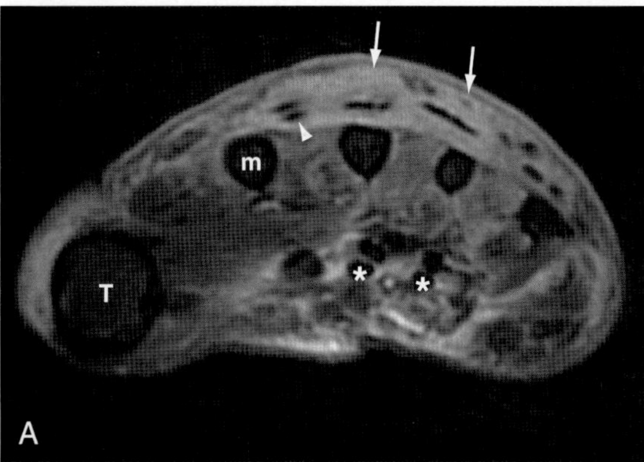

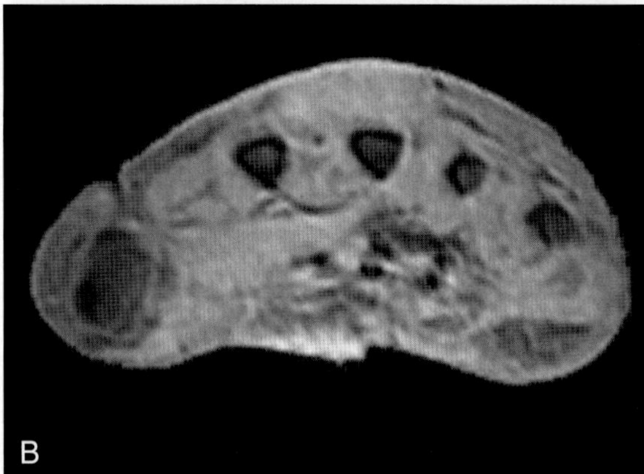

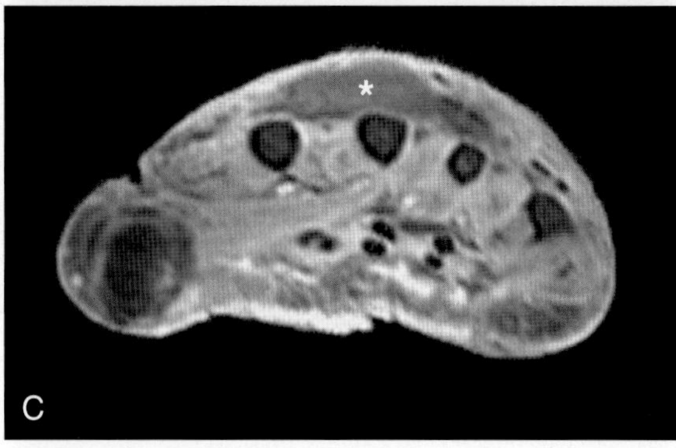

FIGURE 19-11. 67-year-old diabetic woman with *S. aureus* septic wrist extensor tenosynovitis following IV placement. **A,** T2-weighted MRI demonstrates T2 bright signal along the extensor tendons *(arrows)*. The normal dark tendons are easily seen (*arrowhead* on index tendon). The metacarpals are dark *(m)*. The low signal *(dark)* tendons in the carpal tunnel *(*)* are also seen. **B,** T1-weighted fat-suppressed image obtained before contrast injection (compare with **C**) shows nearly isointense signal (compared with muscle) of the affected area. **C,** T1-weighted fat-suppressed image after intravenous gadolinium. Peripheral enhancement involving the extensor tendon sheaths of the third, fourth, and, to a lesser extent, the second extensor tendons of the wrist. The central portion of the fluid collection *(asterisk)* does not enhance. MRI in this case documents the presence of fluid collections (tenosynovitis) but not specifically of infection.

immunodeficiency virus (HIV) or varicella. The most common bacterial cause of this soft tissue infection *is S. aureus.* Other less common organisms include *S. pyogenes, Mycobacterium tuberculosis, Mycobacterium avium-intracellulare, Nocardia asteroides, Cryptococcus neoformanes, Toxoplasmosis, Salmonella,* and *Microsporidia.** Pyomyositis is endemic to warm, humid environments and has been described as tropical myositis. The prevalence of this disease has been on the rise in the United States due to HIV epidemics.[21,29,37,42] The higher prevalence in HIV patients has been attributed to IV drug abuse, rhabdomyolysis, and repeated trauma.[24,41] Infection usually involves a single large muscle such as in the thigh, but the disorder can be multifocal up to 40% of the time. Three clinical stages have been described, from early to late findings with increasing degrees of toxicity. Imaging studies aid in the diagnosis and localization of pyomyositis.

Imaging Features

Conventional radiographs

Radiographs are usually negative except for focal pockets of gas in some cases.

Computed tomography

CT scan shows pyomyositis as a rim-enhancing low attenuation mass within enlarged heterogeneous muscle.[20,24,37,38] There is enhancement of thin septations when present. Involved muscle shows less enhancement than normal muscle. Secondary signs of soft tissue cellulitis are expected and support the diagnosis.

> CT of pyomyositis shows muscle enlargement and heterogeneity with a focal rim-enhancing mass.

Magnetic resonance imaging

MRI is the most sensitive modality, showing a lesion with a hyperintense central zone on T2-weighted images and rim-enhancement lesion with central isointense zone on T1-weighted post-gadolinium images.[25,29,37,38,43] Identification of this abscess can determine the need for surgical rather than antibiotic treatment alone. Additional areas of osteomyelitis and septic arthritis can be identified. Early on, diffuse muscle enlargement with heterogeneous T2 signal and slightly hyperintense T1 signal is seen.

Scintigraphy

Ga-67 and In-111 tagged WBCs are helpful to show occult foci of inflammation and localize multiple lesions, which occur in 20% to 40% of patients.[25,26,29,37]

Ultrasound

Ultrasound shows increased echogenicity in areas of inflammation, which decreases as the tissue liquefies,[25,29,38,41] showing a diffuse or focal hypoechoic collection within muscle.[2]

Septic Bursitis

Septic bursitis, as its name implies, is the infection of a bursa.[20,21] A bursa is an enclosed synovium-lined sac that contains fluid and usually develops at a site of friction. The most commonly involved bursae are the olecranon, prepatellar, and subdeltoid.[29,42] A history of prior local trauma is commonly present.[20,21] Patients with malnutrition, systemic disease, or treatment with corticosteroids are at risk. The most common organisms are *S. aureus* and *S. pyogenes.*[21,29]

*References 20, 24, 28, 29, 37, 41-43.

Imaging Features

Radiographs

Radiographs are usually negative but can show soft tissue swelling.

Magnetic Resonance Imaging

T2-weighted images show high signal fluid collection in the location of a bursa[26,29] (Figure 19-12, *A, B*).

HUMAN IMMUNODEFICIENCY VIRUS (HIV)

Patients with HIV present with infections and inflammatory and neoplastic processes. In this chapter, we will be dealing with the infectious complications affecting the musculoskeletal system. Infection is the most common complication in acquired immune deficiency syndrome (AIDS).[24] Infectious processes include soft tissue infections (cellulitis, necrotizing fasciitis, soft tissue abscess, pyomyositis), osteomyelitis, and septic arthritis. Many of these conditions are not specific for HIV infection but can be seen with other immunosuppressive disorders and have been described previously. Cellulitis and soft tissue abscesses seem to be prevalent in HIV patients secondary to decreased immune function.[20,24,25] Pyomyositis is a bacterial myositis that is one of the most common musculoskeletal complications of AIDS and is readily curable.[20,24] Those infections more specific to HIV are detailed below.

Bacillary Angiomatosis Osteomyelitis

Bacillary angiomatosis osteomyelitis is an infection unique to HIV-infected patients and, to a lesser degree, other immune-suppressed individuals.[20,26,44] It is caused by two species of the gram-negative rickettsia-like bacilli: *Bartonella henselae*, which causes cat scratch disease and *Bartonella quintana*, which causes trench fever.[20,37,45-47]

> Bacillary angiomatosis is an infection due to *Bartonella* species and is usually seen in HIV-infected patients.

In immunocompetent patients a self-limited granulomatous lymphadenitis is induced. In HIV patients, the bacterial infection results in vascular proliferation in various organs such as the skin, lymph nodes, central nervous system, bone, and liver.[26,29,48-50] Osteomyelitis due to this disease is found in up to one third of patients who have bacillary angiomatosis.[20,46,48] The long bones are often affected. These foci of osteomyelitis are manifested by extensive destruction of the cortical bone, periostitis, medullary invasion, and soft tissue masses that may resemble cellulitis.

Imaging Features

Radiographs

Radiographically, periosteal reaction, localized osteopenia, and deep soft tissue swelling are seen early in bacillary angiomatosis.

Magnetic Resonance Imaging

Three-phase bone scan and MRI can differentiate osteomyelitis from cellulitis.[20,26,42,51] CT and MRI show the extent of the disease. MRI shows a low signal mass on T1-weighted images that is high in signal on T2-weighted images. Due to its vascular nature, there is intense enhancement of the soft tissue lesion.[20,26,34]

MYCOBACTERIAL INFECTIONS

Mycobacterium TB is the most common infectious organism worldwide, affecting approximately 2 billion people. In the United States, 10 to 15 million patients are infected.[20,52] The rate of TB

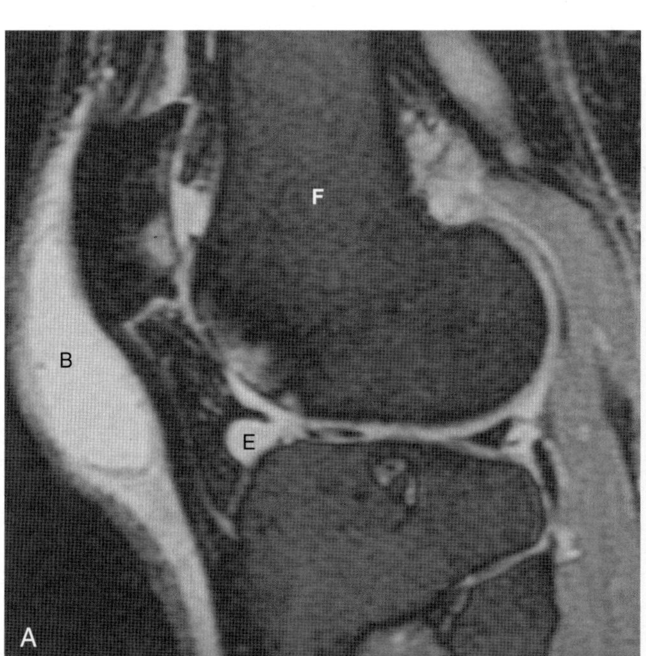

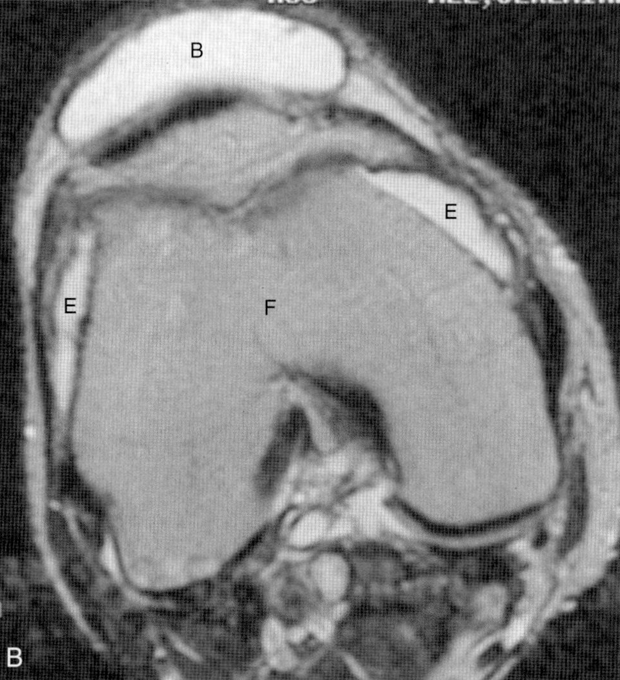

FIGURE 19-12. Prepatellar bursitis in a 62-year-old man with prepatellar swelling. **(A)** Sagittal STIR and **(B)** axial T2-weighted MR images demonstrate a joint effusion *(E)*. A prepatellar fluid collection *(B)* is consistent with prepatellar bursitis and edema extending inferiorly. The distended bursa may or may not be infected. *F*, Femur.

infection is on the rise due to several factors including the AIDS epidemic, a large number of immune-suppressed patients, the development of drug-resistant strains, and an aging population.[20,53] The incidence of TB in AIDS patients is 35 to 500 times the incidence in the general population.[20,34,38,51] Musculoskeletal TB is the fourth most common extrapulmonary presentation of TB. It is found in 1% to 5% of patients who have TB.[54-57] Fewer than 50% of patients with musculoskeletal TB have radiographic evidence of pulmonary TB.

> Because musculoskeletal TB is due to hematogenous spread, the presence of a normal chest radiograph does not exclude musculoskeletal TB.

Although the skeletal lesions of TB are solitary in immunocompetent individuals, the lesions may be multicentric in HIV patients in 30% of cases.[20,55,57,58]

Tuberculous Spondylitis

Infection of the vertebral column is the most common site of musculoskeletal TB involvement.[20,34,38,55,57] The most commonly affected vertebra is the first lumbar vertebra with decreasing frequency of occurrence as one moves cranially or caudally.[53] Spinal TB arises from hematogenous spread of the disease.[20,53,57] It affects more than one vertebral body, usually sparing the posterior vertebral bodies.[20,53] In untreated cases, the tuberculous spondylitis results in progressive inflammation and necrosis of the bone, resulting in vertebral collapse and gibbus deformity.*

> A gibbus deformity is a focal kyphosis that may result from bone destruction from TB infection.

Imaging Features

Conventional radiographs

Radiographically, TB of the spine manifests itself as loss of vertebral height, erosions, and paraspinal masses.[20,53,59]

> Erosion along the anterior aspect of multiple vertebral bodies may be due to tuberculous spondylitis. The differential diagnosis of this finding includes erosion from an aortic aneurysm or adenopathy such as can be caused by lymphoma.

Computed tomography

CT is helpful in the detection of early infection, the visualization of the extent of the disease and focal calcification of paraspinal abscesses, which are pathognomonic for TB.[20,28,57,59]

> Calcified paraspinal masses coupled with vertebral destruction are diagnostic of tuberculous spondylitis.

Magnetic resonance imaging

MRI is the best modality for evaluation of spinal tuberculosis. Vertebral body osteomyelitis and diskitis appear as low signal on T1-weighted images with heterogeneous increased signal on T2-weighted images.[57,60]

Scintigraphy

Increased radiotracer uptake is seen in early stages of spinal TB, but with increased necrosis, technetium, gallium, and indium scans are often negative.[58]

*References 20, 34, 37, 38, 53, 55, 57.

Tuberculous Osteomyelitis

Tuberculous osteomyelitis is related to hematogenous dissemination. It often arises from septic arthritis.[20,34] Any bone may be affected. In the long tubular bones, TB arises in one of the epiphyses and spreads to the adjacent joint. This feature differentiates TB osteomyelitis from pyogenic osteomyelitis, which starts in the metaphysis but generally cannot extend to the epiphysis in children.[53] Tuberculous dactylitis occurs frequently in young children. It is uncommon after age 5. This disease is multifocal in 25% to 35% of cases. It manifests as soft tissue swelling, periostitis, and cyst-like expansion of the bone known as *spina ventosa*.[20,34,53,59] Radiographically, tuberculous osteomyelitis presents as cortical destruction, juxtacortical abscess formation, and medullary destruction.[34,57]

Tuberculous Arthritis

Tuberculous arthritis is the second most common musculoskeletal TB infection.[20,54,55,61,62] Of the extrapulmonary forms of TB, septic arthritis accounts for 1%, seen most often in children and young adults. Risk factors include trauma, alcohol, drug use, intraarticular corriosteroids, and prolonged systemic illness. Spread to the joint is usually hematogenous or contiguous from an adjacent focus. It mostly involves large weight-bearing joints, including the hip and knee, with associated osteomyelitis.[20,34,53]

Imaging Features

Conventional radiographs

On radiography there is juxtaarticular osteoporosis, peripherally located osseous erosions, and gradual narrowing of the joint spaces. This radiographic appearance is known as the *Phemister triad*.[20,34,55] The appearance is similar to rheumatoid arthritis, but when involvement is monoarticular and erosions are poorly defined, the diagnosis of TB should be favored.

> Phemister[62a] incubated cartilage specimens in pus from a pyogenic abscess and in tuberculous pus. The cartilage dissolved quickly in the pyogenic abscess fluid but did not dissolve in the tuberculous fluid, thus showing cartilage loss occurs slowly in tuberculous arthritis. The classic triad of penarticular osteoporosis, marginal erosion, and relative preservation of cartilage spaces in tuberculous arthritis is named *Phemister's triad*.

Computed tomography

CT may help demonstrate kissing sequestra, which are wedge-shaped necrotic foci on either side of the joint. Later changes include extensive joint destruction with sclerosis of the adjacent bones.

Magnetic resonance imaging

MRI shows effusions, periarticular abscess, or synovial hypertrophy.[20,34,53,55]

RHEUMATOLOGIC DISORDERS OF AIDS

The differential diagnosis of infection includes HIV-associated arthritis. Reiter's syndrome is among the most common arthritis seen in patients with HIV.[63,64] The incidence of Reiter's disease is 100 to 200 times more frequent in AIDS patients than in uninfected patients.[51] Reiter's may be the initial presentation of the HIV infection, although it can occur at any stage.[20,65] The typical triad of arthritis, urethritis, and conjunctivitis is not usually seen.[20,43] Feet and ankles are most commonly involved.[25] Enthesopathy, flexor tendinitis, rotator cuff tendinitis, and lateral and medial epicondylitis may occur with this disease.[43] Other arthritides seen in HIV are psoriasis and HIV-associated arthritis.[20]

CANDIDAL SPINAL INFECTION

Although candidemia can be seen in immunocompromised patients, musculoskeletal candidal infection is rare, with candidal vertebral osteomyelitis in particular rarely reported. Hematogenous spread to the spine in adults begins with involvement at the end plates, where blood flow is slow, followed by disk involvement. In children, infection tends to begin in the disk. Patients present weeks to months after the candidemia seeds the spine.

Imaging Features

Radiographs

Radiographs show disk space narrowing with end plate irregularity, and progressive vertebral body destruction.

Computed Tomography

CT has shown end plate destruction, epidural abscess, and loculated low attenuation psoas collections with irregular enhancement, consistent with abscesses.

Magnetic Resonance Imaging

MRI has shown T1 dark, T2 bright disk signal in a narrowed disk space, as well as ring enhancing psoas abscesses, epidural abscesses, and prevertebral soft tissue abscesses. These are nonspecific findings seen in most forms of osteomyelitis.

MRI has notably shown T1 and T2 dark bone marrow, suggesting fibrosis that may reflect a more indolent process. At surgery, the prominent findings are inflammatory necrosing granulomata.[66]

Scintigraphy

Nuclear medicine can offer greater sensitivity earlier by gallium scanning, with In-111 labeled WBC scanning reportedly less sensitive.[66]

ASPERGILLUS SPINAL INFECTION

Fungal infections can be seen in immunocompromised patients, especially aspergillus in boys with chronic granulomatous disease and in patients with AIDS.

Imaging Features

Limited reports suggest CT and MRI appearance of disk spaces and end plates as well as epidural abscesses similar to candidal osteomyelitis. Psoas abscesses have not been specifically described in aspergillus vertebral osteomyelitis.[66]

LYME DISEASE

Lyme borreliosis is an inflammatory condition affecting multiple organ systems including the skin, cardiovascular system, nervous system, eyes, and joints.[67,68] Lyme disease is the most common vector-borne disorder in the United States.[68] It was first encountered in a town in Connecticut by the same name.[53] Geographically, this disorder is centered within the Northeast, upper Midwest, and far West.[53] This condition is not limited to the United States and is found in high numbers in Scandinavia, Germany, Austria, Slovenia, and Sweden.[69] This inflammatory disease is characterized by three stages.[67,69-72] In the first stage, erythema migrans occurs following a tick bite; this finding disappears over a period of weeks.[53,73] In the early dissemination stage, about 2 to 6 months later, the articular manifestations appear. These are characterized by a monoarticular, oligoarticular, or polyarticular process that occurs suddenly and is of short duration.[53,67] Arthralgia and myalgia are common presentations. This process is associated with recurrence and migration to other joints.[53] The most common sites of involvement are the knee, shoulder, and elbow. In stage three, among untreated patients in the United States, approximately two thirds develop intermittent attacks of joint swelling and pain.[67,73] Synovial tissues reveal hypertrophy, vascular proliferation, and infiltration by inflammatory cells. Following a few attacks of arthritis, 10% of patients develop persistent joint inflammation.[74,75]

Imaging Features

Early imaging features include soft tissue swelling and effusion. In untreated cases, a chronic oligoarthritis can develop, which is characterized by juxtaarticular osteoporosis, cartilage loss, and marginal erosions, with evidence of synovitis (Figure 19-13). These findings can also be seen with chronic juvenile arthritis, Reiter's syndrome, and granulomatous infections such as TB.[53]

IMAGING ALGORITHM FOR INFECTION

The following imaging algorithm may be considered following clinical suspicion of infection:

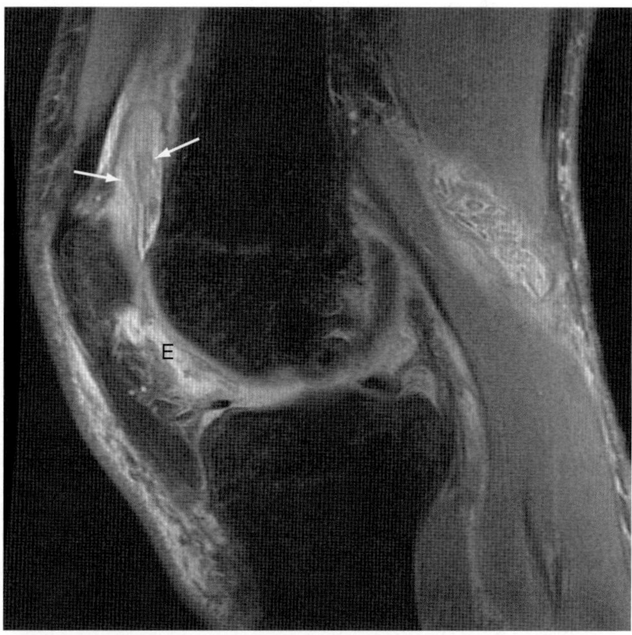

FIGURE 19-13. 51-year-old man with Lyme disease. STIR MRI sequence demonstrates a moderate amount of high signal joint effusion *(E)* and severe synovitis (intermediate signal, *arrows*), consistent with the clinical history of Lyme disease.

Radiographs are always a useful first mode of imaging for identifying radiographic signs of infection and for excluding alternate diagnoses. If positive, Sammak et al. suggest that treatment can then be directly initiated.[19] In the case of diabetic foot, Gold et al. recommend that treatment be instituted if bony changes are identified contiguous with an ulcer, but if osteolysis is seen in the absence of an ulcer, changes should be considered more likely due to neuroarthropathy.[14]

If radiographs are negative, three-phase bone scan is then recommended. If positive with nonviolated bone, Sammak et al. suggest treatment can then be initiated. If positive with violated bone, In-111 or Tc-99m labeled WBC scanning is then recommended to increase the specificity prior to treatment. In-111 WBC imaging is recommended to exclude osteomyelitis in the setting of neuroarthropathy, as it is usually negative with uncomplicated neuroarthropathy.[2] MRI or ultrasound can then be instituted in the absence of response to treatment or as an alternative to scintigraphy (radionuclide imaging being less expensive but MRI being more sensitive with higher spatial resolution).[2] Nuclear scintigraphy is useful for its high sensitivity and for identifying multiple foci of involvement, especially in neonatal osteomyelitis and chronic recurrent multifocal osteomyelitis (CRMO). MRI is useful for its high sensitivity and high spatial resolution in evaluating bones and soft tissues and is most valuable for determining the extent of local chronic infection, evaluating vertebral osteomyelitis, and guiding surgical planning.[2] Ultrasound is useful to show fluid collections in the joints, subperiosteum, and soft tissues and in guiding aspiration. CT is useful to detect gas in the soft tissues. Percutaneous bone biopsy, with care taken to avoid traversing infected ulcers and infecting uninvolved bone, is recommended for diagnostic confirmation and to identify the organism for treatment.

REFERENCES

1. Shirtliff ME, Mader JT: Imaging in osteomyelitis and septic arthritis, *Curr Treat Opt Infect Dis* 5:323-335, 2003.
2. Kothari NA, Pelchovitz DJ, Meyer JS: Imaging of musculoskeletal infections, *Radiol Clin North Am* 39:653-671, 2001.
3. Oudjhane K, Azouz EM: Imaging of osteomyelitis in children, *Radiol Clin North Am* 39:251-266, 2001.
4. Greenspan A: *Orthopedic radiology: a practical approach*, Philadelphia, 2000, Lippincott, Williams and Wilkins, pp 739-774.
5. Tehranzadeh J, Wang F, Mesgarzadeh M: Magnetic resonance imaging of osteomyelitis, *Crit Rev Diag Imaging* 33:495-534, 1992.
6. Restrepo CS, Gimenez CR, McCarthy K: Imaging of osteomyelitis and musculoskeletal soft tissue infections: current concepts, *Rheum Dis Clin North Am* 29:89-109, 2003.
7. Tumeh SS, Aliabadi P, Seltzer SE et al: Chronic osteomyelitis: the relative roles of scintigrams, plain radiographs and transmission computed tomography, *Clin Nucl Med* 13:710-715, 1988.
8. Tehranzadeh J, Wong E, Wang F et al: Imaging of osteomyelitis in the mature skeleton, *Radiol Clin North Am* 39:223-250, 2001.
9. Modic MT, Pflanze W, Feiglin DHI et al: Magnetic resonance imaging of musculoskeletal infections, *Radiol Clin North Am* 24:259-267, 1986.
10. Yang DC, Ratani RS, Mittal PK et al: Radionuclide three-phase whole-body bone imaging, *Clin Nucl Med* 27:419-426, 2002.
11. De Winter F, Vogelaers D, Gemmel F et al: Promising Role of 18-F-Fluoro-D-deoxyglucose positron emission tomography in clinical infectious diseases, *Eur J Clin Microbiol Infect Dis* 21:247-257, 2002.
12. Stumpe KDM, Dazzi H, Schaffner A et al: Infection imaging using whole-body FDG-PET, *Eur J Nucl Med* 27:822-832, 2000.
13. Turpin S, Lambert R: Role of scintigraphy in musculoskeletal and spinal infections, *Radiol Clin North Am* 39:169-189, 2001.
14. Gold RH, Tong DJF, Crim JR et al: Imaging the diabetic foot, *Skeletal Radiol* 24:563-571, 1995.
15. Ledermann HP, Schweitzer ME, Morrison WB: Nonenhancing tissue on MR imaging of pedal infection: characterization of necrotic tissue and associated limitations for diagnosis of osteomyelitis and abscess, *AJR Am J Roentgenol* 178:215-222, 2002.
16. Collins MS, Schaar MM, Wenger DE et al: T1-Weighted MRI characteristics of pedal osteomyelitis, *AJR Am J Roentgenol* 185:386-393, 2005.
17. Ledermann HP, Morrison WB, Schweitzer ME: MR image analysis of pedal osteomyelitis: distribution, patterns of spread, and frequency of associated ulceration and septic arthritis, *Radiology* 223:747-755, 2002.
18. Schmit P, Glorion C: Osteomyelitis in infants and children, *Eur Radiol* 14:L44-L54, 2004.
19. Sammak B, Abd El Bagi M, Al Shahed M et al: Osteomyelitis: a review of currently used imaging techniques, *Eur Radiol* 9:894-900, 1999.

19a. Bouaziz MC, Ladeb MF, Chakroun N, Chaabane S: Spinal brucellosis: a review, *Skeletal Radiol* 37:785-790, 2008.

20. Tehranzadeh J, Ter-Oganesyan RR, Steinbach LS: Musculoskeletal disorders associated with HIV infection and AIDS. Part I: infectious musculoskeletal conditions, *Skeletal Radiol* 33:249-259, 2004.
21. Vassilopoulos D, Chalasani P, Jurado RL et al: Musculoskeletal infections in patients with human immunodeficiency virus infection, *Medicine* 76:284-294, 1997.
22. Espinoza LR, Berman A: Soft tissues and osteo-articular infections in HIV-infected patients and other immunodeficient states, *Baillieres Best Practice Res Clin Rheumatol* 13:115-128, 1999.
23. Casado E, Olive A, Holgado S et al: Musculoskeletal manifestation in patients positive for immunodeficiency virus: correlation with CD4 count, *J Rheumatol* 28:802-804, 2001.
24. Restrepo CS, Lemos DF, Gordillo H et al: Imaging findings in musculoskeletal complications of AIDS, *Radiographics* 24:1029-1049, 2004.
25. Tehranzadeh J, OMalley P, Rafii M: The spectrum of osteoarticular and soft tissue changes in patients with human immunodeficiency virus (HIV) infection, *Crit Rev Diagn Imaging* 37:305-347, 1996.
26. Steinbach LS, Tehranzadeh J, Fleckenstein JL et al: Human immunodeficiency virus infection: musculoskeletal manifestations, *Radiology* 186:833-838, 1993.
27. Barzilai A, Varon D, Martinowitz U et al: Characteristics of septic arthritis in human immunodeficiency virus-infected haemophiliacs versus other risk groups, *Rheumatology* 38:139-142, 1999.
28. Tehranzadeh J, Mesgarzadeh M: Musculoskeletal infection in HIV-positive patients. In Tehranzadeh J, Steinbach LS (eds): *Musculoskeletal manifestation of AIDS*, St Louis, 1994, Warren H Green, pp 3-43.
29. Major N, Tehranzadeh J: Musculoskeletal manifestations of AIDS, *Radiol Clin North Am* 35:1167-1189, 1997.
30. Graif M, Schweitzer ME, Deely D et al: The septic versus nonseptic inflamed joint: MRI characteristics, *Skeletal Radiol* 28:616-620, 1999.
31. Lee DJ, Sartoris DJ: Musculoskeletal manifestation of human immunodeficiency virus infection: review of imaging characteristics, *Radiol Clin North Am* 32:399-411, 1994.
32. Revelon G, Rahmouni A, Jazaerli N et al: Acute swelling of the limbs: magnetic resonance pictorial review of fascial and muscle changes, *Eur J Radiol* 30:11-21, 1999.
33. Brothers TE, Tagge DU, Stutley JE et al: Magnetic resonance imaging differences between necrotizing and non-necrotizing fasciitis of the lower extremity, *J Am Coll Surg* 187:416-421, 1998.
34. Tehranzadeh J, Wong CH: Tuberculosis and other atypical mycobacterial infections in AIDS patients. In Tehranzadeh J, Steinbach LS (eds): *Musculoskeletal manifestation of AIDS*, St Louis, 1994, Warren H Green, pp 63-83.
35. Beltran J: MR imaging of soft tissue infection, *Magn Reson Imaging Clin North Am* 3:743-751, 1995.
36. Struk DW, Munk PL, Lee MJ et al: Imaging of soft tissue infections, *Radiol Clin North Am* 39:277-303, 2001.
37. Biviji AA, Paiement GD, Steinbach LS: Musculoskeletal manifestations of human immunodeficiency virus infection, *J Am Acad Orthop Surg* 10:312-320, 2002.
38. Bureau NJ, Cardinal E: Imaging of musculoskeletal and spinal infections, *Radiol Clin North Am* 39:343-355, 2001.
39. Schmid MR, Kossmann T, Duewell S: Differentiation of necrotizing fasciitis and cellulitis using MR imaging, *Am J Roentgenol* 170:615-620, 1998.
40. Loh NN, Ch'en IY, Cheung LP et al: Deep fascial hyperintensity in soft-tissue abnormalities as revealed by T2-weighted MR imaging, *AJR Am J Roentgenol* 168:1301-1304, 1997.
41. Wu CM, Davis F, Fishman EK: Musculoskeletal complications of the patient with acquired immunodeficiency syndrome (AIDS): CT evaluation, *Semin Ultrasound CT MR* 19:200-208, 1998.
42. Al-Tawfiq JA, Sarosi GA, Cushing HE: Pyomyositis in the acquired immunodeficiency syndrome, *South Med J* 93:330-333, 2000.
43. Plate AM, Boyle BA: Musculoskeletal manifestations of HIV infection, *AIDS Read* 13:62-72, 2003.
44. Husain S, Singh N: Pyomyositis associated with bacillary angiomatosis in patient with HIV infection, *Infection* 30:50-53, 2002.
45. Frean J, Arndt S, Spencer D: High rate of *Bartonella henselae* infection in HIV-positive outpatients in Johannesburg, South Africa, *Trans R Soc Trop Med Hyg* 96:549-550, 2002.
46. Baron AL, Steinbach LS, LeBoit PE: Osteolytic lesions and bacillary angiomatosis in HIV infection: radiologic differentiation from AIDS-related Kaposi sarcoma, *Radiology* 177:77-81, 1990.
47. Gazineo JL, Trope BM, Maceira JP et al: Bacillary angiomatosis: description of 13 cases reported in five reference centers for AIDS treatment in Rio de Janeiro, Brazil, *Rev Inst Med Trop Sao Paulo* 43:1-6, 2001.
48. Koehler JE: *Bartonella*-associated infections in HIV-infected patients, *AIDS Clin Care* 7:97-102, 1995.
49. Cortes EE, Saraceni V, Medeiros D et al: Bacillary angiomatosis and Kaposi's sarcoma in AIDS, *AIDS Patient Care STDS* 14:179-182, 2000.
50. Blanche P, Bachmeyer C, Salmon-Ceron D et al: Muscular bacillary angiomatosis in AIDS, *J Infect* 37:193, 1998.
51. Tehranzadeh J, Tran M: Musculoskeletal imaging in AIDS. In *Medical radiology-diagnostic imaging and radiation oncology. Radiology of AIDS. A practical approach*, Berlin 2001, Springer, pp 169-197.

52. Centers for Disease Control (CDC): *Reported tuberculosis in the United States, 2002.* Atlanta, 2003, US Department of Health and Human Services.
53. Resnick D, Kransdorf MJ (eds): *Bone and joint imaging,* ed 3, Philadelphia, 2005, Elsevier.
54. Soler R, Rodriguez E, Remuinan C et al: MRI of musculoskeletal extraspinal tuberculosis, *J Comput Assist Tomogr* 25:177-183, 2001.
55. Paradisi F, Gimpaolo C: Skeletal tuberculosis and other granulomatous infections, *Baillieres Clin Rheumatol* 13:163-177, 1999.
56. Pertuiset E, Beaudreuil J, Liote F et al: Spinal tuberculosis in adults. A study of 103 cases in developed country, 1980-1994, *Medicine* 78:309-320, 1999.
57. Griffith JF, Kumta SM, Leung PC et al: Imaging of musculoskeletal tuberculosis: a new look at an old disease, *Clin Orthop* 398:32-39, 2002.
58. Watts HG, Lifeso RM: Current concepts review: tuberculosis of bones and joints, *J Bone Joint Surg Am* 78:288-298, 1996.
59. Moore SL, Rafii M: Imaging of musculoskeletal and spinal tuberculosis, *Radiol Clin North Am* 39:329-342, 2001.
60. Arizono T, Oga M, Shiota E et al: Differentiation of vertebral osteomyelitis and tuberculous spondylitis by magnetic resonance imaging, *Int Orthop* 19:319-321, 1995.
61. Jellis JE: Human immunodeficiency virus and osteoarticular tuberculosis, *Clin Orthop* 398:27-31, 2002.
62. Shanley DJ: Tuberculosis of the spine: imaging features, *Am J Roentgenol* 164:659-664, 1995.
62a. Phemister DB: The effect of pressure on articular surfaces in pyogenic and tuberculous arthritides and its bearing on treatment, *Annals of Surgery* 80(4):481-500, 1924.
63. Winchester R, Brancato L, Itescu S et al: Implications from the occurrence of Reiters syndrome and related disorders in association with advanced HIV infection, *Scand J Rheumatol Suppl* 74:89-93, 1988.
64. Cuellar ML, Espinoza LR: Rheumatic manifestations of HIV-AIDS, *Baillieres Best Pract Res Clin Rheumatol* 14:579-593, 2000.
65. Cuellar ML: HIV infection-associated inflammatory musculoskeletal disorders, *Rheum Dis Clin North Am* 24:403-421, 1998.
66. Munk PL, Lee MJ, Poon PY et al: *Candida* osteomyelitis and disc space infection of the lumbar spine, *Skeletal Radiology* 26:42-46, 1997.
67. Singh SK, Girschick HJ: Lyme borreliosis: from infection to autoimmunity, *Clin Microbiol Infect* 10:598-614, 2004.
68. Orloski KA, Hayes EB, Campbell GL et al: Surveillance for Lyme disease: United States, 1992-1998, *MMWR CDC Surveill Summ 2000* 49:1-11, 2000.
69. Stanek G: Lyme disease and related disorders, *Microbiol Sci* 2:231-234, 1985.
70. Steere AC: Lyme disease, *N Engl J Med* 321:586-596, 1989.
71. Weber K, Pfister HW, Reimers CD: Clinical features of Lyme borreliosis: clinical overview. In Weber K, Burgdorfer W (eds): *Aspects of Lyme borreliosis,* Berlin, 1993, Springer, pp 93-104.
72. Hengge UR, Tannapfel A, Tyring SK et al: Lyme borreliosis, *Lancet Infect Dis* 3:489-500, 2003.
73. Strle F, Nadelman RB, Cimperman J et al: Comparison of culture-confirmed erythema migrans caused by *Borrelia burgdorferi sensu stricto* in New York State and by *Borrelia afzelii* in Slovenia, *Ann Intern Med* 130:32-36, 1999.
74. Steere AC, Duray PH, Butcher EC: Spirochetal antigens and lymphoid cell surface markers in Lyme synovitis. Comparison with rheumatoid synovium and tonsillar lymphoid tissue, *Arthritis Rheum* 31:487-495, 1988.
75. Steere AC, Schoen RT, Taylor E: The clinical evolution of Lyme arthritis, *Ann Intern Med* 107:725-731, 1987.

CHAPTER 20

Imaging of Rheumatoid Arthritis

John D. MacKenzie, MD, *and* David Karasick, MD, FACR

Key Facts

- Imaging findings in rheumatoid arthritis (RA) reflect the pathophysiology of the disease.
- Early radiographic findings include fusiform soft tissue swelling and juxtaarticular osteoporosis.
- Later radiographic findings include malalignment, uniform cartilage space narrowing, and bone erosions. Erosions begin near the joint margins ("bare areas") and usually show no repair. Ankylosis is a late finding.
- Cervical spine alignment abnormalities are common and characteristic features of RA and may cause spinal cord compression. The most frequent cervical spine malalignment is anterior subluxation of C1 on C2.
- Computed tomography (CT) is generally reserved for special circumstances, such as evaluation of the skull base and cervical spine, several of the extraskeletal manifestations of the disease, or when magnetic resonance imaging (MRI) is contraindicated.
- MRI and ultrasound are sensitive methods for detecting synovitis, tendon damage, and bone erosion. MRI and ultrasound demonstrate soft tissues better than radiographs or CT.

Rheumatoid arthritis (RA) is a systemic inflammatory disease of unknown etiology that predominantly affects the musculoskeletal system. Identification of the disease and evaluation of its activity are essential in the routine clinical management of patients with this disorder. Imaging plays an important role.

Different facets of RA may be identified and monitored depending on the selected imaging modality. Currently, radiographs, computed tomography (CT), scintigraphy, magnetic resonance imaging (MRI), and ultrasound are the imaging tools available for the clinician who treats patients with RA. Radiographs continue to be the mainstay; however, advanced imaging techniques improve early diagnosis and more accurately monitor therapy and disease progression.

The conventional monitoring of disease activity in RA is assessed with the combination of clinical examination (e.g., joint swelling, tenderness) and measurement of biochemical surrogate markers (e.g., serum C-reactive protein). The need for better strategies, such as imaging, for early detection and disease monitoring has become even more necessary with the current revolution in treatment options for RA. Early aggressive therapy with disease-modifying drugs is now recognized as critical in order to optimize long-term functional outcome and reduce morbidity.[1-3] With the need for early and aggressive therapy, imaging strategies are being developed and adopted that emphasize early diagnosis and accurate monitoring.

> Patients with polyarthritis, minimal physical exam findings, and normal radiographs are candidates for MRI for early diagnosis.

Given the array of imaging tools available, it is important to understand how each modality may help in the diagnosis and management of patients with RA.

An understanding of the way imaging may help in the management of extraarticular complications of RA is equally important. Imaging may also differentiate other conditions from RA. This chapter describes the current and emerging roles of imaging in the management of patients with RA. Suggestions on clinical use for each imaging modality are provided.

GENERAL IMAGING CONSIDERATIONS

Radiographic Findings

Imaging depicts joint derangement and mirrors the pathophysiology of RA. Imaging findings separate the disease into early, classical, and late stages. In the early stage, the nonspecific radiographic findings of periarticular edema, synovial joint distension (due to synovitis and joint effusion), and periarticular osteopenia may be seen. These early stage findings often result from inflammation in and adjacent to the thickened synovium that is infiltrated with inflammatory cells and granulation tissue (pannus).

> *Pannus* means "blanket" and refers to the invasive hyperplastic synovium that develops in RA.

Pannus is a hallmark of RA and contributes to cartilage loss and bone erosions.

As the disease progresses, classic findings include a combination of cartilage space narrowing, erosions, and additional soft tissue thickening in specific joint locations. This combination is characteristic of RA, although mixed connective tissue disease and overlap syndromes may occasionally produce similar findings.

Classic imaging findings represent precise pathologic changes in the joint. The joint space narrowing signifies cartilage loss.

> The term *cartilage space* rather than *joint space* is used in this text to emphasize that cartilage is responsible for most of the thickness of the space between bony articulations, although joint fluid and synovitis may also contribute to this "space."

Erosions are generally irreversible focal and irregular defects in cortical and trabecular bone. The late stages of joint derangement mark a progression of these processes from erosions and cartilage loss to ankylosis or joint subluxation/dislocation and generalized joint destruction. Usually, once the late stages of joint derangement have occurred, the diagnosis of RA is well known.

Other Imaging Modalities

Each imaging modality characterizes certain facets of the underlying joint derangement. This modality-dependent characterization depends on the stage of the disease and the joint structures and pathophysiology best characterized by the imaging technique. There are strengths and limitations to each modality. Although radiographs provide a rapid assessment of global and regional joint involvement by RA, ultrasound and MRI have advantages in characterizing soft tissue structures including synovitis and joint effusion. These are phenomena that tend to occur early in the disease and are not as well demonstrated on radiographs.

OSTEOARTICULAR IMAGING FEATURES (GENERAL AND SPECIFIC JOINTS)

Radiography

Radiography is the initial imaging modality of choice for the workup and monitoring of patients with RA. Radiography is the traditional gold standard for assessment of joint damage.[4,5] As part of the initial evaluation, radiographic findings may confirm the clinical suspicion of RA or may suggest other diagnostic possibilities. Characteristic radiographic findings are part of the American College of Rheumatology (ACR) classification criteria for RA (Box 20-1).[6]

The advantages of radiography include low cost, high availability, possibility of standardization and blinded centralized reading, validated assessment methods, and reasonable reproducibility.[7] Radiography may be used to characterize multiple joints rapidly, and experience with radiography for evaluating rheumatoid patients is well developed. Because of its exquisite resolution and depiction of bony structures, radiography is very good at detecting erosions. Bone demineralization (osteopenia/osteoporosis) may be seen on radiography but not ultrasound or MRI.

Radiographs are often sufficient to provide a global assessment of regional arthritis damage. However, their projectional nature limits three-dimensional (3D) visualization of bony structures and soft tissues. Other disadvantages of radiography include its relative insensitivity to early joint damage and limited assessment of soft tissue abnormalities.

Conventional radiography may help differentiate RA from other joint pathologic entities such as osteoarthritis (OA), psoriatic arthritis, and neoplasms.[5] Also, it may help identify a secondary process affecting the joint of patients with known RA, such as osteomyelitis, septic arthritis, pathologic or stress fractures, and amyloidosis.[8] As noted previously, the radiographic abnormalities of the appendicular joints may be separated into early, classic, and late findings.

BOX 20-1. Classification Tree Criteria for RA

1. Morning stiffness
2. Arthritis of three or more joint areas
3. Arthritis of hand joints (wrist and/or metacarpophalangeal joints)
4. Symmetric arthritis
5. Rheumatoid nodules
6. Serum rheumatoid factor
7. Radiographic erosions typical for RA

From Arnett FC, Edworthy SM, Bloch DA et al: The American Rheumatism Association 1987 revised criteria for the classification of rheumatoid arthritis, *Arthritis Rheum* 31:315-324, 1988.

A diagnosis of RA is established when at least 4 of the 7 criteria are satisfied. Criteria 1 through 4 must have been present for ≥ 6 weeks.

Early Radiographic Findings

The early radiographic findings are nonspecific periarticular soft tissue swelling with a fusiform configuration and periarticular osteopenia (Figure 20-1). Soft tissue swelling occurs from a combination of joint effusion, edema, synovial enlargement (pannus formation), and/or tenosynovitis. Osteopenia typically becomes more generalized as the disease progresses. Initially, the small joints may widen as a result of effusion; however, as cartilage becomes eroded, the cartilage spaces narrow.

Classic Radiographic Findings

Marginal erosions herald classic findings of RA. Erosions usually begin at the intracapsular articular margins—a region of exposed bone between the joint capsule and the start of the cartilage surface. This area of uncovered bone is termed the *bare area* (Figure 20-2).

> The "bare areas" of the joint—areas within the joint capsule that are not covered by thick cartilage—are the earliest sites of erosion in RA.

The mechanism that produces marginal erosions is thought to be a combination of direct mechanical action of the pannus and the action of soluble factors liberated by the pannus that may

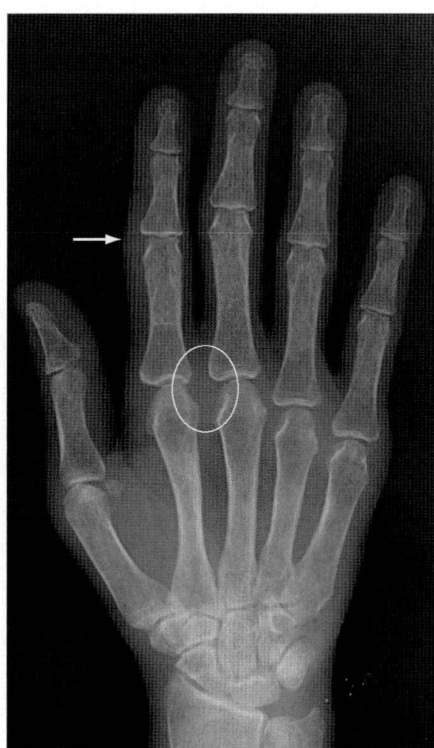

FIGURE 20-1. Early radiographic changes of RA. Posteroanterior radiograph of the hand shows soft tissue swelling at the first PIP *(arrow)* and MCP *(oval)* joints. Osteopenia is demonstrated by generalized thinning of the bone cortices. There is mild erosion of the ulnar styloid and a small cyst in the radial styloid.

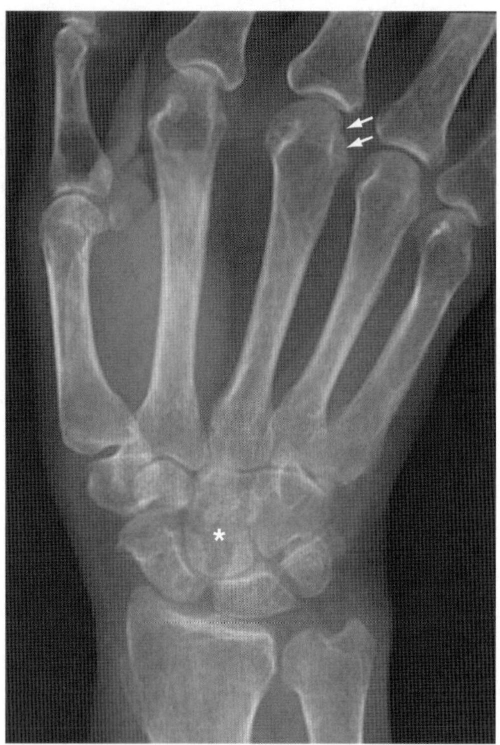

FIGURE 20-2. Hand and wrist changes in RA. Posteroanterior radiograph of the wrist shows periarticular osteopenia, soft tissue swelling, and bare area erosions at the MCP joints, which are most significant at the ulnar side of the third MCP joint in this example *(arrows)*. There is abnormal widening of the scapholunate distance and proximal migration of the capitate *(asterisk)* with narrowing of the scapholunate-capitate cartilage space (SLAC wrist).

stimulate bone loss.[9] Surface resorption may be present along areas of bone that are adjacent to inflamed tissue, such as adjacent to tenosynovitis.

Cartilage loss in RA tends to involve the joint uniformly, instead of along weight-bearing portions of the joint as in OA. For example, axial migration of the femoral head with uniform joint space narrowing is more typical of RA than is superior migration, which is typical of OA (Figure 20-3).

Hypertrophic bone formation, increase in bone mineral density, or repair of erosions is occasionally present in RA and may suggest a favorable treatment effect.[10-12]

> Treatment may result in erosions developing sclerotic margins due to repair.

However, periosteal new bone is uncommon, being more frequent in psoriasis, Reiter's disease, and juvenile RA. Osteophyte formation is one hallmark of OA that is generally easy to distinguish from RA.

Late Radiographic Findings

Continued synovial inflammation coupled with abnormal biomechanics eventually result in significant alteration in joints. Subluxations from ligament, tendon, and joint capsule laxity become more pronounced and may lead to frank dislocations. Once RA progresses to cartilage loss, the altered mechanics predispose to pressure erosions at sites of bone-on-bone rather than cartilage-on-cartilage interfaces.[13]

Progressive loss and obliteration of the cartilage space spreads throughout the joint. This pancompartmental distribution in such joints as the wrist and knee is characteristic of RA and helps differentiate RA from selective compartmental changes encountered in a variety of other articular disease process. Fibroosseous fusion of joints (ankylosis) is a late complication that may occur after complete cartilage loss. The wrist and midfoot bones are the most common locations for fusion. However, ankylosis is a more common feature of juvenile RA than adult RA.

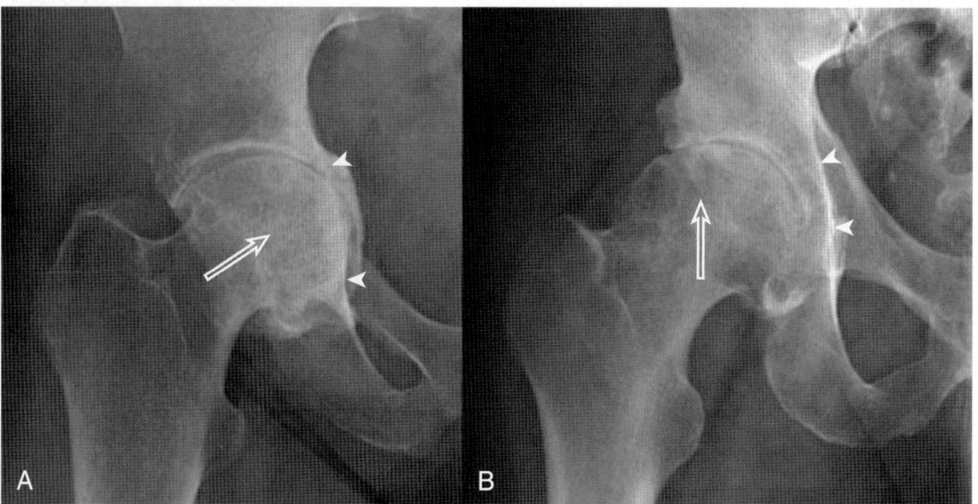

FIGURE 20-3. Arthritic changes in the hip: RA versus OA. RA and OA tend to involve different locations of the hip that may be identified on radiographs. **A,** Cartilage space narrowing in RA is usually uniform and results in axial migration of the hip *(arrow)* and medial migration of the femoral head and acetabulum (acetabular protrusion) with the femoral head located medial to the ilioischial line *(arrowheads)*. A small osteophyte is also present at the superolateral aspect of the femur in **A**, which is likely related to secondary osteoarthritis. **B,** Asymmetric cartilage space narrowing in OA with superior articular narrowing *(arrow)*. No acetabular protrusion is present; the femoral head is located lateral to the ilioischial line *(arrowheads)*.

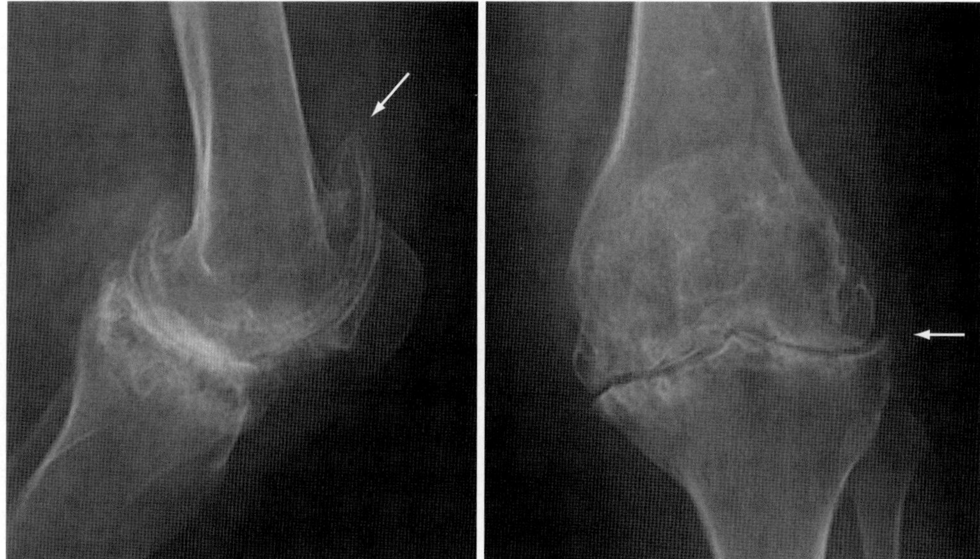

FIGURE 20-4. RA with secondary OA and severe cartilage loss. Radiographs of the knee show severe uniform loss of the cartilage space. The symmetry of medical and lateral compartment narrowing suggests an underlying inflammatory condition. The changes of OA with osteophytes *(arrows)* and subchondral sclerosis are noted. Soft tissue swelling and a suprapatellar knee effusion are also present.

Another late consequence of altered biomechanics in joints affected with RA is secondary OA. Persistent use of a joint with the predisposing anatomic abnormalities of RA may cause the joint to develop osteophyte formation, subchondral sclerosis, and subchondral cysts (Figure 20-4).[14] The result is a mixed picture on radiographs of both the initial and persistent arthritic changes from RA and the subsequent secondary changes from OA.

Distribution of Articular Involvement

Radiographs provide a global assessment of regional arthritis involvement. Although the distribution of radiographic abnormalities in RA is somewhat variable, it is generally symmetrical and polyarticular. RA targets synovial joints; thus the distribution of involvement will correlate with the locations of synovial joints and the synovial lining in the joint. There is a predilection for symmetric involvement of the distal extremities, hands, wrists, and feet, but the elbows, knees, shoulders, and hips are often affected. In the axial skeleton, imaging abnormalities in the articulations of the cervical spine are more often encountered than are changes in the thoracolumbar spine or sacroiliac joints.

Radiographic Appearance in Specific Joints

Hands

Alterations in the hands by RA are well described. These target characteristic locations within certain joints and display characteristic patterns of joint distribution. Soft tissue swelling and periarticular osteoporosis emerge early in the disease and are the indirect signs of synovitis and joint effusion. The index and middle finger metacarpophalangeal (MCP) joints are usually the earliest and most often affected.[15]

> The index and middle finger MCP joints show the earliest features of RA.

As the disease progresses, marginal erosions and concentric loss of the joint space develop and may eventually progress to malalignment and joint ankylosis.

Soft Tissues

Both the character and distribution of soft tissue swelling/effusion in the hands are important in identifying early RA. Although soft tissue abnormalities are better detected with MRI or ultrasound, localization of soft tissue swelling to the proximal interphalangeal (PIP) joints and MCP joints is suggestive of RA even in the absence of bone abnormalities (see Figure 20-1).[16] Fusiform swelling of the PIP joints is characteristic of RA, whereas swelling secondary to OA is often asymmetric, located most often at the distal interphalangeal (DIP) joints, and usually accompanied by osteophytosis. MCP soft tissue swelling/joint effusion may be demonstrated by widening of the MCP joint, bulging of the web spaces, or increased convexity of the marginal soft tissues adjacent to the MCP joints of the thumb, index, and fifth fingers.

Erosions

The joints of the hands affected by soft tissue swelling are also the joints that may be involved by erosions. The earliest bone changes are demonstrated at the bare areas of the radial aspects of the MCP joints where the normal smooth cortex is visible (see Figure 20-2). Bare areas are located at the margins of the joint where bone cortex is relatively unprotected by overlying articular cartilage. This bare area is the region of bone cortex between the thick overlying articular cartilage and the joint capsule.[15] Early marginal erosions are seen on magnification radiographs as localized cortical thinning and a dot-and-dash pattern of cortical disruption. More advanced marginal erosions show loss of cortex with or without preservation of underlying trabeculation.[17,18]

In addition to marginal erosions, compressive (pressure) and superficial surface resorption may occur in the hands.[13] The mechanism of compressive erosion is the collapse of osteoporotic bone as muscular forces pull the articular surfaces together, typically at the MCP joints.[15] Surface resorption occurs at regions of bone adjacent to inflamed tendons, such as at the distal ulna (Table 20-1).

TABLE 20-1. Types of Erosion in RA

Type of Erosion	Cause	Example
Inflammatory marginal	Begin in the bare areas of the joint due to pannus	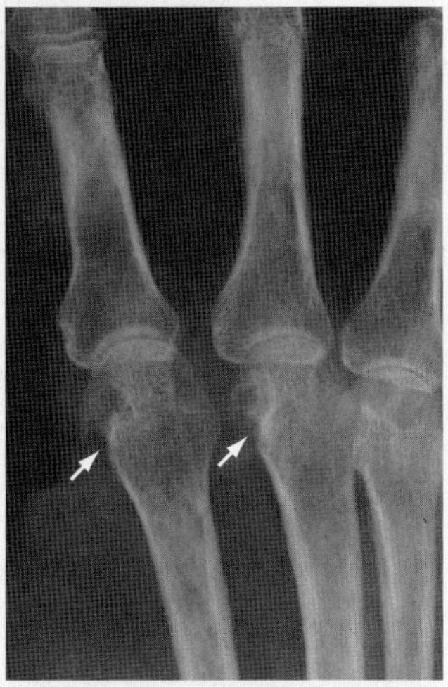
Compressive	Due to collapse of osteoporotic bone usually accompanying malalignment	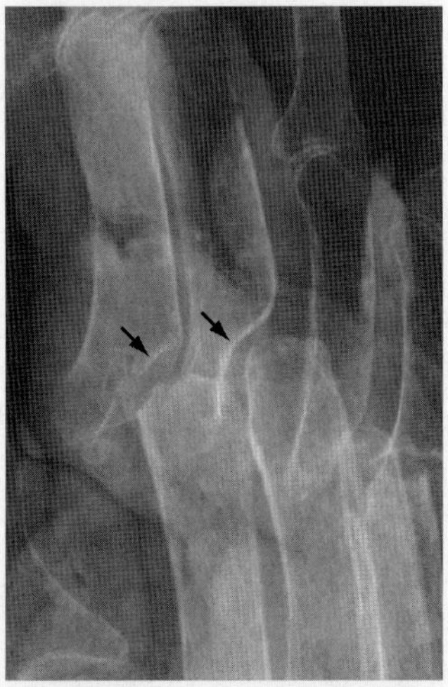
Surface	Erosions occurring beneath inflamed tendons	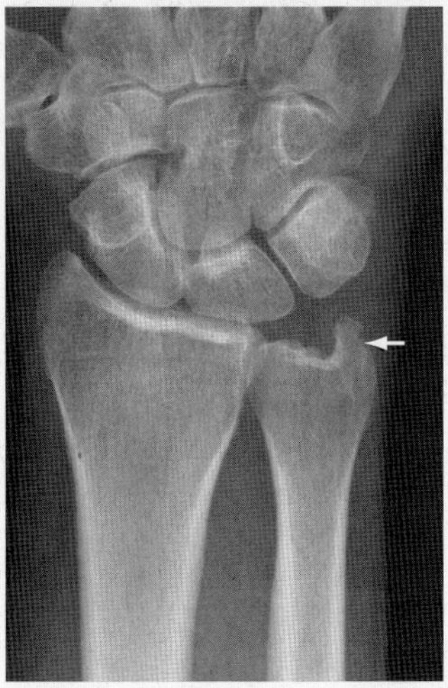

Ankylosis

As destruction of cartilage and bone progresses, the joint space may be destroyed completely. Ankylosis is a fibroosseous fusion of joints after complete cartilage loss and represents the chronic, end-stage sequela of RA.

> Ankylosis is a fibroosseous fusion of joints after complete cartilage loss. It most often affects the carpals and tarsals.

In the hands, ankylosis may occur at the MCP and PIP joints, but fusion is more frequent in the carpal and tarsal bones.

Malalignment

Alignment abnormalities of the hand are common and classic in RA and are attributed to the direct effect of the disease on the articulations, tendons, and ligaments. Common and classic alignment abnormalities include swan-neck, boutonnière and windswept deformities, and flexion/hyperextension-subluxation/dislocations at the thumb.

Swan-neck deformity consists of hyperextension at the PIP joint and flexion at the DIP joint. This deformity results primarily from synovitis of the flexor tendon sheath. With flexion limited at the PIP joint, hyperextension ensues from intrinsic muscle pull. The DIP joint is held in flexion from pull of the flexor profundus tendon.[19]

Boutonnière deformity is a combination of flexion at the proximal interphalangeal and extension at the DIP joints. In patients with the boutonnière deformity, the normal balance between the tendon mechanism and ligamentous restriction is disrupted. Extension is ineffective due to lengthening of the central extensor tendon from capsular distension. The lateral extensor tendon slips fall volar to the axis of motion of the PIP joint and act as flexors of this joint. The extensor tendon slips also produce hyperextension at the DIP joint from increased pull.[19]

Windswept deformity represents one of a variety of MCP and PIP joint deformities. Patients with windswept deformity have symmetric ulnar subluxations and dislocations of the MCP and PIP joints. The windswept deformity affects patients with systemic lupus erythematosus and Jaccoud's arthropathy as well, but these patients lack the characteristic erosions of RA. In hands affected by RA, ulnar deviation and palmar subluxations are common, being found in 25% to 65% and 20% to 68%, respectively.[13]

New Bone Formation

Increased amounts of endosteal bone may form in the distal phalanges. This condition, called *terminal phalangeal sclerosis* or *acral sclerosis,* occurs significantly more frequently in women with RA.[20] Although it may be found in normal individuals, terminal phalangeal sclerosis may also be more frequent in systemic lupus erythematosus (SLE), dermatomyositis, and psoriatic arthritis.

> Sclerosis of the distal phalanges may be seen in RA, SLE, and sarcoidosis but may be a normal finding.

Rarely, repair of erosions may occur[11] and bone density may increase, especially in patients treated with methotrexate or with an anti–tumor necrosis factor antibody.[10]

Wrists

As in the hands, alterations in the wrists due to RA include soft tissue swelling, erosions, joint space narrowing, alignment abnormalities, and ankylosis. These abnormalities also tend to affect particular locations in the joints and tend to be distributed in specific joints that are characteristic for RA. Abnormalities in the wrist are frequently accompanied by involvement in the fingers, either concomitantly or following carpal dominant rheumatoid disease.

Soft Tissues

Soft tissue swelling/edema is depicted on radiographs by obliteration of the fat lines and thickening and increased density of the soft tissues. Soft tissue swelling may be present at any of the compartments of the wrist due to synovial enlargement and/or joint effusion. Intercarpal, carpometacarpal, and radiocarpal joints; overlying tendons; and/or the ligamentous structures may be affected. Soft tissue swelling at the medial aspect of the ulnar styloid is a characteristic early finding in RA and is produced by tenosynovitis of the extensor carpi ulnaris tendon.[16,21] The normal fat lines around the extensor carpi ulnaris on the ulnar side of the wrist and the fat outlining the extensor pollicis brevis and abductor pollicis longus tendons on the radial side may be obscured by soft tissue swelling.

> Infiltration of fat by inflammatory changes obliterates the normal fat lines seen along tendons such as the extensor carpi ulnaris.

Rheumatoid involvement of the tendons coursing through the carpal tunnel may produce carpal tunnel syndrome. Although masses involving the carpal tunnel are better characterized by MRI or ultrasound,[22] radiographs may suggest RA involvement by demonstrating displacement and distortion of the pronator fat line that normally parallels the volar side of the distal radius.[23]

Erosions

Erosions usually involve the intercarpal and radiocarpal articulations symmetrically. As with other joints, bare areas and bony locations adjacent to synovitis are more likely to develop erosions. The ulnar styloid is a particularly common site for erosion.[15]

> The ulnar styloid is a common site for early erosion in RA.

Erosions of the triquetrum and pisiform bones are common in early RA, although the disease can involve any carpal bone. Synovial inflammation at the radiocarpal compartment will erode the radial styloid process and adjacent scaphoid bone. However, there is a normal mild degree of notching at the radial aspect of the scaphoid that must be distinguished from true erosive change.

Ankylosis

Disease progression may lead to pancompartmental changes in the wrist with obliteration of the joint spaces, large osseous erosions, and bony ankylosis. This pancompartmental distribution is characteristic of RA and is extremely unlikely to be the result of other disease processes that are more likely to involve only selected compartments.

Malalignment

Wrist malalignment and deformity generally fall into several well-described patterns of radiocarpal, intercarpal, and radioulnar/distal ulnar malalignment[24]; however, given the intricate relationships and number of ligaments, tendons, and bones at the wrist, the classification of wrist malalignment and deformity should serve primarily as a guide, as there is overlap among the different types. *Radiocarpal malalignment* appears as ulnar and palmar deviation of the proximal carpal row as the carpus slides off the inclined articular surface of the distal radius. Prevalence of radiocarpal malalignment may be as high as 70% of patients with RA.[13] *Intercarpal malalignment* may occur in dorsal or volar directions. Dorsal intercalated segment instability (DISI) results in an increased scapholunate angle (normal, 45 degrees) on lateral radiographs as the scaphoid rotates into a more volar flexed position and the lunate tilts dorsally. The scapholunate angle is reduced in volar intercalated segment instability (VISI) as the lunate rotates into volar flexion and there is volar shift of the capitate. *Inferior radioulnar and distal ulnar malalignment* include dorsal subluxation of the distal ulna and diastasis of the inferior radioulnar compartment. With the end of the ulna subluxed dorsally, patients are predisposed to mechanical rubbing and tenosynovitis of the adjacent extensor compartments and eventual rupture of these tendons. Scapholunate advanced collapse (SLAC) is also seen in RA. With SLAC wrist, the capitate migrates proximally after complete tear of the scapholunate ligament (see Figure 20-2) (Table 20-2).

Feet and Ankles

The radiographic features of soft tissue swelling, erosions, joint space narrowing, alignment abnormalities, and ankylosis found in the hands and wrists are also seen in the feet and ankles. The characteristic and common abnormalities tend to be symmetric, usually affect particular locations in the joints, and distribute among specific joints that are predisposed to synovitis. The metatarsophalangeal (MTP) joints are among the first to be affected by RA.

> The MTP joints are the first sites of involvement in up to 20% of RA patients.

Ten percent to twenty percent of RA patients have the initial manifestation of the disease in the MTP joints.[25]

A classic soft tissue abnormality in the heel is soft tissue thickening in the pre-Achilles' bursa (Figure 20-5). The enlarged pre-Achilles' bursa can be identified as a soft tissue mass located between the posterior superior surface of the calcaneus and the anterior aspect of the distal Achilles' tendon.[16,26] The soft tissue swelling generally precedes erosions at the posterior superior calcaneus adjacent to the Achilles' insertion.[13] Identical findings may be present in ankylosing spondylitis and reactive arthritis (Reiter's disease), but RA is the most common cause of these findings. Plantar calcaneal erosions mimic those seen with psoriasis. Rheumatoid nodules adjacent to the Achilles' and other tendons are better demonstrated with ultrasound or MRI than radiography.

Rheumatoid erosions in the foot and ankle involve similar joints as in the hand and wrist, including the PIP, MTP, intertarsal, and tibiotalar joints. The earliest cortical changes are best demonstrated in the medial aspects of the first through fourth metatarsal heads and the medial and lateral aspects of the fifth metatarsal head bare areas.[27]

> Erosion may occur first at the fifth MTP joint.

At the ankle, uniform cartilage loss with resultant joint space narrowing at the tibiotalar joint has its corollary with the radiocarpal joint. Fibular notch erosion at the distal tibiofibular joint is characteristic for RA (Figure 20-6).[28]

Large Appendicular Joints

Large appendicular joints—the knee, hip, elbow, and shoulder—involved by RA share many radiographic features. The predominant feature of RA in large appendicular joints is uniform and severe cartilage space loss (see Figure 20-4). Progressive destruction of the chondral surface leads to diffuse loss of the cartilage space. Erosions, subchondral cystic lesions, and subchondral sclerosis are often present in the large appendicular joints, but these features are present to a lesser extent than the uniform loss of cartilage space.

Interosseous cystic lesions (or geodes) may occur in the large joints involved by RA.[29,30] These geodes appear on radiographs as lucencies of varying shape and size. Mechanisms for these lesions include intrusion of granulation tissue from the joint through a defect in the cortical bone[15] or formation of rheumatoid nodules within the bone.[29]

Knee

The knee is frequently affected in RA and is often affected early in the disease course. Soft tissue swelling is the most common, but unfortunately nonspecific, finding. Up to 80% of positive knee radiographs in patients with RA may have soft tissue swelling/effusion as the only abnormality.[27]

Effusion will be visible as a soft tissue density in the suprapatellar region on the lateral knee radiograph. Other findings of knee effusion include anterior displacement of the patella on the lateral view and soft tissue density adjacent to the femoral condyles on the anterior view. Synovial enlargement or the combination of synovial enlargement with effusion have similar findings on radiographs (Table 20-3).

> No distinction can be made between joint effusion and pannus on radiographs.

In addition, RA may enlarge popliteal cysts producing soft tissue masses in the posterior aspect of the knee. These cysts may rupture into the calf and cause pseudophlebitis syndrome.

> Rupture of a popliteal cyst in a patient with RA may produce symptoms mimicking phlebitis.

Popliteal cysts can become very large palpable masses that may dissect down the calf and may be confirmed by ultrasound or MRI (Figure 20-7).

As the disease progresses, small erosions on the medial, lateral, and posterior margins of the femoral condyles and tibial plateaus may be observed. Uniform bicompartmental (medial and lateral tibiofemoral) or uniform tricompartmental (including the patellofemoral compartment) joint space narrowing occurs as a consequence of cartilage loss (see Figure 20-4).

> The uniform cartilage loss in RA is in contrast to the asymmetric involvement of knee compartments in OA.

Subchondral erosions and geodes may also develop. As with the hip, superimposed OA may complicate the classical findings of RA in the knee.

Hip

Abnormalities at the hip are much less common than the peripheral joints and tend to be present in patients with long-standing and severe forms of RA. Although soft tissue swelling/joint effusion may be present on radiographs as expansion and increased density of the soft tissues around the femoral neck with obscuration or displacement of the adjacent fat planes or as effacement of the obturator internus muscle fat plane medial to the acetabulum, these findings are unreliable and have been shown to have no value in the detection of joint effusion in adults.[31] The one reliable finding of hip effusion on radiographs is an increase in the tear drop distance (Table 20-4).[32]

TABLE 20-2. Some Hand and Wrist Alignment Abnormalities in RA

Abnormality	Description	Example
Thumb deformities	Boutonniere (hitchhiker's thumb): flexion of the MCP and hyperextension of the IP	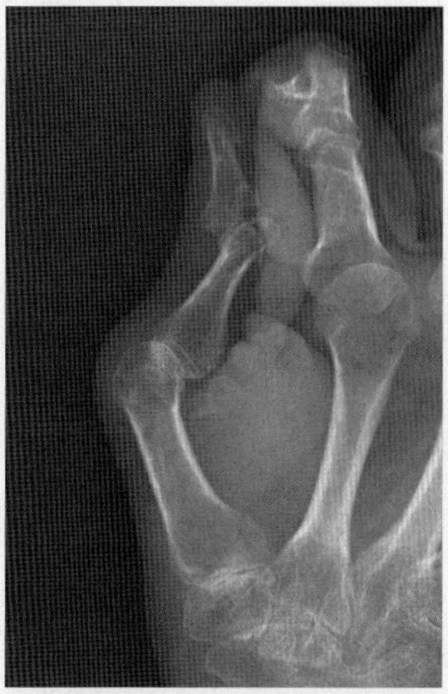
Swan neck deformity	Hyperextension of the PIP joint and flexion of the DIP joint	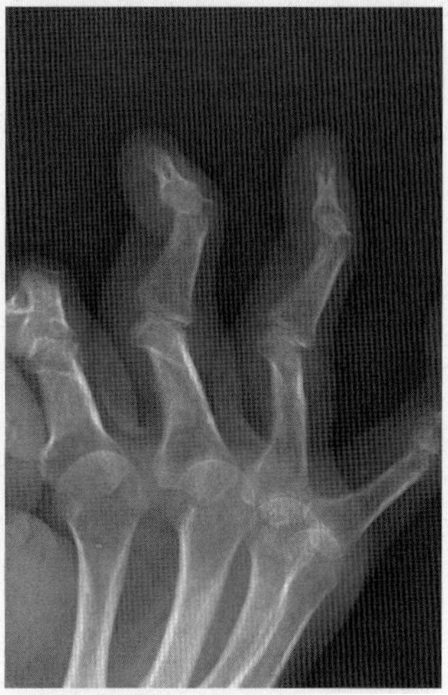
Boutonnière deformity	Flexion of the PIP and hyperextension of the DIP	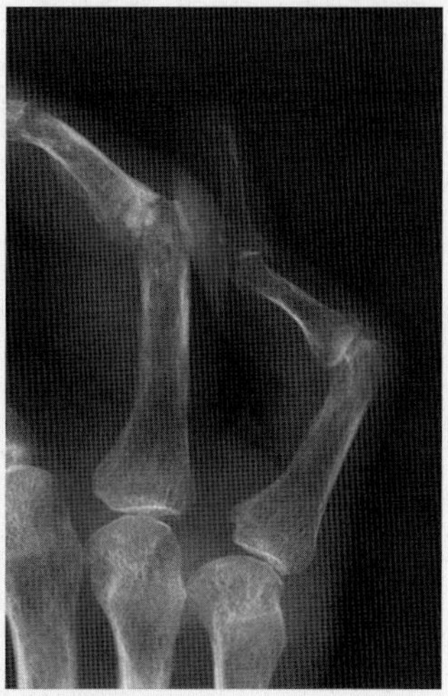

(Continued)

TABLE 20-2. Some Hand and Wrist Alignment Abnormalities in RA—cont'd

Abnormality	Description	Example
Ulnar deviation at the MCPs	Ulnar deviation of the fingers at the MCP joints. May be accompanied by flexion and palmar subluxation of the fingers	
Radial deviation of the hand/wrist	May accompany ulnar deviation of the fingers	
Ulnar translocation of the carpals	The proximal row of carpals migrates in an ulnar–palmar direction	
Scapholunate dissociation	Separation between the scaphoid (S) and lunate (L) on posteroanterior radiograph	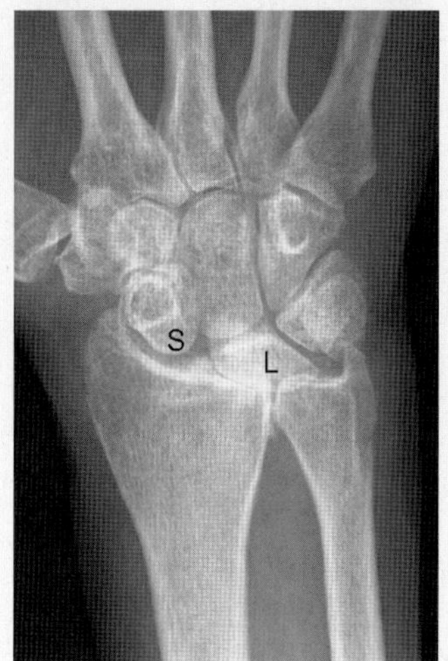

TABLE 20-2. Some Hand and Wrist Alignment Abnormalities in RA—cont'd

Abnormality	Description	Example
DISI (dorsal intercalated segmental instability)	Scapholunate dissociation and volar flexion of the scaphoid with increased scapholunate angle on lateral radiograph (normal angle, 30-60 degrees) C, Capitate; L, lunate; LL, lunate axis; R, radius.	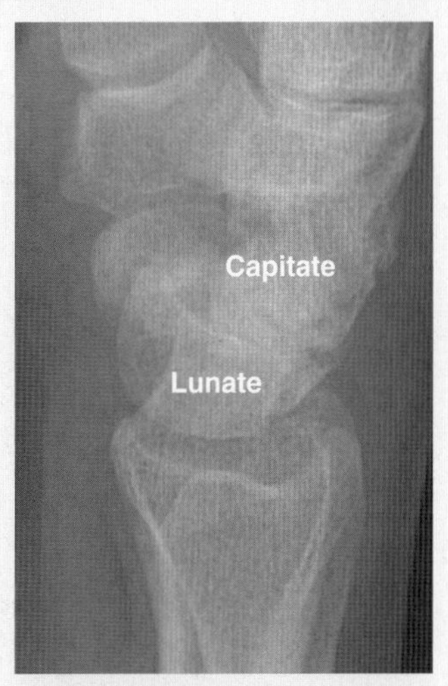
VISI (volar intercalated segmental instability)	Palmar flexion of the lunate and scaphoid. Scapholunate angle < 30 degrees (usually with ulnar migration of the proximal carpal row)	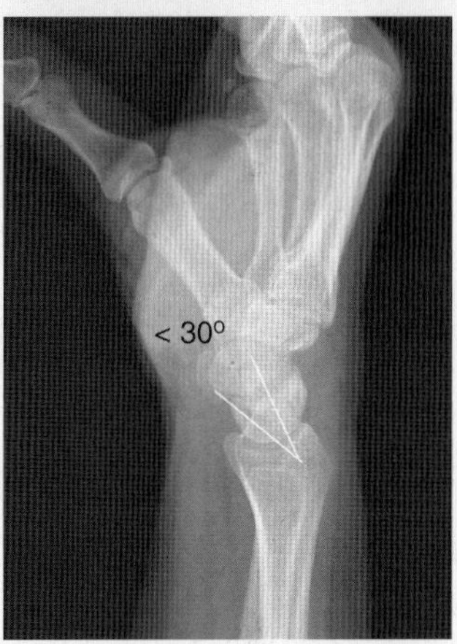
Distal ulnar subluxation	Distal, dorsal subluxation of the ulna, with or without widening of the radioulnar joint. The ulna may impinge on the carpals (impaction) or on dorsal tendons	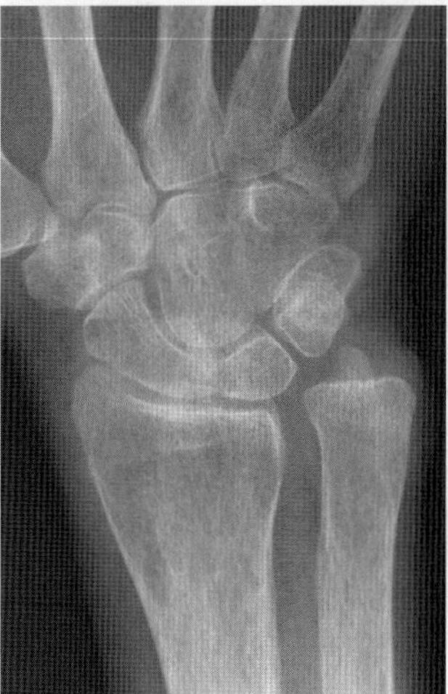

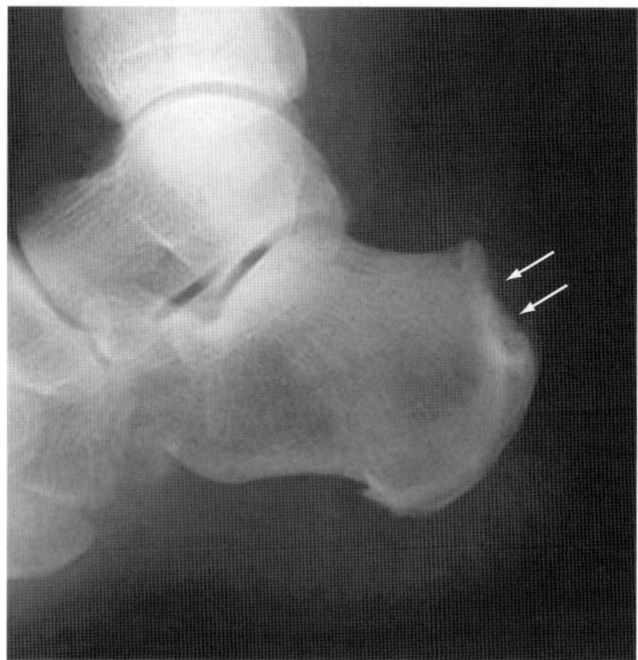

FIGURE 20-5. Heel changes from RA. Lateral radiograph of the heel demonstrates soft tissue prominence at the pre-Achilles' bursa and erosions at the subjacent posterosuperior calcaneus, adjacent to tendon insertion *(arrows).*

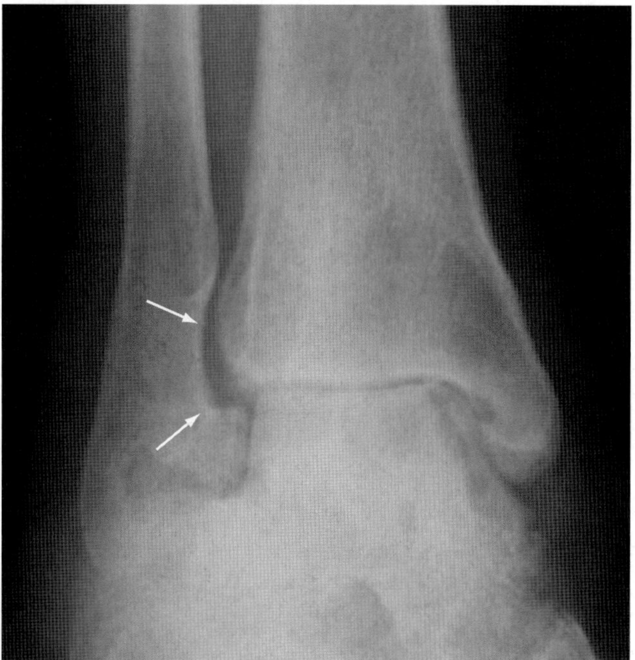

FIGURE 20-6. Ankle erosion from RA. Frontal view of the ankle shows characteristic *fibular notch* erosion at the distal tibiofibular articulation *(arrows).*

The distance between the lateral aspect of the acetabular teardrop shadow on the anteroposterior radiograph and the medial femoral head should be symmetric; differences of only 1 mm between the sides suggest hip joint effusion on the side with the greater measurement (Table 20-4).

TABLE 20-3. The Suprapatellar Pouch as an Indicator of Knee Joint Distension*

Normal suprapatellar pouch	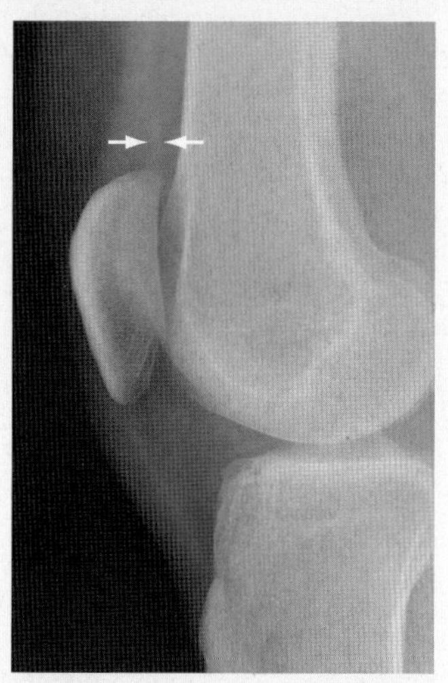
Mild joint distension	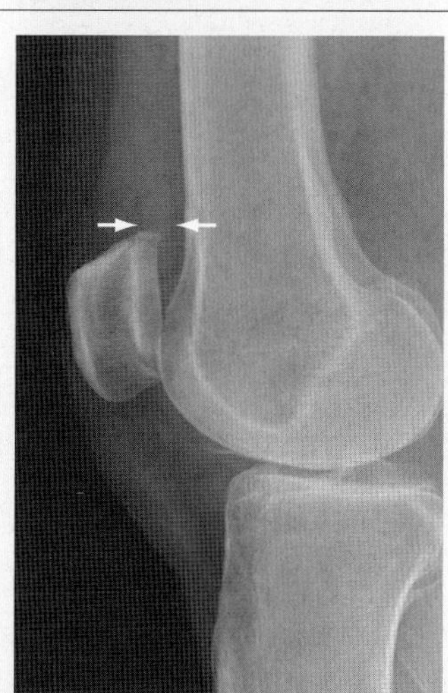
Moderate joint distension	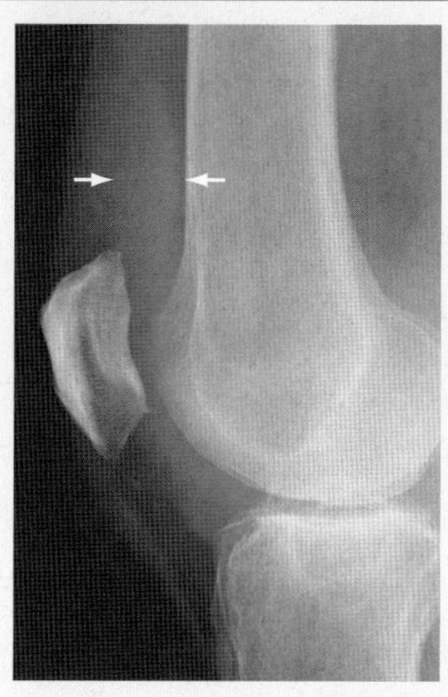

*Effusion with or without pannus.

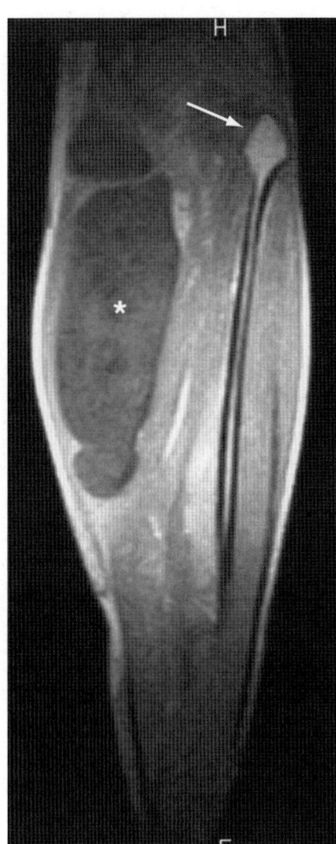

FIGURE 20-7. Large dissecting popliteal cyst. Enhanced coronal T1-weighted MR image (TR/TE = 700/10) of the lower extremity demonstrates a large popliteal cyst *(asterisk)* dissecting in the medial posterior calf. On this posterior image, the fibula *(arrow)* is seen.

Uniform loss of the cartilage space is typically bilateral and symmetric. With uniform loss of the articular cartilage, the femoral head moves along the axis of the femoral neck (termed *axial migration*). Axial migration helps distinguish RA from OA, which tends to cause superior migration with joint space narrowing at the superior weight-bearing portion of the joint. At times it may be difficult to separate RA from OA when features of both conditions are present. Secondary OA in RA occurs, and sometimes OA will develop axial migration; however, the findings in OA tend to be more asymmetric in comparison with the contralateral joint.

TABLE 20-4. The Teardrop Distance for Detection of Hip Joint Effusion

Normal versus widened	
Example	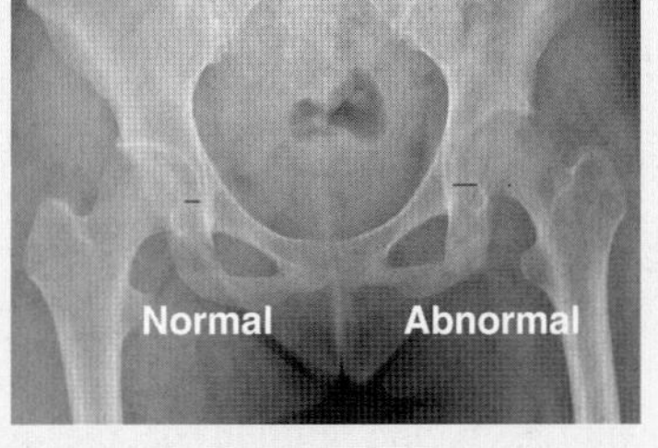

With complete obliteration of the hip cartilage space, the femoral head and acetabulum will protrude into the pelvis (see Figure 20-3). This acetabular protrusion (acetabular protrusio) is generally defined as displacement of the femoral head medial to the acetabular ilioischial line.[33] Severe instances of RA of the hip may lead to fibrous ankylosis.

Patients with RA are at increased risk of osteonecrosis of the femoral head, particularly those patients who are treated with corticosteroids. Several staging systems have been developed that rely on imaging abnormalities to grade severity of osteonecrosis and direct patients for different therapies.[34-36] Radiographic abnormalities in osteonecrosis include cysts and sclerosis, subchondral lucency due to a subchondral fracture (the crescent sign), flattening of the femoral head, cartilage space narrowing with or without acetabular involvement, and finally advanced degenerative changes. When osteonecrosis of the femoral head is suspected but the radiographs are normal or nondiagnostic, MRI or bone scan may indicate osteonecrosis before it is visible radiographically.[37,38]

Elbow

Abnormalities at the elbow are common in RA and, although symmetric, may preferentially affect the dominant arm. A classic radiographic finding that indicates an elbow joint effusion/soft tissue swelling is the fat pad sign (Figure 20-8). On the lateral radiographic view of a normal elbow obtained with the arm flexed at 90 degrees, overlying bony structures obscure fat hidden in the olecranon fossa.

> An intracapsular, extrasynovial fat pad is present both anteriorly and posteriorly along the elbow joint. When this fat pad is visible, joint distension is likely.

When an effusion and/or synovial thickening are present, the fat in the olecranon fossa is displaced dorsally and produces the fat pad sign: abnormal radiolucency (fat) posterior to the distal humerus. The supinator fat (superficial to the supinator muscle) may also be displaced when severe swelling is present. More advanced radiographic changes at the elbow include uniform joint space narrowing, marginal erosions, and eventual osteolysis of large portions of the distal humerus and proximal radius and ulna, often mimicking neuropathic changes.

Shoulder

The primary structures affected by RA in the shoulder include the glenohumeral joint, rotator cuff, and distal end of the clavicle. Progressive cartilage destruction at the glenoid fossa and humeral head leads to diffuse and uniform loss of the glenohumeral joint space (Figure 20-9). Erosions and pseudocysts tend to be located at the superolateral aspect of the humeral head adjacent to the greater tuberosity. Large pressure erosions may develop on the medial aspect of the surgical neck of the humerus from the rubbing and possibly inflammatory change at the adjacent glenoid margin and inferior glenohumeral capsule.

Rotator cuff abnormalities are frequent and tear of the rotator cuff is common in long-standing RA. On radiographs, an indirect sign of rotator cuff tear is the elevation of the humerus in relationship to the glenoid fossa with accompanying narrowing of the space between the humeral head and acromion.

> Narrowing of the acromiohumeral distance to less than 7 mm suggests chronic rotator cuff tear.

Advanced cases may show erosion of the acromion from the acromiohumeral abutment.

Rotator cuff tears are best demonstrated on MRI or ultrasound. Findings on these studies may aid in surgical planning if repair is

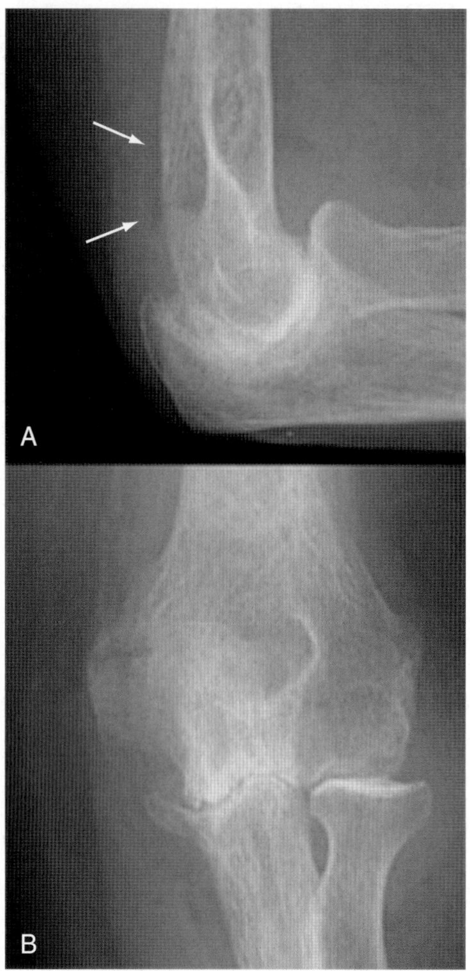

FIGURE 20-8. Posterior fat pad sign and characteristic rheumatoid changes at the elbow. **A,** Lateral radiograph of the elbow demonstrates a lucency *(arrows)* posterior to the distal humerus. This posterior fat pad is revealed because joint effusion or synovial enlargement posteriorly displaces the normally hidden fat in the olecranon fossa, allowing the lucent fat to be visible. In addition, on the frontal view **(B)** severe cartilage loss is demonstrated by uniform narrowing between the trochlea and proximal ulna. Erosions are present along the ulnohumeral and radiocapitellar articulations.

contemplated.[39] In addition, MRI provides a global assessment of the joint including labral abnormalities and synovitis that may be inaccessible for visualization with ultrasound. Inflamed synovial tissue on the undersurface of the rotator cuff tendons adjacent to the greater tuberosity of the humeral head is thought to lead to tendon tears and humeral head erosions and may be visible on MRI.

Erosions of the acromial end of the clavicle may be small or large. Marked tapering and pointing of the distal third of the clavicle may result (see Figure 20-9).[40] Similar changes may occur at the medial end of the clavicle at the sternoclavicular joint. In addition to RA, other causes for resorption or absence of the distal clavicle should be considered, such as hyperparathyroidism, posttraumatic osteolysis, infection, and surgical resection.

Tapering of the distal clavicle may be seen in RA, gout, hyperparathyroidism, posttraumatic osteolysis, and ankylosing spondylitis.

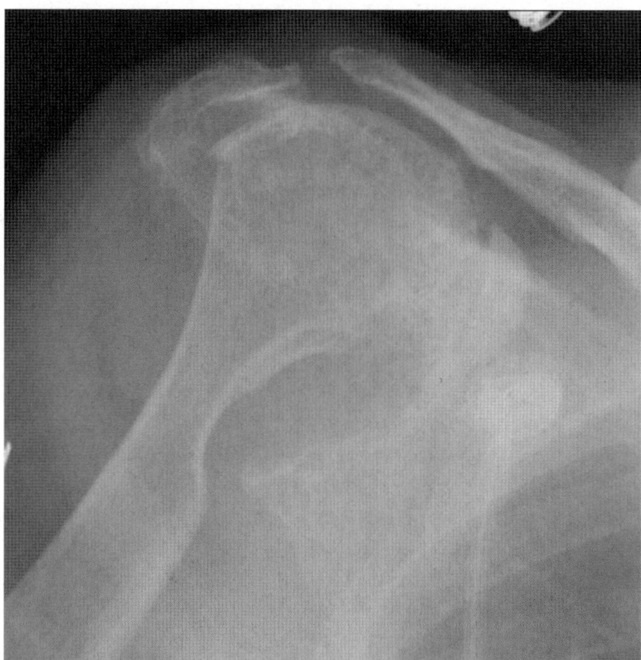

FIGURE 20-9. RA involvement of the shoulder. There is uniform loss of the glenohumeral joint space, in keeping with severe cartilage loss. The glenoid is eroded and deformed. Upward subluxation of the humeral head, resulting from chronic rotator cuff tear has allowed pressure erosion of the medial aspect of the proximal humerus. The tip of the distal clavicle is tapered, thinned, and eroded, characteristic of RA. In addition, the undersurface of the distal clavicle is scalloped, likely the result of direct pressure erosion from the superiorly subluxed humeral head.

Spine

The cervical spine is much more often affected by RA than the thoracic or lumbar spine.[40] Involvement of the cervical spine occurs in up to 70% of all patients with RA.[41] Because the integrity of the transverse ligament may be weakened and the atlantoaxial joints may be eroded, patients are at an increased risk of multidirectional subluxation at the C1-2 level.[42] Furthermore, atlantoaxial impaction (cranial settling) may occur in 5% to 8% of patients with RA.[43]

Subluxation

Anterior subluxation of C1 on C2 is a common and characteristic finding in RA.[44] A small degree of separation is normally present between the anterior arch of C1 (posteroinferior cortex of the anterior arch) and the anterior cortex of the dens of C2. This atlantoaxial interval measures no more than 2.5 mm in adults on the lateral radiograph of the cervical spine, and the interval remains constant with the neck in flexion or extension.[27] The stability of the atlantoaxial interval is maintained primarily by the transverse ligament of the atlas. The transverse ligament runs just posterior to the dens, connected to the lateral masses of the atlas and is in close proximity to synovial bursae located between the dens and the transverse ligament and between the dens and anterior arch of the atlas.

Anterior subluxation of C1 on C2 is documented by a C1-2 interval > 2.5 mm.

RA involvement of the adjacent bursa results in transverse ligament laxity and erosion of the adjacent C1 and dens with subsequent atlantoaxial instability (Figure 20-10). Flexion views

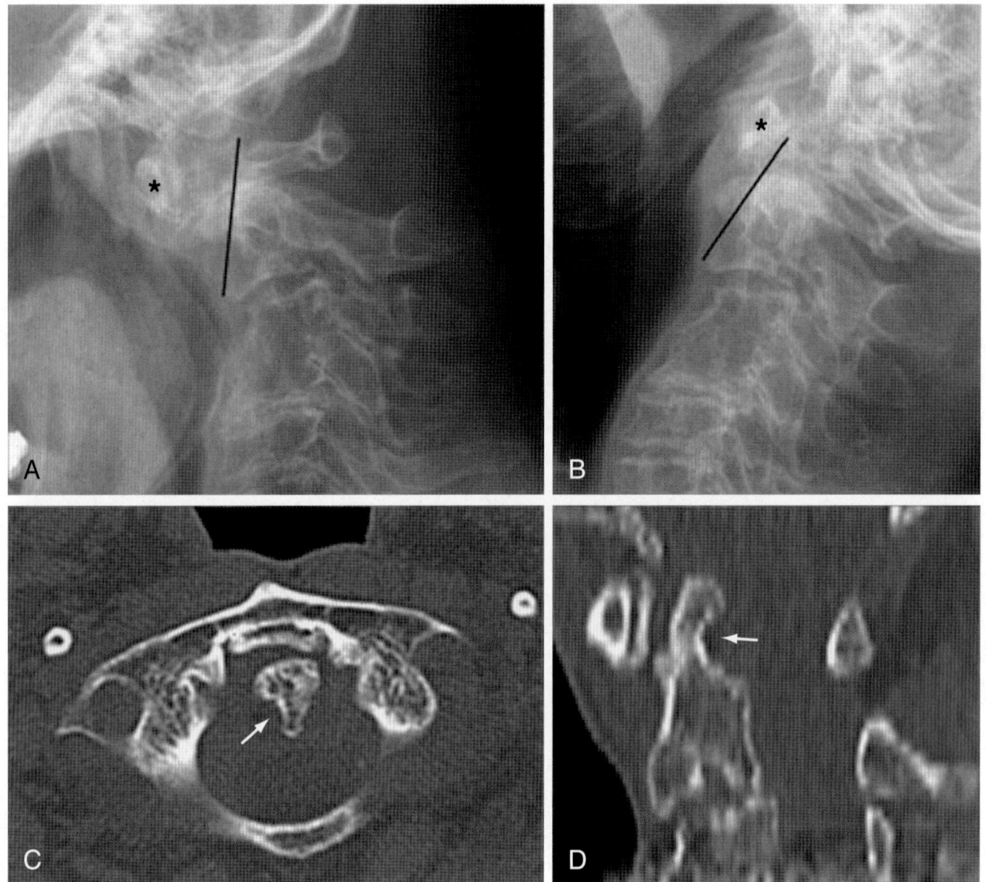

FIGURE 20-10. Anterior atlantoaxial subluxation due to RA. Lateral cervical spine radiographs in flexion **(A)** and extension **(B)** demonstrate anterior subluxation of C1 on C2. The distance between the anterior arch of C1 *(asterisks)* and the odontoid is difficult to measure due to the marked odontoid erosion. A line indicating the anterior aspect of C2 has been used to estimate the anterior surface of the odontoid. The C1-2 distance is wider in flexion than extension. The space for the cervical cord is narrowed on both examinations. The anterior arch of C1 migrates anteriorly on flexion. The tapered and eroded dens *(arrows)* is better shown on the axial CT image **(C)** and the reformatted sagittal CT image **(D)**.

are important to obtain in patients with a clinical suspicion of C1-2 instability, as the atlantoaxial interval may appear normal with the neck in the neutral position (the standard position for a lateral radiograph of the cervical spine).[45] Measurement of the posterior atlantodental interval (PADI) (between the posterior surface of the odontoid and the anterior surface of the posterior arch of C1) seems to correlate better with clinical findings than measurement of the C1-2 interval. PADI measurements < 14 mm suggest the possibility of spinal cord compression[46] (Table 20-5).

CT and MRI may provide additional information regarding the extent of bone erosions, degree of central canal compromise, and integrity of the cervical cord. Because MRI and CT are not routinely performed with the spine flexed, the degree of spinal cord compression may be underestimated from these studies and correlation should be made to lateral radiographs obtained with the neck in flexion and extension.

> Indications for MRI in patients with RA include weakness, spasticity, or other signs of myelopathy or multilevel involvement so that the level for possible surgery can be defined.

In addition to anterior C1-2 subluxation, lateral, rotational, or vertical (superior) subluxation may develop. Subaxial cervical vertebral body subluxation at multiple levels with increased *stepladder* subluxation on flexion views is characteristic but occurs less often than atlantoaxial abnormalities. Patients with OA may also show vertebral body subluxation, but it is usually confined to a single level[47] (Table 20-6).

TABLE 20-5. Radiographic Risk Factors for Spinal Cord Compression

Criteria	
AADI (anterior atlantodental interval)	> 9 mm
PADI (posterior atlantodental interval)	< 14 mm
AAI (atlantoaxial impaction)	
Subaxial canal diameter	< 14 mm
Cervical height index	< 2

From Roche CJ, Eyes BE, Whitehouse GH: The rheumatoid cervical spine: signs of instability on plain cervical radiographs, *Clin Radiol* 57:241-249, 2002.

Atlantoaxial Impaction (Vertical Subluxation)

Atlantoaxial impaction (also called *vertical subluxation*) is the setting of the skull base onto C1 and C1 onto C2 as a consequence of erosion (Figure 20-11).[42] McGregor's line may be used as a

TABLE 20-6. Cervical Subluxations in RA

Subluxation	Description	Example
Anterior subluxation C1-2	Due to damage to the transverse ligament and, in more severe cases, to additional apical and alar ligament damage Anterior C1-2 interval > 2.5 mm *(arrows)* 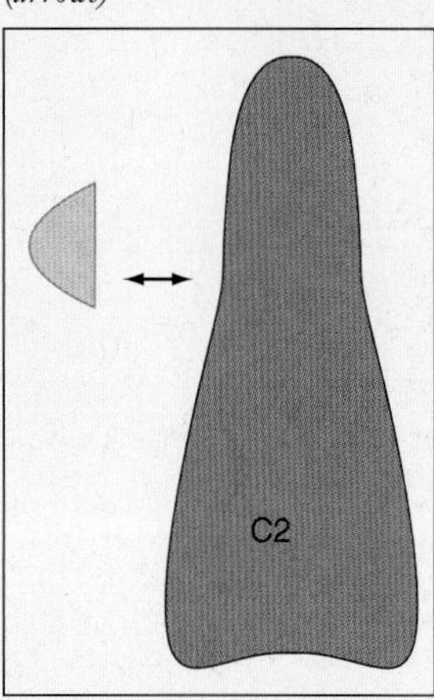	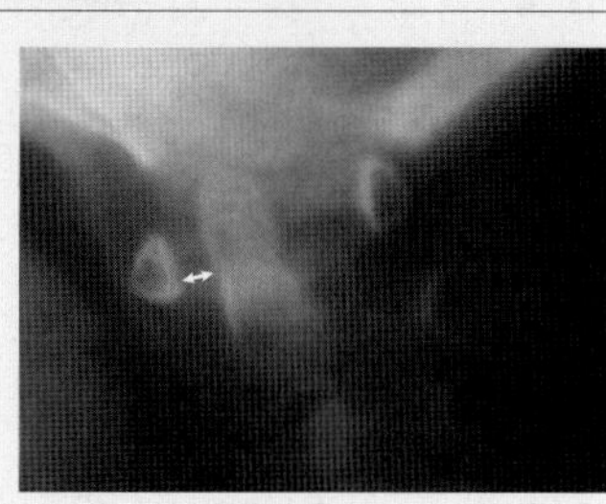
Posterior subluxation C1-2	Usually due to odontoid erosion or fracture *(arrow)*. Posterior margin of anterior arch of C1 *(dashed lines)* behind the anterior margin of the C2 vertebral body 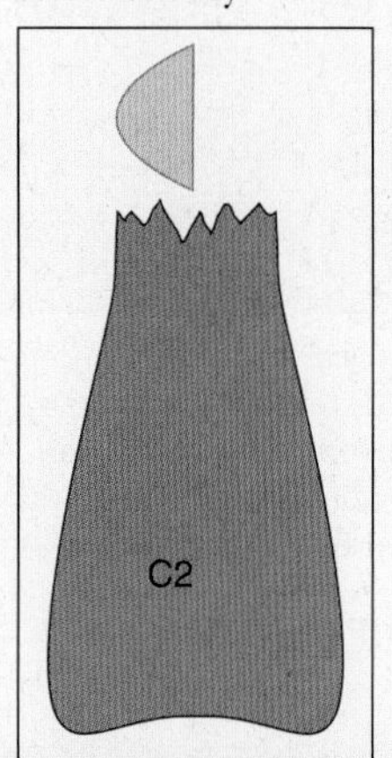	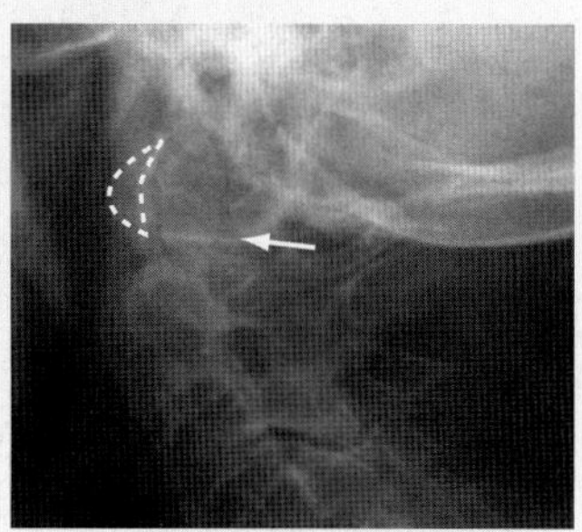
Vertical subluxation (atlantoaxial impaction, AAI)	Settling of C1 on C2 and the occiput on C1 such that the odontoid *(asterisk)* may protrude into the foramen magnum. Abnormal measurements using McGregor's line, Ranawat line, or others (see Table 20-7) 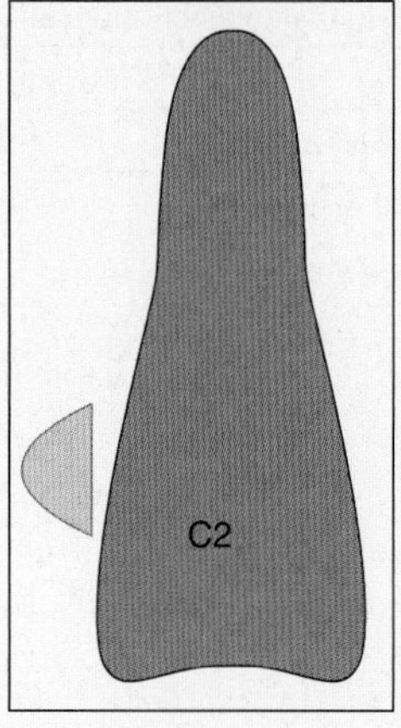	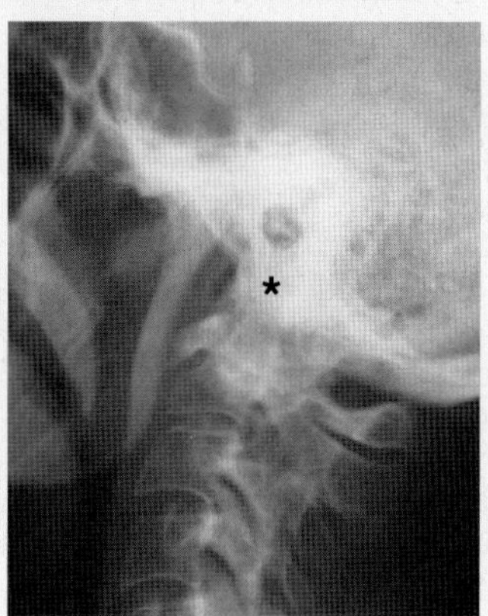

TABLE 20-6. Cervical Subluxations in RA—cont'd

Subluxation	Description	Example
Lateral subluxation C1-2	> 2 mm offset of C1 with relation to C2 on frontal radiograph *(arrow)* 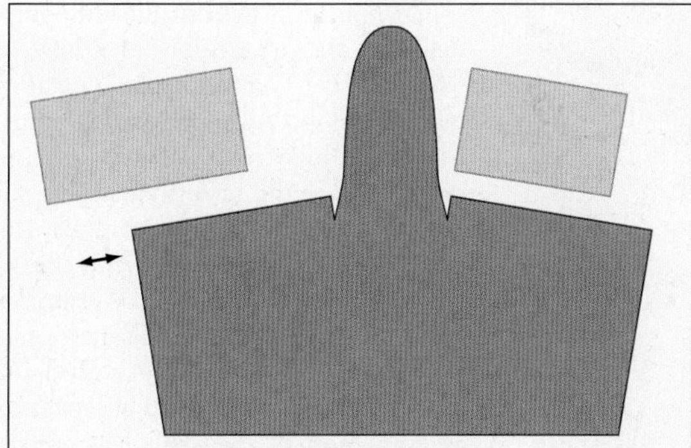	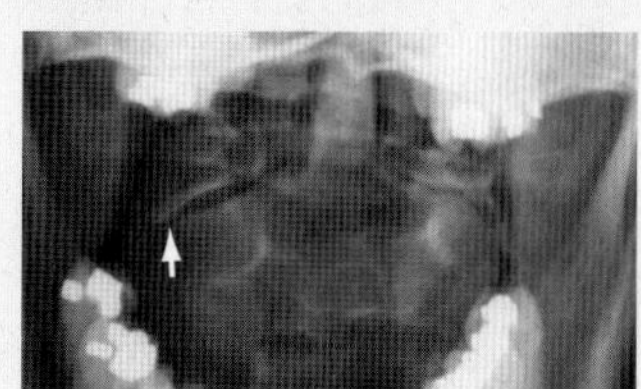
Rotatory C1-2 subluxation	Rotation of C1 on C2 on frontal projection	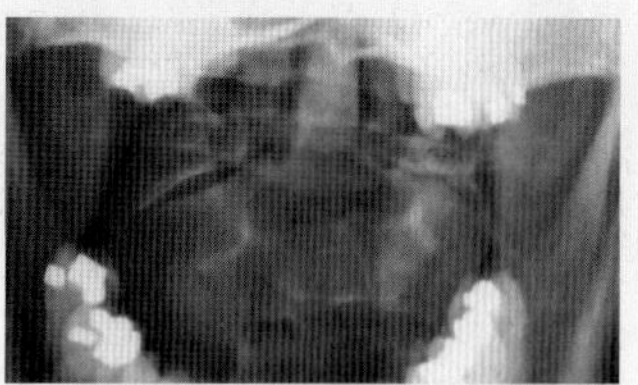
Stepladder subluxation	Multiple subluxations below C2 Offset between levels at the posterior vertebral bodies	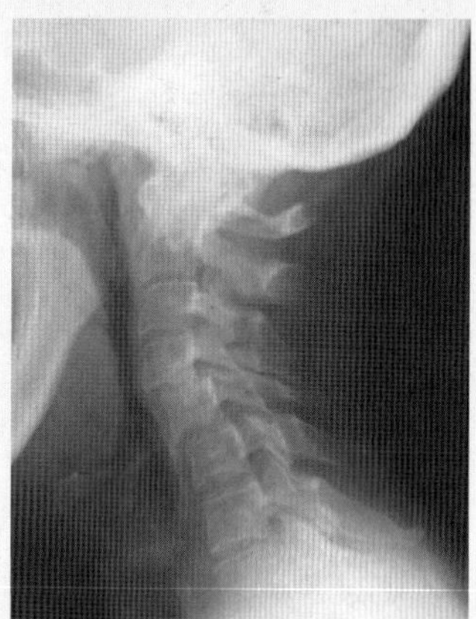
Increased lordosis	Increased lordosis	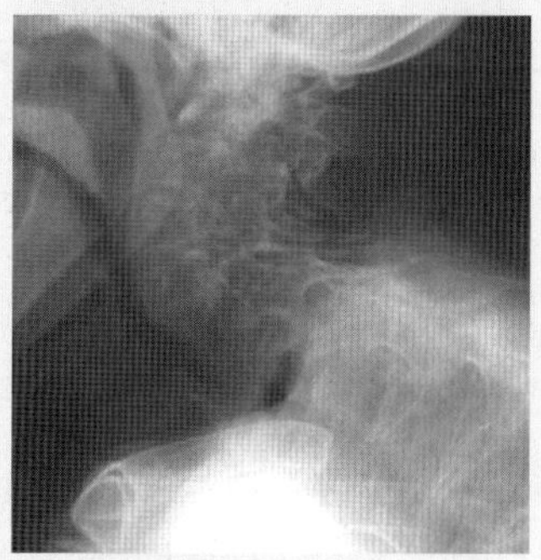

Modified from Bouchaud-Chabot A and Liote F: Cervical spine involvement in rheumatoid arthritis. A review, *Joint Bone Spine* 69:141-154, 2002.

reference to identify atlantoaxial impaction[48] and is drawn on a lateral radiograph from the superior surface of the posterior edge of the hard palate to the most caudal point of the occipital curve. Protrusion of the odontoid process about 1 cm above this line is abnormal and consistent with atlantoaxial impaction.

Originally, McGregor indicated that an odontoid tip > 4.5 mm above his reference line was abnormal; his measurements were performed on a select population, and currently a value of about 1 cm or greater is used to indicate abnormal odontoid position.

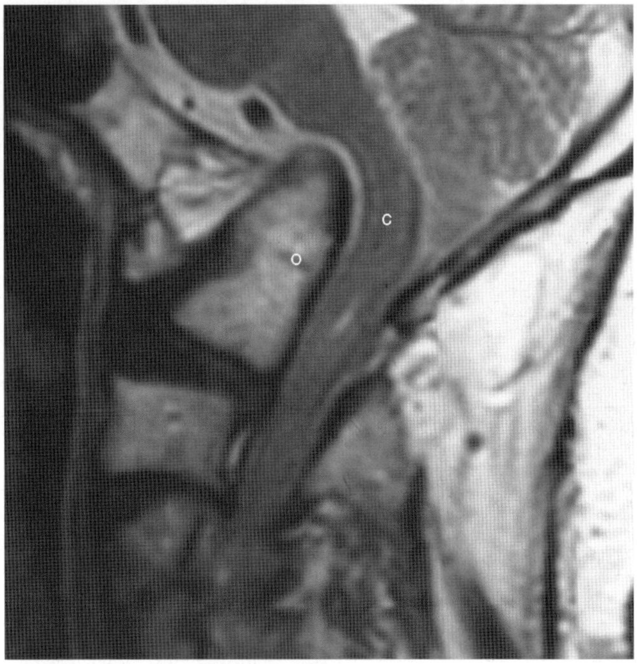

FIGURE 20-11. Atlantoaxial impaction. Sagittal T2-weighted MR image of the cervical spine shows severe settling of the skull base and C1 with superior migration of the dens *(o)* into the cranium. The end result is severe central canal stenosis and severe kinking of the cervical cord *(c)*.

In addition, several other radiographic criteria have been suggested for measuring atlantoaxial impaction[49] (Table 20-7).

In cases where the bony landmarks are obscured by erosion or overlap, settling of the skull may be determined by the relative positions of C1 and C2 on the lateral radiograph.[42] In these situations, articulation of the anterior arch of C1 with the lower half of the dens or body of C2 instead of the more superior portion of the dens will suggest atlantoaxial impaction.

Thoracic and Lumbar Spine

Unlike the characteristic findings in the cervical spine, rheumatoid abnormalities of the thoracic and lumbar spine are relatively uncommon and less distinct. Alterations in the facet joints and irregularity in the subchondral margins of the vertebral bodies with or without sclerosis may be present.[50] Complications of corticosteroid therapy may occur in the thoracic and lumbar spine with osteonecrosis of the vertebral bodies.[51] Although osteonecrosis occurs more often in the femoral head, when osteonecrosis presents in the spine, vertebral body collapse and fragmentation are observed. Spinal rheumatoid nodules may cause myelopathy.[52]

Sacroiliac Joints

Sacroiliac joint involvement by RA is infrequent and mild as opposed to the radiologic abnormalities that characterize sacroiliac joint disease in ankylosing spondylitis. Overlap with ankylosing spondylitis should be suspected in rheumatoid patients who possess the HLA-B27 antigen and have severe sacroiliac joint involvement.[13] Sacroiliac joint abnormalities in RA include erosions that preferentially affect the iliac aspect of the joint and mild joint space narrowing. Unlike ankylosing spondylitis, the distribution in RA tends to be asymmetric. Asymptomatic radiographic abnormalities of the sacroiliac joints may be present in up to 35% of patients with long-standing disease.[13]

Computed Tomography

CT provides 3D information regarding joint structures and their alteration by RA. The strengths of CT are its relatively rapid acquisition time and multiplanar capabilities. The projection superimposition present on radiographs by overlapping structures that may obscure erosions or mimic joint space narrowing is eliminated by CT's multiplanar capabilities. However, the increased radiation dose, additional time required to interpret CT examinations, and high cost in comparison to radiographs have not warranted CT as the primary imaging modality in RA.

As with radiography, contrast among soft tissue structures is limited on CT. Even with the use of intravenous (IV) iodinated contrast material during CT examination, MRI is far superior to CT in visualizing subtle alterations in the soft tissues. Given the advantages of other imaging modalities, CT in the clinical management of RA is generally reserved for special circumstances, such as evaluation of the skull base and cervical spine, several of the extraskeletal manifestations of RA (Table 20-8), or when MRI is contraindicated, such as with a pacemaker or cerebral artery aneurysm clip or when the patient is unable to hold still for the relatively long time of MR image acquisition.

Arthrography

Arthrography has nearly been replaced by MRI and now has a limited role in the evaluation of RA patients. Synovial enlargement and contour irregularity as evidence of synovitis may be seen on arthrography (Figure 20-12). Intraarticular or bursal communication of synovial cysts or cutaneous fistulas draining joints may be delineated during arthrography. Arthrography may be used to document the intraarticular placement of therapeutic agents or gadolinium contrast material for subsequent MR arthrography. Common uses for MR arthrography in patients with RA include documentation of rotator cuff tears and the evaluation of glenoid labral abnormalities (Table 20-8).

Magnetic Resonance Imaging

MRI is superior to other imaging modalities in its ability to resolve soft tissue structures and detect inflammation and abnormalities in the bone marrow. These soft tissue and bone marrow alterations are generally present early in the disease course before radiographic changes are visible. Early detection of disease by MRI may prove invaluable in the initial management of newly diagnosed patients with RA. Early diagnosis of RA is now a high priority, because new disease-modifying therapies show the most promise when used early before irreversible disability has occurred.[1,53]

Although the lack of routine clinical guidelines and high cost currently impede the routine use of MRI in establishing early diagnosis or in monitoring therapy/disease course in RA, MRI is an important area of research. Recently, a grading scheme has been developed to standardize the quantification of synovitis, bone edema, and erosions in the wrist and MCP joints.[54] The grading scheme has been validated in several studies.[55-57]

MRI is also an invaluable tool to address complications and unusual manifestations of RA. In addition to examining the joint manifestations of RA, MRI is useful for targeting complications related to RA pannus and extraskeletal manifestations of RA, such as the degree of cord compression in atlantoaxial subluxation, insufficiency or stress fractures, and tendon abnormalities (see Table 20-8).

Synovitis

Inflammation in the synovium, although subject to some controversy, is considered to be the primary process that leads to joint

TABLE 20-7. Measurements for Identifying Atlantoaxial Impaction (Vertical Subluxation)

Method	Diagram	Normal Values
McGregor's line	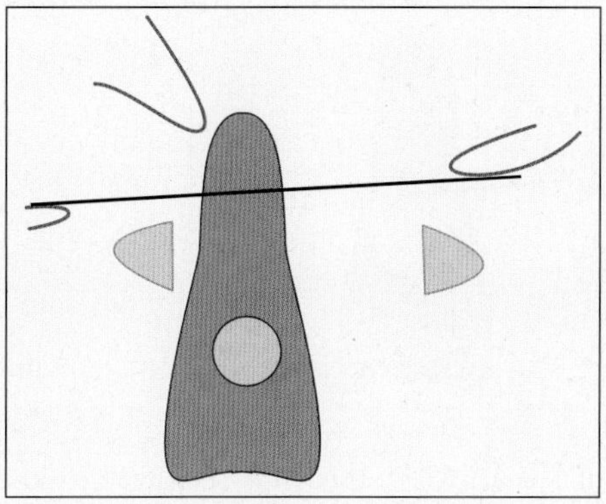	≤ 8 mm men; ≤ 9.7 mm women
Ranawat line	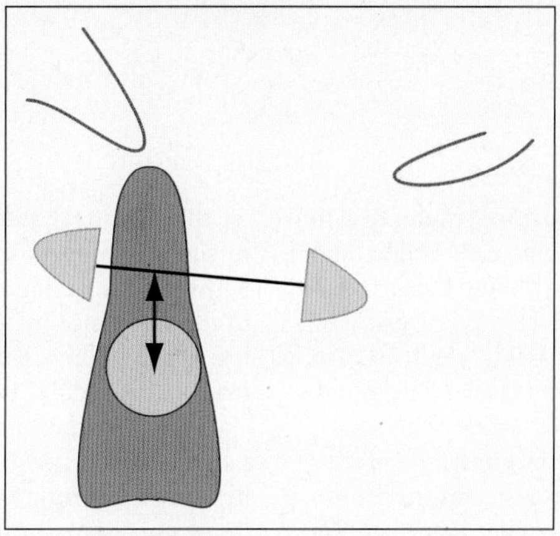	≥ 15 mm men; ≥ 13 mm women
Redlund-Johnell	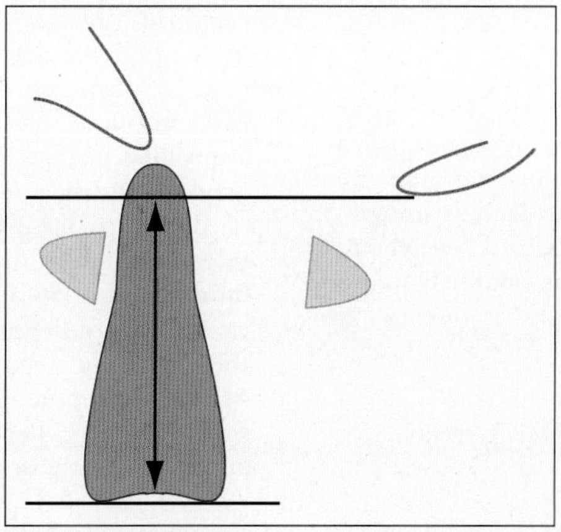	≥ 34 mm men; ≥ 29 mm women

(Continued)

derangement in RA. MRI depicts inflammation by the amount of synovial enlargement and by the degree of synovial edema/blood perfusion. Synovitis may occur at any synovium-lined joint. Synovial inflammation tends to affect the hands, wrists, and feet prior to the more proximal joints (hind feet, ankles, knees, elbows, shoulders, and hips). Studies that examine the utility of MRI for rheumatoid synovitis usually examine alterations in the hands and feet. Synovitis is characterized on MRI by synovial enlargement (pannus) with or without enhancement after IV gadolinium contrast injection.

MRI allows pannus to be differentiated from joint effusion.

Active synovitis shows avid enhancement on fat-suppressed T1-weighted images and is greater in thickness than normal

TABLE 20-7. Measurements for Identifying Atlantoaxial Impaction (Vertical Subluxation)—cont'd

Method	Diagram	Normal Values
Kauppi		Inferior margin of C1 arch lies at or below the level of the top of the C2 sclerotic ring

Figures redrawn from Roche CJ, Eyes BE, Whitehouse GH: The rheumatoid cervical spine: signs of instability on plain cervical radiographs, *Clin Radiol* 57:241-249, 2002.

synovium.[54] Active synovitis should be imaged approximately 6 to 11 minutes after contrast injection to best delineate bright and thickened synovium from the surrounding dark joint fluid. Imaging after this point in time will increase the likelihood of gadolinium contrast material diffusing into the joint fluid, which in turn will create an overestimation of the degree of synovial thickening or pannus volume. Decrease in the degree of active synovitis is believed to represent a favorable treatment response.[58] Inactive pannus will lack avid enhancement after contrast administration and is relatively isointense to skeletal muscle. The quantification of synovial volume has also been evaluated for the diagnosis and monitoring of RA.[59-61]

Bone Marrow Edema

Bone marrow edema is characterized on MRI by high-signal foci with ill-defined margins that are neither erosions nor cysts. Bone marrow edema has no radiographic correlate and is unique to MRI. It is best demonstrated on fat-suppressed T2-weighted or short tau inversion recovery (STIR) images and may indicate increased water or focal increased blood flow in response to external attack by the inflamed synovium.[58] Bone edema can occur in isolation or surround an erosion or geode.

> The term *geode* is sometimes used to refer to large cystic changes in subchondral bone in arthritis.

Common locations for bone marrow edema in the hands and feet include the carpal and tarsal bones and bones adjacent to the MCP joints.[25]

Bone marrow edema may predict future erosion.[62,63] The amount of bone marrow edema has been shown to be greater in patients with established RA than in patients with seronegative spondyloarthropathies.[60]

Bone Erosions

An erosion on MR images is defined as a focal defect in normal bone cortex with or without a defect in the adjacent trabecular bone. Normal cortex is low in signal intensity on both T1-weighted and T2-weighted images and is smoothly marginated by the periosteal soft tissues and bone marrow, which are higher in signal intensity. The tissue inside the erosion may enhance on T1-weighted images after gadolinium administration owing to the presence of inflamed synovium within the defect (Figure 20-13). This enhancement may be used to distinguish erosions from juxtaarticular geodes.[64]

Erosions are more prevalent in wrists affected by RA (97% of patients with known RA versus 14% of controls).[65] Most studies describe a superior sensitivity for the detection of erosions on MR images in comparison with radiography.[66-69] In addition, more erosions may be detected early in the disease course using MRI than using radiography.[63,70,71] A few studies describe comparable sensitivity in erosion detection between radiographic and MRI techniques[71,72]; however, this may be attributable in part to inadequate MRI technique.[73] Multiplanar (axial, coronal, and sagittal planes) acquisition may increase sensitivity, and post-gadolinium imaging may decrease the rate of false-positive erosion detection.[62]

Bone erosions present on MR images may be important predictors of future outcome for patients with RA. Low erosion burden and a low total overall MRI score suggest a better outcome with a decrease in the development of new erosions.[63] Furthermore, bone marrow edema, synovial volume, and overall MRI score appear to predict the development of new bone erosions.[59,63] Once erosions on MRI develop, they persist and appear to be irreversible.[63,72,74]

Juxtaarticular Pseudocysts

These cystic lesions (or pseudocysts because they have no epithelial lining) are fluid-containing structures that develop at juxtaarticular locations in bone.[30] Pathologic processes postulated to form pseudocysts in the bones of patients with RA include migration of synovial fluid under pressure into the adjacent bone (geodes), extension of pannus into bone, and intramedullary rheumatoid nodules.[15,29,30] As with any fluid-containing structure, pseudocysts have low signal on T1-weighted images and high signal on T2-weighted images. MRI more reliably demonstrates juxtaarticular pseudocysts than radiographs.[75-77] No predictive value has been described yet to the presence or absence of pseudocysts in RA.

TABLE 20-8. Complications and Extraarticular Manifestations of RA: Imaging Modality Selection

Location and Clinical Problem	Recommended Modality	Expected Imaging Finding
GENERAL		
Entrapment neuropathy	US, MRI	Mass, nerve enlargement
Stress/insufficiency fracture	R, MRI, NM	Sclerosis, bone edema with or without fracture line, increased activity
Osteomyelitis, septic arthritis	R, MRI*, NM	Erosion, bone edema, sinus tract, enhancement
Osteonecrosis	R, MRI	Sclerosis, serpentine regions of necrosis
Intraarticular bodies	MRI, CT,† US	Fragments, such as of cartilage or rice bodies
Osteopenia/osteoporosis	D	Decreased bone mineral density
Vasculitis	CT*, MRI*, A	Vessel narrowing
UPPER EXTREMITY		
Rotator cuff tear	US, MRI†	Discontinuity of rotator cuff
LOWER EXTREMITY		
Sinus tarsi syndrome	MRI	Synovial proliferation in sinus tarsi
Pes planovalgus	US, MRI	Tendon degeneration/rupture
Achilles' tear	US, MRI	Thickened, with or without disrupted tendon
Plantar fasciitis	US, MRI	Thickened plantar fascia with edema
Popliteal cyst	US, MRI	Large mass in posterior knee/calf
SPINE		
Myelopathy	MRI, CT	Cord compression, cord edema/atrophy, RA nodule
PELVIS		
Iliopsoas bursitis	US, MRI	Enlarged bursa
LUNG		
Pulmonary fibrosis, pneumonitis	R, CT	Consolidation, interstitial thickening, honeycombing
Pleuritis, pleuropericarditis, vasculitis	CT*, US	Pericardial effusion/thickening, vessel narrowing
Rheumatoid nodule	CT	Pulmonary nodule with soft tissue density
Methotrexate lung	R, CT	Parenchymal opacification, interstitial thickening
ABDOMINAL		
Bowel perforation	R, CT*	Free intraperitoneal air, distended bowel with or without wall thickening
Felty's syndrome	US, CT	Enlarged spleen

A, Angiography; *CT*, computed tomography; *D*, densitometry (dual energy x-ray absorptiometry); *MRI*, magnetic resonance imaging; *NM*, nuclear medicine; *R*, radiographs; *US*, ultrasonography.
*Intravenous contrast material is recommended.
†Intraarticular contrast material is recommended.

Rheumatoid Nodules

Rheumatoid nodules are common in RA and appear in approximately 25% of patients.[78] Rheumatoid nodules favor subcutaneous tissues at pressure points, such as adjacent to bony protuberances. The posterior elbow is a common location. Nodules usually have an insidious onset and may persist unchanged for years. MRI shows an irregularly marginated mass in the subcutaneous tissues. Rheumatoid nodules appear isointense to muscle on T1-weighted images and hypointense (solid lesion) or hyperintense (cystic lesion) on T2-weighted images.[79,80] Enhancement characteristics are variable and may show intense or faint solid or ring enhancement.[79,80]

Complications of rheumatoid nodules include ulceration, superinfection, sinus tract formation, and sepsis.[78] Nodules may also appear in the abdominal wall, pleura, and lungs.

Tendons

Tendon abnormalities arising from RA may be demonstrated on MRI and include tendinopathy, tenosynovitis, and partial or complete rupture. The most common tendons referred for imaging evaluation include those about the ankles, wrists, and hands. Tendon involvement as demonstrated by MRI tends to increase with disease progression and is infrequent in early RA.[62,63] Tenosynovitis is shown on MRI by increased fluid in the tendon sheath, sheath thickening, or enhancement (Figure 20-14). Tenosynovitis and tendon tears may be better demonstrated on MR images than by clinical exam.[81]

MRI may demonstrate tendon abnormalities not detectable on clinical examination.

MRI characteristics of tendinopathy and partial rupture usually include fusiform enlargement of the tendon and intrasubstance

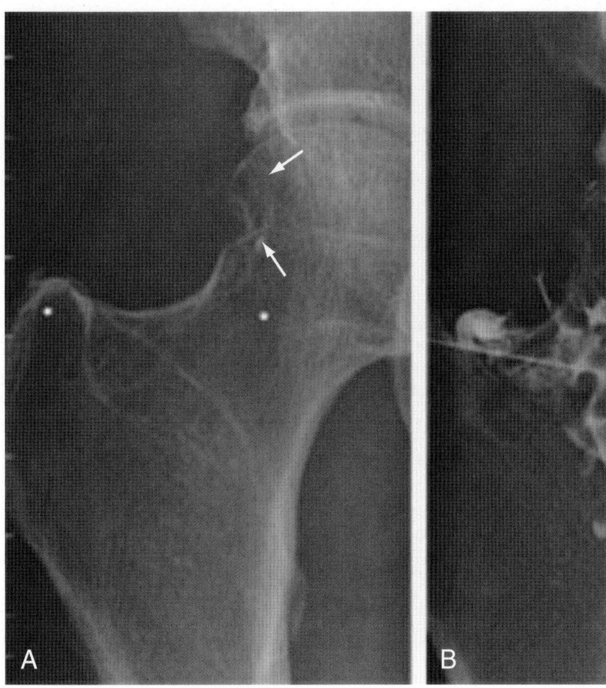

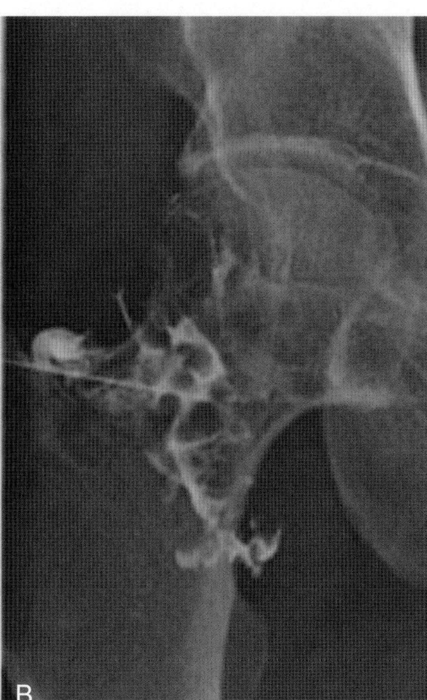

FIGURE 20-12. Hip erosions and synovitis in a patient with 25-year history of RA and acute hip pain evaluated by arthrography. **A,** Erosions are present at the lateral aspect of the femoral head *(arrows).* Metallic BBs mark the site for needle placement for the subsequent arthrogram. **B,** Arthrogram with needle still in place demonstrates multiple round filling defects that represent synovial hypertrophy/ hyperplasia. (Courtesy of R. Klecker, MD, Brigham and Women's Hospital, Boston.)

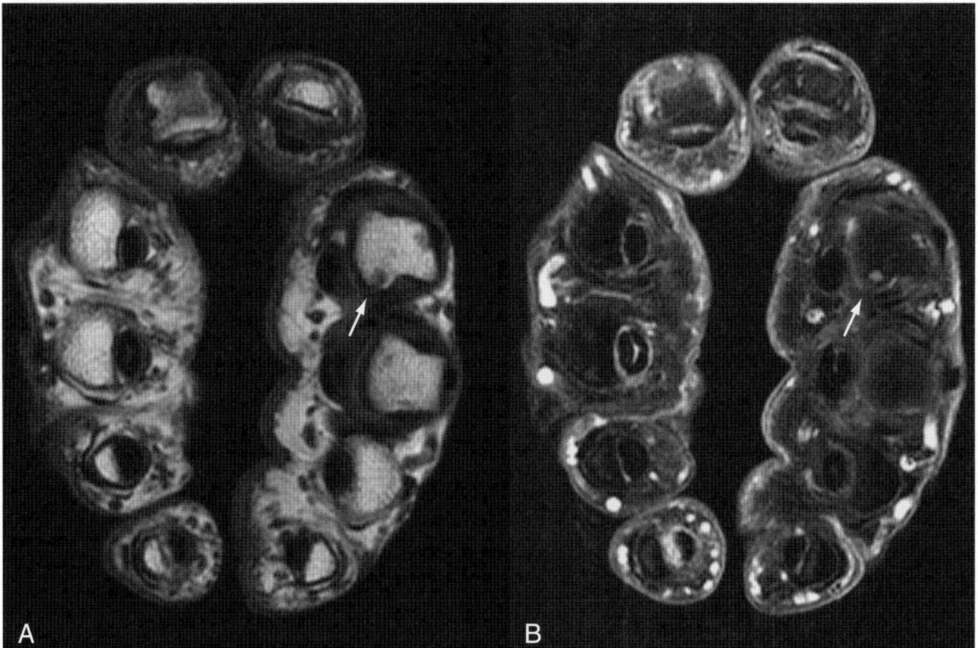

FIGURE 20-13. Erosion and synovitis demonstrated on MRI of a 74-year-old woman with RA and normal radiographs (not shown). **A,** T1-weighted axial image (TR/TE = 437/20) of both hands reveals erosion *(arrow)* at the head of the left index finger metacarpal. **B,** Enhancement in this erosion after IV gadolinium contrast material administration on the fat-suppressed T1-weighted image (TR/TE = 437/20) likely represents infiltrating pannus.

high signal intensity on both T1-weighted and T2-weighted images. When the intrasubstance signal intensity is as bright as fluid on T2-weighted images or there is contour irregularity along the margins of the tendons, tear is likely. Complete tear manifests as complete disruption of the tendon fibers, and the tendon ends may be retracted. Posterior tibial tendon rupture is a well-known complication of RA and may lead to unilateral or bilateral flat foot deformities.[82,83]

> Posterior tibial tendon rupture may lead to a flat foot deformity. The patient will be unable to stand on her toes and will exhibit the "too many toes" sign; when viewed from behind, the toes are visible along the lateral side of the foot.

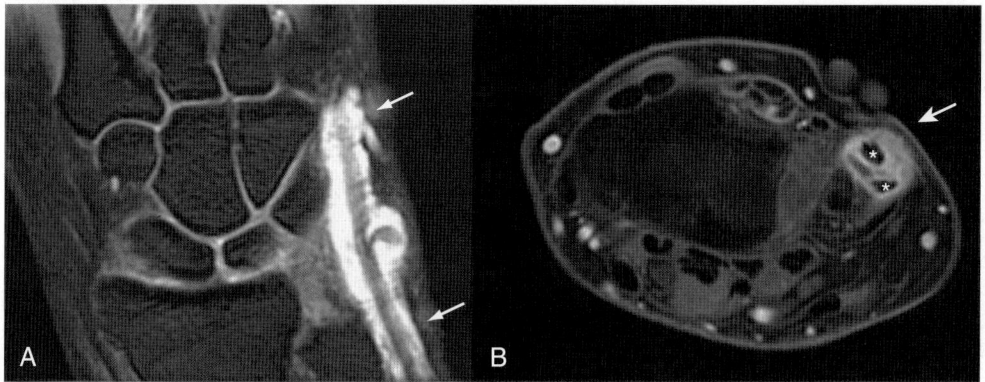

FIGURE 20-14. Tenosynovitis demonstrated on MRI. Coronal **(A)** and axial **(B)** gradient echo (TR/TE = 205/3, flip angle = 90 degrees) fat-suppressed images of the wrist show tendon sheath enhancement *(arrows)*, enlargement, and split tear of the extensor carpi ulnaris tendon *(asterisks)*.

Bursae and Popliteal Cysts

Inflammation of a bursa is common in RA; typical locations for bursitis include the retrocalcaneal, olecranon, iliopsoas, intermetatarsal, and submetatarsal bursae.

> A bursa is an enclosed fluid-filled sac located at points of friction (e.g., between tendon and bone).

Bursitis is a nonspecific finding and can be encountered in seronegative spondyloarthropathies, trauma, infection, or hemorrhage. Bursitis usually appears on MRI as a thick-walled cystic structure, and the cyst wall may enhance after gadolinium contrast material administration.

A popliteal cyst is another structure that arises adjacent to joints and may be involved by RA; however, unlike bursae, popliteal cysts communicate with the knee joint. Popliteal cysts develop by herniation of the synovial membrane through the joint capsule between the semimembranosus tendon and the medial head of the gastrocnemius muscle. Popliteal cysts may become very large and dissect down the posterior calf (see Figure 20-7) and accumulate rice bodies (composed of fibrin). MRI also helps distinguish symptomatic cysts from thrombophlebitis and may identify various complications of enlarged popliteal cysts, such as cyst rupture and compression of venous or neural structures.

Scintigraphy

The possibility of whole body imaging makes scintigraphy a promising candidate for the detection and monitoring of RA. Scintigraphy may be useful for objective and global assessment of disease activity. Although scintigraphy lacks fine spatial resolution, the evaluation of multiple joints or whole body assessment during one imaging session is possible. Abnormal activity on whole body scintigraphy may help target specific joints for evaluation with focused ultrasound or MRI. Cost and administration of radioisotopes are relative barriers to widespread clinical use.

A typical pattern of radiopharmaceutical localization in RA consists of abnormally increased activity in the peripheral joints. Localization to the extremities tends to occur symmetrically and is most prominent in the wrists, MCP and PIP joints of the hands, MTP and interphalangeal joints of the feet, knees, and elbows. Increased uptake may also occur in the cervical spine and temporomandibular joints.

Scintigraphy may detect inflammation or bone turnover at sites of active erosion. Several approaches for evaluating RA have been tested with bone, joint, metabolic, and inflammation-seeking radiopharmaceutical agents. Scintigraphic techniques rely on specific imaging probes to target disease activity. Common radiolabeled probes include bisphosphonates to detect bone turnover and leukocytes to detect inflammation. Molecular probes that may have utility for RA include albumin nanocolloid, immunoglobulins (specific and nonspecific), and ^{18}F-fluoro-deoxy-glucose (F-18-FDG).[84-86]

Ultrasonography

Ultrasonography is a quick, safe, and widely available imaging modality for the assessment of soft tissue and bone involvement by RA. The value of ultrasonography in patents with RA and the number of anatomic sites where ultrasonography is useful for diagnosis, monitoring, and intervention have expanded over recent years. This trend is likely to continue. The low cost of ultrasound in comparison with MRI and the lack of ionizing radiation in comparison with CT or radiography make ultrasound an appealing choice for examining RA changes in joints.

Familiarity with the appearance of RA manifestations on sonographic images and experience of operators in scanning joints have lead to regional and national differences in the application of ultrasound for RA. Another important limitation of ultrasound is its requirement for an acoustic window (a path for ultrasound waves). Restrained positioning of the ultrasound transducer and the inability for sound to penetrate through cortical bone will limit the joint structures that may be visualized by ultrasound.

More common anatomic regions for ultrasound examination in patients with RA include the hands, shoulders, knees, hips, and tendons. Gray-scale ultrasound performed with high-frequency linear array transducers visualizes synovial membrane thickening, bone erosions, and joint effusions. Ultrasound may be used to detect and characterize rheumatoid nodules, enthesopathy, and tendon rupture. Ultrasound may also provide guidance for tissue biopsy, the intraarticular placement of medications, or aspiration of an effusion to help exclude septic arthritis.

Synovitis

Sonography is very sensitive in detecting synovitis and is comparable with MRI for detecting synovitis in the hands.[87,88] Synovial enlargement is defined by its irregular thickening of the synovial membrane and its hypoechogenic texture as compared with intraarticular soft tissue.[89] Increased vascularity in synovium as demonstrated by flow signal on color or power Doppler ultrasound may serve as a

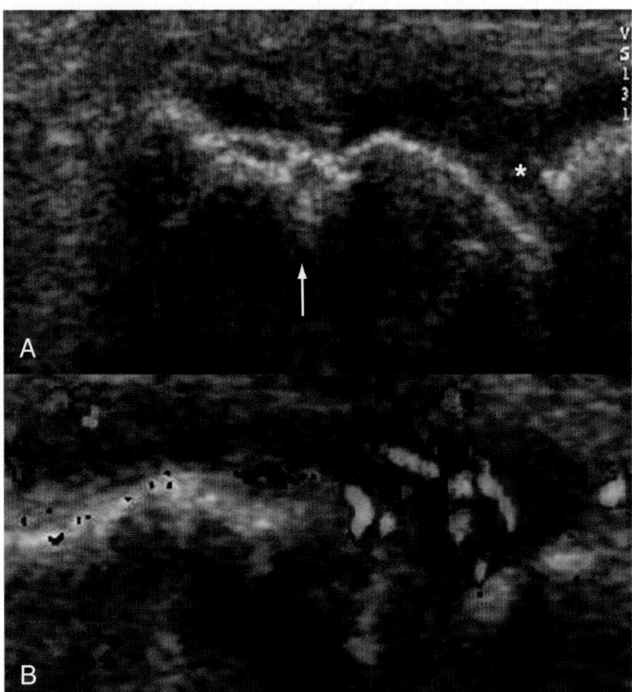

FIGURE 20-15. Erosion and synovitis demonstrated on ultrasound of a 76-year-old woman with RA and normal radiographs (not shown). **A,** Gray-scale image with erosion *(arrow)* adjacent to the MCP joint *(asterisk)*. **B,** The power Doppler image shows flow *(orange)* in the hypoechoic pannus superficial to the erosion. (Courtesy of L. Nazarian, MD, Thomas Jefferson University, Philadelphia.)

marker of proliferative or active synovium (Figure 20-15). Identification of active synovium may improve assessment of disease activity as compared with clinical exam.[88,89]

Erosions

Ultrasonography is a very sensitive method for detection of erosions and may detect more erosions than radiography.[90] An erosion on ultrasound appears as a cortical disruption or defect with an irregular floor (see Figure 20-15). Recording this cortical irregularity on more than one imaging plane (i.e., transverse and longitudinal scan planes) will increase the diagnostic confidence that the visualized defect actually represents an erosion.[89]

Tendon Involvement

As with MRI, sonography is useful to demonstrate tendon involvement by RA. Tendons are usually easily accessible for visualization by ultrasound due to their proximity to the skin. With their regularly aligned and tightly bound connective tissues, normal tendons show a characteristic homogeneous echogenic structure, and rheumatoid changes to this structure are often readily demonstrated by ultrasound. Early stages of inflammation will show alterations in tendon echogenicity due to edema within the tendon fibers.[91,92] Tendon thickening, heterogeneity, and increased tendon fluid are consequences of inflammation that may be visualized on ultrasound. The sequelae of chronic or advanced tendon involvement by RA, such as tendon degeneration and tear, may also be demonstrated with ultrasound.

> Tendon abnormalities are well demonstrated on ultrasound examination.

Documenting rupture of the tibialis posterior tendon as a cause of spontaneous flat foot, pain, and disability is a common indication for ultrasound tendon imaging in RA. Achilles' tendinopathy and partial or complete tendon tears are also amenable to diagnosis with ultrasound.

Extraarticular Imaging of RA

Metabolic Disorders

Several metabolic processes are altered in patients with RA. Alterations in energy and protein metabolism and inflammatory cytokine production appear to lead to accelerated loss of body cell mass.[93] Patients with RA also experience an increased frequency of cardiac disease in comparison with patients with OA; this increase may correlate with decreased insulin sensitivity and serum levels of high-density lipoprotein.[94]

Accelerated bone loss is another common metabolic problem with an associated increase in morbidity from osteoporotic fractures. Two types of bone loss are recognized in patients with RA: the localized periarticular osteopenia due to local disease activity and generalized bone loss. Multiple risk factors likely result in increases in bone loss and include disease duration, reduced mobility, corticosteroid therapy, and menopause.[95] Bone loss in RA may be independent from menopause[96] and glucocorticoid therapy.[2] Routine densitometry is recommended to monitor the rate of bone loss and help in adjusting therapies to prevent osteoporosis.[2] Digital x-ray radiogrammetry is an investigative technique that may be more sensitive than the currently used dual x-ray absorptiometry for detecting early bone losss.[97] Insufficiency fractures that result from osteoporosis may be diagnosed with a multimodality imaging approach.[98]

Rheumatoid Neuropathies

Patients with RA are susceptible to central and peripheral neuropathies.[99] Lesions that affect the brain include rheumatoid nodule formation, infarction, and hemorrhage from vascular disease, as well as amyloidosis. A multimodality imaging approach with CT, CT angiography, MRI, and/or MR angiography is useful to evaluate patients with RA who present with encephalopathy. Spinal cord lesions that directly result from RA include mass effect and infiltration by rheumatoid nodules, hemorrhage, infarction, infection, and vertebral subluxation. MRI targeted to the level of myelopathy, such as the cervical, thoracic, or lumbar spine, will help narrow the diagnostic possibilities.

Peripheral neuropathies in RA may arise from nerve entrapment or vasculitis. Ultrasound and MRI are useful for diagnosis of a mechanical cause for irritation of a specific nerve distribution and potentially guide treatment options. Common sites of peripheral neuropathies in RA include the median nerve (carpal tunnel of the wrist and), ulnar nerve (cubital canal of the elbow and Guyon's canal of the wrist), radial nerve (radial tunnel of the elbow), sciatic/tibia/common peroneal nerve (posterior knee and calf where the tibial nerve can be compressed by a popliteal cyst), and posterior tibial nerve and its medial and lateral plantar branches (tarsal tunnel of the ankle).[100]

Lung Manifestations

Pulmonary involvement is one of the most prevalent extraarticular manifestations of RA, and interstitial lung disease is the most common pulmonary manifestation.[101] Lung manifestations of RA include interstitial lung disease, pleural disease, pulmonary rheumatoid nodules, upper and lower airway obstruction, amyloidosis, vasculitis, and pulmonary hypertension. Patients with RA are also at risk for drug-induced lung disease, such as methotrexate toxicity, and pulmonary infections. Radiographs are usually the first step in identifying pulmonary abnormalities and may be used to follow progression of parenchymal lung disease. A high-resolution CT exam can further characterize findings on radiography as well as reveal additional pathology and fine lung detail.

Felty's Syndrome

The association of RA with chronic neutropenia and splenomegaly has been termed *Felty's syndrome.*[102] Felty's syndrome is considered to be a rare complication of RA (< 1% of patients). The syndrome usually manifests in the fifth, sixth, or seventh decade with arthritis, anemia, adenopathy, leg ulceration, and abnormal skin pigmentation. The destructive arthritis in Felty's syndrome can become severe, and systemic abnormalities such as Sjögren's syndrome may develop. Patients are susceptible to recurrent bacterial infections, particularly in the skin and lungs, presumably from neutropenia and altered neutrophil chemotactic migration.[103] An abdominal ultrasound would be the first step in confirming clinically suspected splenomegaly. Anemia appears to be the result of hemolysis and may improve with splenectomy.

ALGORITHMS AND RECOMMENDATIONS

Where to start when the working diagnosis is RA? Accurate diagnosis is based on clinical criteria, and imaging is one of the parameters used to make the diagnosis. Box 20-1 describes the current ACR classification tree criteria for RA. When four of the seven criteria are met, RA is considered the diagnosis.[6]

The imaging portion of the criteria will likely be modified to incorporate the early detection of arthritis by ultrasound and MRI.[104,105] One proposal for early detection of RA by MRI is to identify patients who present with the clinical suspicion but have normal radiographs and fail to meet the strict classification criteria of rheumatoid arthritis. A decision tree was developed and described by Sugimoto to identify early disease in such patients using MRI.[104] Eventually MRI, ultrasound, and/or scintigraphy may be used for prognosis and serve as a more sensitive baseline to establish the efficacy of new therapies.[105]

Imaging also serves multiple roles outside the diagnosis and monitoring of the primary disease process. Patients with RA are predisposed to a variety of complications in and around the joints that may overlap with the signs and symptoms of RA. Imaging can help identify these abnormalities. Some of the complications in the joint include septic arthritis, osteomyelitis, amyloidosis, and osteoporotic fractures. Given the complications associated with the disease and treatment, there are a multitude of areas where imaging can benefit patients and reduce morbidity. Table 20-8 may serve as a guide in deciding what imaging tests would be the appropriate first step in working up some of the more common complications associated with RA.

References

1. O'Dell JR: Treating rheumatoid arthritis early: a window of opportunity? *Arthritis Rheum* 46:283-285, 2002.
2. Guidelines for the management of rheumatoid arthritis: 2002 update, *Arthritis Rheum* 46:328-346, 2002.
3. Emery P: Treatment of rheumatoid arthritis, *Br Med J* 332:152-155, 2006.
4. Brower AC: Use of the radiograph to measure the course of rheumatoid arthritis. The gold standard versus fool's gold, *Arthritis Rheum* 33:316-324, 1990.
5. Watt I: Basic differential diagnosis of arthritis, *Eur Radiol* 7:344-351, 1997.
6. Arnett FC, Edworthy SM, Bloch DA et al: The American Rheumatism Association 1987 revised criteria for the classification of rheumatoid arthritis, *Arthritis Rheum* 31:315-324, 1988.
7. Sharp JT: Measurement of structural abnormalities in arthritis using radiographic images, *Radiol Clin North Am* 42:109-119, 2004.
8. Hollingsworth JW, Saykaly RJ: Systemic complications of rheumatoid arthritis, *Med Clin North Am* 61:217-228, 1977.
9. Romas E: Bone loss in inflammatory arthritis: mechanisms and therapeutic approaches with bisphosphonates, *Best Pract Res Clin Rheumatol* 19:1065-1079, 2005.
10. Maini SR: Infliximab treatment of rheumatoid arthritis, *Rheum Dis Clin North Am* 30:329-347, vii, 2004.
11. Sharp JT, Van Der Heijde D, Boers Met al: Repair of erosions in rheumatoid arthritis does occur. Results from 2 studies by the OMERACT Subcommittee on Healing of Erosions, *J Rheumatol* 30:1102-1107, 2003.
12. Ikari K, Momohara S: Images in clinical medicine. Bone changes in rheumatoid arthritis, *N Engl J Med* 353:e13, 2005.
13. Resnick D, Kransdorf MJ: *Bone and joint imaging*, Philadelphia, 2005, Elsevier.
14. Solomon L: Patterns of osteoarthritis of the hip, *J Bone Joint Surg Br* 58:176-183, 1976.
15. Martel W, Hayes JT, Duff IF: The pattern of bone erosion in the hand and wrist in rheumatoid arthritis, *Radiology* 84:204-214, 1965.
16. Berens DL, Lockie LM, Lin RK et al: Roentgen changes in early rheumatoid arthritis. Wrists—hands—feet, *Radiology* 82:645-654, 1964.
17. Mall JC, Genant HK, Silcox DC et al: The efficacy of fine-detail radiography in the evaluation of patients with rheumatoid arthritis, *Radiology* 112:37-42, 1974.
18. Guermazi A, Taouli B, Lynch JA et al: Imaging of bone erosion in rheumatoid arthritis, *Semin Musculoskelet Radiol* 8:269-285, 2004.
19. Swanson AB, Swanson GG: Pathogenesis and pathomechanics of rheumatoid deformities in the hand and wrist, *Orthop Clin North Am* 4:1039-1056, 1973.
20. Williams M, Barton E: Terminal phalangeal sclerosis in rheumatoid arthritis, *Clin Radiol* 35:237-238, 1984.
21. Resnick D: Rheumatoid arthritis of the wrist: why the ulnar styloid? *Radiology* 112:29-35, 1974.
22. Buchberger W: Radiologic imaging of the carpal tunnel, *Eur J Radiol* 25:112-117, 1997.
23. Weston WJ: The soft-tissue signs of the enlarged ulnar bursa in rheumatoid arthritis, *J Can Assoc Radiol* 24:282-288, 1973.
24. Linscheid RL, Dobyns JH, Beckenbaugh RD et al: Instability patterns of the wrist, *J Hand Surg Am* 8:682-686, 1983.
25. Boutry N, Flipo RM, Cotten A: MR imaging appearance of rheumatoid arthritis in the foot, *Semin Musculoskelet Radiol* 9:199-209, 2005.
26. Bywaters EG: Heel lesions of rheumatoid arthritis, *Ann Rheum Dis* 13:42-51, 1954.
27. Weissman BN, Sosman JL: The radiology of rheumatoid arthritis, *Orthop Clin North Am* 6:653-674, 1975.
28. Karasick D, Schweitzer ME, O'Hara BJ: Distal fibular notch: a frequent manifestation of the rheumatoid ankle, *Skeletal Radiol* 26:529-532, 1997.
29. Magyar E, Talerman A, Feher M et al: Giant bone cysts in rheumatoid arthritis, *J Bone Joint Surg Br* 56:121-129, 1974.
30. Bullough PG, Bansal M: The differential diagnosis of geodes, *Radiol Clin North Am* 26:1165-1184, 1988.
31. Resnick D, Niwayama G: *Diagnosis of bone and joint disorders*, Philadelphia, 1981, Saunders, pp 123-125.
32. Sweeney JP, Helms CA, Minagi H et al: The widened teardrop distance: a plain film indicator of hip joint effusion in adults, *AJR Am J Roentgenol* 149:117-119, 1987.
33. Hastings DE, Parker SM: Protrusio acetabuli in rheumatoid arthritis, *Clin Orthop Relat Res* 108:76-83, 1975.
34. Steinberg ME, Hayken GD, Steinberg DR: A quantitative system for staging avascular necrosis, *J Bone Joint Surg Br* 77:34-41, 1995.
35. Ficat RP: Idiopathic bone necrosis of the femoral head. Early diagnosis and treatment, *J Bone Joint Surg Br* 67:3-9, 1985.
36. Gardeniers JW: ARCO Committee on Terminology and Staging; Report on the Committee-Meeting at Santiago De Compostela, *ARCO News Lett* 5:79-82, 1993.
37. Mitchell DG, Rao VM, Dalinka MK et al: Femoral head avascular necrosis: correlation of MR imaging, radiographic staging, radionuclide imaging, and clinical findings, *Radiology* 162:709-715, 1987.
38. Mitchell MD, Kundel HL, Steinberg ME et al: Avascular necrosis of the hip: comparison of MR, CT, and scintigraphy, *AJR Am J Roentgenol* 147:67-71, 1986.
39. Thomas T, Noel E, Goupille P et al: The rheumatoid shoulder: current consensus on diagnosis and treatment, *Joint Bone Spine* 73(2):139-143, 2005.
40. Resnick D: Rheumatoid arthritis. In *Diagnosis of bone and joint disorders*, vol 2, Philadelphia, 2002, Saunders, pp 891-987.
41. Park WM, O'Neill M, McCall IW: The radiology of rheumatoid involvement of the cervical spine, *Skeletal Radiol* 4:1-7, 1979.
42. Weissman BN, Aliabadi P, Weinfeld MS et al: Prognostic features of atlantoaxial subluxation in rheumatoid arthritis patients, *Radiology* 144:745-751, 1982.
43. El-Khoury GY, Wener MH, Menezes AH et al: Cranial settling in rheumatoid arthritis, *Radiology* 137:637-642, 1980.
44. Swinson DR, Hamilton EB, Mathews JA et al: Vertical subluxation of the axis in rheumatoid arthritis, *Ann Rheum Dis* 31:359-363, 1972.
45. Martel W: The occipito-atlanto-axial joints in rheumatoid arthritis and ankylosing spondylitis, *Am J Roentgenol Radium Ther Nucl Med* 86:223-240, 1961.
46. Boden S, Dodge L, Bohlmann H et al: Rheumatoid arthritis of the cervical spine: a long-term analysis with predictors of paralysis and recovery, *J Bone Joint Surg Am* 75(9):1282-1297, 1993.
47. Meikle JA, Wilkinson M: Rheumatoid involvement of the cervical spine. Radiological assessment, *Ann Rheum Dis* 30:154-161, 1971.
48. McGregor M: The significance of certain measurements of the skull in the diagnosis of basilar impression, *Br J Radiol* 21:171-181, 1948.
49. Riew KD, Hilibrand AS, Palumbo MA et al: Diagnosing basilar invagination in the rheumatoid patient. The reliability of radiographic criteria, *J Bone Joint Surg Am* 83:194-200, 2001.

50. Heywood AW, Meyers OL: Rheumatoid arthritis of the thoracic and lumbar spine, *J Bone Joint Surg Br* 68:362-368, 1986.
51. Lems WF, Jahangier ZN, Raymakers JA et al: Methods to score vertebral deformities in patients with rheumatoid arthritis, *Br J Rheumatol* 36:220-224, 1997.
52. Levy Y, Stalley P, Bleasel J: Thoracic spinal cord compression by a rheumatoid nodule, *Intern Med J* 34:137-138, 2004.
53. Emery P: The Roche Rheumatology Prize Lecture. The optimal management of early rheumatoid disease: the key to preventing disability, *Br J Rheumatol* 33:765-768, 1994.
54. Ostergaard M, Peterfy C, Conaghan P et al: OMERACT Rheumatoid Arthritis Magnetic Resonance Imaging Studies. Core set of MRI acquisitions, joint pathology definitions, and the OMERACT RA-MRI scoring system, *J Rheumatol* 30:1385-1386, 2003.
55. Lassere M, McQueen F, Østergaard M et al: OMERACT Rheumatoid Arthritis Magnetic Resonance Imaging Studies. Exercise 3: an international multicenter reliability study using the RA-MRI Score, *J Rheumatol* 30:1366-1375, 2003.
56. Conaghan P, Lassere M, Østergaard M et al: OMERACT Rheumatoid Arthritis Magnetic Resonance Imaging Studies. Exercise 4: an international multicenter longitudinal study using the RA-MRI Score, *J Rheumatol* 30:1376-1379, 2003.
57. McQueen F, Lassere M, Edmonds J et al: OMERACT Rheumatoid Arthritis Magnetic Resonance Imaging Studies. Summary of OMERACT 6 MR Imaging Module, *J Rheumatol* 30:1387-1392, 2003.
58. McQueen FM: Magnetic resonance imaging in early inflammatory arthritis: what is its role? *Rheumatology (Oxford)* 39:700-706, 2000.
59. Savnik A, Malmskov H, Thomsen HS et al: MRI of the wrist and finger joints in inflammatory joint diseases at 1-year interval: MRI features to predict bone erosions, *Eur Radiol* 12:1203-1210, 2002.
60. Savnik A, Malmskov H, Thomsen HS et al: Magnetic resonance imaging of the wrist and finger joints in patients with inflammatory joint diseases, *J Rheumatol* 28:2193-2200, 2001.
61. Ostergaard M, Hansen M, Stoltenberg M et al: Magnetic resonance imaging-determined synovial membrane volume as a marker of disease activity and a predictor of progressive joint destruction in the wrists of patients with rheumatoid arthritis, *Arthritis Rheum* 42:918-929, 1999.
62. McQueen FM, Stewart N, Crabbe J et al: Magnetic resonance imaging of the wrist in early rheumatoid arthritis reveals a high prevalence of erosions at four months after symptom onset, *Ann Rheum Dis* 57:350-356, 1998.
63. McQueen FM, Stewart N, Crabbe J et al: Magnetic resonance imaging of the wrist in early rheumatoid arthritis reveals progression of erosions despite clinical improvement, *Ann Rheum Dis* 58:156-163, 1999.
64. Cimmino MA, Bountis C, Silvestri E et al: An appraisal of magnetic resonance imaging of the wrist in rheumatoid arthritis, *Semin Arthritis Rheum* 30:180-195, 2000.
65. Pierre-Jerome C, Bekkelund SI, Mellgren SI et al: The rheumatoid wrist: bilateral MR analysis of the distribution of rheumatoid lesions in axial plan in a female population, *Clin Rheumatol* 16:80-86, 1997.
66. Beltran J, Caudill JL, Herman LA et al: Rheumatoid arthritis: MR imaging manifestations, *Radiology* 165:153-157, 1987.
67. Foley-Nolan D, Stack JP, Ryan M et al: Magnetic resonance imaging in the assessment of rheumatoid arthritis—a comparison with plain film radiographs, *Br J Rheumatol* 30:101-106, 1991.
68. Ostergaard M, Gideon P, Sørensen K et al: Scoring of synovial membrane hypertrophy and bone erosions by MR imaging in clinically active and inactive rheumatoid arthritis of the wrist, *Scand J Rheumatol* 24:212-218, 1995.
69. Gilkeson G, Polisson R, Sinclair H et al: Early detection of carpal erosions in patients with rheumatoid arthritis: a pilot study of magnetic resonance imaging, *J Rheumatol* 15:1361-1366, 1988.
70. Backhaus M, Kamradt T, Sandrock D et al: Arthritis of the finger joints: a comprehensive approach comparing conventional radiography, scintigraphy, ultrasound, and contrast-enhanced magnetic resonance imaging, *Arthritis Rheum* 42:1232-1245, 1999.
71. Lindegaard H, Vallo J, Horslev-Petersen K et al: Low field dedicated magnetic resonance imaging in untreated rheumatoid arthritis of recent onset, *Ann Rheum Dis* 60:770-776, 2001.
72. McQueen FM, Benton N, Crabbe J et al: What is the fate of erosions in early rheumatoid arthritis? Tracking individual lesions using x-rays and magnetic resonance imaging over the first two years of disease, *Ann Rheum Dis* 60:859-868, 2001.
73. Tehranzadeh J, Ashikyan O, Dascalos J: Advanced imaging of early rheumatoid arthritis, *Radiol Clin North Am* 42:89-107, 2004.
74. Klarlund M, Ostergaard M, Jensen KE et al: Magnetic resonance imaging, radiography, and scintigraphy of the finger joints: one year follow up of patients with early arthritis. The TIRA Group, *Ann Rheum Dis* 59:521-528, 2000.
75. Moore EA, Jacoby RK, Ellis RE et al: Demonstration of a geode by magnetic resonance imaging: a new light on the cause of juxta-articular bone cysts in rheumatoid arthritis, *Ann Rheum Dis* 49:785-787, 1990.
76. Gubler FM, Algra PR, Maas M et al: Gadolinium-DTPA enhanced magnetic resonance imaging of bone cysts in patients with rheumatoid arthritis, *Ann Rheum Dis* 52:716-719, 1993.
77. Poleksic L, Zdravkovic D, Jablanovic D et al: Magnetic resonance imaging of bone destruction in rheumatoid arthritis: comparison with radiography, *Skeletal Radiol* 22:577-580, 1993.
78. Kaye BR, Kaye RL, Bobrove A: Rheumatoid nodules. Review of the spectrum of associated conditions and proposal of a new classification, with a report of four seronegative cases, *Am J Med* 76:279-292, 1984.
79. Sanders TG, Linares R, Su A: Rheumatoid nodule of the foot: MRI appearances mimicking an indeterminate soft tissue mass, *Skeletal Radiol* 27:457-460, 1998.
80. Theodorou DJ, Theodorou SJ, Farooki S et al: Disorders of the plantar aponeurosis: a spectrum of MR imaging findings, *AJR Am J Roentgenol* 176:97-104, 2001.
81. Stewart NR, McQueen FM, Crabbe JP: Magnetic resonance imaging of the wrist in early rheumatoid arthritis: a pictorial essay, *Australas Radiol* 45:268-273, 2001.
82. Weishaupt D, Schweitzer ME, Alam F et al: MR imaging of inflammatory joint diseases of the foot and ankle, *Skeletal Radiol* 28:663-669, 1999.
83. Rosenberg ZS, Beltran J, Bencardino JT: From the RSNA Refresher Courses. Radiological Society of North America. MR imaging of the ankle and foot, *Radiographics* 20:S153-S179, 2000.
84. Vorne M, Lantto T, Paakkinen S et al: Clinical comparison of 99Tcm-HMPAO labelled leucocytes and 99Tcm-nanocolloid in the detection of inflammation, *Acta Radiol* 30:633-637, 1989.
85. Liberatore M, Clemente M, Iurilli AP et al: Scintigraphic evaluation of disease activity in rheumatoid arthritis: a comparison of technetium-99m human non-specific immunoglobulins, leucocytes and albumin nanocolloids, *Eur J Nucl Med* 19:853-857, 1992.
86. Brenner W: 18F-FDG PET in rheumatoid arthritis: there still is a long way to go, *J Nucl Med* 45:927-929, 2004.
87. Terslev L, Torp-Pedersen S, Savnik A et al: Doppler ultrasound and magnetic resonance imaging of synovial inflammation of the hand in rheumatoid arthritis: a comparative study, *Arthritis Rheum* 48:2434-2441, 2003.
88. Szkudlarek M, Court-Payen M, Strandberg C et al: Power Doppler ultrasonography for assessment of synovitis in the metacarpophalangeal joints of patients with rheumatoid arthritis: a comparison with dynamic magnetic resonance imaging, *Arthritis Rheum* 44:2018-2023, 2001.
89. Hau M, Schultz H, Tony HP et al: Evaluation of pannus and vascularization of the metacarpophalangeal and proximal interphalangeal joints in rheumatoid arthritis by high-resolution ultrasound (multidimensional linear array), *Arthritis Rheum* 42:2303-2308, 1999.
90. Wakefield RJ, Gibbon WW, Conaghan PG et al: The value of sonography in the detection of bone erosions in patients with rheumatoid arthritis: a comparison with conventional radiography, *Arthritis Rheum* 43:2762-2770, 2000.
91. Gibbon WW: Ultrasound in arthritis and inflammation, *Semin Musculoskelet Radiol* 2:307-320, 1998.
92. Read JW: Musculoskeletal ultrasound: basic principles, *Semin Musculoskelet Radiol* 2:203-210, 1998.
93. Rall LC, Roubenoff R: Rheumatoid cachexia: metabolic abnormalities, mechanisms and interventions, *Rheumatology (Oxford)* 43:1219-1223, 2004.
94. Dessein PH, Joffe BI, Stanwix AE: Effects of disease modifying agents and dietary intervention on insulin resistance and dyslipidemia in inflammatory arthritis: a pilot study, *Arthritis Res* 4:R12, 2002.
95. Bijlsma JW: Bone metabolism in patients with rheumatoid arthritis, *Clin Rheumatol* 7:16-23, 1988.
96. Tourinho TF, Stein A, Castro JA et al: Rheumatoid arthritis: evidence for bone loss in premenopausal women, *J Rheumatol* 32:1020-1025, 2005.
97. Jensen T, Hansen M, Jensen KE et al: Comparison of dual x-ray absorptiometry (DXA), digital x-ray radiogrammetry (DXR), and conventional radiographs in the evaluation of osteoporosis and bone erosions in patients with rheumatoid arthritis, *Scand J Rheumatol* 34:27-33, 2005.
98. Lingg GM, Soltesz I, Kessler S et al: Insufficiency and stress fractures of the long bones occurring in patients with rheumatoid arthritis and other inflammatory diseases, with a contribution on the possibilities of computed tomography, *Eur J Radiol* 26:54-63, 1997.
99. Chang DJ, Paget SA: Neurologic complications of rheumatoid arthritis, *Rheum Dis Clin North Am* 19:955-973, 1993.
100. Hochman MG, Zilberfarb JL: Nerves in a pinch: imaging of nerve compression syndromes, *Radiol Clin North Am* 42:221-245, 2004.
101. Tanoue LT: Pulmonary manifestations of rheumatoid arthritis, *Clin Chest Med* 19:667-685, viii, 1998.
102. Balint GP, Balint PV: Felty's syndrome, *Best Pract Res Clin Rheumatol* 18:631-645, 2004.
103. Howe GB, Fordham JN, Brown KA, Currey HL: Polymorphonuclear cell function in rheumatoid arthritis and in Felty's syndrome, *Ann Rheum Dis* 40:370-375, 1981.
104. Sugimoto H, Takeda A, Masuyama J, Furuse M: Early-stage rheumatoid arthritis: diagnostic accuracy of MR imaging, *Radiology* 198:185-192, 1996.
105. Ostergaard M, Ejbjerg B, Szkudlarek M: Imaging in early rheumatoid arthritis: roles of magnetic resonance imaging, ultrasonography, conventional radiography and computed tomography, *Best Pract Res Clin Rheumatol* 19:91-116, 2005.

CHAPTER 21

Scleroderma and Related Disorders

LEYLA H. ALPARSLAN, MD

KEY FACTS

Musculoskeletal System

- Radiographs can demonstrate the characteristic features of systemic sclerosis including calcinosis, loss of normal distal soft tissue and skin creases, and osteolysis that particularly involves the distal tufts.
- Computed tomography (CT) is useful in demonstrating paraspinal calcifications.
- Magnetic resonance imaging (MRI) is valuable for assessing paraspinal calcifications and their effect on neurologic structures, as well as for identifying areas of inflammatory myopathy.

Pulmonary Involvement

- Radiographs may be normal in early interstitial lung disease.
- High-resolution computed tomography (HRCT) is more sensitive than radiography in the assessment of early interstitial lung disease and is able to differentiate active inflammation from fibrosis.
- Bronchoalveolar lavage (BAL) abnormalities may precede HRCT findings.

Peripheral Vascular System

- Arteriography: Vasospasm and pruning of the small digital vessels are characteristic findings.

Pulmonary Hypertension and Cardiac Involvement

- On posteroanterior erect chest radiographs, the transverse diameter of the right interlobar artery should $\leq$16 mm. Enlargement occurs in pulmonary artery hypertension.
- Right heart catheterization optimally evaluates pulmonary arterial hypertension.
- Myocardial disease can be evaluated using radionuclide imaging, coronary angiography, or cardiac MRI.

Renal Involvement

- Ultrasound and biopsy are used for exclusion of other causes of renal disease.
- Nuclear scans can demonstrate decreased renal blood flow and glomerular filtration rate.

Gastrointestinal System

- Radiographs and CT may show obstruction, pseudoobstruction, volvulus, intestinal perforation, and pneumatosis cystoides intestinalis.
- Barium swallow: Esophageal dilatation, diminished or absent peristalsis in the distal two thirds of the esophagus, and a patulous gastroesophageal junction are typical features. Stricture occurs secondary to chronic gastroesophageal reflux.
- Barium follow through: Delay in transit time with decreased motility, pseudodiverticula, and hidebound appearance.
- Barium enemas are usually avoided because they may result in impaction.
- Scintigraphy: Delayed esophageal transit time and gastric emptying and gastroesophageal reflux are typical features. Delayed scans are useful for detection of pulmonary aspiration.

The term *scleroderma* is derived from the Greek for "hard" *(skleros)* and "skin" *(derma)* and describes a connective tissue disorder of unknown etiology, characterized by thickening and fibrosis of the skin. Although the cutaneous manifestations are the most easily recognized, generalized scleroderma is a systemic disorder affecting virtually every organ system and is more appropriately referred as *systemic sclerosis.*[1]

> Scleroderma can affect virtually every organ system or can be localized.

It is more prevalent in women than men and has a mean onset around age 40 years.

Scleroderma can be classified into disease restricted to the skin (localized scleroderma, including the morphea and linear forms) and systemic disease with visceral organ involvement (systemic sclerosis) (Box 21-1). Systemic sclerosis can be further subclassified based on the extent of involvement. Two main subsets of systemic sclerosis are typically identified: diffuse cutaneous systemic sclerosis and limited cutaneous systemic sclerosis. Diffuse cutaneous systemic sclerosis is characterized by skin thickening of the proximal and distal extremities, the face, and often the trunk; these patients are at increased risk for the development of significant pulmonary, cardiac, and renal disease. Limited cutaneous systemic sclerosis is characterized by skin thickening restricted to the hands and possibly the extremities (distal to the elbows or knees) and may involve the face and neck.[1-3] Visceral involvement occurs late; hence the clinical course is relatively benign. The term *limited cutaneous systemic sclerosis* is preferable to CREST (*c*alcinosis, *R*aynaud's, *e*sophageal dysphagia, *s*clerodactyly, *t*elangiectasia syndrome), because cutaneous manifestations often extend beyond sclerodactyly.[4]

Patients with scleroderma express a variety of serologic markers. These autoantibodies are useful in defining clinical subsets of the disease and provide important prognostic information. For example, anticentromere antibodies are most often seen with limited cutaneous involvement, and affected individuals have a lower frequency of pulmonary fibrosis and a lower mortality despite an increased risk of pulmonary hypertension.[5]

BOX 21-1. Classification of Scleroderma

LOCALIZED
Morphea
Localized
Generalized
Linear
*en coup de saber**

SYSTEMIC SCLEROSIS
Limited cutaneous systemic sclerosis
Diffuse cutaneous systemic sclerosis
Overlap syndromes
Systemic sclerosis *sine scleroderma*†

RAYNAUD'S PHENOMENON
Autoimmune (secondary) Raynaud's phenomenon
Primary Raynaud's phenomenon

*French term that means "cut of the sword." Midline or parasagittal variant of linear scleroderma that manifests in childhood and may occur with defects in underlying facial and skeletal structures.
†Vascular or fibrotic visceral features without skin changes (< 1% cases).

IMAGING IN SYSTEMIC SCLEROSIS

Cutaneous and Musculoskeletal Findings

Cutaneous Involvement

Involvement of the skin is the hallmark of scleroderma, and skin changes usually proceed through three phases: (1) edematous, (2) indurative, and (3) atrophic.[6]

Changes limited to the fingers (sclerodactyly) consist of soft tissue resorption of the fingertips and, later, flexion contractures. Soft tissue resorption is frequently accompanied by calcific deposits and bone resorption. Loss of the normal skin folds at the proximal interphalangeal (PIP) joints can be detected on oblique or lateral radiographs.

Calcinosis

Calcinosis (abnormal deposition of calcium salts in body tissues) occurs in about 25% of patients with scleroderma, usually those with limited cutaneous scleroderma.[7] The cutaneous, subcutaneous, and periarticular calcification is composed of calcium hydroxyapatite (HA) crystal deposits. Calcifications are usually seen at the sites of recurrent microtrauma, such as the finger pads, buttocks, and extensor surfaces of the elbows and forearms[8] (Figure 21-1). Large periarticular calcific deposits can simulate those seen in renal osteodystrophy or tumoral calcinosis.

Clinically, the calcific deposits often present as bothersome subcutaneous lumps that may cause local inflammation due to the release of HA crystals. Superficial calcinosis may result in ulceration of the overlying skin leading to secondary infection.[3] Massive paraspinal calcifications have been reported, leading to pain, stiffness, dysphagia, and spinal cord or nerve root compression.[9,10]

Radiographs can detect and delineate the extent of soft tissue calcifications. Paraspinal calcifications and their effect on neurologic structures are better evaluated by computed tomography (CT) scanning and magnetic resonance imaging (MRI) (Figure 21-2).

Osteolysis

Bony resorption of the phalanges (acroosteolysis) in the hand occurs in 40% to 80% of patients with scleroderma.[11,12] Resorption involves particularly the palmar aspect of the distal phalangeal tufts, leading to penciling or conical deformity of the phalanges (Figure 21-3). In

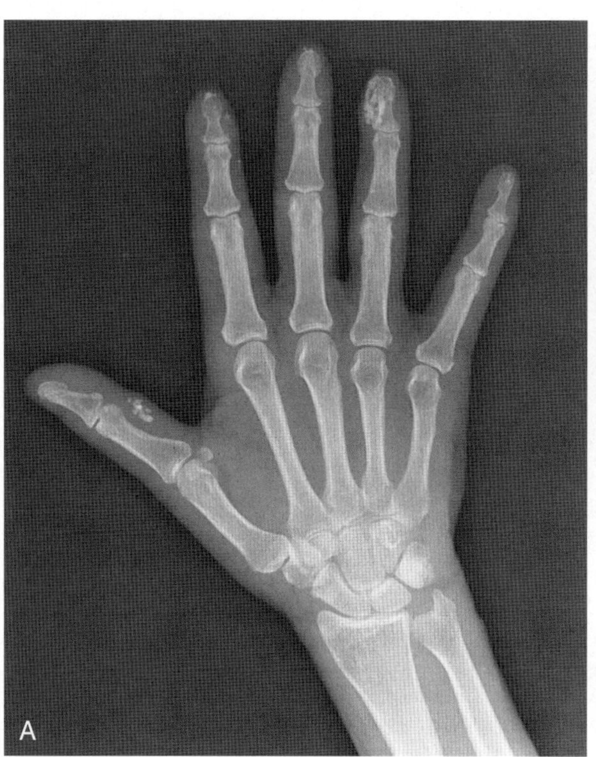

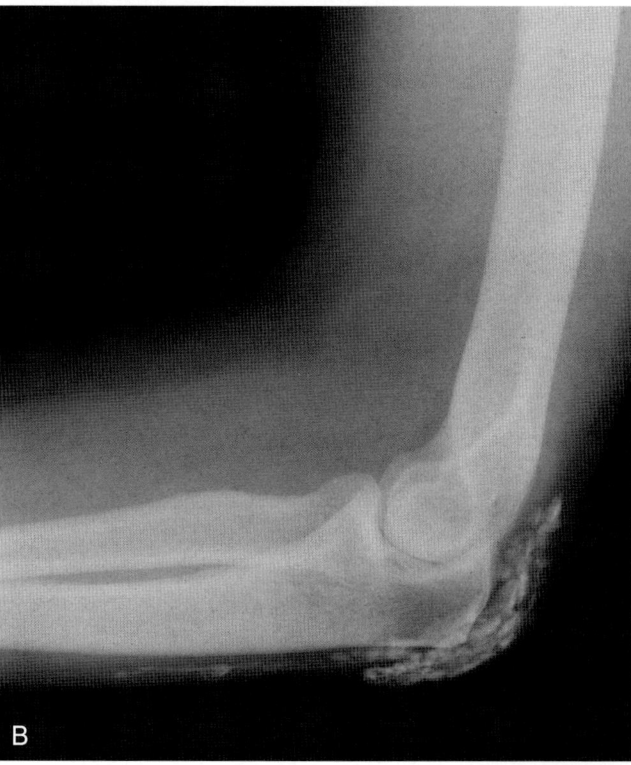

FIGURE 21-1. Calcification in systemic sclerosis. **A,** Soft tissue resorption and soft tissue calcifications of the fingers are present. **B,** Extensive periarticular calcifications are noted along the extensor surface of the elbow.

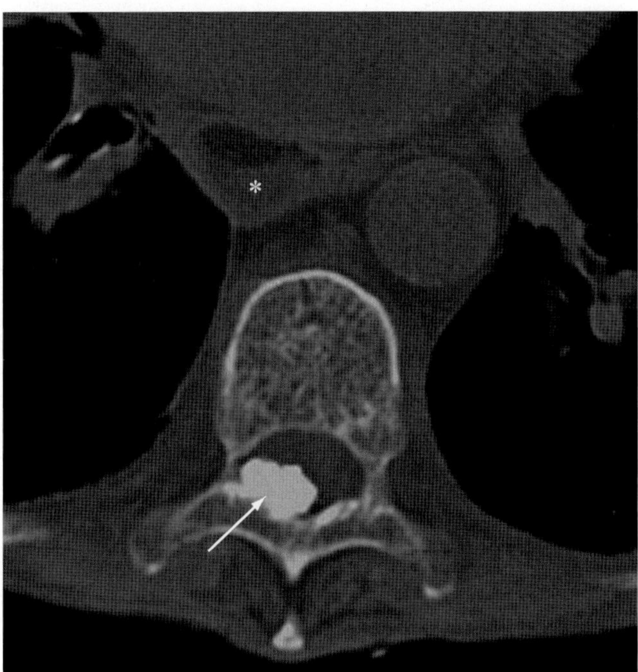

FIGURE 21-2. Spinal calcification. Axial CT scan through lower thoracic spine demonstrates a lobulated calcific mass *(arrow)* in the spinal canal compressing the spinal cord. Note the esophageal dilatation *(asterisk)*.

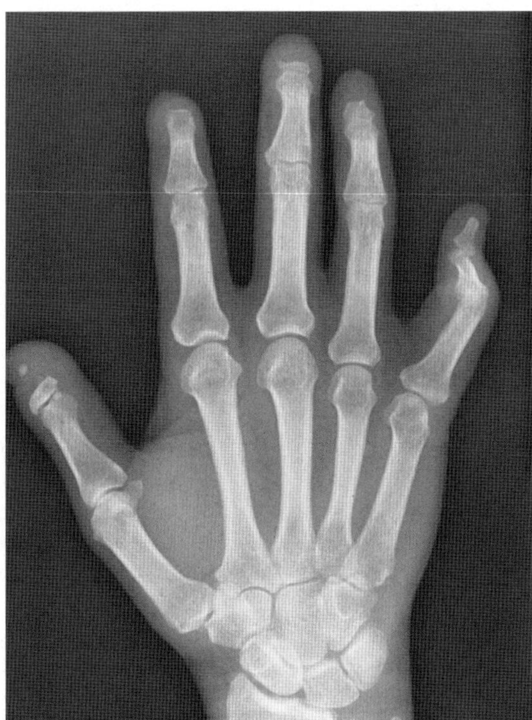

FIGURE 21-3. Acroosteolysis in systemic sclerosis. There has been resorption of part or all of the distal phalanges of each finger. A small calcification or residual bone fragment is seen in the soft tissues of the thumb. The fifth finger shows a boutonnière deformity.

advanced cases, the entire distal phalanx can be destroyed. Resorption of the middle and proximal phalanges, although less common, also occurs. Other sites of bone resorption include the distal ends of the ulna and radius, the clavicle, and mandible, ribs, and humeri.[13-15]

The combination of acroosteolysis and distal soft tissue calcification is typical of scleroderma.

Articular Involvement

Articular abnormalities are very common in patients with systemic sclerosis. The presentation of joint involvement is quite variable, ranging from arthralgia to frank polyarthritis.

Articular changes are usually manifest on radiographs as narrowing of the cartilage space, juxtaarticular osteoporosis, flexion contractures, and thickening of the periarticular soft tissue.[16] Occasionally, radiographic changes may be indistinguishable from those seen in rheumatoid arthritis (RA) and patients may have a detectable rheumatoid factor, frequently believed to represent an overlap syndrome.[17] More than one third of the patients with scleroderma have a positive serologic test for rheumatoid factor.[18] Despite the large percentage of patients with scleroderma who manifest clinical, physical, and laboratory signs of RA, very few show the typical erosive changes of RA on radiographs. This discrepancy in clinical and radiologic findings is most likely due to the underlying pathology of the disease. Early in the clinical course of scleroderma, synovial biopsies show inflammatory reaction with infiltration by lymphocytes and plasma cells—a picture similar to that of RA. In patients with longer disease duration, the synovium is covered and replaced by fibrous tissue. Pannus, which leads to the destructive changes of RA, is notably absent.[16,19,20]

A minority of patients with scleroderma develops erosive changes resembling those occurring in psoriasis or erosive osteoarthritis[16,21] (Figure 21-4). Radiographic abnormalities include erosions involving primarily the distal interphalangeal (DIP) and PIP joints with relative sparing of the metacarpophalangeal (MCP) and wrist joints. Bony ankylosis and pencil-in-cup deformity or ball-in-socket erosions can be observed. Selective involvement of the first carpometacarpal joint with bony resorption and radial subluxation of the first metacarpal has also been reported as a distinctive feature of scleroderma. Associated findings may include intraarticular calcification.

Flexion contractures may occur as a result of fibrosis of the skin, ligaments, and joint capsules, restricting joint mobility. Radiographs of these patients show contractures and periarticular osteopenia without erosions (Figure 21-5). Flexion contractures are particularly seen in the fingers, wrists, elbows, and knees. The fibrosis can also affect the tendons and tendon sheaths, causing tendon friction rubs.[22]

Muscle Involvement

Muscle involvement occurs in most patients with scleroderma and may occur in both the diffuse and limited cutaneous forms of systemic sclerosis.

The patients usually present with one of three forms of myopathy. First, and most commonly, the muscle weakness and wasting are the result of disuse from joint contractures and chronic disease. Second, in about 20% of patients, a chronic myopathy (also called *simple myopathy*) occurs that is characterized by mild muscle weakness and atrophy, minimal elevation of creatine phosphokinase, few or no changes on electromyelography (EMG), and subtle histologic features showing focal replacement of myofibrils with collagen and fibrosis without inflammatory change. This form of myopathy is often unresponsive to antiinflammatory medication.

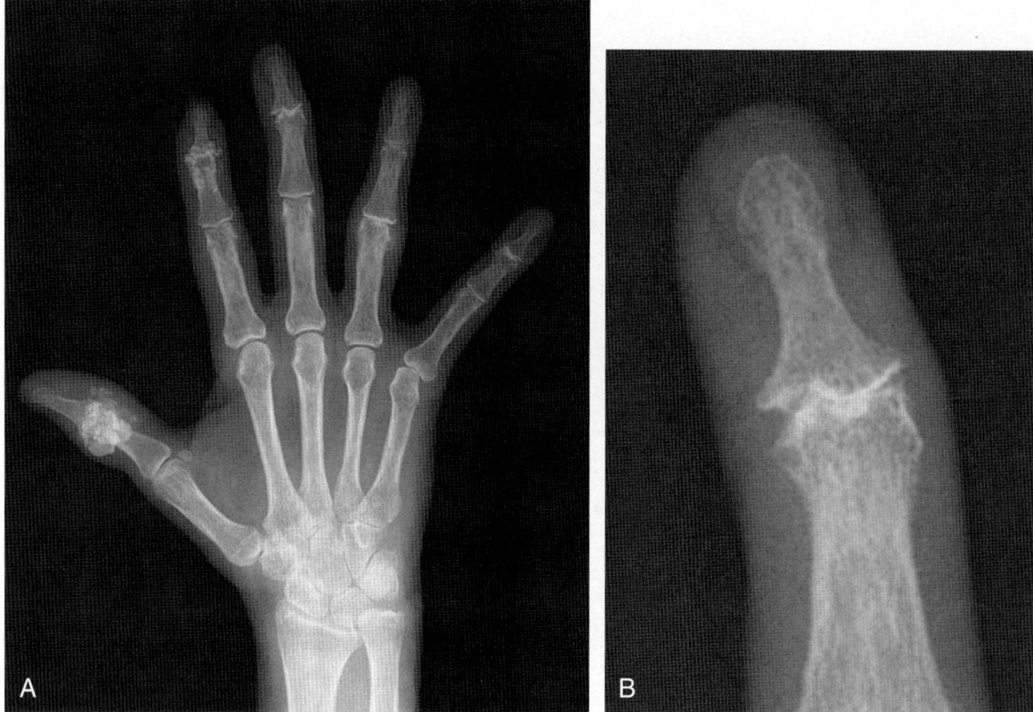

FIGURE 21-4. Systemic sclerosis with distal joint changes. **(A)** Posteroanterior view of the hand and **(B)** coned view of the middle finger. Joint space narrowing and central irregularities at the distal interphalangeal joints resemble the changes of erosive osteoarthritis. Periarticular soft tissue calcifications are present especially at the thumb. Calcifications are not typical features of osteoarthritis.

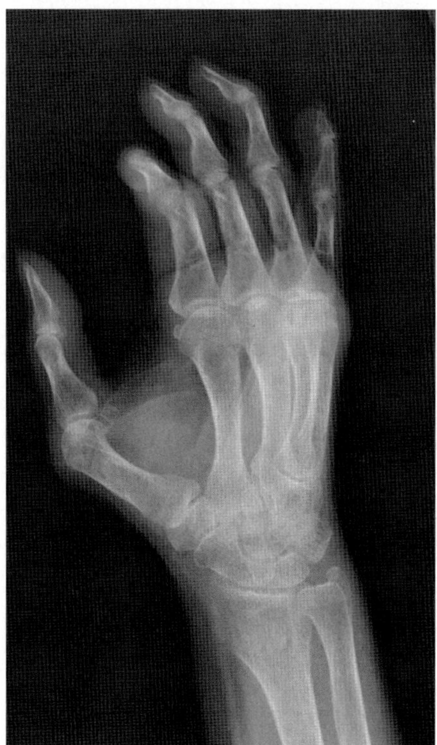

FIGURE 21-5. Flexion contractures. Flexion contractures and osteopenia are present. There is resorption of the distal soft tissues and the distal phalangeal tufts of the thumb, index, and fifth digits.

Third, a minority of patients has an inflammatory myopathy resembling dermatomyositis with significant elevation of creatine phosphokinase and positive EMG changes. Muscle biopsies usually show mononuclear cell infiltrates. In contrast to the noninflammatory myopathy, which is unresponsive to corticosteroid therapy, inflammatory myositis may require treatment with corticosteroids and immunosuppressive drugs.[4,22]

MRI has been demonstrated to be useful in the diagnosis of inflammatory muscle disorders. Areas of increased signal (brightness) on T2-weighted images corresponding to muscle inflammation and fascial thickening have been reported, especially in the hamstring and quadriceps muscles in scleroderma patients with inflammatory myositis.[23] Utilization of MRI for localization of muscle abnormalities prior to muscle biopsy, could decrease sampling errors encountered in "blind" biopsies.

Dental Manifestations

Uniform thickening of the periodontal membrane is a relatively specific finding of scleroderma.[24,25] The thickened membrane creates lucency between the teeth and mandible that is best detected on dental films. The posterior teeth are involved more often than the anterior teeth.

> Thickening of the periodontal membrane on dental radiographs is a relatively specific feature of scleroderma.

Peripheral Vascular System

Raynaud's phenomenon is the earliest and most common clinical manifestation of systemic sclerosis and is characterized by episodes of pallor followed by cyanosis of the distal digits, provoked by cold or emotion. Associated findings include ischemic necrosis, digital ulcerations, and gangrene of digits of the hand or foot. Progressive deficiency in vasodilatory capacity is proposed as a mechanism of Raynaud's phenomenon. The superimposed intimal hyperplasia could result in complete obstruction of small arteries. Similar histopathologic changes are evident in the small arteries and arterioles of affected internal organs.[4,26]

When a patient presents with Raynaud's phenomenon, it is necessary to determine whether there is an underlying connective tissue disease or whether the disorder is primary (idiopathic). Examining the serum autoantibodies and nail fold capillaroscopy are simple, noninvasive procedures that are reliable for detecting patients with secondary Raynaud's phenomenon. The capillaroscopy shows characteristic abnormalities in scleroderma-spectrum disorders, which are enlarged capillary loops, with areas of avascularity and disruption of the normal capillary bed. Areas of hemorrhage may be seen, especially in association with widened capillaries and "bushy" capillaries.[27,28] They appear much like the head of Medusa and are consistently observed in dermatomyositis and in psoriasis.[29]

Arteriography is not usually performed in patients with scleroderma. The characteristic arteriographic findings of Raynaud's phenomenon include vasospasm and pruning of the small digital vessels. Other arteriographic findings are incomplete, poorly formed, or absent palmar arterial arches and ulnar artery. These latter changes may be related to developmental or acquired factors[18,30,31] (Figure 21-6).

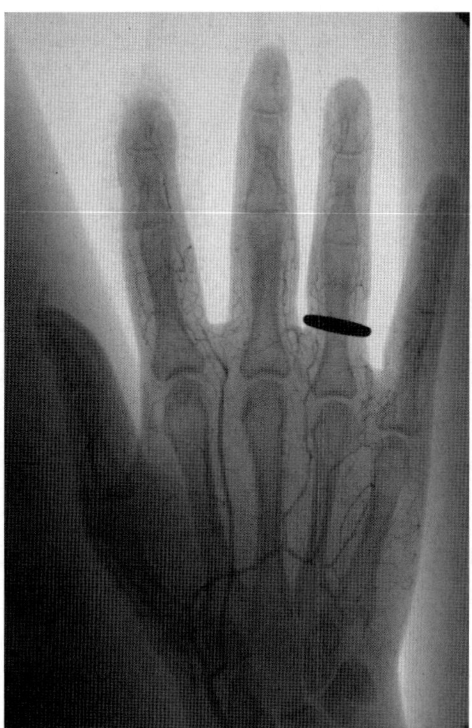

FIGURE 21-6. Angiographic findings of scleroderma. An upper extremity intravenous digital angiogram in a patient with scleroderma and a nonhealing ulcer of the distal index finger demonstrates noncontinuous digital vessels that are fed by a network of collateral vessels. The superficial palmar arch is absent, and the distal ulnar artery is small.

Pulmonary Involvement

Lung disease is the primary cause of mortality in patients with systemic sclerosis.[32] Pulmonary manifestations of scleroderma include interstitial lung disease (ILD), pulmonary hypertension, alveolar hemorrhage, aspiration pneumonitis, bronchiectasis, spontaneous pneumothorax, bronchogenic carcinoma, and pleural disease.

Interstitial Lung Disease

ILD with progressive fibrosis is the most common pulmonary complication of systemic sclerosis with a prevalence of 74% to 100% reported at autopsy.[33,34] Interstitial pulmonary fibrosis occurs more often in patients with diffuse cutaneous systemic sclerosis than in those with the limited form of cutaneous involvement.

Histopathologic features of scleroderma pulmonary fibrosis resemble idiopathic pulmonary fibrosis.[35,36] Alveolar inflammation has been recognized as a primary event. In early stages, alveolar edema with lymphocytic and granulocytic infiltrates occurs. Later, fibrosis is detected involving the interstitium, alveolar septa, and bronchial walls, causing obliteration of alveolar spaces and capillaries.

Patients with pulmonary involvement present with dyspnea, initially with exertion and later at rest and a nonproductive cough. Chest pain, hemoptysis, pleurisy, and fever are uncommon. Pulmonary function tests will be markedly impaired, typically demonstrating a restrictive pattern with proportionate reduction of carbon monoxide transfer factor (DLCO) and forced vital capacity (FVC).[37]

Radiologic Findings

The chest radiograph is abnormal in 25% to 65% of patients with established scleroderma.[35,38,39] As with other fibrosing lung diseases, the interstitial fibrosis of systemic sclerosis can be present despite a normal chest radiograph. The most common radiographic abnormality is a widespread, symmetric, basally predominant reticulonodular pattern that typically starts as a very fine reticular pattern and progresses to coarser reticulation (Figure 21-7). Cystic honeycomb lesions commonly develop in the areas of fibrosis. Serial radiographs may show progressive loss of lung volume manifested by elevation of the diaphragm.[40]

> The chest radiograph is abnormal in as many as 65% of patients with established scleroderma, but interstitial fibrosis may be present even when the radiograph appears normal.

High-resolution computed tomography (HRCT) is more sensitive than radiography in assessing the subtle pulmonary involvement in patients with systemic sclerosis. HRCT not only allows better visualization of the pulmonary parenchyma but also allows differentiation of active inflammation from fibrosis.[41-43] The most common abnormalities seen on HRCT are (1) "ground glass" opacification; (2) a fine reticular pattern, often posterior and subpleural, that is usually associated with traction bronchiectasis and bronchiolectasis; (3) honeycombing with subpleural cysts (1 to 3 cm) (Figure 21-8); (4) lines of various types (septal, subpleural, nonseptal parenchymal lines); and (5) subpleural micronodules.

> HRCT is more sensitive than radiography for detecting pulmonary involvement and may allow differentiation of inflammatory from fibrotic changes.

The areas of ground glass attenuation and poorly defined nodules are usually indicative of active inflammation and are more commonly associated with a cellular biopsy, whereas reticulation, honeycombing, and traction bronchiectasis are irreversible

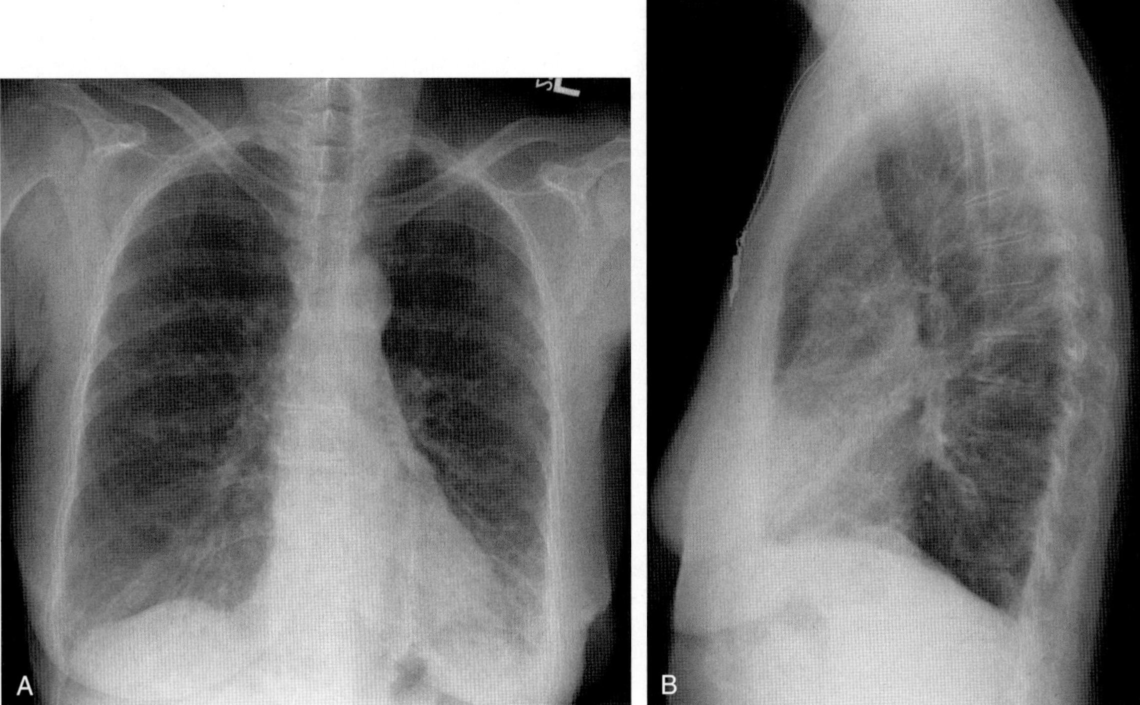

FIGURE 21-7. Interstitial fibrosis. **(A)** Posteroanterior and **(B)** lateral chest radiographs show basilar linear opacities in both lungs, indicating interstitial fibrosis.

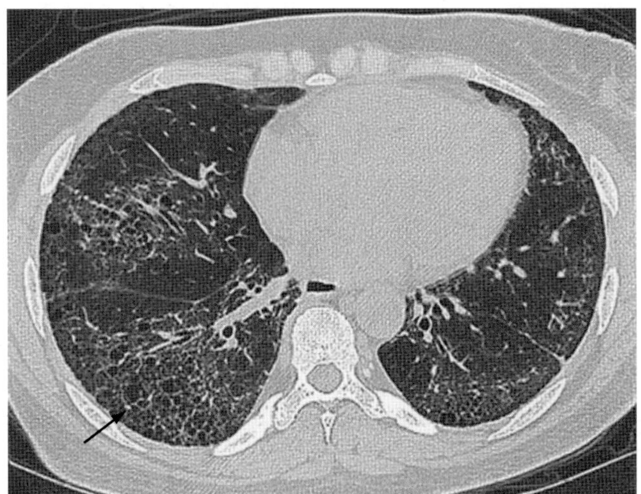

FIGURE 21-8. Pulmonary findings in scleroderma. High-resolution CT scan in a patient with scleroderma shows extensive bibasilar honeycombing *(arrow)* and traction bronchiectasis.

findings. Despite being a sensitive tool for detecting changes of interstitial lung disease, HRCT cannot substitute for bronchoalveolar lavage (BAL) in assessing the inflammatory activity of the alveoli.[44,45]

An increased prevalence (32% to 60%) of enlarged reactive mediastinal lymph nodes has been shown on CT scans of patients with systemic sclerosis.[46-48] Esophageal dilation is also demonstrated in up to 80% of patients on CT.[46]

Nuclear Scans

The usefulness of gallium-67 (Ga-67) scanning in patients with scleroderma is controversial. No correlation has been found between the degree of gallium uptake and the presence and type of symptoms or evidence of alveolitis on bronchoalveolar lavage.[49]

Lung Cancer

Lung cancer incidence is increased 4- to 16-fold in patients with systemic sclerosis compared with the general population and may affect up to 4% of systemic sclerosis patients.[50,51] This is similar to the increased risk observed in patients with idiopathic pulmonary fibrosis. All types of lung cancer may be present, but a slightly higher prevalence of bronchoalveolar cell carcinoma and adenocarcinoma has been reported in some series.[52]

Pulmonary Hypertension and Cardiac Involvement

Pulmonary arterial hypertension (PAH) may occur in systemic sclerosis as a result of interstitial fibrosis and restrictive lung disease, although a subgroup of patients may develop isolated PAH independent of the degree of pulmonary fibrosis. Isolated PAH occurs almost exclusively in patients with limited scleroderma.[53-58] Cardiac involvement may include myocardial disease, pericardial disease, conduction system disease, or arrhythmias. All cardiac abnormalities are seen more often in diffuse scleroderma.[59]

In general, patients with systemic sclerosis undergo annual Doppler echocardiography (ECG), pulmonary function tests, and

ECG examination for detection of presymptomatic PAH. The definitive diagnosis requires exclusion of other causes of PAH such as thromboembolic disease (by ventilation: perfusion lung scan, spiral CT scan, or pulmonary angiography), and establishment that the mean PA pressure is above 25 mmHg at rest or 30 mmHg with exercise. Although there is a reasonably good correlation between estimated peak PA pressure using Doppler ECG and measurements at right heart catheterization at low and high values, this is not always true between 30 and 50 mmHg and caution must be used. For this reason, right heart catheterization has become mandatory for optimal management of these cases. Noninvasive tools such as gated cardiac MRI hold promise for the future but are not yet widely available.[4]

Classical findings of PAH on chest radiographs are enlargement of the main and hilar pulmonary arteries, which rapidly taper as they course peripherally. The evaluation of the hilar vessels on chest radiographs is usually subjective. An objective assessment of hilar vessel enlargement is the measurement of the diameter of the interlobar artery. On posteroanterior (PA) erect chest radiographs, the normal transverse diameter of the right interlobar artery as it descends adjacent to the bronchus intermedius is $\leq$ 16 mm. Compared with chest radiographs, CT scans allow a more accurate determination of the size of the main pulmonary artery and a diameter > 3 cm on CT is generally abnormal.[60]

> Enlargement of the right interlobar pulmonary artery > 16 mm with rapid tapering distally is indicative of PAH on a standing PA chest radiograph.

Renal Involvement

Renal involvement in scleroderma can be acute and life threatening or insidious and benign. Pathologic changes include connective tissue proliferation and vascular abnormalities, which can impair tissue perfusion and lead to organ dysfunction.

Scleroderma renal crisis is defined as the sudden onset of accelerated arterial hypertension and/or rapidly progressive oliguric renal failure during the course of systemic sclerosis. Recognizing the onset of scleroderma renal crisis as early as possible is vital to improve outcome. Diagnosis and management of renal crisis is essentially clinical. Renal biopsies are usually performed to rule out other possible diagnoses such as acute glomerulonephritis. The blood pressure must be controlled before the biopsy to reduce the risk of bleeding. Ultrasound is usually obtained to exclude an intercurrent renal disease and to determine the site for biopsy. Tc-DTPA or 51Cr-EDTA scans have been used to demonstrate decreased blood flow and renal dysfunction, but these techniques have not been successful in the early identification or prediction of future renal crisis.[61-63]

Gastrointestinal System

The gastrointestinal (GI) tract is the most commonly affected visceral organ system in scleroderma. GI involvement occurs in 75% to 90% of patients with scleroderma, of whom approximately one third have subclinical involvement.[64,65]

The pathologic changes in scleroderma are similar throughout the GI tract, with the muscularis propria being the primary target for the disease. Atrophy and fragmentation of the smooth muscle begins in a patchy distribution. As the disease progresses, collagen infiltration and resultant fibrosis and atrophy become more diffuse.[67,68]

> The muscularis propria is the region of the GI tract primarily affected in scleroderma; patchy atrophy and fragmentation of the smooth muscle are later replaced by diffuse fibrosis and atrophy.

Esophageal Manifestations

The esophagus is involved in 55% to 90% of patients with scleroderma by manometric or radiographic criteria and is characterized by decreased or absent peristalsis in the distal two thirds of the esophagus and reduced lower esophageal sphincter (LES) pressure.[68] Chronic gastroesophageal reflux (GER) predisposes to the development of esophagitis, Barrett's metaplasia, and strictures. The patients suffer from dysphagia, heartburn, and regurgitation.

Diagnosis

Barium swallow may show mild to moderate degrees of esophageal dilatation, diminished or absent peristalsis below the aortic arch, and a widely patulous gastroesophageal junction (Figure 21-9). Esophagitis and/or an esophageal stricture may occur as secondary complications of severe and prolonged gastroesophageal reflux.[69]

> Barium swallow may show esophageal dilatation, diminished or absent peristalsis below the aortic arch, a patulous gastroesophageal junction, esophagitis, and/or an esophageal stricture.

Esophageal manometry (EM) is highly sensitive for the detection of esophageal motility abnormalities, including those seen in scleroderma.[70]

Radionuclide scanning may provide additional information about the presence of delayed transit or gastroesophageal reflux with a radiolabeled Technetium meal. The patient undergoes immediate scanning to document delayed clearance and esophageal reflux of the labeled material. This may be followed by scanning the following morning to document any pulmonary aspiration.[67,71,72]

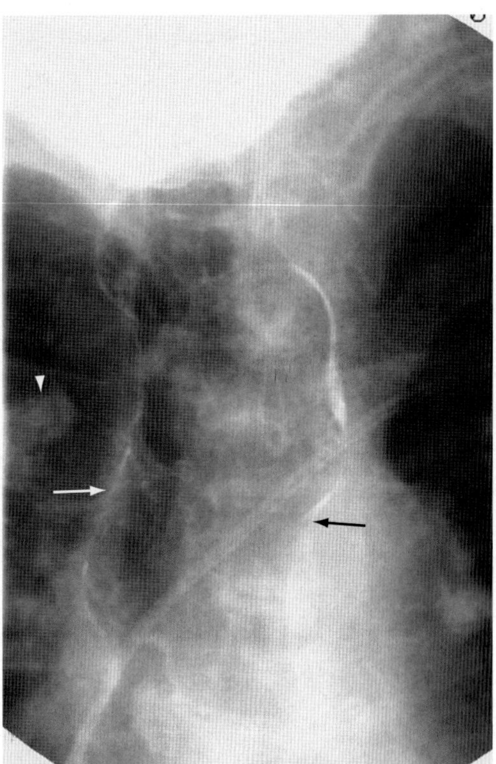

FIGURE 21-9. Esophageal findings in a patient with systemic sclerosis. The barium swallow shows a markedly dilated esophagus *(arrows)*. There was absent peristalsis at fluoroscopy. Soft tissue calcifications *(arrowhead)* are noted.

Gastric and Small Bowel Manifestations

Although involvement of the stomach in scleroderma is uncommon, small bowel involvement has been reported in as many as 50% of patients with scleroderma.[73] Symptoms of nausea, vomiting, abdominal bloating, and constipation may be a result of delayed gastric emptying or small bowel hypomotility. Bacterial overgrowth from intestinal stasis can cause malabsorption and diarrhea.

Barium follow-through studies characteristically show dilation of the duodenum and jejunum without evidence of structural obstruction. There is marked delay in transit time with diminished peristalsis and decreased motility. The small bowel may develop pseudodiverticula, seen as large, broad-based outpouchings. These findings are observed in several neuromuscular disorders of the GI tract, including visceral myopathies and neuropathies, but packing of valvulae conniventes has been demonstrated as a unique radiographic finding that is caused by a combination of dilation and crowded circular folds. This characteristic mucosal fold pattern has been termed a *hidebound* appearance[74] (Figure 21-10).

Intestinal pseudoobstruction is one of the GI complications of advanced scleroderma, presenting as recurring signs of intestinal obstruction in the absence of structural blockage.

> Characteristic findings on barium examination include "pseudoobstruction" of the duodenum, delayed transit time, pseudodiverticula, bowel dilatation, "packing" of the valvulae conniventes (hidebound appearance), and diverticula on the antimesenteric side of the colon.

Acute massive GI bleeding rarely results from GI telangiectasias. *Watermelon stomach* is another term for *gastric antral vascular ectasia* (GAVE), which can be diagnosed by endoscopy.[72]

Colonic and Rectal Manifestations

Colonic involvement in systemic sclerosis has been present on barium enema examinations in 10% to 50% of patients.[64,67] The most common colorectal symptoms are constipation and fecal incontinence. Barium enema may show open-mouth diverticula that are located on the antimesenteric side of the colon. These lesions are true diverticula involving all layers of the bowel wall with smooth muscle atrophy and fibrosis.[75] Other rare reported abnormalities of the colon are ulceration, volvulus, pseudoobstruction, obstruction, and perforation. Barium enemas should be avoided because they may result in impaction; therefore colonoscopy is the preferred procedure for most patients with advanced disease.[73]

> Barium enemas should be avoided in patients with systemic sclerosis because they may result in impaction.

Pneumatosis cystoides intestinalis (PCI) is a relatively uncommon condition seen in association with systemic sclerosis and a variety of other conditions. It is characterized by multiple gas-filled cysts in the walls of the large and small intestines. PCI is usually identified on abdominal CT scans or on radiographs. Occasionally these cysts rupture, producing a pneumoperitoneum without evidence of peritonitis. It is important to recognize pneumatosis as the cause of the pneumoperitoneum in these cases so as to avoid an unnecessary laparotomy.[76,77]

> The gas-filled cysts of pneumatosis cystoides intestinalis may rupture, producing pneumoperitoneum without evidence of peritonitis.

Anal sphincter involvement is common in patients with systemic sclerosis and may lead to fecal incontinence and occasionally rectal prolapse. MRI with a dedicated endorectal coil has been reported to provide excellent visualization of anal sphincter musculature. Endoanal MRI shows forward deviation of the anterior sphincter musculature with descent of rectal air and feces into the anal canal, which is a characteristic finding in patients with scleroderma and fecal incontinence.[80,81] In the incontinent patients, other testing such as anorectal manometric studies or endoanal ultrasound can be obtained.

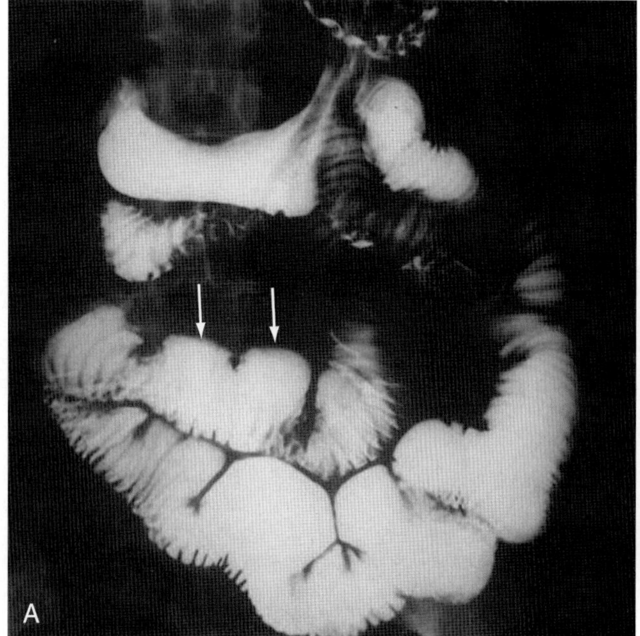

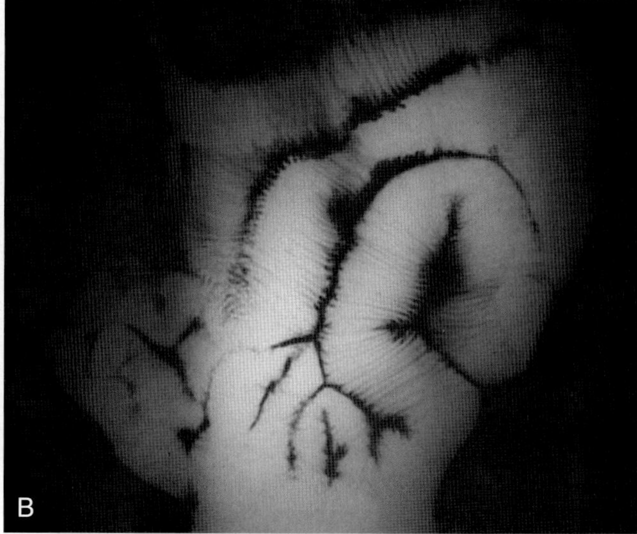

FIGURE 21-10. Scleroderma of the small bowel. **A** and **B,** Sacculations, also known as *pseudodiverticula (arrows),* are seen as large, broad-based outpouchings. The increased number of mucosal folds producing a "hidebound" appearance is a characteristic feature of progressive systemic sclerosis. (Courtesy of P. Clarke, MD, Boston.)

Liver and Biliary Tract

Primary biliary cirrhosis (PBC) is the most common manifestation of hepatobiliary disease in scleroderma. PBC is diagnosed by abnormal liver function tests, especially elevation of alkaline phosphatase, which usually precedes the clinical manifestation of pruritus and jaundice. Liver biopsy shows damage to the small intrahepatic bile ducts and portal inflammation, which eventually leads to fibrosis and cirrhosis.[72]

GRAFT-VERSUS-HOST DISEASE

Graft-versus-host disease (GVHD) is a severe adverse immunologic reaction following allogeneic bone marrow transplantation, induced by the reaction of donor T cells to recipient histoincompatible antigens.

GVHD occurs in either an acute or a chronic form. In the first 100 days following bone marrow transplantation, acute GVHD develops in 25% to 75% of patients and primarily affects the skin, liver, and GI tract.[80,81]

Chronic graft-versus-host disease (cGVHD) occurs in 20% to 45% of patients surviving 6 months beyond transplantation, with approximately 65% of theses cases being preceded by acute GVHD.[79] The disorder usually presents as multiorgan autoimmune disease, including involvement of the skin, GI tract, liver, salivary glands, lymph nodes, mouth, eyes, lungs, and musculoskeletal system (Figure 21-11). Musculoskeletal manifestations include joint contractures, polymyositis, polyserositis, and fasciitis.[82]

cGVHD and scleroderma share clinical characteristics, including skin and internal organ fibrosis. Fibrosis, regardless of the cause, is characterized by extracellular matrix deposition of which

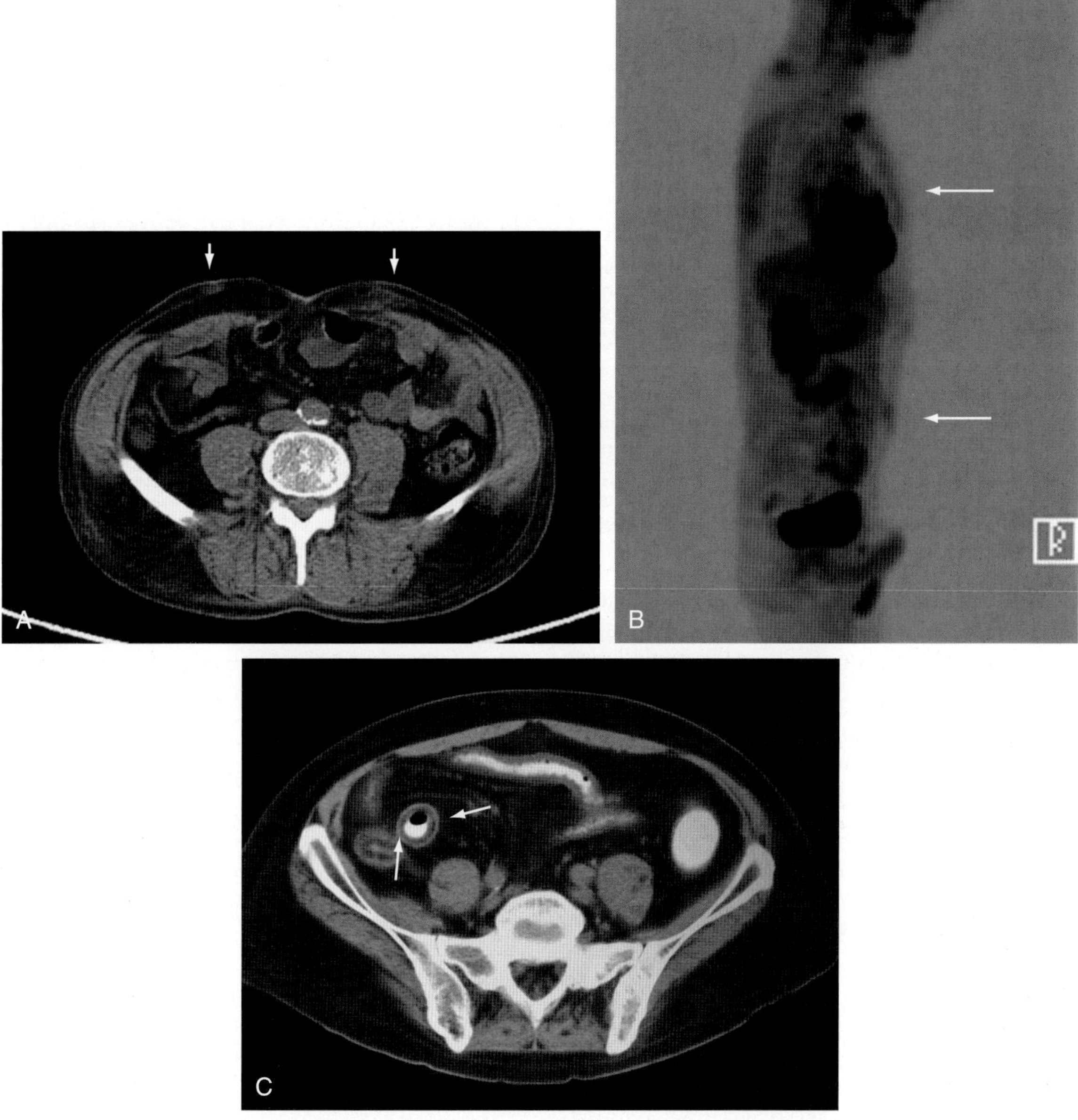

FIGURE 21-11. Graft-versus-host disease. The 56-year-old male in **A** and **B** was status post bone marrow transplantation. He developed biopsy-proven sclerodermatous skin changes of chronic graft-versus-host disease. **A,** Axial CT scan through the lower abdomen shows stranding within the deep subcutaneous fat involving the anterior abdominal wall *(arrows)*. **B,** PET imaging shows mild FDG activity within the subcutaneous tissues anterior to sternum and along the anterior abdominal wall *(arrows)* corresponding to the areas of fibrosing sclerodermatous changes. **C,** CT scan of another patient shows thickening of the walls of the ileum *(arrows)* and cecum.

collagen type I is the major constituent. The progressive accumulation of connective tissue results in destruction of normal tissue architecture and internal organ failure.[83]

Cutaneous involvement in cGVHD can be separated into lichenoid and sclerodermatous forms. Initially, lichenoid cGVHD changes are seen. Clinically this manifests as a spectrum from hyperpigmentation, dryness, and generalized erythema to painful red papules and scattered bullae or vesicles. Rarely, cGVHD will progress from lichenoid type to sclerodermatous form. In one study of 196 patients at risk for cGVHD over a 14-year period, only 3.6% advanced to the generalized sclerodermatous form.[84] With sclerodermatous cGVHD, initially the lichenoid lesions appear to improve; however, increasing hyperpigmentation and induration of the skin results in its becoming inelastic and bound to the deeper structures[85] (Figure 21-11). These advanced fibrosing sclerodermatous changes can be devastating, resulting in contracted and fixed joints with marked impairment of mobility.[86]

In a case report of sclerodermatous cGVHD, stranding within the deep subcutaneous fat involving the anterior abdominal wall was shown with CT imaging. MRI findings included low signal intensity stranding in the subcutaneous fat on T1-weighted images and areas of high signal intensity within the stranding on T2-weighted images, which are thought to represent edema or cellular infiltration and, therefore, areas of active disease.[87]

EOSINOPHILIC FASCIITIS

First described by Schulman,[88] eosinophilic fasciitis (EF) is a rare scleroderma-like fibrosing disorder. In contrast to systemic scleroderma, there is no Raynaud's phenomenon or visceral involvement, and the serologic features characteristic for systemic scleroderma are absent. Clinically, patients present with induration or edema of the extremities. Polyarthralgia and carpal tunnel syndrome have been observed. EF is characterized by inflammation and thickening of the collagen bundles, primarily of the superficial muscle fasciae; peripheral eosinophilia; hypergammaglobulinemia; elevated erythrocyte sedimentation rate; and a favorable response to systemic corticosteroids. The forearms, flanks, and thighs are especially affected in symmetric fashion, whereas the hands and face are usually spared.[89-91]

Several reports have shown that MRI is helpful in identifying this disease, guiding the choice of biopsy site and assessing the response to therapy. MRI findings in active EF are thickening and hyperintensity of the superficial and deep muscle fasciae of the thighs, calves, or arms on T2-weighted and short tau inversion recovery (STIR) sequences with strong enhancement after administration of intravenous contrast agent. A full-thickness epidermis-to-muscle biopsy is essential for definitive diagnosis and distinguishing it from scleroderma, in which signs of inflammation, collagen deposition, and fibrosis are most marked in the skin and superficial dermis.[92,93]

NEPHROGENIC SYSTEMIC FIBROSIS

Nephrogenic systemic fibrosis (NSF), a rare condition linked to the administration of gadolinium chelates in patients with renal failure, was first described in the literature in 2000. It is characterized by fibrotic changes in the skin with a predilection for the peripheral extremities. The trunk can be involved, but the face is usually spared. Because of the skin changes and the occurrence in patients with renal failure, the condition was first termed "nephrogenic fibrosing dermopathy" (NFD). In addition to skin changes, however, systemic manifestations may occur owing to fibrosis of skeletal muscle, lungs, pleura, pericardium, myocardium, kidneys, testes, and dura. The current terminology (nephrogenic systemic fibrosis) reflects this systemic involvement. Because of the risk of developing this condition, care must be utilized in selecting patients for MRI examination with gadolinium contrast. Protocols for doing this vary, and clinicians should consult their imaging providers for screening recommendations.

REFERENCES

1. Loucks J, MD, Pope JE: Osteoporosis in scleroderma, *Semin Arthritis Rheum* 34: 678-682, 2004.
2. Lawrence RC, Helmick CG, Arnett FC et al: Estimates of the prevalence of arthritis and selected musculoskeletal disorders in the United States, *Arthritis Rheum* 41:778, 1998.
3. Subcommittee for Scleroderma Criteria of the American Rheumatism Association Diagnostic and Therapeutic Criteria Committee: Preliminary criteria for the classification of systemic sclerosis (scleroderma), *Arthritis Rheum* 23:581-590, 1980.
4. Black CM, Denton PD: Scleroderma and related disorders in adults and children. In Isenberg DA, Maddison PJ, Woo P et al (eds): *Oxford textbook of rheumatology*, ed 3, Oxford, 2004, Oxford University Press, pp 872-895.
5. Cepeda EJ, Reveilla JD: Autoantibodies in systemic sclerosis and fibrosing syndromes: clinical indications and relevance, *Curr Opin Rheumatol* 16:723-732, 2004.
6. Mitchell H, Bolster MB, LeRoy EC: Scleroderma and related conditions, *Med Clin North Am* 81:129-149, 1997.
7. Robertson LP, Marshall RW, Hickling P: Treatment of cutaneous calcinosis in limited systemic sclerosis with minocycline, *Ann Rheum Dis* 62:267-269, 2003.
8. Boulman N, Slobodin G, Rozenbaum M et al: Calcinosis in rheumatic diseases, *Semin Arthritis Rheum* 34:805-812, 2005.
9. Schweitzer ME, Cervilla V, Manaster BJ et al: Cervical paraspinal calcifications in collagen vascular diseases, *AJR Am J Roentgenol* 157:523-525, 1991.
10. Petrocelli AR, Bassett LW, Mirra J et al: Scleroderma: dystrophic calcification with spinal cord compression, *J Rheumatol* 15:1733-1735, 1988.
11. Yune HY, Vix VA, Klatte AC: Early fingertip changes in scleroderma, *J Am Med Assoc* 215:1113-1116, 1971.
12. Kemp Harper RA, Jackson DC: Progressive systemic sclerosis, *Br J Radiol* 38: 825-834, 1965.
13. Quagliata F, Sebes J, Pinstein ML et al: Long bone erosions and ascites in progressive systemic sclerosis (scleroderma), *J Rheumatol* 9:641-644, 1982.
14. Keats TE: Rib erosions in scleroderma, *AJR Am J Roentgenol* 100:530-532, 1967.
15. Osial TA Jr, Avakian A, Sassouni V et al: Resorption of the mandibular condyles and coronoid process in progressive systemic sclerosis (scleroderma), *Arthritis Rheum* 24:729-733, 1981.
16. Browner AC, Pesnick D, Karlin CK et al: Unusual articular changes of the hand in scleroderma, *Skeletal Radiol* 4:119-123, 1979.
17. Rodnan GP, Medsger TA Jr: The rheumatic manifestations of progressive systemic sclerosis (scleroderma), *Clin Orthop Relat Res* 57:81-93, 1968.
18. Resnick D: Scleroderma (progressive systemic sclerosis). In Resnick D (ed): *Diagnosis of bone and joint disorders*, ed 4, Philadelphia, 2002, Saunders, pp 1194-1220.
19. Clark JA, Winkelman RK, McDuffie FC et al: Synovial tissue changes and rheumatoid factor in scleroderma, *Mayo Clin Proc* 46:97-103, 1971.
20. Rabinowitz JG, Twersky J, Guttadauria M: Similar bone manifestations of scleroderma and rheumatoid arthritis, *AJR Am J Roentgenol* 121:35-44, 1974.
21. Ott AH: Unusual articular abnormalities in scleroderma, *Clin Rheumatol* 13:323-327, 1984.
22. Pope JE: Musculoskeletal involvement in scleroderma, *Rheum Dis Clin North Am* 29:391-408, 2003.
23. Olsen NJ, King LE, Park JH: Muscle abnormalities in scleroderma, *Rheum Dis Clin North Am* 22:783-796, 1996.
24. Stafne EC, Austin LT: A characteristic dental finding in acrosclerosis and diffuse scleroderma, *Am J Orthod* 30:25-28, 1944.
25. Rowell NR, Hopper FE: The periodontal membrane in systemic sclerosis, *Br J Dermatol* 96:15-20, 1977.
26. Kahaleh MB: Raynaud phenomenon and the vascular disease in scleroderma, *Curr Opin Rheumatol* 16:718-722, 2004.
27. Herrick AL, Hutchinson C: Vascular imaging, *Best Pract Res Clin Rheumatol* 18:957-979, 2004.
28. Cutolo M, Grassi W, Matucci Cerinic M: Raynaud's phenomenon and the role of capillaroscopy, *Arthritis Rheum* 11:3023-3030, 2003.
29. LeRoy EC: Systemic sclerosis; a vascular perspective, *Rheum Dis Clin North Am* 22:675-694, 1996.
30. Higgins CB, Hayden WG: Palmar arteriography in acronecrosis, *Radiology* 199: 85-90, 1976.
31. Laws JW, Lillie JG, Scott JT: Arteriographic appearances in rheumatoid arthritis and other disorders, *Br J Radiol* 36:440-447, 1963.
32. Crestani B: The respiratory system in connective tissue disorders, *Allergy* 60:715-734, 2005.
33. D'Angelo WA, Fries JF, Masi AT et al: Pathologic observations in systemic sclerosis (scleroderma): a study of 58 autopsy cases and 58 matched controls, *Am J Med* 46:428-440, 1969.
34. Weaver AL, Divertie MB, Titus JL: Pulmonary scleroderma, *Dis Chest* 54:490-498, 1968.
35. Minai OA, Dweik RA, Arroliga AC: Manifestations of scleroderma pulmonary disease, *Clin Chest Med* 19:713-731, 1998.

36. Harrison NK, Glanville AR, Strickland B et al: Pulmonary involvement in systemic sclerosis: the detection of early changes by thin section CT scan, bronchoalveolar lavage and TC-DTPA clearance, *Respir Med* 83:403-414, 1989.
37. Denton CP, Haddock J, Black CM: Systemic sclerosis. In Isenberg D (ed): *Imaging in rheumatology*, Oxford, 2003, Oxford University Press, pp 300-316.
38. Schurawitzki H, Stiglbauer R, Graninger W et al: Interstitial lung disease in progressive systemic sclerosis: high resolution CT versus radiography, *Radiology* 176:755-759, 1990.
39. Steen VD, Owens GR, Fino GJ et al: Pulmonary involvement in systemic sclerosis (scleroderma), *Arthritis Rheum* 28:759-767, 1985.
40. Silver RM: Clinical problems (the lungs), *Rheum Dis Clin North Am* 22:825-840, 1996.
41. Cheema GS, Quismorio FP Jr: Interstitial lung disease in systemic sclerosis, *Curr Opin Pulmon Med* 7:283-290, 2001.
42. Schurawitzki H, Stiglbauer R, Graninger W et al: Interstitial lung disease in progressive systemic sclerosis: high-resolution CT versus radiography, *Radiology* 176: 755-759, 1990.
43. Wells AU, Hansell DM, Rubens MB et al: High resolution computed tomography as a predictor of lung histology in systemic sclerosis, *Thorax* 47:738-742, 1992.
44. Remy-Jardin M, Remy J, Wallaert B et al: Pulmonary involvement in progressive systemic sclerosis: sequential evaluation with CT, pulmonary function tests, and bronchoalveolar lavage, *Radiology* 188:499-506, 1993.
45. Witt C, Borges AC, John M et al: Pulmonary involvement in diffuse cutaneous systemic sclerosis: bronchoalveolar fluid granulocytosis predicts progression of fibrosing alveolitis, *Ann Rheum Dis* 58:635-640, 1999.
46. Bhalla M, Silver RM, Shepard J et al: Chest CT in patients with scleroderma: prevalence of asymptomatic esophageal dilatation and mediastinal lymphadenopathy, *AJR Am J Roentgenol* 161:269-272, 1993.
47. Garber SJ, Wells AU, duBois RM et al: Enlarged mediastinal lymph nodes in the fibrosing alveolitis of systemic sclerosis, *Br J Radiol* 65:983-986, 1992.
48. Warrick JH, Bhalla M, Schabel SI et al: High resolution computed tomography in early scleroderma lung disease, *J Rheumatol* 18:1520-1528, 1991.
49. Baron M, Feiglin D, Hyland R et al: 67-gallium lung scan in progressive systemic sclerosis, *Arthritis Rheum* 26:969-974, 1983.
50. Abu-shakra M, Guillemin F, Lee P: Cancer in systemic sclerosis, *Arthritis Rheum* 36:460-464, 1993.
51. Hill CL, Nguyen AM, Roder D et al: Risk of cancer in patients with scleroderma: a population based cohort study, *Ann Rheum Dis* 62:728-731, 2003.
52. Guttadauria M, Ellman H, Kaplan D: Progressive systemic sclerosis: pulmonary involvement, *Clin Rheum Dis* 5:151-166, 1979.
53. Trell E, Lindstrom C: Pulmonary hypertension in systemic sclerosis, *Ann Rheum Dis* 30:390-400, 1971.
54. Salerni R, Rodnan GP, Leon DF et al: Pulmonary hypertension in the CREST syndrome variant of progressive systemic sclerosis (scleroderma), *Ann Intern Med* 86:394-399, 1977.
55. Stupi AM, Steen VD, Owens GR et al: Pulmonary hypertension in the CREST syndrome variant of systemic sclerosis, *Arthritis Rheum* 29:515-524, 1986.
56. Ungerer RG, Tashkin DP, Furst D et al: Prevalence and clinical correlates of pulmonary arterial hypertension in progressive systemic sclerosis, *Am J Med* 75:65-74, 1983.
57. Young RH, Mark GJ: Pulmonary vascular changes in scleroderma, *Am J Med* 64: 998-1004, 1978.
58. Yousem SA: The pulmonary pathologic manifestations of the CREST syndrome, *Hum Pathol* 21:467-474, 1990.
59. Coghlan JG, Mukerjee D: The heart and pulmonary vasculature in scleroderma: clinical features and pathobiology, *Curr Opin Rheumatol* 13:495-499, 2001.
60. Boiselle PM: Pulmonary vascular abnormalities. In McLoud TC (ed): *Thoracic radiology*, St Louis, 1998, Mosby, pp 403-419.
61. O'Callaghan CA: Renal manifestations of systemic autoimmune disease: diagnosis and therapy, *Best Pract Res Clin Rheumatol* 18:411-427, 2004.
62. Steen VD: Scleroderma renal crisis, *Rheum Dis Clin North Am* 22:861-878, 1996.
63. Kingdon EJ, Knight CJ, Dustan K et al: Calculated glomerular filtration rate is a useful screening tool to identify scleroderma patients with renal impairment, *Rheumatology* 42:26-33, 2003.
64. Sjogren RW: Gastrointestinal features of scleroderma, *Curr Opin Rheumatol* 8: 569-575, 1996.
65. Cohen S, Laufer I, Snape WJ Jr et al: The gastrointestinal manifestations of scleroderma: pathogenesis and management, *Gastroenterology* 79:155, 1980.
66. D'Angelo WA, Fries JF, Masl AT et al: Pathologic observations in systemic sclerosis (scleroderma). A study of fifty-eight autopsy cases and fifty-eight matched controls, *Am J Med* 49:428, 1969.
67. Young MA, Rose S, Reynold JC: Gastrointestinal manifestations of scleroderma, *Rheum Dis Clin North Am* 22:798-824, 1996.
68. Fulp SM, Castell DO: Scleroderma esophagus, *Dysphagia* 5:204-210, 1990.
69. Luedtke P, Levine MS, Rubesin SE et al: Radiologic diagnosis of benign esophageal strictures: a pattern approach, *Radiographics* 23:897-909, 2003.
70. Spechler SJ, Castell DO: Classification of oesophageal motility abnormalities, *Gut* 49:145-151, 2001.
71. Bestetti A, Carola F, Conciato L et al: Esophageal scintigraphy with a semisolid meal to evaluate esophageal dysmotility in systemic sclerosis and Raynaud's phenomenon, *J Nucl Med* 40:77-84, 1999.
72. Jaovisidha K, Csuka ME, Almagro UA et al: Severe gastrointestinal involvement in systemic sclerosis: report of five cases and review of the literature, *Semin Arthritis Rheum* 34:689-702, 2004.
73. Abu-Shakra M, Guillemin F, Lee P: Gastrointestinal manifestations of systemic sclerosis, *Semin Arthritis Rheum* 24:29-39, 1994.
74. Horowitz AL, Meyers MA: The "hide-bound" small bowel of scleroderma: characteristic mucosal fold pattern, *AJR Am J Roentgenol* 1:332-334, 1973.
75. Compton R: Scleroderma with diverticulosis and colonic obstruction, *Am J Surg* 118:602, 1969.
76. Miercort RD, Merrill FG: Pneumatosis and pseudoobstruction in scleroderma, *Radiology* 92:359-362, 1969.
77. Sequeira W: Pneumatosis cystoides intestinalis in systemic sclerosis and other diseases, *Semin Arthritis Rheum* 19:269-277, 1990.
78. deSouza NM, Williams AD, Wilson HJ et al: Fecal incontinence in systemic sclerosis: assessment of the anal sphincter using high-resolution endoanal MR imaging, *Radiology* 208:529-535, 1998.
79. deSouza NM, Williams AD, Gilderdale DJ: High-resolution magnetic resonance imaging of the anal sphincter using a dedicated endoanal receiver coil, *Eur Radiol* 9:436-443, 1999.
80. Ferrara JLM, Deeg HL: Graft versus host disease, *N Engl Med J* 324:667-674, 1991.
81. Soubani AO, Miller KB, Hassoun PM: Pulmonary complications of bone marrow transplantation, *Chest* 109:1066-1077, 1996.
82. Beredjiklian PK: Orthopaedic manifestations of chronic graft-versus-host disease, *J Pediatr Orthop* 18:572-575, 1998.
83. Pines M, Synder D, Shai Y et al: Halofuginone to treat fibrosis in chronic graft-versus-host disease and scleroderma, *Biol Blood Marrow Transplant* 9:417-425, 2003.
84. Chosidow O, Bagot M, Vernant J et al: Sclerodermatous chronic graft-versus-host disease: analysis of seven cases, *J Am Acad Dermatol* 26:49-55, 1992.
85. Shulman H, Sale G, Lerner K et al: Chronic cutaneous graft-versus-host disease in man, *Am J Pathol* 92:545-570, 1978.
86. Woscoff A, Lascano AR, DePablo AB et al: Sclerodermatous changes of chronic graft-versus-host disease treated with PUVA, *Int J Dermatol* 35:656-658, 1996.
87. Dumford K, Anderson JC: CT and MRI findings in sclerodermatous chronic graft vs. host disease, *J Clin Imaging* 25:138-140, 2001.
88. Shulman LE: Diffuse fasciitis with eosinophilia: a new syndrome? *Trans Assoc Am Physicians* 88:70, 1975.
89. Kent LT, Cramer SF, Moskowitz RW: Eosinophilic fasciitis: clinical, laboratory, and microscopic considerations, *Arthritis Rheum* 24:677-683, 1981.
90. Michet CJ Jr, Doyle JA, Ginsburg WW: Eosinophilic fasciitis: report of 15 cases, *Mayo Clin Proc* 56:27-34, 1981.
91. Lakhanpal S, Ginsburg WW, Michet CJ et al: Eosinophilic fasciitis: clinical spectrum and therapeutic response in 52 cases, *Semin Arthritis Rheum* 17:221-231, 1988.
92. Baumann F, Bruhlmann, Andreisek et al: MRI for diagnosis and monitoring of patients with eosinophilic fasciitis, *AJR Am J Roentgenol* 184:169-174, 2005.
93. Moulton SJ, Kransdorf MJ, Ginsburg WW et al: Eosinophilic fasciitis: spectrum of MRI findings, *AJR Am J Roentgenol* 184:975-978, 2005.
94. Kuo PH, Kanal E, Abu-alfa AK, Cowper SE: Gadolinium based contrast agents and nephrogenic systemic fibrosis, *Radiology* 242:647, 2007.

CHAPTER 22

Systemic Lupus Erythematosus and Related Conditions and Vasculitic Syndromes

BARBARA N. WEISSMAN, MD, HALE ERSOY, MD, LIANGGE HSU, MD, JOHN BRAVER, MD, *and* ANDETTA HUNSAKER, MD

KEY POINTS

- A classic imaging feature of systemic lupus erythematosus (SLE) is deforming arthritis without erosion.
- Avascular necrosis may be present in asymptomatic patients with SLE.
- Antiphospholipid syndrome may be a primary disorder or be associated with other diseases, especially SLE. Imaging reveals thrombosis of affected vessels and its sequela.
- Kawasaki disease presents special imaging considerations because it affects children and long-term follow-up is necessary. Echocardiography is a standard evaluation technique for this disorder. Magnetic resonance imaging (MRI) allows both the coronary artery lumen and wall to be evaluated without ionizing radiation and may be a useful technique. Computed tomography (CT) arteriography is useful but radiation exposure can be similar to that of coronary artery catheterization.
- Takayasu's arteritis affects the aorta, its proximal branches and pulmonary arteries but not muscular arteries. Because inflammation of the vessel wall is a characteristic early feature, MRI, CT, and positron emission tomography CT may be useful. Later disease causes vessel stenoses or occlusions.
- Giant cell arteritis can be diagnosed by arterial biopsy. Recently ultrasound findings have been described that may provide an alternative to biopsy.

SYSTEMIC LUPUS ERYTHEMATOSUS

Definition and Criteria for Diagnosis

Systemic lupus erythematosus (SLE) is an autoimmune disorder that results in inflammation, deposition of immune complexes, vasculitis, and vasculopathy.[1] It affects about 40 individuals per 100,000 population in North America, and more than 80% of cases occur in women of childbearing age.[2] African-Americans and Hispanics are at increased risk of being affected.[1]

The 1982 American College of Rheumatology (ACR) revised criteria for the classification of SLE allow the diagnosis to be made with 96% sensitivity and 96% specificity. Four or more of the 11 described criteria needed to be present to establish the diagnosis with this accuracy.[3] These criteria have been further revised (Table 22-1).

> The diagnosis of SLE can be made with 96% sensitivity and 96% specificity using the revised ACR criteria.

Antinuclear antibodies are present in more than 95% of patients (although these may also be present in low titers in other disorders). Antibodies to native or double-stranded DNA and to Sm (anti-Smith antibody) are more specific for the diagnosis of SLE.[2] Almost one third of SLE patients also have antiphospholipid antibody, which may cause thromboembolic complications including stroke, portal vein thrombosis, thrombophlebitis and pulmonary embolism, and repeated midtrimester abortions[2] (see Antiphospholipid Syndrome, below).

> Almost one third of patients with SLE have antiphospholipid antibody, which may cause thromboembolic complications.

Musculoskeletal Manifestations

Musculoskeletal manifestations of SLE include arthritis, avascular necrosis, soft tissue calcification, changes in the terminal tufts of the fingers, and tendon rupture.

Arthritis

Joint involvement is one of the earliest and most common manifestations of SLE.[4] Thus it may precede other features of the disease.[5] A higher incidence of deforming arthritis has been found with increased disease duration, a positive rheumatoid factor, and antibodies to U1 RNP.[5,6] Patients with deforming arthritis have a higher frequency of sicca symptoms and lower incidence of facial erythema and photosensitivity.[5] Longer disease duration and late onset disease have been noted in patients with radiologic abnormalities of the hands and feet.[6,7]

> Approximately 90% of patients with SLE have joint manifestations.[8,9]

TABLE 22-1. The 1997 Update of the 1982 American College of Rheumatology Revised Criteria for Classification of Systemic Lupus Erythematosus

Criterion	Definition
1. Malar rash	Fixed erythema, flat or raised, over the malar eminences, tending to spare the nasolabial folds
2. Discoid rash	Erythematous raised patches with adherent keratotic scaling and follicular plugging; atrophic scarring may occur in older lesions
3. Photosensitivity	Skin rash as a result of unusual reaction to sunlight, by patient history or physician observation
4. Oral ulcers	Oral or nasopharyngeal ulceration, usually painless, observed by physician
5. Nonerosive Arthritis	Involving two or more peripheral joints, characterized by tenderness, swelling, or effusion
6. Pleuritis or Pericarditis	a. Pleuritis—convincing history of pleuritic pain or rubbing heard by a physician or evidence of pleural effusion *OR* b. Pericarditis—documented by ECG or rub or evidence of pericardial effusion
7. Renal disorder	a. Persistent proteinuria $>$ 0.5 g/day or $>$ 3+ if quantitation not performed *OR* b. Cellular casts—may be red cell, hemoglobin, granular, tubular, or mixed
8. Neurologic disorder	a. Seizures—in the absence of offending drugs or known metabolic derangements, such as uremia, ketoacidosis, or electrolyte imbalance *OR* b. Psychosis—in the absence of offending drugs or known metabolic derangements, such as uremia, ketoacidosis, or electrolyte imbalance
9. Hematologic disorder	a. Hemolytic anemia—with reticulocytosis *OR* b. Leukopenia—less than 4000/mm^3 on 2 or more occasions *OR* c. Lymphopenia—less than 1500/mm^3 on 2 or more occasions *OR* d. Thrombocytopenia—less than 100,000/mm^3 in the absence of offending drugs
10. Immunologic disorder	a. Anti-DNA antibody to native DNA in abnormal titer *OR* b. Anti-Sm—presence of antibody to Sm nuclear antigen *OR* c. Positive finding of antiphospholipid antibodies on: 1. an abnormal serum level of IgG or IgM anticardiolipin antibodies, 2. a positive test result for lupus anticoagulant using a standard method, or 3. a false-positive test result for at least 6 months confirmed by Treponema pallidum immobilization or fluorescent treponemal antibody absorption test.
11. Positive antinuclear antibody	An abnormal titer of antinuclear antibody by immunofluorescence or an equivalent assay at any point in time and in the absence of drugs

Retrieved October 18, 2008, from http://www.rheumatology.org/publications/classification/SLE/1997UpdateOf1982RevisedCriteriaClassificationSLE.asp?aud=mem

A symmetric polyarthritis that most often involves the hands and knees is typical.[8] Arthritis is typically out of proportion to clinically evident synovitis and is episodic, polyoligoarticular, and migratory.[2] The presence of a nonerosive arthritis involving two or more joints is, in fact, one of the clinical criteria used for establishing the diagnosis and is 86% sensitive and 37% specific.[3] Effusions are usually not as large as in rheumatoid arthritis (RA) and not as inflammatory. Labowitz and Schumacher described the synovial fluid as clear to slightly turbid with good viscosity and fewer than 3000/mm^3 white blood cells with mononuclear cells usually predominating.[8]

Radiography

Investigation of hand radiographs in 59 patients with SLE has shown radiographic abnormalities in 34 patients, although the most common features were nonspecific periarticular osteopenia or soft tissue swelling.[7] Erosion is a less common finding in SLE than in RA owing to a lack of aggressive pannus on histologic examination in SLE.

Deformity without Erosion

Deforming arthritis without erosion is a classic feature of SLE and is seen in up to 35% of patients[5,10,11] (Figure 22-1). This pattern is similar to that seen in postrheumatic fever arthritis (termed *Jaccoud's arthropathy*)[14] but is unlike that seen in RA, in which erosion is a characteristic feature.[4] The deformities that occur in lupus are not due to destructive synovitis.[5] Instead they are thought to be a consequence of low-grade inflammation of the synovial membrane and capsule resulting in ligamentous laxity and muscular imbalance.

> Deforming arthritis without erosion is a classic feature of SLE.

Weissman et al. found deformity of the hands to be most common at the proximal interphalangeal joints.[7] Thumb interphalangeal hyperextension and swan neck deformity, ulnar deviation, and metacarpophalangeal (MCP) subluxations of the fingers were noted. Ulnar deviation is the earliest of these features.[10] Thumb deformities begin as passively correctable flexion deformity at the

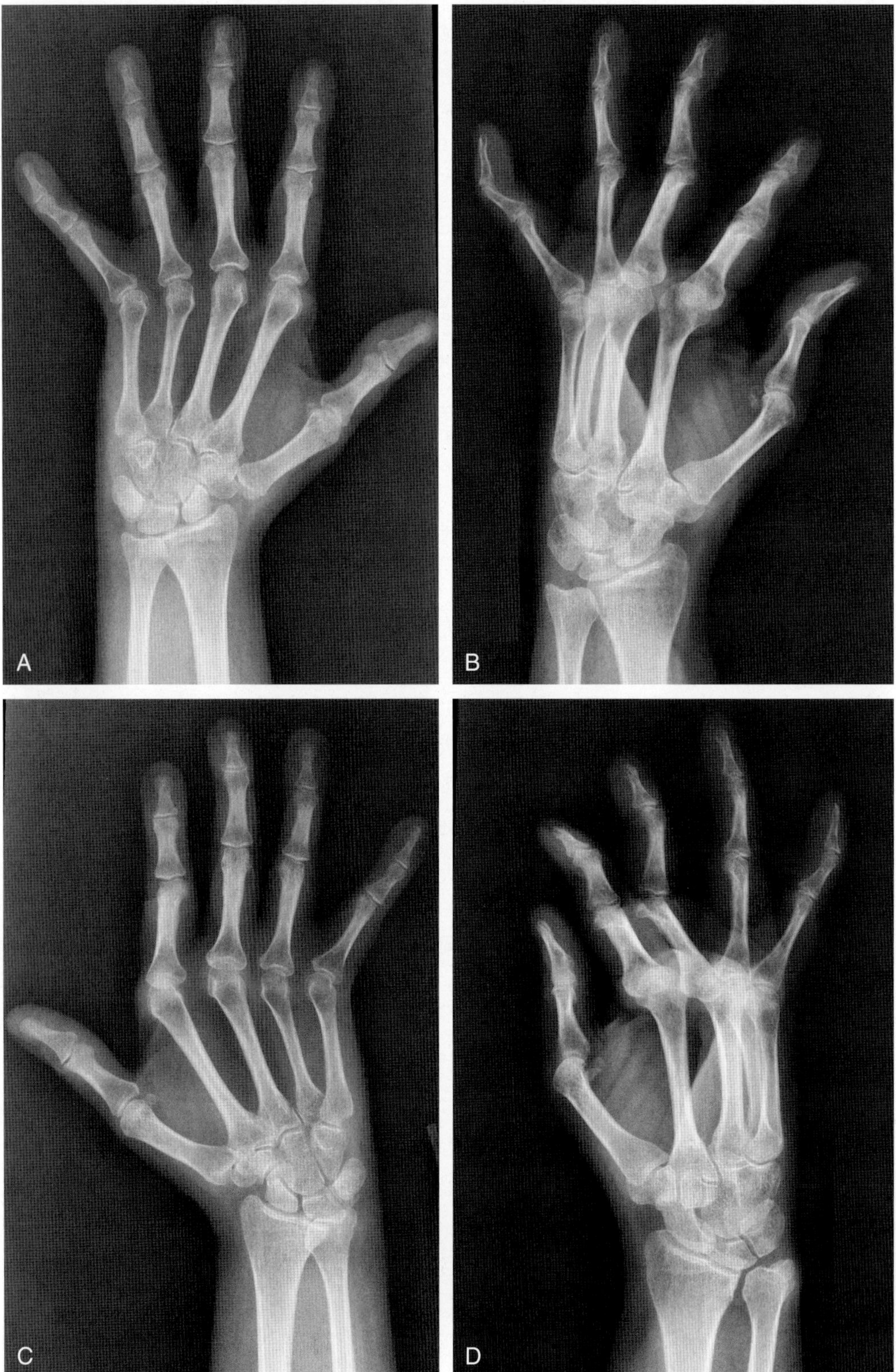

FIGURE 22-1. Finger deformities in SLE. **A,** Posteroanterior (PA) radiograph of the left hand. **B,** Oblique radiograph of the left hand. **C,** PA radiograph of the right hand. **D,** Oblique radiograph of the right hand showing finger deformities without apparent erosions. The correctable nature of the deformity is confirmed by the increased deformity on the oblique views in comparison to the PA radiographs, for which the hands are positioned flat on the cassette.

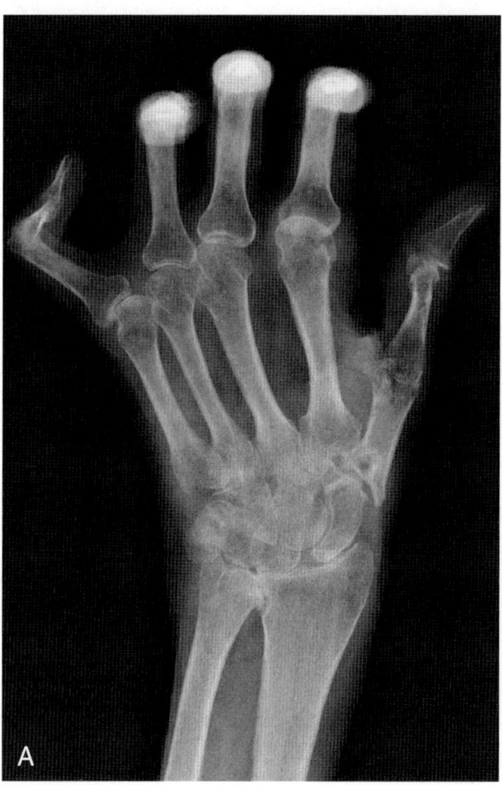

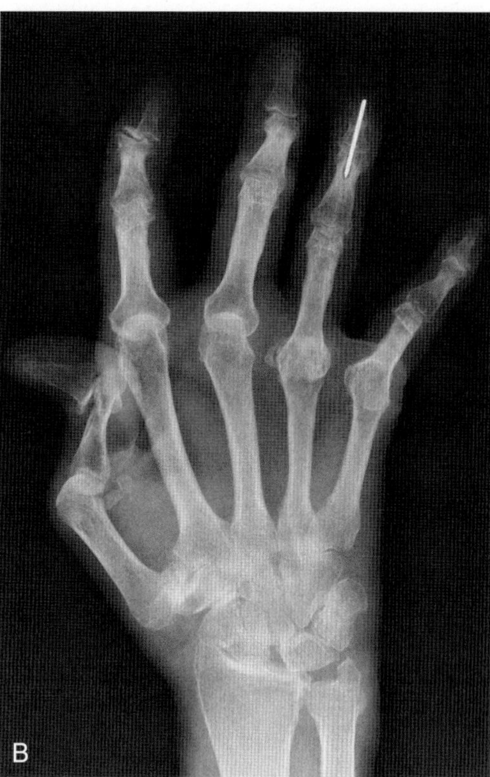

FIGURE 22-2. Thumb and finger deformities in SLE. **A,** Posteroanterior (PA) radiograph of the left hand shows fixed flexion deformities of the fingers. Marked bone loss is seen at the thumb metacarpal base. There is cartilage narrowing in the wrist. **B,** PA radiograph of the right hand shows hyperextension and subluxation of the thumb interphalangeal joint. Degenerative changes are seen at the thumb carpometacarpal articulation with flexion at the MCP joint. Subluxation is present at the index through fifth finger MCP joints. Cartilage space narrowing is noted in the wrist. Incidentally noted are degenerative changes ("gull wing" deformities) at the index finger distal interphalangeal (DIP) joint and attempted surgical fusion of the ring finger DIP.

MCP joint with hyperextension at the interphalangeal joint[12] (Figure 22-2). Later, if the carpometacarpal joint becomes unstable, and subluxation or dislocation and adduction of the thumb metacarpal occur, flexion develops at the intraphalangeal joint with hyperextension at the MCP joint.[12] This is important because treatment will require stabilization of the carpometacarpal joint before other joints are addressed.[12]

Spronk et al. developed an index to describe the severity of these deformities[10] (Table 22-2). Individuals with a score of more than 5 were classified as having Jaccoud's arthropathy.[10] In addition to finger deformities, scapholunate dissociation and ulnar translocation of the carpals may be seen. Changes in the feet consist of hallux valgus and subluxation of the metatarsophalangeal joints.[4]

The absence of erosive disease after 2 years may suggest the diagnosis of SLE over RA.

van Vugt et al. reviewed 176 patients with SLE and found a deforming arthropathy (diagnosed as any deviation of a metacarpal/finger axis) in the hands of 17 patients.[4] Cases of deforming arthropathy were subclassified as follows:

1. An erosive form ("rhupus") demonstrating features simulating RA. This was identified in 3 of 17 patients.
2. Jaccoud's arthropathy ("lupus hand") based on the index described by Spronk was seen in 8 of 17 patients.[10] Coexistence of Jaccoud's arthropathy and the antiphospholipid syndrome (APS) was noted.
3. Mild deforming arthropathy was seen in 6 of 17 patients.

TABLE 22-2. Index for Establishing the Diagnosis of Jaccoud's Arthropathy; Characteristics of Seven Patients Assigned as Having Jaccoud's Arthropathy

	Jaccoud's Index	
	Number of Affected Fingers	Points Assigned
Ulnar drift (> 20 degrees)	1–4	2
	5–8	3
"Swan neck" deformities	1–4	2
	5–8	3
Limited MCP joint extension	1–4	1
	5–8	2
Boutonniere deformities	1–4	2
	5–8	3
Z deformity	1	2
	2	3

Jaccaud's arthropathy was considered present if the score of the index exceeded 5 points.

With permission from: Spronk PE, ter Borg EJ, Kallenberg CG: Patients with systemic lupus erythematosus and Jaccoud's arthropathy: a clinical subset with an increased C reactive protein response? *Ann Rheum Dis* 51:358-361, 1992 (Table 2).

Erosive Arthritis

Although not the classical picture of SLE, approximately 1% to 2% of patients with the disorder develop an erosive arthritis resembling RA (termed *rhupus*)[4]. This may be due to the coexistence of the diseases or may represent a subset of lupus patients.

Bywaters described hook deformities at the MCP joints.[13] These have the radiographic appearance of corticated erosions, and no active pannus is seen in these areas on pathologic examination.[13] As in RA, erosive changes may also occur due to remodeling (compressive erosion) or due to chronic changes from adjacent inflamed tendons.[4] Reilly et al. found ulnar styloid erosions (postulated to be due to adjacent tenosynovitis) in 28% of 51 cases of SLE.[6]

Richter Cohen et al. found erosive changes in 5% of hand or foot radiographs of 200 SLE patients with a minimum follow-up of at least 2 years (or until death). Erosive disease was seen especially in nonwhite women, and there was greater renal involvement and more widespread or severe disease in those with erosive arthropathy.[14] The authors noted that anti RA-33 antibodies may identify those patients with SLE who are at risk for erosive disease.[14] van Vugt et al. found that lupus patients who displayed erosion were positive for rheumatoid factor.[4]

> Erosive changes occur in a small percentage of patients with SLE. Magnetic resonance imaging (MRI) and ultrasound are generally more sensitive for finding erosion than is radiography.

MRI of Joints in SLE

MRI allows all portions of the joint and the periarticular soft tissues to be evaluated and is more sensitive for erosion than are radiographs. MRI evaluation of the hands of 14 patients with SLE by Ostendorf et al. showed periarticular capsular swelling in all cases, joint effusion in 7, and "edematous tenosynovitis" (fluid signal in tendon sheaths) in 6.[11] Even in patients with deforming Jaccoud's arthropathy of long duration or with higher seroactivity, there was no synovial membrane hypertrophy to indicate "active synovitis," and only 1 patient showed mild synovial hypertophy.[11]

MRI is apparently unable to differentiate patients with early SLE from those with early RA.[15] Thus Boutry et al. compared the MRI findings in patients with inflammatory arthralgias later shown to have RA, SLE, or Sjogren's syndrome. Radiographs showed no erosion. No significant difference was found among the groups in terms of global scores for synovitis, bone lesions, and tenosynovitis.[15] The soft tissues adjacent to the joints of patients with SLE did not show abnormalities (such as has been seen in disorders such as psoriatic arthritis and reactive arthritis).[15] Erosions were seen in SLE as well as in RA (Figure 22-3).

Ultrasound of Joints in SLE

High-resolution ultrasound allows real-time assessment of joints and surrounding soft tissues at low cost and with no ionizing radiation. However, ultrasound examination requires an operator experienced in examinations of these musculoskeletal structures.

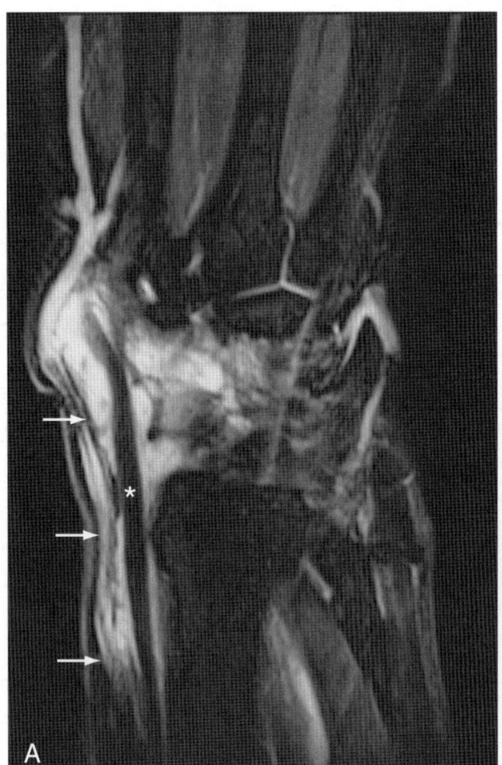

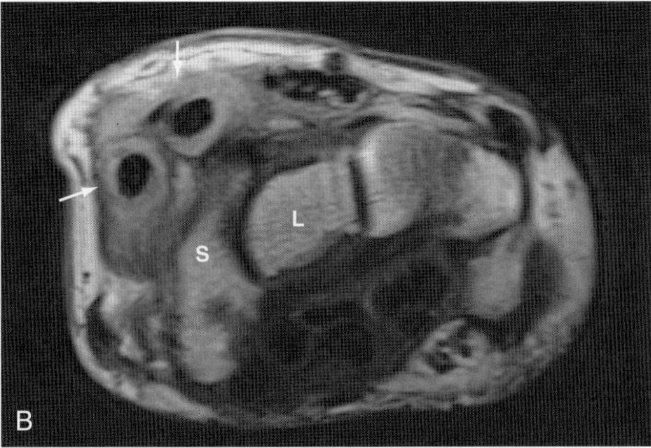

FIGURE 22-3. Synovitis and erosion on MRI of a 70-year-old woman with SLE and wrist swelling of uncertain cause clinically. **A,** Coronal inversion recovery (STIR) image shows marked swelling (high signal, *arrows*) on the radial side of the wrist. The extensor carpi radialis longus tendon *(asterisk)* is surrounded by the swelling. **B,** The axial proton density image of the wrist at the level of the scaphoid *(S)* shows intermediate signal swelling *(arrows)* surrounding the tendons of the second compartment. The dorsal aspect of the wrist is up. *L,* Lunate.

(Continued)

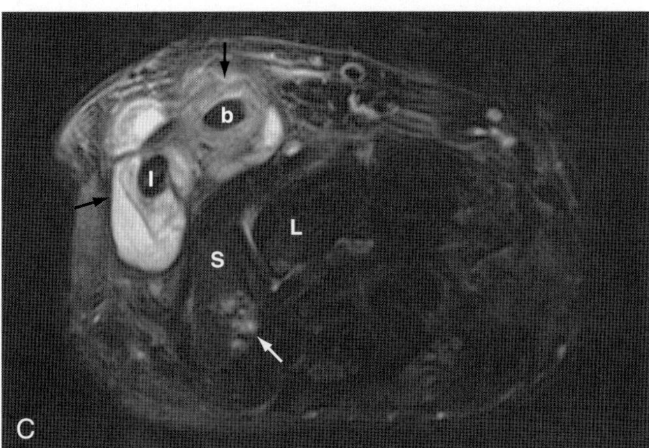

FIGURE 22-3—cont'd. **C,** Axial fat-suppressed T2-weighted image at the level of the lunate *(L)* and scaphoid *(S)*. The bright fluid and intermediate signal tenosynovitis around the extensor carpi radialis longus *(l)* and brevis *(b)* tendons *(arrows)* are well seen. Erosions of the scaphoid *(white arrow)* are noted. The appearance is indistinguishable from rheumatoid arthritis.

Power Doppler is complementary, allowing hyperemia to be detected.[16] Using these techniques, effusion, synovitis and tenosynovitis, tendon rupture, and bone erosion can be detected. Ultrasound is more sensitive for erosion than radiography and can be more sensitive than clinical examination. Evaluation of 17 patients with SLE and clinically involved hands found abnormalities on ultrasound, including tenosynovitis, tendon rupture, and erosions in the second or third MCP joints when no erosion was demonstrated on radiographs.[16] Wrist evaluation in patients with SLE has shown a high incidence of synovitis and tenosynovitis using ultrasound.[17]

> Ultrasound can detect effusion, synovitis and tenosynovitis, tendon rupture, and bone erosion and is generally more sensitive than radiography or clinical examination for these findings.

Calcification

Periarticular calcification occasionally occurs in patients with SLE.[7] Generally, when considering the causes of periarticular calcification, it is helpful to divide them into metabolic causes (abnormal calcium and/or phosphate levels) or dystrophic conditions (due to underlying tissue damage such as an underlying inflammatory process). A third category, idiopathic calcification, contains the specific entity of "tumoral calcinosis."[18] Among the causes of dystrophic calcification are progressive systemic sclerosis, mixed connective tissue disease, dermatomyositis and polymyositis, and SLE.

Calcium deposits in the skin (calcinosis cutis) may also occur in SLE[18,19] (Figure 22-4). Differential considerations for calcinosis cutis may also be grouped into metastatic, dystrophic, and idiopathic categories, as well as iatrogenic causes.[20]

> Causes of periarticular calcification can be grouped into (1) metabolic abnormalities (abnormal calcium and/or phosphate levels),[18] (2) dystrophic calcification (due to underlying tissue damage such as an underlying inflammatory process), and (3) idiopathic calcification.

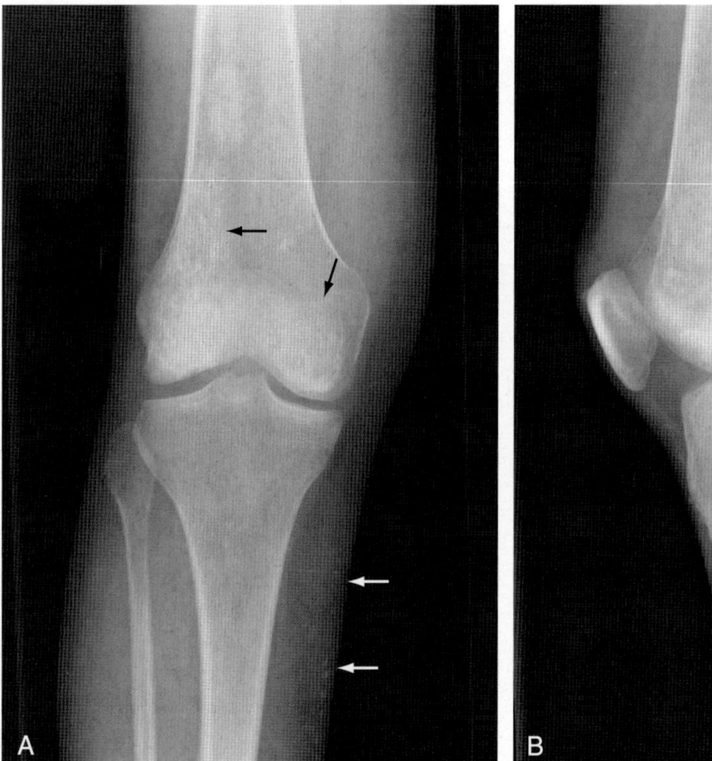

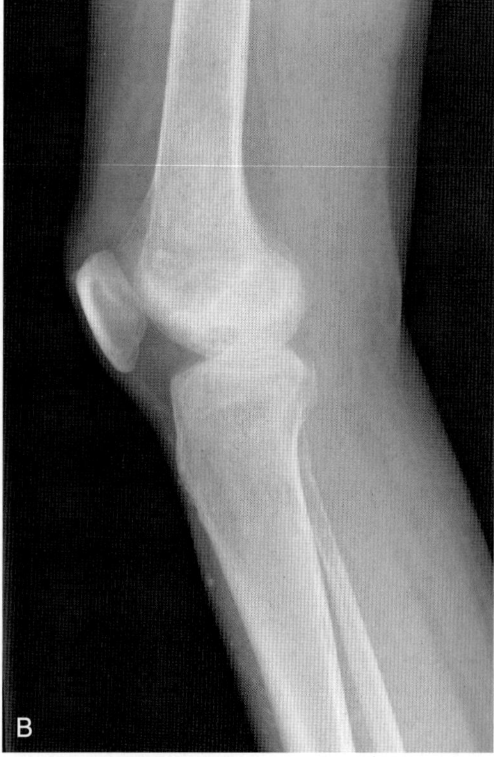

FIGURE 22-4. SLE with AVN and calcinosis cutis. **A,** Anteroposterior and **(B)** lateral radiographs of the knee show areas of increased opacity in the femur *(black arrows)* consistent with extensive infarction. There are scattered calcifications that are located superficially *(white arrows)*, indicating calcinosis cutis.

Cystic Changes

Well-defined radiolucent areas can be seen especially in the metacarpal heads and carpal bones of patients with SLE. Leskinen et al. found these lucencies in 41% of 125 patients with the disorder, and multiple lesions may be seen.[21] The lesions are surrounded by a thin sclerotic rim of normal bone and may enlarge, increase in number and be associated with erosions. They are, however, nonspecific findings that may quite often be seen in unaffected individuals.[7]

Tuft Resorption

Tuft resorption or periarticular calcification is seen in patients with SLE who have Raynaud's phenomenon.[7] Tuft resorption is a nonspecific finding and occurs also in conditions such as scleroderma, hyperparathyroidism, and psoriatic arthritis. These conditions can usually be differentiated on the basis of clinical and radiologic findings.

Acral Sclerosis

Osteosclerosis of the terminal tufts of the fingers is a nonspecific finding seen primarily in RA, scleroderma, dermatomyositis, and sarcoidosis as well as in normal individuals[22] (Figure 22-5). This abnormality was seen in 10 of the 59 (16.9%) SLE patients examined by Weissman et al. and was accompanied by Raynaud's phenomenon in only 4 patients.[7] Braunstein et al. found acral sclerosis in 12% of individuals with SLE presenting over the age of 50 years and in 10% of those presenting earlier in life.[23]

Tendon Rupture

Tendon rupture is an uncommon sequela of SLE. It most likely is the result of inflammatory changes within the tendon[4] but may also occur due to corticosteroid injections or trauma.[17]

Osteonecrosis (Avascular Necrosis)

The association of SLE and avascular necrosis (AVN) was initially reported in 1960 by Dubois and Cozen.[24] All but 1 of the 11 patients described had received corticosteroids, but in 5 patients it had been months or years since corticosteroid administration. The hips, knees, and shoulders are most commonly affected, although AVN of the small bones can also occur (Figure 22-6). AVN can develop within the first months of initiation of high-dose corticosteroid treatment.[25]

Only 5% to 10% of patients with AVN become symptomatic; therefore diagnosis cannot be based on the presence of symptoms.[25] Jaovisidha et al. prospectively evaluated 11 patients with newly diagnosed SLE treated with corticosteroids. Despite being asymptomatic, MRI demonstrated AVN in 4 of 22 hips (2 of 11 patients).[25] Early treatment may prevent collapse of the femoral head, and this suggests a role for screening studies such as MRI.[25] Risk factors for asymptomatic AVN are said to be African-American ethnicity, Raynaud's phenomenon, migraine headaches, and a maximum corticosteroid dose of at least 30 mg/day.[25] Duration of treatment and cumulative dose seemed to relate to the development of clinically occult AVN in the study of Jaovisidha et al.[25] The presence of bone marrow edema on MRI has been shown to correlate with the development of symptoms and the disappearance of edema with subsidence of symptoms.

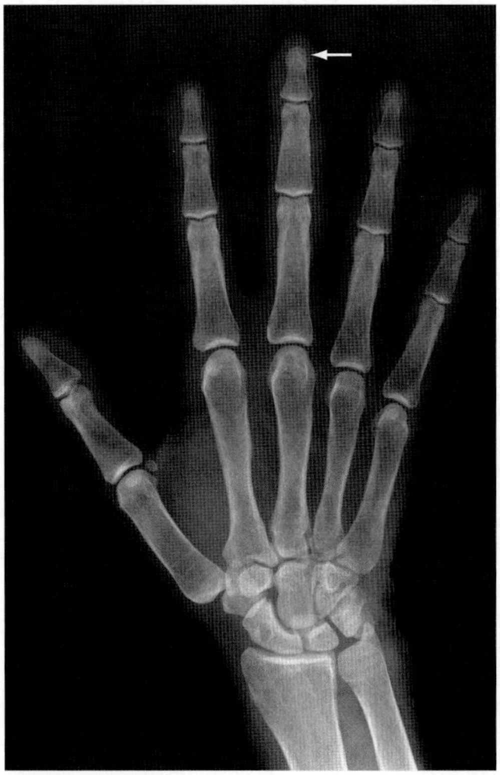

FIGURE 22-5. Acral sclerosis in a patient with SLE. Posteroanterior radiograph of the fingers shows increased density of the terminal phalanges *(arrow)*.

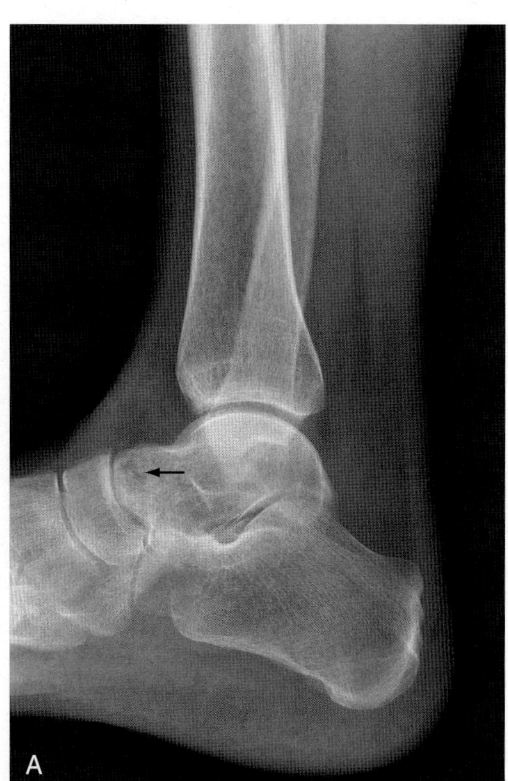

FIGURE 22-6. AVN involving the ankle and hindfoot. **A,** Radiograph of the ankle shows slight lucency of the talar head *(arrow)* but no other abnormality of bone density.

(Continued)

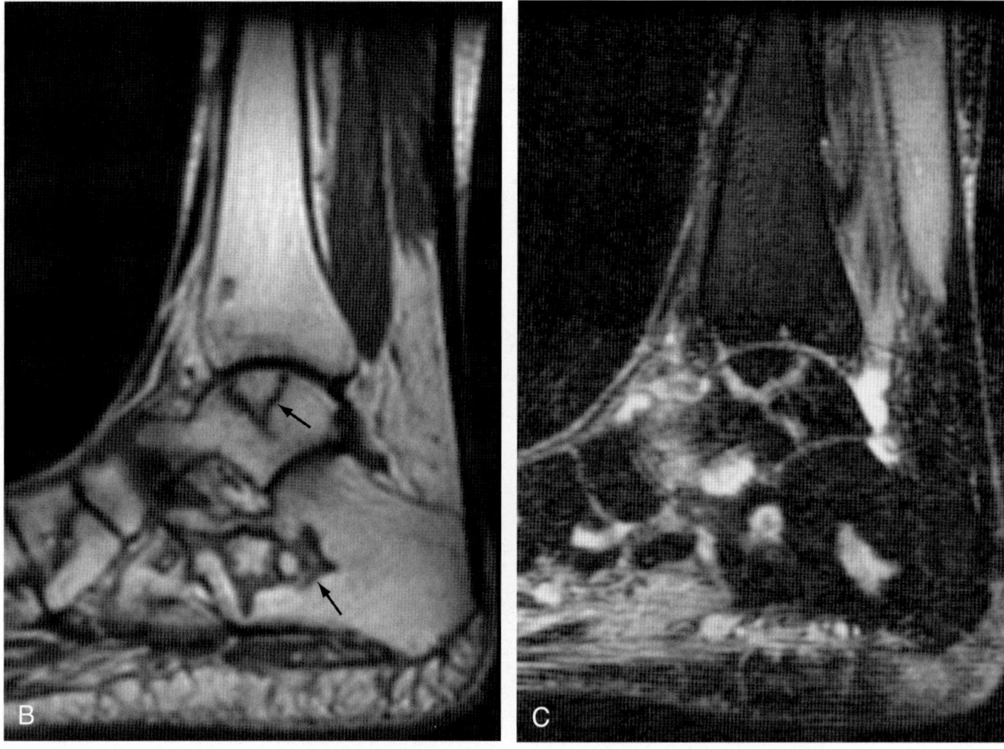

FIGURE 22-6—cont'd. **B,** Sagittal T1-weighted and **(C)** sagittal STIR images show multiple infarcts *(arrows)* including an infarct with edema of the talar head.

This finding has also been correlated with subsequent femoral head collapse[26] (Figure 22-7). In patients with symptomatic AVN, collapse of the femoral head usually occurs within 2 years.[25]

> MRI is useful in detecting early AVN, as changes on MRI may be visible before structural alterations (e.g., crescent sign, collapse) are evident. AVN may be present without symptoms.

Gastrointestinal Manifestations

Gastrointestinal (GI) manifestations of SLE are common[28] and may affect any portion of the GI tract beginning with the mouth.[1] Underlying causes of GI abnormalities include vasculitis, obliterative vascular thrombosis causing bowel ischemia, immune complex deposition producing an inflammatory response, and treatment complications.[1,27] Abdominal pain occurs in up to 40% of patients with SLE and may be due to serositis, pancreatitis, bowel ischemia, or perforation.[1]

Esophagus

Esophageal symptoms include dysphagia (incidence as high as 13%) and heartburn (incidence as high as 50%).[27] Disordered esophageal motility is common, with decreased or absent peristalsis

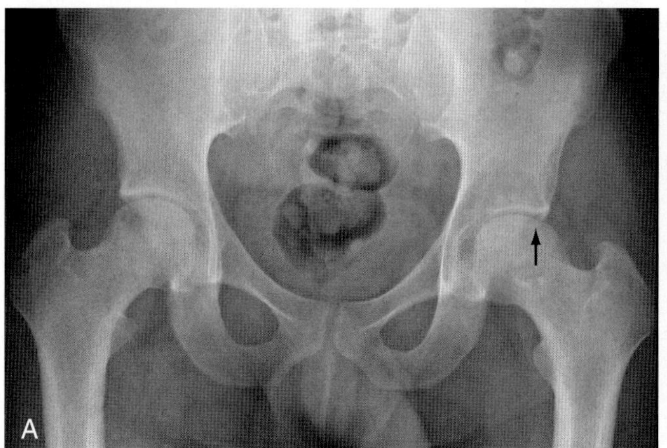

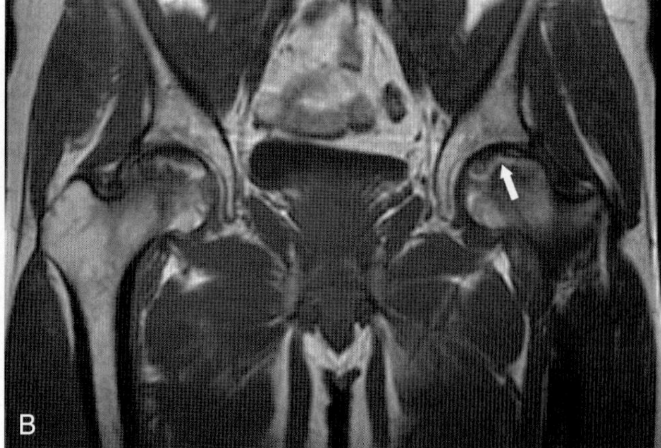

FIGURE 22-7. AVN of the hips in a patient with SLE. **A,** Anteroposterior radiograph of both hips shows cyst-like changes in the right femoral head. There is no definite collapse. On the left, there are areas of slight lucency and sclerosis in the femoral head and neck. A subchondral lucent line (the crescent sign, *arrow*) is seen with overlying flattening of the femoral head. **B,** Coronal T1-weighted image through the femoral heads shows replacement of the normal marrow fat of both the right and left *(arrow)* epiphyses.

(Continued)

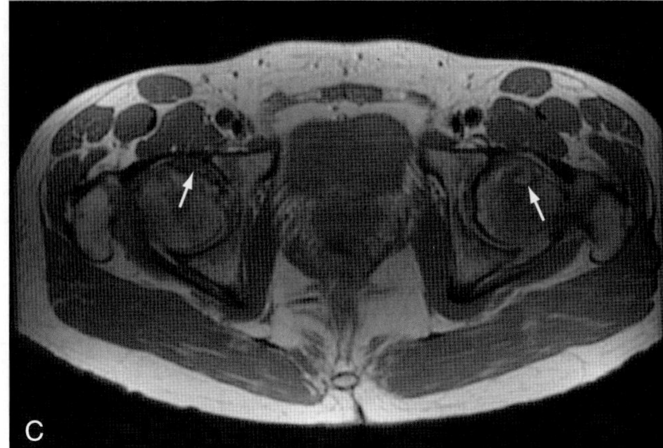

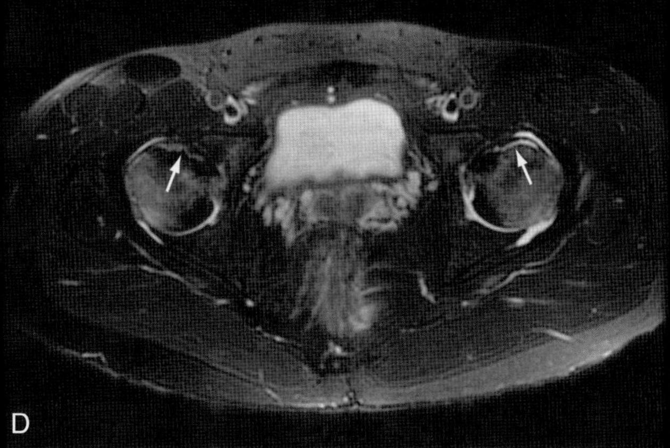

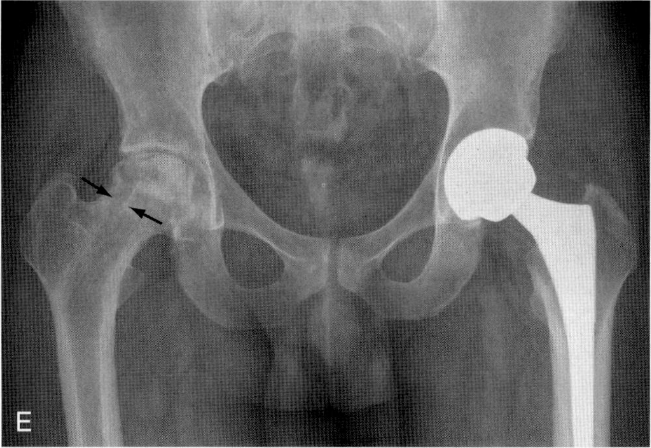

FIGURE 22-7—cont'd. **C,** Axial proton density image through the femoral heads shows the areas of abnormality to be positioned anteriorly, a location typical for avascular necrosis. The margins of the abnormal areas are better delineated *(arrows)* on the MRI than on the radiograph. **D,** Axial STIR image through the femoral heads shows the "double line" sign of AVN on the right with a dark line and an inner bright line *(arrows)*. There is diffuse edema of the femoral head. On the left, a subchondral crescent sign (fracture) is seen *(arrow)* with separation of the anterior cortex from the underlying bone. There is diffuse bone marrow edema. **E,** Radiograph obtained 11 months after total hip replacement on the left and core decompression on the right. The tract *(arrows)* from the core decompression is seen. However, there has developed flattening of the right femoral head since the first radiograph **(A)** 1 year before.

especially in the lower third of the esophagus.[27] Possible causes of dysmotility include an inflammatory reaction in the esophageal muscles, ischemic vasculitic damage of the Auerbach plexus, or involvement of the vagus nerve.[28] Symptoms may also be due to medications including nonsteroidal antiinflammatory medications[27] or bisphosphonates. Esophageal ulceration or perforation may occur.[1] Barium study can demonstrate abnormal motility and mucosal irregularity or ulceration associated with reflux[1] (Figure 22-8).

Stomach and Duodenum

NSAIDs and corticosteroids alone and particularly in combination may cause ulcer disease.[27] In addition, high-dose corticosteroids may mask the early clinical signs of a perforated ulcer, necessitating vigilance on the part of the clinician and the imager.[27] Double-contrast upper GI series can demonstrate ulcers.[1]

Small and Large Bowel

Small-vessel vasculitis may lead to ischemic enteritis, bowel infarction with bleeding and/or perforation, and peritonitis. Clinical presentation is variable and nonspecific, and important and ominous physical findings may be masked by treatment with corticosteroids or immunosuppressant medications.[27] Lee et al. noted enteritis (vasculitis) to be the most common cause of acute abdominal pain in patients with SLE.[29]

Radiographs may show "thumbprinting" due to mural edema or hemorrhage but are less sensitive than computed tomography (CT) for the diagnosis of ischemia.[1] Radiographs may also show free intraperitoneal air, pneumatosis cystoides intestinalis, ileus, or a pseudo-obstruction pattern.[27] Gas in the portal venous system is an ominous sign.

Byun et al. note the importance of CT scanning for detecting the cause of GI symptoms and identifying complications such as perforation. These authors evaluated the CT findings in 33 patients (39 examinations) with SLE and acute abdominal pain.[30] The diagnosis of ischemic bowel disease was made if at least three of the following signs were seen: bowel wall thickening, target sign, dilatation of intestinal segments, engorgement of mesenteric vessels, or increased attenuation of mesenteric fat.[30] The areas of wall thickening could be multiple and did not necessarily correspond to a vascular territory (as would be true in large vessel disease).

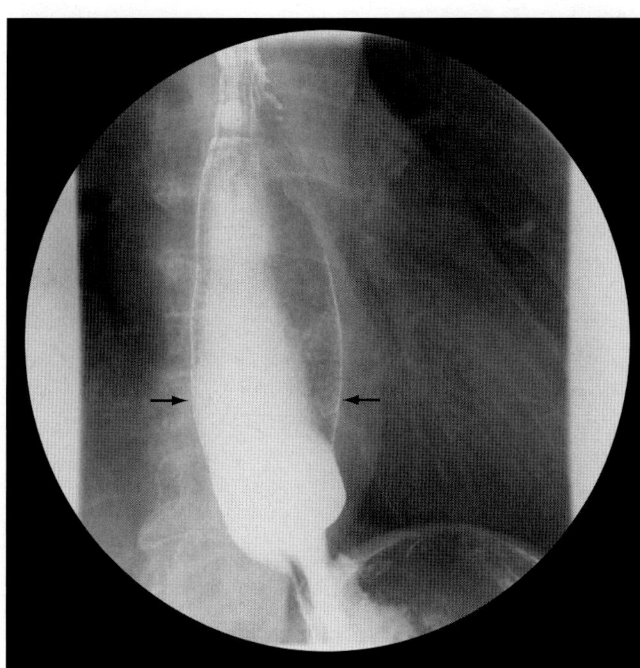

FIGURE 22-8. Esophageal dysmotility in a 76-year-old woman with CREST (calcinosis, Raynaud's, esophageal dysmotility, sclerodactyly, telangiectasia) and a feeling of food sticking in her throat. This fluoroscopic image from a double-contrast barium swallow examination shows a markedly dilated distal esophagus *(arrows)*. Tertiary contractions were noted proximally. No ulceration was detected.

The target sign in contrast-enhanced CT consists of thickened bowel wall with three layers: contrast-enhanced inner and outer layers and an interposed layer of decreased attenuation that is thought to be due to edema.[31] It is a nonspecific finding in ischemia because it is seen in several "benign" conditions such as Crohn's disease. It is not usually a feature of malignancy.[31]

Ulcerative colitis, Crohn's disease, collagenous colitis, celiac disease, and protein losing enteropathy may occur in SLE patients.[27] Infectious colitis is a particularly important complication of SLE because it may be fatal, and this should be excluded before high-dose corticosteroid or immunosuppressive treatment is begun.[27] Colon perforation may occur due to arteritis or diverticula, and the resulting pneumoperitoneum can be confirmed on upright or decubitus radiographs or on CT.[27]

Gallbladder

Acalculous colicystitis may result from periarterial fibrosis and acute vasculitis. Ultrasonography or contrast-enhanced CT can show the resultant gallbladder wall thickening, as well as pericholecystic fluid.[1]

Pancreatitis

Pancreatitis occurs in up to 28% of patients with SLE and is most often associated with active involvement in other organs. Findings on CT or ultrasound of acute pancreatitis are summarized by Lalani et al.[1] as peripancreatic edema, phlegmon formation, infiltration of mesenteric fat, and sometimes enlargement of the affected portion of the gland. The pancreatic margins become indistinct. Chronic pancreatitis is common and may be asymptomatic. The gland saponifies and calcification forms within the ducts, which are irregularly narrowed and dilated on CT or ultrasound.[1]

Renal Manifestations

Most patients with SLE have renal involvement.[1] Lupus nephritis results from autoantibodies cross-reacting with glomerular surface antigens, mesangial matrix, or basement membranes, resulting in the deposition of immune complexes in the subepithelial and subendothelial layers of the glomeruli.[1] Liberation of cytokines and glomerular necrosis and fibrosis ensue.[1] As with other causes of medical renal disease, affected kidneys in SLE are hyperechoic on ultrasound examination and may be small.

Central Nervous System Manifestations

Central nervous system (CNS) abnormalities in SLE occur in approximately 40% of patients.[1] They range from cognitive dysfunction and psychiatric disorders to seizures and strokes.[32] Cognitive dysfunction is usually mild but is present in up to 30% of patients.[2] Some instances of psychiatric symptoms may also be caused by high-dose corticosteroid treatment. Because lupus can involve any region of the nervous system such as the brain, meninges, spinal cord, and peripheral nerves, patients may present with stroke, demyelinating syndromes, headache, chorea, long tract signs, aseptic meningitis, myelopathy, Guillain-Barre syndrome, plexopathy, cranial and/or peripheral neuropathy, myasthenia gravis, autonomic disorder, or migraine.[32] Lupus-related stroke occurs more often in young patients about 35 years old. Etiologies of stroke include coagulopathy associated with lupus anticoagulant, small vessel vasculitis, embolization from Libman-Sacks endocarditis, or even hypertension secondary to renal disease.[32] In addition, accelerated atherosclerosis related to corticosteroid usage may be a contributing factor.[1]

The diagnosis of SLE should be considered in any young patient who presents with stroke.[1]

Infarcts in SLE are often small, involving deep or subcortical white matter, although occasionally they can be large and territorial (Figure 22-9). Arterial or venous thrombosis, seen especially in patients with APS, can lead to serious morbidity and mortality.[1]

Patients with neuropsychiatric disorders should be worked up to exclude underlying causes such as infection, medication effects, or metabolic disorders such as uremia or hypertensive encephalopathy.[33] CT and MRI are useful imaging modalities to assist in the evaluation of these patients. Both unenhanced CT or MRI with GRE and diffusion sequences are particularly applicable for the assessment of hemorrhage and stroke (Figures 22-10 to 22-12). A contrast study, in turn, will help detect infectious or inflammatory etiologies such as meningitis, abscess, or vasculitis.[1]

Some of the CNS findings seen in SLE are shown in Table 22-3. MRI has shown reduction of both gray and white matter volume in patients with SLE as compared with controls.[34] Other MRI techniques such as magnetization transfer and diffusion weighted imaging (DWI) help to understand and define different aspects of the disease process.[35] DWI in conjunction with apparent diffusion coefficient (ADC) maps describe the freedom (Brownian motion) of protons in water molecules to move within their environment (termed *diffusivity*).[35-37] Normally, diffusion is relatively impeded by physical barriers such as myelin sheaths.[37] In cerebral ischemia, restricted diffusivity is thought to be caused by a relative decrease in extracellular water as it shifts to the intracellular space due to failure of sodium potassium pumps. This results in low ADC values with concurrent increased signal on DWI images[37] (see Figures 22-11 and 22-12). In vasogenic edema, protons move freely along white matter fibers with increased ADC values and normal signal on

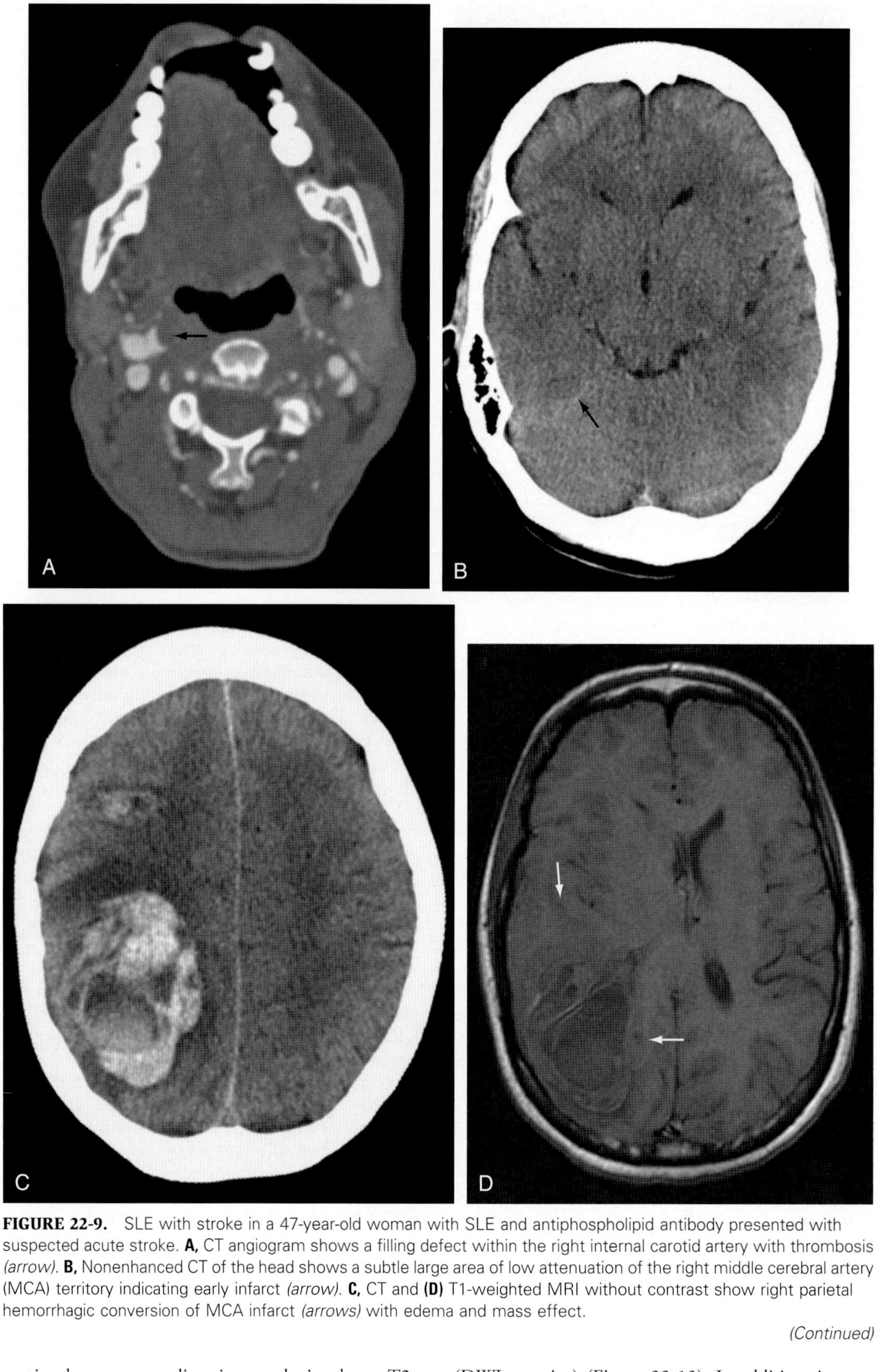

FIGURE 22-9. SLE with stroke in a 47-year-old woman with SLE and antiphospholipid antibody presented with suspected acute stroke. **A,** CT angiogram shows a filling defect within the right internal carotid artery with thrombosis *(arrow)*. **B,** Nonenhanced CT of the head shows a subtle large area of low attenuation of the right middle cerebral artery (MCA) territory indicating early infarct *(arrow)*. **C,** CT and **(D)** T1-weighted MRI without contrast show right parietal hemorrhagic conversion of MCA infarct *(arrows)* with edema and mass effect.

(Continued)

DWI.[37] There is also corresponding increased signal on T2-weighted and fluid attenuated inversion recovery (FLAIR) sequences due to the increased water content.[37] DWI is especially important in differentiating lupus patients with ischemic changes (DWI positive) from those who have hypertensive encephalopathy (DWI negative) (Figure 22-13). In addition, increased diffusivity has been found in patients with neuropsychiatric SLE thought to be related to demyelination or increased CSF space secondary to atrophy from the underlying disease process, corticosteroid usage, and, perhaps, neuronal/axonal damage.[35]

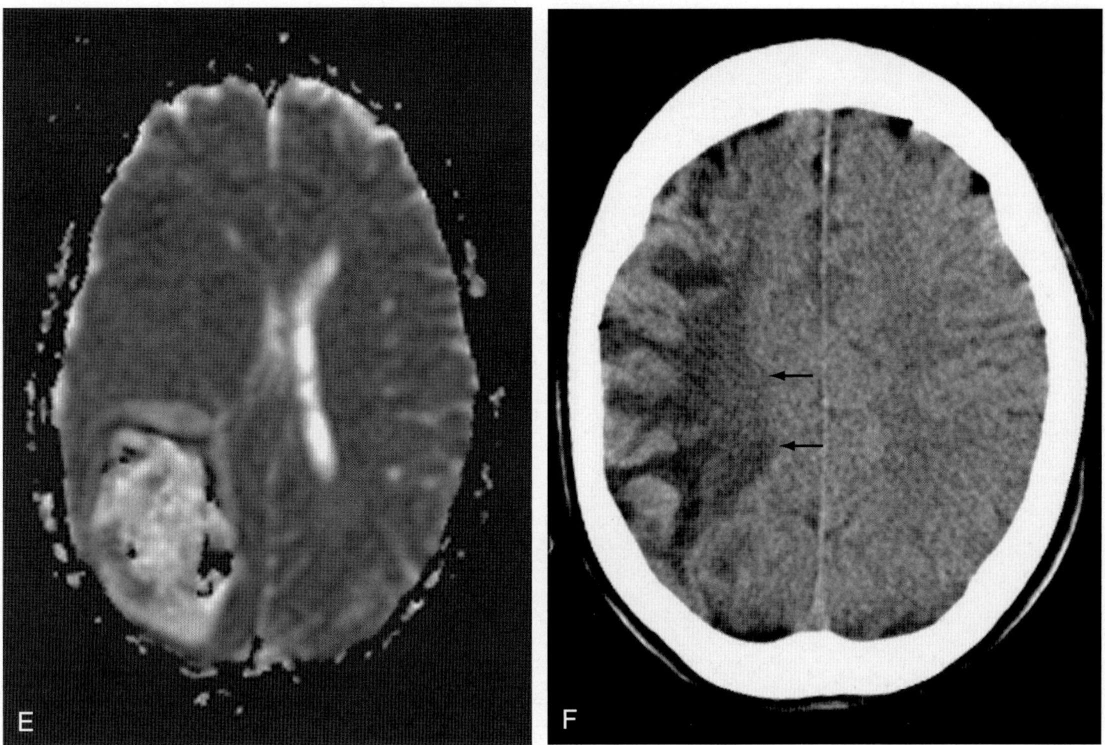

FIGURE 22-9—cont'd. **E,** Diffusion-weighted image again shows heterogeneous signal of hemorrhagic right parietal infarct. **F,** Follow-up noncontrast CT several years later obtained for seizure evaluation demonstrates chronic low attenuation encephalomalacic changes *(arrows)* of the prior hemorrhagic MCA infarct.

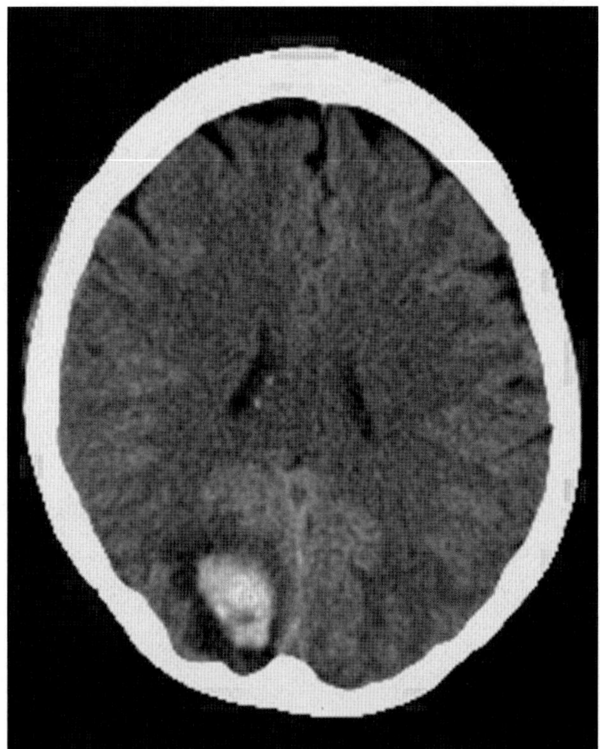

FIGURE 22-10. Hemorrhage. Nonenhanced axial CT image shows high attenuation in the right parietal occipital junction, indicating hemorrhage. The adjacent ring of low (dark) signal indicates edema.

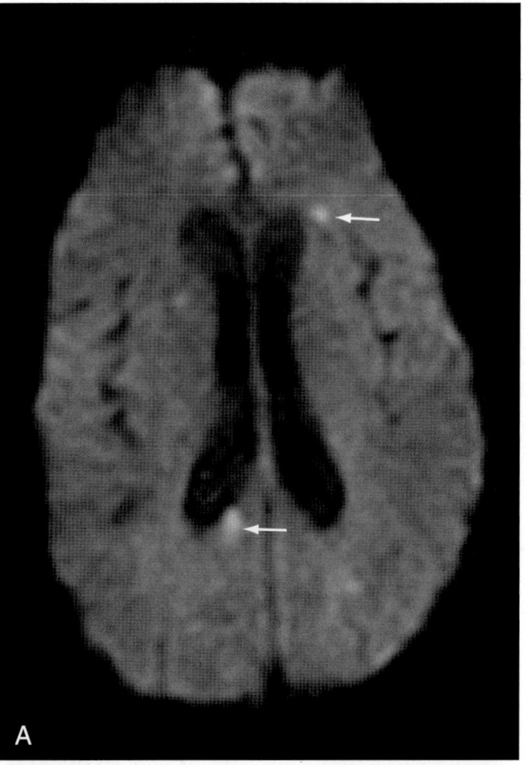

FIGURE 22-11. Small vessel disease in a 68-year-old woman with SLE. **A,** DWI shows multiple small periventricular and subcortical foci of restricted diffusion *(arrows)* consistent with small infarcts.

(Continued)

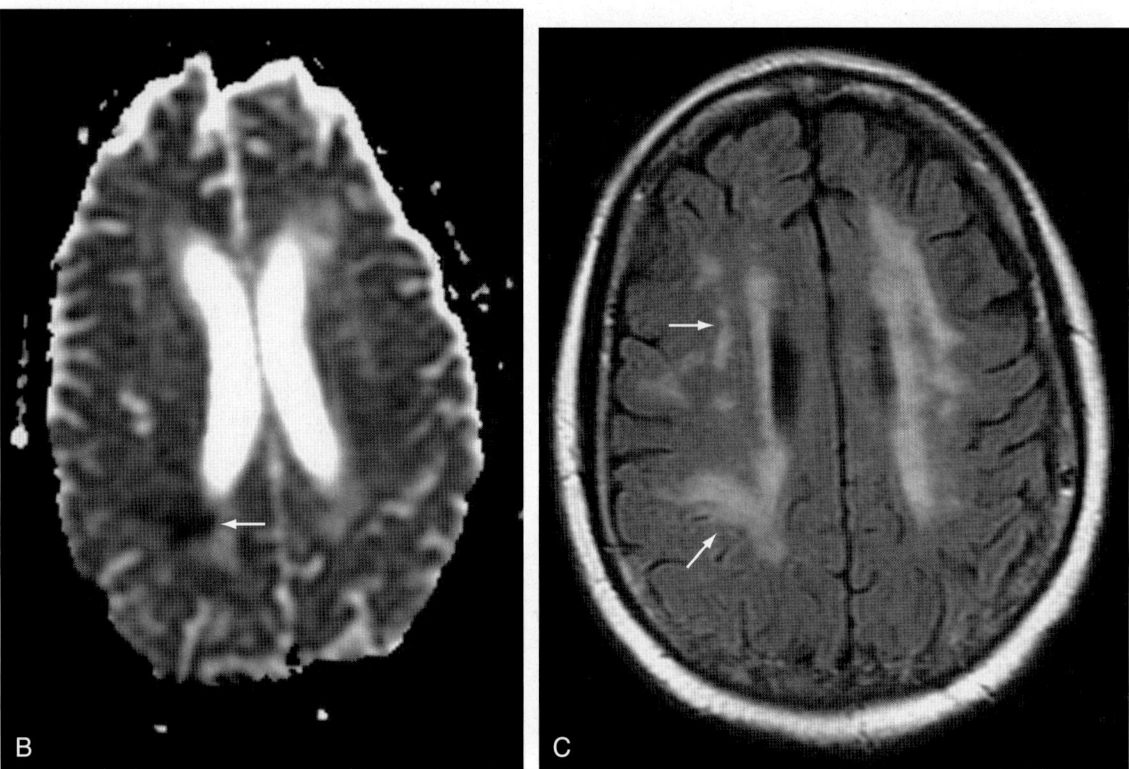

FIGURE 22-11—cont'd. **B,** Corresponding ADC map shows the dark parietal lesion *(arrow)*. **C,** Chronic small vessel disease is shown as high signal *(arrows)* on the FLAIR sequence.

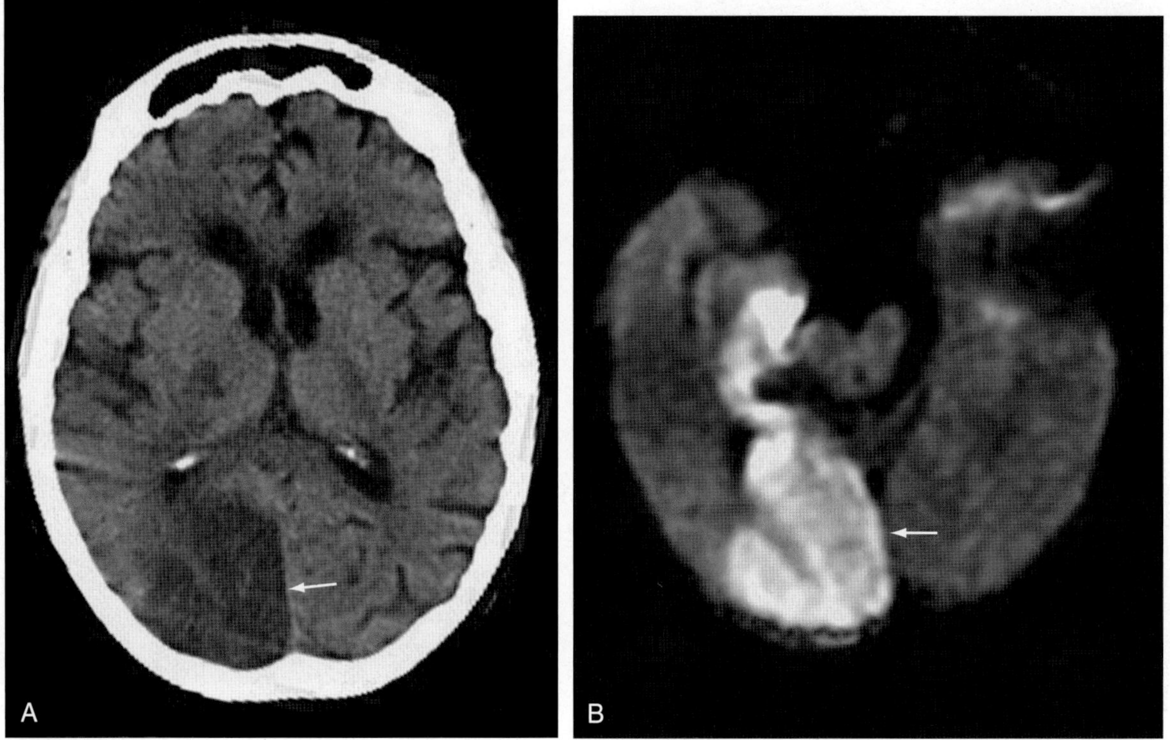

FIGURE 22-12. Large vessel disease. **A,** Noncontrast CT shows low-attenuation right posterior carotid artery (PCA) infarct *(arrow)* without hemorrhage. **B,** DWI shows the corresponding acute right PCA infarct.

TABLE 22-3. Brain CT and MRI Findings in SLE

Location of Lesion	Finding on CT/MRI	Example
Small vessel disease	Small cortical or deep gray matter infarcts	
Large vessel disease	Infarcts in large vessel territory	
Occlusion of dural venous sinuses and deep cerebral veins	CT: Increased attenuation of affected sinus Contrast-enhanced CT: "delta sign" due to thrombus outlined by contrast; edema/infarction low-attenuation areas in thalamus, basal ganglia, or white matter MRI: T1-weighted: abnormal flow, increased signal in sagittal sinus *(arrows)*	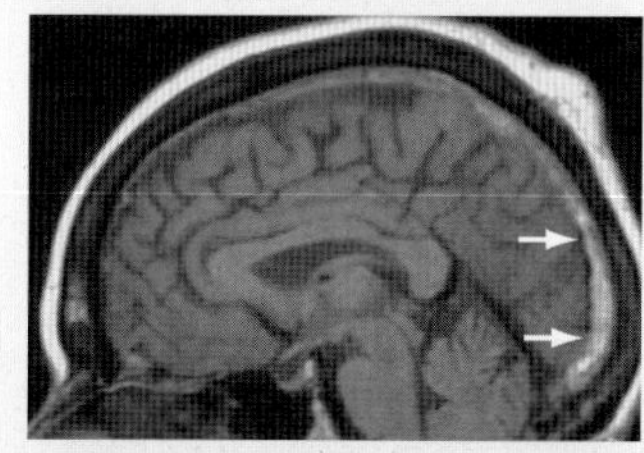
Intracranial hemorrhage	CT: Increased attenuation of blood; intracranial aneurysms due to fibrinoid necrosis of vessel walls	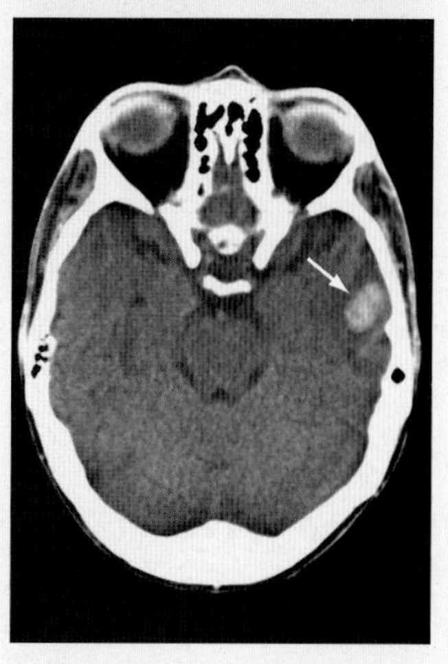

(Continued)

TABLE 22-3. Brain CT and MRI Findings in SLE—cont'd

Location of Lesion	Finding on CT/MRI	Example
Abscess	CT: Low-attenuation mass with peripheral enhancing rim MRI: Rim enhancing mass with surrounding edema (example)	
Vasculitis[1]	Small focal areas of abnormal T2 signal with or without associated punctate linear enhancement Irregularity of vessels on angiogram (example)	
Posterior reversible leukoencephalopathy syndrome[39]	T2 and FLAIR: Hyperintense signal in bilateral occipital, parietal, and temporal white matter with sparing of cortex (example) DWI: Lack of restricted diffusion, increased ADC values due to vasogenic edema[103]	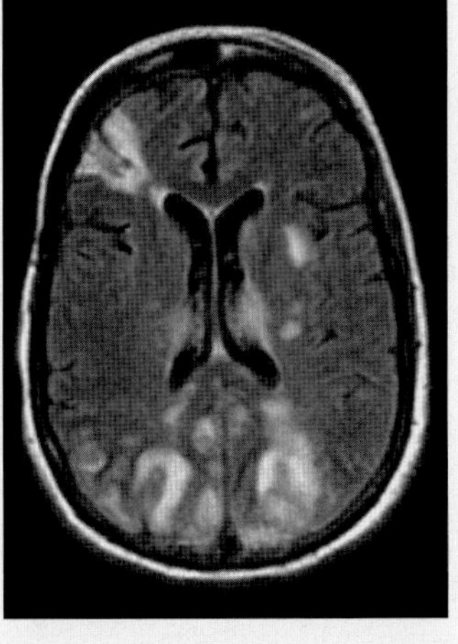

From Lalani TA, Kanne JP, Hatfield GA et al: Imaging findings in systemic lupus erythematosus, *Radiographics* 24:1069-1086, 2004.

In patients with SLE, abscesses may result from Libman-Sacks endocarditis. The edema usually seen associated with abscesses may not be as obvious owing to the suppressive effects of corticosteroids.[1] Venous sinus thrombosis is evident on CT or MRI as increased attenuation or signal, respectively, in the vessel. A so-called delta sign after contrast administration occurs as the thrombus is outlined by contrast. Venous infarcts may also be associated with hemorrhage.

Posterior Reversible Encephalopathy Syndrome

Posterior reversible encephalopathy syndrome (PRES) (also called *reversible posterior leukoencephalopathy syndrome* [RPLS]) may occur in patients with SLE. The syndrome is characterized by clinical findings of rapid onset of headache, seizures, hypertension, altered mental status and bilateral cortical blindness, and imaging findings indicating vasogenic edema of the posterior circulation, particularly bilateral parietooccipital white matter and, occasionally, cerebellar involvement. These findings often resolve after appropriate treatment of hypertension and seizures. Sometimes, however, when treatment is delayed, PRES can progress to frank ischemia involving both gray and white matter with or without associated hemorrhage or enhancement.[37]

The cause of this condition is not certain but is thought to be secondary to underlying endothelial injury exacerbated by a sudden rise in blood pressure that exceeds the autoregulatory capacity of the cerebral vessels; this leads to fluid extravasation and subsequent vasogenic edema.[37] The imaging findings are reflective of the leakiness of the involved vasculature (see Figure 22-13).

In SLE patients, studies have shown that hydrogen-1 MR spectroscopy may be of value. The spectroscopy findings in one study were

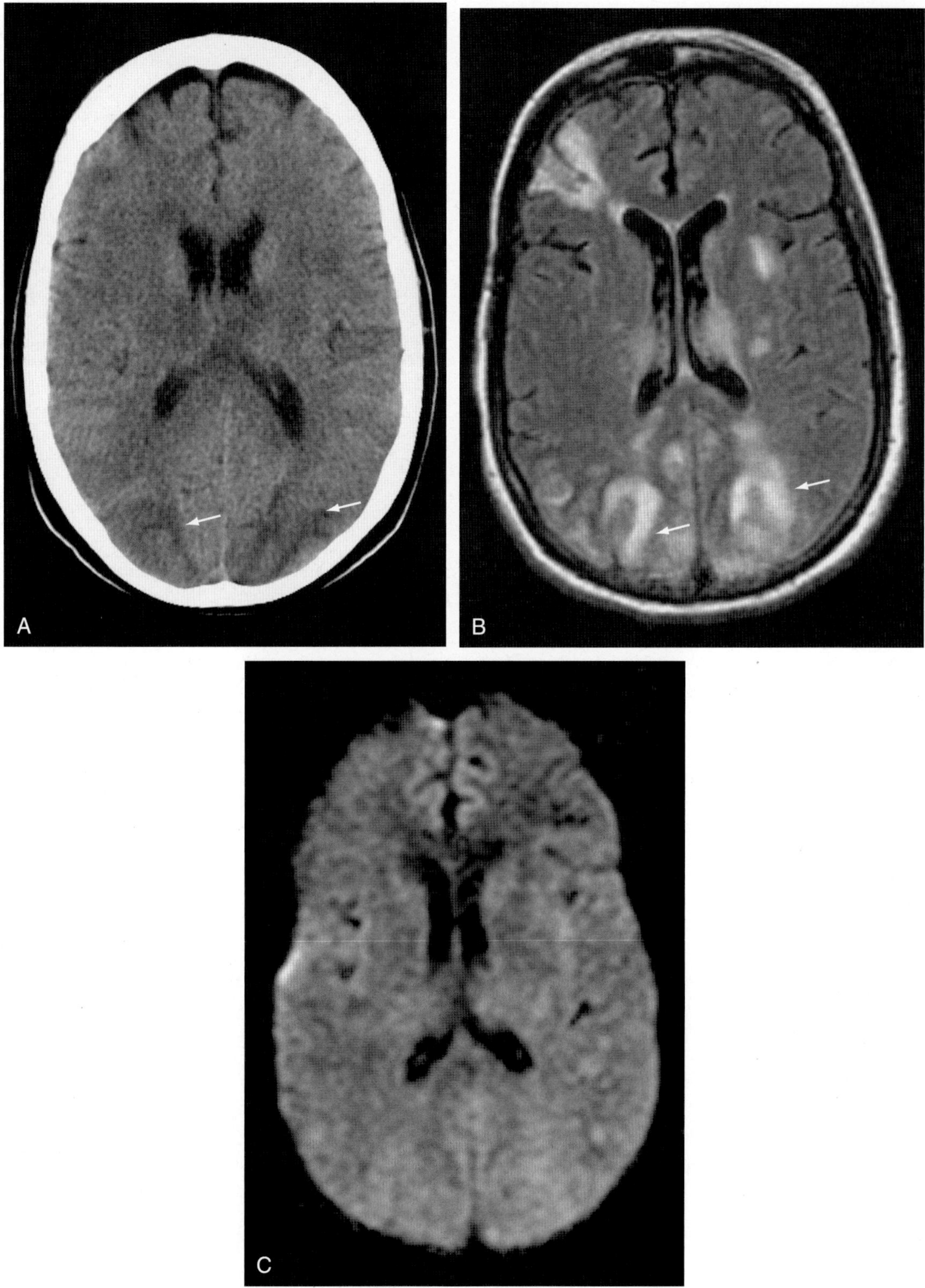

FIGURE 22-13. PRES in a diabetic patient without SLE. **A,** Noncontrast CT shows symmetric and bilateral low attenuation in the parietal occipital subcortical white matter *(arrows)*. **B,** Corresponding MRI FLAIR image reveals increased signal in these regions *(arrows)* as well as other areas of abnormality. **C,** These abnormal areas do not show restricted diffusion, consistent with vasogenic edema and not ischemic changes.

thought to mirror the cerebral metabolic disturbance related to the severity of neuropsychiatric symptoms rather than the MRI findings.[38] Others have also attempted using Tc-99m ECD (ethyl cysteinate dimmer) and SPECT imaging to assess regional cerebral blood flow as a means of documenting changes before and after treatment.[39]

Cardiovascular Involvement

Cardiac involvement may take the form of valvular abnormalities, Libman-Sacks endocarditis, myocarditis, pericarditis, premature coronary atherosclerosis (that may be related to corticosteroid treatment), and coronary arteritis.[2] Pulmonary venous thromboembolic complications may cause pulmonary hypertension and right heart failure, although pulmonary hypertension can exist independent of clots.

Involvement of the cardiac valves is seen in 18% to 74% of the patients and is considered the most common cardiac manifestation of SLE. Valvular involvement is particularly common in antiphospholipid antibody positive patients.[1] Postulated pathogeneses of the development of endocarditis are fibrinoid degeneration of the valvular leaflets, vasculitis, and corticosteroid-related valvulopathy. Valvular involvement in SLE can range from leaflet thickening to Libman-Sacks endocarditis, which is characterized by the presence of small, sterile, pink vegetations that are associated with inflammation.[1] Valvular disease is not related to disease severity, disease activity, or disease duration. The most commonly involved valve is the mitral, followed by the aortic. Hemodynamically significant lesions require immediate diagnosis and surgical repair. Structural abnormalities may predispose to thrombus formation and bacterial endocarditis.

Symptomatic pericarditis occurs in about 25% of SLE patients and asymptomatic pericardial involvement in more than half of the cases.[40] Pericardial effusion and/or inflammation (pericarditis) may be the presenting manifestation of SLE. Cardiac tamponade and constrictive pericarditis rarely result. Relatively large effusions can be detected on radiographs by the "water bottle" shape of the heart on the frontal projection or by separation of the substernal and epicardial fat planes by more than 2 mm (some authors say 4 mm) on the lateral or frontal radiograph (Figure 22-14).[41]

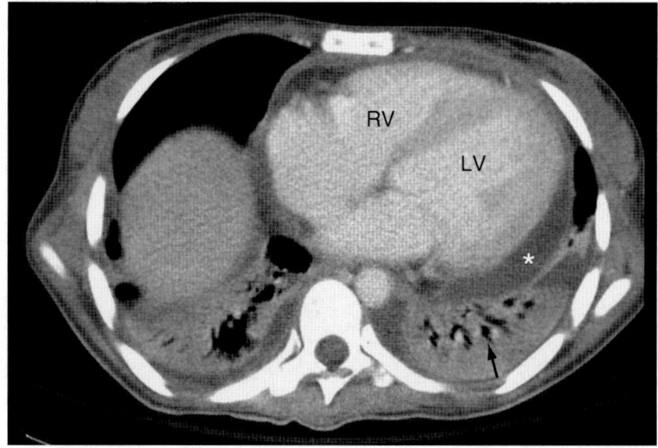

FIGURE 22-15. CT of pericardial effusion. CT scan shows a rind of fluid attenuation *(asterisk)* around the heart. The left *(LV)* and right *(RV)* ventricles and the atria are well seen. There is pulmonary consolidation with air bronchograms *(arrow)* at the lung bases.

Echocardiography (ECG), CT, and MRI are more sensitive for detecting small effusions (Figures 22-15 and 22-16). CT attenuation measurement is useful for initial characterization of pericardial fluid. Pericardial fluid in SLE is usually exudative. Nonhemorrhagic fluid has water density on CT, low signal intensity on T1-weighted spin echo (SE) MR images, and high signal intensity on gradient echo (GRE) cine MR images. Conversely, hemorrhagic effusion is characterized by high density on CT, hyperintense signal on T1-weighted SE MR images, and hypointense signal on GRE cine images. The normal pericardium is primarily composed of fibrous tissue and thus is hypodense on CT images and has low signal intensity on both T1-weighted and T2-weighted MR images. In subacute forms of pericarditis, the thickened pericardium has moderate to high signal intensity on SE images. Post-contrast enhancement in the visceral and parietal

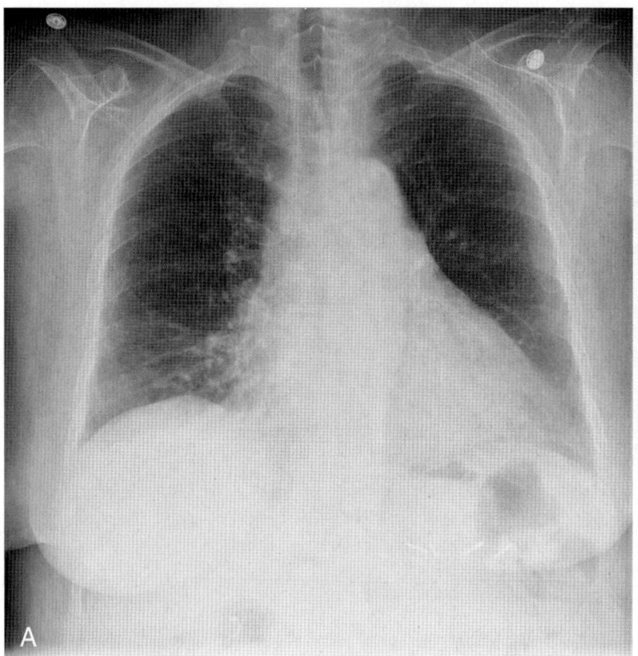

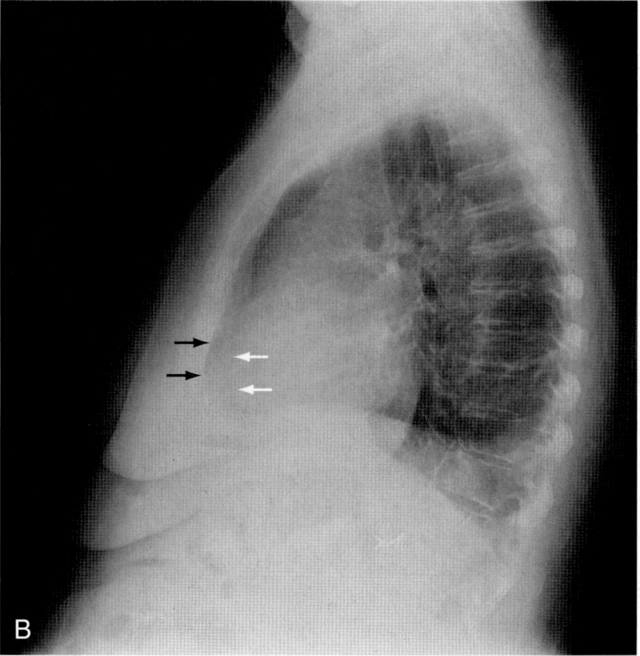

FIGURE 22-14. The "oreo cookie" sign of pericardial effusion. **A,** Posteroanterior radiograph shows the heart to be large. Surgical clips are present from prior splenectomy. **B,** On the lateral radiograph there is separation of the retrosternal *(black arrows)* and epicardial *(white arrows)* fat pads, consistent with a pericardial effusion (the "oreo cookie" sign).

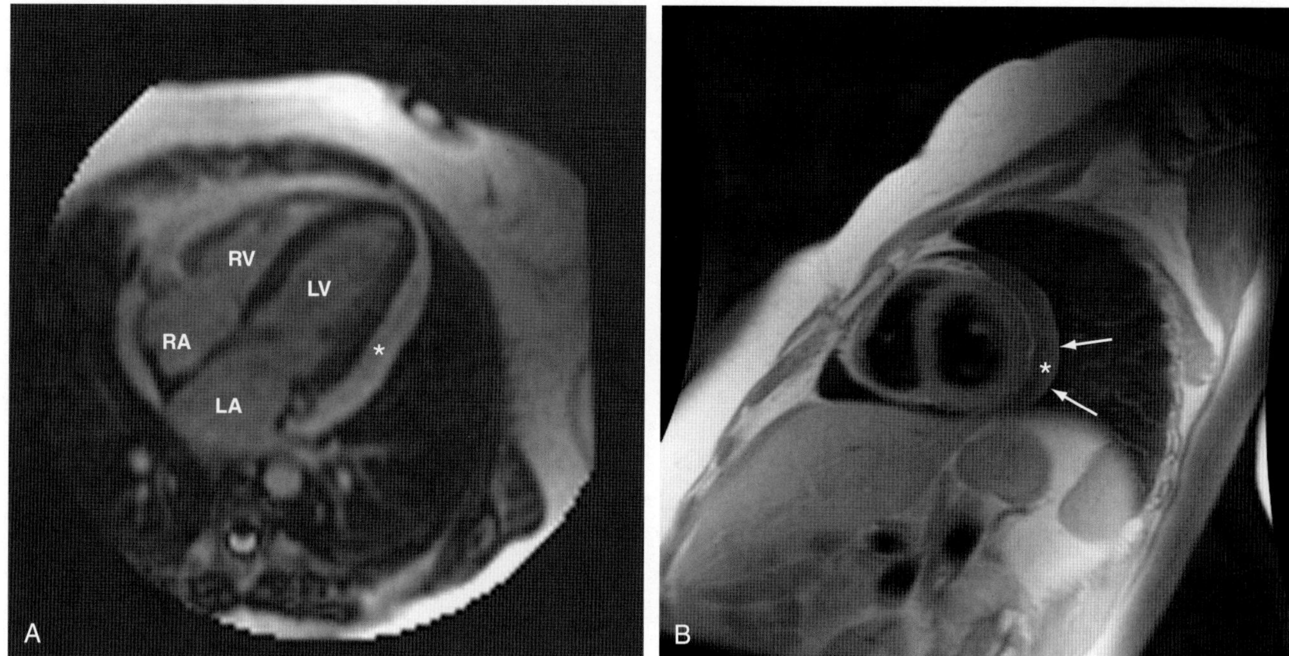

FIGURE 22-16. MRI of pericardial effusion in a 50-year-old patient with a history of SLE endocarditis, pericardial effusion, and chest wall pain. The MRI was performed to evaluate the degree of pericardial thickening. **A,** A four-chamber SSFP (single shot free precession) MR image of the heart shows the bright signal surrounding the heart *(asterisk)*, indicating a pericardial effusion. *LA,* Left atrium; *LV,* left ventricle; *RA,* right atrium; *RV,* right ventricle. **B,** Direct sagittal T1-weighted double inversion recovery image shows the intermediate signal effusion *(asterisk)* around the heart. The pericardial thickness is normal (< 4 mm) *(arrows* on parietal pericardium).

layers of the pericardium and possibly the epicardium on CT and T1-weighted MR images suggests active inflammation. Cine MRI has a reported accuracy of 93% for differentiation between constrictive pericarditis and restrictive cardiomyopathy on the basis of an depiction of abnormally thickened pericardium (4 mm) (Table 22-4).

> Pericardial effusion can be detected and characterized (e.g., hemorrhagic), and thickening of the pericardium can be assessed on CT or MRI.[42]

SLE myocarditis is characterized by myositis associated with perivascular infiltration by neutrophils and lymphocytes, as well as

TABLE 22-4. Cardiovascular Imaging Findings in SLE

Area Involved	Manifestations	Imaging Findings
Myocardium	Myocarditis Left ventricular dysfunction Heart failure	Echo and cine MRI: Global systolic or diastolic left ventricular dysfunction, cardiomegaly MRI: Increased T2 relaxivity in active disease, patchy contrast enhancement in the outer levels of myocardium on IR-GE images
Pericardium	Pericardial effusion Constrictive pericarditis/heart failure	Radiograph: Effusion (positive fat pad sign, “water bottle” heart) Echo: Effusion (but cannot demonstrate pericarditis) CT/MRI: Effusion, abnormal thickening, and enhancement of pericardial layers on T1-weighted images
Valves	Libman-Sacks endocarditis Valvular dysfunction Systemic emboli Subacute bacterial endocarditis	Echo and MRI: Valvular leaflet thickening, valvular vegetations associated with Libman-Sacks endocarditis (1–4 mm granular lesions), flow abnormality through the involved valve on 2D phase contrast MR images, thrombus
Coronary arteries	Unstable angina Myocardial infarction Ischemic cardiomyopathy Sudden death	Conventional and CT coronary angiography: Coronary artery calcifications, occlusive atherosclerotic plaques, coronary aneurysms IVUS: Plaque characterization ECG-gated CT: High calcium scores are predictive for future ischemic events SPECT: Myocardial perfusion defects
Aorta/ Carotid	Hypertension Stroke Peripheral occlusive arterial disease Complications associated with aortic aneurysm and dissection	US/CTA/MRA: Plaques, intimal-medial thickening in carotid arteries; aortic aneurysm/ dissection

intimal proliferation and hyalinization of the intramyocardial small vessels. Myocarditis is diagnosed by the presence of symptoms of heart failure and left ventricular (LV) dysfunction, with or without cardiac dilatation. Patients with active SLE have higher end diastolic volumes than those with inactive SLE or controls. Increased signal intensity on T2-weighted MR images indicates myocardial edema and thus inflammation. Although not specific for SLE myocarditis, increased T2 relaxation values can be a sensitive indicator of active myocardial involvement, even in the absence of clinical criteria. The T2 relaxation value of the myocardium returns to normal in inactive SLE.[43]

MRI can detect active inflammatory myocarditis. Necrotic areas associated with myocarditis demonstrate contrast enhancement on inversion recovery gradient echo (IR-GRE) pulse sequences. With this technique, selective suppression of normal myocardial signal allows markedly increased contrast between normal and enhancing myocardium.

> In contrast to myocardial infarction, foci of enhancement are typically located in the outer myocardial layers, sparing the subendocardium.

In myocarditis, the regions of contrast enhancement are usually in a patchy distribution typically located in the outer myocardial layer, which is different from the typical subendocardial scar tissue enhancement that is seen in myocardial infarction.

Steady-state free precession (SSFP) pulse sequence is commonly used for functional imaging of the heart. This imaging technique allows ventricular wall motion assessment, ventricular volume measurements, and cardiac valve evaluation.

Premature atherosclerosis of the coronary arteries can be seen in SLE and may be associated with vasculitis (fibrinoid necrosis, infiltration by neutrophils and lymphocytes) and induced by corticosteroid treatment. Positive antiphospholipid antibodies may accelerate the atherogenesis and increase the thrombus burden. Inflammation of plaques may lead to plaque vulnerability and, thus, increased risk of thrombus burden due to the rupture, unstable angina, myocardial infarction, and sudden death in the absence of significant (> 50%) luminal stenosis. Coronary aneurysms may suggest vasculitis.

> Neither conventional nor CT angiography can assess plaque vulnerability.

Coronary angiography is the gold standard for demonstrating obstructive atherosclerotic lesions. ECG-gated multislice CT coronary angiography is a recently introduced coronary imaging technique that has 98% negative predictive value in detecting occlusive lesions of the coronary arteries. However, neither conventional nor CT angiography can assess plaque vulnerability. Intravascular ultrasonography (IVUS) is an invasive imaging modality, but it can identify atheromatous plaques in angiographically normal appearing vessels, and can define plaque characteristics which are important in determining plaque stability (i.e., the amount of fibrosis and calcification). Coronary calcium scoring with ECG-gated CT is a highly accepted scanning technique for predicting future ischemic events.

> Coronary calcium scoring with ECG-gated CT is a highly accepted scanning technique for predicting future ischemic events.

In one series, Tc-99m sestamibi myocardial perfusion SPECT imaging identified myocardial perfusion abnormalities in both symptomatic (22 abnormal of 25 patients) and asymptomatic (8 abnormal of 25 patients) patients with SLE.[44] Control patients showed no abnormalities.

Aortic and Carotid Involvement

Recent research has demonstrated reduced elasticity of the arterial walls (sclerosis) in patients with SLE. This functional disturbance can contribute to the atherosclerotic process, which may be already accelerated due to the inflammatory-mediated intimal-medial thickening, and high prevalence of the traditional risk factors seen in SLE.[45,46] Aortic aneurysm has been reported.[47]

Pulmonary and Pleural Involvement

The most common cause for chest pain is costochondritis.

Unilateral or bilateral pleural effusions, often with pericardial effusion, are typical chest imaging manifestations of SLE.[48] They are, however, nonspecific.

> Pleural effusions are the most common pleuropulmonary manifestation of SLE.[1]

Pulmonary findings are less frequent.[7] Analysis of 1000 patients followed for 10 years with SLE revealed lung involvement overall in 3% at onset and an additional 7% on follow-up. Bacterial pneumonias, opportunistic infections, emboli, congestive heart failure, uremia, disseminated intravascular coagulation, pulmonary hemorrhage, or acute lupus pneumonitis may occur.[2,49] Lupus pneumonitis is a diagnosis of exclusion. It is seen on radiographs as patchy consolidation, usually involving the lung bases, often with pleural effusion.[1] Areas of opacification on radiographs may also be seen with hemorrhage, pneumonia, or edema.[48] Patients with acute pulmonary hemorrhage are typically acutely ill and have hemoptysis, fever, cough, and hypoxemia.[1] Recurrent atelectasis and decreased lung volume may occur in patients with SLE, possibly as a consequence of phrenic neuropathy.[2] Repeated pneumonia can result in bronchiectasis.[1]

Interstitial pneumonitis and pulmonary artery hypertension are more often seen in overlap syndromes than in SLE (Figure 22-17). Chronic interstitial pneumonitis and fibrosis are uncommon.[49] A reticular pattern that involves mainly the lower lung zones may be seen on radiographs in patients with SLE and interstitial fibrosis.[49] High-resolution CT scanning is useful in characterizing pulmonary abnormalities that may occur in SLE and is much more sensitive in detecting these changes than are radiographs.[49]

> High resolution CT is recommended when clinical features and pulmonary function tests are abnormal but radiographs are normal.[1]

Kim et al. found that ground-glass attenuation and consolidation may reflect interstitial pneumonitis and fibrosis, acute lupus pneumonitis, hemorrhage or, occasionally, cryptogenic organizing pneumonia (COP). Interstitial changes were usually mild and focal and honeycombing was uncommon.[49] Lalani et al. note that irreversible lung disease and pulmonary fibrosis are characterized by architectural distortion, honeycombing, and subpleural thickening, whereas acute alveolitis (which can be reversed with corticosteroid treatment) shows ground-glass opacity.[1]

Pulmonary artery hypertension is usually associated with antiphospholipid antibody syndrome (due to recurrent pulmonary emboli) or chronic interstitial lung disease.[1]

MIXED CONNECTIVE TISSUE DISEASE

Mixed connective tissue disease (MCTD) is a variant of SLE that is characterized by swelling of the fingers and hands, Raynaud's phenomenon, myositis, arthritis, lung disease, lymphadenopathy,

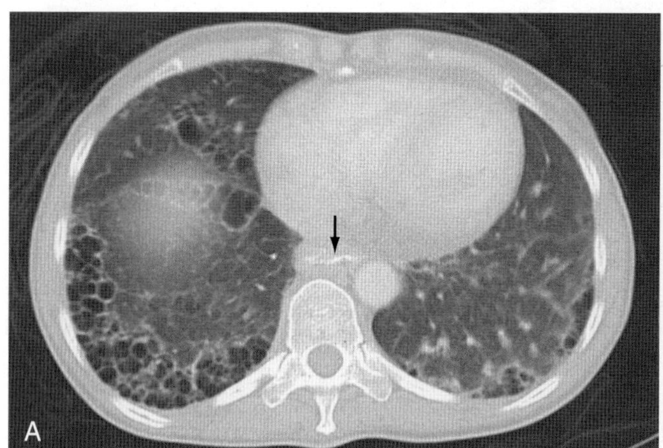

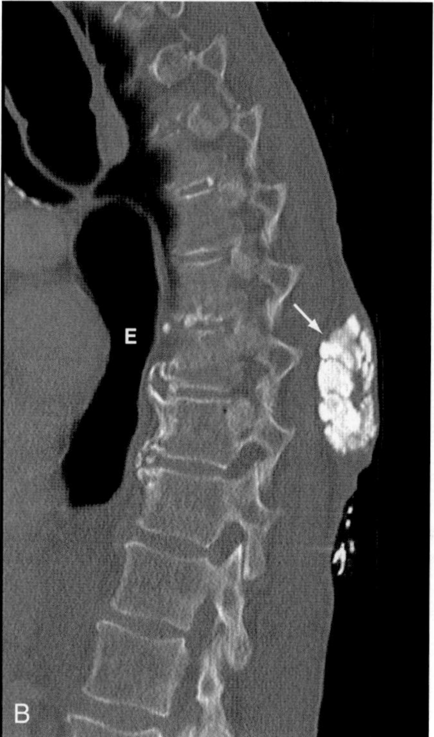

FIGURE 22-17. Scleroderma SLE overlap. **A,** CT scan through the lung bases shows a honeycomb pattern. The contrast-containing esophagus is slightly dilated *(arrow)*. **B,** There is subcutaneous calcification *(arrow)* and esophageal distension *(E)* consistent with scleroderma.

and antibodies to U1-RNP (ribonuclear protein). These patients have a lower incidence of nephritis and CNS manifestations than patients with SLE and antibodies to native DNA.[2]

Imaging features of SLE, polymyositis, progressive systemic sclerosis, and RA or psoriatic arthritis may be present.[50] Radiographic manifestations in the hands of patients with MCTD may be normal or show features of SLE, progressive systemic sclerosis, or RA.[51,52] Thus tuft erosion, distal soft tissue atrophy, periarticular calcification, distal calcification, and alignment abnormalities may occur.[50,53] Often findings consist of nonspecific soft tissue swelling, soft tissue atrophy, juxtaarticular osteopenia, cartilage space narrowing, subluxation, and tuft resporption.[51] O'Connell and Bennett noted the presence of asymmetric, small, punched-out erosions in 12 of 20 patients with MCTD.[50] They concluded that, in individuals with clinical and radiologic features of overlap syndrome, the finding of small, asymmetric, punched-out erosions should suggest a diagnosis of MCTD (Figure 22-18). Changes in the feet are less prominent than those in the hands.[53] Unilateral temporomandibular joint erosive arthritis and erosion of the proximal humerus and femoral head have been noted.[53]

Pulmonary features of MCTD include interstitial fibrosis, decreased lung capacity, subsegmental collapse, and consolidation. Pulmonary arterial vasculitis with pulmonary emboli and pulmonary hypertension has been reported. Pericardial effusion may occur[50] (Figure 22-19). Mediastinal adenopathy is a rare finding and may be accompanied by pulmonary arterial hypertension.[54] High-resolution CT scanning has shown the most frequent pattern of MCTD to be interlobular septal thickening followed by honeycombing (cystic spaces with thickened walls). The findings are those that occur in progressive systemic sclerosis, SLE, and polymyositis/dermatomyositis but with different frequency.[55]

GI findings are those associated with progressive systemic sclerosis, such as pseudodiverticula on the antimesenteric border of the colon and esophageal dilatation.[50] Parotid atrophy may occur, as in Sjogren's syndrome.

ANTIPHOSPHOLIPID SYNDROME

APS is an autoimmune disorder in which arterial or venous thrombosis, recurrent fetal loss, and elevated titers of antiphospholipid antibodies (lupus anticoagulant [LA] and anticardiolipin [aCL] antibodies) occur.[56] It is the most common cause of vascular thrombosis in children.[56] Rarely, catastrophic APS can occur in which multiorgan vascular thrombosis leads to multiorgan failure.[57]

Although APS may be a primary disorder, it may also be associated with autoimmune or other diseases, the most common of which is lupus. aCL antibodies are present in 12% to 30% and LA antibodies in 15% to 34% of patients with SLE.[58] Fifty percent to 70% of patients with SLE and antiphospholipid antibodies will develop this syndrome if followed for 20 years.[58] The diagnosis of APS is made on the basis of a combination of clinical and laboratory findings (Boxes 22-1 and 22-2). Imaging findings are those of thrombosis, most often deep venous thrombosis of the legs, pulmonary emboli, strokes, and coronary occlusions.[58] Adrenal hemorrhage may occur.[59]

KAWASAKI DISEASE

Kawasaki disease is an acute inflammatory vasculitis of as yet unknown cause but thought most likely to be of infectious etiology in a genetically susceptible individual.[60-62] It is the most common cause of multisystem vasculitis in children and has replaced rheumatic fever as the leading cause of acquired cardiovascular disease in children in the United States.[60] Clinical features of Kawasaki disease include fever, desquamative skin rash, bilateral nonpurulent conjunctival injection, erythema of the lips and oral mucosa, redness and swelling of the extremities, and cervical lymphadenopathy.[7,63] The disease especially affects the coronary arteries and results in ectasia or aneurysms in 15% to 25% of untreated children. The patients are at increased risk of coronary thrombosis and ischemia, even sudden death.[64] Aneurysms may also occur in

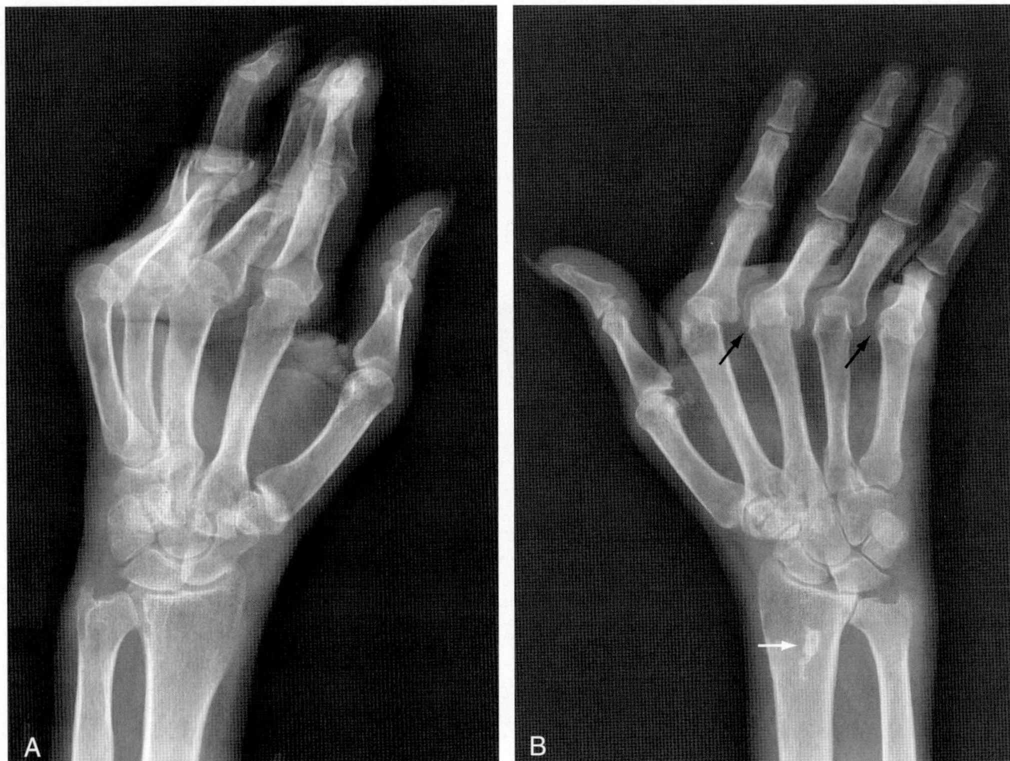

FIGURE 22-18. Hand findings of MCTD. **A,** Posteroanterior (PA) radiograph of the left hand shows periarticular soft tissue swelling and diffuse osteoporosis. There are "swan neck" deformities, especially of the fifth finger, with MCP flexion and subluxation. **B,** PA radiograph of the right hand shows swelling about the joints. Small well-defined erosions *(black arrows)* are present. An infarct is seen in the distal radius *(white arrow)*.

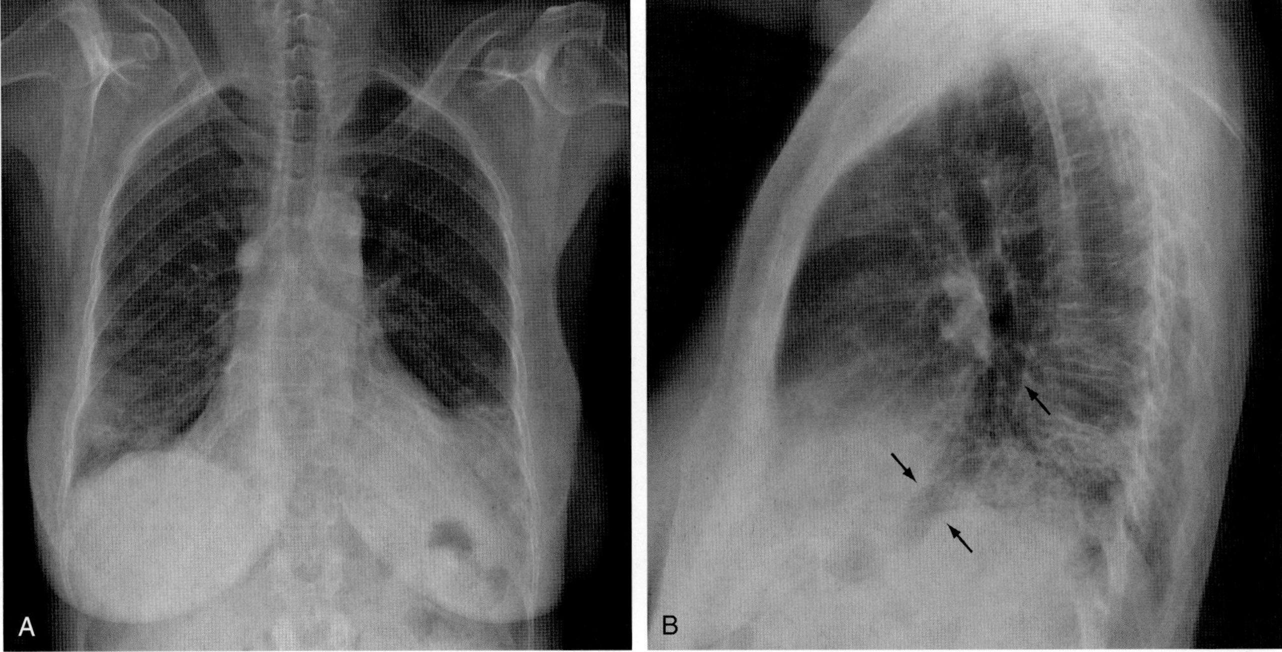

FIGURE 22-19. Chest findings in MCTD. **A,** Posteroanterior radiograph shows increased density in the lung bases. **B,** Lateral radiograph shows gas in the esophagus *(arrows)*.

(Continued)

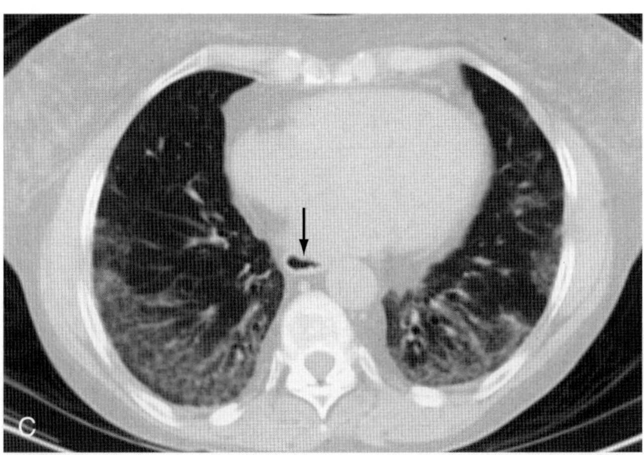

FIGURE 22-19—cont'd. **C,** The CT image better defines the peripherally located pulmonary opacities. There is dilatation of the esophagus *(arrow)*.

BOX 22-1. Radiographic Musculoskeletal Features of SLE

Finger and thumb deformities
Toe deformities
Osteopenia
Cartilage space narrowing
Cystic changes
Subluxations
Periarticular calcification
Acral sclerosis
Tuft resorption
Soft tissue swelling
Soft tissue atrophy
Joint ankylosis
Erosions
Avascular necrosis
Subcutaneous nodules

From Lawless OJ, Whelton JC: Proceedings: deforming hand arthritis in systemic lupus erythematosus, *Arthritis Rheum* 17:323, 1974; Reilly PA, Evison G, McHugh NJ et al: Arthropathy of hands and feet in systemic lupus erythematosus [see comment], *J Rheumatol* 17:777-784, 1990; and Weissman BN, Rappoport AS, Sosman JL et al: Radiographic findings in the hands in patients with systemic lupus erythematosus, *Radiology* 126:313-317, 1978.

BOX 22-2. International Consensus Statement on Preliminary Criteria for the Classification of the Antiphospholipid Syndrome*

CLINICAL CRITERIA

Vascular thrombosis

- One or more clinical episodes of arterial, venous, or small-vessel thrombosis, occurring within any tissue or organ

Complications of pregnancy

- One or more unexplained deaths of morphologically normal fetuses at or after the 10th week of gestation; *or*
- One or more premature births of morphologically normal neonates at or before the 34th week of gestation; *or*
- Three or more unexplained consecutive spontaneous abortions before the 10th week of gestation

LABORATORY CRITERIA†

aCL antibodies

- aCL immunoglobulin G or immunoglobulin M antibodies present at moderate or high levels in the blood on two or more occasions at least 6 weeks apart‡

LA antibodies

- LA antibodies detected in the blood on two or more occasions at least 6 weeks apart, according to the guidelines of the International Society on Thrombosis and Hemostasis§

*A diagnosis of definite APS requires the presence of at least one of the clinical criteria and at least one of the laboratory criteria. No limits are placed on the interval between the clinical event and the positive laboratory findings.

†The following antiphospholipid antibodies are currently not included in the laboratory criteria: aCL IgA antibodies, anti-beta-2-glycoprotein I antibodies, and antiphospholipid antibodies directed against phospholipids other than cardiolipin (e.g., phosphatidylserine, phosphatidylethanolamine) or against phospholipid-binding proteins other than cardiolipin-bound beta-2-glycoprotein I (e.g., prothrombin, annexin V, protein C, protein S).

‡The threshold used to distinguish moderate or high levels of anticardiolipin antibodies from low levels has not been standardized and may depend on the population under study. Many laboratories use 15 or 20 international "phospholipid" units as the threshold separating low from moderate levels of aCL antibodies. Others define the threshold as 2.0 or 2.5 times the median level of aCL antibodies or as the 99th percentile of anticardiolipin levels within a normal population. Until an international consensus is reached, any of these three definitions seems reasonable.

§Guidelines are from Brandt JT, Trplett DA, Alving B et al: Criteria for the diagnosis of lupus anticoaguiants: an update, *Thromb Haemost* 74:1185-1190, 1995.

With permission from Levine JS, Branch DW, Rauch J: The antiphospholipid syndrome [see comment], *N Engl J Med* **346**:752-763, 2002. (See Table 1.)

nonparenchymal muscular arteries such as the celiac artery.[65] Aneurysms may rupture, thrombose, or become stenotic.[66] Giant aneurysms (> 8 mm) are considered of greatest concern.[67,68] Larger aneurysms may calcify, shrink, and become occluded.

The diagnosis of Kawasaki disease is based on clinical findings, inflammation on laboratory analysis, and exclusion of other conditions. The presence of 5 days of fever and four of the five principal clinical features establishes the diagnosis (Box 22-3). Patients with fever for 5 days and fewer than four principal features can be diagnosed as having Kawasaki disease when coronary artery disease is detected by two-dimensional echocardiography (2DE) or coronary angiography. An algorithm has been developed to facilitate diagnosis.[65]

An incomplete form of Kawasaki disease may also occur and demonstrate coronary artery damage.[62] Sonobe et al. evaluated 15,857 cases of Kawasaki disease.[69] Incomplete Kawasaki disease was defined as the presence of four or fewer principal symptoms of the Japanese diagnostic guidelines and was present in 18.4% of the series. Coronary artery abnormalities were present in 14.2% of patients with the complete disease and 18.4% of patients with the incomplete form of the disease.[69]

Treatment options have been reviewed by an American Heart Association (AHA) panel.[65] In the acute phase, treatment is directed toward reducing inflammation in the coronary artery wall and preventing coronary thrombosis, whereas long-term therapy in individuals who develop coronary aneurysms is aimed at preventing myocardial ischemia or infarction. The use of high-dose intravenous immunoglobulin given in the acute phase of the disease has reduced the prevalence of aneurysms by fivefold.[64] Specific treatment regimens are discussed by Newburger and Fulton.[64]

BOX 22-3. Epidemiological Case Definition (Classic Clinical Criteria) of Kawasaki I

Fever persisting at least 5 days
Presence of at least 4 principal features:
1. Changes in extremities
   Acute: Erythema of palms, soles; edema of hands, feet
   Subacute: Periungual peeling of fingers, toes in weeks 2 and 3
2. Polymorphous exanthem
3. Bilateral bulbar conjunctival injection without exudate
4. Changes in lips and oral cavity: Erythema, lips cracking, strawberry tongue, diffuse injection of oral and pharyngeal mucosae.
5. Cervical lymphadenopathy (> 1.5-cm diameter), usually unilateral

Exclusion of other diseases with similar findings.

Excerpted from Newburger JW, Takahashi M, Gerber MA, et al: Diagnosis, treatment, and longterm management of Kawasaki disease. A statement for health professionals from the Committee on Rheumatic Fever, Endocarditis, and Kawasaki Disease, Council on Cardiovascular Disease in the Young, American Heart Association: Circulation, 110:2747-2771, 2004 by permission.

Cardiac Imaging

Imaging findings in Kawasaki disease include coronary artery aneurysms, ectasia, stenosis, calcification, collateral circulation, abnormal left ventricular function, myocardial infarction, heart failure, valve abnormalities, and pericardial effusion.[70,71]

Echocardiography (ECG)

According to the AHA panel, ECG is the preferred imaging modality for cardiac assessment because there is no ionizing radiation, it is noninvasive, and it has high sensitivity and specificity for the detection of abnormalities of the proximal left main and right coronary arteries (the areas of most frequent involvement)[65] (Box 22-4). Criteria for the diagnosis of an enlarged artery have been described, but more recent recommendations include body surface area–adjusted coronary dimensions as a more sensitive measurement technique.[65] ECG is, however, strongly operator dependent, and in adolescents the exam is apparently less satisfactory due to a poor acoustic window in this age group.[70]

BOX 22-4. Echocardiography: Advantages and Disadvantages

ADVANTAGES
No ionizing radiation
Noninvasive
Proximal left main and right coronary well seen

DISADVANTAGES
Less satisfactory in adolescents
Operator dependent
Sedation necessary in young children
Poor ability to assess obstructive lesion
Poor for distal coronary arteries

Magnetic Resonance Imaging

As a noninvasive examination, MR coronary angiography is a promising alternative to catheter angiography for imaging coronary aneurysms and intimal thickness in patients with Kawasaki disease (Figures 22-20 and 22-21). Comparison of whole heart coronary MR angiography to conventional angiography in 5 children (14 aneurysms) with Kawasaki disease found complete

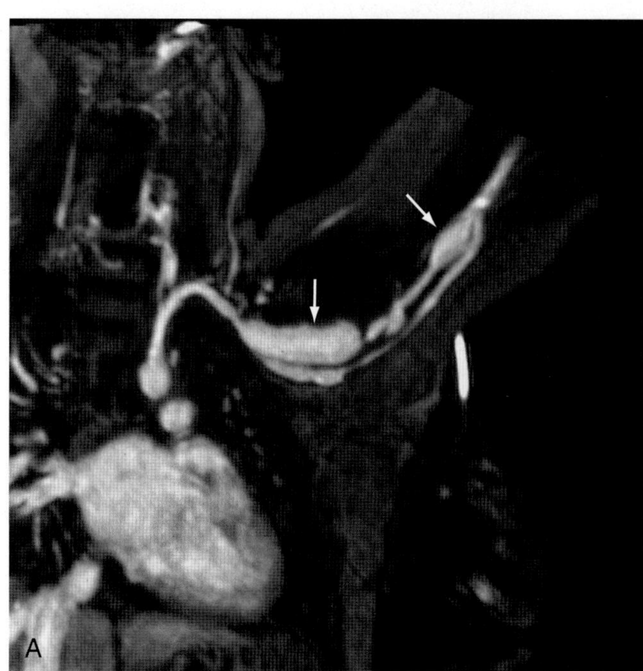

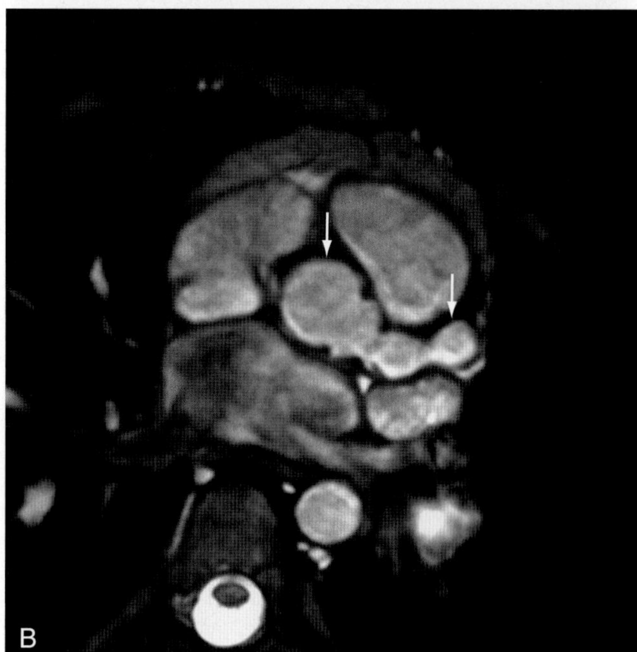

FIGURE 22-20. MRI findings of Kawasaki disease. **A,** Coronal MR angiogram maximum intensity projection (MIP) image shows multiple axillary artery aneurysms *(arrows)*. **B,** Short axis MIP image through the aortic root from a coronary MR angiogram was obtained without contrast administration. The bilobed configuration of the left main and proximal left anterior descending coronary arteries is noted *(arrows)*. (Courtesy Dr. Laureen Sena, Children's Hospital, Boston.)

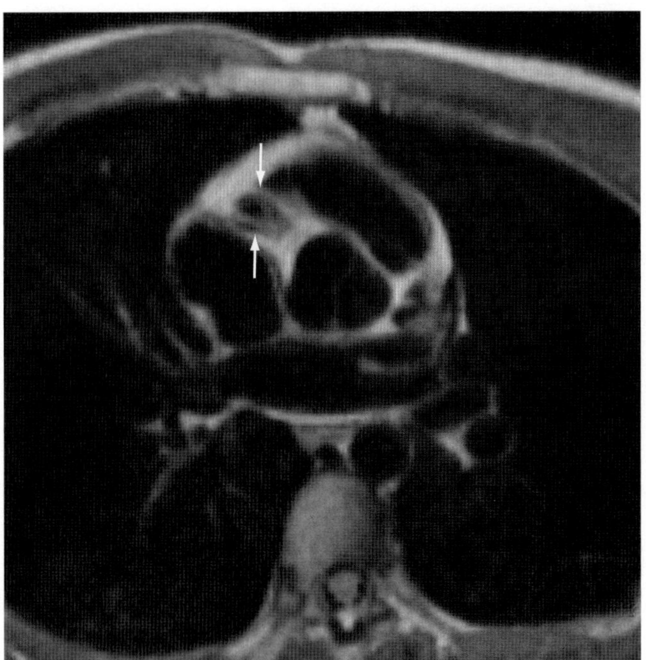

FIGURE 22-21. Kawasaki disease with wall thickening on MR angiography. A "black blood" image through the aortic root shows diffuse thickening of the right coronary artery *(arrows).* (Courtesy Dr. Laureen Sena, Children's Hospital, Boston.)

agreement in the detection of aneurysms and excellent agreement in aneurysm size and location.[66] In addition, using the double inversion recovery (DIR) "black blood" technique, vessel wall thickening can be assessed.[66] Suzuki et al. evaluated noninvasive noncontrast-enhanced free breathing MR coronary angiography in 106 patients with Kawasaki disease.[72] Both "bright blood" images (to evaluate aneurysms) and "black blood" images (to evaluate wall thickness) were performed. Seventy patients had conventional radiographic coronary arteriography for comparison. There was close agreement in the size of aneurysms when the techniques were compared (mean 0.0, 95% confidence interval –1.4 to 1.5). Bright blood imaging provided a sensitivity for occlusion and focal stenosis of 94.2% and 97.2% with a specificity of 99.5% and 97.2% compared with radiographic angiography. The negative predictive values were 99.5% and 97.2%, respectively.[70] Advantages are greatest in young children who are most sensitive to radiation and in whom calcification may not yet have developed.[73] Due to the lack of ionizing radiation and its reproducibility, cardiac MRI and coronary MR angiography are excellent methods for following patients over time.[66] Disadvantages and advantages of coronary MRA and cardiac MRI are summarized in Box 22-5.

Cardiac MRI provides assessment of left ventricular function and myocardial viability, as well as detection of subendocardial myocardial infarctions (Figure 22-22). Modification of techniques allows even young children to be evaluated.[74]

In a study of 16 patients who had coronary angiography, 16-row CT angiography, and MRI, there was 100% agreement between CT and conventional coronary artery catheterization in the detection of aneurysms and stenoses.[73] CT allowed identification of a calcified aneurysm that was not seen on angiography. MRI showed a 93% agreement in the detection of aneurysms; a stenotic lesion was missed on MRI. Ectasia was detected correctly in 90% of CT examinations and 50% of MRI studies. Smaller vessels could not always be evaluated.

BOX 22-5. Coronary MR Angiography and Cardiac MRI

ADVANTAGES

Can evaluate coronary arteries, LV function, myocardial viability
Excellent for aneurysm detection and measurement
Detects stenosis, obstruction
No ionizing radiation
No breath holding required
Can evaluate myocardial perfusion, infarction, scar

DISADVANTAGES

Sedation used for young children
Takes longer than CTA
Relatively low spatial resolution
May use intravascular contrast agent
Severe cardiac motion and respiratory artifacts when gating fails

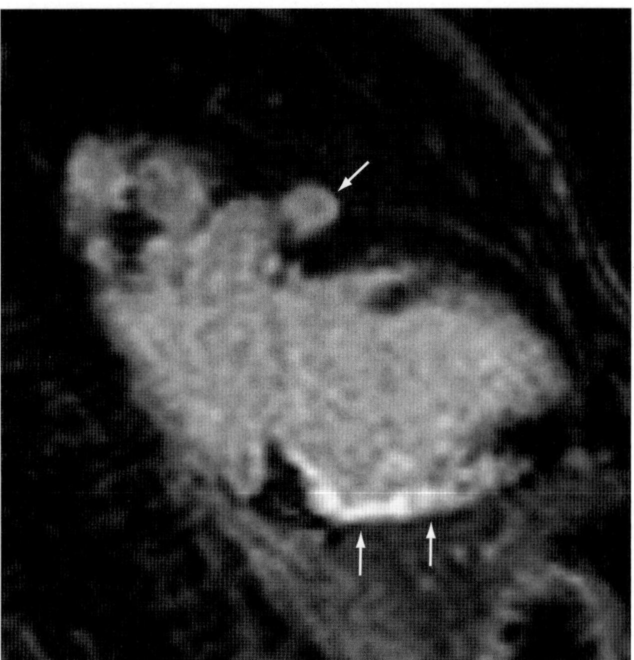

FIGURE 22-22. Acute myocardial infarction demonstrated on MRI in Kawasaki disease. A myocardial delayed enhancement gradient echo vertical long axis view shows involvement of the myocardium (bright signal area, *white arrows*), compatible with infarction. An aneurysm of the left anterior descending artery *(white arrow)* is also seen. (Courtesy Dr. Laureen Sena, Children's Hospital, Boston.)

Computed Tomography

Multislice CT scanning can delineate aneurysms and calcifications.[73,75] Detection of peripheral cardiac aneurysms is better with CT than with ECG.[70,76] CT angiography using a 64-slice scanner has demonstrated high sensitivity (94%) and specificity (97%) for coronary stenosis.[70] Lesions that were not detected were usually located in calcified segments, a finding that may occur in Kawasaki disease. However, coronary CTA may require the use of beta blockers to slow the heart rate.[75,77] Discontinuing anticoagulation is not necessary. Another important consideration in children is

BOX 22-6. Coronary CT Angiography

ADVANTAGES
High spatial resolution
Delineates aneurysms and stenoses
Short scan time
Sensitive for distal coronaries
Delineates mural calcification

DISADVANTAGES
Iodinated contrast used
Beta blocker used to reduce heart rate (low temporal resolution) for some scanners
Relatively high radiation dose
Anesthesia necessary for young children
Calcification may limit evaluation of coronary lumen

the relatively high radiation dose of CTA (approximately equal to or greater than that of conventional angiography), making this test useful primarily as an alternative to invasive angiography[75] (Box 22-6).

SPECT Scanning

Single photon emission computed tomography (SPECT) myocardial perfusion scanning may be helpful in patients with Kawasaki disease. Discordance has been found between dipyridamole stress Tc-99m tetrofosmin SPECT scanning and coronary angiography in patients with Kawasaki disease.[78] Subclinical ischemia may be documented with this technique even when stress testing is otherwise normal, due to the presence of collateral circulation.[50]

Angiography

Catheter angiography provides exquisite imaging of the coronary arteries but it is an invasive procedure, requiring arterial puncture and sedation in young patients (Figure 22-23) (Box 22-7). Other disadvantages of catheter angiography are the relatively high ionizing radiation dose and potentially nephrotoxic iodinated contrast agent administration. Catheter-related complications may occur. Catheter angiography cannot evaluate the vessel wall thickness without using IVUS. On the other hand, interventional procedures, such as balloon angioplasty, can be performed at the time of angiography.

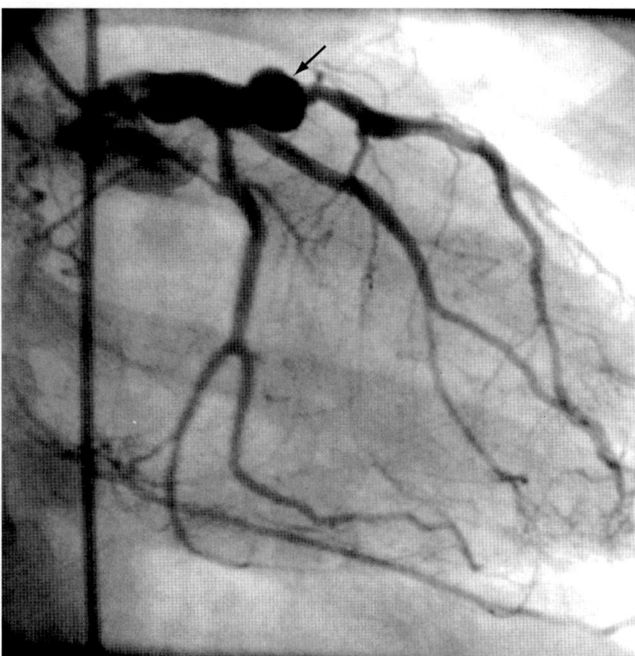

FIGURE 22-23. Angiography in Kawasaki disease. An image from a left coronary angiogram shows aneurysms *(arrow)* of the left main and left anterior descending coronary arteries. (Courtesy Dr. Laureen Sena, Children's Hospital, Boston.)

BOX 22-7. Conventional Coronary Angiography

ADVANTAGES
Gold standard for assessing coronary arteries
Interventions and intravascular ultrasound are possible during the catheterization

DISADVANTAGES
Relatively high radiation dose
Catheterization needed
Sedation in young patients
Use of iodinated contrast
Limited assessment of vessel wall

Recommended Imaging Examinations

The optimal imaging study remains somewhat controversial, as MRI and CT techniques are rapidly improving and larger studies are being performed. Mavrogeni et al. have concluded that ECG is the bedside technique of choice during the acute phase of Kawasaki disease.[70] MRI can be a valuable adjunct and is especially useful in adolescents, in whom ECG may fail to detect coronary artery abnormalities.[70] When MRI is not available, ECG and SPECT can provide anatomic, functional, and perfusion information. Coronary angiography is reserved for patients in need of invasive procedures. These authors believe that CT is of limited value in these patients because of the high radiation dose. However, Arnold et al. note that evaluation of stenotic segments is critical and, in adults, multidetector CT with ECG dose modulation may be a less invasive alternative to conventional coronary angiography for follow-up.[73] They indicate that because stenotic lesions may be missed on MRI, this modality is most suited to younger children in whom radiation sensitivity is greatest and calcification is less likely.[73]

Extracardiac Imaging Abnormalities

Other imaging findings are GI pseudoobstruction, infarction, stricture, or focal colitis.[79] Transient renal enlargement is reported during the acute phase of the disease.[39] Renal scarring may occur and has been assessed by ultrasound and Tc-99m DMSA SPECT scanning.[80] Cerebrovascular disease has also been described.[81] Effusion of atlantoaxial and temporomandibular joints has been documented on MRI.[82]

WEGENER'S GRANULOMATOSIS

Wegener's granulomatosis is necrotizing vasculitis that involves medium and small vessels.[48] Granulomatous lesions typically involve the upper and lower respiratory tract, arteries and veins, and kidneys. Diagnostic criteria were developed in 1990 to distinguish Wegener's granulomatosis from other causes of vasculitis[83] (Table 22-5).

TABLE 22-5. ACR Criteria for the Classification of Wegener's Granulomatosis*

1. Nasal or oral inflammation	Development of painful or painless oral ulcers or purulent or bloody nasal discharge
2. Abnormal chest radiograph	Chest radiograph showing the presence of nodules, fixed infiltrates, or cavities
3. Urinary sediment	Microhematuria (> 5 red blood cells per high power field) or red cell casts in urine sediment
4. Granulomatous inflammation on biopsy	Histologic changes showing granulomatous inflammation within the wall of an artery or in the perivascular or extravascular area (artery or arteriole)

*For purposes of classification, a patient shall be said to have Wegener's granulomatosis if at least 2 of these 4 criteria are present. The presence of any 2 or more criteria yields a sensitivity of 88.2% and a specificity of 92.0%.
With permission from The American College of Rheumatology 1990 criteria for the classification of Wegener's granulomatosis, *Arthritis Rheum* 33:1101-1107, 1990 (Table 3).

Wegener's granulomatosis is characterized by the triad of findings: necrotizing granulomas of the upper and lower respiratory tract, necrotizing vasculitis of arteries and veins, and glomerulonephritis.

Pulmonary disease is common and usually consists of multiple nodules or irregular masses with cavitation in about half the cases.[50] The walls of the cavities are thick and irregular. Unlike septic emboli that occur more at the lung bases, there is no special zonal distribution of these nodules[48] (Figure 22-24).

As summarized by Mayberry et al.,[48] CT demonstrates the irregular nodules and any cavitation. A peribronchovascular distribution is often seen. Peripheral wedge-shaped consolidation (infarcts) may be present. Pleural effusion, pneumonia, or pulmonary hemorrhage producing air-space consolidation may occur. Increased uptake on bone scan has been reported.[84] In addition to pulmonary involvement, tracheal or bronchial mucosal or submucosal granulomatous changes can lead to smooth or nodular wall thickening that may calcify, as well as luminal narrowing, especially in the subglottic region.[48]

Imaging of the paranasal sinuses may show mucosal thickening and opacification, air fluid levels, bone erosion, septal perforation, and occasionally an orbital mass (Figure 22-25). Involvement of the nervous system occurs in the form of peripheral or cranial neuropathy and less often as involvement of the brain and meninges.[85] Mechanisms of nervous system involvement are thought to be (1) contiguous spread from orbital, paranasal, or nasal granulomas; (2) granulomatous vasculitis; (3) a primary necrotizing granulomatous process; and (4) complications from other, non-CNS disease.[85] CT and MRI may show dural thickening and enhancement cerebral infarction, as well as focal areas of increased T2 signal that may include the brainstem.[85] Focal granulomas that are usually located within white matter may show increased T2 signal with homogeneous or ring enhancement after contrast.[85,86] The pituitary and infundibulum can also be involved, leading to clinical manifestations of diabetes insipidus.[87,88]

Cardiac involvement may occur, with pericarditis, coronary arteritis, aortic regurgitation, aortic valvular lesions simulating endocarditis, and thromboembolism reported.[71]

TAKAYASU ARTERITIS

Takayasu arteritis (TA) is one of the most common arteritides involving large vessels.[89] It most often affects young Asian women.[90] Two stages are recognized, an early stage (termed *systemic* or *prepulseless*) of nonspecific clinical findings such as elevated sedimentation rate, fever, or weakness; and a late (occlusive or pulseless) phase with findings related to the vessel stenoses or occlusions.[90]

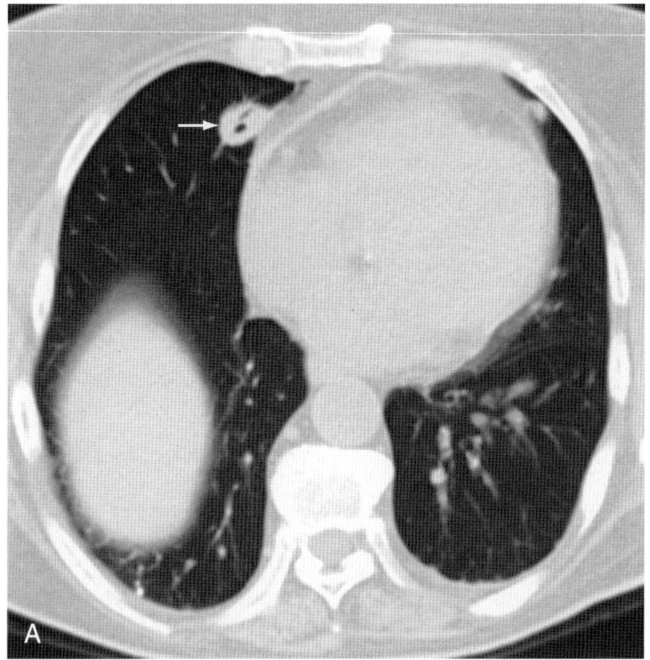

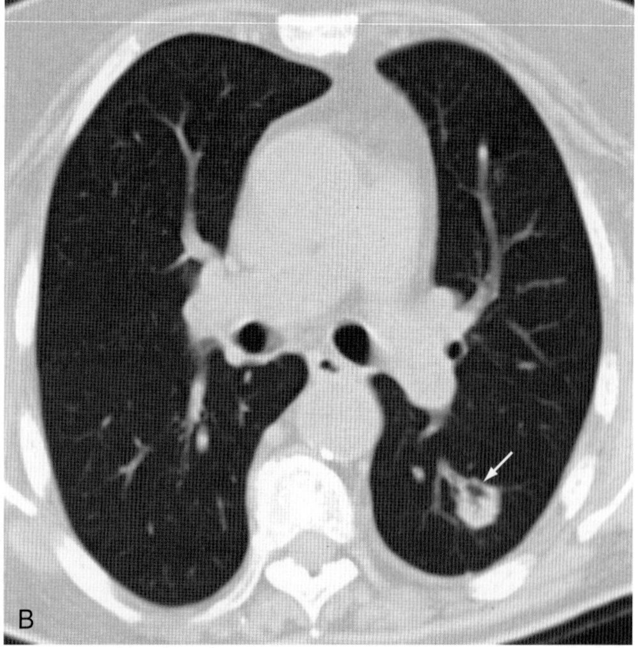

FIGURE 22-24. Wegener's granulomatosis. **A,** CT scan demonstrates a cavitating pulmonary nodule *(arrow)*. **B,** Another cavitating pulmonary nodule is seen *(arrow)*.

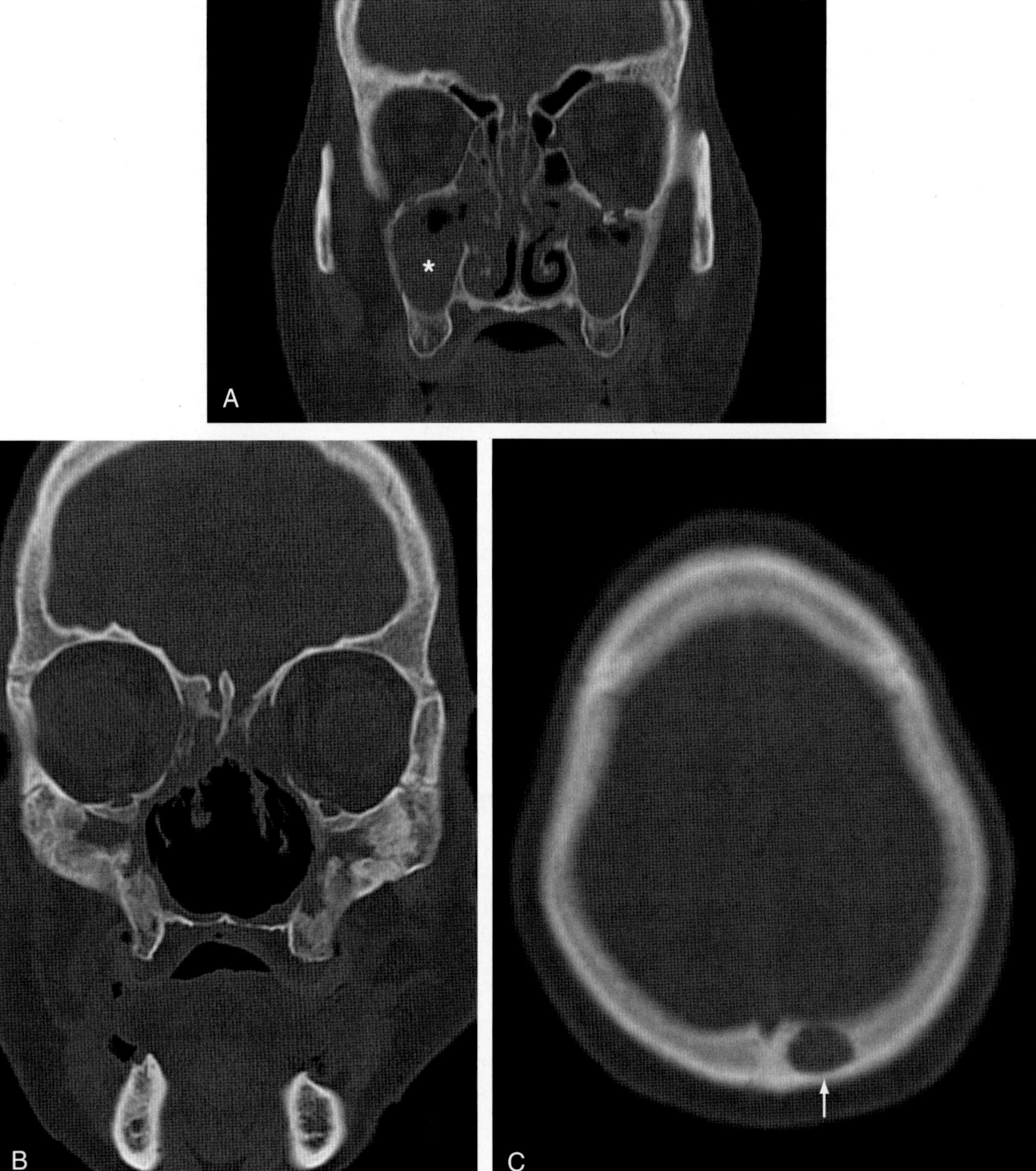

FIGURE 22-25. Wegener's granulomatosis. **A,** CT of the sinuses shows near-complete opacification of the right maxillary antrum *(asterisk)* and the ethmoid sinuses. Bone destruction is present. **B,** There is complete destruction of the nasal septum. **C,** A nonspecific osteolytic calvarial lesion *(arrow)* is noted.

TA is a panarteritis characterized by inflammatory wall thickening that evolves into a fibrotic stage with associated aneurysms, stenosis, and occlusion. The thoracic aorta is typically involved, but the abdominal aorta and the proximal parts of visceral branches may be affected. Late involvement can be subclassified (Figure 22-26). Pulmonary and coronary arteries can be affected, resulting in aneurysms or, less commonly, stenoses. Fistulas can develop between the pulmonary artery and bronchial arteries, coronary arteries, or aorta.[91]

Imaging Findings

Radiographs in early-stage disease may show subtle findings with loss of sharp definition of the aorta and a wavy aortic contour. In this stage, newer imaging techniques that allow evaluation of the vessel wall are especially useful. Radiography in late-stage disease may demonstrate an undulating appearance to the aorta and linear calcifications of the aortic arch and descending aorta. Cardiomegaly, decreased pulmonary vessels, and rib notching due to collateral vessels may be seen.[90]

Many of the principles of advanced imaging described above apply to the evaluation of vascular involvement in TA. Pipitone et al. have provided a comprehensive summary of the utility of the various imaging modalities in the evaluation of large vessel vasculitis.[89] Angiography demonstrates vessel lumens and can reveal smooth long segment stenoses, occlusions, and aneurysms that may occur in this disorder but does not directly evaluate wall changes (Figures 22-27 and 22-28). CT angiography and MRI allow the vessel wall as well as the lumen to be evaluated (Figures 22-29 through 22-32). Circumferential increased

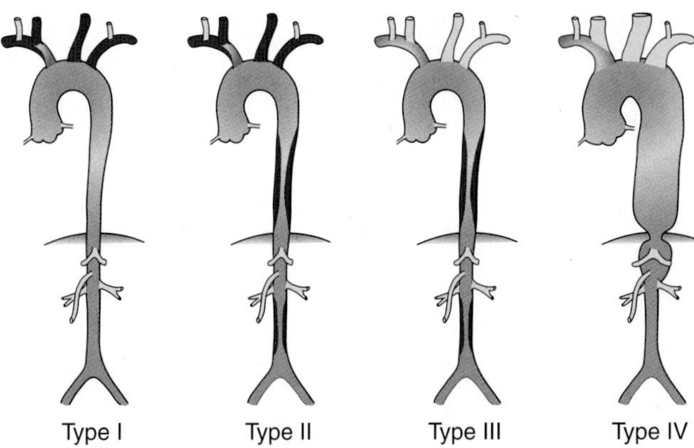

FIGURE 22-26. Angiographic types of late-phase TA. (Redrawn with permission from Endo M, Tomizawa Y, Nishida H et al: Angiographic findings and surgical treatments of coronary artery involvement in Takayasu arteritis, *J Thoracic Cardiovasc Surg* 125:570-577, 2003. [Figure 9].)

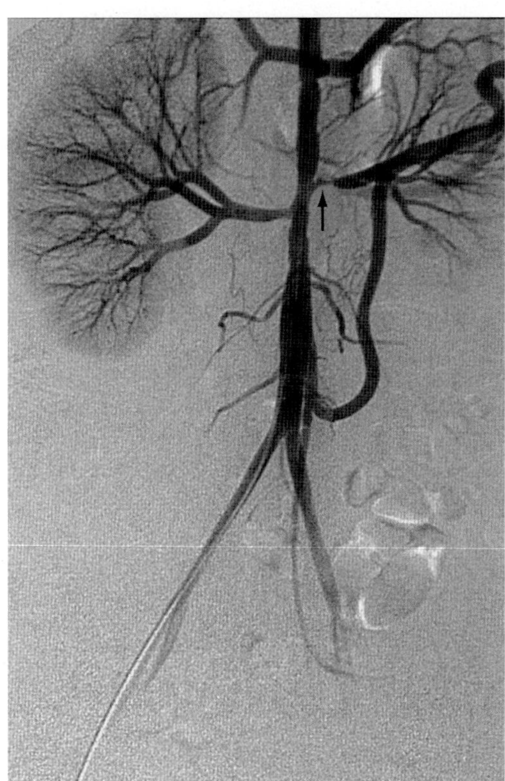

FIGURE 22-27. Takayasu arteritis. A subtraction image of an aortogram in a 25-year-old woman evaluated for hypertension shows a long segment of irregular narrowing of the aortic lumen. There is stenosis of the renal arteries, particularly on the left *(arrow)*.

thickness on DIR "black blood" imaging sequence, increased signal on T2-weighted sequences due to the edema, and post-gadolinium enhancement of the vessel wall on T1-weighted spin echo or DIR sequences are indicators of wall inflammation[89] (see Figures 22-29 and 22-31). A "double ring" appearance on contrast-enhanced CT consists of a poorly enhanced inner ring of swelling of the intima and an enhancing outer ring due to active medial and adventitial inflammatory changes.

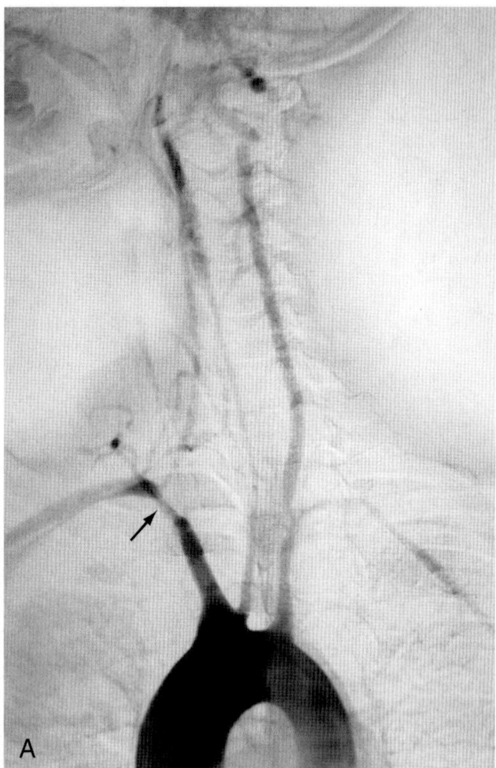

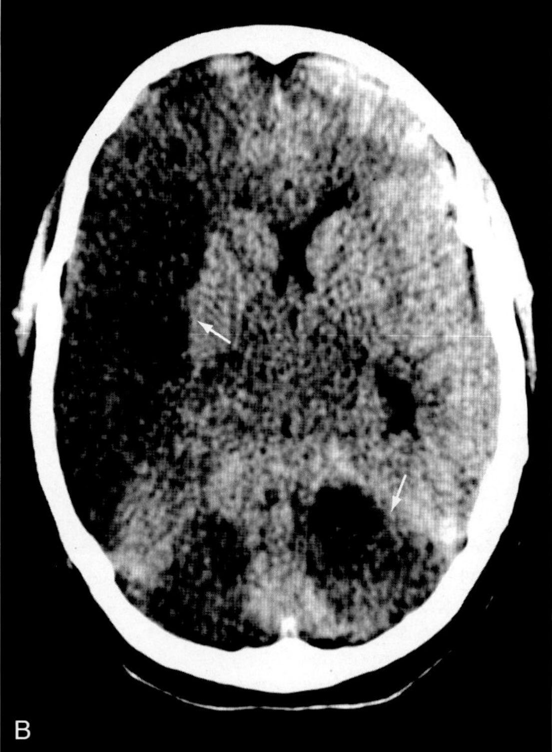

FIGURE 22-28. Takayasu arteritis. **A,** The aortogram shows narrowing of the proximal right subclavian artery *(arrow)* and more diffuse narrowing of the right common carotid, left proximal vertebral, and left subclavian arteries. **B,** The CT scan of the brain shows large areas of decreased attenuation, consistent with extensive infarcts *(arrows)*.

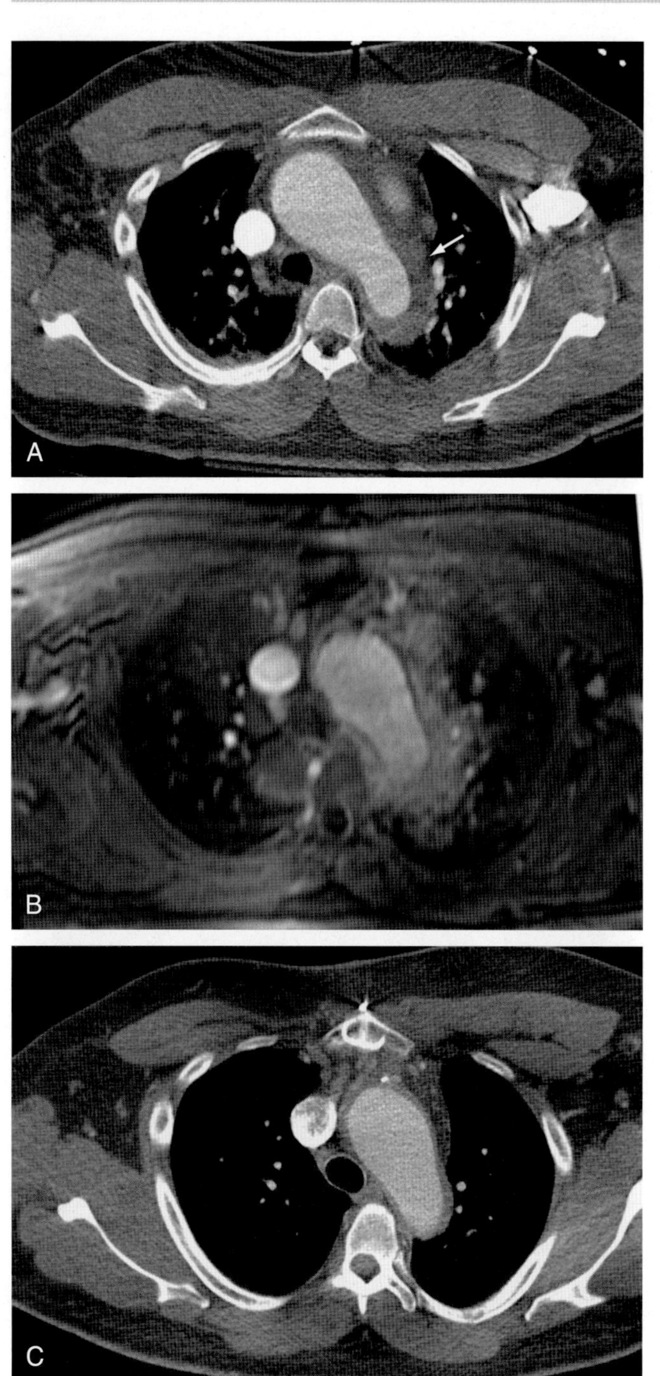

FIGURE 22-29. Takayasu arteritis (TA) in a 38-year-old man. **A,** Contrast-enhanced CT study demonstrated aortic arch aneurysm with significant wall thickening and perivascular soft tissue stranding of the arch and the proximal descending aorta. **B,** Post-gadolinium fat-suppressed T1-weighted gradient echo image demonstrates enhancement of the vessel wall and the perivascular soft tissue associated with active vasculitis. The patient underwent resection and grafting of an ascending aortic aneurysm. Pathology on the aortic specimen demonstrated findings of aortitis consistent with TA. The patient was treated with approximately 6 months of prednisone. **C,** Follow-up CT angiogram shows considerable improvement of the vascular findings.

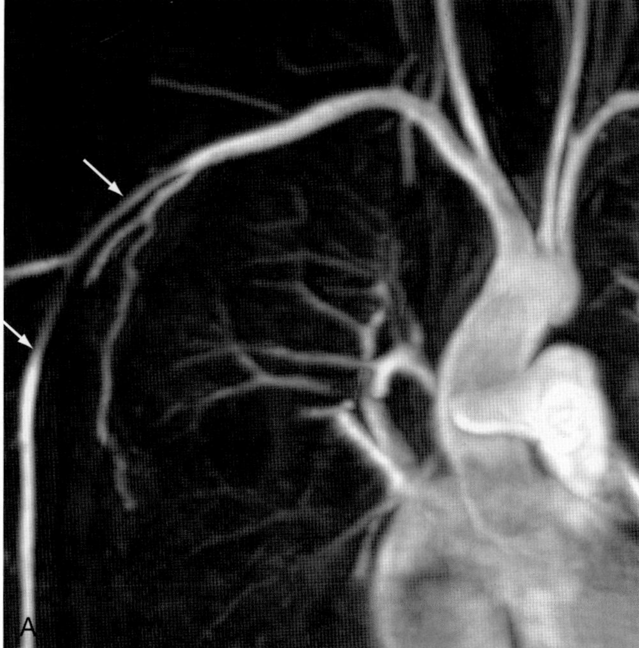

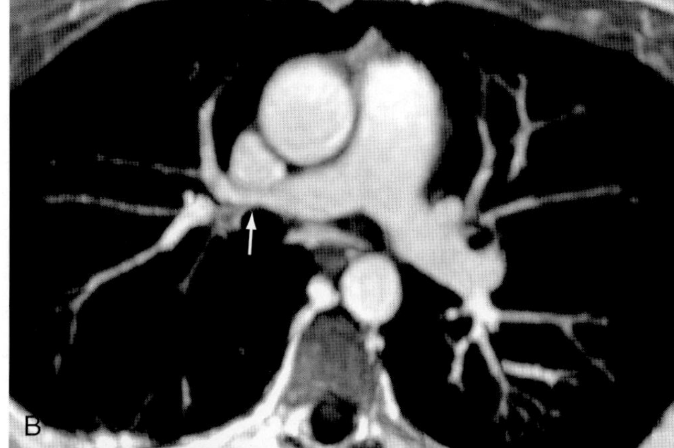

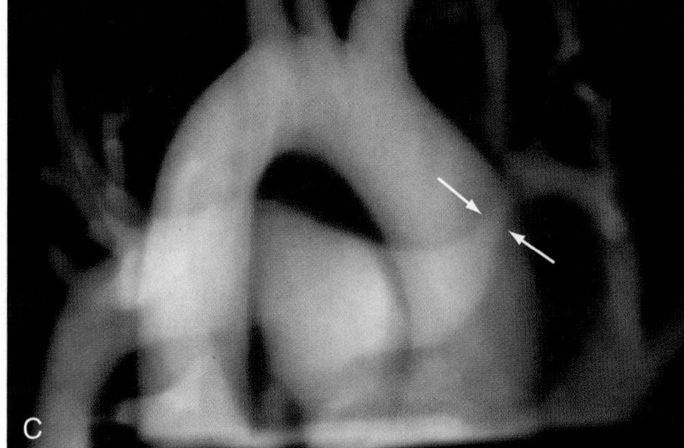

FIGURE 22-30. Takayasu arteritis (TA). This 23-year-old female with a history of deep venous thrombosis was referred for MR angiography of the chest. **A,** Coronal MIP image of the 3D MR angiography demonstrates smooth long segment stenosis of the right axillary artery *(arrows)*. **B,** Post-contrast T1-weighted gradient echo image and **(C)** Sagittal oblique volume rendered 3D image show right pulmonary artery stenosis *(arrows)* that developed secondary to TA.

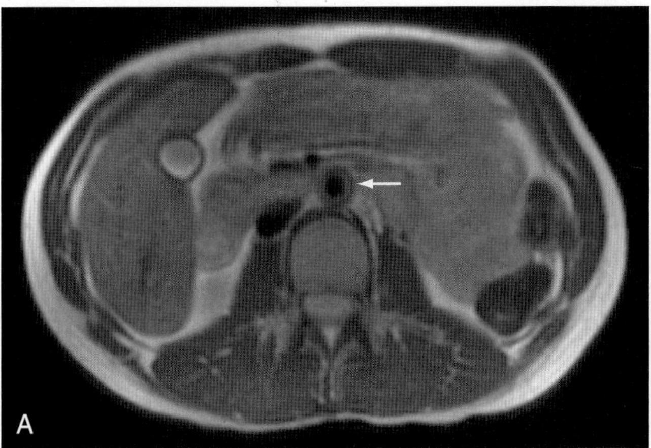
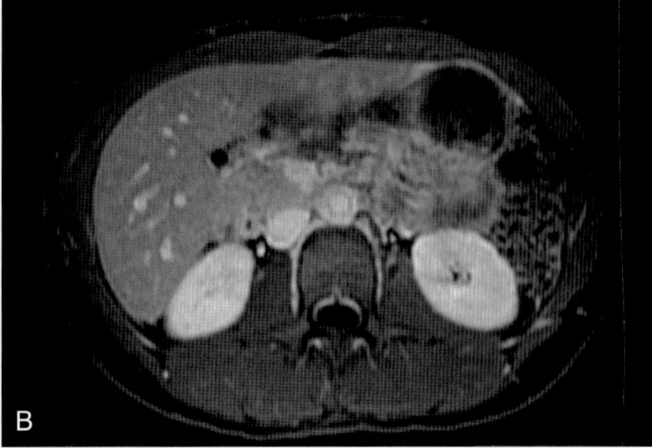

FIGURE 22-31. Takayasu arteritis. **A,** T2-weighted double inversion recovery image demonstrates circumferential thickening of the aortic wall *(arrow)*. **B,** Corresponding post-contrast fat suppressed T1-weighted image reveals the contrast enhancement in the thickened wall of the aorta indicating active inflammation.

A "double ring" appearance of the vessel wall is seen on contrast-enhanced CT in vessels affected by TA. This finding consists of a poorly enhanced inner ring due to swelling of the intima and an enhancing outer ring due to active medial and adventitial inflammatory changes.

Ultrasound is operator dependent but is capable of assessing vessel anatomy, wall changes, and luminal flow. A hyperechoic vessel wall has been demonstrated. PET scanning may show active inflammation of the vessel wall (see Figure 22-32).

Calcification of the ascending aorta may be seen in syphilis, whereas calcification related to TA involves the aortic arch and descending aorta.

Subclinical myocardial involvement without significant coronary artery occlusive disease is not rare. This combination can be demonstrated as exercise-induced thallium-201 myocardial scintigraphic perfusion abnormalities, without significant coronary stenosis on angiography.[92] Pericardial effusion is uncommon but may be the initial manifestation of TA.

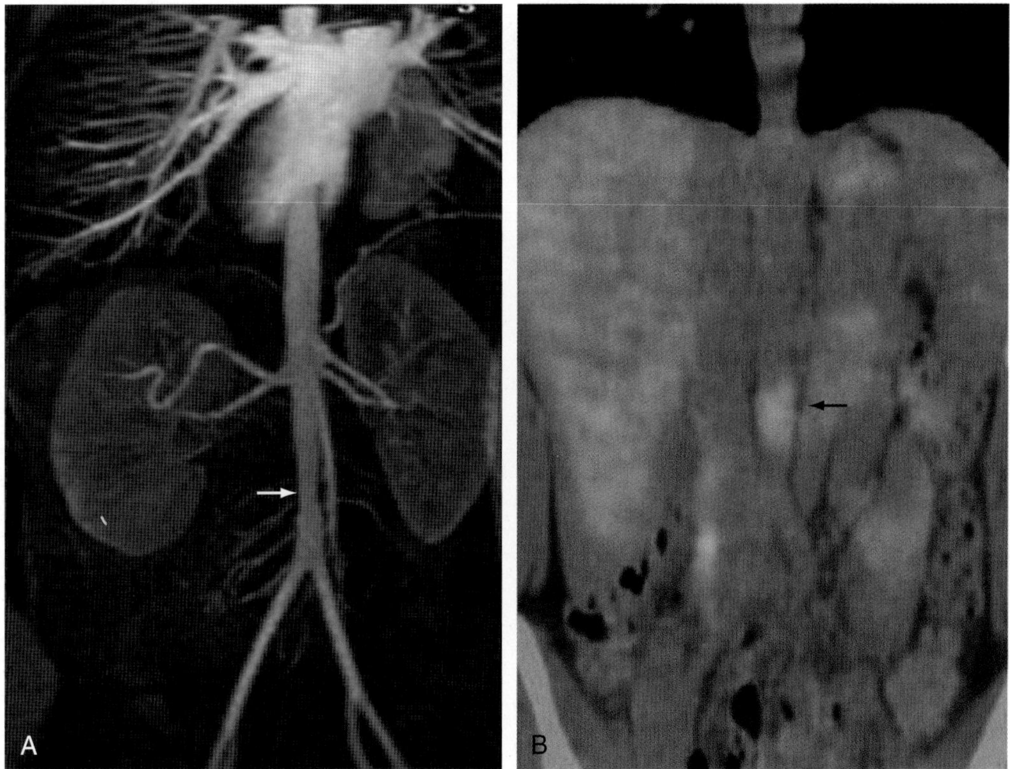

FIGURE 22-32. Takayasu aortitis in a 28-year-old female. **A,** 3D gadolinium-enhanced MR angiogram demonstrates long segment stenosis in the infrarenal aorta *(arrow)*. **B,** Corresponding area demonstrates FDG uptake on PET/CT *(arrow)*.

(Continued)

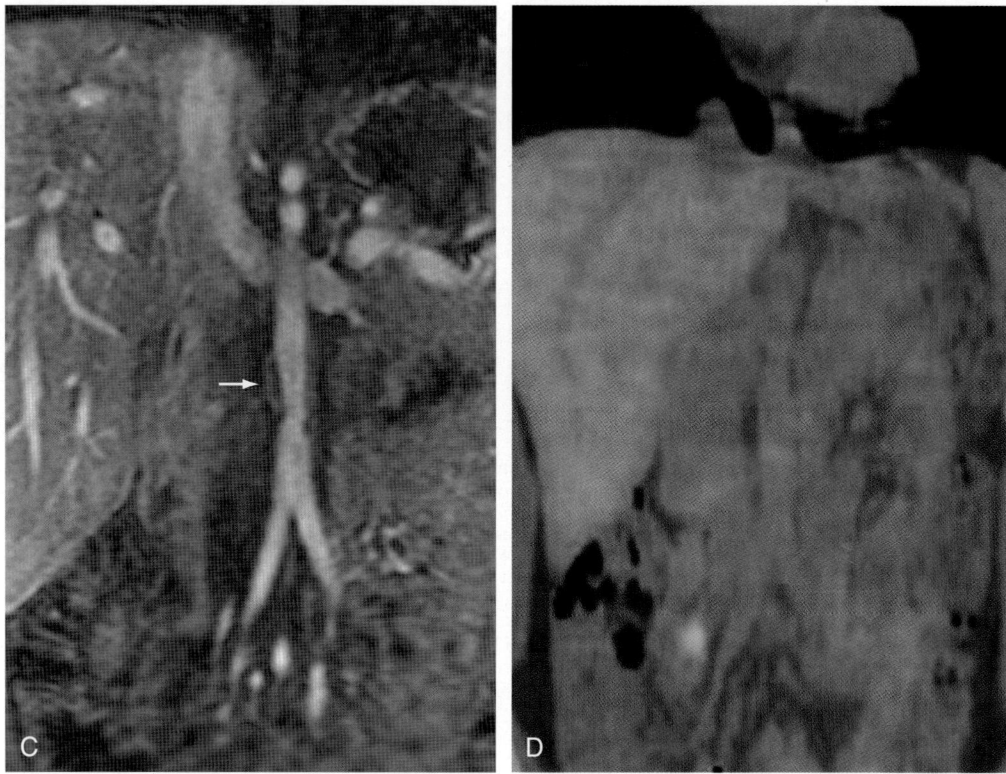

FIGURE 22-32—cont'd. C, Follow-up MR angiogram after 1 year of treatment reveals wall thickening *(arrow)* in the infrarenal aorta without contrast enhancement, indicative of the inactive fibrotic phase. **D,** On PET/CT there is no FDG avid area identified, confirming the inactive phase of the disease.

GIANT CELL ARTERITIS

Giant cell arteritis (GCA), also called *temporal* or *granulomatous arteritis*, is a disease of older patients that can lead to blindness. It is diagnosed on the bases of clinical, laboratory, and histologic findings. Patients are at considerably increased risk of developing thoracic aortic aneurysm and aortic dissection. GCA rarely causes cardiac problems such as coronary arteritis or pericarditis. The diagnosis is made by fulfilling three of five criteria as proposed by the ACR: age at onset > 50 years, new onset of localized headache, temporal-artery tenderness or decreased pulse, erythrocyte sedimentation rate ≥ 50 mm per hour, and abnormal artery biopsy.[93]

Imaging Findings

Temporal artery biopsy is diagnostic, but imaging findings have recently been proposed that may play a significant role in diagnosis, obviate biopsy, and facilitate follow-up. On gray-scale ultrasound, a characteristic finding of temporal arteritis is a diffusely and circumferentially thickened hypoechoic (dark) arterial wall or halo.[94,95] Turbulent flow and stenosis can be detected on color and spectral Doppler ultrasound of affected vessels.[94,95] Wall thickening may resolve after treatment.[95]

MRI evaluation of vessel wall inflammation on contrast-enhanced high-resolution images yielded a sensitivity of 80.6% and a specificity of 97.0% for the diagnosis in comparison with the final rheumatologist's diagnosis (including histology and laboratory tests) in the study by Bley et al. Histology alone resulted in a sensitivity of 77.8% and specificity of 100%[96] (Figure 22-33). A metaanalysis has shown weighted sensitivity of 55% and specificity of 94% compared with the ACR criteria.[89] Pipitone et al.[89] conclude that while a positive halo sign strongly supports the diagnosis of GCA in the correct clinical setting, the absence of the sign does not exclude it.

FDG (18-fluorodeoxyglucose) PET scans show increased uptake in areas of inflammation but cannot demonstrate vessel wall morphology or flow.[89]

POLYARTERITIS NODOSA

Polyarteritis nodosa (PAN) is a necrotizing arteritis of medium and small arteries that does not involve arterioles, capillaries, or venules. Areas of fibrinoid necrotizing inflammatory change in the vessel walls result in aneurysm formation and, later, with repair, wall thickening that may lead to vascular stenosis or occlusion.[97,98]

The diagnosis is made by fulfilling 3 of 10 proposed ACR criteria, one of which is the presence of aneurysms or occlusions of visceral arteries on arteriography.[99] The kidneys are involved most often (80% to 100%), followed by the heart, (up to 70%), the GI tract (50% to 70%), the liver (50% to 60%), the spleen (45%), and the pancreas (25% to 35%).[100] A classic manifestation of PAN is severe arterial hypertension caused by renal artery vasculitis. Although rare, cardiomyopathy is the most common cardiac manifestation of PAN.[101] Coronary vasculitis causing multiple aneurysms and myocardial infarction has been described in several case reports. Migratory polyarthritis may occur that usually involves the large joints of the lower extremities.

Imaging Findings

Radiographic findings of joint disease are uncommon and nonspecific, consisting of swelling without destructive changes. Periosteal reaction may be seen. In other organs, imaging findings may be due to ischemia. Thus changes such as pneumatosis intestinalis

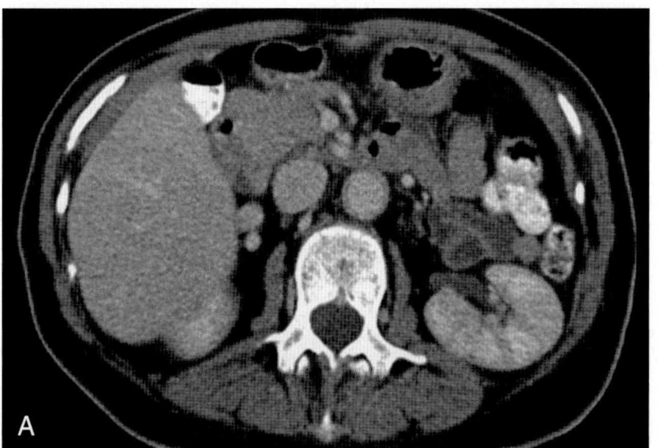

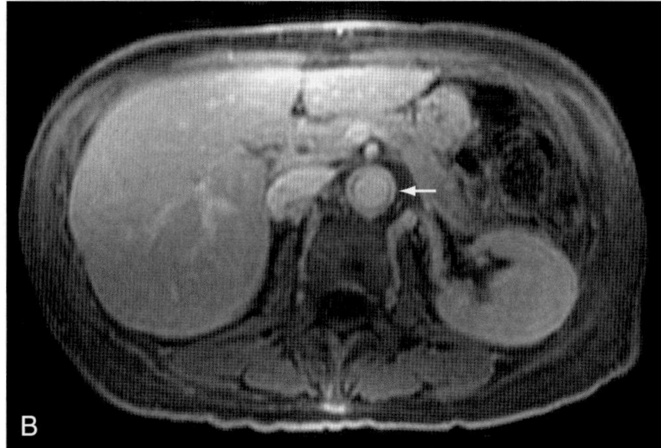

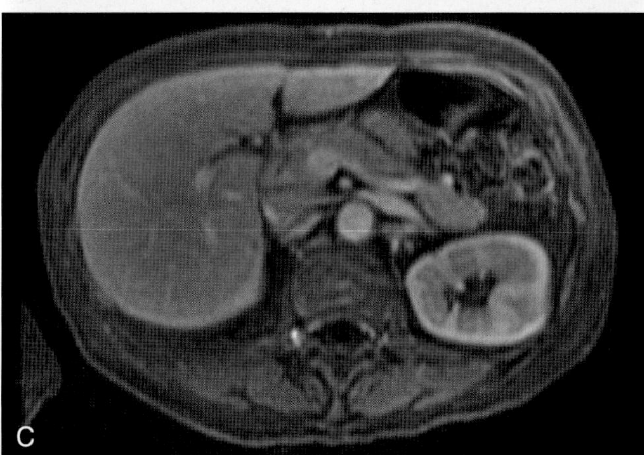

FIGURE 22-33. Gant cell arteritis (GCA) in a 71-year-old female with night sweats, jaw pain, and cheek pain. Initial axial post-contrast CT image **(A)** and axial post-contrast fat-suppressed T1-weighted gradient echo MR image **(B)** demonstrate aortic wall thickening and contrast enhancement *(arrow)*. Left temporal artery biopsy proved active GCA. On follow-up contrast-enhanced MRI study, significant regression of the wall thickening was seen following 1 month of high-dose corticosteroid treatment.

and portal vein gas on CT (or on radiographs) may be seen with bowel involvement.[97] Biopsy of muscle or subcutaneous nodules may provide false-negative results, making demonstration of characteristic angiographic findings important for establishing the correct diagnosis.[100] Angiography shows characteristic findings of multiple, small aneurysms (Figure 22-34). Although the presence of these aneurysms is nearly pathognomonic of PAN, they are

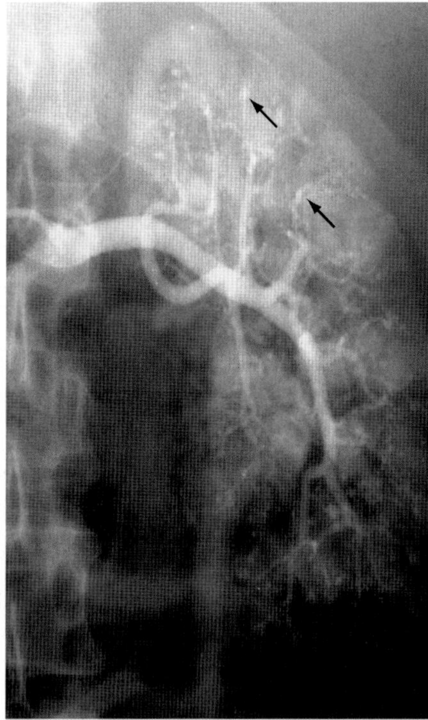

FIGURE 22-34. Polyarteritis nodosa. This renal arteriogram was performed for hypertension. Multiple small aneurysms are noted *(arrows)*. (Courtesy Dr. Richard Baum, Brigham and Women's Hospital, Boston.)

not entirely specific, as patients with heroin and methamphetamine abuse, Wegener's granulomatosis, SLE, diabetes, RA, and (rarely) GCA may show these changes.[97]

References

1. Lalani TA, Kanne JP, Hatfield GA et al: Imaging findings in systemic lupus erythematosus, *Radiographics* 24:1069-1086, 2004.
2. Mills JA: Systemic lupus erythematosus [see comment], *New Engl J Med* 330: 1871-1879, 1994.
3. Tan EM, Cohen AS, Fries JF et al: The 1982 revised criteria for the classification of systemic lupus erythematosus, *Arthritis Rheum* 25:1271-1277, 1982.
4. van Vugt RM, Derksen RH, Kater L et al: Deforming arthropathy or lupus and rhupus hands in systemic lupus erythematosus, *Ann Rheum Dis* 57:540-544, 1998.
5. Alarcon-Segovia D, Abud-Mendoza C, Diaz-Jouanen E et al: Deforming arthropathy of the hands in systemic lupus erythematosus, *J Rheumatol* 15:65-69, 1988.
6. Reilly PA, Evison G, McHugh NJ et al: Arthropathy of hands and feet in systemic lupus erythematosus [see comment], *J Rheumatol* 17:777-784, 1990.
7. Weissman BN, Rappoport AS, Sosman JL et al: Radiographic findings in the hands in patients with systemic lupus erythematosus, *Radiology* 126:313-317, 1978.
8. Labowitz R, Schumacher HR Jr: Articular manifestations of systemic lupus erythematosus, *Ann Intern Med* 74:911-921, 1971.
9. Dubois EL, Tuffanelli DL: Clinical manifestations of systemic lupus erythematosus. Computer analysis of 520 cases, *J Am Med Assoc* 190:104-111, 1964.
10. Spronk PE, ter Borg EJ, Kallenberg CG: Patients with systemic lupus erythematosus and Jaccoud's arthropathy: a clinical subset with an increased C reactive protein response? *Ann Rheum Dis* 51:358-361, 1992.
11. Ostendorf B, Scherer A, Specker C et al: Jaccoud's arthropathy in systemic lupus erythematosus: differentiation of deforming and erosive patterns by magnetic resonance imaging, *Arthritis Rheum* 48:157-165, 2003.
12. Dray GJ: The hand in systemic lupus erythematosus, *Hand Clin* 5:145-155, 1989.
13. Bywaters E: *The relation between heart and joint disease including "rheumatoid heart disease" and chronic post-rheumatic arthritis (type Jaccoud), Brit Heart J* 12:101-131, 1950.
14. Richter Cohen M, Steiner G, Smolen JS et al: Erosive arthritis in systemic lupus erythematosus: analysis of a distinct clinical and serological subset, *Br J Rheumatol* 37:421-424, 1998.
15. Boutry N, Hachulla E, Flipo RM et al: MR imaging findings in hands in early rheumatoid arthritis: comparison with those in systemic lupus erythematosus and primary Sjogren syndrome [see comment], *Radiology* 236:593-600, 2005.
16. Wright S, Filippucci E, Grassi W et al: Hand arthritis in systemic lupus erythematosus: an ultrasound pictorial essay, *Lupus* 15:501-506, 2006.

17. Iagnocco A, Ossandon A, Coari G et al: Wrist joint involvement in systemic lupus erythematosus. An ultrasonographic study, *Clin Exp Rheumatol* 22:621-624, 2004.
18. Olsen KM, Chew FS: Tumoral calcinosis: pearls, polemics, and alternative possibilities, *Radiographics* 26:871-885, 2006.
19. Marzano AV, Kolesnikova LV, Gasparini G et al: Dystrophic calcinosis cutis in subacute lupus, *Dermatology* 198:90-92, 1999.
20. Nunley J, Jones L: *Calcinosis cutis* Feb. 6, 2007. Retrieved Oct. 24, 2008, from http://www.emedicine.com/derm/topic66.htm.
21. Leskinen RH, Skrifvars BV, Laasonen LS et al: Bone lesions in systemic lupus erythematosus, *Radiology* 153:349-352, 1984.
22. McBrine CS, Fisher MS: Acrosclerosis in sarcoidosis, *Radiology* 115:279-281, 1975.
23. Braunstein EM, Weissman BN, Sosman JL et al: Radiologic findings in late-onset systemic lupus erythematosus, *AJR Am J Roentgenol* 140:587-589, 1983.
24. Dubois E, Cozen L: Avascular (aseptic) bone necrosis associated with systemic lupus erythematosus, *J Am Med Assoc* 174:966-971, 1960.
25. Jaovisidha S, Denprechawong R, Suwannalai P et al: Asymptomatic avascular osteonecrosis of the hip in new patients diagnosed as systemic lupus erythematosus in Ramathibodi Hospital, *J Med Assoc Thai* 90:1382-1390, 2007.
26. Iida S, Harada Y, Shimizu K et al: Correlation between bone marrow edema and collapse of the femoral head in steroid-induced osteonecrosis, *AJR Am J Roentgenol* 174:735-743, 2000.
27. Sultan SM, Ioannou Y, Isenberg DA: A review of gastrointestinal manifestations of systemic lupus erythematosus, *Rheumatology* 38:917-932, 1999.
28. Yu KH, Yang CH, Chu CC: Swallowing disturbance due to isolated vagus nerve involvement in systemic lupus erythematosus, *Lupus* 16:746-749, 2007.
29. Lee C-K, Ahn MS, Lee EY et al: Acute abdominal pain in systemic lupus erythematosus: focus on lupus enteritis (gastrointestinal vasculitis), *Ann Rheum Dis* 61: 547-550, 2002.
30. Byun JY, Ha HK, Yu SY et al: CT Features of systemic lupus erythematosus in patients with acute abdominal pain: emphasis on ischemic bowel disease, *Radiology* 211:203-209, 1999.
31. Ahualli J: The target sign: bowel wall, *Radiology* 234:549-550, 2005.
32. Sofat N, Malik O, Higgens CS: Neurological involvement in patients with rheumatic disease, *Q J Med* 99:69-79, 2006.
33. Wong K, Woo EK, Yu YL et al: Neurological manifestations of systemic lupus erythematosus: a prospective study, *Q J Med* 81:857-870, 1991.
34. Appenzeller S, Bonilha L, Rio PA et al: Longitudinal analysis of gray and white matter loss in patients with systemic lupus erythematosus, *Neuroimage* 34:694-701, 2007.
35. Bosma GP, Steens SC, Petropoulos H et al: Multisequence magnetic resonance imaging study of neuropsychiatric systemic lupus erythematosus, *Arthritis Rheum* 50:3195-3202, 2004.
36. Steens SC, Steup-Beekman GM, Bosma GP et al: The effect of corticosteroid medication on quantitative MR parameters of the brain, *AJNR Am J Neuroradiol* 26: 2475-2480.
37. Ishimori ML, Pressman BD, Wallace DJ et al: Posterior reversible encephalopathy syndrome: another manifestation of CNS SLE? *Lupus* 16:436-443, 2007.
38. Lim MK, Suh CH, Kim HJ, et al: Systemic lupus erythematosus: brain MR imaging and single-voxel hydrogen 1 MR spectroscopy, *Radiology* 217:43-49, 2000.
39. Huang HP, Lai YC, Tsai IJ et al: Nephromegaly in children with Kawasaki disease: new supporting evidence for diagnosis and its possible mechanism, *Pediatr Res* 63:207-210, 2008.
40. Moder KG, Miller TD, Tazelaar HD: Cardiac involvement in systemic lupus erythematosus [see comment], *Mayo Clinic Proceed* 74:275-284, 1999.
41. Carsky EW, Mauceri RA, Azimi F: The epicardial fat pad sign: analysis of frontal and lateral chest radiographs in patients with pericardial effusion, *Radiology* 137:303-308, 1980.
42. Masui T, Finck S, Higgins CB: Constrictive pericarditis and restrictive cardiomyopathy: evaluation with MR imaging, *Radiology* 182:369-373, 1992.
43. Singh JA, Woodard PK, Dávila-Román VG et al: Cardiac magnetic resonance imaging abnormalities in systemic lupus erythematosus: a preliminary report, *Lupus* 14:137-144, 2005.
44. Lin CC, Ding HJ, Chen YW et al: Usefulness of technetium-99m sestamibi myocardial perfusion SPECT in detection of cardiovascular involvement in patients with systemic lupus erythematosus or systemic sclerosis, *Int J Cardiol* 92:157-161, 2003.
45. Selzer F, Sutton-Tyrrell K, Fitzgerald SG et al: Comparison of risk factors for vascular disease in the carotid artery and aorta in women with systemic lupus erythematosus, *Arthritis Rheum* 50:151-159, 2004.
46. Thompson T, Sutton-Tyrrell K, Wildman RP et al: Progression of carotid intima-media thickness and plaque in women with systemic lupus erythematosus, *Arthritis Rheum* 58:835-842, 2008.
47. Chang WL, Huang CM, Yang YH et al: Aortic aneurysm in systemic lupus erythematosus, *J Microbiol Immunol Infect* 37:310-312, 2004.
48. Mayberry JP, Primack SL, Muller NL: Thoracic manifestations of systemic autoimmune diseases: radiographic and high-resolution CT findings, *Radiographics* 20:1623-1635, 2000.
49. Kim JS, Lee KS, Koh EM et al: Thoracic involvement of systemic lupus erythematosus: clinical, pathologic, and radiologic findings, *J Comp Assist Tomogr* 24:1, 2000.
50. O'Connell DJ, Bennett RM: Mixed connective tissue disease—clinical and radiological aspects of 20 cases, *Br J Radiol* 50:620-625, 1977.
51. Lawson JP: The joint manifestations of the connective tissue diseases, *Semin Roentgenol* 17:25-38, 1982.
52. Udoff EJ, Genant HK, Kozin F et al: Mixed connective tissue disease: the spectrum of radiographic manifestations, *Radiology* 124:613-618, 1977.
53. Silver, T.M., Farber SJ, Bole GG, et al., Radiological features of mixed connective tissue disease and scleroderma—systemic lupus erythematosus overlap, *Radiology* 120:269-275, 1976.
54. Guit GL, Shaw PC, Ehrlich J et al: Mediastinal lymphadenopathy and pulmonary arterial hypertension in mixed connective tissue disease, *Radiology* 154:305-306, 1985.
55. Saito Y, Terada M, Takada T et al: Pulmonary involvement in mixed connective tissue disease: comparison with other collagen vascular diseases using high resolution CT, *J Comp Assist Tomography* 26:349-357, 2002.
56. Park J, Shin JI, Shin YH et al: Catastrophic antiphospholipid syndrome in a 7-year-old girl, *Clin Rheumatol* 26:6, 2007.
57. Asherson RA: The catastrophic antiphospholipid (Asherson's) syndrome in 2004—a review, *Autoimmun Rev* 4:48-54, 2005.
58. Levine JS, Branch DW, Rauch J: The antiphospholipid syndrome [see comment], *New Engl J Med* 346:752-763, 2002.
59. Provenzale JM, Ortel TL, Nelson RC: Adrenal hemorrhage in patients with primary antiphospholipid syndrome: imaging findings [see comment], *AJR Am J Roentgenol* 165:361-364, 1995.
60. Satou GM, Giamelli J, Gewitz MH: Kawasaki disease: diagnosis, management, and long-term implications, *Cardiol Rev* 15:163-169, 2007.
61. Rowley AH: Finding the cause of Kawasaki disease: a pediatric infectious diseases research priority [comment], *J Infect Dis* 194:1635-1637, 2006.
62. Burns JC: The riddle of Kawasaki disease [see comment], *New Engl J Med* 356:659-661, 2007.
63. Lau AC, Duong TT, Ito S et al: Matrix metalloproteinase 9 activity leads to elastin breakdown in an animal model of Kawasaki disease, *Arthritis Rheum* 58:854-863, 2008.
64. Newburger JW, Fulton DR: Kawasaki disease, *Curr Opin Pediatr* 16:508-514, 2004.
65. Newburger JW, Takahashi M, Gerber MA et al: Diagnosis, treatment, and long-term management of Kawasaki disease: a statement for health professionals from the Committee on Rheumatic Fever, Endocarditis, and Kawasaki Disease, Council on Cardiovascular Disease in the Young, American Heart Association [erratum appears in *Pediatrics* 115:1118, 2005], *Pediatrics* 114:1708-1733, 2004.
66. Greil GF, Seeger A, Miller S et al: Coronary magnetic resonance angiography and vessel wall imaging in children with Kawasaki disease, *Pediatr Radiol* 37:666-673, 2007.
67. Babu-Narayan SV, Cannell TM, Mohiaddin RH: Giant aneurysms of the coronary arteries due to Kawasaki disease—regular review without radiation using cardiovascular magnetic resonance, *Cardiol Young* 16:511-512, 2006.
68. Manghat NE, Morgan-Hughes GJ, Cox ID et al: Giant coronary artery aneurysm secondary to Kawasaki disease: diagnosis in an adult by multi-detector row CT coronary angiography, *Br J Radiol* 79:e133-e136, 2006.
69. Sonobe T, Kiyosawa N, Tsuchiya K et al: Prevalence of coronary artery abnormality in incomplete Kawasaki disease, *Pediatr Int* 49:421-426, 2007.
70. Mavrogeni S, Papadopoulos G, Karanasios E et al: How to image Kawasaki disease: a validation of different imaging techniques, *Int J Cardiol* 124:27-31, 2008.
71. Knockaert DC: Cardiac involvement in systemic inflammatory diseases, *Eur Heart J* 28:1797-1804, 2007.
72. Suzuki A, Takemura A, Inaba R et al: Magnetic resonance coronary angiography to evaluate coronary arterial lesions in patients with Kawasaki disease, *Cardiol Young* 16: 563-571, 2006.
73. Arnold R, Lay S, Ley-Zaporozhan J et al: Visualization of coronary arteries in patients after childhood Kawasaki syndrome: value of multidetector CT and MR imaging in comparison to conventional coronary catheterization, *Pediatr Radiol* 37:998-1006, 2007.
74. Takemura H, Oki T, Murao A et al: [Left ventricular inflow velocity patterns of mitral stenosis by pulsed Doppler echocardiography: comparisons with two cases of left atrial myxoma (author's transl)], *J Cardiography Suppl* 11:703-716, 1981.
75. Aggarwala G, Iyengar N, Burke SJ et al: Kawasaki disease: role of coronary CT angiography, *Int J Cardiovasc Imaging* 22:803-805, 2006.
76. Peng Y, Zeng J, Du Z et al: Usefulness of 64-slice MDCT for follow-up of young children with coronary artery aneurysm due to Kawasaki disease: initial experience, *Eur J Radiol* 2007. Online 27 December 2007.
77. Gelmez S, Saygili A, Tutar E et al: Coronary artery evaluation in Kawaski disease by dual source muti-detector coronary angiography in children, *Anadolu Kardiyol Derg* 10:E9-E10, 2008.
78. Fu YC, Shiau YC, Tsai SC et al: Discordance between dipyridamole stress technetium-99m tetrofosmin single photon emission computed tomography and coronary angiography in patients with Kawasaki disease, *Int J Cardiovasc Imaging* 18: 357-362, 2002.
79. Thapa R, Pramanik S, Chakrabartty S: Kawasaki disease: unusual manifestations and complications, *J Pediatr Child Health* 43:93-95, 2007.
80. Wang JN, Chiou YY, Chiu NT et al: Renal scarring sequelae in childhood Kawasaki disease, *Pediatr Nephrol* 22:684-689, 2007.
81. Muneuchi J, Kusuhara K, Kanaya Y et al: Magnetic resonance studies of brain lesions in patients with Kawasaki disease, *Brain Develop* 28:30-33, 2006.
82. Jen M, Brucia LA, Pollock AN et al: Cervical spine and temporomandibular joint arthritis in a child with Kawasaki disease, *Pediatrics* 118:e1569-e1571, 2006.
83. Leavitt L, Fauci AS, Bloch DA et al: The American College of Rheumatology 1990 criteria for the classification of Wegener's granulomatosis, *Arthritis Rheum* 33:1101-1107, 1990.
84. Kuyvenhoven JD, Ommeslag DJ, Ackerman CM et al: Lung uptake on technetium-99m-MDP bone scan in Wegener's vasculitis, *J Nucl Med* 37:857-858, 1996.
85. Provenzale JM, Allen NB: Wegener granulomatosis: CT and MR findings, *AJNR Am J Neuroradiol* 17:785-792, 1996.

86. Azuma N, Katada Y, Nishimura N et al: A case of granuloma in the occipital lobe of a patient with Wegener's granulomatosis, *Mod Rheumatol* 2008, in press.
87. Czarnecki EJ, Spickler EM: MR demonstration of Wegener granulomatosis of the infundibulum, a cause of diabetes insipidus. *AJNR Am J Neuroradiol* 16(4 Suppl):968-970, 1995.
88. Katzman GL, Langford CA, Sneller MC et al: Pituitary involvement by Wegener's granulomatosis: a report of two cases, *AJNR Am J Neuroradiol* 20:519-523, 1999.
89. Pipitone N, Versari A, Salvarani C: Role of imaging studies in the diagnosis and follow-up of large-vessel vasculitis: an update, *Rheumatology* 47:403-408, 2008.
90. Matsunaga N, Hayashi K, Sakamoto I et al: Takayasu arteritis: protean radiologic manifestations and diagnosis, *Radiographics* 17:579-594, 1997.
91. Endo M, Tomizawa Y, Nishida H et al: Angiographic findings and surgical treatments of coronary artery involvement in Takayasu arteritis, *J Thoracic Cardiovasc Surg* 125:570-577, 2003.
92. Kato T, Kakuta T, Maruyama Y et al: QT dispersion in patients with Takayasu arteritis, *Angiology* 51:751-756, 2000.
93. Hunder GG, Bloch DA, Michel BA et al: The American College of Rheumatology 1990 criteria for the classification of giant cell arteritis, *Arthritis Rheum* 33:1122-1128, 1990.
94. Lockhart ME, Robbin ML: Case 58: giant cell arteritis, *Radiology* 227:512-515, 2003.
95. Schmidt WA, Kraft HE, Vorpahl K et al: Color duplex ultrasonography in the diagnosis of temporal arteritis [see comment], *N Engl J Med* 337:1336-1342, 1997.
96. Bley TA, Uhl M, Carew J et al: Diagnostic value of high-resolution MR imaging in giant cell arteritis, *AJNR Am J Neuroradiol* 28:1722-1727, 2007.
97. Rhodes ES, Pekala JS, Gemery JM et al: Case 129: polyarteritis nodosa, *Radiology* 246:322-326, 2008.
98. Jennette JC, Falk RJ, Andrassy K et al: Nomenclature of systemic vasculitides. Proposal of an international consensus conference, *Arthritis Rheum* 37:187-192, 1994.
99. Lightfoot RW Jr, Michel BA, Bloch DA et al: The American College of Rheumatology 1990 criteria for the classification of polyarteritis nodosa, *Arthritis Rheum* 33:1088-1093, 1990.
100. Jee KN, Ha HK, Lee IJ et al: Radiologic findings of abdominal polyarteritis nodosa [see comment], *AJR Am J Roentgenol* 174:1675-1679, 2000.
101. Guillevin L, Lhote F, Gayraud M et al: Prognostic factors in polyarteritis nodosa and Churg-Strauss syndrome. A prospective study in 342 patients, *Medicine* 75:17-28, 1996.
102. Lawless OJ, Whelton JC: Proceedings: deforming hand arthritis in systemic lupus erythematosus, *Arthritis Rheum* 17:323, 1974.
103. Mak A, Chan BP, Yeh IB et al: Neuropsychiatric lupus and reversible posterior leucoencephalopathy syndrome: a challenging clinical dilemma, *Rheumatology* 47:256-262, 2008.

CHAPTER 23

Seronegative Spondyloarthropathies and SAPHO Syndrome

JOEL RUBENSTEIN, MD, FRCPC

KEY POINTS

- Seronegative spondyloarthropathies are interrelated chronic inflammatory rheumatic diseases that include ankylosing spondylitis (AS), reactive arthritis, psoriatic spondyloarthropathy, spondyloarthropathy associated with inflammatory bowel disease (IBD), and undifferentiated spondyloarthropathy.
- Seronegative spondyloarthropathies are characterized by sacroiliitis with or without spondylitis, peripheral oligoarthritis, enthesitis, dactylitis, and inflammation of nonarticular structures.
- These disorders occur in genetically predisposed individuals and are triggered by environmental factors.
- HLA-B27 is present in up to 95% of patients of European ancestry with AS and is seen in the majority of patients with reactive arthritis, spondylitis associated with IBD, and psoriatic spondylitis.
- Bilateral, symmetric sacroiliac involvement is characteristic of AS but may be seen in any of these disorders and occasionally in other conditions.
- Unilateral or asymmetric sacroiliitis suggests psoriatic arthritis or reactive arthritis. Infection should be excluded in cases of unilateral sacroiliitis.
- Magnetic resonance imaging is preferred over conventional radiography and computed tomography because of its ability to detect early inflammatory changes.
- Spondylitis begins at the discovertebral junctions, resulting in erosions, squaring, "shining corners," and, eventually, bony bridging (syndesmophytes).
- Complications of AS include acute spine fracture, chronic discovertebral lesions, and cauda equina syndrome.
- Psoriatic arthritis typically involves the distal interphalangeal joints with erosion or ankylosis. New bone formation occurs adjacent to the erosions. Osteoporosis is atypical. Periosteal reaction may occur along the phalanges and bony prominences. A "sausage digit" is a characteristic feature.
- The radiographic features of enteropathic spondyloarthropathy are identical to those of ankylosing spondylitis.

The seronegative spondyloarthropathies are a group of heterogeneous, interrelated chronic inflammatory rheumatic diseases that include ankylosing spondylitis (AS), reactive arthritis, psoriatic spondyloarthropathy, spondyloarthropathy associated with inflammatory bowel disease (enteropathic) (IBD), and undifferentiated spondyloarthropathy.[1]

> Seronegative spondyloarthropathies include AS, IBD, reactive arthritis, psoriatic spondylitis, and undifferentiated spondyloarthropathy.

These diseases are characterized by sacroiliitis with or without spondylitis, peripheral joint oligoarthritis, enthesitis, dactylitis, and inflammation of nonarticular structures (e.g., skin, gastrointestinal [GI] tract, eye, and heart).

Although knowledge of the cellular and molecular mechanisms of inflammation in these diseases is incomplete, the data suggest they are multifactorial processes occurring in genetically predisposed individuals, which are triggered by environmental factors. Thus our current understanding of the spondyloarthropathies converges along three lines of investigation: (1) clinical and epidemiologic studies, in which diagnostic imaging has played an important role; (2) genetic and immunologic studies, focusing on an inherited predilection to developing spondyloarthropathy; and (3) studies of infectious agents that may act as the environmental triggers for the development of spondyloarthropathy.

An unresolved entity that also appears linked to the seronegative spondyloarthropathies is SAPHO syndrome (*s*ynovitis, *a*cne, *p*ustulosis, *h*yperostosis, and *o*steitis), in which a significant number of patients fulfill accepted criteria for spondyloarthropathy but do not usually have the genetic predispositions found in patients with the other seronegative spondyloarthropathies.[1]

> SAPHO: *s*ynovitis, *a*cne, *p*ustulosis, *h*yperostosis, and *o*steitis.

CLINICAL DATA AND EPIDEMIOLOGY

The anatomic and clinical reports at the end of the nineteenth century by von Bechterew,[2] Strumpell,[3] and Marie[4] are generally credited as the first significant descriptions of AS, and these reports served to establish AS as a distinct disease entity.

Over the course of the twentieth century, our understanding of AS has been further augmented by the evolution of radiographic techniques. In 1937, Andersson[5] described discovertebral destructive changes representing a spondylodiscitis identified on radiographic examinations of two patients with AS. In 1952, Romanus[6] reported on the radiographic appearance of vertebral margin erosions of bone followed by sclerosis and ossification occurring in patients with AS. In 1956, Forestier et al.[7] described additional radiographic manifestations of AS, including sacroiliitis and syndesmophyte formation. These reports showed the importance of the imaging features of AS, which today remain integral to the diagnosis and staging of the spondyloarthropathies. In the latter half of the twentieth century, the development of more sophisticated imaging techniques such as computed tomography (CT) and magnetic resonance imaging (MRI) has led to numerous reports of improved image sensitivity and specificity for the diagnosis of spondyloarthropathies.

In North America during the midportion of the twentieth century, the concepts of "rheumatoid spondylitis" and "rheumatoid variant" were used to indicate that AS was thought to be a variant of rheumatoid arthritis (RA) affecting the spine. During this same period, there were also clinical, radiographic, and epidemiologic reports showing relationships between AS and other types of arthritis. In 1960, Graham[8] was among the first to suggest that AS was a separate entity from RA. In 1974, Moll et al.[9] suggested that the "rheumatoid variants" were discrete entities and introduced the concept of the "seronegative spondyloarthropathies" on the basis of overlapping clinical and radiologic features within a number of different diseases that shared clinical features distinct from RA. Specific characteristics that were noted to distinguish the spondyloarthropathies from RA were seronegativity for rheumatoid factor, absence of nodules, and radiologic evidence of sacroiliitis. The original grouping of spondyloarthropathies included AS, Reiter's syndrome (i.e., reactive arthritis), psoriatic arthritis, juvenile spondyloarthropathy, and arthritis associated with inflammatory bowel disease (IBD); Whipple's disease and Behçet's syndrome were also incorporated into this grouping but were subsequently excluded.

In 1990, Amor et al.[10] proposed a classification of the spondyloarthropathies using various criteria with a scoring system to establish a diagnosis of spondyloarthritis. In 1991 the European Spondyloarthropathy Study Group (ESSG)[11] broadened these criteria for diagnosis to accommodate undifferentiated forms of spondyloarthropathy (i.e., patients who manifest features of, but fail to fulfill criteria for, the other spondyloarthropathies) and included findings such as seronegative oligoarthritis, dactylitis or polyarthritis of the lower extremities, and heel pain due to enthesitis, which had been ignored in previous epidemiologic studies. In addition, patients with acute anterior uveitis[12] and HLA-B27 positive individuals with spondylitic heart disease (i.e., complete heart block and/or aortic regurgitation)[13] were considered to be within the spectrum of the seronegative spondyloarthropathies. Using these criteria, one epidemiologic study reported undifferentiated spondyloarthropathy to be second in frequency only to AS.[14]

GENETICS AND IMMUNOLOGY

Identification of the human leukocyte antigen (HLA)[15,16] in the 1950s was the initial important step leading to characterization of the human major histocompatibility complex (MHC), later shown to be located on chromosome 6 and responsible for encoding the histocompatibility antigens that are divided into Class I, II, and III genes. This work would subsequently provide a foundation for understanding the genetic predispositions of individuals who develop spondyloarthropathies. A clear correlation has now been documented between patients with spondyloarthropathy and the presence of HLA-B27,[17] which is present in up to 95% of patients of European ancestry with AS,[18] 70% with reactive arthritis,[19] 70% with spondylitis associated with IBD,[20] 60% with psoriatic spondylitis, and 50% with acute anterior uveitis occurring without other features of spondylarthropathy.[12] Studies have also shown a remarkable familial aggregation of these disorders; 20% of HLA-B27 positive relatives of patients with ankylosing spondylitis are ultimately affected[17] and a concordance rate as high as 63% has been shown in identical twins versus 23% in nonidentical twins.[21,22] These statistics, however, provide only limited insight into the complex genetic factors influencing the development of the spondyloarthropathies: Fewer than 5% of individuals who are HLA-B27 positive will develop a spondyloarthropathy,[23] and multiple other MHC genes (e.g., HLA-DRB1) and molecular subtypes of HLA-B27 have now been implicated in the development of AS, including HLA-B*2705, HLA-B*2704, and HLA-B*2707.[17]

> Fewer than 5% of HLA-B27-positive individuals develop spondyloarthropathy.

In contrast to patients with AS who have a high frequency of HLA-B27, patients with psoriatic arthritis have a higher frequency of HLA-B17, HLA-B39, and HLA-Cw6.[1]

ASSOCIATED INFECTIOUS AGENTS

In 1916, Reiter[24] described a syndrome of non-gonococcal urethritis, peripheral arthritis, and conjunctivitis following dysentery. This account presaged subsequent interest in the role of infection in the etiology of the spondyloarthropathies. Subsequent reports by Bauer et al.[25] and Paronen[26] documented a more specific relationship between the development of Reiter's syndrome and prior genitourinary or GI infections. In 1969, Ahvonen et al.[27] reported on patients with arthritis following GI infection with *Yersinia enterocolitica* and proposed the concept of reactive arthritis. Other bacteria implicated in the development of reactive arthritis include genitourinary infections with *Chlamydia trachomatis* and enteric infections with gram-negative organisms such as *Shigella, Salmonella,* and *Campylobacter.*[28] Additional evidence of this association is the finding of antigens for *Salmonella, Yersinia,* and *Chlamydia* in synovial tissue and fluid from patients with reactive arthritis.[29,30] In 1978, Ebringer et al.[31] implicated enteric *Klebsiella pneumoniae* infection as a trigger in the pathogenesis of AS, although this has never been confirmed, and a more recent report by Stebbings et al.[32] implicated *Bacteroides* as a trigger for AS.

There has also been considerable speculation about the etiologic role of infection to explain the association between AS and IBD, presumably resulting from breakdown of the mucosal barrier of the gut allowing intestinal bacteria to stimulate the immune system.[33] This association is more common than past reports would indicate and, in particular, it has been shown that over 50% of patients with spondyloarthropathy have evidence of silent IBD documented by endoscopic examination.[34] Furthermore, de Vlam et al.[35] reported that 30% of 103 patients with either ulcerative colitis or Crohn's disease had symptoms of inflammatory back pain, 90% fulfilled diagnostic criteria for spondyloarthropathy, and 18% had asymptomatic sacroiliitis.

Multiple reports have drawn attention to important links among immunity, infectious agents, and psoriasis. Prinz[36] has shown that, in some patients, psoriasis vulgaris is the result of a sterile antibacterial skin reaction initiated by streptococcal T cells that cross-react against epidermal autoantigens. Not surprisingly, human immunodeficiency virus (HIV) has also been reported in association with psoriatic arthritis, reactive arthritis, and patients with undifferentiated spondyloarthropathy,[37-38] and McGonagle et al.[39] have shown that patients with HIV have a tenfold increased frequency for developing psoriatic arthritis.

SAPHO SYNDROME

In 1987, Chamot et al.[40] suggested the acronym SAPHO to describe a group of 85 patients with pustular acne and hyperostotic inflammation of bone. The characteristic feature of this syndrome is osteitis, usually with negative bacterial cultures, with or without skin lesions.[41,42] Reports of other entities with an association between cutaneous disease and musculoskeletal inflammation that are likely part of the spectrum of SAPHO syndrome include: sternocostoclavicular hyperostosis,[43] pustulotic arthroosteitis,[44] chronic recurrent multifocal osteomyelitis with pustulosis palmaris et plantaris,[45,46] acne conglobata with spondyloarthropathy, and hidradenitis suppurativa.[47-48] Of related interest is a study of clinical subsets in patients with psoriatic arthritis in which 2% of patients showed features of SAPHO syndrome.[49] Maugars et al.[50] have suggested that psoriasis is the "link" between SAPHO and the spondyloarthropathies.

SAPHO more commonly affects women than men and the clinical course is variable, with some patients experiencing continuous bone and joint symptoms, whereas others may show intermittent episodes of disease. Although individuals with SAPHO syndrome have only a slightly increased incidence of HLA-B27, a significant number of patients exhibit diagnostic criteria for seronegative spondyloarthropathy, with a reported frequency of spondylodiscitis between 9% and 32%.[51] The spine is second only to the sternocostoclavicular area as the most common site of involvement in adults, and spondylodiscitis may, in fact, be the initial presentation of SAPHO syndrome.[52,53]

Like other spondyloarthropathies, an association between infection and the development of SAPHO syndrome has been proposed. Although bacterial cultures are usually negative, there have been multiple reports documenting *P. acnes* as a cause of discitis, osteitis, and arthritis, supporting a potential link between this organism and SAPHO syndrome.[54-55]

OSTEOARTICULAR FEATURES AND IMAGING

Ankylosing Spondylitis

AS is the most common inflammatory spondyloarthropathy and represents the prototype for all the other spondyloarthropathies. The diagnosis of AS requires clinical suspicion and astute patient assessment, with medical imaging subsequently playing an important role in confirming the diagnosis.

Patients with AS usually present with back pain and stiffness in adolescence or early adult life, typically commencing in the second or third decade of life,[56] but onset after age 45 may occur. In fact, diagnosis after the age of 45 is not uncommon because symptoms are often insidious and the diagnosis may be overlooked.[57] To further complicate this issue, it has been suggested that late-onset undifferentiated spondyloarthropathy occurs more frequently than AS after the age of 50 and that late-onset spondyloarthropathy is not rare.[58]

Men are two to three times more commonly affected than women, although the prevalence in women has likely been underestimated in many reports because women tend to have less severe involvement of the spine and more symptoms affecting the knees, wrists, ankles, hips, and pelvis.[59-60] The clinical picture with juvenile onset of disease is also different from that of adult onset by the more frequent occurrence of peripheral joint disease.[59]

A long-term follow-up study by Carette et al.[61] showed that the natural history of AS is generally established in the first 10 years of disease and that the presence of peripheral joint involvement, especially of the hip, portends a poorer prognosis.

The imaging hallmark of AS is sacroiliitis, and radiographic studies remain the first line of investigation, looking for both the destructive and proliferative changes of bone associated with structural joint damage.[62]

Sacroiliitis is recognized as the earliest feature of AS. During the initial course of the illness, sacroiliac disease may be asymmetrical, or occasionally unilateral, but with time, the distribution customarily evolves to produce bilateral, symmetric involvement.[63]

> Bilateral, symmetric sacroiliitis is characteristic of AS but not specific.

Both the synovial and ligamentous portions of the sacroiliac (SI) joints are affected, although in the earlier stages of the disease, the iliac side of the joint classically shows greater alteration than the sacral side. The initial manifestations include periarticular osteopenia with ill-definition of the joint margins accompanied by subchondral sclerosis, primarily on the iliac side of the joint; the joint space may also appear variably widened, although discrete erosions may be difficult to identify.

> Erosions involve the iliac sides of the SI joint first.

As the process becomes more advanced, subchondral sclerosis becomes evident on both sides of the joint, erosions become more distinct, and narrowing of the joint space may occur with areas of incomplete bony bridging. The end stage of this process is complete ankylosis of the SI joints, often with loss of the bony eburnation observed in earlier stages of the disease. Other features that may be seen in the pelvis and hips that frequently accompany these findings are ossification of the SI and lumbosacral ligaments, abnormalities of the pubic symphysis, hip arthritis and inflammatory enthesopathy of the iliac crests, ischial tuberosities and femoral trochanters (Table 23-1).

Based on these features, the New York criteria[23] were developed for grading sacroiliitis and are as follows: 0 = normal; 1 = suspicious (no definite abnormality); 2 = minimal (loss of definition of the SI margins, some sclerosis, minimal erosions) (Figure 23-1); 3 = moderate (sclerosis on both sides of the SI joints, indistinct margins, erosions, joint space loss) (Figure 23-2); and 4 = severe (ankylosis) (Figure 23-3).

With the advent of effective treatment for AS, the need to measure structural damage and its progression has become essential. As a result, other radiographic scoring methods, such as the Bath Ankylosing Spondylitis Radiology Index,[64] the Stoke Ankylosing Spondylitis Spine Score (SASSS),[65] and the modified SASSS (M-SASSS),[66] have been developed and tested to evaluate radiographic evidence of disease progression. One recent study concluded that the M-SASSS is the most appropriate for scoring disease progression, but a 2-year radiographic study of these scoring methods in patients with AS concluded that, although these methods are moderately to excellently reliable, change was too small to be reliably detected in the 2-year time frame.[67]

Although scintigraphy may occasionally be helpful for evaluation of unilateral sacroiliitis, its role is limited because it has low sensitivity and specificity and generally does not alter decisions about disease probability.[68]

For patients in whom clinical suspicion of early disease is high, yet radiographic studies are negative or equivocal, computed tomography (CT) and magnetic resonance imaging (MRI) are important in documenting the presence or absence of sacroiliitis. Prior to the introduction of MRI, Kozin et al.[69] showed that CT is more sensitive than radiography and is equally specific for identifying sacroiliitis (Figure 23-4). In HLA-B27 patients with clinical evidence of sacroiliitis, 50% of these individuals had negative or equivocal radiographs whereas only 19% had negative CT images for sacroiliitis. Fam et al.[70] also found that CT improved delineation of the SI joints in early AS and revealed more abnormalities and higher grades of sacroiliitis than conventional radiography (Figure 23-5). Similarly, CT showed the presence of asymptomatic sacroiliitis in 32% of 65 patients with known IBD, compared with conventional radiography, which was positive for sacroiliitis in only 18% of patients.[71] More recent investigation has shown that CT is equally as accurate as MRI in defining erosions of the SI joints but is ineffective in detecting synovial inflammation; thus MRI permits differentiation between active and chronic sacroiliitis.[72]

MRI has proven even more valuable than CT in the early detection of inflammation and destructive changes involving the spine and SI joints, and it is generally preferred over conventional radiography and CT because of its ability to detect the early

TABLE 23-1. Imaging Findings of AS

Feature	Findings	Example
Romanus lesion	Erosions of the anterior superior or inferior margins of the vertebrae, at the discovertebral junctions. These are early features of AS	
Shiny corners	Sclerosis of the superior or inferior margins of a vertebra seen on a lateral radiograph associated with reactive bone formation at the site of prior erosion/inflammation (Romanus lesion)	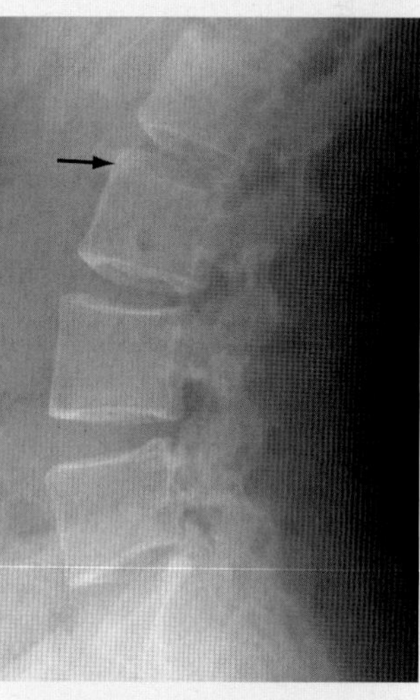
Squaring	Corner erosion leads to a straight anterior contour of the anterior surface of the vertebra	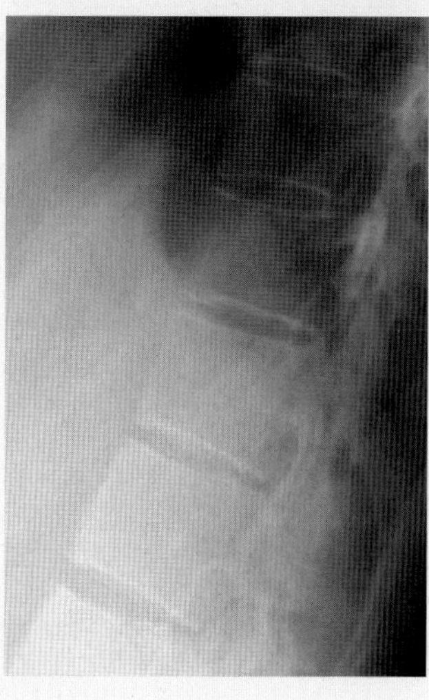

(Continued)

TABLE 23-1. Imaging Findings of AS—cont'd

Feature	Findings	Example
Syndesmophyte	Bony bridging extending from the margin of one vertebra to the next	
Bamboo spine	Vertebral fusion with syndesmophytes leads to an undulating vertebral contour	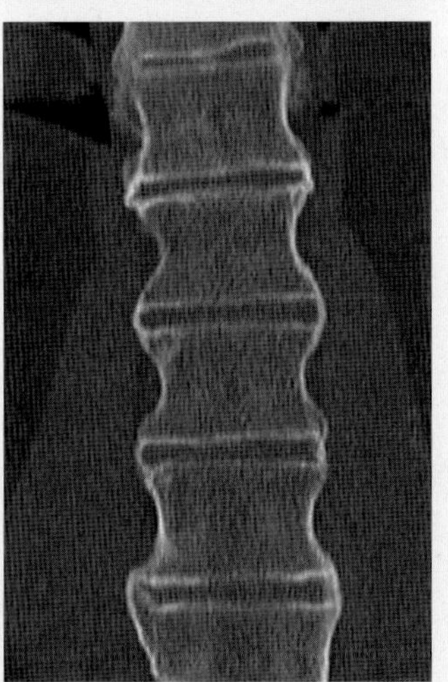
"Pseudarthrosis"	Extensive discovertebral destruction with disruption of previously fused posterior elements	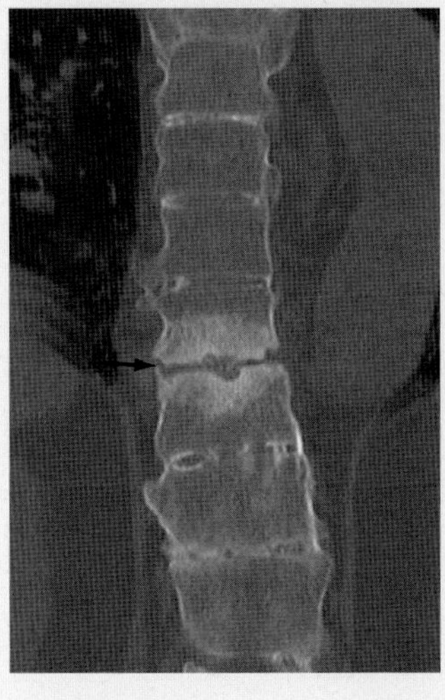

(Continued)

TABLE 23-1. Imaging Findings of AS—cont'd

Feature	Findings	Example
"Trolley track" sign	Three parallel radiodense bands seen on frontal radiographs due to fusion of the apophyseal joint capsules and the interspinous and supraspinous ligaments	
"Dagger" sign	Central radiodense line visible on frontal radiographs connecting the spinous processes	
Enthesopathy	New bone formation at sites of ligament or tendon insertion on bone	

Portions of this table modified from Resnick D: *Diagnosis of bone and joint disorders*, ed 4, Philadelphia, 2002, Saunders, p 1033.

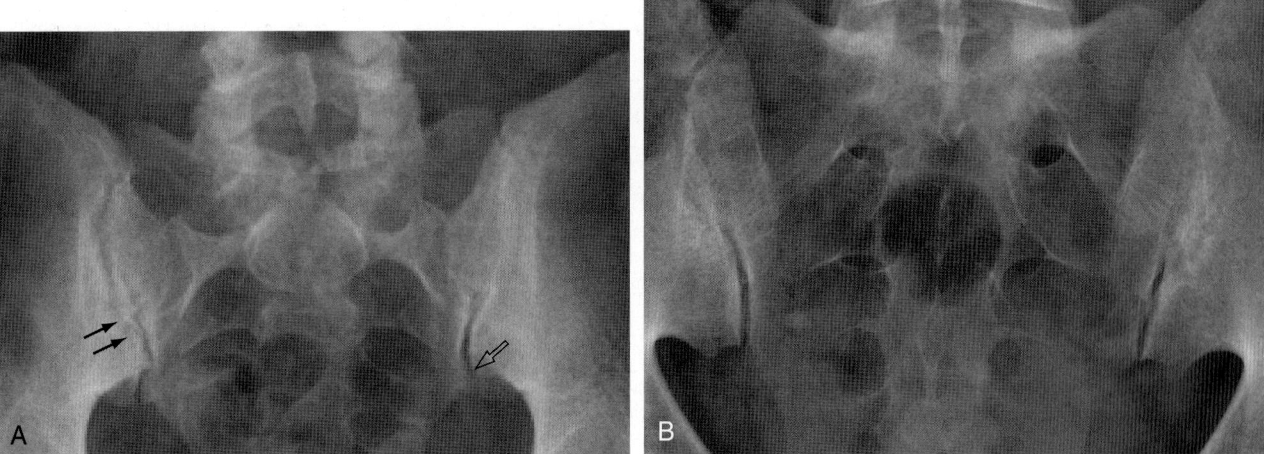

FIGURE 23-1. Grade II sacroiliitis. **A,** Subchondral iliac sclerosis with subtle erosions on the right *(arrows)* and loss of definition of the margins of the anterior portion of the left SI joint *(open arrow)* are noted. **B,** The normal appearance of the SI joints is shown for comparison.

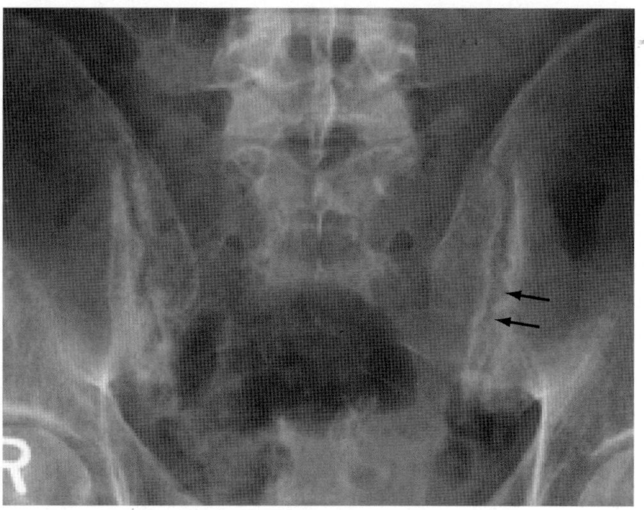

FIGURE 23-2. Grade III sacroiliitis in a patient with AS. Sclerosis of the iliac and sacral sides of the joints is present with distinct erosions on the left *(arrows)* and ill-defined joint margins on the right. The left SI joint appears wide as a consequence of the erosion. The right SI joint is partially fused inferiorly.

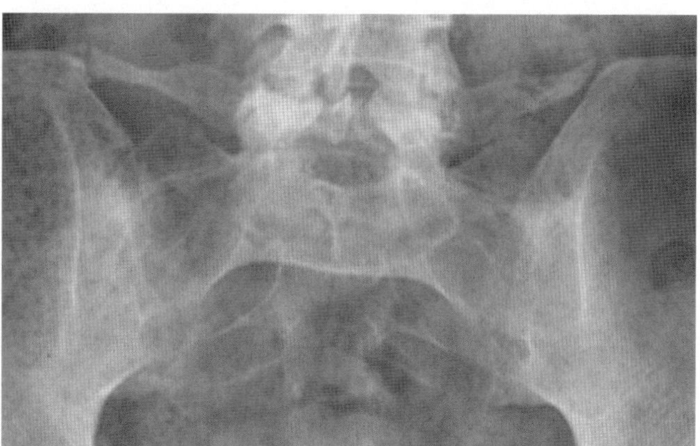

FIGURE 23-3. Grade IV sacroiliitis. Ankylosis of both SI joints is present.

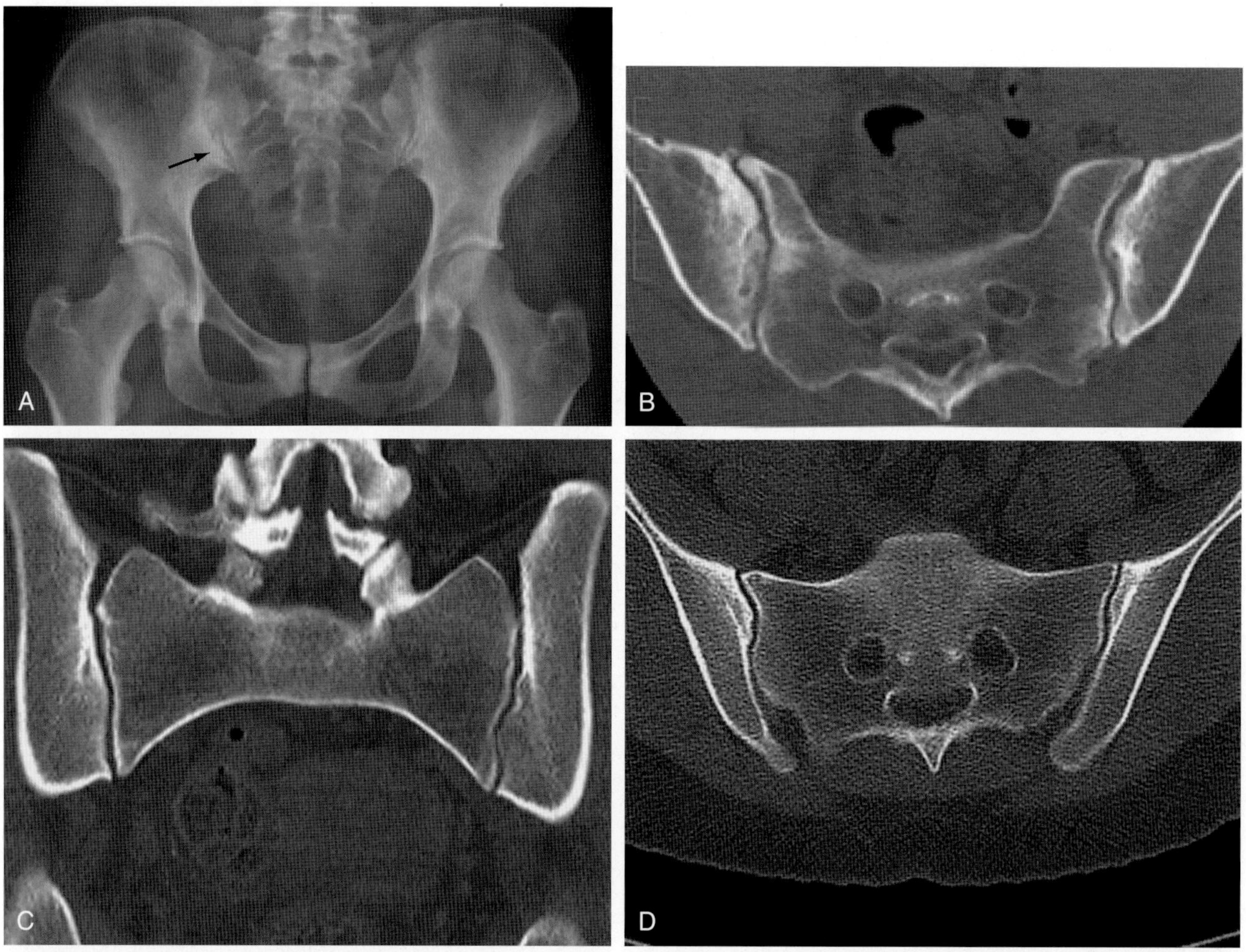

FIGURE 23-4. Osteitis pubis and grade I sacroiliitis. **A,** Florid subchondral sclerosis and erosions of the pubic symphysis are present. There is subtle subchondral sclerosis and loss of definition of the SI joint margins on the right *(arrow)*. Unlike the findings in this case, the SI joint findings in the spondyloarthritides are usually more severe than the changes in the pubic symphysis. **B,** Axial CT of the SI joints. Asymmetric sacroiliitis is present with subchondral sclerosis and erosions that are more marked on the right. **C,** A reformatted CT scan in another patient for comparison shows the normal SI joints in the coronal plane. **D,** A normal axial CT image of the SI joints is shown for comparison. Note the absence of subchondral sclerosis and the sharp line of the white subchondral bone.

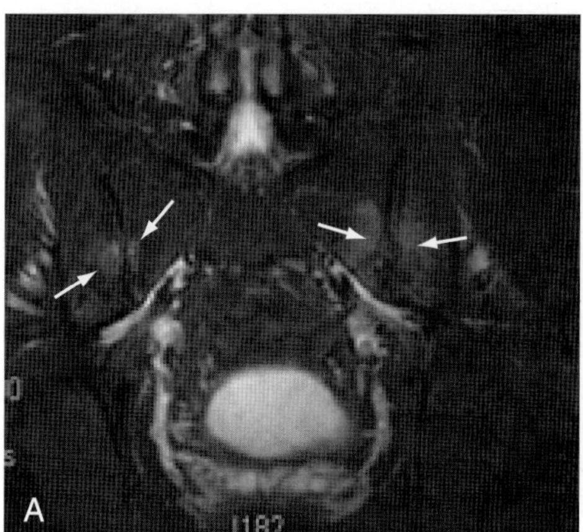

FIGURE 23-5. Grade III sacroiliitis shown on CT. Axial CT through the SI joints shows joint space narrowing with partial bony ankylosis *(arrows)* developing on the right.

inflammatory changes of bone and synovium (Figure 23-6).[73,74] An understanding of the normal MRI appearance of the SI joints is mandatory for accurate interpretation of abnormalities affecting these joints, and axial images provide superior delineation of the normal anatomy and abnormalities of the SI joints.[75] MRI findings in early disease show that sacroiliitis is most often bilateral, affects the iliac side of the joint more frequently than the sacral side, and the inflammation is most frequent in the dorsocaudal parts of the synovial joint and bone marrow.[76] A prospective study comparing radiography, quantitative SI scintigraphy, and MRI for the detection of sacroiliitis in 44 patients with inflammatory low back pain found MRI to be the most sensitive imaging technique (i.e., 95% sensitivity compared with 48% for scintigraphy and 19% for conventional radiography).[77] Thus MRI combined with various scoring techniques has now become an integral part of more recent studies and clinical trials that seek to quantify disease activity and measure response to treatment (Figure 23-7).[78]

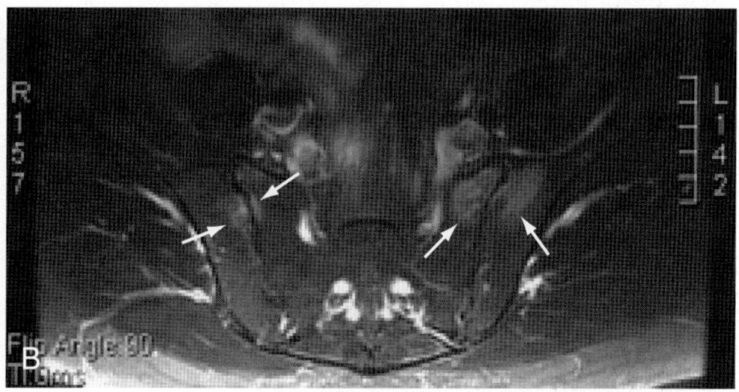

FIGURE 23-6. SI edema consistent with active inflammation. **A,** Coronal STIR image reveals areas of subchondral iliac and sacral edema *(arrows)* plus increased signal in both SI joints, compatible with acute inflammatory disease. **B,** An axial fat-suppressed T2-weighted fast spin echo image demonstrates subchondral iliac and sacral fluid signal edema (*arrows*).

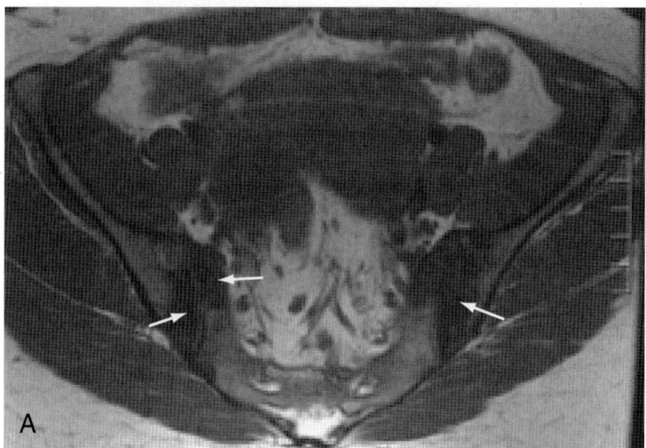

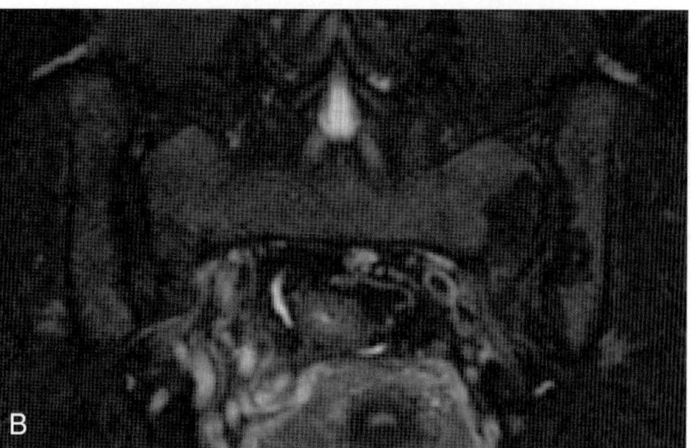

FIGURE 23-7. Chronic sacroiliitis. **A,** An axial T1-weighted fast spin echo image reveals subchondral low (dark) signal *(arrows)* involving the iliac and sacral margins of both sacroiliac joints related to bony sclerosis, compatible with chronic sacroiliitis. **B,** Coronal STIR image. Areas of subchondral iliac and sacral low (dark) signal are present related to subchondral sclerosis due to chronic sacroiliitis. Note also the absence of increased intraarticular signal.

The most commonly employed MR pulse sequences for identifying inflammatory disease in the spine are short tau inversion recovery (STIR) images in the coronal plane and gadolinium-enhanced, T1-weighted, fat-saturated images in the axial and coronal planes; unenhanced T1-weighted and fat-suppressed T2-weighted images have also been included in several studies. One investigation showed that more spinal lesions were detected with the STIR sequence but that reader reliability was better with the gadolinium-enhanced sequences.[79]

MRI methods for grading SI disease reflect those previously developed with the New York criteria and include assessment of erosions, bony sclerosis, and joint space width; however, additional features that can be evaluated include bone marrow edema and gadolinium contrast enhancement. In a recent study by Puhakka et al.,[80] scores for disease severity were obtained by grading each finding as: 0 = normal, 1 = minimal, 2 = moderate, or 3 = severe. An overall score for joint destruction was obtained as the sum of the scores for erosions, sclerosis, and joint width. Similarly, an overall score for inflammation was obtained as the sum of scores for bone marrow edema and gadolinium contrast enhancement of the marrow and joint space. These two overall scores were then considered reflections of chronicity and acuity of disease, respectively. Another important conclusion made by this report was the greater sensitivity of MRI in detecting disease progression during the 1-year period of the study compared with the sensitivity of radiographs, which require about 4 years of follow-up to detect progression.

In the spine, abnormalities first appear at the thoracolumbar and lumbosacral junctions and later progress along the remainder of the spine (Figure 23-8). Osteitis is the earliest expression of spinal involvement, manifesting as focal areas of bone erosion at the discovertebral margins. When accompanied by productive new bone filling the concavity of the anterior vertebral surface, the vertebrae assume a squared appearance, most notably in the lumbar spine (Figure 23-9). Sclerosis develops with healing of the erosions, producing the so-called "shiny corner" sign.

Early findings of spondylitis are "shining" corners and vertebral squaring.

This bone formation then extends along the discovertebral margin, forming vertically oriented ossification of the annulus fibrosus, referred to as *syndesmophytes*. This pattern of ossification can further extend along the anterior longitudinal ligament, as well as the paravertebral soft tissues (Figure 23-10).

Patients with AS may develop cauda equina syndrome, and previous myelographic studies have shown the presence of arachnoid diverticula in these patients associated with a capacious dural sac.[81,82] Although myelography is rarely performed in modern clinical practice, it should be noted that laminar erosions related to these diverticula may be identified with CT and MRI.

Cauda equina syndrome (low back pain, sciatica, leg weakness, sensory disturbance, loss of bladder and bowel function, and saddle anesthesia) may occur in AS.

A report by Braun et al.[83] showed that the thoracic spine is a more common site of spinal disease than either the lumbar or cervical spine. They emphasized that recognition of this factor is important because most radiographic scoring systems do not include this spinal segment, and they added that intrarater and interrater variation of radiographic interpretations was greatest in the thoracic spine. As a result, Braun et al.[83] concluded that the

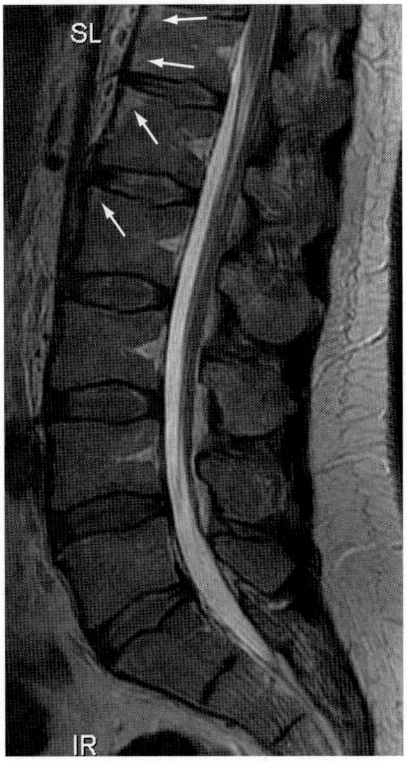

FIGURE 23-8. AS with vertebral inflammation. A sagittal T2-weighted fast spin echo image shows areas of increased signal at the anterior margins of the vertebral end plates from T12 to L2 *(arrows)* related to acute inflammation.

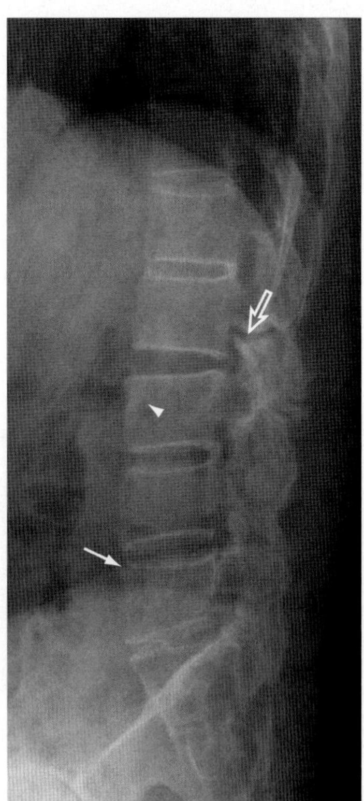

FIGURE 23-9. AS with vertebral fracture after a fall. Squaring of the lumbar vertebrae is present with erosion at the anterior margin of the L5 superior end plate *(arrow)* and "shiny corner" *(arrowhead)* due to osteitis at the anterior-superior margin of L3. There is extensive facet ankylosis with straightening of the normal lumbar lordosis. Widening of the L2-3 disk space and a fracture *(open arrow)* through the posterior elements at this level is noted.

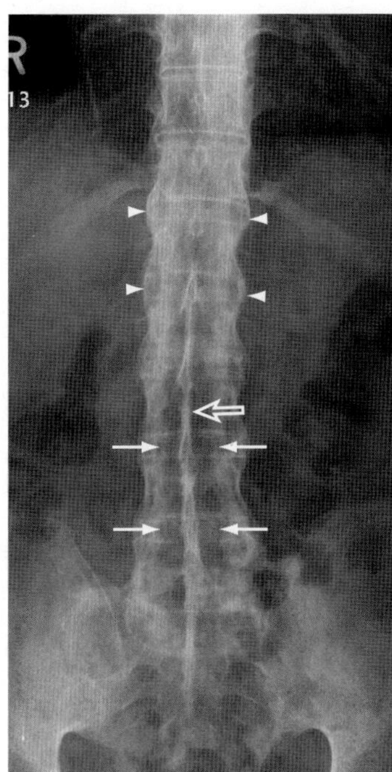

FIGURE 23-10. Advanced AS. There is ankylosis of the sacroiliac joints and syndesmophyte formation *(arrowheads)* along the length of the visualized portions of the thoracolumbar spine. Ossification of the interspinous ligaments (*open arrow*, the "dagger sign") and apophyseal joint capsules ("trolley-track sign," *arrows*) are noted.

thoracic spine is best assessed by MRI, which has an essential role in defining chronic changes in the thoracic spine.

The most serious complication of AS is spine fracture, which can occur, even with minor trauma, due to the rigidity and osteopenia that develop in the spinal column (Figure 23-11).[84] The most frequent sites for fracture are the cervical spine, with the risk of quadriplegia, and the thoracolumbar junction.[85] Fractures that develop in AS patients are associated with high morbidity and mortality rates.[86]

Patients with AS may also develop sclerosis and destructive changes of the discovertebral junction, usually unrelated to infection, and these changes have been termed *Andersson lesions*, named after the investigator who originally described them (Figure 23-12).

> Development of new pain in a patient with late-stage AS suggests "pseudarthrosis." Demonstration of a defect in the posterior elements, as well as anteriorly, helps confirm abnormal motion.

Although the etiology of this abnormality remains controversial, various explanations have been proposed, including inflammation, a persistent motion segment (pseudarthrosis), fracture, and infection.[87-88]

The hip, shoulder, and knee are the most important sites of peripheral arthritis in AS. In the hip, one of the earliest features of arthritis is the development of osteophyte formation at the margin of the femoral head often associated with joint space loss and variable subchondral cystic changes (Figure 23-13).

> Hip disease is common and appears radiographically as combined RA and osteoarthritis.

In the majority of patients, the hip disease is bilateral and symmetric.

Shoulder disease, like that of the hip, is most commonly bilateral. Rosen[89] has described a characteristic erosion occurring at the superolateral margin of the humeral head in patients with AS,

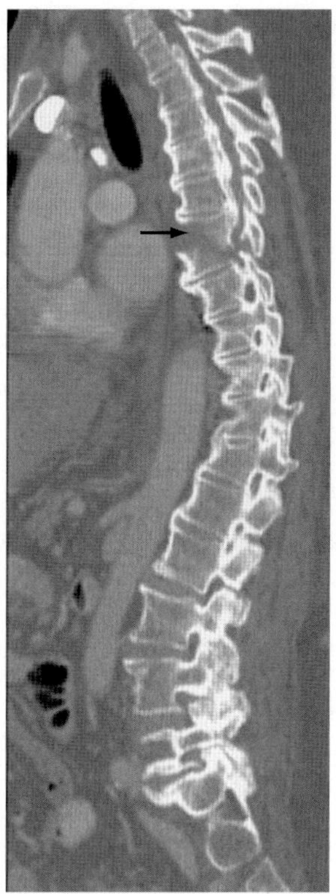

FIGURE 23-11. Acute fracture of an ankylosed spine. Sagittal reformatted CT image of the thoracolumbar spine in a patient with long-standing AS shows an acute fracture at T7 *(arrow)* following a fall.

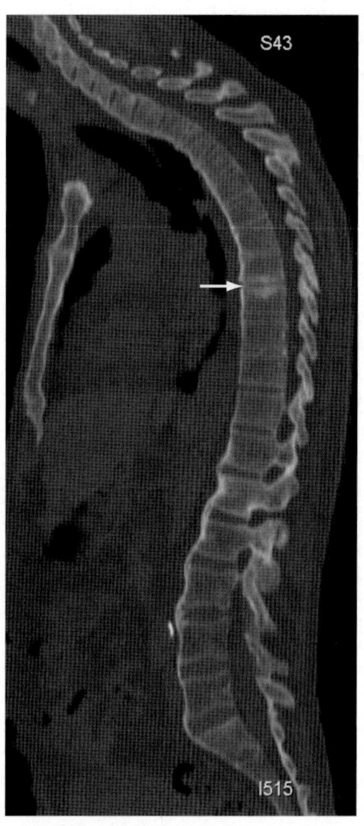

FIGURE 23-12. AS with spondylodiscitis. Sagittal reformatted CT image of the thoracolumbar spine in a patient with long-standing AS demonstrates sclerosis on either side of the disk consistent with spondylodiscitis (Andersson lesion) at T7-8 *(arrow)*.

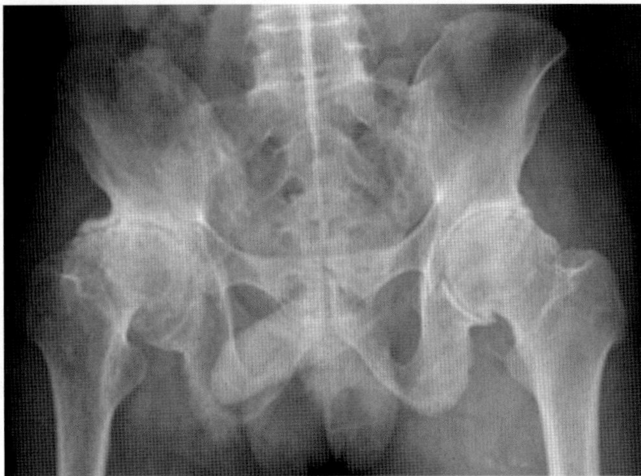

FIGURE 23-13. Hip involvement in AS. There is ankylosis of the SI joints and fusion of the spinous processes. Bilateral hip disease is present with concentric joint space narrowing on the left and prominent femoral osteophytes. The combination of diffuse cartilage loss (such as is seen in RA) and osteophytes is typical of AS. The superior cartilage loss on the right (with very large osteophytes) is more typical of osteoarthritis.

similar to that seen in RA. Other features that may be present include osteopenia and concentric joint space loss.

When the knees are affected, the disease tends to be bilateral and symmetric with features similar to those in the hip and shoulder (i.e., osteopenia, effusions, and subchondral cysts, with visible erosions and joint space narrowing later in the process). Enthesitis at the patellar margins is another feature that may accompany the articular alterations.

Reactive Arthritis and Spondyloarthropathy

Reactive arthritis represents an episode of aseptic peripheral arthritis that develops within 1 month of a primary infection elsewhere in the body, most commonly from genitourinary or enteric infections.[90,91] Less commonly, respiratory tract infections may also cause reactive arthritis, but evidence for this is inconclusive.[92]

The arthritis is typically acute in onset, asymmetric, and oligoarticular and may be associated with a variety of extraarticular features (e.g., conjunctivitis, iritis, urethritis, lesions of the skin and mucous membranes). The arthritis typically lasts for 4 to 5 months but may persist for much longer, and recurrent attacks are not unusual. At presentation, the knee and ankle are the most commonly affected joints, and heel pain is often a prominent feature, with tenderness in the region of the pre-Achilles' bursa and along the plantar aspect of the calcaneus at the insertion of the plantar fascia.

Reiter's syndrome consists of the triad of arthritis, urethritis, and conjunctivitis, but most patients with reactive arthritis do not present with this classic triad. Between 15% and 30% of these patients develop sacroiliitis or spondylitis, and the majority of these individuals have either a family history of spondyloarthropathy or are HLA-B27 positive.[93]

Sacroiliitis and syndesmophyte formation are more common in patients with previous genitourinary-related arthritis than in those with previous enteric-related arthritis, but the radiographic features of the inflammation are similar in both groups of patients.[94]

> The term *syndesmophyte* classically describes the bony bridging in the spine in AS but has been used more generally to describe the bridging in any of the spondyloarthropathies.

The inflammatory arthropathy that occurs in the appendicular skeleton may produce a variety of radiographic features. Soft tissue swelling is an early feature and may be associated with joint effusions and an inflammatory enthesopathy, most commonly seen in the ankle and hindfoot; in addition, dactylitis is a well-described characteristic that may occur in the digits of the hands and feet. In the synovial joints, erosions may be observed initially at the joint margins but can progress to involve more extensive portions of the articular surface. The marginal erosions are often distinguishable from those occurring in RA because they tend to be fuzzy due to associated bony proliferation that is characteristic of the seronegative arthropathies. Subchondral sclerosis and bony ankylosis are additional findings that are typical of the seronegative arthropathies but are rare in RA.

Patients with HIV may also develop findings suggesting a reactive arthritis or undifferentiated spondyloarthropathy; however, with the advent of effective antiviral medication, these conditions now appear to be less common in developed countries but have shown a dramatic increase in numbers in Africa.[38,95]

Psoriatic Spondyloarthropathy

Patients with psoriasis who have peripheral arthritis are also at increased risk to develop inflammatory disease of the spine, although the reported incidence of spondylitis is quite variable. Two separate studies showed sacroiliitis in 25% of such patients,[96,97] yet a third series documented spondylitis in 78% of 221 patients.[98]

In these individuals, the spinal disease may be indistinguishable from AS; however, McEwen et al.[99] described features that occur more often in association with psoriatic spondylitis. These include unilateral or asymmetric sacroiliitis, asymmetric syndesmophytes, nonmarginal syndesmophytes that do not develop along consecutive vertebrae (Figure 23-14), paravertebral ossification that may become large and bulky, and more frequent involvement of the cervical spine.

> Psoriatic spondylitis may exhibit bulky, asymmetric bony bridging that develops from the centers of the vertebral bodies ("nonmarginal").

The bulky nonmarginal syndesmophytes that do occur typically develop at the site of previous erosions along the surface of the vertebrae.

The mechanism whereby bulky syndesmophytes develop in the cervical spine of patients with psoriatic spondylitis appears related to persistent motion of the zygapophyseal joints. Involvement of the apophyseal joints occurs much less frequently than it does in AS, and de Vlam et al.[100] have shown that classic marginal syndesmophytes develop at levels where zygapophyseal fusion had occurred, but more massive, nonmarginal syndesmophytes develop where posterior fusion is not present.

Similar to observations about the role of MRI in AS, Williamson et al.[101] studied 103 patients with psoriatic arthritis and found that MRI commonly identified sacroiliitis that was difficult to detect clinically and best correlated with the duration of disease.

Other features that typify psoriatic spondylitis are atlantoaxial subluxation that is often accompanied by erosions of the odontoid, ligamentous calcification, and ankylosis of the apophyseal joints.[102,103] Of additional interest is work suggesting that peripheral arthritis is frequently more severe in patients who have spondylitis associated with their appendicular disease.[104]

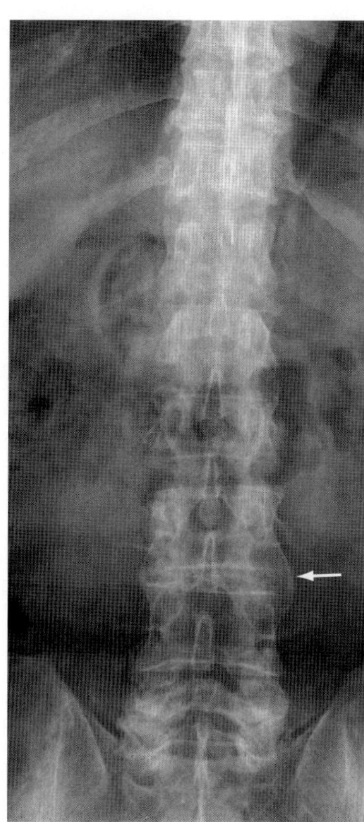

FIGURE 23-14. Psoriatic spondylitis. Bulky, asymmetric nonmarginal ossification (on the left at L3-4, *arrow*) is typical of psoriatic spondylitis. The SI joints are fused.

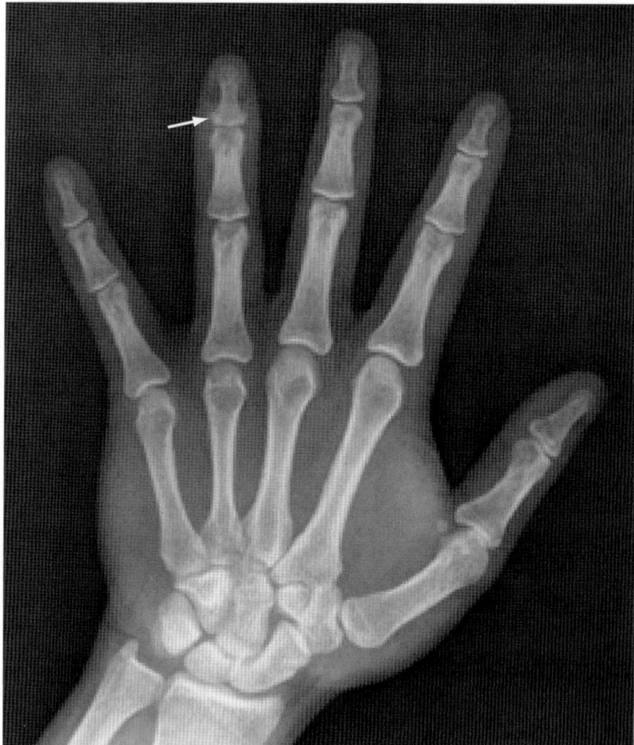

FIGURE 23-15. Psoriatic arthritis. There is soft tissue swelling about the distal interphalangeal joint of the ring finger with indistinct marginal erosions *(arrow)* and associated bony proliferation.

Psoriatic arthritis affects the hands almost twice as frequently as the feet. Moll and Wright[105,106] described several features of peripheral psoriatic arthritis that are typical and serve to distinguish it from RA. Osteoporosis is generally absent in psoriatic arthritis until the disease is advanced, and the presence of polyarthritis is often associated with involvement of the distal interphalangeal joints. Asymmetric oligoarticular involvement is another common pattern of disease that may also affect the wrist, although isolated wrist disease is infrequently seen in the absence of disease in the interphalangeal and metacarpophalangeal joints. A severe, deforming pattern of disease may also occur with bony ankylosis and malalignment that may ultimately progress to an arthritis mutilans.

An "opera glass" *(main en lorgnette)* deformity may result from extensive juxtaarticular bone loss with redundant soft tissues.

In contrast to RA, dactylitis is also a well-recognized manifestation of psoriatic arthritis.

The swollen "sausage digit" is a characteristic finding of psoriatic arthritis.

Like RA, the erosions occur at the joint margins, but in psoriatic arthritis these erosions become ill-defined due to associated bony proliferation (Figure 23-15). This bony proliferation may be identified at the joint margins, as well as along the shafts of the small bones of the hands and feet.

Bony proliferation occurs adjacent to the erosions of psoriatic arthritis.

In the feet, the interphalangeal and metatarsophalangeal joints are most frequently affected, particularly in the great toe. Of interest, an "ivory phalanx" has been described as an uncommon but fairly specific finding; the osteosclerosis is related to endosteal and periosteal bone formation that occurs in the great toe of patients with psoriatic arthritis.[107]

An "ivory phalanx" refers to the sclerotic appearance of the phalanges of the great toes and is seen in psoriatic arthritis and Reiter's syndrome.

Inflammatory enthesopathy, indistinguishable from that occurring in reactive arthritis and classically affecting the hindfoot and ankle, is another characteristic feature of psoriatic arthritis.

Enteropathic Spondyloarthropathy

Enteropathic spondyloarthropathy refers to the occurrence of spondyloarthritis in patients with either ulcerative colitis or Crohn's disease. In addition, peripheral arthritis occurs more commonly in patients with enteropathic arthritis than in patients with primary AS and reportedly develops in 50% to 70% of these patients.

Previous studies have shown that approximately 25% of patients with enteropathic arthritis also have sacroiliitis that may or may not be associated with spondylitis and that the activity of the spinal inflammation generally appears independent of the bowel disease activity (Figure 23-16).[108]

Spine involvement in enteropathic arthropathy is not related to the activity of the bowel disease, whereas the activity of peripheral joint involvement may be.

The clinical and radiographic features of the spondyloarthropathy in these patients are virtually indistinguishable from those of AS.

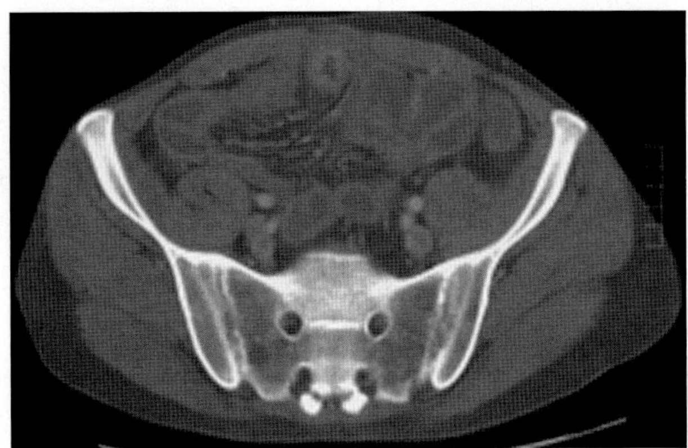

FIGURE 23-16. Enteropathic sacroiliitis. Axial CT of the abdomen shows fused SI joints and distended small bowel loops related to partial bowel obstruction in a patient with Crohn's disease and spondylitis.

The peripheral arthritis in patients with enteropathic spondyloarthropathy tends to be monoarticular or oligoarticular and more commonly involves the lower extremities, most often the knee. Nonspecific features of joint inflammation are usually present, consisting of soft tissue swelling and joint effusions. The arthritis is usually self-limited but may be migratory.

Undifferentiated Spondyloarthropathy

Undifferentiated spondyloarthropathy is a term reserved for patients who manifest features of a spondyloarthropathy but do not fulfill criteria for the other well-defined spondyloarthropathies. According to Zeidler et al.,[109] this terminology represents a provisional diagnosis for distinguishing such patients from those who have other rheumatic inflammatory diseases. These authors conclude that a small percentage of these individuals will subsequently develop a well-defined spondyloarthropathy, others will never develop a well-defined spondyloarthropathy, some represent overlap syndromes, and some may represent entities to be defined in the future.

Dubost and Sauvezie[110] were the first to draw attention to late-onset undifferentiated spondyloarthropathy in 10 male patients over the age of 50 who were HLA-B27 positive and presented with an oligoarthritis and inflammatory pitting edema of the lower extremities but only mild axial skeletal findings. Other reports have cautioned about the potential for confusing the spinal findings of late-onset spondyloarthropathy with diffuse idiopathic skeletal hyperostosis (DISH).[111,112]

SAPHO Syndrome

In adults, the most common site of disease in this syndrome is the upper anterior chest wall, affecting 70% to 90% of patients.

> Sclerosis and arthritis of the sternoclavicular, manubriosternal, and/or costosternal joints is typical of SAPHO syndrome.

The typical findings that occur consist of osteosclerotic lesions, hyperostosis, and arthritis of the sternoclavicular, manubriosternal and costosternal articulations (Figure 23-17).[113,114]

The next most frequently involved site is the spine, affecting approximately one third of patients, occurring most commonly in the dorsal spine and least commonly in the cervical spine.[115] In the spine, abnormalities consist of spondylodiscitis, diffuse vertebral hyperostosis, syndesmophyte formation, paravertebral ligamentous ossification, and sacroiliitis that is most frequently unilateral.

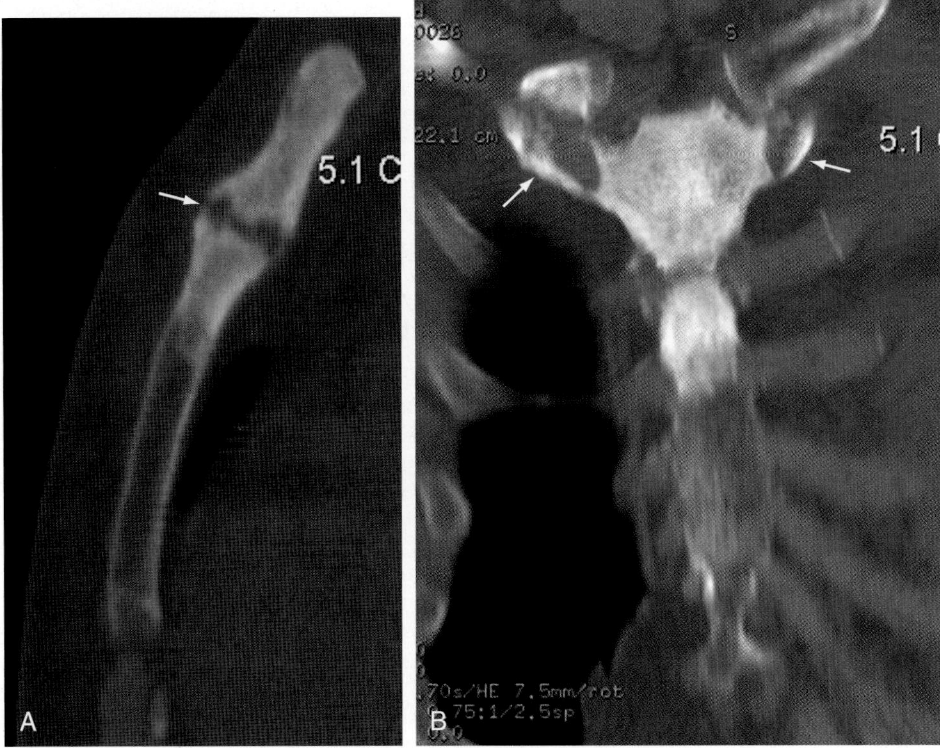

FIGURE 23-17. SAPHO syndrome. **A,** Sagittal reformatted CT of the sternum in SAPHO syndrome. There is dense sclerosis of the manubrium and upper body of the sternum with erosion of the manubriosternal joint *(arrow)*. **B,** Coronal reformatted CT of the same patient showing the bony sclerosis and ossification of the costoclavicular ligaments *(arrows)*.

Radiographically, these imaging features can simulate the presence of infection or neoplasm. MRI shows abnormal areas of marrow signal in the vertebral bodies and posterior elements that may be focal or diffuse, as well as abnormal signal in the intervertebral disks and paravertebral soft tissues.[116,117] Toussirot et al[53] observed that MRI identified vertebral body signal alterations that had no corresponding radiographic abnormality, concluding that MRI was more useful in defining the extent of the inflammatory process in patients with SAPHO, as well as in being able to distinguish active from inactive disease.

Osteosclerotic and osteolytic changes with periostitis may also develop in the long bones, along with a nondestructive peripheral arthritis. In the appendicular skeleton, the radiographic features include periostitis, cortical thickening, and endosteal new bone with resultant narrowing of the medullary canal.[118] Inflammatory enthesopathy is also a described feature of this entity.[52]

In contrast to adults, the long bones are the most common sites of disease in children, followed by the clavicle and the spine.[43]

EXTRAARTICULAR FEATURES AND IMAGING

The seronegative spondyloarthropathies are associated with a wide spectrum of extraarticular clinical manifestations, although imaging plays a relatively small role in the diagnosis of these features. Organ systems that may be involved include the skin, gastrointestinal tract, eye, heart, lung, kidney, and GI tract.[119]

Ankylosing Spondylitis

An association between AS and IBD is well documented, and the presence of occult mucosal inflammation in the bowel of patients with AS has been detected in more than 50% of AS patients.[120]

The most common extraarticular feature of AS is acute anterior uveitis, which may be the presenting symptom.[121] At presentation, the involvement is usually unilateral with the inflammation subsiding in a few weeks, but there is a tendency for recurrence, often in the contralateral eye.

Cardiac involvement is not uncommon and most frequently consists of aortic root inflammation that can lead to aortic incompetence.[122] Extension of the inflammation into the conduction system may result in partial or complete heart block.

Apical pulmonary fibrosis with bullous changes has been reported as an uncommon and usually late complication of AS (Figure 23-18), but high-resolution CT suggests that this process may be underrecognized with conventional radiography.[123]

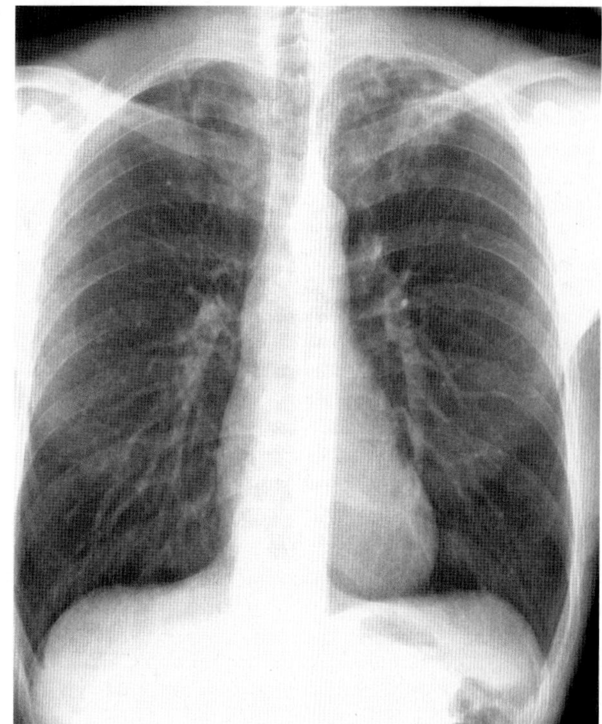

FIGURE 23-18. Pulmonary changes in AS. Fibrotic changes are present in the apices of both lungs in a patient with long-standing AS. The differential diagnosis for this appearance includes tuberculosis but was excluded in this patient.

Apical pulmonary fibrosis may be a late complication of AS.

Renal disease can occur in AS, usually presenting with proteinuria and microscopic hematuria. Amyloidosis may underlie these findings, although this is less frequently seen than in the past due to use of effective antiinflammatory therapies.[124] Immunoglobulin (Ig) A nephropathy has also been reported in patients with AS.[125]

Reactive Arthritis and Spondyloarthropathy

Keratodermia blennorrhagicum, also referred to as *pustulosis palmoplantaris,* is clinically and histologically indistinguishable from pustular psoriasis but is typically confined to the palms and soles and is usually associated with other characteristic features of reactive arthritis such as urethritis and conjunctivitis. Circinate balanitis produces a serpiginous inflammatory lesion of the glans penis and is another feature classically associated with reactive arthritis. A variety of oral lesions have also been described, ranging from painless shiny patches on the tongue, palate, and mucosa to oral ulcerations.

Using ileocolonoscopy, Mielants et al.[126] identified lesions similar to ulcerative colitis or Crohn's disease in patients with an established diagnosis of reactive arthritis.

Inflammatory ocular lesions are classic clinical features of reactive arthritis and may occur in one or both eyes. Conjunctivitis and acute anterior uveitis are the most common abnormalities and may be the initial clinical presentation.

Cardiac involvement is usually not a significant feature of reactive arthritis, although conduction abnormalities have been described.[127]

Pulmonary and renal involvement are not prominent features of reactive arthritis.

Psoriatic Spondyloarthropathy

The papulosquamous lesions of psoriasis are sharply demarcated inflammatory plaques with a silvery scale, most frequently occurring over the extensor surfaces of the knees and elbows, but also commonly seen on the ears, in the scalp, over the presacral area, and on the palms and soles. If large numbers of neutrophils are in the plaques, they may appear as pustular psoriasis. Nail abnormalities, such as pitting and onycholysis, are also common.

Ocular inflammation, including conjunctivitis and iritis, is a recognized feature of psoriatic arthritis.

Oral ulcers, aortic valve incompetence, and urethritis have been observed but are uncommon with psoriatic disease compared with the other seronegative spondyloarthropathies.

Enteropathic Spondyloarthropathy

Erythema nodosum may be present in up to 25% of these patients, is most commonly seen in association with active peripheral arthritis, and tends to parallel the activity of the bowel inflammation. Pyoderma gangrenosum has also been described in association with IBD but occurs less frequently than erythema nodosum.

The frequency of AS associated with IBD is variable, with reports as high as 25% in ulcerative colitis and ranging from 2% to 7% with Crohn's disease.[128] In these patients, the imaging features in the spine and SI joints are indistinguishable from those classically seen in AS.

The most common ocular disease associated with IBD is acute anterior uveitis, which is typically unilateral and short lived at presentation but frequently recurs.

Aortic incompetence has been described in association with IBD, similar to that found in patients with classic AS.

Nephrolithiasis, particularly oxalate stones, are a recognized complication of Crohn's disease.

> Calcium oxalate stones are opaque on radiographs or noncontrast CT.

Amyloidosis has been described, primarily with Crohn's disease and, when it develops, is ultimately fatal in most cases.

SAPHO Syndrome

A variety of cutaneous lesions have been described with this syndrome. Palmoplantar pustulosis is the most common skin disease associated with SAPHO and produces sterile pustules on the palms of the hands and on the soles of the feet. Severe forms of acne have also been described, consisting of acne conglobata, hidradenitis suppurativa, and acne fulminans. Palmoplantar pustulosis is reported in over 50% of patients with SAPHO, whereas acne is present in less than 20% of cases.[129] Pustular psoriasis, which may be difficult to distinguish from palmoplantar pustulosis, has also been described in association with SAPHO syndrome.

ALGORITHMS AND RECOMMENDATIONS

One of the critical issues in dealing with the seronegative spondyloarthropathies has been defining the various disease processes encompassed by this designation; this, in turn, has lead to the development of a variety of diagnostic criteria. AS represents the prototype spondyloarthropathy, and an historical review of the various classification systems for AS shows the evolution of the criteria and emphasizes the central role that diagnostic imaging plays in these systems.

In 1961 the Rome criteria were formulated and allowed the diagnosis of AS to be made if radiographic evidence of sacroiliitis was present in association with one or more of five clinical criteria, *or* if four out of the five clinical criteria were present. In 1966 the New York criteria were formulated as a modification of the Rome criteria, deleting two of the previous five clinical criteria (i.e., thoracic pain and stiffness, history of iritis or its sequelae) and requiring radiographic evidence of grade 3-4 sacroiliitis with one or more clinical criteria *or* grade 3-4 unilateral sacroiliitis *or* grade 2 bilateral sacroiliitis with various combinations of the three clinical criteria (i.e., limitation of spinal motion, pain in the dorsolumbar or lumbar spine, limited chest expansion). In 1984 the modified New York criteria were proposed to incorporate more specific features of inflammatory back pain with the previously stated imaging criteria for sacroiliitis and created a grading system for definite and probable disease; these criteria remain today as the most widely used for the clinical diagnosis of AS.[130] Note that the modified New York criteria, which are diagnostic criteria, should be distinguished from the ESSG criteria mentioned previously, which are an epidemiologic tool for population surveys and allow patients to be classified as having a spondyloarthropathy, even though they may not have a specific diagnosis.

> The criteria for the diagnosis of spondyloarthropathy include radiographic criteria and do not use advanced imaging modalities.

Even with careful implementation of the modified New York criteria and the ESSG criteria, reports have shown there may be delays of up to 9 years in making the diagnosis of an inflammatory spondyloarthropathy.[131,132] In the past, because of the lack of effective therapeutic measures, adverse outcome attached to this delay was limited. More recently, however, with the advent of effective treatments such as the tumor necrosis factor (TNF) blockers (e.g., etanercept, infliximab),[133,134] the early, reliable diagnosis of AS has become an important and relevant issue because of convincing evidence that these agents produce a prompt and dramatic reversal of most features of AS. In this regard, MRI is useful in detecting articular inflammation, as well as following resolution of juxtaarticular bone marrow edema after treatment with TNF inhibitors.[135,136] In addition, Lee et al.[137] studied 19 patients with AS to determine the correlation between MRI and laboratory markers of disease activity and found that synovial enhancement with gadolinium did correlate with laboratory inflammatory markers (i.e., ESR) of AS.

The success of anti-TNF agents has also given rise to requests for identifying and following inflammation of the entire spine, as well as the SI joints. A recent review comparing MRI and conventional radiography has shown that syndesmophytes are best appreciated with radiography, ankylosis is equally defined by radiography and MRI, and all other features of AS (e.g., erosions, diskitis, enthesitis) are better delineated with MRI.[138]

Rudwaleit et al.[139] have proposed an algorithm for the diagnosis of spondyloarthropathies that includes early diagnosis in patients with chronic low back pain who do not have radiographic evidence of sacroiliitis. Although the overlapping features of these entities may interfere with distinguishing the various spondyloarthropathies, particularly in the early stages of disease, this factor does not usually affect treatment.[140] Thus current concepts suggest that patients with seronegative spondyloarthropathies represent a spectrum of the same disease, and the imaging findings in any given individual are an indicator of disease severity and duration rather than of different disease entities.

The initial step in the algorithm is to decide if the patient has inflammatory back pain[11] (i.e., lumbar, thoracic or cervical pain with at least four of the following five features: onset before age 45; insidious onset; improved by exercise; associated with morning stiffness; and, duration of at least 3 months). In patients who do not have features of inflammatory back pain, less than a 2% probability exists that they have a spondyloarthropathy.

For patients with evidence of inflammatory back pain, there is a 14% probability that they have an inflammatory spondyloarthropathy and the next step is to obtain radiographs of the SI joints and spine, as well as assessment of other clinical and laboratory features of spondyloarthropathy: enthesitis, dactylitis, uveitis, positive family history, IBD, alternating buttock pain, psoriasis, asymmetric arthritis, positive response to NSAIDs, and the presence of acute phase reactants (i.e., ESR, CRP). If the radiographs are positive, a diagnosis of AS is confirmed. If the radiographs are negative, but three of the stated features are present, a diagnosis of axial spondyloarthropathy can be made with 80% to 95% probability.

If one or two of these features are present, there is a diagnostic probability of 35% to 70%, and if none of the features are present, the probability is 14%. For these patients, determination of the HLA-B27 status is indicated at this juncture: if positive in patients with one or two features of spondyloarthropathy, the diagnostic probability is 80% to 90%; if negative, the probability is < 10% and alternate diagnoses should be entertained.

In individuals with chronic low back pain who prove to be HLA-B27 positive but who have no clinical or laboratory features of spondyloarthropathy, MRI is key to distinguishing those patients with inflammatory spondyloarthropathy from those with other disease. When MRI is positive in these patients, there is an 80% to 95% probability that they have an inflammatory spondyloarthropathy, whereas a negative MRI correlates with < 15% probability of inflammatory spondyloarthropathy.

SUMMARY

In summary, the seronegative spondyloarthropathies are a group of related chronic inflammatory diseases that show strong evidence of a common genetic predisposition, which is likely triggered by various infectious agents. Each of these diseases shows variable expression of specific musculoskeletal features, including axial skeletal disease, enthesitis, and peripheral arthritis, as well as inflammatory processes affecting the eye, skin, and bowel. For many years, diagnostic imaging has played an important role in documenting the presence and extent of disease in patients with these spondyloarthropathies. The advent of newer therapeutic agents that are effective in the treatment of early disease has also made imaging modalities such as MRI important for early diagnosis, as well as for following the response of these diseases to modern treatment modalities.

REFERENCES

1. Nash P, Mease PJ, Braun J et al: Seronegative spondyloarthropathies: to lump or split? *Ann Rheum Dis* 64(Suppl II): ii9-ii13, 2005.
2. von Bechterew WL: Steifigkeit der Wirbelsaule und ihre Verkrummung als besondere Erkrankungsform, *Neurol Centralbl* 12:426-434, 1893.
3. Strumpell A: Bemerkungen uber die chronisch-ankylosierende Entzundung der Wirbelsoule und der Huftergelenke, *Dtsch Nervenheilk* 11:338-342, 1897.
4. Marie P: Sur la spondylose rhizomelique, *Rev Medecine* 18:285-315, 1898.
5. Andersson O: Rontgenbilden vid spondylarthritis ankylopoetica, *Nord Med Tidskr* 14:2000, 1937.
6. Romanus R, Yden S: Destructive and ossifying spondylitic changes in rheumatoid ankylosing spondylitis (pelvospondylitis ossificans), *Acta Orthop Scand* 22:88-99, 1952.
7. Forestier J, Jacqueline F, Rotes-Querol J (eds): *Ankylosing spondylitis: clinical considerations, roentgenology, pathologic anatomy, treatment*, Springfield, Ill, 1956, Charles C. Thomas.
8. Graham W: Is rheumatoid arthritis a separate entity? *Arthritis Rheum* 3:88-90, 1960.
9. Moll JM, Haslock I, Macrae IF: Associations between ankylosing spondylitis, psoriatic arthritis, Reiter's disease, the intestinal arthropathies and Behcet's syndrome, *Medicine* 53:343-364, 1974.
10. Amor B, Dougados M, Jijijawa M: Criteres de classification des spondylarthropathies, *Rev Rhum* 57:85-89, 1990.
11. Dougados M, van der Linden S, Juhlin R et al: The European spondylarthroapthy study group. Preliminary criteria for the classification of spondylarthropathies, *Arthritis Rheum* 34:1218-1227, 1991.
12. Martin TM, Smith JR, Rosenbaum JT: Anterior uveitis: current concepts of pathogenesis and interactions with spondylarthropathies, *Curr Opin Rheumatol* 14:337-341, 2002.
13. Bergfeldt L: HLA-B27-associated cardiac disease, *Ann Intern Med* 127:621-629, 1997.
14. Braun J, Bollow M, Remlinger G et al: Prevalence of spondylarthropathies in HLA-B27 positive and negative blood donors, *Arthritis Rheum* 41:58-67, 1998.
15. Dausset J, Nenna A: Presence of leuko-agglutinin in the serum of a case of chronic agranulocytosis, *Comptes Rendus Seances Soc Biologie Filiales* 146:1539-1541, 1952.
16. van Rood JJ, Eernisse JG, van Leeuwen A: Leukocyte antibodies in sera of pregnant women. *Nature* 181:1735-1736, 1958.
17. Reveille JD, Arnett FC: Spondyloarthritis: update on pathogenesis and management, *Am J Med* 118:592-603, 2005.
18. Brown MA, Wordsworth BP, Reveille JD: Genetics of ankylosing spondylitis, *Clin Exp Rheumatol* 20:S43-S49, 2002.
19. Ekman P, Kirveskari J, Granfors K: Modification of disease outcome in Salmonella-infected patients by HLA-B27, *Arthritis Rheum* 43:1527-1534, 2000.
20. Arnett FC: Seronegative spondyloarthropathies. In Dale DC, Federman DD (eds): *ACP Medicine, 2004-2005.* New York, 2004, Web MD, pp 1350-1361.
21. Brown MA, Laval SH, Brophy S et al: Recurrence risk modeling of the genetic susceptibility to ankylosing spondylitis, *Ann Rheum Dis* 59:883-886, 2000.
22. Brown MA, Kennedy LG, MacGregor AJ et al: Susceptibility to ankylosing spondylitis in twins: the role of genes, HLA, and the environment, *Arthritis Rheum* 4:1823-1828, 1997.
23. Van der Linden SM, Valkenburg HA, de Jongh BM et al: The risk of developing ankylosing spondylitis in HLA-B27 positive individuals. A comparison of relatives of spondylitis patients with the general population, *Arthritis Rheum* 27:241-249, 1984.
24. Reiter H: Uber eine bisher unerkannte Spirochateninfektion (Spirochaetosis arthritica), *Dtsch Med Wochenschr* 42:1535-1536, 1916.
25. Bauer W, Engleman EP: A syndrome of unknown etiology characterized by urethritis, conjunctivitis and arthritis (so-called Reiter's disease), *Trans Assoc Am Physicians* 57:307-313, 1942.
26. Paronen I: Reiter's disease. A study of 344 cases observed in Finland, *Acta Med Scand* 131:1-114, 1948.
27. Ahvonen P, Sievers K, Aho K: Arthritis associated with *Yersinia enterocolitica* infection, *Acta Rheumatol Scand* 15:232-253, 1969.
28. Granfors K, Marker-Hermann E, De Keyser P et al: The cutting edge of spondyloarthropathy research in the millennium, *Arthritis Rheum* 46:606-613, 2002.
29. Gerard HC, Branigan PJ, Schumacher HR Jr et al: Synovial chlamydia trachomatis in patients with reactive arthritis/Reiter's syndrome are viable but show aberrant gene expression, *J Rheumatol* 25:734-742, 1998.
30. Nikkari S, Rantakokko K, Ekman P et al: Salmonella-triggered reactive arthritis: use of polymerase chain reaction, immunocytochemical staining and gas chromatography-mass spectrometry in the detection of bacterial components from synovial fluid, *Arthritis Rheum* 42:84-89, 1999.
31. Ebringer RW, Cawdell DR, Cowling P et al: Sequential studies in ankylosing spondylitis. Association of *Klebsiella pneumoniae* with active disease, *Ann Rheum Dis* 37:146-151, 1978.
32. Stebbings S, Munro K, Simon MA et al: Comparison of the faecal microflora of patients with ankylosing spondylitis and controls using molecular methods of analysis, *Rheumatology* 41:1395-1401, 2002.
33. Mielants H, Veys EM, Joos R et al: HLA antigens in seronegative spondyloarthropathies. Reactive arthritis and arthritis in ankylosing spondylitis: relation to gut inflammation, *J Rheumatol* 14:466-471, 1987.
34. Leirisalo-Repo M, Turunen U, Stenman S et al: High frequency of silent inflammatory bowel disease in spondyloarthropathy, *Arthritis Rheum* 37:23-31, 1994.
35. de Vlam K, Mielants H, Cuvelier C et al: Spondyloarthropathy is underestimated in inflammatory bowel disease: prevalence and HLA association, *J Rheumatol* 27:2860-2865, 2000.
36. Prinz JC: Psoriasis vulgaris—a sterile antibacterial skin reaction mediated by cross-reactive T cells? An immunological view of the pathophysiology of psoriasis, *Clin Exp Dermatol* 26:326-332, 2001.
37. Winchester R, Bernstein DH, Fischer HD et al: The co-occurrence of Reiter's syndrome and acquired immunodeficiency, *Ann Intern Med* 106:19-26, 1987.
38. Solinger AM, Hess EV: Rheumatic diseases and AIDS—is the association real? *J Rheumatol* 20:678-683, 1994.
39. McGonagle D, Reade S, Marzo-Ortega H Gibbon W et al: Human immunodeficiency virus associated spondyloarthropathy: pathogenic insights based on imaging findings and response to highly active antiretroviral treatment, *Ann Rheum Dis* 60:696-698, 2001.
40. Chamot A, Benhamou Cl, Kahn MF et al: Le syndrome acne pustulose hyperostose osteite (SAPHO), *Rev Rhum* 43:187-196, 1987.
41. Hayem G, Bouchaud-Chabot A, Benali K et al: SAPHO syndrome: a long term follow up study of 120 cases, *Semin Arthritis Rheum* 293:159-171, 1999.
42. Earwaker JWS, Cotton A: SAPHO: syndrome or concept? Imaging findings, *Skeletal Radiol* 32:311-327, 2003.
43. Ongchi DR, Fleming MG, Harris CA: Sternocostoclavicular hyperostosis: two cases with differing dermatologic syndromes, *J Rheumatol* 17:1415-1418, 1990.
44. Prevo RL, Rasker JJ, Kruijsen MWM: Sternocostoclavicular hyperostosis or pustulotic arthroosteitis, *J Rheumatol* 16:1602-1605, 1989.
45. Gideon A, Holthusen W, Masel L: Subacute and chronic symmetrical osteomyelitis, *Ann Radiol* 15:329-342, 1972.
46. Bjorksten B, Gustavson KH, Eriksson B et al: Chronic recurrent multifocal osteomyelitis and pustulosis palmoplantaris, *J Pediatr* 932:227-231, 1978.
47. Windom RE, Sandford JP, Ziff M: Acne conglobata and arthritis, *Arthritis Rheum* 4:632-635, 1961.
48. Houben HH, Lemmens JA, Boerbooms AM: Sacroiliitis and acne conglobata, *Clin Rheumatol* 4:86-89, 1985.
49. Veale D, Rogers S, Fitzgerald O: Classification of clinical subsets in psoriatic arthritis, *Br J Rheumatol* 33:133-138, 1994.
50. Maugars Y, Berthelot JM, Ducloux JM et al: SAPHO syndrome: a followup study of 19 cases with special emphasis on enthesis involvement, *J Rheumatol* 22:135-141, 1995.

51. Toussirot E, Dupond JL, Wendling D: Spondylodiscitis in SAPHO syndrome. A series of eight cases, *Ann Rheum Dis* 56:52-58, 1997.
52. Kotilainen P, Gullichesen RE, Saario R et al: Aseptic spondylitis as the initial manifestation of the SAPHO syndrome, *Eur Spine J* 6:327-329, 1997.
53. Perez C, Hidalgo A, Olier J et al: MR imaging of multifocal spondylodiskitis as the initial manifestations of SAPHO syndrome, *AJR Am J Roentgenol* 171:1431-1432, 1998.
54. Crouzet J, Caudepierre P, Aribi EH et al: Two cases of discitis due to *Propionibacterium acnes*, *Rev Rhum* 65:68-71, 1998.
55. Kooijmans-Coutinho MF, Markusse HM, Dijkmans BAC: Infectious arthritis caused by *Propionibacterium acnes*: a report of two cases, *Ann Rheum Dis* 48:851-852, 1989.
56. Braun J, Sieper J: Inception cohorts for spondyloarthropathies, *Z Rheumatol* 59:117-121, 2000.
57. Feldtkeller E: Age at disease onset and delayed diagnosis of spondyloarthropathies, *Z Rheumatol* 58:21-30, 1999.
58. Olivieri I, Salvarani C, Cantini F et al: Ankylosing spondylitis and undifferentiated spondyloarthropathies: a clinical review and description of a disease subset with older age at onset, *Curr Opinion Rheum* 13:280-284, 2001.
59. Hill HF, Hill AG, Bodmer JG: Clinical diagnosis of ankylosing spondylitis in women and relation to presence of HLA-B27, *Ann Rheum Dis* 35:267-270, 1976.
60. Resnick D, Dwosh IL, Goergen TG et al: Clinical and radiographic abnormalities in ankylosing spondylitis: a comparison of men and women, *Radiology* 119:293-297, 1976.
61. Carette S, Graham D, Little H et al: The natural disease course of ankylosing spondylitis, *Arthritis Rheum* 26:186-190, 1983.
62. Van der Heijde D: Quantification of radiological damage in inflammatory arthritis: rheumatoid arthritis, psoriatic arthritis and ankylosing spondylitis, *Best Pract Res Clin Rheumatol* 18:847-860, 2004.
63. Resnick D: Ankylosing spondylitis. In Resnick D (ed): *Diagnosis of bone and joint disorders*, Philadelphia, 2002, Saunders, pp 1030-1033.
64. MacKay K, Mack C, Brophy S et al: The Bath Ankylosing Spondylitis Radiology Index (BASRI): a new, validated approach to disease assessment, *Arthritis Rheum* 41:2263-2270, 1998.
65. Averns HL, Oxtoby J, Taylor HG et al: Radiological outcome in ankylosing spondylitis: use of the Stoke Ankylosing Spondylitis Spine Score (SASSS), *Br J Rheumatol* 35:373-376, 1996.
66. Wanders AJB, Landewe RBM, Spoorenberg A et al: What is the most appropriate radiologic scoring method for ankylosing spondylitis? A comparison of the available methods based on the outcome measures in rheumatology clinical trials filter, *Arthritis Rheum* 50:2622-2632, 2004.
67. Spoorenberg A, de Vlam K, van der Linden S et al: Radiological scoring methods in ankylosing spondylitis. Reliability and change over 1 and 2 years, *J Rheumatol* 31:125-132, 2004.
68. Goei HS, Lemmens AJ, Goedhard G et al: Radiological and scintigraphic findings in patients with a clinical history of chronic inflammatory back pain, *Skeletal Radiol* 14:243-248, 1985.
69. Kozin F, Carrera GF, Ryan LM et al: Computed tomography in the diagnosis of sacroiliitis, *Arthritis Rheum* 24:1479-1485, 1981.
70. Fam AG, Rubenstein JD, Chin-Sang H et al: Computed tomography in the diagnosis of early ankylosing spondylitis, *Arthritis Rheum* 28:930-937, 1985.
71. McEniff N, Wustace S, McCarthy C et al: Asymptomatic sacroiliitis in inflammatory bowel disease. Assessment by computed tomography, *Clinical Imaging* 19:258-262, 1995.
72. Puhakka KB, Jurik AG, Egund N et al: Imaging of sacroiliitis in early seronegative spondylarthropathy. Assessment of abnormalities by MR in comparison with radiography and CT, *Acta Radiol* 44:218-229, 2003.
73. Puhakka KB, Jurik AG, Schiottz-Christensen B et al: Magnetic resonance imaging of sacroiliitis in early seronegative spondylarthropathy. Abnormalities correlated to clinical and laboratory findings, *Rheumatology* 43:234-237, 2004.
74. Yu W, Feng F, Dion E et al: Comparison of radiography, computed tomography and magnetic resonance imaging in the detection sacroiliitis accompanying ankylosing spondylitis, *Skeletal Radiol* 27:311-320, 1998.
75. Puhakka KB, Egund N, Melsen F et al: MR imaging of the normal sacroiliac joint with correlation to histology, *Skeletal Radiol* 33:15-28, 2003.
76. Muche B, Bollow M, François RJ et al: Anatomic structures involved in early- and late-stage sacroiliitis in spondylarthritis: A detailed analysis by contrast-enhanced magnetic resonance imaging, *Arthritis Rheum* 48:1374-1384, 2003.
77. Blum U, Buitrago-Tellez C, Mundinger A et al: Magnetic resonance imaging (MRI) for detection of active sacroiliitis—a prospective study comparing conventional radiography, scintigraphy and contrast enhanced MRI, *J Rheumatol* 23:2107-2115, 1996.
78. Braun J, Baraliakos X, Golder W et al: Magnetic resonance imaging examinations of the spine in patients with ankylosing spondylitis, before and after successful therapy with infliximab: evaluation of a new scoring system, *Arthritis Rheum* 48:1126-1136, 2003.
79. Baraliakos X, Hermann KG, Landewe R et al: Assessment of acute spinal inflammation in patients with ankylosing spondylitis by magnetic resonance imaging (MRI): a comparison between contrast enhanced T1 and short-tau inversion recovery (STIR) sequences, *Ann Rheum Dis* 64:1141-1144, 2005.
80. Puhakka KB, Jurik AG, Schiottz-Christensen B et al: MRI abnormalities of sacroiliac joints in early spondyarthropathy: a 1-year follow-up study, *Scand J Rheumatol* 33:332-338, 2004.
81. Rosenkranz W: Ankylosing spondylitis: cauda equine syndrome with multiple spinal arachnoid cysts. Case report, *J Neurosurg* 34:241-243, 1971.
82. Milde EJ, Aarli J, Larsen JL: Cauda equine lesions in ankylosing spondylitis, *Scand J Rheumatol* 6:118-122, 1977.
83. Braun J, Baraliakos X, Golder W et al: Analysing chronic spinal changes in ankylosing spondylitis: a systematic comparison of conventional x rays with magnetic resonance imaging using established and new scoring systems, *Ann Rheum* 63:1046-1055, 2005.
84. Mitra D, Elvins DM, Speden DJ et al: The prevalence of vertebral fractures in mild ankylosing spondylitis and their relationship to bone mineral density, *Rheumatology* 39:85:89, 2000.
85. Tico N, Ramon S, Garcia-Ortun F et al: Traumatic spinal cord injury complicating ankylosing spondylitis, *Spinal Cord* 36:349-352, 1998.
86. Shih TT, Chen PQ, Li YW et al: Spinal fractures and pseudoarthrosis complicating ankylosing spondylitis: MRI manifestation and clinical significance, *J Comput Assist Tomogr* 25:164-170, 2001.
87. Wu PC, Fang D, Ho EKW et al: The pathogenesis of extensive discovertebral destruction in ankylosing spondylitis, *Clin Orthop* 230:154-161, 1988.
88. Agarwal AK, Reidbord HE, Kraus DR et al: Variable histopathology of discovertebral lesion (spondylodiscitis) of ankylosing spondylitis, *Clin Exp Rheumatol* 8:67-69, 1990.
89. Rosen PS: A unique shoulder lesion in ankylosing spondylitis: clinical comment, *J Rheumatol* 7:109-110, 1980.
90. Hughes RA, Keat AC: Reiter's syndrome and reactive arthritis: a current view, *Semin Arthritis Rheum* 24:190-210, 1994.
91. Sieper J, Rudwaleit M, Braun J et al: Diagnosing reactive arthritis: role of clinical setting in the value of serologic and microbiologic assays, *Arthritis Rheum* 46:319-327, 2002.
92. Hannu T, Puolakkainen M, Leirisalo-Repo M: *Chlamydia pneumoniae* as a triggering infection in reactive arthritis, *Rheumatology* 38:411-414, 1999.
93. Keat A: Reactive arthritis, *Adv Exp Med Biol* 455:201-206, 1999.
94. Mannoja A, Pekkola J, Hamalainen M et al: Lumbosacral radiographic signs in patients with previous enteroarthritis or uroarthritis, *Ann Rheum Dis* 64:936-939, 2005.
95. Mody GM, Parke FA, Reveille JD: Articular manifestations of human immunodeficiency virus infection, *Best Pract Res Clin Rheumatol* 17:265-287, 2003.
96. Gladman DD, Shuckett R, Russell ML et al: Psoriatic arthritis (PsA)—an analysis of 220 patients, *Q J Med* 62:127-141, 1987.
97. Torre Alonso JC, Rodriguez Perez A, Arribas Castrillo JM et al: Psoriatic arthritis (PA): a clinical, immunological and radiological study, *Br J Rheumatol* 30:245-250, 1991.
98. Battistone MJ, Manaster BJ, Reda DJ et al: The prevalence of sacroiliitis in psoriatic arthritis: new perspectives from a large, multicenter cohort. A Department of Veterans Affairs Cooperative Study, *Skeletal Radiol* 28:196-201, 1999.
99. McEwen C, Di Tatu D, Lingg C et al: A comparative study of ankylosing spondylitis, and spondylitis accompanying ulcerative colitis, regional enteritis, psoriasis and Reiter's disease, *Arthritis Rheum* 14:291-318, 1971.
100. de Vlam K, Mielants H, Verstaete KL et al: The zygapophyseal joint determines morphology of the enthesophyte, *J Rheumatol* 27:1732-1739, 2000.
101. Williamson L, Dockerty JL, Dalbeth N et al: Clinical assessment of sacroiliitis and HLA-B27 are poor predictors of sacroiliitis diagnosed by magnetic resonance imaging in psoriatic arthritis, *Rheumatology* 43:85-88, 2004.
102. Salvarani C, Macchioni P, Cremonesi T et al: The cervical spine in patients with psoriatic arthritis: a clinical, radiological and immunogenetic study, *Ann Rheum Dis* 51:73-77, 1992.
103. Laiho K, Kauppi M. The cervical spine in patients with psoriatic arthritis, *Ann Rheum Dis* 61:650-652, 2002.
104. Taccari E, Spadaro A, Riccieri V: Correlations between peripheral and axial radiological changes in patients with psoriatic polyarthritis, *Rev Rhum* 63:17-23, 1996.
105. Moll JM, Wright V: Family occurrence of psoriatic arthritis. *Ann Rheum Dis* 32:181-201, 1973.
106. Moll JM, Wright V: Psoriatic arthritis, *Semin Arthritis Rheum* 3:55-78, 1973.
107. Resnick D, Broderick TW: Bony proliferation of terminal toe phalanges in psoriasis: the "ivory" phalanx, *J Can Assoc Radiol* 28:187-189, 1977.
108. Smale S, Natt RS, Orchard TR et al: Inflammatory bowel disease and spondyloarthropathy, *Arthritis Rheum* 44:2728-2736, 2001.
109. Zeidler H, Mau W, Khan MA: Undifferentiated spondyloarthropathies, *Rheum Dis Clin North Am* 18:187-202, 1992.
110. Dubost JJ, Sauvezie B: Late onset peripheral spondyloarthropathy, *J Rheumatol* 16:1214-1217, 1989.
111. Yagan R, Khan MA: Confusion of roentgenographic differential diagnosis of ankylosing hyperostosis (Forestier's disease) and ankylosing spondylitis. In Khan MA (ed): *Ankylosing spondylitis and related spondyloarthropathies. Spine: state of the art review*, Philadelphia, 1990, Hanley & Belfus, pp 561-575.
112. Olivieri I, Oranges GS, Sconosciuto F et al: Late onset peripheral seronegative spondyloarthropathy: report of two additional cases, *J Rheumatol* 20:390-393, 1993.
113. Boutin RD, Resnick D: The SAPHO syndrome: an evolving concept for unifying several idiopathic disorders of bone and skin, *AJR Am J Roentgenol* 170:585-591, 1998.
114. Cotton A, Flipo RM, Mentre A et al: SAPHO syndrome, *Radiographics* 15:1147-1154, 1995.
115. Tohme-Noun C, Feydy A, Belmatoug N et al: Cervical involvement in SAPHO syndrome: imaging findings with a 10-year follow-up, *Skeletal Radiol* 28:103-106, 1999.
116. Nachtigal A, Cardinal E, Bureau NJ et al: Vertebral involvement in SAPHO syndrome: MRI findings, *Skeletal Radiolo* 28:163-168, 1999.
117. Akisue T, Yamamoto T, Marui T et al: Lumbar spondylodiskitis in SAPHO syndrome: multimodality imaging findings, *J Rheumatol* 29:1100-1101, 2002.

118. Kahn MF, Khan MA: The SAPHO syndrome, *Baillieres Clin Rheumatol* 8:333-362, 1994.
119. Gladman D: Spondyloarthropathies. In Lahita R, Weinstein A (eds): *Educational review manual in rheumatology*, ed 2 (revised), New York, 2002, Castle Connolly Graduate Medical, 2002, pp 1-26.
120. De Keyser, Baeten D, Van Den Bosch F et al: Gut inflammation and spondyloarthropathies, *Curr Rheumatol Rep* 4:525-532, 2002.
121. Banares A, Hernandez-Garcia C, Fernandez-Gutierrez B et al: Eye involvement in the spondyloarthropathies, *Rheum Dis Clin North Am* 24:771-784, 1998.
122. Lautermann D, Braun J: Ankylosing spondylitis—cardiac manifestations, *Clin Exp Rheumatol* 20 (Suppl 28):S11-S15, 2002.
123. Turetschek K, Ebner W, Fleischmann D et al: Early pulmonary involvement in ankylosing spondylitis: assessment with thin-section CT, *Clin Radiol* 55:632-636, 2000.
124. Strobel ES, Fritschka E: Renal diseases in ankylosing spondylitis: review of the literature illustrated by case reports, *Clin Rheumatol* 17:524-530, 1998.
125. Lai KN, Li PKT, Hawkins B et al: IgA nephropathy associated with ankylosing spondylitis: occurrence in women as well as in men, *Ann Rheum Dis* 48:435-437, 1989.
126. Mielants H, Veys EM: The gut and reactive arthritis, *Rheumatol Eur* 24:9-11, 1995.
127. Lahesmaa-Rantala R, Toivanen A: Clinical spectrum of reactive arthritis. In Toivanen A, Toivanen P (eds): *Reactive arthritis*, Boca Raton, Fla, 1988, CRC Press, pp 1-13.
128. Gravallese EM, Kantrowitz FG. Arthritic manifestations of inflammatory bowel disease, *Am J Gastroenterol* 83:703-709, 1988.
129. Hayem G, Bouchaud-Chabot A, Benali K et al: SAPHO syndrome: a long term follow up study of 120 cases, *Semin Arthritis Rheum* 293:159-171, 1999.
130. Van der Linden SM, Valkenburg HA, Cats A: Evaluation of diagnostic criteria for ankylosing spondylitis. A proposal for modification of the New York criteria, *Arthritis Rheum* 27:361-368, 1984.
131. Braun J, Sieper J, Bollow M: Imaging of sacroiliitis, *Clin Rheumatol* 19:51-57, 2000.
132. Underwood MR, Dawes P: Inflammatory back pain in primary care, *Br J Rheumatol* 34:1074-1077, 1995.
133. Braun J, Sieper J, Breban M et al: Anti-tumour necrosis factor alpha therapy for ankylosing spondylitis: international experience, *Ann Rheum Dis* 61(Suppl III): iii51-iii60, 2002.
134. Gorman JD, Sack KE, David JC: Treatment of ankylosing spondylitis by inhibition of tumor necrosis factor alpha, *N Engl J Med* 346:1349-1356, 2002.
135. Rudwaleit M, Khan MA, Sieper J: The challenge of diagnosis and classification in early anykylosing spondylitis, *Arthritis Rheum* 52:1000-1008, 2005.
136. Baraliakos X, Davis J, Tsuji W et al: Magnetic resonance imaging examinations of the spine in patients with ankylosing spondylitis before and after therapy with the tumor necrosis factor alpha receptor fusion protein etanercept, *Arthritis Rheum* 52:1216-1223, 2005.
137. Lee W-H, McCauley TR, Lee S-H et al: Sacroiliitis in patients with ankylosing spondylitis: association of MR findings with disease activity, *Magn Res Imaging* 22:245-250, 2004.
138. Hermann K-G, Althoff CE, Schneider U et al: Spinal changes in patients with spondyloarthritis: comparison of MR imaging and radiographic appearances, *Radiographics* 25:559-570, 2005.
139. Rudwaleit M, van der Heijde D, Khan MA et al: How to diagnose axial spondylarthritis early, *Ann Rheum Dis* 63:535-543, 2004.
140. Khan MA: Update on spondyloarthropathies, *Ann Intern Med* 136:895-907, 2002.

CHAPTER 24

Imaging Investigation of Arthritis in Children

ANDREA SCHWARTZ DORIA, MD, PHD, MSC, *and* PAUL BABYN, MDCM

KEY FACTS

- Juvenile idiopathic arthritis (JIA) comprises arthritides of unknown etiology that begin before age 16 years and that persist for greater than 6 weeks.
- Ultrasonography is a very useful modality in children because of its ability to detect joint effusions and pannus and measure cartilage thickness, all without ionizing radiation.
- Magnetic resonance imaging (MRI) can document erosion not visible on radiographs and can determine the presence and activity (vascularity) of pannus.
- Complications of JIA include growth abnormalities, amyloidosis, uveitis (especially in patients with oligoarticular disease), and the macrophage activation syndrome.
- *Enthesitis-related arthritis* refers to arthritis accompanied by enthesitis (inflammation at the sites of attachment of ligaments or tendons to bone). Also included are those conditions with either arthritis or enthesitis plus two of the following: (1) sacroiliac joint tenderness and/or inflammatory spinal pain; (2) presence of HLA-B27; (3) family history of HLA-B27–positive disease; (4) acute anterior uveitis; or (5) onset of arthritis in a boy older than 8 years.
- The diagnosis of psoriatic arthritis in children includes children with arthritis and psoriasis or those with arthritis and at least two of the following: (1) dactylitis; (2) nail pitting or onycholysis; or (3) family history of psoriasis in a first-degree relative. Girls are most often affected.
- Arthritis occurs in about 10% of patients with inflammatory bowel disease. The sacroiliitis and spondylitis may progress despite control of the bowel disease. The peripheral joint disease activity mirrors the activity of the bowel disease.
- Suspicion of a septic joint generally requires aspiration. Radiographs are usually performed for initial evaluation. MRI is usually more sensitive than computed tomography or scintigraphy for the detection of changes suggesting septic arthritis.
- Transient synovitis of the hip is an acute, self-limited condition of unknown origin and is most commonly seen in boys between the ages of 3 and 6 years. It usually affects one joint but can be bilateral in up to 5% of cases. Ultrasound, rather than radiography, may be the method of choice for initial evaluation.
- Hemophilic arthropathy produces fairly specific findings on imaging studies. Low-signal synovitis is due to hemosiderin within the hypertrophied synovium and is a characteristic but not an entirely specific feature of the disease.

Imaging often plays a key role in establishing the presence of arthropathy, determining its extent, and defining the specific diagnosis. Previously, radiography was the principal method used to evaluate and follow bone damage in patients with inflammatory arthritis. More recently the use of magnetic resonance imaging (MRI) and ultrasonography have gained wider acceptance due to their multiplanar capabilities. Arthrography is not commonly used in imaging of arthritis in children because less invasive modalities are available that also have the ability to image both bone and soft tissue abnormalities.

Most synovial joints undergo significant osseous development and maturation in early childhood. In the newborn, extensive unossified epiphyseal cartilage limits radiographic joint assessment because the unossified cartilage cannot be distinguished from adjacent soft tissues. Epiphyseal cartilage transforms to bone with increasing age, narrowing the radiographic joint space to the thickness of the opposing layers of articular cartilage.

Normal articular soft tissue components have a similar radiographic density and cannot be clearly differentiated from each other or from adjacent muscles, fascia, tendons, ligaments, nerves, or vessels by radiography. However, displacement of fat deposits in fascial and intermuscular planes assists in the determination of joint effusions in the elbow, knee, and ankle.

This chapter discusses the imaging modalities that are currently available for evaluation of children with arthropathy, including ultrasonography and MRI, and presents the imaging features of common causes of acute and chronic arthritis.

INFLAMMATORY ARTHRITIS

Juvenile Idiopathic Arthritis

The term *juvenile idiopathic arthritis* (JIA) comprises arthritides of unknown etiology that begin before age 16 years and that persist for greater than 6 weeks.[1] Classification into subtypes (systemic, oligoarthritis, polyarthritis with negative and positive rheumatoid factors, psoriatic arthritis and enthesitis-related arthritis, other arthritis) within this overall term is based on the clinical characteristics of the disease rather than on any understanding of the underlying pathology.[2]

JIA is the most important rheumatic disease affecting children and one of the most common chronic diseases of childhood. Although JIA may be self-limited with a majority of patients having no active synovitis in adulthood, many children have significant joint complications.[3]

In JIA the synovium is the target tissue for inflammation. Early in the disease course the affected joints are clinically swollen, stiff, painful, and warm and show limited motion. There is synovial proliferation and infiltration by inflammatory cells including polymorphonuclear leukocytes, lymphocytes, and plasma cells and increased secretion of synovial fluid with development of synovial thickening and pannus formation. Inflammation of synovial coverings of tendons and bursa, which can also be affected, can lead to periostitis. With prolonged inflammation, destruction of cartilage, adjacent bone erosions, and even joint ankylosis may be seen.

Imaging

Osteoarticular Imaging Features

Imaging can be used to determine whether arthritis is indeed present, establish a specific diagnosis, and determine the extent of disease. It may also be used to determine disease activity, detect disease complications, evaluate disease progression, and judge efficacy of drug treatment.[4]

Radiography

Radiographs of symptomatic areas should be obtained at initial presentation to exclude other differential diagnoses and assist in the diagnosis of arthritis (Box 24-1). In early arthritis, radiography is often of limited utility, as the inflamed synovium, soft tissue changes, and cartilage erosions that precede bone erosions are not well seen.[5] Initial radiographs are often nonspecific, reflecting early response of the soft tissues and bones to inflammation with soft tissue swelling, osteopenia, joint effusions, and periosteal reaction (Figure 24-1). The osteopenia is initially periarticular, becoming more diffuse with time. Rarely one sees the band-like pattern observed in leukemia. Periosteal reaction is commonly seen in the phalanges, metacarpals (see Figure 24-1), and metatarsals but can also occur in the long bones.

BOX 24-1. Radiographic Features of JIA

ALIGNMENT
Atlantoaxial subluxation
Coxa valga

BONE DENSITY
Juxtaarticular osteoporosis
Diffuse osteoporosis (late)
Metaphyseal lucencies (rarely)
Periosteal reaction adjacent to affected small joints

CARTILAGE SPACES
Erosions (late), may appear corticated
Cartilage space narrowing (late)
Ankylosis (especially spine, wrists)

DISTRIBUTION
Monarticular, pauciarticular, or polyarticular

GROWTH ABNORMALITIES
Affected small bones are shorter than normal
Overgrowth (lengthening) of affected long bones
Advanced maturation of affected epiphyses
Large epiphyses
Micrognathia (may have mandibular notching)
Protrusio acetabuli
Fused cervical vertebrae
Angular carpals
Square patella
Intercondylar notch widening (also a feature of hemophilia)

SOFT TISSUES
Effusions and joint distension
Nodules
Periarticular calcification (probably due to corticosteroid injections)

Soft tissue nodules can be noted, as may periarticular calcification (see Figure 24-1), although this usually is a consequence of prior intraarticular corticosteroid injection therapy. Joint space narrowing and erosions (see Figure 24-1) are typically later radiographic findings seen 2 years or so after the disease onset. However, in rheumatoid factor–positive polyarthritis and in up to one third of patients with systemic arthritis, early erosive disease can occur. Abnormalities in growth and maturation may be present, leading to accelerated osseous growth, altered maturation, and enlarged epiphyses (see Figure 24-1).

Late sequelae of JIA are not uncommon and include epiphyseal deformity, abnormal angular carpal bones, widening of the intercondylar notch of knees, and premature fusion of the growth plate with brachydactyly (see Figure 24-1). Growth disturbances are more frequent if the onset of the disease is precocious. Other changes include large cyst-like well-corticated erosions, which may be lobulated. Joint space narrowing and osseous erosions are less frequent in JIA than in the adult-onset disease and are usually late manifestations.[6]

> Cartilage space narrowing and bone erosion are less frequent and are later findings in JIA than in adult rheumatoid arthritis (RA).

At the hip protrusio acetabuli (see Figure 24-1), premature degenerative changes, coxa magna, and coxa valga can be seen.[7] Joint space loss can progress to ankylosis particularly in the apophyseal joints of the cervical spine and in the wrist (see Figure 24-1). Subluxation of the joints especially at the wrist (see Figure 24-1) may be evident, and atlantoaxial subluxation may also occur. Growth disturbance of the temporomandibular joint may lead to micrognathia and abnormalities of the temporomandibular disk.

Radiographic Scales Available for Assessment of JIA

Despite the limited sensitivity of conventional radiography to early disease, it remains the standard practice technique used for assessment of responsiveness of therapy for JIA in many pediatric centers around the world. Most radiographic classification systems that are currently available to assess the degree of joint destruction in JIA are in fact targeted to changes of RA in adults.[8-12] Pettersson & Rydholm's[10] classification method for JIA is objective, is highly reproducible, and correlates well with the clinical status of the disease, but the authors evaluated only a small sample of children with JIA (n = 15) with this scoring system by the time the method was first described. Steinbrocker et al.[12] proposed a four-stage scoring system for evaluation of RA. This system has low sensitivity and reproducibility in part because of the vague description of the changes that qualify for each stage. Although no correlations have been found between hand radiographic findings, which were thought to have prognostic implications,[13-15] and patient functional disability using this system,[16] this scoring system is the oldest and simplest method described. The methods that are most widely used for assessment of rheumatoid arthritis are the Larsen

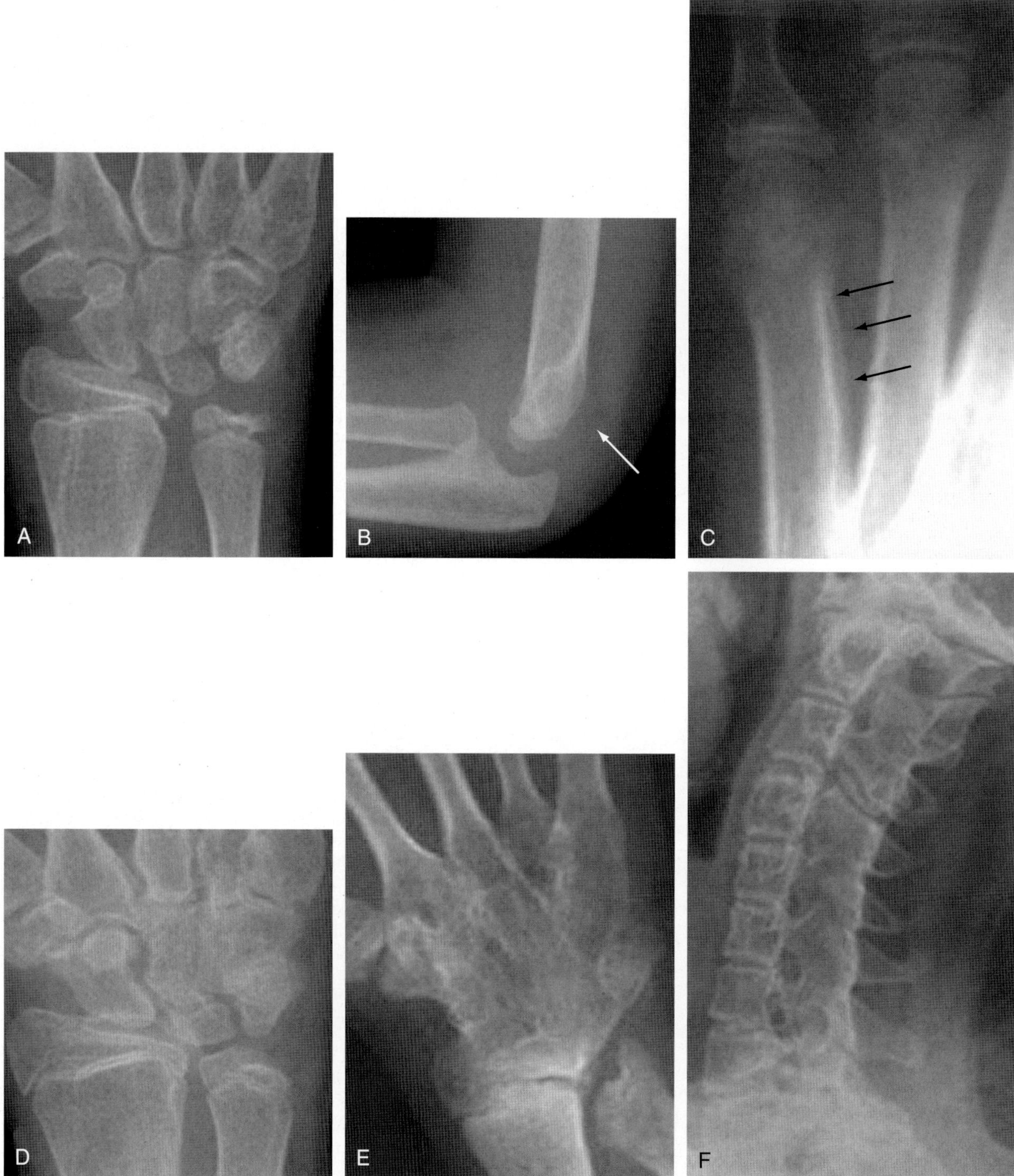

FIGURE 24-1. Radiographic features of JIA. **A** to **C,** Early features of JIA. **A,** Frontal view of the wrist demonstrates periarticular osteopenia and cartilage space narrowing. **B,** Lateral radiograph of the elbow showing displacement of the posterior fat pad *(arrow)*, indicating joint effusion. **C,** Oblique radiograph of the foot shows a line of increased density paralleling the fifth metacarpal *(arrows)*, indicating periostitis. **D** to **H,** Late sequelae of JIA include joint damage and growth abnormalities. **D,** Frontal view of the wrist shows severe joint space narrowing. There is an angular appearance to the individual carpal bones. **E,** Frontal view of the wrist shows ankylosis with coarse trabeculae across the intercarpal and carpometacarpal joints. **F,** There is segmental fusion of the C2-3 and C4-7 facet joints. *(Continued)*

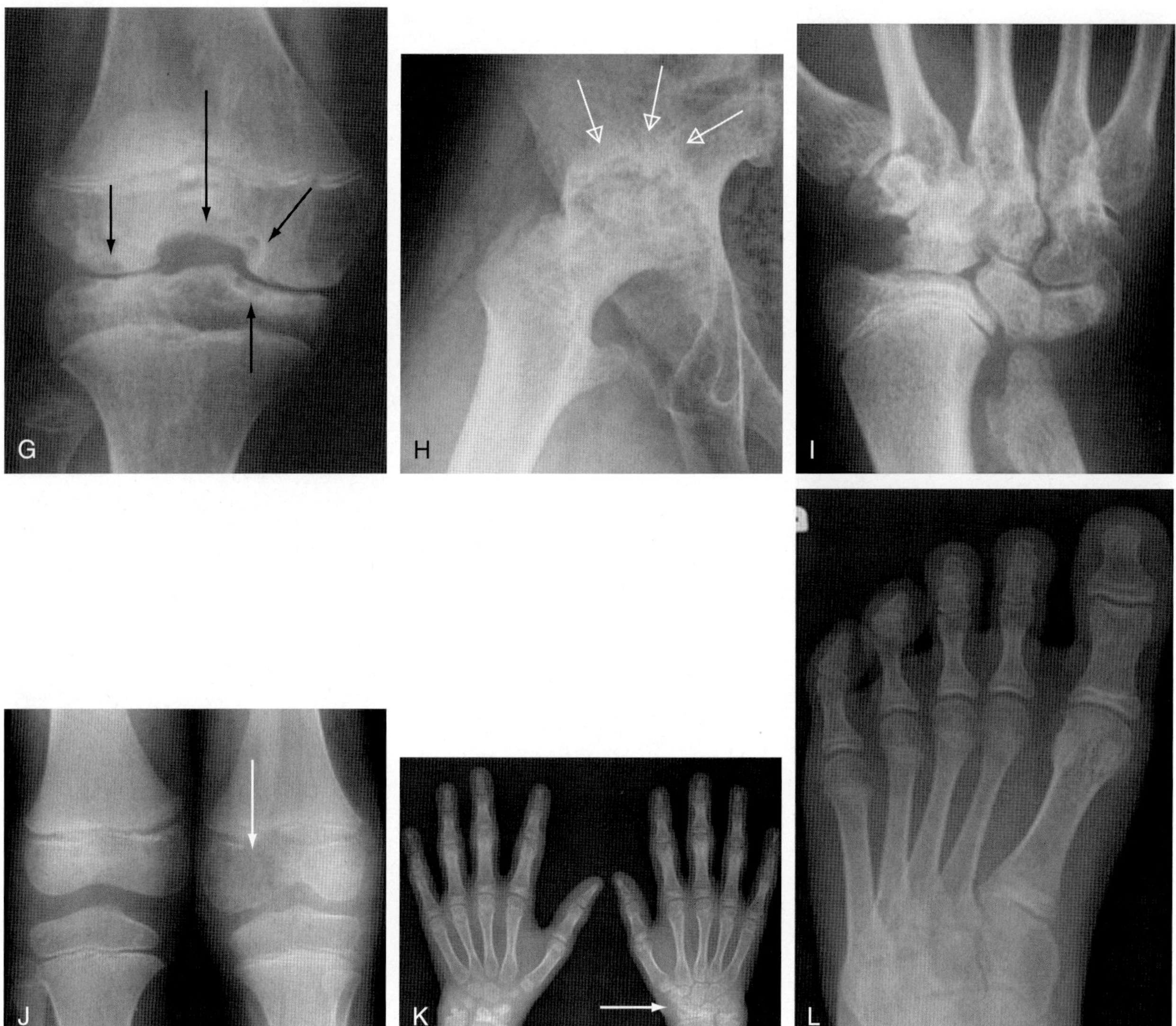

FIGURE 24-1—cont'd. **G,** Anteroposterior (AP) view of the knee shows subchondral cysts and erosions *(small arrows)*. There is widening of the trochlear notch *(long arrow)*. **H,** There is severe hip cartilage loss with subchondral cysts *(arrows)*. There is significant acetabular roof sclerosis and the appearance of "protrusio acetabuli". **I,** Frontal view of the wrist shows that the carpal bones have subluxed toward the ulnar side of the wrist. The ulna is short due to early epiphyseal fusion. **J,** There is overgrowth of the femoral *(arrow)* and tibial epiphyses on the left as compared with the right with advanced bone maturation on the affected side. **K,** Frontal view of the hands and wrists shows increased maturation of the carpals on the left *(arrow)* as compared with the right. **L,** Premature fusion of the growth plates of the toes has resulted in brachydactyly. Figures D and G reprinted with permission from Babyn PS, Doria AS: Radiologic investigation of rheumatic diseases, *Rheum Dis Clin North* 33(3):403-440, 2007.

(Continued)

and Sharp scoring systems with their modifications.[9,17,18] Larsen et al.[9] reported a six-graded scoring system based mainly on erosive damage on standard reference radiographs. It is recommended by the European League against Rheumatism (EULAR). In contrast to Steinbrocker's system, Larsen's method has proved to be of high reproducibility, despite the fact that the changes noted between two radiographic examinations may not qualify the joint for an increase in stage. The Sharp system assigns separate scores for erosions and joint space narrowing, which are combined to provide the final score.

Ultrasonography

Ultrasonography is widely used in assessing the pediatric musculoskeletal system largely because of its ability to visualize cartilage, which is abundant in the immature skeleton and the absence of ionizing radiation.

> Ultrasonography can be used to detect joint effusion, cartilage thickness, and synovitis without ionizing radiation.
> Ultrasound guidance can be used to guide joint aspiration.

Although total joint assessment is often hindered by acoustic barriers,[19] ultrasonography can be used to assess articular cartilage thickness and to detect synovial thickening, joint effusions, and associated synovial cysts.[19-21] Ultrasonography is very sensitive in detecting joint effusion in the hips (Figure 24-2) and shoulders, where radiographs are insensitive. Ultrasonographic scoring systems have been recently developed for assessment of finger joint synovitis in RA of adults.[22] Ultrasonography can also be used

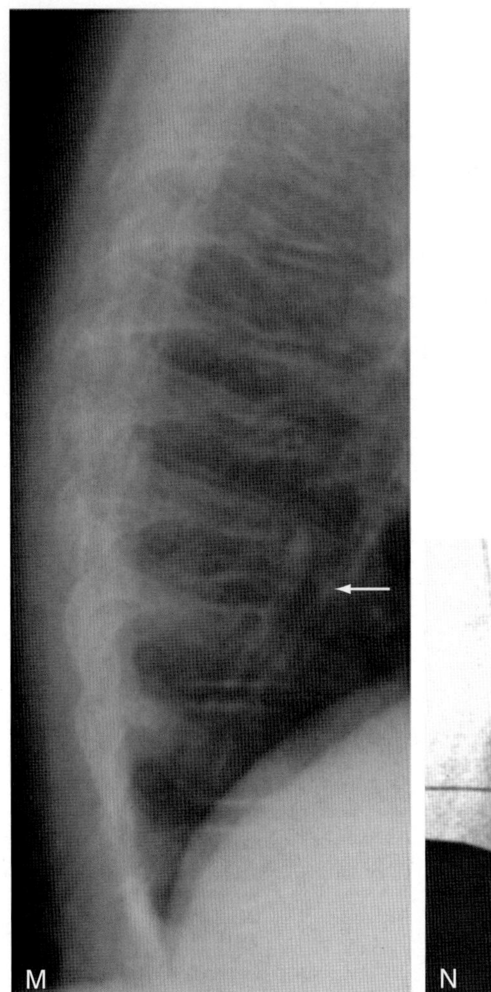

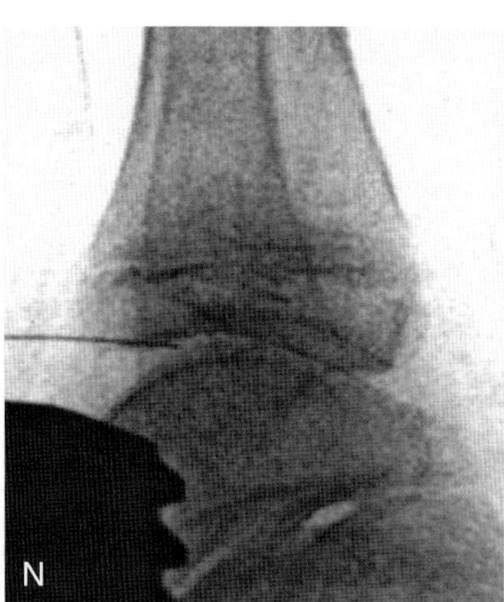

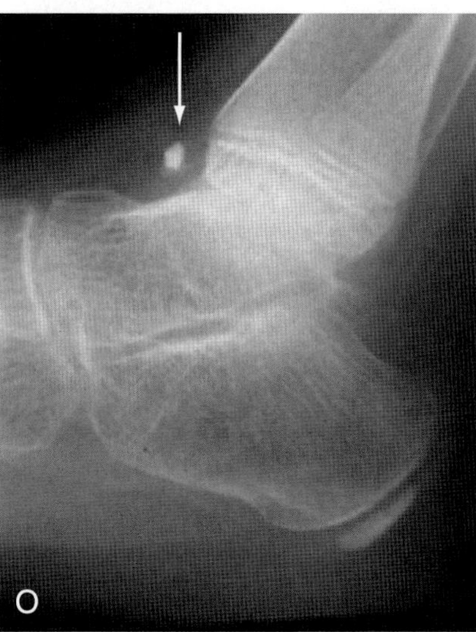

FIGURE 24-1—cont'd. M, Chronic systemic corticosteroid therapy for treatment of JIA may result in vertebral collapse *(arrow)*. **N,** Fluoroscopic image shows needle position for intraarticular administration of corticosteroids. **O,** Follow-up radiograph shows that a calcific focus *(arrow)* has developed at the site of injection.

to assess tendon sheath synovial proliferation (see Figure 24-2) and bursal hypertrophy,[23] to evaluate soft tissue nodules (see Figure 24-2), and to guide joint aspiration or injection. Although previous studies in JIA have shown that MRI is superior to ultrasonography to evaluate erosions in the articular cartilage of knees,[24,25] ultrasonography seems to be more sensitive than conventional radiography and clinical assessment, as demonstrated in adult RA.[26-29] Power Doppler shows promise in evaluating the amount and activity of pannus.[21,30-32]

A novel ultrasonographic technique uses intravascular microbubble contrast agents to improve the Doppler signal intensity. Preliminary results of the use of contrast agents in JIA[33] have shown a potential application for the technique in subclinical cases (see Figure 24-2); however, the lack of standardized interpretation, increased cost, and greater invasiveness have somewhat limited the use of the technique in clinical practice.

Magnetic Resonance Imaging

With MRI one can directly image synovial proliferation, joint fluid, pannus formation, and erosion of cartilage and bone (Figure 24-3). MRI is suitable to assess disease severity or progression and plays an increasing role in diagnosis and outcome assessment of the disease.[21] Uncomplicated joint fluid has usually dark signal on T1-weighted and bright signal on T2-weighted images (see Figure 24-3).[34] Other findings in JIA include popliteal cysts (see Figure 24-2) and meniscal hypoplasia (see Figure 24-3) or atrophy.

MRI enhancement of the synovium can be used for early detection of synovial proliferation, which precedes destructive changes. Normal synovium is thin and shows slight enhancement. Proliferating synovium on MRI without contrast appears as intermediate soft tissue density on T1-weighted and T2-weighted sequences (see Figure 24-3). It may have slightly higher signal intensity than adjacent fluid on unenhanced T1-weighted images.[21,34] Pannus appears as thickened intermediate to dark signal intensity on T2-weighted images best seen when outlined by bright signal joint fluid. Its variable signal intensity reflects its different amounts of fibrous tissue and hemosiderin.

Synovial thickening may be difficult to define without contrast. Contrast enhancement improves visualization of the thickened synovium especially with the use of fat suppression techniques, which allows the proliferating synovium to be seen in regions normally devoid of synovium appearing as enhancing linear, villous, or nodular tissue.[5,21] Images should be obtained immediately after contrast injection, as diffusion of contrast from the synovium into the joint fluid occurs over time. Hypervascular inflamed pannus enhances significantly, whereas fibrous inactive pannus shows much less enhancement.[21]

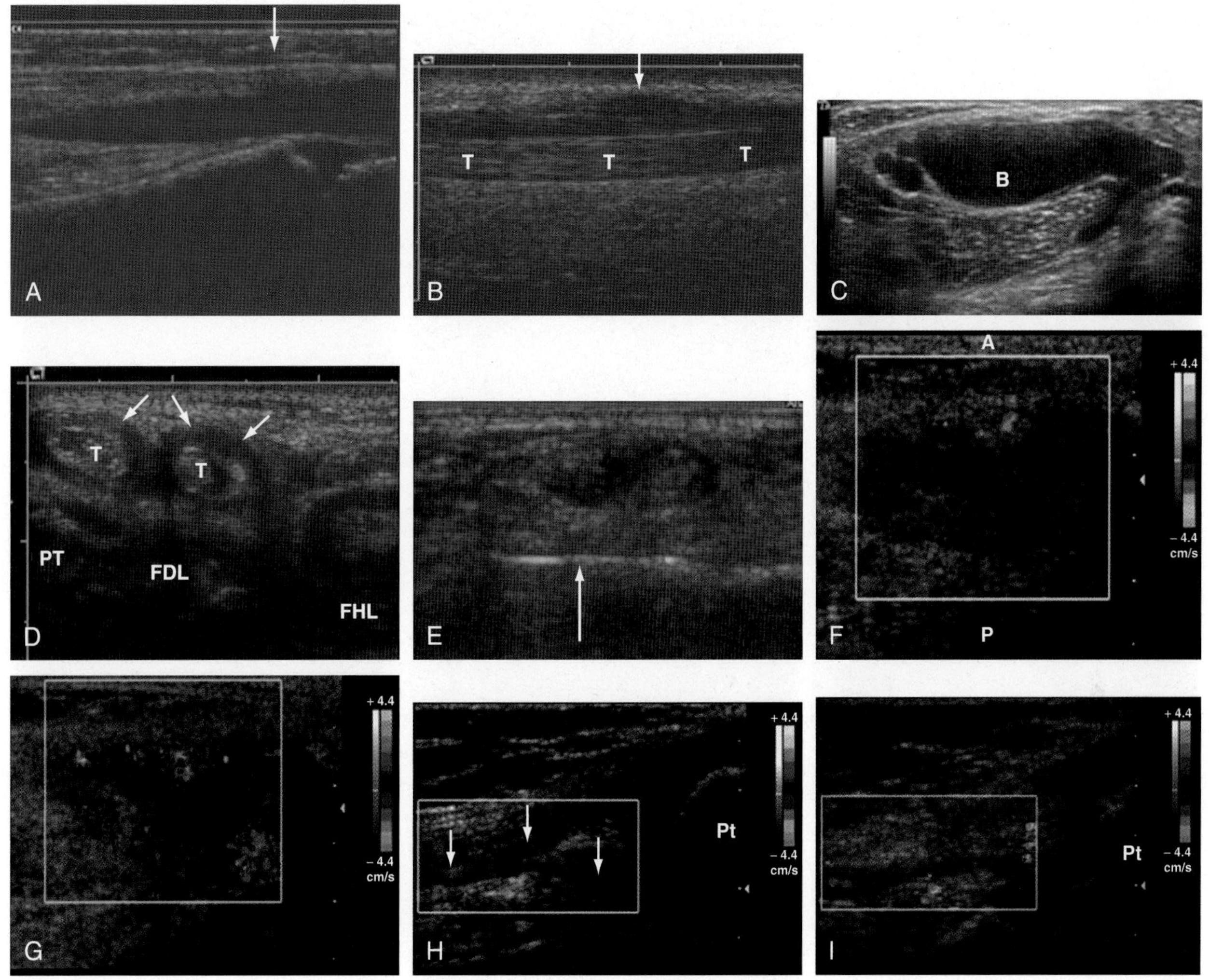

FIGURE 24-2. Ultrasound findings in JIA. **A,** Sagittal scan through the anterior aspect of the knee joint shows the anechoic joint effusion *(arrow)*. **B,** A rheumatoid nodule *(arrow)* is seen on this sagittal scan through the Achilles' tendon *(T)*. **C,** The loculated anechoic structure is a Baker's cyst *(B)* in the popliteal fossa. **D,** An axial scan through the medial posterior aspect of the right ankle shows echogenic tendons surrounded by anechoic fluid indicating tenosynovitis of the posterior tibialis *(PT)*, flexor digitalis longus *(FDL)*, and flexor hallucis longus *(FHL)* tendons. *T,* Tendon. **E,** The transverse gray scale sonogram shows a needle *(arrow)* at the region of tenosynovitis of the left wrist of a 12-year-old girl with polyarticular JIA during the intraarticular injection of corticosteroids. **F** to **I,** Unenhanced and contrast-enhanced longitudinal sonographic scans of JIA patients with clinical (**F,** unenhanced; **G,** enhanced) and subclinical (**H,** unenhanced; **I,** contrast-enhanced) synovitis (*A,* anterior plane; *P,* posterior plane; *Pt,* patella). The colored areas indicate increased blood flow within hypertrophied synovium. Figures F-I are reprinted with permission from Doria AS, Kiss MH, Lotito APN, et al: Juvenile rheumatoid arthritis of the knee: evaluation with contrast-enhanced color Doppler US, *Pediatr Radiol* 31(7):524-531, 2001.

MR images obtained shortly after IV contrast injection demonstrate enhancement of hypervascular-inflamed synovium (pannus) but less enhancement of fibrotic, inactive synovial tissue, thus allowing disease activity to be assessed.

Quantitative techniques may be used to determine synovial volume.[35,36] MRI is more sensitive than clinical evaluation in detecting temporomandibular joint involvement, demonstrating inflammatory change in the absence of clinical symptoms. There is marked variation in the appearance of the intraarticular disk with age, and a flattened disk should only be considered pathologic in the older child (Figure 24-4).[37,38]

Hemosiderin deposition can occur in JIA but is more often seen in disorders typically accompanied by hemarthrosis, including pigmented villonodular synovitis, hemophilic arthropathy, synovial hemangioma, and posttraumatic synovitis. Gradient echo sequences are most sensitive in detecting hemosiderin deposition within the synovium with signal loss occurring due to increased magnetic susceptibility.

Hemosiderin containing synovitis appears very low in signal (black) on all MRI sequences, and this is accentuated on gradient echo sequences.

With prolonged synovial inflammation, as in JIA or tuberculosis, well-defined intraarticular nodules termed "rice bodies" (because of their characteristic macroscopic appearance) can be noted. Rice bodies likely arise from detached fragments of hypertrophied synovial villi and may lead to painless swelling of the joint.[39] On MRI, rice bodies have dark signal on T2-weighted images (see Figure 24-3) owing to their fibrous tissue composition and are associated with joint effusion, synovial hypertrophy, and synovial enhancement after gadolinium administration.[39]

"Rice bodies" are intraarticular nodules that may develop in JIA or tuberculosis.

Cartilage evaluation is important, as cartilage is one of the earliest sites of damage and destruction in JIA. In the immature

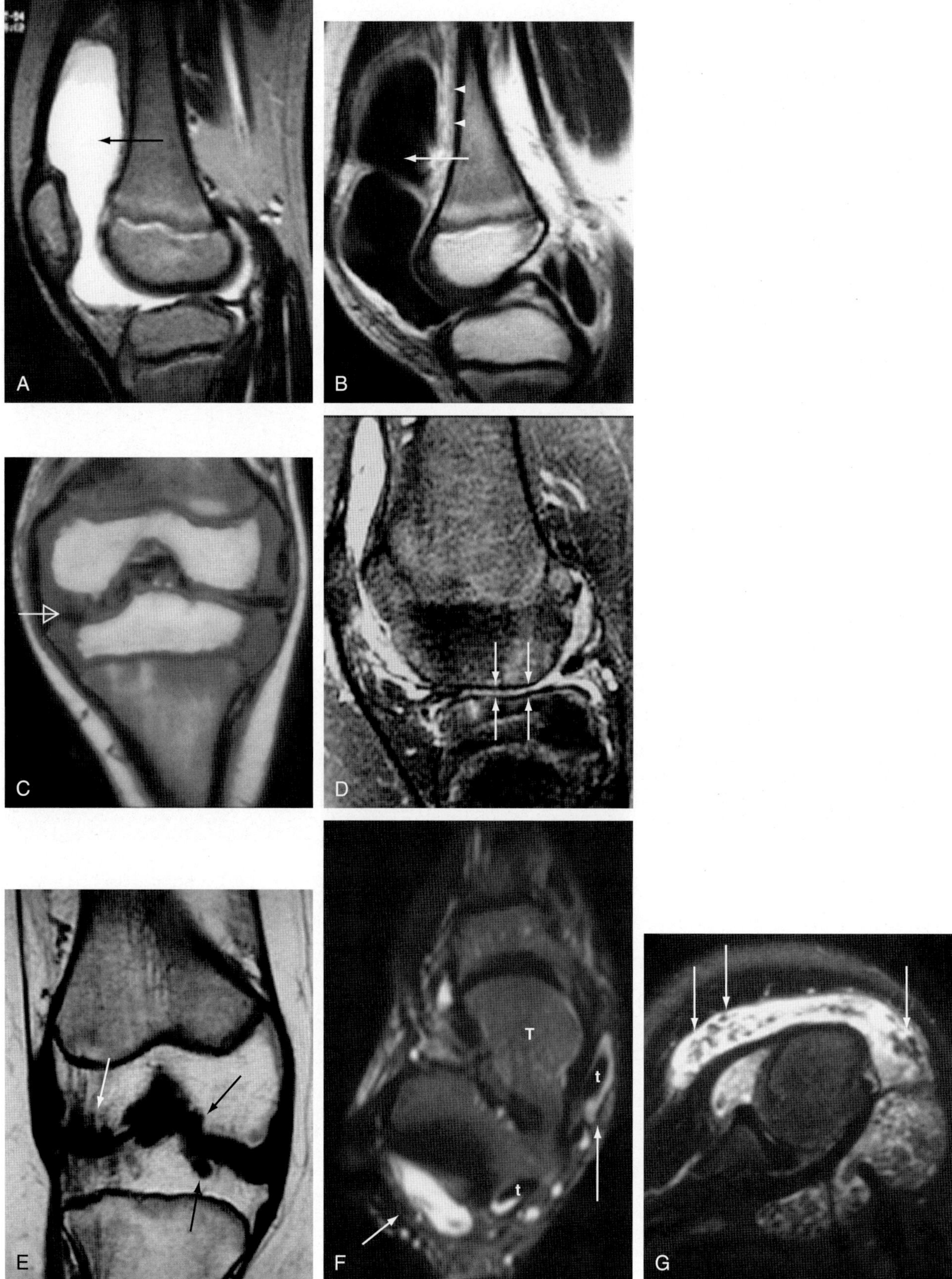

FIGURE 24-3. Characteristic MRI findings of JIA. **A,** Sagittal T2-weighted image with fat saturation shows the high-signal intensity joint effusion *(arrow)*. **B,** Sagittal T1-weighted image post-intravenous gadolinium administration. The unopacified joint effusion is dark *(arrow)*. The gadolinium has enhanced the hypertrophied synovium *(arrowheads)* along the edge of the distended bursa. **C,** A coronal T1-weighted MR image demonstrates meniscal hypoplasia *(arrow)*. Intermediate-signal intensity pannus is seen at the joint. **D,** Sagittal T2-weighted FSE image with fat saturation shows joint space narrowing *(arrows)*. **E,** Coronal T1-weighted spin echo MR image shows erosions *(arrows)*. **F,** Axial T2-weighted image of the hindfoot with fat saturation shows fluid (tenosynovitis, bright, *arrows*) around the dark tendons *(t)*. *T,* Talus. **G,** Axial T2-weighted image with fat saturation of the shoulder shows a distended subacromial subdeltoid bursa with small low-signal bodies (rice bodies, *arrows*).

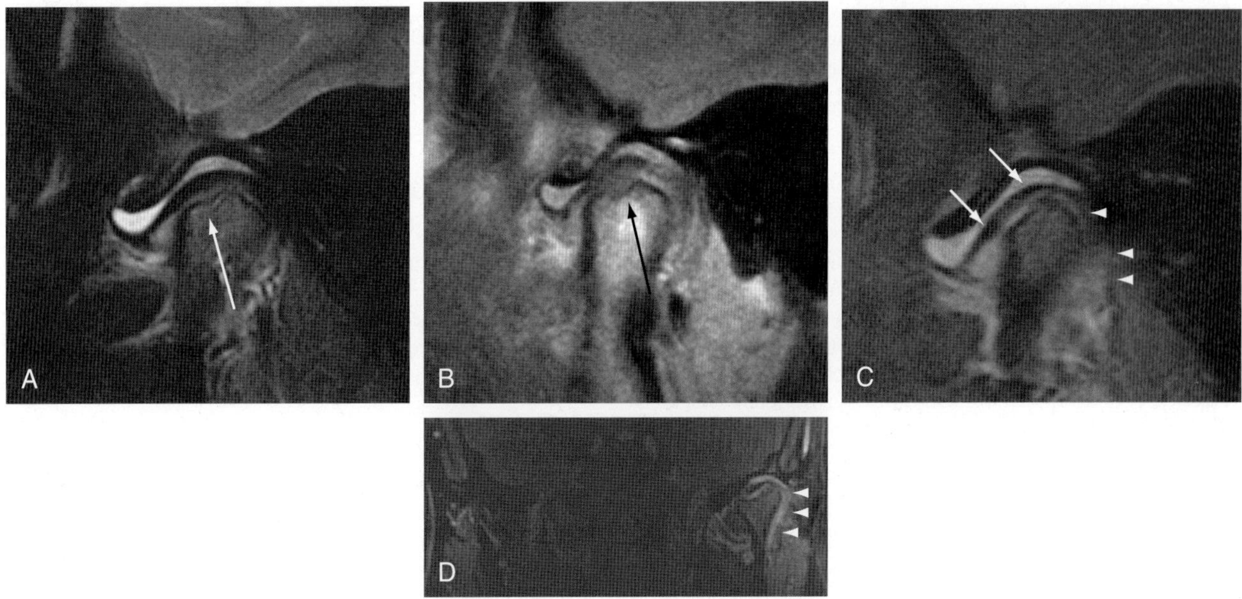

FIGURE 24-4. Temporomandibular joint changes in JIA. A 14-year-old girl with JIA presented with left temporomandibular joint pain and decreased range of mandibular motion. **A,** Sagittal T2-weighted FSE MRI (closed-mouth position) and **(B)** sagittal proton density spin echo (attempted open-mouth position) show cortical erosions of the mandibular condyle *(long arrows)*. **C,** Gadolinium-enhanced sagittal T1-weighted image shows that the temporomandibular joint disk has lost its typically bowtie-shape configuration *(small arrows)* and was noted to be minimally displaced anteriorly (not well seen on the provided images) upon maneuvers to open the mouth. Enhancement of the synovium and perisynovial tissues *(arrowheads)* is seen. **D,** T1-weighted coronal MR image shows significant enhancement of the synovium and perisynovial tissues on the left side.

skeleton, hyaline and epiphyseal cartilage are better distinguished from each other on fast spin echo (FSE) T2-weighted and fat-suppressed proton density sequences. Cartilage is of bright signal on both of the aforementioned sequences, hyaline cartilage having the highest intensity. The articular cartilage should be assessed for areas of altered signal, thinning, erosions, and deep cartilage loss that may extend to the subchondral bone (see Figure 24-3). The fat-suppressed three-dimensional spoiled gradient-recalled echo imaging (3D-SPGR) provides excellent contrast between cartilage, which is of bright signal, compared with adjacent structures.[5,40-42] The development of fast imaging methods with increased signal-to-noise ratio (SNR) efficiency and higher cartilage-synovial fluid contrast, such as driven equilibrium Fourier transform (DEFT),[43,44] dual-echo steady-state (DESS) imaging,[45,46] Dixon water-fat separation technique,[47] and steady-state free precession (SSFP) imaging[48,49] have improved the MRI evaluation of cartilage morphology. The advent of 3-Tesla clinical MRI scanners has improved the signal-to-noise and contrast-to-noise ratio efficiencies of the images, enabling detailed identification of very early cartilage abnormalities in adults.[50,51] Further investigation in the pediatric population should follow.

Scintigraphy

Bone scintigraphy affords high sensitivity but has low specificity for assessment of arthritis because of its lack of spatial resolution.[52] Although previous studies in adults[53-55] have shown that scintigraphy is effective at detecting synovial inflammation and that scintigraphic evidence of synovitis correlates well with later progression of joint erosions in RA, MRI has replaced to a certain extent nuclear studies[21] in the investigation of JIA. Radiotracer accumulation in synovitis depends on increased blood flow, enlargement of the vascular pool, and capillary leak. The radionuclide detection of the active soft tissue inflammatory process of arthritis consists of rapid early transit of activity on angiographic images and enhanced concentration of soft tissue phase activity on blood pool images. Multiphase (angiographic, soft tissue, and delayed) bone scintigraphy with 99mTc methylene diphosphonate (Tc-99m MDP) or hydroxymethylene diphosphonate (Tc-99m HDP) have been considered the preferred imaging technique for differentiation of soft tissue and bone abnormalities[56] and may be useful in excluding serious infection or neoplasm in children with nonspecific arthritic symptoms.

> Bone scintigraphy may be useful for excluding serious infection or tumor in children with nonspecific arthritic symptoms.

Similarly, a few studies in adults[57] have demonstrated the ability of positron emission tomography (PET) to detect inflammation of the synovium; however, very little information is available in children, and clinical implications of potential findings are not clear at this point.

Bone Densitometry

Osteopenia is a well-recognized radiographic finding in JIA as a consequence of chronic corticosteroid therapy. The technique of dual energy x-ray absorptiometry (DXA) permits regional bone and whole body measurement of bone mineral content and bone mineral density. Using a low-radiation-dose scan beam, the computer-generated images are not of diagnostic use. They are used for gross anatomic detail and allow for the selection of regions of interest that will be analyzed by computer. Normative values in children are becoming available[58]; however, overall there is a paucity of appropriate reference databases for osteoporosis. In addition, no formal guidelines are currently available at this point to define pediatric osteoporosis. This is in large part related to reservations that clinicians have about the diagnostic significance of reduced bone mineral density measurements for children and adolescents, in contrast to what these changes mean for adults. As a result, many advocate that the current diagnosis of pediatric osteoporosis should be based on multiple rather than single tests of bone health. Alternative methods for assessment of bone densitometry include quantitative computed tomography (QCT) and quantitative ultrasonography (QUS).[59]

Investigational MRI Techniques for Assessment of Pediatric Osteoporosis

Micro-MRI–based virtual bone biopsy: This imaging modality seeks to acquire images at a resolution sufficient to visualize individual bony trabeculae and to obtain quantitative information in the form of structural parameters similar to those of histomorphometry.[60,61] This method consists of bracelet-style MR receive-only radiofrequency phased array surface coils that detect the raw data, MR scanner software that enhances the SNR, and image processing software that uses special algorithms to transform the data into highly detailed, 3D models of bone microarchitecture. The in-plane image resolution with this technique is approximately 156 μm, which is similar to the dimensions of the bony trabeculae (78 to 200 μm).[62]

Measurement of R_2* of the trabecular bone marrow: This method is based on the rate for the decay of the free induction signal, which is sensitive to the local magnetic field inhomogeneities induced by the trabeculae in the marrow spaces. Reduced bone density lowers R_2*, which is also a function of trabecular orientation relative to the magnet's static field.[63,64]

Measurement of trabecular bone volume fraction: This technique is based on the attenuation of the spin echo amplitude because of the fractional occupation of the imaging voxel by bone (which does not generate a signal). Its resolution is not sufficient to discriminate the individual elements of the bone.[65,66]

Sagittal Laser Optical Tomography

Optical methods that rely on transillumination measurements have emerged as potential new tools for detecting joint inflammation in JIA.[67,68] This investigational technique uses low-level, nonionizing near-infrared radiation. It constitutes a low-cost joint imaging modality with a potential application in JIA for distinguishing joints that have been affected by synovitis versus those that have not.

Extraarticular Findings

Rarely retroperitoneal fibrosis may be associated with autoimmune disorders or idiopathic arthritis.[69] Cross-sectional imaging with ultrasonography, CT, or MRI may demonstrate the retroperitoneal fibrosis directly and identify any associated vascular and ureteral narrowing.

Anemia caused by poor dietary intake, by chronic gastrointestinal blood loss due to drug treatment, or by the chronic disease process may be a significant problem in JIA.[1] Oligoarticular arthritis is associated with chronic uveitis, which is asymptomatic and may therefore go underdetected.[70]

> Chronic uveitis is asymptomatic and is most often found in patients with oligoarticular arthritis. Thus periodic ophthalmologic examination is warranted in patients with oligoarticular disease.

Systemic JIA is associated with amyloidosis, which leads to significant morbidity and mortality.[71] Radiolabeled serum amyloid P component scintigraphy and turnover studies were shown to be useful complementary tools in the diagnosis, screening, and quantitative monitoring of amyloidosis in JIA[72]; however, in practice, other non–radiation-bearing imaging techniques are more frequently used in JIA. Systemic JIA has also been associated with the "macrophage activation syndrome," which may be related to intercurrent viral illness, uncontrolled disease activity, and the use of certain drugs such as gold and sulphasalazine. This syndrome is characterized by fever, hematocytopenia, hepatic dysfunction, encephalopathy, and disseminated intravascular coagulation.[73]

> The macrophage activation syndrome is characterized by fever, hematocytopenia, hepatic dysfunction, encephalopathy, and intravascular coagulation.

Cross-sectional imaging including Doppler ultrasonography of the hepatic vasculature and head CT and MRI are adjunct tools for assessment of potential complications. Ultrasonography and CT may be used to identify extraarticular complications such as hepatosplenomegaly or serositis (Figure 24-5).

New MRI Techniques

Perfusion-weighted imaging (PWI): Used to assess blood flow and residual tissue perfusion in ischemic areas by estimating the physiologic properties of the synovial microvessels, including blood/plasma volume and transendothelial permeability of the contrast agent.[74,75] It uses intravenously administered paramagnetic contrast agents and is based on a dynamic process that quantifies the blood supply to a given region of interest during the transit of the contrast material. Potential roles of this technique in the developing skeleton are to recognize maturation patterns of cartilaginous enhancement in order to rule out pathologic processes such as epiphyseal ischemia, inflammation, edema, and revascularization[76]; to quantify and to monitor synovial inflammation[76]; and to direct therapeutic scheduling for RA according to enhancement patterns.[77]

Delayed gadolinium-DTPA^{2-}-enhanced T1-weighted imaging (dGEMRIC): A technique sensitive to quantification of cartilage proteoglycan content.[78-81] Proteoglycans, collagen, and water play critical roles in the mechanical function of cartilage.[82] Due to negatively charged glycosaminoglycan (GAG) side chains, proteoglycans attract cations and water into the tissue, causing a swelling pressure. These interactions result in a poroelastic, mechanically resilient tissue that enables smooth joint movements and load bearing during locomotion. The dGEMRIC technique utilizes the negative charge of the paramagnetic MR contrast agent, which is assumed to distribute into the cartilage inversely to the fixed charge density of negatively charged GAGs.[78] Thus T1 relaxation time in the presence of the contrast agent is approximately linearly related to the GAG content.

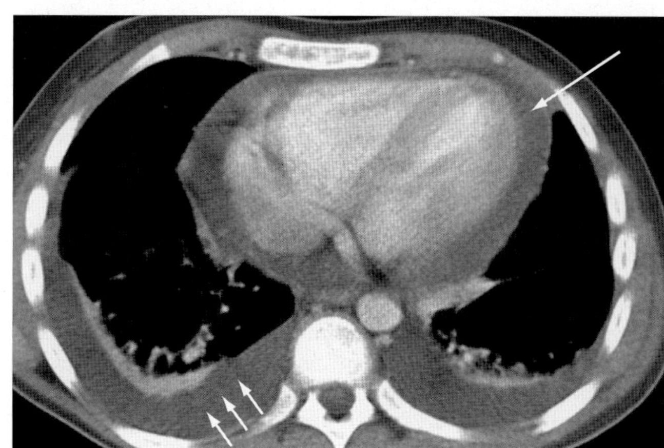

FIGURE 24-5. Pericardial and pleural effusions. CT may be of help for characterization of extraarticular findings of JIA, such as serositis represented by pericardial *(long arrow)* and pleural *(short arrows)* effusions. Dependent atelectasis is noted adjacent to the effusions.

Blood oxygen level dependent (BOLD) MRI: A noninvasive diagnostic technique that assesses the concentration of oxyhemoglobin and deoxyhemoglobin at the capillary level during functional activation by comparing the response of the tissue to vasodilatory (hyperoxia) and nonvasodilatory (normoxia) stimulus. An activated (hyperoxic) state increases the concentration of oxyhemoglobin, thus reducing the concentration of deoxyhemoglobin, which serves as an intrinsic, oxygen-sensitive, paramagnetic marker.[83,84] This technique may detect temporal changes in the synovial response of the joint to a stimulus.[85]

T2-relaxation time mapping: This technique of evaluation of the superficial cartilage has been shown to be sensitive to the integrity of the collagen network. Spatial variation of T2 correlates with the 3D arrangement of the collagen fibrils as revealed by polarized microscopy.[86,87] While cartilage degeneration is known to involve progressive disruption of the collagen network,[88] T2 measurements may characterize the structural integrity of the cartilaginous tissue and quantitatively assess the degree of cartilaginous degeneration as previously shown in the pediatric population.[89]

Recommendations for Imaging

Assessment of disease activity is important for monitoring treatment efficacy and predicting outcome. Histopathologic evidence of persistent synovitis and radiologic deterioration has been observed in patients assumed clinically and biochemically to have inactive disease.

Radiography can be used to quantify joint destruction and assess disease treatment with absence of change and lack of progression implying treatment success.[10] In children who received methotrexate, no interval carpal length narrowing was found in responders compared with the progressive worsening seen in nonresponders.[90] Although joint space narrowing and erosion scores did not improve, some patients did show improvement in carpal length.

Intraarticular corticosteroids can be used to temporarily suppress local joint inflammation.[36] Following injection of intraarticular corticosteroids, periarticular calcification can be noted. Other changes related to intraarticular therapy seem uncommon even with repeated joint injections.[91]

Ultrasonography may also be a useful means to noninvasively follow changes in synovitis with therapy.[25] Ultrasonography may play a role in supporting clinical suspicion of disease activity in clinically mild or silent joints and in deciding upon discontinuation of therapy.[19] Increases in synovial thickening and synovial fluid accompany clinical worsening; however, the significance of residual synovial thickening and effusion seen on ultrasonography in asymptomatic patients remains unclear. It may represent active silent disease or inactive fibrous pannus in a quiescent phase. Following intraarticular therapy for JIA in the hips and knees, decrease in synovial effusion, synovial proliferation, and adenopathy has been noted on ultrasonography.[20]

Contrast-enhanced MRI can be used to quantitatively monitor synovial membrane volumes, effusion volumes, and cartilage and bone erosion scores. Synovial membrane volume may reflect the degree of edema, dilated vessels, and cellular infiltration in the synovial membrane and may be a measure of synovial inflammatory activity. Synovial volume, however, may also reflect the cumulated synovial proliferative disease activity and appears to correlate with duration of clinical remission.[21,36] Several studies have indicated a close relationship between the rate of contrast enhancement and inflammatory activity with the enhancement rate apparently decreasing after intraarticular corticosteroid administration and remaining low during clinical remissions and increasing prior to the return of symptoms, which indicates subclinical increase in synovial inflammatory activity. However, there may be regions of marked heterogeneity in rate of synovial enhancement, so the use of small regions of interest may be a limitation. Cases of clinical relapse show increased enhancement back to pretreatment levels.[92]

Enthesitis-Related Arthritis

This diagnostic subgroup comprises those children with arthritis and enthesitis (inflammation at the site of attachment of ligaments or tendons to bone). Also included are those with either arthritis or enthesitis plus two of the following: (1) sacroiliac (SI) joint tenderness and/or inflammatory spinal pain; (2) presence of HLA-B27; (3) family history of HLA-B27–positive disease; (4) acute anterior uveitis; or (5) onset of arthritis in a boy older than 8 years. A family history of psoriasis would lead to exclusion from this category.[1] Other entities related to the seronegative spondyloarthropathies include the arthritis associated with hyperostosis, acne and/or palmar pustulosis, Whipple's disease, and Behçet's disease.[93] These disorders affect the axial and extraaxial joints. Synovitis and enthesitis are recognized as major target areas of inflammation. Enthesitis is commonly present especially at the insertions of the Achilles' tendon, plantar fascia, and patellar and quadriceps tendons. The juvenile form of enthesitis is more common than the adult form.[93,94] This group of disorders affects boys more often than girls, begins in late childhood or early adolescence (mean age of onset, 10 to 12 years; range, 3 to 15 years), and typically involves fewer than four joints. A family history is often present (30%) as is the HLA-B27 antigen (90%).[95]

Osteoarticular Imaging Features

Radiographic findings are common amongst all the spondyloarthropathies and are similar to JIA with the exception of sacroiliitis and enthesitis, which are more specific for spondyloarthropathy.

Peripheral Skeleton

Radiography

Radiography typically shows asymmetric involvement of the large joints of the lower limb; in other words, the hip, ankle, knee, and tarsal joints (Box 24-2). The small joints are less frequently

BOX 24-2. Radiographic Features of Spondyloarthropathies

PERIPHERAL JOINTS

Asymmetric involvement of large lower limb joints
Involvement of great toe interphalangeal joint
New bone at the margins of erosions
Affected joints: swelling, effusion, epiphyseal overgrowth, erosions, osteopenia, cartilage space narrowing, and rarely fusion
Dactylitis: swelling and periosteal new bone of fingers or toes
Periosteal new bone (e.g., metatarsals, proximal femur)
Entheses
Especially tibial tubercle and calcaneus
Swelling, erosion, new bone formation

SACROILIITIS

Radiographic changes delayed until late teens
Asymmetric involvement may occur early, then symmetric
Erosions occur first on the iliac side of SI joint
"Pseudowidening" occurs due to erosion
Sclerosis and finally ankylosis develop

affected; however, the interphalangeal joint of the hallux is often involved at presentation.[96] Radiographs are usually normal initially but later may demonstrate soft tissue swelling, effusion, ossification and epiphyseal overgrowth, erosions (Figure 24-6), osteopenia, joint space narrowing, or erosion and rarely fusion.[96] Erosions are typically associated with irregular bone apposition at joint margins, referred to as "whiskering" (see Figure 24-6). Rapid joint destruction can be noted.[97] With hip involvement, these proliferative changes are noted at the junction of the femoral head and neck. Dactylitis may be seen with soft tissue swelling and periosteal reaction along the shaft of metacarpals, metatarsals, or phalanges. In juvenile ankylosing spondylitis, extraaxial arthritis usually involves one or more large joints of the lower extremities (e.g., hips, knees, ankles) along with the sacroiliitis.

Enthesitis usually involves the calcaneal and tibial tuberosities and may present with soft tissue swelling at the insertion sites of tendons, localized osteopenia and bone erosion, and/or spur formation particularly at the site of insertion of the Achilles' tendon into the calcaneus, plantar aponeurosis (see Figure 24-6), or patella. Periostitis may be seen involving areas of linear subperiosteal new bone formation such as the shafts of metatarsals and proximal femur.

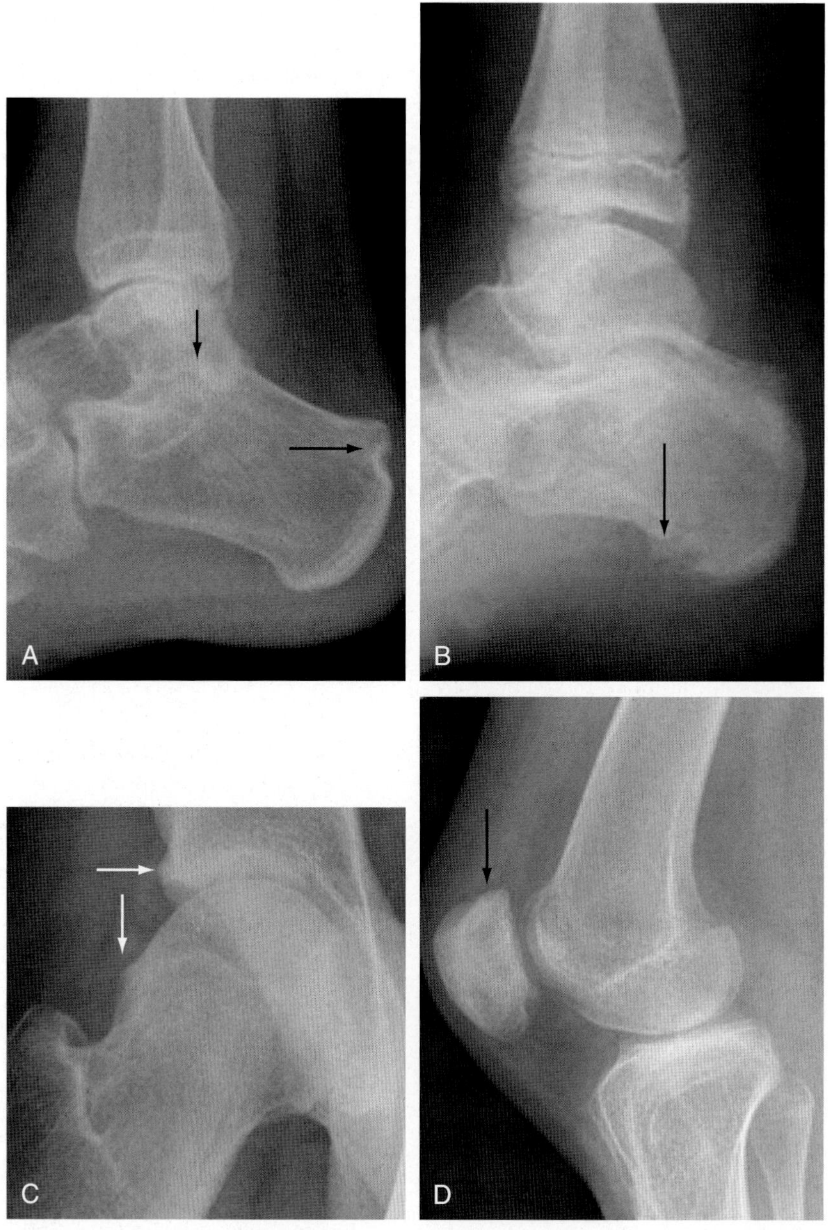

FIGURE 24-6. Radiographic changes in the peripheral skeleton in juvenile spondyloarthropathy. **A,** Lateral radiograph of the ankle shows loss of the posterior subtalar joint space consistent with partial fusion of this joint *(short arrow)*. A small radiolucent erosion with sclerotic borders is present at the superior posterior aspect of the calcaneus near the insertion of the insertion of the Achilles' tendon *(long arrow)*. This is most likely an erosion due to bursitis. **B,** Lateral radiograph of the ankle in another patient demonstrates plantar calcaneal bone overgrowth *(arrow)*. **C,** An anteroposterior view of the hip shows localized bone apposition at the lateral aspect of the acetabular fossa and along the femoral neck ("whiskering") *(arrows)*. **D,** Lateral radiograph of the knee shows sclerosis of the patella *(arrow)*. Figures A, B, and C reprinted with permission from Babyn PS, Doria AS: Radiologic investigation of rheumatic diseases, *Rheum Dis Clin North Am* 33(3):403-440, 2007.

Ultrasonography

Gray scale ultrasound of enthesitis may show loss of the normal fibrillar echotexture of the tendon, blurring of tendon margins, and irregular fusiform thickening.[76,98] The ability of color and power Doppler ultrasonography to assess low-velocity blood flow in small vessels (e.g., synovium) allows a clear depiction of minimal increases of perfusion in inflammatory conditions such as enthesitis.[99] Power Doppler ultrasonography (PDS) denotes the amplitude of the Doppler signal, which is determined by the volume of blood flow present.[100] This technique is best suited for evaluating low-velocity flow in small vessels (e.g., synovium) and is particularly useful for measuring and detecting changes in joints and soft tissues as a consequence of inflammation, which is the case in enthesitis.[101] Recently, D'Agostino et al. evaluated peripheral enthesitis with PDS[99] and reported the ability of PDS to demonstrate a response to treatment with infliximab[102] in young adults presenting with inflammatory heel pain. Tse et al.[103] also demonstrated the ability of color/power Doppler ultrasonography to show increased vascularity at the cortical bone insertion of enthesis and along the adjacent synovium (Figure 24-7)

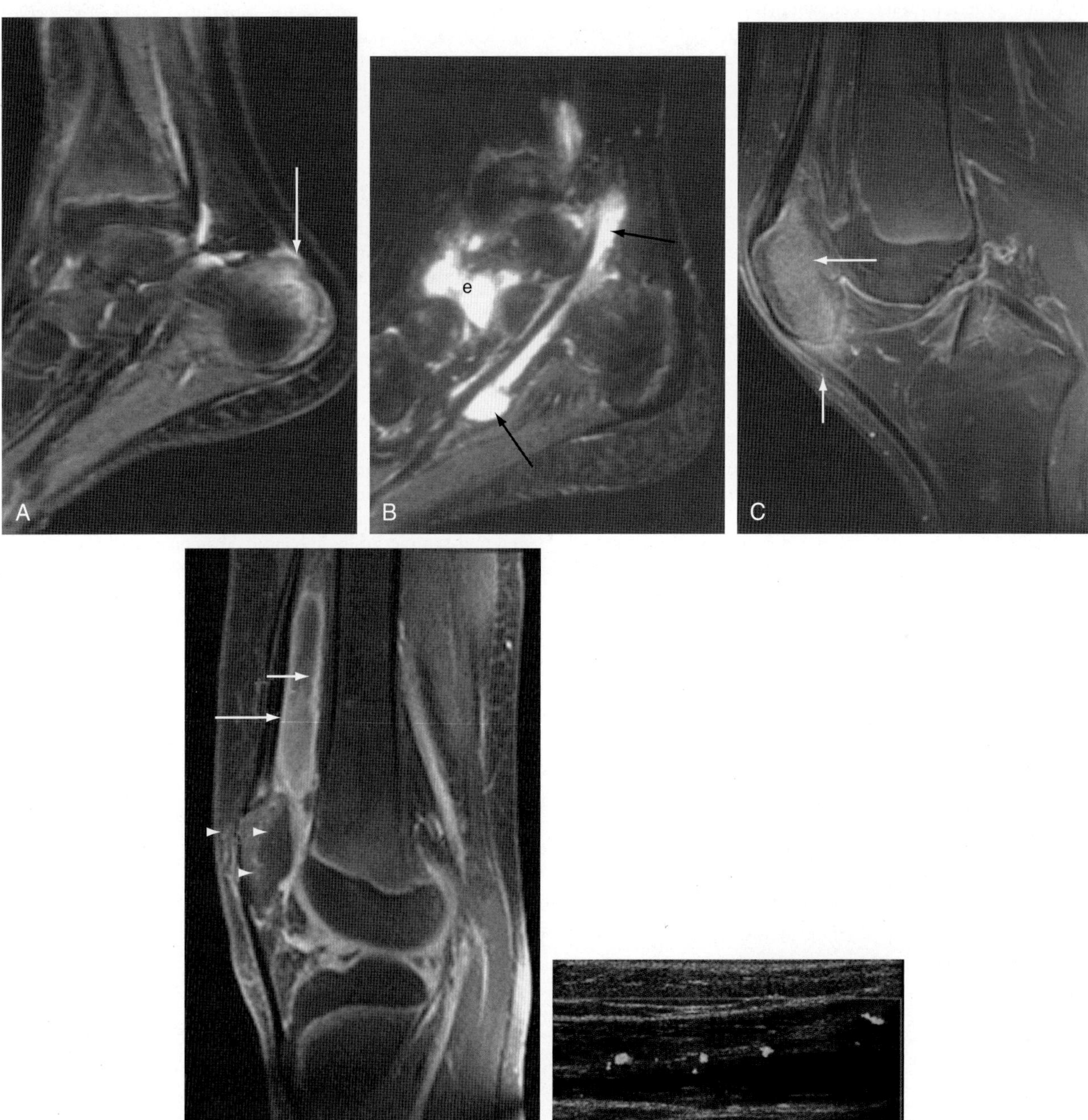

FIGURE 24-7. MRI features of enthesitis-related arthritis in adolescents. **A,** Sagittal STIR image of the ankle demonstrates bone marrow edema along the posterior aspect of the calcaneus at the insertion of the Achilles' tendon *(arrow)*. **B,** Sagittal STIR image of the ankle shows high signal intensity between the tarsal bones suggesting effusion *(e)* and fluid within the tendon sheaths *(arrows)* suggestive of inflammation. **C,** Contrast-enhanced sagittal T1-weighted spin echo image shows increased signal intensity of the patella *(long arrow)* and the proximal aspect of the patellar tendon *(short arrow)*, consistent with inflammation. **D,** Contrast-enhanced T1-weighted image of the knee (same patient as **C**) shows associated synovial hypertrophy (white, *long arrow*), joint effusion (dark, *short arrow*) and increased patellar signal intensity *(arrowheads)* indicating enthesitis. **E,** The corresponding color Doppler ultrasound scan of the patient in **D** shows mild hyperemia of the synovium of the suprapatellar bursa of the knee. Figure A reprinted with permission from Babyn PS, Doria AS: Radiologic investigation of rheumatic diseases, *Rheum Dis Clin North Am* 33(3):403-440, 2007.

in children with spondyloarthropathy, suggesting that this technique may add valuable information to gray scale ultrasonography.[104-106]

Magnetic Resonance Imaging

With MRI one may see bone marrow edema (see Figure 24-7), tenosynovitis (see Figure 24-7), granulation tissue, or cortical erosion at the site of enthesitis.

Scintigraphy

An abnormal pattern of uptake consisting of increased tissue-phase activity in an enthesis distribution with a normal or similarly distributed mild increase in activity on delayed images is seen in patients with enthesitis.[56] Once the existence of an inflammatory process has been established at the entheses, its response to therapy should be assessed clinically, because radionuclide remission can lag behind clinical improvement.[107]

Axial Skeleton

Radiography

In juvenile enthesitis-related arthritis, changes in the spine and SI joints are not frequently seen until the latter part of the second decade.[96] Occasionally there may be localized osteitis, erosions, and sclerosis, particularly at vertebral margins (Figure 24-8). Syndesmophytes are rarely seen in children.[2,93]

> Radiographic spine and SI joint changes in juvenile enthesitis-related arthritis are typically not present until the late teens.

Rarely atlantoaxial subluxation can be present.[108]

Radiographs may demonstrate unilateral or bilateral sacroiliitis with indistinct articular margins, pseudowidening, erosions, and reactive sclerosis (see Figure 24-8), particularly on the iliac side of the joint. Radiography shows asymmetric sacroiliac joint changes in the initial phase of the disease but eventually the classic bilateral, symmetric joint involvement can be seen (see Figure 24-8). Initially there is joint space widening with erosions and reactive sclerosis. Eventually the joint space becomes narrowed and ankylosed. Diffuse osteopenia of the pelvic bones is also seen as a late change.[96]

Magnetic Resonance Imaging

MRI demonstrates early changes in the SI joints and spine and is especially sensitive for evaluation of subchondral bone abnormalities not shown on other types of imaging,[109] as well as bone marrow edema. The administration of gadolinium-DTPA chelates improves the detection of early sacroiliitis.[110] On MRI, periarticular low signal may be seen on T1-weighted images with high signal on T2-weighted images from inflammatory changes in bone marrow, whereas low signal will be seen with bone sclerosis. MRI may also demonstrate changes in articular cartilage with erosions.

Computed Tomography

Sacroiliitis may be demonstrated on either CT or MRI at an earlier stage compared with radiography.[93] CT scan of the SI joints is useful in demonstrating erosive disease not evident on radiographs. On CT, angled scans through the SI joint should be used to lower the radiation dose.[93]

Scintigraphy

Bone scintigraphy can overcome the difficulty in recognizing early SI abnormalities on radiography.[56] However, because there is normally a higher concentration of physiologic activity in the SI joints, mild to moderate increases in the radioisotope uptake may sometimes evade visual detection. In addition, because bilateral and symmetrically enhanced SI uptake can occur in juvenile ankylosing spondylitis, quantitative analysis at the SI joints is usually necessary. Asymmetric uptake is more common in childhood spondyloarthropathies other than juvenile ankylosing spondylitis.

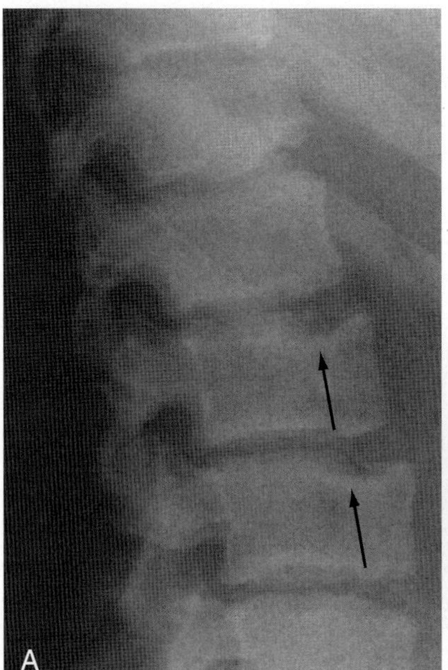

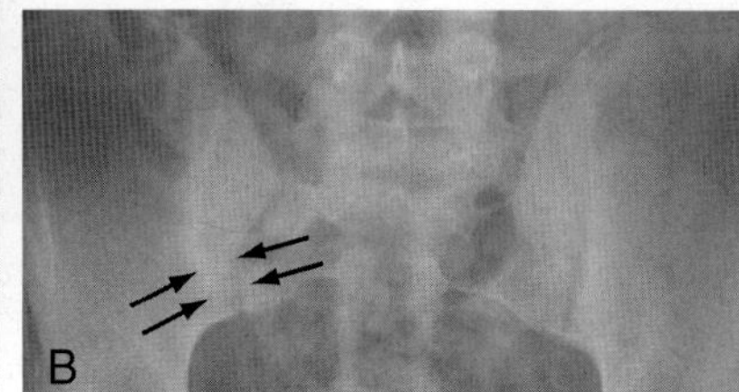

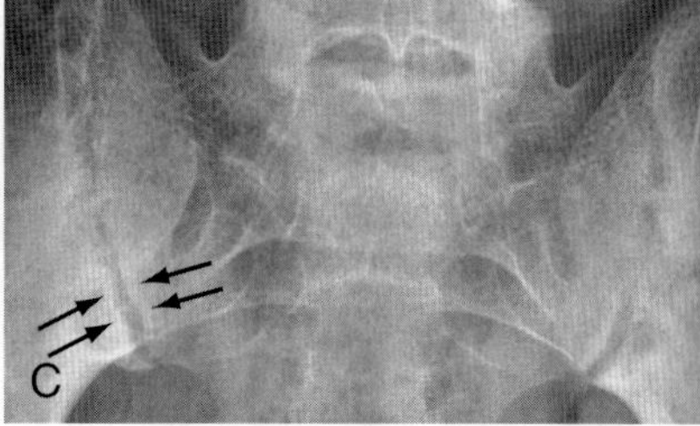

FIGURE 24-8. Radiographic findings in the axial skeleton of enthesitis-related arthritis. **A,** Lateral radiograph of the spine shows sclerosis and irregularity of the endplates of multiple thoracic vertebrae *(arrows)*. **B,** Mild and **(C)** prominent diffuse sclerosis and irregularity of the sacroiliac joints with cartilage space widening *(arrows)*.

Psoriatic Arthritis

The term "psoriatic arthritis" includes children with arthritis and psoriasis or those with arthritis and at least two of the following: (1) dactylitis; (2) nail pitting or onycholysis; or (3) family history of psoriasis in a first-degree relative.[1] The mean age of onset of this disease is 9 to 10 years. It affects primarily young girls (2.5:1 ratio)[111] with a positive family history of the disease. In approximately half of patients, the characteristic rash precedes arthritis by months or years; in the remainder, arthritis is the initial manifestation, with psoriasis appearing later. The most common form of pediatric psoriatic arthritis is asymmetric with pauciarticular joint involvement.[112]

Peripheral Skeleton

Radiography

Radiographs obtained in the initial phase of the disease may be normal or show juxtaarticular osteoporosis. Characteristic radiographic features of psoriatic arthritis include joint erosions, joint space narrowing, bony proliferation including periarticular and shaft periostitis, osteolysis including "pencil-in-cup" deformity, acroosteolysis (Figure 24-9), spur formation, and ankylosis[113] (Box 24-3). The bone erosions tend to be larger and more asymmetric than those seen in JIA; however, in some cases the

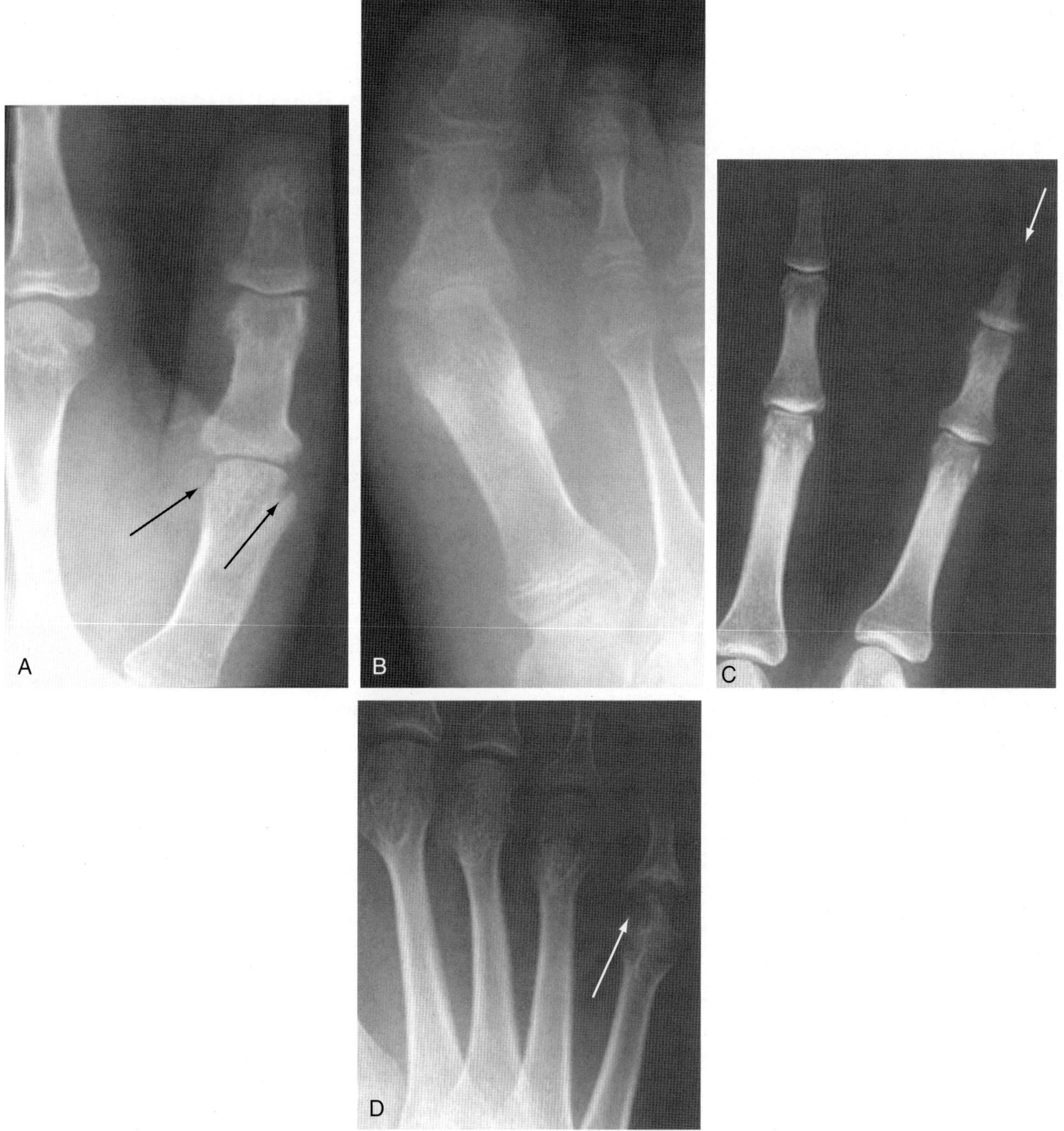

FIGURE 24-9. Two children with psoriatic arthritis. **A,** Selected image of the thumb shows joint erosions *(arrows)* and cartilage space narrowing. **B,** Anteroposterior (AP) radiograph of the great toe shows joint space narrowing. **C,** AP radiograph of the fingers shows acroosteolysis *(arrow)*. **D,** AP radiograph of the foot shows a "pencil in cup" deformity of the fifth toe metatarsophalangeal joint *(arrow)*.

BOX 24-3. Radiographic Features of Juvenile Psoriatic Arthritis

Asymmetric involvement
Periosteal reaction along bones adjacent to affected joints
Distal joint erosion (leading to "pencil in cup" deformity or ankylosis)
Erosion of distal phalangeal tufts (acroosteolysis)
Erosion with new bone formation at the margins
Nonspecific erosion and cartilage space narrowing
Enthesitis (erosion and new bone at entheses)
"Sausage digit"
Asymmetric sacroiliitis
Nonmarginal vertebral bony bridging

radiographic features may be indistinguishable from those of pauciarticular JIA.[114] The characteristic late changes seen at the distal interphalangeal joints are uncommon in children.[96]

Ultrasonography

Enthesitis at the Achilles' tendon is identified by ultrasonography in a much higher frequency than on clinical examination in patients with psoriasis.[115] Ultrasonography may also be a useful tool in the assessment of tenosynovitis (Figure 24-10) or dactylitis.[116] Previous studies[117] showed that gray scale ultrasound is more sensitive than clinical examination for detection of abnormalities in hands and wrists of psoriatic patients and that power Doppler signals correlate significantly with the number of swollen joints. Also, gray scale and color/power Doppler ultrasonography (see Figure 24-10) seem to be reliable tools for measurement of joint response to therapy with biologic agents.[118]

Magnetic Resonance Imaging

In psoriatic arthritis, MRI demonstrates erosive changes, joint space narrowing, ligament disruption, and tenosynovitis (see Figure 24-10).[119] Dactylitis is characteristic and is caused by inflammation of the flexor tendon sheath. Soft tissue edema and synovial proliferation in sausage-like digits is best seen on contrast-enhanced T1-weighted MR images (see Figure 24-10) that can clearly demonstrate dactylitis as a manifestation of the disease. Severe erosions can be seen particularly in the digits.[93] MRI may also be used to evaluate the responsiveness of therapy as noted by a significant reduction in gadolinium uptake following treatment with infliximab.[120]

> "Sausage" digits are seen in patients with psoriatic arthritis and reactive arthritis (Reiter's disease). These swollen fingers or toes result from tenosynovitis, soft tissue edema, and synovial proliferation.

Axial Skeleton

Radiography

Sacroiliitis and vertebral involvement typically manifest later on during the progression of the disease. The sacroiliitis of juvenile psoriasis is usually asymmetric at onset and resembles that of reactive arthritis (Reiter's syndrome).[96] Syndesmophytes, paraspinal calcification, and atlantoaxial subluxation are rare in children.[114] Syndesmophytes occur in both psoriatic arthritis and ankylosing spondylitis, but in psoriatic arthritis they may be paramarginal and typically do not appear in consecutive vertebrae.[113]

Computed Tomography

CT may be useful in assessing spine disease but has little role in the assessment of peripheral joints.[113] Previous studies have shown that CT is as accurate as MRI for assessment of erosions in the SI joints but is not as effective for identifying synovial inflammation.[121] CT may also help guide SI joint injection.[113]

Scintigraphy

Bone scintigraphy was widely used in the past for assessment of psoriatic arthritis, but it has been replaced by ultrasound and MRI techniques.[121a] It can be used to diagnose sacroiliitis and enthesitis and to detect inflammatory changes in situations where radiography is normal.[122]

OTHER FORMS OF ARTHRITIS

Inflammatory Bowel Disease

Arthritis is the most common extraintestinal manifestation of inflammatory bowel disease (IBD). Approximately 10% of children with IBD have arthritis.[111,112] The symptoms of arthritis may precede or follow the clinical diagnosis of IBD. Two distinct patterns of arthritis may be present: the more frequently seen peripheral arthritis or the less common sacroiliitis and spondylitis. Peripheral arthritis usually is pauciarticular and involves knees, ankles, wrists, and less often, hands and shoulders. The typical peripheral arthritis directly reflects the clinical activity of the bowel disease and remits as the intestinal inflammation diminishes.[114] Sacroiliitis and spondylitis may progress regardless of control of the underlying bowel disease.

> Peripheral arthritis activity varies directly with the activity of the IBD, whereas sacroiliitis and spondylitis may progress despite control of the bowel disease.

Radiography

Radiographic findings of peripheral arthropathy include soft tissue swelling, joint effusions, periostitis, enthesitis, and erosive changes.[96] Osteoporosis and growth retardation can be additional manifestations of the disease related to corticosteroid therapy.

Septic Arthritis

Acute purulent infection of the joints is more common in infancy and early childhood[5] due to the greater blood flow to the joints during the active stages of growth. The usual cause is hematogenous dissemination related to an upper respiratory infection or pyoderma. Infection may also spread from adjacent osteomyelitis, cellulitis, abscess, or traumatic joint invasion.[5] In children, septic arthritis develops commonly from osteomyelitis in metaphyses that are intraarticular, such as the hip.[5,123,124] The diagnosis of the obvious septic joint is not much of a challenge, although time to diagnosis is critical to avoid a poor outcome such as destruction of the femoral head, degenerative arthritis, or permanent deformity.

The vast majority of septic arthritides are monoarticular with the most commonly affected joints being the knee, hip, and ankle.[124] In septic arthritis, bacterial contamination causes hypertrophy and edema of the synovium. In infants with septic arthritis, distension of the joint capsule may result in pathologic dislocation particularly in the hip or shoulder. Joint space narrowing results from cartilage destruction by proteolytic enzymes. There may be associated bone erosion and destruction or periosteal reaction.[125]

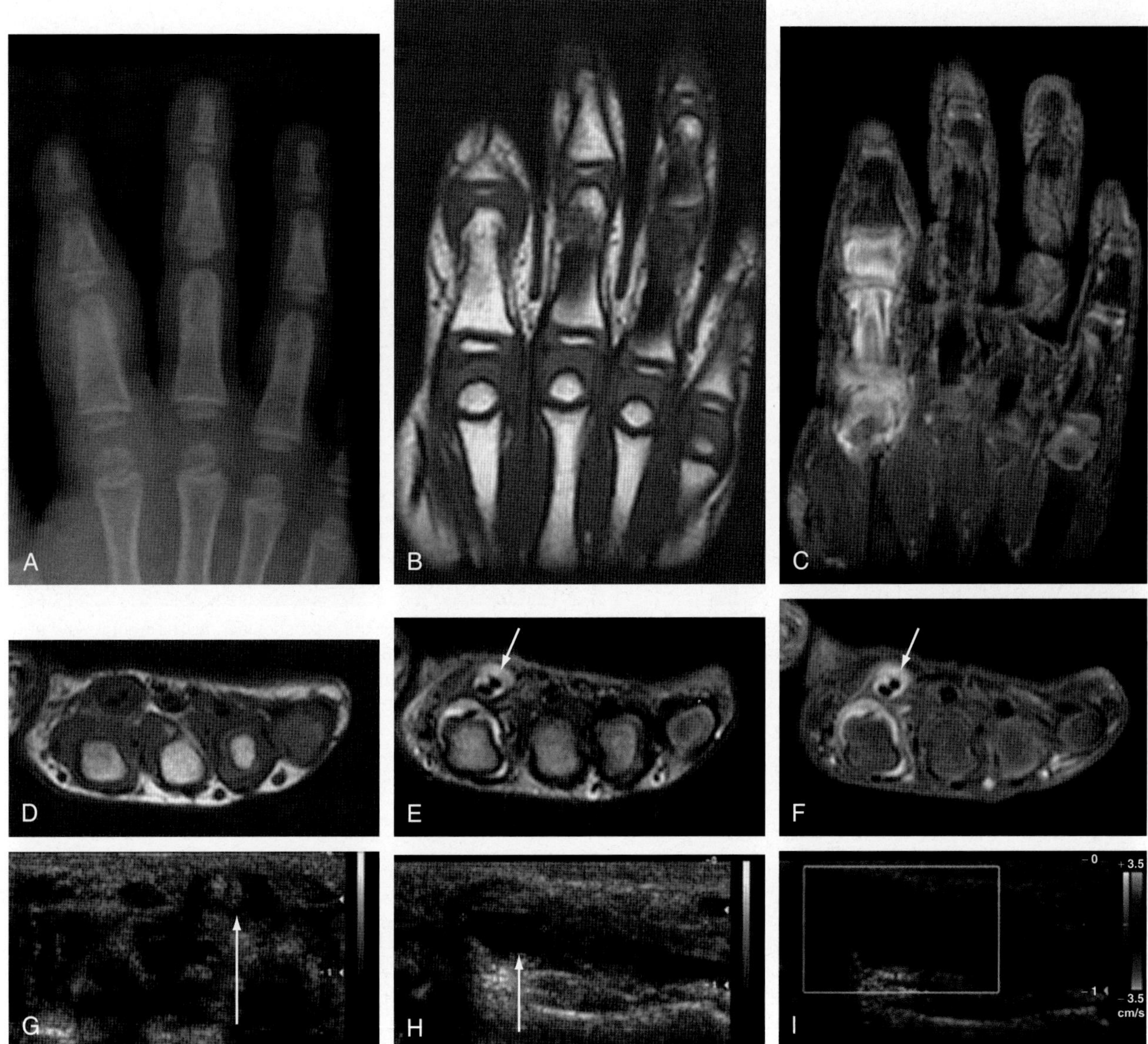

FIGURE 24-10. Psoriatic arthritis. This 20-month-old girl experienced left index finger swelling. **A,** Radiograph of the fingers shows soft tissue swelling of the proximal interphalangeal (PIP) joint of the second digit. The adjacent proximal phalanx and, to a lesser extent, the middle phalanx of this finger show periosteal reaction. The PIP joint space appears mildly narrowed. **B,** Unenhanced coronal T1-weighted spin echo MR image. There is intermediate signal soft tissue distending the PIP joint. **C,** Contrast-enhanced T1-weighted MR image. There is enhancement of the synovial tissue of the distended PIP and metacarpophalangeal joints. **D,** Unenhanced axial T1-weighted spin echo, **(E)** axial T2-weighted FSE, and **(F)** contrast-enhanced T1-weighted images **(D** to **F)** through the metacarpals (displayed with the palm up). These images show abnormal enhancement and circumferential synovial thickening and effusion involving the sheath of the flexor digitorum superficialis and profundus tendons (tenosynovitis, *arrow*). **G,** Axial gray scale ultrasound, **(H)** longitudinal gray scale ultrasound of the index finger, and **(I)** color Doppler ultrasonographic images show tenosynovitis of the second digit of the left hand *(arrows)* with mild synovial hyperemia. The hypoechoic area *(arrows)* corresponds to the fluid within the tendon sheath around the echogenic tendons.

Pus in the joint increases intraarticular pressure and may result in osteonecrosis of the epiphysis.[124] Other sequelae include angular deformities, leg length discrepancy, and ankylosis. Prompt diagnosis of septic arthritis is essential in infants and children to prevent complications.

Radiography

The classic radiographic findings of acute septic arthritis are soft tissue swelling (Figure 24-11), rapid joint space loss (Figure 24-12), and erosions with relative preservation of mineralization (Box 24-4). These findings indicate advanced irreversible destruction of the joint with progression to ankylosis (Figures 24-12 and 24-13) but are not specific for infection. Early radiographic findings of joint effusion may be detected in the knee, ankle, or elbow but radiographs are less sensitive for detecting effusion in the shoulder, hip, or SI joints.[126]

> If there is a question of septic arthritis, joint aspiration is necessary.

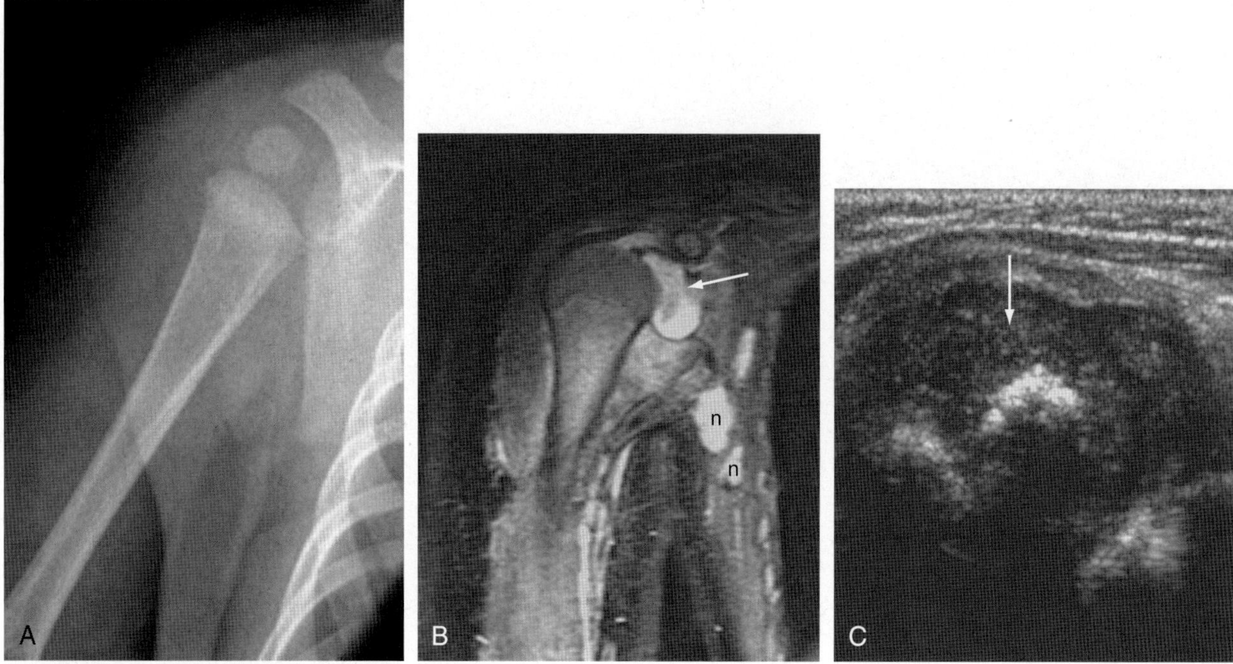

FIGURE 24-11. Septic arthritis. This young boy presented with fever, pain and swelling of the right shoulder. **A,** The frontal view of the right shoulder demonstrates soft tissue swelling overlying the humeral-scapular joint. **B,** Coronal inversion recovery image of the shoulder shows high signal intensity joint effusion *(arrow)* and extensive inflammation of the adjacent soft tissues. Enlarged axillary lymph nodes are identified *(n)*. **C,** An axial ultrasound scan of this shoulder shows the presence of debris within the joint effusion *(arrow)*, suggesting the purulent nature of the fluid.

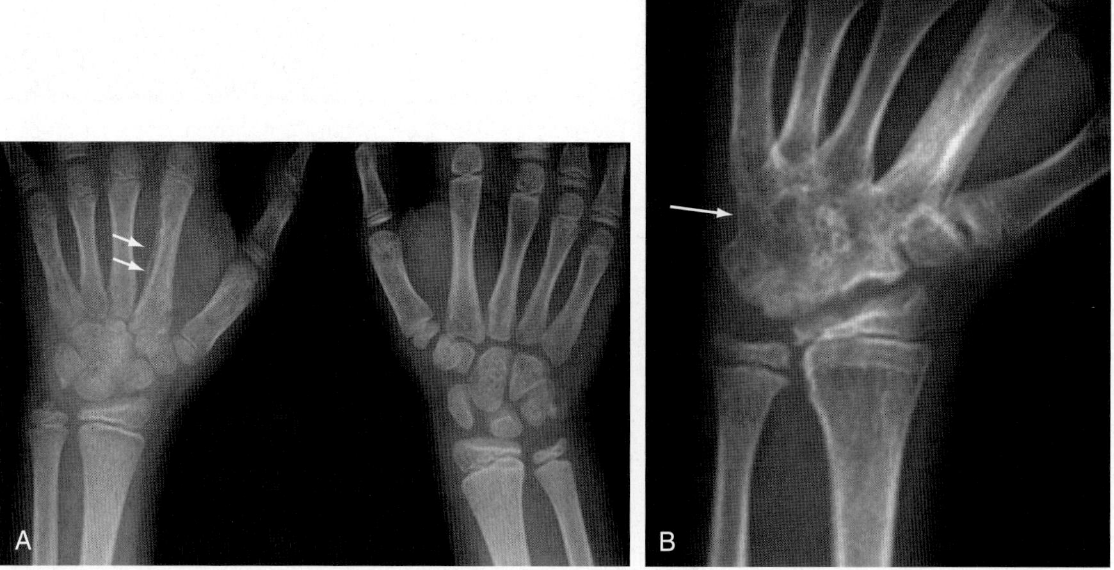

FIGURE 24-12. Septic arthritis and osteomyelitis. **A,** This 9-year-old girl presented with fever and pain in the left wrist for 1 month. The frontal radiograph of the hands shows soft tissue swelling at the carpal region of the left hand, irregularity and sclerosis along the cortex of the left second metacarpal *(arrows)*, a permeative pattern of the bone marrow of the left fifth metacarpal, and joint space reduction between the carpal bones. The bone changes suggest osteomyelitis. **B,** The frontal radiograph of the left wrist of another patient who had an unfavorable progression of septic arthritis with progression to ankylosis of the carpal bones *(arrow)* is shown. Note the marked thickening of the second metacarpal, likely due to previous osteomyelitis.

BOX 24-4. Radiographic Features of Septic Arthritis in Children

Effusion
Rapid loss of cartilage space
Erosions

Ultrasonography

Ultrasound, CT, and MRI are sensitive in demonstrating joint effusion (see Figures 24-11 and 24-13) but cannot distinguish infected from noninfected joint effusion, and aspiration is still necessary for diagnosis. Ultrasonography or CT can be used for guiding diagnostic aspiration or drainage of the joint.

The absence of a joint effusion does not completely exclude a septic joint.

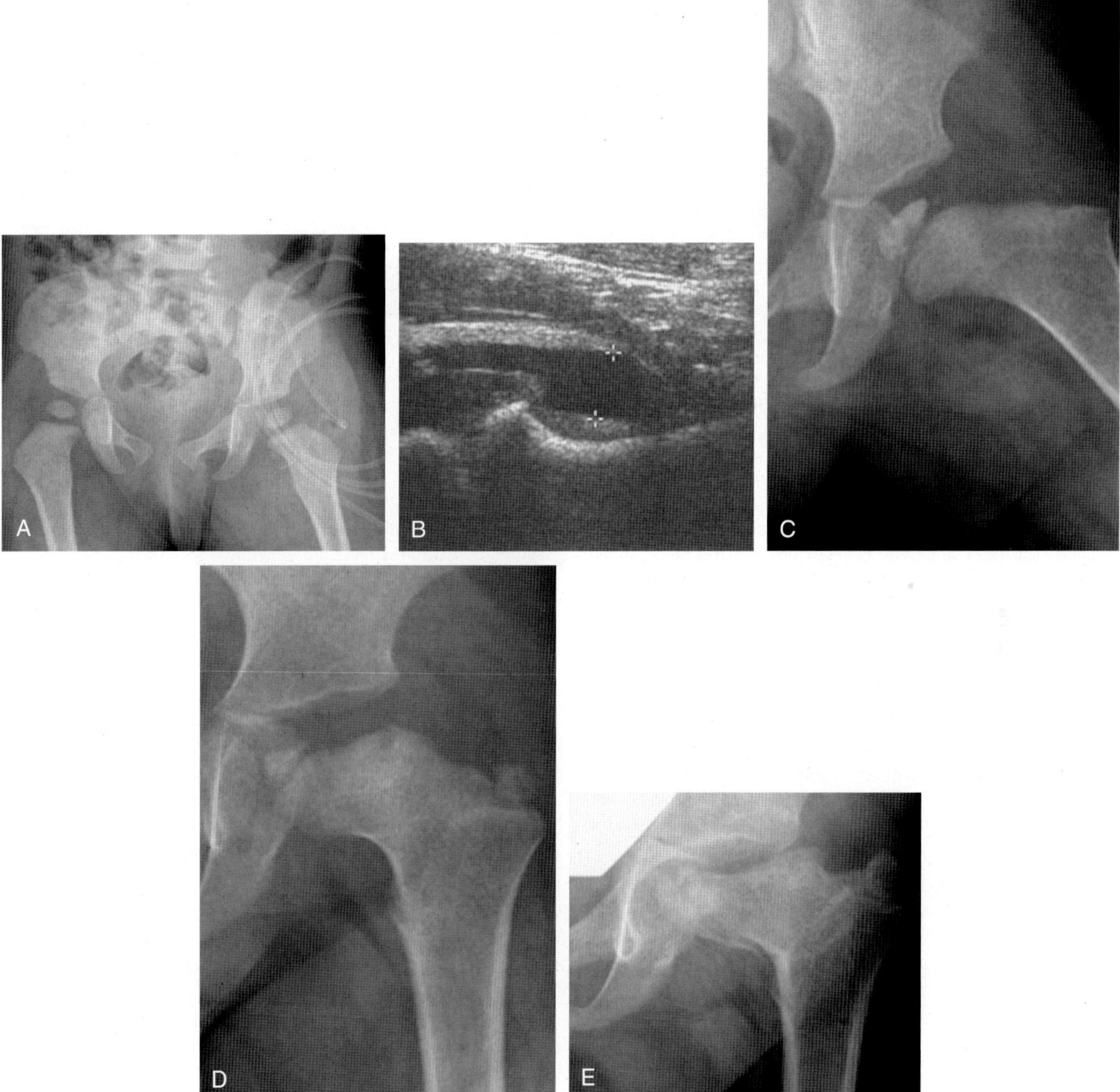

FIGURE 24-13. Septic arthritis. Young girl presenting with left hip pain and fever. **A,** Comparison of the distances from the proximal femur to the teardrop shadow of the acetabulum on each side shows a larger measurement on the left consistent with effusion. There is adjacent soft tissue swelling. **B,** The sagittal ultrasound scan of the proximal left hip shows a large joint effusion within the anterior synovial recess of the hip with associated thickening of the capsule. The surgical-histopathologic diagnosis was septic arthritis. **C** to **E,** Follow-up radiographs obtained 1 **(C)**, 2 **(D)**, and 4 **(E)** years after the acute episode of septic arthritis demonstrate associated avascular necrosis with subsequent fragmentation and destruction of the proximal femoral epiphysis, broadening of the femoral neck, and consequent coxa vara/magna, which resulted in limb length discrepancy and hip instability.

Magnetic Resonance Imaging

MRI may be used to demonstrate early bone erosions and cartilage destruction (Box 24-5). In addition to joint effusions (see Figure 24-11), associated findings include synovial thickening and enhancement, septations, and debris within the joint.[34,127] Uncomplicated septic arthritis may cause abnormal signal within the marrow on both sides of the joint secondary to reactive edema, which may be difficult to be differentiated from osteomyelitis.[5,123,127] A secondary complication of septic arthritis includes soft tissue abscess, which demonstrates localized fluid collection with peripheral enhancement following gadolinium enhancement. Edema within periarticular structures or fluid collections in tendon sheaths will also show bright signal on T2-weighted images.[34] MRI is helpful for assessment of infection of the axial skeleton including the pelvis and spine. Septic sacroiliitis in children is uncommon but can present with nonspecific clinical symptoms such as back pain and can mimic diskitis, septic hip, intrapelvic and extrapelvic abscess, psoas abscess, osteomyelitis of the ilium, pyelonephritis, or appendicitis.[128]

MRI features of septic sacroiliitis include dark signal intensity on T1-weighted images and bright signal intensity on T2-weighted/short tau inversion recovery (STIR) images of the joint space and of the periarticular muscle tissue, as well as anterior and/or posterior subperiosteal infiltration.[128,129] Bone marrow edema and inflammatory changes of adjacent muscle tissue may be evident. Advanced stages of septic sacroiliitis can include demonstration of erosions, contrast enhancement, sequestration, and abscess formation. Subperiosteal infiltration is a specific sign not seen in other inflammatory causes of sacroiliitis.

In other inflammatory causes of sacroiliitis, such as the seronegative spondyloarthropathies, contrast enhancement of the intraarticular spaces, erosions, and anterior and posterior enhancement of the capsule and bone marrow edema may be seen. Sequestration and abscess formation do not typically occur in spondyloarthropathy-associated sacroiliitis. The late changes often encountered in the seronegative spondyloarthropathies, including subchondral sclerosis and transarticular bone bridges, are not typically found in septic sacroiliitis.

Computed Tomography

CT can demonstrate displacement or thinning of the periarticular fatty tissue layer, edema of adjacent muscles, and abscess formation. CT may be the best modality for evaluating certain joints such as the sternoclavicular joint.[126] However, MRI provides better soft tissue contrast and has been shown to be more sensitive than CT or skeletal scintigraphy.

> MRI is generally more sensitive than CT or scintigraphy for the detection of changes suggesting septic arthritis. In the sternoclavicular joints, however, CT may be a better choice.

CT-guided puncture of the SI joint may be needed when blood culture fails to isolate the pathogen. MRI can also be used to assess progression or regression at follow-up, recognizing that MR findings will be delayed relative to clinical improvement.[128,129]

BOX 24-5. MRI Features of Septic Arthritis

Effusion and periarticular edema
Synovial thickening, joint debris
Erosion
Abscesses
Bone marrow edema on either side of the joint

Scintigraphy

Radiographs are normal early on, whereas skeletal scintigraphy using T99M-MDP may reveal elevated tracer uptake within 2 to 6 days after the onset of clinical symptoms. Radionuclide imaging is therefore more sensitive than radiographs for the diagnosis of septic arthritis and osteomyelitis and may be used to localize the site of infection. In septic arthritis there is increased articular activity in the blood flow and blood pool phases, and there may be uptake in the juxtaarticular bones on the delayed phase due to hyperemia.[126] Increased intraarticular pressure from joint effusion may result in reduced radionuclide uptake within the epiphysis due to ischemia.

> Avascular necrosis may be a sequela of joint infection with capsular distension. The lack of blood flow will result in decreased epiphyseal isotope uptake on bone scan (a "cold" epiphysis) or in decreased epiphyseal enhancement on post-contrast MRI.

Transient Synovitis

Pain in the hip, also known as *irritable hip*, is a common presentation. Transient synovitis is the most common cause of childhood hip pain and can be mimicked by a number of more serious hip disorders including Legg-Calve-Perthes' disease, slipped capital femoral epiphysis, juvenile chronic arthritis, septic arthritis, and malignancy.[93] This disorder is acute, self-limiting, and of unknown origin and is most commonly seen in boys between the ages of 3 and 6 years. It usually affects one joint but can be bilateral in up to 5% of cases.[93] Although the clinical manifestation of septic arthritis of the hip may be similar to that of transient synovitis, pain and fever are generally more pronounced in septic arthritis. Various strategies for the workup of children with hip pain have been proposed, some based on clinical signs and laboratory findings, whereas others rely on imaging and aspiration of the hip joint. Imaging is usually performed with conventional radiography and/or ultrasound. It has been proposed that radiography should not be used in the primary evaluation of most children with hip pain, as it is generally normal or shows only subtle findings of joint effusion. Exceptions should be made in infants younger than 1 year and in children older then 8 years because of the lower incidence of transient synovitis in these age groups along with the higher risk of child abuse and septic arthritis in infancy and the occurrence of slipped capital femoral epiphysis in the older age group[93] (Box 24-6).

Radiography

Radiography is indicated in patients with a history of trauma, in patients with symptoms lasting more than 2 to 3 weeks to exclude Legg-Calve-Perthes' disease, and in patients with suspected septic arthritis for documentation and follow-up of possible osteomyelitis.[11]

Ultrasonography

Ultrasonography is a sensitive and noninvasive method of detecting hip joint effusion in transient synovitis.[129a,b] It is performed by scanning along the anterior aspect of the femoral neck, as this is where fluid tends to accumulate within the hip joint (Figure 24-14).[129b] However, the role of ultrasonography is uncertain, changing

BOX 24-6. Evaluation of Hip Pain in Children

Ultrasound is suggested for initial evaluation of most children with hip pain (exceptions below).
Radiography is the first imaging technique in patients < 1 year.
Radiography is the first imaging technique in children > 8 years old.
Radiography is suggested if there is a history of trauma.
Radiography is suggested if symptoms last > 2-3 weeks.
Radiography is suggested if there is a suspicion of septic arthritis or osteomyelitis (although radiographic findings tend to occur late in the course of the disease).

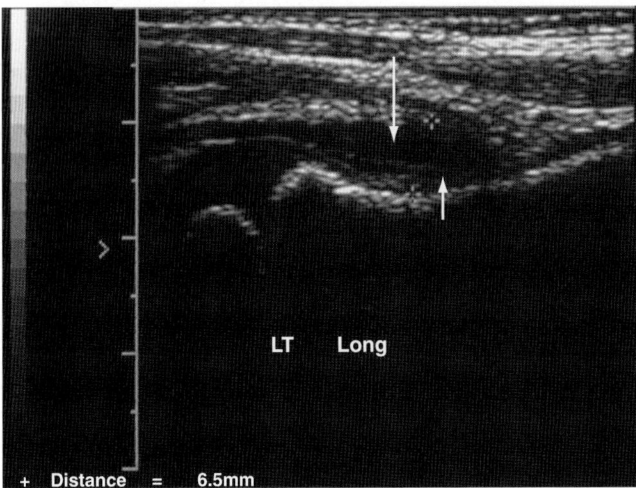

FIGURE 24-14. Transient synovitis of the hip. Sagittal scan of the anterior aspect of the proximal left femur in a 1.5-year-old boy with fever, pain, and difficulty moving the left lower extremity for 1 week shows synovial hypertrophy *(short arrow)* and joint effusion (black, *long arrow*) within the anterior synovial recess of the left hip. This patient was diagnosed as presenting with transient synovitis of the left hip.

management in fewer than 1% of cases in large series. Aspiration is required if infection is a consideration.[127]

Scintigraphy, MRI, CT, Arthrography

Other modalities such as bone scans, CT, and MRI are not initially used in evaluation of irritable hips because of their higher cost and limited benefit. On MRI there is evidence of joint effusion but no evidence of bone abnormality.[127,129]

NONINFLAMMATORY ARTHRITIS

Hemophilic Arthropathy

Hemophilia is an X-linked recessive disorder characterized by abnormality of the coagulation mechanism. It may be secondary to a deficiency in factor VIII as in classic hemophilia (hemophilia A) or secondary to a deficiency of factor IX in Christmas disease (hemophilia B).[130] Hemarthrosis occurs in approximately 75% to 90% of patients with hemophilia.[131] The most commonly affected joints are the knees, elbows, and ankles. Hemorrhage may be secondary to trauma or may occur spontaneously.[132] Recurrent hemarthrosis leads to breakdown of extravasated blood products from synovial vessels, which concur to the development of synovial inflammation and proliferation.[133] The age of onset and frequency of hemarthrosis is determined by the level of factor deficiency, which can be severe (factor VIII or IX baseline activity $\leq$ 1%), moderate (residual activity 2% to 5%), or mild (residual activity > 5%).[134] The breakdown of extravasated blood from synovial vessels ultimately leads to synovitis, cartilage loss, and subchondral bone irregularity. With hyperemia and prolonged inflammation, epiphyseal overgrowth, early growth plate fusion, and fibrosis of ligaments can be seen.[135] Medical imaging of joints in children with hemophilia is important for detecting abnormalities, staging their severity, and following the effects of treatment.

Radiography

Radiographic changes depend on the age of the patient at the time of the bleed, the site of the bleed, and the acuteness/chronicity of disease. Deposition of iron in the synovium leads to increased soft tissue density around joints. The radiographic changes may be identical to JIA, but clinical findings and typical joint involvement help distinguish these entities (Box 24-7). Radiodense joint effusions and subchondral changes (Figure 24-15) are commonly seen in hemophilic arthropathy. In the knee, classic radiographic findings include squaring of the femoral condyles and patella and widened intercondylar notch.[136]

Ultrasonography

Ultrasound may provide a useful complementary modality in evaluating musculoskeletal involvement of joints in children with hemophilia. It is easily accessible and does not require sedation. It is also sensitive for soft tissue changes such as effusions and synovial hyperplasia. However, it is user dependent. Previous studies have evaluated ultrasonographic images of joints of hemophilic children with regard to the imaging features,[137,138] degree of severity of arthropathy,[139] and responsiveness to treatment[139a] and have shown a potential role of ultrasound for assessment of hemophilic arthropathy, most notably in its early stage. Further validation of ultrasonography as an outcome measure to guide response to treatment and to enable follow-up of children under prophylaxis is required.

Magnetic Resonance Imaging

MRI may be used to determine whether hemarthrosis has occurred so that therapy with coagulation factors can be administered to prevent chronic joint damage.[130,131] Acute hemarthrosis and chronic joint effusion may be indistinguishable with low signal on T1-weighted images and high signal on T2-weighted images.[133] Subacute hemarthrosis has usually high signal on both T1-weighted and T2-weighted images (Figure 24-16) related to the presence of extracellular methhemoglobin.[133] The synovial thickening often has areas of low signal on T1-weighted and T2-weighted images related to fibrosis or hemosiderin deposition.[133] Gadolinium better delineates the extent of synovial thickening, which shows less enhancement compared with rheumatoid arthritis. This is likely secondary to hypovascular connective tissue and hemosiderin deposition within the synovium.[140] MRI detects early localized or more diffuse changes within cartilage. Gradient echo imaging is helpful for evaluation of hemosiderin and cartilage abnormalities.[131] Subchondral cysts (see Figure 24-16) may result from intraosseous bleeding, and rarely pseudotumors may develop secondary to hemorrhage in bone or the periarticular soft tissues. Signal characteristics are variable depending on the age of the hematoma.[137]

BOX 24-7. Imaging Features of Hemophilia

RADIOGRAPHS

Joint effusion (dense effusion reflects hemosiderin deposition)
Squaring of femoral condyles
Wide intercondylar notch
Overgrowth of epiphyses
Subchondral cysts
Cartilage space narrowing

MRI

Intraarticular hemorrhage or effusion
(Acute hemorrhage or effusion: low signal on T1-weighted images, high signal on T2-weighted images; subacute hemorrhage: high signal on T1-weighted and T2-weighted images)
Low signal synovial proliferation with minimal contrast enhancement
Subchondral cysts, larger "pseudocysts"
Hematomas

Currently Available Imaging Scales for Assessment of Hemophilic Arthropathy

In order to follow progression of joint disease more systematically, two radiographic scoring systems for imaging children's joints with hemophilic arthropathy were developed in the 1970s. The Arnold-Hilgartner scale[141] is a progressive metric in which the stage of disease is given according to the worst findings in the joint. The Pettersson scale[142] is an additive scoring system in which the presence of different radiographic findings are weighted and added to form a final sum in keeping with the stage of disease.

Improved therapy has led to the need for more sensitive tools such as MRI. Of the several other MRI scales, two scoring systems[143,144] have been most widely used. The Denver MRI scale is a progressive metric in which the most severe change in the joint determines the score, mirroring the Arnold-Hilgartner radiographic scale. The European MRI scoring scheme gives a final score in the shape of four concatenated numerical values where each value is based on a progressive metric specific to an aspect of the disease, mirroring the Pettersson radiographic scale and separating the different pathologic components. More recently, the international MRI expert working group of the International Prophylaxis Study Group (IPSG) has presented a scoring method that includes a combined 10-step progressive scale and a 20-step additive scale, encompassing both the progressive and additive concepts (Figure 24-17), in an effort to facilitate international comparison of data.[144a]

Computed Tomography

Hemophilic pseudotumors constitute an uncommon and severe complication of hemophilia that may affect intraarticular[145] or extraarticular[146] regions; however, they tend to occur in adults.[148] CT and MRI have important roles in detecting pseudotumors, especially in the pelvis.[137,148] CT is useful in detecting both the extent of soft tissue masses and the involvement of bone. Pseudotumors contain coagulated blood and are surrounded by a thick wall. Contrast-enhanced CT is useful in determining the thickness of the wall. In the acute stage, the center of the pseudotumor is hypodense on CT, but the periphery is isodense and indistinguishable from surrounding muscle.[149]

Scintigraphy

Investigational studies have used blood pool imaging to evaluate the effectiveness of radiosynovectomy using ^{90}Y citrate colloid,[150,186] Re sulfide colloid,[150] or ^{32}P colloidal suspension[151] injected into the joints of patients with hemophilic synovitis. Follow-up examinations with soft tissue scintigraphy using methylene diphosphonate (MDP) demonstrated significant joint improvement and a 3-month pain relief following radiosynovectomy[151]; however, further clinical validation is required.

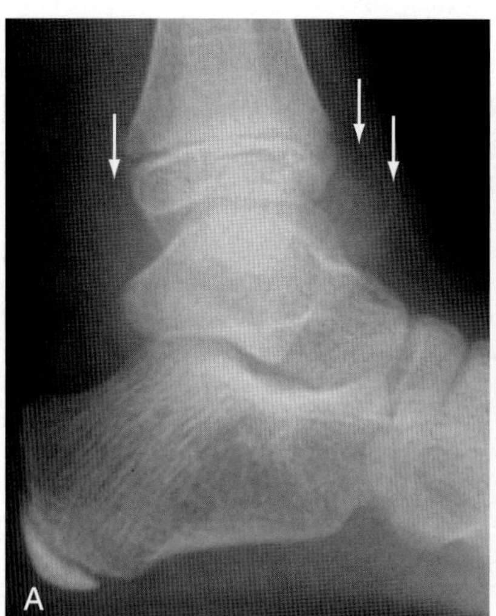

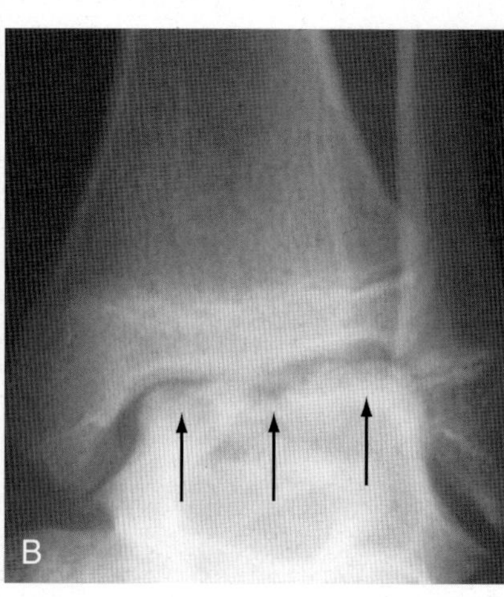

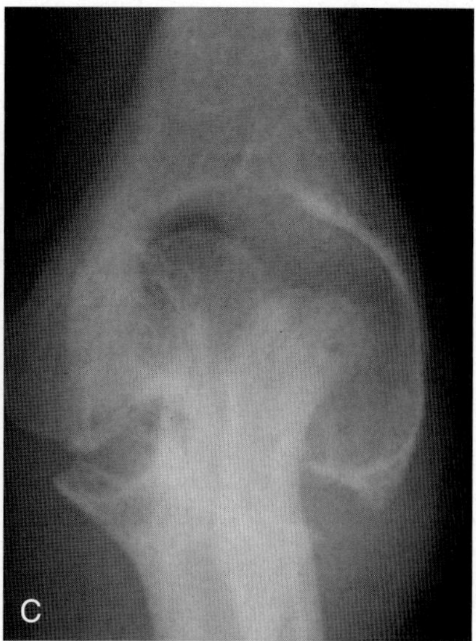

FIGURE 24-15. Radiographic findings of hemophilic arthropathy. **A,** A lateral radiograph shows bulging of the anterior and posterior ankle joint recesses due to joint effusion/hemarthrosis *(arrows)*. **B,** An anteroposterior (AP) radiograph of the ankle shows subchondral cysts, erosions of the talar dome *(arrows)*, and cartilage space narrowing. **C,** An AP radiograph of the elbow shows marked joint destruction and epiphyseal overgrowth.

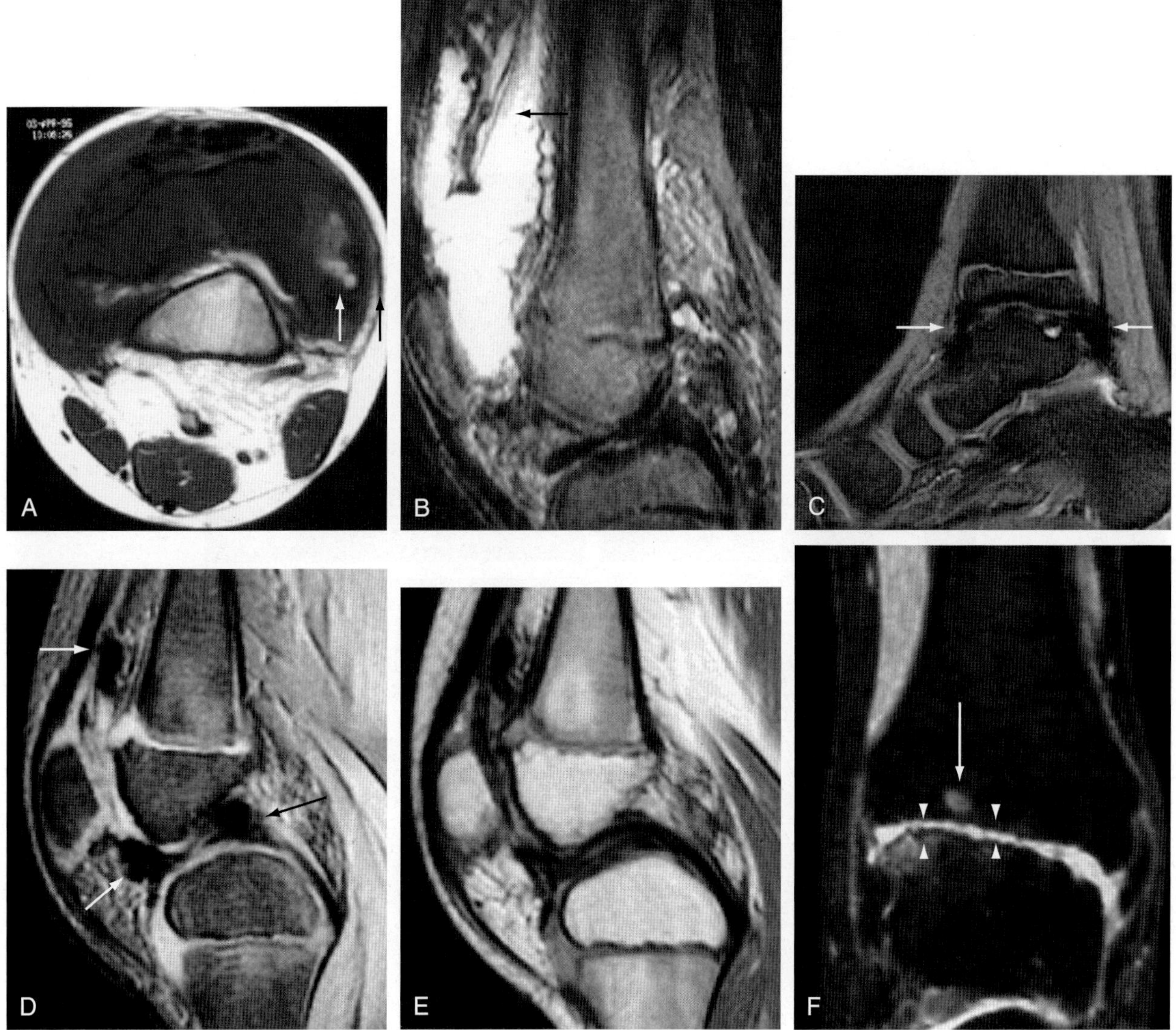

FIGURE 24-16. MRI findings in hemophilia. MRI has the advantage over conventional radiography in the ability to demonstrate hemarthrosis and its sequelae. **A,** T1-weighted axial image of the knee shows hemarthrosis as documented by high signal intensity *(arrows)* on both the T1-weighted and **(B)** T2-weighted image with fat suppression. (*Arrows* represent areas of extracellular methemoglobin.) **C,** Multiphase gradient recalled image of the ankle demonstrates the low signal intensity of hemosiderin deposition. **D,** Multiphase gradient recalled sagittal image of the knee shows the low signal intensity of hemosiderin *(arrows)* resulting from chronic bleeding into the joint. **E,** T1-weighted image of the knee (same patient as in **D**) shows the low signal hemosiderin deposits but not as well as on the gradient recalled images. **F,** A fat-suppressed T1-weighted image of the ankle provides better assessment of cartilage loss *(arrowheads)* and subchondral changes *(arrow)*.

Extraarticular Findings: Intracranial Bleeding/Abdominal Bleeding

Bleeding into extraarticular anatomic structures may be life threatening, especially if it affects the central nervous system. Orbital subperiosteal hemorrhage may develop from the orbital extension of a subgaleal hemorrhage. CT scan of the brain and orbits may easily lead to the correct diagnosis.[152]

In hemophilic pseudotumors, CT and MRI are helpful to guide therapeutic procedures such as local radiotherapy[145] in intracranial[153] and extracranial[146] locations.

Intraabdominal hemorrhage may include bleeding into choledochal cysts[154] and intramural ureteral[155] and retroperitoneal[156] hemorrhage. Ultrasound may suggest the presence of hemorrhagic content within a choledochal cyst, which can be confirmed by MRI. CT may help detecting the extension of the hemorrhage and dissection of the ureteral layers longitudinally,[155] the potential extension of the bleeding into the kidneys,[156] and the need for surgical intervention.

AUTOIMMUNE CONNECTIVE TISSUE DISEASES

Joint findings are generally limited in connective tissue disorders. In juvenile dermatomyositis (JDM), a multisystem disorder primarily affecting blood vessels, there may be joint effusions but erosions are not typically found. MRI may be used to confirm myositis either in those with JIA, dermatomyositis, or mixed connective tissue disorders.

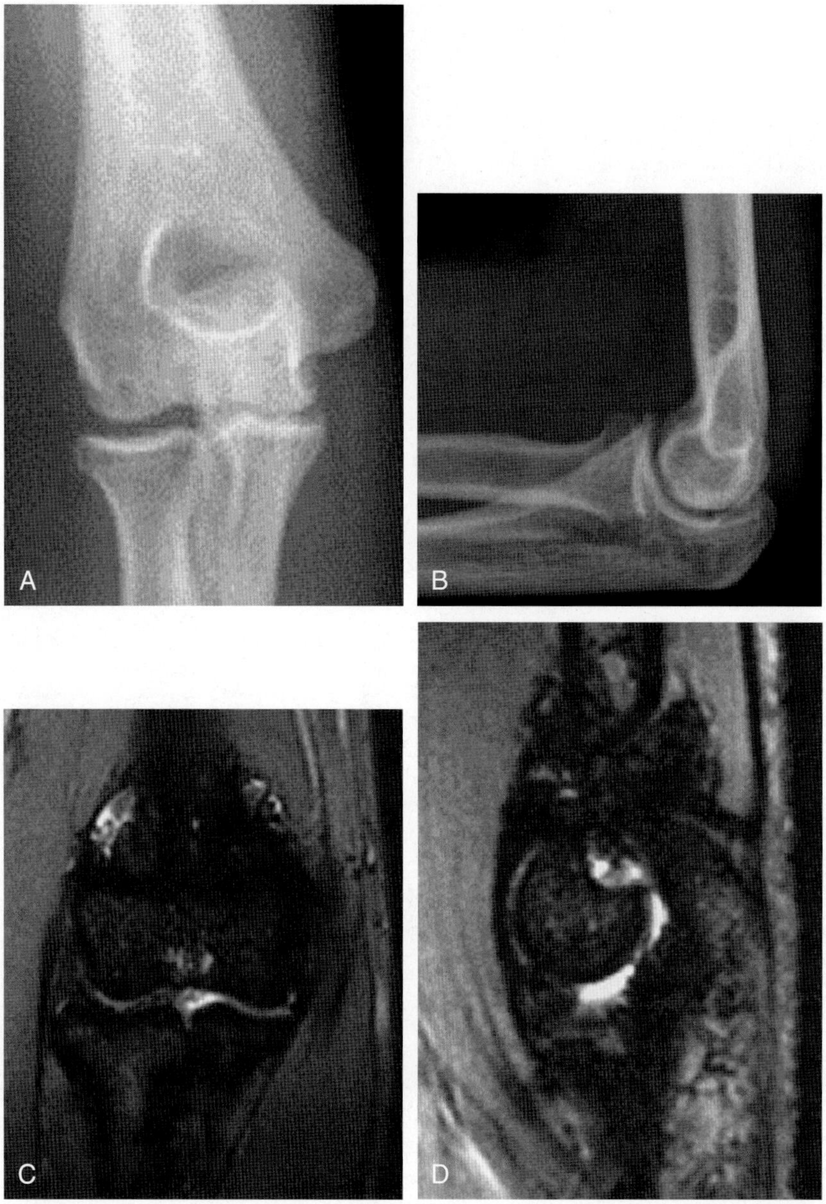

FIGURE 24-17. MRI of hemophilia. MRI has better sensitivity than conventional radiography for evaluation of soft tissue and osteochondral changes. **A,** Anteroposterior and **(B)** lateral radiographs of the left elbow of a 16-year-old hemophilic boy. These radiographs received a score of 1 (slightly enlarged epiphysis) according to the Pettersson scoring system and a score of 2 (overgrowth of epiphysis; no cysts; no narrowing of cartilage space) according to the Arnold-Hilgartner scoring system. **C,** Coronal and **(D)** sagittal gradient echo images of the elbow received a score of 10 (> 50% cartilage loss = 10; large hemosiderin deposition = 6; synovial hypertrophy = 6; mild effusion = 1; full surface erosions = 8) according to the progressive component of the Compatible MRI Scale and a score of 8 (large synovial hypertrophy = 3; hemosiderin deposition = 1; subchondral bone changes = 2 including any surface erosion and erosion in at least one bone; cartilage loss = 2 including any loss of joint cartilage height and full-thickness loss in at least one bone).

Juvenile Dermatomyositis

JDM is an autoimmune inflammatory myopathy characterized by diffuse nonsuppurative inflammation of muscle fibres and skin.[157] The inflammatory infiltrates are predominantly perivascular or in the interfascicular septa or around the fascicles.[158] It most commonly presents between the ages of 5 and 14 years.[159] Clinical findings include severe proximal muscle weakness, fatigue, heliotrope rash (pink-purple rash on the face and knuckles), and underlying vasculitic changes.[159,160]

Musculoskeletal System

Radiography

In the acute stage of JDM, radiologic changes are minimal. However, incipient soft tissue swelling and subcutaneous edema (Figure 24-18) represented by blurring of fatty tissue planes can be noted in the proximal appendicular skeleton in some cases. The muscles of the scapular and pelvic girdles are most frequently affected and their involvement is typically symmetric (Figure 24-19).[161,162] In chronic disease, radiographs demonstrate

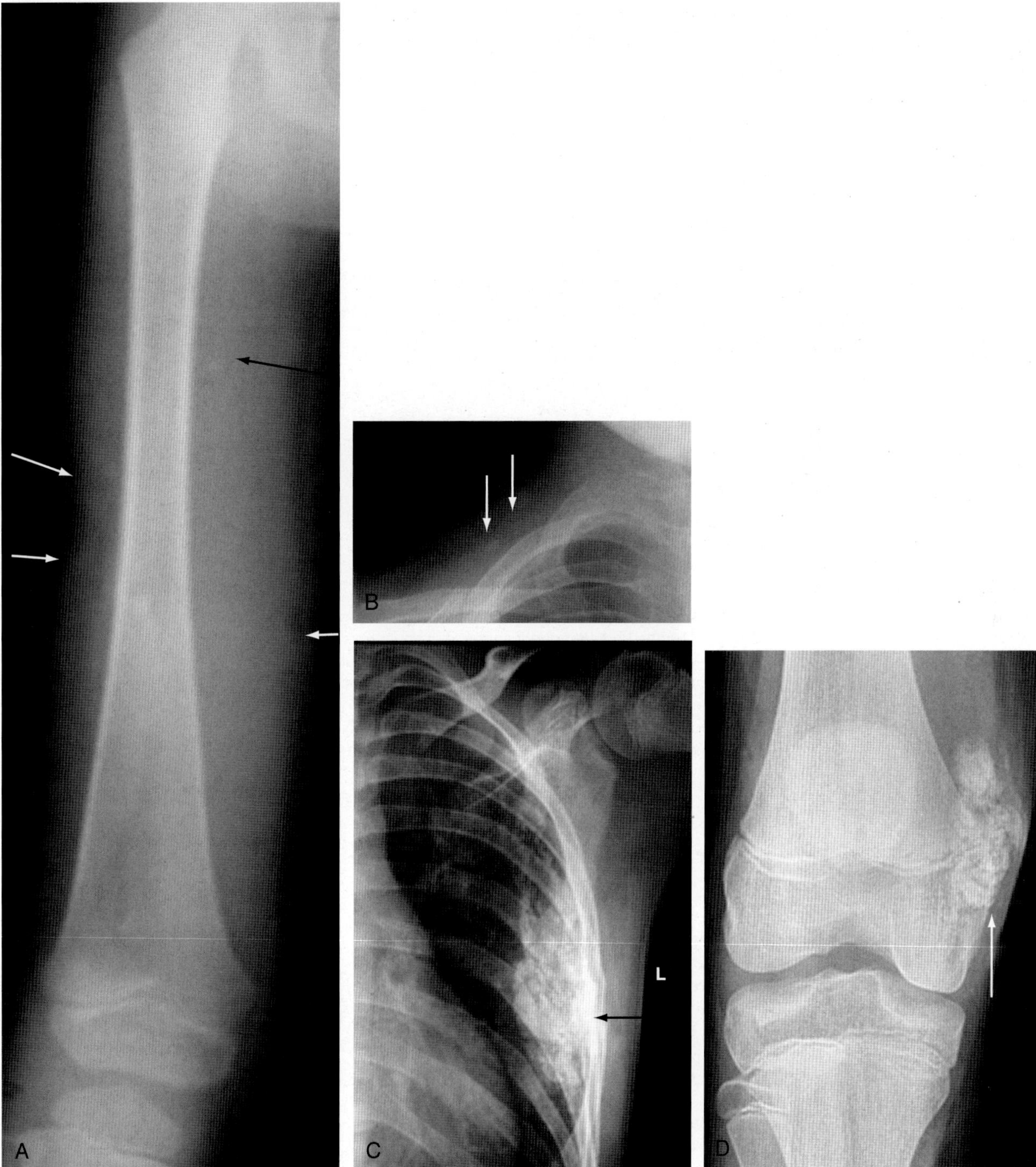

FIGURE 24-18. Juvenile dermatomyositis. The different stages of evolution of the radiographic features of juvenile dermatomyositis are shown. **A,** Frontal radiograph of the left femur demonstrates scattered calcific deposits *(arrows)* in the soft tissues of the thigh. **B,** Anteroposterior (AP) radiograph of the supraclavicular region shows scattered calcifications *(arrows)* in the soft tissues of the right shoulder girdle. **C,** AP radiograph of the chest shows massive deposits of calcium in the soft tissues of the left lateral chest wall. **D,** AP radiograph of the knee shows large deposits of calcium along the medial aspect of the left knee joint *(arrow).*

loss of soft tissue bulk secondary to muscle atrophy. There may also be marked osteoporosis of the long bones and vertebral bodies. The most characteristic finding of chronic disease, however, is the deposition of calcium in the soft tissues (see Figure 24-19), which is identified in 25% to 50% of the cases.[163] The calcium deposits may present as subcutaneous plaques, nodules, periarticular calcific foci, and large clumps or sheets of calcium within the musculature or subcutaneous tissue.[164] The arthritis associated with JDM is usually transient and nondeforming in nature.[164]

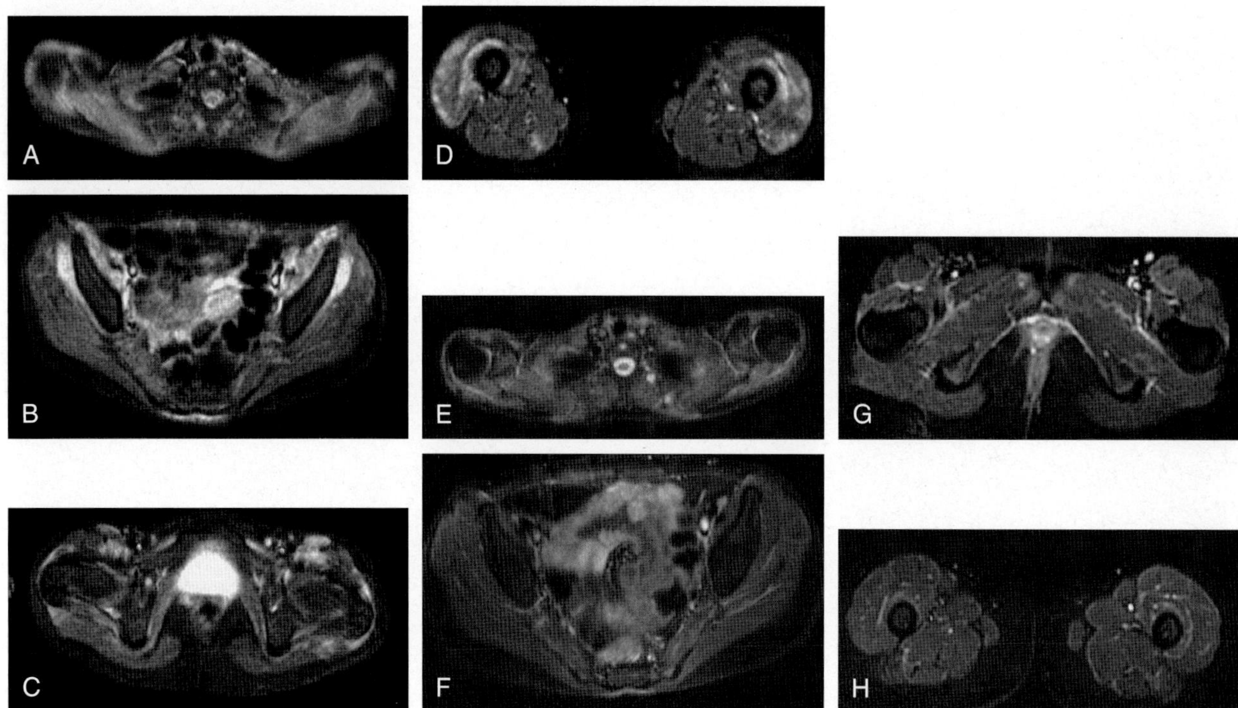

FIGURE 24-19. MRI of active and quiescent dermatomyositis. **A** to **D**, Axial inversion recovery images in a 15-year-old boy with active juvenile dermatomyositis. **A**, Axial image through the shoulder girdle shows diffuse increased signal intensity involving the sternocleidomastoid, triceps, long and short heads of the biceps, infraspinatus, subscapularis, teres minor, deltoid, and spinal muscles bilaterally. **B**, Axial image through the pelvis shows increased signal in the iliacus and gluteus minimus muscles. **C**, Axial image through the hips shows gluteus minimus and intermedius increased signal. **D**, Axial image through the distal femurs shows increased signal especially in the vastus lateralis and intermedius muscles bilaterally. **E** to **H**, Corresponding MR images obtained 3 years later, during remission of the disease, demonstrate a remarkable reduction in the signal intensity within the musculature of the shoulder girdle, pelvic girdle, and thigh.

Ultrasonography

Ultrasonographic scanning of the involved musculature shows diffusely increased echogenicity of the soft tissues and acoustic shadowing within the musculature in regions that correspond to calcium deposits. Histopathologically, muscle lipomatosis significantly correlates to muscle echogenicity.[158] Other sonographic findings that may be seen in JDM include atrophy, decreased muscular bulk, and soft tissue fasciculation as well as tenosynovitis and soft tissue nodularities.[165]

Magnetic Resonance Imaging

Ultrasonography and MRI have a similar capacity to demonstrate the features of inflammatory muscle disease, but MRI is more sensitive for the detection of edema, representing inflammation in the acute phase of the disease. Although both MRI and ultrasonography allow guided biopsy and aspiration of muscle abnormalities,[166-169] ultrasonography has the advantage over MRI of not requiring sedation for younger children. MRI reveals increased water content (edema) within infarcted muscles as a result of the vasculitis.[170] This intramuscular edema is depicted as increased signal intensity on T2-weighted and STIR MR images (see Figure 24-19). In fact, T2-relaxation time can be used as a quantitative measure of muscle inflammation (see Figure 24-19) and correlates well with other measures of disease activity.[171] Note, however, that because physical exercise can induce changes that mimic inflammation at MRI of muscle, children with JDM should be at rest at least 30 minutes before acquisition of MR images to assess disease activity.[172]

In chronic disease, focal areas of low signal intensity are usually seen on all MRI sequences, which represent calcific and fibrotic foci. Focal areas of increased signal intensity on T1-weighted images representing partial fatty replacement of muscles and tenosynovitis-related changes may also be identified on MRI.[171,173]

Computed Tomography

Although CT does not detect inflammatory changes in muscle tissue, it is the modality of choice for identifying calcifications in soft tissues, which are characteristically associated with JDM.[158] It also allows quantification of muscle atrophy and fatty replacement in deep muscles.

Scintigraphy

Whole body ^{201}Tl-chloride and 99m-Tc muscle scintigraphy is a potentially useful tool to investigate occult muscle groups affected by dermatomyositis; however, further investigation in the pediatric population is required.[174] Furthermore, bone scans with 99m-Tc-MDP can function as auxiliary tools to evaluate calcinosis in patients with JDM.[175]

New MRI Techniques

Magnetic Resonance Spectroscopy

P-31 magnetic resonance spectroscopy (MRS) has emerged as an imaging modality able to characterize metabolic abnormalities in vivo and to localize nonhomogeneous inflammation in JDM patients.[159] It uses the same technology as conventional MRI to determine noninvasively the biochemical composition of tissues and is sensitive to the different atomic nuclei of biologic tissues. Data are usually displayed as spectra with peaks reflecting the chemical structure and concentration of individual metabolites. Studies in humans have used phosphorus (^{31}P-MRS)[176] for evaluation of biochemical abnormalities in JDM.[159,177]

Biochemical abnormalities in JDM are probably related to decreased delivery of energy substrates and oxygen expressed by reduced levels of ATP and phosphocreatine within the muscle region of interest. The decreases in capillary bed volume and cytochrome oxidase activity in the mitochondria would result in focal ischemic muscle damage, perifascicular atrophy, and necrosis.[178,179] Previous studies[159,177] showed defective oxidative phosphorylation in the mitochondria of diseased JDM muscles, which was in accordance with clinical symptoms. An additional potential role of this technique is to monitor joints after the disappearance of inflammation and normalization of serum levels of muscle enzymes.[179a]

Diffusion Tensor Imaging

Diffusion-weighted imaging (DWI) allows recording the translational movement (Brownian motion) of water molecules and the free water diffusion that occurs in all tissues through the MR software.[180,181] It is based on the suppression of signal intensity of free diffusing water. The degree of diffusion is dependent on viscosity, barriers to free movement, and temperature. With the use of a paramagnetic tridimensional gradient it is possible to record the magnetic signal coming from water protons during reduced or increased molecular movement in damaged tissues. The degree of water proton mobility can be quantified by a parameter known as *apparent diffusion coefficient* (ADC).[176] Diffusion tensor imaging (DTI) is a more sophisticated form of DWI and allows determination of the directionality as well as the magnitude, form, trend, and integrity of a particular anatomic region.[176] With this technique, diffusion-sensitizing gradients are applied in at least six different directions in space (not only in three, as seen on DWI), allowing detection of directionality as well as evaluation of the extent of water diffusion. In the future, this technique may find a definite clinical application in assessing the in vivo structure of the musculature,[182-184] which could be used as an adjunct diagnostic tool for JDM and in depicting the architecture of the zones of cartilage.[185] This could be helpful in the follow-up of JIA and hemophilic arthropathy.

Foreign Body Synovitis

Foreign body synovitis usually presents with a monoarticular synovitis (Figure 24-20) and may be suggested by the presence of a puncture wound. However, there is often a delay in diagnosis, especially if there is no history of injury and the foreign body is difficult to detect. Wood splinters, especially plant thorns such as palm or blackthorn, may produce a chronic synovitis or tendinitis. Extraction of the foreign body is essential for recovery, and identification of the foreign body by imaging will allow a localized synovectomy.[186] Plant thorns have slightly higher density than soft tissue and may be detected on CT. Non-radiopaque foreign bodies may also be identified with ultrasound or MRI.

> Foreign bodies that are not opaque on radiographs may be detected on ultrasound or MRI.

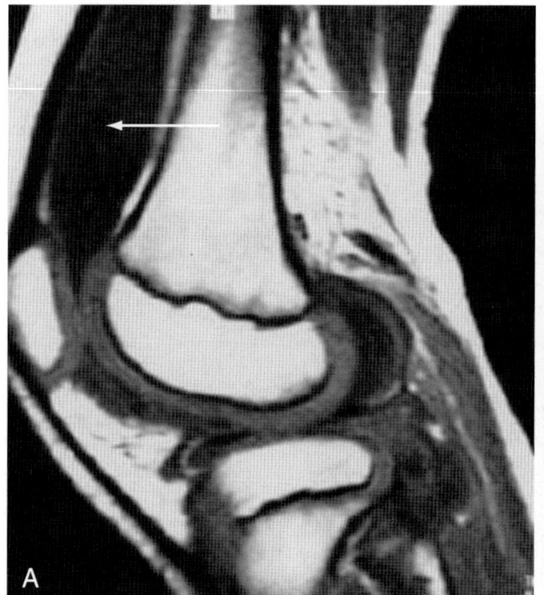

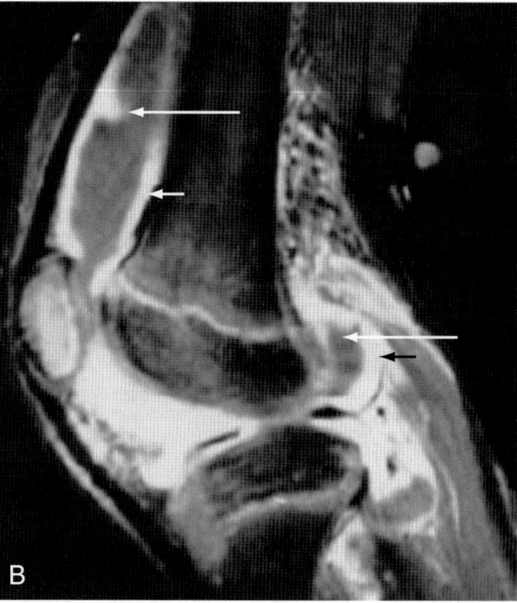

FIGURE 24-20. Thorn-induced synovitis. Ten-year-old boy with chronic right knee swelling for 3 months. Synovial biopsy showed granulomatous inflammation and the presence of birefringent material of plant origin. **A,** Unenhanced and **(B)** contrast-enhanced fat-suppressed sagittal T1-weighted images of the right knee show a moderate joint effusion (dark, *long arrows*) and enhanced synovium *(short arrows)* at the suprapatellar and posterior recesses of the knee. Figure B reprinted with permission from Babyn PS, Doria AS: Radiologic investigation of rheumatic diseases, *Rheum Dis Clin North Am* 33(3):403-440, 2007.

REFERENCES

1. Davidson J: Juvenile idiopathic arthritis: a clinical overview, *Eur J Radiol* 33: 128-134, 2000.
2. Petty RE, Southwood TR, Baum J et al: Revision of the proposed classification criteria for juvenile idiopathic arthritis: Durban, 1997, *J Rheumatol* 25:1991-1994, 1998.
3. Schanberg LE, Sandstrom MJ: Causes of pain in children with arthritis, *Rheum Dis Clin North Am* 25:31-53, vi, 1999.
4. Kaye JJ: Arthritis: roles of radiography and other imaging techniques in evaluation, *Radiology* 177:601-608, 1990.
5. Gylys-Morin VM: MR imaging of pediatric musculoskeletal inflammatory and infectious disorders, *Magn Reson Imaging Clin N Am* 6:537-559, 1998.
6. Cohen PA, Job-Deslandre CH, Lalande G et al: Overview of the radiology of juvenile idiopathic arthritis (JIA), *Eur J Radiol* 33:94-101, 2000.
7. Patriquin HB, Camerlain M, Trias A: Late sequelae of juvenile rheumatoid arthritis of the hip: a follow-up study into adulthood, *Pediatr Radiol* 14:151-157, 1984.
8. Kellgren JH, Jefrey MR, Ball J: The epidemiology of chronic rheumatism. In Kellgren JH, Jefrey MR, Ball J (eds): *Atlas of standard radiographs of arthritis*, Oxford, 1963, Blackwell Scientific Publications.
9. Larsen A, Dale K, Eek M: Radiographic evaluation of rheumatoid arthritis and related conditions by standard reference films, *Acta Radiol Diagn (Stockh)* 18:481-491, 1977.
10. Pettersson H, Rydholm U: Radiologic classification of knee joint destruction in juvenile chronic arthritis, *Pediatr Radiol* 14:419-421, 1984.
11. Sharp JT, Lidsky MD, Collins LC et al: Methods of scoring the progression of radiologic changes in rheumatoid arthritis. Correlation of radiologic, clinical and laboratory abnormalities, *Arthritis Rheum* 14:706-720, 1971.
12. Steinbrocker O, Traeger CH, Batterman RC: Therapeutic criteria in rheumatoid arthritis, *J Am Med Assoc* 140:659-662, 1949.
13. Brook A, Corbett M: Radiographic changes in early rheumatoid disease, *Ann Rheum Dis* 36:71-73, 1977.
14. Brook A, Fleming A, Corbett M: Relationship of radiological change to clinical outcome in rheumatoid arthritis, *Ann Rheum Dis* 36:274-275, 1977.
15. Regan-Smith MG, O'Connor GT, Kwoh CK et al: Lack of correlation between the Steinbrocker staging of hand radiographs and the functional health status of individuals with rheumatoid arthritis, *Arthritis Rheum* 32:128-133, 1989.
16. Kaye JJ, Fuchs HA, Moseley JW et al: Problems with the Steinbrocker staging system for radiographic assessment of the rheumatoid hand and wrist, *Invest Radiol* 25:536-544, 1990.
17. Scott DL, Houssien DA, Laasonen L: Proposed modification to Larsen's scoring methods for hand and wrist radiographs, *Br J Rheumatol* 34:56, 1955.
18. van der Heijde D: How to read radiographs according to the Sharp/van der Heijde method, *J Rheumatol,* 26:743-745, 1999.
19. Cellerini M, Salti S, Trapani S et al: Correlation between clinical and ultrasound assessment of the knee in children with mono-articular or pauci-articular juvenile rheumatoid arthritis, *Pediatr Radiol* 29:117-123, 1999.
20. Eich GF, Halle F, Hodler J et al: Juvenile chronic arthritis: imaging of the knees and hips before and after intraarticular steroid injection, *Pediatr Radiol* 24:558-563, 1994.
21. Lamer S, Sebag GH: MRI and ultrasound in children with juvenile chronic arthritis, *Eur J Radiol* 33:85-93, 2000.
22. Scheel AK, Hermann KG, Kahler E et al: A novel ultrasonographic synovitis scoring system suitable for analyzing finger joint inflammation in rheumatoid arthritis, *Arthritis Rheum* 52:733-743, 2005.
23. Ruhoy MK, Tucker L, McCauley RG: Hypertrophic bursopathy of the subacromial-subdeltoid bursa in juvenile rheumatoid arthritis: sonographic appearance, *Pediatr Radiol* 26:353-355, 1996.
24. El Miedany YM, Housny IH, Mansour HM et al: Ultrasound versus MRI in the evaluation of juvenile idiopathic arthritis of the knee, *Joint Bone Spine* 68:222-230, 2001.
25. Sureda D, Quiroga S, Arnal C et al: Juvenile rheumatoid arthritis of the knee: evaluation with US, *Radiology* 190:403-406, 1994.
26. Backhaus M, Burmester GR, Sandrock D et al: Prospective two year follow up study comparing novel and conventional imaging procedures in patients with arthritic finger joints, *Ann Rheum Dis* 61:895-904, 2002.
27. Grassi W, Filippucci E, Farina A et al: Ultrasonography in the evaluation of bone erosions, *Ann Rheum Dis* 60:98-103, 2001.
28. Wakefield RJ, Gibbon WW, Conaghan PG et al: The value of sonography in the detection of bone erosions in patients with rheumatoid arthritis: a comparison with conventional radiography, *Arthritis Rheum* 43:2762-2770, 2000.
29. Weidekamm C, Koller M, Weber M et al: Diagnostic value of high-resolution B-mode and doppler sonography for imaging of hand and finger joints in rheumatoid arthritis, *Arthritis Rheum* 48:325-333, 2003.
30. Filippucci E, Farina A, Carotti M et al: Grey scale and power Doppler sonographic changes induced by intra-articular steroid injection treatment, *Ann Rheum Dis* 63:740-743, 2004.
31. Karmazyn B, Bowyer SL, Schmidt KM, et al: Ultrasonography of metacarpophalangeal joints in children with juvenile rheumatoid arthritis, *Pediatr Radiol* 37(5): 475-482, 2005.
32. Newman JS, Laing TJ, McCarthy CJ et al: Power Doppler sonography of synovitis: assessment of therapeutic response—preliminary observations, *Radiology* 198:582-584, 1996.
33. Doria AS, Kiss MH, Lotito AP et al: Juvenile rheumatoid arthritis of the knee: evaluation with contrast-enhanced color Doppler ultrasound, *Pediatr Radiol* 31:524-531, 2001.
34. White EM: Magnetic resonance imaging in synovial disorders and arthropathy of the knee, *Magn Reson Imaging Clin N Am* 2:451-461, 1994.
35. Doria AS: Comparative analysis between three-dimensional and bi-dimensional assessment in magnetic resonance imaging—clinical applications in knees in juvenile rheumatoid arthritis (JRA), *Radiol Bras* 33:129-137, 2000.
36. Ostergaard M, Stoltenberg M, Gideon P et al: Changes in synovial membrane and joint effusion volumes after intraarticular methylprednisolone. Quantitative assessment of inflammatory and destructive changes in arthritis by MRI, *J Rheumatol* 23:1151-1161, 1996.
37. Kuseler A, Pedersen TK, Herlin T et al: Contrast enhanced magnetic resonance imaging as a method to diagnose early inflammatory changes in the temporomandibular joint in children with juvenile chronic arthritis, *J Rheumatol* 25:1406-1412, 1998.
38. Taylor DB, Babyn P, Blaser S et al: MR evaluation of the temporomandibular joint in juvenile rheumatoid arthritis, *J Comput Assist Tomogr* 17:449-454, 1993.
39. Chung C, Coley BD, Martin LC: Rice bodies in juvenile rheumatoid arthritis, *AJR Am J Roentgenol* 170:698-700, 1998.
40. Disler DG, McCauley TR, Wirth CR et al: Detection of knee hyaline cartilage defects using fat-suppressed three-dimensional spoiled gradient-echo MR imaging: comparison with standard MR imaging and correlation with arthroscopy, *AJR Am J Roentgenol* 165:377-382, 1995.
41. Disler DG: Fat-suppressed three-dimensional spoiled gradient-recalled MR imaging: assessment of articular and physeal hyaline cartilage, *AJR Am J Roentgenol* 169: 1117-1123, 1997.
42. Recht MP, Piraino DW, Paletta GA et al: Accuracy of fat-suppressed three-dimensional spoiled gradient-echo FLASH MR imaging in the detection of patellofemoral articular cartilage abnormalities, *Radiology* 198:209-212, 1996.
43. Gold GE, Fuller SE, Hargreaves BA et al: Driven equilibrium magnetic resonance imaging of articular cartilage: initial clinical experience, *J Magn Reson Imaging* 21:476-481, 2005.
44. Hargreaves BA, Gold GE, Lang PK et al: MR imaging of articular cartilage using driven equilibrium, *Magn Reson Med* 42:695-703, 1999.
45. Eckstein F, Sittek H, Milz S et al: The morphology of articular cartilage assessed by magnetic resonance imaging (MRI). Reproducibility and anatomical correlation, *Surg Radiol Anat* 16:429-438, 1994.
46. Mosher TJ, Pruett SW: Magnetic resonance imaging of superficial cartilage lesions: role of contrast in lesion detection, *J Magn Reson Imaging* 10:178-182, 1999.
47. Reeder SB, Wen Z, Yu H et al: Multicoil Dixon chemical species separation with an iterative least-squares estimation method, *Magn Reson Med* 51:35-45, 2004.
48. Duerk JL, Lewin JS, Wendt M et al: Remember true FISP? A high SNR, near 1-second imaging method for T2-like contrast in interventional MRI at .2 T, *J Magn Reson Imaging* 8:203-208, 1998.
49. Vasanawala SS, Hargreaves BA, Pauly JM et al: Rapid musculoskeletal MRI with phase-sensitive steady-state free precession: comparison with routine knee MRI, *AJR Am J Roentgenol* 184:1450-1455, 2005.
50. Eckstein F, Charles HC, Buck RJ et al: Accuracy and precision of quantitative assessment of cartilage morphology by magnetic resonance imaging at 3.0T, *Arthritis Rheum* 52:3132-3136, 2005.
51. Kornaat PR, Reeder SB, Koo S et al: MR imaging of articular cartilage at 1.5T and 3.0T: comparison of SPGR and SSFP sequences, *Osteoarthritis Cartilage* 13:338-344, 2005.
52. Imhof H, Nobauer-Huhmann IM, Gahleitner A et al: Pathophysiology and imaging in inflammatory and blastomatous synovial diseases, *Skeletal Radiol* 31:313-333, 2002.
53. Barrera P, van der Laken CJ, Boerman OC et al: Radiolabelled interleukin-1 receptor antagonist for detection of synovitis in patients with rheumatoid arthritis, *Rheumatology (Oxford)* 39:870-874, 2000.
54. Jamar F, Houssiau FA, Devogelaer JP et al: Scintigraphy using a technetium 99m-labelled anti-E-selectin Fab fragment in rheumatoid arthritis, *Rheumatology (Oxford)* 41:53-61, 2002.
55. Mottonen TT, Hannonen P, Toivanen J et al: Value of joint scintigraphy in the prediction of erosiveness in early rheumatoid arthritis, *Ann Rheum Dis* 47:183-189, 1988.
56. Harcke HT, Mandell GA, Cassell IL: Imaging techniques in childhood arthritis, *Rheum Dis Clin North Am* 23:523-544, 1997.
57. Roivainen A, Parkkola R, Yli-Kerttula T et al: Use of positron emission tomography with methyl-11C-choline and 2-18F-fluoro-2-deoxy-D-glucose in comparison with magnetic resonance imaging for the assessment of inflammatory proliferation of synovium, *Arthritis Rheum* 48:3077-3084, 2003.
58. Faulkner RA, Bailey DA, Drinkwater DT et al: Regional and total body bone mineral content, bone mineral density, and total body tissue composition in children 8-16 years of age, *Calcif Tissue Int* 53:7-12, 1993.
59. Genant HK, Engelke K, Fuerst T et al: Noninvasive assessment of bone mineral and structure: state of the art, *J Bone Miner Res* 11:707-730, 1996.
60. Link TM, Majumdar S, Augat P et al: In vivo high resolution MRI of the calcaneus: differences in trabecular structure in osteoporosis patients, *J Bone Miner Res* 13:1175-1182, 1998.
61. Wehrli FW, Hwang SN, Ma J et al: Cancellous bone volume and structure in the forearm: noninvasive assessment with MR microimaging and image processing, *Radiology* 206:347-357, 1998.
62. Jara H, Wehrli FW, Chung H et al: High-resolution variable flip angle 3D MR imaging of trabecular microstructure in vivo, *Magn Reson Med* 29:528-539, 1993.
63. Chung H, Wehrli FW, Williams JL et al: Relationship between NMR transverse relaxation, trabecular bone architecture, and strength, *Proc Natl Acad Sci U S A* 90:10250-10254, 1993.

64. Yablonskiy DA, Reinus WR, Stark H et al: Quantitation of T2′ anisotropic effects on magnetic resonance bone mineral density measurement, *Magn Reson Med* 37:214-221, 1997.
65. Fernandez-Seara MA, Song HK, Wehrli FW: Trabecular bone volume fraction mapping by low-resolution MRI, *Magn Reson Med* 46:103-113, 2001.
66. Machann J, Raible A, Schnatterbeck P et al: Osteodensitometry of human heel bones by MR spin-echo imaging: comparison with MR gradient-echo imaging and quantitative computed tomography, *J Magn Reson Imaging* 14:147-155, 2001.
67. Hielscher AH, Klose AD, Scheel AK et al: Sagittal laser optical tomography for imaging of rheumatoid finger joints, *Phys Med Biol* 49:1147-1163, 2004.
68. Scheel AK, Backhaus M, Klose AD et al: First clinical evaluation of sagittal laser optical tomography for detection of synovitis in arthritic finger joints, *Ann Rheum Dis* 64:239-245, 2005.
69. Tsai TC, Chang PY, Chen BF et al: Retroperitoneal fibrosis and juvenile rheumatoid arthritis, *Pediatr Nephrol* 10:208-209, 1996.
70. Cabral DA, Petty RE, Malleson PN et al: Visual prognosis in children with chronic anterior uveitis and arthritis, *J Rheumatol* 21:2370-2375, 1994.
71. David J, Vouyiouka O, Ansell BM et al: Amyloidosis in juvenile chronic arthritis: a morbidity and mortality study, *Clin Exp Rheumatol* 11:85-90, 1993.
72. Hawkins PN, Richardson S, Vigushin DM et al: Serum amyloid P component scintigraphy and turnover studies for diagnosis and quantitative monitoring of AA amyloidosis in juvenile rheumatoid arthritis, *Arthritis Rheum* 36:842-851, 1993.
73. Stephan JL, Zeller J, Hubert P et al: Macrophage activation syndrome and rheumatic disease in childhood: a report of four new cases, *Clin Exp Rheumatol* 11:451-456, 1993.
74. Bhujwalla ZM, Artemov D, Glockner J: Tumor angiogenesis, vascularization, and contrast-enhanced magnetic resonance imaging, *Top Magn Reson Imaging* 10: 92-103, 1999.
75. Neeman M, Provenzale JM, Dewhirst MW: Magnetic resonance imaging applications in the evaluation of tumor angiogenesis, *Semin Radiat Oncol* 11:70-82, 2001.
76. Brunelle F, Strife JL (eds): *Contrast enhancement in pediatric musculoskeletal MR imaging: rationale and opinion*, Milan, 2001, Springer-Verlag.
77. Doria AS, Noseworthy MD, Oakden W: Dynamic contrast-enhanced MRI quantification of synovium microcirculation in experimental arthritis, *Pediatr Radiol* 33(Suppl 1):S92, 2003.
78. Bashir A, Gray ML, Burstein D: Gd-D, *Magn Reson Med* 36:665-673, 1996.
79. Bashir A, Gray ML, Hartke J et al: Nondestructive imaging of human cartilage glycosaminoglycan concentration by MRI, *Magn Reson Med* 41:857-865, 1999.
80. Nieminen MT, Rieppo J, Silvennoinen J et al: Spatial assessment of articular cartilage proteoglycans with Gd-DTPA-enhanced T1 imaging, *Magn Reson Med* 48:640-648, 2002.
81. Nissi MJ, Toyras J, Laasanen MS et al: Proteoglycan and collagen sensitive MRI evaluation of normal and degenerated articular cartilage, *J Orthop Res* 22:557-564, 2004.
82. Bader DL, Kempson GE, Egan J et al: The effects of selective matrix degradation on the short-term compressive properties of adult human articular cartilage, *Biochim Biophys Acta* 1116:147-154, 1992.
83. Brasch RC, Li KC, Husband JE et al: In vivo monitoring of tumor angiogenesis with MR imaging, *Acad Radiol* 7:812-823, 2000.
84. Lythgoe DJ, Williams SC, Cullinane M et al: Mapping of cerebrovascular reactivity using BOLD magnetic resonance imaging, *Magn Reson Imaging* 17:495-502, 1999.
85. Doria AS: Functional angiogenic process in an antigen-induced arthritis model: correlative BOLD MR imaging (fMRI) of the stages of synovitis along the time course of the disease, *Pediatr Radiol* 32(Suppl 1):S52, 2002.
86. Nieminen MT, Rieppo J, Toyras J et al: T2 relaxation reveals spatial collagen architecture in articular cartilage: a comparative quantitative MRI and polarized light microscopic study, *Magn Reson Med* 46:487-493, 2001.
87. Xia Y, Moody JB, Alhadlaq H et al: Imaging the physical and morphological properties of a multi-zone young articular cartilage at microscopic resolution, *J Magn Reson Imaging* 17:365-374, 2003.
88. Buckwalter JA, Mankin HJ: Articular cartilage, part II: degeneration and osteoarthrosis, repair, regeneration, and transplantation, *J Bone Joint Surg Am* 79:612-632, 1997.
89. Dardzinski BJ, Laor T, Schmithorst VJ et al: Mapping T2 relaxation time in the pediatric knee: feasibility with a clinical 1.5-T MR imaging system, *Radiology* 225:233-239, 2002.
90. Harel L, Wagner-Weiner L, Poznanski AK et al: Effects of methotrexate on radiologic progression in juvenile rheumatoid arthritis, *Arthritis Rheum* 36:1370-1374, 1993.
91. Sparling M, Malleson P, Wood B et al: Radiographic followup of joints injected with triamcinolone hexacetonide for the management of childhood arthritis, *Arthritis Rheum* 33:821-826, 1990.
92. Smith HJ: Contrast-enhanced MRI of rheumatic joint disease, *Br J Rheumatol* 35 (Suppl 3):45-47, 1996.
93. Azouz EM, Duffy CM: Juvenile spondyloarthropathies: clinical manifestations and medical imaging, *Skeletal Radiol* 24:399-408, 1996.
94. Bollow M, Braun J, Kannenberg J et al: Normal morphology of sacroiliac joints in children: magnetic resonance studies related to age and sex, *Skeletal Radiol* 26:697-704, 1997.
95. Carty H: *Imaging children*, Edinburgh, 1994, Churchill Livingstone.
96. Hanlon R, King S: Overview of the radiology of connective tissue disorders in children, *Eur J Radiol* 33:74-84, 2000.
97. Jacobs JC, Berdon WE, Johnston AD: HLA-B27-associated spondyloarthritis and enthesopathy in childhood: clinical, pathologic, and radiographic observations in 58 patients, *J Pediatr* 100:521-528, 1982.
98. Kamel M, Eid H, Mansour R: Ultrasound detection of heel enthesitis: a comparison with magnetic resonance imaging, *J Rheumatol* 30:774-778, 2003.
99. D'Agostino MA, Said-Nahal R, Hacquard-Bouder C et al: Assessment of peripheral enthesitis in the spondylarthropathies by ultrasonography combined with power Doppler: a cross-sectional study, *Arthritis Rheum* 48:523-533, 2003.
100. Bude RO, Rubin JM: Power Doppler sonography, *Radiology* 200:21-23, 1996.
101. Wakefield RJ, Brown AK, O'Connor PJ et al: Power Doppler sonography: improving disease activity assessment in inflammatory musculoskeletal disease, *Arthritis Rheum* 48:285-288, 2003.
102. D'Agostino MA, Breban M, Said-Nahal R et al: Refractory inflammatory heel pain in spondylarthropathy: a significant response to infliximab documented by ultrasound, *Arthritis Rheum* 46:840-841, 2002.
103. Tse SM, Burgos-Vargas R, Laxer RM: Anti-tumor necrosis factor alpha therapy leads to improvement of both enthesitis and synovitis in children with enthesitis-related arthritis, *Arthritis Rheum* 52(7):2103-2108, 2005.
104. Balint PV, Kane D, Wilson H et al: Ultrasonography of entheseal insertions in the lower limb in spondyloarthropathy, *Ann Rheum Dis* 61:905-910, 2002.
105. Lehtinen A, Taavitsainen M, Leirisalo-Repo M: Sonographic analysis of enthesopathy in the lower extremities of patients with spondylarthropathy, *Clin Exp Rheumatol* 12:143-148, 1994.
106. Lehtinen A, Leirisalo-Repo M, Taavitsainen M: Persistence of enthesopathic changes in patients with spondylarthropathy during a 6-month follow-up, *Clin Exp Rheumatol* 13:733-736, 1995.
107. Tannenbaum H, Rosenthall L, Arzoumanian A: Quantitative scintigraphy using radiophosphate and radiogallium in patients with rheumatoid arthritis, *Clin Exp Rheumatol* 5:17-21, 1987.
108. Foster HE, Cairns RA, Burnell RH et al: Atlantoaxial subluxation in children with seronegative enthesopathy and arthropathy syndrome: 2 case reports and a review of the literature, *J Rheumatol* 22:548-551, 1995.
109. Ahlstrom H, Feltelius N, Nyman R et al: Magnetic resonance imaging of sacroiliac joint inflammation, *Arthritis Rheum* 33:1763-1769, 1990.
110. Bollow M, Braun J, Biedermann T et al: Use of contrast-enhanced MR imaging to detect sacroiliitis in children, *Skeletal Radiol* 27:606-616, 1998.
111. Schaller JG: Ankylosing spondylitis and other arthropathies. In Behrman RE, Kliegman RM, Arvin AM (eds): *Nelson's textbook of pediatrics*, Philadelphia, 1996, Saunders, pp 670-672.
112. Buchmann RF, Jaramillo D: Imaging of articular disorders in children, *Radiol Clin North Am* 42:151-168, vii, 2004.
113. Ory PA, Gladman DD, Mease PJ: Psoriatic arthritis and imaging, *Ann Rheum Dis* 64(Suppl 2):ii55-ii57, 2005.
114. Cassidy JT, Petty RE: Spondyloarthropathies. In Cassidy JT, Petty RE (eds): *Textbook of paediatric rheumatology*, Philadelphia, 1995, Saunders, pp 224-259.
115. De Simone C, Guerriero C, Giampetruzzi AR et al: Achilles tendinitis in psoriasis: clinical and sonographic findings, *J Am Acad Dermatol* 49:217-222, 2003.
116. Kane D, Greaney T, Bresnihan B et al: Ultrasonography in the diagnosis and management of psoriatic dactylitis, *J Rheumatol* 26:1746-1751, 1999.
117. Milosavljevic J, Lindqvist U, Elvin A: Ultrasound and power Doppler evaluation of the hand and wrist in patients with psoriatic arthritis, *Acta Radiol* 46:374-385, 2005.
118. Fiocco U, Ferro F, Vezzu M et al: Rheumatoid and psoriatic knee synovitis: clinical, grey scale, and power Doppler ultrasound assessment of the response to etanercept, *Ann Rheum Dis* 64:899-905, 2005.
119. Stoller DW, Brody GA: The wrist and hand. In Stoller DW (ed): *MRI in orthopaedics and sports medicine*, Philadelphia, 1997, Lippincott Raven, p 968.
120. Antoni C, Dechant C, Hanns-Martin Lorenz PD et al: Open-label study of infliximab treatment for psoriatic arthritis: clinical and magnetic resonance imaging measurements of reduction of inflammation, *Arthritis Rheum* 47:506-512, 2002.
121. Puhakka KB, Jurik AG, Egund N et al: Imaging of sacroiliitis in early seronegative spondylarthropathy. Assessment of abnormalities by MR in comparison with radiography and CT, *Acta Radiol* 44:218-229, 2003.
121a. Ory PA, Gladman DD, Mease PJ: Psoriatic arthritis and imaging. *Ann Rheum Dis* 64(2):55-57, 2005.
122. Grigoryan M, Roemer FW, Mohr A et al: Imaging in spondyloarthropathies, *Curr Rheumatol Rep* 6:102-109, 2004.
123. Brower AC: Septic arthritis, *Radiol Clin North Am* 34:293-309, x, 1996.
124. Jaramillo D, Treves ST, Kasser JR et al: Osteomyelitis and septic arthritis in children: appropriate use of imaging to guide treatment, *AJR Am J Roentgenol* 165:399-403, 1995.
125. Mitchell M, Howard B, Haller J et al: Septic arthritis, *Radiol Clin North Am* 26:1295-1313, 1988.
126. Forrester DM, Feske WI: Imaging of infectious arthritis, *Semin Roentgenol* 31:239-249, 1996.
127. Lee SK, Suh KJ, Kim YW et al: Septic arthritis versus transient synovitis at MR imaging: preliminary assessment with signal intensity alterations in bone marrow, *Radiology* 211:459-465, 1999.
128. Sandrasegaran K, Saifuddin A, Coral A et al: Magnetic resonance imaging of septic sacroiliitis, *Skeletal Radiol* 23:289-292, 1994.
129. Sturzenbecher A, Braun J, Paris S et al: MR imaging of septic sacroiliitis, *Skeletal Radiol* 29:439-446, 2000.
129a. Marchal GJ, Van Holsbeeck MT, Raes M et al: Transient synovitis of the hip in children: role of US, *Radiology* 162:825-828, 1987.
129b. Robben SG, Lequin MH, Diepstraten AF et al: Anterior joint capsule of the normal hip and in children with transient synovitis: US study with anatomic and histologic correlation, *Radiology* 210:499-507, 1999.
130. Yulish BS, Lieberman JM, Strandjord SE et al: Hemophilic arthropathy: assessment with MR imaging, *Radiology* 164:759-762, 1987.

131. Rand T, Trattnig S, Male C et al: Magnetic resonance imaging in hemophilic children: value of gradient echo and contrast-enhanced imaging, *Magn Reson Imaging* 17:199-205, 1999.
132. Rodriguez-Merchan EC: Effects of hemophilia on articulations of children and adults, *Clin Orthop Relat Res* 328:7-13, 1996.
133. Baunin C, Railhac JJ, Younes I et al: MR imaging in hemophilic arthropathy, *Eur J Pediatr Surg* 1:358-363, 1991.
134. Hilgartner MW: Current treatment of hemophilic arthropathy, *Curr Opin Pediatr* 14:46-49, 2002.
135. Nuss R, Kilcoyne RF, Geraghty S et al: Utility of magnetic resonance imaging for management of hemophilic arthropathy in children, *J Pediatr* 123:388-392, 1993.
136. Kottamasu SR: Bone changes in diseases of the blood and blood-forming organs. In Kuhn JP, Slovis TL, Haller JO (eds): *Caffey's pediatric diagnostic imaging,* Philadelphia, 2004, Elsevier, pp 2417-2435.
137. Hermann G, Gilbert MS, Abdelwahab IF: Hemophilia: evaluation of musculoskeletal involvement with CT, sonography, and MR imaging, *AJR Am J Roentgenol* 158:119-123, 1992.
138. Merchan EC, De Orbe A, Gago J: Ultrasound in the diagnosis of the early stages of hemophilic arthropathy of the knee, *Acta Orthop Belg* 58:122-125, 1992.
139. Klukowska A, Czyrny Z, Laguna P et al: Correlation between clinical, radiological and ultrasonographical image of knee joints in children with haemophilia, *Haemophilia* 7:286-292, 2001.
139a. Wallny T, Brackmann HH, Semper H et al: Intra-articular hyaluronic acid in the treatment of haemophilic arthopathy of the knee, *Haemophilia* 6(5):566-570, 2000.
140. Nagele M, Kunze V, Hamann M et al: [Hemophiliac arthropathy of the knee joint. Gd-DTPA-enhanced MRI; clinical and roentgenological correlation], *Rofo* 160:154-158, 1994.
141. Arnold WD, Hilgartner MW: Hemophilic arthropathy. Current concepts of pathogenesis and management, *J Bone Joint Surg Am* 59:287-305, 1977.
142. Pettersson H, Ahlberg A, Nilsson IM: A radiologic classification of hemophilic arthropathy, *Clin Orthop Relat Res* (149):153-159, 1980.
143. Lundin B, Pettersson H, Ljung R: A new magnetic resonance imaging scoring method for assessment of haemophilic arthropathy, *Haemophilia* 10:383-389, 2004.
144. Nuss R, Kilcoyne RF, Rivard GE et al: Late clinical, plain x-ray and magnetic resonance imaging findings in haemophilic joints treated with radiosynoviorthesis, *Haemophilia* 6:658-663, 2000.
144a. Lundin B, Babyn P, Doria AS: The International Prophylaxis Study Group. Compatible scales for progressive and additive MRI assessments of haemophilic arthropathy. *Haemophilia* 11(2):109-115, 2005.
145. Issaivanan M, Shrikande MP, Mahapatra M et al: Management of hemophilic pseudotumor of thumb in a child, *J Pediatr Hematol Oncol* 26:128-132, 2004.
146. Steele NP, Myssiorek D, Zahtz GD et al: Pediatric hemophilic pseudotumor of the paranasal sinus, *Laryngoscope* 114:1761-1763, 2004.
147. Kerr R: Imaging of musculoskeletal complications of hemophilia, *Semin Musculoskelet Radiol* 7:127-136, 2003.
148. Keller A, Terrier F, Schneider PA et al: Pelvic haemophilic pseudotumour: management of a patient with high level of inhibitors, *Skeletal Radiol* 31:550-553, 2002.
149. Hermann G, Yeh HC, Gilbert MS: Computed tomography and ultrasonography of the hemophilic pseudotumor and their use in surgical planning, *Skeletal Radiol* 15:123-128, 1986.
150. Turkmen C, Zulflkar B, Taser O et al: Radiosynovectomy in hemophilic synovitis: correlation of therapeutic response and blood-pool changes, *Cancer Biother Radiopharm* 20:363-370, 2005.
151. Soroa VE, del H, V, Giannone C et al: Effects of radiosynovectomy with p-32 colloid therapy in hemophilia and rheumatoid arthritis, *Cancer Biother Radiopharm* 20:344-348, 2005.
152. Oh JY, Khwarg SI: Orbital subperiosteal hemorrhage in a patient with factor VIII and factor XII deficiency, *J Pediatr Ophthalmol Strabismus* 41:367-368, 2004.
153. Libby EN, White GC: Cranial pseudotumour in haemophilia, *Haemophilia* 10:186-188, 2004.
154. Stein M, Oates E: Hemorrhage into a choledochal cyst in a hemophiliac child, *Pediatr Radiol* 20:118-119, 1989.
155. Ameri A, Martin R, Vega R et al: Successful management of intramural ureteral hemorrhage in a patient with factor VIII deficiency and high-titer inhibitor, *J Thromb Haemost* 2:2273, 2004.
156. Ylmaz S, Oren H, Irken G et al: Life-threatening mediastinal-retroperitoneal hemorrhage in a child with moderate hemophilia A and high inhibitor titer: successful management with recombinant activated factor VII 5, *J Pediatr Hematol Oncol* 27:400-402, 2005.
157. Pachman LM: Juvenile dermatomyositis. Pathophysiology and disease expression, *Pediatr Clin North Am* 42:1071-1098, 1995.
158. Reimers CD, Fleckenstein JL, Witt TN et al: Muscular ultrasound in idiopathic inflammatory myopathies of adults, *J Neurol Sci* 116:82-92, 1993.
159. Park JH, Niermann KJ, Ryder NM et al: Muscle abnormalities in juvenile dermatomyositis patients: P-31 magnetic resonance spectroscopy studies, *Arthritis Rheum* 43:2359-2367, 2000.
160. Chan WP, Liu GC: MR imaging of primary skeletal muscle diseases in children, *AJR Am J Roentgenol* 179:989-997, 2002.
161. Ozonoff MB, Flynn FJ Jr: Roentgenologic features of dermatomyositis of childhood, *Am J Roentgenol Radium Ther Nucl Med* 118:206-212, 1973.
162. Steiner RM, Glassman L, Schwartz MW et al: The radiological findings in dermatomyositis of childhood, *Radiology* 111:385-393, 1974.
163. Sullivan DB, Cassidy JT, Petty RE: Dermatomyositis in the pediatric patient, *Arthritis Rheum* 20(2 Suppl):327-331, 1977.
164. Cassidy JT, Petty RC: Juvenile dermatomyositis. In Cassidy JT, Petty RE (eds): *Textbook of paediatric rheumatology,* Philadelphia, 1995, Saunders, pp 323-364.
165. Rose AL: Childhood polymyositis. A follow-up study with special reference to treatment with corticosteroids, *Am J Dis Child* 127:518-522, 1974.
166. Bureau NJ, Cardinal E, Chhem RK: Ultrasound of soft tissue masses, *Semin Musculoskelet Radiol* 2:283-298, 1998.
167. Reimers CD, Finkenstaedt M: Muscle imaging in inflammatory myopathies, *Curr Opin Rheumatol* 9:475-485, 1997.
168. Fornage BD: The case for ultrasound of muscles and tendons, *Semin Musculoskelet Radiol* 4:375-391, 2000.
169. Yosipovitch G, Beniaminov O, Rousso I et al: STIR magnetic resonance imaging: a noninvasive method for detection and follow-up of dermatomyositis, *Arch Dermatol* 135:721-723, 1999.
170. Hernandez RJ, Keim DR, Sullivan DB et al: Magnetic resonance imaging appearance of the muscles in childhood dermatomyositis, *J Pediatr* 117:546-550, 1990.
171. Maillard SM, Jones R, Owens C et al: Quantitative assessment of MRI T2 relaxation time of thigh muscles in juvenile dermatomyositis, *Rheumatology (Oxford)* 43:603-608, 2004.
172. Summers RM, Brune AM, Choyke PL et al: Juvenile idiopathic inflammatory myopathy: exercise-induced changes in muscle at short inversion time inversion-recovery MR imaging, *Radiology* 209:191-196, 1998.
173. Huppertz HI, Kaiser WA: Serial magnetic resonance imaging in juvenile dermatomyositis—delayed normalization, *Rheumatol Int* 14:127-129, 1994.
174. Wu Y, Seto H, Shimizu M et al: Extensive soft-tissue involvement of dermatomyositis detected by whole-body scintigraphy with 99mTc-MDP and 201TL-chloride 2, *Ann Nucl Med* 10:127-130, 1996.
175. Bar-Sever Z, Mukamel M, Harel L et al: Scintigraphic evaluation of calcinosis in juvenile dermatomyositis with Tc-99m MDP 1, *Clin Nucl Med* 25:1013-1016, 2000.
176. Govoni M, Castellino G, Padovan M et al: Recent advances and future perspective in neuroimaging in neuropsychiatric systemic lupus erythematosus, *Lupus* 13:149-158, 2004.
177. Cea G, Bendahan D, Manners D et al: Reduced oxidative phosphorylation and proton efflux suggest reduced capillary blood supply in skeletal muscle of patients with dermatomyositis and polymyositis: a quantitative 31P-magnetic resonance spectroscopy and MRI study, *Brain* 125:1635-1645, 2002.
178. Banker BQ: Dermatomyositis of childhood, ultrastructural alterations of muscle and intramuscular blood vessels, *J Neuropathol Exp Neurol* 34:46-75, 1975.
179. Woo M, Chung SJ, Nonaka I: Perifascicular atrophic fibers in childhood dermato myositis with particular reference to mitochondrial changes, *J Neurol Sci* 88:133-143, 1988.
180. Moritani T, Shrier DA, Numaguchi Y et al: Diffusion-weighted echo-planar MR imaging of CNS involvement in systemic lupus erythematosus, *Acad Radiol* 8:741-753, 2001.
181. Warach S, Chien D, Li W et al: Fast magnetic resonance diffusion-weighted imaging of acute human stroke, *Neurology* 42:1717-1723, 1992.
182. Damon BM, Ding Z, Anderson AW et al: Validation of diffusion tensor MRI-based muscle fiber tracking, *Magn Reson Med* 48:97-104, 2002.
183. Galban CJ, Maderwald S, Uffmann K et al: A diffusion tensor imaging analysis of gender differences in water diffusivity within human skeletal muscle, *NMR Biomed* 18:489-498, 2005.
184. Sinha S, Lucas-Quesada FA, Sinha U et al: In vivo diffusion-weighted MRI of the breast: potential for lesion characterization, *J Magn Reson Imaging* 15:693-704, 2002.
185. Filidoro L, Dietrich O, Weber J et al: High-resolution diffusion tensor imaging of human patellar cartilage: feasibility and preliminary findings, *Magn Reson Med* 53:993-998, 2005.
186. Maillot F, Goupille P, Valat JP: Plant thorn synovitis diagnosed by magnetic resonance imaging, *Scand J Rheumatol* 23:154-155, 1994.

CHAPTER 25

Pediatric Developmental and Chronic Traumatic Conditions, the Osteochondroses, and Childhood Osteoporosis

MARC J. LEE, MD, JEANNETTE M. PEREZ-ROSSELLO, MD, *and* BARBARA N. WEISSMAN, MD

KEY FACTS

- Although clinically useful, bone age measurements may be imperfect due, for example, to methodologic problems and the applicability of standard reference guides to the patient assessed.
- Structural scoliosis involves both lateral and rotational deformity of the vertebral column and, by definition, has a fixed component. Postural scoliosis is due to causes extrinsic to the spine itself.
- Leg length discrepancy can be quantified using special radiographic techniques. The process of limb lengthening can correct the disparity and its progress can be followed using radiography or ultrasound.
- Growth of the femoral head and acetabulum is an interdependent process, Early treatment of developmental dysplasia is necessary to avoid permanent morphologic changes that may predispose to premature osteoarthritis and severe morbidity. Hip sonography is more sensitive than physical exam for mild forms of dysplasia.
- Tarsal coalition (fusion of tarsal bones) affects about 1% of the population and is a cause of rigid flat foot deformity. The bridging tissue may be bone, cartilage, or fibrous tissue.
- Specific patterns of skeletal injury can identify instances of nonaccidental trauma.
- Slipped capital femoral epiphysis occurs in adolescence and is usually diagnosed on radiographs. Computed tomography or magnetic resonance imaging (MRI) may be helpful in diagnosis and in demonstrating complications such as chondrolysis, early fusion of the growth plate, or osteonecrosis.
- A lag of several months may occur before radiographs are positive in patients with Legg-Calve-Perthes' disease. Bone scintigraphy and MRI may show abnormalities earlier in the disease. Several radiographic, scintigraphic, and MRI findings are useful in determining prognosis.
- Imaging appearances may help differentiate physiologic bowing from Blount's disease.
- Interpretation of bone densitometry in children is not identical to that in adults. In children, for example, comparison is usually made to age-, gender-, and race-matched controls (the Z score) rather than to peak bone mass (the T score).

In this chapter, we present the imaging indications, workup, and characteristics of several important and commonly encountered congenital and developmental conditions, as well as of the sequelae of chronic trauma that occur during development. Also discussed are the idiopathic abnormalities collectively referred to as the *osteochondroses*, resulting from disordered ossification in the growing child. Nonaccidental trauma is included given the utmost importance of recognizing this condition, whereas the broad topic of acute accidental skeletal injuries is not included. Finally, we discuss the rapidly emerging field of osteoporosis and bone density measurement in children. Because many of these conditions may first manifest or have sequelae in the adult, there will be some overlap with the adult population and findings mentioned elsewhere in this book.

Emphasis is placed on appropriate indications, the most commonly employed imaging modalities, utilization of advanced imaging techniques, and technique limitations. Imaging findings that can be readily recognized, particularly on radiographs, are emphasized, especially because many of these entities can be diagnosed using this standard modality. Specific mention is made of those findings that affect clinical management. Where possible, algorithms of imaging workup are included to facilitate diagnostic evaluation.

CONGENITAL AND DEVELOPMENTAL ANOMALIES

Assessment of Skeletal Maturity

Determining an individual's skeletal or bone age, in contrast with the chronological age, is important in understanding whether a child is growing appropriately, a metric commonly used in the fields of pediatric orthopedics, endocrinology, and forensics[1] (Box 25-1 and Box 25-2). Bone age is generally determined by comparing radiographs of the individual with those catalogued from a reference "normal" population. Because skeletal maturity follows a reproducible pattern of changes over time involving appearance of ossification centers, alterations of osseus contours, and timing and closure of the growth plates,[2] skeletal age can be

BOX 25-1. Generalized Causes of Advanced Skeletal Maturation

ENDOCRINE
Sexual precocity:
- Idiopathic
- Tumors, brain (hypothalamus, pineal, other):
- Tumors, other (liver, sex glands, adrenal):
  - Premature thelarche
  - Premature adrenarche

Medication with sex hormones
Thyroid:
- Hyperthyroidism

CONGENITAL DISORDERS
Acrodysostosis
Beckwith-Wiedemann syndrome
Cerebral gigantism
Cockayne syndrome
Fibrous dysplasia (McCune-Albright)
Lipodystrophy
Marshall syndrome
Pseudohypoparathyroidism
Weaver syndrome

OTHER CONDITIONS
Large children
Obesity
Idiopathic

BOX 25-2. Generalized Causes of Retarded Skeletal Maturation

ENDOCRINE DISORDERS
Thyroid:
- Hypothyroidism

Adrenal:
- Addison's disease
- Cushing's disease
- Steroid therapy

Gonadal:
- Hypogonadism

Pituitary:
- Panhypopituitarism
- Growth hormone deficiency
- Laron dwarfism
- Pituitary giantism

CHROMOSOMAL DISORDERS
Trisomy 21
Trisomy 18
XO
XXXXY
Most other chromosomal disorders

OTHER CONGENITAL CONDITIONS
Most bone dysplasias
Most types of primordial dwarfism (e.g., Silver syndrome)
Most congenital malformation syndromes

OTHER CONDITIONS
Congenital heart disease
Constitutional
Chronic illness (any)
Diabetes mellitus (pediatric)
Inflammatory bowel disease
Intrauterine growth retardation
Legg-Perthes
Malnutrition
Maternal deprivation
Neurogenic disorders
Renal failure
Rickets

estimated by comparison with standards that have been developed from such reference populations.

The two most commonly utilized methods are the Greulich and Pyle method and the Tanner-Whitehouse method. The Greulich and Pyle method is the most commonly used in the United States.[1,2] It should be remembered that the determination of skeletal age is an inexact science,[3] with radiographs the mainstay of estimation.

Indications for Imaging to Determine Skeletal Maturation

There are myriad reasons why it may be necessary to determine a child's skeletal maturation, including for the diagnosis and treatment of abnormalities of growth and maturation (e.g., a child too short or tall for age), approximation of expected adult height in the setting of a growth abnormality, evaluation of endocrinopathies (particularly involving the gonads, pituitary, and thyroid), timing and course of treatment with hormonal therapy, and timing of orthopedic surgical procedures such as correction of limb length discrepancy and scoliosis.[2,4,5] From an orthopedic standpoint, the bone age is critical and the chronological age essentially irrelevant for evaluation and management decisions. Bone age determinations at two separate timepoints are recommended when major therapeutic decisions are contemplated.[3,6]

Technique

The method of Greulich and Pyle involves only a single posteroanterior (PA) radiograph of the left hand and wrist, which is compared with standard radiographs in the atlas.

> Bone age is usually determined by comparison of a radiograph of the left hand and wrist with a standard atlas of images. Normal values are within two standard deviations of chronological age.

The atlas images were derived from children of each representative age as based on a prospective study of 1000 healthy Caucasian children of higher socioeconomic status from Cleveland, Ohio, during 1931 to 1942.[2] There are separate male and female standards. The patient's skeletal age is assigned as that being the closest match. A patient's skeletal age is generally considered normal if within two standard deviations of his or her chronological age. The time period constituting two standard deviations is a value that also should be included in the report, as determined by charts from the Brush Foundation that are included within the atlas.[2] As systemic factors and illness may more greatly alter maturation of the carpal than phalangeal bones, heavier weighting is given to the appearance of the tubular bones.[2] The Tanner-Whitehouse method also uses radiographs of the hand and wrist. This technique involves evaluation of the extent of ossification and morphology of 20 bones of the hand and wrist with assignment of a developmental stage to each bone, including the distal radius and ulna (2); the phalanges and metacarpals of the first, third, and fifth rays (11); and the carpal bones excluding the pisiform (7).[2] The sum of the carpal scores is averaged with the sum of the remaining scores to give an overall value that is compared with a plot of standards developed from serial hand and wrist radiographs of 2564 British middle-class children obtained from 1945 to 1958.[2]

Discrepancies between skeletal age and actual chronological age, irrespective of abnormalities such as delayed maturation, can come from natural variation of individuals in their progress of skeletal maturity, as well as discrepancy arising from the method itself[5] (Box 25-3). The accuracy of these standardized methods is the subject of much research, with potential sources of error including systematic errors of the method, such as a real difference between the reference standard population and the actual local population being evaluated, and variability in the interpretation of the radiographs by different individuals.[5]

In addition to differences between boys and girls, other factors may affect evaluation, including racial, regional, and socioeconomic variables that may make comparison between an individual child and the reference standard population inexact.[2] Moreover, standards developed early in the prior century have been questioned as to their validity today, given changes over time in nutrition, the environment, and socioeconomic factors.[2]

Some studies have suggested that the Tanner-Whitehouse method is slightly closer to true chronological age in normal children than the Greulich and Pyle method, but the former is significantly more laborious to perform with less reproducibility between observers and may not be suitable for a general hospital setting. Studies directly comparing these methods report that the Tanner-Whitehouse method gives a more advanced skeletal age than the Greulich and Pyle method[7,8] or vice versa,[5] making it important not to compare skeletal ages that are determined by different techniques. An interesting study that evaluated the actual 26 images of the "standard hands" comprising the Greulich and Pyle atlas with the Tanner-Whitehouse method showed that the Greulich and Pyle method consistently indicated a more advanced skeletal age.[9]

In studies evaluating the accuracy of the Greulich and Pyle method in children of different ethnicities, bone age has been shown to vary according to ethnicity and for different age ranges. For example, in one study of U.S. children, the greatest discrepancies were shown in black and Hispanic girls and in Asian and Hispanic boys in late childhood and adolescence, in whom bone ages were shown to possibly exceed the chronological age by as much as 9 to 11.5 months.[1] In preadolescent Asian boys, bone age lagged behind chronological age by 9.5 months.[1] In a study of children born after 1980 in Los Angeles of either European or African descent, prepubertal children of European descent showed delayed skeletal age compared with those of African descent, whereas postpubertal European-American males had delayed maturation compared with African-American males.[10] In another study evaluating black and white children in the late 1980s in the same geographic region from which the Greulich and Pyle standards were derived, the authors concluded that, particularly for black girls, the standards are not applicable.[11] Such results indicate that some caution is prudent in applying these widely used standards based on Caucasian children to other populations, although no comparable nonwhite, race-specific atlases have been published. The Greulich-Pyle method has been characterized by some orthopedists as limited during puberty owing to many factors, such as lack of standards at certain timepoints (e.g., 14.5 years in boys and 11.5 and 12.5 years in girls) and the few and sometimes subtle changes in the hand and wrist during puberty.[6,12] In the first 2 years of puberty, the Sauvegrain method has been advocated as an alternative technique, based on evaluation of more readily apparent dynamic changes occurring in the elbow.[12] This method is based on evaluation of anteroposterior (AP) and lateral radiographs of the left elbow with assignment of scores based on development of the four ossification centers of the lateral condyle, trochlea, proximal radial epiphysis, and olecranon when compared with a standard diagram.[6,12] A modified version of the Sauvegrain method has been recently proposed as a reproducible method that compares favorably with and can complement the Greulich and Pyle technique.[12]

In Europe, a sonographic version of the Greulich and Pyle atlas has been proposed as a valid possible alternative for evaluating the ossification centers of the hand and wrist.[13] This method avoids ionizing radiation by using a specialized automated ultrasound device that evaluates the distal radial and ulnar epiphyses. This technique has been reported to provide accurate bone age assessment.[14] Sonographic evaluation of ossification of the iliac crest apophysis also has been described as a possible alternative method.[15] These methods are not in general use, however, and their reproducibility in the non-research setting has not yet been reported.

BOX 25-3. Potential Limitations of Bone Age Determinations

Reference population may be incorrect
Standards are too old
Racial and ethnic differences
Socioeconomic differences
Lack of standards at some time points
Variability in image interpretation
Individual variation
Disorders may affect local maturation (e.g., hyperemia)

Scoliosis

Scoliosis, the abnormal lateral curvature of the spine in the coronal plane, can be divided into structural and postural causes. Structural scoliosis involves both lateral and rotational deformity of the vertebral column, may affect the thoracic and/or lumbar spine, and, by definition, has a fixed component. Postural scoliosis is due to causes extrinsic to the spine itself; for example, leg length discrepancy resulting in compensatory curvature, or splinting as in the setting of nerve irritation.

> *Scoliosis* is defined as a lateral curvature of the spine and may be due to structural or postural causes. Structural scoliosis involves both lateral and rotational deformity.

Structural scoliosis is idiopathic in the vast majority of cases, beginning during childhood. In the adolescent age group, idiopathic scoliosis is equal in incidence in girls and boys for minor curves but is nearly 10 times more common in girls than boys for more severe curves that require treatment (Figure 25-1). Idiopathic adolescent scoliosis accounts for the majority of patients

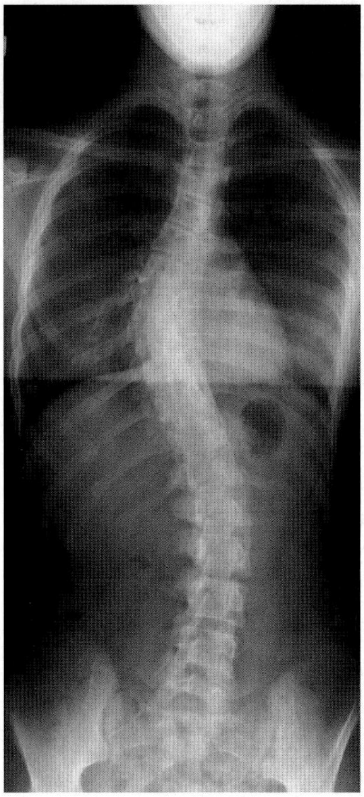

FIGURE 25-1. Idiopathic scoliosis in a 12-year-old female with thoracic dextroscoliosis and compensatory lumbar levoscoliosis.

with scoliosis and is the focus of this section. Less commonly, structural scoliosis is due to one of the other four, smaller etiologic categories (Figure 25-2)[16]: congenital, as from hemivertebrae or fused ribs (Figure 25-3); developmental, such as that due to skeletal dysplasia; neuromuscular/paralytic, as might be due to myelomeningocele, syringomyelia, and spinal cord tumors (Figure 25-4); or secondary, as from growth asymmetry due to prior trauma, infection, or irradiation (Figure 25-5) (Box 25-4).

> Most cases of structural scoliosis are idiopathic and begin during childhood.

The most common treatment of adolescent idiopathic scoliosis involves early identification and conservative management to prevent curve progression.[17] Curves of 30 to 40 degrees in skeletally immature patients have a predilection to progress during adulthood at a rate of approximately 1 degree per year, making a curve of 40 to 50 degrees an important threshold to indicate need for arthrodesis and instrumentation.[17]

Indications for Imaging

Imaging studies play a critical role in the diagnosis, surgical planning, and post-treatment follow-up of scoliosis. Radiographs are the mainstay of evaluation, whereas computed tomography (CT), magnetic resonance imaging (MRI), nuclear medicine exams, and ultrasound are employed in specific circumstances. MRI is the predominant and most useful ancillary imaging modality.[16,18]

Radiography of the spine is indicated in those with alteration in normal alignment on physical exam, for evaluation of curvature progression, follow-up after orthotic or surgical treatment, and in those with a parent or sibling with scoliosis.[19] The patient with scoliosis also may come to clinical attention because of symptoms such as back pain or headache or by way of identification during routine screening programs. In a retrospective series of 2442 patients with idiopathic scoliosis, 23% had back pain at presentation.[18] Scoliosis also may be suspected in high-risk groups, such as patients who have the VATER association (*v*ertebral anomalies, *a*nal atresia, *t*racheoesophageal fistula, *e*sophageal atresia, and *r*enal anomalies/*r*adial ray dysplasia). Milder scoliosis may be an incidental finding on imaging studies performed for other reasons (Box 25-5).

Osteoarticular Imaging

Radiographs are the initial imaging method of choice for diagnostic confirmation and evaluation and possible operative planning. The initial study includes a frontal radiograph of the entire spine obtained while standing without shoes. A gonadal shield is used to minimize radiation exposure. The exam is performed with the x-ray beam directed from posterior to anterior to minimize radiation dose to the breasts and thyroid.[20] A lateral view may be included on initial evaluation to evaluate associated kyphosis and lordosis, and this view also may detect other important abnormalities including spondylolisthesis or canal widening.[16] Frontal views while the patient bends to each side laterally also are typically included on initial evaluation in order to distinguish the degree to which secondary compensatory curvatures are correctable by bending and also may be obtained at the time of preoperative planning.

> Radiation dose to the thyroid and breast tissue is reduced by obtaining PA rather than AP scoliosis radiographs. Gonadal shielding is also employed.

The radiographic study is evaluated to assess degree and type of curvature, as well as whether scoliosis is related to a postural or structural cause. Important abnormalities in the vertebral bodies, ribs, and pelvis can be identified on this study. Although structural scoliosis can be surgically corrected if severe enough, treatment of postural scoliosis is aimed at correction of the underlying etiology. Because the skeletal age is important in determining the likelihood that scoliosis will worsen, its assessment is also important in management. On the scoliosis radiographs, skeletal maturity can be followed by evaluating the degree of ossification of the iliac crest apophysis (Risser's sign), which begins with calcification of the iliac apophysis at the anterior superior iliac spine, progresses posteromedially, and ultimately terminates with fusion of the apophysis to the iliac crest. A PA radiograph of the left wrist and hand is often also requested for bone age determination.[16]

In the coronal plane, curves are classified as cervical, thoracic, lumbar, thoracolumbar, or double curves. Thoracolumbar curves are defined as those with an apex at T12 or L1. Double curves are two separate curves in different regions. Location and apices of the curves are described. Often there is more than one abnormal curvature of the spine. The more severe curve is often the major curve, whereas curves above and below may be compensatory and shown to be correctable on bending views.

> Lateral bending views can demonstrate curves that are correctable.

The Cobb method is universally used to measure the angle of concavity in the frontal plane on radiographs and is based on the principle that the upper and lower vertebra with the greatest tilt in the horizontal plane delimit the curve.[16] The Cobb angle is that formed by a line paralleling the superior end plate of the vertebral body at the top of the curve and a line paralleling the inferior end plate of the vertebra at the bottom of the curve. Often it is easier to

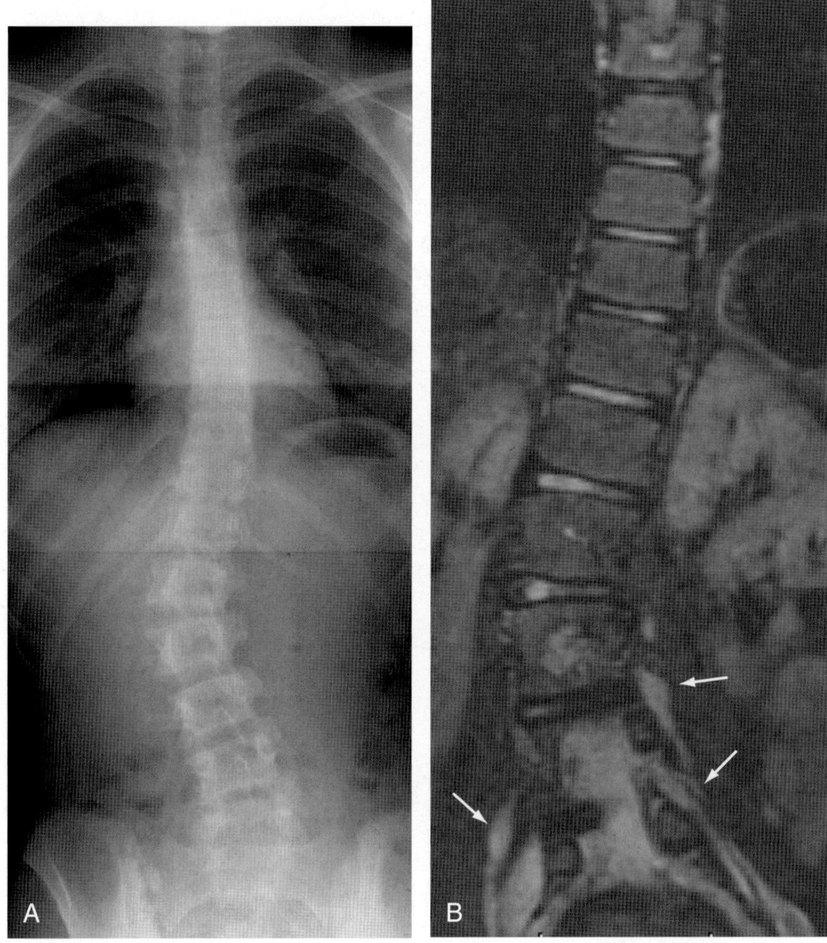

FIGURE 25-2. Developmental scoliosis in an 11-year-old with neurofibromatosis. **A,** PA view of the spine shows lumbar dextroscoliosis. **B,** Coronal T2-weighted MR image shows ectasia of the exiting nerve root sheaths *(arrows).*

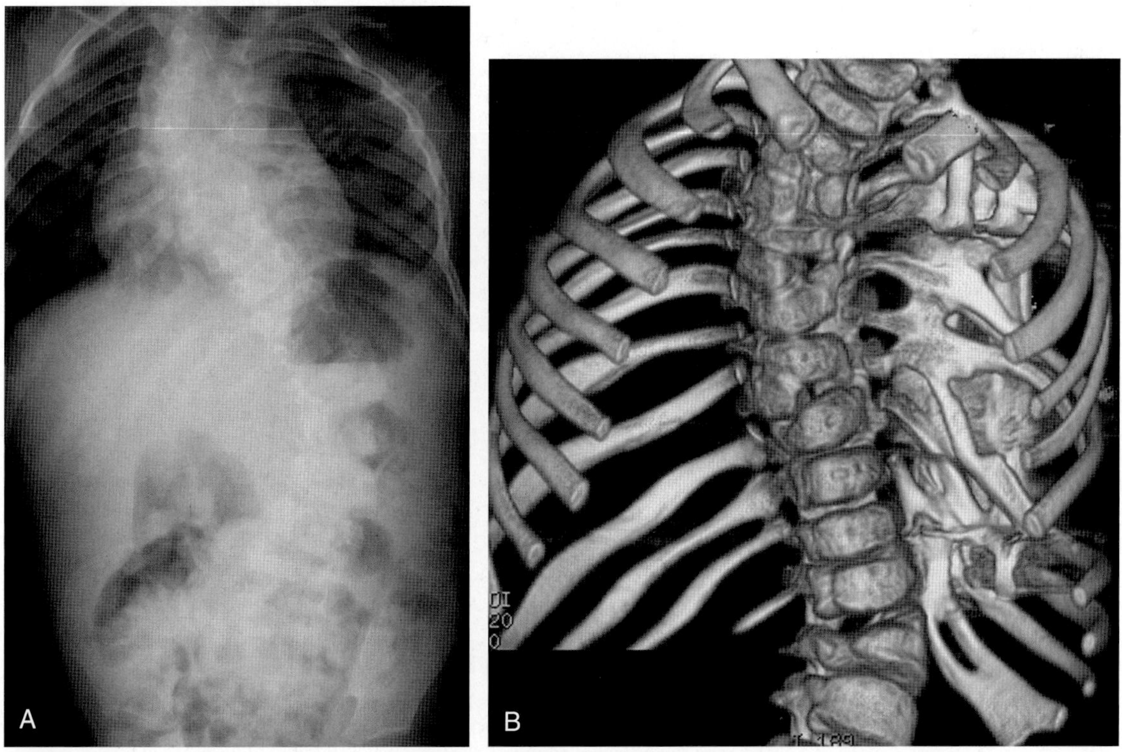

FIGURE 25-3. Congenital scoliosis in a 23-month-old child. **A,** Radiograph of the thoracolumbar spine and **(B)** CT 3D model of the chest show multiple vertebral segmentation and rib anomalies.

(Continued)

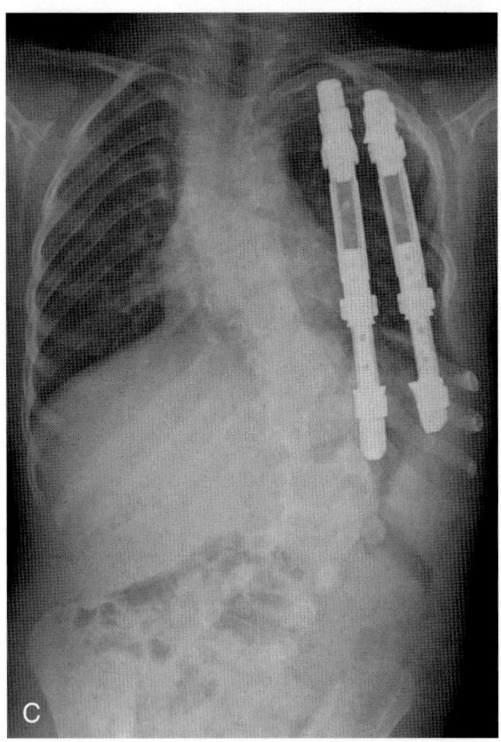

FIGURE 25-3—cont'd. **C,** Placement of VEPTR (vertical expandable prosthetic titanium ribs) to allow better lung growth.

measure the angle by drawing additional lines perpendicular to those above, as illustrated in Figure 25-6. The vertebra at the apex of the curve has the greatest degree of rotation.[16] Rotational deformity of the spine is detected by noting the degree to which the pedicles move away from the edge of the vertebral body and is important for operative planning. The Cobb angle is reported to correlate well with clinical surface measurements using the scoliometer and inclinometer.[16] Normally the spinous process is projected equidistant from each pedicle on the frontal radiograph; rotational deformity can be documented by asymmetry in this appearance.

The typical adolescent idiopathic scoliosis is thoracic or thoracolumbar and convex to the right. Leftward thoracic scoliosis should raise suspicion of an underlying specific etiology.

> A thoracic scoliosis that is convex to the left should raise the suspicion of an underlying abnormality.

Myopathic scoliosis, such as in the setting of muscular dystrophy or cerebral palsy, often has a wide C shape and is related to neuromuscular imbalance, most typically extending from the upper thoracic to lumbar region in association with an oblique orientation of the pelvis.[21]

Serial radiographs are performed to assess worsening deformity under nonsurgical management. Curves tend to worsen and should be followed particularly during the adolescent growth spurt. Following skeletal maturity, scoliosis tends not to progress if it is less than about 30 degrees, although severe scoliosis can progress throughout adulthood.[21] In the postoperative patient,

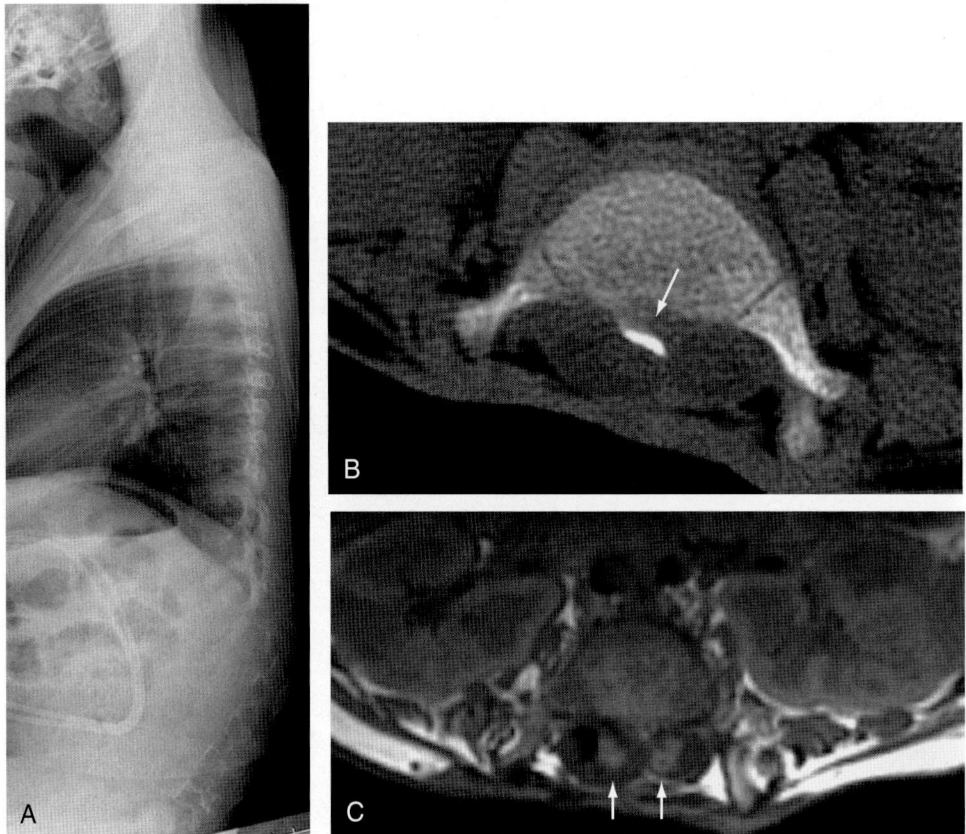

FIGURE 25-4. Seventeen month old with congenital kyphoscoliosis due to diastematomyelia and myelomeningocele. **A,** Sagittal radiograph of the spine shows lumbar kyphosis. **B,** Axial CT images show the bony spur *(arrow)* originating from the posterior aspect of the vertebral body splitting the cord in two. There is incomplete fusion of the posterior elements. **C,** Axial T1-weighted MR image shows the two hemicords *(arrows)*.

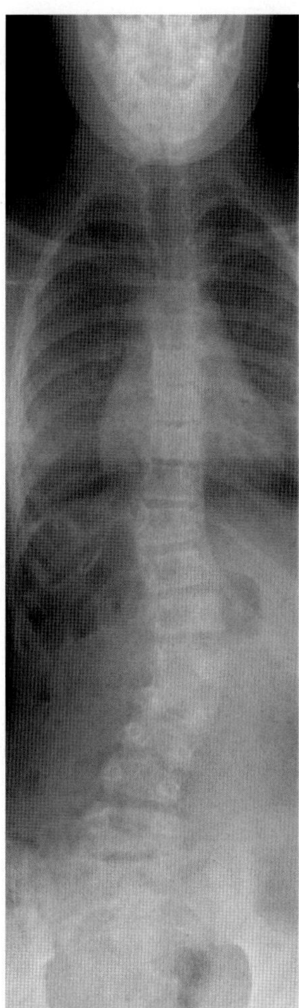

FIGURE 25-5. Secondary scoliosis. Fourteen-year-old with resection of the right kidney due to Wilm's tumor. The patient was treated with radiotherapy and developed a secondary lumbar levoscoliosis. Note also the smaller right ilium.

imaging allows assessment of the degree of scoliotic correction, evaluation of bony fusion, and detection of complications, which include breakage of wires and rods, slippage or fracture of hooks, spondylolysis, and pseudarthrosis.[21] MRI is limited in the postoperative patient, in whom metallic hardware for internal fixation creates susceptibility artifact that obscures the images.

Clinical evaluation plays an important role in deciding when to do advanced imaging studies, most importantly MRI, for evaluation of the neural axis. The use of MRI in the workup of presumed adolescent idiopathic scoliosis is controversial, although many studies support its use in presumed idiopathic scoliosis in the infantile (birth to 3 years) and juvenile (4 to 10 years) subpopulations.[22] Screening in the adolescent population has been reported in a large prospective series to be of low yield as a routine measure.[23] However, many reports advocate MRI in those patients with certain "atypical" clinical findings and symptoms: abnormal neurologic examination (e.g., abnormal reflexes, clonus, weakness, pes cavus), headache and neck pain, back or radicular pain, or rapid progression.[16,18,24-26] Pain as an indicator for MRI is particularly controversial, with some authors noting that it is a common complaint in scoliosis without underlying pathology[18] and negative MRI results are often found when pain is the sole indication for the examination.[25] Of 560 patients in a large series with presumed idiopathic scoliosis and pain, 9% had an underlying pathologic condition.[18]

Radiologic identification of these underlying abnormalities is important in order to identify correctable causes of scoliosis, entities that should be treated before scoliosis is treated, and conditions such as hydrosyringomyelia in which forcible surgical correction may lead to paraplegia.[27] Taken together, these results underscore the importance of thorough history and physical exam, including neurologic exam, in deciding on referral for MRI.

In addition to abnormal clinical findings, abnormal initial radiographic findings that should prompt further evaluation include thinned pedicles, spinal canal widening, unusual curves such as left thoracic or thoracolumbar curves, short-segment scoliosis, rapid progression, and absence of the thoracic apical segment lordosis typically seen with idiopathic scoliosis (i.e., presence of thoracic kyphosis of 20 degrees or greater)[16,18,24,25] (Box 25-6).

In patients with these atypical clinical and radiographic features, MRI findings may include hydrosyringomyelia, spinal cord tumors, tethered cord, Arnold-Chiari malformations, disk protrusion, and dural ectasia.[16,18,24,25] How hydrosyringomyelia and Chiari malformations lead to scoliosis is unknown.

Patients with congenital scoliosis (scoliosis present from birth) also should undergo additional evaluation given a high association with neural axis abnormalities. In this group, diastematomyelia (split spinal cord malformation) is the most frequent intraspinal abnormality[16] (see Figure 25-4). MRI has been shown useful in these patients, with other commonly encountered abnormalities including hydrosyringomyelia, Chiari malformation, spinal cord tumors, and tethered cord.[16]

CT with multiplanar reformations and three-dimensional reconstruction is helpful for further evaluation of scoliosis in selected cases, including in the setting of complex congenital osseus deformity[26] (see Figure 25-3). Such reformations also can be helpful for operative planning. As CT shows osseus detail to better advantage than MRI, some authors suggest localized CT to further characterize bony abnormalities such as segmentation anomalies.[26] CT is also helpful in identification or confirmation of certain bone tumors that may underlie scoliosis such as osteoid osteoma.

Nuclear medicine examinations are of limited use in evaluating scoliosis. Whole body Tc99m-MDP phosphate bone scanning is sometimes used to localize a bony abnormality such as a tumor or infection and may be helpful in specifying a site of abnormality in the young child who indicates back pain but cannot localize the site.[26] Radiographs or axial imaging techniques can be performed subsequently for dedicated evaluation of the abnormal site. Bone scan does play an important role in evaluating the patient in whom infection related to internal fixation hardware is suspected, cases in which both CT and MRI may be limited by hardware artifact.

In the infant, sonography is useful for evaluation of the spinal canal and for evaluation of open and closed dysraphism that may be associated with scoliosis.

Extraarticular Findings

In the patient with congenital scoliosis, particular search should be made for the VATER association. Congenital scoliosis is commonly associated with genitourinary malformations such as unilateral renal agenesis, and all patients with such congenital spine anomalies should have evaluation of the genitourinary system such as with renal sonography.[21]

Developmental scoliosis can be seen in patients with neurofibromatosis, Marfan's syndrome, Ehlers-Danlos syndrome, and mucopolysaccharidoses, in whom additional clinical and rheumatologic stigmata may be encountered. Indeed, in patients with neurofibromatosis type 1, scoliosis is the most common skeletal abnormality[16] (see Figure 25-2). Table 25-1 lists additional findings that may suggest a particular disease or syndrome associated with scoliosis.[16]

BOX 25-4. Etiologic Classification of Structural Scoliosis

IDIOPATHIC
Infantile (0-2 years):
- Resolving
- Progressive

Juvenile (3-10 years)
Adolescent (10 years to skeletal maturity)
Adult

NEUROMUSCULAR
Neuropathic:
- Upper motor neuron:
  - Cerebral palsy
  - Spinocerebellar degeneration:
    - Friedreich ataxia
    - Charcot-Marie-Tooth disease
    - Roussy-Levy syndrome
  - Spinal cord neoplasm
  - Syringomyelia (acquired)
  - Other
- Lower motor neuron:
  - Poliomyelitis and other viral myelitides
  - Spinal muscular atrophy (SMA):
    - Werdnig-Hoffman disease (SMA I & II)
    - Kugelberg-Welander disease (SMA III)

Paralytic myelomeningocele:
- Neuropathic arthrogryposis
- Dysautonomia (Riley-Day syndrome)
- Spinal cord traumatic injury
- Other

Myopathic:
- Myopathic arthrogryposis
- Muscular dystrophy:
  - Duchenne (pseudohypertrophic)
  - Becker
  - Limb-girdle
  - Fascioscapulohumeral
  - Myotonic
- Fiber type disproportion
- Congenital hypotonia

CONGENITAL
Osteopathic vertebral/skeletal anomaly:
- Anomalous formation:
  - Wedge vertebra
  - Hemivertebra
- Anomalous segmentation:
  - Unilateral bar
  - Fused ribs only (extraspinal anomaly)
- Spondylolisthesis associated

Neuropathic:
- Spinal cord anomaly:
  - Tethered cord
  - Syringomyelia (congenital)
  - Diastematomyelia
  - Other
- Spinal dysraphism:
  - Meningocele
  - Myelomeningocele

DEVELOPMENTAL
Skeletal dysplasia (intrinsic defect of bone growth):
- Diastrophic dysplasia
- Spondyloepi(meta)physeal dysplasias

Mucopolysaccharidoses:
- Morquio disease
- Other heteroglycanoses

Other
Skeletal dysostosis (ectodermal/mesodermal):
- Neurofibromatosis
- Marfan's syndrome
- Ehlers-Danlos syndromes
- Other

SECONDARY/MISCELLANEOUS
Postirradiation
Postinfectious (osteopathic and nonviral)
Posttraumatic (osteopathic)
Postsurgical
Secondary to neoplasm (osteopathic, spinal canal, or beyond)
Other

With permission from Oestreich AE, Young LW, Poussaint T: Scoliosis circa 2000: radiologic imaging perspective. 1. Diagnosis and pretreatment evaluation, *Skeletal Radiol* 27:591-605, 1998.

BOX 25-5. Indications for Imaging in Scoliosis

Abnormal alignment on physical examination
Evaluating curvature progression
Posttreatment follow-up
Consider in high-risk groups (VATER association)

Leg Length Discrepancy

Pediatric leg length discrepancy is a clinical manifestation of a broad range of underlying etiologies. Leg length discrepancy is due to a structural inequality in which the femur, tibia, or both are physically shorter on one side. This should be contrasted with functional or apparent discrepancies, in which the leg lengths are actually symmetric but appear dissimilar due to other abnormalities, such as a high-riding congenital hip dislocation, pelvic obliquity, scoliosis, or contractures at the hip, knee, ankle, or foot.[28]

> Leg length discrepancy may be due to structural changes in an extremity; in some cases, equal leg lengths may appear to be disparate (e.g., due to scoliosis, hip dislocation).

True leg length discrepancy may be congenital or acquired, the latter due to trauma or infection, or to neurologic, neoplastic, dysplastic, or inflammatory etiologies (Table 25-2).[29] Asymmetry may be due to either decreased size or inhibited growth of the short limb or, conversely, to overgrowth of the long limb. For example, whereas a malignant tumor may involve and disrupt the physis to cause lower extremity shortening, a hemangioma can result in increased vascularity and, therefore, may stimulate overgrowth. Additionally, etiologies, in a simplified fashion, can be thought of as those that affect the length of the bone without affecting growth (e.g., a healed diaphyseal fracture

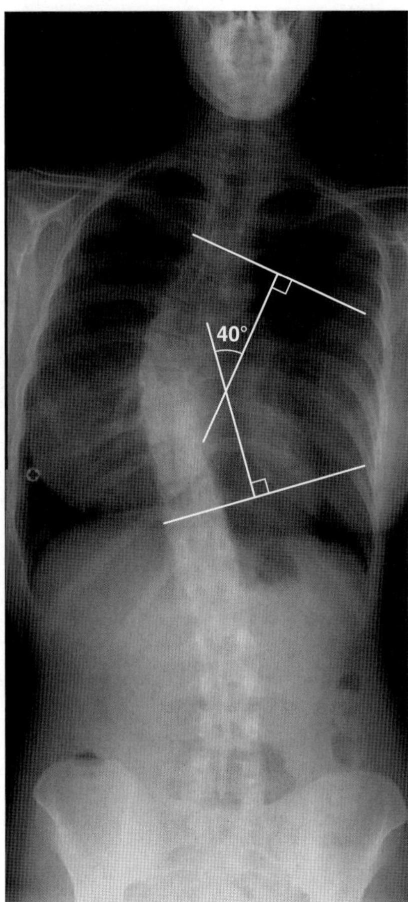

FIGURE 25-6. Cobb angle. Standing PA radiograph. The Cobb angle is the angle formed by the intersecting perpendicular lines to the superior end plate of the most tilted vertebra above the apex of the curve and the inferior end plate of the most tilted vertebra below the apex of the curve. In this case the curve measures 40 degrees.

TABLE 25-1. Diagnostic Guide Based on Findings in Addition to Scoliosis

Additional Findings	Diagnosis
Achondroplastic proportions with normal face and early progression of scoliosis	Spondyloepiphyseal dysplasias
Arachnodactyly, sternum abnormality	Marfan's syndrome
Back pain in adolescent with radiodense vertebral pedicle	Osteoid osteomas
Back pain with other neurologic signs	Osteoblastoma (or canal tumor)
Café-au-lait spots	Neurofibromatosis 1 (or fibrous dysplasia)
Cat-cry in an infant	Cri du chat syndrome
Clubfoot, hitchhiker thumbs, cervical kyphosis	Diastrophic dysplasia
Dislocated hips and abnormal clenched hand	Trisomy 18
Dolichostenomelia, Marfan-like trunk osteoporosis	Homocystinuria
Facies resembling a bird	Seckel syndrome
Interpedicle widening, central opaque spicule, and neurologic symptoms	Diastematomyelia
Kidney surgically absent	Wilms tumor resected, postirradiation changes
Mandible cysts and basal cell tumors, falx calcification	Gorlin's syndrome
Osteoarthrosis out of proportion to age	Ochronosis
Pneumonia, chronic, in an infant	Riley-Day syndrome
Short great toes and palpable masses beneath the skin	Myositis ossificans progressiva
Thoracic paravertebral mass with thinned or spread ribs	Thoracic neuroblastoma
Trunk relatively long with shortened limbs at birth	Metatropic dysplasia
Vertebral bodies with H- or U-shaped flattening, limb shortening at birth, death in a few days	Thanatophoric dysplasia

With permission from Oestreich AE, Young LW, Poussaint T: Scoliosis circa 2000: radiologic imaging perspective. 1. Diagnosis and pretreatment evaluation, *Skeletal Radiol* 27:591-605, 1998.

BOX 25-6. Possible Clinical and Radiographic Findings Indicating MRI Study in Patients with Scoliosis

CLINICAL FINDINGS

"Idiopathic scoliosis" in infants (birth-3 years) and children (4-10 years)
Atypical clinical findings or symptoms
Abnormal neurologic examination (e.g., abnormal reflexes, clonus, weakness, pes cavus)
Headache and neck pain
Back pain (controversial)
Radicular pain
Rapid progression

RADIOGRAPHIC FINDINGS

Thinned pedicles
Widening of spinal canal
Unusual curves
Rapid progression
Thoracic kyphosis ≥ 20 degrees

with overriding fragments) or those affecting growth and perhaps subsequently length (e.g., osteomyelitis affecting the physeal plate).[30] Although there are numerous etiologies, no clear underlying cause is identifiable in a large percentage of cases, which thus are considered idiopathic.[30a] In the case of fracture, the Salter-Harris classification predicts the likelihood of effect on the future growth of the bone.

The Salter-Harris classification of epiphyseal injuries helps predict the affect of a growth plate injury on epiphyseal growth.

Indications for Imaging

The child with leg length discrepancy may come to clinical attention because of an obvious difference in length lengths, gait disorders, lower back or lower extremity pain, or postural problems leading to compensatory scoliosis. Imaging is generally performed

TABLE 25-2. Causes of Leg Length Discrepancy

	Shortening	Overgrowth
Congenital	Femoral deficiencies Congenital coxa vara	Anisomelia (hemihypertrophy and hemiatrophy)
	Congenital deficiencies of the leg	1. Russell-Silver syndrome
	1. Posteromedial bowing of the tibia	2. Klippel-Trenaunay-Weber syndrome
	2. Fibular hemimelia	
	3. Tibial hemimelia	
	4. Congenital pseudarthrosis of the tibia	
	Neurofibromatosis	Vascular malformations
Traumatic	Overriding fractures	Healing fractures causing overstimulation
	Epiphyseal fractures causing growth plate damage	
Infection	Osteomyelitis causing growth plate damage	Osteomyelitis causing overstimulation
	Septic arthritis	
Neurologic	Cerebral palsy	
	Myelodysplasia	
	Poliomyelitis	
Tumors or dysplasias	Malignant tumors	Hemangiomata
	Multiple exostoses	
	Fibrous dysplasia	
	Ollier's disease	
Inflammatory	Rheumatoid arthritis Hemophilia	Rheumatoid arthritis or hemophilia causing overstimulation

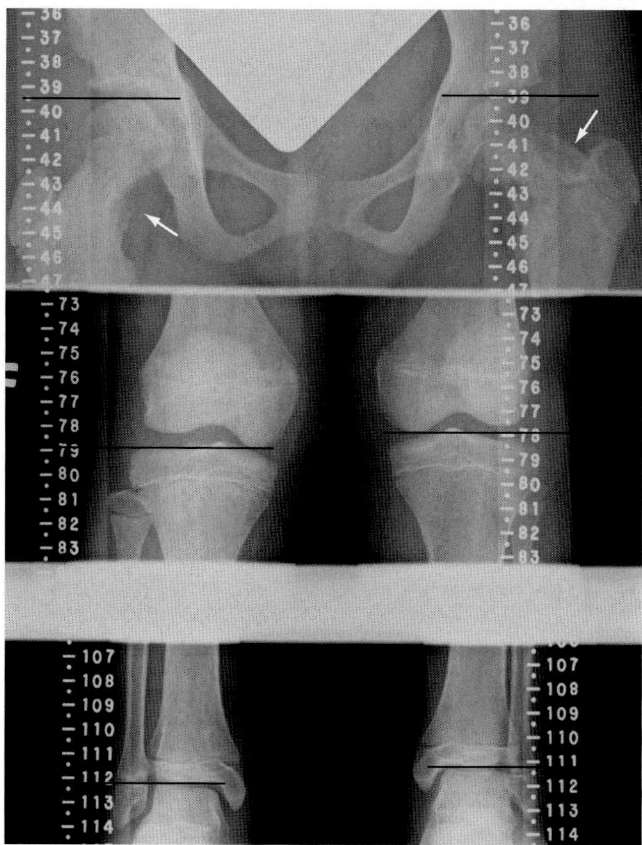

FIGURE 25-7. Scanogram. Nine year old with McCune Albright syndrome. The scanogram shows leg length discrepancy secondary fibrous dysplasia in the proximal femurs *(arrows)*. The right femur measures 39.5 cm; left femur, 39 cm; right tibia, 33 cm; and left tibia, 33 cm.

in these patients after examination that includes clinical measurement of leg lengths and gait analysis and is performed for diagnostic confirmation, assessment of severity, detection of underlying contributory pathology such as tumors, and operative planning. After surgical treatment, serial radiographs to monitor progression and to detect the complications of lengthening procedures are also an important component of management.[31] A discussion is included here on radiographic evaluation of the commonly used Ilizarov bone-lengthening device.

Osteoarticular Imaging

A few radiographic methods are used for measurement of leg length discrepancy.[30] The *teleoradiograph* uses a single exposure of both limbs in their entirety onto a long film with the patient standing, a technique limited by magnification. The teleoradiograph is helpful in young children who cannot remain still for three separate exposures and, thus, cause measurement errors. The *orthoradiograph* avoids magnification error by utilizing three separate exposures, with resultant shorter focus-to-film distance, centered over the hip, knee, and ankle onto a single long film. Similar to the orthoradiograph, the *scanogram*, the most widely used method, utilizes three separate exposures as well, although the film cassette moves beneath the patient between exposures at each station to produce a smaller composite image (Figure 25-7). A *scout view from a CT* scanner may be used for evaluating limb length in non–weight-bearing lower extremities.

On the scanogram or CT, bony landmarks used for measurement are the top of the femoral head, medial femoral condyle, and ankle mortise. A radiopaque ruler on the image is then used to identify the levels of the joints, and comparison with the contralateral side allows assessment of the disparity in length in centimeters. Validity depends on careful patient positioning and may be misleading if there is angular deformity. In many departments, the exam is performed using digital radiography, exposing the patient to less radiation. On this study, particular abnormalities involving affected physeal plates can be noted, as the four physes of the femur and tibia contribute differently to overall leg length, an important factor in management decisions. Serial examinations are typically performed in order to plot growth patterns over time and are analyzed by standardized methods,[28,30] as the treatment goal is chosen according to the discrepancy expected at the time of skeletal maturation rather than the present discrepancy. A bone age radiograph of the hand and wrist is also often performed to help predict the discrepancy at maturation in order to plan treatment, as skeletal age correlates more closely with leg growth than with chronological age.[30]

Although radiographic measurements are considered more accurate, discrepancies in lengths by scanogram should correlate closely with clinically measured true leg lengths as determined with a tape measure from the anterosuperior iliac crest to the medial malleolar tip.[30]

The severity of discrepancy is generally more important than the etiology in choosing one of the following treatment strategies.[30] As a generalized guideline, inequalities of up to 2 cm result in no functional or clinical adversity and are therefore not treated. Between 2 and 6 cm, treatment options include a shoe lift, shortening of the long limb, or arresting growth of the longer limb (epiphysiodesis). From 6 to 20 cm, lengthening is performed of the shorter limb. Greater than 20 cm, a prosthesis is generally used.

Because length discrepancy is more often due to abnormal shortening of one extremity, methods to shorten the longer leg involve operation on the normal leg as a compensatory measure.[28] Epiphysiodesis, which arrests physeal growth on the normal side, allows the other limb to "catch up," is a low-morbidity procedure, and is the most frequently performed procedure for limb equalization.[28] It is usually performed at the distal femur, proximal tibia, or both.[28] It can be performed with removal of a small block of bone across the physis, inverting its orientation and reinserting it; by extraperiosteal staples spanning the physis; or by percutaneous techniques, now the favored method. Bone shortening, an additional technique, is generally performed of the femur and involves removal of bone with internal fixation.

In contrast, leg lengthening can be performed on the shorter leg to equalize lengths,[28,32] the most commonly used method involving partially cutting the bone to be lengthened (corticotomy) and then distracting the ends via an external fixator such as the Orthofix or Ilizarov devices (Figure 25-8). The Orthofix device is a unilateral fixator, while the Ilizarov is a circumferential device. The Ilizarov apparatus is both a strong and adaptable device and benefits from a relatively low rate of complications; avoidance of bone grafting, internal fixation, and multiple operations; and partial to full weight-bearing activity is allowed.[32,33] The Wagner method of limb lengthening is a more involved three-step operation including open mid-diaphyseal osteotomy and external pin fixation and distraction, interposition of bone graft and application of a sideplate and screws, and then removal of internal hardware after bony maturation.[31]

The Ilizarov method is particularly useful for complex deformities and has gained popularity as a method of choice for bone lengthening.[34] It relies on controlled gradual tension-stress over time using an external Ilizarov apparatus, a method of distraction osteogenesis in which new bone is formed between bony surfaces that are pulled apart[32] (Figure 25-9). The Ilizarov apparatus is composed of a circular fixator frame with which distraction and compression forces are achieved by threaded rods. Angular deformities can be corrected by hinge mechanisms. A corticotomy is made with a sleeve of periosteum remaining intact to provide scaffolding onto which new bone can grow. After a latency period of days to allow osteogenesis to commence, distraction by adjustment of the rods is usually performed at 0.25 mm four times per day until the desired length is obtained, and then the frame remains in place until there is adequate consolidation of the new bone.

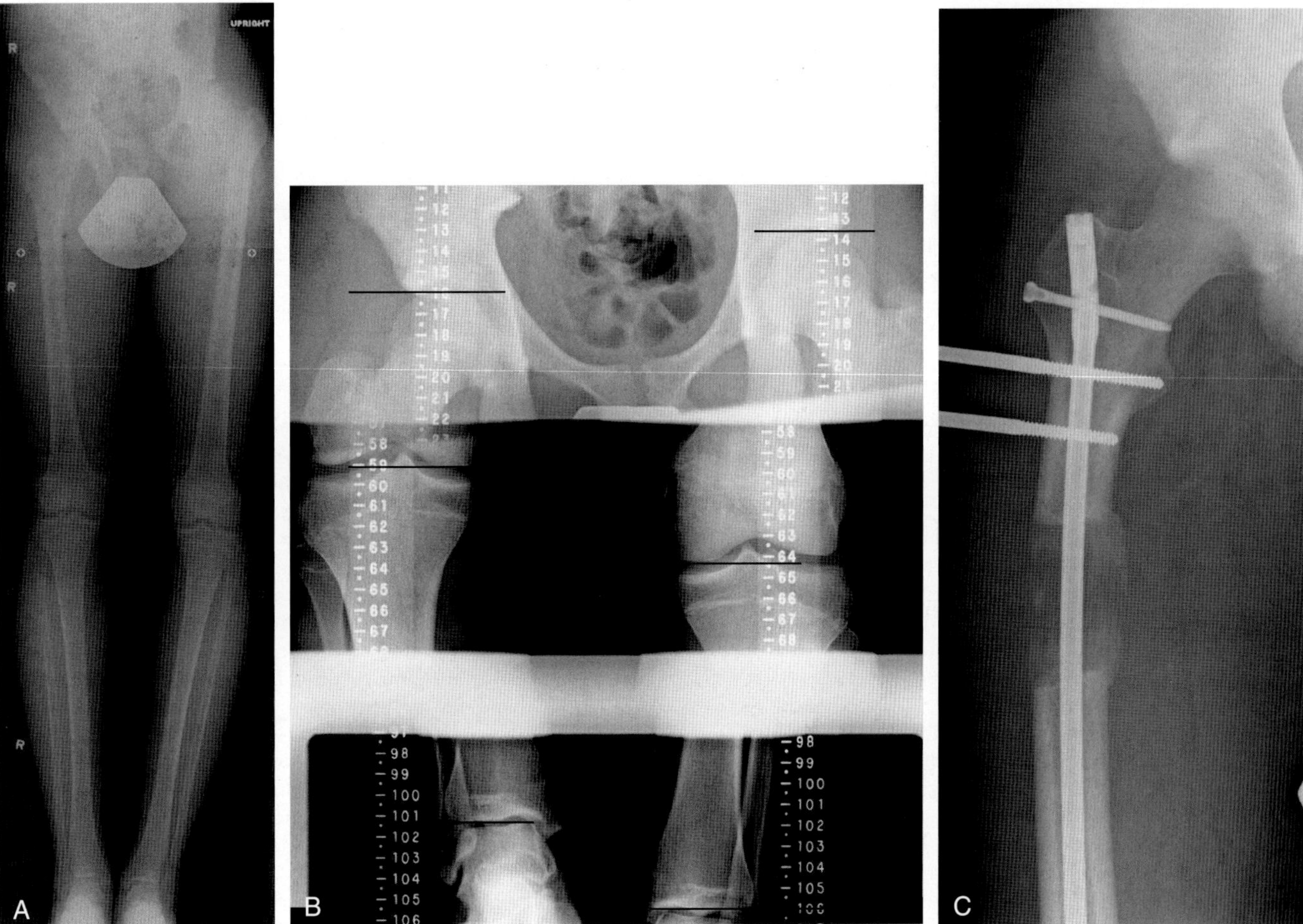

FIGURE 25-8. Sixteen year old with leg length discrepancy secondary to premature closure of the right distal femur physis after a Salter II fracture at 11 years of age. **A,** Teleoradiograph and **(B)** scanogram show the foreshortened right femur. The right femur measures 43 cm and the left femur 51 cm, an 8-cm difference. **C,** Leg lengthening was performed with the Orthofix device. At 3 months of treatment, 7 cm of growth has been achieved.

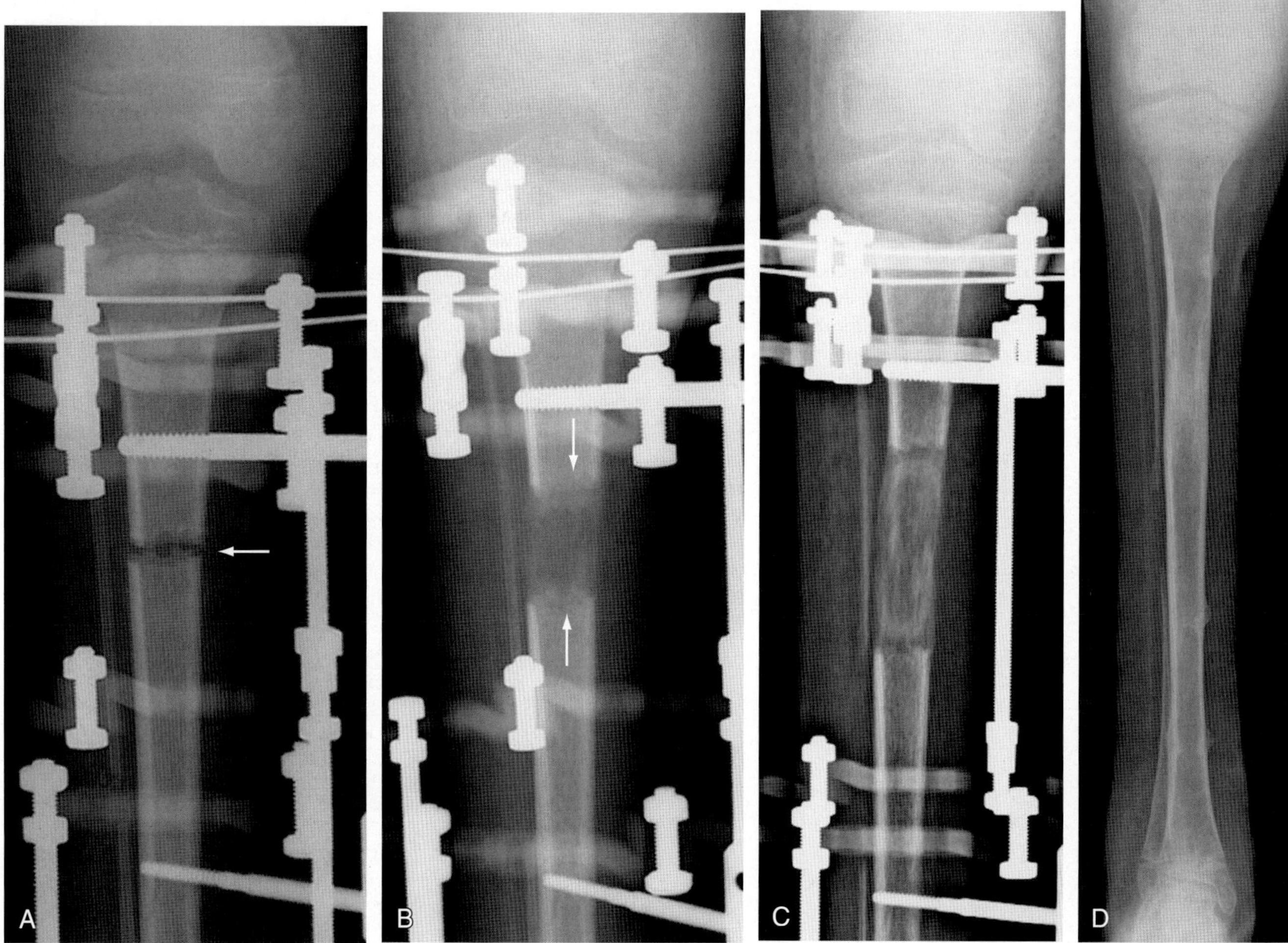

FIGURE 25-9. Ilizarov. Nine year old with leg length discrepancy secondary to a short right tibia due to fibular hemimelia. **A,** Two weeks after osteotomy and distraction there is no new bone formation seen at the osteotomy site *(arrow)*. **B,** At seven weeks, hazy bone formation seen; the bone bridge is 4 cm *(arrows)*. **C,** At 13 weeks there is further distraction and longitudinal growth; the bone bridge is 6.2 cm. **D,** At 10 months, 6.3 cm of lengthening has been achieved.

Radiographs are the standard and most useful imaging exam by which the gap of lengthening and the extent of new bone formation are documented.[33-35] Radiographs are performed at 2- to 4-week intervals after hospital discharge.[30] In the first few weeks of distraction, no new bone is seen radiographically. Thereafter a hazy amorphous opacity develops within the gap, followed by progressively increased density that assumes a longitudinal orientation and, finally, exhibits corticomedullary differentiation.[32,33]

Radiographs should include the entire bone or joint to assess overall alignment of the osteotomized segments, as well as a clear view of the distraction gap. This may require centering the x-ray beam at this site for accurate measurement.[33] Distraction performed too quickly inhibits bone formation, whereas that performed too slowly can precipitate early consolidation. The radiographs allow the orthopedic surgeon to fine-tune the tempo of distraction.[35] A widening lucency within the gap is a sign of distraction performed too quickly. Ultrasound has been reported to show initial bone growth within the gap earlier than radiographs.[34]

The orthopedic surgeon decides when to remove the device based on the correct length of distraction and the radiographic demonstration of new bone that has progressed to early corticomedullary differentiation.[33] However, no standardized radiographic metrics of adequate bony consolidation have been published.[30]

Complications of bone lengthening procedures that can be demonstrated radiographically include displacement, angular deformity, premature or delayed consolidation, fracture or deformity of the new bone within the gap, hardware fracture, pin loosening or infection (evidenced by abnormal surrounding radiolucency), delayed union or non-union, and reflex sympathetic dystrophy.[31,32,35] A sawtooth-like lucency in the center of the new bone may be a sign of either stress fracture or delayed union, with differentiation aided by the presence of pain in the former and by follow-up imaging.[32] Particularly in patients with congenitally short femurs, who have anterior cruciate ligament deficiency and lateral femoral condyle hypoplasia, posterior knee subluxation is a complication. Cystic degeneration within the distraction gap is best demonstrated with ultrasound and may be suspected in the setting of delayed bone formation.[33,34] Believed due to lymphatic or venous congestion, cystic degeneration may require bone grafting.[35]

Complications that have been reported after hardware removal and that are evaluable on radiographs include deformity and fracture of the callus in cases where new bone formation was not yet mature.[32] Long-term follow-up radiographs may be warranted to evaluate for fractures at the lengthened site, as this segment of bone may be weaker than normal for years.[32]

Other complications of lengthening will be radiographically inapparent and include muscle contracture, arthrofibrosis, cartilage damage, motor palsy, hematoma, nerve or vascular injury, and compartment syndrome.[33] Interestingly, hypertension can develop during lengthening and is of unclear cause, resolving with shortening of the distraction gap.[30]

Developmental Dysplasia of the Hip

Developmental dysplasia of the hip (DDH) is a broad term that includes congenital and developmental abnormalities leading to an abnormal relationship of the femoral head and acetabulum, ranging from mild capsular laxity or instability, to subluxation, to irreducible dislocation.[36] Some forms are only shown on imaging studies as mild malformation of the acetabulum. Although the vast majority of cases are present at birth, DDH may not become apparent until months to years later. In part due to the diversity of the conditions encompassed by the term *DDH*, differences in definitions, and the fact that mild dysplasia often resolves on its own, the true incidence is elusive and controversial.[37] Involvement is more commonly unilateral than bilateral.

Growth of the femoral head and acetabulum is an interdependent process, so early treatment is necessary to avoid permanent morphologic changes that may predispose to premature osteoarthritis and severe morbidity.[38] Without normal articulation, the acetabulum will become shallow with increased anteversion and may fill with hypertrophy of a fibrofatty tissue in the joint, called *pulvinar tissue*. Femoral head ossification becomes delayed, and femoral anteversion and coxa valga may result.

> Without the normal articulation, the acetabulum will become shallow.

Indications for Imaging

Most cases of DDH are detectable at birth,[17] and the diagnosis is often a clinical one. On newborn screening exams, the femoral head can be manipulated in and out of the acetabulum of the infant with DDH (Barlow and Ortolani maneuvers). Other important clinical clues, generally seen at a later stage, include asymmetry of thigh or buttock folds, apparent shortening of the femur, and limited hip abduction. After the initial postnatal period, clinical detection may be more difficult due to tightening of the hip capsule and muscular contraction.

> In the newborn, DDH can be detected by manipulation of the femoral head in and out of the acetabulum of the infant with DDH (Barlow and Ortolani maneuvers). Later clinical clues include asymmetry of thigh or buttock folds, apparent shortening of the femur, and limited hip abduction.

Ultrasound is often performed for diagnostic confirmation and to obtain a baseline measure of severity prior to treatment; it is also helpful in cases of indeterminate clinical findings. Early detection allows less invasive treatment and prevents the need for future surgical correction, all the more important because standard harness treatment for DDH discovered early carries a low rate of complications. Hip sonography is more sensitive than physical exam for mild forms of dysplasia.[36,39]

Risk factors for DDH include female gender, first-born child, breech position, positive family history, oligohydramnios, and postural molding conditions such as torticollis or foot deformity.[17,36] DDH is reported to occur in up to 23% of infants of breech presentation.[36] Many of these risk factors appear to be conditions in which in utero positioning is restricted.

Although ultrasound is performed in some European countries such as Switzerland and Germany as part of universal newborn screening, in the United States typically only those with abnormal physical exams or high risk factors are evaluated with imaging.[40] As such, sonography is not recommended by the American Academy of Pediatrics (AAP) as a routine newborn screening exam, as this has not been of proven benefit.[36]

The use and timing of imaging studies is somewhat controversial. In the infant with a normal clinical exam and no risk factors, periodic clinical exam suffices without ultrasound. For a female breech infant, a particularly high-risk group, imaging evaluation is recommended. In the neonate with an abnormal exam, urgent attention including referral to an orthopedic surgeon is warranted. If there is a hip click or equivocal exam but not a positive Barlow or Ortolani sign, these infants should be reexamined in 2 weeks and either referred to an orthopedist if the exam is positive or referred for ultrasound in 2 to 3 weeks or for orthopedic consultation if still inconclusive.[36]

The American College of Radiology regards radiography of both hips in the AP view more appropriate than bilateral ultrasound in patients with clinically suspected DDH who are older than 4 months.[41]

It should be noted that imaging is usually not performed during the first 2 weeks of life due to normal physiologic laxity, since minor evidence of instability detected sonographically most often resolves without treatment.[42] There is no way to differentiate at this early time those who will require treatment from those who will not.[43]

Osteoarticular Imaging Findings

Ultrasonography is the widely accepted method of choice for screening and evaluation of DDH in the newborn for several reasons. First, in infants, the entire proximal femur is composed of cartilage, which is readily visualized by sonography but radiographically imperceptible. Sonography does not use ionizing radiation, and it allows morphometric and dynamic assessment, with direct visualization of the effects of stress maneuvers. Conventional radiographs are used instead once femoral head ossification has occurred, and evaluation can be performed by radiographic reference lines constructed on a frontal view of the pelvis. CT, MRI, and conventional or cross-sectional arthrography are advanced techniques most helpful in preoperative and postsurgical imaging.

Ultrasound is performed in patients younger than 6 months of age and is generally not helpful after 1 year of age due to ossification of the proximal femur. Using a high-frequency linear transducer, a coronal image is obtained of each hip in the supine or lateral position at rest with the ultrasound transducer positioned laterally in the mid-acetabular plane (Figure 25-10). On this view, the alpha angle is measured, described by a line drawn along the iliac wing and a second line that parallels the osseus acetabular roof (Figure 25-11). Normally this angle is 60 degrees or greater in a mature hip, and smaller angles indicate a more shallow osseus acetabulum. Coverage of the femoral head by the acetabulum should be at least 50% in normal cases. The beta angle, less frequently used, is formed by a line drawn along the lateral straight edge of the ilium and the fibrocartilaginous labrum, which should be less than 55 degrees in a mature hip. This angle is an index of cartilaginous acetabular development. In the axial plane with hip flexion, both static and dynamic views are obtained In this plane, subluxation and dislocation are shown to better advantage, and force is applied to the femur similar to the Barlow maneuver while observing the femoral head for abnormal posterior subluxation over the ischium. Dislocation is typically superiorly and laterally.

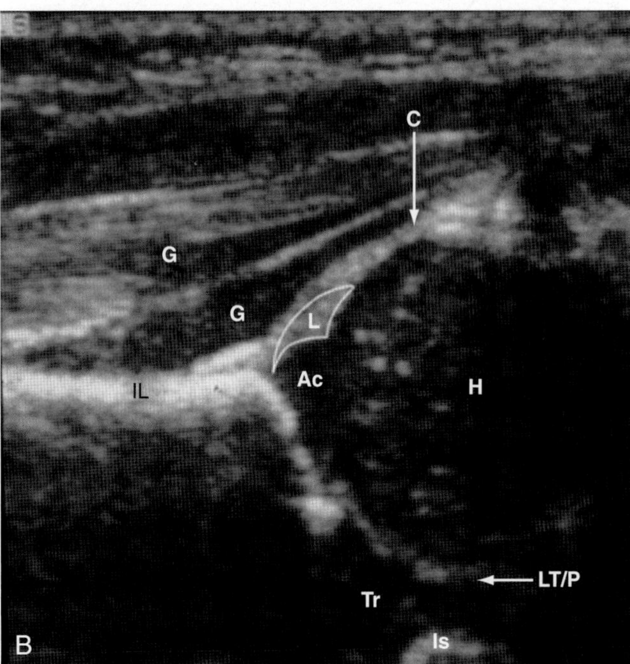

FIGURE 25-10. Coronal ultrasound of the hip. Diagram **(A)** and corresponding ultrasound image **(B)** of the neonatal hip from the AIUM guidelines. *Ac,* Acetabular cartilage; *C,* capsule; *G,* gluteus muscles; *GT,* greater trochanter; *H,* cartilaginous femoral head; *IL,* ilium; *Is,* ischium; *L,* labrum, *LT/P,* ligamentum teres/pulvinar complex; *M,* femoral metaphysis; *Pu,* pubis; *Tr,* triradiate cartilage. (From AIUM practice guideline for the performance of ultrasound examination for detection of developmental dysplasia of the hip, *J Ultrasound Med* 22:1131-1136, 2003, with permission.)

On coronal images, the promontory, that portion of the ilium that begins to deviate medially to form the acetabular roof, is normally sharply angulated. In DDH, it may appear rounded or flattened. In the premature infant, however, this rounded appearance may simply represent immaturity, and a follow-up scan is often helpful.

As normal development of a cup-shaped acetabulum requires the presence of an articulating spherical femoral head, subluxation or dislocation that goes untreated will result in a dysplastic contour of the acetabulum. For this reason, and because it cannot be determined which patients will progress and which will stabilize spontaneously, treatment for all cases of DDH must be initiated early, typically by maintaining the legs in abduction in a Pavlik harness. It is helpful to determine the position of the femoral head while in the harness using ultrasonography. Follow-up sonography can be performed to evaluate progress during harness treatment. Use of ultrasound while under harness treatment appears to maximize the effectiveness of the harness, aiding clinical decisions about adjustments and weaning and alerting the clinician if this treatment modality is failing.[43-45] Stress maneuvers are not performed during treatment.[42]

The proximal femoral ossification center begins to appear between the fourth and seventh months of life, such that radiography becomes more reliable than ultrasound for evaluation. The typical radiograph of a child diagnosed late will show a shallow acetabulum, decreased femoral head coverage, disruption of Shenton's line (a smoothly curved line along the femoral neck and inferior cortex of the superior pubic ramus), and delayed appearance of the proximal femoral ossification center. Several radiographic lines are helpful for radiographic diagnosis of DDH (Figure 25-11).

CT is the standard examination for evaluation of the reduced hip when a plaster cast has been placed after closed or open surgical reduction because of late diagnosis or severe disease.[46] Due to concern about gonadal radiation dose, limited CT with low-dose technique can be performed.[46] CT also has been shown useful in evaluating the morphology of the untreated dysplastic acetabulum in preparation for or after surgery, especially when combined with three-dimensional (3D) reconstructions, given the complex structure of the acetabulum.[38,47] For patients undergoing evaluation for pelvic osteotomy, a procedure to improve the biomechanical forces across the hip joint to minimize development of osteoarthritis, preoperative CT is helpful. CT details the shape, contours, and orientation of the acetabulum and gives information about the fit of the femoral head so that the most appropriate type of osteotomy can be chosen.[38]

In the preoperative setting, MRI provides the additional benefit of illustrating the acetabular labrum, as well as barriers to adequate reduction including an excessively large pulvinar, ligamentum teres thickening, or interposition of the labrum or capsule. Morphology of the acetabulum, femoral head, and femoral and acetabular anteversion also can be characterized.

MRI also has been shown useful to confirm postoperative reduction.[48] In severe cases requiring operative closed or open reduction, a plaster spica cast is placed with the hip in 90 degrees of flexion and controlled abduction. Postoperative imaging is critical to ensure that the hip has not redislocated, and axial gradient echo MRI has been shown useful and avoids the ionizing radiation of CT (Figure 25-12). Radiographs are limited in this setting by overlying plaster material. Ultrasound only can be performed if a window as been cut in the cast, which may weaken it.[48] Osteonecrosis (avascular necrosis, AVN) of the femoral head, a known complication of excessive abduction in a spica cast, is best demonstrated by MRI. To minimize motion artifacts during MRI, some authors suggest performing imaging in the postoperative period while the child is still recovering from anesthesia.[48]

In an adolescent to adult population evaluated for acetabular osteotomy for correction of symptomatic hip dysplasia, a recent study suggests that multidetector CT arthrography may be more sensitive than 3D gradient echo MRI for evaluation of higher-grade articular cartilage lesions with substance loss.[49]

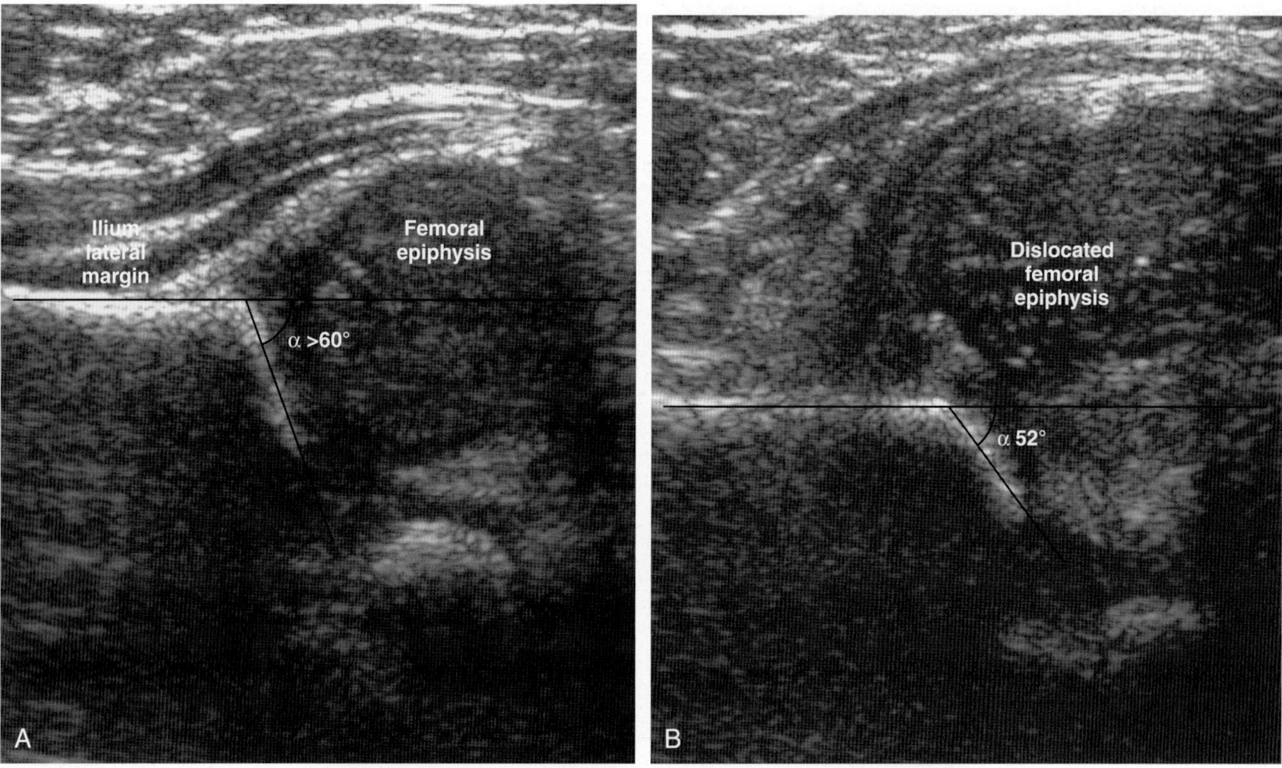

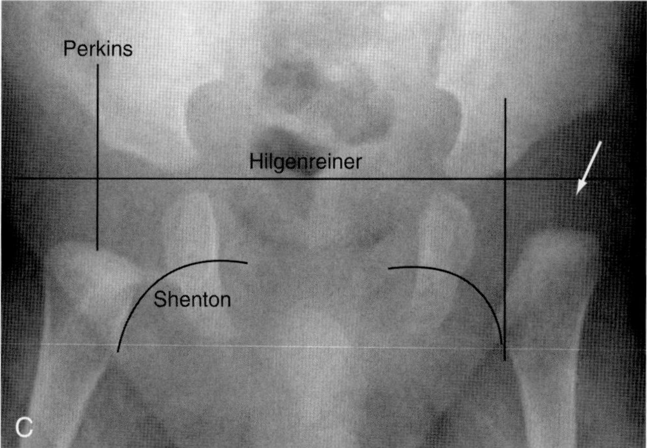

FIGURE 25-11. Infant with developmental hip dysplasia. **A,** Six weeks of age: Ultrasound of the normal right hip shows an alpha angle greater than 60 degrees and more than 50% coverage of the femoral epiphysis by the acetabulum. **B,** Ultrasound of the left hip shows a shallow acetabulum; the alpha angle is 52 degrees. There is superior and lateral dislocation of the femoral epiphysis. **C,** Three months of age: Radiograph of the pelvis shows delayed ossification of the left femoral head with a shallow acetabulum, superior and lateral dislocation of the femoral head *(arrow)*, and disruption of Shenton's arc.

Femoral Anteversion

Femoral anteversion is a developmental deformity in the proximal femur of unknown etiology in which there is increased anterior angulation of the femoral neck with respect to the coronal plane.[50] It is the most common cause of intoeing in children older than 3 years. Normally the femoral neck is directed about 34 to 40 degrees anterior to the femoral shaft at birth, decreasing to 10 to 15 degrees by adolescence.[51] *Abnormal femoral anteversion* refers to abnormally increased anterior angulation of the proximal femur for the child's age. With larger angulations, the entire limb becomes medially rotated in order to maintain the femoral head–acetabular relationship (the synonymous term *medial femoral torsion*).

In the vast majority of cases, abnormal anteversion will correct by early adolescence without intervention. The only treatment, surgical correction with a femoral derotation osteotomy, is generally considered if the deformity is persistent, severe, and produces cosmetic and functional impairment.[52] Performing osteotomy to prevent subsequent osteoarthritis as an adult is considered controversial, as the causal relationship of abnormal anteversion on development of osteoarthritis is in dispute.[53]

Indications for Imaging

The younger child with abnormal femoral anteversion typically is brought to the clinician because of intoeing or because he or she

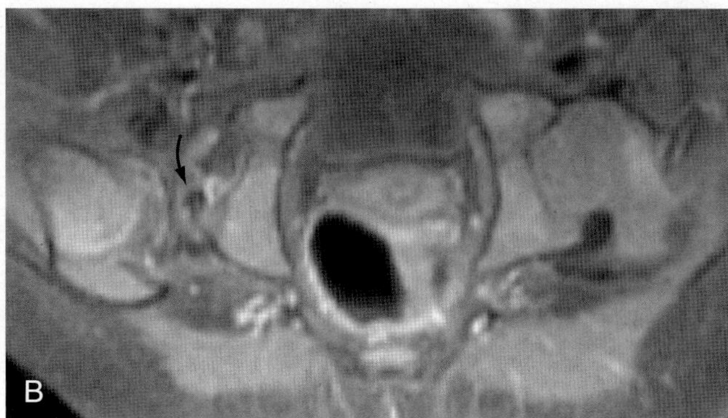

FIGURE 25-12. Spica in a 4 month old who underwent closed reduction and spica cast placement. **A,** Coronal proton density fat-saturated MR image of the pelvis shows persistent superior and lateral dislocation of the right hip. **B,** Axial proton density fat-saturated MR image after IV gadolinium shows interposition of the labrum in the hip joint preventing reduction. The fibrocartilaginous labrum is hypointense in both sequences *(arrows)*.

may trip and fall more often than other children, perceived as clumsiness. Imaging is warranted in the child in whom abnormal anteversion is suspected based on clinical and exam findings and in the postoperative patient after osteotomy.

Anteversion is also associated with several conditions in which the torsion angle may need to be measured for management decisions, including cerebral palsy, poliomyelitis, myelomeningocele, Legg-Calve-Perthes' disease, developmental dysplasia of the hip, and fracture.[51,54-56] The converse situation, retroversion, is seen in slipped capital femoral epiphysis.[51]

Osteoarticular Imaging

In the past, a number of fluoroscopic and radiographic methods were utilized to measure femoral anteversion, including biplane radiography with calculation using trigonometric equations.[50] Currently, CT is the standard method for direct assessment and has been shown to be more accurate and reliable than radiographs.[57] The anteversion angle is measured as the angle that the femoral neck makes with a transverse plane projected through the femoral condyles, viewing the femur on end. Although numerous methods of calculation have been proposed and debated,[51,54,55,58,59] a commonly used and widely cited method is described here.[54] Selected CT slices are obtained from two different scans, one through the femoral neck and the other through the distal femur at the condyles. Proximal images should include the femoral neck at a level including the upper margin of the greater trochanter, whereas distal images should be measured at a level just below the upper pole of the patella near the distal condyles. The angle of anteversion is that angle formed by a line drawn through the femoral neck and a line through the transcondylar axis. The transcondylar line is that which bisects a line tangential to the anterior margin of the condyles and a line tangential to the posterior margins (Figure 25-13).

In patients with cerebral palsy, femoral anteversion is a common problem owing to muscular imbalance and delayed weight bearing.[56] Although many have proposed the need for 3D CT reconstruction for evaluation in these patients in order to compensate for difficulties such as in positioning the spastic patient or for anatomic variables such as an increased shaft-neck angle, this topic is debated.[60]

Because MRI and ultrasound do not involve ionizing radiation, they are tempting alternatives for measurement of anteversion. Although MRI has been reported to yield results similar to those of CT in children and adults, it is not used routinely, perhaps because of its limited availability, increased exam time, and increased cost. Direct measurements performed by ultrasound have been reported to be unreliable in measuring anteversion.[61]

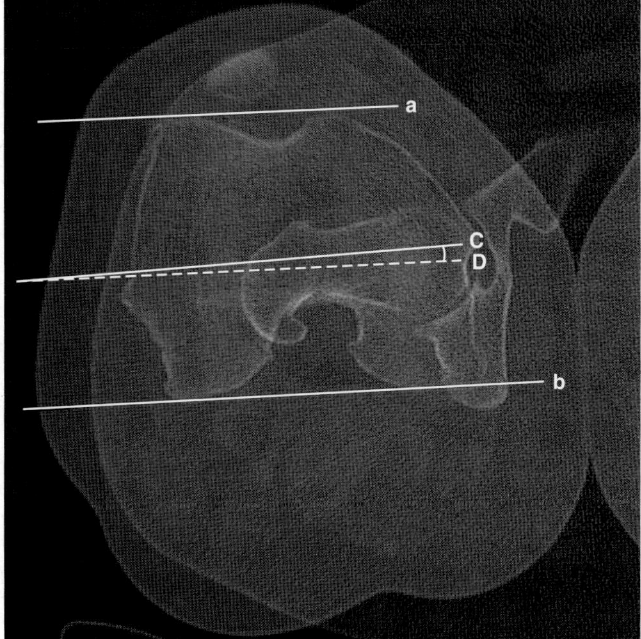

FIGURE 25-13. CT scanning for determining femoral anteversion. CT scans are obtained through the femoral necks and the femoral condyles. The proximal and distal images are superimposed. Axis of the femoral condyle (line C) is the bisector of angle between tangents to anterior (line a) and posterior (line b) margins of the femoral condyles. Line D is the axis of the femoral neck. Femoral torsion is the angle between line C and line D.

Genu Valgum (Knock Knees)

Genu valgum is a common entity that is most often physiologic in nature and part of the normal developmental change in lower extremity alignment that occurs during childhood. The overwhelming majority of cases are physiologic variants that will resolve.[62] Less commonly, focal or systemic pathologic conditions are the culprit, resulting in valgus that is more inclined to progress and require treatment.[62] It is important to understand the normal developmental sequence, which begins with maximal bowing (genu varum) in the newborn period, straightening between 20 and 22 months of age, and then reversal of this configuration into maximum valgus angulation of 10 to 15 degrees at approximately 3 years of age.[62] Then gradual reduction of valgus alignment to the normal "adult" level of 5 to 7 degrees occurs by 6 to 7 years of age. Minimal change in valgus is normally observed during adolescence.[63] By definition, pathologic genu valgum exists when the tibiofemoral angle is more than two standard deviations above normal.[62,64] Several graphs of normal values have been published.[64]

In normal developmental, the knees show maximal bowing (genu varum) in the newborn period, straightening between 20 and 22 months of age, and reversal into maximum valgus angulation of 10 to 15 degrees at approximately 3 years of age, followed by gradual reduction of valgus to the normal "adult" level of 5 to 7 degrees by 6 to 7 years of age.

Pathologic genu valgum can be idiopathic, posttraumatic (from inadequate reduction or physeal damage and growth arrest), metabolic, neuromuscular, postinfectious (from growth plate disruption or hyperemia resulting in asymmetric growth), or from generalized inherited disorders[62] (Figure 25-14). The presence of unilateral valgus deformity should raise suspicion of underlying tumor, infection, prior fracture at the distal femur or proximal tibia, physeal trauma, prior surgery, metaphyseal dysplasia, fibular hemimelia, or multiple epiphyseal dysplasia.[65]

Unilateral valgus deformity requires investigation for an underlying cause.

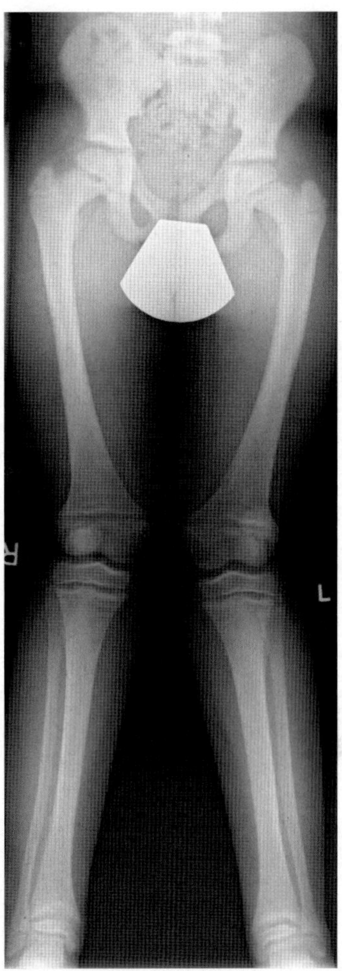

FIGURE 25-14. Genu valgum due to rickets. Ten year old with hypophosphatemic rickets. Radiograph of the lower extremities shows irregularity and cupping of the growth plates resulting in genu valgum.

Indications for Imaging

The child with physiologic valgus will typically be less than 7 years of age, be of normal stature, will have symmetric involvement of the lower limbs, and will have a tibiofemoral angle of under 15 degrees.[62] Assessment of genu valgum on clinical exam includes measurement of the tibiofemoral angle and intermalleolar and intercondylar distances, for which tables of normal ranges have been reported.[64] Clinical assessment should include observation of gait, particularly the stance phase in order to detect presence of a medial thrust at the knee, the presence of which indicates that the medial ligamentous and muscular knee restraints have become insufficient to resist deformity just after heel strike.[65,66] A medial thrust is seen in pathologic but not physiologic states.[66]

In patients with clinical findings compatible with physiologic genu valgum, radiographs are typically not necessary.[62] However, radiographs have been recommended in cases of suspected pathologic genu valgum; for example, when deformity is severe or asymmetric, there are other musculoskeletal abnormalities, there is a positive family history, the tibiofemoral angle is greater than 15 to 20 degrees, or the patient is of short stature[62,63] (Figure 25-15).

Osteoarticular Imaging

A single long-cassette anteroposterior radiograph during weight bearing is obtained of both lower extremities, including the hips, knees, and ankles.[62,63] The image is taken with the knees facing forward, disregarding the positioning of the feet in order to get a true understanding of the mechanical axes.[63] A lateral radiograph may be helpful to detect abnormalities in the sagittal plane if such deformity is suspected.[62] The tibiofemoral angle is measured as the angle formed by lines drawn along the long axes of the femoral and tibial shafts. Specific causes of pathologic valgum should be evaluated, such as angular deformity from prior fracture or physeal injury. Patients with idiopathic genu valgum may show flattening of the lateral femoral condyle.[62]

Clubfoot

Clubfoot, or talipes equinovarus, describes a complicated malalignment of the foot and ankle that is composed of equinus of the hindfoot (fixed plantar flexion of the talus), varus deformity of the heel, and varus deformity of the forefoot.[67,68] There also may be cavus (raised longitudinal arch of the foot) and forefoot adductus, depending on severity.[68]

Clubfoot has been reported to occur two times more commonly in boys than girls and has an overall incidence ranging from 0.6 to 6.8 per 1000, depending on race.[67] Genetics have been reported to play an important role in clubfoot such that the occurrence rate is 17 times higher for first-degree relatives and six times higher for second-degree relatives of affected persons.[67]

There are four main classes of clubfoot.[67] The first class is idiopathic, occurring in otherwise normal children and requiring intensive treatment for resolution. The second class is postural in nature, resolving entirely with manipulation or one or two casts. The third class is neurogenic clubfoot, which occurs in patients with myelomeningocele. The fourth class is that seen in patients with certain syndromes.

Indications for Imaging

Mosca states that the diagnosis of clubfoot can and should be made on clinical grounds alone, with no clear consensus as to the role of radiography in diagnosis and management.[67] Clinical criteria for grading the severity of clubfoot have been described.[69] Radiographs in this setting are limited because there is little ossification in the bones of the newborn foot, and, moreover, there is delayed ossification in the setting of clubfoot.[67] In addition, the ossific nuclei are not located centrally within their cartilage anlagen, making assessment of the true relationships of the structures difficult. Finally, it is arduous to reproducibly position the clubfoot for radiographs, rendering assessment and comparisons difficult.[67,70] Nevertheless, some authors propose that radiographs may be helpful for confirming correction or to assess residual deformity in patients who have undergone treatment; intraoperatively to confirm adequate correction; postoperatively to confirm maintenance of correction; and when there is recurrence or secondary deformity.[67,71]

Osteoarticular Imaging

Radiographic technique and patient positioning for evaluation of clubfoot are very important and the subject of extensive descriptions and controversy, with the foot ideally positioned in as close as possible to the maximally corrected appearance.[72] Radiographs should be focused on the hindfoot, as measurements in this region are the main purpose of this view.[70,72]

On the AP view, in normal individuals, a line drawn along the longitudinal axis of the midtalus should intersect or pass just medial to the first metatarsal, whereas in clubfoot this line will lie more laterally[73,74] (Figure 25-16). A line drawn along the longitudinal axis of the midcalcaneus should normally overlie the fourth metatarsal head but will fall more laterally in clubfoot.[73] The angle formed between these lines, the talocalcaneal angle, will be abnormally small in clubfoot due to hindfoot varus. On the AP radiograph, features that should be evaluated include abnormal medial displacement of the cuboid on the calcaneus, the talocalcaneal angle (typically <20 degrees in clubfoot), and the talus–first metatarsal angle (up to 30 degrees valgus normally and mild to severe varus in clubfoot).[70]

On the lateral radiograph, the normal angle formed by lines drawn through the midtalus and the midaxis of the calcaneus should be acute, whereas in clubfoot these approach parallelism due to the equinus deformity with elevation of the posterior calcaneus[73,74] (Figure 25-16, *B*). A line drawn through the midtalus will coincide with a line drawn through the first metatarsal (in children older than 5 years), whereas in clubfoot these will form an obtuse angle.[73,74] The talocalcaneal (usually <25 degrees in clubfoot) and talar–first metatarsal angles should be measured.[70] A line drawn along the inferior cortical surface of the calcaneal body normally forms an obtuse angle with a line drawn along the inferior fifth metatarsal cortex, an angle that increases in

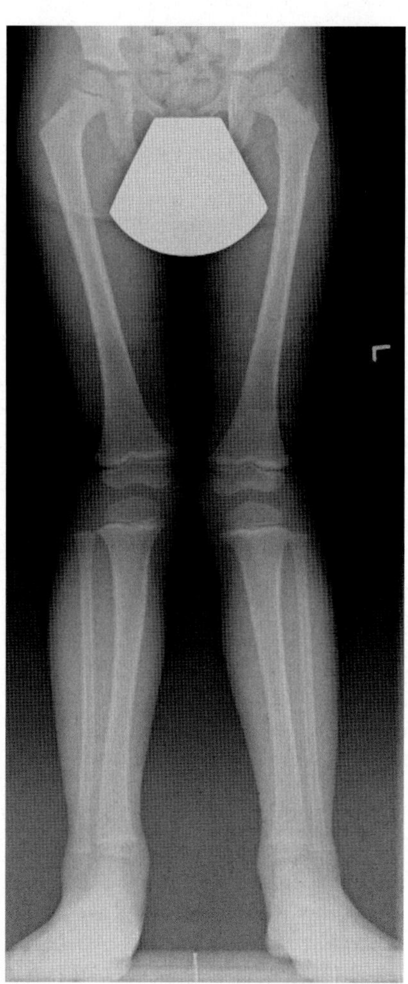

FIGURE 25-15. Four year old with idiopathic genu valgum.

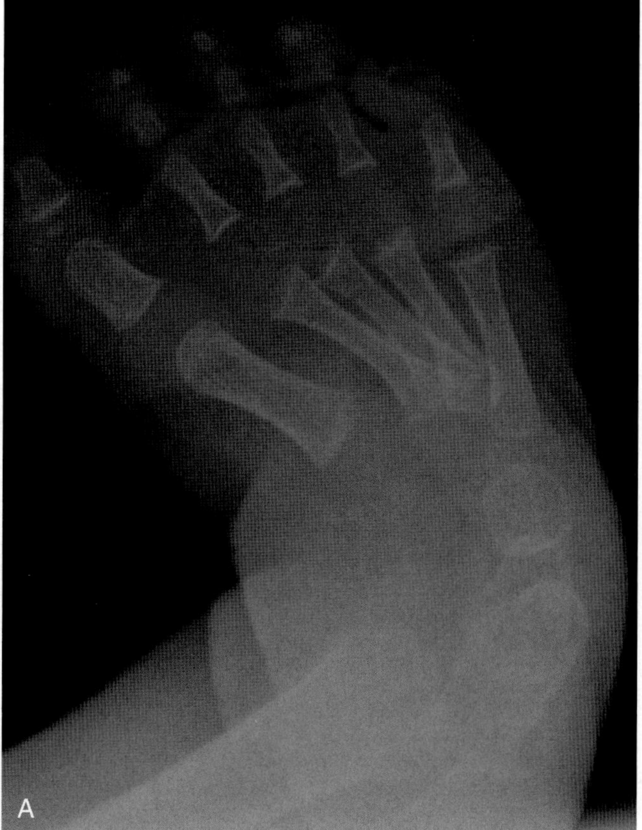

FIGURE 25-16. One year old with clubfoot. Simulated weight-bearing radiographs. **A,** AP view shows hindfoot and forefoot varus. The talus overlaps the calcaneus.

(Continued)

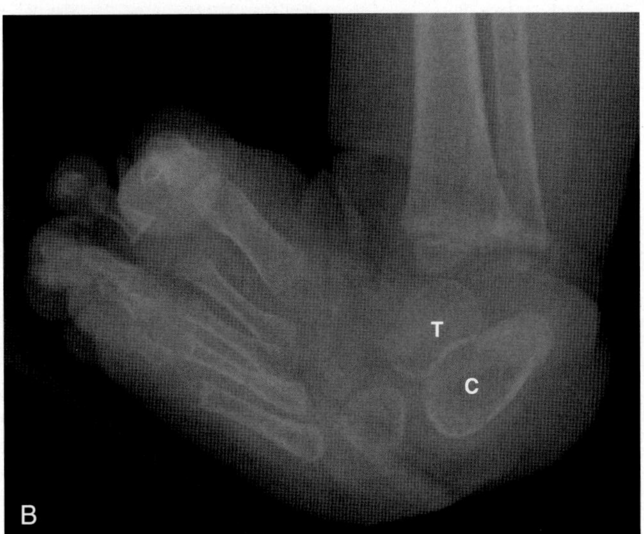

FIGURE 25-16—cont'd. B, Lateral view shows the talus *(T)* and calcaneus *(C)* parallel to each other and stepladder configuration of the metatarsals.

clubfoot.[74] Plantar flexion of the forefoot on the lateral view may be due to contracted soft tissues or to a triangular shape of the navicular[70]. These angles change with age, and graphs depicting the range of normal values in children have been reported.[72,74,75]

Radiographs obtained in long-term follow-up after correction have been reported to show residual abnormalities related to incomplete correction or post-treatment changes, including an inferiorly wedged appearance of the navicular on the lateral view, dorsal displacement of the navicular, flattening of the trochlear surface of the talus, decreased overall length of the talus, shortening of the calcaneus, decreased talocalcaneal angle on both the frontal and lateral views, and lateral wedging of the distal tibial epiphysis.[71] Some of these changes have been postulated as due to sequelae of dorsiflexion during cast correction.[71]

European centers have reported the use of ultrasound for preoperative and postoperative evaluation of clubfoot to evaluate the talonavicular joint, as the navicular can be medially displaced relative to the talar head, and deformity at this joint has important ramifications for the success of treatment.[76,77]

3D analysis based on CT also has been reported for evaluating the complex intraosseus and interosseus relationships that comprise the clubfoot deformity.[78] The talocalcaneal angle is considered an important parameter for evaluating the corrected clubfoot, and CT with 3D reconstruction has been reported to more accurately reveal the talocalcaneal angle than AP radiographs in this population.[79] Hindfoot correction using this measurement was reported to be misleading by radiographs compared with 3D CT in 75% of patients in one study.[79]

MRI is not routinely performed for evaluation of the idiopathic clubfoot.[67] Thus far, reports utilizing MRI have been primarily in a research setting, contributing to understanding of the pathoanatomic relationships in clubfoot.[80,81] Deformities that have been reported include a medial deviation of the talar head and neck, a parallel appearance of the talus relative to the calcaneus, and internal rotation of the calcaneus relative to the talus with resultant lateral deviation of the posterior calcaneus.[80] MRI shows the cartilaginous as well as the ossified structures in order to more fully evaluate alignment of hindfoot and midfoot structures.[80,81] One example of the importance of assessing the cartilage was illustrated by a study showing an abnormally smaller angle due to internal rotation of the cartilaginous talus relative to the bimalleolar plane than in normals, compared with a similar angle when using the osseus talus for measurement.[81] Based on this finding, some authors suggest that preoperative MRI may be helpful when contemplating surgical medial talar de-rotation.[81]

Extraarticular Findings

Clubfoot can be associated with several syndromes, including arthrogryposis, constriction bands (Streeter's dysplasia), prune belly, tibial hemimelia, Mobius syndrome, Pierre Robin syndrome, diastrophic dwarfism, Opitz's syndrome, Larsen's syndrome, and Freeman-Sheldon syndrome.[67]

Although many texts recommend screening hip radiographs in children with idiopathic clubfoot to evaluate for occult but associated developmental dysplasia of the hip, both of which may be related to in utero crowding, the actual rate of hip dysplasia in this population has been reported to be less than 1% in one study.[82]

Tarsal Coalition

Tarsal coalition is abnormal fusion of two tarsal bones. In 90% of cases, fusion occurs between the talus and calcaneus or the calcaneus and the navicular.[83] Coalition is most commonly congenital as the result of failure of segmentation, although it also may be acquired as the sequela of surgery, trauma, infection, or articular disorders. An autosomal dominant inheritance pattern with variable or near-full penetrance has been suggested.[67] It is estimated to affect about 1% of the population and is bilateral in 50% to 60% of cases.[84] The tissue forming the coalition may be osseus, cartilaginous, fibrous, or a combination thereof.

> Tarsal coalition (fusion of tarsal bones) may be fibrous, cartilaginous, or osseous and most often is talocalcaneal or calcaneonavicular.

Indications for Imaging

Tarsal coalition generally becomes symptomatic in adolescence when coalitions tend to ossify.[85,86] Some will present in adulthood. Not uncommonly, the onset of symptoms may coincide with increased stress or trauma.[85] Complaints and findings include vague midtarsal pain, recurrent ankle sprains, worsening pain with activity, eversion of the foot and pain on inversion (peroneal tendon spasm), decreased subtalar movement, and painful flatfoot.[87] These findings and symptoms are not pathognomonic for coalition, and imaging studies are used for diagnosis of coalition and exclusion of differential considerations such as infection, trauma, or arthritis. Finally, coalition may be asymptomatic and discovered incidentally.

Although radiographs are often the initial examination performed in the setting of foot pain, the complicated anatomy of the hindfoot often necessitates advanced imaging techniques, particularly for talocalcaneal coalition. Radiographs alone are more sensitive for detecting calcaneonavicular than talocalcaneal coalition.[88] After radiographs, CT is more commonly used than MRI, although both have high sensitivity and perform better than radiographs alone. The combination of radiographs and CT can identify most coalitions.[85] Bone scan or arthrography is rarely utilized.

Osteoarticular Imaging

Radiography is often the initial evaluation, a study that includes standard AP and lateral weight-bearing views, as well as a 45-degree internal rotation lateral oblique view. If the radiologist is aware of the suspicion of coalition, a special Harris view of the calcaneus is considered the most helpful radiographic view for talocalcaneal fusion, although the technique is somewhat challenging and may require images at multiple degrees of angulation.[89] Several radiographic signs have been described that facilitate identification, although it should be kept in mind that radiographs may appear normal, particularly in cases of talocalcaneal coalition.

In talocalcaneal coalition, abnormal fusion is usually seen at the middle facet of the subtalar joint (Figure 25-18). Much less commonly, fusion may occur at the posterior subtalar joint.[90] Classically described signs, evident on the lateral view, are the C-sign, describing the continuous C-shaped cortical contour of the fused abnormal medial talus with the inferior outline of the sustentaculum tali[91] (Box 25-7), and the "talar beak" sign, an exophytic and often triangular-shaped protuberance at the anterosuperior aspect of the talar head resulting from periosteal elevation with osseus repair due to abnormal subtalar joint motion.[88] Although the C-sign is helpful when present and has a reported sensitivity of 40% to 98%,[92,93] a higher rate of false negative exams has been reported in patients younger than 12 years and in those with posterior rather than middle subtalar fusion.[93] Moreover, the C-sign has been reported to be possibly a specific (although insensitive) marker of flatfoot deformity and may be neither specific nor sensitive for subtalar coalition itself.[94]

Other signs reported helpful in the diagnosis include a short talar neck, nonvisualization of the middle talocalcaneal facet, a dysmorphic-appearing sustentaculum tali, broadening of the lateral process of the talus, posterior subtalar joint narrowing, and a ball-and-socket appearance of the ankle joint.[84,95] In particular, the "absent middle facet" sign on a lateral standing radiograph may be as useful as the C-sign.[92]

BOX 25-7. Radiographic Signs of Tarsal Coalition

TALOCALCANEAL
- C-sign (continuous medial talus and sustentaculum) on lateral view
- Flat foot
- Talar beak
- Short talar neck
- Absent middle facet
- Abnormal sustentaculum tali
- Wide lateral process of the talus
- Narrow subtalar joint
- "Ball and socket" ankle

CALCANEONAVICULAR
- "Anteater" sign
- Broad navicular
- Tapering of the lateral navicular
- Calcaneonavicular fusion or narrow calcaneonavicular joint, cystic changes
- Talar bea
- Short talar neck
- Flat foot

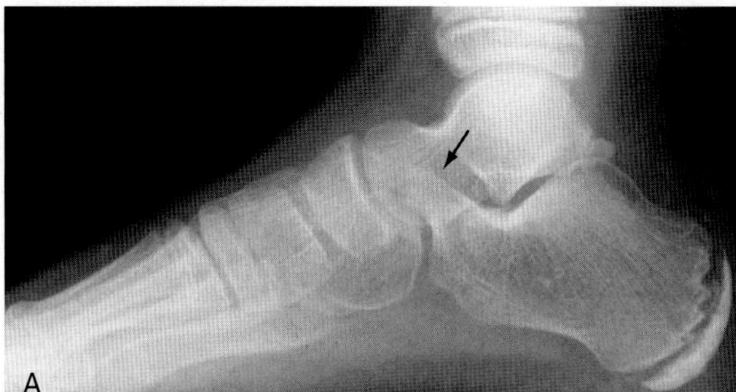

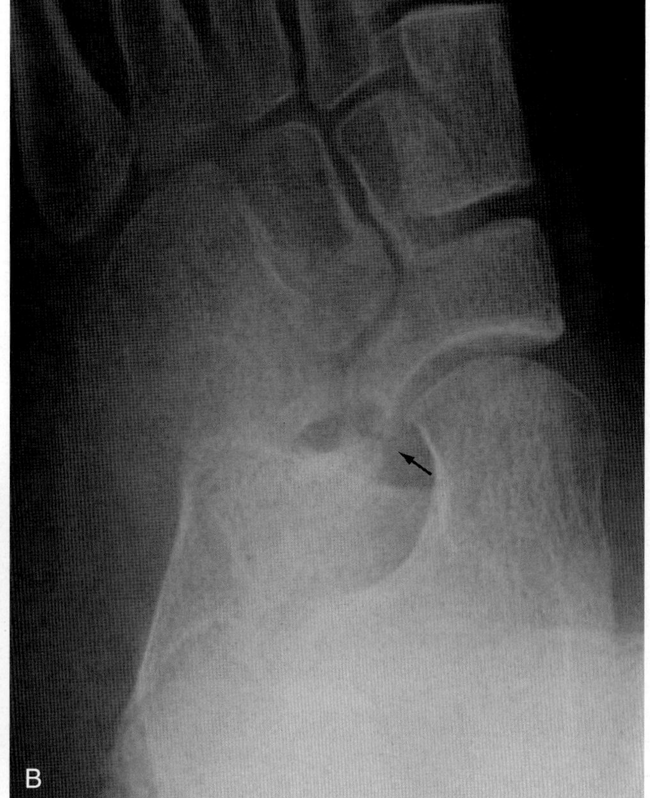

FIGURE 25-17. Nine year old with unilateral calcaneonavicular fibroosseous coalition. **A,** Lateral radiograph of the foot shows a broad, elongated irregular anterior calcaneal process ("anteater" sign, *arrow*). **B,** Oblique radiograph shows the narrow joint, partial osseous bridge and wide and irregular navicular surface *(arrow)*.

In calcaneonavicular coalition, there is fusion between the anterior process of the calcaneus and the navicular bone (see Figure 25-17). The classic sign is the "anteater" sign, so called because of the elongated and broad-tipped anterior calcaneal process simulating an anteater's nose as appreciated on the lateral view. The oblique radiograph is the most helpful for directly visualizing the coalition. In osseus coalition, a bony bar will join the two bones. In nonosseus coalition, the calcaneonavicular gap will be narrowed, the anterior process of the calcaneus will have a flattened and widened contour, and the apposed cortical surfaces may be irregular.[96] Other helpful signs that have been reported and may be seen on the AP view include a broad navicular (wider than the talonavicular joint), tapering of the lateral navicular, and visualization of the calcaneonavicular bar.[95]

The "talar beak" sign and a short talar neck also may be seen in calcaneonavicular fusion and are therefore not specific for talocalcaneal fusion.[95] The talar beak can be differentiated from other entities also occurring at the dorsal talus, including a normal or hypertrophied talar ridge at the insertion of the joint capsule (located over the dorsum of the talar neck, more proximal than a true talar beak) and talar osteophytes seen in the setting of osteoarthritis (at the talar head near the articulation with the navicular).[97] In both calcaneonavicular and talocalcaneal coalitions, pes planus, or flatfoot deformity, may be seen on the lateral view.

CT is performed in the patient with suspected or confirmed coalition based on radiographs, for diagnosis when there is high clinical suspicion and nonsuggestive radiographs, for better assessment of the nature of coalition (osseus, cartilaginous, or fibrous), for evaluation of other sites of coalition in the same or contralateral foot, and for operative planning. CT should include both feet and is obtained with axial (long axis) and coronal (short axis) images.

The coronal (short axis) view shows talocalcaneal coalition to best advantage (Figure 25-18). Although osseus coalition is usually obvious, the only suggestion of nonosseus coalition may be minimal narrowing of a middle facet that does not have its normal medially upward slope.[88] In calcaneonavicular coalition, bony bridging or an abnormal articulation will be seen between a widened anterior calcaneus and the navicular, best seen on the axial (long axis) view (Figure 25-19). Fibrous or cartilaginous coalitions are commonly associated with hypertrophic bony changes and irregularity at apposing surfaces and are often more subtle than frank osseus coalition. Other findings in nonosseus coalition[88] include joint space narrowing, cystic changes, and subchondral sclerosis.[86]

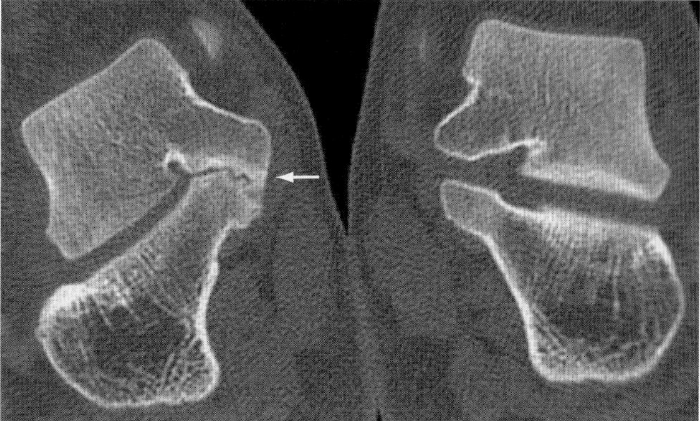

FIGURE 25-18. Eleven year old with unilateral talocalcaneal coalition. CT coronal image shows bony coalition of the right middle talocalcaneal facet *(arrow)*. The left side is normal.

Although CT generally poorly discriminates cartilaginous from fibrous coalition (both substances are of similar soft tissue density), the distinction is not critical for management decisions.[86] From CT images, maps can be constructed to assess the area of the subtalar joint surface involved with coalition, a factor used in determining surgical treatment.[85] Secondary degenerative changes are also important findings and impact surgical decision-making.[88]

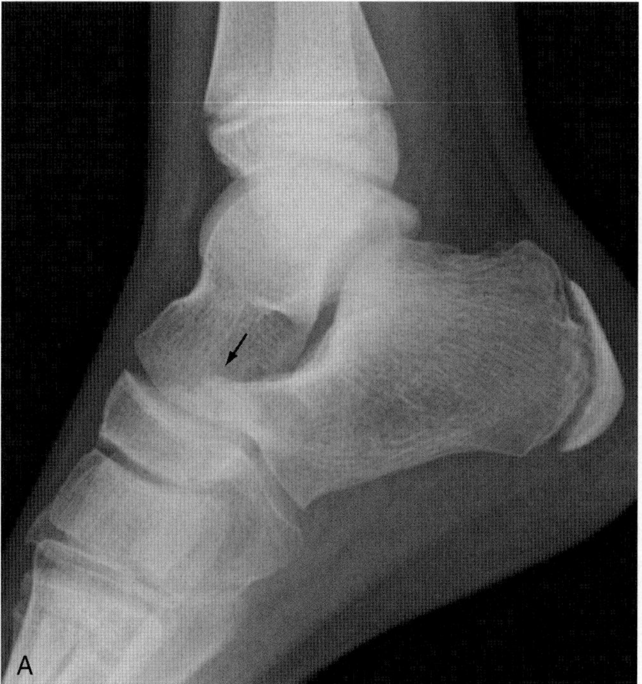

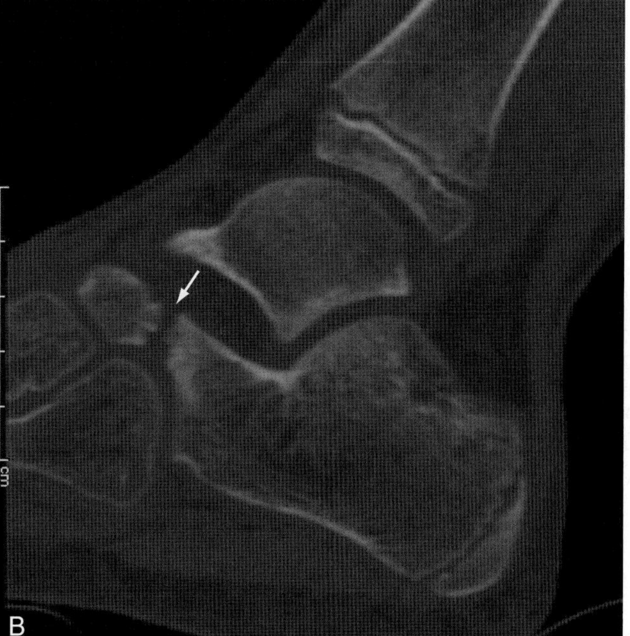

FIGURE 25-19. Eleven year old with unilateral calcaneonavicular coalition. **A,** Lateral radiograph of the foot shows an elongated anterior calcaneal process, the "anteater" sign *(arrow)*. **B,** Sagittal CT image shows the irregularity and narrowing of the calcaneonavicular joint consistent with nonosseous coalition *(arrow)*.

(Continued)

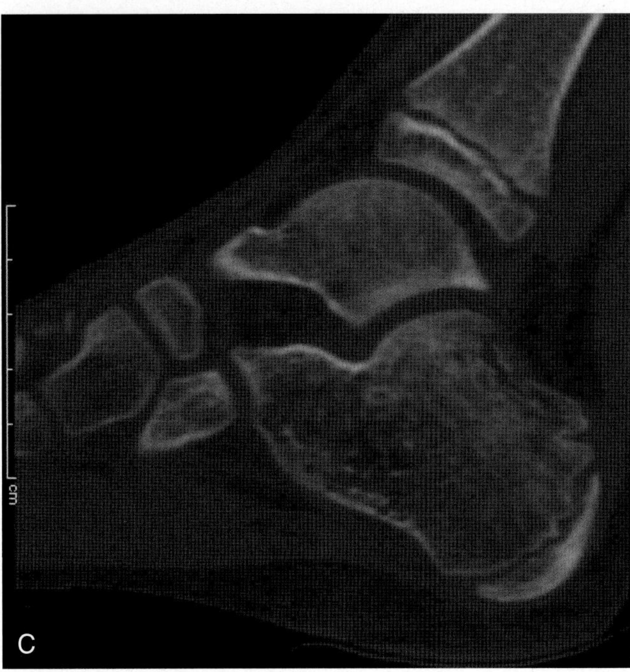

FIGURE 25-19—cont'd. **C,** CT sagittal image of the opposite foot is normal.

CT is generally considered the cross-sectional exam of choice for coalition and is more cost effective than MRI. MRI has a high rate of agreement with CT and can better demonstrate other abnormalities. MRI therefore should be considered for use in patients in whom other causes of pain are also suspected.[86] Osseus coalition will be evidenced by marrow continuity between the involved bones, whereas nonosseus bridging will show an abnormal articulation and reactive changes as in CT (Figure 25-20). MRI is better than CT for determining whether coalition is cartilaginous or fibrous. MRI is more sensitive for detection of fibrous coalition than CT and/or radiographs, which may appear normal or nearly so.[83] As ossification of the coalition occurs during adolescence, MRI may be particularly useful in younger patients. MRI may show marrow edema at the site of a tarsal coalition at the margins of the abnormal articulation, which can be a helpful sign, particularly when other findings are subtle or the diagnosis is not suspected.[88] Generally, MRI is recommended when there is suspected tarsal coalition and radiographs and CT are negative or indeterminate,[85] as may be the case with fibrous coalition.

Bone scintigraphy is generally not particularly helpful during childhood and adolescence due to the presence of normal epiphyseal activity obscuring the affected areas.[83] However, use of specific magnification views has been shown to be positive in children and adolescents with talocalcaneal coalition and can be helpful in the setting of negative or equivocal CT results with high clinical suspicion, especially for nonosseus union.[98] Positive

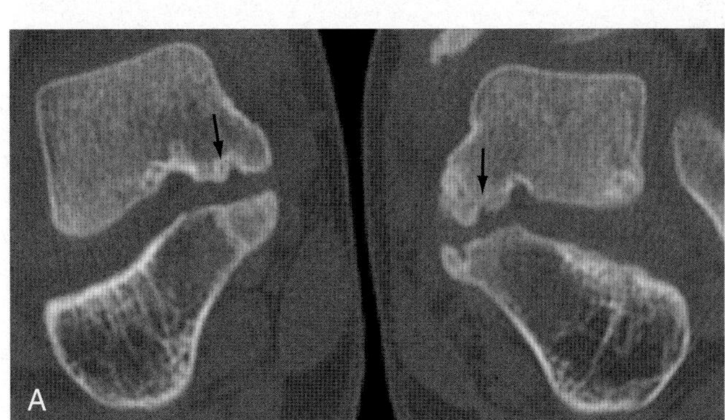

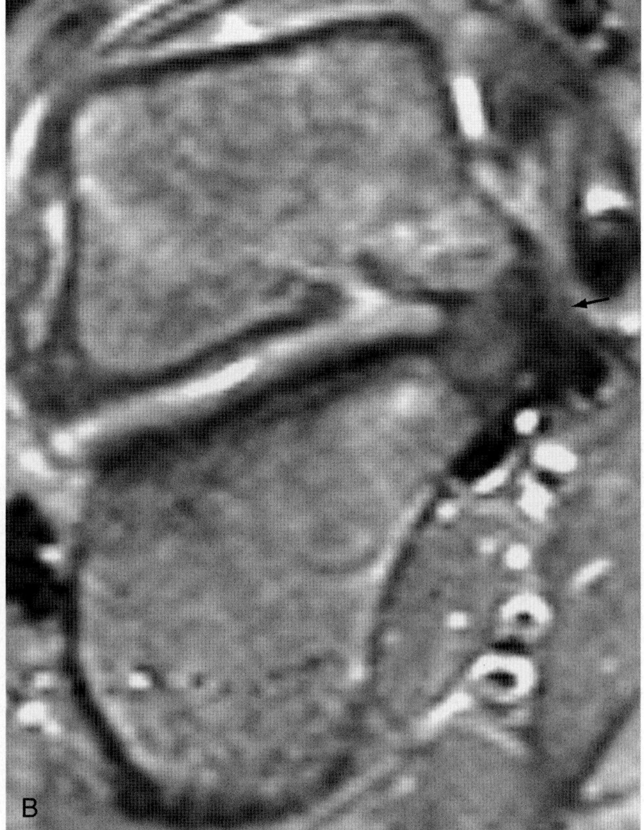

FIGURE 25-20. Six year old with bilateral talocalcaneal fibrous coalition. **A,** Coronal CT image shows irregularity and sclerosis of the articulating surfaces of the middle facets. **B,** Coronal T2-weighted MRI of the right side shows low signal intensity in the joint of the middle facet consistent with fibrous bridging *(arrows)*.

localized uptake has been reported in several cases of subtalar coalition in adolescents and adults.[89,99,100] In those patients in whom comparison was made with CT, CT was also positive or suggestive of the abnormality. In the pediatric population, localized subtalar uptake is nonspecific and could also be due to trauma, synovitis, infection, tumor, chondrolysis, or juvenile rheumatoid arthritis.[98,99]

Extraarticular Findings

Although tarsal coalition is most commonly an isolated finding, it can be associated with other congenital disorders, including fibular hemimelia, clubfoot, Apert's syndrome and Nievergelt-Pearlman's syndrome.[67] These coalitions have a propensity for more extensive subtalar involvement.

TRAUMA

Nonaccidental Trauma

According to available figures from the U.S Department of Health and Human Services, in 2006 an estimated 905,000 children were victims of child abuse and neglect and about 1500 children died. Risk factors include age < 1 year, prematurity, physical disability, low birth rate weight, low socioeconomic status, male sex, multiple birth, and stepchild status.[101]

Although neurologic and visceral injuries are important in the abused child, this section will focus on the musculoskeletal aspects of nonaccidental trauma. Skeletal injuries are infrequently life threatening, but they are common injuries and may be the most specific radiologic indicators of abuse.[36,102] Indeed, fractures are second only to skin lesions in the presentation of physical abuse.[103] Most fractures due to abuse occur in those younger than 3 years.[104]

Indications for Imaging

Imaging is indicated in the infant or child with suspected physical abuse. The skeletal survey[105] allows diagnosis of sites of fracture supporting abuse and detection of fractures in various stages of healing. It is also serves as a record and is often presented as evidence in care and protection cases, criminal proceedings, and other forms of litigation. It affords a global evaluation of the skeleton to allow differentiation of injury due to abuse from developmental changes, anatomic variants, and uncommon syndromes that may simulate abuse. If the examination demonstrates findings suspicious for abuse, a physician is legally required to notify local child protection authorities.

Because of the increased risk of abuse in twins, if one twin is injured, consideration should be given to imaging the other infant twin as well.[36]

According to the AAP Section on Radiology,[36] a skeletal survey is mandatory in suspected physical abuse for those younger than 2 years. For children ages 2 to 5, individualized use of a skeletal survey is recommended based on clinical indicators of abuse. For children older than 5 years, the screening skeletal survey or bone scan is considered of limited value. In these patients, focused radiographs in areas of complaint would be more judicious, given that occult, asymptomatic fractures are considered unlikely.

It should be remembered that because there are myriad fracture types that occur in abused children, the clinical history and purported mechanism of injury and the developmental state of the child must be considered. For example, a spiral fracture of the long bone, which arises from an unusual torsional force, should raise suspicion of abuse in a child who is not yet ambulatory.[106] The same fracture, however, is relatively common in the tibia ("toddler's fracture") once ambulation has begun.

Osteoarticular Imaging

Musculoskeletal injuries are commonly the result of shaking the child, creating forced flexion and extension on the spine and abnormal AP compression of the thoracic cage.[101] Pulling and twisting of the extremities result in long bone fractures, whereas blunt trauma accounts for skull fractures.[101]

The mainstay of diagnosis is the radiographic skeletal survey, a thorough multi-image examination performed with specific technical requirements of the entire axial and appendicular skeleton.[105] A "babygram" or "body gram," which includes the entire body on a single or two radiographs, is not considered of adequate detail for evaluation.[36] Although there are no data specifically analyzing whether digital imaging is comparable to traditional screen-film radiography, a significant percentage of radiology departments have migrated to newer digital technologies for the skeletal survey.[107]

When there is high clinical suspicion of abuse, a follow-up skeletal survey has been suggested approximately 2 weeks after initial evaluation to increase detection of and confidence in fracture diagnosis, especially for rib and metaphyseal fractures, and to add additional information as to the timing of injuries.[108]

Although nearly every type and location of fracture has been reported in nonaccidental trauma,[106] certain types of fractures are seen more commonly and are considered more specific for abuse.[102] Fractures considered of high specificity include the classic metaphyseal lesion, rib fractures (especially posterior), and sternal, scapular, and spinous process fractures (Box 25-8).

The classic metaphyseal lesion is the most specific fracture in abuse and is present in 39% to 50% of abused children younger than 18 months (Figure 25-21, *A*). Considered virtually diagnostic of abuse, it is a subepiphyseal plane of microfractures through the most immature area of mineralized matrix in the metaphysis that, depending on the size and severity of the fragment and orientation on imaging, results in a "bucket handle" lesion, metaphyseal lucency, or corner fracture.[109] This fracture is generally oriented perpendicular to the long axis of the bone and results from traction

BOX 25-8. The Specificity of Skeletal Injuries for Nonaccidental Trauma

HIGH SPECIFICITY
Classic metaphyseal lesions
Rib fractures (especially posterior)
Scapular fractures
Spinous process fractures
Sternal fractures

MODERATE SPECIFICITY
Multiple fractures (especially bilateral)
Fractures of different ages
Epiphyseal separation
Vertebral body fractures and subluxations
Digital fractures
Complex skull fractures

COMMON BUT LOW SPECIFICITY
Subperiosteal new bone formation
Clavicular fractures
Long bone shaft fractures
Linear skull fractures

From Kleinman PK: *Diagnostic imaging of child abuse*, ed 2, St Louis, 1998, Mosby, with permission.

and torsion on the extremity.[101] A disk-like fragment of bone results, thinner centrally, that may either have the shape of a bucket handle or a fractured corner of the metaphysis. These fractures are most commonly present in the humerus, femur, and tibia. They are reported almost solely in children younger than 2 years, who are small enough to be violently shaken.[106]

> The classic metaphyseal lesion is the most specific fracture for abuse and is seen in up to half of abused children younger than 18 months.

Rib fractures, especially posterior rib fractures, are of high specificity and importance in the diagnosis of abuse but are considered unusual even in severe accidental trauma[101] (Figure 25-21, *B*). They are rarely a birth-related event.[110] Unlike in the adult patient, even cardiopulmonary resuscitation (CPR) in children very uncommonly results in rib fractures and does not cause posterior fractures. Resulting from excessive AP compression of the thoracic cage, rib fractures in abuse are most commonly posterior but may occur at all sites, most commonly involve the middle ribs, and are often symmetric.[101] Posterior fractures are believed to be due to the pivoting of the rib head and neck over the vertebral transverse process during compression.[111] Discovery of posterior rib fractures in an otherwise normal infant without explanatory history of severe accidental trauma is highly suspicious for abuse. Adjunctive studies such as oblique chest radiographs, bone scintigraphy, follow-up radiographs, or CT all have been recommended to confirm or increase detection of rib fractures.[101,110]

Scapular and sternal fractures are of high specificity and involve large amounts of force. Scapular fractures most commonly involve the acromion[101] and should be differentiated radiologically from anatomic variants such as the acromiale.

Skull fractures are best detected with radiographs (Figure 25-22). CT may miss fractures that occur along the axial plane of the scan, and bone scan has been shown insensitive in this setting.[112] Fractures in the hands and feet are relatively uncommon in abuse, with one series finding fractures isolated to the metacarpals and proximal phalanges, predominantly of the buckle variety.[113] These fractures are best detected with oblique views or follow-up radiographs.

Discovering fractures in various stages of healing is considered a red flag for abuse, particularly so in the setting of an inconsistent explanatory history. The apparent stage of a fracture may be incongruent with the history provided by the caretaker, which itself can be an important clue to abuse.[104] Although the imaging appearance can suggest a time frame for occurrence, the timing of fracture dating in children evaluated for abuse may be an inexact science.[104,114]

CT and MRI have not been established as indicated for screening for nonaccidental skeletal trauma. MRI may be helpful for suspected epiphyseal separation based on radiographs.[36] CT with multiplanar reformations of the spine may be helpful for further characterization of complex fractures, whereas spine MRI should be performed if injury to the neural axis is suspected.[36]

The use of the radionuclide bone scan as the initial screening test for child abuse is somewhat controversial. It is likely best thought of as a complementary rather than competing examination with the skeletal survey, as has been proposed by some authors. The AAP Section of Radiology proposes that it may be an adjunctive or alternative exam for evaluation and may increase sensitivity for rib fractures, subtle diaphyseal fractures, and early

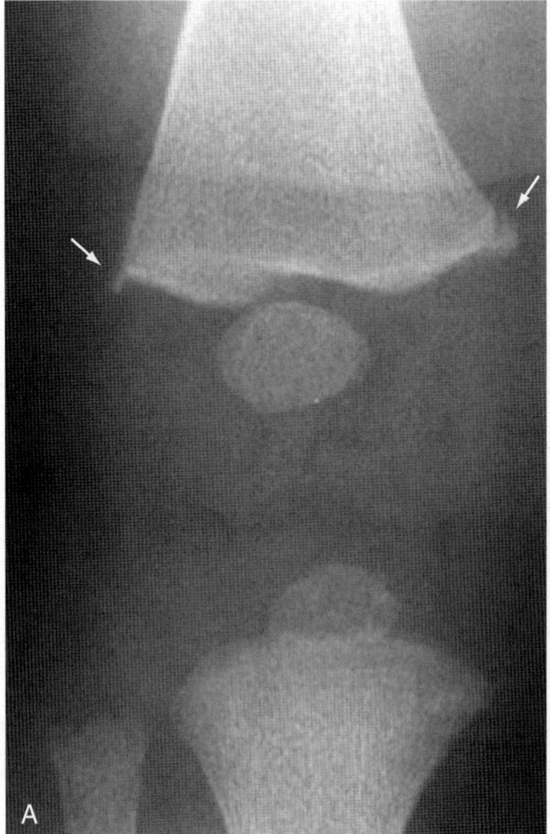

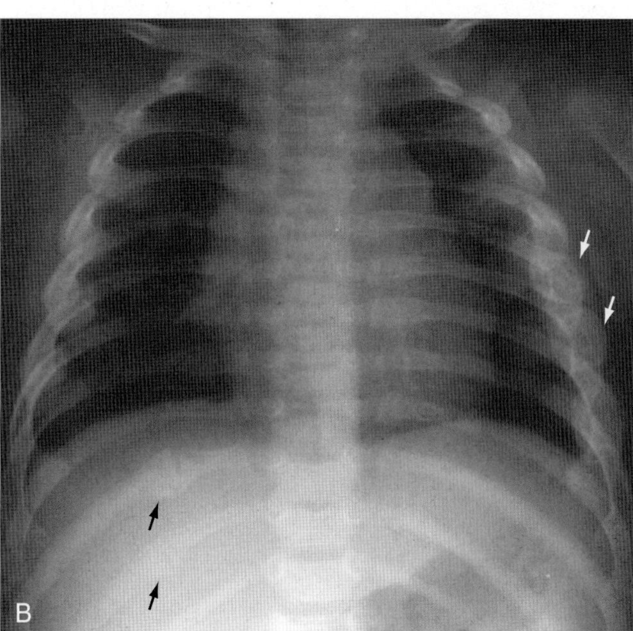

FIGURE 25-21. Two-month-old abused infant. **A,** AP radiograph of the knee shows classic metaphyseal lesions *(arrows)*. **B,** AP radiograph of the chest shows multiple rib fractures *(arrows)*.

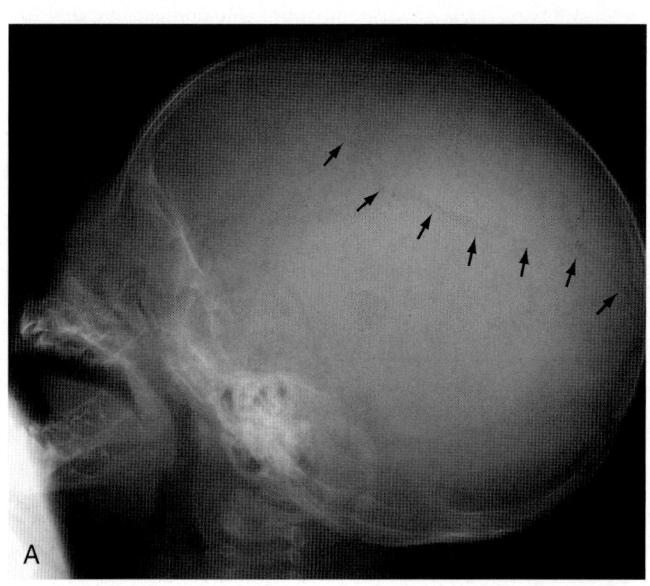

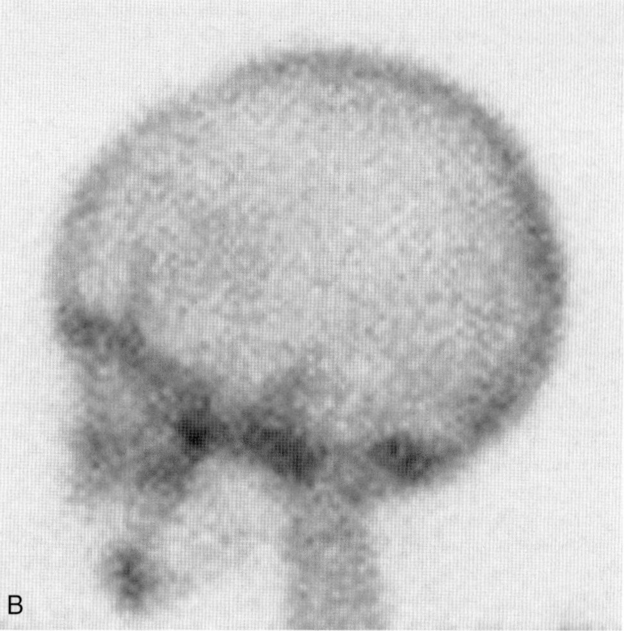

FIGURE 25-22. Two-month-old abused infant. **A,** Lateral radiograph of the skull shows a parietal skull fracture *(arrows)*. **B,** The fracture is not identified by skeletal scintigraphy.

periosteal elevation.[36] Thus bone scan is generally superior to radiographs for detection of rib fractures, periosteal injury, nondisplaced long bone fractures, and occult injuries but may perform less well than radiographs for older healed fractures and nondisplaced skull fractures.

To illustrate, in one retrospective study of 30 children with suspected nonaccidental trauma undergoing both radiography and bone scan examinations, 20% of children had positive findings on bone scan with negative skeletal survey, whereas 10% had radiographic findings and a negative bone scan. Of the radiographically missed injuries, there were four radial or ulnar, two rib, one foot, and one pelvic fracture. Scintigraphically missed injuries were predominantly classic metaphyseal injuries, a potential "blind spot" of the bone scan given normal increased radiotracer activity at the metaphyses in the same area where such fractures occur. However, with modern gamma camera technique, some authors conclude that such lesions should be detectable. The bone scan also may increase the conspicuity of lesions in areas with complex anatomy on radiographs, such as the scapula, pelvis, spine, and ribs. Even if an initial skeletal survey confirms abuse, the bone scan may disclose a more extensive injury pattern that may be important in legal proceedings.[114]

Because the bone scan may remain positive even with old fractures, the timing of injuries is limited from this study alone. If bone scan is used, all positive findings should be investigated further with dedicated radiographs, and two views of the skull should be obtained given the insensitivity of bone scan for cranial fracture.[36]

Extraarticular Findings

Intracranial trauma is an important cause of morbidity and mortality in the abused child, and all infants and children with suspected intracranial injury should be imaged with CT and/or MRI.[36] Noncontrast CT is highly specific and sensitive for detection of extraaxial hemorrhage and, because it is readily and quickly obtained, is important for detection of abnormalities that may require emergent surgical attention.[36] Sonography of the neonatal brain can show parenchymal and extraaxial trauma but is insensitive for small acute subdural hematomas and thus should generally be supplemented with CT or MRI.[36] MRI may show intraparenchymal hemorrhage, contusions, shear injuries, and edema.[36]

Blunt thoracoabdominal trauma should be evaluated with CT, with chest CT performed for detection of pulmonary contusion, pneumothorax, pleural effusion, rib fractures, and vascular or tracheobronchial injuries.[36] These findings are the same as those that may be seen in accidental trauma. Abdominal/pelvic CT is performed for evaluation of solid organ injury. In addition, findings of pancreatitis, duodenal hematoma, and bowel perforation should increase suspicion of abuse.[36]

Spondylolysis

Spondylolysis is a fatigue fracture of the pars interarticularis of the vertebral body arch, estimated to occur in 4% to 6% of the population[115] and more common in males. It has been widely reported that the incidence of this condition is higher in adolescent athletes, in whom spondylolysis is a common cause of low back pain and in whom clinical management and activity restriction can be challenging.[115,116] It predominates at the L5 level (85% to 95%), with L4 the second most common (5% to 15%) and upper lumbar vertebrae much less frequently involved.[115,117] In the majority of cases, defects are bilateral.[117]

Most spondylolytic defects are believed to develop over time during early childhood as the result of chronic mechanical stress, as this entity has not been seen in newborns.[115,118] Although a single traumatic event can complete a developing spondylolysis, acute trauma is not believed to be the sole etiology in most cases.[115] Of primary concern in spondylolysis is the predisposition to spondylolisthesis, anterior slippage of the vertebral body, with resultant spinal stenosis. While most patients fare well with nonsurgical management including rest and antilordotic bracing, spinal fusion is performed in the persistently symptomatic or in those who progress to spondylolisthesis and lumbar instability.[119]

> Spondylolysis (a fatigue fracture of the pars interarticularis) occurs in up to 6% of the population, is often bilateral, and may lead to spondylolisthesis (slipping) of the affected vertebra on the one below.

Indications for Imaging

The majority of cases of spondylolysis are asymptomatic, with low back pain the most common complaint in symptomatic individuals.[115] Pain may be focal and radiate into the buttocks or proximal lower extremities and may be gradual in onset or begin acutely after an event.[115] On physical exam, findings described include hyperlordotic posture with tight hamstrings, as well as reproduction of pain on hyperextension while standing on one leg (ipsilateral to a unilateral pars defect).[115]

Imaging plays an important role in evaluation of the patient with suspected spondylolysis, with radiographs usually performed to document the lesion and any accompanying spondylolisthesis. More sensitive techniques of CT, scintigraphy, and MRI are often used to evaluate the status of the defects and accompanying findings. There are several stages in the progression or healing of the pars defect that can be assessed on imaging studies. MRI and bone scan may allow detection of early changes prior to evidence of abnormality by other techniques, which is important for early treatment, particularly in the adolescent athlete in whom future participation in sports may be limited when the defect is found. Bone scan and MRI also may be important for determining the activity of a lesion and, given the presence of a large percentage of asymptomatic patients, may help to determine when spondylolysis requires treatment. Long-term symptoms of established spondylolysis include chronic low back pain and sciatica.[120]

Osteoarticular Imaging

Radiographs are the first step in evaluation of the young patient with low back pain.[121] A radiographic series including AP and lateral views is standard, with the oblique views used in selected cases as they are a source of relatively high radiation dose.[122,123] Spondylolysis is seen on radiographs as a linear lucency in the region of the pars interarticularis coursing from posterosuperior to anteroinferior. On oblique images, the appearance of the lucency has been likened to the broken neck or collar around the neck of a "Scottie dog" (Figure 25-23). Because of the orientation of the lucency and the fact that the defects are not tangential to the x-ray beam in many instances in these standard views, this study may not demonstrate spondylolysis with certainty. Studies show that two additional special projections may prove more useful, including a spot view of the lumbosacral junction and an AP view with 30 degrees cranial angulation with the x-ray beam centered on the superior aspect of the pubic symphysis.[122,124]

Secondary signs on an AP view include lateral deviation of the spinous process away from an effectively lengthened lamina secondary to a pars defect, as well as reactive sclerosis of a pedicle contralateral to a unilateral pars defect.[125,126]

> A dense pedicle in a child may result from a contralateral pars defect (due to stress changes), an osteoid osteoma (benign lesion), or a malignancy.

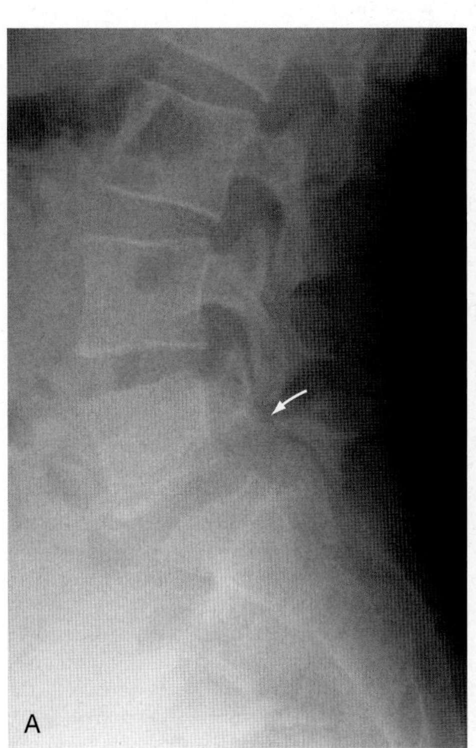

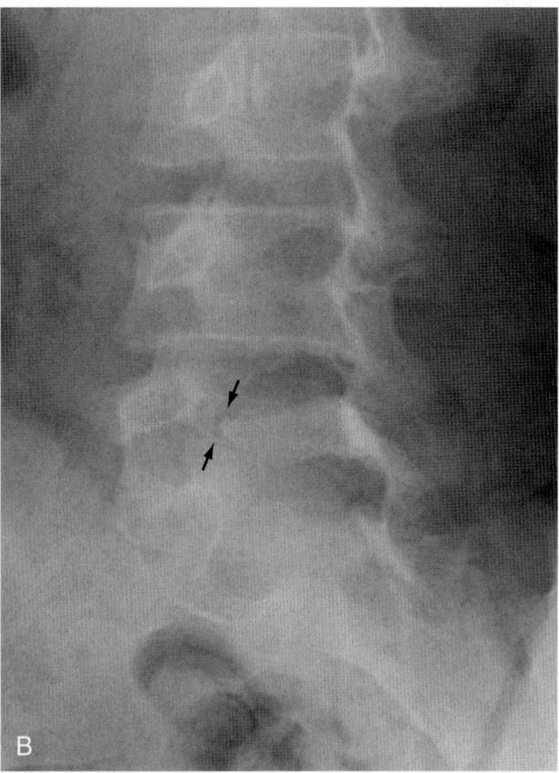

FIGURE 25-23. Fourteen year old with bilateral L5 spondylolysis and spondylolisthesis. **A,** Lateral radiograph of the lumbosacral spine shows the pars defect *(arrow)* and anterior slippage of L5 on S1; grade I spondylolisthesis. **B, C,** Oblique radiographs show the lucencies in the pars interarticularis, through the "Scottie dog" necks *(arrows).*

(Continued)

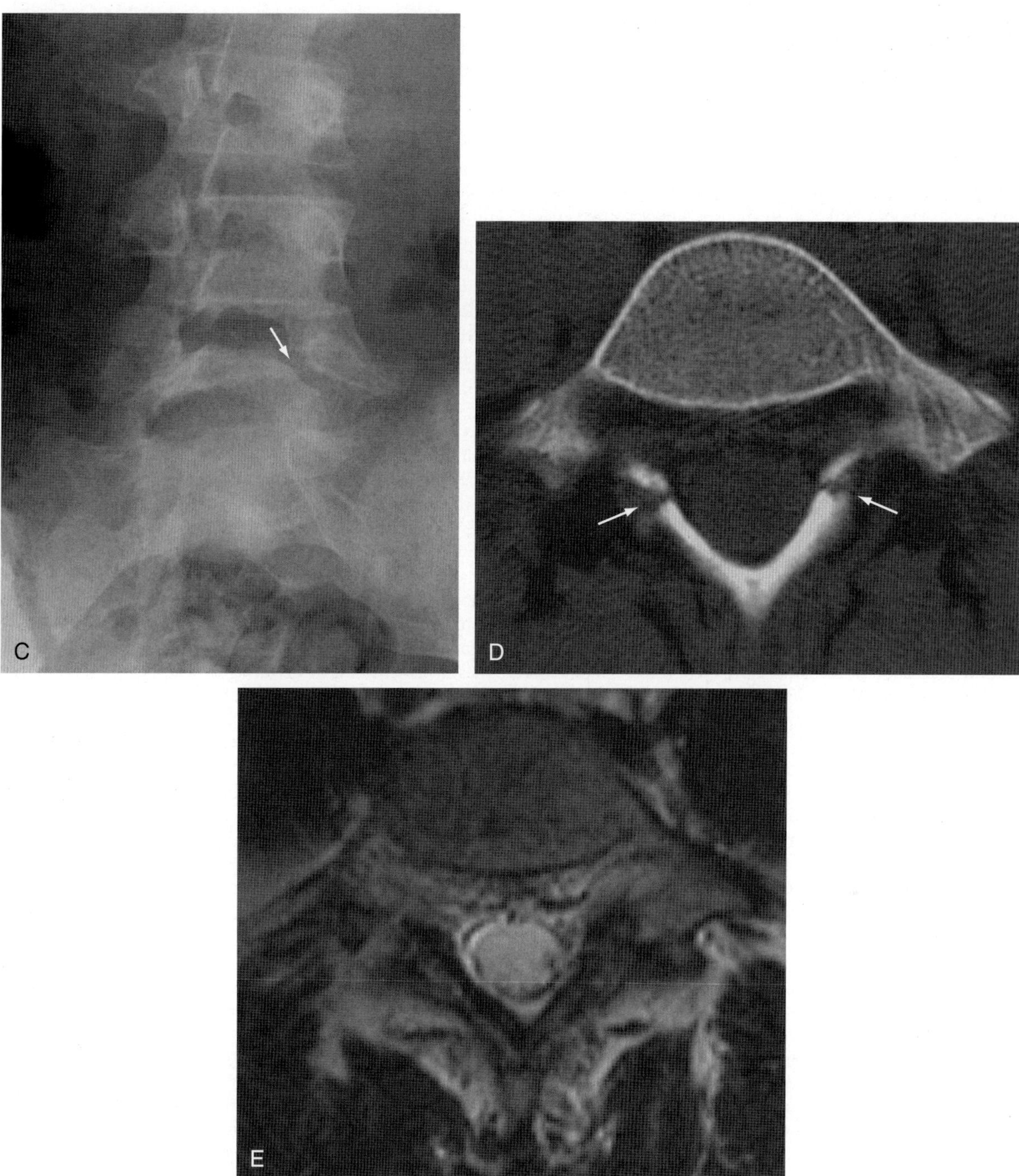

FIGURE 25-23—cont'd. **D,** Axial CT image shows bilateral pars lucencies and irregularity of the fracture margins *(arrows)*. **E,** Axial T2-weighted MR image shows minimal sclerosis in the pars fractures and no significant marrow edema, making the diagnosis with this modality difficult.

Posterior vertebral body wedging may be observed, which may be due to hypoplastic remodeling.[127] The lateral view is the most useful for determining the degree of any associated slippage (spondylolisthesis) in the AP direction, which is graded on a scale from 1 (< 25% slip with relation to the superior surface of the lower vertebral body) to 5 (complete slippage).

CT is currently the most frequently used advanced imaging modality for detection and characterization of spondylolysis and is more sensitive than radiographs[117] (see Figure 25-23, *C*). Therefore negative radiographs with clinical suspicion of spondylolysis warrant a CT scan. On axial images, the earliest change may be osteopenia of the pars interarticularis. As microfractures progress with chronic stress, a frank lucency (discontinuity) may appear. At first glance this lucency may appear similar to a facet joint, but these can be differentiated by the irregular contour of the spondylolysis and its location adjacent to the facets.[128] The defect can be partial or complete, narrow or wide. It will be seen on the axial slice just above the level of the neural foramen.

Associated findings include an elongated AP diameter of the bony canal and, in unilateral cases, hypertrophy of the contralateral neural arch.[128] If there is concomitant spondylolisthesis, a pseudobulging disk may be seen posterior to the slipped vertebra. The apparent disk bulge is usually broad and extends into both neural foramina, termed a "pseudobulge" because it is actually due to uncovering of the disk rather than to disk pathology per se.[117]

A wide spondylitic defect with corticated margins favors established non-union without potential for healing under conservative management.[126] Healed pars defects will manifest as irregularity with sclerosis and no frank fracture line evident, and there may also be elongation and narrowing of the pars.

Reformatted sagittal CT images, similar to a lateral radiograph, are best for showing any associated spondylolisthesis. Because pars defects typically parallel the plane of the L5-S1 disk and fractures are best seen when scanned perpendicular to the fracture plane, some authors propose improved conspicuity by reverse angulation of the CT gantry to acquire images rather than with standard spine technique performed with axial images paralleling the disk space.[126,129]

Bone scan using Tc99m MDP is also commonly used to detect spondylolysis. Although standard planar bone scan images (e.g., whole body bone scan) may show spondylolysis, sensitivity and specificity is increased with use of single photon emission computed tomography (SPECT) views that eliminate overlap, on which focal increased uptake is seen in the posterior elements.[121,130] Bone scan may be most useful for identifying the increased metabolic activity of an acute stress reaction of the pars before there is radiographic or CT abnormality in order to institute early treatment and prevent a complete break, as well as for determining the activity of a lesion seen by other methods.[119,121,126,131] Many authors conclude that radiographic findings without a positive bone scan indicate old injury, and positive scintigrams with normal radiographs denote an early or active abnormality.[119] Therefore a positive bone scan without radiographic abnormality may lead an orthopedist to treat conservatively with a back brace, whereas in a patient with pain and a radiographic as well as a scintigraphic abnormality, treatment may be either a back brace or surgical fusion.[121] Focal uptake on bone scan correlating with radiographic sclerosis contralateral to a frank defect may be due to active, early spondylolysis or to reactive changes.[119] Positivity on bone scan, however, is nonspecific and may be difficult to differentiate from facet osteoarthritis (in older individuals) and from osteoid osteoma or infection in the case of unilateral uptake.[115,126,132] This lack of specificity has led some authors to conclude that the etiology of a positive bone scan should be confirmed by CT.[126] An additional limitation of the bone scan is that chronic, healed lesions may not be shown,[119,131] and early stress reaction may not be differentiated from overt fracture.

> Because other lesions may be responsible for focal increased activity on bone scan (e.g., an osteoid osteoma), radiographic or CT correlation is always necessary.

Many authors conclude that a normal SPECT study effectively excludes spondylolysis as the cause of pain.[121,130] Although definitive studies correlating bone scan positivity with clinical significance and outcome have not been performed, a positive bone scan may provide guidance as to the need for treatment, particularly when other potential etiologies for pain are also identified.

MRI would seem an ideal modality for evaluation given its multiplanar capabilities and lack of ionizing radiation (particularly in adolescent females in whom the ovaries are included in the radiation field on other exams). However, MRI is not widely used as a first-line diagnostic method, and its role is under investigation and not yet well established.[133] In a study directly comparing the accuracy of MRI with CT and SPECT in the adolescent population, the authors concluded that MRI could be used as a first-line imaging modality given its high accuracy.[120] The main limitation of MRI was seen in cases in which CT revealed a partial or incomplete defect, which MRI misgraded. Importantly, that study utilized thin-section 3D gradient echo sagittal images for MRI evaluation, a sequence not standard in routine lumbar spine protocols at most institutions. Moreover, the authors recommended limited CT when MRI shows acute defects or stress reaction to establish a baseline for follow-up, or for indeterminate cases for further evaluation.

On MRI, direct visualization of the pars defect may be difficult, particularly in the absence of spondylolisthesis.[134] The presence of marrow changes and other secondary MRI findings, including increased AP canal diameter and posterior vertebral body wedging, can improve the sensitivity of MRI for diagnosis.[135] Spondylolisthesis is evident on sagittal images, in which case there may be a more horizontal orientation of the neural foramina than normally seen.[135]

Although frank spondylolysis will be evident as an interruption of the marrow and cortex at the pars defect analogous to CT, MRI in some cases will show the additional finding of marrow signal abnormalities adjacent to the defect. These changes may be similar to and progress in the same sequence as the marrow changes in vertebral bodies adjacent to degenerated disks (Modic changes).[134] Some authors surmise that the early marrow changes of decreased signal on T1 and increased signal on T2 without frank spondylolysis may be useful in detecting developing spondylolysis prior to fully developed defects in childhood or adolescence.[134] This may be analogous to the increased uptake seen on bone scan in early cases without radiographic or CT abnormality. However, a positive bone scan and a marrow edema pattern by MRI have not been shown to exactly correlate.[120] In a prospective study of symptomatic children, marrow edema without irregularity or fragmentation has been shown to resolve under conservative management, suggesting the ability to avoid a frank pars defect when the condition is detected and treated at the earliest stage.[133]

On long-term radiographic follow-up, unilateral pars defects are not associated with spondylolisthesis, slip progression slows over the ensuing decades, and there are no clear predictors on initial imaging of the degree of future slippage.[118,127,136] Degenerative disk disease may occur more frequently and earlier in spondylolytic patients with spondylolisthesis.[127] In a study of 185 patients with spondylolysis treated with a brace for 3 to 6 months, healing as evidenced by radiographs and/or CT was shown in a large percentage of early (hairline defect or bony absorption) or progressed lysis (wide defect with small fragments), whereas healing was not seen in cases that had already advanced to sclerosis.[137] In this study, not surprisingly, unilateral defects had a significantly higher chance of healing than bilateral defects.

> Pars defects may heal.

Slipped Capital Femoral Epiphysis

Slipped capital femoral epiphysis (SCFE) is a predominantly posterior but also medial slippage of the proximal femoral epiphysis relative to the metaphysis secondary to weakening of the interposed physis. Thus it is effectively a Salter-Harris type 1 fracture. SCFE is primarily a disorder of the adolescent period during the growth spurt and is more frequent in obese children.[138] Bilaterality is present in about 25% of cases, divided between cases with bilateral involvement at presentation and those with a unilateral slip initially and subsequent contralateral development.[138] When occurring sequentially, the second slip occurs in the vast majority of cases within 18 months of the first.[138] SCFE is more common in boys than girls.[139,140] Although SCFE can be associated with renal osteodystrophy, radiation therapy, and endocrine disorders (e.g., growth hormone deficiency, hypothyroidism), the majority of cases are idiopathic.[138,141] It is a relatively uncommon disorder, estimated to occur in 1 to 7 per 100,000[141] and has been reported to be higher in incidence in African-Americans and Polynesians than Caucasians.[138,142]

> SCFE is a Salter-Harris type 1 fracture through a weakened proximal femoral growth plate. It occurs primarily in adolescent boys, is more common in obese children and African-Americans, and is bilateral in about 25% of cases (initially or usually within 18 months).

SCFE can be divided clinically into those patients who are able to ambulate (stable) and, less commonly, those unable to ambulate (unstable). Temporally, SCFE can be classified as acute (symptoms < 3 weeks in duration), chronic (symptoms > 3 weeks), or acute on chronic.[141] These classifications have important implications for treatment and prediction of outcome,[138] as AVN occurs much more frequently in unstable SCFE and in the acute cases.[141]

Treatment is aimed at preventing further slip. The most widely accepted management for stable acute and chronic SCFE is in situ fixation using a single cannulated screw, at which time reduction is not attempted because of the risk of provoking AVN and ability of the proximal femur to remodel.[141] Management of unstable and more severe SCFE remains controversial.[141,143] The main complications of SCFE are premature osteoarthritis, chondrolysis, and AVN, the latter two seen primarily after treatment.[138,141]

Indications for Radiographs

SCFE is the most common hip disorder of the adolescent.[140,144] The patient may complain of hip or thigh pain, a change in range of motion of the hip, and a gait abnormality or limp.[138,145] Because of referred pain, patients may also complain of distal thigh or knee pain,[141,144] a presentation not intuitively related to the hip that, consequently, has been shown to have a higher incidence of delayed diagnosis.[146] The most commonly encountered presentation is that of chronic intermittent pain with antalgic gait and limp and, on exam, an externally rotated limb with mild lower extremity shortening and diminished ability to internally rotate the hip.[138,140]

Early diagnosis may be elusive but is critical in order to institute treatment, as delayed diagnosis is the most important factor associated with a poor outcome.[141] Delayed diagnosis is associated with a greater degree of slip, more frequent treatment complications of osteonecrosis and chondrolysis, and with worse long-term outcomes including pain, osteoarthritis, and limitation of movement.[146] Imaging studies play a critical role in diagnosis and follow-up of SCFE and are particularly important for early diagnosis.

Osteoarticular Imaging

Radiographs are the most widely used method of evaluation and the modality of choice for initial detection of SCFE.[144] A standard series includes an AP view of the pelvis and a lateral view of the hip. In the acute patient who is unable to ambulate, the frog-leg lateral view should be avoided, as it has the potential to increase displacement during positioning for the study.[138] Therefore some authors advocate a true lateral radiograph rather than the frog-leg view if pain is the predominant symptom.[144]

> In the acute patient who is unable to ambulate, the frog-leg lateral view should be avoided, as it has the potential to increase epiphyseal displacement during positioning for the study.

In SCFE, the proximal femoral epiphysis slips medially, posteriorly, and inferiorly in relation to the metaphysis, and early detection depends on delineating slight displacement in one or all of these directions. In the earliest stages, there may be physeal widening with accompanying demineralization.[144] As many slips are initially posterior, the lateral view may be more revealing than the frontal projection. Abnormality may be seen on the lateral view as slight uncovering of the lateral aspect of the femoral neck at the epiphyseal plate and on the AP view as overlap of the femoral head and the proximal femoral neck.[147] In the normal hip, the lateral aspect of the femoral head overhangs the femoral neck on a frontal view, such that a line (Klein's line) drawn along the superior/lateral aspect of the femoral neck will intersect the femoral head. However, with increased severity of slip medially, there will be failure of the line to intersect the femoral head.[147] A true lateral view may be the most helpful in demonstrating the posterior displacement of the femoral head, although this view is frequently of limited diagnostic quality in the obese patient.[138]

Other early radiographic signs include widening and irregularity of the epiphyseal plate, metaphyseal irregularity, and an apparent decreased height of the femoral head on the AP view[138,140,147] (Figure 25-24). In more advanced cases, there also may be remodeling of the femoral neck and a metaphyseal "crow's beak"[147] (Box 25-9).

The degree of slip can be measured as the absolute length of slip from the superior femoral neck to the displaced head, the percentage of the diameter of the metaphysis/neck at the physis, or the head-neck or head-shaft angle (angle of the epiphysis in relation to the

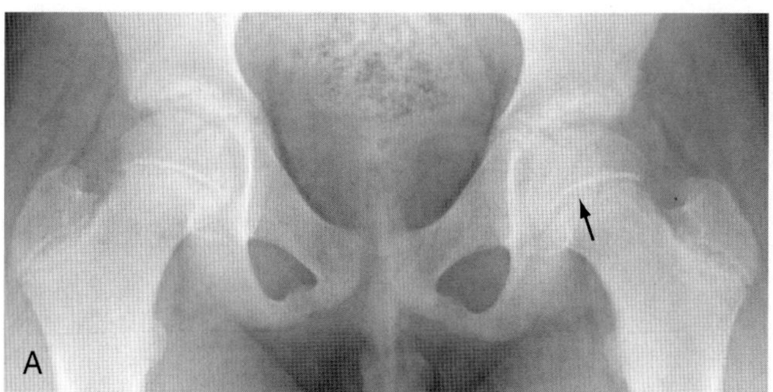

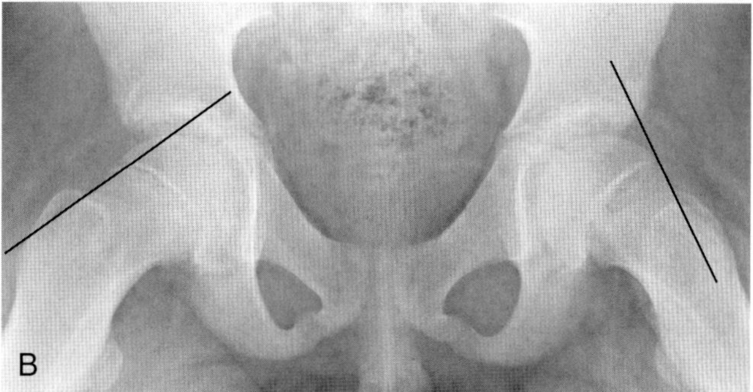

FIGURE 25-24. Thirteen year old with left slipped capital femoral epiphysis. **A,** AP view of the pelvis shows irregularity and widening of the left physis *(arrow)*. **B,** Frog-leg lateral view of the pelvis shows mild posteromedial slip of the left femoral epiphysis; the line of Klein does not intersect the femoral head.

BOX 25-9. Findings of SCFE on Radiographs

Epiphyseal widening
Femoral epiphysis medial, posterior, inferior in relation to metaphysis
Overlap of head and neck on AP view
Uncovering of lateral femoral neck on lateral view
Klein's line along the superolateral femoral neck does not intersect the femoral head
Decreased apparent height of femoral head
Metaphyseal irregularity
Metaphyseal "crow's beak"

femoral neck or shaft) with comparison to a standard or the contralateral normal side.[143,147,148] Schemes defining mild, moderate, or severe slip vary by author and have not been standardized.[149]

In the patient with a history of SCFE, the complication of chondrolysis (cartilage degeneration) is most commonly seen within 1 year of epiphyseal separation and is important to recognize as a risk factor for ensuing osteoarthritis. It is defined as rapid loss of at least 50% of the cartilaginous thickness and may involve both the acetabular and femoral surfaces.[144] It may cause increased pain and decreased range of motion.[144] Radiographically, it may manifest as periarticular osteopenia, diffuse or superior joint space narrowing, erosions, flattening, and thinning or disappearance of the subchondral bone.[150,151] In the absence of prior radiographs for assessment of interval change, a joint space < 3 mm should suggest chondrolysis.[144] Other complications that can be detected on radiographs include hardware failure, osteonecrosis, slip progression, limb length discrepancy due to early physeal fusion, and secondary osteoarthritis.[144]

Complications of SCFE include chondrolysis (seen as cartilage space narrowing), osteonecrosis, progression of slip, failure of hardware, early physeal fusion, and osteoarthritis.

Ultrasound has been proposed for diagnosis of SCFE,[148,152-154] although it is generally believed to add little information above that provided by radiographs alone[138] and has not been widely utilized. With an anterior longitudinal transducer position, step-off at the physis distorts the anterior outline due to posterior slip of the epiphysis. Also, shortening of the proximal femur can be measured as a decreased distance from the anterior acetabular rim to the proximal metaphysis at its exposed aspect.[148,152-154] Joint effusion is also a frequent accompanying finding.[148,152-154] In one small series, ultrasound had a sensitivity similar to MRI.[152]

CT can be a useful adjunct to radiographs when the diagnosis is uncertain[139] and, with 3D images, can be a useful tool for surgical planning when femoral osteotomy is contemplated. CT also may be useful to evaluate the position of fixation screws to check for protrusion of the screw tip into the joint space, a situation that may increase the risk of chondrolysis. CT has not been evaluated for its accuracy in the diagnosis of SCFE,[142] although changes have been described in that disorder including physeal widening and irregularity, metaphyseal irregularity or scalloping, and posterior metaphyseal beaking.[140] CT appears more accurate than radiographs for quantifying the degree of slip[149] and also may be useful to evaluate accompanying early physeal closure in severe slips.[138]

MRI has been used to demonstrate the changes of early SCFE,[140] revealing globular or diffuse widening of the physis that is best depicted on axial and coronal T1 sequences. Synovitis and bone marrow edema with high signal in the marrow on T2-weighted images may be present.[140] The widening of the physis often has a dome-shaped appearance with its greatest width centrally.[155] In one small series, the unstable slips were associated with increased T2 signal in the physis.[155]

MRI may be able to show "pre-slip," an early stage of presumed SCFE without changes on conventional radiographs or CT.[139,140,152,156] In the cases that have been reported, MRI revealed distortion and widening of the physis and/or bone marrow edema adjacent to the physis without femoral head slippage and then, subsequently, confirmed slippage.[156] Pre-slip has also been presumed in a series showing physeal widening on T1 in asymptomatic hips contralateral to known SCFE, instigating prophylactic pinning.[155] A hyperintense physis on T2* images and a joint effusion also have been reported in a few cases of presumed pre-slip in a different small series of patients.[152]

Early "preslip" changes may be present on MRI and could be helpful in cases of high clinical suspicion with normal radiographs.

Apart from the case of pre-slip, diagnosis usually can be made on radiographs, and MRI is expensive and of limited availability. Thus, although MRI is not considered a test of choice for routine diagnosis of SCFE, it may be performed in the patient with hip pain for exclusion of a number of other entities, and the exam may suggest the diagnosis of pre-slip. It may also prove useful in cases with high clinical suspicion but negative radiographs. MRI is clearly useful for assessment of the complications of chondrolysis and osteonecrosis.[140]

Radionuclide bone scan has not been shown to be particularly useful for the primary diagnosis of SCFE, as either normal or increased uptake on bone scan may be seen in the proximal femoral epiphysis at presentation, even with a severe slip.[157] In SCFE, greater uptake than normal is present at the physeal plate and contiguous metaphysis as a result of increased metabolic activity from repair. This abnormal uptake may be slight, allowing detection only by virtue of the asymmetry found when comparison is made with a contralateral normal hip.[158] In the few small series that have been performed, concurrent radiographic findings were also diagnostic, further limiting the value of the nuclear medicine examination.[157-159]

Bone scintigraphy may be useful, however, for determining the integrity of femoral head vascularity and the status of the physis. Following manipulation or surgery, decreased radionuclide uptake can be seen in the femoral head as a sign of vascular compromise. Also, a possible role of bone scintigraphy for evaluating vascular integrity of the femoral head at the time of presentation in the case of acute or severe slip has been suggested.[140,157-159] In addition, bone scintigraphy may provide helpful information for management decisions, such as in the case of chronic slip when the aggressiveness of treatment may depend on whether the slip is still active and the growth plate is open or closed.[159]

OSTEOCHONDROSES

Legg-Calvé-Perthes' Disease

Legg-Calvé-Perthes' disease (LCPD) is an "osteochondrosis" resulting from idiopathic osteonecrosis of the femoral head with ensuing flattening and collapse. LCPD has an estimated cumulative incidence of 1 in 1200 children less than 15 years of age, affecting approximately 1 in 740 males.[160] Males are affected more commonly than girls by a factor of 4 or 5 to 1.[160,161] LCPD affects children between 3 and 12 years of age and is bilateral in about

15% of patients.[162] Bilaterality is rare in girls and is distinctly sequential rather than synchronous.[163] LCPD is considered rare in African-American children.[163]

Although the exact inciting factor is unknown, interruption of the vascular supply to the femoral head is involved in the pathogenesis.[162] LCPD progresses through the stages of necrosis, resorption and fragmentation, reossification, and then remodeling, stages that are evident on imaging examinations.[161] Signs and symptoms often present weeks to months after the actual onset of osteonecrosis, such that radiographs may not show abnormalities for the first 5 months of symptoms.[114]

> LCPD results from osteonecrosis of the femoral head. It usually affects boys between the ages of 3 and 12 years old. Radiographic findings may be delayed for several months.

Indications for Imaging

The child with LCPD often presents with pain, limp, and limited range of motion, and the diagnosis should be considered in all children presenting with acute and chronic hip symptoms. The imaging and clinical manifestations of LCPD are broad and have been studied extensively. Myriad modalities have been used to evaluate different aspects of the condition, particularly as they relate to prognosis. Radiographs are the initial and main diagnostic study, although findings appear somewhat late. As surgery is most effective when performed before radiographic signs develop,[164] bone scan and MRI have emerged as important adjuncts for both confirmation of an early diagnosis and prognostication. Early treatment helps to minimize the significant sequela of osteoarthritis, related to ensuing joint deformity and incongruity between the femoral head and acetebulum.[165]

Osteoarticular Imaging

Conventional radiographs are the primary method of diagnosis, classification, and assessment of the clinical course in LCPD,[161,162] with standard exams including an AP view of the pelvis and frog-leg lateral views of both hips. In the earliest stage, radiographs will be normal.[166] Subsequently, radiographic features follow the pathologic stages.[161] Initial findings will include an ossific nucleus that appears smaller than normal as well as more dense due to osteopenia of the surrounding bone, apparent medial joint space widening due to cartilaginous overgrowth, and a subchondral radiolucent zone called the "crescent sign," indicating trabecular fracture (Box 25-10). The frog-leg lateral view is often most helpful for detecting the linear or crescentic subchondral fracture at the upper margin of the femoral head ossification center.

In the fragmentation stage, the bony epiphysis fragments and the previously dense avascular bone are replenished by lucent granulation tissue. In the reparative stage, bone formation will occur in areas of prior lucency and fragmentation. Finally, in the remodeling phase, the femoral head and metaphysis remodel until skeletal maturity, with sequelae including femoral head deformity, leg length discrepancy, and overgrowth of the greater trochanter. Typically, the femoral head appears large (coxa magna) and may have an irregular and flattened shape. Later stages also may reveal metaphyseal "cystic" radiolucencies, which are of uncertain etiology (Figure 25-25).

Several radiographic signs suggest a less favorable outcome and a femoral head that is at risk of collapsing.[167,168] These "head-at-risk" signs include: Gage's sign (a radiolucent, osteoporotic V pointing medially at the lateral aspect of the epiphysis and metaphysis on a frontal radiograph), calcifications lateral to the epiphysis (calcified extruded cartilage), lateral subluxation of the femoral head, and a horizontal growth plate. Metaphyseal cyst-like radiolucencies are also findings that suggest a poor prognosis.[169]

BOX 25-10. Radiographic Features of Legg-Calvé-Perthes' Disease

Normal early in disease
Ossific nucleus small and more dense
Medial joint space widening due to cartilage overgrowth
Crescent sign due to subchondral fracture
Fragmentation of the bony epiphysis
Femoral head deformity, coxa magna
Leg length discrepancy
Overgrowth of greater trochanter
Metaphyseal cystic changes

"HEAD AT RISK" SIGNS

Gage's sign
Calcifications lateral to the epiphysis
Lateral subluxation of the femoral head
Horizontal growth plate
Metaphyseal cyst-like lucencies

Multiple classification systems have been proposed to aid prognostication. One commonly cited system grades the extent of epiphyseal involvement.[167] In group 1, only the anterior portion of the epiphysis is involved with no evidence of collapse. In group 2, in addition to anterior involvement, there is collapse and sequestration of fragments. Group 3 includes those with almost entire epiphyseal involvement and collapse. In group 4, the entire epiphysis is involved with total collapse. Unfortunately, this classification is not useful in the earliest stages and has been criticized for its poor interobserver reproducibility.[166,170]

Bone scintigraphy has been used for staging LCPD and is the traditional gold standard for early diagnosis, recommended by some authors when initial radiographs show no "head-at-risk" signs but the diagnosis is suspected clinically.[164] Bone scintigraphy has been reported to have both high sensitivity and specificity for the diagnosis of LCPD.[171] It is particularly useful for staging the extent of bone necrosis, an important prognostic factor; radiographs are limited in demonstrating the true extent of necrosis until the resorptive phase is completed.[162,172-174] Both AP and frog-leg views are standard, and magnification using pinhole collimation is critical.[161,175] Early necrosis will present as a photopenic defect with lack of radiotracer uptake as a consequence of decreased vascularity in the femoral head. This defect can be seen even when radiographs are normal.[171,175] As vascularity is reestablished at the periphery, the defects will become smaller with increased marginal uptake.[171,174] The initial photopenic defect may be of variable size at diagnosis; in early cases, smaller defects are often seen only anterolaterally,[173] and these are associated with less severe radiological changes and better outcome.[174]

In studies utilizing serial bone scans, several important prognostic signs have been observed on scans after approximately 5 months of disease. At this time, vascularity in the epiphysis has begun to fill in.[164,165] On anterior images, the presence of a "lateral column," a tongue of radiotracer uptake in the lateral capital femoral epiphysis, was highly associated with a good final outcome, avoidance of head-at-risk signs, and proclivity for conservative management.[164,165] The lateral column is believed to be a sign of early and rapid revascularization via recanalization, allowing healing prior to the morphologic changes that result in deformity.[164,165,175] Conversely, extension of radiotracer activity centrally from the base of the epiphysis ("mushrooming" or

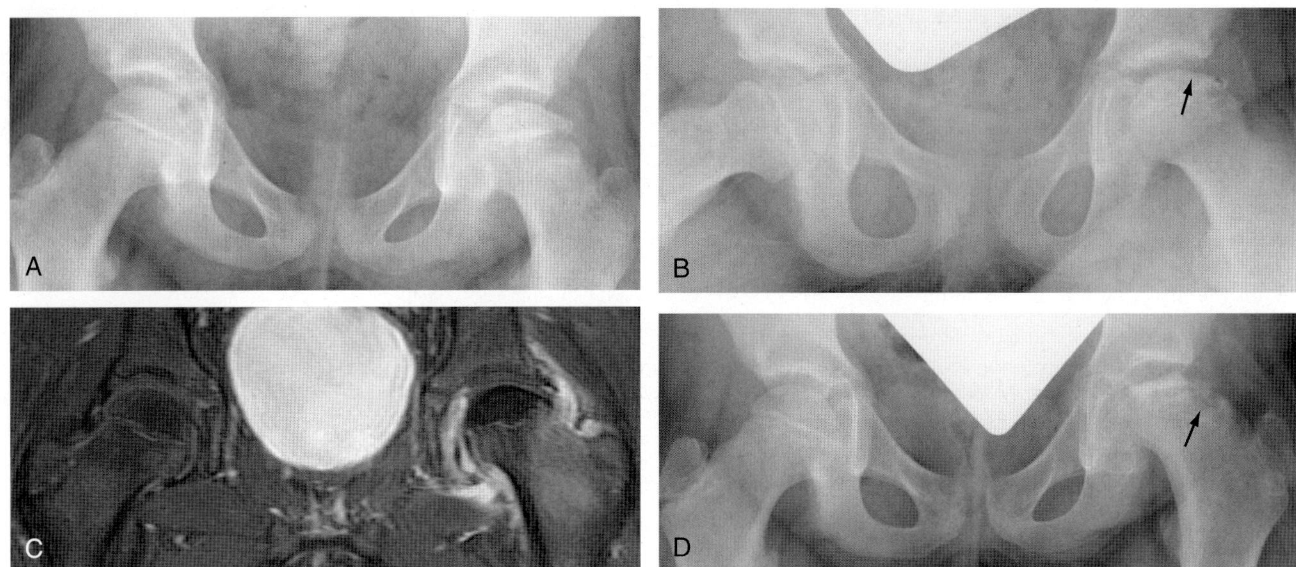

FIGURE 25-25. Eleven year old with left Legg-Calvé-Perthes' disease. **A,** Early stage: AP radiograph of the pelvis shows a sclerotic and small left femoral epiphysis. **B,** Frog-leg view of the hips shows a subchondral lucency representing a fracture, the crescent sign *(arrow)*. **C,** Coronal T1-weighted MR image with fat saturation after gadolinium enhancement shows hypertrophy of the synovium of the left hip causing joint space widening. There is no enhancement of the left femoral epiphysis, which therefore appears darker than the normal right side. **D,** Late stage: AP radiograph of the pelvis shows a flattened, sclerotic femoral epiphysis, a widened femoral neck, and cystic metaphyseal radiolucency *(arrow)*.

"base filling") highly predicted poor outcome and generally indicates that more aggressive treatment is warranted.[164,165,175] This pattern is postulated to be secondary to neovascularity rather than simply revascularization, with new vessels growing through the physis to the femoral head leading to slower healing and a predisposition to complications such as collapse.[165,166] These pathways of vascularity precede the radiographically evident loss of femoral head containment by about 3 months.[166] A less frequently observed sign is abnormally increased uptake at the metaphyseal growth plate, also a sign of poor prognosis.[164]

> Bone scanning may be useful for early diagnosis as well as for providing a prognostic tool in patients with SCFE.

MRI has emerged as a powerful tool for evaluation and prognostication, although its role is still under active investigation.[176] It is sensitive for diagnosis and has been shown to be as sensitive as bone scan for early diagnosis.[177] MRI has been shown superior to both radiographs and bone scan for assessing the extent of femoral head necrosis.[161,162,178-180] The location of the necrotic zone can be well characterized relative to the main weight-bearing aspect of the joint, and this is important for surgical planning.[181] Lateral subluxation and the shape of the femoral head can be accurately assessed on MRI.[161] Acetabular and epiphyseal cartilage and the shape of the femoral head can be assessed as well as or better than with arthrography[161,182-186] and is less invasive. MRI also can be useful for postoperative imaging after osteotomy to evaluate the femoral head shape as it remodels to its spheric configuration. Radiographic demonstration of this remodeling is delayed.[186]

The pattern of epiphyseal necrosis and revascularization has been studied with subtraction MRI using intravenous gadolinium contrast. MRI results are comparable with those of bone scintigraphy, but MRI has an advantage by being free of ionizing radiation.[176] Necrosis is demonstrated as decreased enhancement in the involved segment (all or part of the epiphysis) and may be abnormal even when radiographs are negative. Revascularization is accurately depicted as well as or better than scintigraphy, with the lateral column and base filling patterns evidenced by increased T2 signal and early increased and persisting enhancement compared with the unaffected side. Some authors recommend MRI for early diagnosis and at 4 to 6 months after presentation for the prognostic value of these revascularization pathways.[176]

Dynamic MRI in an open magnet system performed with the lower extremities in multiple positions can show femoral head containment and articular congruency as well as arthrography, including demonstration of "hinge abduction," an important feature that must be relieved during surgery, in which a severely flattened femoral head abuts the lateral acetabular margin on abduction and thereby forces it out of the acetabulum.[184,187] Therefore dynamic MRI can substitute for arthrographic pretreatment evaluation. Finally, MRI can show transphyseal bone bridging and metaphyseal extension of physeal cartilage (metaphyseal lucencies appearing as "cysts" radiographically), signs predicting growth arrest.[188]

CT is not sensitive for identification of early infarction as shown by bone scan or MRI, but it has been used to reveal the morphologic changes in LCPD for determining the extent of disease and for surgical planning and follow-up.[139] CT is more sensitive than radiography for delineating the anatomic changes of LCPD.[189] An asymmetric femoral epiphysis, joint effusion, and the crescentic lucency indicating subchondral collapse, as well as later changes of fragmentation and irregularity of the epiphysis and femoral neck deformities, are best illustrated on coronal or volume-rendered 3D reformatted images.[139]

Conventional arthrography has been used for diagnosis and assessment. Although arthrography has been reported to show lateral subluxation variably better or worse than a standard AP radiograph depending on the research study, it does not appear indicated for determining this head-at-risk sign if the initial radiographs show this finding.[190] Arthrography is useful for evaluating the thickness and contour of articular cartilage, including loss of sphericity, flattening, and irregularity, findings that predict outcome and subsequent osteoarthritis.[161,190] An additional advantage of this real-time technique is that it allows dynamic examination to determine how much abduction or rotation is needed for the acetabulum to contain the femoral head, a critical goal of therapy and important for choosing the type of brace or surgical procedure needed.[162,190]

Ultrasound is not used routinely for evaluation, although it may demonstrate synovial thickening in LCPD. It can be useful to exclude hip effusion at presentation that may suggest an alternative diagnoses such as toxic synovitis.[161]

Although not used for routine diagnosis, angiography has been studied in patients with LCPD, showing a devascularized epiphysis with obstruction to flow involving the superior capsular artery, a branch of the medial femoral circumflex artery (the main blood supply to the epiphysis).[191] In the revascularization stage, dilated superior and inferior capsular arteries have been demonstrated, with the interface of these territories possibly affecting the location of the sequestrum.[191]

Extraarticular Findings

Femoral head fragmentation and collapse can occur in multiple specific entities or in conditions that cause osteonecrosis and should be distinguished from the idiopathic osteonecrosis of LCPD. These other conditions include hypothyroidism, sickle cell anemia, Gaucher's disease, and multiple epiphyseal and spondyloepiphyseal dysplasias.[162] Stigmata of these conditions may be evident on exam or on imaging of other coexistent skeletal abnormalities. Meyer's dysplasia, a normal developmental variant, also can cause a fragmented appearance, but it can often be distinguished from LCPD because of its frequent bilateral involvement, lack of sclerosis and metaphyseal changes, and coalescence of fragments over time into a normal femoral head.[163] It is also often an incidental finding in an asymptomatic child.

Osgood-Schlatter's Disease

Osgood-Schlatter's disease (OSD) is a nonarticular osteochondrosis at the site of the patellar tendon's attachment to the apophysis of the tibial tuberosity;[192] it is generally a benign and self-limited process. Although trauma has been considered the etiology of OSD since its first description,[193] there remains some controversy as to whether it represents increased strain and tendinitis of the patellar tendon or avulsion of the cartilage and/or bone of the tibial tuberosity.[194-196] OSD occurs in the adolescent when the tongue-shaped apophysis of the tibial tubercle is undergoing ossification.[197] It occurs more often in boys and generally between 11 and 15 years of age.[198] It is a problem frequently seen in the adolescent athlete.[199] Bilateral involvement occurs in about 25% of cases.[163]

> OSD is likely a posttraumatic condition involving the patellar attachment on the tibial tubercle, frequently seen in the adolescent athlete and bilateral in about 25% of cases.

Indications for Imaging

The diagnosis of OSD is generally clinical.[200] Patients typically complain of pain at the tibial tubercle, which may be prominent to palpation, accompanied by overlying soft tissue swelling and tenderness.[198] The knee joint itself will be normal on examination.[198] Radiographic examination may be considered in unilateral cases given that rarely infection or neoplasm will involve the tibial tubercle,[197] but imaging is often not necessary with a typical clinical history and pain localized only to the tibial tubercle.[198] Radiographs are not considered indicated in bilateral cases with characteristic clinical features.[198] Radiographs may be performed if symptoms are acute in onset to rule out fracture,[198,201] particularly acute tibial tuberosity avulsion seen as a sports-related injury in the setting of active extension or passive flexion of the knee against a contracted quadriceps.[200] Radiographs are the mainstay of image confirmation, although features on CT, MRI, ultrasound, and bone scan are also described here.

Osteoarticular Imaging

Radiographs of the knee are typically the initial imaging exam, with the lateral view most important. Several radiographic stages of OSD have been described.[202,203] Early findings are related to soft tissue changes and will include increased density on both sides of the patellar tendon and at the inferior angle of Hoffa's fat pad, as well as indistinct margins and enlargement of the tendon itself. Subsequently, anterior to the tibial tuberosity, there may be one or more avulsed calcified or ossified fragments or a thin, shell-like calcification (Figure 25-26). Occasionally, a "donor site" for the avulsed fragment can be seen at the anterior aspect of the tuberosity. With time, these displaced osseus fragments can enlarge and either may remain isolated or fuse with each other or with the subjacent tibial tuberosity. Soft tissue swelling typically subsides over time. As a fragmented appearance of the tibial tuberosity can be a normal ossification pattern during development in asymptomatic individuals,[204] the presence of soft tissue swelling is considered fundamental to the radiographic diagnosis of this condition.

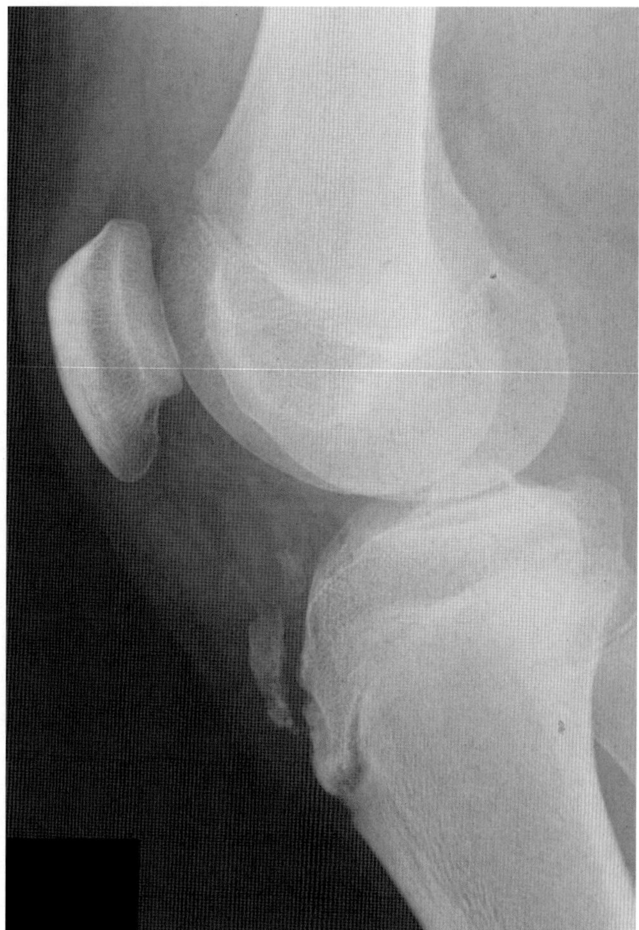

FIGURE 25-26. Fourteen year old with OSD. Lateral radiograph of the knee shows irregularity of the tibial tuberosity, two avulsed ossified fragments from the tibial tuberosity, thickening of the patellar tendon, and soft tissue swelling in Hoffa's fat pad.

Fragmentation of the tibial tubercle with accompanying soft tissue swelling are the typical radiographic features of OSD.

In a large study with average follow-up of about 2.5 years, the most common outcome was only residual mild deformity of the tibial tuberosity with resolution of soft tissue swelling, whereas other outcomes included normal radiographs, a very prominent tibial tuberosity, or presence of separate ossicles often accompanied by persistent soft tissue swelling and ligamentous thickening.[202] In many patients with unfused ossicles, persistent pain has been reported.[202,203]

On CT the patellar tendon will be characteristically abnormally thickened and exhibit decreased density of its substance near the tibial insertion.[196] Ossicles present anterior to the tibial tuberosity and swelling of the deep infrapatellar bursa posterior to the insertion of the patellar tendon also may be present.[196]

Studies of MRI in OSD have reported variable findings. In one study of 17 affected knees, all cases had abnormal signal within an enlarged patellar tendon, and common additional findings included superficial and deep infrapatellar bursitis.[196] Ossicles were more difficult to see on MRI than CT. Osseus changes included marrow edema in the tibial tuberosity and tibial epiphysis but are less frequently seen than soft tissue changes (Figure 25-27).

A more recent investigation of 40 knees followed by serial MRI exams over the course of OSD revealed progressive findings related to the tibial tuberosity, including edema signal within the secondary ossification center, fragmentation of the secondary ossification center, and then superior displacement and complete separation of the avulsed fragment.[205] Patellar tendon thickening was a finding characterizing the late stages and not seen early in the course of disease, leading the authors to conclude that the avulsion was the primary abnormality and tendinous changes were secondary.[205] In some cases, patients diagnosed with OSD clinically had normal initial MRI exams.[205]

In a study comparing imaging appearances before and after treatment, it has been noted that both soft tissue and osseus changes on CT and MRI improved over time, although findings persisted even after pain relief.[196] Fusion of ossicles was also demonstrated in many of the patients after relief of pain.

Ultrasound has been studied for its utility in diagnosis, with reports generated primarily from outside the United States, where ultrasound is performed more frequently for evaluating the musculoskeletal system. Demonstrated features include pretibial swelling in early cases, a fragmented and hypoechoic appearance of the ossification center, diffuse thickening and increased echogenicity of the patellar tendon near its insertion, and a fluid collection in

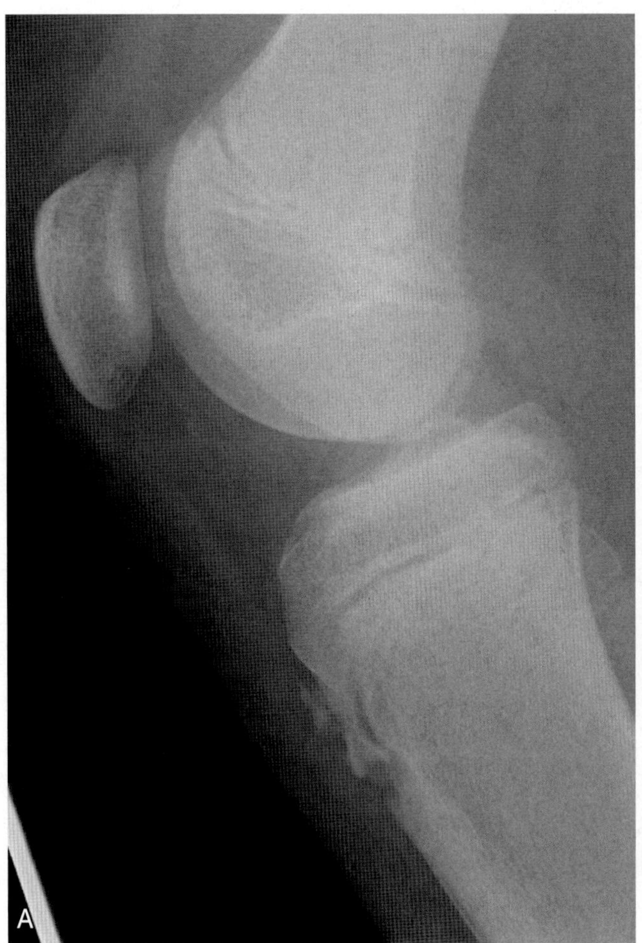

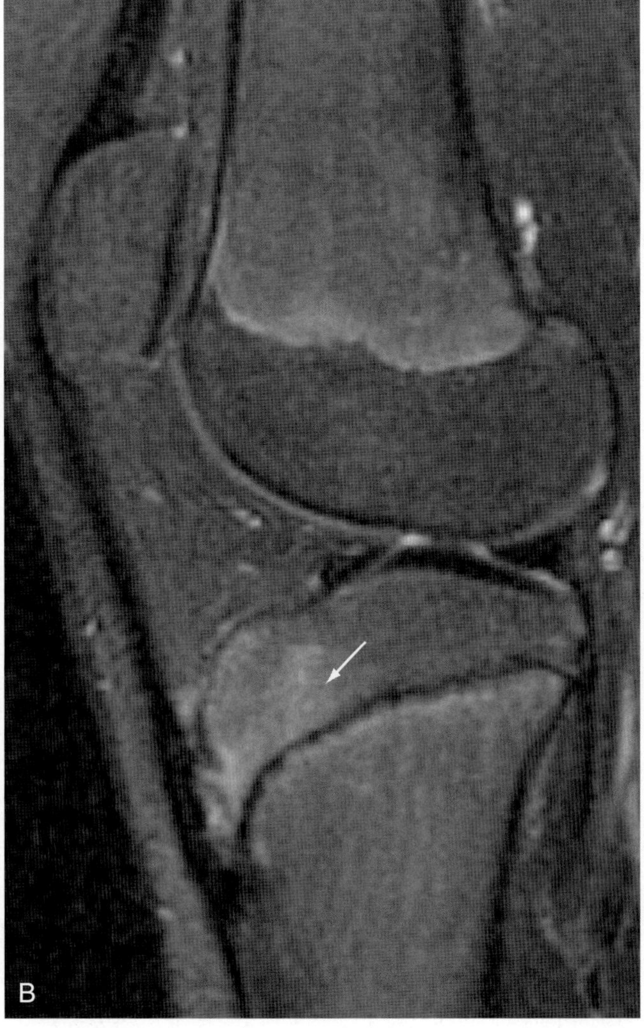

FIGURE 25-27. MRI findings of OSD. Ten year old with OSD. **A,** Lateral radiograph of the knee shows fragmentation of the tibial tuberosity. **B,** Sagittal STIR MR image of the knee shows marrow edema *(arrow)* in the tibial tubercle and normal signal intensity in the patellar tendon.

the retrotendineal soft tissue (deep infrapatellar bursitis).[201,206-208] Ultrasound may show the early changes prior to any radiographic abnormality.[206]

Literature on the use of bone scintigraphy for diagnosis of OSD is scant. In a study in which triphasic bone scan was performed in 10 patients, all patients had normal scans except for one patient who showed increased tracer on the blood flow phase to the affected side without abnormal uptake on delayed bone phase images.[196] A case report of a 21-year-old patient with delayed maturation reported increased uptake at the tibial tuberosity with concomitant radiographic findings of OSD.[209]

Blount's Disease and Physiologic Bowing

Genu varum, referred to colloquially as "bowlegs," is a not uncommon finding in children and is most frequently "physiologic" with excellent outcome and no need for treatment. Of the remaining pathologic etiologies causing genu varum, Blount's disease is the most common[210] and will be discussed in greatest detail here. Other pathologic causes include achondroplasia, vitamin D–resistant rickets, renal osteodystrophy, and osteogenesis imperfecta.[210] Blount's disease results from growth disturbance that is localized to the medial tibial physis, characterized by an abrupt varus deformity at the proximal tibia.[211] Mechanical factors are implicated in its development, although the exact cause is unknown.[212] Unlike physiologic bowing, Blount's disease is progressive and will uncommonly correct itself,[210] therefore making the differentiation between these entities critical, as the physiologic genu varum present at birth disappears in the first to second year of life.[213]

> Blount's disease results from growth disturbance that is localized to the medial tibial physis, characterized by an abrupt varus deformity at the proximal tibia. This disorder is usually identified at the onset of walking and is not self-correcting.

Blount's disease has two predominant peaks of incidence, a more common infantile form (onset < 5 years of age) and an adolescent form.[210] The infantile form generally has onset from 1 to 3 years of age and is commonly first noticed at the onset of walking,[212] with the greatest progression seen within the first 4 years of life.[214]

Indications for Imaging

In the toddler, physiologic genu varum predominates as the most common cause of varus alignment. During normal development, infantile genu varum follows as part of a sequence from varus to excessive genu valgum, which is then gradually corrected to the adult valgus pattern.[210,213] Developmental or physiologic bowing is an exaggeration of the varus deformity and is centered at the knee. Because the physiologic genu varum present at birth disappears in the first to second year of life,[213] varus angulation seen after 2 years of age is generally considered abnormal.[215] Physiologic genu varum is an exaggeration of genu varum that corrects itself later than normal.[216] Some orthopedists believe that radiographs are not necessary in a child of normal stature with exam consistent with physiologic bowing and that these children can be managed with period examinations and reassurance.[210] That said, exaggerated physiologic bowing may be difficult to clearly distinguish from Blount's disease clinically and radiographically, and, indeed, several authors have proposed that they may actually be a spectrum of the same condition.[216,217]

Clinical factors that may point to an etiology other than physiologic bowing include family history of varus malalignment or short stature, abnormal attainment of developmental milestones, history of progression, and, on exam, limb shortening, short stature, or abrupt angulation[210] The findings of deformity localized to the proximal tibia, posteromedial instability of the knee on mild flexion (Siffert-Katz sign), lateral thrust of the affected knee during gait, and internal tibial torsion are clinical signs that have been described in Blount's disease.[212,218] Blount's disease is more common in African Americans and obese children, more common in females in the infantile form and males in the adolescent form, and bilateral in 80% of the infantile patients but usually unilateral in the late-onset form.[210] Although historical and clinical features may be diagnostic of Blount's disease, radiographs are considered critical for diagnosis and assessment of severity.[214]

> Varus angulation seen after 2 years of age is generally considered abnormal.

Osteoarticular Imaging

Radiographs are the primary imaging method for diagnosis and should include weight-bearing AP views of both lower extremities.[215]

Physiologic bowing will be manifest as bowing of the entire lower extremity.[210] With physiologic bowing, there may be a mild medial metaphyseal "beak" at the proximal tibia and distal femur without fragmentation, medial tibial cortical thickening due to buttressing, or tilt of the ankle joint (with the medial aspect more cephalad).[215,216] Physiologic bowing can be diagnosed when there is varus deformity, as determined by the tibiofemoral angle measuring > 10 degrees at 18 months or older.[219] The tibiofemoral angle, however, cannot differentiate severe physiologic bowing from Blount's disease,[219] and a beak-like protuberance at the medial proximal tibia also cannot clearly differentiate the two.[220]

In Blount's disease, the characteristic finding is abrupt angulation of the medial aspect of the upper tibia (Figure 25-28). A general pattern of radiographic progression has been described.[211] The earliest findings are fragmentation at the medial aspect of the proximal tibial metaphysis, medial metaphyseal beaking, and generalized metaphyseal irregularity. Subsequently, there will be progressive medial metaphyseal depression resulting in varus angulation and deepening of the metaphyseal beak. The medial epiphysis will appear sloped downward and enlarge to fill the metaphyseal gap. In later stages the epiphysis will appear to be divided into two parts. In the latest stage, there is osseous fusion across the medial physis. Advanced cases also may show lateral subluxation of the tibia.[215]

> Physiologic bowing will be manifest on standing radiographs as bowing of the entire lower extremity measuring > 10 degrees at 18 months or older. In Blount's disease there is abrupt angulation of the medial aspect of the upper tibia with medial metaphyseal irregularity, deformity, and beaking.

Radiographic staging of infantile Blount's disease is the most common classification system used by orthopedic surgeons[210,220a] (Figure 25-29). Although progression through these stages may not be discrete, the scheme serves as a general framework to guide treatment.[210] No staging classification has been proposed for the late-onset or adolescent forms.[212]

The characteristic radiographic changes of Blount's disease are rarely manifest prior to 2 years of age.[212] One measurement that has been proposed to help differentiate physiologic bowing from infantile Blount's disease before significant radiographic sequelae of Blount's disease are evident is the metaphyseal-diaphyseal angle on a frontal radiograph, created by a line drawn along the transverse plane of the proximal tibial metaphysis and a line perpendicular to the long axis of the tibial diaphysis.[219] A measurement > 11 degrees has been posited as indicative of Blount's disease with high association with the future development of its more characteristic radiographic stigmata.[219] However, a

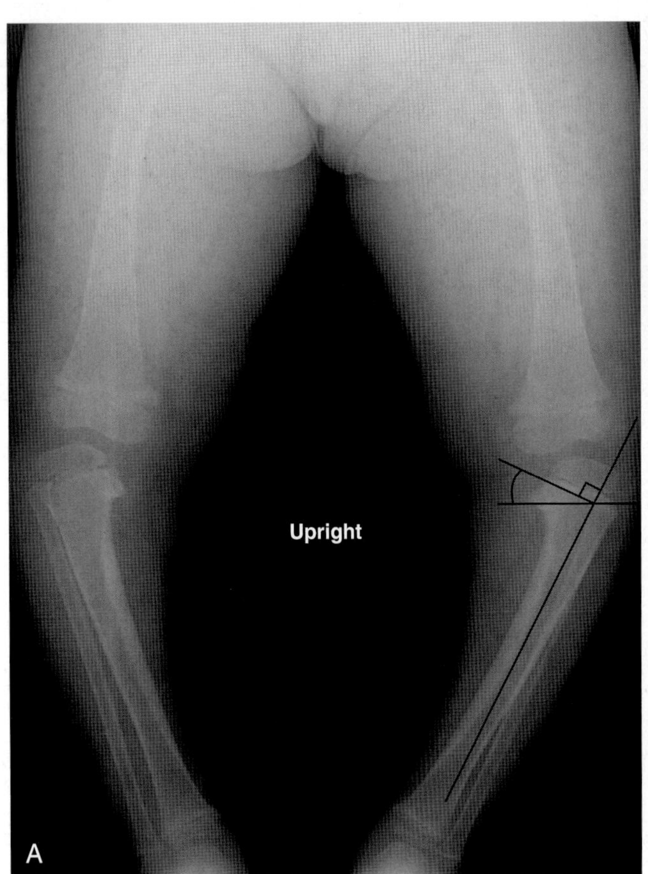

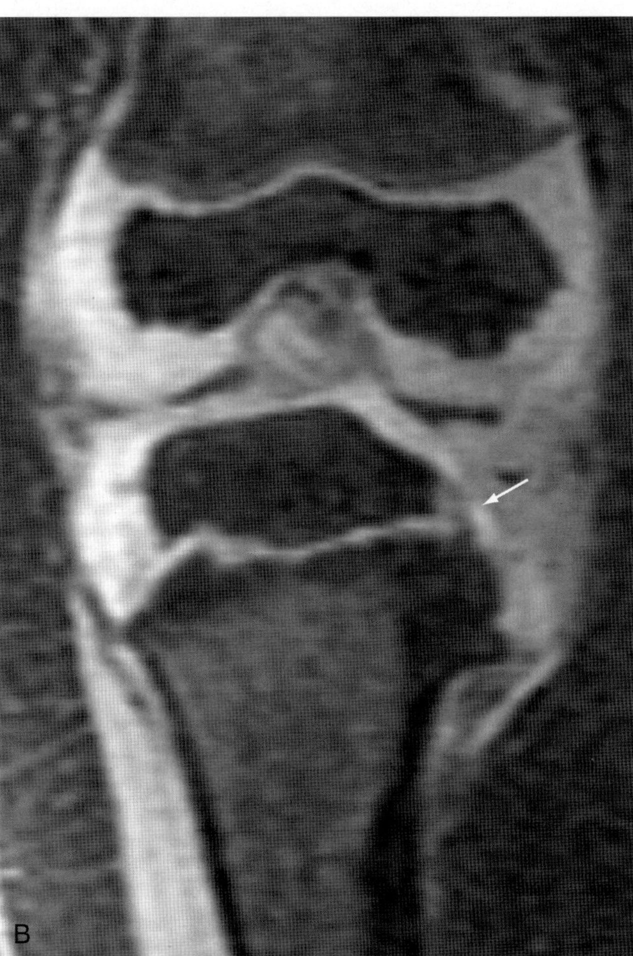

FIGURE 25-28. Two year old with Blount's disease. **A,** Standing radiograph shows bilateral genu varum, beaking and fragmentation of the medial tibial metaphyses, and thickening of the medial tibial diaphyses. The metaphyseal-diaphyseal angle is more than 11 degrees as documented on the left. **B,** Right and **(C)** left coronal 3D-SPGR MRI with fat suppression show the low-signal medial physeal bridges *(arrow)*. The low-signal secondary centers of ossification are contrasted with the adjacent higher-signal cartilage *(c)*.

(Continued)

subsequent study has shown that this degree of angulation may not be as reliable a criterion in younger patients and should not be utilized as the sole criterion for diagnosis.[218] These authors proposed 9 degrees or less as a discriminator for physiologic bowing and 16 degrees or more for Blount's disease (9 to 16 degrees being intermediate) in order to achieve less than 5% false-negative and false-positive rates.[218] Subsequent studies have further called into question the utility of the metaphyseal-diaphyseal angle,[220,221] and therefore, although an important metric of proximal tibial deformity, it should not be used a sole criterion for diagnosis.

MRI is the advanced modality most used in the evaluation of Blount disease. A characteristic finding is a sloped or stair-like deformity of the medial physis.[221] Other findings that have been described include: delayed medial epiphyseal ossification with cartilaginous enlargement compensating for metaphyseal collapse; medial epiphyseal fragmentation; widening, depression, and irregularity of the growth plate, particularly posteromedially; widening of the lateral growth plate; depression and irregularity of the medial tibial plateau; a metaphyseal beak of varying signal intensity; small intrusions of cartilage into the metaphysis; edema of the medial tibial epiphysis and metaphysis; enlargement of the medial meniscus with occasional abnormal intrameniscal signal; varus alignment; and bone bridging in advanced cases.[217,221-223] Medial meniscal hypertrophy is of unknown cause but has been postulated as a compensatory finding from abnormal forces.[222]

MRI shows to advantage the shape of the cartilaginous and bony epiphysis, which may have important implications for treatment. It also adds information regarding the articular surfaces, which may provide information as to prognosis.[222] MRI is particularly useful for evaluation of the physis prior to planned bone bridge resection and for surgical planning.[222] Physeal bony bridging can be well demonstrated on MRI and is particularly conspicuous when a fat-suppressed 3D spoiled gradient-recalled echo sequence (3D SPGR) is used. On these images, the low-signal bony bridge is contrasted with the contiguous high-signal physeal cartilage.[222]

Studies have been performed to evaluate MRI for delineating the risk that severe physiologic bowing will progress to Blount's disease. One study found that an undulated appearance of the posteromedial physis or high T2 signal in the epiphyseal cartilage was associated with a more protracted course of severe physiologic bowing, although none of the study patients subsequently developed Blount's disease.[221] In a second study, abnormally increased T2 signal was present in the medial epiphysis in patients with physiologic bowing that improved, whereas the additional initial findings of medial physeal depression, physeal widening, and abnormal signal in the medial perichondrium prognosticated development of Blount's disease in a significant number of patients.[217] The increased signal in the epiphysis in physiologic bowing is postulated to be a mechanical stress response.[217]

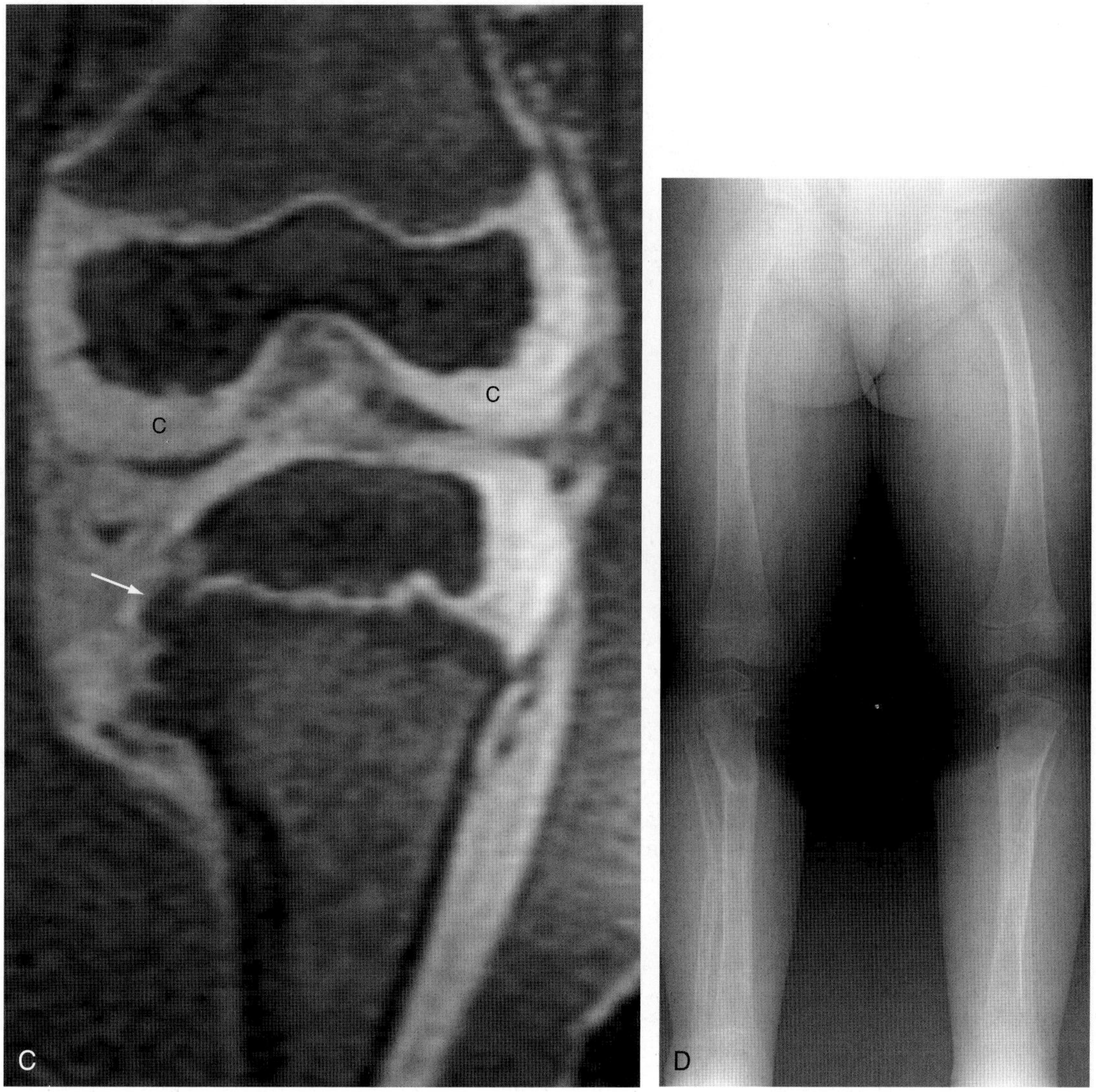

FIGURE 25-28—cont'd. **D,** Standing radiograph shows improved alignment after bilateral tibial and fibular osteotomies.

CT can show changes similar to those identified radiographically, with coronal reformatted images the most helpful for appreciating the varus deformity. CT can be useful for demonstrating the physeal bridge that may develop, particularly in infantile Blount's disease.[210]

Freiberg's Infraction

Freiberg's infraction, first described in 1914,[224,224a] is a primary articular osteochondrosis[192] that usually affects the second metatarsal head. It occurs most commonly in adolescent girls and is the only osteochondrosis predominating in females.[67] Third metatarsal head involvement is the next most common site, followed by the fourth metatarsal head.[67,225,226] Second metatarsal involvement may be the most common because it is often the longest metatarsal and may be subject to the greatest forces during ambulation and weight bearing.[224,226,227] Although the condition usually starts during adolescence, it may be recognized in the adult.[224,228] Unilateral involvement comprises over 90% of cases,[67] and the condition can also occur in more than one digit in the same foot, although this is not common.

The exact cause is controversial; proposed etiologies include trauma and repeated stress, high-heel shoes, and vascular anomalies.[67,224] In the adult, an association with diabetes mellitus has been reported; these patients are theorized to be at risk secondary to neuropathic weakness of the intrinsic muscles of the foot leading to altered mechanics.[229]

Indications for Imaging

The typical presentation is an adolescent, especially a girl, with forefoot pain that is relieved by rest and worsened with weight bearing. Pain, decreased range of motion, swelling, and tenderness centered at the metatarsophalangeal joint are the typical clinical indicators of the disorder.[67,230] Symptoms may precede radiographic changes by several weeks, and initial radiographs may be normal.[225,230]

> Freiberg's infraction affects a metatarsal head, usually the second, producing pain, swelling and tenderness of the affected metatarsophalangeal joint. Typically, adolescent girls are affected. The resulting metatarsal head flattening may persist into adulthood.

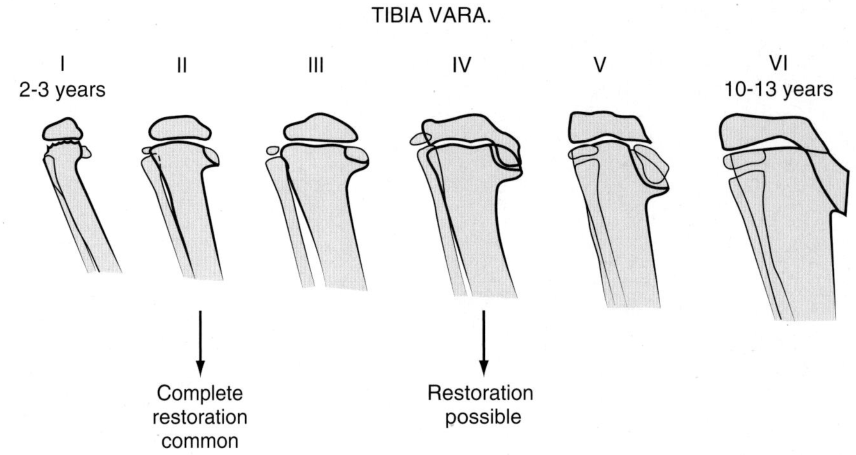

TIBIA VARA.

I 2-3 years | II | III | IV | V | VI 10-13 years

Complete restoration common

Restoration possible

FIGURE 25-29. The six stages of tibia vara, as described by Langenskiöld Stage I (seen in children up to age 3 years) is characterized by medial and distal beaking of the metaphysis and irregularity of the entire metaphysis. Stage II (seen in children aged 2½ to 4 years) is characterized by a sharp lateromedial depression in the ossification line of the wedge-shaped medial metaphysis. Complete restoration is common in this stage. Stage III (seen from ages 4 to 6 years) is characterized by deepening of the metaphyseal beak, which gives the appearance of a step in the medial metaphysis. Stage IV (seen from ages 5 to 10 years) is characterized by enlargement of the epiphysis, which occupies the medial metaphyseal depression. Restoration is still possible in this stage. Stage V (seen from ages 9 to 11) is characterized by a cleft in the epiphysis, which gives the appearance of a double epiphysis; the articular surface of the medial tibia is deformed, sloping distally and medially from the intercondylar region. Stage VI (seen from ages 10 to 13) is characterized by closure of the medial proximal tibial physis, with a normal lateral physis. Langenkiöld described his findings on the basis of his observations of Finnish children; changes in African-American children tend to occur at a younger age. (With permissions from J Am Acad Orthop Surg. 1995 Nov;3 (6):326-335 "Genu Varum in Children; Diagnosis and Treatment. Brooks WC, Gross RH.)

Osteoarticular Imaging

Radiographs are the typical exam on which the diagnosis is based, with AP and oblique views revealing a spectrum of findings depending on the pathologic stage. Findings are said to be essentially pathognomonic for this condition.[163] Early findings will include sclerosis, mild flattening, and cystic lucencies in the metatarsal head, accompanied by widening of the adjacent joint. Later, the condition progresses to produce an osteochondral fragment, further flattening and sclerosis of the metatarsal head, and periostitis of the contiguous metaphysis and diaphysis. In the advanced stage, intraarticular loose bodies, premature growth plate closure, deformity, metatarsal head enlargement, and widening of the proximal phalangeal base may be seen (Figure 25-30). Secondary osteoarthritis may ensue.

In early disease, MRI studies reveal low signal intensity in the metatarsal head on T1-weighted images with corresponding increased signal on T2 and short tau inversion recovery (STIR) sequences (see Figure 25-20, *B*). These are nonspecific findings, however, and could also indicate a stress response. In more advanced disease, flattening of the metatarsal head will be evident, and sclerosis will be indicated by low-signal intensity marrow on all series.[231] An additional finding that may be seen is a serpentine low-signal intensity line around an area of necrosis in the metatarsal head on T1-weighted images. However, osteonecrosis manifesting as low signal intensity on both T1- and T2-weighted images in the affected metatarsal head without the demarcating interface that characterizes osteonecrosis elsewhere, such as the femoral head, has been described.[232]

Although nonspecific, bone scintigraphy may localize a patient's pain to the metatarsal head. Focally increased uptake has been reported in the metatarsal head in both the early and late stages.[227] Pinhole collimation to produce high-resolution magnification images has been reported to be particularly helpful in the early phase, in which there may be focal photopenia with decreased radionuclide uptake suggesting AVN associated with a surrounding collar of increased uptake.[227]

Kohler's Disease

Kohler's disease is a self-limited osteochondrosis affecting the tarsal navicular bone.[192] The navicular bone comprises the apex of the arch of the foot, with resultant compressive forces during weight bearing predisposing it to vascular compromise.[67] It affects children between 4 and 9 years of age[233] and is seen in boys four times more frequently than girls.[67] It is unilateral in about 75% of cases.[163] Distinction should be made between this entity and spontaneous osteonecrosis that may occur in the adult, in whom it is known as Mueller-Weiss syndrome. Mueller-Weiss syndrome is typically bilateral, more common in women, more severe in course, and characterized by a comma-shaped navicular that thins laterally due to collapse.[234]

> Kohler's disease is a self-limited disorder of the navicular in children 4 to 9 years old. Medial and dorsal midfoot pain and radiographic evidence of sclerosis, fragmentation, and flattening of the navicular will be noted. Reconstitution to normal appearances occurs on follow-up.

Indications for Imaging

The diagnosis of Kohler's disease depends on both clinical and radiographic findings.[67] Clinically, the child may have an antalgic limp and characteristically favors walking on the lateral border of the foot.[67,233] Pain will be localized to the dorsomedial midfoot. There may be local

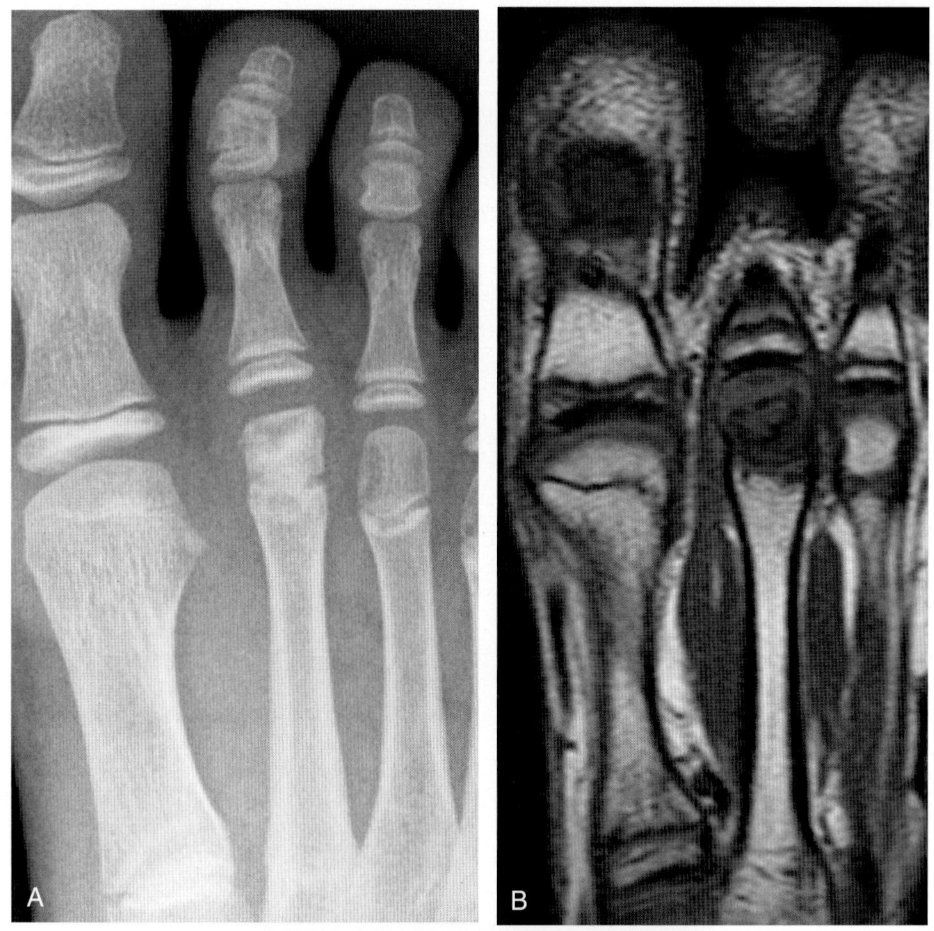

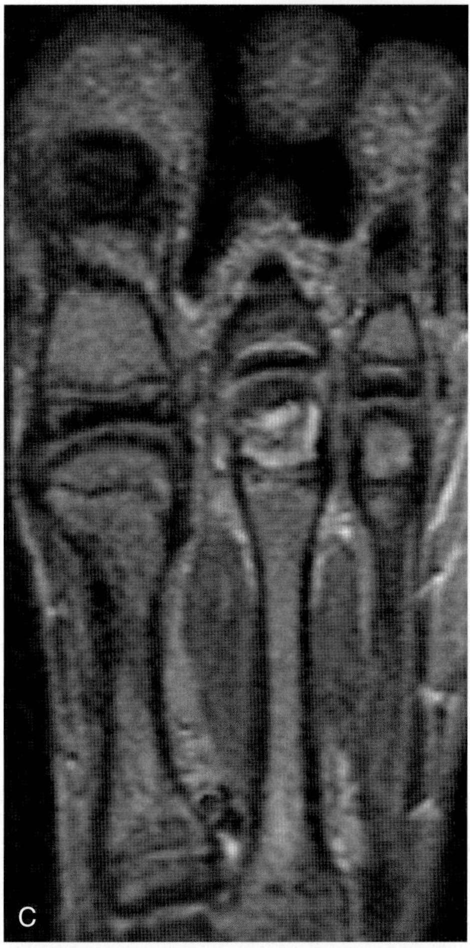

FIGURE 25-30. Eleven year old with Freiberg's infraction. **A,** AP radiograph of the foot shows sclerosis and flattening of the second metatarsal head with associated widening of the MTP joint. MRI shows **(B)** low signal intensity on T1-weighted sequence and **(C)** high signal intensity on STIR sequence.

signs of swelling, redness, warmth, and tenderness, signs that may falsely suggest infection or inflammatory arthropathy.[67] Infection is unlikely in this location in the absence of a history of penetrating trauma.[67] If infection is possible, however, laboratory evaluation with C-reactive protein, sedimentation rate, and complete blood count should be performed.[67] Radiographs are the primary modality for evaluation of Kohler's disease, although use of bone scan also has been described.[238,239] MRI features are also mentioned.[196,238]

Osteoarticular Imaging

Foot radiographs are the most commonly utilized examination, revealing sclerosis, fragmentation, and flattening in the proximal-distal dimension[235,236] (Figure 25-31). Adjacent soft tissue swelling also may be present.[237] The navicular may have a similar appearance with multiple ossification centers during normal development, emphasizing the importance of corroborative symptomatology in order to make the diagnosis.[67,163,237] Comparison with a prior radiograph that showed a normal navicular bone can increase diagnostic confidence.[238] As changes may be subtle, comparison with images of the contralateral foot also may be helpful.

Studies of long-term radiographic follow-up averaging over 30 years from initial diagnosis have shown an excellent prognosis, with most cases, regardless of treatment type, revealing reconstitution of the navicular over the course of months to give a normal appearance or slight enlargement and no evidence of osteoarthritis or cartilage-space narrowing.[235,236]

Bone scan has been shown in case reports to reveal decreased activity in the tarsal navicular in blood pool and delayed bone phase images in the setting of Kohler's disease,[238,239] with return of normal radiotracer uptake on resolution of symptoms.[238] Use of pinhole collimation can improve resolution of the small bones of the foot to aid diagnostic accuracy.[238]

On MRI, osteonecrosis of the tarsal navicular may appear as low signal intensity on T1- and T2-weighted images.[196,238]

Panner's Disease

Panner's disease is an articular osteochondrosis characterized by osteonecrosis of the capitellum of the humerus. It was initially described in 1927 and noted for its resemblance to Legg-Calvé-Perthes' disease in the hip.[240] Panner's disease affects young children most typically between 5 and 10 years of age. This is during the time of active ossification of the capitellum[241] with the capitellum only supplied by end-arteries that enter from posteriorly, rendering it vulnerable in these skeletally immature individuals.[242] Panner's disease is considered a benign, self-limited process that resolves with rest.[241,243] It occurs predominantly in the dominant elbow, especially in throwing athletes and gymnasts, and is considered rare.[244] It affects males almost exclusively.

Panner's disease should not be confused with the related entity of osteochondritis dissecans, a more common problem that also involves the capitellum with osteochondral injury at its anterolateral aspect, perhaps from repetitive trauma.[241] Osteochondritis dissecans may be distinguishable by the presence of loose bodies within the joint, older age at onset, and a more prolonged clinical course than is seen in Panner's disease.[241,243,244] Although radiographic appearances are somewhat similar, Panner's disease is differentiated from osteochondritis dissecans mainly on the basis of the patient's age, as the latter occurs in

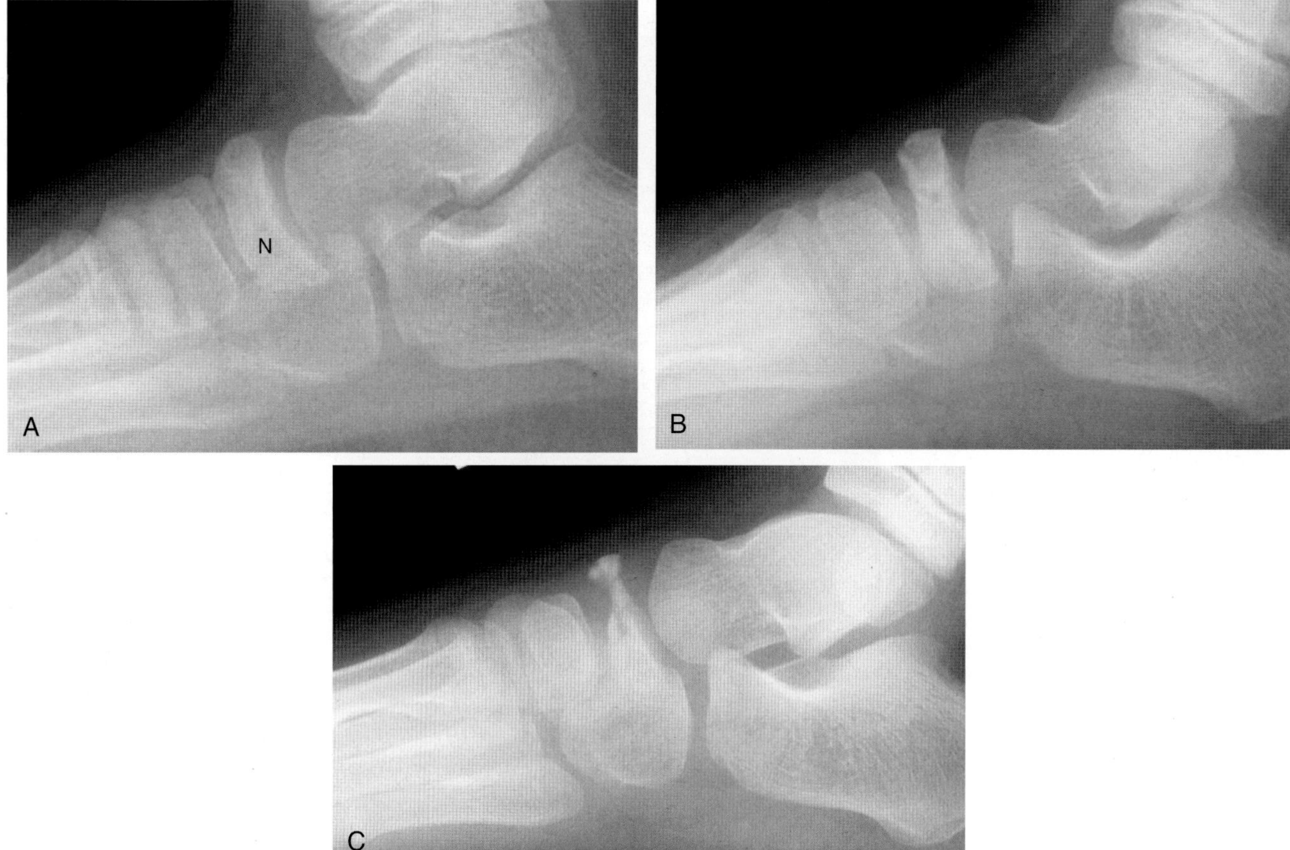

FIGURE 25-31. Eight year old with Kohler's disease. **A,** Initial lateral radiograph of the foot shows sclerosis of the navicular bone *(N)*; **(B)** 9 months later there is fragmentation; and **(C)** 13 months later there is flattening and further sclerosis.

adolescents and adults when the capitellum is completely ossified.[163] Panner's disease produces findings of osteonecrosis in the capitellum in children 5 to 10 years old. Panner's disease is a self-limited condition and should be distinguished from osteochondritis dissecans, which occurs in adolescents and adults.

> Panner's disease is self-limited, whereas osteochondritis is an osteochondral injury with a more prolonged course.

The term "Little Leaguer's elbow" was originally used to describe traumatic avulsion injury of the medial epicondylar epiphysis,[245] although it is now commonly used to more broadly incorporate several different disorders involving the lateral elbow, including both Panner's disease and osteochondritis dissecans.[242,244]

Indications for Imaging

Clinical symptoms of Panner's disease typically include tenderness, swelling, decreased range of motion, and pain.[241,242] Pain is often maximal over the radiocapitellar joint. Symptoms are often present for weeks and may be exacerbated by activity and ameliorated by rest.[244] Age > 10 years and evidence of locking may be more suggestive of osteochondritis dissecans.[244] When a lateral elbow abnormality is suspected, radiographs are the initial exam of choice.[244]

Osteoarticular Imaging Findings

Radiographs should include AP, external oblique, and lateral views of the elbow. In Panner's disease, radiographs will show multiple changes in the capitellum, including osteopenia with radiolucency, ill-defined cortical margins, increased density, fissuring, and fragmentation[242,244] (Figure 25-32). Joint effusion with elevation of the anterior and posterior fat pads also may be seen.[244]

With conservative treatment, reossification with reconstitution of the capitellum is typical, with follow-up radiographs often reverting to normal and persistent deformity, such as flattening of the capitellum, being uncommon.[242,244,246] Osteochondral loose bodies do not form in Panner's disease.[241] In patients presenting at an advanced stage, radiographs will show collapse, radial head overgrowth related to hyperemia from repair, and joint incongruity predisposing to osteoarthritis.[246]

Because of its generally self-limited course, MRI is not commonly performed in patients with Panner's disease.[241] Early changes of marrow edema may be seen as decreased signal in the chondroepiphysis on T1- and increased signal on T2-weighted images, findings that may be present before radiographic abnormalities are evident[242,244] (Figure 25-32, *B*). Later stages have an appearance similar to osteonecrosis as in other sites in the skeleton.[242]

Although bone scan is not routinely performed for diagnosis due to its nonspecificity,[244] scintigraphy has been shown to demonstrate focally increased radiotracer uptake at the elbow on blood pool and static bone phase images in patients with Panner's disease.[247]

Sever's Disease

Calcaneal apophysitis, also known as *Sever's disease*, is the most common cause of heel pain in athletes aged 5 to 11 years.[248] The disorder is self-limited with resolution of symptoms usually in 3 to 6 weeks with conservative treatment such as icing, stretching, activity modification, or orthotics.[248] The significance of various radiographic findings has been discussed, as the normal appearance of the calcaneal apophysis can be varied. Thus radiographs even in normal children may show sclerosis of the calcaneal apopyhses.[249] Volpon and de Carvalho Filho evaluated lateral radiographs and optical densitometry of the heels of 392 children and 69 children with calcaneal apophysitis. Sclerosis could not be used as a differentiating feature because the density of the primary and secondary ossification centers were actually less dense in affected individuals than in controls. Greater fragmentation of the secondary ossification center was found in the apophysitis group (Figure 25-33). This suggested that the condition was due to stress during a vulnerable period rather than a vascular insult. The condition affects only those children with open apophyses that are visible radiographically.

> Sever's disease is likely a stress-related condition that causes heel pain most commonly in athletes aged 5 to 11 years. Radiographs show fragmentation of the calcaneal apophysis. MRI may show bone marrow edema signal in the apophysis.

OSTEOPOROSIS IN CHILDREN

Osteoporosis and Bone Densitometry

Knowledge about osteoporosis in childhood is rapidly accumulating. Numerous congenital and acquired conditions compromise skeletal health in the child, with the ramifications of low bone mineral density ranging from asymptomatic states to chronic bone pain, fractures, and progressive skeletal deformity.[250] It is widely written that a key factor influencing postmenopausal or involutional osteoporosis is the amount of skeletal mass acquired during adolescence and early adulthood.[251-253] Put in other terms, senile osteoporosis may be a disease that begins in childhood.[252,253]

Disorders associated with low bone mass include genetic conditions such as Ehlers-Danlos, osteogenesis imperfecta, and Marfan syndrome; diseases of malabsorption including celiac disease, cystic fibrosis, and inflammatory bowel disease; endocrine disorders including hypogonadal states, hyperthyroidism, and hyperparathyroidism; immobilization as from paraplegia or cerebral palsy; chromosomal abnormalities, primarily Turner's and Klinefelter's syndromes; and other conditions such as idiopathic juvenile osteoporosis and idiopathic scoliosis.[250,253,254] Chronic oral glucocorticoid administration is another important predisposing factor.[254] Causes of osteoporosis in patients with anorexia nervosa include undernutrition and hypogonadism.[254] Idiopathic juvenile osteoporosis is a rare entity of unknown cause in which osteoporosis develops in a previously healthy child and in whom no identifiable clinical or laboratory cause is found.[253]

Although the motivation for performing bone density measurements in children are the same as in adults—to predict fracture, decide who needs treatment, and assess response to treatment— performance and interpretation of these tests is more challenging in children.[250] There is a lack of defined association between bone density measurements in children and a clinical outcome measurement (e.g., hip fracture, as used in adults), and the risks of osteoporosis and fractures later in life also remain to be clearly defined.[253]

Indications for Imaging

The goal of measuring bone density is to identify children who are at risk for fracture before the fracture occurs.[250] Fracture that occurs in the setting of minimal or no trauma provides clinical evidence of low bone mass.[250] Although consensus statements recommend baseline dual-energy x-ray absorptiometry (DXA) studies by age 18 in patients with cystic fibrosis and survivors of childhood cancer, formal recommendations for other at-risk populations are generally lacking.[250] In other patients who are at increased risk for bone disease, the decision to order a bone densitometry study can be informed by disease severity, bone pain, dose and duration of exposure to potentially harmful medications, and recurrent fractures or prior fractures with minimal trauma.[250] Formal assessment of bone density also may be indicated in patients believed

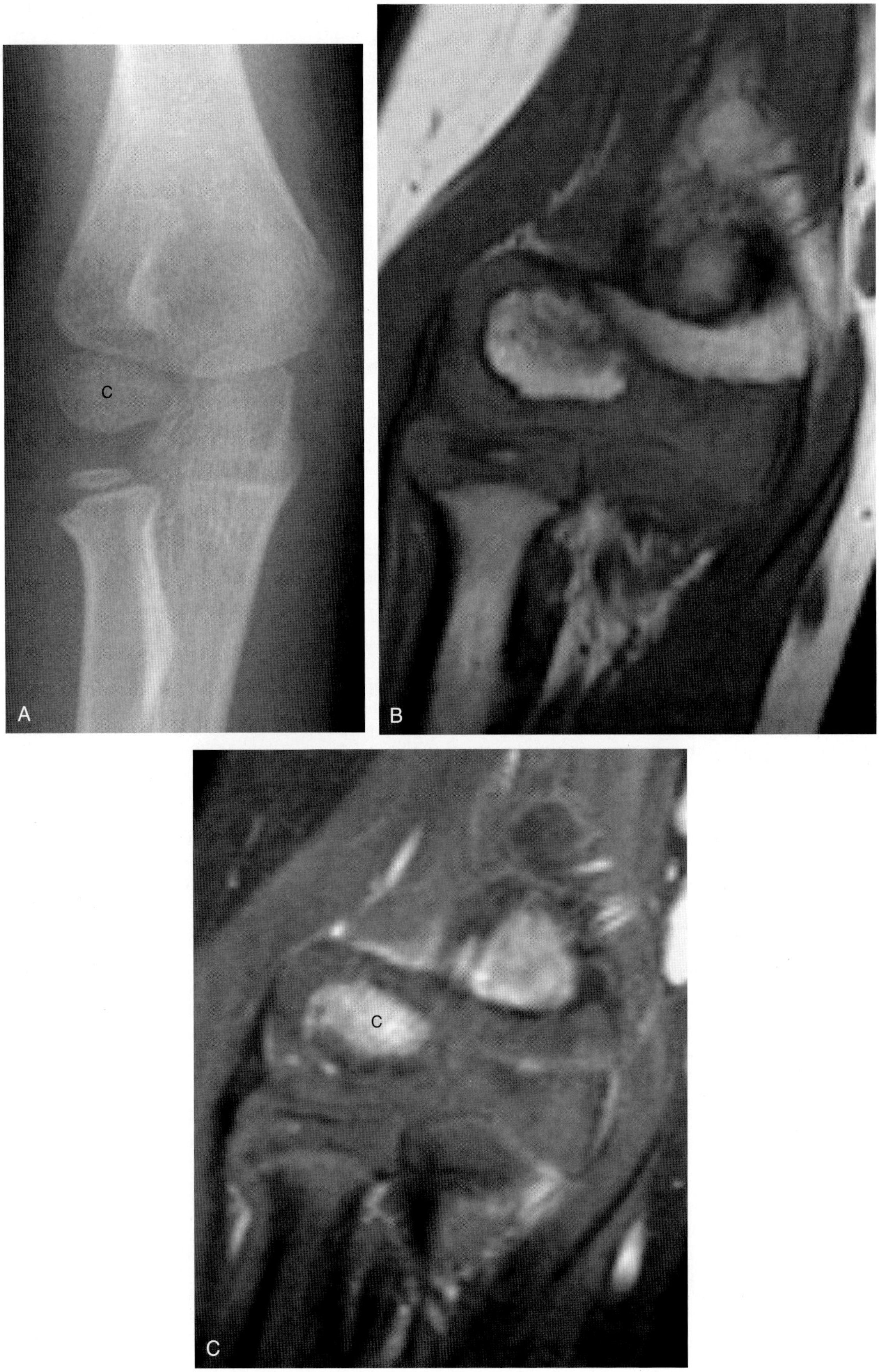

FIGURE 25-32. Four year old with Panner's disease. **A,** Coronal radiograph of the elbow shows osteopenia of the capitellum *(C)*. **B,** MRI shows low signal intensity on T1-weighted sequence and **(C)** high signal intensity in the capitellum *(C)* on STIR sequence.

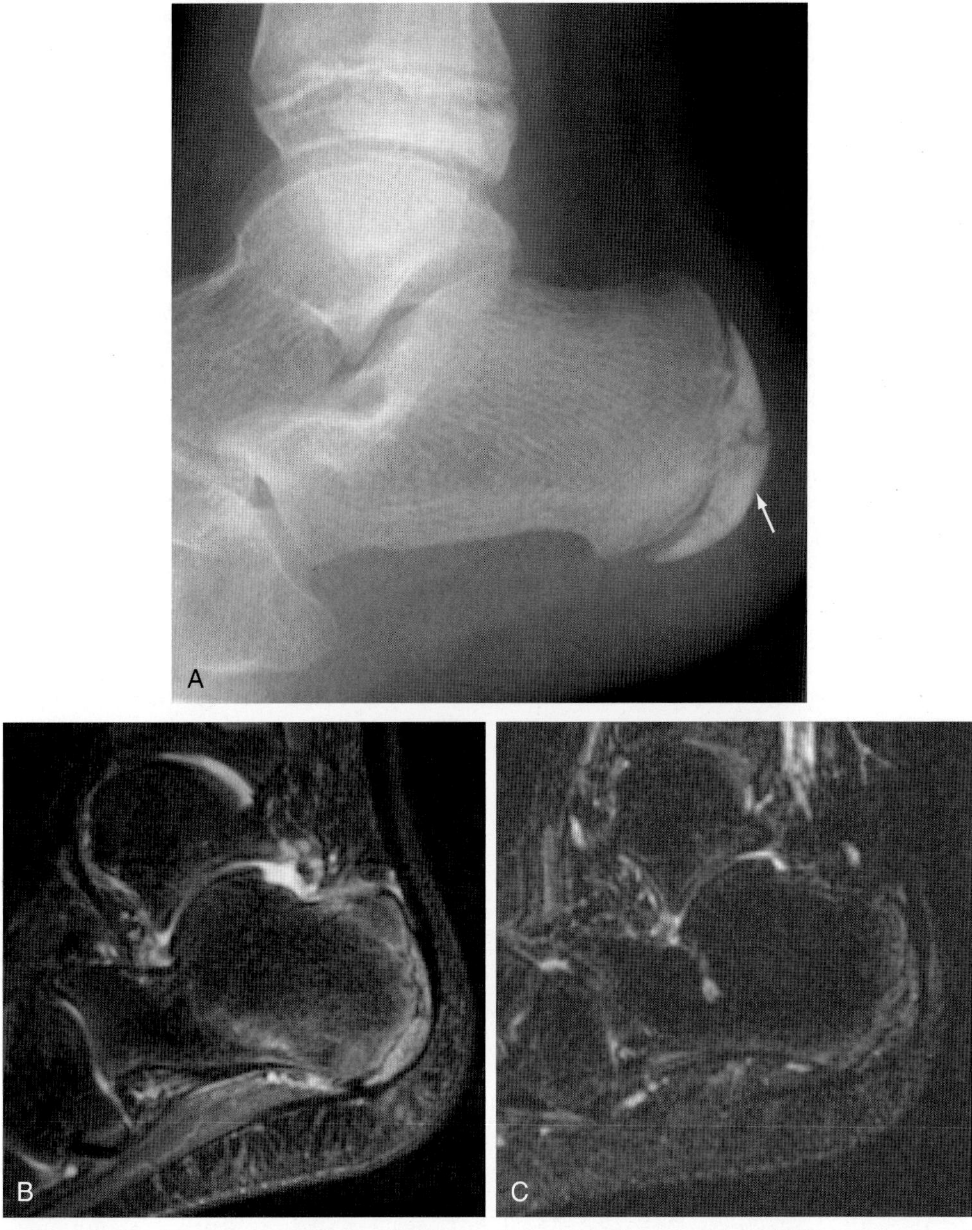

FIGURE 25-33. Nine year old with Sever's disease. **A,** Lateral radiograph of the ankle shows the normal dense apophysis of the calcaneus *(arrow)*. **B,** MRI shows hyperintensity of the calcaneal apophysis and associated soft tissue inflammation. **C,** MRI of the normal opposite calcaneus.

to have osteopenia on conventional radiographs as an incidental finding.[250]

Finally, some authors advocate that a baseline densitometry study, preferably a total body DEXA scan, be obtained in children to be placed on chronic medications known to compromise bone density, such as oral corticosteroids, diuretics, antimetabolites such as methotrexate, and anticonvulsants.[255] As opposed to treatment with oral corticosteroids, inhaled corticosteroids for treatment of childhood asthma have been reported in several studies to have no adverse affect on bone density unless taken at high doses for long periods.[256-260]

The skeletal site to be studied by DXA is determined by the clinical question to be answered. For example, entities of sex steroid deficiency and glucocorticoid excess generally result in greater trabecular than cortical bone loss, whereas growth hormone deficiency or hyperparathyroidism favors loss of cortical bone.[250] As such, scanning sites predominating in trabecular bone, such as the spine and hip, are preferred in the former, whereas scanning the whole body may be more useful in the latter.[250]

Once an initial densitometry study has been performed, some authors recommend that follow-up studies be performed no more frequently than once per year, or every 6 months if the child has a condition that might rapidly mobilize calcium stores or severely affect gut absorption of calcium.[255]

The American College of Radiology regards as the most appropriate radiologic exams for assessment of osteoporosis in the child with a significant clinical risk factor (undefined) both the DXA of the lumbar spine in the frontal projection and DXA of the proximal femur, as well as quantitative CT (QCT) of the thoracolumbar spine (adjusted for body size) although of higher radiation dose.[261]

Osteoarticular Imaging

Several methods are clinically available for the noninvasive assessment of central, peripheral, and total body bone density, all of which are more sensitive than conventional radiographs for the detection of deficient bone density.[250]

DEXA is generally regarded as the method of choice and is the most widely used method for clinical evaluation in children because it is precise, fast, and widely available and involves low radiation exposure.[250,255,262] Radiation exposure from this study is estimated as equivalent to that of a roundtrip transcontinental plane flight.[250] This technique can be compared with reference data for the whole body, lumbar spine, and proximal femur.[250] In most children, the PA lumbar spine (L1-4 or L2-4) is preferred because of the precision, speed, and availability of normative data for this area.[250]

In this technique, an x-ray source is used as a generator of photons at two energies, which are passed through the subject and then measured after exiting the region of interest (see also Chapter 6 on Osteoporosis). The attenuation values are then converted into a bone mineral content. DXA studies report bone mass as bone mineral content in grams, which can be divided by the projected area of bone analyzed to give a bone mineral density in grams per square centimeter.[263] Results in children should then be reported as a Z-score, which is the number of standard deviations from the mean for age- and gender-matched controls.[250] Unlike in adults, a T-score should not be used in patients younger than 20 years, as this score is the number of standard deviations from the mean for healthy adults at peak bone mass.[250]

> Bone density measurements in individuals less than 20 years of age should be reported as Z-scores. Normal measurements are within two standard deviations of age- and gender-, matched controls.

The International Society for Clinical Densitometry advises that the World Health Organization criteria for osteoporosis should not be applied to children, in whom the diagnosis of osteoporosis should not be made on the basis of densitometry alone.[264] This statement is based on the insufficient evidence that exists in the pediatric population to define the standard deviation criteria for osteopenia and osteoporosis.[265] Rather, the Society advises using terms such as "low bone density for chronological age" if the Z-score is below –2.0.[264]

The interpretation of DXA scans in children is more complex than in adults because the bone size, geometry, and mineral content change over time.[250] Multiple factors that affect measurement should be considered when comparing results with a normative population, including age, sex, weight, ethnicity, body and bone size, and pubertal status.[262,265-272] Among the variables that have been reported include a larger size of bones in the axial skeleton

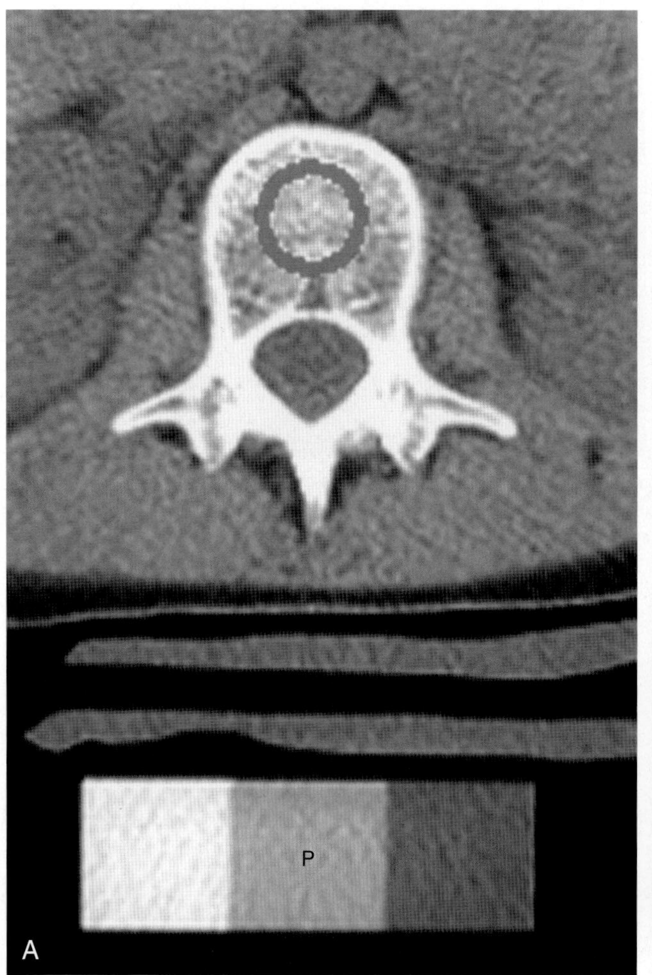

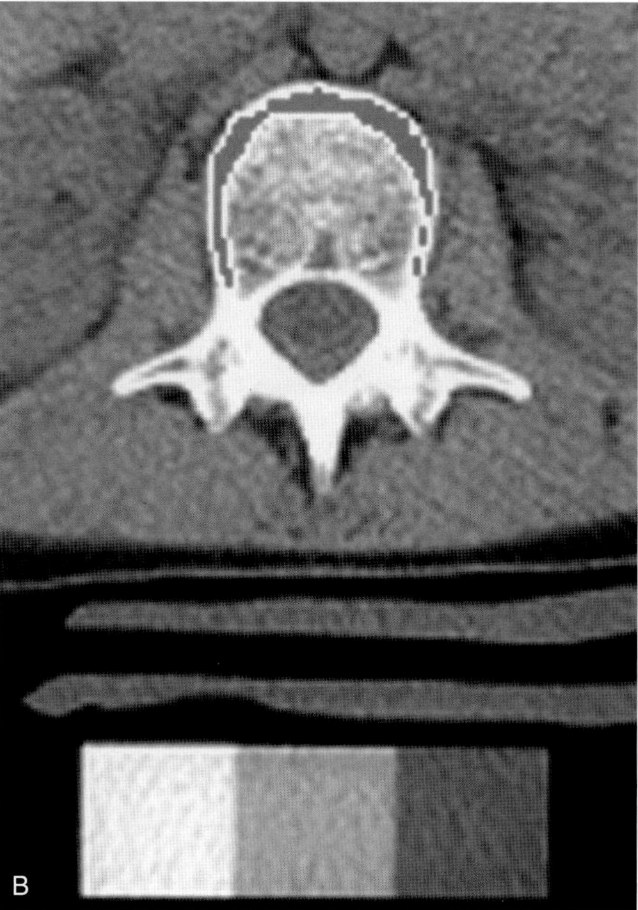

FIGURE 25-34. QCT axial images of a lumbar vertebral body. Regions of interest are drawn to calculate **(A)** the trabecular bone density and **(B)** the cortical bone density. The patient is lying on a reference phantom *(P)*.

in boys than girls and larger bones in heavier children,[273] a marked increase in spinal bone density during puberty,[268,271,274] and higher bone density in black compared with white children.[263,275] Higher bone densities also have been reported in the axial and appendicular skeleton in more physically active children.[267,269,276]

Because DXA measurements are based on a two-dimensional depiction of a 3D structure, increasing bone size with growth over time can cause an apparent, and erroneous, increase in the calculated bone density despite an actual bone density that remains constant over serial measurements.[255,263] That said, there are no agreed-upon standards yet for making many of these corrections, such that any modifications for these factors should be noted in the report.[264] The International Society for Clinical Densitometry also advises that serial measurements in the same patient be done on the same machine using the same scanning modes, software, and analysis method.[264]

Inexperience with these pediatric issues in osteoporosis on behalf of those interpreting studies may lead to overdiagnosis of osteoporosis. In a small series from the National Institutes of Health, 88% of studies had at least one error of interpretation, including use of a T-score to diagnose osteoporosis, using a reference database that disregards gender and ethnic differences, an incorrect bone map, and disregard for short stature.[272]

Quantitative CT is a second method of measurement and is based on comparison of bone to a series of known densities within a phantom (Figure 25-34). The CT is performed on a clinical CT scanner with comparison to a liquid or solid bone mineral phantom using special software.[263] Special smaller QCT scanners are also available but are limited to use in the peripheral skeleton.[263] QCT is able to measure true volumetric bone density, can be utilized for both the peripheral and central skeleton, and can distinguish between cortical and trabecular bone, but it is less available, more expensive, and, importantly, requires a radiation exposure about 10 times that of DXA.[250] Its main advantage over DXA is that it can measure the size and density of bone without the influence of body size.[263,277]

Quantitative ultrasound (QUS) is another method available, benefiting from its lack of ionizing radiation, low cost, and portability, but suffering from less precision than DXA, limitation to the peripheral skeleton, and fewer available reference normative data.[250] This technique relies on changes in the energy and velocity of sound waves as they pass through bone.[263] Bone measurements are obtained mainly from the calcaneus but also the patella, phalanges, and tibia.[263] Because measurements do not strongly correlate with those obtained from other modalities, QUS cannot serve as a surrogate for other methods of measurement.[263] Heel ultrasound measurements are reported to correlate only modestly with DXA measurements in children and young adults.[250]

Extraarticular Findings

The differential considerations in a child with generalized osteopenia and vertebral compression fracture include the uncommon initial presentation of leukemia. Signs of bone marrow failure, such as fatigue and anemia, often provide clues to the underlying diagnosis.[278]

References

1. Ontell FK, Ivanovic M, Ablin DS et al: Bone age in children of diverse ethnicity [see comment], *AJR Am J Roentgenol* 167: 1395-1398, 1996.
2. Zerin JM, Hernandez RJ: Approach to skeletal maturation, *Hand Clin* 7:53-62, 1991.
3. Cundy P, Paterson D, Morris L et al: Skeletal age estimation in leg length discrepancy, *J Pediatr Orthop* 8:513-515, 1988.
4. Berst MJ, Dolan L, Bogdanowicz MM et al: Effect of knowledge of chronologic age on the variability of pediatric bone age determined using the Greulich and Pyle standards, [see comment], *AJR Am J Roentgenol* 176:507-510, 2001.
5. Cole AJ, Webb L, Cole TJ: Bone age estimation: a comparison of methods, *Br J Radiol* 61:683-686, 1988.
6. Dimeglio A: Growth in pediatric orthopaedics, *J Pediatr Orthop* 21:549-555, 2001.
7. Roche AF, Davila GH, Eyman SL: A comparison between Greulich-Pyle and Tanner-Whitehouse assessments of skeletal maturity, *Radiology* 98:273-280, 1981.
8. Bull RK, Edwards PD, Kemp PM et al: Bone age assessment: a large scale comparison of the Greulich and Pyle, and Tanner and Whitehouse (TW2) methods, *Arch Dis Child* 81:172-173, 1999.
9. Buckler JM: Comparison of systems of estimating skeletal age, *Arch Dis Child* 52:667-668, 1977.
10. Mora S, Boechat MI, Pietka E et al: Skeletal age determinations in children of European and African descent: applicability of the Greulich and Pyle standards, *Pediatr Res* 50:624-628, 2001.
11. Loder R, Estle DT, Morrison K et al: Applicability of the Greulich and Pyle skeletal age standards to black and white children of today, *Am J Dis Child* 147:1329-1333, 1993.
12. Dimeglio A, Charles YP, Daures JP et al: Accuracy of the Sauvegrain method in determining skeletal age during puberty, *J Bone Joint Surg Am* 87:1689-1696, 2005.
13. Bilgili Y, Hizel S, Kara SA et al: Accuracy of skeletal age assessment in children from birth to 6 years of age with the ultrasonographic version of the Greulich-Pyle atlas, *J Ultrasound Med* 22:683-690, 2003.
14. Mentzel HJ, Vilser C, Eulenstein M et al: Assessment of skeletal age at the wrist in children with a new ultrasound device, *Pediatr Radiol* 35:429-433, 2005.
15. Wagner UA, Diedrich V, Schmitt O: Determination of skeletal maturity by ultrasound: a preliminary report [see comment], *Skeletal Radiol* 24:417-420, 1995.
16. Oestreich AE, Young LW, Young Poussaint T: Scoliosis circa 2000: radiologic imaging perspective. I. Diagnosis and pretreatment evaluation, *Skeletal Radiol* 27:591-605, 1998.
17. Weinstein SL, Dolan LA, Spratt KF et al: Health and function of patients with untreated idiopathic scoliosis: a 50-year natural history study [see comment], *J Am Med Assoc* 289:559-567, 2003.
18. Ramirez N, Johnston CE, Browne RH: The prevalence of back pain in children who have idiopathic scoliosis, *J Bone Joint Surg Am* 79:364-368, 1997.
19. American College of Radiology: *ACR practice guideline for the performance of radiography for scoliosis in children*, 151-155, 2004.
20. American College of Radiology: *ACR practice guideline for the performance of radiography for scoliosis in children*, 151-155, 2006.
21. Ozonoff M: Spinal anomalies and curvatures. In Resnick D, Kransdorf FM (eds): *Bone and joint imaging*, Philadelphia, 2005, WB Saunders, pp 1326-1334.
22. Gupta P, Lenke LG, Bridwell KH: Incidence of neural axis abnormalities in infantile and juvenile patients with spinal deformity. Is a magnetic resonance image screening necessary? *Spine* 23:206-210, 1998.
23. Do T, Fras C, Burke S et al: Clinical value of routine preoperative magnetic resonance imaging in adolescent idiopathic scoliosis. A prospective study of three hundred and twenty-seven patients [see comment], *J Bone Joint Surg Am* 83:577-579, 2001.
24. Barnes PD, Brody JD, Jaramillo D et al: Atypical idiopathic scoliosis: MR imaging evaluation, *Radiology* 186:247-253, 1993.
25. Davids JR, Chamberlin E, Blackhurst DW: Indications for magnetic resonance imaging in presumed adolescent idiopathic scoliosis, *J Bone Joint Surg Am* 86:2187-2195, 2004.
26. Wright N: Imaging in scoliosis, *Arch Dis Child* 82:38-40, 2000.
27. Nokes SR, Murtagh FR, Jones JD 3rd et al: Childhood scoliosis: MR imaging, *Radiology* 164:791-797, 1987.
28. Siffert RS: Lower limb-length discrepancy, *J Bone Joint Surg Am* 69:1100-1106, 1987.
29. Dahl MT: Limb length discrepancy, *Pediatr Clin North Am* 43:849-865, 1996.
30. Moseley C: Leg length discrepancy. In Morrissy RT, Weintstein SL (eds): *Pediatric orthopaedics*, Philadelphia, 2001, Lippincott, Williams and Wilkins, pp 1105-1150.
31. Walker CW, Aronson J, Kaplan PA et al: Radiologic evaluation of limb-lengthening procedures, *AJR Am J Roentgenol* 156:353-358, 1991.
32. Vade A, Eissenstat R: Radiographic features of bone lengthening procedures, *Radiology* 174:531-537, 1990.
33. Young JW, Kovelman H, Resnik CS et al: Radiologic assessment of bones after Ilizarov procedures, *Radiology* 177:89-93, 1990.
34. Blane CE, Herzenberg JE, DiPietro MA: Radiographic imaging for Ilizarov limb lengthening in children, *Pediatr Radiol* 21:117-120, 1991.
35. Aronson J: Limb-lengthening, skeletal reconstruction, and bone transport with the Ilizarov method, *J Bone Joint Surg Am* 79:1243-1258, 1997.
36. American Academy of Pediatrics: Clinical practice guidelines: early detection of developmental dysplasia of the hip. Committee on Quality Improvement, Subcommittee on Developmental Dysplasia of the Hip, *Pediatrics* 105:896-905, 2000.
37. Bialik V, Blazer S, Sujov P et al: Developmental dysplasia of the hip: a new approach to incidence, *Pediatrics* 1:93-99, 1999.
38. Gillingham BL, Sanchez AA, Wenger DR: Pelvic osteotomies for the treatment of hip dysplasia in children and young adults, *J Am Acad Orthop Surg* 7:325-337, 1999.
39. Harcke HT: Developmental dysplasia of the hip: a spectrum of abnormality, *Pediatrics* 103:152, 1999.
40. Woolacott NF, Puhan MA, Steurer J et al: Ultrasonography in screening for developmental dysplasia of the hip in newborns: systematic review, *Br Med J* 330:1413, 2005.
41. American College of Radiology: *Developmental dysplasia of the hip—child. ACR appropriateness criteria*, 1-7, 2005.
42. AIUM practice guideline for the performance of the ultrasound examination for detection of developmental dysplasia of the hip, *J Ultrasound Med* 22:1131-1136, 2003.

43. Harcke HT: The role of ultrasound in diagnosis and management of developmental dysplasia of the hip [comment], *Pediatr Radiol* 25:225-227, 1995.
44. Harcke HT: Imaging methods used for children with hip dysplasia, *Clin Orthop Rel Res* (434):71-77, 2005.
45. Taylor GR, Clarke NM: Monitoring the treatment of developmental dysplasia of the hip with the Pavlik harness. The role of ultrasound, *J Bone Joint Surg Br* 79:719-723, 1997.
46. Eggli KD, King SH, Boal DK et al: Low-dose CT of developmental dysplasia of the hip after reduction: diagnostic accuracy and dosimetry, *AJR Am J Roentgenol* 163:1441-1443, 1994.
47. Lafferty CM, Sartoris DJ, Tyson R et al: Acetabular alterations in untreated congenital dysplasia of the hip: computed tomography with multiplanar re-formation and three-dimensional analysis, *J Comput Assist Tom* 10:84-91, 1986.
48. McNally EG, Tasker A, Benson MK: MRI after operative reduction for developmental dysplasia of the hip [see comment], *J Bone Joint Surg Br* 79:724-726, 1997.
49. Nishii T, Tanaka H, Nakanishi K et al: Fat-suppressed 3D spoiled gradient-echo MRI and MDCT arthrography of articular cartilage in patients with hip dysplasia, *AJR Am J Roentgenol* 185:379-385, 2005.
50. Budin E, Chandler E: Measurement of femoral neck anteversion by a direct method, *Radiology* 69:209-213, 1957.
51. Mesgarzadeh M, Revesz G, Bonakdarpour A: Femoral neck torsion angle measurement by computed tomography, *J Comp Assist Tomography* 11:799-803, 1987.
52. Staheli LT, Lippert F, Denotter P: Femoral anteversion and physical performance in adolescent and adult life, *Clin Orthop Relat Res* (129):213-216, 1977.
53. Hubbard DD, Staheli LT, Chew DE et al: Medial femoral torsion and osteoarthritis, *J Pediatr Orthop* 8:540-542, 1988.
54. Hernandez RJ, Tachdjian MO, Poznanski AK et al: CT determination of femoral torsion, *AJR Am J Roentgenol* 137:97-101, 1981.
55. Sugano N, Noble PC, Kamaric E: A comparison of alternative methods of measuring femoral anteversion, *J Comp Assist Tomography* 22:610-614, 1998.
56. Morrell DS, Pearson JM, Sauser DD: Progressive bone and joint abnormalities of the spine and lower extremities in cerebral palsy, *Radiographics* 22:257-268, 2002.
57. Kuo TY, Skedros JG, Bloebaum RD: Measurement of femoral anteversion by biplane radiography and computed tomography imaging: comparison with an anatomic reference, *Investigative Radiol* 38:221-229, 2003.
58. Mahboubi S, Horstmann H: Femoral torsion: CT measurement, *Radiology* 160:843-844, 1986.
59. Hoiseth A, Reikeras O, Fonstelien E: Evaluation of three methods for measurement of femoral neck anteversion. Femoral neck anteversion, definition, measuring methods and errors, *Acta Radiol* 30:69-73, 1989.
60. Davids JR, Marshall AD, Blocker ER et al: Femoral anteversion in children with cerebral palsy. Assessment with two- and three-dimensional computed tomography scans, *J Bone Joint Surg Am* 85:481-488, 2003.
61. Lausten GS, Jorgensen F, Boesen J: Measurement of anteversion of the femoral neck. Ultrasound and computerised tomography compared [see comment], *J Bone Joint Surg Br* 71:237-239, 1989.
62. White G, Mencio G: Genu valgum in children: diagnostic and therapeutic alternatives, *J Am Acad Orthop Surg* 3:275-283, 1995.
63. Schoenecker P, Rich M: The lower extremity. In Morrissy RT, Weinstein SL: *Pediatric orthopaedics,* Philadelphia, 2001, Lippincott, Williams and Wilkins, pp 1059-1104.
64. Heath CH, Staheli LT: Normal limits of knee angle in white children—genu varum and genu valgum, *J Pediatr Orthop* 13:259-262, 1993.
65. Herring JA, Kling TF Jr: Genu valgus, *J Pediatr Orthop* 5:236-239, 1985.
66. Kling TF Jr, Hensinger RN: Angular and torsional deformities of the lower limbs in children, *Clin Orthop Relat Res* (176):136-147, 1983.
67. Mosca V: The foot. In Morrissy RT, Weinstein SL: *Pediatric orthopaedics,* Philadelphia, 2001, Lippincott, Williams and Wilkins, pp 1150-1215.
68. Ritchie GW, Keim HA: Major foot deformities their classification and x-ray analysis, *J Can Assoc Radiol* 19:155-166, 1968.
69. Dimeglio A, Bensahel H, Souchet P et al: Classification of clubfoot, *J Pediatr Orthop Br* 4:129-136, 1995.
70. Cummings RJ, Davidson RS, Armstrong PF et al: Congenital clubfoot [see comment], *J Bone Joint Surg Am* 84:290-308, 2002.
71. Miller JH, Bernstein SM: The roentgenographic appearance of the "corrected clubfoot", *Foot Ankle* 6:177-183, 1986.
72. Simons GW: A standardized method for the radiographic evaluation of clubfeet, *Clin Orthop Relat Res* (135):107-118, 1978.
73. Davis LA, Hatt WS: Congenital abnormalities of the feet, *Radiology* 64:818-825, 1955.
74. Templeton AW, McAlister WH, Zim ID: Standardization of terminology and evaluation of osseous relationships in congenitally abnormal feet, *Am J Roentgenol Rad Ther Nucl Med* 93:374-381, 1965.
75. Vanderwilde R, Staheli LT, Chew DE et al: Measurements on radiographs of the foot in normal infants and children, *J Bone Joint Surg* 70:407-415, 1988.
76. Tolat V, Boothroyd A, Carty H et al: Ultrasound: a helpful guide in the treatment of congenital talipes equinovarus, *J Pediatr Orthop B* 4:65-70, 1995.
77. Hamel J, Becker W: Sonographic assessment of clubfoot deformity in young children, *J Pediatr Orthop B* 5:279-286, 1996.
78. Johnston CE 2nd, Hobatho MC, Baker KJ et al: Three-dimensional analysis of clubfoot deformity by computed tomography, *J Pediatr Orthop B* 4:39-48, 1995.
79. Ippolito E, Fraracci L, Farsetti P et al: Validity of the anteroposterior talocalcaneal angle to assess congenital clubfoot correction, *AJR Am J Roentgenol* 182:1279-1282, 2004.
80. Downey D, Drennan J, Garcia J: Magnetic resonance image findings in congenital talipes equinovarus, *J Pediatr Orthop B* 12(2):224-228, 1992.
81. Cahuzac JP, Baunin C, Luu S et al: Assessment of hindfoot deformity by three-dimensional MRI in infant club foot, *J Bone Joint Surg Br* 81:97-101, 1999.
82. Westberry DE, Davids JR, Pugh LI: Clubfoot and developmental dysplasia of the hip: value of screening hip radiographs in children with clubfoot, *J Pediatr Orthop* 23:503-507, 2003.
83. Wechsler RJ, Scweitzer ME, Deely DM et al: Tarsal coalition: depiction and characterization with CT and MR imaging, *Radiology* 193:447-452, 1994.
84. Resnick D, Kransdorf M: Additional congenital or heritable anomalies and syndromes. In: Resnick D, Kransdorf M (editors): *Bone and joint imaging,* ed 3, Philadelphia, 2005, WB Saunders, pp 1135-1355.
85. Gessner A, Kumar S, Gross G: Tarsal coalition in pediatric patients, *Semin Musculoskelet Radiol* 3:239-246, 1999.
86. Emery KH, Bisset GS 3rd, Johnson ND et al: Tarsal coalition: a blinded comparison of MRI and CT, *Pediatr Radiol* 28:612-616, 1998.
87. Sullivan JA: Pediatric flatfoot: evaluation and management, *J Am Acad Orthop Surg* 7:44-53, 1999.
88. Newman JS, Newberg AH: Congenital tarsal coalition: multimodality evaluation with emphasis on CT and MR imaging, *Radiographics* 20:321-332, 2000; quiz 526-527.
89. Goldman AB, Pavlov H, Schneider R: Radionuclide bone scanning in subtalar coalitions: differential considerations, *AJR Am J Roentgenol* 138:427-432, 1982.
90. Kim SH: The C sign, *Radiology* 223:756-757, 2002.
91. Lateur LM, Van Hoe LR, Van Ghillewe KV et al: Subtalar coalition: diagnosis with the C sign on lateral radiographs of the ankle, *Radiology* 193:847-851, 1994.
92. Liu PT, Roberts CC, Chivers FS et al: "Absent middle facet": a sign on unenhanced radiography of subtalar joint coalition, *AJR Am J Roentgenol* 181:1565-1572, 2003.
93. Taniguchi A, Tanaka Y, Kadono K et al: C sign for diagnosis of talocalcaneal coalition [see comment], *Radiology* 228:501-505, 2003.
94. Brown RR, Rosenberg ZS, Thornhill BA: The C sign: more specific for flatfoot deformity than subtalar coalition, *Skeletal Radiol* 30:84-87, 2001.
95. Crim JR, Kjeldsberg KM: Radiographic diagnosis of tarsal coalition, *AJR Am J Roentgenol* 182:323-328, 2004.
96. Lysack JT, Fenton PV: Variations in calcaneonavicular morphology demonstrated with radiography, *Radiology* 230:493-497, 2004.
97. Resnick D: Talar ridges, osteophytes, and beaks: a radiologic commentary, *Radiology* 151:329-332, 1984.
98. Mandell GA, Harcke HT, Hugh J et al: Detection of talocalcaneal coalitions by magnification bone scintigraphy, *J Nucl Med* 31:1797-1801, 1990.
99. de Lima RT, Mishkin FS: The bone scan in tarsal coalition: a case report, *Pediatr Radiol* 26:754-756, 1996.
100. Deutsch AL, Resnick D, Campbell G: Computed tomography and bone scintigraphy in the evaluation of tarsal coalition, *Radiology* 144:137-140, 1982.
100a. http://www.acf.hhs.gov/programs/cb/pubs/cm06/chapter3.htm#child (accessed November 24, 2008.)
101. Nimkin K, Kleinman PK: Imaging of child abuse, *Radiol Clin North Am* 39:843-864, 2001.
102. Kleinman P: *Diagnostic imaging of child abuse,* ed 2, St Louis, 1998, Mosby, p 439.
103. Kocher MS, Kasser JR: Orthopaedic aspects of child abuse, *J Am Acad Orthop Surg* 8:10-20, 2000
104. Prosser I, Maguire S, Harrison SK et al: How old is this fracture? Radiologic dating of fractures in children: a systematic review, *AJR Am J Roentgenol* 184:1282-1286, 2005.
105. American College of Radiology: *Suspected physical abuse: child ACR appropriateness criteria,* 1-4, 2005. http://acsearch.acr.org/variantlist.aspx?topicid=68777 (accessed November 23, 2008.)
106. Kleinman PK: Skeletal trauma: general considerations. In Corra E (editor): *Diagnostic imaging of child abuse,* ed 2, St Louis, 1998, Mosby, pp 8-25.
107. Kleinman PL, Kleinman PK, Savageau JA: Suspected infant abuse: radiographic skeletal survey practices in pediatric health care facilities, *Radiology* 233:477-485, 2004.
108. Kleinman PK, Nimkin K, Spevak M et al: Follow-up skeletal surveys in suspected child abuse, *AJR Am J Roentgenol* 167:893-896, 1996.
109. Kleinman PK, Marks SC, Blackbourne B: The metaphyseal lesion in abused infants: a radiologic-histopathologic study, *AJR Am J Roentgenol* 146:895-905, 1986.
110. Lonergan, G.J., Baker AM, Morey MK et al: From the archives of the AFIP. Child abuse: radiologic-pathologic correlation, *Radiographics* 23:811-845, 2003.
111. Kleinman PK, Schlesinger AE: Mechanical factors associated with posterior rib fractures: laboratory and case studies, *Pediatr Radiol* 27:87-91, 1997.
112. Merten DF, Radkowski MA, Leonidas JC: The abused child: a radiological reappraisal, *Radiology* 146:377-381, 1983.
113. Nimkin K, Kleinman PK: Imaging of child abuse, *Pediatr Clin North Am* 44:615-635, 1997.
114. Conway JJ, Collins M, Tanz RR et al: The role of bone scintigraphy in detecting child abuse, *Semin Nucl Med* 23:321-333, 1993.
115. Standaert CJ, Herring SA: Spondylolysis: a critical review, *Br J Sports Med* 34: 415-422, 2000.
116. El Rassi G, Takemitsu M, Woratanarat P et al: Lumbar spondylolysis in pediatric and adolescent soccer players, *Am J Sports Med* 33:1688-1693, 2005.
117. Teplick JG, Laffey PA, Berman A et al: Diagnosis and evaluation of spondylolisthesis and/or spondylolysis on axial CT, *AJNR Am J Neuroradiol* 7:479-491, 1986.
118. Beutler WJ, Fredrickson BE, Murtland A et al: The natural history of spondylolysis and spondylolisthesis: 45-year follow-up evaluation, *Spine* 28:1027-1035, 2003; discussion 1035.
119. Papanicolaou N, Wilkinson RH, Emans JB et al: Bone scintigraphy and radiography in young athletes with low back pain, *AJR Am J Roentgenol* 145: 1039-1044, 1985.

120. Campbell RS, Grainger AJ, Hide IG et al: Juvenile spondylolysis: a comparative analysis of CT, SPECT and MRI, *Skeletal Radiol* 34:63-73, 2005.
121. Bellah RD, Summerville DA, Treves ST et al: Low-back pain in adolescent athletes: detection of stress injury to the pars interarticularis with SPECT, *Radiology* 180:509-512, 1991.
122. Libson E, Bloom RA: Anteroposterior angulated view. A new radiographic technique for the evaluation of spondylolysis, *Radiology* 149:315-316, 1983.
123. Libson E, Bloom RA, Dinari G et al: Oblique lumbar spine radiographs: importance in young patients, *Radiology* 151:89-90, 1984.
124. Amato M, Totty WG, Gilula LA: Spondylolysis of the lumbar spine: demonstration of defects and laminal fragmentation, *Radiology* 153:627-629, 1984.
125. Araki T, Harata S, Nakano K et al: Reactive sclerosis of the pedicle associated with contralateral spondylolysis, *Spine* 17:1424-1426, 1992.
126. Harvey CJ, Richenberg JL, Saifuddin A et al: The radiological investigation of lumbar spondylolysis, *Clin Radiol* 53:723-728, 1998.
127. Saraste H: Long-term clinical and radiological follow-up of spondylolysis and spondylolisthesis, *J Pediatr Orthop* 7:631-638, 1987.
128. Grogan JP, Hemminghytt S, Williams AL et al: Spondylolysis studied with computed tomography, *Radiology* 145:737-742, 1982.
129. Hession P, Butt W: Imaging of spondylolysis and spondylolisthesis, *Eur Radiol* 6:284-290, 1996.
130. Collier BD, Johnson RP, Carrera GF et al: Painful spondylolysis or spondylolisthesis studied by radiography and single-photon emission computed tomography, *Radiology* 154:207-211, 1985.
131. Pennell RG, Maurer H, Bonakdarpour A: Stress injuries of the pars interarticularis: radiologic classification and indications for scintigraphy, *AJR Am J Roentgenol* 145:763-766, 1985.
132. Gelfand MJ, Strife JL, Kereiakes JG: Radionuclide bone imaging in spondylolysis of the lumbar spine in children, *Radiology* 140:191-195, 1981.
133. Cohen E, Stuecker RD: Magnetic resonance imaging in diagnosis and follow-up of impending spondylolysis in children and adolescents: early treatment may prevent pars defects, *J Pediatr Orthop B* 14:63-67, 2005.
134. Ulmer JL, Elster AD, Mathews VP et al: Lumbar spondylolysis: reactive marrow changes seen in adjacent pedicles on MR images, *AJR Am J Roentgenol* 164:429-433, 1995.
135. Ulmer JL, Mathews VP, Elster AD et al: MR imaging of lumbar spondylolysis: the importance of ancillary observations, *AJR Am J Roentgenol* 169:233-239, 1997.
136. Danielson BI, Frennered AK, Irstam LK: Radiologic progression of isthmic lumbar spondylolisthesis in young patients, *Spine* 16:422-425, 1991.
137. Morita T, Ikata T, Katoh S et al: Lumbar spondylolysis in children and adolescents, *J Bone Joint Surg Br* 77:620-625, 1995.
138. Kehl D: Slipped capital femoral epiphysis. In Morrissy RT, Weinstein SL (editors): *Lovell and Winter's pediatric orthopaedics*, ed 5, New York, 2001, Lippincott, pp 999-1033.
139. Fayad LM, Johnson P, Fishman EK: Multidetector CT of musculoskeletal disease in the pediatric patient: principles, techniques, and clinical applications, *Radiographics* 25:603-618, 2005.
140. Umans H, Liebling MS, Moy L et al: Slipped capital femoral epiphysis: a physeal lesion diagnosed by MRI, with radiographic and CT correlation, *Skeletal Radiol* 27:139-144, 1998.
141. Uglow MG, Clarke NM: The management of slipped capital femoral epiphysis [see comment], *J Bone Joint Surg Br* 86:631-635, 2004.
142. Billing L, Bogren HG, Wallin J: Reliable X-ray diagnosis of slipped capital femoral epiphysis by combining the conventional and a new simplified geometrical method, *Pediatr Radiol* 32:423-430, 2002.
143. Boyer DW, Mickelson MR, Ponseti LV: Slipped capital femoral epiphysis. Long-term follow-up study of one hundred and twenty-one patients, *J Bone Joint Surg Am* 63:85-95, 1981.
144. Boles CA, el-Khoury GY: Slipped capital femoral epiphysis, *Radiographics* 17:809-823, 1997.
145. Flynn JM, Widmann RF: The limping child: evaluation and diagnosis, *J Am Acad Orthop Surg* 9:89-98, 2001.
146. Kocher MS, Bishop JA, Weed B et al: Delay in diagnosis of slipped capital femoral epiphysis, *Pediatrics* 113:e322-e325, 2004.
147. Klein A, Joplin RJ, Reidy JA et al: Roentgenographic features of slipped capital femoral epiphysis, *Am J Roentgenol Rad Ther Nucl Med* 66:361-374, 1951.
148. Kallio PE, Lequesne GW, Paterson DC et al: Ultrasonography in slipped capital femoral epiphysis. Diagnosis and assessment of severity, *J Bone Joint Surg Br* 73:884-889, 1991.
149. Cohen MS, Gelberman RH, Griffin PP et al: Slipped capital femoral epiphysis: assessment of epiphyseal displacement and angulation, *J Pediatr Orthop* 6:259-264, 1986.
150. Sartoris DJ, Resnick D: Radiologic vignette: primary disorders of articular cartilage in childhood, *J Rheumatol* 15:812-819, 1988.
151. El-Khoury GY, Mickelson MR: Chondrolysis following slipped capital femoral epiphysis, *Radiology* 123:327-330, 1977.
152. Magnano G, Lucigrai G, De Filippi C et al: Diagnostic imaging of the early slipped capital femoral epiphysis, *Radiol Med (Torino)* 95:16-20, 1998.
153. Castriota-Scanderbeg A, Orsi E: Slipped capital femoral epiphysis: ultrasonographic findings, *Skeletal Radiol* 22:191-193, 1993.
154. Terjesen T: Ultrasonography for diagnosis of slipped capital femoral epiphysis. Comparison with radiography in 9 cases, *Acta Orthop Scand* 63:653-657, 1992.
155. Futami T, Suzuki S, Seto Y et al: Sequential magnetic resonance imaging in slipped capital femoral epiphysis: assessment of preslip in the contralateral hip, *J Pediatr Orthop B* 10:298-303, 2001.
156. Lalaji A, Umans H, Schneider R et al: MRI features of confirmed "pre-slip" capital femoral epiphysis: a report of two cases, *Skeletal Radiol* 31:362-365, 2002.
157. Strange-Vognsen H, Wagner A, Dirksen K et al: The value of scintigraphy in hips with slipped capital femoral epiphysis and the value of radiography and MRI after 10 years, *Acta Orthop Belg* 65:33-38, 1999.
158. Gelfand MJ, Strife JL, Graham EJ et al: Bone scintigraphy in slipped capital femoral epiphysis, *Clin Nucl Med* 8:613-615, 1983.
159. Smergel EM, Harcke HT, Pizzutillo PD et al: Use of bone scintigraphy in the management of slipped capital femoral epiphysis, *Clin Nucl Med* 12:349-353, 1987.
160. Molloy MK, MacMahon B: Incidence of Legg-Perthes disease (osteochondritis deformans), *New Engl J Med* 275:988-990, 1966.
161. Gross G, Articolo G: Legg-Calve-Perthes disease: imaging evaluation and management, *Semin Musculoskelet Radiol* 3:379-391, 1999.
162. Kaniklides C: Diagnostic radiology in Legg-Calve-Perthes disease, *Acta Radiol* 406 (Suppl):1-28, 1996.
163. Resnick D, Kransdorf M: Osteochondroses. In Resnick D, Kransdorf M (editors): *Bone and joint imaging*, ed 3, Philadelphia, 2005, Saunders, pp 1089-1107.
164. Comte F, De Rosa V, Zekri H et al: Confirmation of the early prognostic value of bone scanning and pinhole imaging of the hip in Legg-Calve-Perthes disease, *J Nucl Med* 44:1761-1766, 2003.
165. Tsao AK, Dias LS, Conway JJ et al: The prognostic value and significance of serial bone scintigraphy in Legg-Calve-Perthes disease, *J Pediatr Orthap* 17: 230-239, 1997.
166. Conway JJ: A scintigraphic classification of Legg-Calve-Perthes disease, *Semin Nucl Med* 23:274-295, 1993.
167. Catterall A: The natural history of Perthes' disease, *J Bone Joint Surg Br* 53:37-53, 1971.
168. Murphy RP, Marsh HO: Incidence and natural history of "head at risk" factors in Perthes' disease, *Clin Orthop Relat Res* (132):102-107, 1978.
169. Kaniklides C, Sahlstedt B, Lönnerholm T et al: Conventional radiography and bone scintigraphy in the prognostic evaluation of Legg-Calve-Perthes disease, *Acta Radiol* 37:561-566, 1996.
170. Herring J, Kim H, Browne R: Legg-Calve-Perthes disease. Part I: classification of radiographs with use of the modified lateral pillar and Stulberg classifications, *J Bone Joint Surg Am* 86:2103-2120, 2004.
171. Bok B, Cavailloles F, Lonchampt MF et al: Bone scintigraphy in the diagnosis, prognosis, and follow-up of Legg-Calve-Perthes' disease, *Ann Radiol* 26:665-669, 1983.
172. Danigelis JA: Pinhole imaging in Legg-Perthes disease: further observations, *Semin Nucl Med* 6:69-82, 1976.
173. Danigelis JA, Fisher RL, Ozonoff MB et al: 99m-to-polyphosphate bone imaging in Legg-Perthes disease, *Radiology* 115:407-413, 1975.
174. Fisher RL, Roderique JW, Brown DC et al: The relationship of isotopic bone imaging findings to prognosis in Legg-Perthes disease, *Clin Orthop Relat Res* (150):23-29, 1980.
175. Conway J: A scintigraphic classification of Legg-Calve-Perthes disease, *Semin Nucl Med* 23:274-295, 1993.
176. Lamer S, Dorgeret S, Khairouni A et al: Femoral head vascularisation in Legg-Calve-Perthes disease: comparison of dynamic gadolinium-enhanced subtraction MRI with bone scintigraphy, *Pediatr Radiol* 32:580-585, 2002.
177. Ranner G, Ebner F, Fotter R et al: Magnetic resonance imaging in children with acute hip pain, *Pediatr Radiol* 20:67-71, 1989.
178. Henderson R, Renner JB, Sturdivant MC et al: Evaluation of magnetic resonance imaging in Legg-Perthes disease: a prospective, blinded study, *J Pediatr Orthop B* 10:289-297, 1990.
179. Uno A, Hattori T, Noritake K et al: Legg-Calve-Perthes disease in the evolutionary period: comparison of magnetic resonance imaging with bone scintigraphy, *J Pediatr Orthop* 15:362-367, 1995.
180. Oshima M, Yoshihasi Y, Ito K et al: Initial stage of Legg-Calve-Perthes disease: comparison of three-phase bone scintigraphy and SPECT with MR imaging, *Eur J Radiol* 15:107-112, 1992.
181. Bluemm RG, Falke TH, Ziedses des Plantes BG Jr et al: Early Legg-Perthes disease (ischemic necrosis of the femoral head) demonstrated by magnetic resonance imaging, *Skeletal Radiol* 14:95-98, 1985.
182. Hochbergs P, Geckerwall NE, Jonsson K et al: Femoral head shape in Legg-Calve-Perthes disease. Correlation between conventional radiography, arthrography and MR imaging, *Acta Radiol* 35:545-548, 1994.
183. Ecklund K, Jaramillo D: Patterns of premature physeal arrest: MR imaging of 111 children [see comment], *AJR Am J Roentgenol* 178:967-972, 2002.
184. Jaramillo D, Galen TA, Winalski CS et al: Legg-Calve-Perthes disease: MR imaging evaluation during manual positioning of the hip–comparison with conventional arthrography, *Radiology* 212:519-525, 1999.
185. Rush BH, Bramson RT, Ogden JA: Legg-Calve-Perthes disease: detection of cartilaginous and synovial change with MR imaging, *Radiology* 167:473-476, 1988.
186. Egund N, Wingstrand H: Legg-Calve-Perthes disease: imaging with MR, *Radiology* 179:89-92, 1991.
187. Weishaupt D, Exner GU, Hilfiker PR et al: Dynamic MR imaging of the hip in Legg-Calve-Perthes disease: comparison with arthrography, *AJR Am J Roentgenol* 174:1635-1637, 2000.
188. Jaramillo, D., Kasser JR, Villegas-Medina OL et al: Cartilaginous abnormalities and growth disturbances in Legg-Calve-Perthes disease: evaluation with MR imaging, *Radiology* 197:767-773, 1995.
189. Weisz I, Bialik V, Adler O et al: Some observations on the use of computerised tomography in Legg-Calve-Perthes' disease, *AJR Am J Roentgenol* 43:402-404, 1988.
190. Gallagher JM, Weiner DS, Cook AJ: When is arthrography indicated in Legg-Calve-Perthes disease? *J Bone Joint Surg Am* 65:900-905, 1983.

191. Theron J: Angiography in Legg-Calve-Perthes disease, *Radiology* 135:81-92, 1980.
192. Siffert RS: Classification of the osteochondroses, *Clin Orthop Relat Res* (158):10-18, 1981.
193. Osgood RB: Lesions of the tibial tubercle occurring during adolescence, *Clin Orthop Relat Res* (286):4-9, 1993.
194. Ogden JA, Southwick WO: Osgood-Schlatter's disease and tibial tuberosity development, *Clin Orthop Relat Res* (116):180-189, 1976.
195. Cohen B, Wilkinson R: The Osgood Schlatter lesion: a radiological and histological study, *Am J Surg* 95:731-742, 1958.
196. Rosenberg ZS, Kawelblum M, Cheung YY et al: Osgood-Schlatter lesion: fracture or tendinitis? Scintigraphic, CT, and MR imaging features, *Radiology* 185:853-858, 1992.
197. D'Ambrosia R, MacDonald G: Pitfalls in the diagnosis of Osgood-Schlatter Disease, *Clin Orthop Relat Res* 110:206-209, 1975.
198. Bush M: Sports medicine in children and adolescents. In Morrissy RT, Weisnstein SL (editors): *Pediatric orthopaedics*, Philadelphia, 2001, Lippincott, Williams and Wilkins, pp 1273-1318.
199. Bowers JK: Patellar tendon avulsion as a complication of Osgood-Schlatter's disease, *Am J Sports Med* 9:356-359, 1981.
200. Stevens S, Beaupre G, Carter D: Computer model of endochondral growth and ossification in long bones: biological and mechanobiological influences, *J Orthop Res* 17:646-653, 1999.
201. Blankstein A, Cohen I, Heiman Z et al: Ultrasonography as a diagnostic modality and therapeutic adjuvant in the management of soft tissue foreign bodies in the lower extremities, *IMAJ Israel Med Assoc J* 3:411-413, 2001.
202. Ehrenborg G, Lagergren C: Roentgenologic changes in the Osgood-Schlatter disease, *Acta Chir Scan* 121:315-327, 1961.
203. Hulting B: Roentgenologic features of fracture of the tibial tuberosity (Osgood-Schlatter's disease), *Acta Radiol* 48:161-174, 1957.
204. Ogden JA: Radiology of postnatal skeletal development. X. Patella and tibial tuberosity, *Skeletal Radiol* 11:246-257, 1984.
205. Hirano A, Fukubayashi T, Ishii T et al: Magnetic resonance imaging of Osgood-Schlatter disease: the course of the disease, *Skeletal Radiol* 31:334-342, 2002.
206. De Flaviis L, Nessi R, Scaglione P et al: Ultrasonic diagnosis of Osgood-Schlatter and Sinding-Larsen-Johansson diseases of the knee, *Skeletal Radiol* 18:193-197, 1989.
207. Lanning P, Heikkinen E: Ultrasonic features of the Osgood-Schlatter lesion, *J Pediatr Orthop* 11:538-540, 1991.
208. Carr JC, Hanly S, Griffin J et al: Sonography of the patellar tendon and adjacent structures in pediatric and adult patients, *AJR Am J Roentgenol* 176:1535-1539, 2001.
209. Namey TC, Daniel WW: Scintigraphic study of Osgood-Schlatter disease following delayed clinical presentation, *Clin Nucl Med* 5:551-553, 1980.
210. Brooks W, Gross R: Genu varum in children: diagnosis and treatment, *J Am Acad Orthop Surg* 3:326-335, 1995.
211. Langenskiold A: Tivia vara: (osteochondrosis deformans tibiae); a survey of 23 cases, *Acta Chir Scan* 103:22, 1952.
212. Bradway JK, Klassen RA, Peterson HA: Blount disease: a review of the English literature, *J Pediatr Orthop* 7:472-480, 1987.
213. Shopfner CE, Coin CG: Genu varus and valgus in children, *Radiology* 92:723-732, 1969.
214. Langenskiold A: Tibia vara: osteochondrosis deformans tibiae. Blount's disease, *Clin Orthop Relat Res* (158):77-82, 1981.
215. Cheema JI, Grissom LE, Harcke HT: Radiographic characteristics of lower-extremity bowing in children, *Radiographics* 23:871-880, 2003.
216. Hansson LI, Zayer M: Physiological genu varum, *Acta Orthop Scand* 46:221-229, 1975.
217. Mukai S, Suzuki S, Seto Y et al: Early characteristic findings in bowleg deformities: evaluation using magnetic resonance imaging, *J Pediatr Orthop* 20:611-615, 2000.
218. Feldman MD, Schoenecker PL: Use of the metaphyseal-diaphyseal angle in the evaluation of bowed legs [see comment], *J Bone Joint Surg Am* 75:1602-1609, 1993.
219. Levine AM, Drennan JC: Physiological bowing and tibia vara. The metaphyseal-diaphyseal angle in the measurement of bowleg deformities, *J Bone Joint Surg Am* 64:1158-1163, 1982.
220. Eggert P, Viemann M: Physiological bowlegs or infantile Blount's disease. Some new aspects on an old problem, *Pediatr Radiol* 26:349-352, 1996.
221. Iwasawa T, Inaba Y, Nishimura G et al: MR findings of bowlegs in toddlers, *Pediatr Radiol* 29:826-834, 1999.
222. Craig J, Holsbeeck MV, Zaltz I: The utility of MR in assessing Blount disease, *Skeletal Radiol* 31:208-213, 2002.
223. Ducou le Pointe H, Mousselard H, Rudelli A et al: Blount's disease: magnetic resonance imaging, *Pediatr Radiol* 25:12-14, 1995.
224. Frieberg A: Infraction of the second metatarsal bone: a typical injury, *Surg Gynecol Obstet* 19:191-193, 1914.
225. Omer GE Jr: Primary articular osteochondroses, *Clin Orthop Relat Res* (158):33-40, 1981.
226. Gauthier G, Elbaz R: Freiberg's infraction: a subchondral bone fatigue fracture. A new surgical treatment, *Clin Orthop Relat Res* (142):93-95, 1979.
227. Mandell GA, Harcke HT: Scintigraphic manifestations of infraction of the second metatarsal (Freiberg's disease), *J Nucl Med* 28:249-251, 1987.
228. Peh WC: Freiberg's infraction, *Am J Orthop* 30:878, 2001.
229. Nguyen VD, Keh RA, Daehler RW: Freiberg's disease in diabetes mellitus, *Skeletal Radiol* 26:425-428, 1991.
230. Mizel M, Yodlowski ML: Disorders of the lesser metatarsophalangeal joints, *J Am Acad Orthop Surg* 3:166-173, 1995.
231. Ashman CJ, Klecker RJ, Yu JS: Forefoot pain involving the metatarsal region: differential diagnosis with MR imaging, *Radiographics* 21:1425-1440, 2001.
232. Rosenberg Z, Beltran J, Bencardino J: From the RSNA Refresher Courses. Radiological Society of North America. MR imaging of the ankle and foot, *Radiographics* S153-S179, 2001.
233. Sherry D, Malleson P: Nonrheumatic musculoskeletal pain. In Cassidy JT, Petty RE (editors): *Textbook of pediatric rheumatology*, ed 4, Philadelphia, 2001, Saunders, pp 362-380.
234. Haller J, Sartoris DJ, Resnick D et al: Spontaneous osteonecrosis of the tarsal navicular in adults: imaging findings, *AJR Am J Roentgenol* 151:355-358, 1988.
235. Ippolito E, Ricciardi Pollini PT, Falez F: Kohler's disease of the tarsal navicular: long-term follow-up of 12 cases, *J Pediatr Orthop* 4:416-417, 1984.
236. Borges JL, Guille JT, Bowen JR: Kohler's bone disease of the tarsal navicular, *J Pediatr Orthop* 15:596-598, 1995.
237. Weston WJ: Kohler's disease of the tarsal scaphoid, *Austral Radiol* 22:332-337, 1978.
238. McCauley RG, Kahn PC: Osteochondritis of the tarsal navicula: radioisotopic appearances, *Radiology* 123:705-706, 1977.
239. Gips S, Ruchman RB, Groshar D: Bone imaging in Kohler's disease, *Clin Nucl Med* 22:636-637, 1997.
240. Panner H: An affection of the capitulum humeri resembling Calve-Perthes disease of the hip, *Acta Radiol* 8:617-618, 1927.
241. Kijowski R, Tuite M, Sanford M: Magnetic resonance imaging of the elbow. Part I: normal anatomy, imaging technique, and osseous abnormalities, *Skeletal Radiol* 33:685-697, 2004.
242. Stoane JM, Poplausky MR, Haller JO et al: Panner's disease: x-ray, MR imaging findings and review of the literature, *Comp Med Imaging Graphics* 19:473-476, 1995.
243. Sofka CM, Potter HG: Imaging of elbow injuries in the child and adult athlete, *Radiol Clin North Am* 40:251-265, 2002.
244. Kobayashi K, Burton KJ, Rodner C et al: Lateral compression injuries in the pediatric elbow: Panner's disease and osteochondritis dissecans of the capitellum, *J Am Acad Orthop Surg* 12:246-254, 2004.
245. Brogdon B, Crow N: Little leaguer's elbow, *Am J Roentgenol Radium Ther Nucl Med* 83:671-675, 1960.
246. Daniel WW: Panner's disease [see comment], *Arthritis Rheum* 32:341-342, 1989.
247. Sty JR, Boedecker R: Panner's disease (osteonecrosis of the capitellum), *Clin Nucl Med* 3:117, 1978.
248. Cassas K, Cassettari-Wayhs A: Childhood and adolescent sports-related overuse injuries, *Am Fam Physician* 73:1014-1022, 2006.
249. Volpon J, Filho G: Calcaneal apophysitis: a quantitative radiographic evaluation of the secondary ossification center, *Arch Orthop Trauma Surg* 122:338-341, 2002.
250. Bachrach LK: Osteoporosis and measurement of bone mass in children and adolescents, *Endocrin Metabol Clin North Am* 34:521-535, 2005.
251. Theintz G, Buchs B, Rizzoli R et al: Longitudinal monitoring of bone mass accumulation in healthy adolescents: evidence for a marked reduction after 16 years of age at the levels of lumbar spine and femoral neck in female subjects, *J Clin Endocrin Metabol* 75:1060-1065, 1992.
252. Loro ML, Sayre J, Roe TF et al: Early identification of children predisposed to low peak bone mass and osteoporosis later in life, *J Clin Endocrin Metabol* 85:3908-3918, 2000.
253. Saggese G, Baroncelli GI, Bertelloni S: Osteoporosis in children and adolescents: diagnosis, risk factors, and prevention, *J Pediatr Endocrinol* 14:833-859, 2001.
254. Osteoporosis prevention, diagnosis and therapy. NIH Consensus Statement, *J Am Med Assoc* 285:785-795, 2001.
255. Ponder SW: Clinical use of bone densitometry in children: are we ready yet? [comment], *Clin Pediatr* 34:237-240, 1995.
256. Konig P, Hillman L, Cervantes C et al: Bone metabolism in children with asthma treated with inhaled beclomethasone dipropionate, *J Pediatr* 122:219-226, 1993.
257. Kinberg KA, Hopp RJ, Biven RE et al: Bone mineral density in normal and asthmatic children, *J Allergy Clin Immunol* 94:490-497, 1994.
258. Hopp RJ, Degan JA, Biven RE et al: Longitudinal assessment of bone mineral density in children with chronic asthma, *Ann Allergy Asthma Immunol* 75:143-148, 1995.
259. Martinati LC, Bertoldo F, Gasperi E et al: Effect on cortical and trabecular bone mass of different anti-inflammatory treatments in preadolescent children with chronic asthma, *Am J Respir Crit Care Med* 153:232-236, 1996.
260. Agertoft L, Pederson S: Bone mineral density in children with asthma receiving long-term treatment with inhaled budesonide, *Am J Respir Crit Care Med* 157:178-183, 1998.
261. American College of Radiology, E.P.o.P.I., ACR Appropriateness Criteria: Osteoporosis and Bone Mineral Density. *American College of Radiology*, 1998 (rev. 2001).
262. Southard RN, Morris JD, Mahan JD et al: Bone mass in healthy children: measurement with quantitative DXA, *Radiology* 179:735-738, 1991.
263. Gilsanz V: Bone density in children: a review of the available techniques and indications, *Eur J Radiol* 26:177-182, 1998.
264. Lewiecki EM, Binkley N, Bilezikian J et al: Official positions of the international society for clinical densitometry, *J Clin Endocrinol Metab* 89:3651-3655, 2004.

265. Wren TA, Liu X, Pitukcheewanont P et al: Bone acquisition in healthy children and adolescents: comparisons of dual-energy x-ray absorptiometry and computed tomography measures, *J Clin Endocrinol Metab* 90:1925-1928, 2005.
266. Lu PW, Briody JN, Ogle GD et al: Bone mineral density of total body, spine, and femoral neck in children and young adults: a cross-sectional and longitudinal study, *J Bone Miner Res* 9:1451-1458, 1994.
267. Kroger H, Kotaniemi A, Vainio P et al: Bone densitometry of the spine and femur in children by dual-energy x-ray absorptiometry [erratum appears in *Bone Miner* 17:429, 1992], *Bone Miner* 17:75-85, 1992.
268. Kroger H, Kotaniemi A, Kröger L et al: Development of bone mass and bone density of the spine and femoral neck—a prospective study of 65 children and adolescents, *Bone Miner* 23:171-182, 1993.
269. Rubin K, Schirduan V, Gendreau P et al: Predictors of axial and peripheral bone mineral density in healthy children and adolescents, with special attention to the role of puberty [see comment], *J Pediatr* 123:863-870, 1993.
270. Molgaard C, Thomsen BL, Prentice A et al: Whole body bone mineral content in healthy children and adolescents [see comment], *Arch Dis Child* 76:9-15, 1997.
271. Glastre C, Braillon P, David L et al: Measurement of bone mineral content of the lumbar spine by dual energy x-ray absorptiometry in normal children: correlations with growth parameters, *J Clin Endocrinol Metab* 70:1330-1333, 1990.
272. Gafni RI, Baron J: Overdiagnosis of osteoporosis in children due to misinterpretation of dual-energy x-ray absorptiometry (DEXA), *J Pediatr* 144:253-257, 2004.
273. Gilsanz V, Kovanlikaya A, Costin G et al: Differential effect of gender on the sizes of the bones in the axial and appendicular skeletons [erratum appears in *J Clin Endocrinol Metab* 82:2274, 1997], *J Clin Endocrinol Metab* 82:1603-1607, 1997.
274. Gilsanz V, Skaggs DL, Kovanlikaya A et al: Differential effect of race on the axial and appendicular skeletons of children [see comment], *J Clin Endocrinol Metab* 83:1420-1427, 1998.
275. Bell NH, Shary J, Stevens J et al: Demonstration that bone mass is greater in black than in white children, *J Bone Miner Res* 6:719-723, 1991.
276. Slemenda CW, Miller JZ, Hui SL et al: Role of physical activity in the development of skeletal mass in children, *J Bone Miner Res* 6:1227-1233, 1991.
277. Wren TA, Liu X, Pitukcheewanont P et al: Bone densitometry in pediatric populations: discrepancies in the diagnosis of osteoporosis by DXA and CT, *J Pediatr* 146:776-779, 2005.
278. Bertuna G, Famà P, Lo Nigro L et al: Marked osteoporosis and spontaneous vertebral fractures in children: don't forget, it could be leukemia, *Med Pediatr Oncol* 41:450-451, 2003.

CHAPTER 26

Crystal Diseases

CATHERINE C. ROBERTS, MD, *and* ETHAN M. BRAUNSTEIN, MD*

KEY FACTS

Gout

- Clinically significant attacks may occur many years before radiographic changes are evident.
- Radiographs classically show well-defined erosions with overhanging edges and sclerotic borders.
- Soft tissue nodules (tophi) may calcify or ossify.
- Classically, gout involves the first metatarsophalangeal joint.
- Lesions of gout are randomly distributed in the hand.
- Osteoporosis is not a feature of gout.
- Gout occurs concomitantly with calcium pyrophosphate dihydrate deposition (CPPD) in 40% of patients.

CPPD Disease

- CPPD disease may be a secondary finding in patients with gout, primary hyperparathyroidism, or hemochromatosis.
- CPPD disease may mimic gout (then termed *pseudogout*), infection, or neuropathic arthropathy.
- Calcification of hyaline and fibrocartilage structures (chondrocalcinosis) is a hallmark of the disorder although not pathognomonic.
- The arthropathy of CPPD disease commonly involves the second and third metacarpophalangeal, radiocarpal, and patellofemoral joints.
- CPPD disease causes "drooping" osteophytes and prominent subchondral cysts.

Hydroxyapatite Deposition Disease (HADD)

- HADD may be acutely symptomatic and cause fever, increased C-reactive protein, and increased erythrocyte sedimentation rate.
- Crystals are beyond the resolution of light microscopy, making pathologic diagnosis cumbersome in routine clinical work.
- HADD typically appears on radiographs as amorphous globular calcifications in and around joints.
- HADD most commonly involves the shoulder.
- HADD may mimic malignancy when it causes erosion of adjacent bone and bone marrow edema.

Several types of crystals may deposit in joints. Crystal deposition may lead to symptoms, such as those due to inflammation or may be asymptomatic.

> Crystal deposition may be symptomatic or asymptomatic.

Gout, calcium pyrophosphate dihydrate deposition (CPPD) disease, and calcium hydroxyapatite deposition disease (HADD) are common examples. Deposition of these respective crystals in and around joints will produce changes typical of each disease.

GOUT

Writing about gout in 1683, Thomas Sydenham captured the baffling nature of the disease at that time: "Either men will think that the nature of gout is wholly mysterious and incomprehensible, or that a man like myself, who had suffered from it thirty-four years, must be of a slow and sluggish disposition not to have discovered something respecting the nature and treatment of a disease so peculiarly his own."[1]

Gout has been known since antiquity. Early descriptions deemed it an affliction of wealthy adult men, but its cause (an extracellular urate supersaturation that results in the deposition of monosodium urate crystals [MSU] in the tissues) was not identified until the last half of the 20th century.

> Extracellular urate supersaturation leads to monosodium urate crystal deposition.

Crystal deposition incites a complex inflammatory response[2] that damages the tissue. The accumulation of these crystals may be idiopathic, a result of enzyme deficiencies, or the consequence of a myriad of disease states (e.g., renal disease, hyperparathyroidism, hypoparathyroidism, myeloproliferative disorders, diuretic use). A diet rich in red meat, seafood, and liquor also increases the incidence of gout.[3] Saturnine gout is caused by chronic ingestion of homemade liquor (i.e., moonshine) contaminated with lead[4] (Table 26-1).

Clinically, gout may take the form of intermittent acute attacks of a red, swollen, painful joint or chronic arthropathy. White men who are middle aged to elderly are most commonly affected. Gout is uncommon in children and teenagers but may affect some young persons.[5,6]

> Gout is very uncommon in premenopausal women and is common in transplant patients.[6a]

Diagnosis is based on the presence of hyperuricemia (although the concentration of serum uric acid may be within normal

*We extend special thanks to Ann E. McCullough, MD, for assistance with questions about laboratory fluid analysis and to Patrick T. Liu, MD; F. Spencer Chivers, MD; and William W. Daniel, MD, for contributing cases. Editing, proofreading, and reference verification were provided by the Section of Scientific Publications, Mayo Clinic, Rochester, Minn.

TABLE 26-1. Some Causes of Gout

Cause	Frequency	Examples
Uric acid overproduction	10%	Primary: Idiopathic, Lesch-Nyhan syndrome (HGPRT deficiency) Secondary: Increased cell turnover (hematologic malignancies, psoriasis, Paget's disease, chemotherapy), increased purine intake (alcohol), accelerated ATP degradation (alcohol, muscle overexertion)
Uric acid underexcretion	90%	Primary: Idiopathic Secondary: Renal insufficiency, inhibition of tubular urate secretion (ketoacidosis and lactic acidosis), enhanced tubular reabsorption (diuretics, and dehydration), drugs (cyclosporine, pyrazinamide, ethambutol, low-dose ASA), lead, alcohol

From Agudelo CA, Wise CM: Gout: diagnosis, pathogenesis, and clinical manifestations, *Curr Opin Rheumatol* 13:234-239, 2001.
ASA, aspirin; *ATP*, adenosine triphosphate; *HGPRT*, hypoxanthine phosphoribosyltransferase.

limits),[7,8] clinical history, radiographic findings, MSU crystal identification, or rapid symptom resolution after colchicine therapy.

Most individuals with hyperuricemia do not develop clinical gout.

MSU forms needle-shaped crystals that exhibit strong negative birefringence under polarized light microscopy (Figure 26-1). When oriented parallel to the compensator, the crystals appear yellow, whereas they appear blue when oriented perpendicularly.

MSU crystals are negatively birefringent.

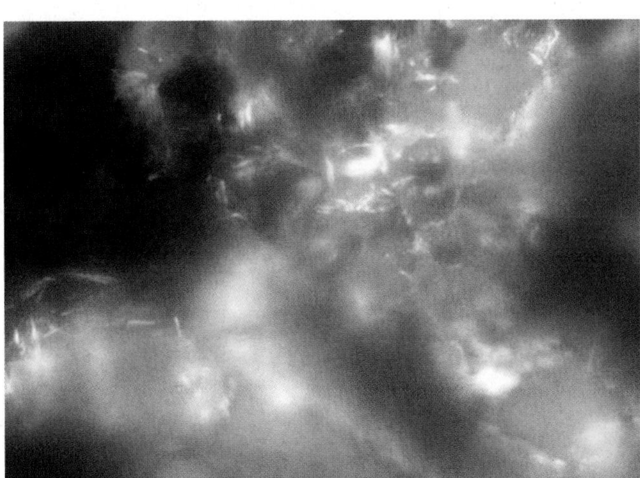

FIGURE 26-1. Needle-shaped MSU crystals under polarized light microscopy.

The crystals may be intracellular (e.g., within neutrophils) or extracellular. A secondary finding is an elevated white blood cell count in synovial fluid caused by the crystal-induced inflammation.

Osteoarticular Imaging Features

Radiographs

Radiographic findings of gout are pathognomonic (Figure 26-2) (Box 26-1). Round to oval intraarticular or paraarticular erosions have well-defined sclerotic borders, giving them a punched-out appearance. The bone adjacent to the erosions may extend outward to produce an "overhanging margin."

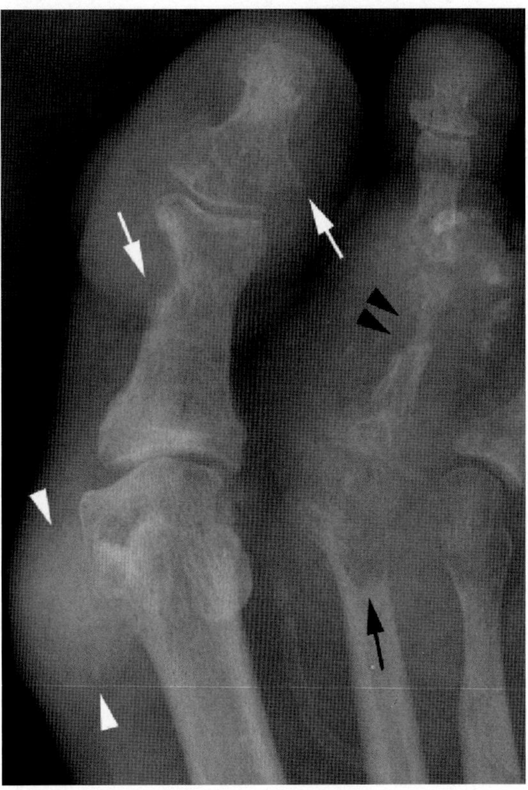

FIGURE 26-2. Gout. An AP radiograph of the foot shows multiple findings typical of gout. Well-defined intraarticular and paraarticular erosions have overhanging edges *(white arrows)*. The first MTP joint is involved with a large adjacent tophus *(white arrowheads)*. An intraosseous tophus *(black arrow)* is noncalcified. Erosions are present remote from a joint *(black arrowheads)* due to pressure from overlying tophi.

BOX 26-1. Radiographic Features of Chronic Tophaceous Gout

Normal or near-normal bone density
Normal alignment
Asymmetric joint involvement
Soft tissue masses that may calcify or ossify
Cartilage spaces may remain normal
Intraarticular and extraarticular erosions
Erosions have sclerotic bases and "overhanging margins"

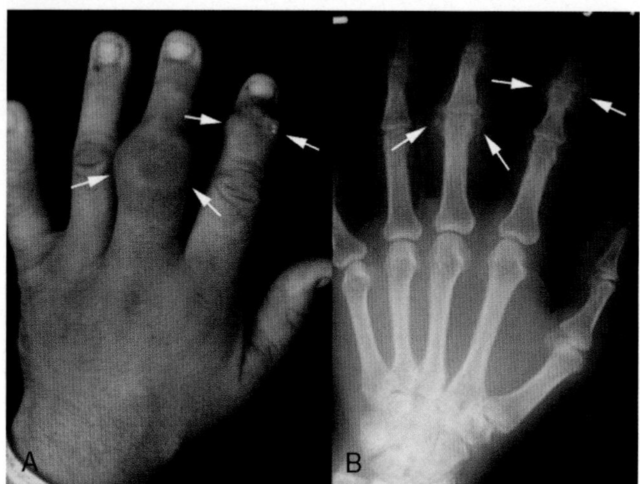

FIGURE 26-3. Gout. **A,** Photograph of the left hand showing reddened, periarticular tophi at the third digit proximal interphalangeal joint and second digit distal interphalangeal joint *(arrows)*. **B,** The corresponding PA radiograph shows the nodular appearance due to partially calcified tophi *(arrows)*.

Erosions classically have sclerotic bases and new bone formation ("the overhanging margin of gout").

Additional productive changes include enlargement of the phalangeal bases. Bone density in gout is normal unless disuse osteoporosis supervenes. The joint spaces are often well preserved until late in the disease, and the relative lack of cartilage destruction may help differentiate gout from other erosive arthropathies. Soft tissue tophi may be of homogeneous increased density or may contain focal calcification, which is more common in patients with altered calcium metabolism. The tophi cause a nodular appearance (Figure 26-3). They are more common in patients who have had gout for many years or who have responded poorly to treatment.[9]

Gout is asymmetric and polyarticular. Unfortunately, these typical radiographic changes are not visible until about 10 years after clinical presentation and early diagnosis is largely clinical.[10] Advanced changes of gout (Figure 26-4) are seldom observed now because of improved diagnosis and treatment.

Gout most commonly affects the feet. In more than half of patients, the initial sign is acute inflammation of the first metatarsophalangeal (MTP) joint.[11] The other MTP joints, interphalangeal joints, midfoot, and hindfoot may also be involved. In the hand, the distal interphalangeal, proximal interphalangeal, and intercarpal joints are often involved. The bones may enlarge because of reactive new bone formation (Figure 26-5). When this occurs in the phalangeal bases or the ulnar styloid process, it produces a mushroom appearance. Within the elbow, the olecranon may be eroded with tophus formation in the overlying bursa (Figure 26-6).

Large joints, such as the knee, are less commonly affected than are the small joints of the feet and hands. Within the knee, marginal erosions (Figure 26-7) and involvement of the prepatellar bursa are typical. Within the pelvis, the sacroiliac joints may be markedly eroded (Figure 26-8). Spinal involvement is seldom observed. However, gout in the spine has been reported in vertebral bodies, intervertebral disks,[12,13] posterior elements,[14,15] and facets.[16] Because gout in the spine is so rare, infection and neoplasm are often diagnostic alternatives.[16]

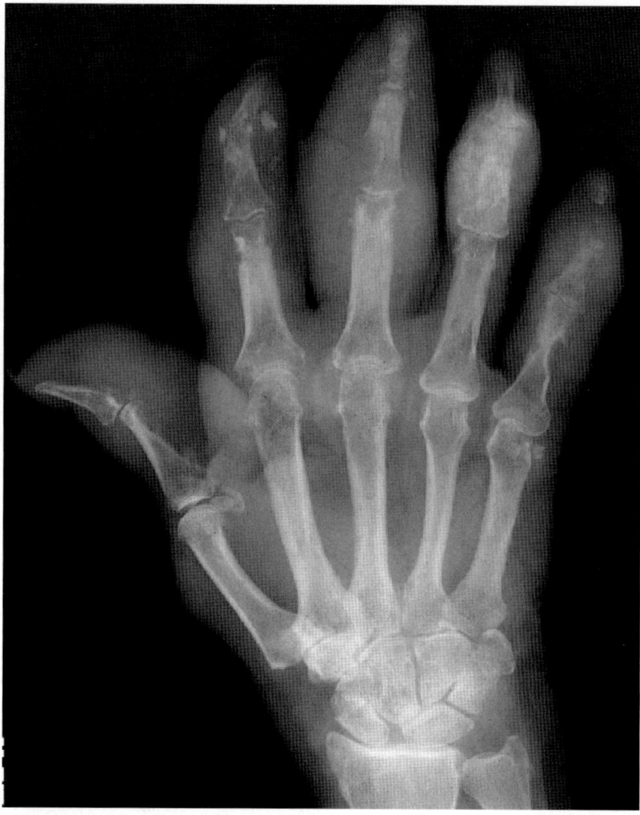

FIGURE 26-4. Gout. PA radiograph of the hand in a 63-year-old woman. This patient was erroneously thought to have rheumatoid arthritis and was treated with antirheumatoid drugs for 10 years. Note the marked soft tissue swelling, numerous erosions with overhanging margins, and soft tissue calcifications.

Focal collections of crystals (i.e., tophi) occur in the synovium, ligaments,[17] tendons,[18] and bursae.[19] When tophi are intraosseous, they have a predilection for the patella[20] and almost never calcify, in contrast to the soft tissue tophi that sometimes[21] contain calcifications.

Lytic lesions of the patella are usually benign.[21a]

Intraosseous tophi may have an aggressive appearance simulating that of a malignancy.[22,23] Extraarticular tophi tend to occur in the olecranon bursa, the prepatellar bursa, and the dorsum of the foot. Pressure from tophi can produce extraarticular erosions and mass effect on adjacent neurovascular structures, resulting in carpal tunnel syndrome[24] or paraplegia.[25] Erosion of bone and soft tissues by tophi sometimes leads to pathologic fracture[26] or tendon rupture.[27]

Conditions associated with nontraumatic tendon rupture include gout, systemic lupus erythematosus, rheumatoid arthritis, obesity, Ciprofloxacin use, and diabetes.

Urate crystals can also penetrate the cartilage and extend into the medullary canal, producing small, circular, calcified deposits in the bone. Punctate intraosseous calcifications that collect in the subchondral bone can mimic bone infarcts and enchondromas.

Gout sometimes coexists with other articular disorders (e.g., osteoarthritis, CPPD disease). When radiographic findings of multiple entities occur together, diagnosis may be difficult, especially when gout coexists with infection.[28]

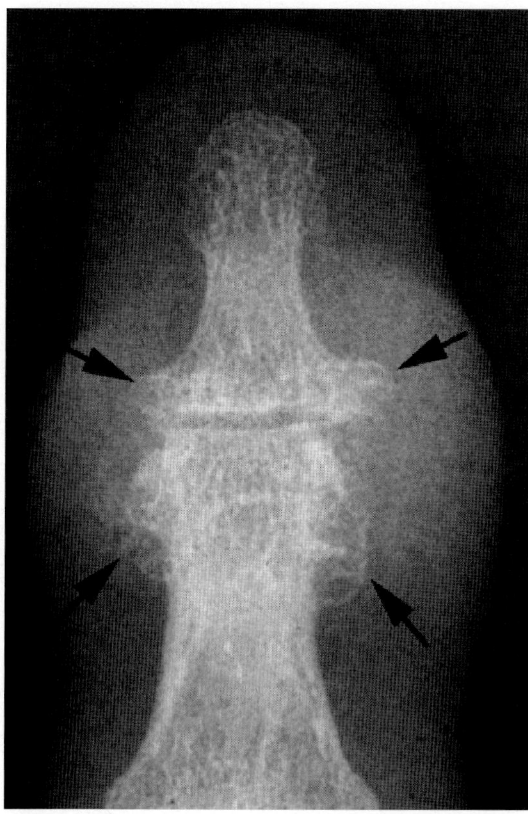

FIGURE 26-5. Gout. PA radiograph of the second distal interphalangeal joint demonstrates proliferative bone formation *(arrows)*, enlarging the bone around the joint. Soft tissue swelling is due to tophi. The bone changes are similar to osteoarthritis proliferation.

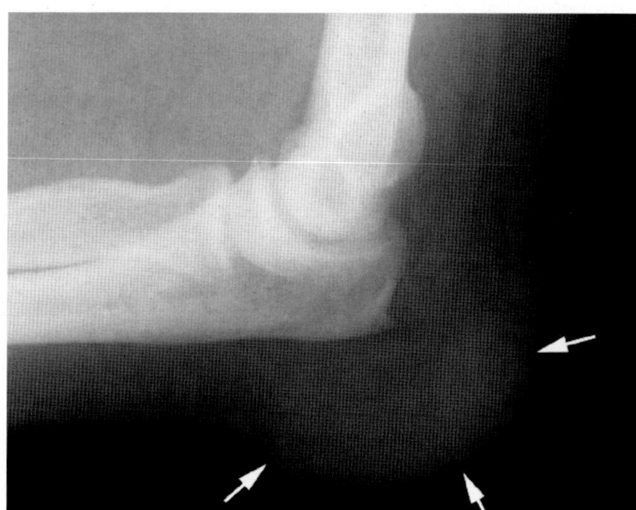

FIGURE 26-6. Gout. Lateral radiograph of the elbow with a large mass *(arrows)* of faintly increased density located dorsal to the olecranon, corresponding to a gouty tophus in the olecranon bursa. There are no bone erosions in this case.

Computed Tomography

Erosions and soft tissue tophi show up clearly on computed tomography (CT) (Figure 26-9). MSU crystals have a characteristic density of 160 Hounsfield units (HU).[29] This measurement is substantially lower than that of calcium, which is 450 HU. CT can be especially helpful in defining abnormalities in areas such as the spine that have multiple overlapping structures on radiographs.

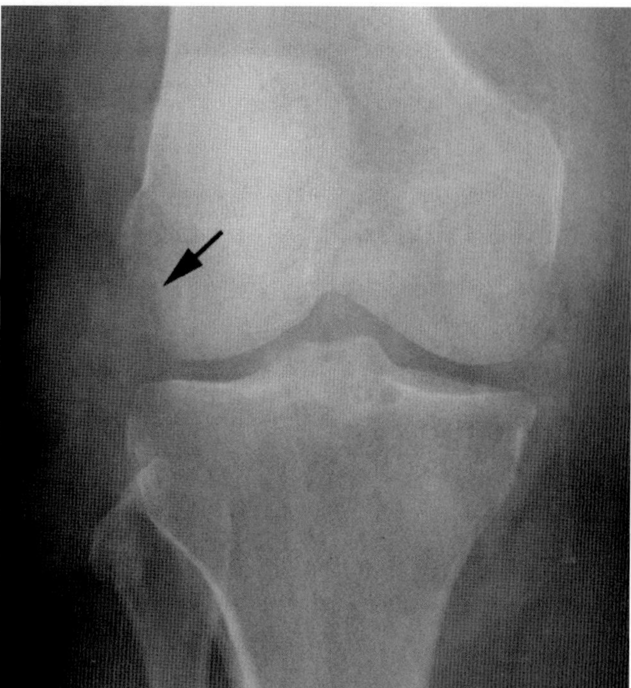

FIGURE 26-7. Gout. AP view of the knee showing a marginal erosion *(arrow)* and faintly increased density of soft tissues in a patient with gout.

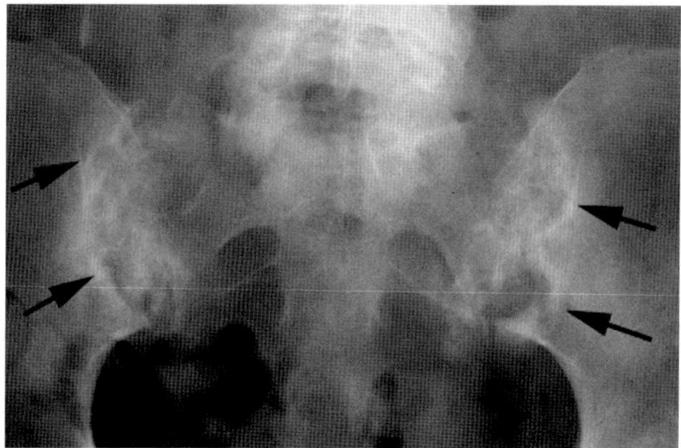

FIGURE 26-8. Gout involving the sacroiliac joints. An AP view of the pelvis demonstrates large gout erosions with sclerotic borders *(arrows)* involving sacroiliac joints.

Magnetic Resonance Imaging

Magnetic resonance imaging (MRI) is helpful in evaluating the extent of gout, especially in the spine,[30] but it has limited diagnostic usefulness.

> MRI has limited diagnostic value in patients with gout but demonstrates the degree of bone and soft tissue involvement better than radiographic or clinical examination.

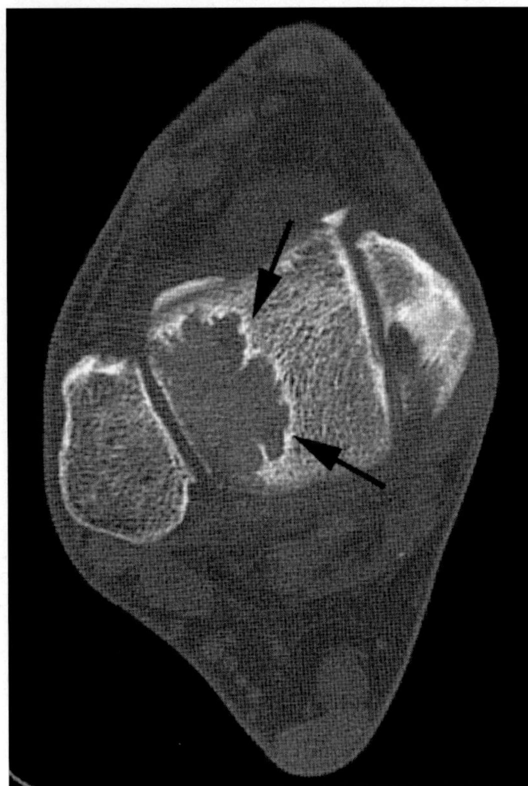

FIGURE 26-9. Gout. Axial unenhanced CT through the talar dome in a 44-year-old man. A well-defined erosion with sclerotic border *(arrows)* is present. Biopsy confirmed gout. This lesion had increased radiotracer uptake on bone scan (not shown).

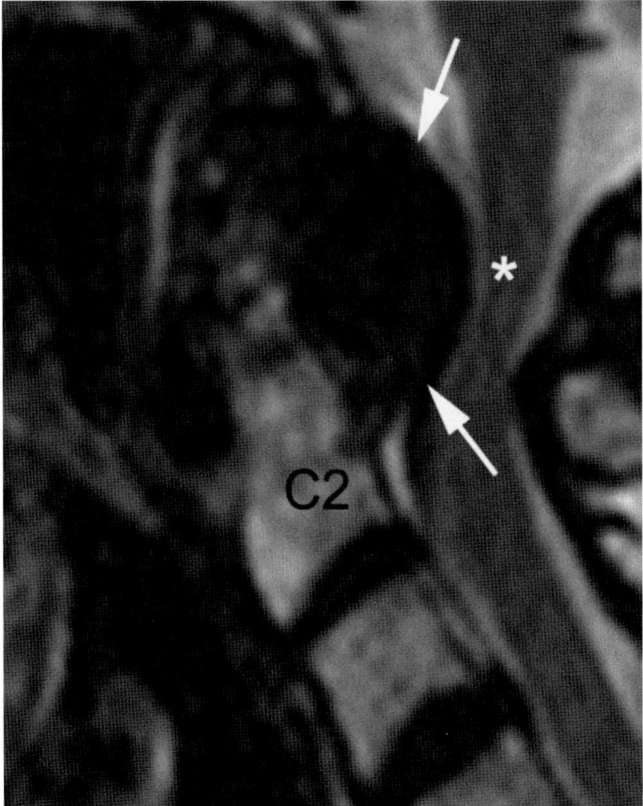

FIGURE 26-10. Gouty tophus producing spinal cord compression. Sagittal T2-weighted MRI through the upper cervical spine demonstrates a low signal mass dorsal to the dens *(arrows)*. This was causing spinal cord compression *(asterisk)*. Pathologic examination confirmed a gouty tophus. Most tumors show increased signal on T2-weighted images.

A tophus may have low to intermediate signal on T1-weighted images and a variable low to high signal on T2-weighted images (Figure 26-10).

> Tophi demonstrate intermediate signal on T1-weighted images and variable signal on T2-weighted images.

Tophi may show homogeneous, inhomogeneous, or only peripheral enhancement (Figure 26-11). Some tophi may contain focal fluid collections.[31] The varied appearance of gout on MRI may be related to the amount of calcium within a tophus.[32] MRI is useful, however, for identifying tophi that are not clinically evident.[33]

Scintigraphy

In active gout, radionuclide bone scanning shows nonspecific increased radiotracer uptake. Neoplasm, trauma, and infection can have a similar appearance. Gout can mimic infection clinically and radiographically.[34] Unfortunately, even three-phase bone scanning, which usually has a high specificity for infection, may produce false-positive findings because of gout.[35] Tophi are hypermetabolic on positron emission tomography (PET).[36] A case report using PET imaging of an intraosseous patellar tophus identified metabolic activity that was less than that of malignancy, which suggests a possible role for PET in differentiating gout from neoplasm.[37] Indium 111-labeled leukocyte imaging can sometimes help differentiate gout from infection, but there have been false-positive cases.[38] Cases of infection typically show increased uptake on indium-labeled white blood cells scans. Increased radiotracer uptake is seen in inflamed joints including those with crystal disease when imaged using Tc-99m ciprofloxacin. This technique has been proposed as a method for monitoring response to treatment.[39] Cases that are healing typically exhibit decreasing uptake.

Arthrography

Conventional arthrography has little use in the diagnosis or follow-up of gout. Fluoroscopy can guide joint aspiration for crystal analysis, and the injection of contrast material may ensure accurate intraarticular needle placement.

Ultrasonography

Ultrasound is useful for guiding joint aspirations and biopsy. It can also be used to identify joint effusions and alterations of the surrounding soft tissue structures, such as tendons[40,41] and ligaments. On Doppler ultrasound, tophi have a nonspecific heterogeneous appearance with a hypervascular rim.[29] After tophi are identified, they are easy to measure with ultrasound, which can be useful for follow-up.[42] Ultrasound is also helpful for assessing renal complications of hyperuricemia.[43]

Extraarticular Imaging Features

Gouty tophi may occur in many soft-tissue sites, including cartilaginous involvement of the nose[44] and the helix of the ear.[45] Hyperuricemia may also affect the kidneys, causing nephrolithiasis and chronic urate nephropathy. Urate calculi are typically opaque

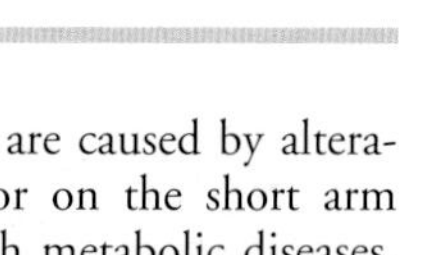

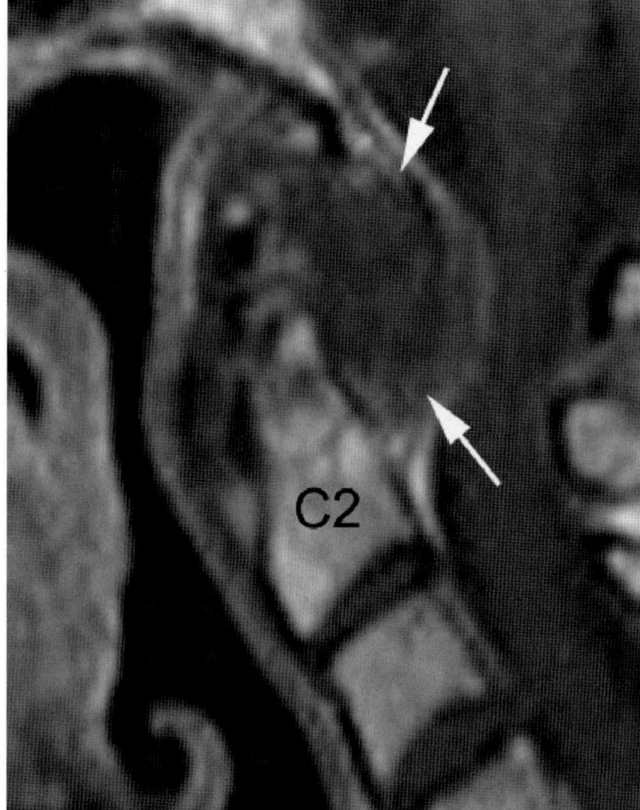

FIGURE 26-11. Gouty tophus. Sagittal T1-weighted, gadolinium-enhanced MRI through the upper cervical spine. The tophus dorsal to the dens *(arrows)* showed mild inhomogeneous internal enhancement and moderate peripheral enhancement. The imaging appearance was nonspecific, and surgery was necessary for diagnosis and treatment.

on noncontrast CT examinations. Tophi in the corpus cavernosum may cause erectile dysfunction. Reflex sympathetic dystrophy has been reported as a complication of gout.[46] One case report described a gouty tophus that tracked alongside the iliopsoas muscle and mimicked an intrapelvic abscess.[47]

Algorithms and Recommendations

In cases suspected of gout, survey radiographs should include anteroposterior (AP), oblique, and lateral views of the feet and a posteroanterior (PA) view of the hands. Symptomatic areas should also be imaged with radiographs. When gout is suspected but not clearly defined, CT or MRI may be of use, especially for imaging the spine.[46]

> In acute monarthritis, radiographs should be considered prior to arthrocentesis to assess for fracture, especially if there is a history of trauma or risk factors for osteoporosis.[6a]

CPPD DISEASE

In CPPD disease, crystal deposition is usually idiopathic but also may be hereditary or associated with several underlying diseases.

> Some causes of CPPD disease include familial, hyperparathyroidism, hemochromatosis, ochronosis, or hypophosphatasia.

The two familial forms of CPPD disease are caused by alterations on the long arm of chromosome 8 or on the short arm of chromosome 5.[48] CPPD is associated with metabolic diseases, such as hyperparathyroidism, hemochromatosis, ochronosis, or hypophosphatasia.[49] In cases with intermittent acute attacks of joint pain mimicking the clinical presentation of gout, CPPD disease is referred to as *pseudogout.*

> Clinical manifestations of CPPD disease include asymptomatic, pseudorheumatoid, pseudogout, pseudoneuropathic, pseudoosteoarthritis.[49a]

Although cartilage calcification (chondrocalcinosis) is most commonly associated with CPPD deposition disease, other crystals (e.g., dicalcium phosphate dihydrate or calcium hydroxyapatite)[50] may precipitate in cartilage to produce chondrocalcinosis. Calcium pyrophosphate dihydrate crystals are rod shaped or rhomboid and, on polarized light microscopy, have positive birefringence (blue when parallel to the compensator axis).

> CPPD crystals are smaller and less brightly refringent on polarized light microscopy compared with MSU crystals and may, therefore, often missed.[6a]

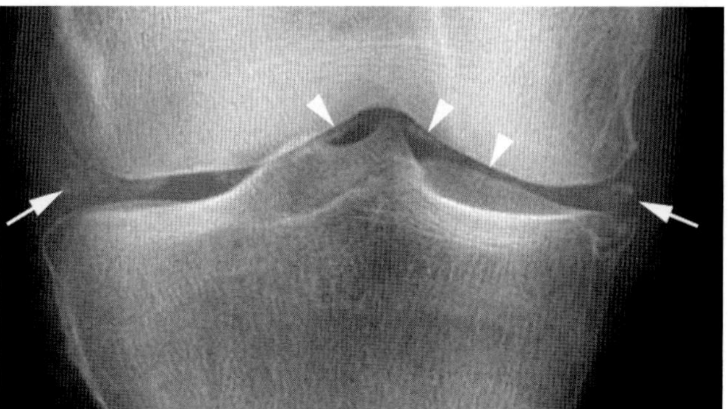

FIGURE 26-12. Chondrocalcinosis. An AP radiograph of the knee demonstrates globular calcification in the meniscal fibrocartilage *(arrows)* and linear calcification in the articular cartilage *(arrowheads)*.

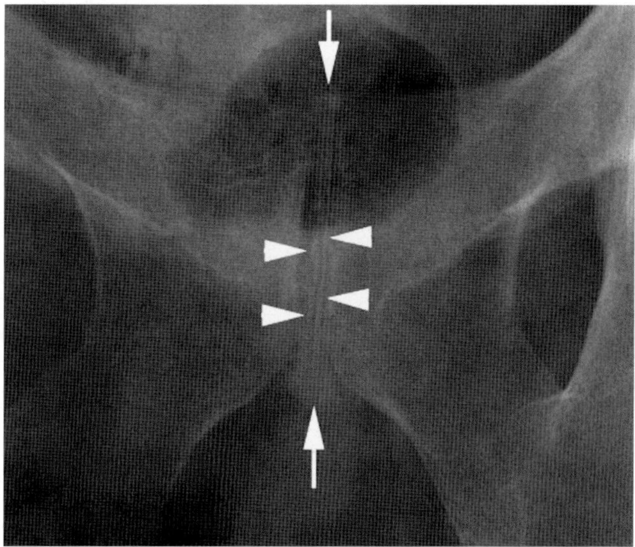

FIGURE 26-13. Chondrocalcinosis. A coned AP view of the pelvis demonstrates linear chondrocalcinosis of symphysis pubis *(arrowheads)* and faint calcification within the superior and inferior joint recesses *(arrows)*.

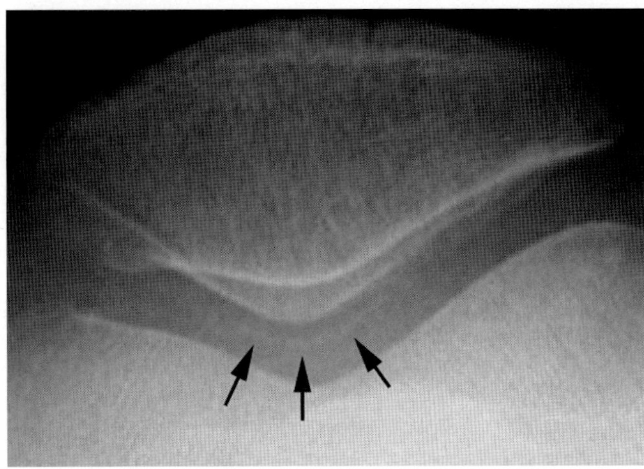

FIGURE 26-14. Chondrocalcinosis. A tangential patellar radiograph demonstrates the fine linear appearance of hyaline cartilage chondrocalcinosis *(arrows)*.

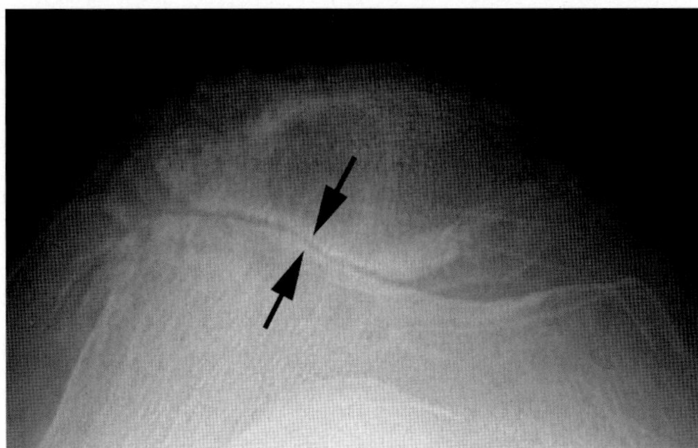

FIGURE 26-15. CPPD disease with marked patellofemoral cartilage loss. A tangential patellar view shows advanced narrowing of the patellofemoral joint *(arrows)*. A patellar cyst is persent. The tibiofemoral joint compartments in this patient were normal.

Osteoarticular Imaging Features

Radiographs

Radiographs are the most important imaging tests in the evaluation of CPPD disease. The hallmark finding is chondrocalcinosis of hyaline cartilage or fibrocartilage (Figure 26-12). Chondrocalcinosis of fibrocartilage is most commonly observed in the knee menisci, wrist triangular fibrocartilage complex, symphysis pubis (Figure 26-13), and acetabular labrum.

> Essentially all patients with chondrocalcinosis may be discovered if radiographs of three sites: the knees, wrists, and pelvis (pubic symphysis) are obtained.

Crystals may also collect in tendons,[51] ligaments, synovium, bursae, and joint capsules. Chondrocalcinosis in hyaline cartilage parallels the underlying bone and appears as thin linear deposits (Figure 26-14). Crystal deposition in cartilage causes accelerated cartilage breakdown[52] and a radiographic appearance that mimics degenerative joint disease. Changes may be so severe that they mimic neuropathic or Charcot-like destruction of the joint.[53] Joint changes are typically bilateral and symmetric.

The key differentiating factor between CPPD disease and degenerative joint disease is the location of the joint changes.

> CPPD disease typically affects the radiocarpal, patellofemoral, and second and third MCP joints.

CPPD disease tends to affect areas not typically involved by degenerative joint disease (e.g., the radiocarpal, patellofemoral, second and third MCP joints, and the shoulder and elbow). The lack of erosion differentiates CPPD disease from gout and rheumatoid arthritis. The lack of osteopenia differentiates CPPD disease from septic arthritis and rheumatoid arthritis.

The most commonly affected joint is the knee, where cartilage space narrowing and osteophytes may involve all three compartments. Severe changes in the patellofemoral joint are suggestive of CPPD disease (Figure 26-15), particularly when found in isolation.

> Isolated patellofemoral cartilage space narrowing suggests CPPD arthropathy.

Chondrocalcinosis is commonly found in the menisci and less commonly in the articular cartilage. CPPD disease in the hip should be suspected when large subchondral cysts are present. Labral chondrocalcinosis may be subtle (Figure 26-16).

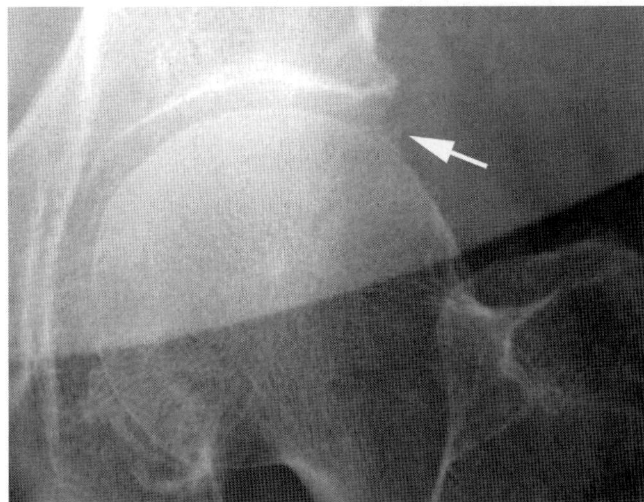

FIGURE 26-16. Chondrocalcinosis. An AP radiograph of the hip shows faint calcification of the acetabular labrum *(arrow)*. There is no significant narrowing of the hip joint.

> Large subchondral cysts suggest CPPD arthropathy.

Changes evident on radiographs in the radiocarpal joint include chondrocalcinosis, cartilage space narrowing, and scapholunate dissociation. Chondrocalcinosis is most common in the lunotriquetral ligament (Figure 26-17) and the triangular fibrocartilage complex.[54] Narrowing of the radiocarpal and scaphotrapeziotrapezoid joint spaces is common. When the scaphoid and lunate bones dissociate, the capitate can migrate proximally, producing the scapholunate advanced collapse (SLAC) wrist deformity (Figure 26-18). This deformity is not pathognomonic for CPPD disease, however. It may also be caused by trauma, infection, neuropathy, amyloid deposition, or rheumatoid arthritis. The scaphoid can erode into the distal radius, producing a stepladder appearance. Changes in the second and third MCP joints include joint space narrowing and hook-like or "drooping" osteophytes from the radial aspect of the metacarpal heads (Figure 26-19). Similar osteophytes occur with

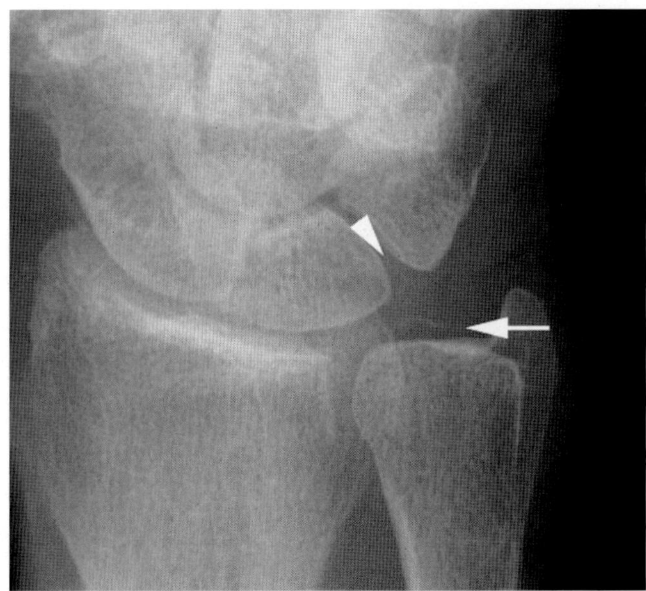

FIGURE 26-17. Chondrocalcinosis. An oblique radiograph of the wrist demonstrates chondrocalcinosis of the triangular fibrocartilage complex *(arrow)* and lunotriquetral ligament *(arrowhead)*.

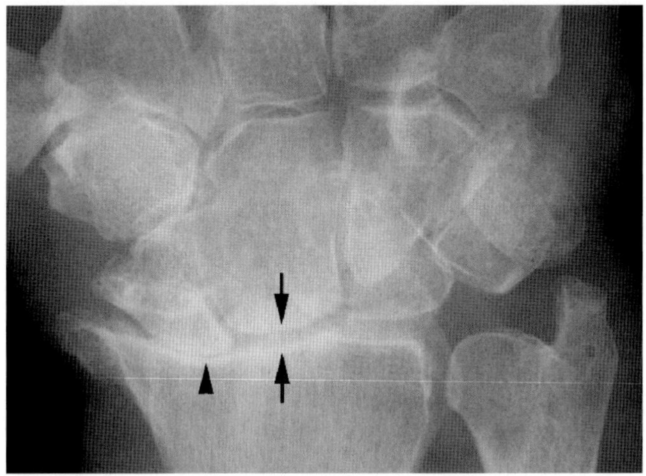

FIGURE 26-18. Scapholunate advanced collapse (SLAC) wrist. A PA radiograph of the wrist shows SLAC. The capitate has migrated proximally and articulates with the distal radius *(arrows)*. The proximal pole of the scaphoid is eroding into the distal radius *(arrowhead)*.

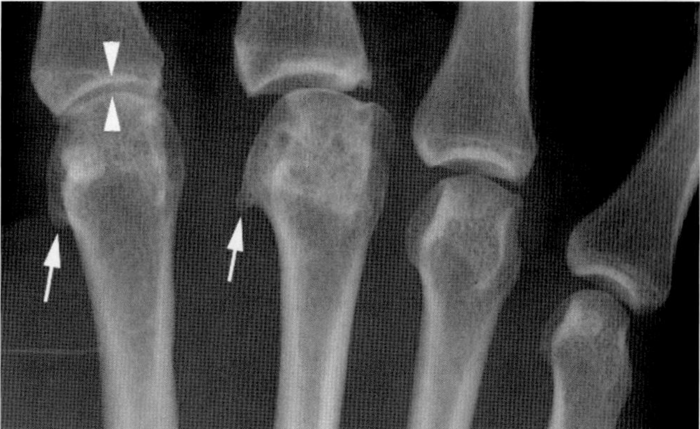

FIGURE 26-19. CPPD arthropathy. PA radiograph of the MCP joints demonstrates hook-like osteophytes extending from the radial aspect of the second and third metacarpal heads *(arrows)*. The second MCP joint is moderately narrowed *(arrowheads)*.

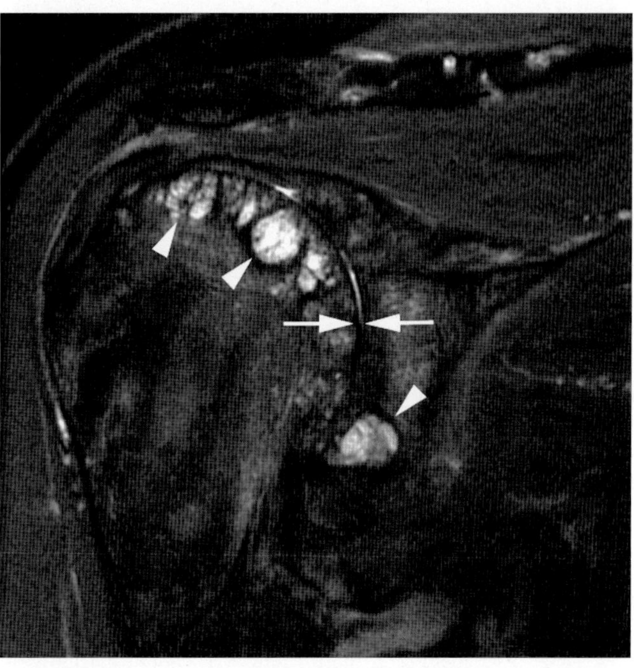

FIGURE 26-20. CPPD arthropathy. Coronal oblique, T2-weighted fat-suppressed MRI of the shoulder demonstrates prominent subchondral cystic change *(arrowheads)* and a markedly narrowed joint space *(arrows)*.

hemochromatosis when there is secondary intra-articular deposition of CPPD crystals.[55] The interphalangeal joints tend to be uninvolved in CPPD disease but often are affected in osteoarthritis, which is common and can coexist with any entity.

In the shoulder and elbow, any changes that resemble degenerative joint disease should raise the suspicion of CPPD disease, because these joints rarely show radiographic evidence of severe degenerative change.

> Degenerative changes in the shoulder or elbow raise the possibility of CPPD disease.

Osteophytes may extend from the inferomedial humeral head and the inferolateral glenoid. A subtle line of chondrocalcinosis can sometimes be identified in the cartilage covering the humeral head. Subchondral cysts may line the articular surface of the humeral head in a "string-of-pearls" configuration (Figure 26-20). Tendon calcification in CPPD disease is typically more linear or punctate than in calcium HADD, which tends to be globular and amorphous.

Spinal CPPD deposition disease is uncommon; it involves the ligamentum flavum[56,57] of the posterior spinal canal. Less commonly, it involves the intervertebral disks[58] and facet joints.[59] When crystal deposition is nodular, it may cause mass effect on the spinal cord and exiting nerve roots, resulting in cord compression[60-63] and radiculopathy.[64] The term *crowned dens syndrome* refers to CPPD deposition surrounding the top and sides of the odontoid process. This syndrome may cause acute neck pain and can mimic other entities, such as meningoencephalitis,[65] temporal arteritis, and bone metastases.[66]

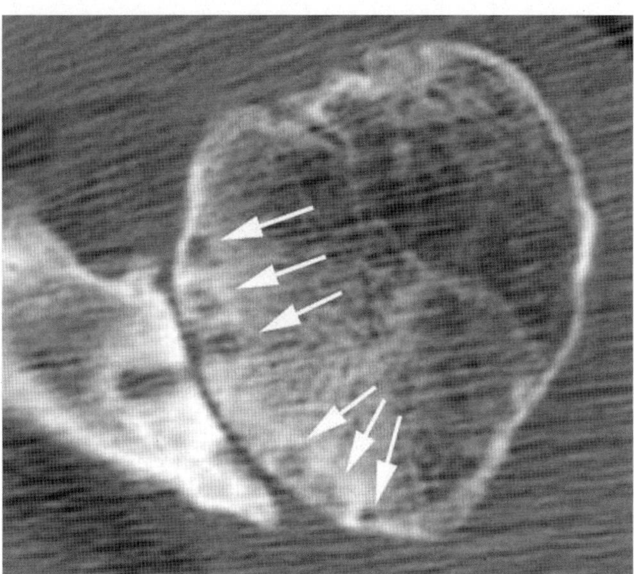

FIGURE 26-21. CPPD arthropathy. An axial CT scan through the shoulder well demonstrates joint space narrowing and subchondral cysts in a "string of pearls" configuration *(arrows).*

Other regions of CPPD involvement in the body include the acromioclavicular,[67] sternoclavicular, sacroiliac,[68] and temporomandibular joints.[69-71]

Computed Tomography

CT well demonstrates calcifications, articular surface deformities, and subchondral cysts (Figure 26-21). However, CT is not typically used in the evaluation of a painful joint. CT is more commonly used for preoperative planning for joint replacement, because its more detailed demonstration of joint changes can help in selecting and guiding surgical intervention.[72]

Magnetic Resonance Imaging

Whether MRI is more or less sensitive than radiographs in detecting the calcification caused by CPPD disease has been debated.[73,74] Typically, calcium has low signal on MRI sequences that, theoretically, would be obscured within other structures also having a normally low signal (e.g., menisci, tendons). However, chondrocalcinosis in the menisci has increased signal on T1-weighted, proton density-weighted, and inversion recovery sequences.[75] In some cases, this increased signal can simulate a meniscal tear.[76]

CPPD disease can mimic a meniscal tear on MRI.

MRI sequences tailored to image cartilage, particularly gradient recalled echo, best demonstrate linear low-signal calcification within the intermediate signal intensity cartilage.[73] Tumoral CPPD deposits can be T2 hyperintense and show peripheral enhancement.[77] MRI is useful for evaluation of associated soft tissue abnormalities, such as rotator cuff tears (Figure 26-22) or fluid collections.

Scintigraphy

Before arthropathy changes are visible radiographically, radionuclide bone scintigraphy shows radiotracer uptake in joints. Unfortunately, this radiotracer uptake is nonspecific and would not facilitate differentiation of CPPD arthropathy from other types of inflammatory or degenerative arthritis.

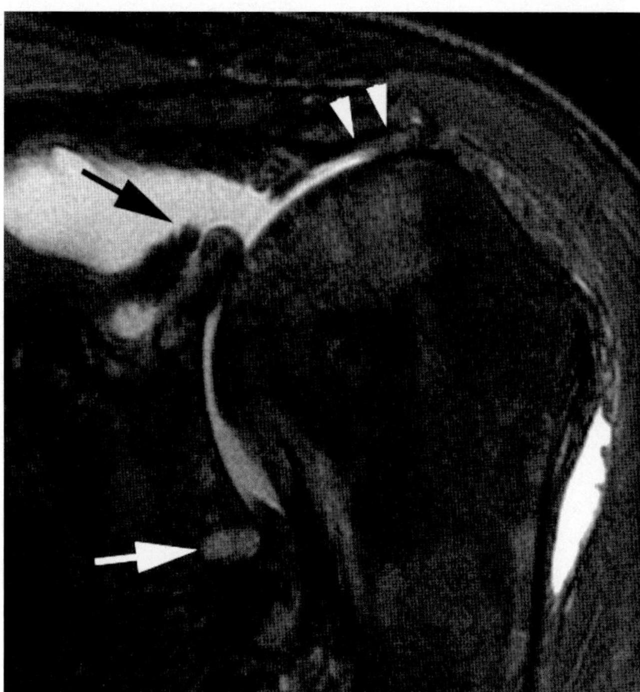

FIGURE 26-22. Rotator cuff tear accompanying CPPD arthropathy. Coronal oblique, T2-weighted, fat-suppressed MRI of the shoulder. There is a full-thickness tear of the supraspinatus tendon, which is retracted to the level of the glenoid *(black arrow).* The humeral head is superiorly subluxed and erodes the undersurface of the acromion *(arrowheads).* Subchondral cysts in the glenoid *(white arrow)* were seen more prominently on additional images.

Arthrography

Conventional arthrography is of limited utility in the diagnosis of CPPD arthropathy. Fluoroscopy may be informative when used to guide and confirm joint aspiration. The aspirated joint fluid can be evaluated by microscopy to identify the presence of positively birefringent calcium pyrophosphate dihydrate crystals.

Ultrasonography

High-frequency ultrasound transducers can detect CPPD deposits in cartilage, which appear as linear hyperechoic foci in the hypoechoic cartilage. Ultrasound can be helpful in evaluating subtle changes in the patellofemoral joint,[78] an area that can be difficult to assess radiographically. A recent study suggests that ultrasonography is at least as sensitive and as specific as radiographs for detection of CPPD calcifications.[79] Despite its potential usefulness, however, ultrasound is not commonly employed for evaluation of CPPD arthropathy, probably because it is relatively time consuming and user dependent. In the future, ultrasound may gain more widespread use for detection of changes in cartilage before they become apparent radiographically.

Extraarticular Imaging Features

CPPD crystals may be deposited focally in the soft tissues, producing large soft tissue masses mimicking gout (tophaceous pseudogout). These masses usually form adjacent to a joint but may be remote from any joint. The patient may lack other changes of CPPD crystal deposition. The masses have a nonspecific appearance and may raise suspicion of malignancy.[80-83] Biopsy is necessary in these cases to exclude neoplasm.

Algorithms and Recommendations

Survey imaging for CPPD disease should be primarily radiographic, with images that include the symptomatic joints. Projections most likely to show changes caused by CPPD crystal deposition are the AP and lateral knees, the PA wrists, and the AP pelvis. CT and ultrasonography are sensitive in detecting calcifications that may be subtle or not visible on radiographs. Whether MRI is sensitive enough to detect CPPD deposits is questionable. For preoperative planning, radiographs and CT are the most useful techniques.

HYDROXYAPATITE DEPOSITION DISEASE

HADD involves crystal deposition in the soft tissues in and around joints. Its pathogenesis is unknown.[84] HADD may cause acute pain, but the calcium deposits in this common disease are asymptomatic in more than two thirds of patients, according to a classic 1941 study.[85]

> More than two thirds of patients with HADD are asymptomatic.

Although laboratory findings are usually normal, HADD may cause fever, increased concentrations of C-reactive protein, and an increased erythrocyte sedimentation rate.[86] HADD is responsible for what is commonly termed *calcific tendinitis.* Other terms, such as *calcific periarthritis, peritendinitis* or *periarthritis calcarea,* and *hydroxyapatite rheumatism,* have also been used to describe this entity.[87] It may affect single or multiple joints, but involvement of a single joint is more common. Most cases of HADD are found in adults, but children and infants may also be affected.[88,89] Treatment usually focuses on symptom alleviation.

Although HADD has a typical appearance on radiographs, actual identification of the crystals is difficult because hydroxyapatite crystals are beyond the resolution of light microscopy. Aggregates of hydroxyapatite crystals may appear as nonbirefringent collections on light microscopy, but the appearance is nonspecific. Definitive diagnosis is based on electron microscopy or electron diffraction studies, neither of which is practical for clinical use. Alizarin red S stain can screen for hydroxyapatite but is also nonspecific because it also stains any calcium,[90] including other types of calcium crystals such as calcium pyrophosphate dihydrate.

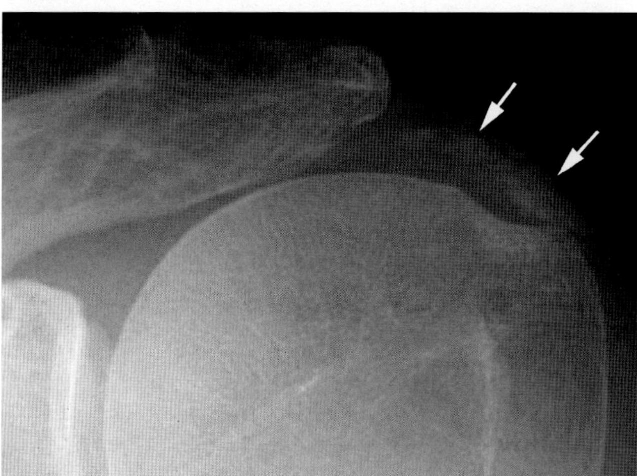

FIGURE 26-23. Hydroxyapatite deposition disease (HADD). An externally rotated radiograph of the shoulder shows the cloud-like appearance of calcium hydroxyapatite in the supraspinatus tendon *(arrows).*

Osteoarticular Imaging Features

Radiographs

The calcifications in HADD are more cloudlike (Figure 26-23) than the linear and punctate calcifications of CPPD disease. HADD calcifications can be differentiated from dystrophic or heterotopic ossification by the lack of trabeculation and the lack of a cortical rim. Calcifications associated with acute symptoms tend to be poorly defined and less dense than chronic calcifications. Cartilage calcification (chondrocalcinosis) in HADD is uncommon but may be present. It is not clear whether the chondrocalcinosis is caused by HADD or the coexistence of multiple crystal types in a single joint.[91,92] Erosion of adjacent bone may occur. Tendinous, capsular, ligamentous,[93] synovial, or bursal deposits of hydroxyapatite may be found in and around any joint. They have also been documented in many tendons remote from joints.[94] The most commonly affected joint is the shoulder. Within the shoulder, the supraspinatus tendon is most likely to show hydroxyapatite deposition, but it may also affect any other portion of the rotator cuff, joint capsule, or periarticular soft tissues. Calcifications near the greater tuberosity on an external rotation radiograph are within the supraspinatus tendon (Figure 26-24). Calcifications in the infraspinatus tendon or teres minor tendon overlap the humeral head on external rotation and then project near the middle and inferior facets of the greater tuberosity on internal rotation. Subscapularis tendon calcifications are observed best on axillary views. When calcifications project onto the superior glenoid on an AP radiograph, they are usually in the origin of the long head of the biceps tendon. Calcifications in the pectoralis major origin or deltoid insertion project over the proximal humeral shaft.

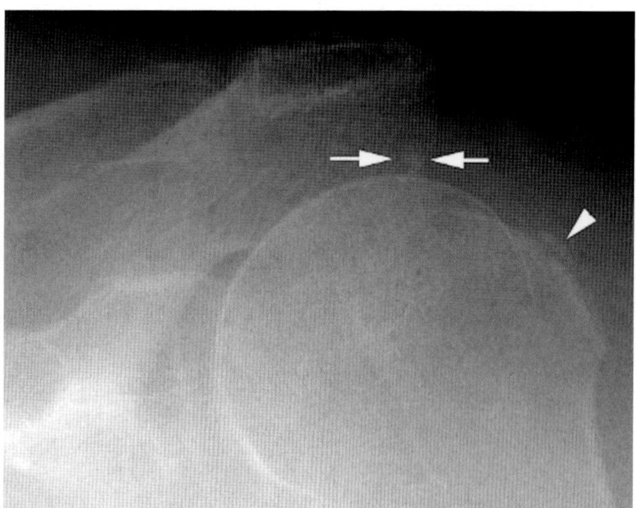

FIGURE 26-24. Hydroxyapatite deposition disease (HADD). An external rotation view of the shoulder shows two calcifications typical for hydroxyapatite deposition within the rotator cuff. The calcification above the humeral head *(arrows)* is within the supraspinatus tendon. The calcification adjacent to the inferior facet of the greater tuberosity *(arrowhead)* is within the infraspinatus tendon.

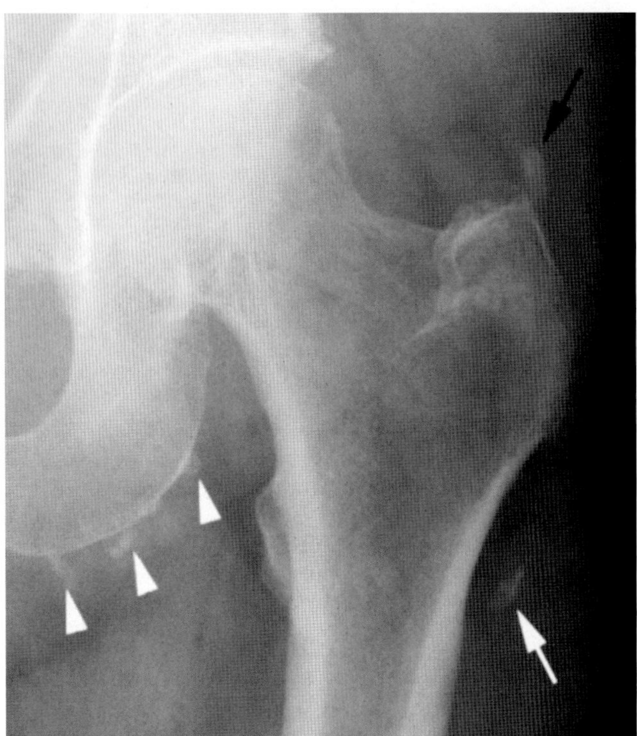

FIGURE 26-25. Hydroxyapatite deposition disease (HADD). An AP radiograph of the hip demonstrates calcification in multiple locations. Calcifications adjacent to the greater trochanter *(black arrow)* are within the gluteus minimus or medius tendons. Calcifications near the proximal femoral shaft *(white arrow)* are within the gluteus maximus (better seen on the lateral view). Calcifications adjacent to the ischium *(arrowheads)* are within the common hamstring origin.

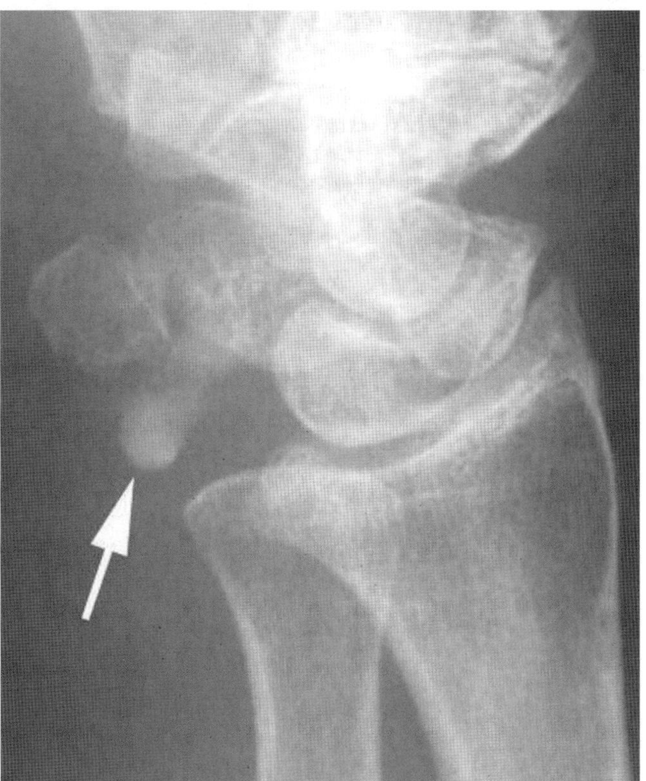

FIGURE 26-26. Hydroxyapatite deposition disease (HADD). Reverse oblique radiograph of the wrist shows hydroxyapatite deposition within the flexor carpi ulnaris tendon *(arrow)* near the attachment to the pisiform bone along the volar aspect of the wrist.

"Milwaukee shoulder" refers to advanced destruction of the glenohumeral joint along with a chronic, large rotator cuff tear associated with intraarticular hydroxyapatite crystals.[95,96]

> "Milwaukee shoulder" or "cuff tear arthropathy" refers to a large rotator cuff tear, glenohumeral damage, and joint/bursal distension and intraarticular hydroxyapatite crystals.

This condition may be a crystalline-induced arthropathy, although the exact cause is controversial.

The hip is the second most common site of HADD involvement.[50] Calcifications adjacent to the greater trochanter involve the gluteus minimus and gluteus medius tendons (Figure 26-25). Calcifications along the proximal femoral shaft typically involve the gluteus maximus tendon.

Within the hand and foot, the flexor carpi ulnaris (Figure 26-26) and the flexor hallucis longus and brevis are common regions of involvement. Depending on the location, HADD in the wrist may produce carpal tunnel syndrome.[97] Achilles' tendon calcifications have several causes, including HADD. Hydroxyapatite may deposit around the first MTP joint, producing a clinical presentation similar to gout[98] (i.e., a red, warm, acutely painful joint) that is called *pseudopodagra.* It occurs in men[99] and women aged 30 to 40 years old, with a female predominance.[100] Radiographically, pseudopodagra appears as calcific deposits around the joint, without bone erosion.

In the elbow, the origins of the common flexor and common extensor tendons are the most involved regions. Bursal and collateral ligament hydroxyapatite deposits are also found.

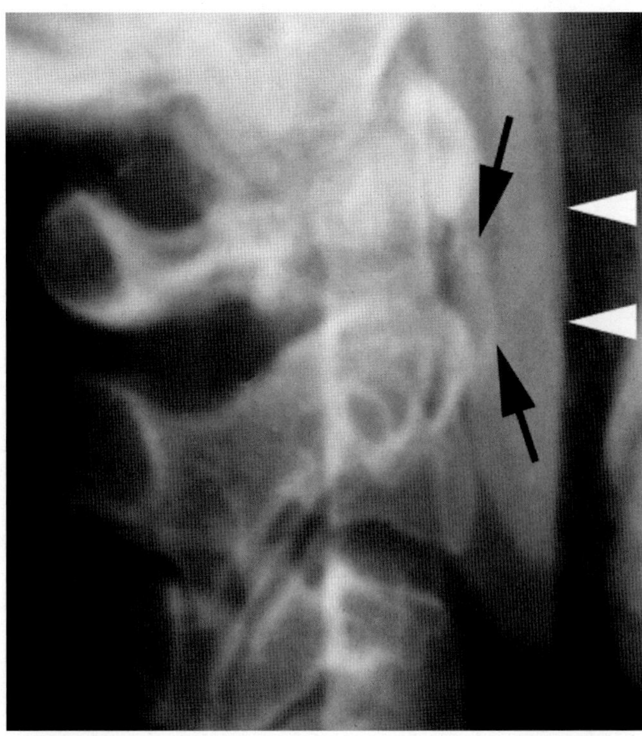

FIGURE 26-27. HADD (calcific tendinitis) of the longus colli. A lateral view of the cervical spine shows an amorphous calcification lying inferior to the anterior arch of C1 *(arrows).* The prevertebral soft tissues are swollen *(arrowheads).*

HADD in the spine is found in three typical locations: (1) within the longus colli muscle, (2) surrounding the dens, and (3) within the intervertebral disks.[86] The anterosuperior portion of the longus colli muscle is most commonly involved.

> Symptoms of longus colli calcific tendinitis include pain, stiffness, and odynophagia. Calcification and swelling on radiographs can confirm the diagnosis.

Spinal HADD appears as a globular calcification of the prevertebral soft tissues anterior to C1 and C2 (Figure 26-27). CT can confirm the location of the calcified deposit, and MRI can exclude a retropharyngeal abscess or discitis. Calcifications surrounding the dens produce the crowned dens syndrome, which, as previously discussed, may be caused by HADD or CPPD disease.

> Crowned dens syndrome: Neck pain associated with calcification surrounding the odontoid process.

Calcifications within the intervertebral disks tend to be symptomatic in children and asymptomatic in adults.[86]

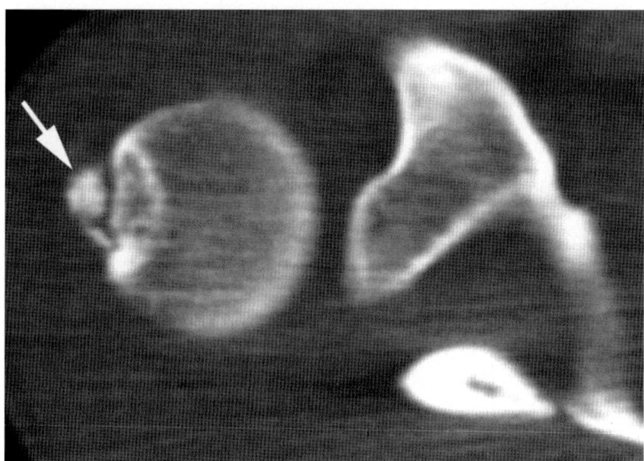

FIGURE 26-28. Hydroxyapatite deposition disease (HADD). An axial CT of the shoulder shows a globular calcification *(arrow)* at the lateral aspect of the humeral head. The underlying bone is either eroded or deformed from prior trauma.

> Disk calcification in children is likely to indicate the site of symptoms.

The ligaments and apophyseal joints may also be calcified. Paraspinal HADD masses can narrow the spinal canal,[101] causing a symptomatic radiculopathy or neuropathy. Paraspinal HADD may also be symptomatic due to the inflammatory response elicited by the crystals.

The differential diagnosis of calcifications in and around joints is broad. Other conditions that may mimic HADD include calcifications associated with collagen vascular diseases, small foci of tumoral calcinosis in metabolic disorders, and metastatic calcification caused by hypervitaminosis D, hypoparathyroidism, or sarcoidosis.

> Periarticular calcifications may be seen in hypervitaminosis D, hypoparathyroidism, milk alkali syndrome, calcinosis universalis, and renal osteodystrophy.

Computed Tomography

Calcifications of HADD show up well on CT scans, which can be useful in initial diagnosis, especially in the spine where overlapping bone may obscure findings.[102] CT is particularly helpful when calcifications are associated with bone erosion (Figure 26-28). In some cases, erosions and calcifications may simulate malignancy such as synovial sarcoma. Malignancy is also a diagnostic possibility if the calcification and erosion occur in a region where calcific tendinitis is uncommonly found.[103] When malignancy is suspected, CT or MRI may confirm the lack of a soft tissue mass. CT can also be used to further evaluate the "flame-like"[104] or "comet tail" appearance of calcifications, which is commonly[105] but not always[106] present with HADD.

> "Comet tail" calcification is characteristic of HADD and may be helpful in establishing the correct diagnosis when erosion is present.

Magnetic Resonance Imaging

MRI best evaluates secondary findings sometimes observed with HADD, such as fluid collections, synovitis, capsular thickening, or soft tissue or bone marrow edema. Hydroxyapatite crystal deposition in tendons has low signal on T1-weighted and T2-weighted images. Sometimes there is surrounding edema, which appears on MRI as a rim of increased signal on T2-weighted images (Figure 26-29). The crystal deposits can erode into the adjacent bone.[107-109] High signal on fluid-sensitive images may be present in adjacent bone marrow, even without any erosions.[110,111]

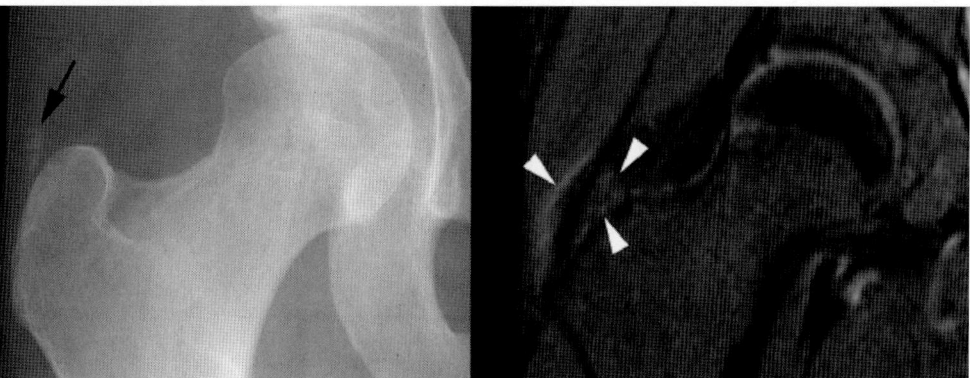

FIGURE 26-29. HADD in a 42-year-old woman with acute onset of hip pain. An AP radiograph and coronal T2-weighted, fat-suppressed MRI of the hip show calcification *(arrow)* and surrounding edema *(arrowheads)* consistent with gluteus medius calcific tendinitis.

Scintigraphy

Bone scintigraphy has limited use in the diagnosis of HADD. Although inflammation surrounding acute calcific deposits produces increased radiotracer uptake,[112] this finding is nonspecific. Similar findings have been observed with infection, neoplasm, or other causes of inflammation.

Arthrography

Arthrography or fluoroscopy can be used to guide joint aspiration but rarely adds additional diagnostic information because hydroxyapatite crystals are so difficult to identify definitively. Arthrography can provide information about related joint structures, such as the presence of a rotator cuff tear in the shoulder or a ligamentous injury in the wrist.

Ultrasonography

Calcifications in tendons and cartilage are visible on ultrasound, and ultrasound may be more sensitive than radiography for detection of early calcifications. An additional use for ultrasound is treatment of calcific tendinitis with high-energy extracorporeal shock waves.[113]

Extraarticular Imaging Features

Hydroxyapatite crystals may produce soft-tissue masses similar to the tophaceous pseudogout masses caused by CPPD disease. The exact crystal composition of both of these masses has been questioned,[114] because it is difficult to accurately identify basic calcium crystals with the pathologic methods routinely used in clinical settings.

Algorithms and Recommendations

Radiography is the mainstay of diagnosis. The symptomatic joint or area of the body should be imaged and carefully evaluated for the presence of calcific deposits. However, the presence of calcification alone does not necessarily indicate that it is the cause of pain. Poorly defined, low-density areas of calcification with adjacent blurring of soft tissue planes are more likely to be symptomatic. In patients who have bone erosion detected on radiographs, CT or MRI can be used to confirm the lack of a soft tissue mass, thereby excluding malignancy. MRI can best evaluate secondary findings, including edema in the soft tissues and bone marrow.

REFERENCES

1. Sydenham T: On gout. In Latham RG (translator): *The works of Thomas Sydenham*, London, 1850, The Sydenham Society, pp 123-162.
2. Dalbeth N, Haskard DO: Mechanisms of inflammation in gout, *Rheumatology (Oxford)* 44:1090-1096, 2005.
3. Choi HK, Curhan G: Gout: epidemiology and lifestyle choices, *Curr Opin Rheumatol* 17:341-345, 2005.
4. Podgorski MR, Ibels LS, Webb J: Case report 445: bilateral acromioclavicular gouty arthritis with pseudo-tumor of the outer end of the right clavicle: saturine gout, *Skeletal Radiol* 16:589-591, 1987.
5. Garagiola DM, Clark SA, Colyer RA et al: Case report 536: chronic tophaceous gout in a 17-year-old male, *Skeletal Radiol* 18:377-379, 1989.
6. Yun CH, Shih SL, Fang YK et al: Juvenile intraosseous gout of the calcaneus, *Pediatr Radiol* 35:899-901, 2005.

6a. Todd D, Helfgott SM: Personal communication, Department of Rheumatology Brigham and Women's Hospital, Boston, Massachusetts. September 23, 2008.

7. Rott KT, Agudelo CA: Gout, *J Am Med Assoc* 289:2857-2860, 2003.
8. Terkeltaub RA: Clinical practice: gout, *N Engl J Med* 349:1647-1655, 2003.

8a. Martel W: The overhanging margin of bone: a roentgenologic manifestation of gout, *Radiology* 91:755, 1968.

9. Gerster JC, Landry M, Duvoisin B et al: Computed tomography of the knee joint as an indicator of intraarticular tophi in gout, *Arthritis Rheum* 39:1406-1409, 1996.
10. Bloch C, Hermann G, Yu TF: A radiologic reevaluation of gout: a study of 2,000 patients, *AJR Am J Roentgenol* 134:781-787, 1980.
11. Gentili A: Advanced imaging of gout, *Semin Musculoskelet Radiol* 7:165-174, 2003.
12. Yen PS, Lin JF, Chen SY et al: Tophaceous gout of the lumbar spine mimicking infectious spondylodiscitis and epidural abscess: MR imaging findings, *J Clin Neurosci* 12:44-46, 2005.
13. Duprez TP, Malghem J, Vande Berg BC et al: Gout in the cervical spine: MR pattern mimicking diskovertebral infection, *AJNR Am J Neuroradiol* 17:151-153, 1996.
14. Hsu CY, Shih TT, Huang KM et al: Tophaceous gout of the spine: MR imaging features, *Clin Radiol* 57:919-925, 2002.
15. Cabot J, Mosel L, Kong A et al: Tophaceous gout in the cervical spine, *Skeletal Radiol* 34:803-806, 2005.
16. Barrett K, Miller ML, Wilson JT: Tophaceous gout of the spine mimicking epidural infection: case report and review of the literature, *Neurosurgery* 48:1170-1172, 2001.
17. Melloni P, Valls R, Yuguero M et al: An unusual case of tophaceous gout involving the anterior cruciate ligament, *Arthroscopy* 20:e117-e121, 2004.
18. Bond JR, Sim FH, Sundaram M: Radiologic case study: gouty tophus involving the distal quadriceps tendon, *Orthopedics* 27:18, 90-92, 2004.
19. Buckwalter KA, Swan JS, Braunstein EM: Evaluation of joint disease in the adult hand and wrist, *Hand Clin* 7:135-151, 1991.
20. Uri DS, Martel W: Radiologic manifestations of the crystal-related arthropathies, *Semin Roentgenol* 31:229-238, 1996.
21. Resnick D: Gouty arthritis. In Resnick D (editor): *Diagnosis of bone and joint disorders. Volume 2: Articular diseases*, Philadelphia, 2002, Saunders, pp 1519-1559.

21a. Kransdorf MJ,Moser RP Jr, Vinh' TN et al: Primary tumors of the patella. A review of 42 cases. *Skeletal Radiol*18:365-371, 1989.

22. Liu SZ, Yeh L, Chou YJ et al: Isolated intraosseous gout in hallux sesamoid mimicking a bone tumor in a teenaged patient, *Skeletal Radiol* 32:647-650, 2003.
23. Recht MP, Seragini F, Kramer J et al: Isolated or dominant lesions of the patella in gout: a report of seven patients, *Skeletal Radiol* 23:113-116, 1994.
24. Chen CK, Chung CB, Yeh L et al: Carpal tunnel syndrome caused by tophaceous gout: CT and MR imaging features in 20 patients, *AJR Am J Roentgenol* 175:655-659, 2000.
25. Magid SK, Gray GE, Anand A: Spinal cord compression by tophi in a patient with chronic polyarthritis: case report and literature review, *Arthritis Rheum* 24:1431-1434, 1981.
26. Espinosa-Morales R, Escalante A: Gout presenting as non-union of a patellar fracture, *J Rheumatol* 24:1421-1422, 1997.
27. Hung JY, Wang SJ, Wu SS: Spontaneous rupture of extensor pollicis longus tendon with tophaceous gout infiltration, *Arch Orthop Trauma Surg* 125:281-284, 2005.
28. Yu KH, Luo SF, Liou LB et al: Concomitant septic and gouty arthritis: an analysis of 30 cases, *Rheumatology (Oxford)* 42:1062-1066, 2003.
29. Gerster JC, Landry M, Dufresne L et al: Imaging of tophaceous gout: computed tomography provides specific images compared with magnetic resonance imaging and ultrasonography, *Ann Rheum Dis* 61:52-54, 2002.
30. Oostveen JC, van de Laar MA: Magnetic resonance imaging in rheumatic disorders of the spine and sacroiliac joints, *Semin Arthritis Rheum* 30:52-69, 2000.
31. Morrison WB, Ledermann HP, Schweitzer ME: MR imaging of inflammatory conditions of the ankle and foot, *Magn Reson Imaging Clin N Am* 9:615-637, 2001.
32. Yu JS, Chung C, Recht M et al: MR imaging of tophaceous gout, *AJR Am J Roentgenol* 168:523-527, 1997.
33. Yu KH, Lien LC, Ho HH: Limited knee joint range of motion due to invisible gouty tophi, *Rheumatology (Oxford)* 43:191-194, 2004.
34. Rousseau I, Cardinal E E, Raymond-Tremblay D et al: Gout: radiographic findings mimicking infection, *Skeletal Radiol* 30:565-569, 2001.
35. Pickhardt PJ, Shapiro B: Three-phase skeletal scintigraphy in gouty arthritis: an example of potential diagnostic pitfalls in radiopharmaceutical imaging of the extremities for infection, *Clin Nucl Med* 21:33-39, 1996.
36. Bancroft LW, Peterson JJ, Kransdorf MJ: Cysts, geodes, and erosions, *Radiol Clin North Am* 42:73-87, 2004.
37. Sato J, Watanabe H, Shinozaki T et al: Gouty tophus of the patella evaluated by PET imaging, *J Orthop Sci* 6:604-607, 2001.
38. Palestro CJ, Vega A, Kim CK et al: Appearance of acute gouty arthritis on indium-111-labeled leukocyte scintigraphy, *J Nucl Med* 31:682-684, 1990.
39. Appelboom T, Emery P, Tant L et al: Evaluation of technetium-99m-ciprofloxacin (Infection) for detecting sites of inflammation in arthritis, *Rheumatology (Oxford)* 42:1179-1192, 2003.
40. Aslam N, Lo S, McNab I: Gouty flexor tenosynovitis mimicking infection: a case report emphasizing the value of ultrasound in diagnosis, *Acta Orthop Belg* 70: 368-370, 2004.
41. Ho CF, Chiou HJ, Chou YH et al: Peritendinous lesions: the role of high-resolution ultrasonography, *Clin Imaging* 27:239-250, 2003.
42. Nalbant S, Corominas H, Hsu B et al: Ultrasonography for assessment of subcutaneous nodules, *J Rheumatol* 30:1191-1195, 2003.
43. Tchacarski V, Nicolov D: Ultrasonic changes in primary gouty nephropathy, *Int Urol Nephrol* 24:649-655, 1992.
44. Hughes JP, Di Palma S, Rowe-Jones J: Tophaceous gout presenting as a dorsal nasal lump, *J Laryngol Otol* 119:492-494, 2005.
45. Monu JU, Pope TL Jr: Gout: a clinical and radiologic review, *Radiol Clin North Am* 42:169-184, 2004.
46. Zucchi F, Varenna M, Binelli L et al: Reflex sympathetic dystrophy syndrome following acute gouty arthritis, *Clin Exp Rheumatol* 14:417-420, 1996.
47. Chen CH, Chen CK, Yeh LR et al: Intra-abdominal gout mimicking pelvic abscess, *Skeletal Radiol* 34:229-233, 2005.

48. Netter P, Bardin T, Bianchi A et al: The ANKH gene and familial calcium pyrophosphate dihydrate deposition disease, *Joint Bone Spine* 71:365-368, 2004.
49. Bencardino JT, Hassankhani A: Calcium pyrophosphate dihydrate crystal deposition disease, *Semin Musculoskelet Radiol* 7:175-185, 2003.
49a. McCarty DJ: Crystal deposition joint disease, *Ann Rev Med* Feb:279-288, 1974.
50. Steinbach LS: Calcium pyrophosphate dihydrate and calcium hydroxyapatite crystal deposition diseases: imaging perspectives, *Radiol Clin North Am* 42:185-205, 2004.
51. Waguri-Nagaya Y, Kubota Y, Sekiya I et al: Extensor tendon rupture related to calcium pyrophosphate crystal deposition disease, *Rheumatol Int* 21:243-246, 2002.
52. Masuda I: Calcium crystal deposition diseases: lessons from histochemistry, *Curr Opin Rheumatol* 16:279-281, 2004.
53. Helms CA, Chapman GS, Wild JH: Charcot-like joints in calcium pyrophosphate dihydrate deposition disease, *Skeletal Radiol* 7:55-58, 1981.
54. Yang BY, Sartoris DJ, Djukic S et al: Distribution of calcification in the triangular fibrocartilage region in 181 patients with calcium pyrophosphate dihydrate crystal deposition disease, *Radiology* 196:547-550, 1995.
55. Adamson TC 3rd, Resnik CS, Guerra J Jr et al: Hand and wrist arthropathies of hemochromatosis and calcium pyrophosphate deposition disease: distinct radiographic features, *Radiology* 147:377-381, 1983.
56. Hodge JC, Ghelman B, DiCarlo EF et al: Calcium pyrophosphate deposition within the ligamenta flava at L2, L3, L4, and L5, *Skeletal Radiol* 24:64-66, 1995.
57. Muthukumar N, Karuppaswamy U: Tumoral calcium pyrophosphate dihydrate deposition disease of the ligamentum flavum, *Neurosurgery* 53:103-108, 2003.
58. Hayashi M, Matsunaga T, Tanikawa H: Idiopathic widespread calcium pyrophosphate dihydrate crystal deposition disease in a young patient, *Skeletal Radiol* 31:246-250, 2002.
59. Fujishiro T, Nabeshima Y, Yasui S et al: Pseudogout attack of the lumbar facet joint: a case report, *Spine* 27:E396-E398, 2002.
60. Rivera-Sanfeliz G, Resnick D, Haghighi P et al: Tophaceous pseudogout, *Skeletal Radiol* 25:699-701, 1996.
61. Srinivasan A, Belanger E, Woulfe J et al: Calcium pyrophosphate dihydrate deposition disease resulting in cervical myelopathy, *Can J Neurol Sci* 32:109-111, 2005.
62. Griesdale DE Jr, Boyd M, Sahjpaul RL: Pseudogout of the transverse atlantal ligament: an unusual cause of cervical myelopathy, *Can J Neurol Sci* 31:273-275, 2004.
63. Baty V, Prost B, Jouvet A et al: Acute spinal cord compression and calcium pyrophosphate deposition disease: case illustration, *J Neurosurg* 99(Suppl 2):240, 2003.
64. Paolini S, Ciappetta P, Guiducci A et al: Foraminal deposition of calcium pyrophosphate dihydrate crystals in the thoracic spine: possible relationship with disc herniation and implications for surgical planning: report of two cases, *J Neurosurg Spine* 2:75-78, 2005.
65. Sato Y, Yasuda T, Konno S et al: Pseudogout showing meningoencephalitic symptoms: crowned dens syndrome, *Intern Med* 43:865-868, 2004.
66. Wu DW, Reginato AJ, Torriani M et al: The crowned dens syndrome as a cause of neck pain: report of two new cases and review of the literature, *Arthritis Rheum* 53:133-137, 2005.
67. Tshering Vogel DW, Steinbach LS, Hertel R et al: Acromioclavicular joint cyst: nine cases of a pseudotumor of the shoulder, *Skeletal Radiol* 34:260-265, 2005.
68. el Maghraoui A, Lecoules S, Lechevalier D et al: Acute sacroiliitis as a manifestation of calcium pyrophosphate dehydrate crystal deposition disease, *Clin Exp Rheumatol* 17:477-478, 1999.
69. Marsot-Dupuch K, Smoker WR, Gentry LR et al: Massive calcium pyrophosphate dihydrate crystal deposition disease: a cause of pain of the temporomandibular joint, *AJNR Am J Neuroradiol* 25:876-879, 2004.
70. Lambert RG, Becker EJ, Pritzker KP: Case report 597: calcium pyrophosphate deposition disorder (CPPD) of the right temporomandibular joint, *Skeletal Radiol* 19:139-141, 1990.
71. Smolka W, Eggensperger N, Stauffer-Brauch EJ et al: Calcium pyrophosphate dihydrate crystal deposition disease of the temporomandibular joint, *Oral Dis* 11:104-108, 2005.
72. Sartoris DJ, Resnick D, Bielecki D et al: Computed tomography with multiplanar reformation and three-dimensional image reconstruction in the preoperative evaluation of adult hip disease, *Int Orthop* 12:1-8, 1988.
73. Abreu M, Johnson K, Chung CB et al: Calcification in calcium pyrophosphate dihydrate (CPPD) crystalline deposits in the knee: anatomic, radiographic, MR imaging, and histologic study in cadavers, *Skeletal Radiol* 33:392-398, 2004.
74. Beltran J, Marty-Delfaut E, Bencardino J et al: Chondrocalcinosis of the hyaline cartilage of the knee: MRI manifestations, *Skeletal Radiol* 27:369-374, 1998.
75. Kaushik S, Erickson JK, Palmer WE et al: Effect of chondrocalcinosis on the MR imaging of knee menisci, *AJR Am J Roentgenol* 177:905-909, 2001.
76. Burke BJ, Escobedo EM, Wilson AJ et al: Chondrocalcinosis mimicking a meniscal tear on MR imaging, *AJR Am J Roentgenol* 170:69-70, 1998.
77. Zunkeler B, Schelper R, Menezes AH: Periodontoid calcium pyrophosphate dihydrate deposition disease: "pseudogout" mass lesions of the craniocervical junction, *J Neurosurg* 85:803-809, 1996.
78. Sofka CM, Adler RS, Cordasco FA: Ultrasound diagnosis of chondrocalcinosis in the knee, *Skeletal Radiol* 31:43-45, 2002.
79. Frediani B, Filippou G, Falsetti P et al: Diagnosis of calcium pyrophosphate dihydrate crystal deposition disease: ultrasonographic criteria proposed, *Ann Rheum Dis* 64:638-640, 2005.
80. Sissons HA, Steiner GC, Bonar F et al: Tumoral calcium pyrophosphate deposition disease, *Skeletal Radiol* 18:79-87, 1989.
81. Biankin S, Jaworski R, Mawad S: Tumoural calcium pyrophosphate dihydrate crystal deposition disease presenting clinically as a malignant soft tissue mass diagnosed on fine needle aspiration biopsy, *Pathology* 34:336-338, 2002.
82. Lambrecht N, Nelson SD, Seeger L et al: Tophaceous pseudogout: a pitfall in the diagnosis of chondrosarcoma, *Diagn Cytopathol* 25:258-261, 2001.
83. Olin HB, Pedersen K, Francis D et al: A very rare benign tumour in the parotid region: calcium pyrophosphate dihydrate crystal deposition disease, *J Laryngol Otol* 115:504-506, 2001.
84. Resnick D: Calcium hydroxyapatite crystal deposition disease. In Resnick D (editor): *Diagnosis of bone and joint disorders. Volume 2: Articular diseases*, Philadelphia, 2002, Saunders, pp 1619-1657.
85. Bosworth BM: Calcium deposits in the shoulder and subacromial bursitis: a survey of 12,122 shoulders, *J Am Med Assoc* 116:2477-2482, 1941.
86. Feydy A, Liote F, Carlier R et al: Cervical spine and crystal-associated diseases: imaging findings, *Eur Radiol* 16:459-468, 2006.
87. Garcia GM, McCord GC, Kumar R: Hydroxyapatite crystal deposition disease, *Semin Musculoskelet Radiol* 7:187-193, 2003.
88. Rush PJ, Wilmot D, Shore A: Hydroxyapatite deposition disease presenting as calcific periarthritis in a 14-year-old girl, *Pediatr Radiol* 16:169-170, 1986.
89. Stenstrom R, Gripenberg L: Acute bursitis calcarea trochanterica in an infant, with perforation into the hip joint demonstrated by arthrogram, *Pediatr Radiol* 7:51-52, 1978.
90. Theil KS: Body fluid analysis. In McClatchey KD (editor): *Clinical laboratory medicine*, Baltimore, 1994, Williams & Wilkins, pp 549-567.
91. Halverson PB, Ryan LM: Triple crystal disease: monosodium urate monohydrate, calcium pyrophosphate dihydrate, and basic calcium phosphate in a single joint, *Ann Rheum Dis* 47:864-865, 1988.
92. Constantin A, Bouteiller G: Acute neck pain and fever as the first manifestation of chondrocalcinosis with calcification of the transverse ligament of the atlas: five case-reports with a literature review, *Rev Rhum Engl Ed* 65:583-585, 1998.
93. Anderson SE, Bosshard C, Steinbach LS et al: MR imaging of calcification of the lateral collateral ligament of the knee: a rare abnormality and a cause of lateral knee pain, *AJR Am J Roentgenol* 181:199-202, 2003.
94. Hayes CW, Conway WF: Calcium hydroxyapatite deposition disease, *Radiographics* 10:1031-1048, 1990.
95. McCarty DJ, Halverson PB, Carrera GF et al: "Milwaukee shoulder:" association of microspheroids containing hydroxyapatite crystals, active collagenase, and neutral protease with rotator cuff defects. I. Clinical aspects, *Arthritis Rheum* 24:464-473, 1981.
96. Antoniou J, Tsai A, Baker D et al: Milwaukee shoulder: correlating possible etiologic variables, *Clin Orthop Relat Res* (407):79-85, 2003.
97. Verfaillie S, De Smet L, Leemans A et al: Acute carpal tunnel syndrome caused by hydroxyapatite crystals: a case report, *J Hand Surg Am* 21:360-362, 1996.
98. Mines D, Abbuhl SB: Hydroxyapatite pseudopodagra in a young man: acute calcific periarthritis of the first metatarsophalangeal joint, *Am J Emerg Med* 14:180-182, 1996.
99. Goupille P, Valat JP: Hydroxyapatite pseudopodagra in young men, *AJR Am J Roentgenol* 159:902, 1992.
100. Fam AG, Stein J: Hydroxyapatite pseudopodagra in young women, *J Rheumatol* 19:662-664, 1992.
101. Munday TL, Johnson MH, Hayes CW et al: Musculoskeletal causes of spinal axis compromise: beyond the usual suspects, *Radiographics* 14:1225-1245, 1994.
102. De Maeseneer M, Vreugde S, Laureys S et al: Calcific tendinitis of the longus colli muscle, *Head Neck* 19:545-548, 1997.
103. Kraemer EJ, El-Khoury GY: Atypical calcific tendinitis with cortical erosions, *Skeletal Radiol* 29:690-696, 2000.
104. Mizutani H, Ohba S, Mizutani M et al: Calcific tendinitis of the gluteus maximus tendon with cortical bone erosion: CT findings, *J Comput Assist Tomogr* 18: 310-312, 1994.
105. Hayes CW, Rosenthal DI, Plata MJ et al: Calcific tendinitis in unusual sites associated with cortical bone erosion, *AJR Am J Roentgenol* 149:967-970, 1987.
106. Cahir J, Saifuddin A: Calcific tendonitis of pectoralis major: CT and MRI findings, *Skeletal Radiol* 34:234-238, 2005.
107. Chan R, Kim DH, Millett PJ et al: Calcifying tendinitis of the rotator cuff with cortical bone erosion, *Skeletal Radiol* 33:596-599, 2004. [Erratum in Skeletal Radiol 34:61, 2005.]
108. Flemming DJ, Murphey MD, Shekitka KM et al: Osseous involvement in calcific tendinitis: a retrospective review of 50 cases, *AJR Am J Roentgenol* 181:965-972, 2003.
109. Thomason HC 3rd, Bos GD, Renner JB: Calcifying tendinitis of the gluteus maximus, *Am J Orthop* 30:757-758, 2001.
110. Bui-Mansfield LT, Moak M: Magnetic resonance appearance of bone marrow edema associated with hydroxyapatite deposition disease without cortical erosion, *J Comput Assist Tomogr* 29:103-107, 2005.
111. Yang I, Hayes CW, Biermann JS: Calcific tendinitis of the gluteus medius tendon with bone marrow edema mimicking metastatic disease, *Skeletal Radiol* 31:359-361, 2002.
112. Hutton CW, Maddison PJ, Collins AJ et al: Intra-articular apatite deposition in mixed connective tissue disease: crystallographic and technetium scanning characteristics, *Ann Rheum Dis* 47:1027-1030, 1988.
113. Jakobeit C, Winiarski B, Jakobeit S et al: Ultrasound-guided, high-energy extracorporeal–shock-wave treatment of symptomatic calcareous tendinopathy of the shoulder, *ANZ J Surg* 72:496-500, 2002.
114. Grant GA, Wener MH, Yaziji H et al: Destructive tophaceous calcium hydroxyapatite tumor of the infratemporal fossa: case report and review of the literature, *J Neurosurg* 90:148-152, 1999.

CHAPTER 27

Gaucher's Disease

ANDREW A. WADE, MD, and DANIEL I. ROSENTHAL, MD

KEY POINTS

- Gaucher's disease is an autosomal recessive condition.
- Deficiency of beta glucosidase leads to accumulation of glucosylceramide in lysosomes of monocyte/macrophage lineage.
- Hepatosplenomegaly and replacement of bone marrow are typically present; central nervous system changes occur in some cases.
- Musculoskeletal findings include marrow replacement, osteopenia, focal lytic lesions ("Gaucheromas"), acute focal bone disease (osteonecrosis, osteomyelitis or pseudoosteomyelitis, fracture), and Erlenmeyer flask deformity of the femurs.
- Magnetic resonance imaging (MRI) shows homogeneous or patchy low-signal intensity marrow on both T1-weighted and T2-weighted imaging sequences.
- Marrow "reconversion" occurs with replacement of the proximal marrow and formation of red marrow further peripherally.
- MRI is the most effective method of identifying acute infarction.
- Bone scans are more useful than MRI for distinguishing acute infarcts from acute osteomyelitis, as photopenia is present in the first 3 days after infarction.

Gaucher's disease (GD) is due to a genetic deficiency of the enzyme beta glucosidase.

> GD is an autosomal recessive condition characterized by a deficiency of beta glucosidase.

This functional deficit results in accumulation of a cell membrane metabolite, glucosylceramide, in lysosomes of cells of the monocyte/macrophage lineage.[1] The condition is named for Philippe Gaucher, a French dermatologist who first described the clinical syndrome. GD is the most common of the lysosomal storage diseases and results in a high frequency of skeletal symptoms.

More than 300 mutations that may result in clinical GD have been identified; seven alleles account for the majority of nucleotide substitutions, four of which are responsible for approximately 90% of cases. Inheritance is autosomal recessive. The condition is widely distributed in the population but is particularly prevalent among the Ashkenazi Jews, in whom 1 in 14 may be carriers.[2]

Diagnosis of GD is typically made by enzyme assay, DNA analysis, bone marrow biopsy, spleen or liver biopsy, or some combination of these four methods.[3] Of these, assay for glucocerebrosidase activity of peripheral blood leukocytes is considered to be the most efficient and reliable means of diagnosis.[2]

> Diagnosis is confirmed by assay for glucocerebrosidase in leuckocytes.

However, GD was recognized prior to the introduction of enzyme assay by its clinical features, which are the result of accumulation of glucosylceramide in cells of the reticuloendothelial system. Apoptosis is inhibited in these cells, and their relative immortality leads to accumulation of characteristic Gaucher cells, causing hepatosplenomegaly and replacement of normal marrow elements. The severity of disease is widely variable. In general, the younger the age at presentation, the more severe the condition.

> In general, the younger the age at presentation, the more severe the condition.

In rare instances, severely affected individuals have been identified as early as the second trimester of pregnancy by the presence of polyhydramnios, hydrops fetalis with bilateral hydrothorax, hepatosplenomegaly, arthrogryposis, absent fetal movements, and thickened skin.[4]

The presence and degree of central nervous system (CNS) involvement has been used to delineate three more-or-less distinct clinical forms of the disease.[5] The most prevalent form of GD (type 1) lacks primary involvement of the CNS (Box 27-1).

Traditionally, this has been referred to as the "adult type"; however, 66% of individuals with Type 1 GD manifest symptoms in childhood.[6] The most severe variants of type 1 GD may cause death at an early age due to visceral and hematologic manifestations, although the more common forms are compatible with a normal life expectancy.

Type 2 is characterized by onset in infancy with severe CNS involvement and death in early childhood. Type 3 demonstrates milder CNS involvement with onset in adolescence or early adulthood and a more indolent course.[3]

OSTEOARTICULAR IMAGING FEATURES

Skeletal complications appear slowly over time, and therefore skeletal manifestations are less characteristic of the more fulminant forms of the disease. However, when skeletal disease is present in the more severe clinical forms, the same spectrum of radiographic findings is seen as in type 1 disease. Vertebral compression fractures and osteonecrosis of the long bones occur frequently.[7]

For many patients with type 1 disease, the skeletal manifestations are probably the most disabling aspect. Although some affected individuals can be asymptomatic with neither radiographic, scintigraphic, nor histologic evidence of bone involvement, this is the exception. Findings from the International Collaborative Gaucher Group Registry, an international database of more than 2600 patients, show that nearly all patients with GD have radiologic evidence of skeletal involvement, and the majority has a history of serious skeletal complications.

BOX 27-1. Types and Characteristics of GD

TYPE 1 (ADULT TYPE)
No CNS involvement

TYPE 2
Infantile onset
Severe CNS disease
Death in childhood

TYPE 3
Adolescent or early adult onset
Milder CNS involvement

The skeleton is not affected uniformly but rather tends to have focal or multifocal manifestations, and sometimes much of the skeleton is preserved. These observations suggest that bone is affected because of collections of Gaucher cells scattered throughout its substance. It is possible that local effects may be the result of a toxic process around these foci. Alternatively, the storage of glucocerebroside in tissue macrophages may disturb the generation of competent osteoclasts and thus result in a failure to maintain a healthy skeleton.[8]

Patients commonly experience nonspecific bone pain, and some suffer from intermittent episodes of severe pain (bone crises) similar to those seen in sickle cell disease. Up to 20% have impaired mobility.[9]

Radiographically demonstrable involvement results from five basic processes:

1. Marrow replacement
2. Generalized osteopenia
3. Skeletal resorption due to adjacent heavily involved marrow leading to focal lytic lesions
4. Acute focal bone disease including:
   - Osteonecrosis, especially collapse of the femoral head
   - Osteomyelitis and "pseudoosteomyelitis"
   - Fractures
5. The Erlenmeyer flask deformity, a characteristic (but not universally present) modeling abnormality of the distal femur

> The Erlenmeyer flask deformity is the characteristic modeling abnormality of the distal femurs in patients with GD.

Bone Marrow Replacement

Marrow replacement is the most universally present skeletal manifestation of GD. Normal bone marrow becomes infiltrated by cellular elements containing foam cells (macrophages packed with glucocerebroside). This feature is impossible to recognize on radiographs and is extremely subtle on CT scans but quite obvious on MRI. Marrow affected by GD characteristically demonstrates either homogeneous or patchy low-signal intensity on both T1-weighted and T2-weighted imaging sequences.[10] These signal alterations presumably reflect the combined effects of replacement of marrow fat and the highly structured microtubular arrays in which the glucocerebroside accumulates.

During normal development, the maximal extent of red marrow occurs at the ninth month in utero. Subsequently the red marrow is progressively replaced by yellow or fatty marrow, beginning in the distal parts of the appendicular skeleton and proceeding proximally corresponding with increases in the marrow signal on T1-weighted images.

By age 6, adult levels of fat content (40% to 45%) are reached in the posterior ilium.[11] By age 10, marrow signal intensity in most pelvic sites is similar to that of adults, although fatty replacement remains ongoing throughout life. Most normal epiphyseal centers have fatty marrow throughout life, speculatively because the physiologic requirement for red marrow is declining by the time in childhood that ossification of the secondary centers occurs.[12] Therefore the normal pattern of marrow conversion is centripetal, except for the fact that the secondary centers do not participate.

In GD, the process of fatty marrow conversion is reversed, with accumulation of GD-affected tissue beginning in the axial skeleton and proceeding into the proximal and then the distal long bones. The epiphyses are relatively spared, although with advanced disease they too are affected (Figure 27-1).[13]

> Gaucher tissue is deposited first in areas of red marrow, which leads to reconversion of peripheral yellow marrow to hematopoietic marrow.

This pattern of disease progression is thought to reflect the availability of the macrophages that serve as reservoirs for the glucocerebroside accumulation. Such macrophages are primarily found in red marrow, and therefore areas of residual red marrow tend to be affected first. Replacement of the proximal marrow induces hematopoiesis with formation red marrow further peripherally, and Gaucher accumulation follows. This reverse process is known as *reconversion* and may also be seen in other marrow-replacing disorders.[14]

Several approaches have been devised to quantify the extent of marrow replacement. Simple scales based upon the known pattern of disease progression and visual determination of the presence of disease have been developed by Rosenthal and Hermann

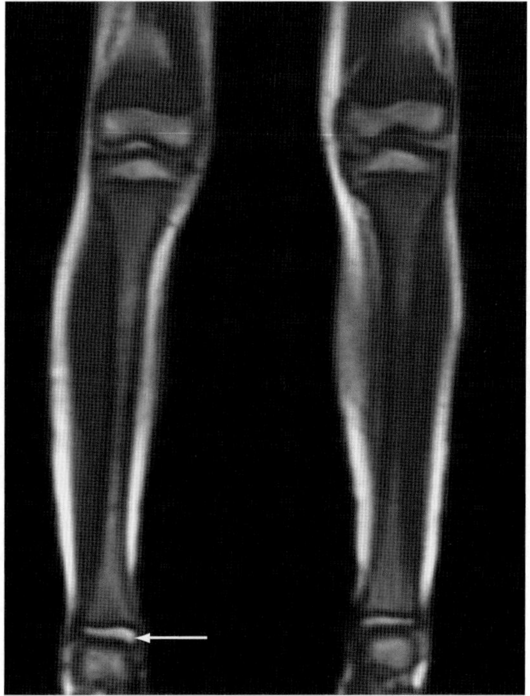

FIGURE 27-1. Marrow involvement. T1-weighted MRI of the legs showing lack of marrow fat in the tibial shaft, indicating replacement of normal fatty marrow by Gaucher tissue. There is relative preservation of the normal fat signal in the epiphysis *(arrow)*.

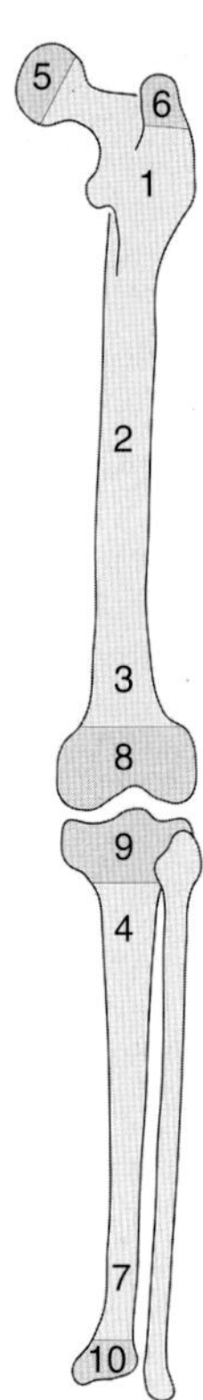

FIGURE 27-2. Sites of marrow involvement. Line drawing of the long bones of the lower extremity. The lower-numbered regions tend to show involvement of marrow by GD before the higher-numbered areas. Therefore the highest-numbered site of involvement may serve as a sort of semi-quantitative severity score.

(Figure 27-2).[15,16] These scales are valuable because the extent of marrow replacement is related to the other indices of disease severity, indicates the probability of skeletal symptoms, and may help to guide the need for therapy.[17]

Because the vertebral marrow appears darker than expected on T1-weighted images due to absence of fat, one "semi-quantitative" approach to determine whether the marrow is affected by GD is to compare vertebral body signal intensity to disk brightness. If the normalized vertebra to disk ratio (NVDR) is taken to be 1.0 in controls (95% confidence limits 0.70 to 1.30), for untreated patients with GD the ratio is below 0.7.[18]

> Gaucher vertebrae are darker than normal on T1-weighted images due to the absence of fat.

It is also possible to calculate a truly quantitative value for the extent of marrow disease, which is inversely related to the remaining volume percent of fat (fat fraction). Fat fraction is generally calculated using the technique of quantitative chemical shift imaging. It is decreased severalfold in GD patients compared with normal individuals.[19]

A correlation has been demonstrated between fat fraction of axial bone marrow as calculated by Dixon quantitative chemical shift imaging (Dixon QCSI) and bone complications. There is an 85% increase in risk of bone complication for every decrement of 0.1 in the fat fraction. Furthermore, fat fractions are significantly lower in GD patients who have undergone splenectomy than in those who have not. The latter observation supports the clinical impression that removal of the splenic "reservoir" may worsen the skeletal disease.[20] Other studies have also demonstrated a correlation between fat fraction and clinical disease severity, although not always with bone complications.[15]

> Splenectomy may worsen bone disease.

Radioisotope scans have also been used to evaluate the marrow changes of GD. Whole body scans performed using inhaled xenon-133 have been shown to correlate with the extent of skeletal disease.[15] The extent of marrow involvement as determined by Tc-99m sulfur colloid correlated well with the clinical and radiologic changes of the skeleton, but a normal pattern was found in the early stages of the disease. Tc-99m sestamibi (MIBI) has also been utilized for direct visualization of glycolipid deposits in the bone marrow. Although MIBI scanning is a sensitive technique for detecting bone marrow deposits, there is no clear correlation between the observed uptake and clinical disease. Some studies suggest that MIBI scans are inadequate for early identification of patients at high risk for skeletal complications or for the follow-up of patients treated with enzyme replacement.[21] Others have found that a semiquantitative scintigraphic score was highly correlated with an overall clinical severity score index (SSI) and with various parameters contributing to the SSI, either positively or negatively. Scintigraphic score is most highly correlated with measurements of serum chitotriosidase, an overall biochemical marker of disease severity. Enzyme replacement therapy (ERT)-naive patients showed high correlation of the scintigraphic score with the clinical SSI, with a radiographically based score, and with serum chitotriosidase. In the ERT-treated patients, the scintigraphic score was correlated with the clinical SSI, with hepatomegaly, and with hemoglobin.[22]

Osteopenia

Patients with GD are usually found to have osteopenia at all sites. It is typically manifested on radiographs as cortical thinning and may also be measured by dual-energy x-ray absorptiometry (DXA). Low levels of bone density in GD are associated with serum markers of accelerated bone turn over and breakdown, suggesting that the osteopenia of type 1 GD is associated with increased bone resorption.[23]

The severity of osteopenia is related to overall disease severity and is correlated with genotype, the more severely affected N370S/84GG having lower density than milder N370S/N370S. As in individuals without GD, density typically declines as a function of age.[24] DXA has been advocated for following response to therapy for children with GD, although absolute measurements do not correlate with severity of disease.[2]

Unlike DXA and radiography, quantitative CT (QCT) can be used to detect the amount of reduction in purely trabecular bone. However, in patients with GD the observed reduction has been unimpressive. Presumably in patients with GD cortical bone loss predominates, suggesting that the role for quantitative CT is limited. In addition, when performed using conventional single-energy methods, replacement of normal marrow fat with Gaucher cells tends to artifactually elevate the apparent bone mass. Although rarely performed because of technical complexity, dual-energy CT measurements more accurately reflect the degree of bone loss.[25]

Focal Gaucher Deposits

Focal accumulation of Gaucher cells may result in osteolytic lesions (Figure 27-3). These are typically asymptomatic unless infarction or fracture supervenes. Extraosseous GD may occur

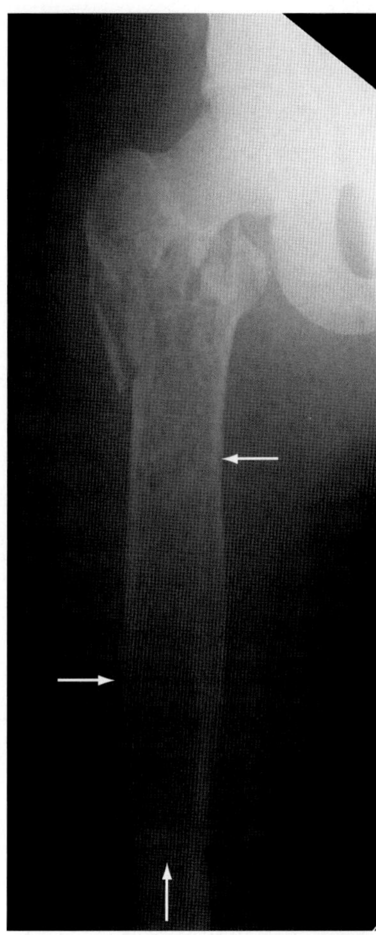

FIGURE 27-3. A radiograph of the right femur demonstrates a pathologic fracture through a large lytic lesion of the proximal femoral shaft *(arrows).*

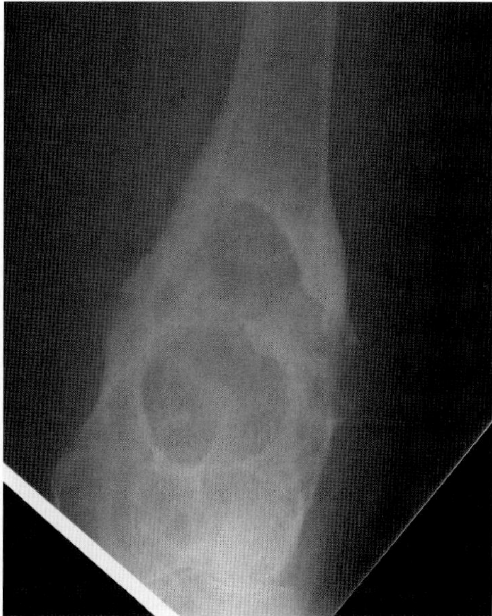

FIGURE 27-4. A radiograph of the distal femur demonstrates an expanded space-occupying lesion arising within the marrow and extending into the soft tissues. This pseudoneoplastic manifestation has been termed a "Gaucheroma."

when focal marrow deposits grow so large that they violate the cortex. Such focal deposits, commonly referred to as "Gaucheromas," might simulate malignancy (Figure 27-4).

> Gaucheromas are mass-like extensions of Gaucher marrow deposits into the soft tissues.

This differential may occasionally become problematic in view of the increased risk of multiple myeloma in patients with GD. In one rare instance, an extraosseous Gaucher cell accumulation even produced a monoclonal immunoglobulin (Ig) G kappa gammopathy, further simulating a myeloma.[26] Gaucheromas tend to be very slowly progressive.[27] In some instances the connection to the bone, although always present, may be subtle.[28]

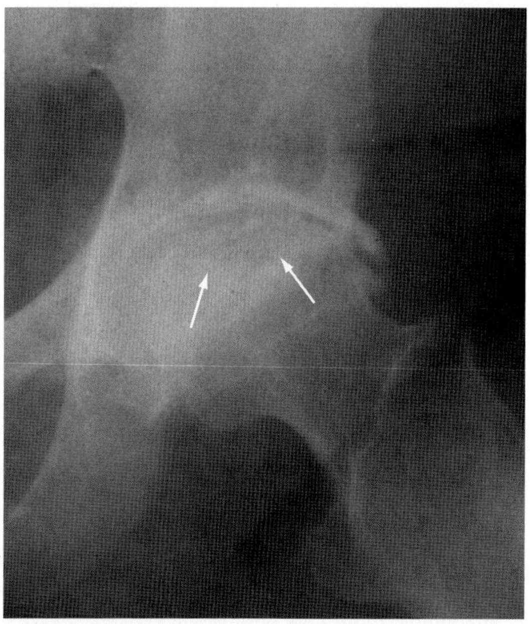

FIGURE 27-5. A radiograph of the left hip in the "frog-leg" lateral position demonstrates typical osteonecrosis *(arrows)* with collapse of the articular cortex. Osteoarthritic changes, including a lucent cyst in the acetabulum and lateral osteophytes, are noted.

Osteonecrosis

Osteonecrosis is extremely common in patients with GD. As in unaffected individuals, it manifests in one of two clinical forms depending upon the anatomic site. Osteoarticular necrosis affects the ends of bone and leads to a clinical syndrome that usually results in collapse of the articular cortex and destruction of the adjacent joint (Figure 27-5). Medullary necrosis affects the shaft or metaphysis of the bones. Medullary necrosis, although often painful, usually resolves without clinical sequelae other than residual imaging changes within the affected bones. Following an episode of infarction due to small vessel disease, the bone marrow appears diffusely sclerotic. If larger territories are affected, the infarcted area may appear as a focal lucency surrounded by a calcified or partially calcified margin. During an episode of acute pain caused by osteonecrosis, radiographs and CT may be normal, but MRI demonstrates bright signal within the affected marrow on T2-weighted images (Figure 27-6).[16,29] As in patients without GD, scintigraphy may reveal osteonecrosis as a focal area of diminished perfusion.[30]

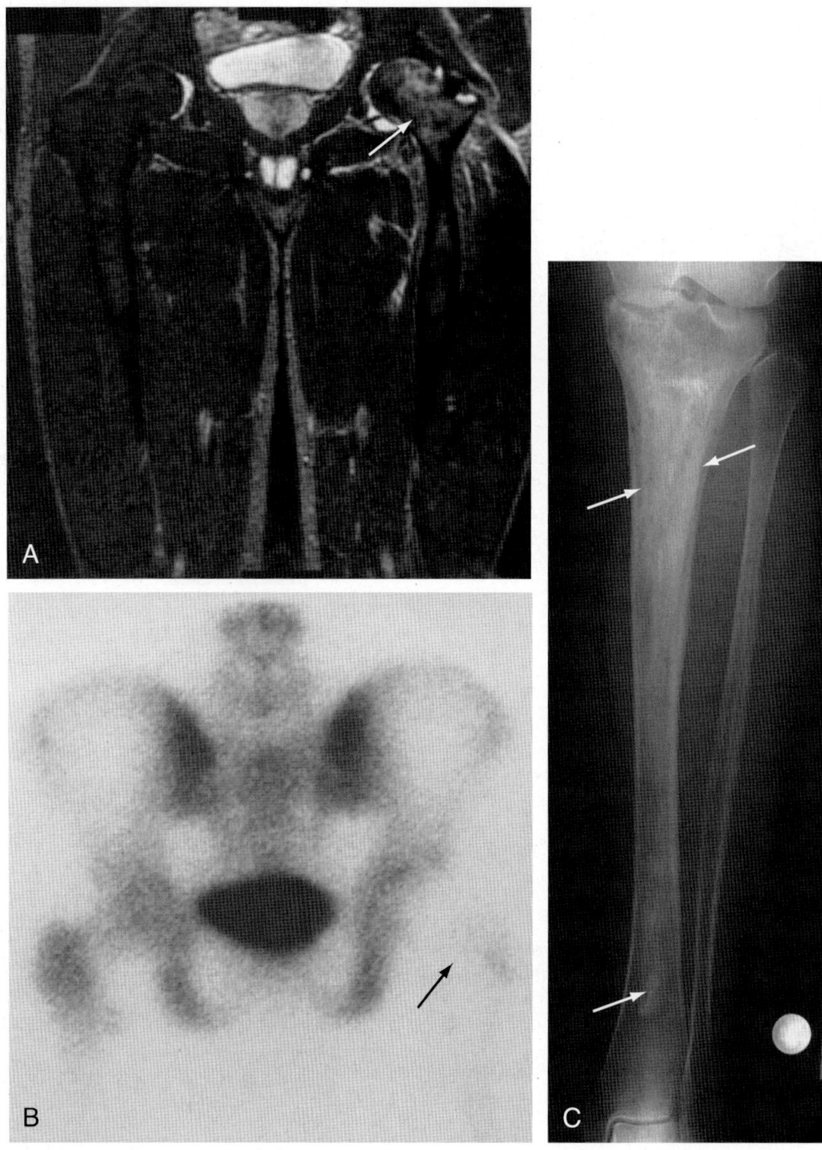

FIGURE 27-6. Infarction. **A,** T2-weighted MR image of the hips shows increased signal within the marrow of the left femoral head and neck *(arrow)*, representing edema due to acute infarction (bone "crisis"). **B,** A radioisotope bone scan demonstrates complete lack of uptake in the proximal left femur *(arrow)*. **C,** A radiograph of the tibia demonstrates old areas of medullary necrosis. The boundaries of the necrotic area are demarcated by a sclerotic interface *(arrows)*.

Central depression of multiple vertebral end plates may be seen in the spine, similar to findings observed in patients with sickle cell disease (Figure 27-7).

H-shaped vertebrae may be seen in sickle cell disease or GD.

As in that disorder, this finding presumably is due to osteonecrosis of bone beneath the endplate.[31,32]

Osteomyelitis and Pseudoosteomyelitis

Patients with GD are at an increased risk for osteomyelitis and infections in general. However, the presence of signs and symptoms consistent with osteomyelitis may also occur due to marrow infarction, resulting in a syndrome that has been termed *pseudoosteomyelitis.*

Marrow infarction may mimic osteomyelitis clinically.

It can be difficult to distinguish osteomyelitis clinically from pseudoosteomyelitis. Photopenia on bone scan performed within 1 to 3 days of presentation is suggestive of pseudoosteomyelitis.[33]

As previously mentioned, increased T2 marrow signal may be present during the acute phase of avascular episodes, and no specific feature on MRI can differentiate between pseudoosteomyelitis and pyogenic osteomyelitis. Clinical correlation is essential.[10]

Fractures

Fractures are relatively common in patients with GD. Insufficiency fractures may occur due to generalized osteopenia, and pathologic fractures may occur due to weakened skeletal areas at sites

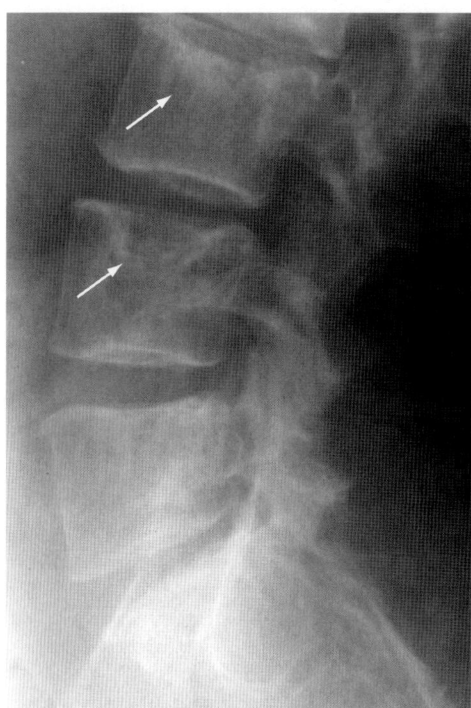

FIGURE 27-7. H-shaped vertebrae. A lateral radiograph of the lumbar spine demonstrates multiple end plate deformities. The fractures have the characteristic step-like or "square shoulder" appearance resulting in the H shape that is due to end plate infarction and is best known as a manifestation of sickle cell disease *(arrows)*.

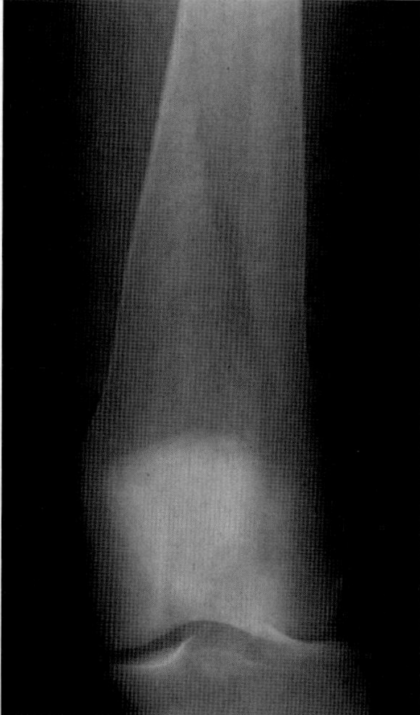

FIGURE 27-8. Erlenmeyer flask deformity. A radiograph of the distal femur demonstrates the typical (but not invariably present) Erlenmeyer flask deformity. Note the triangular widened appearance of the distal femur, due to the dysfunction of osteoclasts in the metaphyseal "cut-back" zone.

of focal osteolysis (see Figure 27-3). Marrow insufficiency, especially thrombocytopenia, may complicate surgical treatment of such fractures.[34]

Erlenmeyer Flask Deformity

The Erlenmeyer flask deformity is a well-known and characteristic feature of GD, representing undertubulation of the femur due to failure of bone resorption in the "cut-back" zone of the distal metaphysis (Figure 27-8). The Erlenmeyer flask deformity is not unique to GD, as it may also be seen in disorders associated with osteoclast failure due to a variety of causes (e.g., osteopetrosis) and may be associated with certain other rare marrow-packing diseases such as mannosidosis, a glycoprotein storage disease of lysosomes due to specific absence of alpha-D-mannosidase.[35]

The Erlenmeyer flask deformity can be strikingly obvious or extremely subtle in patients with GD. In our experience, its presence does not necessarily reflect either disease severity or local marrow involvement.

Some Controversial Features

Notching of the medial aspect of the proximal humeral metaphysis, in some cases contributing to pathologic fracture, has been reported in GD and in other infiltrative marrow processes such as leukemia, Niemann-Pick, Hurler's disease and metastatic neuroblastoma, although it has also been observed in normal patients. We therefore believe that this finding represents a normal variant.[36-39]

A few small series have reported an overall increase in the number of malignancies in patients with GD. However, a recent study of the Gaucher Registry reveals an increase in incidence of multiple myeloma, but no significant increase in risk for cancers of the breast, prostate, colon and rectum, lung, and hematologic malignancies other than myeloma.[40,41]

EXTRASKELETAL IMAGING FINDINGS

Accumulation of glucocerebroside in the lysosomes of visceral macrophages gives rise to multiple systemic manifestations, including hepatosplenomegaly, anemia, thrombocytopenia, growth retardation, and skeletal disease.

A variety of soft tissue manifestations may be detected by imaging. In some of the severe forms of the disease, pulmonary infiltrates and thoracic lymph node enlargement are the predominant imaging findings.[7]

Chest imaging may also demonstrate pulmonary findings in some patients with type 1 disease. Radiographs tend to show a reticular pattern, and high-resolution CT demonstrates interlobular septal and intralobular interstitial thickening, irregular interfaces at the pleural surfaces, and ground-glass appearance, corresponding to both alveolar and interstitial components of the pulmonary involvement.[42]

Enlargement of the liver and spleen is almost universal in patients with GD.

Hepatosplenomegaly is almost universal in GD disease.

CT, ultrasound, or MRI may be used to assess organ volume, as well as volume changes after treatment (Figure 27-9). CT is fast and accurate but entails radiation exposure. MRI is more reproducible than ultrasound though more expensive, and neither of these uses ionizing radiation.[2] Imaging of patients following institution of ERT can demonstrate an initial dramatic decline and sustained decreases in organ size in pediatric patients.[43]

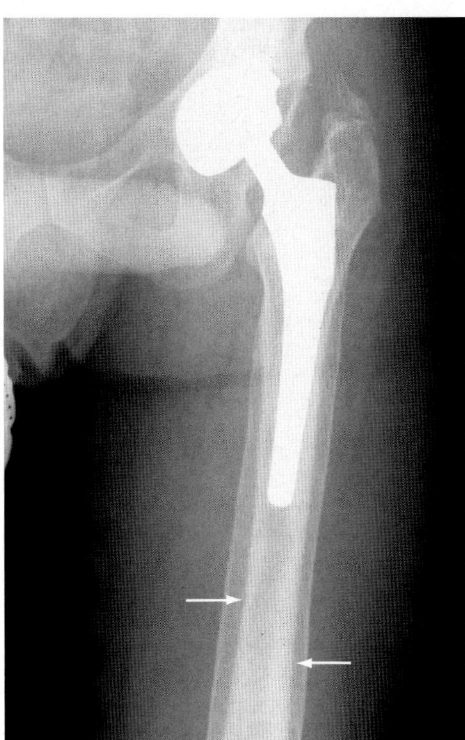

FIGURE 27-9. Osteonecrosis. A radiograph of the hip demonstrates a total joint replacement performed because of osteonecrosis. In addition, there is a striking "bone-within-bone" appearance of the femur due to massive necrosis of the femoral shaft *(arrows)*.

In addition to organomegaly, about 5% of patients have focal splenic or hepatic lesions that can be hypoechoic, hyperechoic, or mixed on ultrasound and presumably represent areas of infarction or fibrosis related to previous infarction.[43] Similar focal changes can also be demonstrated by CT.[44]

Liver scintigraphy also demonstrates various degrees of organ enlargement and inhomogeneous uptake. Focal defects may represent liver involvement with GD, but as is the case in individuals without GD, focal defects can be caused by other conditions such as metastatic carcinoma. Like ultrasound, scintigraphy can be useful in detecting splenic infarction and in following enlargement of the spleen after partial splenectomy.[30]

Hypersplenism leading to thrombocytopenia and moderate immunocompromise is a frequent complication of GD, often requiring splenectomy. Partial splenic embolization may be performed to avoid the increased risk of serious infectious complications and deterioration of the disease associated with operative splenectomy.[45]

Cardiac involvement is rare in GD. The few affected individuals have been mostly adults with pericardial changes. However, thickened, relatively immobile mitral and aortic valves have also been seen, resulting in significant mitral regurgitation. Therefore echocardiographic investigation of patients with suspected cardiac involvement with GD is recommended.[46]

Brain involvement in the severe, neuronopathic forms may be demonstrated by single photon emission computed tomography (SPECT) brain scans with Tc-99m hexamethylpropyleneamine-oxime (HMPAO). Multifocal hypoperfusion of the brain has been shown to correlate with neurologic abnormalities, and extensive hypoperfusion foretells clinical deterioration. Progressive cerebral atrophy in the frontal and temporal lobes has been demonstrated on serial brain MRI.[14]

TREATMENT

Enzyme Replacement

Prior to the development of ERT, treatment for GD was mainly symptomatic relief. Primary treatment with glucocerebrosidase allows removal of the lipid metabolite whose accumulation causes the pathology. Alglucerase is a mannose-terminated form of human placenta-derived glucocerebrosidase, which was developed to treat patients with GD. Subsequently, in vitro methods of protein production have led to the synthetic replacement imiglucerase, which is more predictable with respect to composition.[48]

After initiation of intravenous enzyme therapy, improvements become evident within 6 months. Patients have increased hemoglobin levels and platelet counts and decreased incidence of epistaxis and bruising. Hepatosplenomegaly is decreased, and skeletal symptoms improve. Children gain height, and most patients can resume work and daily activities. ERT is well tolerated, with few mild adverse reactions reported.[49,50]

Imaging can be used to track the progress of improvement with ERT. MRI was used to demonstrate return of marrow fat in treated individuals.[19] Subsequently, response to ERT has been repeatedly observed as a quantitative increase in signal intensity on T1-weighted images, even when it is not perceptible as a change in the pattern of marrow involvement.[51]

The first objective evidence that ERT with alglucerase might be effective for treatment of bone disease was the report of one child treated for 2 years. Bone biopsies showed a progressive return to normal marrow and cortical thickness.[52] However, whether enzyme replacement produces demonstrable changes in skeletal lesions remains controversial. In our own work, the lipid composition of bone marrow, determined by direct chemical analysis, began to improve after 6 months of treatment, at which time noninvasive imaging studies showed no significant changes. By 42 months, improvement in marrow composition was demonstrable on all noninvasive, quantitative imaging modalities (magnetic resonance score, quantitative xenon scintigraphy, and quantitative chemical shift imaging).

Imaging studies may take years to show improvement in bone.

Quantitative chemical shift imaging, the most sensitive technique, demonstrated a dramatic normalization of the marrow fat content in all patients. Net increases in either cortical or trabecular bone mass, as assessed by combined cortical thickness measurements and dual-energy QCT, respectively, also occurred.[53] Other studies have also demonstrated modest improvement in patients treated for 2 years or more,[50] and there have been a number of anecdotal reports of improvement.[54] However, in some studies there was little benefit of ERT, possibly due to the patients' splenectomized state.[55]

ERT in Children

For pediatric patients with GD, ERT has the potential to prevent the development of serious, irreversible skeletal complications. Symptomatic children treated with ERT experience significant increases in skeletal growth and bone mineral density.

Treatment in childhood may prevent skeletal complications of GD.

ERT therefore has the potential to prevent serious skeletal complications such as fractures and vertebral compression later in life.[56] Therefore very few, if any, children diagnosed by signs and symptoms should go untreated.[57]

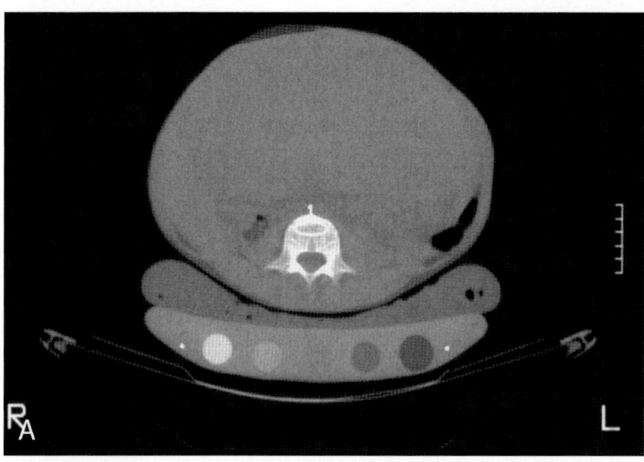

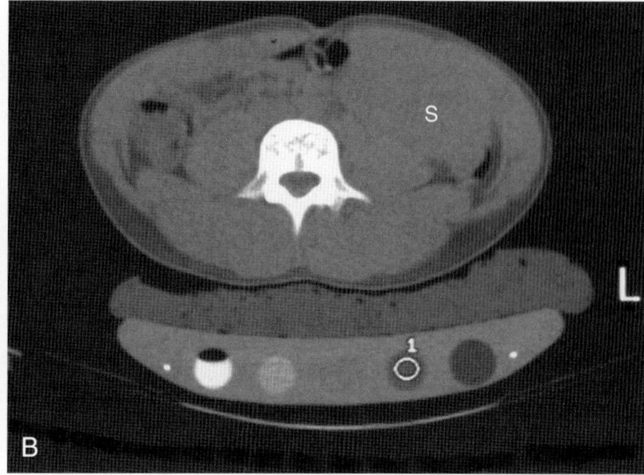

FIGURE 27-10. Hepatosplenomegaly with improvement on treatment. **A,** CT scan of a 16-year-old boy demonstrates massive hepatosplenomegaly. The spleen is so large that it occupies almost the entire visible area. Note the extreme paucity of subcutaneous tissues. Severely affected patients often appear malnourished. **B,** Three years after initiation of enzyme replacement, the spleen *(S)* has markedly decreased in size, and there has been an increase in subcutaneous fat. The patient is lying on a bone density phantom, which explains the circular areas of different density beneath the patient.

Surgical Interventions

Surgical interventions continue to be required in the era of ERT. Osteonecrosis of the joints—particularly the hips but also the knees and shoulders—and pathologic fractures of the long bones are common manifestations. Surgical interventions such as joint arthroplasties remain important adjuvant treatments in this population. In view of the hematologic problems and increased risk of infection, presurgical hematologic profiling and antibiotic cover are equally critical.[58]

Total hip arthroplasty in this condition has been reported to result in aseptic loosening of the components soon after operation, perhaps because many patients are young. Osteotomy may be an alternative to arthroplasty for such individuals[59] (Figure 27-10).

Bone marrow transplantation has been successful in a small number of patients (although attended with the usual problems), suggesting that, in advanced GD, bone marrow transplant may be an option if an HLA-identical related or unrelated donor is available.[60,61]

Algorithms and Recommendations

ERT for GD is among the costliest of all drug regimens. Alternative approaches to lowering the cost of treatment include the use of lower dosages[50,62] and pharmacologic alternatives to ERT.[63]

It is unclear when in the course of disease ERT should be implemented. In the opinion of some experts, it is important that patients be monitored closely and that ERT be initiated prior to development of irreversible skeletal complications such as infarction and fibrosis.[64] Some evidence indicates that the vulnerable period is during childhood, adolescence, or early adulthood when there is the greatest risk of progression. There is a marked tendency for stabilization thereafter, which suggests that GD in most of the patients is not a relentless progressive disorder but a rather stable disorder during adulthood.[65]

GD may stabilize in adulthood.

Because of the great cost and controversy, consensus recommendations have been devised for a comprehensive schedule of monitoring of all relevant aspects to confirm the achievement, maintenance, and continuity of the therapeutic response.[66,67]

The current recommendations for ERT suggest that adults at increased risk of complications and all affected children should begin therapy with an intravenous infusion of 60 units/kg every 2 weeks. Lower-risk adults may begin at a dose of 30 to 45 units/kg every 2 weeks. Following clinical improvement, dose decreases may be considered in 15% to 25% increments every 3 to 6 months in higher-risk adults and children, with a minimum recommended maintenance dose of 30 units/kg every 2 weeks; lower-risk adults can be maintained at a minimum of 20 units/kg every 2 weeks.[68]

Specialized quantitative imaging techniques played an important role in the efforts to understand the pathophysiology of the disease and the effects of therapy. However, these complex methods are probably not justified in the routine care of patients who can be followed based upon clinical and laboratory findings with imaging studies as indicated by specific symptoms.

REFERENCES

1. Brady RO, Kanfer JN, Shapiro D: Metabolism of glucocerebrosides. II. Evidence of an enzymatic deficiency: Gaucher's disease, *Biomed Biophys Res Commun* 18:221-225, 1965.
2. Charrow J, Andersson HC, Kaplan P et al: Enzyme replacement therapy and monitoring for children with type 1 Gaucher disease: consensus recommendations, *J Pediatr* 144:112-120, 2004.
3. Charrow J, Andersson HC, Kaplan P et al: The Gaucher Registry: demographics and disease characteristics of 1698 patients with Gaucher Disease, *Arch Intern Med* 160:2835-2843, 2000.
4. Sarfati R, Hubert A, Dugue-Marechaud M et al: Prenatal diagnosis of Gaucher's disease type 2. Ultrasonographic, biochemical and histological aspects, *Prenat Diagn* 20:340-343, 2000.
5. Mankin HJ, Rosenthal DI, Xavier R: Gaucher disease: new approaches to an ancient disease, *J Bone Joint Surg Am* 83:748-762, 2001.
6. Grabowski GA, Andria G, Baldellou A et al: Pediatric non-neuronopathic Gaucher disease: presentation, diagnosis and assessment. Consensus statements, *Eur J Pediatr* 163:58-66, 2004.
7. Hill SC, Damaska BM, Tsokos M et al: Radiographic findings in type 3b Gaucher disease, *Pediatr Radiol* 26:852-860, 1996.
8. Stowens DW, Teitelbaum SL, Kahn AJ et al: Skeletal complications of Gaucher disease, *Medicine* 64:310-322, 1985.
9. Wenstrup RJ, Roca-Espiau M, Weinreb NJ et al: Skeletal aspects of Gaucher disease: a review, *Br J Radiol* 75(Suppl 1):A2-A12, 2002.
10. Cremin BJ, Davey H, Goldblatt J: Skeletal complications of type I Gaucher disease: the magnetic resonance features, *Clin Radiol* 41:244-247, 1990.

11. Dawson KL, Moore SG, Rowland JM: Age-related marrow changes in the pelvis: MR and anatomic findings, *Radiology* 183:47-51, 1992.
12. Waitches G, Zawin JK, Poznanski AK: Sequence and rate of bone marrow conversion in the femora of children as seen in MR imaging: are accepted standards accurate? *AJR Am J Roentgenol* 162:1399-1406, 1994.
13. Rosenthal DI, Scott JA, Barranger J, Mankin HJ, Saini S, Brady TJ, et al. Evaluation of Gaucher disease using magnetic resonance imaging, *J Bone Joint Surg Am* 68:802-808, 1986.
14. Baur A, Stabler A, Lamerz R et al: Light chain deposition disease in multiple myeloma: MR imaging features correlated with histopathological findings, *Skeletal Radiol* 27:173-176, 1998.
15. Rosenthal DI, Barton NW, McKusick KA et al: Quantitative imaging of Gaucher disease, *Radiology* 185:841-845, 1992.
16. Hermann G, Shapiro RS, Adbelwahab IF et al: MR imaging in adults with Gaucher disease type I: evaluation of marrow involvement and disease activity, *Skeletal Radiol* 22:247-251, 1993.
17. Terk MR, Esplin J, Lee K et al: MR imaging of patients with type I Gaucher's disease: relationship between bone and visceral changes, *AJR Am J Roentgenol* 165:599-604, 1995.
18. Vlieger EJP, Maas M, Akkerman EM et al: The application of the vertebra-disc ratio in a population of patients with Gaucher's disease, *Proc Intl Soc Mag Reson Med* 8:21-31, 2000.
19. Johnson LA, Hoppe BE, Gerard EL et al: Quantitative chemical shift imaging of vertebral bone marrow in patients with Gaucher disease, *Radiology* 182:451-455, 1992.
20. Maas M, Hollak CEM, Akkerman EM et al: Quantification of skeletal involvement in adults with type I Gaucher disease: fat fraction measured by Dixon quantitative chemical shift imaging as a valid parameter, *AJR Am J Roentgenol* 179:961-965, 2002.
21. Aharoni D, Krausz Y, Elstein D et al: Tc-99m sestamibi bone marrow scintigraphy in Gaucher disease, *Clin Nucl Med* 27:503-509, 2002.
22. Mariani G, Filocamo M, Giona F et al: Severity of bone marrow involvement in patients with Gaucher's disease evaluated by scintigraphy with 99mTc-sestamibi, *J Nucl Med* 44:1253-1262, 2003.
23. Fiore CE, Barone R, Pennisi P et al: Bone ultrasonometry, bone density, and turnover markers in type 1 Gaucher disease, *J Bone Miner Metab* 20:34-38, 2002.
24. Pastores GM, Wallenstein S, Desnick RJ et al: Bone density in type 1 Gaucher disease, *J Bone Miner Res* 11:1801-1807, 1996.
25. Rosenthal DI, Mayo-Smith W, Goodsitt MM et al: Bone and bone marrow changes in Gaucher disease: evaluation with quantitative CT, *Radiology* 170:143-146, 1989.
26. Kaloterakis A, Cholongitas E, Pantelis E et al: Type I Gaucher disease with severe skeletal destruction, extraosseous extension, and monoclonal gammopathy, *Am J Hematol* 77:377-380, 2004.
27. Hermann G, Shapiro R, Abdelwahab IF et al: Extraosseous extension of Gaucher cell deposits mimicking malignancy, *Skeletal Radiol* 23:253-256, 1994.
28. Poll LW, Koch JA, vom Dahl S et al: Type I Gaucher disease: extraosseous extension of skeletal disease, *Skeletal Radiol* 29:15-21, 2000.
29. Bisagni-Faure A, Dupont AM, Chazerain P et al: Magnetic resonance imaging assessment of sacroiliac joint involvement in Gaucher's disease, *J Rheumatol* 19:1984-1987, 1992.
30. Israel O, Jerushalmi J, Front D: Scintigraphic findings in Gaucher's disease, *J Nucl Med* 27:1557-1563, 1986.
31. Hansen GC, Gold RH: Central depression of multiple vertebral end-plates: a "pathognomonic" sign of sickle hemoglobinopathy in Gaucher's disease, *AJR Am J Roentgenol* 129:343-344, 1977.
32. Colhoun EN, Cassar-Pullicino V, McCall IW et al: Unusual disco-vertebral changes in Gaucher's disease, *Br J Radiol* 60:925-928, 1987.
33. Bilchik TR, Heyman S: Skeletal scintigraphy of pseudo-osteomyelitis in Gaucher's disease. Two case reports and a review of the literature, *Clin Nucl Med* 17:279-282, 1992.
34. Goldblatt J, Keet P, Dall D: Spinal cord decompression for Gaucher's disease, *Neurosurgery* 21:227-230, 1987.
35. DeFriend DE, Brown AEM, Hutton CW, Hughes PM: Mannosidosis: an unusual cause of a deforming arthropathy, *Skeletal Radiol* 29:358-361, 2000.
36. McHugh K, Olsen EOE, Vellodi A: Gaucher disease in children: radiology of non-central nervous system manifestations, *Clin Radiol* 59:117-123, 2004.
37. Li JK, Birch PD, Davies AM: Proximal humeral defects in Gaucher's disease, *Br J Radiol* 61:579-583, 1988.
38. Ozonoff MB, Ziter FMJ: The upper humeral notch. A normal variant in children, *Radiology* 113:699-701, 1974.
39. Pastores GM, Hermann G, Norton K et al: Resolution of a proximal humeral defect in type-1 Gaucher disease by enzyme replacement therapy, *Pediatr Radiol* 25:486-487, 1995.
40. Rosenbloom BE, Weinreb NJ, Zimran A et al: Gaucher disease and cancer incidence: a study from the Gaucher Registry, *Blood* 105:4569-4572, 2005.
41. Bohm P, Kunz W, Horny HP et al: Adult Gaucher disease in association with primary malignant bone tumors, *Cancer* 91:457-462, 2001.
42. Aydin K, Karabulut N, Demirkazik F et al: Pulmonary involvement in adult Gaucher's disease: high resolution CT appearance, *Br J Radiol* 70:93-95, 1997.
43. Patlas M, Hadas-Halpern I, Abrahamov A et al: Spectrum of abdominal sonographic findings in 103 pediatric patients with Gaucher disease, *Eur Radiol* 12:397-400, 2002.
44. Hainaux B, Christophe C, Hanquinet S et al: Gaucher's disease. Plain radiography, US, CT and MR diagnosis of lungs, bone and liver lesions, *Pediatr Radiol* 22: 78-79, 1992.
45. Thanopoulos BD, Frimas CA, Mantagos SP et al: Gaucher disease: treatment of hypersplenism with splenic embolization, *Acta Paediatr Scand* 76:1003-1007, 1987.
46. Saraclar M, Atalay S, Kocak N et al: Gaucher's disease with mitral and aortic involvement: echocardiographic findings, *Pediatr Cardiol* 13:56-58, 1992.
47. Lin DS, Lin SP, Liang DC et al: Technetium-99m-HmPAO brain SPECT in infantile Gaucher's disease, *Pediatr Neurol* 20:66-69, 1999.
48. Mankin HJ, Rosenthal DI, Xavier R: Gaucher disease current concepts review, *J Bone Joint Surg Am* 83:748-762, 2001.
49. Whittington R, Goa KL: Alglucerase. A review of its therapeutic use in Gaucher's disease, *Drugs* 44:72-93, 1992.
50. Beutler E, Demina A, Laubscher K et al: The clinical course of treated and untreated Gaucher disease. A study of 45 patients, *Blood Cells Mol Dis* 21:86-108, 1995.
51. Poll LW, Koch JA, vom Dahl S et al: Magnetic resonance imaging of bone marrow changes in Gaucher disease during enzyme replacement therapy: first German long-term results, *Skeletal Radiol* 30:496-503, 2001.
52. Barton NW, Brady RO, Dambrosia JM et al: Dose-dependent responses to macrophage-targeted glucocerebrosidase in a child with Gaucher disease, *J Pediatr* 120:277-280, 1992.
53. Rosenthal DI, Doppelt SH, Mankin HJ et al: Enzyme replacement therapy for Gaucher disease: skeletal responses to macrophage-targeted glucocerebrosidase, *Pediatrics* 96:629-637, 1995.
54. Pastores GM, Hermann G, Norton KI et al: Regression of skeletal changes in type 1 Gaucher disease with enzyme replacement therapy, *Skeletal Radiol* 25:485-488, 1996.
55. Schiffmann R, Mankin H, Dambrosia JM et al: Decreased bone density in splenectomized Gaucher patients receiving enzyme replacement therapy, *Blood Cells Mol Dis* 28:288-296, 2002.
56. Bembi B, Ciana G, Mengel E et al: Bone complications in children with Gaucher disease, *Br J Radiol* 75(Suppl 1):A37-A44, 2002.
57. Baldellou A, Andria G, Campbell PE et al: Paediatric non-neuronopathic Gaucher disease: recommendations for treatment and monitoring, *Eur J Pediatr* 163:67-75, 2004.
58. Itzchaki M, Lebel E, Dweck A et al: Orthopedic considerations in Gaucher disease since the advent of enzyme replacement therapy, *Acta Orthop Scand* 75:641-653, 2004.
59. Iwase T, Hasegawa Y, Iwata H: Transtrochanteric anterior rotational osteotomy for Gaucher's disease. A case report, *Clin Orthop Relat Res* (317):122-125, 1995.
60. Ringden O, Groth CG, Erikson A et al: Ten years' experience of bone marrow transplantation for Gaucher disease, *Transplantation* 59:864-870, 1995.
61. Starer F, Sargent JD, Hobbs JR: Regression of the radiological changes of Gaucher's disease following bone marrow transplantation, *Br J Radiol* 60:1189-1195, 1987.
62. Figueroa ML, Rosenbloom BE, Kay AC et al: A less costly regimen of alglucerase to treat Gaucher's disease, *New Engl J Med* 327:1632-1636, 1992.
63. Ciana G, Cuttini M, Bembi B: Short-term effects of pamidronate in patients with Gaucher's disease and severe skeletal involvement, *N Engl J Med* 337:712, 1997.
64. Pastores GM, Patel MJ, Firooznia H: Bone and joint complications related to Gaucher disease, *Curr Rheumatol Rep* 2:175-180, 2000.
65. Zimran A, Kay A, Gelbart T et al: Gaucher disease. Clinical, laboratory, radiologic, and genetic features of 53 patients, *Medicine (Baltimore)* 71:337-353, 1992.
66. Charrow J, Esplin JA, Gribble TJ et al: Gaucher disease: recommendations on diagnosis, evaluation, and monitoring, *Arch Intern Med* 158:1754-1760, 1998.
67. Pastores GM, Weinreb NJ, Aerts H et al: Therapeutic goals in the treatment of Gaucher disease, *Semin Hematol* 41(4 Suppl 5):4-14, 2004.
68. Andersson HC, Charrow J, Kaplan P et al: Individualization of long-term enzyme replacement therapy for Gaucher disease [erratum appears in *Genet Med* 7:460, 2005], *Genet Med* 7:105-110, 2005.

CHAPTER 28

Hemochromatosis, Wilson's Disease, Ochronosis, Fabry Disease, and Multicentric Reticulohistiocytosis

Barbara N. Weissman, MD

Key Facts

Hemochromatosis

- Most cases are due to a mutation that results in increased iron absorption from the gut.
- Secondary hemochromatosis is due to iron overload from other conditions such as multiple blood transfusions.
- Cirrhosis, diabetes, bronze coloration of the skin, hypogonadism, cardiomyopathy, and arthropathy may result.
- A distinctive arthropathy may occur that resembles osteoarthritis but typically involves the metacarpophalangeal (MCP) joints and other joints not typically affected by osteoarthritis. Chondrocalcinosis, hook-like osteophytes at the MCP joints, and cystic changes may be present.
- Hepatocellular carcinoma occurs in approximately 30% of cases.
- Magnetic resonance imaging (MRI) and computed tomography can detect abnormal iron accumulation in involved abdominal organs and the heart.

Ochronosis

- Alkaptonuria is produced by a defect in the metabolism of homogentisic acid leading to darkening of the urine when exposed to air or reducing agents.
- *Ochronosis* refers to the connective tissue manifestations of alkaptonuria.
- Early degeneration and later calcification of the lumbar spine and dorsal spine intervertebral cysts are characteristic. Findings similar to ankylosing spondylitis may occur.

Wilson's Disease

- Wilson's disease is a rare, autosomal recessive disease leading to copper deposition, especially in the brain, corneas, and liver.
- Characteristic findings may be seen in the central nervous system on MRI.

Fabry Disease

- This disease is an X-linked condition in which there is decreased activity of the lysosomal enzyme, α galactosidase A, leading to the accumulation of neutral glycosphingolipids, especially globotriaosylceramide (Gb3).
- Chronic renal insufficiency, arterial hypertension, atherosclerosis, cerebrovascular complications, and cardiac involvement may lead to a shortened life span and decreased quality of life.

Multicentric Reticulohistiocytosis

- This condition is also known as lipoid dermatoarthritis.
- Characteristic red-brown skin nodules may occur after the arthritis is manifest.
- Radiographic features include symmetrical, well-defined erosions of interphalangeal joints without osteoporosis or periosteal reaction. Eventually arthritis mutilans may result.
- Diagnosis is confirmed by the characteristic histologic findings.
- Accompanying malignant lesions should be excluded.

HEMOCHROMATOSIS

Hemochromatosis results from excess iron deposition in the body due either to a genetic cause (primary) or to iron overload from other conditions (secondary). The primary form is an autosomal recessive condition. The responsible "hemochromatosis gene," HFE, was identified in 1996,[1] and most cases are due to a mutation of this gene resulting in a base change at position 282 of the HFE protein (C282Y). Other gene mutations may also result in hereditary hemochromatosis. Secondary hemochromatosis is due to iron overload from other conditions such as multiple blood transfusions, sickle cell anemia, or increased iron ingestion.

The condition "bronzed diabetes" was first reported in 1865; in 1889, von Recklinghausen reported 12 patients with iron deposition in most organs.[2] The primary form is fairly frequent with approximately 5 of every 1000 persons of northern European descent being homozygous for the C282Y mutation.[1]

> Hemochromatosis is the most common genetic disease in populations of European ancestry.[3]

Hereditary hemochromatosis results in increased absorption of iron from the gastrointestinal tract. Normal iron stores are about 5 g, and symptoms occur when iron stores reach 15 to 20 g.[2]

Iron is deposited especially in the liver and pancreas and to a lesser degree in the endocrine glands and heart. Iron is also found in the synovial cells of the joints.[4]

Hereditary hemochromatosis results in increased iron absorption from the gastrointestinal tract and deposition of iron in the liver, pancreas, and heart.

Clinical features of hemochromatosis include cirrhosis, diabetes, bronze coloration of the skin (due to melanin in the basal layer),[4] hypogonadism, cardiomyopathy, and arthropathy.[5] However, due to earlier detection, the classic triad of cirrhosis, bronze skin, and diabetes has become rare in adult-onset disease.[1] Symptoms typically begin between the ages of 50 and 60 years. Men are much more commonly affected, probably due to the protective effect of menses and childbirth on iron overload.[2] Most often, fatigue, malaise, and arthralgia—sometimes with hepatomegaly or slightly elevated aminotransferase levels—are the presenting findings in middle-aged adults. Juvenile-onset disease may be manifested by hypogonadotrophic hypogonadism or unexplained heart failure.[1]

The classic triad of hemochromatosis consists of diabetes, cirrhosis, and bronze skin.

The diagnostic evaluation of patients suspected of having adult-onset hereditary hemochromatosis is reviewed by Pietrangelo[1] and Adams.[3] Markers of iron overload and subsequent genetic testing can confirm the diagnosis.[1] Diagnosis can also be confirmed on liver biopsy showing parenchymal iron distribution with a periportal to central gradient and an iron index above 1.9 (hepatic iron concentration in micromoles per gram of liver dry weight divided by the age in years).[1]

Liver cancer (especially hepatocellular carcinoma) is the cause of death in up to 45% of patients with genetic hemochromatosis.[5]

The presence of hepatocellular carcinoma should suggest the possibility of underlying hemochromatosis.

Bone and Joint Disease

Arthropathy occurs in up to half of patients with hemochromatosis and may be the presenting feature of the disease.[2] The severity of the arthropathy is not correlated with the amount of intraarticular iron or with total iron stores.[5] Pathologic examination of the synovium in cases of hemochromatosis shows hemosiderin in the synovial lining cells but no synovial proliferation.[2] In contrast, other disorders in which iron deposition occurs (such as hemophilia or and pigmented villonodular synovitis) show iron deposited in the deep macrophages.

Pathologic examination allows differentiation of iron deposition due to bleeding disorders from that seen in hemochromatosis.

As summarized by Papakonstantinou et al.,[5] cartilage damage in hemochromatosis is precipitated by iron or calcium pyrophosphate or apatite crystals. Iron increases cartilage stiffness and leads to fragmentation at the area of greatest stress, which is the tidemark between the calcified and noncalcified cartilage. This area of splitting is different from the subchondral fractures seen in avascular necrosis or the changes of osteoarthritis.

In 1964, Schumacher[7] reported a distinctive pattern of arthritis in patients with hemochromatosis[7] (Table 28-1). The hands and wrists (especially the proximal interphalangeal [PIP] and metacarpophalangeal [MCP] joints) are most often involved. The hips, shoulders, knees, elbows, and ankles may also be affected.[2]

TABLE 28-1. Distinctive Features of Hemochromatosis Arthropathy (HA)

Versus Osteoarthritis	Versus Rheumatoid Arthritis
Earlier onset of HA	Negative latex fixation
Greater PIP and MCP involvement	Normal globulins
Demineralization	No inflammation on synovial biopsy
Cystlike changes	Involvement of DIP joints
	No inflammatory episodes
	No nodules
	No vasomotor changes

From Schumacher HR Jr: Hemochromatosis and arthritis, *Arthritis Rheum* 7:41-50, 1964.

Radiographic Features

Chondrocalcinosis occurs on radiographs in up to 30% of patients with hemochromatosis.[2] It is usually seen in the knees (hyaline cartilage and menisci), the pubic symphysis, the wrists, and the intervertebral disks.

Hands and Wrists

Both hemochromatosis and idiopathic calcium pyrophosphate disease (CPPD)–related arthropathy produce changes of osteoarthritis in joints that are usually not affected by this condition. The radiocarpal and midcarpal joints and the MCP joints are typically involved in these conditions (Figure 28-1). Diffuse cartilage space narrowing is seen instead of the typically asymmetrical narrowing that characterizes primary osteoarthritis. Intraarticular and periarticular calcifications may occur in either condition.[8]

The presence of osteoarthritic changes in a rheumatoid distribution should suggest the possibility of CPPD or hemochromatosis arthropathy.

Despite many similar features, there are subtle clues that may allow the diagnosis of hemochromatosis to be suggested over idiopathic CPPD. A blinded review of the hand and wrist radiographs of 26 patients with idiopathic CPPD arthropathy and 26 patients with hemochromatosis revealed some of these subtle differences in appearance (Table 28-2). The most prominent differentiating feature is the involvement of all of the MCP joints including the fourth and fifth and the larger hook-like osteophytes in patients with hemochromatosis.

Knee

Chondrocalcinosis and predominance of patellofemoral cartilage space narrowing may be seen (Figure 28-2; See also Figure 8-25).

Hip

Hip disease is thought to be common and severe in patients with hemochromatosis. Imaging features resemble osteoarthritis or CPPD arthropathy and include concentric joint space narrowing, subchondral lucencies, sclerosis, and osteophytes.[5]

Axford et al.[9] reviewed the radiographs of 112 patients with genetic hemochromatosis and arthritis. Twenty-eight (25%) of the 112 patients had hip abnormalities detected on radiographs. Osteoarthritis and chondrocalcinosis (12/28) or osteoarthritis alone (9/28, 32%) were the most common findings. Chondrocalcinosis without accompanying findings was seen in five patients (5/28).

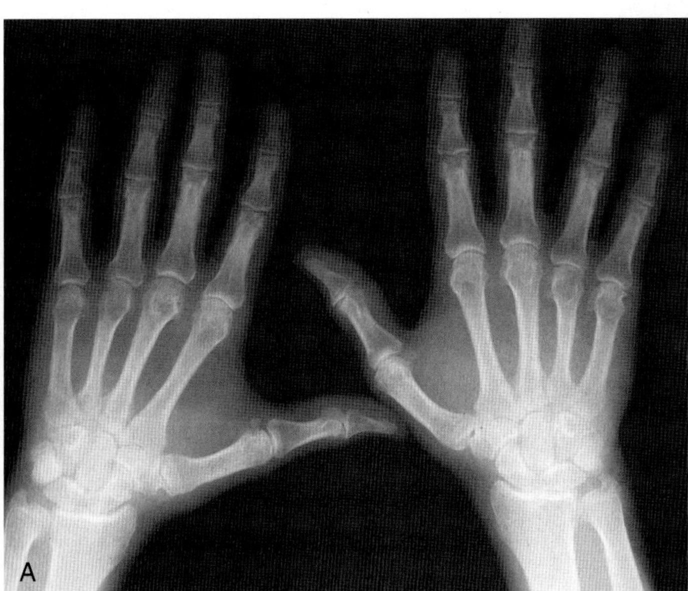

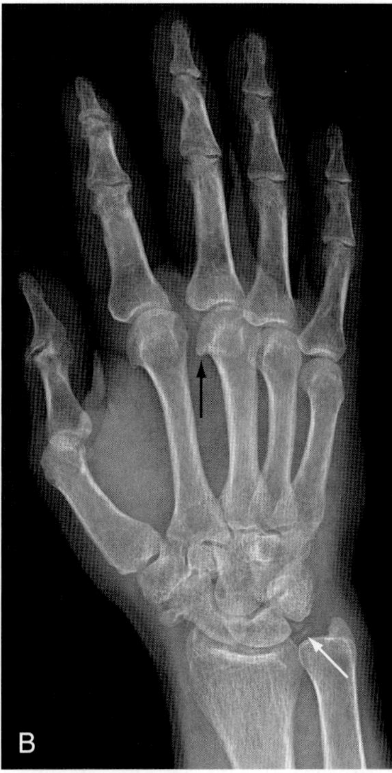

FIGURE 28-1. Hemochromatosis. **A,** Posteroanterior radiograph of the hands shows cartilage space narrowing and hook-like osteophytes at most of the MCP joints. While the features resemble osteoarthritis, the distribution with prominent MCP changes makes primary osteoarthritis unlikely. Involvement of most of the MCP joints helps suggest the diagnosis of hemochromatosis over that of CPPD-related arthropathy. (Courtesy of Piran Aliabadi, MD, Boston.) **B,** Oblique radiograph of the hand in another patient shows hook-like osteophytes predominantly at the index and middle *(black arrow)* MCP joints (a distribution that may be seen with CPPD-related arthropathy). There is calcification of the triangular fibrocartilage and synovium *(white arrow).*

TABLE 28-2. Features Useful in Distinguishing Idiopathic CPPD from Hemochromatosis Arthropathy

Feature	Idiopathic CPPD Arthropathy	Hemochromatosis
MCP narrowing	Second and third MCP	Every MCP including four and five
Osteophytes	Small	Larger hook-like osteophytes from the radial aspects of metacarpal heads
Scapholunate dissociation	More often	Less often
MCP versus RC involvement	Both MCP and RC	May have MCP without RC
Chondrocalcinosis	More often at thumb CMC Otherwise same distribution	Less often at CMC Otherwise same distribution

From Pietrangelo A: Hereditary hemochromatosis—a new look at an old disease, *N Engl J Med* 350:2383-2397, 2004. [See comment.]
CMC, Carpometacarpal; *RC,* radiocarpal.

In two patients, an unusual arthropathy was described with small osteophytes, cartilage space narrowing, and a wedge-shaped area of subchondral lucency. No patient demonstrated the subchondral cyst formation that is thought to be typical of hemochromatosis involving other joints (Box 28-1).

In a case described by Papakonstantinou et al.,[5] subchondral lucencies were the result of articular cartilage growing into the subchondral bone rather than subchondral cyst formation.

Axial migration of the femoral head (cartilage loss along the axis of the femoral neck) with osteophytes suggests arthropathy associated with CPPD or hemochromatosis.

MRI may show prominent cystic changes (See Figure 8-16D and E).

Ankle and Hindfoot

Although involvement of the ankle and hindfoot is unusual in hemochromatosis, occasionally patients with the disorder present with symmetrical pain and swelling of the ankles.[10] Radiographic findings are those of osteoarthritis, although this distribution should suggest an underlying cause (e.g., rheumatoid arthritis, prior trauma) (Figure 28-3). Magnetic resonance imaging (MRI) has shown synovial thickening in addition to the features of osteoarthritis.[10]

Symmetrical ankle/hindfoot pain and swelling in relatively young men is occasionally a clinical manifestation of hemochromatosis.

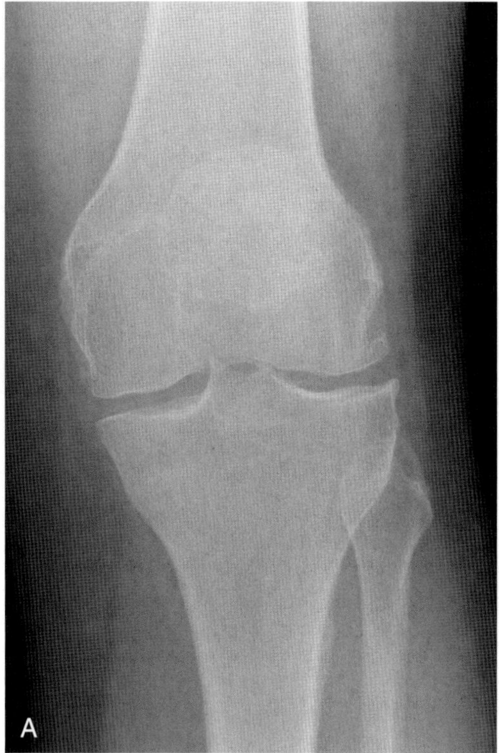

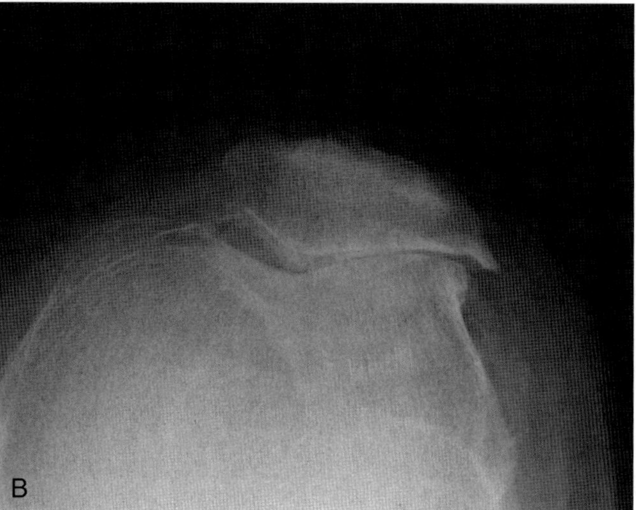

FIGURE 28-2. Hemochromatosis. **A,** An anteroposterior radiograph of the knee shows osteophytic lipping from the joint margins but no cartilage space narrowing. No chondrocalcinosis is seen in this case. **B,** The tangential patellar view shows severe patellofemoral cartilage space narrowing. This distribution of cartilage loss (with much greater severity at the patellofemoral joint than the femorotibial articulation) should suggest CPPD-related arthropathy or hemochromatosis.

BOX 28-1. Features of Hip Arthropathy in Hemochromatosis

Symmetrical cartilage loss
Axial migration of the femoral head
Subchondral lucencies
Osteophytes
Subchondral sclerosis
Diffuse osteopenia
Bone marrow edema on MRI
Subchondral cyst-like areas on MRI
Subchondral crescent with fluid signal on MRI

MRI Features

Generally, the quantity of intraarticular iron is not adequate in the joint or synovium of patients with hemochromatosis to produce signal changes such as are seen in solid organs in patients with this disorder.[5] The exception is a case reported by Moore et al.[11] in which a periarticular susceptibility artifact in the wrist was described that decreased as the patient was successfully treated.

MRI of Hip

Papakonstantinou et al.[5] correlated MRI findings with gross pathologic and histologic examination in a patient with hemochromatosis. No decrease in signal intensity was present to indicate the presence of iron and histologic examination did not disclose the presence of iron. The imaging findings were nonspecific, although the separation of cartilage at the tidemark on histologic examination suggested the diagnosis.

Nonosseous Imaging Features

Imaging findings generally depend on the presence of iron and the sequelae of iron deposition (e.g., micronodular cirrhosis). Excess iron in genetic hemochromatosis is deposited in hepatocytes, pancreatic acinar cells, the myocardium, joints, endocrine glands, and skin.[12] The cells of the RES are unable to store the excess iron.

Computed Tomography

Computed tomography (CT) findings in hemochromatosis include increased density to the liver, hepatomegaly, cirrhosis, and hepatocellular carcinoma[4] (Table 28-3). Increased iron deposition in the liver produces a white appearance on non–contrast-enhanced CT scans.

Normally, the mean CT number of the liver is 24.9 ± 4.6, and is higher than that of the spleen (mean 21.1 ± 4).[13] The liver spleen difference in CT numbers is 3.8 ± 2.1. In hemochromatosis, the liver density will be > 70 Hounsfield units.[13]

In hemochromatosis, the density of the liver will be > 70 HU and the liver-spleen difference will be greater than normal.

Since the density of the spleen does not increase in iron overload (parenchymal organs rather than the reticuloendothelial system are affected), the liver–spleen difference will be larger than

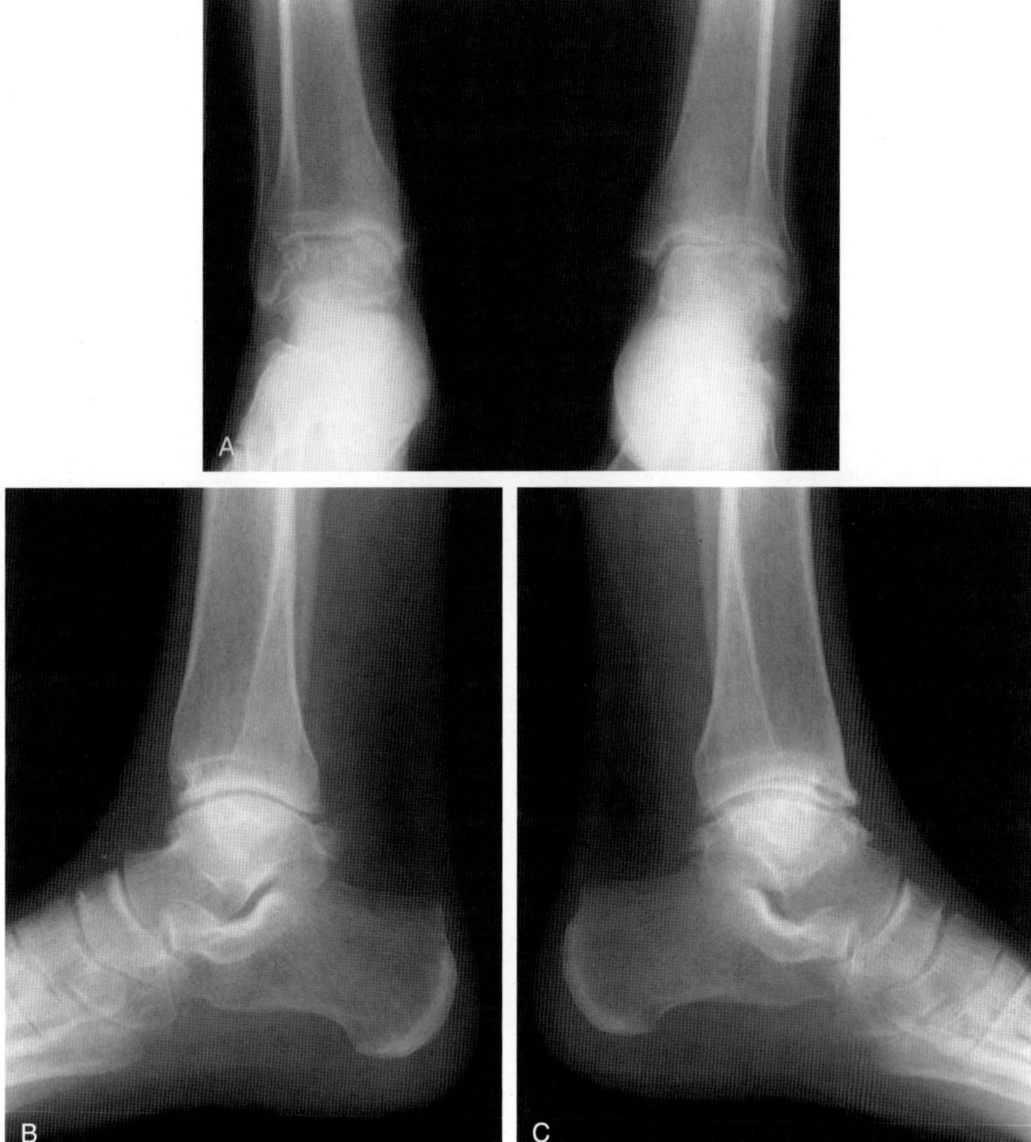

FIGURE 28-3. Ankle changes in hemochromatosis. **A,** Anteroposterior radiograph of both ankles shows subchondral sclerosis with cartilage-space narrowing, especially on the left. Both lateral views of the left **(C)** and right **(B)** ankles show osteophytes from the joint margins. While the changes are consistent with osteoarthritis, the symmetry and location at the tibiotalar joints should suggest an underlying condition.

normal.[4] CT is nearly 100% accurate in detecting iron overload that is five times upper normal levels and about 60% sensitive for detecting iron overload that is 2.5 times the upper limit of normal.[4] Normal CT liver values do not completely exclude the possibility of iron overload.[6] Dual-energy CT has correlated with hepatic iron content measured by liver biopsy.[14]

> Hepatocellular carcinoma occurs in about 30% of patients with hemochromatosis and is a significant cause of mortality in this condition.

Hepatocellular carcinoma may also occur in patients previously unsuspected of having hemochromatosis.[6] The tumor usually appears as a space occupying hypodense mass in contrast to the hyperdense liver on non-contrast CT examination. Lwakatare et al.,[6] however, reported a patient in whom even contrast-enhanced CT examination did not identify the tumor, whereas MRI and contrast-enhanced ultrasonography did. In a liver demonstrating iron overload, a non–iron-containing area should be suspected of being an area containing hepatocellular carcinoma.[6]

Other causes of increased density in the liver include treatment with iodine-containing drugs such as amioderone, or glycogen storage disease.[4]

MRI Compared to CT

Overall, MRI is more sensitive and more specific than CT for detecting elevated liver iron concentrations.[15] The paramagnetic effects of iron produce a low-signal-intensity liver on T1-weighted MRI and especially low signal intensity on T2-weighted and

TABLE 28-3. CT and MR Imaging Features of the Liver in Hemochromatosis

CT	White liver on noncontrast study
	Liver density > 70 HU
	Liver-to-spleen ratio increased
	Hepatomegaly
	Micronodular cirrhosis
	Hepatocellular carcinoma
MRI	Low signal on T1W and T2W image

T2*-weighted sequences.[16] (The interested reader is referred to the article by Pomerantz and Siegelman[16] for a more thorough discussion of these findings.) Other entities that produce diffuse low signal on MRI sequences are supermagnetic contrast administration, Wilson's disease, and Osler-Weber-Rendu disease.

> MRI is more sensitive and specific than CT for the detection of iron in the liver.

Quantification of liver iron using noninvasive MRI techniques could offer a clinically relevant alternative to serial liver biopsies. However, relatively low concentrations of iron and relatively large amounts of iron are problematic. Unlike CT, MRI does not provide absolute values; ratios of tissue-to-tissue signal on the same image or calculating a liver index such as T2 relaxation time from a set of images obtained without changing RF parameters can be used for quantification.[15] The ratio of signal intensity on T2-weighted images of the liver to that of the paraspinal muscles of < 0.5 is a predictor of hepatic iron concentrations more than five times the upper limit of normal.[17]

Several MRI techniques have been explored, which are summarized by St Pierre et al.[18] as follows: (1) signal-intensity–ratio methods based on T2 contrast, (2) signal-intensity–ratio methods based on T2* contrast, (3) relaxometry methods based on T2 measurement, and (4) relaxometry methods based on T2* measurement.[18]

In 1994, Gandon et al.[15] reported the quantification of hepatic iron with MRI (using the comparison of liver to fat or liver to muscle ratios on gradient echo sequences) and were able to detect liver iron concentrations of 80 to 300 μM/g.[15] Using this method and a mathematic model, Alustiza et al.[19] generated liver iron concentrations and compared them to biopsy results. For estimated hepatic iron concentrations of > 85 μM/g, the positive predictive value for hemochromatosis was 100%. For concentrations of < 40 μM, the negative predictive value was 100%.

St Pierre et al.[18] reported a noninvasive technique for the measurement and imaging of liver iron concentration in vivo using measurement of tissue proton-transverse relaxation rates (R2) obtained on 1.5T clinical MRI scanners. High sensitivity and specificity were found compared to biopsy-documented liver iron concentrations of clinically significant amounts. The authors noted that the 20-minute scan allowed higher specificity and sensitivity over a greater range of liver iron concentrations than other MRI-based methods available at the time. Custom-designed software is necessary, however.

Similar CT and MRI appearances due to iron deposition occur in other affected organs such as the pancreas and heart. Iron overload detected in the pancreas suggests advanced disease.[16] Myocardial iron can be detected on MRI and can be more accurate than myocardial biopsy, which is subject to sampling error and false negative results.[16,20] Iron stored as ferritin or hemosiderin interacts with hydrogen nuclei in the vicinity in tissue water to shorten the relaxation times T1, T2, and T2*, which produce low signal on corresponding MRI.[21] When T2* values are less than 20 msec, left ventricle (LV) systolic function has been shown to decline.[21] The presence of cardiac involvement has prognostic implications and may be a contraindication to orthotopic liver transplantation or suggest the need for combined heart and liver transplantation.[16]

Secondary Hemochromatosis

Secondary hemochromatosis is the result of excess iron administration, usually from multiple transfusions or rarely from excessive ingestion.[22] The term *hemosiderosis* is sometimes used synonymously with hemochromatosis, but it specifically refers to extracellular ferric iron deposition.[23]

Damaged transfused red blood cells are taken up by the reticuloendothelial cells of the bone marrow and spleen and the Kupffer cells of the liver.[23] The iron is stored as hemosiderin.[23] The reticuloendothelial system (RES) can store about 10 g of iron (equivalent to about 40 units of blood). Thereafter, excess iron is deposited in the parenchymal tissues as in primary hemochromatosis.[23] Unlike the deleterious effects seen with parenchymal iron deposition, iron deposited in the RES does not lead to organ fibrosis or hepatocellular carcinoma.[24] Treatment with iron chelation is used to prevent the sequelae of parenchymal iron deposition (such as diabetes).[16]

> Iron deposition in hemosiderosis occurs in the reticuloendothelial cell of the bone marrow and spleen and the Kupffer cells of the liver, and it does not usually lead to the complications seen in hemochromatosis.

Magnetic Resonance Imaging

The characteristic MRI appearance of patients with RES iron overload is low signal intensity in the liver and spleen on spin echo T2-weighted or T2*-weighted, gradient-echo images with a normal pancreas (specificity = 93%)[24] (Figure 28-4). In hemosiderosis, liver iron concentration is between 36 and 80 μM/gram.[19] In hemosiderosis, the affected bone marrow is low in signal (dark).[23] Normally in adults, because of the increasing vertebral marrow fat, the vertebrae appear brighter than the intervertebral disks, especially on T1-weighted images.[25] In contrast, when hemosiderosis is present, the vertebral marrow will be darker than the disks. In patients with chronic anemia (e.g., sickle cell anemia), the vertebral marrow will reconvert to red marrow.[23] This marrow contains less fat and will appear low to intermediate in signal intensity on T1-weighted images but should increase in signal on T2-weighted images (unlike hemochromatosis, which exhibits low signal marrow on both sequences).[23]

> The distribution of iron deposition in transfusion-related hemosiderosis differs from that of primary hemochromatosis. In hemosiderosis, the spleen and bone marrow primarily show low signal on MRI (Tables 28-4 and 28-5).

WILSON'S DISEASE

Hepatolenticular degeneration (Wilson's disease) is a rare, autosomal-recessive disease characterized by impaired trafficking of copper in hepatocytes leading to copper deposition in various tissues and organs, especially the brain, corneas, and liver.[26] The disorder is characterized clinically by liver disease, neurologic symptoms, and greenish-brown corneal rings (Kayser-Fleisher rings).[26] Liver disease

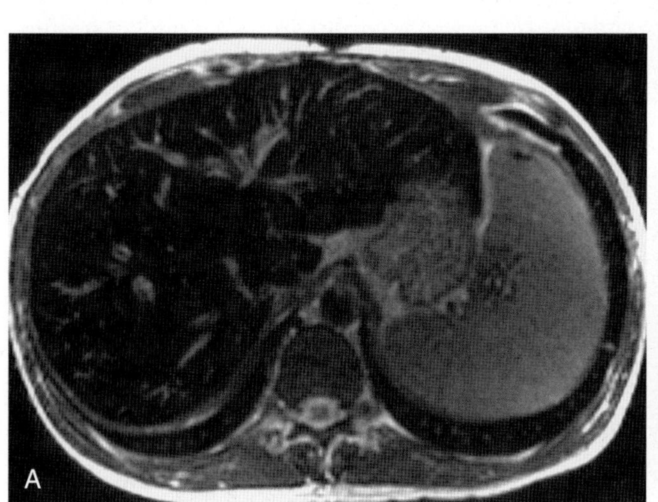

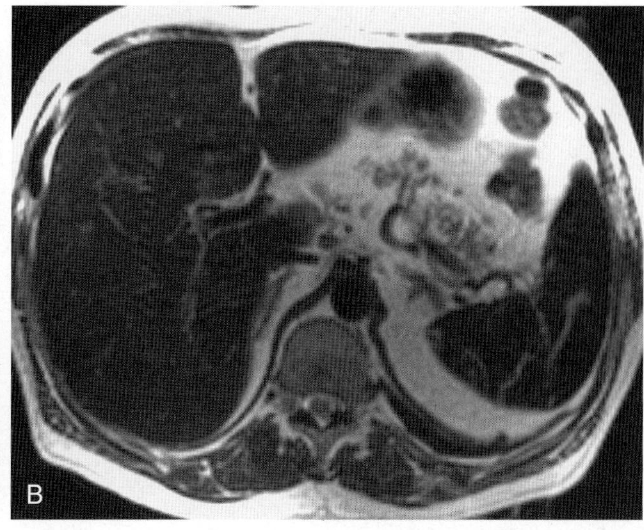

FIGURE 28-4. MRI of hemochromatosis and hemosiderosis. **A,** Hemochromatosis. T2-weighted image shows the liver to be abnormally low in signal. **B,** Hemosiderosis. This patient with leukemia shows the effects of multiple transfusions with low signal intensity in the liver and spleen on this T-2 weighted image. (Courtesy Koenraad Mortele, MD and Cheryl Sadow, MD, Brigham and Women's Hospital Boston, MA.)

TABLE 28-4. Abdominal Imaging Features in Primary Hemochromatosis, Secondary Hemochromatosis (Hemosiderosis) and Cirrhosis from Other Causes

	Liver	Spleen	Pancreas	Bone Marrow
Hemosiderosis	Low signal[a]	Low signal	Normal	Low signal
Hemochromatosis	Low	Normal	Low	Normal
Cirrhosis	Mildly low	Normal	Normal	Normal

[a]T2W signal intensity.
From Siegelman ES, Mitchell DG, Rubin R, et al: Parenchymal versus reticuloendothelial iron overload in the liver: distinction with MR imaging, *Radiology* 179:361-366, 1991. [See comment.]

TABLE 28-5. Differential Features of Bone Marrow Signal in Hemosiderosis

	T1-weighted	T2-weighted	GRASS
Normal adult	Brighter than disks[a]	Intermediate[a]	
Hemosiderosis	Low signal	Low signal	Low signal
Marrow fibrosis with Sickle cell anemia	Patchy low signal	Patchy low signal	
Myelofibrosis	Low signal	Low signal	Not as low signal

[a]Vande Berg, Malghem J, Lecouvete FE, et al.[25]

and neuropsychiatric abnormalities are the most common presenting features.[26] Diagnosis can be made when two of the following are present: Kayser-Fleisher rings, typical neurologic findings, and low serum ceruloplasmin.[26]

> Symptoms and MRI abnormalities of Wilson's disease can be reversed with chelation.

Musculoskeletal Manifestations

Skeletal changes in Wilson's disease result from (1) osteoporosis or osteomalacia and (2) degenerative changes in joints[27] (Figure 28-5). A postulated mechanism for the genesis of osteoporosis and osteomalacia is hyperphosphaturia, which leads to hypophosphatemia. The cause of degenerative changes is uncertain but may be due to chronic injury[27] or to copper deposition.[28] Synovial thickening with plasma cell and lymphocytic infiltration and copper pigment deposition has been reported.[27]

Large joints, particularly the shoulders and hips, or less often the hands and wrists, are affected.[28] Imaging features include marginal bone fragments, intraarticular bodies, calcification of joint capsules or tendons, and squaring of the metacarpal heads.[28] CPPD may be manifested by chondrocalcinosis on radiographs and arthropathy. As in other patients with CPPD, subchondral cyst formation may be prominent[27] (Box 28-2).

> The presence of CPPD-related arthropathy in a young patient suggests the possibility of Wilson's disease, among other conditions (Box 28-3).

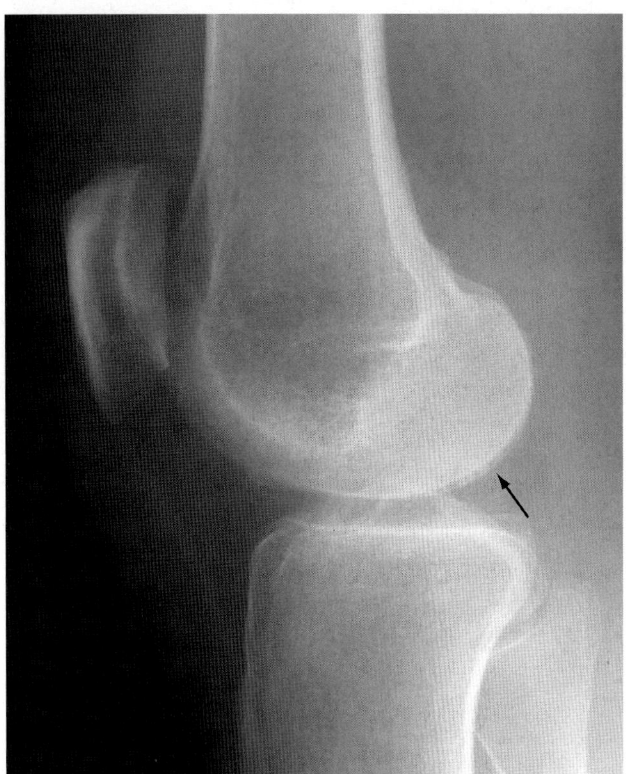

FIGURE 28-5. Wilson's disease. Lateral radiograph of the knee shows a rim of irregular calcifications around the condyles *(arrow)*.

BOX 28-2. Musculoskeletal Features of Wilson's Disease

Osteoporosis
Osteomalacia
Cystic changes and resorption of the lamina dura mimicking hyperparathyroidism
Premature osteoarthritis of large joints
Chondrocalcinosis
Chondromalacia patellae

Modified from Balint G, Szebenyi B: Hereditary disorders mimicking and/or causing premature osteoarthritis, *Best Pract Res Clin Rheumatol* 14:219-250, 2000.

BOX 28-3. Causes of Calcium Pyrophosphate Arthropathy (CPPD) in a Young Patient

Hyperparathyroidism
Hemochromatosis
Wilson's disease
Hypophosphatasia
Hypomagnesemia

From Hammoudeh M, Siam AR: Pseudogout in a young patient, *Clin Rheumatol* 17:242-245, 1998.

Liver

Copper is deposited particularly in the periportal areas of the liver and along the hepatic sinusoids. This deposition provokes inflammation, acute hepatitis, and fatty changes.[12] The chronic active hepatitis that develops leads to hepatic fibrosis and macronodular cirrhosis. Nonspecific hepatomegaly, fatty changes, and cirrhosis may be seen. Since copper has a high atomic number, the liver appears hyperdense on noncontrast CT scans in some cases.[12]

On MRI, prior to the onset of severe cirrhosis, nodules may be seen that are hyperintense on T1-weighted images and hypointense on T2-weighted images.[12] Akhan et al. reported a patient with liver nodules (chronic parenchymal liver disease with dysplastic changes) that enhanced with contrast in the arterial phase.[30]

Ultrasound findings are usually nonspecific increases in echogenicity of the liver, irregular contour, and a small right lobe.[30] Round nodules resembling metastatic lesions may be seen.

> A dense liver may be seen on unenhanced CT in patients with Wilson's disease due to the high atomic number of copper.

Neurologic Findings

Neurologic symptoms include dysarthria, dyspraxia, ataxia, and Parkinson-like extrapyramidal signs.[26] MRI is used to gauge the extent of disease, and resolution of the signal changes may occur following treatment.[31] Sinha et al.[31] found that all (93) symptomatic patients demonstrated abnormal MRI examinations, whereas presymptomatic patients[7] had normal studies. MRI findings in Wilson's disease include atrophy of the cerebrum, brainstem, and cerebellum and abnormal signal intensity, especially in the putamen, caudate, and midbrain.[31] Characteristic features include hypointensity of the globus pallidus on T2-weighted images, the unusual but diagnostic "face of giant panda" sign (hyperintense signal in the tegmentum and hypointense signal in the red nuclei on T2-weighted images), and striatal hyperintensity on T1-weighted images.[32]

> Deposition of heavy metal (iron or copper) may produce the low signal intensity seen on MRI examinations in patients with Wilson's disease.[33]

A smaller "face of the miniature panda" in the pontine tegmentum may also be seen with relative hypointensity in the medial longitudinal fasiculi and central tegmental tracts (the "eyes of the panda") and hyperintensity of the opening of the fourth ventricle (the nose and mouth of the panda).[34] Central pontine myelinosis and the bright claustral sign may be present.[31]

> The "face of the giant panda" is an unusual but characteristic midbrain appearance that may be present on MRI in patients with Wilson's disease.

Positron-emission tomography (PET) scanning has been used for assessing the effects of treatment on the glucose metabolism of the brain.[35]

OCHRONOSIS

Alkaptonuria is produced by a defect in the metabolism of homogentisic acid (a product of the metabolism of tyrosine and phenylalanine) that leads to darkening of the urine when exposed to air or reducing agents. The term *ochronosis* refers to the connective tissue manifestations of alkaptonuria, including changes produced in hyaline cartilage, tendons, ligaments, and muscles owing to the accumulation of homogentisic acid polymers. This pigment is blue-black macroscopically and ochre in color on microscopic examination.[36]

> Ochronosis refers to the connective tissue manifestations of alkaptonuria and is so named because of the ochre (yellow/brown) color of the deposited pigment as seen during microscopic examination.

The condition is rare, affecting 1 in 250,000 to 1,000,000 and results from autosomal recessive mutations of the HGO gene on chromosome 3q.[37] There are several mechanisms by which damage to connective tissues results from alkaptonuria. As summarized by Keller et al.,[37] absence of homogentisic acid oxidase (which is primarily in the liver and kidneys) leads to accumulation of homogentisic acid (HGA). HGA can be excreted in the kidneys, but with increasing age and decreasing renal function HGA accumulates. HGA is polymerized to ochronotic pigment. Connective tissue damage may be due to several mechanisms. The HGA can bind to connective-tissue macromolecules, affecting its structural integrity, or it may function as a chemical irritant. Also, an oxidative byproduct (benzoquinoneacetate [BQA]) or its derivatives may be responsible for alterations in tissue. BQA may bind to connective tissue and alter its structure. Free radical formation and inhibition of lysyl hydroxylase are other mechanisms producing tissue damage. The weakened connective tissue is prone to damage-producing inflammation that exacerbates the process.[37]

Common clinical manifestations of ochronosis are shown in Box 28-4.

Musculoskeletal Findings

Pigment is deposited in articular cartilage, ligaments, and menisci, causing loss of elasticity and susceptibility to mechanical damage.[38] Arthropathy usually develops after the fourth decade and is manifested by chronic joint stiffness and pain. The spine, knees, hips, and shoulders are affected.[38]

The most incapacitating complication of alkaptonuria is ochronotic arthropathy, which typically affects the spine, knees, and hips.

BOX 28-4. Common Clinical Manifestations of Ochronosis

Darkening of the urine on exposure to air or reducing agents
Dark pigmentation of pinnae, nasal ala, and sclera
Degenerative disk disease, disk calcification, vertebral osteoporosis, bony bridging, back pain and stiffness
Degenerative hip and knee disease
Cardiac valve calcification and stenosis and coronary artery calcification
Renal stones
Prostate stones

From Keller JM, Macaulay JM, Nercessian OA, et al: New developments in ochronosis: review of the literature, *Rheumatol Int* 25:81-85, 2005.

Radiographs of involved joints show degenerative changes with cartilage space loss, prominent subchondral sclerosis, small cysts, and periarticular calcification.[38] Osteophytes are less prominent than in osteoarthritis generally, and the severity of damage is greater than would be expected for the patient's age.[38]

Spine

Widespread disk degeneration is seen with dense disk calcification (Figure 28-6). Dorsolumbar changes predominate in contrast to the lumbosacral involvement seen in the usual cases of degenerative disk disease.[38] Multilevel disk narrowing with osteopenia and end-plate sclerosis may be seen, usually in younger adults. On MRI, prolapsed disks, which are low in signal on both T1-weighted and T2-weighted images, may be seen.[36,39]

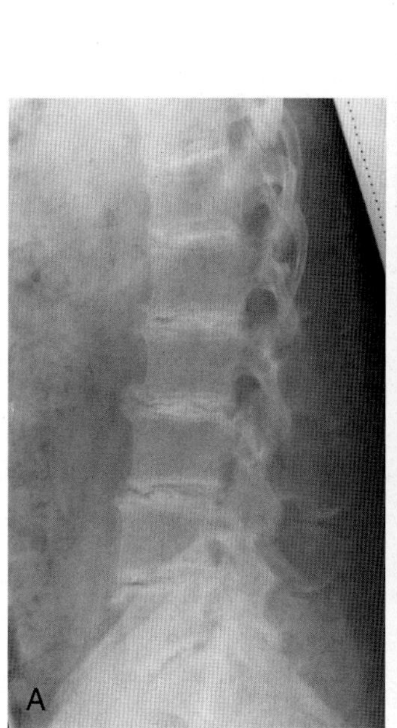

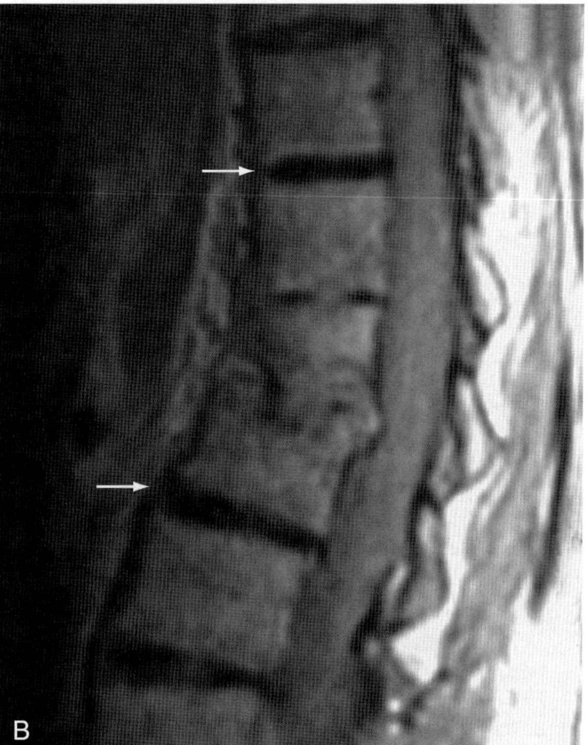

FIGURE 28-6. Disk calcification in ochronosis. **A,** Lateral radiograph of the lumbar spine shows calcification at each intervertebral disk with accompanying disk-space narrowing and gas (vacuum disks). **B,** Sagittal proton density MRI of the lumbar spine in another patient shows the intervertebral disks to be narrow and very low in signal *(arrows)*. The destruction at the T12-L1 level is due to an infection.

MRI may show low-signal disks on T1-weighted and T2-weighted images.

Some patients with advanced spine changes of ochronosis have findings resembling ankylosing spondylitis (Figure 28-7) (Box 28-5). Squaring and syndesmophyte formation may be seen in ochronosis.[40] Typically the sacroiliac (SI) joints are not fused, allowing differentiation from AS, but as in a case reported by Balaban et al.,[40] SI joint erosion and narrowing may occur. In that patient, however, the facet joints remained normal (unlike the expected fusion that occurs in ankylosing spondylitis).

FABRY DISEASE

Fabry disease is an X-linked condition in which there is decreased activity of the lysosomal enzyme α-galactosidase A.[41] This deficit leads to the accumulation of neutral glycosphingolipids especially globotriosylceramide (Gb3). This substance accumulates in lysosomes leading to cell death and organ failure and is prominent in the endothelium and media of small vessels, renal tubules and glomeruli, cardiac muscle and conducting fibers, autonomic ganglia, and cortical and brainstem structures.[42,43] Enzyme replacement therapy is available, and imaging may be a useful method of judging its efficacy.[41]

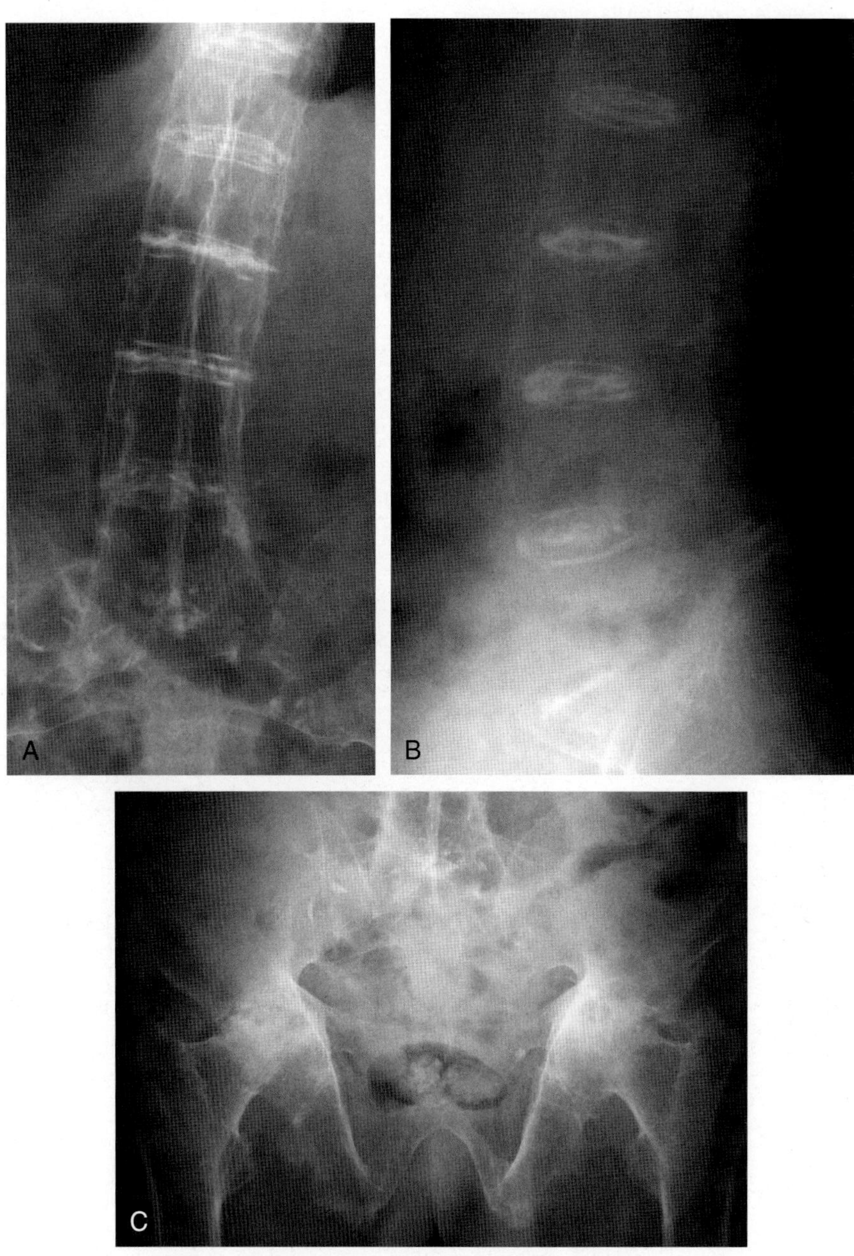

FIGURE 28-7. Changes of ankylosing spondylitis accompanying ochronosis. **A,** Anteroposterior radiograph of the lumbar spine shows calcification of each lumbar disk. **B,** The lateral radiograph confirms the calcification in the intervertebral disks and shows the bony bridging (syndesmophytes) spanning the intervertebral disks to advantage. There is marked osteopenia. **C,** An anteroposterior radiograph of the pelvis shows fusion of the sacroiliac (SI) joints, marked enthesopathy at the ischial tuberosities, and severe hip joint cartilage space narrowing. Although in this case the SI joints are fused, the typical appearance of ochronosis with ankylosing spondylitis changes shows the SI joints to remain open.

BOX 28-5. Spine Manifestations of Ochronosis

Multilevel narrow disks in the lumbar spine with end-plate sclerosis and osteopenia.
Changes begin in lumbar spine.
Multilevel prolapsed disks with low signal on T1-weighted and T2-weighted images.
Calcified disks.
Vertebral squaring and syndesmophytes, bamboo spine.
Apophyseal joints unfused (unlike ankylosing spondylitis).
SI joints may have erosion but typically are uninvolved.

Clinical Manifestations

Symptoms are more severe in men than in heterozygous women.[41] Affected individuals have a relatively shorter life span than unaffected individuals owing to the combination of chronic renal insufficiency, arterial hypertension, atherosclerosis, cerebrovascular complications, and cardiac involvement.[44] Symptoms and signs include acroparesthesia, angiokeratoma in a swimsuit distribution, corneal opacities ("cornea verticillata"), and hypohydrosis leading to heat and exercise intolerance[41] (Table 28-6). Ischemic strokes may occur at an early age and have a predilection for the vertebrobasilar system.[45]

Imaging of Central Nervous System

MRI has been helpful for diagnosis and monitoring treatment. Some of the MRI features in the central nervous system are shown in Table 28-7. White matter lesions are the most frequent abnormalities[45] (Figure 28-8).

> Isolated increased signal in the pulvinar on T1-weighted images should suggest Fabry disease.

Isolated increased signal in the pulvinar on T1-weighted images is a characteristic feature of Fabry disease and increases in frequency with increasing age.[11] In one series, corresponding increase in CT attenuation suggested that the finding was consistent with calcification.[11]

TABLE 28-6. Clinical Manifestations of Fabry Disease

Systemic	Fever Exercise and Heat Intolerance
Renal	Proteinuria Tubular dysfunction Abnormal urinalysis Arterial hypertension End-stage renal disease
Neurologic	Acroparesthesias Hypohidrosis with reduced saliva and tear formation Tinnitus, vertigo, headache Cerebrovascular accidents Psychosocial and psychiatric disease, including suicide
Skin	Angiokeratomas Lymphedema Angioma Telangiectasias
Eyes	Corneal dystrophy (cornea verticillata) Vessel tortuosity
Gastrointestinal	Intestinal dysmotility Cramps, nausea, vomiting
Cardiac	Hypertrophic infiltrative cardiomyopathy Bradyarrhythmia Abnormal mitral and aortic valves
Reproductive	Male infertility

Modified from Table 1, Kampmann C, Wiethoff CM, Perrot A, et al: The heart in Anderson Fabry disease, *Z Kardiol* 91:786-795, 2002.

> Substances that may cause increased signal on T1-weighted images include fat, calcium (chondrocalcinosis), manganese, methemoglobin, and melanin.[11]

> Disorders causing calcification of the deep gray nuclei are HIV, hypercalcemia, hypocalcemia, postirradiation, postinfarct, postinflammatory changes, and Fahr syndrome.

TABLE 28-7. MRI Findings of Fabry Disease Involving the Central Nervous System

Location	Finding	Postulated Cause
White matter	Asymmetrical, widespread deep nodules, especially frontal and parietal, hyperintense on T2W or T2 flair. Rare before 20s, usual after mid-50s Cerebral volume loss.	Ischemia or demyelinization
Grey matter	Nodules as in white matter.	May be ischemic lesions or lacunar infarcts
Deep gray nuclei	Symmetrical hyperintensity on T1W, especially lateral pulvinar. "Pulvinar sign." No corresponding calcifications on CT.	Possibly microvascular calcification
Ischemic and hemorrhagic stroke	Large and small vessel strokes with deep small vessel infarcts or lacunae in the basal ganglia.	Large and small vessel disease
Vascular abnormalities	Dolico-ectasia (vessels tortuous and dilated). Especially in posterior circulation and in large vessels.	Glycolipid deposited in vessel walls; weakening of involved large vessels

From Moore DF, Altarescu G, Herscovitch P, et al: Increased signal intensity in the pulvinar on T1-weighted images: a pathognomonic MR imaging sign of Fabry disease, *Am J Neuroradiol* 24:1096-1101, 2003; Lidove O, Klein I, Lelieure JD, et al: Imaging features of Fabry disease, *AJR Am J Roentgenol* 186:1184-1191, 2006; and Ginsberg L, Manara R, Valentine AR, et al: Magnetic resonance imaging changes in Fabry disease, *Acta Paediatr Suppl* 95:57-62, 2006. [See comment.]

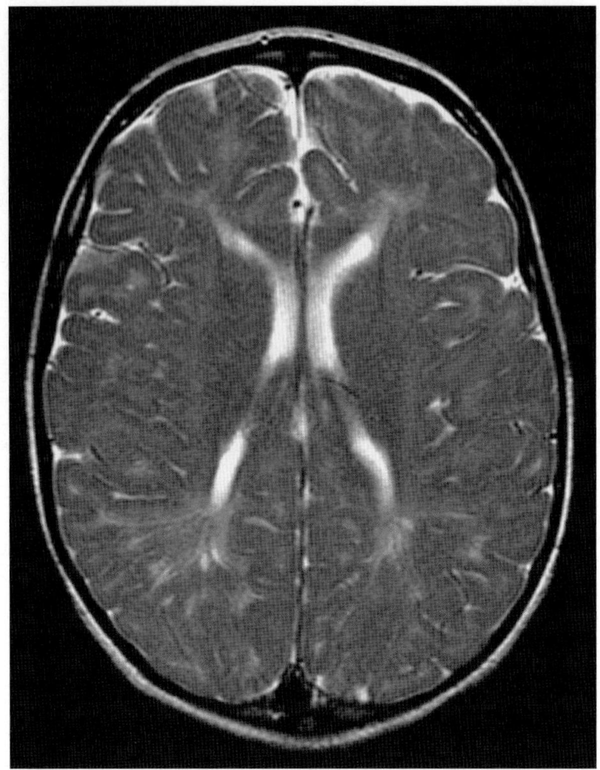

FIGURE 28-8. Fabry Disease. This axial T2-weighted MRI image shows anterior and posterior increased signal in the white matter. This finding is nonspecific. (Courtesy Caroline Robson, MD.)

PET scanning has shown increased cerebral blood flow in the posterior circulation.[11] MRI has been shown to be a more sensitive measure of disease progression (which may occur even during treatment) than neurologic examination.[46] Spectroscopy and diffusion tensor imaging have demonstrated abnormalities in regions thought to be normal on MRI.[43,45]

Musculoskeletal Manifestations

There are minimal musculoskeletal findings of this disorder. Avascular necrosis may occur.[41]

Cardiac

Involvement of the heart is frequent and can be assessed and followed using MRI.[47] Abnormalities include LV hypertrophic infiltrative cardiomyopathy, valve abnormalities, arrhythmias, conduction abnormalities, and coronary artery disease.[44] Valve changes are thought to be due to lipid accumulation and fibrosis. Abnormalities increase with age.[44] A variant of the condition affects primarily the heart, and this should be considered in patients with LV hypertrophy.[44]

Lidove et al.[41] have reviewed the imaging findings in Fabry disease and enumerated specific MRI sequences and postprocessing that they felt were necessary for evaluation. Myocardial fibrosis occurs, which is most prominent in the basal inferolateral wall. MRI examination shows LV hypertrophy with thick hyperenhancing bands in men and patchy nodular involvement in women.[41] Unlike myocardial infarction, the involvement is not subendocardial. Valve thickening may occur. MRI demonstrates the above changes, and postprocessing allows LV mass, end-diastolic and end-systolic volumes, LV ejection fraction, and LV mass to be determined.

Renal

Renal involvement leads to proteinuria and renal failure may occur, typically after the fourth decade in men.[41] Cortical or parapelvic cysts are the most common finding.

> Multiple renal sinus cysts in a patient with renal disease should suggest the possibility of Fabry disease.

Ries et al.[48] found parapelvic cysts of variable size in half of 24 patients with Fabry disease but in only 7% of control patients. The prevalence of cysts increased with patient age. Other findings are noted in Box 28-6.

Pulmonary

The pathogenesis of pulmonary involvement is uncertain. Cough, wheezing, and dyspnea may occur. Radiographs may be normal, although hyperinflation, bullae or bibasilar opacities, and interstitial prominence have been reported.[49] Kim et al.[49] reported a patient who exhibited a CT pattern of mixed areas of ground-glass opacity and hyperlucent areas due to air trapping, with changes most prominent in the upper lobes. The CT appearance improved and the pulmonary symptoms lessened on enzyme replacement therapy.

Monitoring Treatment

The classical form of Fabry's disease affects both the quality of life, leading to chronic renal failure in most patients, and its duration, leading to a reduced survival by 15 to 20 years compared to unaffected individuals.[44] Imaging, particularly MRI, may be useful in monitoring the effects of treatment.[41] Central nervous system lesions may persist, worsen, or disappear on MRI after treatment. Areas of slightly increased T2 signal seen early in the course of treatment in the deep grey nuclei have been attributed to edema.[41] LV mass is a useful measure of prognosis and treatment efficacy. Valve thickening should also be monitored.

MULTICENTRIC RETICULOHISTIOCYTOSIS

Multicentric reticulohistiocytosis (MCRH) is a rare systemic condition that primarily affects the skin and synovium, resulting in an erosive, deforming polyarthritis.[50] There are several synonyms for this disorder, including lipoid dermatoarthritis and lipoid rheumatism.[50] The disorder is categorized as one of the non–Langerhans cell histiocytoses.[51]

Clinical Features and Incidence

Caucasians predominate among affected individuals, and two or three times as many females as males have the disorder.[50] The polyarthritis is symmetrical, may involve multiple joints, and may precede the appearance of the typical skin nodules by 6 or more years.[51]

BOX 28-6. Renal Imaging Findings in Fabry Disease

Cortical or Parapelvic Cysts
Increased echogenicity on ultrasound
Decreased cortical thickness with normal renal size
Decreased corticomedullary differentiation on MRI

There is no specific laboratory test for MCRH, and histology is necessary to confirm the diagnosis.

Interphalangeal involvement is typical and the distal interphalangeal (DIP) joints in particular may be involved.

> Conditions with prominent DIP joint involvement include osteoarthritis, psoriatic arthritis, and MCRH.[52]

Rapid progression of joint damage is a clinical hallmark and results in "arthritis mutilans" in about half of patients with MCRH. Bone loss at the interphalangeal joints causes an "opera glass" or "concertina" deformity.[50,51]

The characteristic skin nodules are tan to reddish-brown and are especially prominent near the ears, nasal bridge, scalp, dorsal aspects of the hands, and nail beds.[50,51]

> The small masses around the nail folds, called "coral beads," are a typical clinical sign of MCRH.[51]

Severe facial involvement may lead to a deformity known as *leonine facies.* Other tissues may also be involved, including the oral mucosa, lungs, larynx,[53] pleura, hilar lymph nodes, pericardium, liver, perirenal fat and muscle, stomach, and endocardium.[51,53-55] Systemic manifestations such as weight loss, malaise, and fever are common.[51]

Although the cause is unknown, a reactive process is postulated. Several conditions have been found in association with MCRH, including autoimmune diseases, mycobacterial infection, hypothyroidism, diabetes, and especially malignancy.[51,56] Almost one third of patients have or develop a malignancy.[51]

> The possibility of a malignancy should be excluded in all cases of MCRH.[51]

Histologic Features

The nodules or synovitis are characterized by granulomas with minimal accompanying inflammation.[50] The hallmark of the skin and subcutaneous nodules is the presence of multinucleate, lipid-laden histiocytes.[50] The nuclei within the giant cells are bizarre in appearance and are arranged centrally or peripherally.[57] The cytoplasm of the mononuclear histiocytes and multinucleated, foreign body–type giant cells is described as "ground glass," eosinophilic, and PAS (periodic acid–Schiff) positive. Masses in other locations demonstrate the same histologic features.

Affected synovium has exhibited positive staining for interleukin-1Beta (IL-1B, IL-6) and tumor necrosis factor alpha. Abundant cytokine production was also noted.[58] These factors can stimulate bone resorption,[58] and their presence has suggested that treatment with bisphosphonates or anti TNF-alpha might be appropriate.[59]

Radiographic Features

Radiographic features are characteristic and may be diagnostic (Figure 28-9). These include the following (Box 28-7):

- Bilateral symmetrical arthritis, particularly involving the interphalangeal joints
- Uncalcified nodules of the skin subcutaneous tissues and tendon sheaths
- Sharply circumscribed erosions that begin marginally and progress centrally leading to juxtaarticular bone loss
- Atlantoaxial involvement
- Minimal symptoms despite severe disease
- Minimal or absent osteoporosis
- Minimal or absent periosteal reaction[51,52,57,60-63]

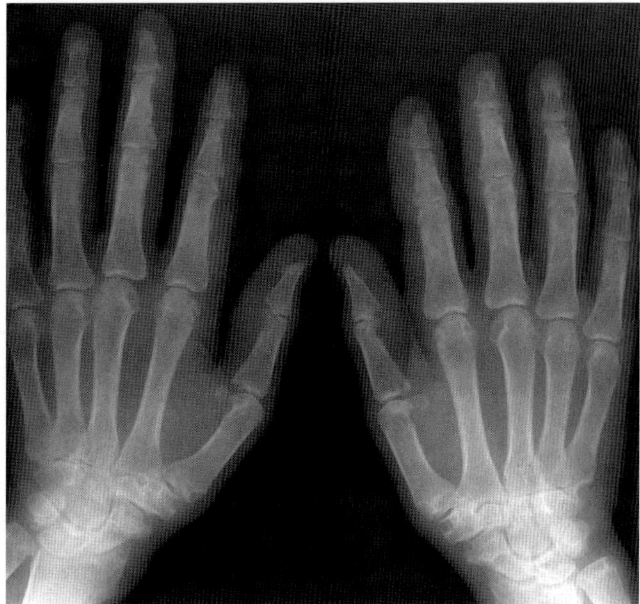

FIGURE 28-9. Multicentric reticulohistiocytosis. Posteroanterior radiograph of both hands and wrists shows well-defined erosions in the wrists *(arrows).* There is erosion of the distal interphalangeal joints and resorption of the terminal tufts, best seen in the thumbs. The soft tissues of the fingers appear enlarged and slightly lobulated in contour. (Courtesy of Piran Aliabadi, MD, Boston.)

BOX 28-7. Radiographic Features of MCRH

- Bilateral symmetrical involvement
- Interphalangeal involvement, especially distal interphalangeal joints
- Uncalcified soft tissue nodules
- Sharply delineated erosions that begin at margins of a synovial joint and progress centrally
- Rapid progression of damage
- Absent or minimal osteoporosis
- Absent or minimal periosteal reaction
- Atlantoaxial involvement (may be rapid and severe)
- "Opera-glass" deformities
- Lytic skull lesions[63]
- Pathologic fracture of femur[58]
- Temporomandibular joint involvement in 10%[53]
- Sacroiliac joint erosion

The radiographic features are thought to be highly suggestive of the disorder. Furthermore, because the skin lesions are often a delayed feature, radiographic findings may be important in establishing the diagnosis.

> In patients with reticulohistiocytosis, polyarthritis precedes the development of skin changes by an average of 3 years.[50]

Differential diagnosis radiographically includes several conditions (Table 28-9). Psoriatic arthritis, in particular, may produce similar radiographic findings with interphalangeal involvement that may result in extensive bone loss in the absence of osteoporosis. However, fluffy periosteal reaction about the erosions (producing the "mouse ears" appearance) or bony ankylosis that are

TABLE 28-9. Differential Diagnosis of the Radiographic Features of MCRH

Disease	Differentiating Features from MR
Psoriatic arthritis	Asymmetrical, periosteal reaction produces fluffy margins to the erosions. Bony ankylosis may occur. Most patients have skin lesions and no nodules.
Gout	Distribution is asymmetrical, and damage is slowly progressive. Nodules may calcify or ossify.
Rheumatoid arthritis	Osteoporosis is typical. Distal joint involvement is not typical.
Sarcoidosis	Lace-like pattern of bone destruction is typical and not a feature of MCRH.
Dialysis arthropathy	Distal joints may be affected; the history is typical.
Osteoarthritis	Osteophytes are typical in osteoarthritis.
Fibroblastic rheumatism	Symmetrical arthritis (prominent DIP involvement), sclerodactyly and "flesh-colored" skin nodules are present. Raynaud's is usually present. Sclerodactyly and Raynaud's are not features of MCRH.[64]

characteristic features of psoriatic arthritis are not seen in MCRH. Also, the nodules that are so characteristic of MCRH are not present in psoriatic arthritis.

Scinigraphic Features

Suga et al.[65] reported abnormal uptake of gallium-67 citrate in the soft tissues around the symmetrically involved joints and in the superficial and deep muscles of the chest wall, neck, back, and perineum, as well as in hilar and mediastinal lymph nodes. Isotope uptake in muscles was more apparent than abnormalities seen on contrast-enhanced CT examination of the same subject.

CT Features

CT examination of a proven supraglottic MCRH mass lesion showed the mass to enhance after intravenous contrast.[53] In another case report, CT showed a nodule of MCRH to appear as a nonspecific 8 × 4–cm mass of reduced attenuation in the serratus anterior muscle.[55] The mass demonstrated early and intense rim enhancement and conformed to the shape of the chest.

MRI Features

A few reports of the MRI appearance of MCRH of the knee have been published.[66,67] Yamada et al.[67] reported knee imaging in a patient with MCRH to reveal bulky intraarticular masses that were intermediate in signal intensity on T1-weighted images and relatively high in signal on T2-weighted images. Small interspersed areas of low signal intensity on both T1-weighted and T2-weighted images were confirmed histologically to be due to hemosiderin deposition.

Treatment

The treatment of MCRH has not been established, and the interested reader is referred to a review by Trotta et al.[51] for an overview of treatment options. Because of the severity of the arthritis and the disfiguring skin manifestations, the need for aggressive therapy is usually emphasized, although an intermittent course is possible and quiescence may occur spontaneously.[53] Underlying malignancy and active tuberculosis should be excluded prior to treatment.[60] Immunosuppressive drugs, especially methotrexate and cyclophosphamide, cytotoxic agents, anti-TNF alpha agents, and alendronate have been used.[51] Corticosteroids alone do not appear to control the disease.[51]

REFERENCES

1. Pietrangelo A: Hereditary hemochromatosis—a new look at an old disease, *N Engl J Med* 350:2383-2397, 2004. [See comment.]
2. Tanglao EC, Stern MA, Agudelo CA: Case report: arthropathy as the presenting symptom in hereditary hemochromatosis, *Am J Med Sci* 312:306-309, 1996.
3. Adams P: Review article: the modern diagnosis and management of haemochromatosis, *Alim Pharmacol Ther* 23:1681-1691, 2006.
4. Jager HJ, Mehring U, Gotz GF, et al: Radiological features of the visceral and skeletal involvement of hemochromatosis, *Eur Radiol* 7:1199-1206, 1997.
5. Papakonstantinou O, Mohana-Borges A, Campell L, et al: Hip arthropathy in a patient with primary hemochromatosis: MR imaging findings with pathologic correlation, *Skel Radiol* 34:180-184, 2005.
6. Lwakatare F, Hayashida Y, Yamashita Y: MR imaging of hepatocellular carcinoma arising in genetic hemochromatosis, *Magn Reson Med Sci* 2:57-59, 2003.
7. Schumacher HR Jr: Hemochromatosis and arthritis, *Arthritis Rheum* 7:41-50, 1964.
8. Adamson TC 3rd, Resnick CS, Guerra J Jr, et al: Hand and wrist arthropathies of hemochromatosis and calcium pyrophosphate deposition disease: distinct radiographic features, *Radiology* 147:377-381, 1983.
9. Axford JS, Bomford A, Revell P, et al: Hip arthropathy in genetic hemochromatosis. Radiographic and histologic features, *Arthritis Rheum* 34:357-361, 1991.
10. Schmid H, Struppler C, Braun GS, et al: Ankle and hindfoot arthropathy in hereditary hemochromatosis, *J Rheumatol* 30:196-199, 2003.
11. Moore DF, Ye F, Schiffmann R, et al: Increased signal intensity in the pulvinar on T1-weighted images: a pathognomonic MR imaging sign of Fabry disease, *Am J Neuroradiol* 24:1096-1101, 2003.
12. Mortele KJ, Ros PR: MR imaging in chronic hepatitis and cirrhosis, *Semin Ultrasound CT MR* 23:79-100, 2002.
13. Piekarski J, Goldberg HI, Royal SA, et al: Difference between liver and spleen CT numbers in the normal adult: its usefulness in predicting the presence of diffuse liver disease, *Radiology* 137:727-729, 1980.
14. Chapman RW, Williams G, Bydder G, et al: Computed tomography for determining liver iron content in primary haemochromatosis, *BMJ* 280:440-442, 1980.
15. Gandon Y, Guyader D, Heautot JF, et al: Hemochromatosis: diagnosis and quantification of liver iron with gradient-echo MR imaging, *Radiology* 193:533-538, 1994.
16. Pomerantz S, Siegelman ES: MR imaging of iron depositional disease, *Magn Reson Imaging Clin North Am* 10:105-120, 2002.
17. Bonkovsky HL, Slaker DP, Bills EB, et al: Usefulness and limitations of laboratory and hepatic imaging studies in iron-storage disease, *Gastroenterology* 99:1079-1091, 1990.
18. St Pierre TG, Clarke PR, Chua-anusorn W, et al: Noninvasive measurement and imaging of liver iron concentrations using proton magnetic resonance, *Blood* 105:855-861, 2005.
19. Alustiza JM, Artetxe J, Castiella A, et al: MR quantification of hepatic iron concentration, *Radiology* 230:479-484, 2004.
20. Ptaszek LM, Price ET, Hu MY, et al: Early diagnosis of hemochromatosis-related cardiomyopathy with magnetic resonance imaging, *J Cardiovasc Magn Reson* 7:689-692, 2005.
21. Cheong B, Huber S, Muthupillai R, et al: Evaluation of myocardial iron overload by T2* cardiovascular magnetic resonance imaging, *Texas Heart Inst J* 32:448-449, 2005.
22. Burke DM, McCartney WH, Lesesne HR, et al: Secondary hemochromatosis: diagnosis by MRI, *Am Fam Physician* 43:771, 1991.
23. Hennemeyer C, Sundaram M: Radiologic case study. Post-transfusioal reticuloendothelial system iron overload of sickle cell disease secondary hemochromatosis, *Orthopedics.* Apr;23:(4):303, 398-400, 2000.
24. Siegelman ES, Mitchell DG, Rubin R, et al: Parenchymal versus reticuloendothelial iron overload in the liver: distinction with MR imaging, *Radiology* 179:361-366, 1991. [See comment.]
25. Vande Berg BC, Malghem J, Lecouvete FE, et al: Magnetic resonance imaging of normal bone marrow, *Eur Radiol* 8:1327-1334, 1998.
26. Kitzberger R, Madl C, Ferenci P: Wilson disease, *Metab Brain Dis* 20:295-302, 2005.
27. Kataoka M, Tsumura H, Itonga I, et al: Subchondral cyst of the tibia secondary to Wilson disease, *Clin Rheumatol* 23:460-463, 2004.
28. Balint G, Szebenyi B: Hereditary disorders mimicking and/or causing premature osteoarthritis, *Best Pract Res Clin Rheumatol* 14:219-250, 2000.
29. Hammoudeh M, Siam AR: Pseudogout in a young patient, *Clin Rheumatol* 17:242-245, 1998.
30. Akhan O, Akpinar E, Oto A, et al: Unusual imaging findings in Wilson's disease, *Eur Radiol* 12(Suppl 3):S66-S69, 2002.

31. Sinha S, Taly AB, Ravishanker S, et al: Wilson's disease: cranial MRI observations and clinical correlation, *Neuroradiology* 48(9):613-621, 2006.
32. Hitoshi S, Iwata M, Yoshikawa K: Mid-brain pathology of Wilson's disease: MRI analysis of three cases, *J Neurol Neurosurg Psychiatry* 54:624-626, 1991.
33. Kuruvilla A, Joseph A: "Face of the giant panda" sign in Wilson's disease: revisited, *Neurol India* 48(4):395-396, 2000.
34. Jacobs DA, Markowitz CE, Liebeskind DS, et al: The "double panda sign" in Wilson's disease, *Neurology* 61:969, 2003.
35. Cordato DJ, Fulham MJ, Yiannikas C: Pretreatment and posttreatment positron emission tomographic scan imaging in a 20-year-old patient with Wilson's disease, *Mov Disord* 13:162-166, 1998.
36. Choudhury R, Rajamani SS, Rajshekhar V: A case of ochronosis: MRI of the lumbar spine, *Neuroradiology* 42:905-907, 2000.
37. Keller JM, Macaula YW, Nercesslan OA, et al: New developments in ochronosis: review of the literature, *Rheumatol Int* 25:81-85, 2005.
38. Hamdi N, Cooke TD, Hassan B: Ochronotic arthropathy: case report and review of the literature, *Int Orthop* 23:122-125, 1999.
39. Izzo L, Caputo M, Costi U, et al: Risonanza magnetica e radiologia tradizionale nelle localizzazioni vertebrali dell'artropatia ocronotica alcaptonurica, *Giornale Chirurgia* 26:78-82, 2005.
40. Balaban B, Taskaynatar M, Yasar E, et al: Ochronotic spondyloarthropathy: spinal involvement resembling ankylosing spondylitis, *Clin Rheumatol* 25:598-601, 2006.
41. Lidove O, Klein I, Lelievre JD, et al: Imaging features of Fabry disease, *AJR Am J Roentgenol* 186: 1184-1191, 2006.
42. MacDermot KD, Holmes A, Miners AH: Anderson-Fabry disease: clinical manifestations and impact of disease in a cohort of 98 hemizygous males, *J Med Genet* 38: 750-760, 2001.
43. Fellgiebel A, Mazanek M, Whybra C, et al: Pattern of microstructural brain tissue alterations in Fabry disease: a diffusion-tensor imaging study, *J Neurol* 253:780-787, 2006.
44. Kampmann C, Wiethoff CM, Perrot A, et al: The heart in Anderson Fabry disease, *Z Kardiol* 91:786-795, 2002.
45. Ginsberg L, Manara R, Valentine AR, et al: Magnetic resonance imaging changes in Fabry disease, *Acta Paediatr Suppl* 95:57-62, 2006. [See comment.]
46. Jardim L, Vedolin L, Schwartz IV, et al: CNS involvement in Fabry disease: clinical and imaging studies before and after 12 months of enzyme replacement therapy, *J Inherit Metab Dis* 27:229-240, 2004.
47. Bhatia GS, Leahy JF, Connolly DL, et al: Severe left ventricular hypertrophy in Anderson-Fabry disease, *Heart* 90:1136, 2004.
48. Ries M, Bettis KE, Choyke P, et al: Parapelvic kidney cysts: a distinguishing feature with high prevalence in Fabry disease, *Kidney Int* 66:978-982, 2004.
49. Kim W, Pyeritz RE, Bernhardt BA, et al: Pulmonary manifestations of Fabry disease and positive response to enzyme replacement therapy, *Am J Med Genet Part A* 143:377-381, 2007.
50. Gold RH, Metzer AL, Mirra JM, et al: Multicentric reticulohistiocytosis (lipoid dermato-arthritis). An erosive polyarthritis with distinctive clinical, roentgenographic and pathologic features, *Am J Roentgenol Radium Ther Nucl Med* 124:610-624, 1975.
51. Trotta F, Castellino G, Lo Monaco A: Multicentric reticulohistiocytosis, *Best Pract Res Clin Rheumatol* 18:759-772, 2004.
52. Brodey PA: Multicentric reticulohistiocytosis: a rare cause of destructive polyarthritis, *Radiology* 114:327-328, 1975.
53. Malhotra R, Pribitkin EA, Bough ID, et al: Upper airway involvement in multicentric reticulohistiocytosis, *Otolaryngol Head Neck Surg* 114:661-664, 1996.
54. Fast A: Cardiopulmonary complications in multicentric reticulohistiocytosis. Report of a case, *Arch Dermatol* 112:1139-1141, 1976.
55. Kamel H, Gibson G, Cassidy M: Case report: the CT demonstration of soft tissue involvement in multicentric reticulohistiocytosis, *Clin Radiol* 51:440-441, 1996.
56. Maki DD, Caperton EM, Griffiths HJ: Radiologic case study. Multicentric reticulohistiocytosis, *Orthopedics* 18:77, 1995.
57. Gold RH, Bassett LW, Seeger LL: The other arthritides. Roentgenologic features of osteoarthritis, erosive osteoarthritis, ankylosing spondylitis, psoriatic arthritis, Reiter's disease, multicentric reticulohistiocytosis, and progressive systemic sclerosis, *Radiol Clin North Am* 26:1195-1212, 1988.
58. Nakamura H, Yoshino S, Shiga H, et al: A case of spontaneous femoral neck fracture associated with multicentric reticulohistiocytosis: oversecretion of interleukin-1beta, interleukin-6, and tumor necrosis factor alpha by affected synovial cells, *Arthritis Rheum* 40: 2266-2270, 1997.
59. Kovach BT, Calamia KT, Walsh JS, et al: Treatment of multicentric reticulohistiocytosis with etanercept, *Arch Dermatol* 140:919-921, 2004. [See comment.]
60. Campbell DA, Edwards NL: Multicentric reticulohistiocytosis: systemic macrophage disorder, *Baillieres Clin Rheumatol* 5:301-319, 1991.
61. Wright GD, Doherty M: Unusual but memorable. Multicentric reticulohistiocytosis, *Ann Rheum Dis* 56:134, 1997.
62. Scutellari PN, Orzincolo C, Trotta F: Case report 375: Multicentric reticulohistiocytosis, *Skel Radiol* 15:394-397, 1986.
63. Ho SG, Yu RC: A case of multicentric reticulohistiocytosis with multiple lytic skull lesions, *Clin Exp Dermatol* 30:515-518, 2005.
64. Romas E, Finlay M, Woodruff T: The arthropathy of fibroblastic rheumatism, *Arthritis Rheum* 40:183-187, 1997. [See comment.]
65. Suga K, Ogasawara N, Motoyama K, et al: Ga-67 scintigraphic findings in a case of multicentric reticulohistiocytosis, *Clin Nucl Med* 27:144-145, 2002.
66. Baghestani S, Khosravi F, Dehghani-Zahedani M, et al: Multicentric reticulohistiocytosis presenting with papulonodular skin eruption and polyarthritis, *Eur J Dermatol* 15:196-200, 2005.
67. Yamada T, Kurohori YN, Kashiwazaki S, et al: MRI of multicentric reticulohistiocytosis, *J Computer Assisted Tomogr* 20:838-840, 1996.

CHAPTER 29

Paget's Disease, Fibrous Dysplasia, Sarcoidosis, and Amyloidosis of Bone

HAKAN ILASLAN, MD, *and* MURALI SUNDARAM, MD, FRCR

KEY FACTS

Paget's Disease

- The cause of Paget's disease is not known.
- Patients are frequently asymptomatic.
- It is often an incidental finding on imaging studies.
- It is usually seen after the fourth decade.
- The pelvis, femora, tibia, vertebra, and sacrum are favored locations.
- Three phases are distinguishable: lytic, intermediate, and sclerotic.
- Involvement may be monostotic or polyostotic and asymmetric.
- The "blade of grass" appearance and involvement that include the end of a bone usually allow the lytic phase of Paget's disease to be correctly identified on radiographs.
- Thickened cortices and trabeculae are typical features.
- Preservation of normal marrow fat is a characteristic finding of the lytic phase of Paget's disease on magnetic resonance imaging (MRI) and allows it to be distinguished from most tumors.
- Paget's bone may not be hypermetabolic on positron emission tomography scanning (unlike many tumors).
- Complications of Paget's disease include fractures (incomplete or complete), benign or malignant tumors, and degenerative arthritis.
- MRI is usually reliable in separating secondary sarcoma from uncomplicated Paget's disease.

Fibrous Dysplasia

- Designated a neoplasm in the World Health Organization classification
- All ages affected; there is no racial/ethnic predilection.
- Monostotic lesions are more common than polyostotic.
- Most common benign lesion of a rib.
- McCune Albright syndrome (polyostotic fibrous dysplasia, café-au-lait spots and hyperfunctioning endocrinopathies).
- Mazabraud's syndrome consists of a soft-tissue myxoma and fibrous dysplasia.
- Malignancy is very rare.
- Low-grade central osteosarcoma is often misdiagnosed as fibrous dysplasia.

Sarcoidosis

- More common in blacks.
- Nonspecific synovitis; ankle synovitis should suggest the diagnosis.
- Bone lesions, lytic or sclerotic; lacy pattern in the phalanges.
- MRI demonstrates marrow lesions.
- Vertebral destruction is rare.

PAGET'S DISEASE

Paget's bone disease has been present for at least a thousand years. Human remains found in Lancashire, England dated to about 900 C.E. clearly show the characteristic osseous changes that are now recognized as Paget's disease. The disorder is named for Sir James Paget who, in 1877, provided a description so perceptive that it holds true today: "It begins in middle age or later, is very slow in progress—no other trouble than those which are due to change of shape, size and direction of the diseased bones."[1]

Etiology

The cause of Paget's disease remains unknown. Of the proposed causes, a viral etiology has some support.[2]

> The cause of Paget's disease is uncertain but likely involves genetic and environmental factors; a virus may play a role.[3]

Clinical Features

Paget's disease is common in Western society and is found in about 1% of the U.S. population over 40 years of age.[4] It appears that there has been a decline in the prevalence and severity of the disorder in recent years.[5] It usually affects individuals over the age of 40 years.[6] The disease appears to be uncommon in China, the Indian subcontinent, and Africa. Most patients with Paget's disease are asymptomatic,[7] and the disease is most frequently encountered as incidental findings on imaging studies.

Unlike other metabolic disorders, Paget's disease is unusual in that it may be monostotic or polyostotic and asymmetric.

Imaging

Virtually any bone can be affected by Paget's disease. It predominates in the pelvis, sacrum, lumbar segment of the vertebral column, calvarium, and long bones with a preference for the ends of long bones (Figures 29-1 through 29-3).

Except in the tibia, Paget's disease always involves the end of a bone.

The disease has three distinct phases: lytic, intermediate, and sclerotic (Figure 29-4). Exacerbation of the lytic phase may be encountered after the intermediate and sclerotic phases have set in. The purely lytic phase of the disease is the rarest manifestation, and only 1% to 2% of patients with Paget's disease clinically exhibit a purely lytic stage of involvement[8] (Figure 29-5). Because of the aggressive radiographic appearance of the lytic phase of Paget's disease, its relative rarity as the sole imaging finding, and the advanced age of the typical patient, the lytic phase is often confused with malignant disorders such as metastasis or lymphoma. A clue to the diagnosis of lytic Paget's disease on the radiograph of long bones is the involvement of the end of the bone and the "blade of grass" appearance in which the advancing edge of the lesion has a sharply defined, tapered contour (Table 29-1).

Technetium bone scintigraphy demonstrates a marked increase in radio-tracer accumulation. Although the marked uptake is consistent with a malignant disease process, the distribution of uptake often allows the correct diagnosis to be made. Magnetic resonance imaging (MRI), however, may permit more accurate characterization than the radiograph and suggest the correct diagnosis.

Lytic Paget's disease may be differentiated from other disorders by MRI; there is preservation of fatty marrow in lytic Paget's disease but replacement of marrow fat by tumor.

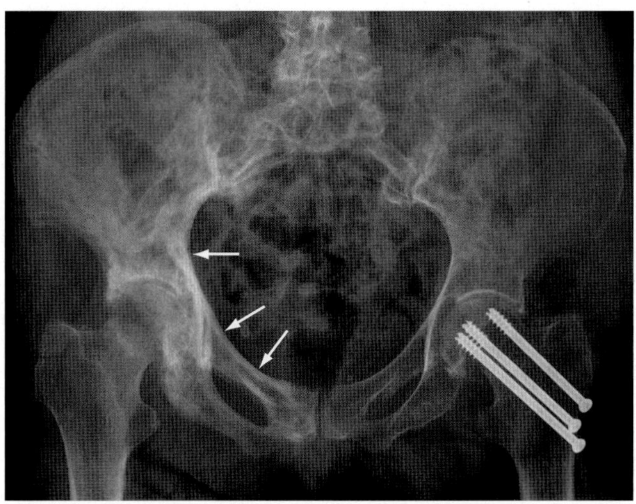

FIGURE 29-1. Paget's disease of the pelvis. Anteroposterior (AP) pelvis radiograph shows the intermediate/sclerotic phase of Paget's disease involving the right acetabulum, pubis, and ischium with thickened trabecula, cortices, and iliopectineal line *(arrows)*. The left hip was pinned for a previous fracture unrelated to Paget's disease.

In purely lytic Paget's disease, fatty marrow signal is preserved on MRI even in the presence of a radiographic lytic lesion[9] (Figure 29-5). This finding of fatty marrow preservation in osteolytic Paget's disease is entirely in keeping with the histologic appearance of resorbed bone. The destruction of bone is caused by resorption, not infiltration; hence the preservation of marrow fat signal on MRI. Because of its aggressive nature and the need to exclude a more ominous disease, MRI ought to be performed when there is difficulty in distinguishing the "osteoporosis" of resorptive changes from the infiltration of a malignant disease

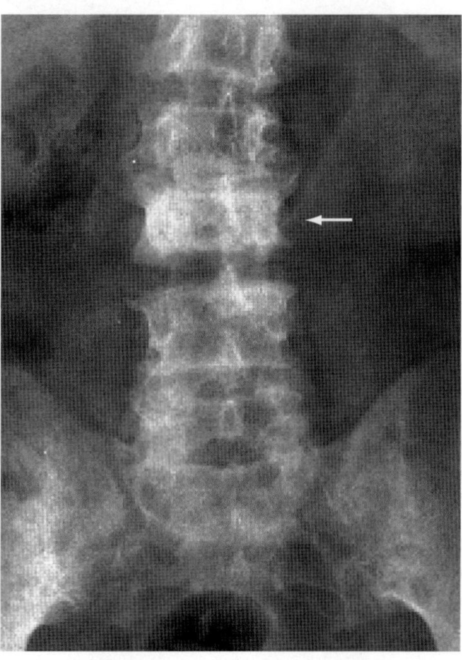

FIGURE 29-2. Vertebral involvement in Paget's disease. AP radiograph of the lumbar spine shows an enlarged and sclerotic L3 vertebra *(arrow)* with intact pedicles consistent with Paget's disease.

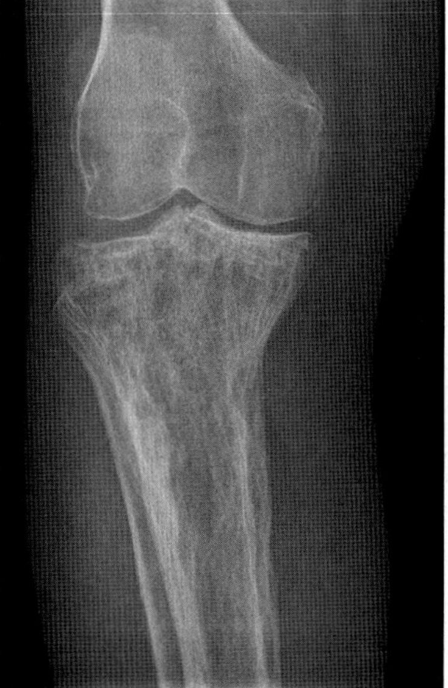

FIGURE 29-3. Characteristic long bone appearance of Paget's disease in the tibia. The coarse trabecular pattern and thickened cortices extend distally from the end of the bone. The femur, by contrast, shows normal bone architecture.

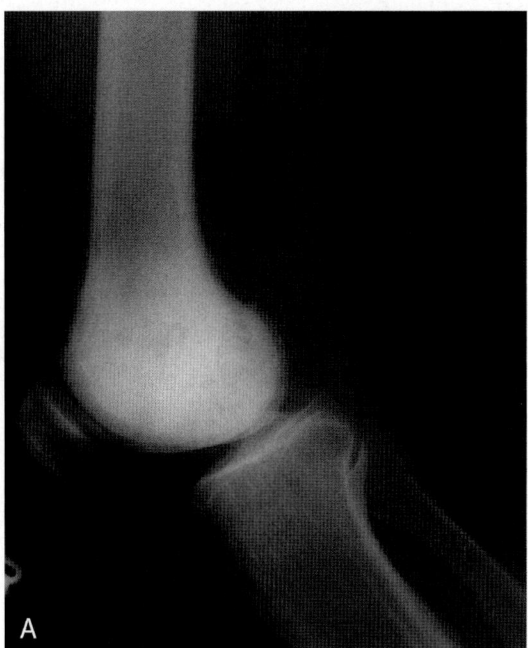

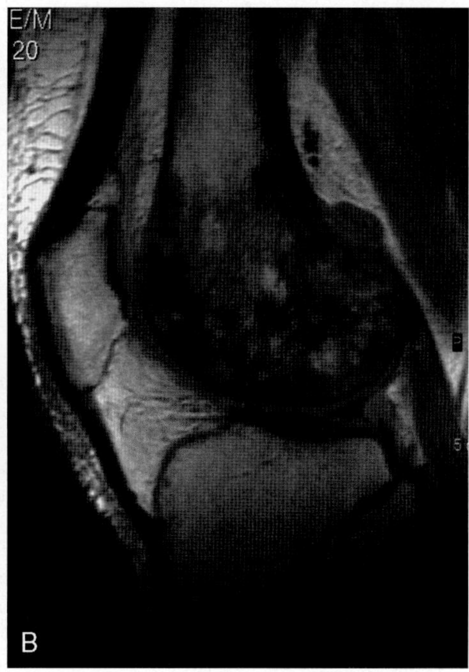

FIGURE 29-4. Biopsy proven sclerotic phase of Paget's disease mimicking osteosarcoma. **A,** A lateral radiograph of the knee shows marked sclerosis of the distal femur. The characteristic cortical and trabecular thickening observed in Paget's disease are not well seen, raising the possibility of another lesion, especially osteosarcoma. **B,** A sagittal T1-weighted MRI (TR=506 msec, TE=16 msec) shows low-signal intensity with small islands of residual, fatty marrow signal (bright signal). The retained fat suggests Paget's disease, because typically, there is no marrow fat signal identifiable within a sarcoma.

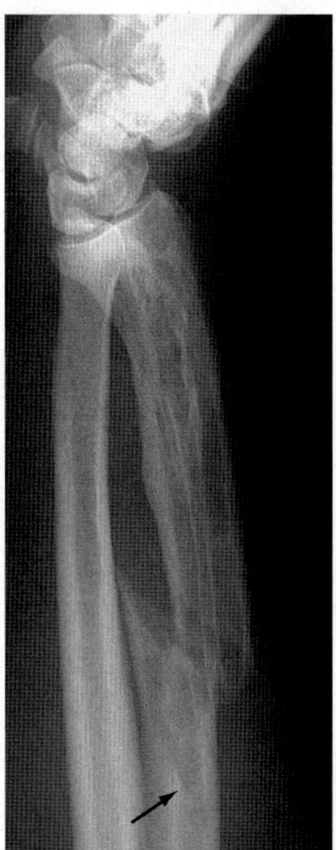

FIGURE 29-5. Lytic Paget's disease of the distal radius with a fracture. AP forearm radiograph shows thickened cortices and trabecula extending to the end of the bone. The sharply tapering end of the lucency *(arrow)* has a "blade of grass" appearance that is typical of Paget's disease.

process on radiographs (Figure 29-6). Although a bone biopsy would resolve the issue, the procedure should be avoided because of the risk of fracture.[10,11]

> Bone biopsy should be avoided if possible in lytic Paget's disease due to the risk of fracture.

An important variation in the location of lytic Paget's disease to be borne in mind is that although an exclusively diaphyseal location is exceptional, it may be observed in the tibia (Figures 29-7 and 29-8).

Intermediate and Sclerotic Phases

The intermediate phase is characterized by sclerosis, lysis, and thickened trabecula and cortices; it is the stage most frequently encountered radiographically and does not usually present a diagnostic problem (Figures 29-1 through 29-3). The sclerotic phase of Paget's disease is an advanced, late intermediate phase. As a consequence of the reparative process, an involved vertebra may become diffusely sclerotic—the so-called "ivory vertebra" (Figure 29-9). If the vertebra is enlarged and dense, the diagnosis of Paget's disease should be suggested.

> The differential diagnosis of a dense vertebra includes metastasis and lymphoma. If the vertebra is enlarged, Paget's disease should be favored.

Often a dense vertebra from Paget's disease is not expanded and has to be distinguished from a sclerotic metastasis (usually from prostate or breast cancer). In this situation, the signal characteristics of MRI may not be helpful since the signal may be low on

TABLE 29-1. Radiographic Signs of Paget's Disease

"Osteoporosis circumscripta"	Lytic Paget's disease involving the calvarium.	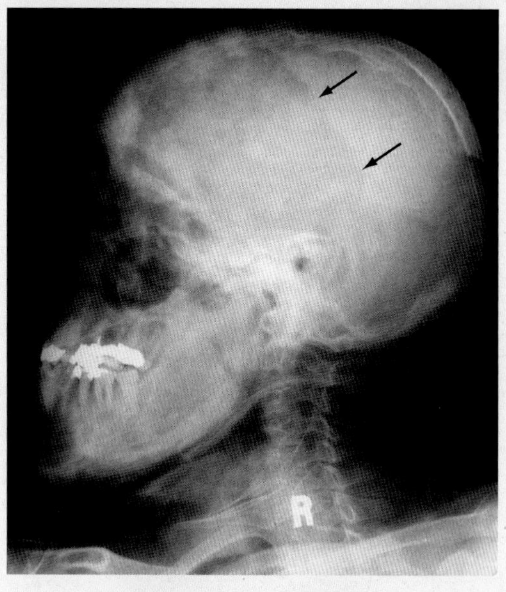
"Blade of grass"	Tapered leading edge of lytic Paget's disease in a long bone.	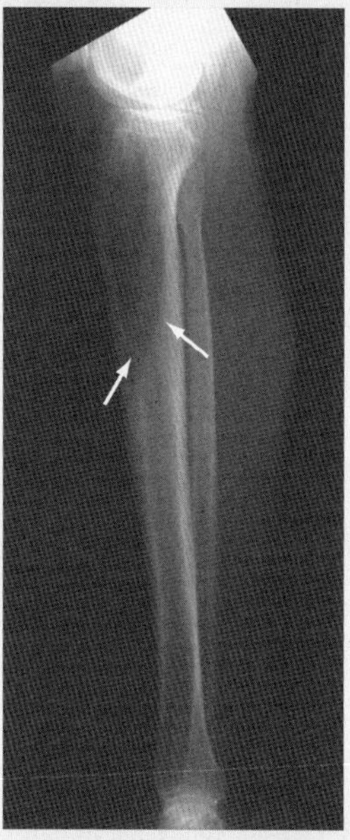
"Cotton-wool"	The areas of sclerosis in the skull. The skull is usually thickened, helping to differentiate this from metastatic disease.	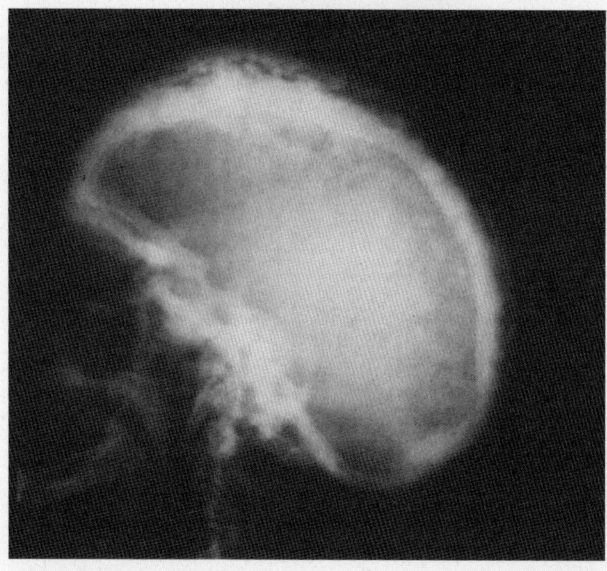

(Continued)

TABLE 29-1. Radiographic Signs of Paget's Disease—cont'd

"Picture frame"	The thickened outline of a vertebra affected by Paget's disease due to the presence of peripherally located, thickened trabecula.	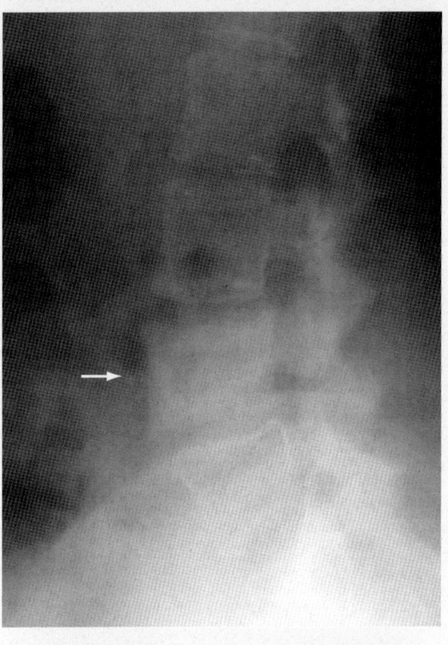
Ivory vertebra	A diffusely dense vertebral body.	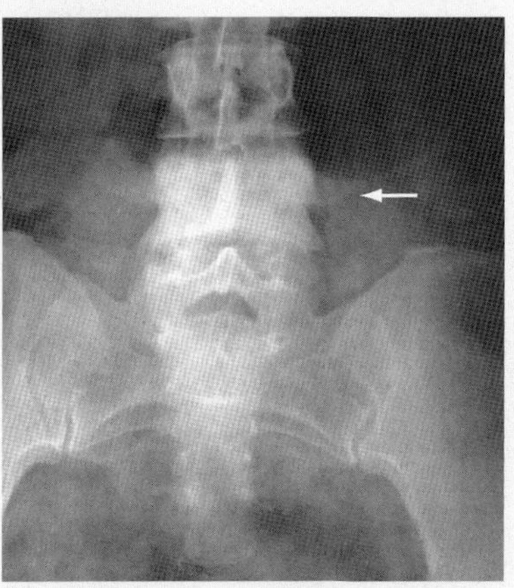
Basilar invagination	Relative upward protrusion of the bony structures around the foramen magnum.	
Platybasia	Flattening of the skull base.	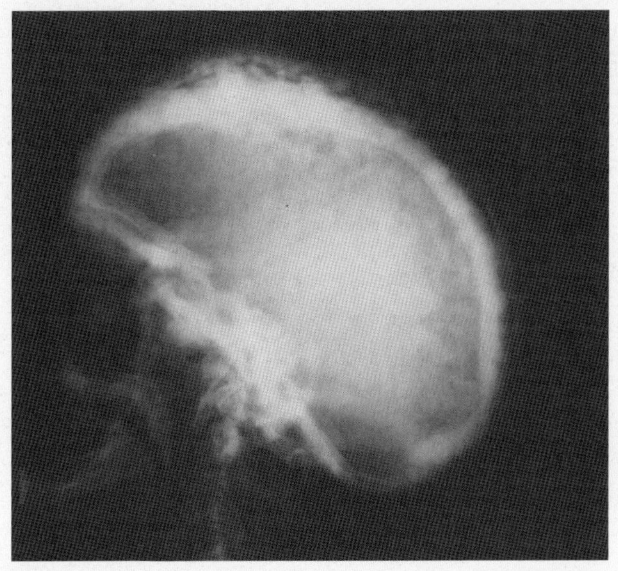

(Continued)

TABLE 29-1. Radiographic Signs of Paget's Disease—cont'd

"Brim sign"	Thickening of the bony cortex of the iliopectineal line in the pelvis.	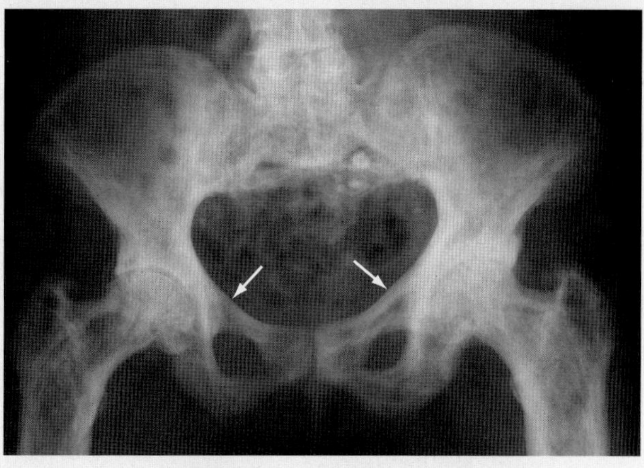
Fissure fractures	Incomplete fractures involving the convex side of a long bone.	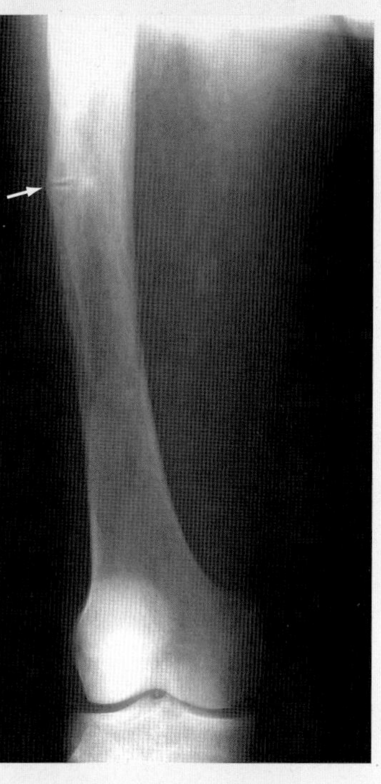

all pulse sequences due to the sclerosis. The presence of a soft tissue mass would favor a malignant etiology.

Complications of Paget's Disease

Musculoskeletal complications of Paget's disease include fractures, degenerative arthritis, and benign or malignant neoplasms.

Fractures

Fractures may be insufficiency fractures or complete fractures. Cortical insufficiency fractures, particularly in the femur and tibia, are more common than complete fractures. Insufficiency fractures may appear as single or multiple horizontal radiolucent lines favoring the convex aspects of bone, which distinguishes them from osteomalacic Looser zones that favor the concave aspects of long bones.

> Insufficiency fractures in long bones involved by Paget's disease involve the convex side of the bone.

Complete fractures are typically transverse and usually non-comminuted. They may occur spontaneously or follow minor trauma. These fractures may be seen in vertebrae and long bones with the subtrochanteric femur being the most common location.

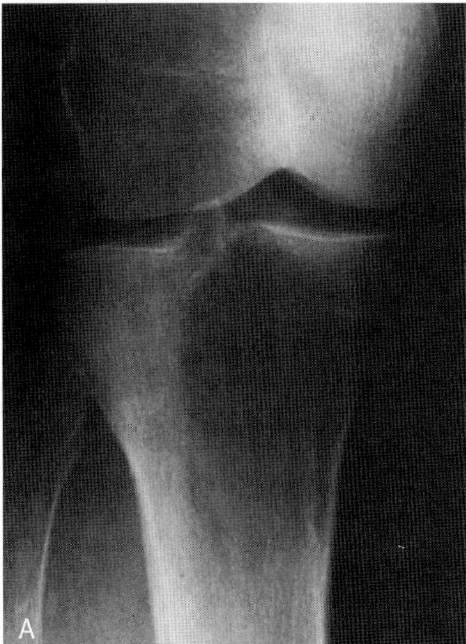

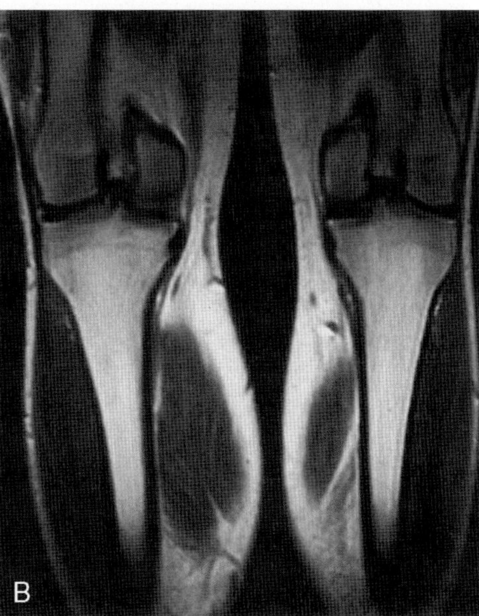

FIGURE 29-6. Lytic Paget's disease in a 69-year-old male mimicking malignancy. The radiograph shows a "lytic" subarticular lesion. The absence of a sclerotic margin to the lesion or the typical features of Paget's disease are suggestive of a malignant disease process. A T1-weighted coronal MRI (TR 500 msec, TE 13 msec) shows preservation of fatty marrow signal, which would preclude a bone neoplasm, benign or malignant and is seen in osteolytic Paget's disease.

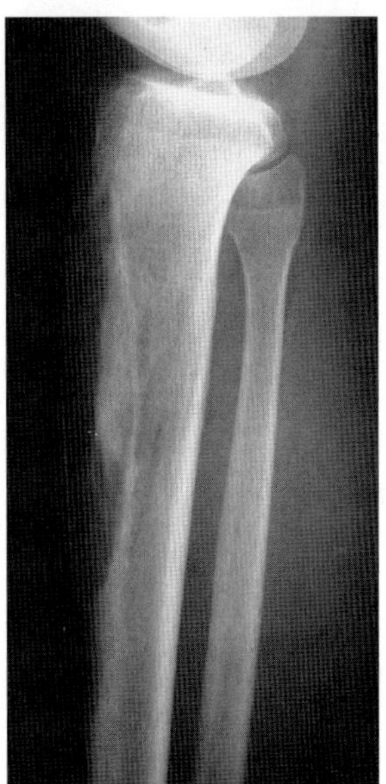

FIGURE 29-7. Diametaphyseal Paget's sparing the end of the bone and involving the tibial tubercle. In all other long bones, Paget's disease extends to the end of the bone. (Courtesy of T. Moore, MD, University of Nebraska Medical Center.)

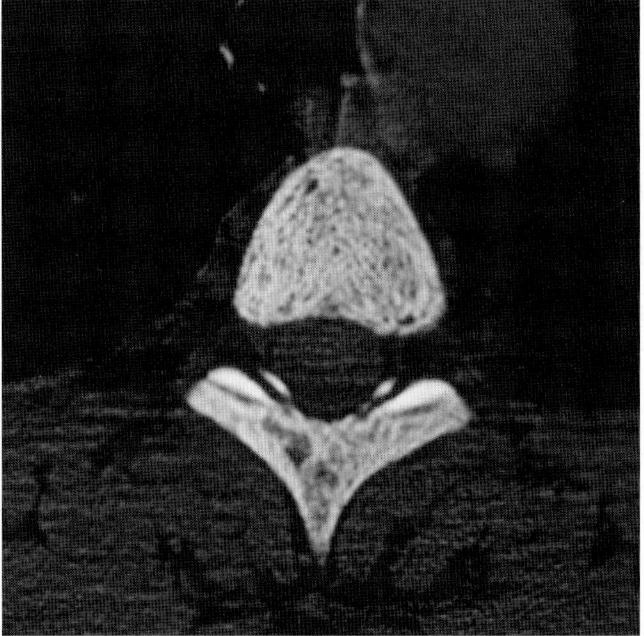

FIGURE 29-8. Ivory vertebra in Paget's disease. A CT image shows a dense but unexpanded vertebra with involvement of the body and posterior elements. Because the characteristic vertebral enlargement and cortical and trabecular thickening Paget's disease were not present, a biopsy was performed and proved the diagnosis of an "ivory" vertebra due to Paget's disease.

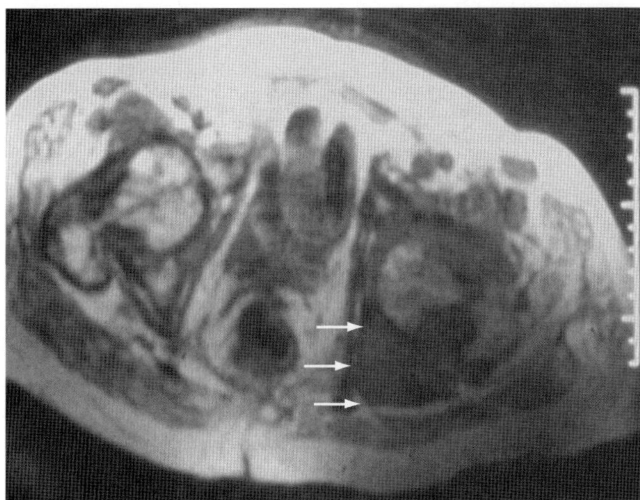

FIGURE 29-9. Paget's sarcoma of the acetabulum. A T1-weighted transverse MRI showing marrow replacement of the left acetabulum *(arrows)* due to Paget's sarcoma. The coarse trabecular pattern and fatty marrow preservation on the right are typical of uncomplicated Paget's disease.

Fractures occurring as a result of Paget's disease are typically transverse, whereas traumatic fractures have varied configurations.

Neoplasms

Although uncommon, the most dreaded and serious complication of Paget's disease is sarcomatous degeneration. The prevailing view is that sarcomatous degeneration affects about 1% of patients with Paget's disease.[12] MRI usually permits the differentiation of sarcomatous degeneration from uncomplicated Paget's disease or the intermediate phase of Paget's disease exacerbated by the lytic phase[13] (Figure 29-10). In addition, MRI is useful for tumor staging. Metastatic disease, myeloma, and lymphoma may also be superimposed on pre-existing Paget's disease.

A rare benign tumor associated with Paget's disease is a giant cell tumor. Interestingly, this tumor has been found to have a familial pattern and geographic cluster in Italian Americans whose ancestral roots were in a small town called Avellino.[14] These tumors have been known to decrease in size after treatment with corticosteroids.

Giant cell tumors in Paget's disease have been treated with corticosteroids.

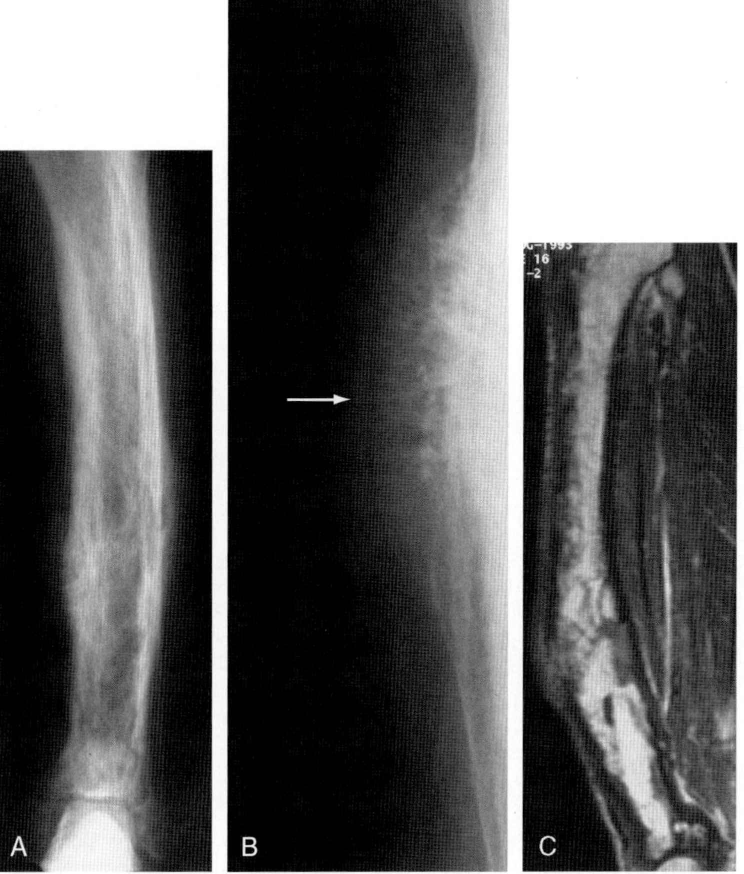

FIGURE 29-10. Aggressive periosteal reaction mimicking a sarcoma. AP radiograph **(A)** and coned view **(B)** of the distal tibia show marked aggressive periosteal reaction *(arrow)* with a soft tissue mass reminiscent of a sarcoma. **C,** Sagittal T1-weighted MRI (TR 630 msec, TE 15 msec) shows preservation of marrow signal intensity precluding a sarcoma. (Courtesy of Mark Davies, FRCR Royal Orthopedic Hospital, Birmingham England.)

Pseudosarcomas in Paget's Disease

Periosteal proliferation from Pagetic bone can produce a soft tissue mass that clinically mimics a sarcoma.[15] MRI effectively demonstrates these changes and marrow signal is usually preserved, distinguishing it from a sarcoma.[13]

Rapid Osteolysis

This phenomenon may be observed in patients with an immobilized Paget's fracture. Because sarcomas in Paget's disease are often lytic, the development of osteolysis is a cause for concern (Figure 29-11). Although we are not aware of MRI having been performed in this setting, we believe that the MRI findings will be those of osteoporosis. Thus, in a patient with an immobilized fracture through Paget's bone, the lack of marrow infiltration especially on the T1-weighted sequences, could preclude the need for a biopsy.

> Diffuse osteolysis may be observed in Paget's bone in patients whose fractures have been immobilized.

Degenerative Arthritis

The hip and knee are the most frequent sites affected by degenerative arthritis in Paget's disease. Whether there is a direct cause–effect relationship is unclear. Recent reviews of hip and knee arthroplasties in these patients report successful outcomes.[16,17]

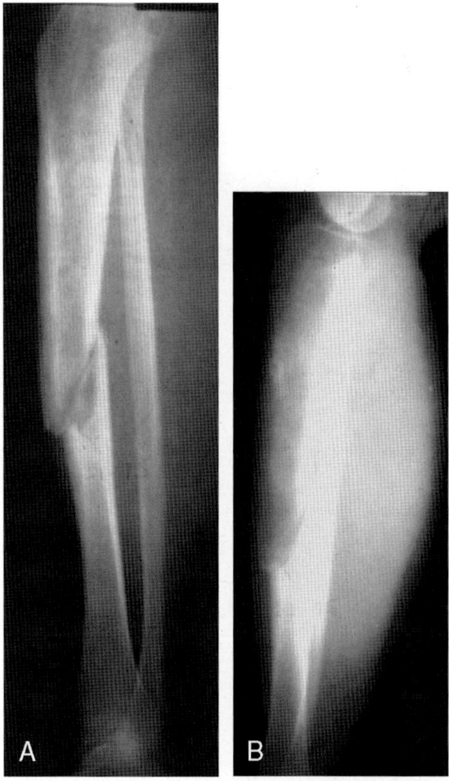

FIGURE 29-11. Tibial fracture through lytic tibial Paget's disease. **A,** Initial radiograph shows a fracture of the tibia through Paget's bone. **B,** Eight weeks later, a radiograph shows progression of aggressive osteolysis secondary to immobilization. (Courtesy of T. Moore, MD, University of Nebraska Medical Center.)

Treatment

Indications

In a review of Paget's disease, Whyte[4] outlines the following indications for treatment:

- Symptoms resulting from active bone lesions (bone pain, headache with skull involvement, back pain due to Pagetic radiculopathy or arthropathy, other neurologic syndromes, fissure fractures)
- Prophylaxis, even in asymptomatic patients, when affected sites and their metabolic hyperactivity suggest risk from progression and complications, such as fracture in weight-bearing long bones or nerve compression
- Elective surgery planned for a Pagetic site (such as total hip replacement)
- Hypercalcemia resulting from immobilization

Pharmacologic treatment of Paget's disease usually consists of a bisphosphonate or salmon calcitonin as delineated in the above review.[4]

Imaging following Medical Therapy for Paget's Disease

Location of the lesion, symptoms, and elevated serum alkaline phosphatase and urinary hydroxyproline levels have all influenced the use of therapeutic agents. Bisphosphonates are designed to inhibit bone resorption by inhibiting osteoclastic activity, leading to pain relief and biochemical response. Radiographic improvement especially after calcitonin use has been reported.[18] Scintigraphy has advantages over radiography in monitoring treatment response because changes of reduced radionuclide accumulation are easier to appreciate than are subtle radiographic changes and the radionuclide technique lends itself to quantitative assessment.[19]

Fluorine-18-FDG PET scanning of 18 asymptomatic patients with established Paget's disease revealed that the majority[14] of patients showed no uptake; uptake seen in the remainder of patients correlated with serum alkaline phosphatase elevation.[20] Authors of a more recent study of 14 patients undergoing 18^{F}-Fluoride PET scanning for monitoring bisphosphonate therapy found that baseline uptake of F18-fluoride by Pagetic bone was higher than in normal bones. These authors concluded that the maximum standard uptake value (SUV max) correlated well with biochemical markers of untreated active Paget's disease but correlated poorly in those with treated Paget's disease. Thus, markers returned to normal but SUV max was above normal.[21] These authors also concluded that SUV max alone would be sufficient for PET scanning in Paget's disease without the need for dynamic acquisition of arterial blood sampling.

Extraskeletal Complications

Systemic complications of Paget's disease are rare and include hypercalcemia (hyperparathyroidism should be excluded), increased cardiac output (atypically with heart failure), aortic valve, endocardial and arterial calcification, nephrolithiasis, or Peyronie's disease.[4] Compression of blood vessels or nerves may occur.

OSTEOFIBROUS DYSPLASIA

Osteofibrous dysplasia is almost always seen only in the tibia and fibula and predominantly involves the cortices. Some reports have suggested that this entity may be related to adamantinoma, a low-grade malignancy, because of some shared histologic features and because some cases of osteofibrous dysplasia may progress to adamantinoma. This is a controversial subject and remains under review.[22] For practical purposes, osteofibrous dysplasia is seen in the first two decades of life, while adamantinoma is seen in the third decade or after. Bone deformity with bowing of the tibia is a feature of osteofibrous dysplasia and is not usually seen with adamantinoma. Adamantinoma may rarely metastasize. Surgery for osteofibrous dysplasia is for cosmetic reasons, while biopsy and excision are mandatory for adamantinoma.

FIBROUS DYSPLASIA

The World Health Organization classifies fibrous dysplasia as a tumor of undefined neoplastic nature based on reports of clonal chromosomal aberrations.[23] Activating mutations in the GNAS1 gene have been demonstrated in both the monostotic and polyostotic forms of the disease.[24] Fibrous dysplasia (FD) is a benign, medullary fibroosseous lesion that may involve one (monostotic) or more bones (polyostotic), is encountered worldwide in children and adults, and affects all racial/ethnic groups and with an equal gender distribution. The monostotic form is six times more common than polyostotic fibrous dysplasia.

Clinical Features

The disease is usually clinically silent and is a frequently diagnosed incidental radiographic or MRI finding (Figure 29-12). Fracture or pain (usually attributed to microfracture) brings the lesion to clinical attention. The polyostotic form usually manifests earlier in life due to deformity, pain, or fracture. The McCune-Albright syndrome (MAS) is a sporadically occurring disorder that usually affects females and consists of polyostotic fibrous dysplasia (FD), café-au-lait spots, and hyperfunctioning endocrinopathies. MAS is encountered in about 3% of patients with polyostotic fibrous dysplasia[25] (Figure 29-13).

McCune-Albright syndrome usually affects females and comprises polyostotic FD, café-au-lait spots, and hyperfunctioning endocrinopathies.

The association of intramuscular myxoma and FD is known as Mazabraud's syndrome[26] (Figure 29-14). The myxomas may be seen in the monostotic and polyostotic forms of the disease.

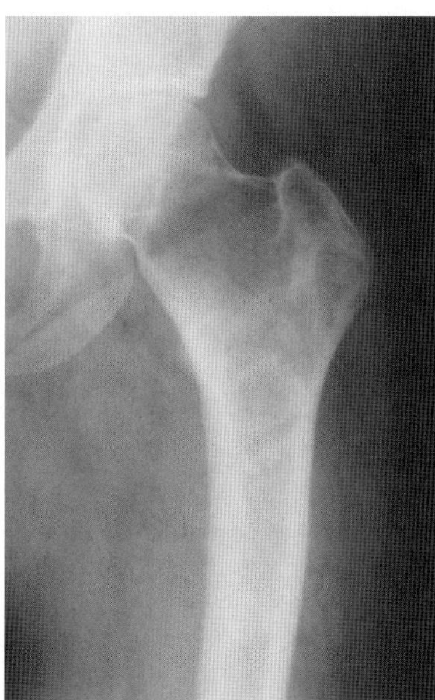

FIGURE 29-12. Fibrous dysplasia. AP radiograph of the left femur shows an expansile, osteolytic, well-marginated lesion in the femoral neck, and faint sclerosis in the subtrochanteric region.

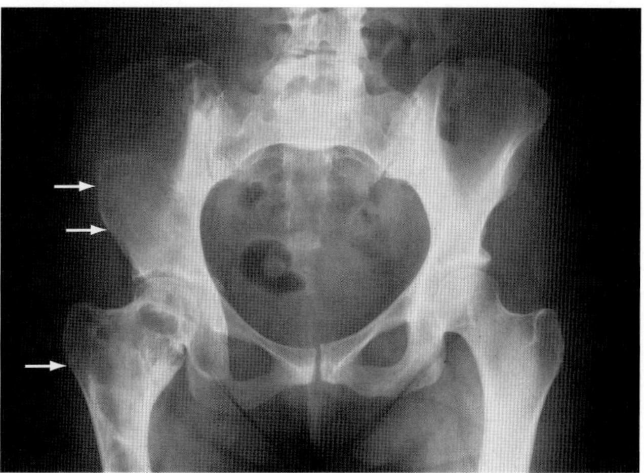

FIGURE 29-13. McCune-Albright syndrome in a 9-year-old female. Polyostotic fibrous dysplasia is present involving the right ilium, ischium, and proximal femur *(arrows)*. There is varus deformity of the femur. Endocrinopathy was also present consistent with McCune-Albright syndrome.

Mazabraud's syndrome comprises intramuscular myxomas and FD.

Malignancy arising *de novo* in FD is an exceptional occurrence.

Imaging Features

The most common sites of involvement are the ribs, femur, tibia, and humerus (Figure 29-15).

Fibrous dysplasia is the most frequent benign lesion of ribs.

Unilateral fusiform enlargement of one or more ribs is characteristic. Involvement of the hands or vertebrae is uncommon (Figure 29-16). Craniofacial involvement affects half of all patients with polyostotic disease and 10% of those with monostotic disease. The polyostotic form may have a characteristic monomelic distribution, a feature that it shares with Ollier's disease (enchondromatosis) (Figure 29-13).

FD may involve the femur alone, but when the ilium is involved, the femur is usually also involved. This may help in differential diagnosis of an ilial lesion.

The radiographic features of FD are varied and include patterns that may be lucent, sclerotic, mixed, or resembling ground glass, and a small percentage show calcification (Table 29-2). The presence of calcification in FD has led to the redundant pathologic term *fibrocartilaginous dysplasia*, which, in fact, is identical in its biologic behavior to conventional FD.[27]

The MRI features of FD reflect the heterogeneity of its histologic composition, which may include fibrovascular tissue, cysts, and secondary aneurysmal bone cysts. An expansile lesion of FD usually reflects the development of secondary aneurysmal bone cyst—a diagnosis readily made by correlating MRI with radiographic findings. Although malignancy in nonirradiated FD is rare, the malignancy that can be mistaken for FD on imaging and histology is a low-grade central osteosarcoma. A critical imaging distinction between the two entities that has bearing on the histologic interpretation is that in FD, cortical destruction or effacement with a contiguous soft tissue mass should not be

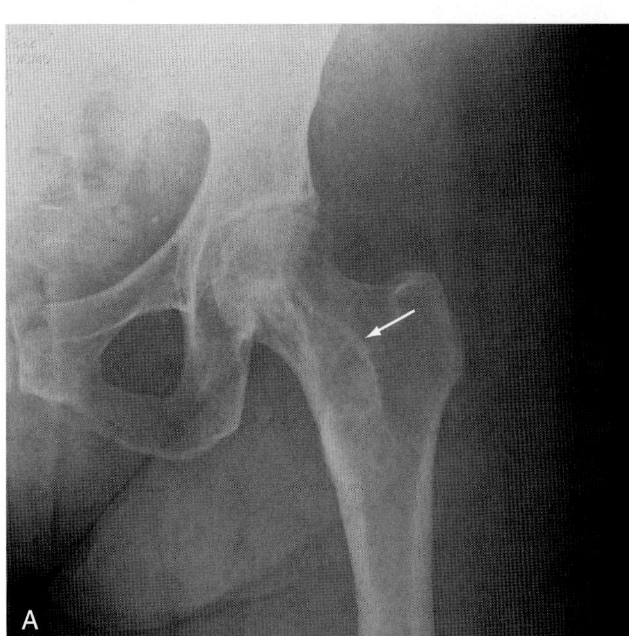

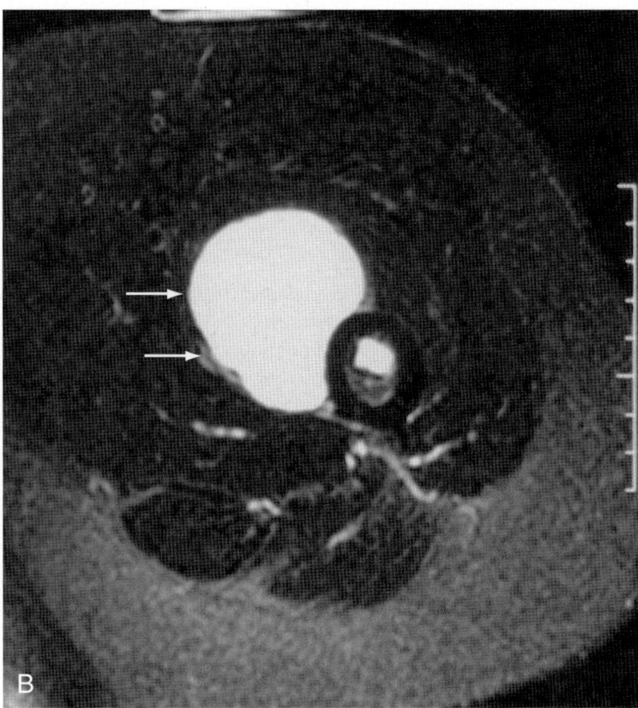

FIGURE 29-14. Mazabraud's syndrome. **A,** AP radiograph of the femur shows a lucent lesion with a rim of sclerosis *(arrow)* consistent with fibrous dysplasia. **B,** MRI shows the soft tissue myxoma *(arrows)*.

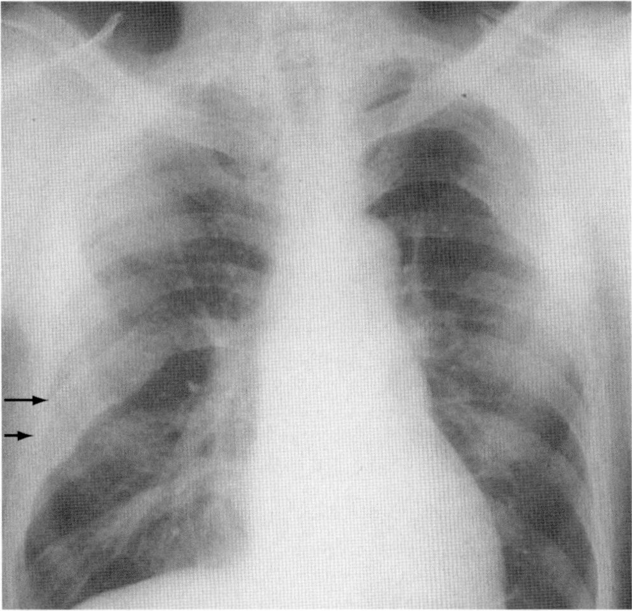

FIGURE 29-15. Fibrous dysplasia of the ribs. PA chest radiograph shows long expansile lesions *(arrows)* with "ground-glass" appearance involving multiple ribs. Fibrous dysplasia is considered the most common benign neoplasm of the ribs.

encountered. Such an appearance should raise the possibility of a low-grade central osteosarcoma.[28]

The soft tissue mass of intramuscular myxoma that is associated with FD of bone, constituting Mazabraud's syndrome, may be adjacent to the osseous abnormality, but it is not associated with cortical destruction or contiguity with the medullary cavity. On MRI, the myxomas of Mazabraud's syndrome have virtually identical features to conventionally encountered myxomas[29] (Figure 29-14).

FD is primarily a radiographic diagnosis that rarely needs confirmatory advanced imaging study. The widespread use of MRI for joint problems has resulted in FD being encountered as an incidental finding, and recognition of its varied MRI features and correlation with radiographs could prevent unnecessary biopsies.

SARCOIDOSIS

Sarcoidosis of the musculoskeletal system is an uncommon diagnosis and accordingly is infrequently considered in routine practice by musculoskeletal radiologists in contradistinction to their chest colleagues. In the United States, sarcoidosis most often affects African Americans, while in the United Kingdom it is a rare disease in blacks and common in whites.

Sarcoidosis may affect bones or joints. Although acute and chronic polyarthritis are well-recognized clinical symptoms of sarcoidosis, no predictable or recognizable radiographic pattern of articular sarcoidosis has emerged.

> The clinical findings of ankle arthritis, especially if bilateral, or erythema nodosum should raise the possibility of sarcoidosis and prompt radiographic examination of the chest.

Bone changes in sarcoidosis are usually associated with chest abnormalities (adenopathy or interstitial lung disease). The advent of MRI has brought to our attention axial, long bone, and muscle sarcoidosis rarely encountered in the preMRI era[30-32] and some unexpected presentations of sarcoidosis.[33]

Imaging

The radiographic lattice-like or honeycombed appearance in the phalanges is the most familiar radiographic sign of osseous

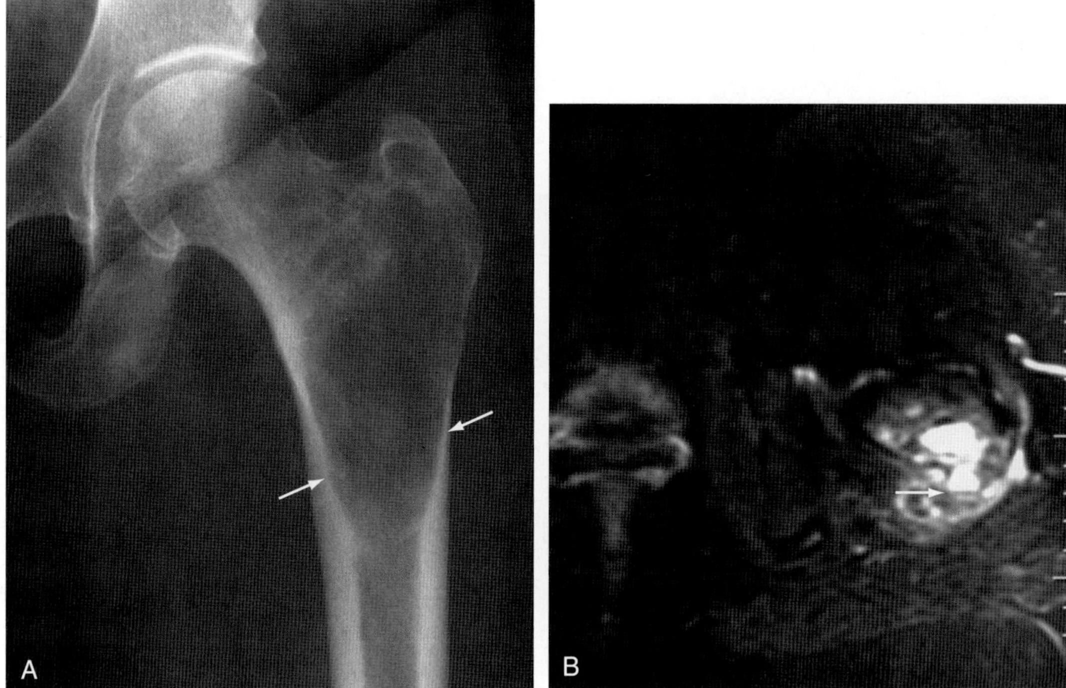

FIGURE 29-16. Fibrous dysplasia with secondary aneurysmal bone cyst. **A,** AP radiograph shows osteolysis and expansion *(arrows)* in a common location for fibrous dysplasia. **B,** Axial T2-weighted fat-suppressed MRI shows fluid–fluid levels of a secondary aneurysmal bone cyst *(arrow).* Because of pain and possible impending fracture, the lesion was operated on. Histology confirmed the imaging diagnosis.

TABLE 29-2. Radiographic Features of Fibrous Dysplasia

Tubular bones	Intramedullary Predominantly diaphyseal Central or eccentric Solitary or multiple lesions Often radiolucent or "ground glass" Fusiform expansion of bone Intralesional calcification or ossification Femoral bowing ("shepherd's crook" deformity)
Ribs	May be unilateral Fusiform enlargement Long lesion
Skull	Expansile lesions Sclerosis of the skull base and sphenoid wings Donut lesions (lucent lesion with sclerotic rim)

sarcoidosis. The soft tissues may appear thickened. Sclerotic or lytic lesions that mimic metastases may also be seen.

In a prospective MRI series performed on patients with sarcoidosis and musculoskeletal symptoms, 17 of 40 patients who were imaged had intramedullary lesions (Figure 29-17). In nine patients who had large bones involved, the lesions were multiple and indistinguishable from metastases or multiple myeloma. Interestingly, none of the large bone lesions showed cortical destruction in this series, although extraosseous disease was evident when small bones were involved. The joint findings were

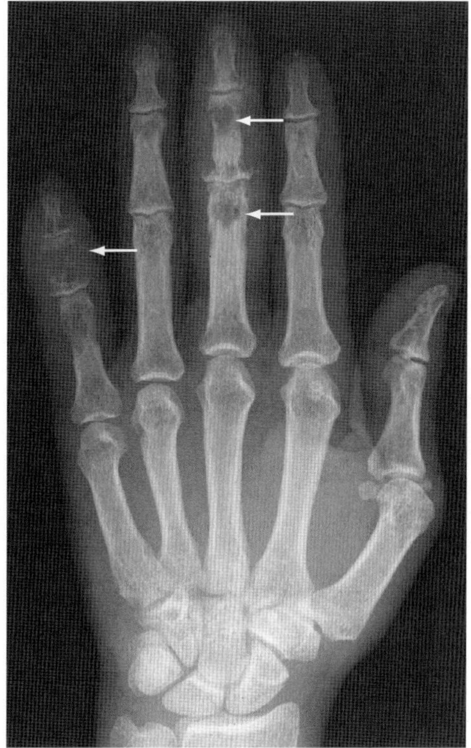

FIGURE 29-17. Sarcoid involving the phalanges. A radiograph of the hand shows lytic lesions *(arrows)* of the phalanges. There is marked accompanying soft tissue swelling.

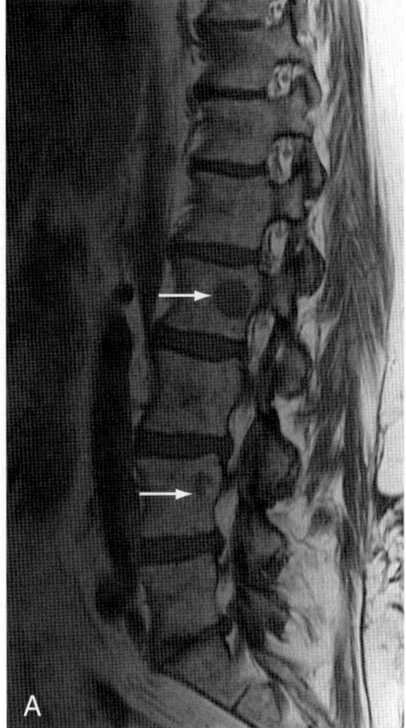

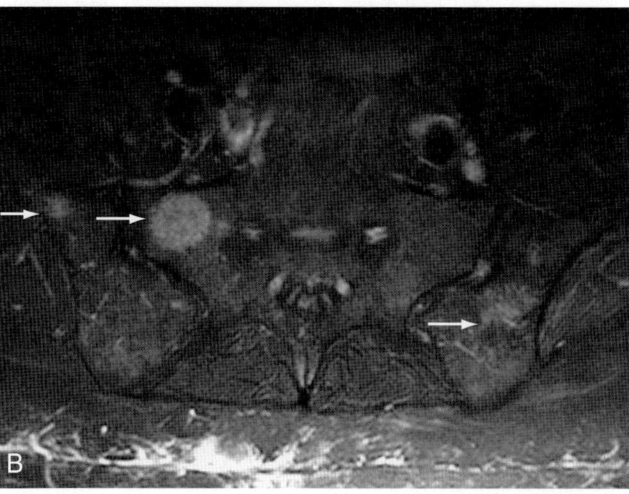

FIGURE 29-18. MRI features of vertebral sarcoid. Sagittal T1-weighted MRI of spine **(A)** and axial fluid sensitive sequence through the sacrum **(B)** show multiple ovoid lesions *(arrows)* indistinguishable from metastasis or multiple myeloma. Biopsy revealed noncaseating granulomas consistent with sarcoidosis. (Courtesy of Mark Kransdorf, MD, Mayo Clinic, Jacksonville, Fla.)

felt to be relatively nonspecific (Figure 29-18). Muscle involvement was uncommon and ranged from an edemalike pattern to intramuscular nodules.

Sarcoidosis of the vertebral column is rare.[34] Osteosclerotic or osteolytic lesions may be seen on radiographs, mimicking metastases or multiple myeloma, particularly when the patient is elderly. Exceptionally, vertebral sarcoidosis may be destructive with a soft tissue mass[35] unlike its long-bone counterparts.

Extraarticular Features

Central Nervous System

Sarcoidosis involves the central nervous system (CNS) in 5% to 10% of patients. MRI with gadolinium can reveal basal leptomeningeal enhancement, the most characteristic appearance of CNS sarcoidosis. Other findings include small enhancing granulomas located superficially in the brain substance, as well as deep and superficial white matter lesions resembling those of multiple sclerosis.

Pulmonary

In about 90% of cases, a chest radiograph reveals an abnormal finding, including lymphadenopathy, parenchymal opacities, or both.[35] Based on the chest radiographic appearance, sarcoidosis is staged as follows:

Stage 0—normal chest radiograph
Stage I—nodal enlargement only
Stage II—nodal enlargement and parenchymal opacity
Stage III—parenchymal opacity without adenopathy or fibrosis
Stage IV—lung fibrosis

Some classifications consider fibrotic and nonfibrotic opacities together as stage III.[36] Most of the patients with sarcoidosis (45% to 65%) are at stage I at the time of presentation. The stage at presentation correlates with prognosis: the higher the stage, the lower would be the chance of resolution of symptoms and radiographic abnormalities without treatment.[37] Patients at stage 0 usually have remarkable extrathoracic disease such as uveitis or skin abnormalities. Computer tomography (CT) can be helpful in detecting lung disease in patients at stage 0 with reduced vital capacity or lung-diffusing capacity.

Lymphadenopathy, the most common intrathoracic finding in sarcoidosis, is seen in 75% to 80% of patients at some point during the illness. Hilar, right paratracheal, aortopulmonary, and subcarinal regions are common sites of intrathoracic lymphadenopathy. Aortopulmonary adenopathy produces a characteristic local convexity in the aortopulmonary window.[38] Both the more proximal tracheobronchial and the more distal bronchopulmonary nodes are enlarged in sarcoidosis, and the latter is a characteristic finding.

> Symmetric adenopathy is a diagnostic finding in sarcoidosis and is not usually seen in other diseases, such as tuberculosis, lymphoma, amyloidosis, or metastases.

Sometimes adenopathy on the right side may appear more prominent than the left. Unilateral hilar lymphadenopathy may be observed in 3% to 5% of patients, which is about twice as common on the right as on the left. In this situation, further investigation is necessary to rule out the possibility of malignancy, primary or AIDS-related tuberculosis, or fungal infection. Mediastinal lymphadenopathy is not a prominent or sole finding in sarcoidosis, and alternative diagnoses should be considered. Subcarinal adenopathy can be significant and result in dysphagia or airway obstruction.

As parenchymal changes develop in patients presenting at stage I (i.e., enlarged lymph node only), adenopathy usually begins to shrink. This can be a valuable feature in the differentiation of sarcoidosis from lymphoma and carcinoma in which adenopathy progresses in parallel with parenchymal involvement.[39]

Calcification can occur in diseased nodes, and its morphology on chest radiographs is nonspecific. Eggshell calcification is seen peripherally in some patients and is a valuable diagnostic finding, occurring in sarcoidosis and silicosis.[40] It is uncommonly seen in histoplasmosis, blastomycosis, amyloidosis, and lymphoma (postirradiation).[35] CT can provides more detailed information about the nodal calcifications.

In almost half of patients with sarcoidosis, parenchymal disease is radiographically observed at the time of presentation and can be classified into reversible and nonreversible (fibrotic) and mixed types. Reversible changes include three major patterns and may present alone or in combination.[39]

- Reticulonodular opacities
- Alveolar opacities
- Large nodular sarcoidosis

High-resolution CT scanning can effectively show parenchymal opacities, and specific findings are often present that allow the diagnosis of sarcoidosis with high accuracy.

Other Pulmonary Findings

Narrowing of the airways may occur due to nodal compression, extrinsic scarring, or endobronchial granulomas and fibrosis.[35] Lobar or segmental collapse is rarely seen and most commonly affects the middle lobe. Chest radiographs usually underestimate the extent of airway involvement in sarcoidosis.[38] Sarcoid effusions, classically lymphocyte-rich exudates, more often develop in the context of the extensive pulmonary disease. They are usually small in size and commonly unilateral.[35]

AMYLOIDOSIS

Amyloid was so named by the German pathologist Rudolf Virchow in 1854 because he incorrectly believed the waxy substance to be starchlike because of its staining affinity for iodine. Amyloid is, in fact, a group of proteins made up of beta-pleated sheets of amino acids, which on electron microscopy are seen as fibrils of 8- to 10-mm diameter. Apple green birefringence under polarizing microscopy of tissue stained with Congo red is a characteristic finding.

There are several varieties of amyloidosis. Primary systemic amyloidosis is often associated with a monoclonal plasma cell dyscrasia, and secondary amyloidosis is associated with an underlying inflammatory or infectious process (e.g., Crohn's disease, juvenile rheumatoid arthritis, chronic osteomyelitis, and systemic lupus erythematosus).[41] A solitary lesion of amyloid is termed an amyloidoma.

Another type of systemic amyloidosis (beta-2 microglobulin amyloid) is usually related to chronic hemodialysis and became clinically frequent in this select population.[42-44] Beta-2 microglobulin amyloid commences after 6 to 7 years of dialysis with a predilection for joints, typically the wrists and shoulders, and after 15 years of dialysis, amyloidosis is almost universal.[45-50] Recently, the incidence of this type of amyloid has decreased.

Imaging

Goldman and Bansal discussed the imaging manifestations of AL and beta-2 microglobulin amyloid (the most frequently encountered types).[51] Osseous, articular (including carpal tunnel syndrome), diffuse marrow, diffuse myopathy, localized nodular soft tissue deposits, and destructive spondylitis were described.

Articular

Amyloid involvement of bursae and joints produces synovial thickening. Involvement of capsular and pericapsular structures produces soft tissue swelling on radiographs and may lead to joint subluxation and erosion of articular or paraarticular bone.[52] Osteopenia is found. The cartilage spaces remain normal, helping to differentiate these findings from rheumatoid arthritis. The shoulders, hips, elbows, and knees are most often affected, and usually involvement is bilateral. Pathologic fractures may occur.[52]

> Pathologic fracture of the femoral neck may be a presenting feature of amyloid arthropathy in patients on chronic hemodialysis.

The development of multiple cyst-like lesions in the carpals of patients on dialysis is often attributed to amyloid, especially if the patient is not hypercalcemic and is unlikely to have brown tumors. These changes may progress to a destructive arthropathy (Figure 29-19).

Amyloid tissue is echogenic on ultrasound and can be distinguished from the adjacent anechoic fluid in the joint or bursa. On MRI, amyloid shows synovial masses that are characteristically low in signal on T2-weighted images[53] (Figure 29-20). While the MRI signal is identical to the masses seen in patients with pigmented villonodular synovitis (PVNS), involvement of more than one joint is very unusual in PVNS and much more consistent with amyloidosis.

The clinical diagnosis of carpal tunnel syndrome in patients on dialysis is common and is attributed to amyloid deposition. The need for imaging is rare. If required, either ultrasound or MRI could be used for evaluating the carpal tunnel. Ultrasound is a quicker and significantly less expensive examination. MRI shows the abnormal tissue within the carpal tunnel surrounding and displacing the tendons.[51]

Marrow

Marrow involvement results in osteopenia, vertebral collapse,[52] or lytic lesions. A large osteolytic lesion of amyloid would need to be distinguished from a plasmacytoma, an osteolytic metastasis, or a brown tumor. Biochemical values may permit differentiation from a brown tumor, but usually a histologic diagnosis is required to distinguish an "amyloidoma" from a plasmacytoma or metastasis (Figure 29-21). However, amyloidomas may exhibit low signal on T1-weighted and T2-weighted images, which is in contrast to

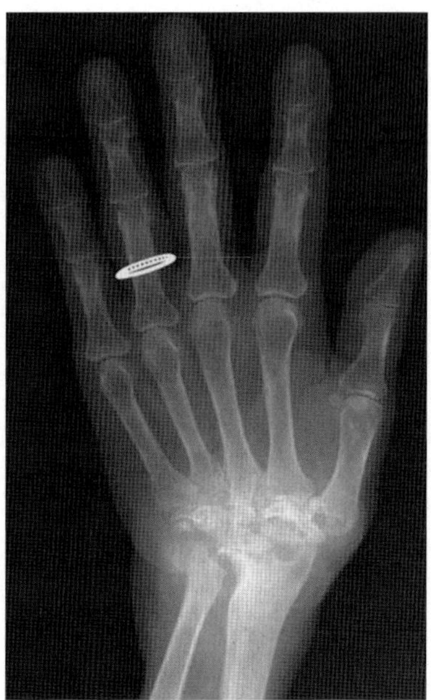

FIGURE 29-19. Destructive arthropathy of the carpus from amyloid. There are marked erosion and bone loss of the carpals, distal ulna, and radius with soft tissue swelling.

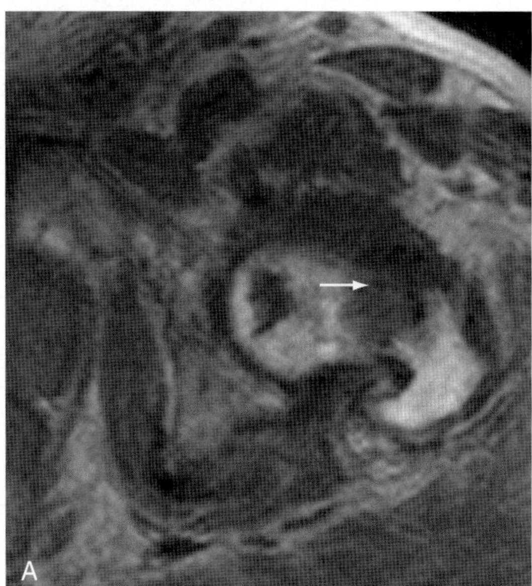

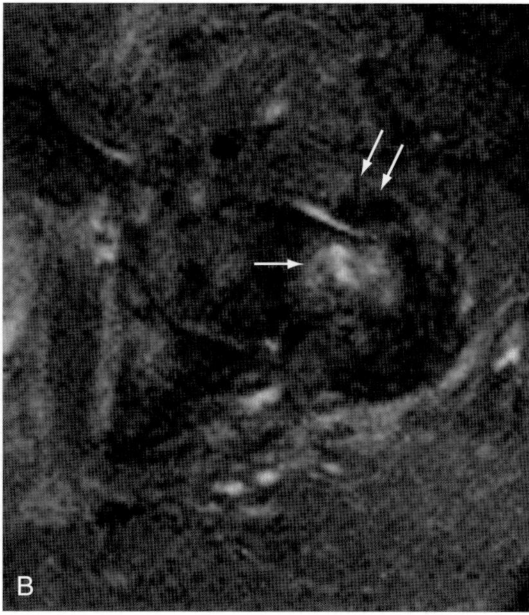

FIGURE 29-20. Biopsy-proven amyloidosis of the hips. Axial T1W **(A)** and T2-weighted **(B)** fat-suppressed MRIs of the left hip demonstrate large cystic erosions (*arrows*) of the femoral neck. The low signal of the thickened capsule on T2-weighted images *(arrows)* is characteristic (but not specific) of amyloid.

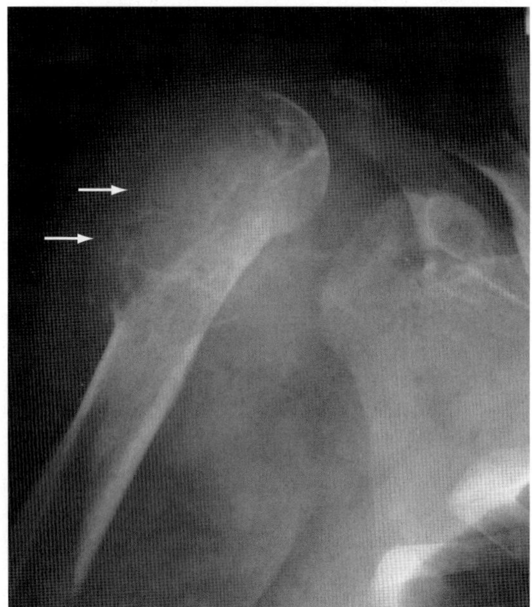

FIGURE 29-21. Amyloidoma. The large destructive lesion of the humerus was proven to be due to an "amyloidoma" *(arrows)*, but the appearances are indistinguishable from a plasmacytoma or lytic metastatic lesion. An extensive soft tissue component is likely responsible for increasing the distance between the humeral head and the glenoid.

most other masses that are bright on T2-weighted images.[51] Solitary masses of amyloid (amyloidomas) are reported in the spine.[54]

Muscle

Myopathy presents with muscle stiffness and enlargement.[51] The muscles appear enlarged on MRI with indistinct boundaries. The subcutaneous fat shows a reticulated pattern of decreased signal intensity.[51]

Discovertebral

Discovertebral destruction in patients on chronic hemodialysis has been termed *renal spondyloarthropathy.* The cause may be multifactorial. Since the virtual elimination of aluminum-induced bone disease, the most likely causes for this condition, in the absence of infection, are hyperparathyroidism and amyloidosis. A helpful MRI sign of a noninfectious cause for a destructive spondyloarthropathy in a patient on dialysis is a discovertebral lesion that is dark on T2-weighted pulse sequences.[55]

REFERENCES

1. Paget J: On a form of chronic inflammation of bones (osteitis deformans), *Med Chir Trans* 60:37, 1877.
2. Mills BG, Singert FR: Nuclear inclusions in Paget's disease of bone science, *Science* 194:201, 1976.
3. Siris ES: Paget's disease of bone, *J Bone Miner Res* 13:1061-1065, 1998.
4. Whyte MP: Paget's disease of bone, *N Engl J Med* 355:593-600, 2006.
5. Cundy T: Is Paget's disease of bone disappearing? *Skeletal Radiol* 35:350-351, 2006.
6. Schmorl G: Ueber Osteitis deformans Paget, *Virchows Arch* 283:694, 1932.
7. Siris ES: Indications for medical treatment of Paget's disease of bone, In Singer FR, Wallach S (eds): *Paget's Disease of Bone*, Amsterdam, 1991, Elsevier.
8. Eisman JA, Martin J: Osteolytic Paget's disease, *J Bone Joint Surg* 68A:112-117, 1968.
9. Sundaram M, Khanna G, El-Khoury GY: T1-weighted MR imaging for distinguishing large osteolysis of Paget's disease from sarcomatous degeneration. *Skeletal Radiol* 30:378-383, 2001.
10. Seaman WB: The roentgen appearance of early Paget's disease, *AJR Am J Roentgenol* 66(4):587-594, 1951.
11. Jacobs P: Osteolytic Paget's disease, *Clin Radiol* 25:138-144, 1974.
12. Greditzer HG III, Mcleod RA, Unni KK et al: Bone sarcomas in Paget's disease, *Radiology* 146:327, 1983.
13. Kaufmann GA, Sundaram M, McDonald DJ: Magnetic resonance imaging in symptomatic Paget's disease, *Skeletal Radiol* 20:413, 1991.
14. Tins BJ, Davies AM, Mangham DC: MR imaging of pseudosarcoma in Paget's disease of bone. A report of two cases, *Skeletal Radiol* 30:161, 2001.
15. McNairn JDK, Damron TA, Landas SK et al: Benign tumefactive soft tissue extension from Paget's disease of bone simulating malignancy, *Skeletal Radiol* 30:157, 2001.
16. Gabel GT, Rand JA, Sion FH: Total knee arthroplasty for osteoarthrosis in patients who have Paget's disease of bone at the knee, *J Bone Joint Surg Am* 73:739, 1991.
17. Ludkowski P, Willis-McDonald J: Total arthroplasty in Paget's disease of the hip. A clinical review and review of the literature, *Clin Orthop* 255:160, 1991.
18. Maldagne B, Malghem J: Dynamic radiologic patterns of Paget's disease of bone, *Clin Orthop* 217:126, 1987.
19. Vellenga CJLR, Pauwels EKJ, Bijvoet OL et al: Bone scintigraphy in Paget's disease treated with combined calcitonin and diphosphonate (EHDP), *Metab Bone Dis Relat Res* 4:103, 1982.

20. Cook GJ, Maisey MN, Fogelman I: Fluorine-18-FDG PET in Paget's disease of bone, *J Nucl Med* 38:1495-1497, 1997.
21. Installe J, Nzeusseu A, Bol A et al: 18F-fluoride PET for monitoring therapeutic response in Paget's disease of bone, *J Nucl Med* 46(10):1650-1658, 2005.
22. Schubert F, Siddlek J, Harper JS: Diaphyseal Paget's disease: an unusual finding in the tibia, *Clin Radiol* 35:71-74, 1984.
23. Siegal G, Dal Cin P, Aranjo ES: Fibrous dysplasia in WHO classification of tumors. In Fletcher CDM, Unni KK, Mertens F (eds): *Pathology and genetics of tumors of soft tissue and bone*, Lyon, 2002, IARC Press, pp 341-342.
24. Cohen M: Fibrous dysplasia is a neoplasm, *Am J Med Genet* 98:290-293, 2001.
25. Albright F, Butler AM, Hampton AO et al: Syndrome characterized by osteitis fibrosa disseminate, areas of pigmentation and endocrine dysfunction with precocious puberty in females: report of five cases, *N Engl J Med* 216:726-748, 1937.
26. Mazabraud A, Semat P, Roze R: A propos de l'association de fibromyxomes des tissues mous a la dysplasie fibreus des os, *Presse Med* 75:2223, 1965.
27. Kyriakos M, McDonald DJ, Sundaram M: Fibrous dysplasia with cartilaginous differentiation ("fibrocartilaginous dysplasia"): a review, with an illustrative case followed for 18 years, *Skeletal Radiol* 33:51-62, 2004. (Review.)
28. Andresen KJ, Sundaram M, Unni KK et al: Imaging features of low-grade central osteosarcoma of the long bones and pelvis, *Skeletal Radiol* 33:373-379, 2004.
29. Sundaram M, McDonald DJ, Merenda G: Intramuscular myxoma—a rare but important association with fibrous dysplasia of bone, *AJR Am J Roentgenol* 153:107-108, 1989.
30. Moore SL, Terrstein A, Golimbu C: MRI of sarcoidosis patients with musculoskeletal symptoms, *AJR Am J Roentgenol* 185:154-159, 2005.
31. Rayner CK, Burnet SP, McNeil JD: Osseous sarcoidosis: a magnetic resonance imaging diagnosis, *Clin Exp Rheumatol* 20:546-548, 2002.
32. Otake S, Ishigaki T: Muscular sarcoidosis, *Semin Musculoskelet Radiol* 5:167-170, 2001.
33. Fujimoto H, Shimofusa R, Shimoyama K et al: Sarcoidosis presenting as prepatellar bursitis, *Skeletal Radiol* 35:58-60, 2005.
34. Sundaram M, Place H, Shauffer WO et al: Progressive destructive vertebral sarcoid leading to surgical fusion, *Skeletal Radiol* 28:717-722, 1999.
35. Vogler III JB, Kim JH: Metabolic and endocrine disease of the skeleton. In Grainger RG, Allison DJ, Adam A et al (eds): *Grainger & Allison's Diagnostic Radiology: A Textbook of Medical Imaging*, 4th ed, London, 2001, Churchill Livingstone, pp 1925-1966.
36. DeRemee RA: The roentgenographic staging of sarcoidosis. Historic and contemporary perspectives, *Chest* 83:128-133, 1983.
37. Lynch JP III, Kazerooni EA, Gay SE: Pulmonary sarcoidosis, *Clin Chest Med* 18:755-785, 1997.
38. Miscellaneous diffuse lung diseases. In Hansell DM, Armstrong P, Lynch DA, Mcadams HP (eds): *Imaging of Diseases of the Chest*, 4th ed, St. Louis, 2005, Mosby, pp 631-710.
39. Kirks DR, McCormick VD, Greenspan RH: Pulmonary sarcoidosis. Roentgenologic analysis of 150 patients, *Am J Roentgenol Radium Ther Nucl Med* 117:777-786, 1973.
40. Gross B, Schneider HJ, Proto AV: Eggshell calcification of lymph nodes: an update, *AJR Am J Roentgenol* 135:1265-1268, 1980.
41. Georgiades CS, Neyman EG, Barish MA et al: Amyloidosis: review and CT manifestations, *RadioGraphics* 24:405-416, 2004.
42. Beyjo F, Yamada H, Odani S et al: A new form of amyloid protein associated with chronic hemodialysis was identified as beta 2-microglobulin, *Biochem Biophys Res Commun* 129:701-706, 1985.
43. Gorevic PD, Casey TT, Stoen WJ et al: Beta 2 microglobulin is an amyloidogenic protein in man, *J Clin Invest* 76:2425-2429, 1985.
44. Hirahama T, Skinnet M, Cohen AS et al: Histochemical and immunohistochemical characterization of amyloid associated with chronic hemodialysis as beta-2-microglobulin, *Lab Invest* 53:705-709:1985.
45. Cameron JS: Dialysis artheropathy, amyloidosis and beta-2 microglobulin, *Pediatr Nephrol* 1:224-229, 1987.
46. Kleinman RS, Cobson JW: Amyloid syndromes associated with hemodialysis, *Kidney Int* 35:567-575, 1989.
47. Roch RM: Dialysis related amyloidosis (nephrology forum), *Kidney Int* 41:1416-1429, 1992.
48. Charra B, Calmard E, Laurent G: Chronic renal failure treatment duration and mode: their relation to the late dialysis periarticular syndrome, *Blood Purif* 6:117-124, 1988.
49. Floege J, Ehlerding G: B2-microglobulin associated amyloidosis, *Nephron* 72:9-26, 1996.
50. de Strihou CVY, Judoul M, Malghem J et al: Effect of dialysis membrane and patients age on signs of dialysis related amyloidosis. Report of the working party on dialysis amyloidosis, *Kidney Int* 39:1012-1019, 1991.
51. Goldman AB, Bansal M: Amyloidosis and silicone synovitis, *Radiol Clin North Am* 34:375-393, 1996.
52. Weinfeld A, Stern MH, Marx LH: Amyloid lesions of bone, *AJR Am J Roentgenol* 108:799-805, 1970.
53. Aoki Y, Kaneda K, Miyagi N et al: Popliteal amyloidoma presenting with leg ischemia in a chronic dialysis patient, *Skeletal Radiol* 29:717-720, 2000.
54. Nas K, Arslen A, Ceviz A et al: Spinal cord compression by amyloidoma of the spine, *Yonsei Med J* 43:681-685, 2002.
55. Leone A, Sundaram M, Cerase A et al: Destructive spondyloarthropathy of the cervical spine in long-term hemodialyzed patients: a five-year clinical radiological prospective study, *Skeletal Radiol* 30:431-441, 2001.

CHAPTER 30

Imaging of Total Joint Replacement

BARBARA N. WEISSMAN, MD

KEY FACTS

- Total joint replacement is a highly successful method for providing pain relief from various arthritic conditions.
- Radiographs remain the standard technique for evaluating the position and integrity of joint replacements.
- Joint aspiration is critical for identifying infection following joint replacement but is not infallible.
- Technical modifications have permitted computed tomography and magnetic resonance imaging to become important methods for the assessment of prosthetic complications such as granuloma formation.
- Combined white blood cell and marrow imaging (indium 111 WBC/technetium 99m sulfur colloid) is the standard imaging examination for identifying infected joint prostheses.

TOTAL HIP REPLACEMENT

Joint replacement surgery is one of the great success stories of modern medicine. Results of total hip replacement are excellent, producing marked improvement in physical function, social interaction, and overall health.[1] Modern prostheses are expected to last more than 15 years.[2] The foundation for this success was the introduction by Sir John Charnley of the cemented metal to polyethylene prosthesis in the early 1960s.[3] Currently, over 600,000 hip replacements are performed in Europe each year.[4] A total of 202,500 primary total hip arthroplasties were performed in the United States in 2003, and it is estimated that by 2030, the demand for these operations will grow by 174% to 572,000.[5]

Indications

Joint replacement is generally considered for patients 65 years of age or older.[6] Candidates for total hip replacement usually have arthritis with disabling hip pain and functional limitation in spite of adequate medical therapy (Table 30-1).[7] Patients 65 years of age or older suffering pain that interferes with sleep or activities and is unresponsive to 3 to 6 months of conservative treatment (such as anti-inflammatory medication) may be candidates for joint replacement.[6] In patients aged 55 to 65, a longer course of conservative treatment is usually warranted before joint replacement is considered.[6] Recent investigations seek to further improve these prostheses and techniques to allow use of prostheses in younger individuals who may have greater physical demands and the desire for early return to work.[4] Some areas of investigation, include optimizing implant positioning, decreasing wear, preserving bone and minimally invasive surgery.[2,4]

Types of Prostheses

Initial hip prostheses consisted of a metallic femoral component and a high density polyethylene acetabular component (Figure 30-1). Contemporary prostheses are modular including a separate femoral head and sometimes a separate femoral neck or proximal body, thus allowing adjustments to provide optimal biomechanics. The acetabular liner is inserted with a metal backing that provides the irregular surface for bone ingrowth. These metal-backed bone ingrowth acetabular components have shown lower rates of radiographic loosening at 10 years compared with cemented acetabular components.[8]

Preserving Bone: Surface Replacements

Surface replacements have shorter femoral component stems allowing less bone to be resected and are, therefore, important options for younger patients. The current generation of surface replacements has a metal-to-metal articulation (not metal to high density polyethylene as older surface replacements) (Figure 30-2). As summarized by Eingartner, problems may include adverse reactions to metal ion release (from wear), reduced acetabular options if revision surgery is necessary, a more invasive initial surgical procedure, and the danger of femoral neck fracture.[4] Indications for surface replacement may include active younger patients (males < 65, women < 60) with good bone quality[4] (Table 30-2).

Proper patient selection (including radiologic evaluation of the proximal femur for bone density, shape, biomechanics and focal bone defects) and attention to operative details are important for achieving optimal results of surface replacement.[9] Shmalzried et al. noted a suboptimal femoral shape for surface replacement to be characterized by a broad, short, femoral neck with a femoral head neck diameter ratio of less than 1.2 cm or neck length less than 2 cm.[9] Poor biomechanics included limb length discrepancy greater than 1 cm or neck-shaft angle less than 120 degrees. Low bone density would increase the risk of postoperative femoral neck fracture and cysts larger than 1 cm in diameter are poor prognostic factors.

The cause of most surface replacement failures is femoral component loosening.[10] Femoral neck fractures may complicate surface replacement procedures and can be minimized by attention to technical details including avoiding notching of the lateral femoral neck.[10,10a] Postoperative radiographs should, therefore, be scrutinized for metaphyseal radiolucencies, femoral neck notching, change in component position, and femoral fractures.

Fixation of Components

Methyl methacrylate cement was used by Charnley to provide stress transmission from the components to bone. “Bone

TABLE 30-1. Selected Indications and Contraindications for Total Hip Replacement

Indications	Unremitting pain
Contraindications/relative contraindications	Active infection
	Vascular insufficiency
	Paralysis
	Severe obesity
	Prior surgical joint fusion

From Berquist TH: Imaging of joint replacement procedures, *Radiol Clin North Am* 44:419-437, 2006.

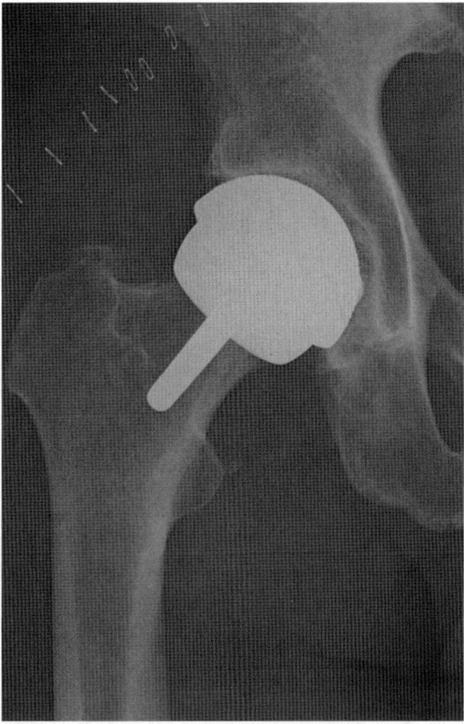

FIGURE 30-2. Surface replacement. This prosthesis has a metal-to-metal articulation with porous coated surfaces for bone ingrowth. Minimal femoral bone needs to be resected. The surgery was recent and skin staples are in place.

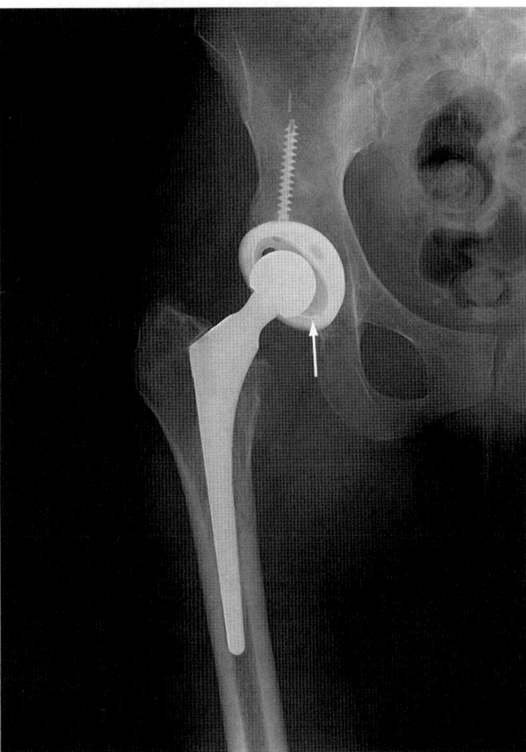

FIGURE 30-1. Uncomplicated bone ingrowth total hip arthroplasty. The nonopaque acetabular liner is marked by a thin circular wire about its rim *(arrow)*. The acetabular metal backing has an irregular surface adjacent to the bone for bone ingrowth. A fixation screw maintains stability so that bone ingrowth can occur.

TABLE 30-2. Possible Indications and Contraindications for Surface Replacement

Indications	Young active patients (women < 60, men < 65) with good bone stock
Contraindications	Metal allergy
	Renal insufficiency
	Dysplasia
	Osteonecrosis
	Femoral neck deformity

From Eingartner C: Current trends in total hip arthroplasty, *Ortop Traumatol Rehabil* 9:8-14, 2007.

ingrowth" fixation was later developed in which an irregular prosthetic surface allows bone to grow between the surface irregularities (pores) to provide fixation that was both durable and adaptable to changes in stress (Figure 30-3). For this to occur, certain geometric properties of the surface pores are necessary and there must be relatively little motion between the implant and the bone during healing. The term "osseointegration" is sometimes used to describe bone ingrowth fixation. Osseointegration refers to the stable anchorage of an implant achieved by direct bone-to-implant contact; since fibrous tissue may be present around bone ingrowth components this designation may or may not be entirely accurate.[11]

Coating the bone ingrowth surfaces with hydroxyapatite was developed to provide initial stability to allow bone ingrowth without the presence of a fibrous tissue interface (osseointegration). This coating is not visible on radiographs.

Hybrid fixation describes the situation in which a cemented femoral component is paired with a bone ingrowth acetabular component (Figure 30-3, *B*). Acetabular component stability is improved with bone ingrowth fixation as compared to cement fixation. Hybrid fixation is used most often in patients over the age of 65.[4] Two bone ingrowth femoral stem designs are currently used most often, components with a straight stem and extensive surface coating for bone ingrowth and components with a tapered stem and proximal coating.[10] Loosening rates for both types of components used in the last decade are extremely low.

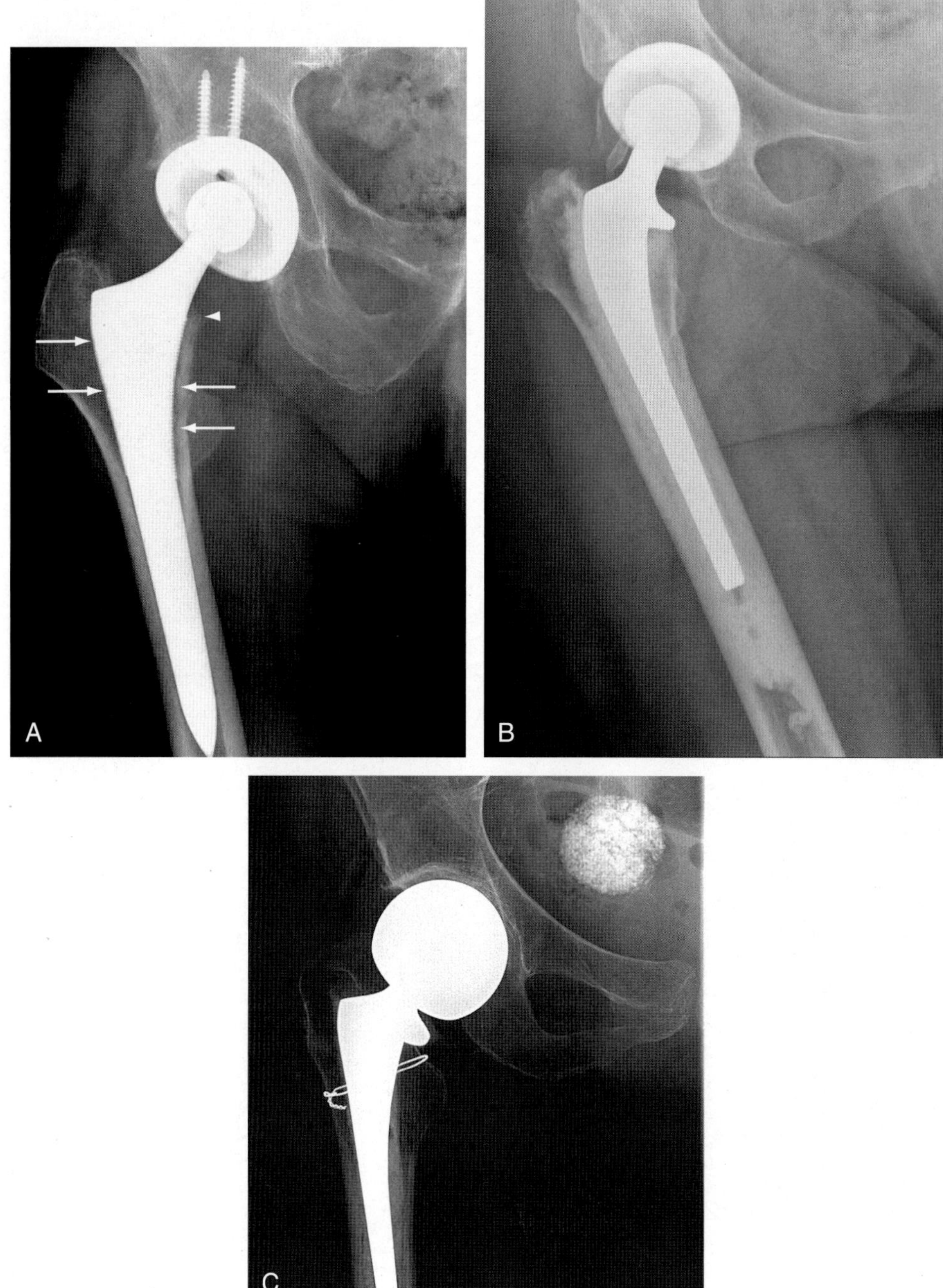

FIGURE 30-3. Component fixation. **A,** Bone ingrowth fixation. The irregular surfaces for bone ingrowth *(arrows)* are evident. Bone extends to and between these femoral surface irregularities and those of the acetabular component. Slight osteopenia of the medial femoral cortex *(arrowhead)* is consistent with "stress shielding," and is further evidence that bone ingrowth has occurred. **B,** Hybrid fixation. There is a bone ingrowth acetabular component and a cemented femoral component. A small amount of heterotopic bone is present. **C,** Bipolar total hip prosthesis. The acetabular component is not fixed to the acetabulum allowing motion to occur at this site. An inner articulation is present between the femoral component and the acetabulum. Thus, there are two sites for hip motion. The round pelvic calcification is likely a calcified uterine fibroid.

In *bipolar prostheses,* the acetabular component is not fixed to the acetabulum (Figure 30-3, *C*). Theoretically (but not always actually), motion can occur between the femoral component and the acetabulum and between the acetabular component and the native acetabulum.

Articular Surfaces (Decreasing Wear)

Highly cross-linked polyethylene is the most common liner surface for total hip replacements today. This liner results in decreased wear when compared to conventional polyethylene components and possibly a decrease in osteolysis. A 10-fold decrease in mean

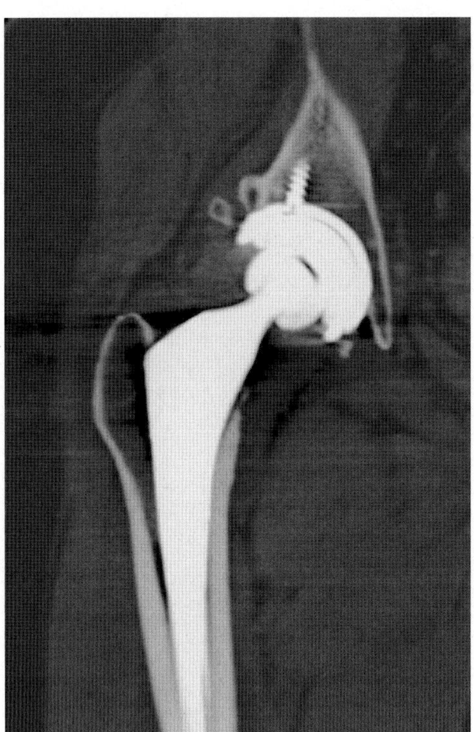

FIGURE 30-4. Ceramic articulation. This reformatted CT scan shows that the femoral head and acetabular liner of this prosthesis are nonmetallic and denser than soft tissue. The interface between the components is difficult to see, a normal finding. The acetabular metal backing and the fixation screw are well seen.

liner wear per year has been noted (0.20 for conventional polyethylene liners versus 0.02 mm/year).[10] Particle size is also different compared to conventional polyethylene components.

Ceramic-on-ceramic bearings have been developed (Figure 30-4). Intermediate-term data have shown a low rate of femoral osteolysis.[10] Fracture of the femoral head or chipping of the acetabular liner and audible squeaking have been reported, however.[4a,10]

Decreasing wear of articular surfaces is an important factor in increasing prosthetic life and reducing complications.

Metal-on-metal bearings also have the potential advantage of decreasing wear. However, as noted by Huo, controversy continues regarding the safety of metal-on-metal bearing surfaces, particularly with regard to release of metal ions and the potential for hypersensitivity reactions.[10] Delayed hypersensitivity reactions may be the cause of early osteolysis in some patients with these prostheses.[10]

Minimally Invasive Surgery

The term "minimally invasive surgery" may refer the use of a traditional surgical approach but with minimal skin and soft tissue incision (minimal incision technique),[12] or it may refer to a technique using two incisions.[13] Minimally invasive techniques attempt to shorten the hospital stay and postoperative recovery time by decreasing the extent of soft tissue disruption (usually including a smaller skin incision).[4,14] Although more rapid improvement in function has been noted[13] after 3 months, no advantage to these techniques is documented.[4] Overall, the cost of the two incision technique and the standard technique are not significantly different.[10] Complication rates appear greater with the two-incision technique, but tend to decrease with experience.

Imaging of Total Hip Replacement

Preoperative Assessment

Preoperative imaging is essential for determining the degree of cartilage and bone damage and for preoperative planning. Generally, at the Brigham and Women's Hospital, an anteroposterior radiograph of the pelvis and anteroposterior and "frog lateral" views of the affected hip that includes at least the proximal third of the femur are obtained for these assessments. A magnification marker placed alongside the hip at the level of the bone allows for correction of radiographic magnification and for any enlargement or minification of digital images. A pelvic baseline such as the biischial line facilitates evaluation of leg-length discrepancy (Figure 30-5). The position of the native acetabulum can be determined (using the Ranawat triangle method).[15] Areas of bone deficiency should be looked for and can be filled using grafts or specialized components. Computed tomography (CT) can be used to evaluate bone stock in questionable cases. Wide femoral canals, as assessed by a calcar-to-canal isthmus ratio, may not be suitable for bone ingrowth femoral components.[6] As noted above, the shape and angulation of the femoral head and neck, the degree of cyst formation and leg-length disparity are considerations in selecting patients for surface replacement.

Postoperative Radiographs

Timing

An initial postoperative radiograph is indicated in all patients, and must include the bone past the tip of the femoral stem since this area is prone to fracture. As indicated in the American College of Radiology appropriateness criteria, the schedule for obtaining radiographs in asymptomatic individuals thereafter is uncertain.[16] Lifelong follow-up is recommended, however, even in asymptomatic patients since osteolysis may occur without symptoms.

Initial radiographs and serial radiographs may be critical for detecting complications, including infection, wear, and osteolysis.

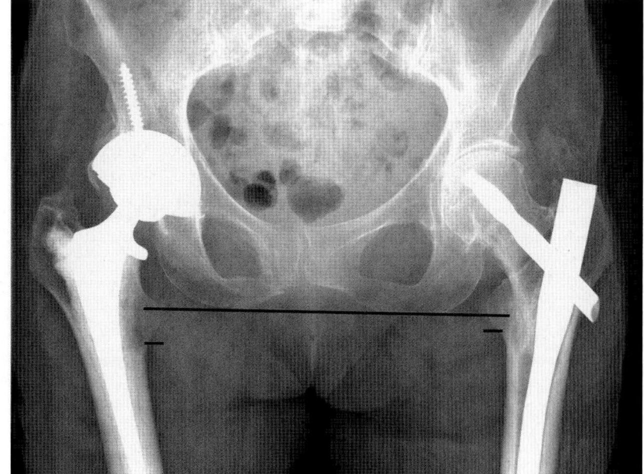

FIGURE 30-5. Leg length comparison. This patient underwent a hybrid right total hip arthroplasty and previous internal fixation of a left intertrochanteric fracture that has healed. Comparison of the distances between each lesser trochanter and the biischial baseline allows comparison of leg lengths. In this case, the right leg is longer. Ideally the patient should not be rotated for this assessment, but in this case, slight patient rotation is present.

TABLE 30-3. Radiographic Appearances of Conventional Total Hip Replacements

	Usual Appearance	Abnormal Appearances
Acetabular component position	Inclination angle usually 45 degrees; (range 35 to 55 degrees)	
Acetabular polyethylene liner	Femoral head is normally centered within acetabulum	Thinning of distance from femoral head to lateral acetabulum suggests wear or liner disruption
Acetabular screws	Do not project more than slightly into pelvis	Rarely, protruding screws may be associated with vascular or visceral injury. CT suggested if suspected.
Acetabular fixation	< 2-mm lucency around acetabular cement Remodeling around bone ingrowth component	2 mm or more cement–bone interface, change in position of component indicate loosening.
Femoral component position	Stem tip usually centrally located or directed medially (valgus)	Varus position is not optimal
Femoral fixation	Cement: Close apposition/interdigitation of cement and bone. Bone ingrowth: interdigitation of bone with the prosthetic bone ingrowth surface, "spot welds," stress shielding. Stable 1-mm lucency may indicate fibrous ingrowth.	Cement: 2 mm or more of lucency especially if along entire cement mantle, cement fracture, change in component position indicate loosening. Development of metal–cement lucency laterally. Bone ingrowth: 2 mm or more of lucency along bone ingrowth surface, progressive shedding of surface beads, settling after 1 year or > 1 cm indicate loosening.
Adjacent bone	Stress shielding—Bone resorption occurs in unstressed areas (e.g., medial femoral cortex) after bone ingrowth stabilizes component. Stress shielding does not progress after 1–2 years	Fracture: Marked sclerosis at tip of prosthesis may indicate loosening. Focal lucent lesions (granulomas)
Soft tissues	Gas resorbs shortly postoperatively	Heterotopic bone may be visible within weeks

Stulberg et al. proposed CT scanning to help determine the extent and location of silent osteolysis and to guide medical and surgical treatment.[17] An initial CT scan is advocated 7 to 10 years postoperatively to establish a baseline; additional CT scans should be done on the basis of the appearance of the original scan. The decision to operate on a patient with extensive acetabular osteolysis is based on the likelihood that a well-fixed cup may become loose during the patient's lifetime.

Reporting

A standard system of reporting the radiographic results after total hip replacement has been proposed.[18] Positioning of components is assessed as shown in Table 30-3 and Figure 30-6. When describing the periprosthetic regions of a total hip arthroplasty, the nomenclature of DeLee and Charnley is used for the acetabulum (zones I to III) and that of Gruen et al. is used for the proximal femur (regions 1 to 7)[19,20] (Figure 30-7).

Fixation

Cemented Components

Methyl methacrylate cement is made radiopaque so that its distribution and interdigitation with trabeculae can be evaluated on radiographs. Optimally, cement should fill the space between the femoral component and the proximal medial cortex and extend past the tip of the femoral stem by about 2 cm (Figure 30-8). Thin (1 to 2 mm) lucencies may develop along the cement bone interface owing to the presence of fibrous tissue.

Uncemented Components

Bone ingrowth fixation attempts to allow bone to grow into the irregular surface (pores) of the components to provide a lasting bond between them. Fibrous tissue ingrowth also occurs to some extent and may provide stability but is not ideal. When bone ingrowth occurs, stress from weight bearing is transmitted through the relatively rigid prosthesis resulting in decreased stress on some areas of bone (such as the proximal medial femur). This process is called stress shielding, and the decrease in bone density that results indicates bone ingrowth has occurred. The bone loss usually stops at 1[21] or 2[22] years after surgery, and increasing bone loss after that time is worrisome for other processes (such as granuloma formation).

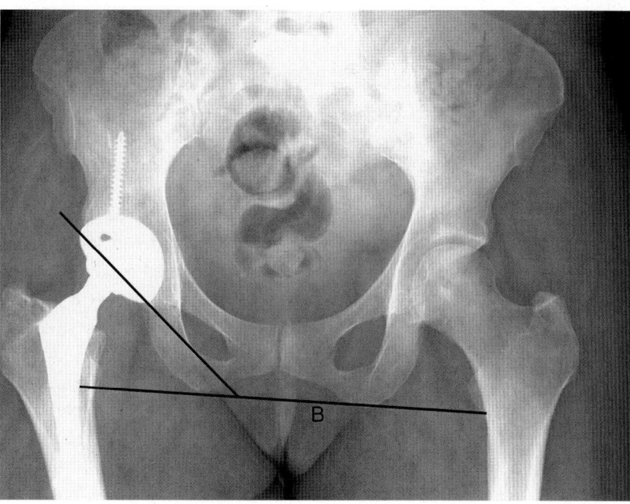

FIGURE 30-6. Acetabular inclination. The tilt of the acetabular component is measured with relation to a baseline, B, drawn through the ischia.

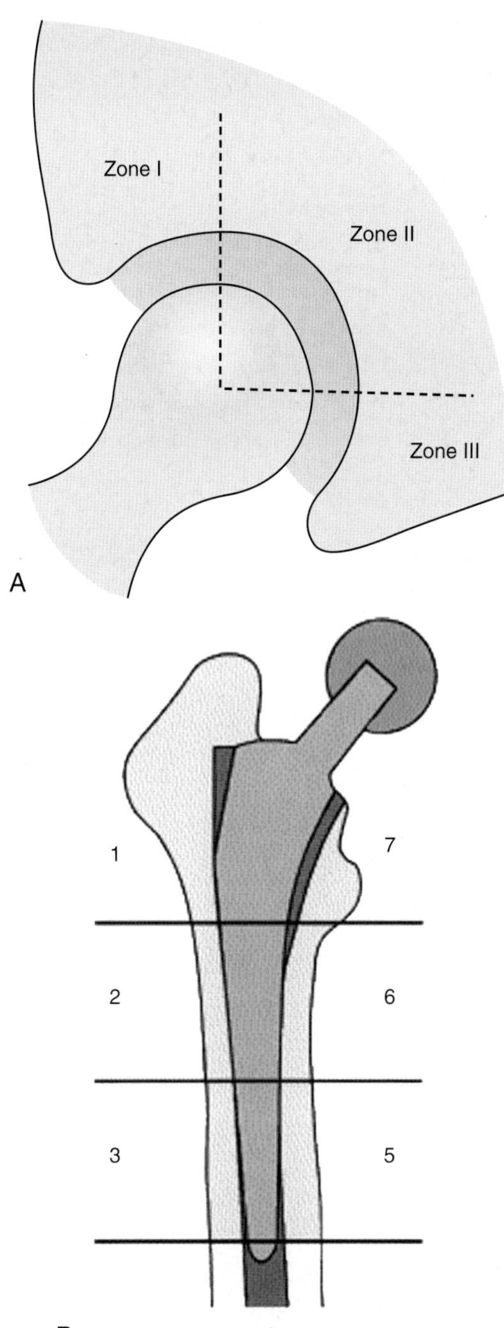

FIGURE 30-7. Nomenclature for describing interfaces. Interface locations are described according to DeLee and Charnley for the acetabulum (zones I to III, **A**) and Gruen et al. for the proximal femur (regions 1 to 7, **B**). Additional numbering of zones on the lateral projection has been described.

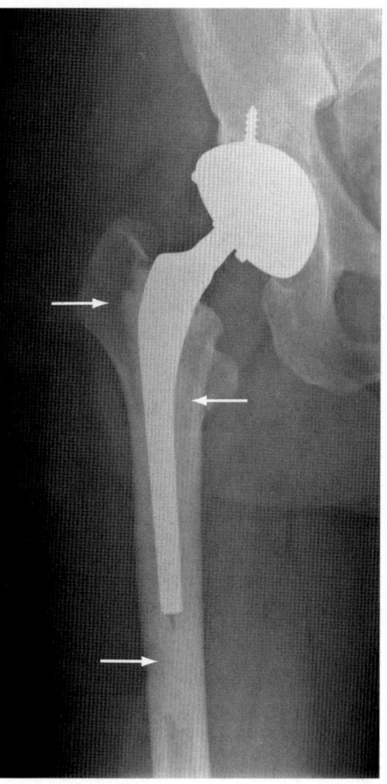

FIGURE 30-8. Hybrid total hip prosthesis. This anteroposterior radiograph of the right hip shows a hybrid total hip replacement (a bone ingrowth acetabular component and a cemented femoral component). The opaque cement *(arrows)* extends past the tip of the femoral stem and fills the femoral canal and medial intertrochanteric region. No loosening is seen. The femoral head is not seen due to the overlying metal backing of the acetabular component; however, judging by the femoral head neck junction, the femoral head is centrally positioned within the acetabulum.

Acetabular Component

Moore et al. compared radiographic appearances of bone ingrowth acetabular components with findings at revision surgery[23] and found five signs useful in determining stable fixation (Figure 30-9):

- Absence of radiolucent lines
- Presence of a superolateral buttress
- Medial bone stress-shielding
- Radial trabeculae
- Inferomedial buttress

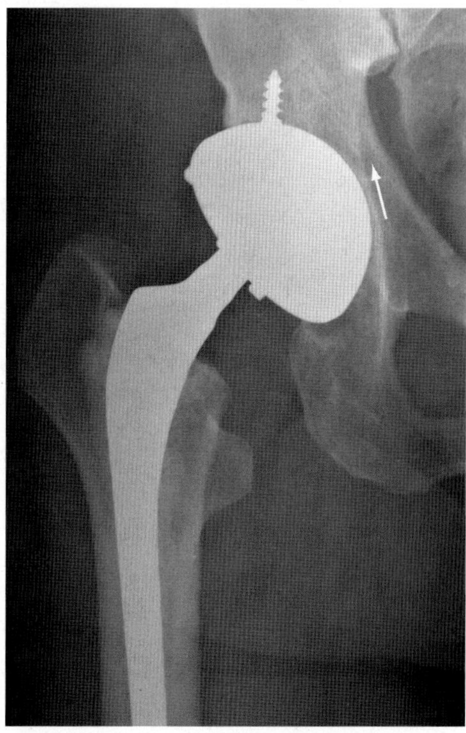

FIGURE 30-9. Normal bone ingrowth acetabular component. This acetabular component shows signs of osseointegration with no lucent lines present, developing superolateral sclerosis, medial osteopenia (stress shielding), and remodeling of trabeculae *(arrow)*.

Ninety-seven percent of the cups with three or more of these signs were stable at the time of revision surgery whereas 83% of the cups with two or fewer signs were loose[23] (Table 30-4).

Femoral Component

Radiographs are useful in documenting femoral component fixation. Three appearances have been described for assessing fixation of bone ingrowth stems. Although described for extensively coated components these findings are usually applied to proximally coated components as well.

In stable fixation by bone ingrowth, bone extends to and between the prosthetic surface beads. Areas of increased endosteal bone density ("spot welds") develop usually at the junction of the smooth and bone ingrowth surfaces. The cortices proximally become less dense due to stress shielding. No sclerotic lines ("demarcation lines") are present along the bone ingrowth portion of the stem (although they may be seen along the smooth portion of the stem). These findings are visible by 1 year after surgery (Figure 30-10).

In stable fixation by fibrous tissue, thin sclerotic lines develop along the bone ingrowth area but no change in component position occurs. Kaplan et al.[21] noted this finding in 79% of cases, usually within the first year after surgery.[24]

TABLE 30-4. Radiographic Findings That May Be Seen in Uncomplicated Bone Ingrowth Prostheses

Location	Finding
Femoral component	No lucent lines
	Stress shielding
	Thin proximal lucent line along bone ingrowth surface especially laterally (usually 1-2 mm) with a thin adjacent sclerotic line
	Endosteal sclerosis ("spot weld")
	Focal cortical thickening (may also be abnormal)
	Periosteal reaction due to stress changes
	Settling of stem of < 1 cm occurring < 1 year after surgery
Acetabular component	No lucent lines
	Superolateral, inferomedial buttressing
	Medial stress shielding
	Radial trabeculae

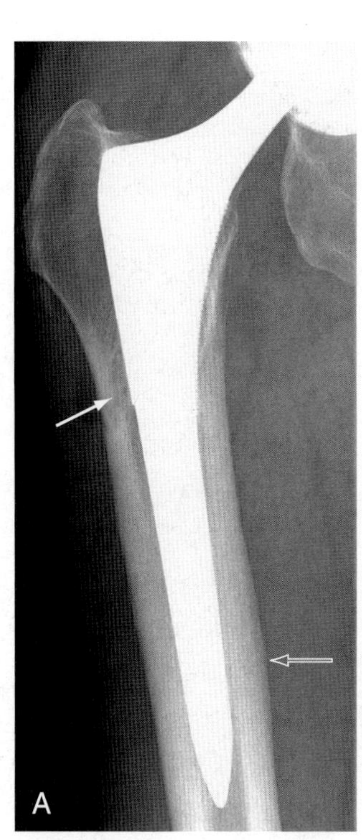

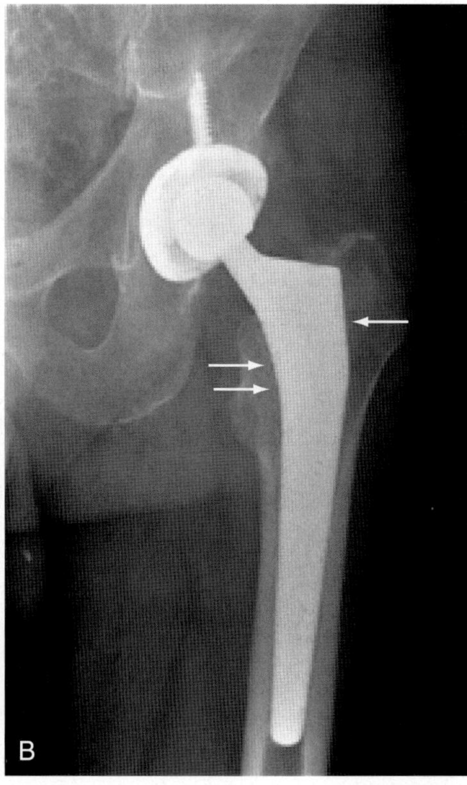

FIGURE 30-10. Femoral bone ingrowth and femoral fibrous ingrowth. **A,** Bone ingrowth. Several years after insertion of this prosthesis for damage due to avascular necrosis, there is evidence of bone ingrowth about the femoral component. No lucent lines are seen along the irregular surfaces for bone ingrowth. There has been reorientation of trabeculae and focal endosteal thickening is developing ("spot weld," *arrow*) at the junction of the bone ingrowth and smooth surfaces. There are thinning and rounding of the medial femoral cortex and osteopenia of the proximal femur indicating "stress shielding." Cortical thickening has occurred due to the transmission of stress to the femoral shaft through the prosthesis *(open arrow)*. **B,** Presumed fibrous ingrowth. This follow-up radiograph 1 year after a bone ingrowth total hip replacement shows that thin lucencies have developed along the bone ingrowth prosthetic surfaces *(arrows)*. These may indicate that fibrous ingrowth has occurred, but further follow-up (at least 2 years) is advised to be certain that these lucent lines do not widen.

Unstable fixation, or widening of a lucent zone along the bone ingrowth surface shows.[25] Continued displacement of surface beads suggests loosening. Settling of bone ingrowth components may occur early in the course but settling greater than 1 cm, especially if it continues more than 1 year after surgery, has a strong association with implant failure.[26]

Lucent lines may develop along the nonbone ingrowth (smooth) surface of a femoral component due to the differences in stiffness between the bone and the prosthesis. This may occur even with well-fixed components. Screws may be inserted to fix the acetabular component while bone ingrowth is occurring. Acetabular screw penetration into the pelvis should be noted. Oblique radiographs may be helpful in delineating this.[27] Screws that are perpendicular to the acetabular surface in the posterior quadrants usually are safe while those fixed perpendicular in the anterior quadrants are generally thought unsafe. If there is any question about screw position and its relation to vital structures, CT is performed.

Arthrography

Intra-articular contrast injection is usually performed as an adjunct to joint aspiration to allow the intra-articular needle position to be confirmed. Normally, injected arthrographic contrast fills a small smooth joint capsule and fills little, if any, of the cement bone interface.

> Contrast injection into the joint is recommended as a good practice to confirm needle position and define any abnormality of the joint (e.g., fistulae, bursae, or synovitis) whenever aspiration is performed.

Anesthetic Arthrography

The injection of anesthetic into the joint may be helpful in clarifying the origin of hip pain. Pain relief suggests an intra-articular source whereas absence of relief is considered nonspecific.

> Anesthetic injection into the hip joint may help determine the source of hip pain. Pain relief suggests an intra-articular source whereas absence of relief is considered nonspecific.

Scintigraphy

Increased radionuclide uptake may be seen on bone scans "normally" following total hip arthroplasty, but gradually decreases over a period of 6 to 12 months.[28]

Computed Tomography

While CT scanning is traditionally limited by the presence of metal hardware, newer multichannel scanners and attention to technical parameters have made this technique of considerable value for assessing prosthetic complications (Figure 30-11). Reformatted images reconstructed from the original axial data set provide images in the sagittal and coronal planes analogous to standard radiographic projections.

> Improvements in CT have made this an important technique for evaluating prostheses.

Technical factors for imaging of hip prostheses differ from standard body imaging techniques. Those suggested by Buckwalter et al. are shown in Table 30-5.[29] The radiation dose of these CT scans can be relatively high, and this should be considered when selecting imaging studies for younger individuals.

Normally, CT confirms the metallic femoral head to be centered in the acetabular liner (see Figure 30-11). Ceramic components are of homogeneous density (less dense than metal) and the interface between the acetabular and femoral components should be nearly imperceptible.[29] Bone should be closely apposed to the cement. Any lucent lines along the cement should be thin. Stable uncemented acetabular components should normally

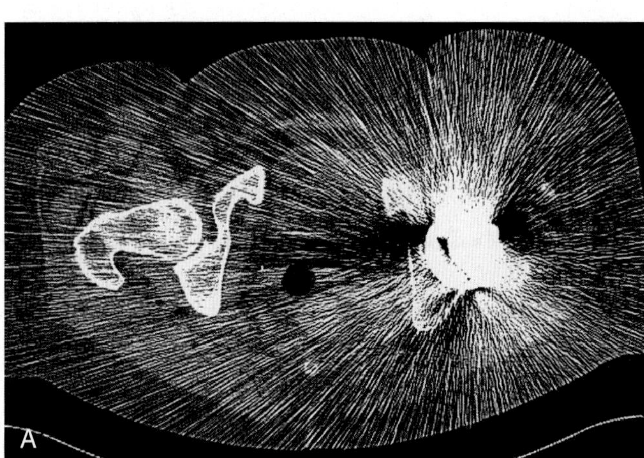

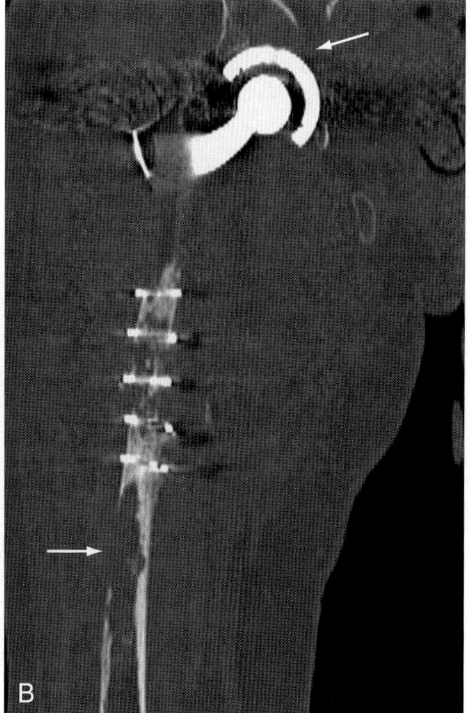

FIGURE 30-11. CT scanning. **A,** Image of a pelvis performed on an old CT scanner shows marked artifact. **B,** A reformatted CT at the level of the joint shows the femoral head centered in the acetabulum. Lytic metastatic lesions in the acetabulum and femur *(arrows)* are well seen despite the adjacent metal artifact.

(Continued)

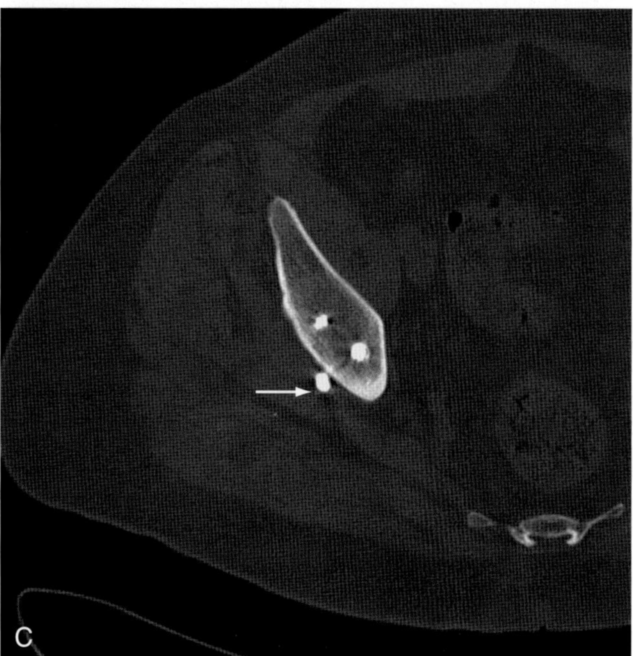

FIGURE 30-11—cont'd. **C,** An axial CT image in another patient shows a screw *(arrow)* extending past the bony cortex posteriorly but no impingement on nerves or vessels.

confirm trabecular bone adjacent to the irregular bone ingrowth surfaces of the prosthesis.[29]

CT is very useful in evaluating screw position, acetabular position in the sagittal plane (see Figure 30-11, *C*) and granuloma formation. CT is extremely helpful in identifying and quantifying areas of osteolysis. Radiographs underestimate the degree and size of osteolytic bone destruction. Evaluation of surgically produced lytic lesions in a cadaver model with a hip replacement in place showed the sensitivity for detecting lesions was 51.7% for radiographs, 74.7% for CT, and 95.4% for MRI (using specific protocols for CT and MRI to decrease meal artifact).[30]

TABLE 30-5. Technical Factors Suggested for Multichannel CT Scanning

Parameter	Recommended Value
Pitch[a]	Low (0.3 if possible)
kVp	140
mAs	35-450 if one THR
	450-600 if bilateral THRs
Focal spot	Small if possible
Dose modulation	Off
Detector array	Small
Scanned area	Tops iliac crests to tip of femoral stem (and cement if present)
Reconstruction algorithm	Standard or soft tissue
FOV	Both sides included
Spacing	3-mm contiguous
Reconstructions	
Axial of hip	160-220-mm FOV, mid-pelvis down
	1-1.5 mm thick, 50% overlap
	Soft image reconstruction filter
Sagittal and coronal reformations (two sets)	Femoral stem, acetabulum, proximal femoral component
	1.5 mm thick
	Use hip images for source

Buckwalter KA, Parr JA, Choplin RH, et al: Multichannel CT imaging of orthopedic hardware and implants, *Semin Musculoskel Radiol* 10:86-97, 2006.

Magnetic Resonance Imaging

Despite the fact that metal is a basic part of most total joint replacements and that metal induces artifacts on MRI, MRI can be used effectively in patients after total joint replacement especially if certain technical modifications are used.

> Improved techniques have made MRI a useful modality for assessing joint prostheses. MRI is particularly helpful to assess patients with unexplained pain after joint replacement or to further assess abnormalities identified on other imaging studies.[31]

Naraghi and White have reviewed the problems and the methods of improving MRI in patients with joint replacement.[31] As they explain, a homogeneous magnetic field and gradients are required for MR imaging.

Metallic components become magnetized to some degree when placed in a magnetic field (magnetic susceptibility); this results in inhomogeneities in the local field, producing artifacts.[31] This magnetization and, therefore, the artifact, is less in low magnetic fields and with certain metals such as titanium. Metal-induced artifacts include intra-voxel dephasing, misregistration, diffusion-related signal loss, and slice thickness variation.[31] The artifacts related to the presence of metallic components can be minimized using various techniques, depending on the type of artifact (Table 30-6). The tissues around the acetabular components are

TABLE 30-6. Methods of MRI Artifact Reduction in Presence of Metallic Hardware

Artifact	Artifact Reduction Modification
Intravoxel dephasing	Use SE and FSE in lieu of GRE
Misregistration	Broaden receiver bandwidth
	Use higher-frequency encoding strength
	Orient long axis of implant with B 0 (main magnetic field)
	Orient frequency encoding along long axis of implant
	Use lower magnetic field strength
	View angle tilting
Diffusion-related signal loss	Use FSE and short TE sequences
	Reduce interecho spacing
Slice thickness variation	Reduce slice thickness
	Increase matrix size
	Use 3D technologies
Nonhomogeneous fat saturation	Use STIR instead of spectral fat saturation
	Use modified three-point Dixon technique

FSE, Fast spin echo; *GRE,* gradient echo; *SE,* spin echo; *STIR,* short tau inversion recovery; *TE,* echo time.
With permission, from Naraghi AM, White LM: Magnetic resonance imaging of joint replacements, *Semin Musculoskel Radiol* 10:98-106, 2006.

generally less well demonstrated than those around the femoral component.[32]

Complications of Total Hip Replacement

Loosening

Component loosening may be secondary to infection or to a reaction to particulate debris, usually small polyethylene liner wear particles. Late aseptic loosening is the most common reason for implant failure.[33] Features of loosening that can be seen on radiographs are shown in Table 30-7. Stumpe et al. diagnosed loosening (without infection) when at least one of the following criteria was present: migration (of less than 2 mm within 6 to 12 months), periprosthetic lucency (in a smooth [linear] fashion) 2 mm or greater in diameter, periosteal reaction (of the solid type), and/or cement fracture.[28]

> Late loosening of hip prostheses, often due to osteolysis from wear particles, is the most frequent reason for failure of total hip prostheses.

Differentiation of septic from aseptic loosening is difficult or impossible on radiographs. Absence of the sclerotic line (demarcation line) that is usually seen separating a lucent zone from the adjacent bone may be an indication of infection. In addition, rapid progression on serial radiographs is suggestive of infection.[28]

> Differentiation of septic from aseptic loosening is difficult or impossible on radiographs.

Currently, arthrography is not often used at our hospital for the diagnosis of component loosening (although it is often used as an adjunct to joint aspiration). CT or scintigraphy is more likely to be performed. For the most accurate detection of loosening on arthrography, high injection pressure and subtraction techniques are most helpful. Using these techniques, Maus et al. found a sensitivity of 96%, and specificity of 92% for the diagnosis of femoral loosening and a sensitivity of 97% and specificity of 68% for acetabular loosening.[34] Arthrography indicates loosening following cemented total hip replacement if contrast at the cement bone interface extends past the intertrochanteric line of the femur for standard components or halfway down the stem for long-stemmed

TABLE 30-7. Radiographic Features of Component Loosening

Component Fixation	Finding	Example
Cement	Change in component position *(open arrow)*	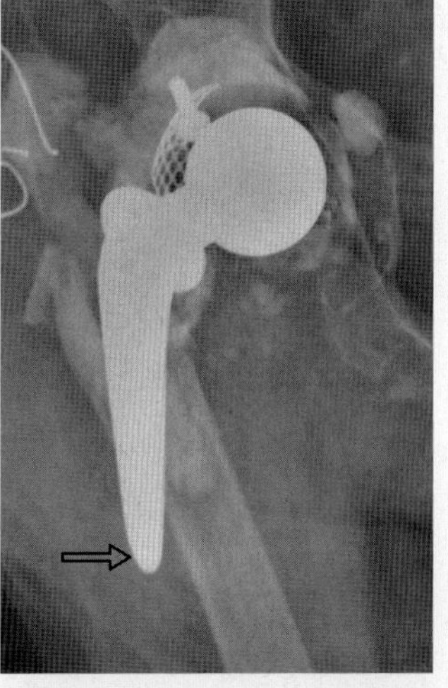
	2 mm or more linear lucency at cement–bone interface (definite loosening is present if 100% of interface is involved as in this example)	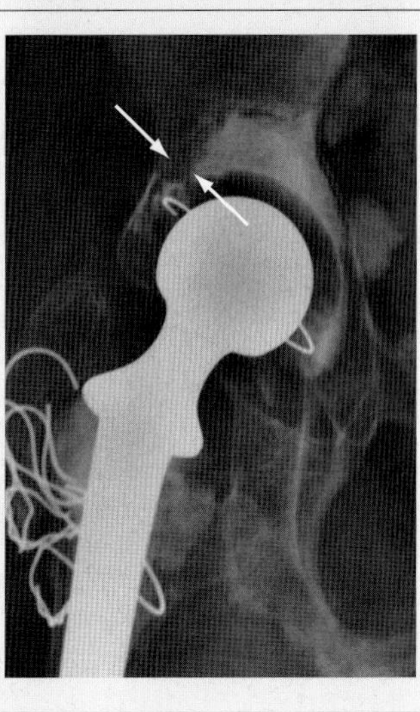

(Continued)

TABLE 30-7. Radiographic Features of Component Loosening—cont'd

Component Fixation	Finding	Example
	Cement fracture	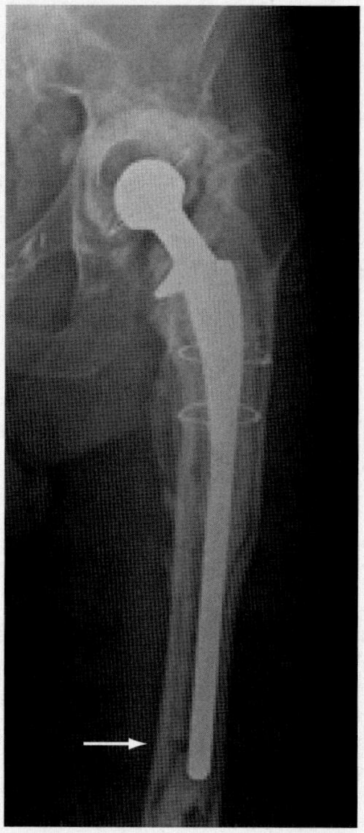
Uncemented components	Settling of femoral component > 1 cm or for > 1 year	
	Linear lucency along cement bone interface of 2 mm or more	
	Progressive shedding of surface beads	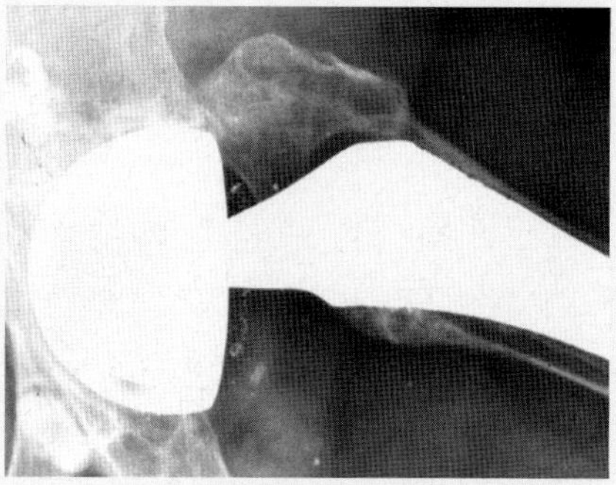

components.[34] Acetabular component loosening is more likely if the contrast fills the entire cement bone interface, is in zones I and II or II and III, or if the contrast is thicker than 2 mm in any region.

The value of arthrography for the detection of loosening of bone ingrowth components is less clear than for cemented components as contrast may insinuate along portions of the prosthetic interface even if bone ingrowth is present in other areas.

Scintigraphy is useful for detecting loosening of total hip replacements. Generally focal areas of increased uptake after 1 year are thought to indicate loosening while diffuse uptake suggests infection; unfortunately, the patterns are not specific and patients with focal uptake may also have infection[35] (Figure 30-12).

On MRI, loosening has been demonstrated as a nonenhancing linear area of low T1 signal and high T2 signal paralleling the femoral component[34] (Figure 30-13).

Wear and Osteolysis

Periprosthetic osteolysis is the major long-term complication of total hip arthroplasty.[36] Harris notes it also to be "the major cause of acetabular component loosening, necessitating revision of acetabular components, a major contributor to loosening of femoral

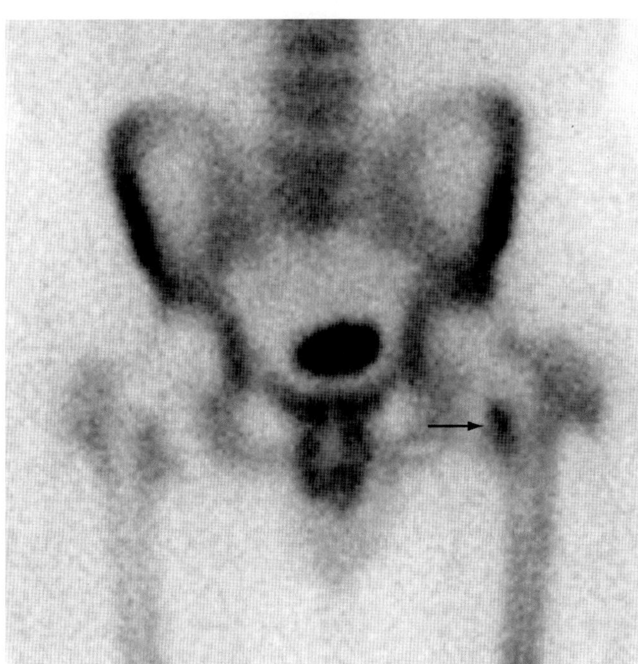

FIGURE 30-12. Femoral component loosening demonstrated on bone scan. Anterior image from a technetium 99m bone scan demonstrates focal uptake around the left total hip prosthesis *(arrow)*. The blood flow and blood pool images were normal. The right hip also has a prosthesis as evidenced by decreased uptake in the femoral head and neck but no increased uptake is seen.

components, and the single most important process behind pathologic fractures of the femur and pathologic fractures of the acetabulum following total hip arthroplasty."[36] It is most often the result of a reaction to particles generated by wear of the ultra-high molecular-weight polyethylene acetabular liner. Development of alternative articulating surfaces (metal on metal, ceramic on ceramic and highly cross-linked polyethylenes) have decreased the prevalence of osteolysis and could eliminate it.[36]

Measuring Wear

As noted above, the major cause of component failure is particle disease due most often to polyethylene wear and the subsequent development of periprosthetic osteolysis.[37] Thinning of the acetabular liner due to wear can be evaluated on radiographs since it eventually leads to a visible asymmetry in the position of the metallic femoral head within the acetabular component. Usually the femoral head shifts superolaterally in the acetabulum as wear increases (Figure 30-14). Several methods have been developed to quantify the amount of wear from radiographs.[38] In 1973, Charnley and Cupic reported wear at 9 to 10 years by evaluating a single radiograph.[39] Comparison of measurements on initial and follow-up radiographs is thought to be more accurate than a single measurement.[38,40]

These methods assess wear in the superior and lateral dimension, termed "linear" wear, and this has been shown to correlate with osteolysis.[41] Study of 235 Charnley low friction arthroplasties by Sochart followed 74 to 364 months showed that total wear averaged 2.1 mm (range, 0 to 7.2 mm), and the average wear rate was 0.11 mm per year, with the wear rate of revised components being twice that of surviving ones.[37] For every additional millimeter of wear, the risk of acetabular revision in any 1 year increased by 45% and for the femur increased by 32%.

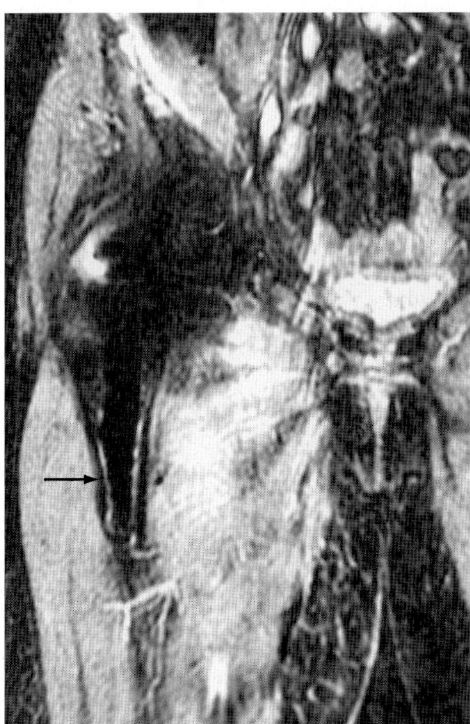

FIGURE 30-13. Presumed loosening of femoral component on MRI. This coronal STIR image shows a zone of increased signal *(arrow)* around the femoral component strongly suggesting loosening. No surgical confirmation is available.

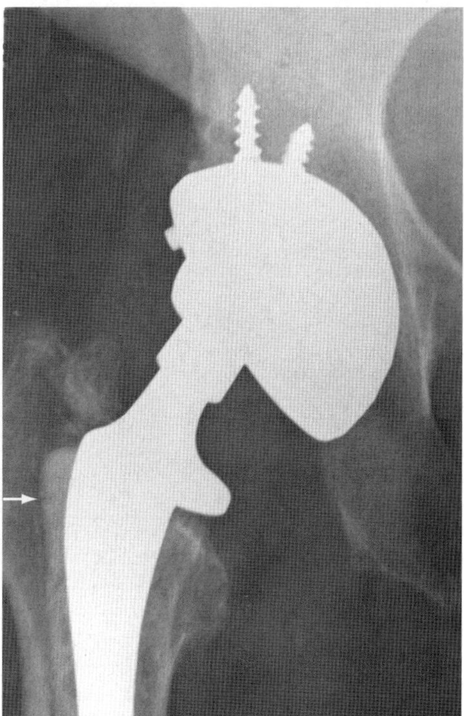

FIGURE 30-14. Acetabular wear. The femoral head is eccentrically positioned within the acetabular component. A lucency is seen along the femoral cement/bone interface laterally *(arrow)*. This is wider than 2 mm and suggests proximal femoral component loosening.

Measurement of wear in the anteroposterior dimension from lateral radiographs can also be done providing a three-dimensional (3D) assessment.

Digital imaging and computer-aided analysis provides greater accuracy and reproducibility.[42] Using weight-bearing radiographs to assess wear (rather than standard supine radiographs), has shown that measured vertical wear is significantly greater when radiographs are taken weight-bearing. Also, calculations of rates of linear wear of the acetabular component were significantly underestimated when radiographs were taken supine.[43]

Wear of the acetabular liner leads to an asymmetrical position of the femoral head.

Evaluating Osteolysis

Osteolysis occurs and progresses without clinical symptoms, making detection by imaging essential.[17] Unfortunately, radiographs are insensitive for the detection of osteolytic lesions generally, including those resulting from focal granulomatous lesions (Figure 30-15).

A study of cadavers with bilateral total hip replacements and surgically created bone defects has confirmed radiography to be limited in its ability to detect areas of pelvic osteolysis (sensitivity 51.7%). Lesions of the posterior rim and ischium are most difficult to identify.[30] Both MRI (using a specific protocol) and CT scanning with metal reduction techniques had better sensitivity (74.7% for CT and 95.4% for MRI) than radiography. Sensitivity improved with larger lesions; MRI was best for detecting small (< 3 cm) periacetabular lesions. Most of the underestimation of osteolytic lesions is in the detection of smaller lesions that may not be of clinical relevance. A strong correlation has been noted between the two-dimensional size and the 3D volume estimate of the lesions.

When evaluating radiographs or CT scans for areas of osteolysis, several points are helpful. Comparison with preoperative radiographs is useful to be sure that lucent areas seen postoperatively are not remnants of preoperative cysts. Lytic lesions should be described as to location and approximate size. Buckwalter notes that small cyst-like lucent lesions may be present normally at unoccupied screw holes possibly due to synovial fluid under pressure entering these areas[29] although areas of osteolysis usually demonstrate a communication to the joint space.[44] Cyst-like areas due to particle disease may extend into the soft tissues.[29]

Foreign body granulomatous reaction with hyperplastic capsules can produce positive 18-F-fluorodeoxyglucose (FDG) positron emission tomography (PET) scans that can mimic infection.[28]

Granulomas may mimic infection on PET scanning.

MRI is more sensitive for the detection of osteolysis than is radiography or CT. Osteolysis has been characterized on MRI as a localized periprosthetic intraosseous mass that is low in signal on T1-weighted images and low to intermediate in signal on

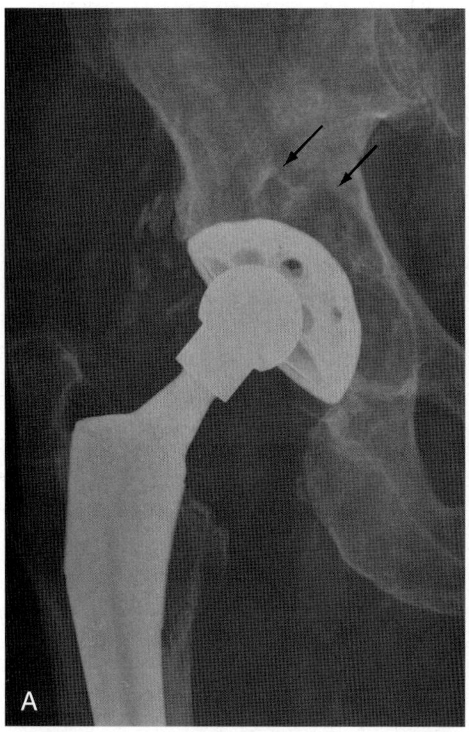

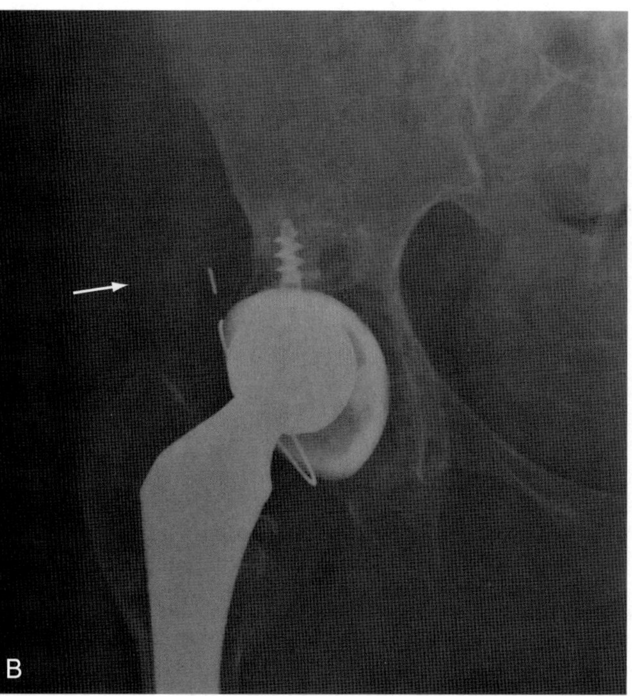

FIGURE 30-15. Wear with granuloma formation. **A,** This bone ingrowth prosthesis shows no lucent zones along the bone ingrowth areas of the femoral component to indicate loosening. However, lobulated lucencies have developed around the acetabular component *(arrows)* consistent with extensive granuloma formation. The femoral head is shifted laterally and superiorly in the acetabular component indicating wear of the acetabular liner. The resulting shedding of polyethylene particles has led to the granuloma formation. **B,** Wear with metal synovitis. This patient had juvenile rheumatoid arthritis (JRA) treated with a total joint replacement many years before. There has been wear of the acetabular liner resulting in the femoral head being shifted superiorly and laterally within the acetabular component. The titanium metal backing has been eroded as evidenced by the increased density of the joint fluid *(arrow)*, indicating metal within the joint (metal synovitis). Lucent areas around the proximal femoral component are due to granuloma formation. Note the thin femoral shaft due to the JRA.

T2-weighted images with a heterogeneous appearance. Peripheral and patchy internal enhancement is noted after intravenous contrast.[45] A hypointense margin surrounds these lesions. Synovitis due to particle disease may also be seen before other imaging techniques demonstrate abnormalities.[46]

Osteolytic defects and wear with stable components are treated with liner replacement and bone grafting.[10] Follow-up CT examinations have shown a decrease in lesion size, confirming the efficacy of this treatment.[47]

Fracture

Intraoperative fractures most often occur during broaching of the femoral canal.[10] Periprosthetic fractures later are uncommon complications but are more frequent after revision than primary total hip replacement.[10] These fractures are typically difficult to treat.

Dislocation

Dislocation continues to be a cause of early revision.[10] Ali Khan et al. reviewed 6774 total hip replacements from multiple centers and found dislocation occurred in 2.1%.[48] Component malposition such as an acetabular component that is too vertical or too anteverted or a femoral component that is too anteverted is often present.[48] Other predisposing factors include the surgical approach and the presence of neurologic disorders.

Radiographs are usually diagnostic. Blocks to reduction may be identified. Also, complications following reduction (including incomplete reduction, fracture, dissociation of components) are occasionally seen (Figure 30-16).

Infection

Two-thirds of periprosthetic hip infections develop during the first year after surgery.[28] The diagnosis of postoperative infection can be difficult on clinical and on imaging evaluation, yet the results are critical since treatment differs if infection is found.

Aspiration for Joint Infection

Joint aspiration is the most important examination if infection of a joint replacement is suspected in spite of the fact that both false-positive and false-negative results are reported (sensitivity 50% to 93% and specificity of 82% to 97%).[16] Levitsky et al. noted cultures to be superior to three-phase bone scan or sedimentation rate to detect infection in total hip replacements.[49] A prospective study of 202 patients prior to revision surgery, however, showed that no patient with infection had both negative C-reactive protein (CRP) and sedimentation rate.[50] A more recent series of 220 patients (235 hip arthropathies) confirmed that no hip was infected if the erythrocyte sedimentation rate was < 30 mm/hr and the C-reactive protein was < 10 mg/dL.[50a] In one series, aspiration of the joint (excluding patients on antibiotics) yielded 0.86 sensitivity, 0.94 specificity, 0.67 positive predictive value (PPV), and 0.98 negative predictive value (NPV).[50] In addition to culturing joint fluid, contrast injected at arthrography may show irregular collections extending from an infected joint (that may need separate aspiration) or demonstrate fistulae (Figure 30-17).

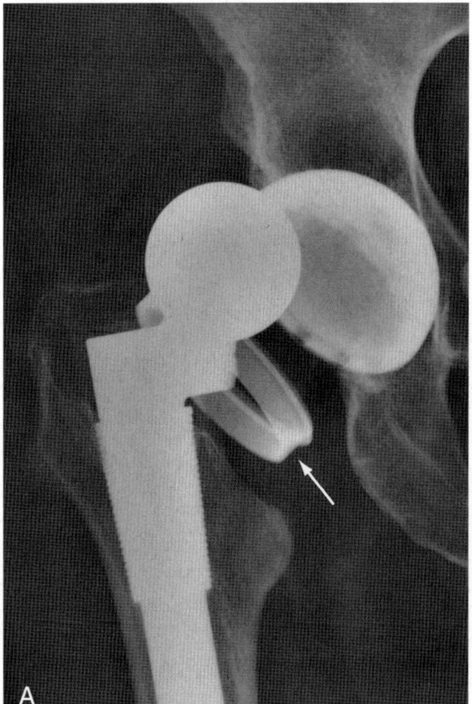

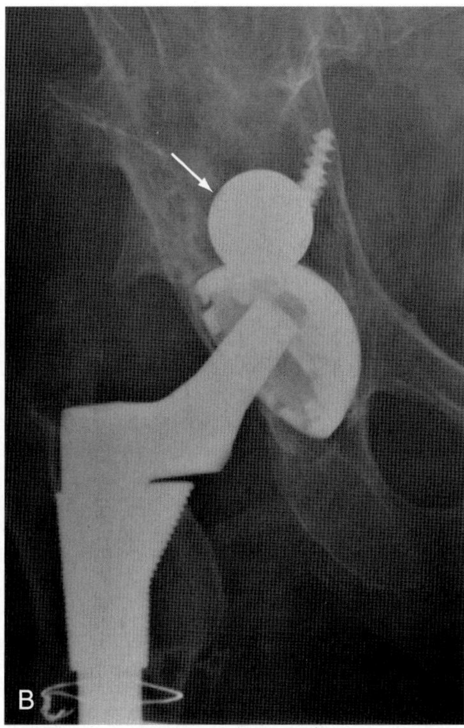

FIGURE 30-16. Dislocation in three patients. **A,** This patient had numerous prior dislocations leading to revision and placement of a constrained acetabular component with a metal ring peripherally to resist dislocation. However, dislocation has recurred and the restraining ring *(arrow)* has become displaced from the acetabular liner rim where it is normally located. **B,** Disengagement of the femoral head after reduction of a hip dislocation. This follow-up anteroposterior radiograph of the hip shows that the femoral head *(arrow)* has become displaced from the femoral neck of the prosthesis.

(Continued)

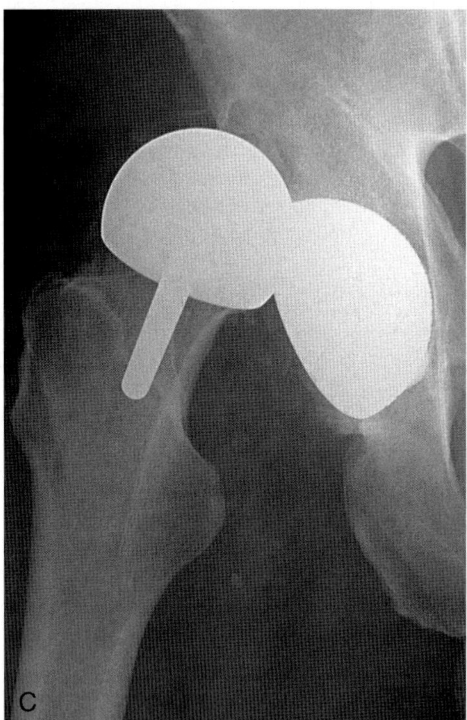

FIGURE 30-16—cont'd. **C,** Dislocated surface prosthesis. This 51-year-old man underwent a surface replacement for osteoarthritis. Following a fall, dislocation of the femoral component has occurred.

Radiography

Radiographs are generally inaccurate diagnostic tools for the detection of infection following total joint replacement.[35] Infection may be present even if radiographs are normal.[51] Serial radiographs are more useful than isolated examinations. Infection is suggested if there is rapid change in component position (prosthetic migration) on serial radiographs (at least 2 mm within 6 to 12 months), rapidly progressive periprosthetic osteolysis, and/or irregular periprosthetic osteolysis.[28] Using these criteria to evaluate 35 patients suspected of having septic loosening, Stumpe and colleagues correctly diagnosed infection by one reader in eight of nine patients and by a second reader in seven of nine patients with infection.[28] However, false-positive findings were seen in 13 cases by the first reader and nine cases by the second reader. Periosteal reaction may also be seen around infected joints (Box 30-1).

Computed Tomography

CT may be useful in detecting infection although joint aspiration is always necessary if infection is suspected. Evaluation using helical CT has shown that periosteal new bone formation was always associated with infection (100% specificity) but had only 16% sensitivity. Soft tissue findings were more accurate. Fluid collections in muscles and perimuscular fat had a 100% PPV value and the absence of joint distension a 96% NPV.[52]

Radionuclide Scanning

Technetium-99-m bone scans are thought to be sensitive but not specific for postoperative infection.[35] Unfortunately however, negative bone scan does not completely exclude infection.

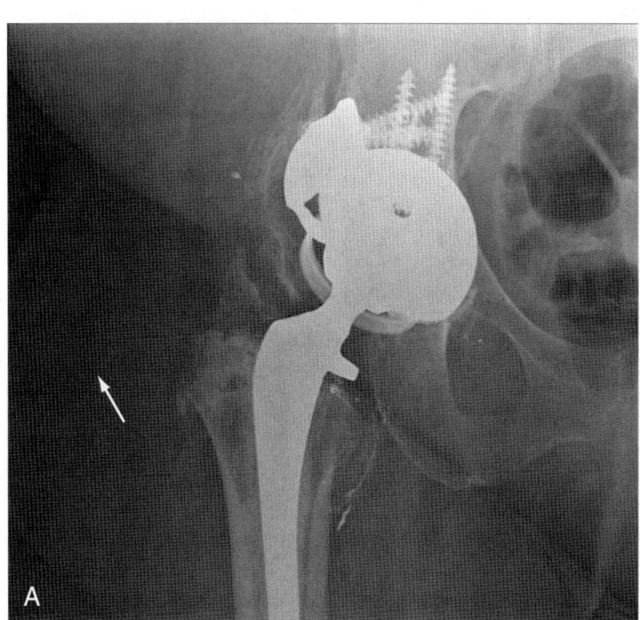

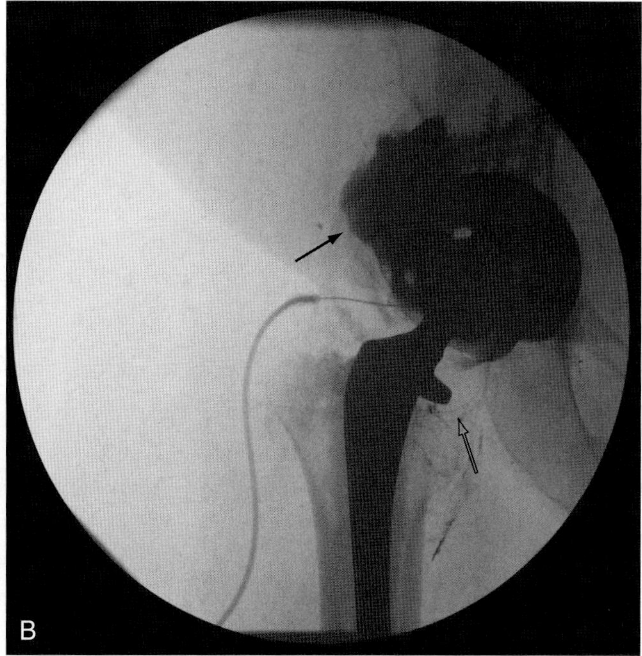

FIGURE 30-17. Infection. **A,** This patient underwent prior revision surgery. There is a hybrid prosthesis with a constrained acetabular component. Periarticular calcifications are noted. A soft tissue abscess with gas *(arrow)* is seen. **B,** A spot film from the arthrogram shows contrast extending along the lateral aspect of the acetabular component *(arrow)* but no definite loosening. There is filling of lymphatic channels medially *(open arrow)*. A small tract extends toward the abscess but does not appear to connect to it.

(Continued)

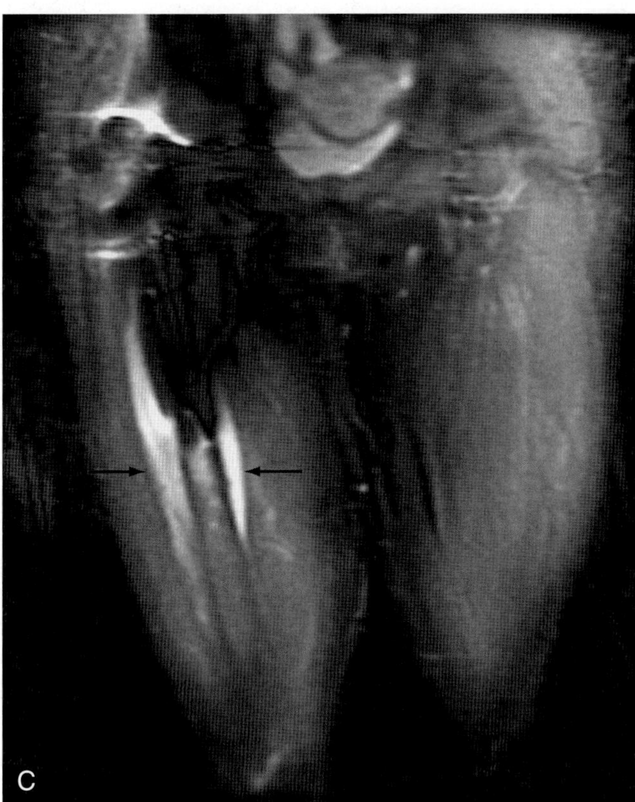

FIGURE 30-17—cont'd. C, MRI of infection. This patient had recurrent infection. The STIR image shows marked edema like signal *(arrows)* along the femur and within the femoral canal distal to the prosthesis. Infection was proven at surgery and the prosthesis was removed.

BOX 30-1. Radiographic Features Suggesting Infection after Total Hip Replacement

Rapid change in component position
Rapid development of periprosthetic osteolysis
Poorly defined areas of osteolysis
Periosteal reaction (especially irregular)
Absence of sclerotic demarcation line

Indium-111–labeled white blood cells (WBCs) accumulate at the site of a number of inflammatory processes, including acute osteomyelitis, acute exacerbations of chronic osteomyelitis, septic arthritis, abscesses, and rheumatoid arthritis. The sensitivity of the indium WBC scans for infection decreases as the chronicity of the infection increases. Sensitivities for the diagnosis of infection after total joint replacement range from 50% to 100% and specificities from 45% to 100%.[53]

The best radionuclide technique for the diagnosis of an infected joint replacement is the combined indium-111–labeled leukocyte/technetium-99-m sulfur colloid marrow scan. This combination allows correction for the abnormal leukocyte accumulation that may occur due to either displacement of marrow at the time of component insertion or stimulation of the reconversion of yellow to red marrow.[28] An incongruent pattern (absent bone marrow uptake in the face of accumulation of leukocytes) is highly accurate for diagnosing prosthesis infection. Examination of 40 hips with histopathologic and microbiologic confirmation showed the sensitivity of these combined scans to be 1.00, specificity 0.88, accuracy 0.93, PPV 0.82, and NPV 1.00.[54] However, this technique has drawbacks including being labor intensive, requiring the handling of blood products, expense and inconvenience to the patient.

> Combined indium-111 (^{111}In) and technetium-99-m (^{99m}Tc) sulfur colloid marrow imaging currently provide the highest sensitivity and specificity for the assessment of infected total hip replacements.[28]

Leukocytes may also be labeled with Tc-99-m stannous colloid providing advantages such as decreased cost, better imaging characteristics and greater availability.[55] Tc99-m stannous colloid labels both granulocytes and monocytes, which could improve detection of chronic infections associated with total joint replacement.

PET Scanning

Fluorine 18-FDG PET scanning has been reported to provide high sensitivity and specificity for the diagnosis of infection. Zhuang et al. noted that because of elevated glycolytic activity, inflammatory cells such as neutrophils and activated macrophages have increased FDG uptake at sites of inflammation and infection.[56] These authors examined 38 hip prostheses in patients with unexplained chronic hip pain. The PET scan identified 9 of 10 infections and excluded infection in 25 of 28 joints without infection (90% sensitivity, 89.3% specificity, and 89.5% accuracy). The test proved more accurate for detecting infections associated with hip prostheses than for detecting infections associated with knee prostheses (sensitivity, specificity, and accuracy of PET for detecting infection associated with knee prostheses were 90.9%, 72.0%, and 77.8%, respectively). Love et al. compared the results of F18-FDG imaging with indium-111–labeled leuckocyte/Tc-99-m sulfur colloid in patients with failed joint replacements and concluded that coincidence detection–based FDG imaging was less accurate than combined leukocyte marrow imaging.[54] Stumpe et al. found FDG PET scanning to be less sensitive than either radiography or bone scanning and less specific than three-phase bone scanning for the diagnosis of periprosthetic infection.[28] Foreign body granulomas may produce false positive results for infection,[28] as there is overlap between the histologic features of septic and aseptic loosening (granulomatous disease).

Quantitative evaluation (maximal standard uptake values) has indicated a significant difference in the FDG uptake at the soft tissue prosthesis interface in infected as compared to non-infected joints. Quantitative methods may, therefore, be useful adjuncts to standard image evaluation.[57]

Magnetic Resonance Imaging

On MRI, areas of infection are more poorly defined than areas of osteolysis due to granulomatous disease and demonstrate surrounding edema.[46]

Other Studies

Analysis of gene expression patterns in the WBCs in synovial fluid is a promising modality for diagnosing postoperative infection and distinguishing it from other causes of inflammation.[10]

Muscle and Tendon Injury

Gluteal muscle avulsion has been demonstrated on MRI in patients with otherwise unexplained pain after total hip replacement.[58] Fatty atrophy of the gluteus medius and the posterior half of the gluteus minimus are not usually seen findings in asymptomatic patients.[59]

Evaluation Prior to Revision Surgery

Prior to revision, radiographs are reviewed to determine the degree of bone loss due to osteolysis. Perforation of the medial acetabular wall is suspected if there is ballooning or discontinuity of Kohler's line (the ilioischial line) or the iliopubic line that was not present on initial postoperative radiographs.[60] In these cases, CT can be done for further evaluation.

Removal of acetabular components and cement may be associated with damage to major vessels and evaluation of the position of intrapelvic screws and their relationships to vital structures may be helpful in surgical planning.[27] Angled and oblique radiographs are also helpful but standard anteroposterior radiographs may miss important screw penetration.[27] Contrast enhanced CT can define these relationships preoperatively.[61]

Joint aspiration may be performed to identify infection prior to revision. Joint aspiration is the best test for identifying infection. The sensitivity of preoperative aspiration for infection ranges from 50% to 93% and the specificity from 82% to 97% (thus, both false-positive and false-negative studies occur). The indications for arthrography prior to revision surgery remain uncertain. Spangehl et al. suggest that an elevated sedimentation rate, CRP, or clinical suspicion of infection are indications for the procedure.[50,62]

KNEE PROSTHESES

Total knee prostheses have been clinically used since the late 1960s. A total of 402,100 primary total knee arthroplasties and 32,700 revision knee arthroplasties were performed in 2003, and it is estimated that by 2030, the demand for total knee arthroplasties will grow by 673% to 3.48 million.[63]

Patient satisfaction is greater than 90%, and there is a reported survival of the implants of greater than 90% at 10 to 15 years.[64] Nonetheless, failures do occur and it is thought that the demand for revision surgery will double by 2015.[63] Sharkey reviewed the causes of failure of 212 consecutive, revision total knee replacements from September 1997 to October 2000.[64] The most common causes of failure were polyethylene wear (25%), aseptic loosening (24.1%), instability (21.2%), infection (17.5%), arthrofibrosis (14.6%), malalignment or malposition (11.8%), and extensor mechanism deficiency (6.6%). Early failure (before 2 years) was due in 50% of cases to instability, malalignment, malposition, or failure of fixation. The most common cause of failure in the early group was infection (25.4%). Late revision was usually the result of wear, loosening, or instability.

> Total knee replacement is a highly successful procedure with long-term high levels of component retention and patient satisfaction.

Types of Prostheses

A "total knee" arthroplasty resurfaces the femoral and tibial sides of the joint, or more often, the femoral, tibial, and patellar surfaces. Patellofemoral replacement without femorotibial replacement or replacement of patellofemoral and one femorotibial compartment may also be performed, but these procedures are uncommon. Most total knee prostheses are "unconstrained" or "partially constrained," providing little inherent knee stability (Figure 30-18).

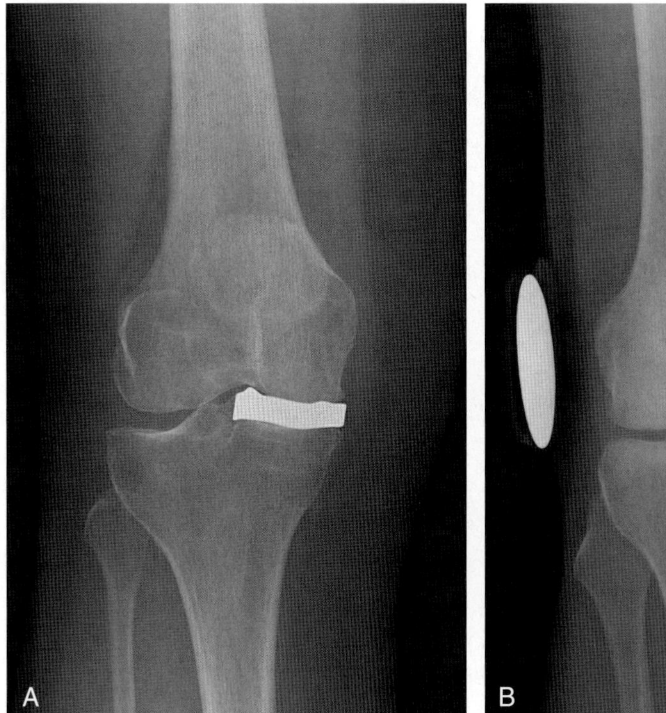

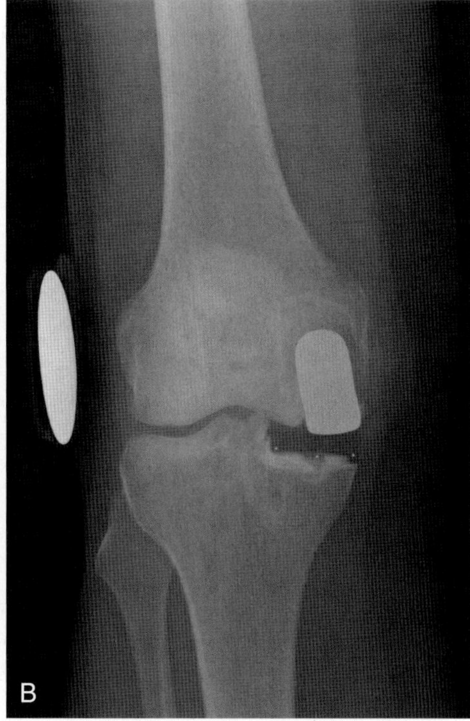

FIGURE 30-18. Knee prostheses. **A,** ConforMIS spacer knee prosthesis. This prosthesis comprises a spacer between the bones filling in the defect left from thinned cartilage. Based on MRI examination, the component is designed to conform to the cartilage defect. It is not fixed to bone or cartilage. **B,** Medial unicondylar prosthesis. The cemented non–metal-backed tibial component and the cemented metallic femoral component are seen without evidence of tibial lucent lines to indicate component loosening. Revision was necessary, however, because of instability. The metallic disk laterally is a magnification marker of known size.

(Continued)

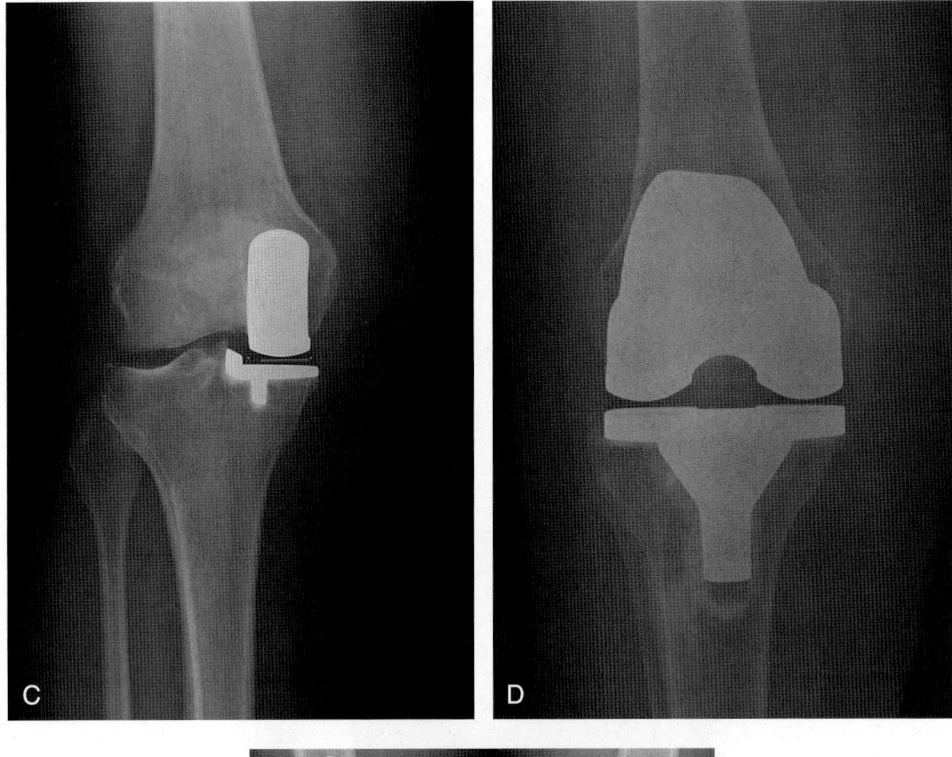

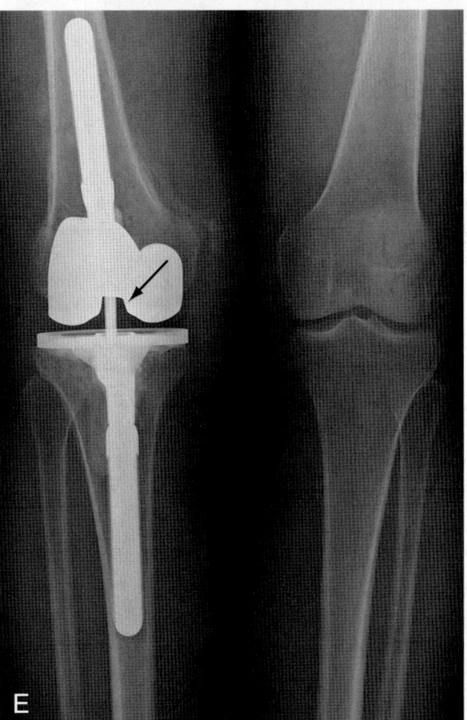

FIGURE 30-18—cont'd. **C,** Mobile bearing unicondylar prosthesis. Osteoarthritic damage was largely confined to the medial compartment. A unicondylar prosthesis was inserted with cemented femoral and tibial components and a polyethylene articular surface that can move on the metal backing. This increased motion should decrease wear of the liner. **D,** Unconstrained total knee prosthesis. The anteroposterior view shows the cemented metal backed tibial component, polyethylene articular surface and metal femoral component. **E,** Constrained total knee prosthesis. This prosthesis has a central articulation *(arrow)* that helps maintain stability. Periosteal reaction along the femur is the consequence of a previously treated infection.

Some of these prostheses sacrifice the posterior cruciate ligament ("cruciate sacrificing" prostheses), while other designs retain the patient's native posterior cruciate ligament ("cruciate retaining"). The anterior cruciate ligament is routinely sacrificed at surgery even if it was not previously damaged. A posterior-stabilized prosthesis is a cruciate-sacrificing prosthesis in which a cam in the femoral intercondylar notch engages a post on the tibial side as the knee flexes.[65] In patients with ligamentous laxity, constrained prostheses may be used that provide inherent stability but limit motion.

All these prostheses contain articulations between a metallic femoral component and a high density polyethylene tibial surface. The tibial polyethylene is usually attached to a metal tibial tray (used to distribute stress to the underlying bone). In "meniscal-bearing" or "mobile-bearing" designs, the polyethylene articular surface can rotate somewhat on the underlying metal similar to having a meniscus present. Patellar components are currently polyethylene with no metal backing. A "unicondylar" prosthesis ("unicompartmental" arthroplasty) resurfaces the bones of either the medial or lateral femorotibial compartment in patients with minimal damage elsewhere in the knee. Mobile bearing unicondylar prostheses are also available. Most total knee prostheses are cemented.

> Several types of knee prostheses are available to accommodate knees in which only one compartment is damaged to those in which involvement is greater or the knee is unstable.

Positioning

The expected positioning of knee prosthetic components is shown in Table 30-8.

TABLE 30-8. Evaluating Positioning of Total Knee Components on Radiographs

	Anteroposterior Projection	Lateral Projection	Tangential Patellar View	Standing View of Both Legs
Femoral	Femoral component 97 or 98 degrees to femoral shaft 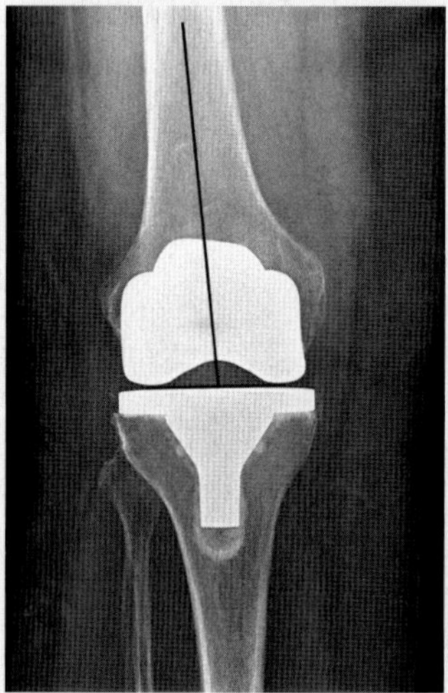	Femoral component perpendicular to femoral shaft 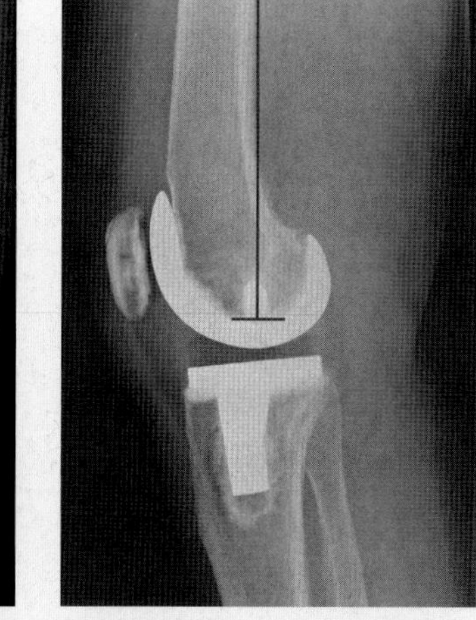		
Tibial	Tibial tray 90 degrees to tibial shaft 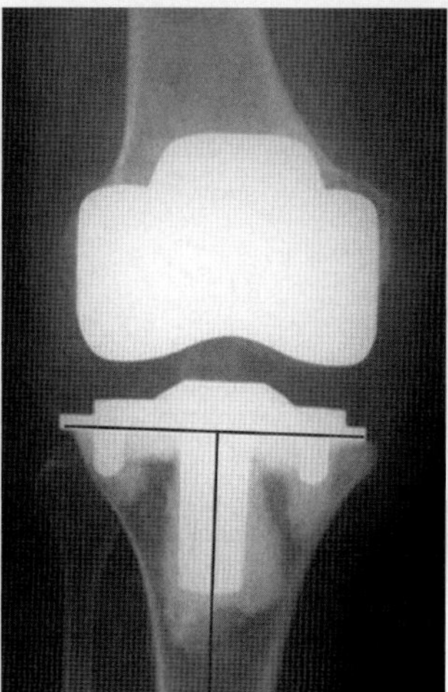	Tibial tray 90 degrees to tibial shaft (or tilted slightly downward posteriorly) 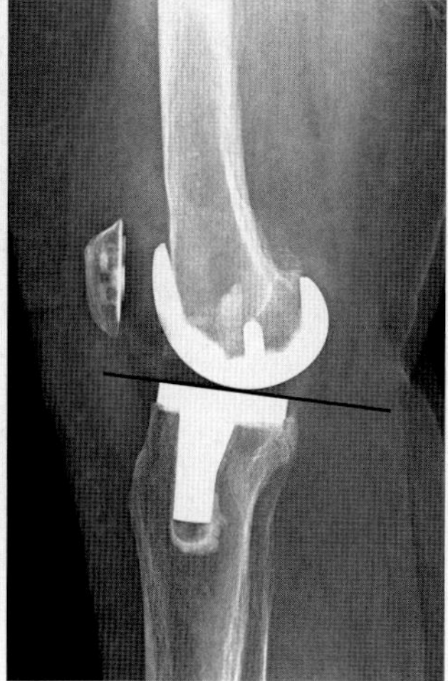		

(Continued)

TABLE 30-8. Evaluating Positioning of Total Knee Components on Radiographs —cont'd

	Anteroposterior Projection	Lateral Projection	Tangential Patellar View	Standing View of Both Legs
				Mechanical axis (mid-femoral head to mid-tibial plafond) passes through center of knee 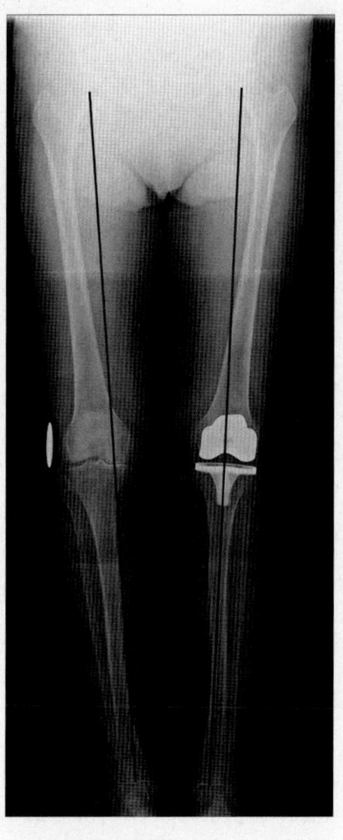
Patella		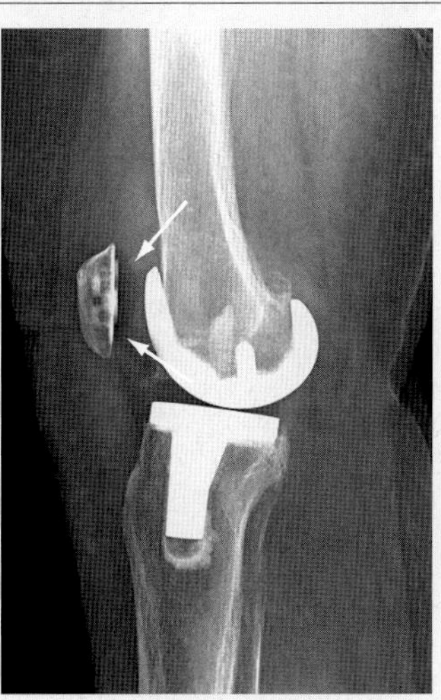	Centered on femur, not tilted or dislocated Thickness same as preoperative	

(Continued)

TABLE 30-8. Evaluating Positioning of Total Knee Components on Radiographs —cont'd

	Anteroposterior Projection	Lateral Projection	Tangential Patellar View	Standing View of Both Legs
Interfaces	Close apposition of bone to prosthesis or bone to cement			
Bone		Diffuse lucency around femoral component may be due to stress shielding		
Soft tissue		Joint effusion should be decreasing		

Routine Radiography

Immediate postoperative imaging is usually unnecessary if the procedure was uncomplicated. Baseline radiographs are usually performed at the first postoperative visit.[66] One study assessed the effectiveness of radiographs obtained upon admission to a rehabilitation facility following hip or knee arthroplasty.[67] This retrospective chart review examined 209 patients admitted after total knee replacement and found two (0.95%) with abnormal findings on radiographs. There was no change in hospital stay or medical intervention in these patients. While this type of study has some limitations, the conclusion that routine radiography upon admission to a rehabilitation facility after knee replacement surgery is not cost-effective seems justified.

Follow-up radiographs are evaluated for component position, knee alignment, thickness of the articular liner, and the presence of lucent lines. Standard nomenclature can be used to describe the periprosthetic interfaces[68] (Figure 30-19).

Computed Tomography

In addition to alignment in the coronal and sagittal planes, rotational alignment of the femoral and tibial components is important. Anterior knee pain, patellofemoral instability and excessive wear of the polyethylene articular surfaces may result from rotational malalignment.[69]

There are several methods of determining the proper degree of *femoral* component rotation at the time of surgery; including the relationship to the transepicondylar axis of the femur, the posterior femoral condyles, or a vertical midtrochlear line.[69] There are also several methods of determining the correct *tibial* component rotation at the time of surgery including using anatomical landmarks (such as the tibial tubercle, the posterior condylar line of the tibia, and the malleolar axis of the ankle) or a range of motion technique in which the tibial trial component is allowed to orient itself with relation to the femoral component while the knee is flexed and extended, and this position is used for the permanent component.[69]

Postoperatively, both CT and MRI can evaluate the rotational alignment of the tibial and femoral components and the relationship between them. The method of Berger et al. is used at The Brigham and Women's Hospital to evaluate component rotation. CT scans are obtained perpendicular to the femoral and then perpendicular to the tibial axis using a lateral scout view for planning. Imaging is performed from proximal to the femoral component to below the tibial tubercle[70,71] (Figure 30-20).

Combined Component Rotation

The combined component rotation is the sum of the femoral and tibial component rotational angles. Internal rotation is added as a negative value and external rotation as a positive angle.

Relationship of Femoral and Tibial Components

Uehara et al. evaluated rotational mismatch between femoral and tibial components.[72] A baseline for the anteroposterior axis of each component was drawn based on the epicondylar axis for the femur and the medial third of the tibial tuberosity. The angle between these lines was used to determine the rotational mismatch.

Complications

Loosening

In one series, loosening was a cause of revision in 34% of cases revised 2 years or more after implant insertion.[64] A wide (2 mm or more) or increasing lucent zone around the prosthesis interface or a change in component position indicates loosening[73] (Figure 30-19) (Box 30-2). Duff et al. defined loosening on radiographs by the presence of prosthetic fracture, cement fracture, periprosthetic fracture, or gross component migration.[74] The wide bands of lucency suggesting component loosening are separated from the adjacent bone by a thin dense line (demarcation line) as is seen in total hip arthroplasty.

Radiographs

Evaluation of lucent lines requires that they be seen in profile. Fluoroscopy can accomplish this and, therefore, facilitate the detection of loosening.[75] However, necessary time and expense limit the use of routine fluoroscopic assessment.

A more diffuse decrease in density, especially prominent beneath the anterior or posterior flanges of the femoral component

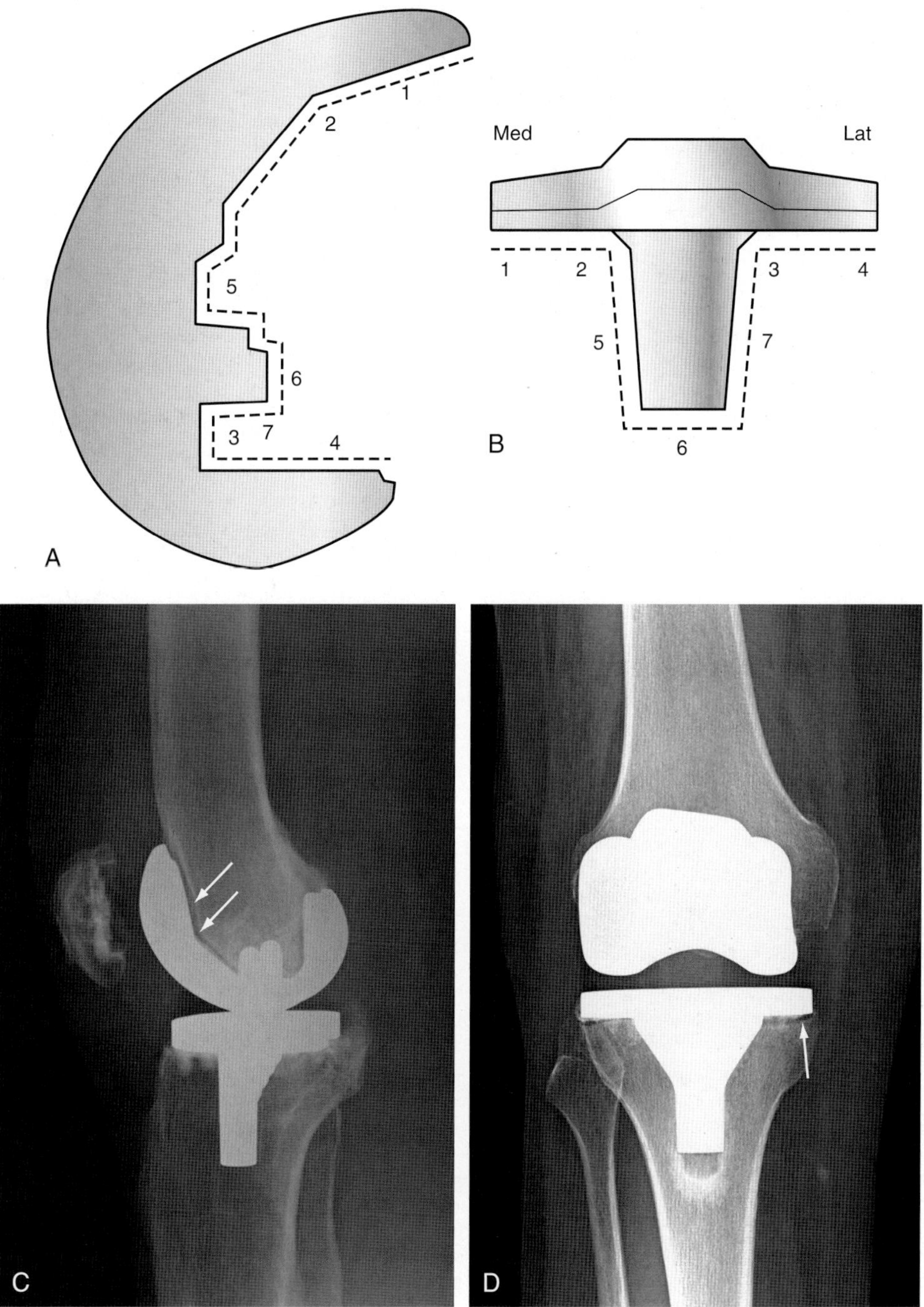

FIGURE 30-19. Cement bone interfaces and loosening. **A,**The standard nomenclature used for location of periprosthetic lucencies is shown for the femoral and **B,** tibial components. **C,** Femoral component loosening. The lateral radiograph shows extensive lucent zones along the cement bone interface of the femoral component *(arrows)*. Considerable joint distension is present. The femoral component was loose at surgery. **D,** Tibial lucent lines. A 2-mm thick lucent line is noted under the medial *(arrow)* and lateral aspects of the tibial tray at the cement bone interface. Additional lucency along the central stem would be even more suggestive of loosening.

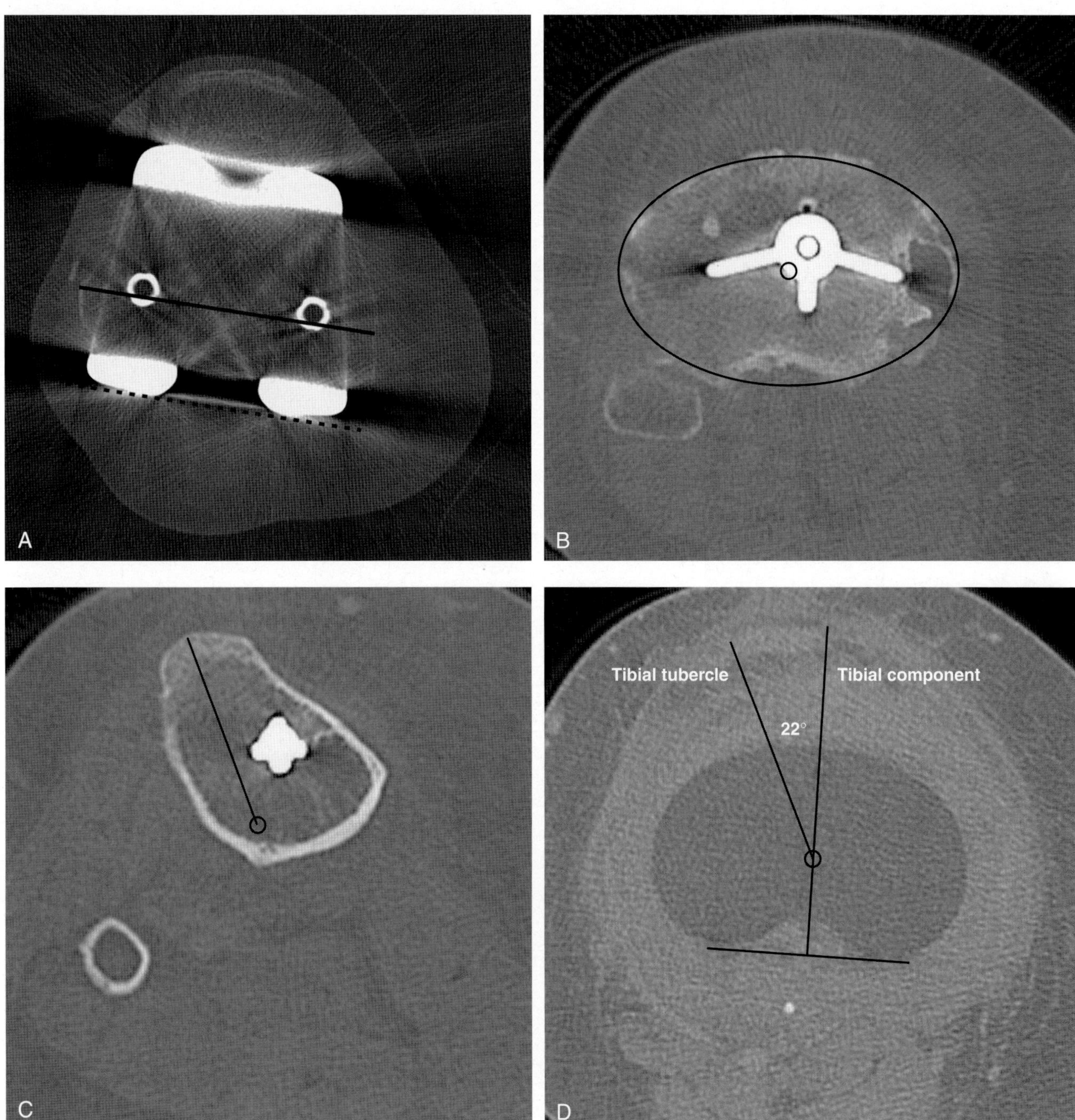

FIGURE 30-20. Analysis of component rotation on CT after Berger et al. **A,** Femoral component rotation. The CT slice that passes through the femoral epicondyles is used to assess femoral component rotation. The transepicondylar axis is constructed by connecting the prominence of the lateral epicondyle to the center of the trough between the prominences of the medial epicondyle *(solid line)*. The posterior condylar line is drawn along the posterior aspects of the medial and lateral posterior condylar surfaces *(dashed)*. Ideally the femoral component is parallel to this line or in external rotation. The angle between these lines is measured. If the angle opens medially, the component is in internal rotation. Since women normally have a posterior condylar angle of 3.1 (± 1.2) degrees of internal rotation, this angle is subtracted from any measured internal rotation to determine the degree of "excessive internal rotation." **B,** Tibial component rotation. A CT scan is obtained through the tibia below the prosthesis. This allows the center of the tibia to be defined, establishing a reference point. In this case, lucent granulomas are present. **C,** The center reference point in **B** is transposed onto the image showing the most prominent portion of the tibial tubercle and the axis is drawn between these two points. **D,** On the image through the articular polyethylene, a line is drawn along the posterior surface of the polyethylene liner and a perpendicular is drawn to that. The tibial tubercle axis from **C** is superimposed on the image and the angle measured. Eighteen degrees (the normal rotation of the tibia is 18 ± 2.6 degrees) are subtracted from the measured internal rotation to determine the "excessive internal rotation."

BOX 30-2. Findings Suggesting Loosening of a Total Knee Prosthesis

- Progressive widening of a lucent zone
- > 2 mm lucency at cement–bone interface
- Lucency at metal–cement interface
- Metal bone lucency

From Math KR, et al: Imaging of total knee arthroplasty, *Semin Musculoskel Radiol* 10:47-63, 2006.

or under the tibial tray, may develop due to a shift in stress away from these areas (stress shielding). No demarcation lines are seen delimiting these areas so confusion with criteria for loosening is unlikely.

Bone Scintigraphy

Bone scintigraphy is most helpful many years after surgery since positive bone scans are noted in 20% of asymptomatic knees a year after surgery and in 12.5% of individuals 2 years postoperatively.[76] Generally, increased isotope uptake on the static scan but not on the blood pool scan is thought more likely to be due to loosening than infection. Evaluation of 80 symptomatic total knee prostheses found that the method distinguished abnormal (loosening or infection) from normal patients with a sensitivity of 92.3% (and specificity 75.9%) but was unable to distinguish between these two abnormal conditions. The NPV of 95% made a normal scan reassuring.[77]

Infection

Infection occurs in 1% to 4% of total knee replacements,[78] and is more common in older patients and in patients with prior surgery.[74] In one series, infection was responsible for 25.4% of early revisions and 7.8% of revisions performed more than 2 years after the initial surgery.[64] Duff et al. noted that the diagnosis of infection was not obvious in more than half of knees prior to revision arthroplasty.[74] *Staphylococcus epidermidis* and *Staphylococcus aureus* are the most common causative organisms.[74]

Clinical Features

Pain is the most common presenting symptom but is nonspecific.[79] Night pain or pain at rest are typical of infection, whereas pain on weight bearing is more consistent with mechanical loosening.[79] Early acute infections after total knee arthroplasty are usually clinically evident and manifested by pain, swelling, fever, systemic symptoms, and erythema. Low-grade or chronic infections may be more difficult to identify.[74] A knee may be infected without the presence of fever, chills, erythema, or swelling.[74] Treatment of deep periprosthetic infections is related to the time of presentation (Table 30-9).

Laboratory findings are often nonspecific. Peripheral leukocyte counts are not elevated in most patients with infected prostheses.[74] Sedimentation rates are abnormal in patients with infection but the finding may also be seen in uninfected patients, limiting the value of the test.[74] C-reactive protein (CRP) is significantly higher in patients with infection compared to those with aseptic loosening (sensitivity 79% for hip and knee prostheses) although a normal level does not exclude infection.[78] A large multicenter study found CRP and joint aspiration to be the most useful tools to diagnose infection.[80]

Radiographs

Duff et al. found radiographs not to be helpful since loosening, periostitis, focal osteolysis, and radiolucent lines were seen in infected and uninfected knees[74] (see Figures 30-17, Figure 30-21). Most importantly, infection may be present with a "normal" radiograph.

Infection may not be detectable on radiographs.

Aspiration

Knee joint aspiration has been found to be extremely useful in the diagnosis of infection after total joint arthroplasty. Duff et al. found a sensitivity, specificity, and accuracy of 100% for aspiration in a series of 43 knees with pain, instability, loosening, or suspected infection undergoing surgical revision.[74] Antibiotics were discontinued for 2 to 3 weeks before aspiration.[74] Virolainen et al. found joint aspiration to be 100% specific and 75% sensitive for the diagnosis of infection and to be the best test for the diagnosis of infection in a group of total hip and knee replacement patients.[78] Bach et al. found early aspiration to lead to a significant reduction in the duration of treatment and a better outcome.[81] Multiple aspirations may be necessary, however, to obtain a positive culture. Barrack et al. noted that, in contrast to aspiration of total hip replacements where false positive results are more common, aspirations of knee joints are more often falsely negative.[82] At least 2 weeks off antibiotics is recommended before the aspiration is performed (with careful clinical monitoring for sepsis), but as long as a month may be necessary for cultures of aspirated fluid to become positive. Therefore, when the CRP level is greater than 10 mg/l, repeat joint aspiration or biopsy is suggested.

Bone Scan

It is usually stated that bone scintigraphy is useful for excluding infection but of limited value in detecting it.[83] Thus, sensitivity is

TABLE 30-9. Classification of Deep Periprosthetic Infection

Type	Timing	Definition	Treatment
1	Positive intraoperative culture	Two or more positive intraoperative cultures	Appropriate antibiotics
2	Early postoperative	Infection occurring within first month after surgery	Attempt debridement with salvage of prosthesis
3	Acute hematogenous	Hematogenous seeding of previously well-functioning prosthesis	Attempt at debridement with salvage or removal of prosthesis
4	Late (chronic) infection	Chronic indolent course; infection present for > 1 month	Removal of prosthesis

With permission from Leone JM, Hanssen AD: Management of infection at the site of a total knee arthroplasty, *J Bone Joint Surg Am* 87:2335-2348, 2005.

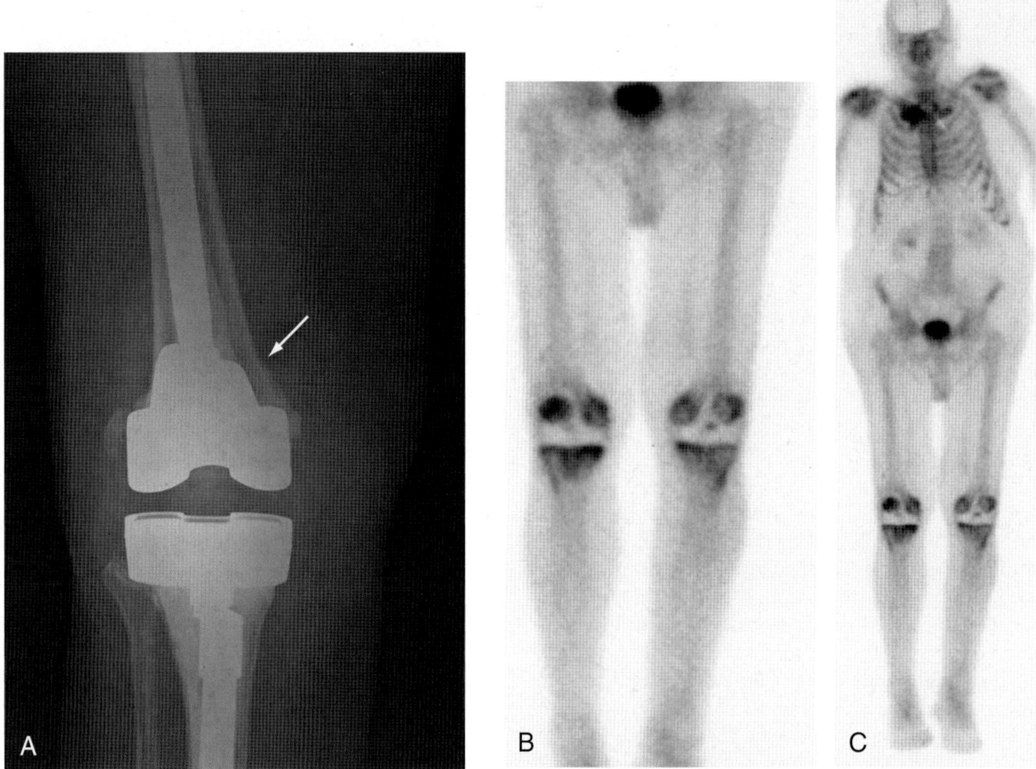

FIGURE 30-21. Infected total knee prosthesis. **A,** This AP radiograph shows no evidence of component loosening. There is mild periosteal reaction medially *(arrow)*. The prosthesis was infected. **B,** Blood pool images from another patient with rheumatoid arthritis and bilateral total knee prostheses shows diffuse increase in activity around each knee. The radiographs were negative for loosening or periosteal reaction. **C,** The static bone scan shows increased activity bilaterally. Both knees were proven to be infected.

high and specificity is low. Loosening is thought to be most likely if the blood pool phase is normal, and there is increased uptake on the delayed (static) scan, whereas infection is more likely if there is increased uptake on both blood pool and delayed images.[77]

Indium Scan for Diagnosis of Periprosthetic Infection

Labeling leukocytes with indium-111 requires that the patient's venous blood sample be drawn and the WBCs isolated and labeled with indium-111 oxine and then reinjected intravenously prior to scanning.[84] Accurate interpretation requires comparison of the indium isotope uptake to activity on bone scan; a positive indium scan for infection generally requires increased indium-111 uptake either in a different distribution (an "incongruent" scan) or in greater intensity than on the bone scan.[84] Using these criteria and surgical confirmation, Scher et al. evaluated patients with loose or painful total knee replacements, and found a sensitivity of 88%, specificity of 78%, PPV 75%, and NPV of 90% for infection. The examination was not recommended routinely because of the expense, complexity, and limited sensitivity and specificity, PPV, and accuracy. In equivocal cases and when an experienced musculoskeletal pathologist it not available to interpret the frozen section, a negative indium scan may be helpful to suggest the absence of infection.[84] A positive indium scan for infection generally requires increased indium-111 uptake either in a different distribution (an "incongruent" scan) or in greater intensity than on the bone scan.

Use of indium scanning may lead to a high false positive rate thought to be due to marrow packing.[83] The addition of technetium-99-m–labeled sulfur colloid has been investigated to reduce this. However, Joseph et al. found that low sensitivity and the potential for false-negative results made this combination of scans of limited utility for the diagnosis of prosthetic infection; it was therefore no longer used in their institution. In that group of 22 total knee prostheses evaluated and later operated upon, there was a sensitivity of 66%, specificity of 100%, 100% PPV, 88% NPV, and 91% accuracy. The addition of blood pool and flow assessment decreased the number of false negative scans (sensitivity of 83%, specificity 94%, PPV of 83%, and NPV 94%). However, overall, the performance of the indium/colloid scan protocol was thought to be of limited clinical utility for assessing patients with a painful prosthesis and these examinations are no longer routinely used by this group for this assessment.[83] Evaluation of combined indium-111–labeled leukocyte and Tc-99-m sulfur colloid marrow scanning by Love and colleagues revealed more optimistic results. In 19 total knee replacements with a final diagnosis confirmed by histologic and microbiologic examinations, this scan combination yielded a sensitivity, specificity and accuracy of 1.00.[54]

> Some authors find the combined indium/colloid scan protocol to be of limited clinical utility for assessing patients with a painful total knee prosthesis.

Study of a small series of total knee arthroplasties using indium-111 IgG found the sensitivity of this agent for infection to be high but its specificity low (sensitivity 100%, specificity 50%). Bernard et al. performed a literature review and a multicenter trial of various clinical laboratory, radiologic, and scintigraphic methods for the diagnosis of hip and knee infections.[80] Scans using tagged white cells or radiolabeled immunoglobulin demonstrated a sensitivity of 74% and specificity of 76% for the diagnosis of infection and literature review indicated sensitivity of 38% to 100% and specificity of 41% to 100%. These studies were therefore not recommended as routine for differentiating mechanical failure from occult infection in painful loose total joints.[80]

FDG Positron Emission Tomography

Elevated glycolytic activity causes inflammatory cells such as neutrophils and activated macrophages to be FDG avid at sites of inflammation and infection.[56] Thus, FDG PET imaging may be useful for detection of infection after joint replacement. The examination is much faster and less expensive than combined bone marrow and indium scintigraphy.[56] In one series, the use of FDG PET scanning showed no advantage when combined with bone scanning over HMPAO-labeled WBC scan and bone scanning.[85] However, study of 36 painful knee prostheses examined using 18F-FDG PET scanning showed identification of 10 of 11 infected cases, but false-positive results in 7 cases (sensitivity of 90.9%, specificity of 72%, and accuracy of 77.8% for the detection of infection).[56] This was lower accuracy than for assessment of hip prostheses. The cause for the high number of false-positive knee cases was not known. Overall, FDG PET scan had a sensitivity of 95% and specificity of 72.7% in the evaluation of 64 prosthetic implants.[86]

Algorithm

Virolainen et al. recommend that, if arthroplasty patients have pain in a prosthetic joint without clear radiologic evidence of loosening, bone scans, and preoperative joint aspirations should be undertaken. The same tests should be implemented if radiologic evidence of loosening is accompanied by one or more of the following criteria: elevated CRP level, radiologic evidence of infection, and loosening within the first 5 years after implantation. In case of infection, a delayed two-stage reconstruction should be managed.[78]

Wear

The polyethylene articular surface of a total knee arthroplasty may undergo true wear, deformation, and creep that lead to a decrease in the thickness of the polyethylene that may be clinically referred to as "wear".[87] Several methods have been used to study the thickness of the polyethylene and thus the extent of wear.

Collier et al. examined single-leg, standing frontal radiographs of the knees for assessment of polyethylene thickness.[87] Measuring the minimum distance from the metallic femoral condyle to a line through the top surface of the baseplate at its widest dimension resulted in 87% of measurements being within 1 mm of the known implant thickness. However, accuracy decreased for evaluation of polyethylene thickness in patients with wear requiring revision.

Because of the tilt of the tibial component in some cases, fluoroscopy has been used to align radiographs perpendicular to the joint surface. This allows measurement of the thickness of the polyethylene liner so that decreases in liner thickness (indicating wear) can be measured. Correction for magnification is made using the known diameter of a portion of the tibial component. In vivo assessment has shown repeatability (precision) of these measurements to be 0.2 mm with a 99% confidence level.[88] The major source of variation is angulation of the tube in the craniocaudal direction.

Varus/valgus stress has been added to the fluoroscopic examination to improve evaluation of polyethylene thickness. The coefficient of variation for repeat examination was 3.4% in one series.[89]

Oblique posterior femoral condylar radiographs have been recommended as a method to evaluate the posterior condyles after total knee replacement.[90] This method was thought to be especially helpful when a posterior stabilized prosthesis is in place.

Sonography is under investigation for evaluating the thickness of polyethylene liners[91] but is not in general use.

Eventually, the tibial polyethylene liner is worn through and the metal of the femoral condyle will articulate with the metal backing of the tibial component. The abraded metal (titanium from the tibial tray) can be seen on radiographs by its high density in the joint and synovial lining (the "metal line sign")[92] (Figure 30-22).

Computed Tomography

Math et al.[73] recommend using CT examination in patients with painful total knee arthroplasties and equivocal radiographs. CT was particularly recommended for evaluation of:

- Extent and width of lucent zones that may be less apparent on radiographs (loosening).
- Painful total knee arthroplasties with normal or equivocal radiographs and increased uptake on all three phases of a bone scan to look for osteolysis.
- Assessing rotational alignment of the femoral component.
- Detection of subtle or occult periprosthetic fractures.[65,73]

Osteolysis

Osteolysis due to wear particles may be visible on radiographs. These lesions appear as focal areas of lucency with well-defined margins. CT is more sensitive than radiography for detection of granulomas (Figure 30-23). There is less experience with MRI.

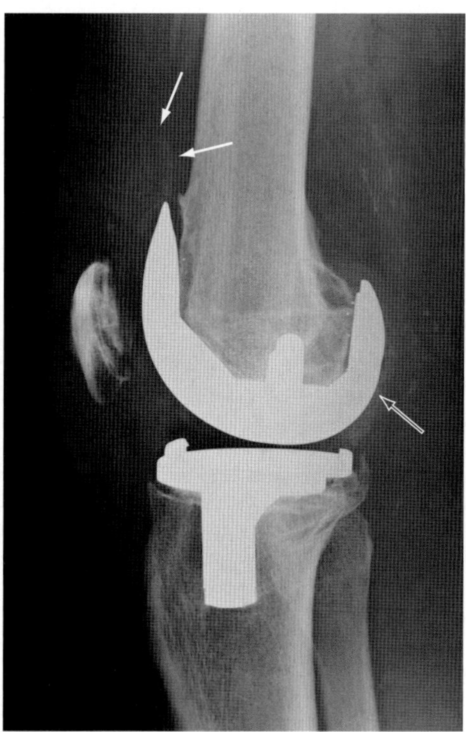

FIGURE 30-22. Wear with metal synovitis and loosening. The lateral radiograph shows soft tissue swelling in the suprapatellar pouch with a thin rim of increased density *(arrows)* consistent with metal debris in the synovial lining. This is evidence of wearing through of the articular polyethylene liner with metal-on-metal wear. Metal is also seen posteriorly in the joint *(open arrow)*.

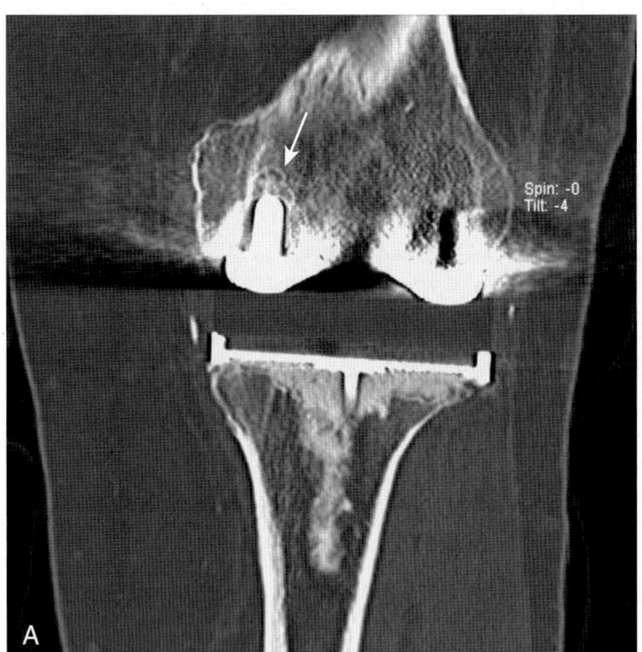

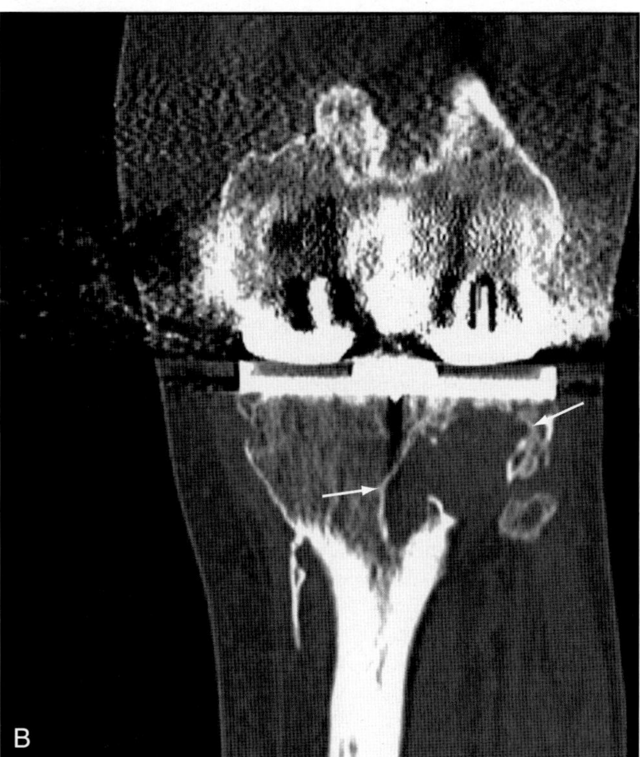

FIGURE 30-23. CT of granulomatous disease. **A,** A coronal CT scan shows a small, well-defined area of lucency adjacent to the medial femoral condyle consistent with granuloma formation. The articular polyethylene is well seen on this image and shows no visible defects. No loosening of the tibial component is seen although a very thin lucent line is present along the cement bone interface laterally. **B,** A coronal CT scan of another patient shows a large lucency (granuloma) with sclerotic margins *(arrows)* under the tibial component and disrupting the lateral tibial cortex. No component loosening is seen.

Magnetic Resonance Imaging

Improved pulse sequences and techniques have facilitated evaluation of the periprosthetic soft tissues and bone allowing demonstration of focal osteolysis and inflammatory synovitis, as well as ligament and tendon abnormalities[91] (Figure 30-24).

Patellar Complications

Anterior knee pain occurs in 10% to 20% of postoperative patients and may occur whether or not the patella is resurfaced. Patellar complications include subluxation, dislocation, fracture, component loosening, impingement, and osteonecrosis.

Radiographs are usually satisfactory for the diagnosis of patellar complications (Figure 30-25). Patients with tibial-component or combined femoral and tibial-component internal rotation have a greater risk of anterior knee pain making assessment of component rotation by CT imaging an important examination in these individuals.[71]

Patellar fractures occur in up to 3.8% of patients, most within the first postoperative year.[93] Many are asymptomatic highlighting the importance of radiography for their identification. Risk factors include older age, osteonecrosis, lateral release, surgical technique, prosthetic malalignment, and improper patellar resection. Transverse fractures are thought to be associated with patellar maltracking, while vertical fractures often occur through a fixation hole. Patellar stress fractures may occur when there is extensive resection of the patella with disruption of the blood supply due to a lateral release and fat pad excision.[94]

Fractures

Stress fractures of the tibia may be associated with axial malalignment, component malposition, tibial tubercle osteotomy, component loosening, or weakening of the medial tibia from pinholes used for component positioning.[94] Rheumatoid arthritis, osteoporosis, and neurologic disorders are other potential predisposing factors.

TOTAL SHOULDER REPLACEMENT

The glenohumeral joint is the most frequently symptomatic of the shoulder joints and the one usually addressed in shoulder replacement (TSR) surgery. The modern era of total shoulder replacement began in the early 1950s with the introduction of a humeral head prosthesis by Neer et al.[95] The Neer II prosthesis was an unconstrained prosthesis that included a polyethylene glenoid component.[96] Modifications of this unconstrained TSR provide different fixation designs and a modular design allowing use of prosthetic heads of variable diameter and neck length. The third-generation device has stems of variable inclination and the option to offset the head.[96]

Approximately 7000 total shoulder replacements were performed yearly in the United States from 1996 to 2002, markedly increased from previous years.[97] The procedure has been shown to provide significant and long-lasting improvement in pain, range of motion, and strength.[98] Survivorship analysis performed on 320 shoulders (1974 to 1988) yielded 85% of implants in place at 20 years.[98] Long-term studies do show a decrease in patient satisfaction and increases in

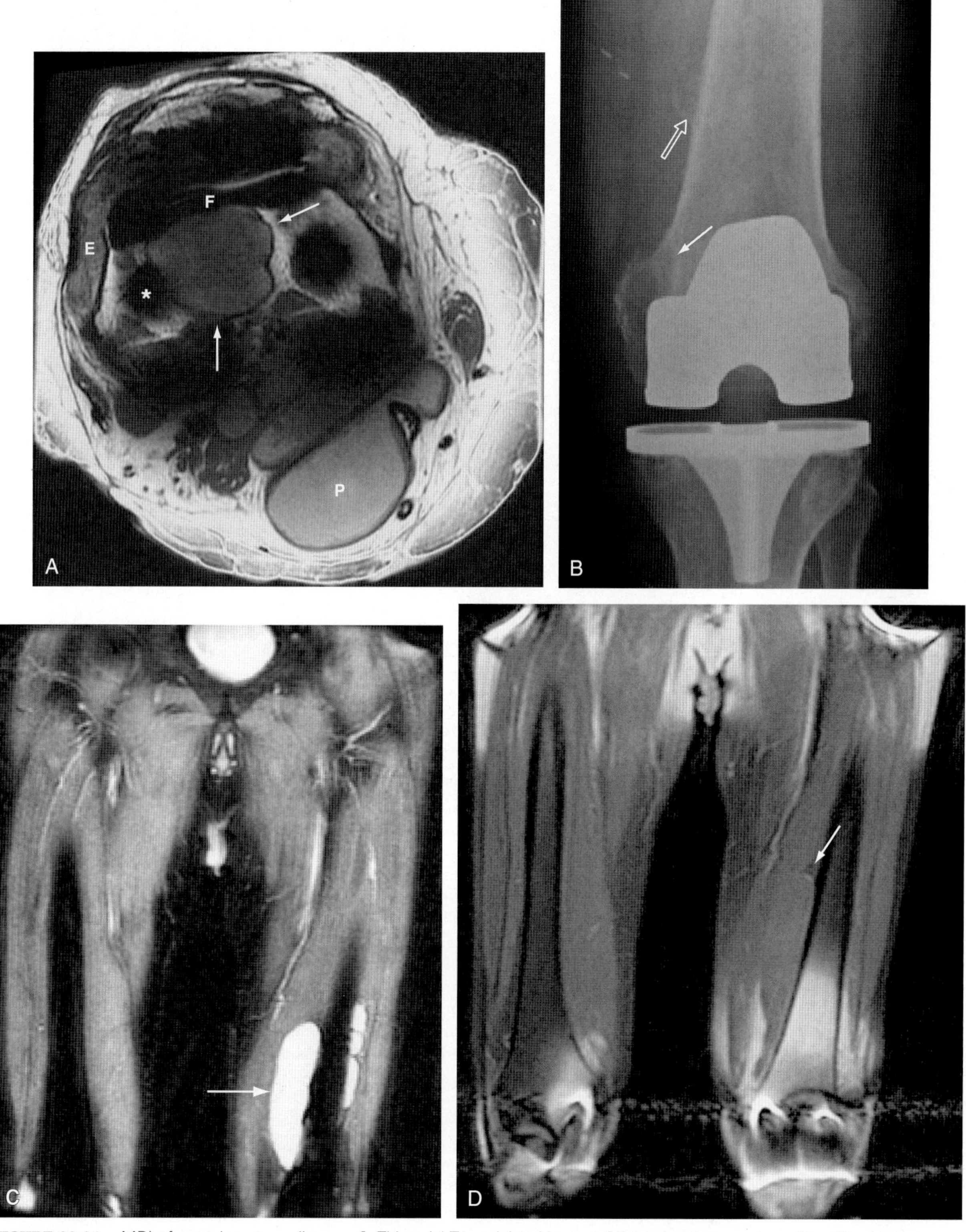

FIGURE 30-24. MRI of granulomatous disease. **A,** This axial T1-weighted image of the knee shows some artifact from the metallic femoral component. However, the large granuloma *(arrows)* between the fixation lugs *(asterisk)* and behind the anterior flange of the femoral component *(F)* is well seen. A large popliteal cyst *(P)* and fluid in the joint *(E)* are noted. **B,** Radiograph of the knee of another patient many years after a total knee prosthesis shows a lucency in the medial femur *(arrow)* consistent with a granuloma. There is periosteal reaction *(open arrow)* and scalloping of the medial cortex consistent with a mass. **C,** STIR image from the MRI shows increased signal in the lesions *(arrow)* and no abnormality in the adjacent marrow. **D,** A post contrast fat suppressed T1-weighted image shows only slight peripheral enhancement *(arrow)* of the lesion. This would be unusual for a tumor. Hematoma or granuloma were considered possibilities and revision surgery confirmed extensive granuloma formation.

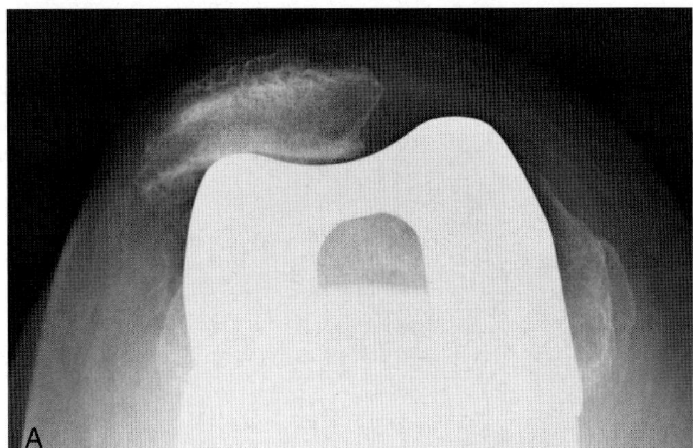

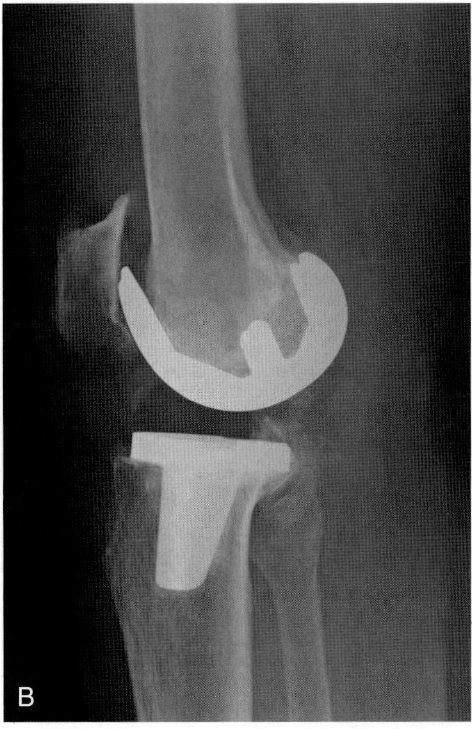

FIGURE 30-25. Femoral component malposition. **A,** The tangential patellar view shows lateral subluxation of the patella. The patella has not been resurfaced. **B,** The lateral radiograph shows a flexed position of the femoral component.

glenoid erosion (hemiarthroplasties) and glenoid component loosening (total shoulder replacement) with time.[99]

Types of Shoulder Prostheses

Several options for surgical replacement of the shoulder joint have been developed as listed in Table 30-10.

Hemiarthroplasty

Hemiarthroplasty involves replacement of only the humeral side of the joint. The choice to replace the glenoid is controversial.[100] Hemiarthroplasty is less expensive and a shorter operation with less blood loss than total shoulder arthroplasty (TSA).[97] Revision of a hemiarthroplasty to a total shoulder replacement is expensive and the results may be less satisfactory than those achieved with primary TSA.[97] Comparison of humeral hemiarthroplasty to total shoulder replacement has generally shown better function and subjective assessment for patients with TSA.[101] Glenoid component loosening, however, may complicate total shoulder replacement especially in the long term.

When massive cuff tears are present, the upward subluxation of the humeral head may lead to eccentric stresses and early glenoid loosening.[102] Review of 40 previously reported studies of total shoulder replacement and hemiarthroplasties showed high satisfaction rates for both procedures.[99] As summarized by Werner et al., although partial pain relief may be provided by hemiarthroplasty, function may be poor and the procedure is reserved for elderly individuals with low demands.[103] Reported complications of TSA and hemiarthroplasty are shown in Table 30-11.

Bipolar Shoulder Replacement

The bipolar total shoulder replacement, as in the bipolar hip replacement, consists of an inner metal-to-polyethylene bearing and an outer articulation between the native glenoid and the metal shell. Theoretically, the inner motion should protect the glenoid from wear. Radiographic evaluation of head motion has, however, shown that the bipolar device actually acted as a unipolar prosthesis.[104]

Reverse Total Shoulder

The reverse total shoulder prosthesis has been used in the United States since 2004.[105] These prostheses are reverse ball and socket configurations that allow the deltoid muscle to power the shoulder in situations in which rotator cuff function is largely absent.[106] They are considered salvage procedures that are used in patients with irreparable loss of the rotator cuff and severe arthritis coupled with severe loss of shoulder function.[106] Adequate glenoid bone must be present to seat the prosthesis.[97] Simovitch et al. note that in addition to the overhead elevation that can be restored using this prosthesis, external rotation is necessary for activities of daily living.[106] Marked fatty infiltration of the teres minor muscle (demonstrable on CT or MRI preoperatively) is associated with less postoperative external rotation and a poorer clinical outcome.[106]

Long-term follow-up has confirmed (with revision as the end point) prosthetic survival of 91%, but significantly poorer results in patients with diagnoses other than cuff tear arthropathy.[102] Evaluation of the Delta III prosthesis by Werner et al. noted major and minor complications in 50% of patients and reoperation was performed in a third of patients.[103] Ideally, patients undergoing these procedures are elderly and the surgeon experienced.[106] Indications and contraindications to reverse shoulder prostheses are shown in Boxes 30-3 and 30-4.

Imaging Evaluation

Preoperative Assessment

Preoperative investigation usually consists of radiographs to evaluate the degree of cartilage loss and bone erosion. CT scanning can help document the degree of glenoid bone loss such as may occur

TABLE 30-10. Types of Shoulder Arthroplasties

Type of Prosthesis	Characteristics	Example
Hemiarthroplasty	The humeral head is replaced. The glenoid may be reamed.	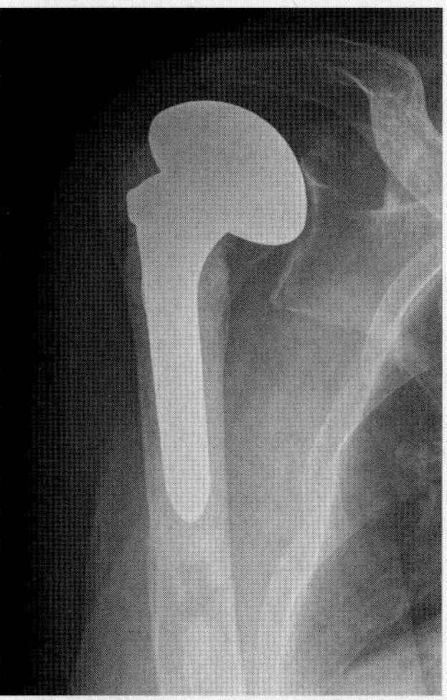
Conventional (Neer type) total shoulder	Metal humeral head articulates with a polyethylene glenoid component (in this case metal-backed)	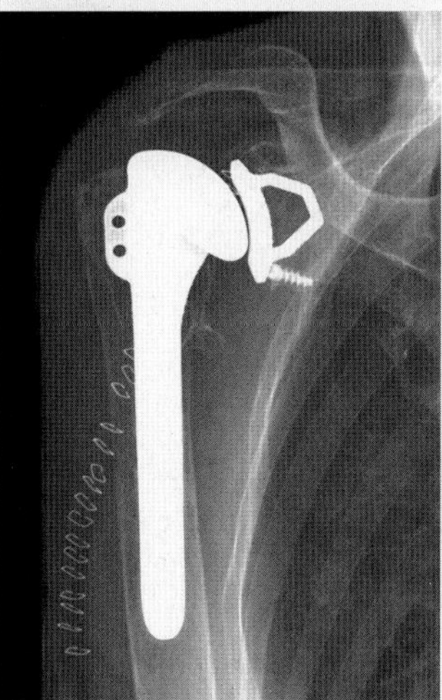
Reverse prosthesis	Medializes the center of rotation of the shoulder. The deltoid provides overhead elevation in cases in which severe rotator cuff damage is present.	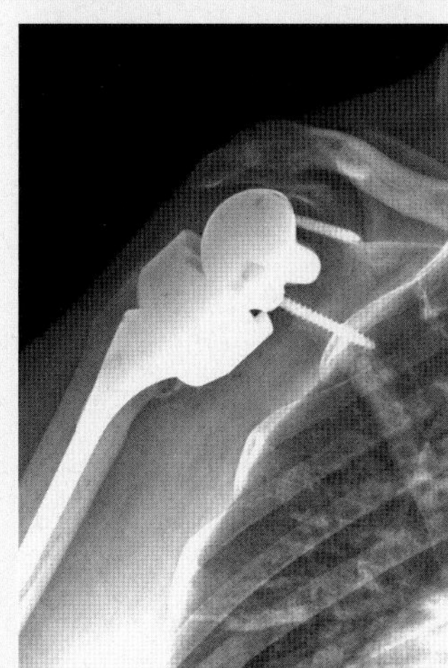 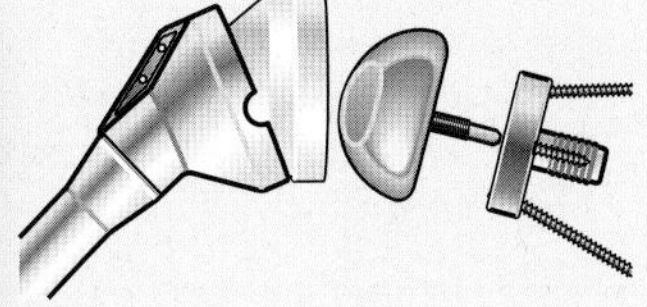

TABLE 30-11. Complications of Unconstrained Total Shoulder Replacement and Humeral Hemiarthroplasty

Complication	Total Shoulder Replacement (%)	Hemiarthroplasty (%)
Infection	0.9	0.4
Instability	5	20
Proximal migration	11	38
Glenoid erosion		22 (increases with time)
Persistent severe pain	9	9
Glenoid loosening component	59% lucent lines, 9% radiographic loosening, 2% revised for loosening	
Humeral component loosening	3.6	3.6

Data from van de Sande MA, Brand R, Rozing PM: Indications, complications, and results of shoulder arthroplasty, *Scand J Rheumatol* 35:426-434, 2006.

BOX 30-3. Potential Indications for Reverse Total Shoulder Prosthesis

- 70 years of age or older
- Low functional demands
- Rotator cuff tear arthropathy (irreparable cuff tear, pain, arthritis, minimal function)
- Failed shoulder arthroplasty

Guery J, Favard L, Sirveaux F, et al: Reverse total shoulder arthroplasty. Survivorship analysis of eighty replacements followed for five to ten years, *J Bone Joint Surg Am* 88:1742-1747, 2006; and Rockwood CA Jr: The reverse total shoulder prosthesis. The new kid on the block, *J Bone Joint Surg Am* 89:233-235, 2007. [Comment.]

BOX 30-4. Contraindications for Reverse Total Shoulder Prosthesis

Nonfunctioning deltoid muscle
Active infection
Excessive glenoid bone loss
Severe neurologic deficiencies
Refusal to modify postoperative physical activities
Metal allergy

With permission, from Frankle M, Siegal S, Pupello D, et al: The reverse shoulder prosthesis for glenohumeral arthritis associated with severe rotator cuff deficiency. A minimum two-year follow-up study of sixty patients, *J Bone Joint Surg Am* 87:1697-1705, 2005.

in rheumatoid arthritis and osteoarthritis and any subluxation of the humeral head. Normally the glenoid is retroverted from 0 to 10 degrees and this can be assessed on the axial CT images.[107] CT may also be useful to evaluate any fatty replacement of muscles such as described by Goutallier et al[108] (Table 30-12). Poorer clinical outcomes, due to limited external rotation of the shoulder are found after reverse TSR if there is Goutallier grade 3 or 4 fatty infiltration of the teres minor muscle[109] (see Table 30-12).

TABLE 30-12. Goutallier Grading of Fatty Infiltration of Rotator Cuff Muscles

Stage	Degree of Fatty Replacement
0	No fatty infiltration
1	Some fatty streaks
2	Less fat than muscle
3	Equal muscle and fat
4	More fat than muscle

Note: This grading system can be used for sagittal non fat suppressed MRI images as well as for CT imaging.

Adapted from Goutallier D, Postel JM, Bernageau J, et al: Fatty muscle degeneration in cuff ruptures. Pre- and postoperative evaluation by CT scan, *Clin Orthop Rel Res* 304:78-83, 1994.

Postoperative Radiographic Assessment

Fluoroscopy can be used to ensure adequate radiographic positioning so that the components are seen in profile.[107] However, the posterior oblique view with the humerus in external rotation (Grashey projection) usually is adequate to show the components in profile without the need for fluoroscopy. This view is supplemented by axillary and outlet views and additional projections if necessary.

As in other joints, radiolucent lines are used as markers of component fixation although their clinical significance is not clear. Pfahler et al. found an adverse effect on functional outcome when lucent lines were present.[101] Radiographs (or CT scans) are assessed for the presence, extent and thickness of radiolucent lines and, as expected, CT scans show a higher prevalence of these lines and better inter- and intra-observer reliability in their assessment than radiography.[107] In one series, postoperative pain was significantly associated with the CT scores for radiolucent lines but not with the radiographic scores.[107] Glenoid lucent zones have been reported in up to 100% of cases.[97]

Lucent lines present on the immediate postoperative radiographs are thought to indicate inadequate initial fixation that may contribute to loosening. Later development of lucent zones, especially when they are wider than 2 mm or extensive, suggest component loosening. Component migration, tilt, or a complete radiolucent line of 1.5 mm or more have been suggested as indicators of glenoid loosening.[110] Several schemes have been proposed for evaluation of lucent lines.[107,111]

MR Imaging of Total Shoulder Arthroplasty

MRI is more limited after total shoulder replacement than total hip arthroplasty because the shoulder is not located in the center of the magnet where the field is homogeneous. Also, the configuration of the prosthetic components leads to artifact.[31] The rotator cuff can be imaged and tears of the subscapularis have been identified.

Complications

Complications of total shoulder replacement are shown in Table 30-13. Complications may take many years to present and long term follow-up is essential.[98] Loosening of the glenoid component is usually reported as the major cause of failure of total

TABLE 30-13. Reported Complications of Unconstrained Total Shoulder Replacement from 1996 to 2005

Complication	Percentage of All Shoulders
Component Loosening	6.3
Glenoid	5.3
Humerus	1.1
Instability	4.9 (Figure 30-26)
Periprosthetic fracture	1.8
Intraoperative	1.1
Postoperative	0.7
Rotator cuff tear	1.3
Neural injury	0.8
Infection	0.7
Deltoid detachment	0.08

Adapted from Bohsali KI, Wirth MA, Rockwood CA Jr: Complications of total shoulder arthroplasty, *J Bone Joint Surg Am* 8:2279-2292, 2006.

shoulder arthroplasty.[107] Review by Bohsali et al. found glenoid loosening to account for 32% of all complications of unconstrained total shoulder replacements.[97] However, review of the complications of total shoulder arthroplasties performed between 1990 and 2000 by Chin et al. found that revision due to loosening is rare at an average follow up time of 4.3 years.[112]

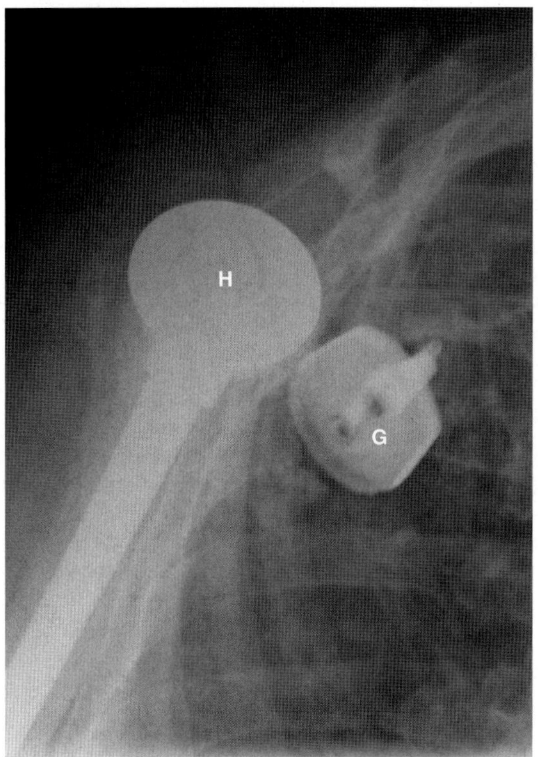

FIGURE 30-26. Dislocated total shoulder prosthesis. This scapular Y view normally shows the humeral head and the glenoid to be superimposed. In this case, the humerus *(H)* is posteriorly dislocated with relation to the glenoid component *(G)*.

Infection

Infections occur in fewer than 1% of patients and are more likely to occur in susceptible individuals (e.g., patients with rheumatoid arthritis, systemic lupus erythematosus, diabetes mellitus or those undergoing chemotherapy). Infections are classified by the interval after surgery in which they present; acute cases within 3 months, subacute, 3 months to 1 year, and late, more than 1 year.[97] Most patients with infection present with pain. Treatment includes removal of the prosthesis sometimes with placement of an antibiotic impregnated spacer before reinsertion of a prosthesis or as a permanent alternative. Imaging findings are usually nonspecific.[97]

Fractures

Periprosthetic humeral fractures are uncommon.[113] The location and configuration of the fracture are considerations in determining treatment.[113] Periprosthetic humeral fractures have been classified by Wright and Cofield[114] as follows:

A: Located at the tip of the prosthesis and extending proximally

B: Located at the tip, minimal or no proximal extension, but variable distal extension

C: Located distal to the tip

Type C fractures can be treated nonoperatively.

Radiographic Evaluation of Reverse Prostheses

The Delta III prosthesis consists of several components and all but the polyethylene inlay are visible on radiographs. As in other shoulder prostheses, images are evaluated for component position and the presence or absence of radiolucent lines. The posterior oblique, external rotation positioning for the anteroposterior radiograph allows the retroverted humeral component (< 20 degrees) to be seen in profile.[103] The glenoid base plate is placed so that its inferior border is flush with the inferior rim of the glenoid.

Notching of the scapular neck (probably by mechanical pressure from the polyethylene cup) occurred in 96% of patients in one series[103] (Box 30-5). It may be graded by severity with severe notching thought to indicate loosening by some authors. Werner et al. found no corresponding clinical features or complication associated with this finding. The notching appeared early in the postoperative course and the size of the bony lesion stabilized by 1 year after surgery in 79% of cases.

BOX 30-5. Complications of Reverse Total Shoulder Prostheses That Can Be Evaluated on Radiographs

- Instability
- Infection
- Humeral fracture
- Glenoid loosening
- Humeral loosening
- Humeral disassembly
- Glenoid disassembly
- Scapular or acromial fracture
- Scapular notching

OTHER JOINTS

Many of the concepts discussed above are applicable to small joint arthroplasty as well. Some additional concepts that are of importance in imaging evaluation of the small joints are included here. A more complete review can be found in an article by Lecomte et al.[115]

Types of Prostheses

In addition to metal to polyethylene joint replacement, silicone rubber and pyrolytic carbon components are used in small joint replacement.

Silicone rubber prostheses are used exclusively for small joint arthroplasty. They function as spacers around which a fibrous capsule develops. Therefore, the integrity of the implant is less important once the fibrous capsule has formed. These implants are not rigidly fixed and the stems piston within the bone.

On radiologic examination, silicone rubber prostheses are slightly radiodense with their single or double stems barely visible. Metal coverings (grommets) may be used to protect them. Sclerotic lines are almost always observed around the prostheses and may be a favorable sign.[116] Mechanical wear of silicone prostheses may lead to shedding of particles into the joint which incites a foreign body granulomatous reaction. This "silicone synovitis" typically presents at 2 to 5 years after surgery and may clinically mimic a low grade infection (Figure 30-27). This complication is seen most frequently in the wrist and first carpometacarpal (CMC) joint, and rarely around finger implants, which are subjected to less stress. It is also seen following great toe metatarsophalangeal replacement. Silicone debris has been identified in distal lymph nodes.[117] The radiographic findings of silicone synovitis include cyst like lucencies that tend to enlarge with time. Fragmentation or deformity of the implant may be seen. Osteopenia is less prominent than in cases of infection and this may help distinguish these conditions.[118,119] MR imaging can show the deformed prosthesis (which is low in signal on all pulse sequences) and the granulomas to advantage.

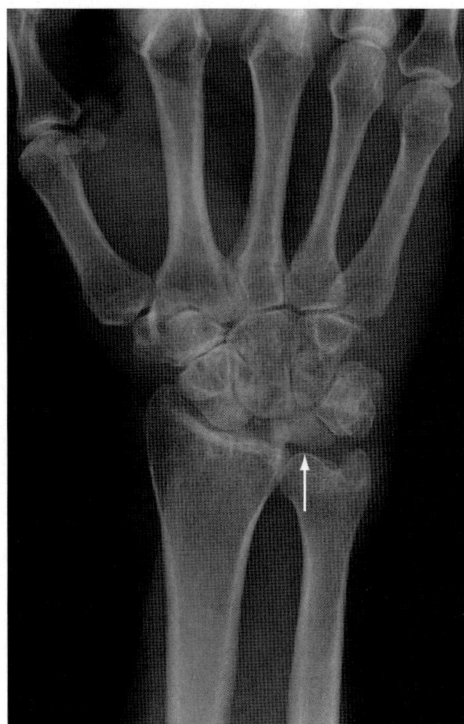

FIGURE 30-27. Silicone synovitis. The posteroanterior view of the wrist in a patient following insertion of a lunate prosthesis shows deformity of the surface of the prosthesis *(arrow)*. There are numerous small cystlike changes in the carpals and ulnar styloid. The bone density is only mildly decreased, and there is only mild cartilage space narrowing. (With permission, from Lecomte AR, Singh SK, Fitzgerald B, Weissman, BN: Small joint arthroplasty, *Semin Musculoskel Radiol* 10:64-78, 2006.)

Pyrolytic carbon is a synthetic material that is deposited onto a high-strength graphite substrate. The qualities of the material are very similar to those of cortical bone. These implants are designed for insertion without cement.

Radiographic Assessment of Small Joint Arthroplasty

As in other joints, radiographs obtained in the immediate postoperative period are used to evaluate component position and exclude dislocation or fracture. On follow-up examinations, radiographs allow assessment of (1) component position, (2) component articulation, (3) component interfaces, and (4) the soft tissues. Also, as in all joints, the comparison to prior radiographs improves the ability to evaluate subtle changes.

Hinges on implants should be evaluated for evidence of asymmetry that could indicate wear or disruption. Nonconstrained prostheses are scrutinized for subluxation or dislocation. Radiographic evidence of prosthetic loosening is defined by a lucent line at least 2 mm wide around a cemented component or along the bone ingrowth surfaces, or change in component position over time.[120] Settling of silicone rubber MCP prostheses may occur, however, without clinical consequence.

MCP Joints

The MCP joint is a ball-and-socket joint with three axes of motion, flexion to 80 or 90 degrees, rotation and medial-lateral deviation. The primary indication for MCP arthroplasty is joint destruction with painful fixed deformity that cannot be corrected with soft tissue reconstruction alone. Contraindications include vasculitis, poor skin condition, or inadequate bone stock.[121] Extensive erosion of the metacarpal head and proximal phalanx and excessive fatty replacement of the cancellous bone are relative contraindications.[121]

Silicone

Silicone implants are usually used to replace the index through fifth finger MCP joints in patients with rheumatoid arthritis. Reports generally showed favorable patient satisfaction with improved motion, correction of deformity, improved joint stability and an increased sense of well-being,[122] although these results tend to worsen with time.[123]

Radiographic Findings

The prosthesis is slightly radiodense and the rectangular shaped hinge portion of the prosthesis parallels and lies adjacent to the cut bone surfaces (Figure 30-28). Recurrent deformity, implant fracture or infection with swelling and periosteal reaction can be detected on radiographic examination.

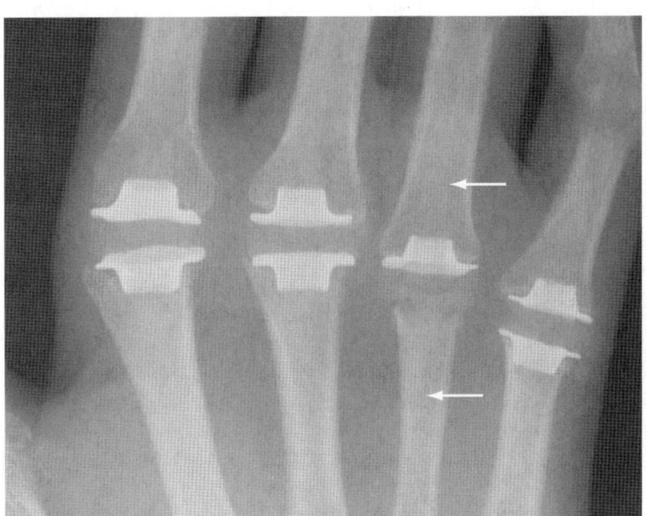

FIGURE 30-28. Silicone MCP prostheses. The MCP prostheses are difficult to see. The stems are faintly seen in the metacarpals and proximal phalanges *(arrows)*. Metallic grommets are present at all but the ring finger metacarpal.

Wrist

The major indication for total wrist arthroplasty is rheumatoid arthritis with progressive pain and deformity involving both wrists or multiple upper extremity joints.[124] Absolute contraindications to total wrist arthroplasty include the necessity to weight bear through the joint such as with the use of a crutch or walker, or a severely unbalanced wrist, poor bone quality, marked ulnar or volar translocation on radiographs,[125] lack of sensory or motor function, and infection.[126] There are two major categories of wrist prostheses: the silicone rubber prosthesis, such as the Swanson implant (Wright Medical Technology Inc, Arlington, TN) and various metal to polyethylene prostheses. The Swanson prosthesis is a one piece hinged silicone rubber implant similar to MCP prostheses. The proximal stem is placed within the radius and the distal stem passes through the capitate into the third metacarpal. As with the MCP prostheses, they are slightly denser than soft tissues on radiographs. The component position, carpal height and alignment of the wrist should be assessed and evaluated for change over time. The distal portion of the component should be aligned with the third metacarpal and the proximal portion should be aligned with the ulnar border of the distal radius.[120] In the lateral projection, the carpal bones should be in the neutral position in relation to the radius, but palmar or dorsiflexion is acceptable.[126]

> Wrist prostheses are primarily indicated for patients with rheumatoid arthritis and bilateral wrist involvement.[127]

The most common wrist implants currently consist of a metal metacarpal stem articulating with a metal-backed polyethylene radial stem. The metacarpal stem is fixed into the second or third metacarpal shaft.

In uncomplicated cases, radiographs show the distal stem of the prosthesis centered within the medullary canal in all views. The proximal component should be aligned with the ulnar border of the distal radius. Complications visible on radiographs include deformity due to muscle imbalance, loosening (lucent zones around the components of 2 mm or more or change in component position) metacarpal fracture, component dislocation or dissociation, infection (osteopenia and periostitis), extensor tendon rupture, and radiocarpal subluxation.[127-129]

ELBOW

The primary indication for a total elbow prosthesis is pain relief, especially in patients with rheumatoid arthritis. Secondary indications include severe acute fractures with non-reconstructible articular surfaces or elbow fracture nonunion.[126] Contraindications include prior elbow joint sepsis, fusion, or severe neuromuscular disease.[126] There are of two basic types of prostheses currently in use, unlinked (unconstrained) components and linked (semiconstrained) components (Figure 30-29). Good to excellent clinical results are seen in 85% to 91% of patients undergoing elbow arthroplasties performed predominantly for rheumatoid arthritis.[130-133] Complications include infection, ulnar neuropathy, dislocation, implant loosening, triceps avulsion, and fracture. Subluxation or dislocation is the major complications of the unconstrained prostheses, and loosening is the major complication of constrained prostheses.[126]

ANKLE

Patients with severe ankle osteoarthritis are usually treated with surgical fusion if the subtalar joint remains mobile. Ankle replacement is reserved for older patients with low demands, and multiple joint osteoarthritis or inflammatory arthropathy to relieve unrelenting pain.[126] Active infection, peripheral vascular disease, deficient soft tissues, and Charcot neuropathy are contraindications.[126] In comparison to the marked success of total hip and total knee arthroplasty, total ankle arthroplasty results are disappointing and show high loosening rates.

Most current prostheses replace the three articular surfaces of the tibiotalar joint (the medial, lateral, and superior articular surfaces) and use bone ingrowth fixation. Current prostheses can be grouped into two-component designs (e.g., Agility Ankle [DePuy, Warsaw, IN]) that require fusion of the syndesmosis and three-component designs (e.g., Scandinavian Total Ankle Replacement [STAR], the Buechel-Pappas LCS ankle replacement (Endotec, South Orange, NJ) (Figure 30-30).

Preoperative radiographs and CT may be used to assess the ankle and adjacent joints. If more than 10 degrees of angulation is present in any plane due to supramalleolar malalignment, this should be corrected with a tibial osteotomy prior to ankle replacement surgery.[134] Postoperatively, the tibial component is optimally positioned perpendicular to the long axis of the tibia, parallel to the ground.[126]

Postoperative complications that may be diagnosed on radiographs include malposition of components, degenerative changes in adjacent joints, intraoperative fractures (usually of the medial malleolus), component wear or fracture, subluxation or dislocation, reflex sympathetic dystrophy, fibular impingement and loosening and/or infection: The Buechel Pappas LCS prosthesis is inserted through an anterior window in the tibia, resulting in a cortical discontinuity that should not be mistaken for an anterior tibial fracture. Loosening is identified by a change in component position, including component sinking into the adjacent bone, or by wide lucent interfaces.[120]

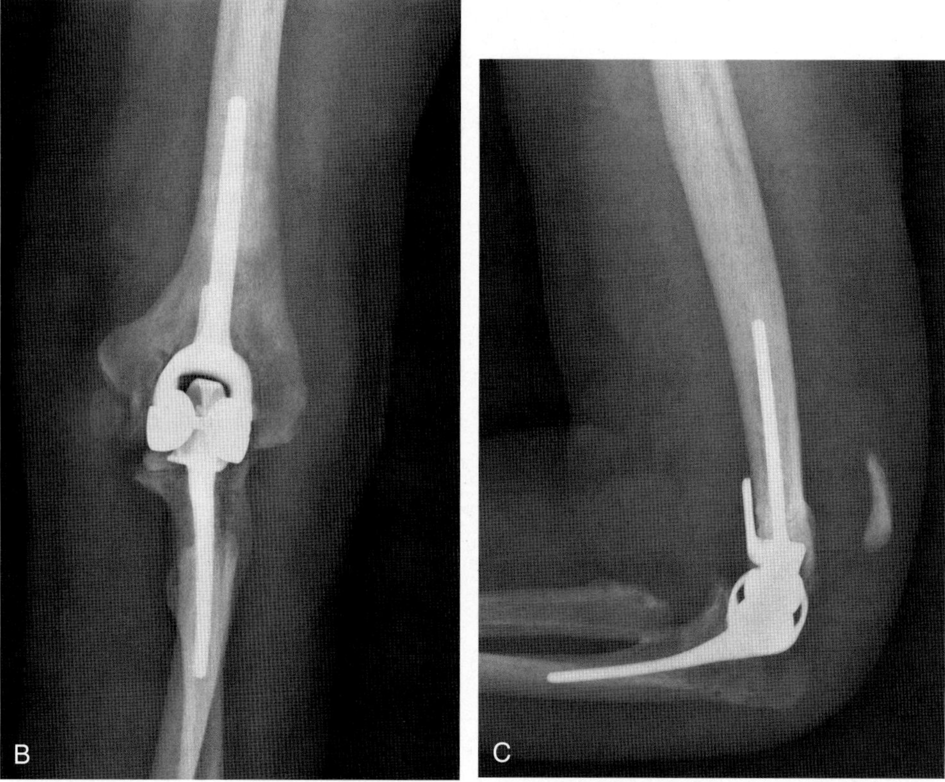

FIGURE 30-29. Elbow prostheses. **A,** Lateral radiograph of an unconstrained total elbow prosthesis shows no dislocation or loosening. (With permission, from Lecomte AR et al: Small joint arthroplasty, *Semin Musculoskel Radiol* 10:64-78, 2006.)**B,** The hinge of this constrained total elbow prosthesis is well seen. **C,** The lateral radiograph shows a large bony fragment, most likely resulting from triceps avulsion.

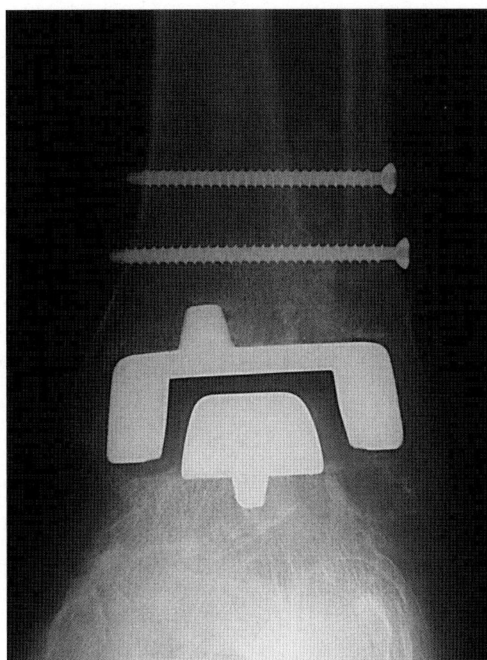

FIGURE 30-30. Total ankle prosthesis. This is a two-component prosthesis. The syndesmosis is fused. (With permission, from Lecomte AR et al: Small joint arthroplasty, *Semin Musculoskel Radiol* 10:64-78, 2006.)

REFERENCES

1. Laupacis A, et al: The effect of elective total hip replacement on health-related quality of life, *J Bone Joint Surg Am* 75:1619-1626, 1993.
2. Huo MH, Parvizi J, Bal BS, Mont M: Specialty update: what's new in total hip arthroplasty, *J Bone Joint Surg* 90:2043-2055, 2008.
3. Charnley J: Arthroplasty of the hip. A new operation, *Lancet* 27:1129-1132, 1961.
4. Eingartner C: Current trends in total hip arthroplasty, *Ortop Traumatol Rehabil* 9:8-14, 2007.
5. Kurtz S, et al: Prevalence of primary and revision total hip and knee arthroplasty in the United States from 1990 through 2002, *J Bone Joint Surg Am* 87:1487-1497, 2005.
6. Berquist TH: Imaging of joint replacement procedures, *Radiol Clin North Am* 44:419-437, 2006.
7. National Institutes of Health: Total Hip Joint Replacement, http://consensus.nih.gov/1982/1982HipReplacement033html.htm, 1982.
8. Illgen R 2nd, Rubash HE: The optimal fixation of the cementless acetabular component in primary total hip arthroplasty, *J Am Acad Orthop Surg* 10:43-56, 2002.
9. Schmalzried TP, et al: Optimizing patient selection and outcomes with total hip resurfacing, *Clin Orthop Rel Res* 441:200-204, 2005.
10. Huo MH, Parvizi J, Gilbert NF: What's new in hip arthroplasty, *J Bone Joint Surg Am* 88:2100-2113, 2006.

10a. Vail TP, Glisson RR, Dominguez, et al: Positron of hip resurfacing component affects strain and resistance to fracture in the femoral neck, *J Bone Joint Surg Am* 90:1951-1960, 2008.

11. Albrektsson T, C. Johansson, Osteoinduction, osteoconduction and osseointegration, *Eur Spine J* 10:S96-S101, 2001.
12. Wojciechowski, P., et al: Minimally invasive approaches in total hip arthroplasty, *Ortop Traumatol Rehabil* 9:1-7, 2007.
13. Dutka, J., et al: Total hip arthroplasty through a minimally invasive lateral approach—our experience and early results, *Ortop Traumatol Rehabil* 9:39-45.
14. Michel, M.C, P. Witschger, MicroHip: a minimally invasive procedure for total hip replacement surgery using a modified Smith-Peterson approach, *Ortop Traumatol Rehabil* 9:46-51, 2007.
15. Weissman BN: Imaging of joint replacement. In Resnick D: *Diagnosis of Bone and Joint Disorders*, 4th edition, Volume II, Saunders. 2002; Philadelphia, pp. 595-644.
16. American College of Radiology: Imaging after Total Hip Arthroplasty, http://www.acr.org/SecondaryMainMenuCategories/quality_safety/app_criteria/pdf/ExpertPanelonMusculoskeletalImaging/ImagingafterTotalHipArthroplastyDoc12.aspx, 1998.
17. Stulberg SD, et al: Monitoring pelvic osteolysis following total hip replacement surgery: an algorithm for surveillance, *J Bone Joint Surg Am* 84-A:116-122, 2002.
18. Johnston RC, et al: Clinical and radiographic evaluation of total hip replacement. A standard system of terminology for reporting results, *J Bone Joint Surg Am* 72:161-168, 1990. [See comment. Erratum appears in *J Bone Joint Surg Am* 73:952, 1991.]
19. DeLee JG, Charnley J: Radiological demarcation of cemented sockets in total hip replacement, *Clin Orthop Rel Res* 1976:20-32, 1976.
20. Gruen TA, McNeice GM, Amstutz HC: "Modes of failure" of cemented stem-type femoral components: a radiographic analysis of loosening, *Clin Orthop Rel Res* 1979:17-27, 1979.
21. Kaplan PA, et al: Bone-ingrowth hip prostheses in asymptomatic patients: radiographic features, *Radiology* 169:221-227, 1988.
22. Engh CA, Bobyn JD, Glassman AH: Porous-coated hip replacement. The factors governing bone ingrowth, stress shielding, and clinical results, *J Bone Joint Surg Br* 69:45-55, 1987.
23. Moore MS, et al: Radiographic signs of osseointegration in porous-coated acetabular components, *Clin Orthop Rel Res* 444:176-183, 2006.
24. Cameron HU, Pilliar RM, Macnab I: The rate of bone ingrowth into porous metal, *J Biomed Mater Res* 10:295-302, 1976.
25. Engh CA, Massin P, Suthers KE: Roentgenographic assessment of the biologic fixation of porous-surfaced femoral components, *Clin Orthop Rel Res* 1990:107-128, 1990. [See comment. Erratum appears in *Clin Orthop* 1992:310-312, 1992.]
26. Kattapuram SV, et al: Porous-coated anatomic total hip prostheses: radiographic analysis and clinical correlation, *Radiology* 174:861-864, 1990.
27. Galat DD, Petrucci JA, Wasielewski RC: Radiographic evaluation of screw position in revision total hip arthroplasty, *Clin Orthop Rel Res* 2004:124-129, 2004.
28. Stumpe KD, Nötzli HP, Zanetti M, Kamel EM: FDG PET for differentiation of infection and aseptic loosening in total hip replacements: comparison with conventional radiography and three-phase bone scintigraphy, *Radiology* 231:333-341, 2004.
29. Buckwalter KA, Parr JA, Choplin HR, et al: Multichannel CT imaging of orthopedic hardware and implants, *Semin Musculoskel Radiol* 10:86-97, 2006.
30. Walde TA, Weiland DE, Leung SB, et al: Comparison of CT, MRI, and radiographs in assessing pelvic osteolysis: a cadaveric study, *Clin Orthop Rel Res* 2005:138-144, 2005.
31. Naraghi AM, White LM: Magnetic resonance imaging of joint replacements, *Semin Musculoskel Radiol* 10:98-106, 2006.
32. White LM, Kim JK, Mehta M, et al: Complications of total hip arthroplasty: MR imaging-initial experience, *Radiology* 215:254-262, 2000.
33. Crawford RW, Murray DW: Total hip replacement: indications for surgery and risk factors for failure, *Ann Rheum Dis* 56:455-457, 1997.
34. Maus TP, Berquist TH, Bender CE, et al: Arthrographic study of painful total hip arthroplasty: refined criteria, *Radiology* 162:721-727, 1987.
35. Aliabadi P, Tumeh SS, Weissman BN, et al: Cemented total hip prosthesis: radio graphic and scintigraphic evaluation, *Radiology* 173:203-206, 1989.
36. Harris WH: Conquest of a man-made, worldwide human disease, *Orthopaedic Journal at Harvard Medical School Online* 6, 2001, http://www.orthojournalhms.org/volume6/manuscripts/ms16.htm.
37. Sochart DH: Relationship of acetabular wear to osteolysis and loosening in total hip arthroplasty, *Clin Orthop Rel Res* 1999:135-150, 1999.
38. Clarke JC, Black K, Rennie C, et al: Can wear in total hip arthroplasties be assessed from radiographs? *Clin Orthop Rel Res* 1976:126-142, 1976.
39. Charnley J, Cupic Z:, The nine and ten year results of the low-friction arthroplasty of the hip, *Clin Orthop Rel Res* 1973:9-25, 1973.
40. Amstutz HC, Campbell P, Kossovsky N, et al: Mechanism and clinical significance of wear debris-induced osteolysis, *Clin Orthop Rel Res* 1992:7-18, 1992.
41. Shih CH, Lee PC, Chen JH, et al: Measurement of polyethylene wear in cementless total hip arthroplasty, *J Bone Joint Surg Br* 79:361-365, 1997.
42. Devane PA, Bourne RB, Rorabeck CH, et al: Measurement of polyethylene wear in metal-backed acetabular cups. I. Three-dimensional technique, *Clin Orthop Rel Res* 1995:303-316, 1995.
43. Smith PN, Ling RS, Taylor R: The influence of weight-bearing on the measurement of polyethylene wear in THA, *J Bone Joint Surg Br* 81:259-265, 1999.
44. Kitamura N, et al: Diagnostic features of pelvic osteolysis on computed tomography: the importance of communication pathways, *J Bone Joint Surg Am* 87:1542-1550, 2005.
45. Mason MD, Zlatkin MB, Esterhai JL, et al: Chronic complicated osteomyelitis of the lower extremity: evaluation with MR imaging, *Radiology* 173:355-359, 1989.
46. Potter HG, Nester BJ, Sofka CM, et al: Magnetic resonance imaging after total hip arthroplasty: evaluation of periprosthetic soft tissue, *J Bone Joint Surg Am* 86-A: 1947-1954, 2004.
47. Puri L, Lapinski B, Wixson RL, et al: Computed tomographic follow-up evaluation of operative intervention for periacetabular lysis, *J Arthroplasty* 21:78-82, 2006.
48. Ali Khan MA, Brakenbury PH, Reynolds IS: Dislocation following total hip replacement, *J Bone Joint Surg Br* 63-B:214-218, 1981.
49. Levitsky KA, Hozack WJ, Balderston RH, et al: Evaluation of the painful prosthetic joint. Relative value of bone scan, sedimentation rate, and joint aspiration, *J Arthroplasty* 6:237-244, 1991.
50. Spangehl MJ, Masri BA, O'Connell JX, et al: Prospective analysis of preoperative and intraoperative investigations for the diagnosis of infection at the sites of two hundred and two revision total hip arthroplasties, *J Bone Joint Surg Am* 81: 672-683, 1999.

50a. Schinsky MF, Della Valle CJ, Sporer SM, Paprosky WG: Perioperative testing for joint infection in patients undergoing revision total hip arthroplasty, *J Bone Joint Surg* 90:1869-1875, 2008.

51. Tigges S, Stiles RG, Roberson JR: Complications of hip arthroplasty causing periprosthetic radiolucency on plain radiographs, *AJR Am J Roentgenol* 162: 1387-1391, 1994.

52. Cyteval C, Hamm V, Sarrabere MP, et al: Painful infection at the site of hip prosthesis: CT imaging, *Radiology* 224:477-483, 2002.
53. Harris WH, Barrack RL: Contemporary algorithms for evaluation of the painful total hip replacement, *Orthopaed Rev* 22:531-539, 1993.
54. Love C, Marwin SE, Tomas MB, et al: Diagnosing infection in the failed joint replacement: a comparison of coincidence detection 18F-FDG and 111In-labeled leukocyte/99 mTc-sulfur colloid marrow imaging, *J Nucl Med* 45: 1864-1871, 2004.
55. Chik KK, Magee MM, Bruce WJ, et al: Tc-99m stannous colloid-labeled leukocyte scintigraphy in the evaluation of the painful arthroplasty, *Clin Nucl Med* 21: 838-843, 1996.
56. Zhuang H, Duarte PS, Pourdehnad M, et al: The promising role of 18F-FDG PET in detecting infected lower limb prosthesis implants, *J Nucl Med* 42:44-48, 2001.
57. Iruvuri S, Chryssikos T, Alzeair S, et al: FDG activity in patients with painful hip prosthesis and quantitative analysis, *J Nucl Med* 48:282P, 2007.
58. Twair A, Ryan M, O'Connell M, et al: MRI of failed total hip replacement caused by abductor muscle avulsion, *AJR Am J Roentgenol* 181:1547-1550, 2003.
59. Pfirrmann CW, Notzli HP, Dora C, et al: Abductor tendons and muscles assessed at MR imaging after total hip arthroplasty in asymptomatic and symptomatic patients, *Radiology*. 235:969-976, 2005. [See comment.]
60. Walde TA, Mohan V, Leung S, et al: Sensitivity and specificity of plain radiographs for detection of medial-wall perforation secondary to osteolysis, *J Arthroplasty* 20: 20-24, 2005.
61. Fehring TK, Guilford WB, Baron J: Assessment of intrapelvic cement and screws in revision total hip arthroplasty, *J Arthroplasty* 7:509-518, 1992.
62. Somme D, Ziza JM, Desplaces N, et al: Contribution of routine joint aspiration to the diagnosis of infection before hip revision surgery, *Joint Bone Spine* 70:489-495, 2003.
63. Kurtz S, Ong K, Lau E, et al: Projections of primary and revision hip and knee arthroplasty in the United States from 2005 to 2030, *J Bone Joint Surg Am* 89: 780-785, 2007.
64. Sharkey PF, Hozack WJ, Dorr LD, et al: The bearing surface in total hip arthroplasty: evolution or revolution, *Instructional Course Lectures* 49:41-56, 2000.
65. Clarke HD, Math KR, Scuderi GR: Polyethylene post failure in posterior stabilized total knee arthroplasty, *J Arthroplasty* 19:652-657, 2004.
66. American College of Radiology: Imaging after Total Knee Arthroplasty, http://www.acr.org/SecondaryMainMenuCategories/quality_safety/app_criteria/pdf/ExpertPanelon-MusculoskeletalImaging/ImagingafterTotalKneeArthroplastyDoc13.aspx, 2006.
67. Lee AJ, Lim SS, Kong Y, et al: Cost-effectiveness of screening x-rays at admission to acute rehabilitation after joint replacement surgery: a retrospective chart review, *Am J Phys Med Rehabil* 80:276-279, 2001.
68. Ewald FC: The Knee Society total knee arthroplasty roentgenographic evaluation and scoring system, *Clin Orthop Rel Res* 1989:9-12, 1989.
69. Ikeuchi M, Yamanaka N, Okanoue Y, et al: Determining the rotational alignment of the tibial component at total knee replacement: a comparison of two techniques, *J Bone Joint Surg Br* 89:45-49, 2007.
70. Berger RA, Crossett LS, Jacobs JJ, et al: Malrotation causing patellofemoral complications after total knee arthroplasty, *Clin Orthop Rel Res* 1998:144-153, 1998.
71. Barrack RL, Schrader T, Bertot AJ, et al: Component rotation and anterior knee pain after total knee arthroplasty, *Clin Orthop Rel Res* 2001:46-55, 2001.
72. Uehara K, Kadoya Y, Kobayashi A, et al: Bone anatomy and rotational alignment in total knee arthroplasty, *Clin Orthop Rel Res* 2002:196-201, 2002. [See comment.]
73. Math KR, Zaidi SF, Petchprapa C, et al: Imaging of total knee arthroplasty, *Semin Musculoskel Radiol* 10:47-63, 2006.
74. Duff GP, Lachiewicz PF, Kelley SS: Aspiration of the knee joint before revision arthroplasty, *Clin Orthop Rel Res* 1996:132-139, 1996.
75. Mintz AD, Pilkington CA, Howie DW: A comparison of plain and fluoroscopically guided radiographs in the assessment of arthroplasty of the knee, *J Bone Joint Surg Am* 71:1343-1347, 1989.
76. Duus BR, Boeckstyns M, Stadeager C: The natural course of radionuclide bone scanning in the evaluation of total knee replacement—a 2-year prospective study, *Clin Radiol* 41:341-343, 1990.
77. Smith SL, Wastie ML, Forster I: Radionuclide bone scintigraphy in the detection of significant complications after total knee joint replacement, *Clin Radiol* 56:221-224, 2001.
78. Virolainen P, Lähteenmäki H, Hiltuner A, et al: The reliability of diagnosis of infection during revision arthroplasties, *Scand J Surg* 91:178-181, 2002.
79. Leone JM, Hanssen AD:, Management of infection at the site of a total knee arthroplasty, *J Bone Joint Surg Am* 87:2335-2348, 2005.
80. Bernard L, Lubbeke A, Stern R, et al: Value of preoperative investigations in diagnosing prosthetic joint infection: retrospective cohort study and literature review, *Scand J Infect Dis* 36:410-416, 2004.
81. Bach CM, Sturmer R, Nogler M, et al: Total knee arthroplasty infection: significance of delayed aspiration, *J Arthroplasty* 17:615-618, 2002.
82. Barrack RL, Jennings RW, Wolfe MW, et al: The Coventry Award. The value of preoperative aspiration before total knee revision, *Clin Orthop Rel Res* 1997:8-16, 1997.
83. Joseph TN, Mujtaba M, Chen AL, et al: Efficacy of combined technetium-99 m sulfur colloid/indium-111 leukocyte scans to detect infected total hip and knee arthroplasties, *J Arthroplasty* 16:753-758, 2001.
84. Scher DM, Pak K, Lonner JH, et al: The predictive value of indium-111 leukocyte scans in the diagnosis of infected total hip, knee, or resection arthroplasties, *J Arthroplasty* 15:295-300, 2000.
85. Van Acker F, Nuyts J, Maes A, et al: FDG-PET, 99 mtc-HMPAO white blood cell SPET and bone scintigraphy in the evaluation of painful total knee arthroplasties, *Eur J Nucl Med* 28:1496-1504, 2001.
86. Crymes WB Jr, Demos H, Gordon L: Detection of musculoskeletal infection with 18F-FDG PET: review of the current literature, *J Nucl Med Technol* 32:12-15, 2004.
87. Collier MB, Jewett BA, Engh CA Jr: Clinical assessment of tibial polyethylene thickness: comparison of radiographic measurements with as-implanted and as-retrieved thicknesses, *J Arthroplasty* 18:860-866, 2003.
88. Hide IG, Grainger AJ, Wallace IW, et al: A radiological technique for the assessment of wear in prosthetic knee replacements, *Skel Radiol* 29:583-586, 2000.
89. Sanzen L, Sahlstrom A, Gentz CF, et al: Radiographic wear assessment in a total knee prosthesis. 5- to 9-year follow-up study of 158 knees, *J Arthroplasty* 11: 738-742, 1996.
90. Miura H, Matsuda S, Mawatari T, et al: The oblique posterior femoral condylar radiographic view following total knee arthroplasty, *J Bone Joint Surg Am* 86-A: 47-50, 2004.
91. Sofka CM, Adler RS, Laskin R: Sonography of polyethylene liners used in total knee arthroplasty, *AJR Am J Roentgenol* 180:1437-1441, 2003.
92. Weissman BN, Scott RD, Brick GW, et al: Radiographic detection of metal-induced synovitis as a complication of arthroplasty of the knee, *J Bone Joint Surg Am* 73:1002-1007, 1991.
93. Chun KA, Ohashi K, Bennette DL, et al: Patellar fractures after total knee replacement, *AJR Am J Roentgenol* 185:655-660, 2005.
94. Brumby SA, Carrington R, Zayontz S, et al: Tibial plateau stress fracture: a complication of unicompartmental knee arthroplasty using 4 guide pinholes, *J Arthroplasty* 18:809-812, 2003.
95. Neer C, Brown TJ, Mclaughlin H: Fracture of the neck of the humerus with dislocation of the head fragment, *Am J Surg* 85:252-258, 1953.
96. Kelly IG, Foster RS, Fisher WD: Neer total shoulder replacement in rheumatoid arthritis, *J Bone Joint Surg Br* 69:723-726, 1987.
97. Bohsali KI, Wirth MA, Rockwood CA Jr: Complications of total shoulder arthroplasty, *J Bone Joint Surg Am* 88:2279-2292, 2006.
98. Deshmukh AV, Koris M, Zurakowski D, et al: Total shoulder arthroplasty: long-term survivorship, functional outcome, and quality of life, *J Shoulder Elbow Surg* 14:471-479, 2005.
99. van de Sande MA, Brand R, Rozing PM: Indications, complications, and results of shoulder arthroplasty, *Scand J Rheumatol* 35:426-434, 2006.
100. Lo IK, Litchfield RB, Griffin S, et al: Quality-of-life outcome following hemiarthroplasty or total shoulder arthroplasty in patients with osteoarthritis. A prospective, randomized trial, *J Bone Joint Surg Am* 87:2178-2185, 2005.
101. Pfahler M, Jena F, Neyton L, et al: Hemiarthroplasty versus total shoulder prosthesis0000 results of cemented glenoid components, *J Shoulder Elbow Surg* 15:154-163, 2006.
102. Guery J, Favard L, Sirveaux F, et al: Reverse total shoulder arthroplasty. Survivorship analysis of eighty replacements followed for five to ten years, *J Bone Joint Surg Am* 88:1742-1747, 2006.
103. Werner CM, Steinmann PA, Gilbart M, et al: Treatment of painful pseudoparesis due to irreparable rotator cuff dysfunction with the Delta III reverse-ball-and-socket total shoulder prosthesis, *J Bone Joint Surg Am* 87:1476-1486, 2005.
104. Stavrou P, Slavotinek J, Krishnan J: A radiographic evaluation of birotational head motion in the bipolar shoulder hemiarthroplasty, *J Shoulder Elbow Surg* 15: 399-401, 2006.
105. Frankle M, Siegal S, Pupello D, et al: The reverse shoulder prosthesis for glenohumeral arthritis associated with severe rotator cuff deficiency. A minimum two-year follow-up study of sixty patients, *J Bone Joint Surg Am* 87:1697-1705, 2005.
106. Rockwood CA Jr: The reverse total shoulder prosthesis. The new kid on the block, *J Bone Joint Surg Am* 89:233-235, 2007. [Comment.].
107. Yian EH, Werner CM, Nyffeler RW, et al: Radiographic and computed tomography analysis of cemented pegged polyethylene glenoid components in total shoulder replacement, *J Bone Joint Surg Am* 87:1928-1936, 2005.
108. Goutallier D, Postel JM, Bernageau J, et al: Fatty muscle degeneration in cuff ruptures. Pre- and postoperative evaluation by CT scan, *Clin Orthop Rel Res* 1994: 78-83, 1994.
109. Simovitch RW, Helmy N, Zumstein MA, et al: Impact of fatty infiltration of the teres minor muscle on the outcome of reverse total shoulder arthroplasty, *J Bone Joint Surg Am* 89:934-939, 2007.
110. Edwards TB, Boulahia A, Kempf JF, et al: The influence of rotator cuff disease on the results of shoulder arthroplasty for primary osteoarthritis: results of a multicenter study, *J Bone Joint Surg Am* 84-A(12):2240-2248, 2002.
111. Lazarus MD, Jensen KL, Southwarth C, et al: The radiographic evaluation of keeled and pegged glenoid component insertion, *J Bone Joint Surg Am* 84-A:1174-1182, 2002.
112. Chin PY, Sperling JW, Cofield RH, et al: Complications of total shoulder arthroplasty: are they fewer or different? *J Shoulder Elbow Surg* 15:19-22, 2006.
113. Kumar S, Sperling JW, Haidukewych GH, et al: Periprosthetic humeral fractures after shoulder arthroplasty, *J Bone Joint Surg Am* 86-A:680-689, 2004.
114. Wright TW, Cofield RH:, Humeral fractures after shoulder arthroplasty. *J Bone Joint Surg Am* 77:1340-1346, 1995.
115. Lecomte AR, Singh, Fitzgerald B, et al: Small joint arthroplasty. *Semin Musculoskel Radiol* 10:64-78, 2006.
116. Cracchiolo A 3rd, Weltmer JB, Jr, Lian G, et al: Arthroplasty of the first metatarsophalangeal joint with a double-stem silicone implant. Results in patients who have degenerative joint disease failure of previous operations, or rheumatoid arthritis, *J Bone Joint Surg Am* 74:552-563, 1992.
117. Nalbandian RM: Synovitis and lymphadenopathy in silicone arthroplasty implants, *J Bone Joint Surg Am* 65:280-281, 1983.

118. Boles CA, Daniel WW, Adams BD, et al: Hand and wrist, *Radiol Clin North Am* 33:319-354, 1995.
119. Christie AJ, Pierret G, Levitan J: Silicone synovitis, *Semin Arthritis Rheum* 19: 166-171, 1989.
120. Weissman BN, Simmons BP, Thomas WH: Replacement of "other" joints, *Radiol Clin North Am* 33:355-373, 1995.
121. Abboud JA, Beredjiklian PK, Bozentka DJ: Metacarpophalangeal joint arthroplasty in rheumatoid arthritis, *J Am Acad Orthop Surg* 11:184-191, 2003.
122. Bieber EJ, Weiland AJ, Volenec-Dowling S: Silicone-rubber implant arthroplasty of the metacarpophalangeal joints for rheumatoid arthritis, *J Bone Joint Surg Am* 68:206-209, 1986.
123. Goldfarb CA, Stern PJ: Metacarpophalangeal joint arthroplasty in rheumatoid arthritis. A long-term assessment, *J Bone Joint Surg Am* 85-A:1869-1878, 2003. [See comment.]
124. Levadoux M, Legre R: Total wrist arthroplasty with Destot prostheses in patients with posttraumatic arthritis, *J Hand Surg Am* 28:405-413, 2003.
125. Simmons B, Millender L, Nalebuff E: Surgery of the hand. In Sledge CB, Harris ED, Rudy S et al (eds): *Arthritis and Surgery*, Philadelphia, 1994, WB Saunders, pp . 706-737.
126. Taljanovic MS, Jones MD, Hunter TB, et al: Joint arthroplasties and prostheses, *Radiographics* 23:1295-1314, 2003.
127. Jolly SL, Ferlic DC, Clayton ML, et al: Swanson silicone arthroplasty of the wrist in rheumatoid arthritis: a long-term follow-up, *J Hand SurgJ Hand Surg Am* 17:142-149, 1992. [See comment.]
128. Meuli HC, Total wrist arthroplasty. Experience with a noncemented wrist prosthesis, *Clin Orthop Rel Res* 1997:77-83, 1997.
129. Menon J: Total wrist replacement using the modified Volz prosthesis, *J Bone Joint Surg Am* 69:998-1006, 1987.
130. Ruth JT, Wilde AH: Capitellocondylar total elbow replacement. A long-term follow-up study, *J Bone Joint Surg Am* 74:95-100, 1992.
131. Morrey BF, Adams RA: Semiconstrained arthroplasty for the treatment of rheumatoid arthritis of the elbow, *J Bone Joint Surg Am* 74:479-490, 1992.
132. Pritchard RW: Total elbow joint arthroplasty in patients with rheumatoid arthritis, *Semin Arthritis Rheum* 21:24-29, 1991.
133. Ewald FC, Simmons ED, Jr, Sullivan, JA, et al: Capitellocondylar total elbow replacement in rheumatoid arthritis. Long-term results, *J Bone Joint Surg Am* 75:498-507, 1993. [Erratum appears in *J Bone Joint Surg Am* 75:1881, 1993.]
134. Conti SF, Wong YS: Complications of total ankle replacement, *Clin Orthop Rel Res* 2001:105-114, 2001.

Section III

Imaging of Metabolic Conditions

CHAPTER 31

Imaging Evaluation of Osteoporosis

JUDITH E. ADAMS, MBBS, FRCR, FRCP

KEY FACTS

- Osteoporosis is the most common metabolic bone disease and affects one in three women and one in five men over 50 years of age.
- Osteoporotic fractures are associated with considerable morbidity, mortality, and social and health-care costs.
- Effective therapies are available to reduce future fracture risk.
- Radiographic features (osteopenia, thinned cortex, reduced number, and thickness of trabeculae) may be present before fractures occur.
- Vertebral fractures are the most common osteoporotic fracture.
- Thirty percent to 50% of vertebral fractures may be present without symptoms.
- Vertebral fractures are powerful predictors of future fracture (vertebral five times; hip two times).
- The presence of vertebral fracture should be clearly and accurately reported by radiologists, and should stimulate further investigation/management.
- Other imaging techniques (magnetic resonance imaging [MRI], radionuclide imaging, and computed tomography) are helpful in identifying fractures that are occult on radiographs and in differentiating whether fractures are acute/chronic or due to other causes.
- MRI allows bone marrow edema present in reflex sympathetic dystrophy or migratory osteoporosis to be detected.
- Dual energy x-ray absorptiometry (hip, spine) is a quantitative method for confirming the diagnosis of osteoporosis.

Metabolic bone diseases affect bone as a tissue; all bones are involved histologically, but radiologic features are not always present. A variety of nutritional, biochemical, genetic, endocrine, and biochemical disorders can result in metabolic bone diseases.[1,2]

Osteoporosis is the most common of the metabolic bone diseases and is now defined as "a systemic skeletal disease characterized by low bone mass and microarchitectural deterioration of bone tissue, with a consequent increase in bone fragility and susceptibility to fracture."[3]

> Osteoporosis is the most common metabolic bone disease.

Not only is the amount of bone tissue reduced (quantitative abnormality of bone), but also the structural integrity and biomechanical strength of bone are compromised by reduction in number, thickness, and connectivity of trabeculae.[4] Bones become brittle and fracture with little, or no, trauma (insufficiency [fragility] fractures), and these fractures are the cardinal clinical feature of osteoporosis. This is in contrast to rickets and osteomalacia in which there is a qualitative abnormality of bone (reduced mineral to osteoid ratio), the bones are soft and bend, and Looser zones may be present as a diagnostic radiologic feature (see Chapter 35).

> Osteoporosis is characterized by a reduction in the number, thickness, and connectivity of trabeculae leading to reduced bone strength.

EPIDEMIOLOGY

Osteoporosis poses a significant public health problem, and in the Western world one in two women and one in five men over the age of 50 years will suffer a fracture in their lifetime.[5] In the past 20 years there have been significant advances in knowledge of the epidemiology, pathophysiology, and treatment of osteoporosis.[6] The fractures that occur in osteoporosis result in considerable morbidity and mortality for patients and incur large social and health care costs. The risk of fracture increases independently with advancing age and reduction in bone mass; approximately 70% of bone strength is related to bone mineral density (BMD).

> Seventy percent of bone strength is related to bone density, and bone density can be measured by techniques such as dual energy x-ray absorptiometry (DXA) scanning.

The incidence of fracture varies with the population being studied; in Britain, 60,000 hip fractures, 50,000 wrist fractures, and 120,000 vertebral fractures occur per year,[5] with associated health care costs of approximately £2 billion. In the United States, the age-adjusted incidence of insufficiency fractures in both men and women is 25% higher than in Britain and other areas of Europe, and the estimated cost of managing these fractures was $17 billion in 2001. The incidence of hip fracture has doubled over the past three decades, and it is predicted to continue to rise beyond what would be predicted from increased longevity in populations, particularly in the Far East.

Following hip or vertebral fracture, mortality at 5 years is about 20% greater than that expected, and mortality rate is highest in men aged over 75 years who have comorbidities. Most of the excess deaths occur in the first 6 months after hip fracture. One year after hip fracture, 40% of patients are unable to walk independently, 60% have difficulty with one essential activity of daily living, 80% are restricted in other living activities (e.g., driving, shopping), and 27% will be admitted to a nursing home for the first time.[6]

Vertebral fractures are the most common type of osteoporotic fracture and may occur in the absence of, or after only minimal, trauma. In the United States, it is estimated that 25% of women aged over 50 years will have a vertebral fracture, and this will rise to 33% in those over 75 years.[7] In Europe, there is a similar prevalence of 20% in women over 50, and a strong age dependency.[6] In men, a prevalence of 20% over the age of 50 is found, but as more of these were present at an earlier age, traumatic events are presumed to be the etiology.[8]

> Vertebral fractures are the most common type of osteoporotic fracture. Hip fractures are the most life threatening.

BONE PHYSIOLOGY

Bones have an outer cortical (compact) shell and inner trabecular (net-like cancellous) bone tissue, which enable the skeleton to be light but strong. The relative amounts of each type of bone vary by skeletal site (Table 31-1),[9,10] and both contribute to bone strength. In research studies, quantitative measurements made in various anatomic sites and by different methods (DXA, quantitative computed tomography [QCT], and quantitative ultrasound [QUS]) may give complementary information about the amount and rates of change of the various bone components in diseases and with therapies.

Bone—which is composed of a matrix of collagen fibers, mucopolysaccharides, and inorganic crystalline mineral matrix (calcium hydroxyapatite)—is hard and strong and remains metabolically active throughout life (bone turnover), being continuously resorbed (by osteoclasts) and formed (by osteoblasts). This process can be modified by many factors, and bones consequently model and remodel throughout life from birth to maturity, maintaining their basic shape, repairing following fracture and responding to physical forces (i.e., mechanical loading). The overall strength of a bone is related to its hardness and other physical properties, size, shape, and architectural arrangement of the compact and trabecular bone.[4]

> Bone is a dynamic tissue, with bone resorption and bone production (bone turnover) occurring throughout life.

Bone formation (osteoblastic activity) and bone resorption (osteoclastic activity) constitute bone turnover, a process that takes place on bone surfaces and continues throughout life. Trabecular bone has a greater surface-to-volume ratio than compact bone, is about eight times more metabolically active, and therefore has a larger turnover than cortical bone. In adult life and under normal circumstances, bone formation and resorption are linked in a consistent sequence; precursor cells are activated to form osteoclasts, which erode a fairly constant amount of bone. After a period of time (about 3 to 4 months), the bone resorption stops and osteoblasts are recruited to fill the eroded space with new bone tissue. Under normal circumstances, this osteoblastic and osteoclastic activity is coupled and constitutes the basal multicellular unit (BMU). There will be numerous BMUs throughout the skeleton at different stages of this cycle, and the amount of bone in the skeleton at any moment in time depends on peak bone mass attained during puberty and adolescence and the balance between bone resorption and formation. If there is uncoupling of this process, with either excessive osteoclastic resorption or defective osteoblastic function, then there is a net loss of bone (osteoporosis). Increased activation frequency of resorption units results in high bone turnover states (hyperparathyroidism, postmenopausal bone loss, Paget's disease). Therapy with bisphosphonates reduces the activation of resorption units by inhibiting osteoclastic function, and the consequent reversal of the mineral deficit contributes to the increase in BMD that occurs with such therapy.

TABLE 31-1. Approximate Ratios of Cortical to Trabecular Bone by Anatomic Skeletal Site

Anatomic Site	Cortical/Trabecular Ratio
Whole body	80/20
Hip	60/40
Lumbar spine	50/50
Distal radius	95/5
Ultra distal radius	40/60
Calcaneus	5/95

> Normally, bone turnover is coupled so that bone production and destruction are balanced; uncoupling results from excessive resorption or defective bone production.

The bones grow during the first two decades of life with a pubertal spurt during adolescence. Skeletal maturity is achieved at an earlier age in girls (16 to 18 years) than in boys (18 to 20 years). Following attainment of skeletal maturity, a period of consolidation follows during which peak bone mass is achieved. For cortical bone, this is reached at about 35 years of age and a little earlier for trabecular bone. Although the long bones grow in length at the metaphyses, they are remodeled in shape during development by endosteal resorption and periosteal apposition. The size and shape of the skeleton and its individual bones are determined by genetic factors,[11] but they are influenced by endocrine and local growth factors, nutrition, and physical activity.[11-14] Remodeling allows the skeleton to adjust to mechanical forces to which it is exposed. There is considerable variation in skeletal size and weight both within and between race/ethnic groups.[12] Dark-skinned people tend to have larger and heavier bones than whites, and some Asian groups tend toward a small skeletal mass and size.[13] Although genetic factors are important, they are modified by environmental differences such as diet and physical activity.[14]

The amount of bone in the skeleton at any moment in time depends on peak bone mass and the balance between bone resorption and formation. Osteoporosis is not a single disease entity but an end result of many disease processes.[15] It may result from defective skeletal accretion during bone growth and development in childhood and adolescence or defective osteoblastic function (e.g., in glucocorticoid therapy). Alternatively, it can result from disease processes in which bone resorption exceeds new bone formation, resulting in a net loss of bone mass and consequent compromise in skeletal strength.

> Postmenopausal bone loss is usually due to excessive bone resorption.

Bone can also be lost focally in specific anatomic regions, such as occurs in periarticular regions in the inflammatory arthritides (e.g., metacarpal and proximal interphalangeal joints in rheumatoid arthritis). This loss of bone is related to hyperemia and the release of cytokines, which stimulate local osteoclastic bone resorption. This is perhaps more appropriately described as "osteopenia" than osteoporosis.

In the past, treatment of established osteoporosis was limited and unsatisfactory and consisted mainly of hormone replacement therapy [HRT] for postmenopausal osteoporosis. However, in recent years the introduction of bone protective therapies (bisphosphonates, selective estrogen receptor modulators [SERMs], strontium ranelate) and the anabolic agent teriparatide (parathyroid hormone) have been shown to result in modest increases in bone mineral density (incremental changes of 6% to 12%) and, more importantly, reduce future fractures to a much greater extent (reductions of 40% to 70%).[16-18] Treatment strategies have generally favored prevention of osteoporosis by maximizing peak bone mass, minimizing age-related and postmenopausal bone loss (HRT in premature menopause), and avoidance of risk factors (e.g., smoking, excessive alcohol) with adequate dietary intake of calcium and vitamin D (for supplementation, this is achieved by 1 g of elemental calcium and 800 units vitamin D) and regular weight-bearing physical activity. Bisphosphonates are increasingly being used to treat osteoporosis due to a variety of causes in children as well.[19]

Compliance and persistence with oral bone-protective therapies taken daily is relatively poor, being approximately 50% at 1 year. This situation has been improved with the introduction of monthly dosing with certain bisphosphonates and intravenous administration of others. It is with the latter, rather than with oral preparations, which are being given for hypercalcemia in patients with metastatic cancer, that reports have emerged of the uncommon complication of osteonecrosis of the jaw.[20]

Adequate analgesia should be given to manage pain during an acute fracture episode or appropriately as improves the quality of life thereafter for those severely affected by osteoporosis; physiotherapy may also be helpful.

CLASSIFICATION AND CAUSES OF OSTEOPOROSIS

Osteoporosis can be generalized, involving the whole skeleton, or regional, in which only a segment, or focal area, of the skeleton is affected. There are many etiologies of both types of osteoporosis.

Generalized Osteoporosis

This may be primary (Box 31-1) in origin or secondary to other disorders (Table 31-2), which either reduce acquisition of peak adult bone mass or increase age-related bone loss. Osteoporosis can occur in adults and children (Box 31-2).

Primary Osteoporosis

Idiopathic juvenile osteoporosis (IJO)[21] is a rare, self-limiting disease in prepubertal children aged 8 to 14 years who have previously been healthy. For a period of about 2 to 4 years, growth arrest and fractures occur, with loss of both cortical and trabecular bone and a wide spectrum of severity. Only one or two vertebral fractures are present in mild disease, but in more severe cases fractures involve all vertebrae and the extremities, particularly the metaphyseal region of the distal tibia. In a few patients, these can result in severe kyphoscoliosis, deformities of the extremities, and even death from respiratory failure due to deformity of the thorax. The disease is reversible and remits spontaneously, with the residue of only a mild or moderate kyphosis, short stature, and some bone deformity following fractures. Investigations indicate uncoupling of bone turnover with increased resorption and decreased formation. The condition must be differentiated from osteogenesis imperfecta (no blue sclerae) and other forms of juvenile osteoporosis. Other important differential diagnoses in children with vertebral fractures are hypercortisolism (e.g., Cushing's disease or systemic glucocorticoid therapy) and leukemia (Box 31-2) (Figure 31-1).

BOX 31-1. Primary Osteoporosis

- Idiopathic juvenile
- Osteoporosis of young adults
- Osteogenesis imperfecta
- Postmenopausal (estrogen decline)
- Senile (age related)

TABLE 31-2. Selected Causes of Secondary Osteoporosis

Endocrine	Nutritional
Glucocorticoid excess Estrogen/testosterone deficiency Hyperparathyroidism Hyperthyroidism Growth hormone deficiency (childhood onset)	Intestinal malabsorption Chronic alcoholism Chronic liver disease Vitamin C deficiency (scurvy) Partial gastrectomy
Hereditary	**Hematologic**
Homocystinuria Ehlers-Danlos syndrome Marfan syndrome	Sickle cell disease Thalassemia Gaucher's disease
Other	**Other**
Rheumatoid arthritis Hemochromatosis Long-term heparin therapy	Prolonged bed rest/inactivity Breast cancer therapies (e.g., aromatase inhibitors) Stroke Spinal cord injury

BOX 31-2. Causes of Osteoporosis in Children

PRIMARY OSTEOPOROSIS
- Osteogenesis imperfecta
- Idiopathic juvenile osteoporosis
- Osteoporosis of young adults

SECONDARY OSTEOPOROSIS
- Systemic long-term glucocorticoid therapy
- Hypogonadism, primary or secondary
- Prolonged immobilization (e.g., cerebral palsy, paraplegia)
- Chronic inflammatory disease (e.g., juvenile inflammatory arthritis)
- Chronic liver and inflammatory bowel disease
- Neoplasia and therapy (e.g., leukemia)
- Other, including cystic fibrosis, anorexia nervosa

Osteoporosis of young adults is a heterogeneous condition that occurs in young men and women equally, usually runs a mild course with multiple vertebral fractures occurring over a decade or more, and is associated with height loss. Fractures of metatarsals and ribs are also common, and hip fractures may occur. The cause of the condition is obscure, and it may simply be that inadequate bone mass has been accrued during skeletal growth; some affected individuals may have a mild variant of osteogenesis imperfecta. Exceptionally, osteoporosis may present during pregnancy, but whether this is a causal or coincidental association is unknown.

Osteogenesis imperfecta (OI) or "brittle bone" syndrome, results from mutations affecting either the COL1A1 or COL1A2 genes of type I collagen.[22,23] A number of inherited disorders of connective tissue can result in osteoporosis (Table 31-2).[15] Although the disease is usually apparent at birth or in childhood, more mild forms of the disease may not become apparent until

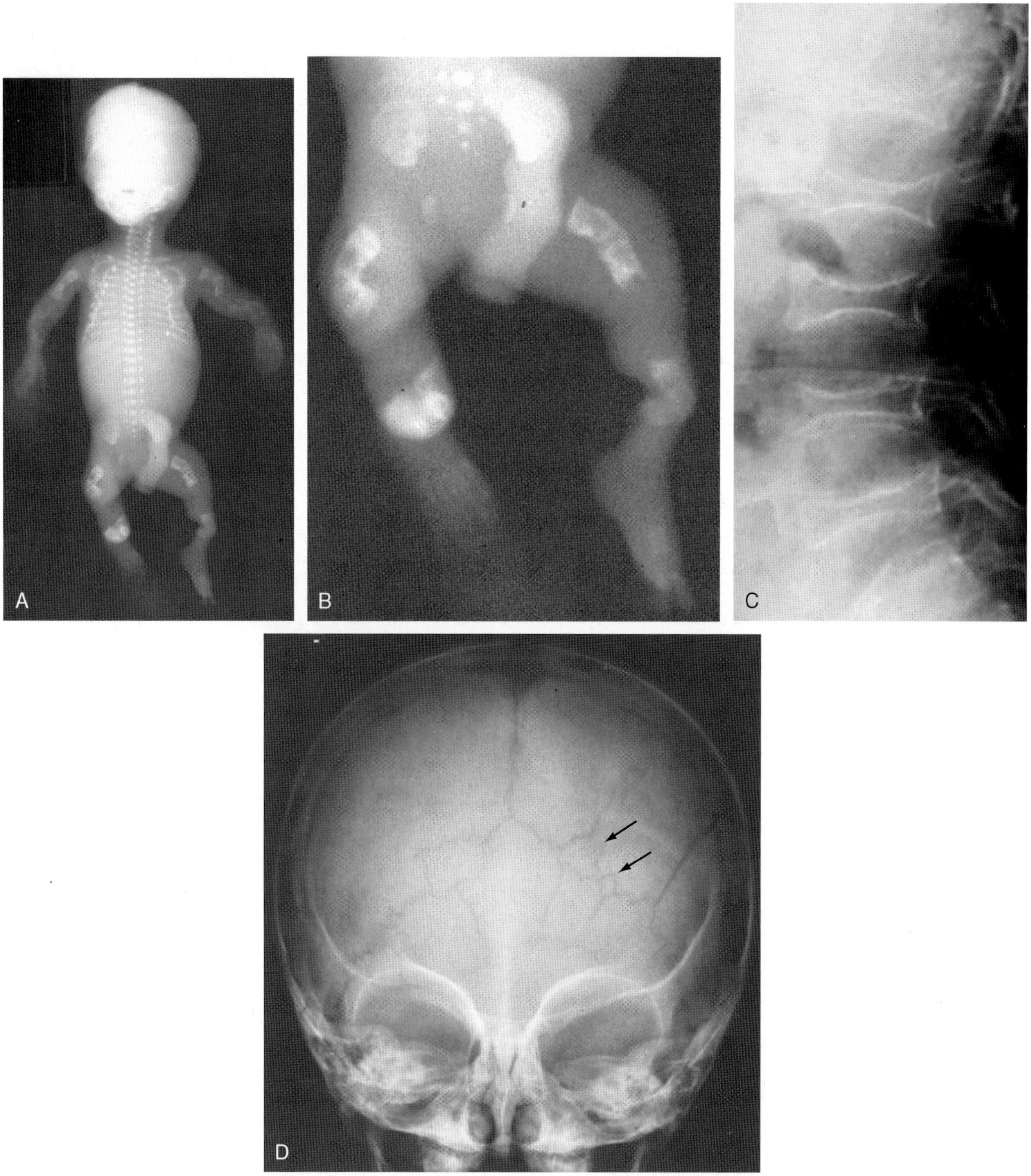

A B C D

FIGURE 31-1. Osteogenesis imperfecta. **A,** "Babygram" of stillborn infant with type II (lethal perinatal) osteogenesis imperfecta showing poor mineralization of the skull and skeleton generally with multiple fractures of the ribs, giving a "beaded" appearance. **B,** Severe deformity of the femora is present giving the "concertina" appearance due to multiple fractures. **C,** Lateral radiograph of the lumbar spine showing severe osteopenia and platyspondyly due to multiple vertebral fractures. The differential diagnoses for vertebral fractures in children include hypercortisolism (e.g., Cushing's disease or systemic glucocorticoid therapy) and leukemia. **D,** The frontal radiograph of the skull showing Wormian (intrasutural) bones *(arrows)*. (**A** and **B** courtesy of Sarah Russell, MD, St Mary's Hospital, Manchester; **C,** courtesy of Moira Cheung, Shriners Hospital for Children, Montreal, Canada. **D** courtesy of Amaka Offiah, MD, Great Ormond Street Hospital, London.)

adulthood, when affected individuals present with insufficiency fractures and osteopenia. A common classification (types I to IV) of OI is one devised by Sillence.[22] (See Chapter 32.) The important characteristics in this classification include blue sclerae, the severity of the disorder, and the mode of inheritance (dominant, recessive, sporadic/new mutation), although accurate classification is difficult because of phenotypic overlap. Subjects who do not have dental involvement are designated as group "A," and those with dentinogenesis imperfecta are designated as group "B."

Type I is the mildest and most prevalent form of OI and may only become apparent in adulthood. There is a history of fractures, generally dating back to childhood. In children the fractures may become radiographically and clinically apparent as the child becomes more active (5 years and older) and may be overt fractures of long bones and vertebrae or microfractures of the metaphyses. If present in infancy, these features may resemble those found in nonaccidental injury.[24] The differential diagnosis can usually be resolved by the presence of associated extraskeletal manifestations of OI (blue sclera, dentinogenesis imperfecta) or a family history of OI, so bone biopsy is seldom required for diagnosis. Stature is short, with only 10% of patients being of normal height; there is joint laxity, blue sclerae, and pre-senile hearing loss. Transmission is by autosomal dominant trait, and radiologically the bones are usually reduced in density, although some patients may have normal bone density. Bones may be narrow and undertubulated (gracile) or normally modeled. Vertebral fractures occur in the fourth decade, and scoliosis, if present, is mild.

Type II (lethal perinatal) OI results in affected infants being small, with deep blue sclerae and short and deformed limbs due to multiple fractures (Figure 31-1). Fractures involve ribs, and death is usually the result of pulmonary insufficiency making survival beyond the first 3 months of life rare. Other complications include brain and spinal cord injury. Radiologically, multiple fractures are present with a characteristic "concertina" deformity of the lower limbs; the ribs may appear "beaded" due to multiple rib fractures (Figure 31-1), which can occur in utero. The cranial vault is severely undermineralized and may be distorted by molding. Wormian (intrasutural) bones in the occipital and parietal region (Figure 31-1) and platyspondyly are noted.

Type III (severe progressive) OI is inherited as an autosomal recessive trait, with fractures usually present at birth and involving long bones, clavicles, ribs, and cranium with resulting deformity. Although size at birth is normal, retardation of growth is evident in the first year of life, and many patients reach only 3 to 4 feet in height in adulthood. As growth proceeds, increasing deformity of the calvaria occurs, with resulting facial distortion, malocclusion, and mild prognathism, basilar invagination, and progressive hearing loss. Sclerae are blue at birth, but this diminishes with age, and sclerae are white in adults. Vertebral fractures occur at an early age (see Figure 31-1,*C*) and contribute to the progressive and severe kyphoscoliosis that develops during childhood. Patients tend to be wheelchair-bound because of the progressive deformities resulting from fractures. Complications include progressive pulmonary insufficiency through distortion of the thorax. Radiologically, the bones may be slender or broad due to recurrent fractures, and epiphyses are abnormal, with expansion and islands of calcified ("popcorn") cartilage.[25] As in other forms of OI, the incidence of fracture declines following puberty.

Type IV (moderately severe) OI is inherited as an autosomal dominant trait and can vary in severity and be confused with either type I or type III OI. There is generally more severe osteopenia and extensive bone deformity than in type I. The sclerae are blue in children, which may persist into adulthood but may also fade to white. Patients are short in stature with abnormal molding of the calvarium and basilar invagination in a high proportion of patients. Bones of the spine and limbs are osteoporotic and dysplastic, resulting in scoliosis and deformity, particularly of the pelvis. Joint laxity can result in dislocation, particularly of the ankle or knee.

Although there is no cure for OI, treatments have been aimed at increasing bone strength to prevent fracture and maintain physical activity. Bisphosphonates, either oral (alendronate) or intravenous (pamidronate, zolendronate), have been demonstrated to increase bone mass, restore vertebrae to their more normal shape, and reduce fractures in small study groups[26,27] (Figure 31-2). If cyclical doses of bisphosphonates are given (e.g., intravenous pamidronate, which is given every 3 months), then sclerotic lines result in the metaphyses of long bones in children (see Figure 31-2).

Postmenopausal (Type I) Osteoporosis

At menopause, estrogen levels fall, and as a consequence all women lose bone at this time, some losing trabecular bone at a rate three times greater than normal (2% to 10% per annum). The bone loss is greatest during the first 4 years after menopause. The condition characteristically becomes clinically evident in women 15 to 20 years after the menopause. Fractures occur in sites of the skeleton rich in trabecular bone, including the vertebrae and distal forearm (Colles fracture) (Figure 31-3). In premature menopause, bone

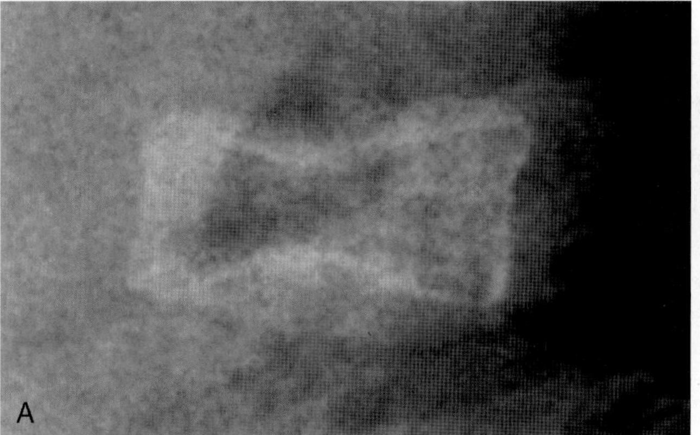

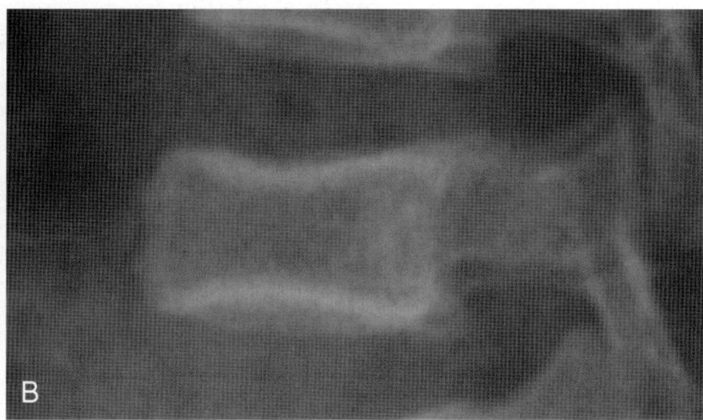

FIGURE 31-2. Bisphosphonate therapy in children. Bisphosphonates are increasingly used to treat osteoporosis in children. **A,** The baseline lateral lumbar radiograph of a child with osteogenesis imperfecta and vertebral fractures who was treated with cyclical intravenous pamidronate every 3 months shows decreased vertebral body height, giving a biconcave appearance. **B,** After treatment, there is some restoration of shape to the vertebral body and thickening of the endplates.

(Continued)

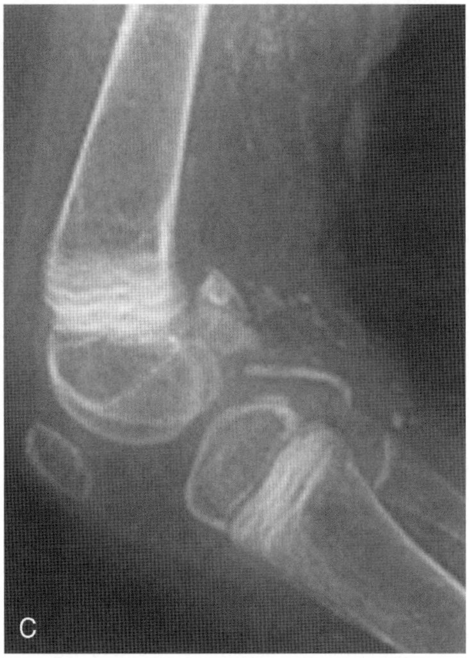

FIGURE 31-2—cont'd. **C,** Such cyclical treatment in a child with osteoporosis secondary to juvenile dermatomyositis caused dense lines in the metaphyses of the long bones. Evident are the radiographic features of osteoporosis including osteopenia (reduced radiographic density), thinned bone cortices, and reduced trabeculae. There is also soft tissue calcification related to juvenile dermatomyositis. (**C** courtesy of Amaka Offiah, MD, Great Ormond Street Hospital, London.)

loss can be prevented by HRT up to the age of natural menopause (approximately 50 years of age). However, it is now believed that HRT should not be used long term after this age for the purpose of bone protective therapy as there are other more specific and effective bone agents now available[16,17,28] and because of the increased risk of breast cancer and cardiovascular events with long-term use of HRT in elderly women.

> HRT should not be used long term after menopause as bone protective therapy as there are other more specific and effective bone agents available and there is increased risk of breast cancer and cardiovascular events.

Senile (type II) osteoporosis occurs in both men and women of 75 years or older and is due to age-related bone loss related to impaired bone formation and secondary hyperparathyroidism that occur with advancing age. The latter is a consequence of reduced calcium absorption from the intestine secondary to decreased production of the active metabolite of vitamin D (1,25$[OH]_2$D) in the kidneys of the elderly. There is reduction in both cortical and trabecular bone, and the syndrome manifests mainly as hip fractures (Figure 31-4) and wedge fractures of the vertebrae. However, fractures may also occur in the proximal tibia, proximal humerus, and pelvis.

Secondary Osteoporosis

Many conditions can result in osteoporosis and may be of endocrine, nutritional, hereditary, hematologic, or other origin (Box 31-2).[29] Radiologically, the appearances may be indistinguishable from involutional (senile) osteoporosis,[30] although some diseases may have specific and diagnostic radiologic features

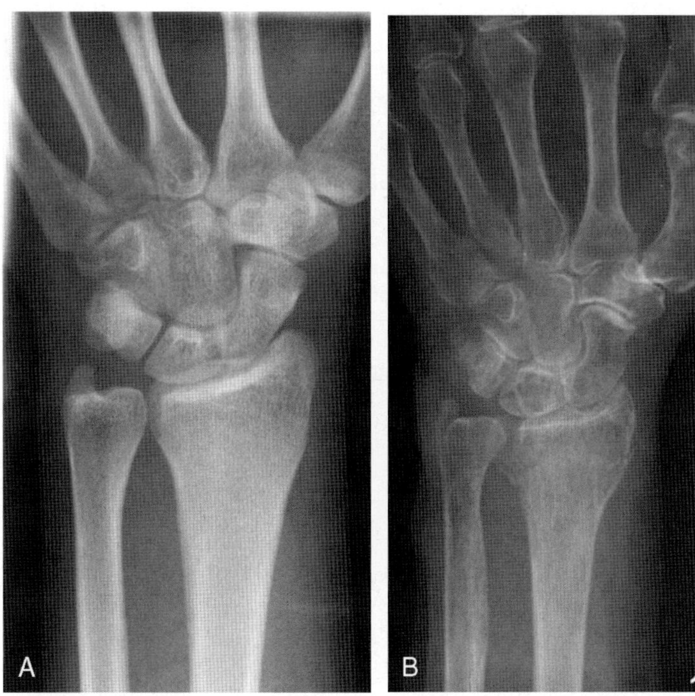

FIGURE 31-3. Postmenopausal (type 1) osteoporosis. **A,** Normal bone density. This posteroanterior radiograph of the wrist in a young patient demonstrates normal radiographic bone density, normal width of bone cortices, and normal trabecular number. **B,** Osteoporosis. The posteroanterior radiograph of the wrist of an elderly woman with a Colles fracture (which occurred after a fall from standing height [low trauma]) shows the radiographic features of osteoporosis, including reduced bone density, thinned bone cortices, and trabecular bone loss.

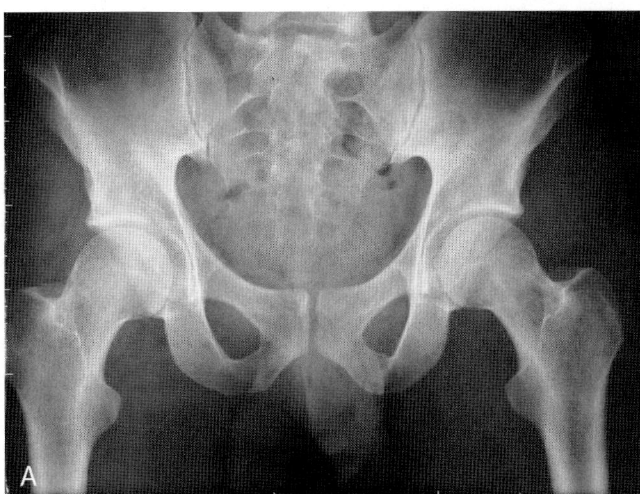

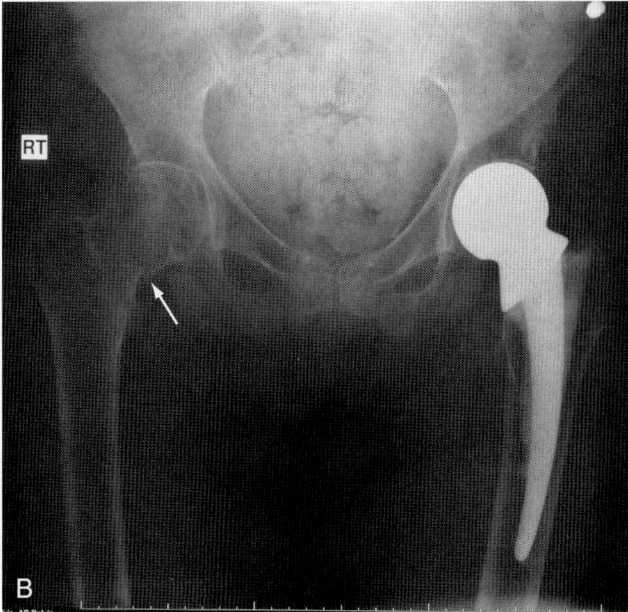

FIGURE 31-4. Senile (type II) osteoporosis. **A,** Pelvic radiographs in a young patient show normal bone density, cortical thickness, and trabecula. **B,** Anteroposterior radiograph of the pelvis of an elderly woman with a transcervical fracture *(arrow)* in the right femur shows the radiographic features of osteoporosis with reduced bone density, thinned cortices, and trabecular loss. The hemiarthroplasty on the left was inserted following a prior hip fracture.

(e.g., subperiosteal erosions of the phalanges in primary hyperparathyroidism). In glucocorticoid excess[31] (endogenous and exogenous), there is reduced bone formation due to a direct effect on the osteoblasts, with increased osteoclastic activity, probably mediated through secondary hyperparathyroidism stimulated by reduced gastrointestinal absorption of calcium. There is also evidence that glucocorticoids induce premature apoptosis of both osteoblasts and osteoclasts. The adverse effect is primarily on trabecular bone, and fractures occur particularly in the vertebrae and ribs; the latter may heal with profuse callus formation.

> Myeloma may produce generalized osteoporosis.

Thyrotoxicosis stimulates catabolic activity and increases osteoclastic bone resorption and may be severe enough to occasionally cause recognizable osteoporosis. Long-term heparin therapy has also been reported to cause osteoporosis, possibly due to release of collagenase from lysosomes. Formation of osseous matrix also requires other substances such as protein and vitamin C (for the formation of collagen). Hence osteoporosis may develop in deficiency states involving lack of proteins (e.g., in starvation or severe malnutrition) or in scurvy. Hematologic disorders can result in osteoporosis; in hemolytic anemias, there is marrow hyperplasia and expansion, which causes change in bone modeling, thinned bone cortex, and a coarse and prominent net-like trabecular pattern (Figure 31-5). Myeloma can cause generalized osteoporosis, but there may also be "punched-out" lytic lesions in bones (see Figure 31-5), particularly in the skull. Finally, a number of other disorders including hepatic disease and chronic alcoholism may cause osteoporosis by various mechanisms, many of which are still not clearly understood at the present time.

REGIONAL OSTEOPOROSIS (OSTEOPENIA)

In some conditions, bone loss may not be generalized but localized to a specific anatomic region (Box 31-3).

Disuse osteoporosis occurs through inactivity and failure to load the skeleton normally[32-34] (Figure 31-6). The growth and development of the skeleton and maintenance of bone health throughout life depends on normal activity and loading of the skeleton. If, for any reason, there is inactivity (e.g., stroke, polio, spinal cord injury), there will be localized osteopenia involving the part of the skeleton affected. Such a process may be acute (e.g., following a fracture) or chronic (e.g., following a stroke, cerebral palsy) (Figure 31-6).

Reflex sympathetic dystrophy (RSD) syndrome (Sudeck's atrophy) is a more severe form of localized osteopenia, which can occur in children or adults and be precipitated by a variety of conditions.[35] (See also Chapter 32.) Fracture is a common cause, but other etiologies include infection, peripheral neuropathy, and tumor or central nervous system abnormality. However, in a significant number of cases, no precipitating cause is found. The causative mechanism is not clearly understood, but it is thought that the precipitating factor results in abnormal neural reflexes traveling along the peripheral nerves and producing localized symptoms. There are consequently sympathetic nervous system influences through increased sensitivity to catecholamines and other neuropeptides that result in pain, soft tissue swelling, and hyperemia.[36] There is excessive bone resorption (probably stimulated by cytokines), which occurs particularly in a periarticular distribution and may simulate malignant disease. Any joint may be affected, with involvement of the shoulder and hand being most common; there may rarely be involvement of multiple joints. RSD tends to be progressive, and atrophic changes may eventually be evident in the skin, which develops a smooth and glistening appearance.

Regional migratory osteoporosis is also known as migratory osteolysis and is an uncommon and self-limiting condition presenting as arthralgia with migration between weight-bearing joints of the lower limb.[37,38] The condition is often associated with generalized osteoporosis and may be the result of microinsufficiency fractures in the subarticular region of the affected joint and can rarely be associated with rapid osteolysis.[39,40] Transient osteoporosis of the hip is the most common site and was originally described in pregnant women[37]; however, it is now known to be just as common in middle-aged men. Clinically, there is hip pain

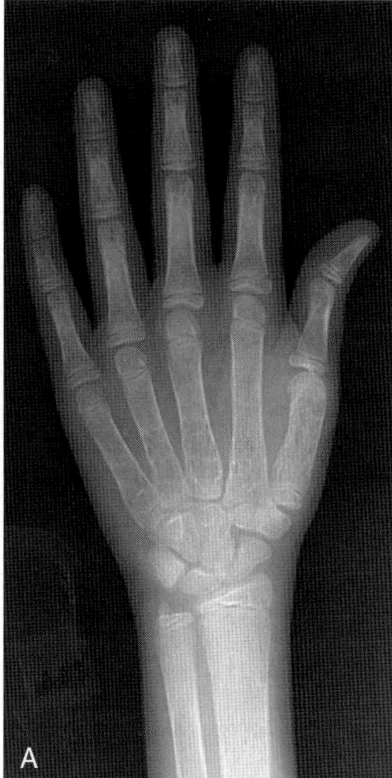

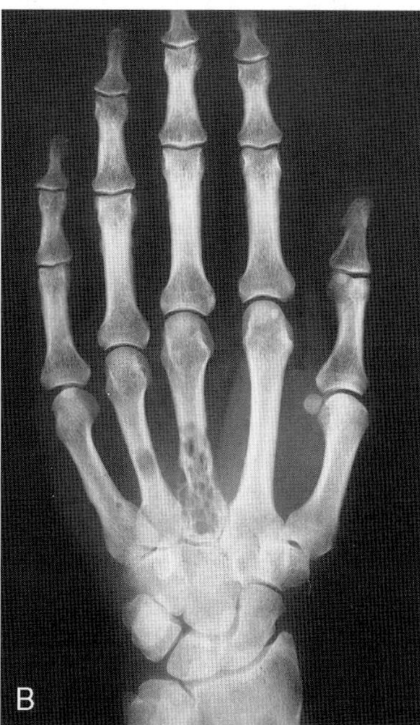

FIGURE 31-5. Hematologic causes of secondary osteoporosis. **A,** Posteroanterior hand radiograph in a child with hemolytic anemia (thalassemia major) showing expansion of the diaphyses of bones, thinned bone cortices, and a coarse and prominent trabecular pattern, all resulting from marrow hyperplasia. **B,** Multiple myeloma can be associated with generalized osteoporosis but may also cause focal osteolytic areas, generally in the skull vault but also in other bones as evident in this hand radiograph showing a multiloculated lytic area in the base of the third metacarpal and a focal single lytic area in the shaft of the fourth metacarpal.

BOX 31-3. Causes of Regional Osteopenia

- Disuse (e.g., stroke, poliomyelitis, cerebral palsy, spinal cord injury)
- Reflex sympathetic dystrophy (Sudeck's atrophy)
- Regional migratory osteoporosis
- Periarticular osteoporosis (e.g., inflammatory arthritis)

with no history of injury; the pain may progress and be sufficiently severe to cause a limp and to restrict movement in the joint affected. An effusion may be present due to a mild and chronic synovitis. Joint aspirations, which are often performed to exclude infection as a cause of the symptoms and signs, are sterile. Recovery usually occurs spontaneously in 6 to 12 months without late sequelae. Symptoms may develop rapidly and then resolve, only to recur again in some other joint. The joint adjacent to the diseased one is usually the next to be affected, but there may be two or more joints symptomatic at the same time.

Periarticular osteoporosis occurs in inflammatory (e.g., rheumatoid arthritis) or some infective arthropathies (Figure 31-7). The reduction in bone density is related to hyperemia and cytokines that stimulate osteoclastic bone resorption.

IMAGING FEATURES

General osteoporosis is characterized by less bone being present than normal, and this will be evident on radiographs as decreased radiodensity of bone and cortical thinning[15,29,30,41,42] (Figures 31-3 and 31-4). A useful descriptive term to use if fractures are not present is *osteopenia.* The radiologic appearances of osteoporosis are essentially the same, irrespective of the cause. Despite the introduction of newer imaging methods (computed tomography [CT], magnetic resonance imaging [MRI]), osteoporosis is still most commonly initially diagnosed on radiographs. However, radiography is relatively insensitive in detecting early bone loss (less than 30% to 40% loss of bone tissue). Bone density on radiographs will be affected by patient size and the radiographic factors used, and visual judgment of bone density on a radiograph is subjective, hence the importance of quantitative, bone densitometry techniques (DXA) for the definitive diagnosis of osteoporosis and identification of those at risk of fracture.

Cortical thinning occurs as a result of endosteal, periosteal, or intracortical (cortical tunneling) bone resorption or a combination of all these. Endosteal resorption is the least specific radiographic finding as it may be evident in many metabolic disorders, including osteoporosis. Intracortical tunneling is slightly more specific, occurring mainly in disorders with rapid bone turnover such as disuse osteoporosis and reflex sympathetic dystrophy (RSD). Subperiosteal resorption is the most specific finding, being diagnostic of hyperparathyroidism.[1,43]

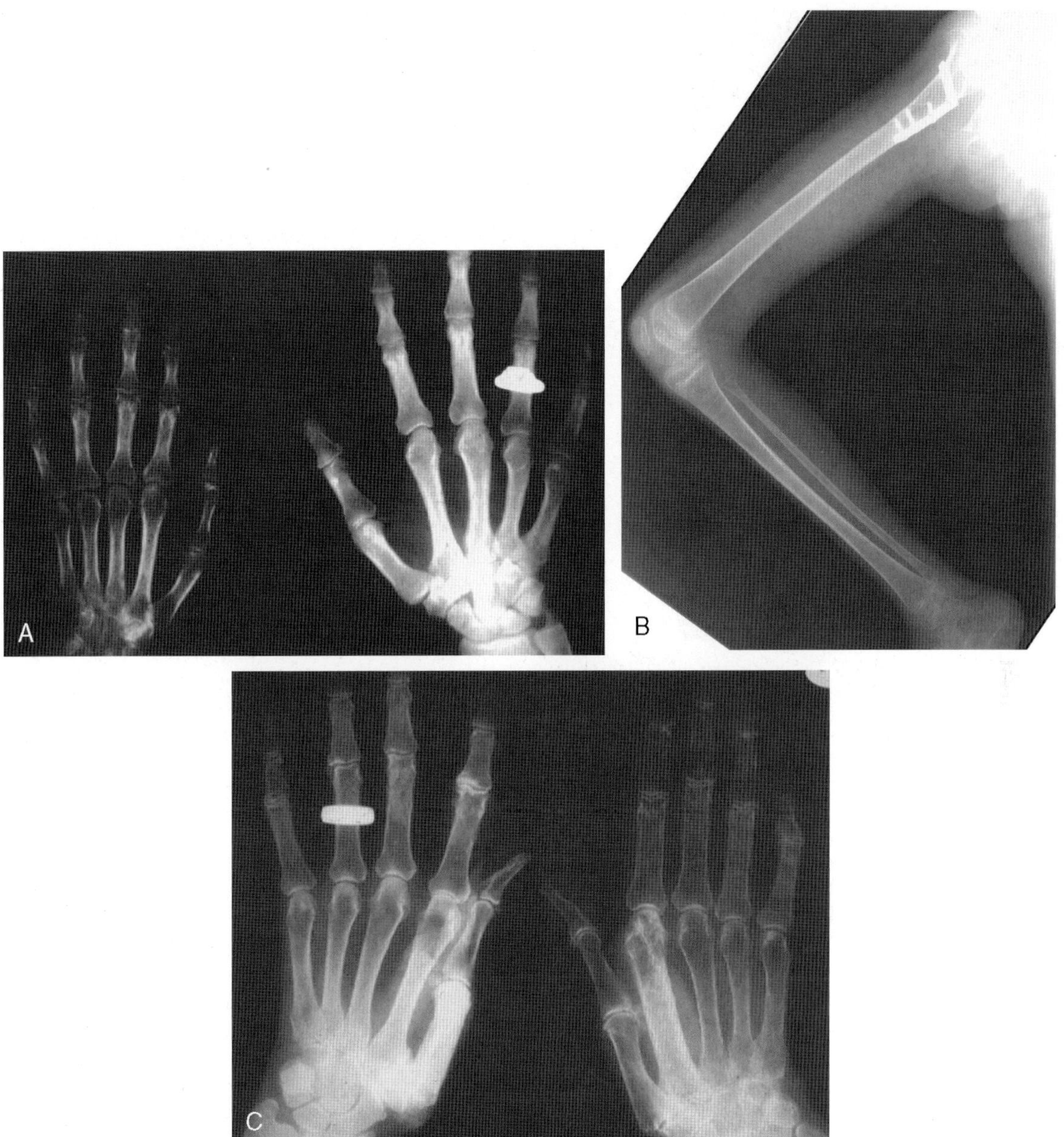

FIGURE 31-6. Focal osteoporosis. Disuse osteoporosis occurs through inactivity and failure to load the skeleton normally. The growth and development of the skeleton, and maintenance of bone health throughout life, depends on normal activity and loading of the skeleton. **A,** Hand radiographs in a patient who had poliomyelitis involving the left arm during childhood. The involved hand is small in size with osteopenic bones. **B,** This child with cerebral palsy has a severely osteopenic and slender tibia and femur. A metal pin and plate fix a previous fracture of the proximal femur. Fractures may be caused in such children simply by handling or physiotherapy. **C,** This elderly patient suffered a right-side stroke, and as a result the bones in the right hand are osteopenic through disuse. There is also Paget's disease involving the right second and left first metacarpals (causing the affected bones to be enlarged with disorganized trabecular pattern and mixed bone sclerosis and osteopenia).

> Subperiosteal bone resorption is a specific feature of hyperparathyroidism.

The radiographic features of generalized osteoporosis predominate in the axial (central) skeleton and proximal long bones, which are rich in trabecular bone. There is resorption and thinning of trabeculae, some of which may be lost completely (see Figures 31-3 and 31-4). The process initially affects secondary trabeculae, and the primary trabeculae may appear more prominent as they are affected at a later stage.

> In generalized osteoporosis, areas of trabecular bone (most prominent in the vertebrae and proximal long bones) are affected earliest.

In the proximal femur, the principal compressive and tensile trabeculae are accentuated, with loss of trabeculae in the area (Ward's) between them, which appears more radiolucent. In some sites, the presence of multiple microfractures and callus formation can cause osteosclerosis on radiographs, which must be distinguished from other more sinister malignant causes

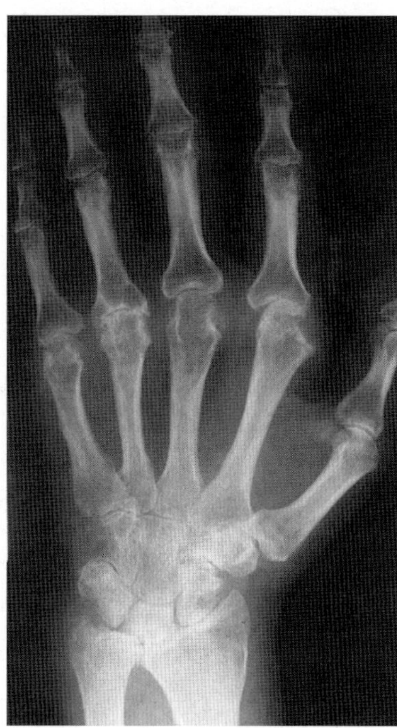

FIGURE 31-7. Periarticular osteoporosis caused by inflammatory arthritis. Posteroanterior hand radiograph in a patient with rheumatoid arthritis. Periarticular osteoporosis occurs in inflammatory arthropathies such as rheumatoid arthritis (RA) and results in juxta-articular focal osteopenia, as is evident in this hand radiograph at the metacarpal/phalangeal and proximal interphalangeal joints. There are erosions in the heads of the metacarpal bones and loss of joint spaces, particularly in the carpus, typical of RA. The reduction in bone density is related to hyperemia and cytokines, which stimulate osteoclastic bone resorption and may be the earliest radiographic feature of RA, preceding evidence of erosions.

(e.g., metastases). Such insufficiency microfractures occur in particular anatomic sites, including the symphysis pubis, the sacrum, pubic rami, and calcaneus[44,45] (Figure 31-8). Other sites involved are the sternum, supra-acetabular area, and elsewhere in the pelvis, femoral neck, and proximal and distal tibia.[39,40] Some of these fractures may be accompanied by considerable osteolysis, particularly those involving the symphysis pubis and pubic rami and may be erroneously diagnosed on radiographs as due to malignant tumor.[40] Other imaging techniques (radionuclide scanning [RNS], CT, and MRI) may help to differentiate insufficiency fractures from other conditions (Figure 31-8). On radionuclide scans there is increased uptake in regions of acute insufficiency fractures; in the sacrum this often gives a characteristic H pattern ("Honda" sign) of radionuclide uptake[46] (Figure 31-8). CT is particularly helpful in defining the fracture lines of insufficiency fractures involving the sacrum (fractures are usually parallel to the sacroiliac joints) and the calcaneus (Figure 31-8). In these sites, fractures may not be identified on radiographs because of the complex anatomy and superimposition of other anatomic structures. MRI is particularly sensitive in identifying insufficiency fractures in the femoral neck before they are evident radiographically, as is RNS.[45,46]

Insufficiency fractures occur in abnormal bone subjected to normal stress.

Insufficiency fractures occur most often in the symphysis pubis, sacrum, pubic rami, and calcaneus. MRI (best over all), bone scan, and CT are helpful in detection and differentiation from other lesions.

Spine

Vertebral fractures are the most common osteoporotic fracture. Early radiographic features of spinal osteoporosis, perhaps related to biomechanical forces through the spine, initially involve the loss of the horizontally oriented secondary trabeculae, and the

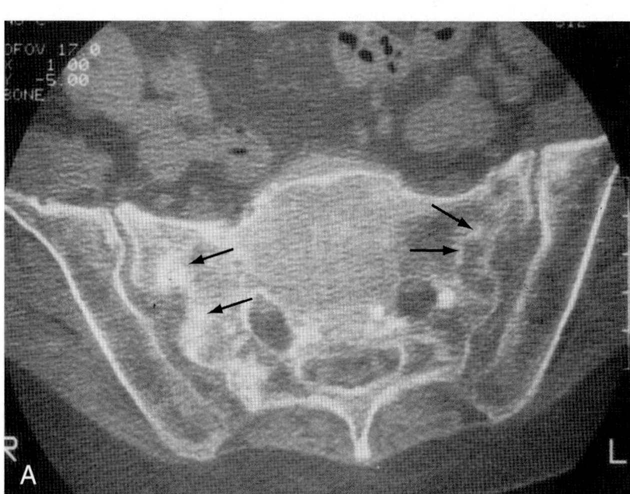

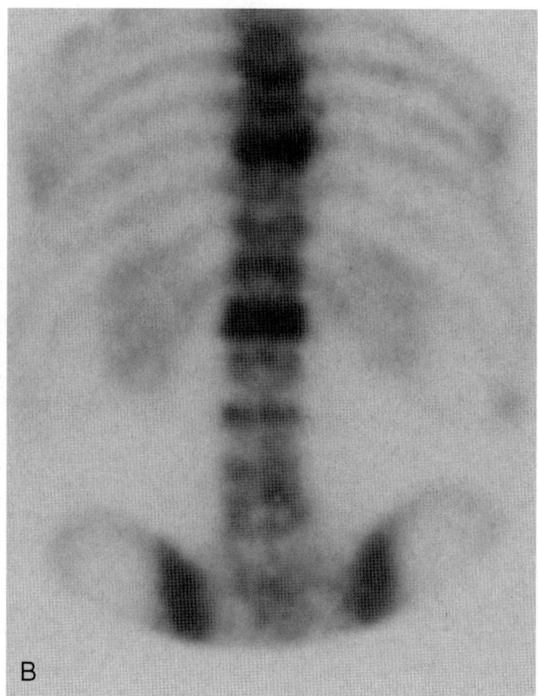

FIGURE 31-8. Insufficiency fractures. In some sites, the presence of multiple microfractures and callus formation can cause osteosclerosis. In other sites, the fractures may not be evident on radiographs. Other imaging techniques may be more sensitive to identification of such fractures. **A,** CT scan demonstrates fractures of the sacral ala *(arrows)*. **B,** Radionuclide bone scan shows increased isotope uptake in insufficiency fractures in both sacral ala and in multiple vertebral fractures (T7, T9, L1, and L3).

vertical trabeculae actually become more prominent and thickened (Figure 31-9), resulting in a vertical "striated" appearance to the vertebral body on lateral spinal radiographs.[1,29,30] This feature is generally seen in several, or all, of the vertebrae when it is related to osteoporosis, in contrast to a similar appearance in a single vertebral body when caused by hemangioma.

Vertebral fractures: the anterior and central mid-portion of the vertebrae withstand compression forces less well than the posterior and outer ring elements of the vertebrae, resulting in wedge or end-plate fractures or, less commonly, crush fractures[47,48] (Figure 31-10). Vertebral fractures have been used as important outcome measures in therapeutic trials in osteoporosis assessing

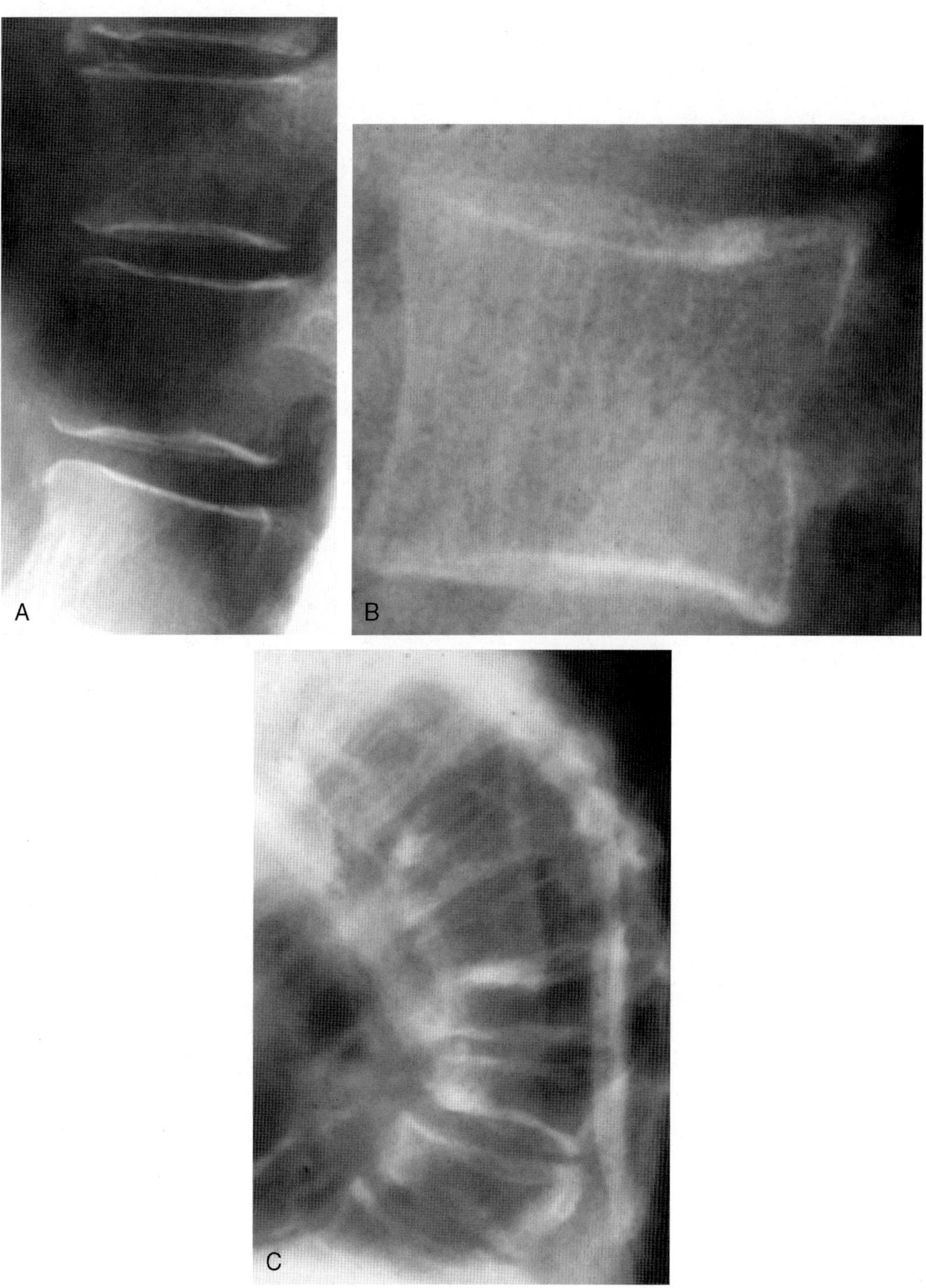

FIGURE 31-9. Spinal osteoporosis. **A,** Normal lateral spinal radiograph. The vertebrae are normal in shape and density. **B,** Osteoporosis. Because of loss of transverse trabeculae, there is increased prominence of vertical trabeculae giving a striated appearance, which is an early radiographic feature of spinal osteoporosis and may be present before vertebral fractures occur. **C,** Osteoporosis with compression fractures. Multiple vertebral fractures are present in the thoracic spine resulting in kyphosis ("dowager" hump). Clinically, there will be a loss in height in affected patients.

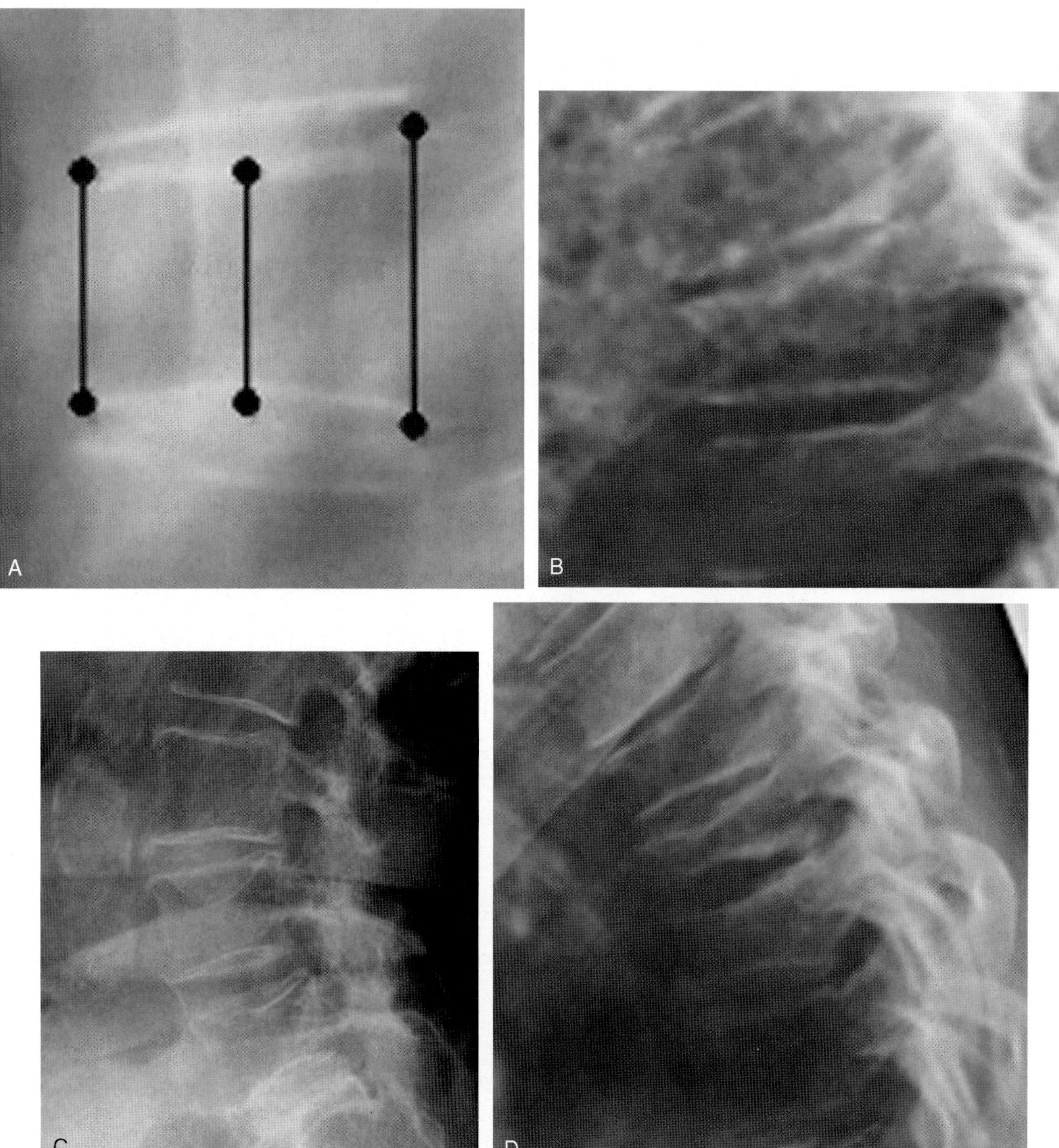

FIGURE 31-10. Types of vertebral fractures and quantitative/semiquantitative assessment: **A,** The six-point vertebral assessment: Points are placed at the anterior, middle, and posterior edges of the vertebral endplates to measure the anterior, mid, and posterior heights of vertebrae, and to quantify change in vertebral body shape. This method has been used in trials assessing the efficacy of osteoporotic therapy. **B,** Vertebral fractures can be described by their shape, as in wedge fracture and endplate fracture. **C,** Note the texture changes below and adjacent to the upper endplates of L4 and L5, indicating fractures of the central portions of the endplates, which are weaker than the outer ring. **D,** Crush fracture. Such fractures can be graded as mild (grade 1, less than 25% deformity), moderate (grade 2, 25% to 40% deformity), and severe (grade 3, greater than 40% deformity), which constitutes the semiquantitative method of vertebral fracture assessment, which is most widely used in pharmaceutical efficacy studies.[52]

drug efficacy. This has demanded reproducible quantitative methods of vertebral fracture assessment (six-point vertebral morphometry), usually from the levels of T4 to L4.[47-51] Such methods require six points to be placed around each vertebral body on the endplates (superior and inferior points of anterior margin, middle endplate, and posterior margin of the vertebra), and several different methods have been devised[47-51] (Figure 31-10). All these methods are time consuming, and although used in pharmaceutical trials, they are not practical in a clinical setting and may not be very reproducible, particularly when only minor deformity is present. Vertebral fractures can be graded as mild (grade 1, less than 25% deformity), moderate (grade 2, 25% to 40% deformity), and severe (grade 3, greater than 40% deformity)[52] (see Figure 31-10). This semiquantitative grading method is most frequently applied at present to define the prevalence and incidence of vertebral fractures in epidemiology studies and pharmaceutical trials of the efficacy of new osteoporosis therapies. The more severe the grade of vertebral fracture, the greater the risk of future fracture. Vertebral fractures are powerful predictors of future fracture (hip X2, vertebral X5),[53,54] a patient with the combination of vertebral fracture and low bone density has a 25-fold increased risk for subsequent vertebral fracture than does a patient with no fracture and high bone density.[55] It is therefore extremely important that, if present, vertebral fractures are accurately and clearly reported by radiologists as fractures, and other terms, such as *deformities,* be avoided. There is evidence that vertebral fractures are under-reported by radiologists, with the result that patients who should be receiving treatment to reduce their risk of future fractures are not being identified.[56,57] Consequently, there has been a joint initiative between the International Osteoporosis Foundation (IOF) and the European Society of Musculoskeletal Radiology (ESSR Osteoporosis Group) to improve the sensitivity and accuracy of reporting of vertebral fractures by radiologists. (An interactive teaching CD is available, or can be downloaded from www.iofbonehealth.org.)

Vertebral fractures are strong predictors of future fracture and should be reported when they are identified even as incidental findings on radiographs.

Vertebral fracture may occur as an acute event related to minor trauma and be accompanied by pain, which generally resolves spontaneously over 6 to 8 weeks. This resolution of symptoms serves to distinguish osteoporotic vertebral fractures from similar events due to more sinister causes, such as metastases, in which the symptoms are more protracted. The clinical symptoms of vertebral fractures include back pain, loss of height, deformity, disability, and limited spinal mobility and are associated with increased mortality. However, between 30% and 50% of vertebral fractures can be present in asymptomatic patients. Osteoporotic fractures occur most commonly in the thoracic and thoracolumbar regions and result in progressive loss of height in affected individuals. Height loss of more than 5 cm is an indication to perform bone mineral density and spinal radiographs to confirm the diagnosis of osteoporosis and identify asymptomatic vertebral fractures. Osteoporotic fractures are uncommon above T7; if fractures are present in this anatomic region, metastases should be considered (Figure 31-11). Wedging of multiple vertebral bodies in the thoracic spine can lead to increased kyphosis ("dowager" hump) (see Figure 31-9), which, if severe, may result in the ribs abutting on the iliac crests and compromise of respiratory function.

Up to 50% of vertebral fractures can be present in asymptomatic patients. Height loss of more than 5 cm is an indication to perform bone mineral density testing and spinal radiographs.

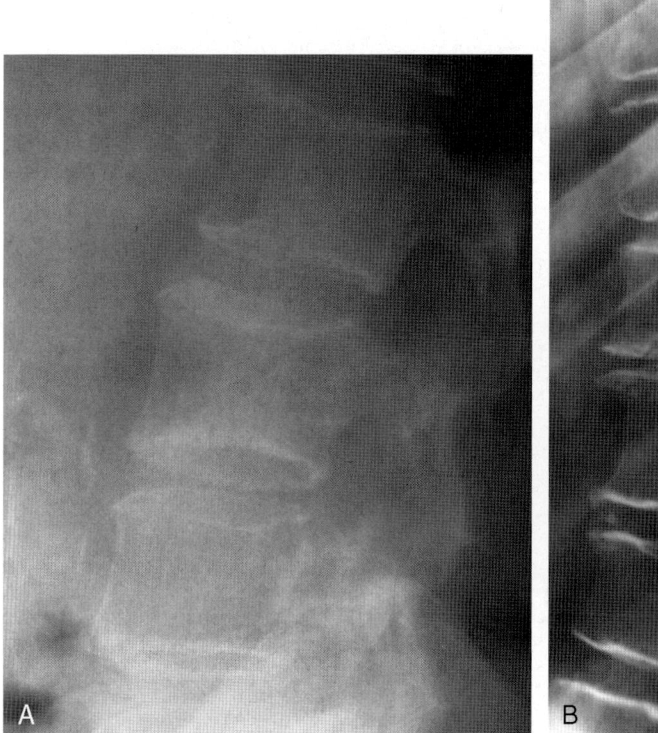

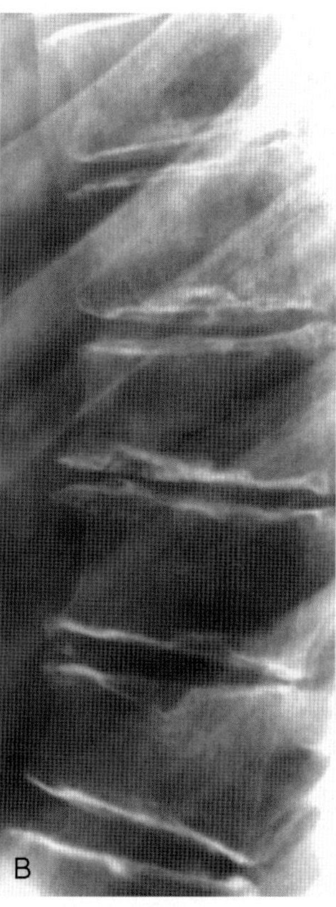

FIGURE 31-11. Differential diagnoses of vertebral fractures **A,** Poor positioning. Good radiographic technique is required when imaging the spine, particularly in the lateral projection. The spine must be parallel to the radiographic table to prevent the vertebrae from appearing to have a biconcave endplate (an artifact due to tilting of the vertebrae, or the divergence of the x-ray beam ("beam can" effect). **B,** Scheuermann's disease causes endplate irregularity, most commonly in the thoracic spine, and involves several adjacent vertebrae.

(Continued)

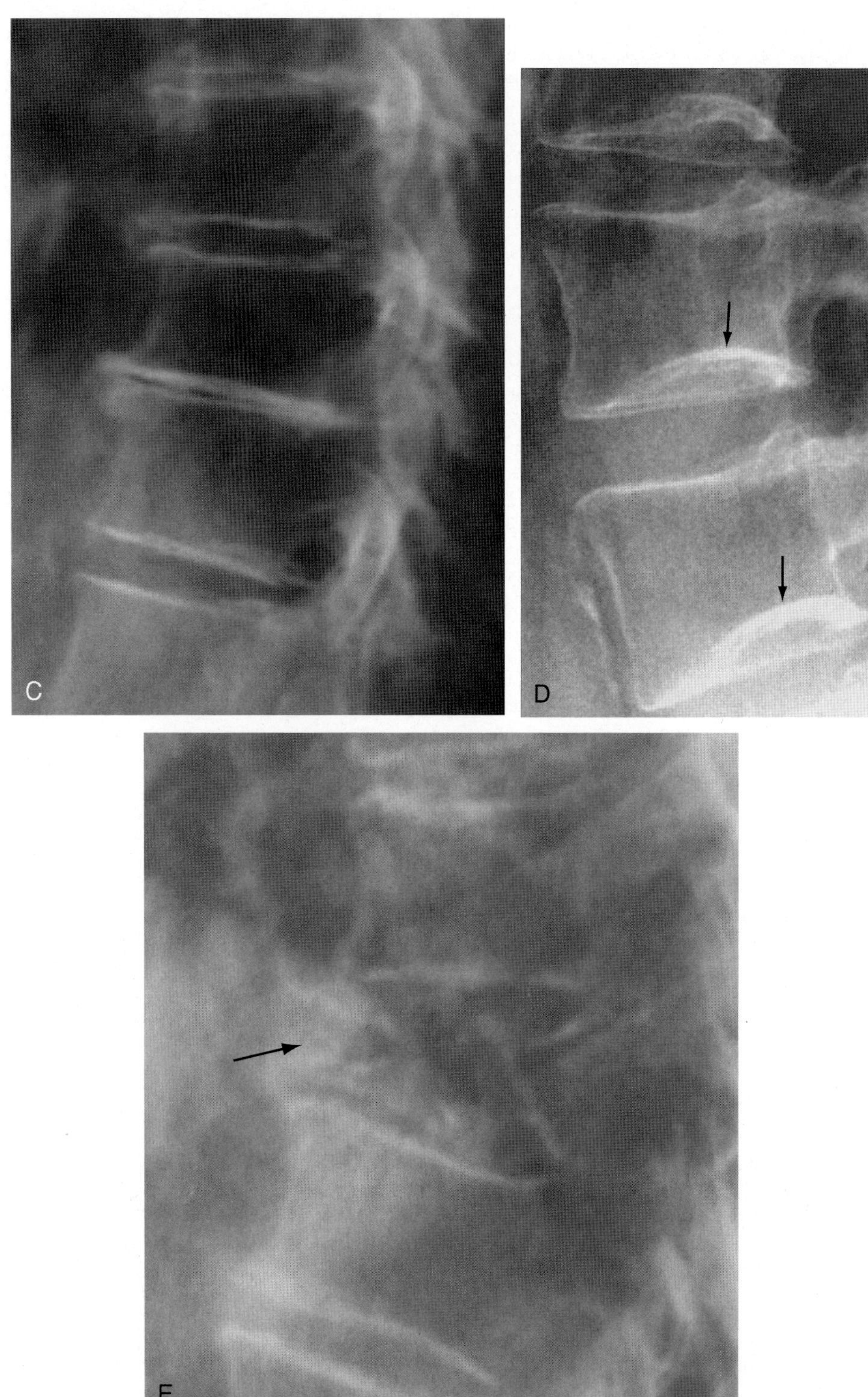

FIGURE 31-11—cont'd. **C,** With spondylosis there may be remodeling of the vertebrae, which appear to have slight anterior wedging and are elongated in their anteroposterior diameter. **D,** Normal variants, such as a "cupid's bow" as illustrated here *(arrows)*, may cause deformities of the vertebra and have to be differentiated from osteoporotic vertebral fracture. The well-defined margins to the endplate, and absence of the texture changes found in endplate fractures enable these normal variations to be recognized. **E,** Vertebral metastasis. Destruction of the vertebral endplate is indicative of a more sinister etiology, such as metastatic disease. Myeloma may give a similar appearance. MRI is helpful in differentiating osteoporotic fractures from tumor if radiographic features are nondiagnostic.

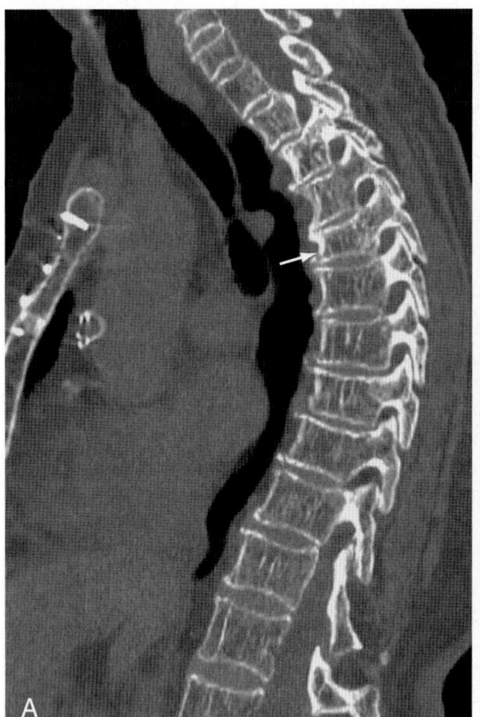

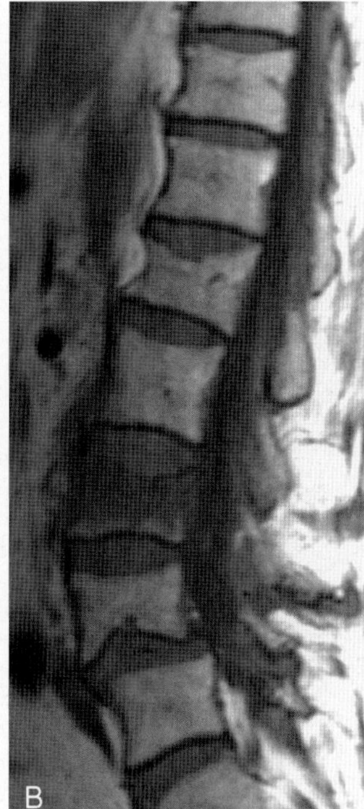

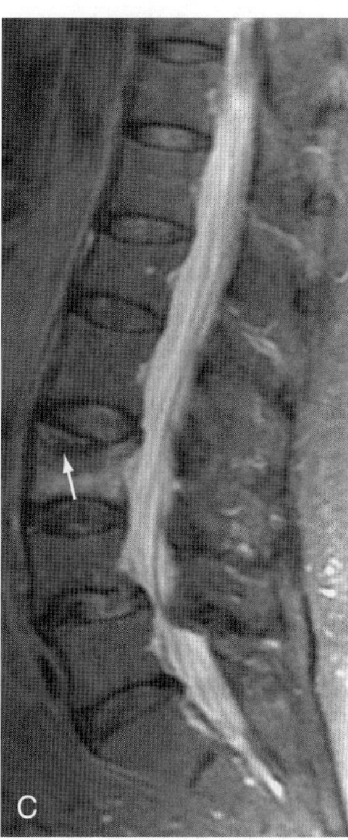

FIGURE 31-12. Alternative imaging methods for vertebral fracture identification and differential diagnosis **A,** CT scanning: A reformatted midline sagittal image from a 3D CT is superior to axial images for identifying vertebral deformity and fractures, as is seen in one of the mid-thoracic vertebral bodies *(arrow)*. Asymptomatic vertebral fractures may be diagnosed fortuitously with this technique. The prominent vertical striations of all vertebrae are indicative of osteoporosis. MRI is helpful in differentiating old vertebral fractures from acute fractures. The fracture deformities of L1 and L4 are not acute, as evidenced by retention of the normal marrow fat signal on both T1-weighted **(B)** and T2-weighted **(C)** images. The acute fracture of L3 has low signal on the T1-weighted image **(B)** and high signal on the T2-weighted image due to replacement of marrow fat signal by edema signal. A low signal fracture line *(arrow)* is visible. (Images courtesy of Thomas Link, MD, University of California, San Francisco.)

Although vertebral fractures are generally associated with change in shape of the vertebrae, this is not always so, and it is important to observe associated subtle density changes adjacent and inferior to the vertebral endplate, which indicate fracture of just the middle portion of the endplate[47,48,51] (see Figure 31-10). However, not all vertebrae that are changed in shape (deformed) are vertebral fractures. Good radiographic techniques are required when imaging the spine, particularly in the lateral projection. The spine must be parallel to the radiographic table to prevent the vertebrae appearing to have a biconcave endplate, which is caused by an artifact of tilting the vertebrae or the divergence of the x-ray beam ("beam can" effect)[58] (see Figure 31-11). Other pathologic conditions (trauma, myeloma, metastases, Scheuermann's disease, Schmorl's nodes, infection, degenerative disease, and congenital anomalies) and normal variants (cupid's bow, short vertebral height) may cause deformities of the vertebra and have to be differentiated from osteoporotic vertebral fracture[48,51] (see Figure 31-11). An algorithm-based approach for the qualitative identification of vertebral fractures (ABQ method) has been proposed to differentiate vertebral fractures from other etiologies of vertebral deformities.[47] Scheuermann's disease causes endplate irregularity, most commonly in the thoracic spine, and it involves several adjacent vertebrae (see Figure 31-11). With spondylosis, there may be change in modeling of the vertebrae, which appear to have slight anterior wedging and are elongated in their anteroposterior diameter (see Figure 31-11). Other imaging methods such as CT (particularly the mid-sagittal reformation from 3D volume imaging now feasible on multidetector spiral CT scanners) (Figure 31-12), MRI (see Figure 31-12), and RNS (see Figure 31-8) can be helpful in this differentiation.[51] MRI is particularly useful in differentiating acute from chronic vertebral fractures, as in the former there is marrow edema. A fracture line that fills with fluid (and demonstrates high signal on T2-weighted images) is useful in differentiating an osteoporotic vertebral fracture from other infiltrating causes of vertebral fracture, such as myeloma and metastases.[59,60]

> MRI may be helpful in distinguishing vertebral fractures due to osteoporosis from those associated with underlying tumor.

Although radiographs are the most widely used method of identifying vertebral fractures, the introduction of fan-beam technology in DXA has enabled good-quality (dual- and single-energy modes) images (posteroanterior and lateral projections) of the thoracic and lumbar spine to be obtained (Figure 31-13). From these instant vertebral assessment (IVA) and morphometric measurements can be made (MXA).[61,62] The advantage of MXA over conventional spinal radiography is a lower radiation dose (1/100th of conventional spine radiographs; 12μSv posteroanterior and lateral single-energy image; 42μSv for dual-energy image [personal communication, Glen Blake, MD, London]), less endplate distortion because the x-ray beam is parallel to the endplate at each vertebral level, and the entire spine is visualized on a single image (see Figure 31-13). It may be feasible in the future for computer vision techniques to be applied to both DXA and radiographic images to automate vertebral fracture identification.[63-65]

Vertebroplasty has selected application in patients with osteoporotic vertebral fracture that are persistently painful (see Chapter 40). Although performed by several medical specialists, radiologists are probably the most appropriate group to perform this image-guided interventional technique, particularly as imaging

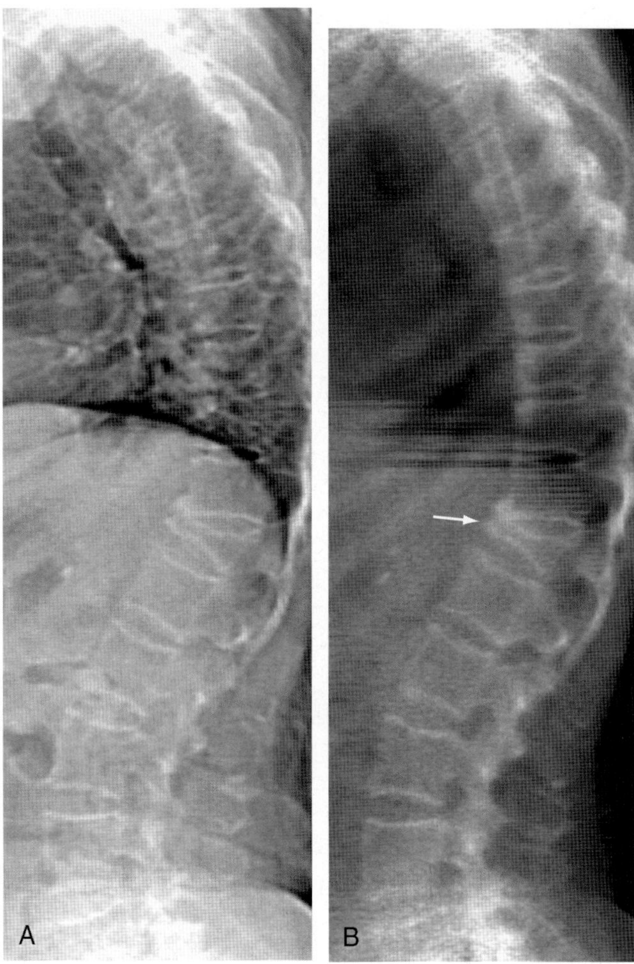

FIGURE 31-13. Spinal imaging using DXA. The introduction of fan beam DXA has enabled good-quality single-energy **(A)** and dual-energy **(B)** lateral images to be obtained of the thoracic and lumbar spine at a considerably lower radiation dose than conventional spinal radiography. There is a grade-3 (severe) crush fracture of T12 *(arrow)* present. The endplates of the thoracic vertebrae are more clearly visualized on the dual-energy images. The resolution of the DXA images is not as good as radiography provides, however.

(radiographs, RNS, CT, and MRI) plays a role in selecting patients appropriate for the procedure.[66] All patients treated by vertebroplasty or kyphoplasty for osteoporotic compression fractures should be under the care of a clinician with special interest in osteoporosis management and on appropriate medical therapy to reduce future fracture risk.

Hands

The hands are often radiographed in metabolic bone disorders; in osteoporosis, the trabecular pattern at the ends of the bones will be reduced in number, and those that remain appear more prominent. Normally, cortical bone appears as a solid white line on a radiograph with a smooth inner (endosteal) and outer (periosteal) surface. In osteoporosis, cortical bone is thinned by endosteal resorption, which causes it to become scalloped and irregular in outline. Within the cortical bone, Haversian systems and Volkmann's canals enlarge and become visible as longitudinal radiolucent striations within the cortex. Before the introduction of modern quantitative bone densitometry techniques such as DXA, measurement of the thickness of the cortex of the second metacarpal of the nondominant hand on a radiograph played an important role in the assessment of skeletal development in children and of osteoporosis in adults.[67,68] However, the reproducibility was limited (coefficient of variation [CV] up to 11%) because the endosteal surface becomes irregular and more difficult to identify with bone resorption. Consequently, longitudinal studies had to extend over a decade or more to assess change with time. Now modern computer vision methods (active shape models [ASMs]) have been applied to automate the measurements made and improve precision to better than a CV of 0.6% (digital x-ray radiogrammetry [DXR]).[69-71] This technique shows potential to provide a simple, inexpensive, and low-radiation method for measuring peripheral bone densitometry and morphometry in children and adults[72,73] and to predict fracture risk in adults.[74]

Thinning of the cortices of the mid-portion of the second metacarpal of the nondominant hand indicates osteoporosis. However, because osteoporosis involves trabecular bone first, this is a late finding.

Other Skeletal Sites

Elsewhere in the skeleton similar changes occur, with reduction in trabecular number and cortical width. The trabecular pattern in the femoral neck has been quantified as an index of osteoporosis (Singh index)[75] to which computer vision techniques can also be applied.[76,77] Fractures that occur in osteoporosis generally heal well with satisfactory callus formation. In some sites, the presence of multiple microfractures and callus formation can cause osteosclerosis on a radiograph, which must be distinguished from other more sinister malignant conditions. Such insufficiency fractures occur in particular anatomic sites, including the symphysis pubis, sacrum, pubic rami, and calcaneus. Other sites involved are the sternum, supra-acetabular area, and elsewhere in the pelvis, femoral neck, and proximal and distal tibia.[38,39,78-80] Some of these fractures may be accompanied by considerable osteolysis, particularly those involving the symphysis pubis, and may be erroneously diagnosed on radiographs as due to malignant tumor.[40] Other imaging techniques (radionuclide, CT, and MRI) may help to differentiate insufficiency fractures from other pathologic entities. On radionuclide scans, there is increased uptake in regions of acute insufficiency fractures. When the sacrum is involved, this often gives a characteristic "H" pattern (Honda sign) of radionuclide uptake[46] (see Figure 31-8). CT is particularly helpful in defining the fracture lines of insufficiency fractures involving the sacrum (fractures usually parallel to the sacroiliac joint) (see Figure 31-8) and in the calcaneus. In these sites, fractures may not be identified on radiographs because of complex anatomy and overlying structures. MRI is particularly sensitive for identifying insufficiency fractures in the femoral neck before they are evident radiographically, as is RNS.[81]

REGIONAL OSTEOPOROSIS

Chronic disuse is characterized by a uniform pattern of bone loss; acute immobilization causes more focal and irregular bone formation and resorption. This results in different patterns of bone loss that include diffuse osteopenia, linear translucent bands, speckled radiolucent areas, and cortical bone resorption.[30]

Reflex Sympathetic Dystrophy Syndrome (Sudeck's Atrophy)

RNS is useful in the diagnosis of this condition, especially if no radiographic abnormality is present, and is reported to have a sensitivity and specificity of over 80%.[30] The predominant feature is

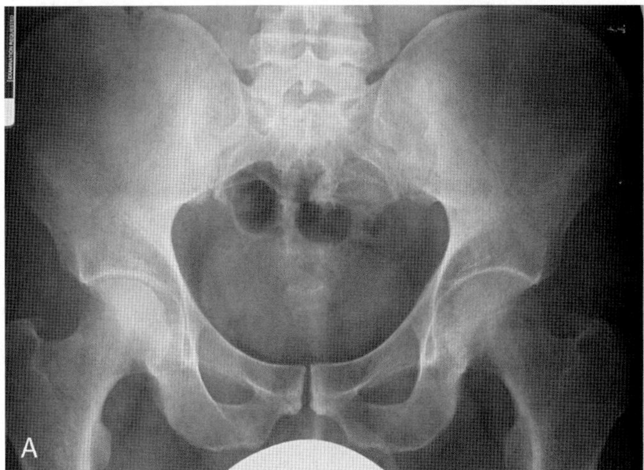

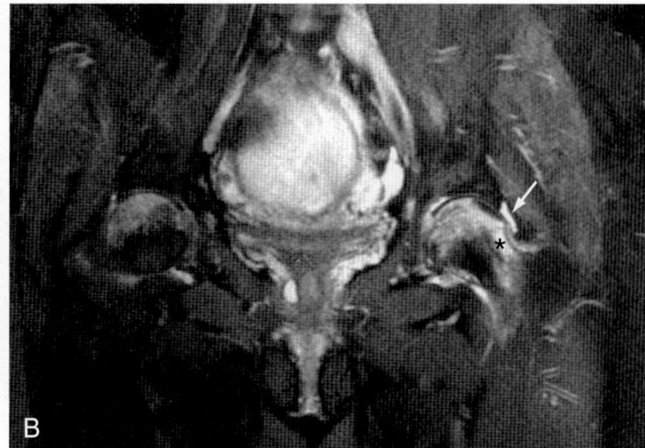

FIGURE 31-14. Regional osteoporosis of the left hip. **A,** Pelvic radiograph of a patient with regional osteoporosis shows osteopenia of the left hip. Radiographs, however, may show no abnormality in this condition. **B,** MRI (fat-suppressed or STIR sequences) are more sensitive in showing the high-signal marrow edema *(asterisk)* in the proximal portion of the left femur, with a small effusion *(arrow)* in the left hip joint. (Images courtesy of Richard Whitehouse, MD, Manchester Royal Infirmary.)

intense and diffuse isotope uptake in the affected bones in the blood flow, blood pool, and static images. MRI may be normal or may show nonspecific soft tissue edema, soft tissue atrophy, or marrow edema. (See Chapters 32.)

Regional osteoporosis is most common in the hip, and on radiographs there is reduction in density of the proximal femur (Figure 31-14). There may be an underlying abnormality of perfusion of the marrow, which is edematous. RNS shows nonspecific increased uptake of isotope in the affected hip. MRI is sensitive in demonstrating the edematous marrow before any radiographic abnormality is present[37,38] (Figure 31-14). The edema-like marrow signal is characterized by decreased signal on T1-weighted images and increased signal on T2-weighted images involving the femoral head and intracapsular portion of the femoral neck. The use of chemical-shift, fat-suppression, and STIR imaging is effective in accentuating the signal changes and improves the detection of marrow edema.[30] A joint effusion may accompany these changes. Focal bone loss and marrow edema can also occur with tumor, arthritis, or infection, which must be excluded before the diagnosis of transient osteoporosis of the hip can be made.

Periarticular osteoporosis is probably the most common form of regional osteoporosis encountered in clinical practice and is related to hyperemia of the inflamed joint and the presence of local cytokines that stimulate osteoclastic bone resorption. Periarticular osteoporosis is a characteristic early feature of rheumatoid arthritis (see Figure 31-7), but a generalized reduction in bone mass can also occur, which involves both compact and trabecular bone and is present in affected adults and children.[82-85] The bone loss might be greater in the hand than other skeletal sites.[86,87] There is generally increased bone resorption, with normal or reduced bone formation. The causes of these changes are complex. Immobilization and glucocorticoid therapy contribute to the osteoporosis.

DIAGNOSIS OF OSTEOPOROSIS USING QUANTITATIVE METHODS

If fractures and specific radiographic features (thinned cortex, reduced trabeculae) are not present, then judging bone density from radiographs is not a precise science. Radiographic osteopenia, however, is a strong predictor of osteoporosis and an indication for DXA bone densitometry.[88]

> Radiographs are insensitive tests for osteoporosis generally, but if osteopenia (decreased radiographic bone density) is seen, DXA testing is indicated.

Currently osteoporosis is defined in terms of axial DXA as a T score (standard deviation [SD] from peak bone mass [PBM]) of −2.5 and less on the recommendation of the World Health Organization (WHO)[89] (see Chapter 6). This definition is not applicable to children who have not yet reached PBM, and a Z score (SD from mean of age-matched BMD) must be used. The size dependency of DXA is a problem in growing children in whom some size corrections have to be applied to results.[90-93] Quantitative computed tomography (QCT) has some advantages over DXA but currently remains largely a research tool with few data on its ability to predict fracture. QCT[1,94] (Figure 31-15) uniquely allows for the separate estimation of trabecular and cortical BMD and provides a true volumetric density in grams per liter (milligrams per cubic centimeter), rather than the "areal" (grams per square centimeter) of DXA. QCT is therefore not size dependent and of particular relevance in children and in diseases that result in small stature (Turner's syndrome, growth hormone deficiency). The 2D QCT technique is generally applied to the lumbar spine. For 2D QCT, a lateral projection radiograph is obtained on the CT scanner and a scanning plane is selected (10-mm slice) through the middle of each vertebral body, generally L1-L3, parallel to the vertebral endplates; thinner (5-mm) sections may be required to avoid including the vertebral endplate in the section scanned (which would cause overestimation of BMD). A low-dose scanning technique (80 kV, 70 mA, 2 seconds) can be used to reduce patient radiation dose.[95] The entry of the basivertebral vein on the transverse axial section confirms the section to be in the midplane of the vertebral body. An oval region of interest to include as much of the vertebral trabecular bone as possible, without including the cortical rim or basivertebral vein, is selected for analysis. QCT is performed with a calibration reference phantom to transform Hounsfield units into bone-mineral equivalent units. These phantoms were initially fluid (K_2HPO_4) but are now made of solid hydroxyapatite material. The results from various types of calibration phantoms are not interchangeable, unless a cross-calibration calculation can be made. In longitudinal studies, it is preferable that the same reference phantom be used.

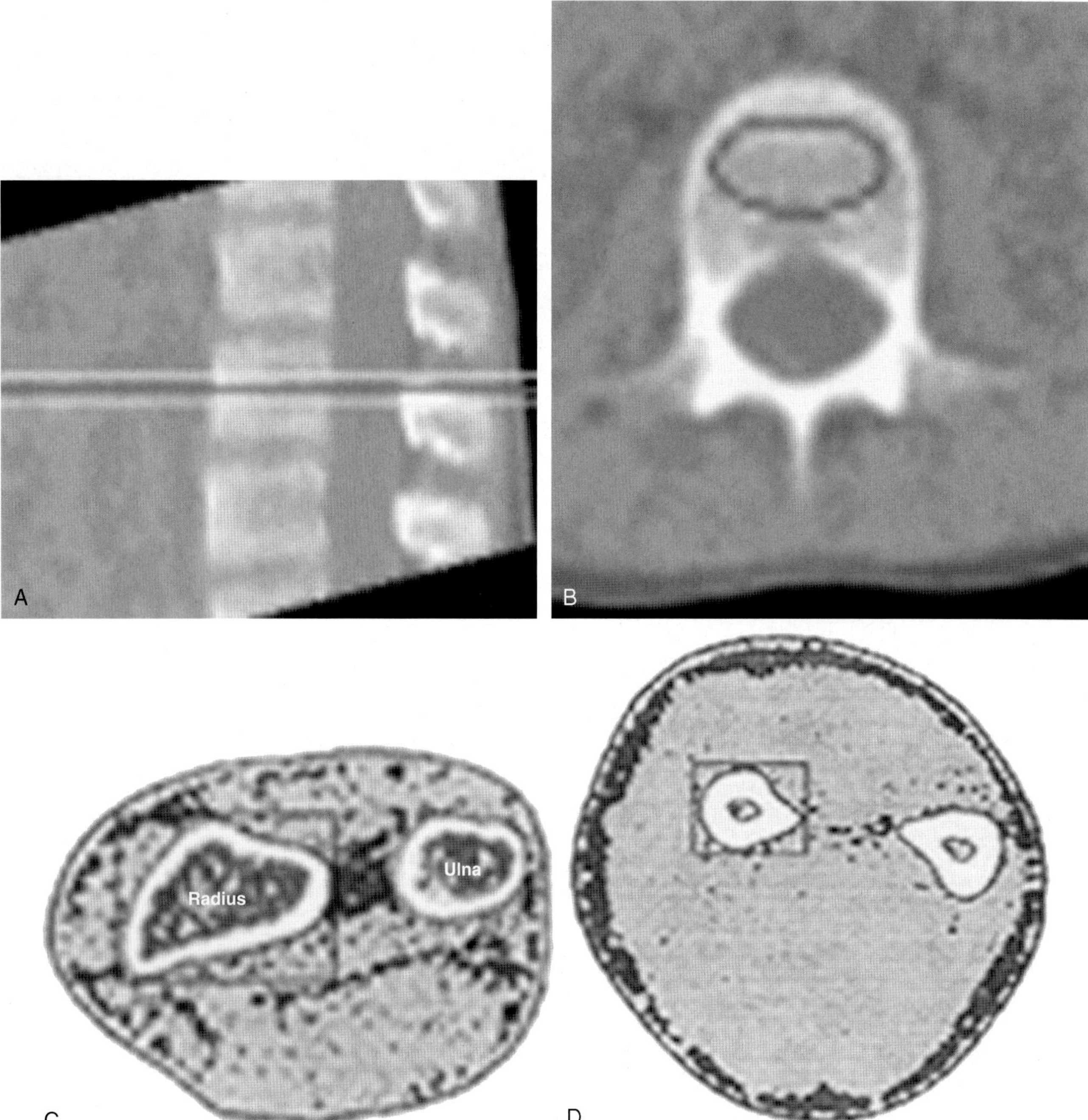

FIGURE 31-15. Quantitative computed tomography (QCT). DXA is the current method of choice for confirming osteoporosis in terms of bone densitometry (WHO T score below −2.5). However, QCT has some advantages over DXA, particularly in research studies, in that it provides a true volumetric density (milligrams per cubic centimeter) rather than an "areal" density (grams per square centimeter), so is not size dependent. **A,** A lumbar spine 3D volume image of L1-L3 shows a level (parallel lines) selected for densitometry evaluation. **B,** QCT also uniquely measures cortical and trabecular bone density separately. This transverse axial section shows the oval region of interest for measuring trabecular bone mineral density in a vertebral body. Peripheral CT scan **(C)** through the distal radius at the "4% distal site" and **D,** CT scan of the mid-shaft of the forearm. Note the thicker cortex of the mid-shaft in comparison to the distal forearm, which has greater amounts of trabecular bone. Scans in the diaphysis of long bones provide measurements of cross-sectional muscle and bone area, from which certain biomechanical parameters (stress-strain index and moment of inertia) can also be extracted to investigate interactions in the "muscle/bone" unit.

Original CT scanners used rotate-translate technology, which permitted only single 2D sections. The recent technical developments in CT of continuous rotation of the x-ray tube and multiple rows of detectors enable rapid 3D-volume scanning (see Figure 31-15). As a consequence, precision has improved (better than CV = 1%), and the method is applicable to measure bone size and density in the hip. The WHO definition of osteoporosis (T score less than −2.5) is *not* applicable to QCT; a Z score of −2.0 and lower is abnormal. Some use the definition of a QCT of 100 mg/cm^3 or below as "osteopenia," and 80 mg/cm^3 or below as "osteoporosis" (personal communication, Dieter Felsenberg, MD PhD, Berlin, Germany).

The WHO definition of osteoporosis (T score less than –2.5) is *not* applicable to QCT.

A QCT Z score of –2.0 and below is abnormal. A QCT measurement of 100 mg/cm^3 or less has been considered osteopenia and 80 mg/cm^3 or below osteoporosis.

Although usually applied to the vertebral trabecular bone, more recently dedicated, small CT scanners (peripheral pQCT) have been developed, which allow separate analysis of cortical and trabecular bone in the nondominant forearm (see Figure 31-15) and in other sites of the skeleton, including the tibia. Measurement of cross-sectional bone and muscle area and certain biomechanical parameters can also be made from these scans.[91,93] These dedicated pQCT scanners use older CT technology (rotate and translate), and each section consequently takes about 1 minute to obtain. The radiation dose from axial (central) QCT is higher than DXA (effective dose equivalent EDE 1 to 6 μSv), but it still compares favorably with conventional radiographic procedures (e.g., lumbar spine radiographs EDE 700 to 1000 μSv). By using a low KV, the dose for QCT (including the initial scout view) will be approximately EDE 90 μSv. The dose from pQCT is extremely low (less than 0.5 μSv).

Other Research Methods

Quantitative ultrasound (QUS) measures broadband ultrasound attenuation (BUA) and speed of sound (SOS) and shows potential in fracture prediction.[96,97] It is predominantly applied to the calcaneus, where it predicts hip fracture risk in elderly women. However, it cannot be used to diagnose osteoporosis as defined by the WHO; it is also temperature sensitive and a poor monitoring tool. QUS has been applied to numerous other skeletal sites (e. g., phalanges). It is not clear how QUS should be used in clinical practice in other patient groups (men, young women, and children).[97,98]

Quantitative magnetic resonance (QMR) has been applied in research to assessing bone density and trabecular bone structure.[99] The diameter of bone trabeculae range from about 50 to 200 μm and can be demonstrated on conventional radiographs, particularly in the appendicular skeleton (hands), where visualization can be enhanced by magnification techniques. More recently, there has been an increase in the research application of high-resolution CT (HR-CT) and HR-MRI for examining trabecular structure in vivo. Micro-CT systems have been developed with increased spatial resolution, but these are generally only applicable to examine small tissue samples in vitro because of the radiation doses required.[99]

SUMMARY OF IMAGING STRATEGIES IN OSTEOPOROSIS

Generalized Osteoporosis

Evidence to suggest osteoporosis on radiographs (thinned cortex, osteopenia, trabeculae reduced in number and thickness) should be noted, and bone densitometry performed to confirm or refute the diagnosis.

Fractures

Fractures are usually diagnosed on radiographs; if no fracture is visualized but clinical symptoms and signs are strongly suggestive of fracture, then MRI (or alternatively, RNS, although less desirable as it involves ionizing radiation) should be performed to confirm occult fractures.

If the patient with fracture is over 50 years of age, review the trauma history. If the fracture occurred from standing height only and with minimal trauma, consider osteoporotic fracture. Look for (and radiologists should report) other radiographic features of osteoporosis (thinned cortex, osteopenia, trabeculae reduced in number and thickness) and perform further investigation (DXA bone densitometry) and management as required (consider referral to physician with expertise in osteoporosis).

If vertebral fractures are present in patients 50 years of age and older, they are strong predictors of future fracture, so they must be designated clearly on radiologic reports as fractures, rather than using other ambiguous terms such as deformities. In these cases, further investigation (DXA) is warranted with treatment as noted in the previous paragraph. To distinguish between osteoporotic vertebral fractures and other causes of vertebral deformities, the following radiographic signs may be helpful:

- Endplate is intact in osteoporotic fractures.
- Texture changes in the vertebral body adjacent to the endplate may suggest osteoporotic fracture of the central portion of the endplate with the outer ring remaining intact.
- Modeling changes and osteophytes indicate spondylosis as a cause for the deformity.[47,48,50]
- Destruction of the endplate suggests metastases, tumor, or myeloma.
- Destruction of a pedicle is seen with metastases.

When features suggest a sinister etiology, then MRI is the method of choice for further evaluation. MRI is also useful for distinguishing between acute (marrow edema) and chronic (marrow fat signal present) vertebral fractures (as is relevant before embarking upon vertebroplasty). RNS can also distinguish between acute (increased isotope uptake "hot spot") and chronic (no abnormal isotope uptake) vertebral fractures. CT can also be helpful in defining bone destruction of a vertebral body and any associated soft tissue paraspinal mass, and the midline sagittal image from 3D-volume CT of the thorax and abdomen is far superior in demonstrating vertebral fractures than transverse axial images.

As radiographs are poor at demonstrating microfractures in the sites that they tend to occur (sacrum, calcaneus), other imaging methods (MRI, CT, and RNS in order of preference) have to be used to confirm their presence.

Regional Osteoporosis

In the inflammatory arthropathies initially the joint involved or the hands and feet are radiographed; periarticular osteopenia may be the earliest radiographic feature to confirm the diagnosis, but other more specific features (e.g., juxta-articular erosions in rheumatoid arthritis) should be sought. Other imaging methods (ultrasound and MRI) are proving to be more sensitive methods for assessing and monitoring disease activity.[100-102]

Affected patients may have generalized osteoporosis as well, which is related to the disease and its treatment (e.g., systemic glucocorticoids), so the comments in the previous section may also apply to these patients.

In reflex sympathetic dystrophy and regional migratory osteoporosis, there may be evidence of radiographic osteopenia, but radiographs may also show no abnormality. MRI is more specific in demonstrating marrow edema and joint effusion that may be present; RNS will show increased uptake of isotope in the bones affected. As migratory osteoporosis may be caused by juxtaarticular microfractures related to systemic osteoporosis, DXA bone densitometry is relevant.

REFERENCES

1. Adams JE: Metabolic and endocrine skeletal disease. In Grainger RG, Allison DJ, Dixon AK (eds): *Grainger and Allison's Diagnostic Radiology: A Textbook of Medical Imaging*, 5th ed, New York, 2007, Elsevier, pp 1083-1113.
2. Adams JE: Metabolic bone disease. In Hodler J, von Schuthess GK, Zollikofer ChL (eds): *Musculoskeletal Diseases: Diagnostic Imaging and Interventional Techniques* New York, 2005, Springer-Verlag, pp 89-105.
3. National Institutes of Health: *Osteoporosis Prevention, Diagnosis and Therapy*, NIH Consensus Statement 17, Bethesda, Md, 2000, NIH.
4. Bouxsein ML, Karasik D: Bone geometry and skeletal fragility, *Curr Osteoporos Rep* 4:49-56, 2006.
5. van Staa TP, Dennison EM, Leufkens HG et al: Epidemiology of fractures in England and Wales, *Bone* 29:517-522, 2001.
6. Sambrook P, Cooper C: Osteoporosis, *Lancet* 367:2010-2018, 2006.
7. Melton LJ, Lane AW, Cooper C et al: Prevalence and incidence of vertebral fracture, *Osteoporos Int* 3:113-119, 1993.
8. O'Neill T, Felsenberg D, Varlow J et al: The prevalence of vertebral fracture in European men and women: the European Vertebral Osteoporosis Study, *J Bone Miner Res* 11:1010-1018, 1996.
9. Eastell R, Wahner HW, O'Fallon WM et al: Unequal decrease in bone density of the lumbar spine and ultradistal radius in Colles' and vertebral fracture syndromes, *J Clin Invest* 83:168-174, 1989.
10. Faulkner KG, Gluer CC, Majumdar S et al: Non-invasive measurements of bone mass, structure and strength: current methods and experimental techniques, *Am J Radiol* 157:1229-1237, 1991.
11. Nelson DA, Kleerekoper M, Parfitt AM: Bone mass, skin color and body size among black and white women, *Bone Miner* 4:257-264, 1988.
12. Gilsanz V, Roe TF, Mora S et al: Changes in vertebral bone mineral density in black girls and white girls during childhood and puberty, *N Engl J Med* 325:1597-1600, 1991.
13. Ralston SH: Genetics of osteoporosis, *Proc Nutr Soc* 66:158-165, 2007.
14. Krall EA, Dawson-Hughes B: Heritable and life-style determinants of bone mineral density, *J Bone Miner Res* 8:1-9, 1993.
15. Marcus R, Feldman D, Kelsey J (eds): *Osteoporosis*, 2nd ed, San Diego, Calif, 2001, Academic Press.
16. Compston J: Guidelines for the management of osteoporosis: the present and the future, *Osteoporos Int* 16:1173-1176, 2005.
17. Poole KE, Compston JE: Osteoporosis and its management, *Br Med J* 333:1251-1256, 2006.
18. Meunier PJ: Anabolic agents for treatment of postmenopausal osteoporosis, *Joint Bone Spine* 68:576-581, 2001.
19. Shaw NJ, Bishop NJ: Bisphosphonate treatment in bone disease, *Arch Dis Child* 90:494-499, 2005.
20. Lam DK, Sandor GK, Holmes HI et al: A review of bisphosphonate-associated osteonecrosis of the jaws and its management, *J Can Dent Assoc* 73:417-422, 2007.
21. Kauffman RP, Overton TH, Shiflett M et al: Osteoporosis in children and adolescent girls: case report of idiopathic juvenile osteoporosis and review of the literature, *Obstet Gynecol Surg* 56:492-504, 2001.
22. Sillence D: Osteogenesis imperfecta: an expanding panorama of variants, *Clin Orthop Rel Res* 59:11-25, 1981.
23. Rauch F, Glorieux FH: Osteogenesis imperfecta, *Lancet* 363:1377-1385, 2004.
24. Gahagan S, Rimsza ME: Child abuse or osteogenesis imperfecta: how can we tell? *Pediatrics* 88:987-992, 1991.
25. Goldman AB, Davidson D, Pavlov H et al: Popcorn calcification: a prognostic sign in osteogenesis imperfecta, *Radiology* 136:351-358, 1980.
26. Glorieux FH: Experience with bisphosphonates in osteogenesis imperfecta, *Pediatrics* 119:S163-S165, 2001.
27. Rauch F, Glorieux FH: Treatment of children with osteogenesis imperfecta, *Curr Osteoporos Rep* 4:159-164, 2006.
28. Meunier PJ, Delmas PD, Eastell R et al: Diagnosis and management of osteoporosis in postmenopausal women: clinical guidelines. International Committee for Osteoporosis Clinical Guidelines, *Clin Ther* 21:1025-1044, 1999.
29. Adams JE: Osteoporosis. In Pope T, Bloem HL, Beltran J, Morrison W, Wilson J (eds): *Imaging of the Musculoskeletal System*, Philadelphia 2008, Saunders Elsevier, pp 1489-1508.
30. Quek ST, Peh WC: Radiology of osteoporosis, *Semin Musculoskelet Radiol* 6:197-206, 2002.
31. van Staa TP, Leufkens HG, Cooper C: The epidemiology of corticosteroid induced osteoporosis: a meta-analysis, *Osteoporos Int* 13:777-787, 2002.
32. Ferretti JL, Cointry GR, Capozza RF et al: Bone mass, bone strength, muscle-bone interactions, osteopenias and osteoporoses, *Mech Ageing Dev* 124:269-279, 2003.
33. Jiang SD, Dai LY, Jiang LS: Osteoporosis after spinal cord injury, *Osteoporos Int* 17:180-192, 2006.
34. Jiang SD, Jiang LS, Dai LY: Mechanisms of osteoporosis in spinal cord injury, *Clin Endocrinol (Oxf)* 65:555-565, 2006.
35. Harden RN, Bruehl SP: Diagnosis of complex regional pain syndrome: signs, symptoms, and new empirically derived diagnostic criteria, *Clin J Pain* 22:415-419, 2006.
36. Pham T, Lafforgue P: Reflex sympathetic dystrophy and neuromediators, *Joint Bone Spine* 70:12-17, 2003.
37. Toms AP, Marshall TJ, Becker E et al: Regional migratory osteoporosis: a review illustrated by five cases, *Clin Radiol* 60:425-438, 2005.
38. vande Berg BC, Lecouvet FE, Maldague B et al: Osteonecrosis and transient osteoporosis of the femoral head. In Davies AM, Johnson K, Whitehouse RW (eds): *Imaging of the Hip and Bony Pelvis—Techniques and Applications*, New York, 2006, Springer, pp 195-216.
39. Yamamoto T, Schneider R, Iwamoto Y et al: Subchondral insufficiency fracture of the femoral head in a patient with systemic lupus erythematosis, *Ann Rheum Dis* 65: 837-838, 2006.
40. Yamamoto T, Schneider R, Iwamoto Y et al: Rapid acetabular osteolysis secondary to subchondral insufficiency fracture, *J Rheumatol* 34:592-595, 2007.
41. Mayo-Smith W, Rosenthal DI: Radiographic appearances of osteopenia, *Radiol Clin North Am* 29: 37-47, 1991.
42. Pitt M: Osteopenic bone disease, *Orthop Clin North Am* 14:65-80, 1983.
43. Adams JE: Radiology of rickets and osteomalacia. In Feldman D, Pike JW, Glorieux FH (eds): *Vitamin D*, 2nd ed, New York, 2005, Elsevier, pp 967-994.
44. Peh W: Imaging of pelvic insufficiency fracture, *Radiographics* 16:335-348, 1996.
45. Peh WCG, Davies AM: Bone trauma: stress fractures, In Davies AM, Johnson K, Whitehouse RW (eds): *Imaging of the Hip and Bony Pelvis—Techniques and Applications*, New York, 2006, Springer, pp 247-266.
46. Hain SF, Fogelman I: Nuclear medicine studies in metabolic bone disease, *Semin Musculoskelet Radiol* 6:323-329, 2002.
47. Jiang G, Eastell R, Barrington NA et al: Comparison of methods for the visualisation of prevalent vertebral fracture in osteoporosis, *Osteoporos Int* 15:887-896, 2004.
48. Ferrar L, Jiang G, Adams J et al: Identification of vertebral fractures: an update, *Osteoporos Int* 16:717-728, 2005.
49. National Osteoporosis Foundation Working Group on Vertebral Fractures: Assessing vertebral fractures, *J Bone Miner Res* 10:518-523, 1995.
50. Guermazi A, Mohr A, Grigorian M et al: Identification of vertebral fractures in osteoporosis, *Semin Musculoskelet Radiol* 6:241-252, 2002.
51. Link TM, Guglielmi G, van Kuijk C et al: Radiologic assessment of osteoporotic fracture: diagnostic and prognostic implications, *Eur Radiol* 15:1521-1532, 2005.
52. Genant HK, Wu CY, van Kuijk C et al: Vertebral fracture assessment using a semi-quantitative technique, *J Bone Miner Res* 8:1137-1148, 1993.
53. Lindsay R, Silverman SL, Cooper C et al: Risk of new vertebral fracture in the year following a fracture, *J Am Med Assoc* 285:320-323, 2001.
54. Black DM, Arden NK, Palermo L et al: Prevalent vertebral fractures predict hip fractures and new vertebral fractures but not wrist fractures. Study of Osteoporotic Fractures Research Group, *J Bone Miner Res* 14:821-828, 1999.
55. Ross PD, Davis JW, Epstein RS et al: Pre-existing fractures and bone mass predict vertebral fracture incidence in women, *Ann Intern Med* 14:919-923, 1991.
56. Gehlbach SH, Bigelow C, Heimisdottir M et al: Recognition of vertebral fracture in a clinical setting, *Osteoporos Int* 11:577-582, 2000.
57. Delmas PD, van de Langerijt L, Watts NB et al: IMPACT Study Group. Underdiagnosis of vertebral fractures is a worldwide problem: the IMPACT study, *J Bone Miner* Res 20:557-563, 2005.
58. Banks LM, van Kuijk C, Genant HK: Radiographic technique for assessing osteoporotic vertebral fracture. In Genant HK, Jergas M, van Kuijk C (eds): *Vertebral Fracture in Osteoporosis*, San Francisco, 1995, University of California Osteoporosis Research Group, pp 131-147.
59. Baur A, Stabler A, Bruning R et al: Diffusion-weighted MR imaging of bone marrow: differentiation of benign versus pathologic compression fractures, *Radiology* 207: 349-356, 1998.
60. Baur A, Stabler A, Arbogast S et al: Acute osteoporotic and neoplastic vertebral compression fractures: fluid sign at MR imaging, *Radiology* 225:730-735, 2003.
61. Rea JA, Steiger P, Blake GM et al: Optimizing data acquisition and analysis of morphometric x-ray absorptiometry, *Osteoporos Int* 8:177-183, 1998.
62. Jiang G, Eastell R, Barrington NA et al: Visual identification of vertebral fractures in osteoporosis using morphometric x-ray absorptiometry, *J Bone Miner Res* 18:933-938, 2003.
63. Smyth PP, Taylor CJ, Adams JE: Vertebral shape: automatic measurement with active shape models, *Radiology* 211:571-578, 1999.
64. Roberts M, Cootes T, Adams JE: Vertebral morphometry: semi-automated determination of detailed vertebral shape from dual-energy x-ray absorptiometry images using active appearance models, *Invest Radiol* 41:849-859, 2006.
65. de Bruijne M, Lund MT, Tanko LB et al: Quantitative vertebral morphometry using neighbor-conditional shape models, *Med Image Anal* 11:503-512, 2007.
66. Peh WC, Gilula LA: Percutaneous vertebroplasty: indications, contraindications, and technique, *Br J Radiol* 76:69-75, 2003.
67. Garn SM, Poznanski AK, Nagy JM: Bone measurement in the differential diagnosis of osteopenia and osteoporosis, *Radiology*,100:509-518, 1971.
68. Barnett E, Nordin BE: The clinical and radiological problem of thin bone, *Br J Radiol* 34:683-692, 1961.
69. Jorgensen JT, Andersen PB, Rosholm A et al: Digital x-ray radiogrammetry: a new appendicular bone densitometric method with high precision, *Clin Physiol* 20:330-335, 2000.
70. Ward K, Cotton J, Adams JE: A technical and clinical evaluation of digital x-ray radiogrammetry, *Osteoporos Int* 14:389-395, 2003.
71. Nielsen SP: The metacarpal index revisited: a brief overview, *J Clin Densitom* 4:199-207, 2001.
72. Black DM, Palermo L, Sorenson T et al: A normative database study for the Pronosco X exposure system, *J Clin Densitom* 4:5-12, 2001.
73. van Rijn RR, Grootfaam DS, Lequin MH et al: Digital radiogrammetry of the hand in a pediatric and adolescent Dutch Caucasian population: normative data and measurements in children with inflammatory bowel disease and juvenile chronic arthritis, *Calcif Tissue Int* 74:342-350, 2004.

74. Bouxsein ML, Palermo L, Yeung C et al: Digital x-ray radiogrammetry predicts hip, wrist and vertebral fracture risk in elderly women: a prospective analysis from the study of osteoporotic fractures, *Osteoporos Int* 13:358-365, 2002.
75. Singh M, Nagrath AR, Maini PS: Changes in trabecular pattern of the upper end of the femur as an index of osteoporosis, *J Bone Joint Surg Am* 52:457-467, 1970.
76. Smyth PP, Adams JE, Whitehouse RW et al: Application of computer texture analysis to the Singh Index, *Br J Radiol* 70:242-247, 1997.
77. Gregory JS, Stewart A, Undrill PE et al: Bone shape, structure, and density as determinants of osteoporotic hip fracture: a pilot study investigation the combination of risk factors, *Invest Radiol* 40:591-597, 2005.
78. De Smet AA, Neff JR: Pubic and sacral insufficiency fractures: clinical course and radiologic findings, *AJR Am J Roentgenol* 145:601-606, 1985.
79. Cooper KL, Beabout JW, McCleod RA: Supra-acetabular insufficiency fractures, *Radiology* 157:15-17, 1985.
80. Manco LG, Schneider R, Pavlov H: Insufficiency fractures of the tibial plateau, *AJR Am J Roentgenol* 140:1211-1215, 1983.
81. Haramati N, Staron RB, Barax C et al: Magnetic resonance imaging of occult fractures of the proximal femur, *Skel Radiol* 23:19-22, 1994.
82. Sinigaglia L, Varenna M, Girasole G et al: Epidemiology of osteoporosis in rheumatic diseases, *Rheum Dis Clin North Am* 32:631-658, 2006.
83. Romas E, Gillespie MT: Inflammation-induced bone loss: can it be prevented? *Rheum Dis Clin North Am* 32:759-773, 2006.
84. Woo P: Systemic juvenile idiopathic arthritis, *Nat Clin Pract Rheumatol* 2:28-34, 2006.
85. Thornton J, Ashcroft DM, Mughal MZ et al: Systematic review of effectiveness of bisphosphonates in treatment of low bone mineral density and fragility fractures on juvenile idiopathic arthritis, *Arch Dis Child* 91:753-761, 2006.
86. Haugeberg G, Emery P: Value of dual-energy x-ray absorptiometry as a diagnostic and assessment tool in early rheumatoid arthritis, *Rheum Dis Clin North Am* 31:715-728, 2005.
87. Jawaid WB, Crosbie D, Shotton J et al: Use of digital x-ray radiogrammetry in the assessment of joint damage in rheumatoid arthritis, *Ann Rheum Dis* 65:459-464, 2006.
88. Ahmed AI, Ilic D, Blake GM et al: Review of 3,530 referrals for bone densitometry measurements of spine and femur: evidence that radiographic osteopenia predicts low bone mass, *Radiology* 207:619-624, 1998.
89. World Health Organization (WHO) Study Group: *Assessment of Fracture Risk and Its Application to Screening for Postmenopausal Osteoporosis*, WHO Technical Report Series 843, Geneva, 1994, World Health Organization.
90. National Osteoporosis Society: *A Practical Guide to Bone Densitometry in Children*, Camerton, Bath, UK, 2004, National Osteoporosis Society.
91. van Rijn RR, Van der Sluis IM, Link TM: Bone densitometry in children: a critical appraisal, *Eur Radiol* 13:700-710, 2003.
92. Sawyer AJ, Bachrach LK, Fung EB (eds): *Bone Densitometry in Growing Patients: Guidelines for Clinical Practice*, 2006, Totowa, NJ, Humana Press.
93. Mughal MZ, Ward K, Adams J: Assessment of Bone status in children by densitometric and quantitative ultrasound techniques. In Carty H, Brunelle F, Stringer DA et al (eds): *Imaging in Children*, 2nd ed, vol 1, New York 2005, Elsevier pp 477-486.
94. Guglielmi G, Lang TF: Quantitative computed tomography, *Semin Musculoskel Radiol* 6:219-227, 2002.
95. Kalender WA: Effective dose values in bone mineral measurements by photon absorptiometry and computed tomography, *Osteoporos Int* 2:282-287, 1992.
96. Boonen S, Nicholson P: Assessment of femoral bone fragility and fracture risk by ultrasonic measurements at the calcaneus, *Age Ageing* 27:231-237, 1998.
97. Stewart A, Reid DM: Quantitative ultrasound in osteoporosis, *Semin Musculoskelet Radiol* 6:229-232, 2002.
98. Engelke K, Gluer CC: Quality and performance measures in bone densitometry, Part 1: errors and diagnosis. *Osteoporos Int* 17:1283-1292, 2006.
99. Link TM, Bauer JS: Imaging of trabecular bone structure, *Semin Musculoskelet Radiol* 6:253-261, 2002.
100. Ostergaard M, McQueen F, Bird P et al: The OMERACT Magnetic Resonance Imaging inflammatory Arthritis Group—advances and priorities, *J Rheum* 34:852-853, 2007.
101. Farrant JM, O'Connor PJ, Grainger AJ: Advanced imaging in rheumatoid arthritis. Part 1: synovitis, *Skel Radiol* 36:269-297, 2007.
102. Farrant JM, Grainger AJ, O'Connor PJ: Advanced imaging in rheumatoid arthritis. Part 2: synovitis, *Skel Radiol* 36:381-389, 2007.

CHAPTER 32

Reflex Sympathetic Dystrophy, Migratory Osteoporosis, and Osteogenesis Imperfecta

KEVIN CARTER, DO, *and* JOEL NIELSEN, DO

KEY FACTS

Reflex Sympathetic Dystrophy

- Clinically, patients with reflex sympathetic dystrophy (RSD) present with intense, prolonged pain, vasomotor disturbances, delayed functional recovery, and trophic changes in the affected extremity that usually following minor trauma.
- Radiographs of RSD are characterized by regional osteoporosis with soft tissue swelling in the affected extremity. In the upper extremity, usually the hand and wrist, and in the lower extremity, the foot and ankle are most often involved.
- Radiographs can differentiate RSD from a primary articular disorder by the absence of significant intraarticular erosions and the preservation of the joint space in RSD.
- Three-phase bone scans are complementary to the clinical history in diagnosing RSD, characterized by increased accumulation of the radiotracer in the juxta-articular region of the affected joint on all three phases, with the delayed images being the most sensitive for confirming the diagnosis.
- Magnetic resonance imaging (MRI) adds very little to the clinical diagnosis of RSD, but it is beneficial in helping to exclude other entities that may present with similar clinical symptoms.

Regional Migratory Osteoporosis

- Clinically, patients with regional migratory osteoporosis (RMO) present with sudden onset of joint pain classically in the lower extremity and usually affecting men in the fourth to fifth decade.
- Diminishing pain in one joint with development of pain in an adjacent joint is typical of RMO.
- Osteoporosis of the affected area with preservation of joint space is typical of the radiographic findings of RMO or transient osteoporosis (TO).
- Classic findings on MRI are a bone marrow edema-like signal in the affected joint and a joint effusion. Findings return to normal following resolution of the patient's symptoms.
- RMO must be differentiated from early osteonecrosis by MRI.

Osteogenesis Imperfecta

- Osteogenesis imperfecta is actually a spectrum of genetic disorders characterized by connective tissue defects. The Sillence type I is the most frequently observed variety and is characterized by blue sclera, ligamentous laxity, and increased tendency to sustain fractures.
- Osteogenesis imperfecta type II is the most severe form of the disease and is characterized by dwarfism and severe bone deformities. Few patients survive beyond the neonatal period.
- Osteogenesis imperfecta is the most common genetic cause for osteoporosis.
- Classically on radiographs, patients may have gracile bones, multiple fractures, and cystic changes at the metaphyses.
- Excessive callus at the healing fracture site may be distinguished from osteosarcoma with CT or MRI, which allows visualization of a fracture line confirming the diagnosis of fracture callus.

Osteoporosis is a very common disorder and the most frequently encountered metabolic bone disease worldwide. Diminished bone mass can result from a failure to reach optimal peak bone mass in early adulthood, increased bone resorption, or decreased bone formation after peak bone mass has been achieved. Numerous conditions can cause a decrease in bone mass; consequently, its distribution can aid in determining the underlying etiology. The distribution of osteoporosis can be divided into a regional and a generalized process. The regional form is confined to a segment of the body and associated with disorders of the appendicular skeleton. Classically, this is seen secondary to disuse or immobilization, but other causes include reflex sympathetic dystrophy and transient regional osteoporosis, which includes regional migratory osteoporosis. Numerous processes can result in generalized osteoporosis, which is primarily manifested in the axial skeleton and in the proximal portions of the appendicular skeleton. Common etiologies associated with the generalized form include senile causes, medications (e.g., corticosteroids and heparin), endocrine abnormalities, malnutrition/deficiency states, alcoholism, and liver disease, among others. The most common genetic cause of generalized osteoporosis is osteogenesis imperfecta. Through the combination of clinical history and laboratory information, as well as imaging findings, both the distribution and the underlying etiology for the development of osteoporosis can usually be determined, allowing for appropriate management and prevention of potentially serious complications.

REFLEX SYMPATHETIC DYSTROPHY

Reflex sympathetic dystrophy (RSD) is a pain syndrome that has various clinical forms, precipitating factors, physiopathologic hypotheses, and diagnostic criteria. It was first described in 1864 by Mitchell and his colleagues[1] in U.S. Civil War soldiers who had suffered gunshot wounds that affected peripheral nerves. These patients went on to develop a persistent, burning pain with progressive trophic changes in the affected limb. More than six dozen different terms have been utilized since the original description to describe RSD in the English, French, and German literature.[2] Some of these include *causalgia, acute bony atrophy, Sudeck's atrophy* or *osteodystrophy, post-traumatic osteoporosis, traumatic angiospasm* or *vasospasm, algodystrophy, reflex dystrophy of the extremities, minor causalgia, postinfarctional sclerodactyly, shoulder-hand syndrome, reflex neurovascular dystrophy,* and *the reflex sympathetic dystrophy syndrome.*[3] In 1994, a new term adopted by the International Association for the Study of Pain—*complex regional pain syndromes* (CRPS)—was intended to be an all-encompassing term for this group of disorders, in which pain that is felt to originate from the sympathetic nervous system is accepted as a common etiology.[4] CRPS are subdivided into type I CRPS (RSD) and type II CRPS (causalgia). The distinction between the two is based on the absence of a documented nerve injury for causalgia. Because the older terminology is still widely used, the term *RSD* will be used herein.

Any neurally related condition that may affect the musculoskeletal system, including a neurologic or vascular insult, may serve as a potential source for developing RSD. Trauma secondary to accidental injury has been described as the most common cause of RSD.[5] These injuries may include sprains, dislocations, fractures, traumatic amputations, crush injuries, contusions, and lacerations or punctures of the extremities.[5] RSD will develop in 1% to 5% of these patients.[6] Almost 28% of patients with a Colles fracture[6] and 30% of patients with a tibial fracture[7] will progress clinically to develop RSD. It is also observed in 1% to 20% of patients following myocardial infarctions[8] and in 12% to 20% of patients following development of hemiplegia.[9] Other reported causes may include infection, cervical osteoarthritis, tendinitis, peripheral neuropathy, herniated disks, use of barbiturates, and antituberculosis drugs, as well as psychological stress.[10] Malignant tumors including those involving the brain, lung, ovary, breast, pancreas, and bladder are also associated with RSD.[11-16] RSD has also been observed during the postoperative recovery period, commonly associated with arthroscopic surgical procedures and prolonged usage of extremity tourniquets.[17]

RSD is observed less frequently in children than in adults. When present, it is more commonly found in girls than boys and will usually involve a lower extremity. It generally develops following a physical injury and may present with unique radionuclide features. The disease process is usually self-limited and benign in nature with no clinical residual.[3]

The pathogenesis of RSD is not completely understood, and no pathophysiologic mechanism has been established. It is thought to be multifactorial in nature. The earliest and most widely accepted theory is that of the "internuncial pool" in which an injury or lesion will produce a painful impulse that travels via afferent pathways to the spinal cord, where a series of reflexes are initiated that spread via that interconnecting pool of neurons. These latter reflexes stimulate the lateral and anterior tracts, provoking efferent pathways that travel to the peripheral nerves producing the local findings of RSD.[3] The International Association for the Study of Pain describes the CRPS as a complex neurologic disease involving the somatosensory, somatomotor, and autonomic nervous systems in various combinations, with distorted information processing of afferent sensory signals to the spinal cord.[19,20] Others have proposed that the pain is caused by activation of sensory fibers by sympathetic efferents.[10] The importance of the involvement of the sympathetic nervous system is further supported by the identification of nerve fibers in the periosteum that are sympathetic in origin and contain vasoactive intestinal peptide, a substance that stimulates bone resorption.[3] Many other biochemical factors have also been proposed as being involved in this mechanism including substance P, histamine, and prostaglandins. Another theory is that minuscule peripheral nerve twigs are damaged in soft tissue injury and these twigs form artificial synapses; this is an attempt to explain why minor trauma may result in RSD.[10]

Vascular abnormalities are well known to occur with RSD and are responsible for some of the changes seen on imaging exams. Many investigators feel that the sympathetic nervous system may also be responsible for these abnormalities; they confirmed their theories through the use of thermographic imaging that showed differences in the temperature of the affected extremities,[18] which is felt to be related to blood flow. This was also confirmed by the significant effect on distal blood flow that occurs following sympathectomy.[3] A different theory suggests that occlusion of the arterioles may initiate changes followed by capillary and venous stasis. This may occur following paralysis due to immobilization by casting or as described earlier, due to prolonged use of tourniquets in the operating room.[3] This occlusion/stasis may result in local shunts that lead to the increased local temperature that is seen during certain phases of the disease.[3] Despite all of these various proposals, the exact mechanism remains unknown.

The clinical signs and symptoms of RSD are variable (Box 32-1). The diagnosis of florid RSD is generally not difficult, although the differential diagnosis is extensive.[21] The diagnosis of a mild or early case is difficult due to the changing clinical features and the subjectivity of the clinical complaints.[21]

> Early diagnosis of RSD is essential because the results of treatment are better when there is early initiation of therapy.

The most well-known form of RSD affects the upper extremity, with a regional distribution involving the distal forearm, wrist, and hand. It may also affect the lower extremity, most often at the foot and ankle. Classically, patients with RSD will present with four consistent clinical characteristics: intense prolonged pain, vasomotor disturbances, delayed functional recovery, and various trophic changes.

> RSD is characterized by four clinical features: intense prolonged pain, vasomotor disturbances, delayed functional recovery, and trophic changes.

RSD is commonly divided into three stages.[22] Not all patients will pass through all three stages. The initial (inflammatory) stage (I) lasts from 1 to 7 weeks and is characterized by diffuse nonfocal pain, inflammation, and edema associated with joint stiffness and decreased range of motion, as well as either hypothermia or hyperthermia. In the second (dystrophic) stage (II), which lasts from 3 to 6 months, the principal clinical findings are pain that decreases

BOX 32-1. Clinical Features of RSD

- History of prior injury may be present
- Distal extremity affected
- Intense pain
- Vasomotor changes
- Delayed recovery
- Trophic changes

over time and is exacerbated with exercise, thickening of the skin and fascia, increased sensitivity of the skin to temperature and pressure changes, and the beginning of muscle atrophy. In the final (atrophic) stage (III), the pain persists and scleroderma-like skin changes occur with continued decrease in the range of motion and increased joint stiffness. Aponeurotic and tendinous retraction may occur in this final stage. The extremity becomes cooler with decreased vascularity. All of the changes in this final stage are irreversible.[23] The final diagnosis of RSD is established by the patient's clinical course and with the aid of the imaging findings[23,24] (Figure 32-1). The majority of cases completely resolve over time with few progressing to the final stage.[23,24]

Imaging

Imaging of the patient with signs and symptoms of RSD is essential in helping to confirm the clinical assessment, as well as rule out potential serious entities that may present in a similar fashion (Table 32-1). Imaging findings often reveal that RSD is a bilateral process, although the patient's symptoms and imaging abnormalities will be much more pronounced on one side than the other. Rarely, a localized form may be observed affecting one joint in an extremity or one of several digits in a hand or foot.[3]

Along with the clinical findings, the radiographs may aid in making the diagnosis of RSD. The most common radiographic findings include soft tissue swelling and regional osteoporosis.[3] The osteoporosis observed in association with RSD is nonspecific and is variably present; reported in 30% to 70% of RSD cases.[25] The early

TABLE 32-1. Imaging Features of RSD

Radiographs	Soft Tissue Swelling
	Trabecular resorption (spotty osteoporosis)
	Subperiosteal resorption (may mimic hyperparathyroidism)
	Endosteal resorption (scalloped appearance to the inner cortex)
	Cortical resorption (striated appearance to cortex)
	Subchondral resorption (mild erosive changes)
	Preservation of the cartilage space
	Usually no or minimal articular erosions
	Occasional insufficiency fractures
Scintigraphy	All phases: Diffuse increased uptake with juxta-articular accentuation.
	Unusual appearance in children.
	All three phases may show areas of decreased uptake ("cold").
MRI	Nonspecific.
	Absent bone marrow edema in RSD, may aid in separating RSD from transient osteoporosis.
	May have joint effusion, skin changes, soft tissue edema, muscle atrophy, normal cartilage.

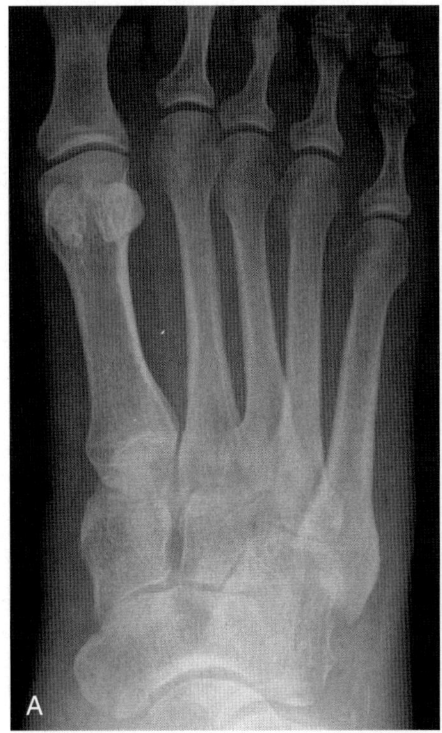

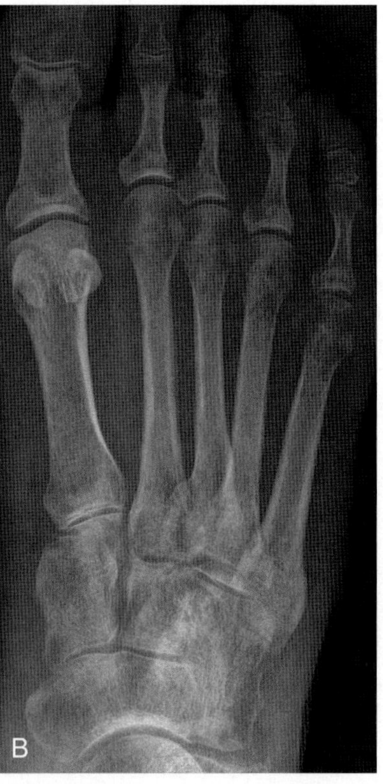

FIGURE 32-1. RSD. This 46-year-old female presented with pain following a minor twisting injury. **A,** Initial AP radiograph shows normal bone density. There is mild soft tissue swelling over the lateral malleolus. A small spur suggests a calcaneal avulsion injury. On lateral radiograph (not shown), a small avulsion fracture was present at the dorsal aspect of the talus. Surgical fusion of the third toe PIP is incidentally noted. **B,** The patient had persistent pain and burning. The AP radiograph at 3-month follow-up shows interval development of patchy osteoporosis consistent with RSD.

findings of RSD are patchy demineralization of the epiphyses and short bones of the affected extremity.[26] Genant and associates[24] have described five types of bone resorption patterns that may occur with RSD, and these are best visualized with fine-detail radiography.[3] These findings include irregular resorption of the trabecular bone in the metaphysis, resulting in patchy or spotty osteoporosis, subperiosteal bone resorption, intracortical bone resorption, endosteal bone resorption, and surface erosions of subchondral and juxtaarticular bone.[24] The subperiosteal resorption is similar to that seen in hyperparathyroidism.[27] Striation and tunneling of the cortical bone are observed with intracortical bone resorption, but these findings are not diagnostic of RSD and may occur with any condition that will result in disuse.[26] The endosteal bone is the region of the greatest bone mineral loss in RSD and results in the initially observed excavation and scalloping at the endosteal surface. As a result, there is subsequent uniform remodeling of the endosteum and widening of the medullary canal.[28] The erosions occurring in the subchondral and juxtaarticular bones result in small periarticular erosions and intraarticular gaps.[28] Once patchy osteopenia is present, the patient has usually already progressed to stage II RSD.

A primary articular disorder may be mistaken for RSD due to the rapid onset and severity of bone resorption that may be observed in the periarticular regions.[30] RSD can be differentiated from other arthritides due to the absence of significant intraarticular erosions and preservation of the joint space; the latter is a key finding in RSD.[3] In rare cases, RSD may be accompanied by insufficiency fractures.[31]

Bone Scintigraphy

Bone scintigraphy is established as a beneficial imaging modality in making the diagnosis of RSD.[32] Bone scintigraphy will demonstrate abnormalities that may be observed prior to recognizing abnormalities on radiographs[32-34] (Figure 32-2).

> In patients with RSD, scintigraphic changes often precede radiographic abnormalities.

Imaging with Tc-99m MDP shows increased accumulation of the radiotracer in the involved bones. This is due to both increased vascularity, as well as rapid ion exchange at the highly vascularized bone surfaces.[35] The classic distribution of the radiotracer is diffuse, with an accentuation of accumulation in the juxtaarticular regions of the involved extremity. This is preceded by hyperemia in a similar distribution, seen on both the immediate postinjection blood flow and the slightly delayed blood pool phases of the exam.[10] With three-phase scanning, the delayed images show this pattern of periarticular accumulation, and this is the most sensitive indicator of the diagnosis[36] (Figure 32-3). Scintigraphic images obtained at different times may show migration of the abnormalities from one side of the joint to another similar to a pattern observed in regional migratory osteoporosis (RMO).[38]

Rarely, decreased accumulation, or "cold" areas may be observed in bone scintigraphy examinations of children.[39] The scintigraphic findings of this "cold" variant include photopenic abnormalities on the delayed scan and hypoxemia on the immediate blood-flow and blood-pool phases of the exam at the affected region. These abnormalities can be recognized in children who have open epiphyses by the incongruence of the involved epiphyseal activity compared with the remote ipsilateral or contralateral normal epiphyseal plate activity.[10]

Magnetic Resonance Imaging

Very little data have been accumulated on MRI findings in patients with RSD. Koch et al. described nonspecific soft tissue changes such as edema and muscle atrophy in RSD patients and concluded that these findings were not helpful in establishing the diagnosis.[22] Multiple other reports have described additional MRI findings that may aid in diagnosing RSD, including contrast enhancement of the involved joint/extremity and at a late stage, skin thinning[38,40,41] (Figure 32-4). Others have stated that an associated effusion in the involved joint is an additional useful sign in detecting RSD in its early stage.[38] Bone marrow edema has been inconsistently seen in association with RSD.[40] This is one of the features that may aid in distinguishing RSD from regional migratory osteoporosis, which typically shows bone marrow edema. The MRI examination is beneficial in confirming the clinical diagnosis of RSD, but it should not be used as the primary imaging modality in making this diagnosis.

> MRI is helpful in excluding entities, such as fracture, that might be confused with reflex sympathetic dystrophy but is of limited use in establishing the diagnosis of RSD.

Differential Diagnosis

Clinically, the diagnosis of RSD may be difficult due to the variable clinical manifestations and the natural history of the disease. Many conditions may mimic the symptoms observed with RSD, including diabetic neuropathy and peripheral nerve damage, as well as cartilage injuries. The misdiagnosis of RSD as one of these other entities will lead to ineffective treatment in the early, more treatable stage, potentially resulting in permanent disability for the patient. Imaging studies may aid in making this diagnosis earlier and help confirm the clinical diagnosis. Based on the imaging findings, the differential diagnosis may include osteomyelitis, various arthritides, hyperparathyroidism, or even a trabecular fracture. Unfortunately, the usual findings observed on radiographs of decreased bone density with soft tissue swelling are nonspecific, and when observed may be a late manifestation of the disease. Bone scintigraphy adds to the diagnostic capability by allowing for earlier diagnoses to be made but is only 60% sensitive.[42] MRI provides little beyond what may already be known clinically, but it does aid in narrowing the differential diagnosis by eliminating such entities as metastasis, bone infarcts, or even an occult fracture. Clinical follow-up remains the gold standard for the diagnosis of RSD with clinical confirmation based upon the patient's response to therapy.[38]

Treatment

The usual treatment consists of control of the patient's symptoms, especially the pain, with nonsteroidal anti-inflammatory drugs. Veldman et al. suggested that early symptoms of RSD are responsive to this conservative treatment.[38] Multiple other agents are being investigated to help in treatment, including vitamin C, clonidine, glucocorticoid therapy, and bisphosphonates, as well as ketamine and spinal cord stimulation.[43,44] Ultimately, the diagnosis and treatment may rest on a nerve block using alpha-adrenergic blocking agents.[38] Physical therapy is necessary to maintain full range of motion of the affected joints.[45] Most patients will completely recover following conservative treatment with no persistent clinical sequela.[3]

REGIONAL MIGRATORY OSTEOPOROSIS

Believed by some to be related to RSD, RMO is a sequential polyarticular arthralgia of the weight-bearing joints, most frequently seen in the lower extremities.[46] It is an uncommon condition, although its incidence is probably underestimated, with many

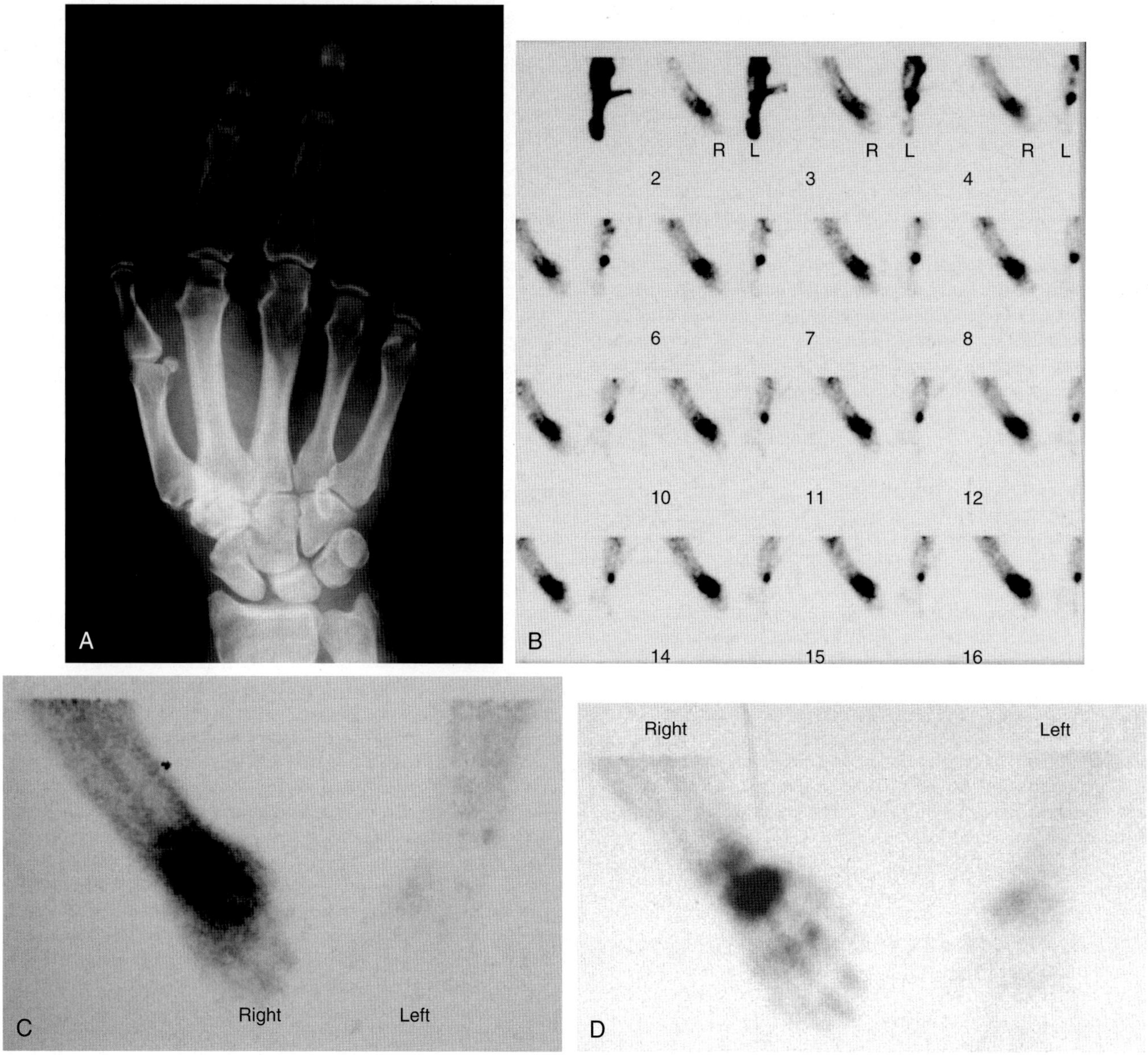

FIGURE 32-2. RSD, scintigraphic findings. This 73-year-old female presented after a minor fall with clinical signs and symptoms of RSD. **A,** Single view of right wrist shows mild soft-tissue swelling without osteopenia or fracture. A Tc 99m 3 phase bone scan was performed with the flow phase demonstrating increased flow to the right wrist **(B)**. Blood pool images **(C)** show increased uptake within the region of the right wrist. On delayed images **(D),** there is asymmetric accumulation of the radiotracer within the bones of the wrist and distal radius and ulna consistent with RSD confirming the clinical suspicions.

cases being labeled as transient osteoporosis of the hip. Along with transient osteoporosis of the hip, it is included in the conditions classified under transient regional osteoporosis. Transient regional osteoporosis is a general term applied to related conditions which are characterized by a sudden onset of joint pain followed by local osteopenia, which progresses to spontaneous healing.[47]

> The *term transient regional osteoporosis* includes the subtypes of transient osteoporosis of the hip and regional migratory osteoporosis. All of these conditions are characterized by sudden onset of joint pain followed by localized osteoporosis and eventual spontaneous healing.

RMO was first described by Duncan et al.[48] in 1967 as a disorder affecting several joints at different times. They labeled this condition *migratory osteolysis.* It is characterized by a transient regional osteoporosis that is migratory in nature. The migratory nature of this process is the major factor that separates this entity from transient osteoporosis of the hip.[49] RMO is an entity that is seen more frequently in men than women and is usually found during the fourth to fifth decade of life.[48]

The etiology of this disease process is unknown and has been extensively debated. McCord et al.[49] reported electromyographic (EMG) abnormalities in regional migratory osteoporosis, but EMG studies have been normal in other reports.[50] Others have proposed that regional migratory osteoporosis and reflex sympathetic dystrophy (RSD) may be closely related or even identical diseases because RSD may precede the clinical onset of regional migratory osteoporosis. They have a similar pattern of osteoporosis early in the course. Radiographically, bilateral extremity joint

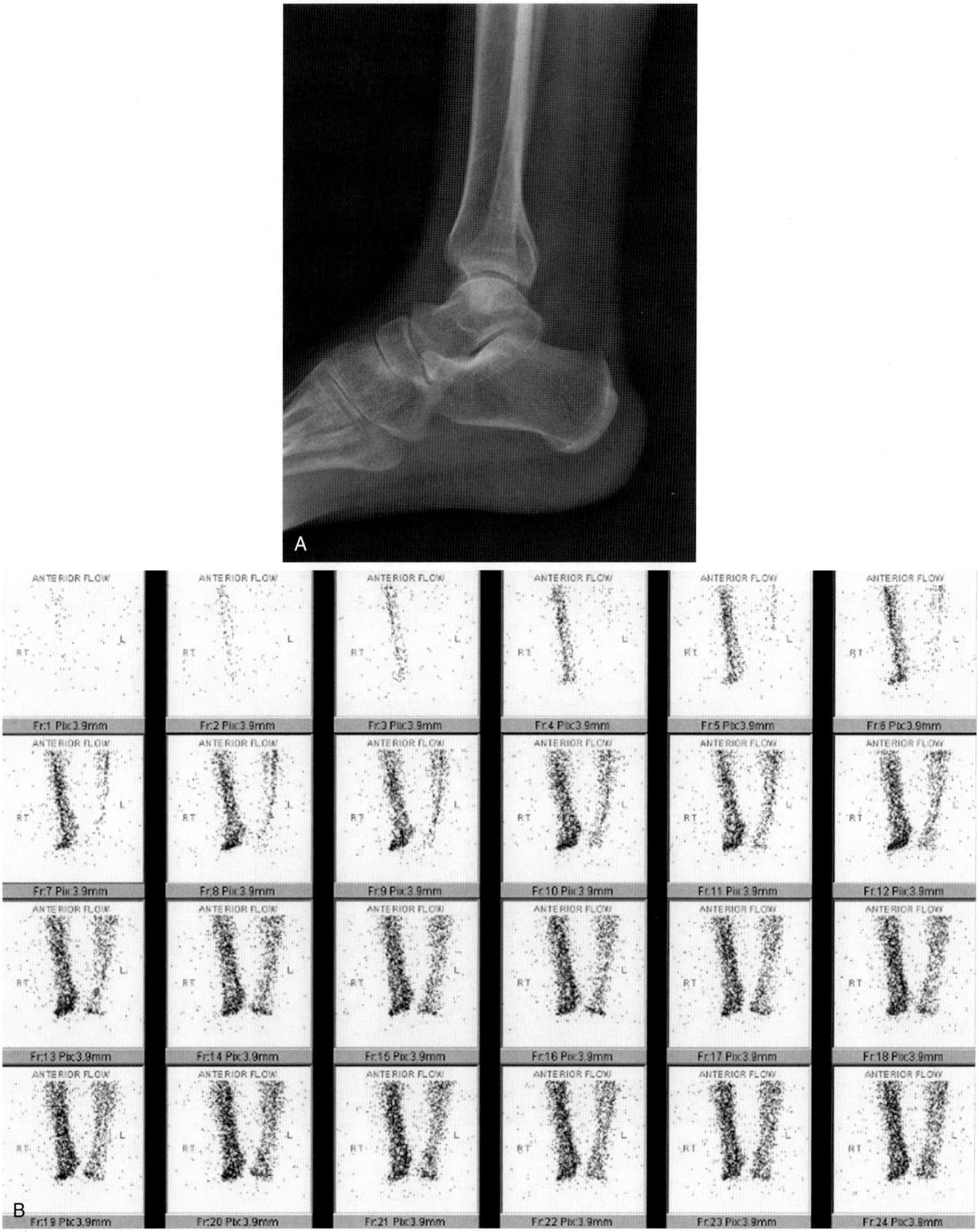

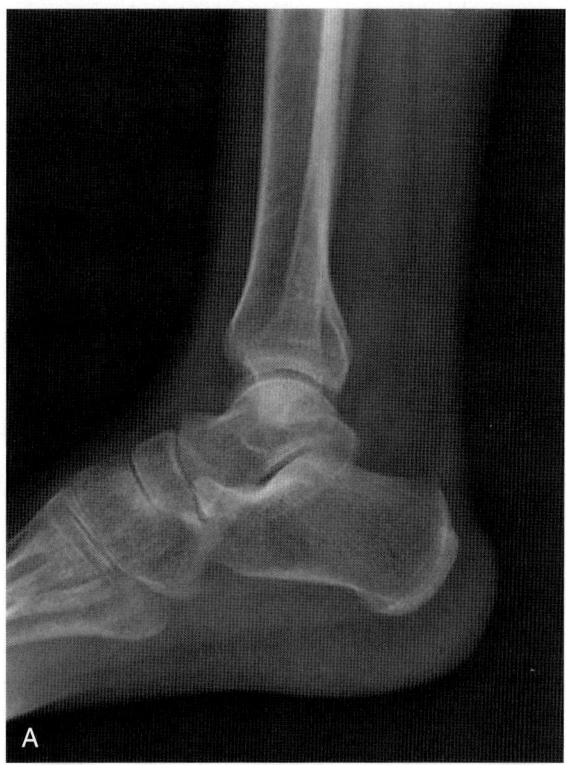

FIGURE 32-3. RSD: scintigraphic findings. This 35-year-old female presented three weeks following a twisting injury of her ankle with continued right ankle pain. A clinical diagnosis was made of reflex sympathetic dystrophy. **A,** Lateral radiograph obtained as part of a three-view series of the ankle showed mild posterior swelling. **B,** The patient had a whole-body bone scan performed. The flow portion of the exam shows increased flow unilaterally to the right lower extremity.

(Continued)

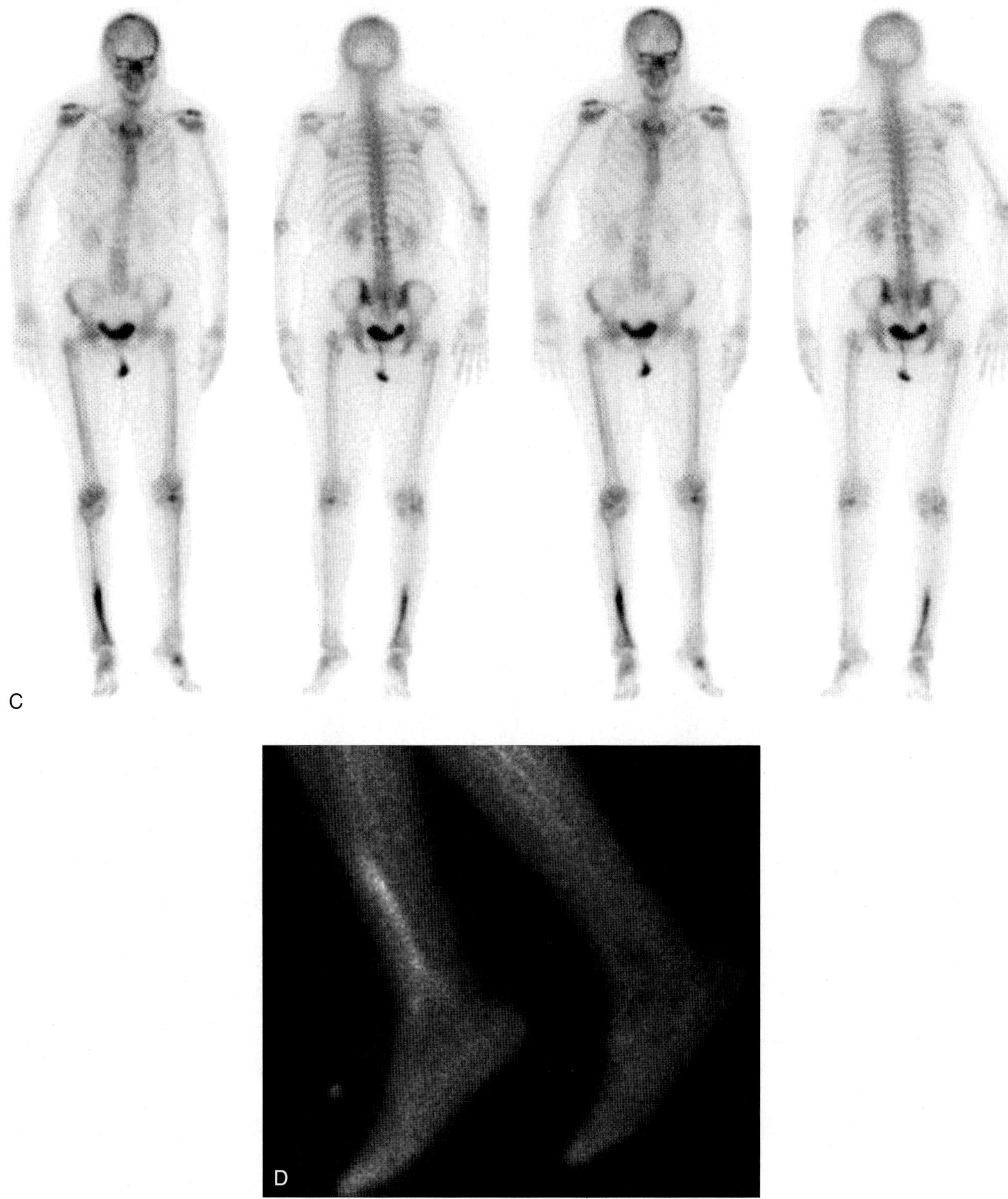

FIGURE 32-3—cont'd. **C** and **D,** The delayed images of the lower extremities show focal uptake in the periarticular region of the distal tibia consistent with the clinical diagnosis of RSD. No fracture was found.

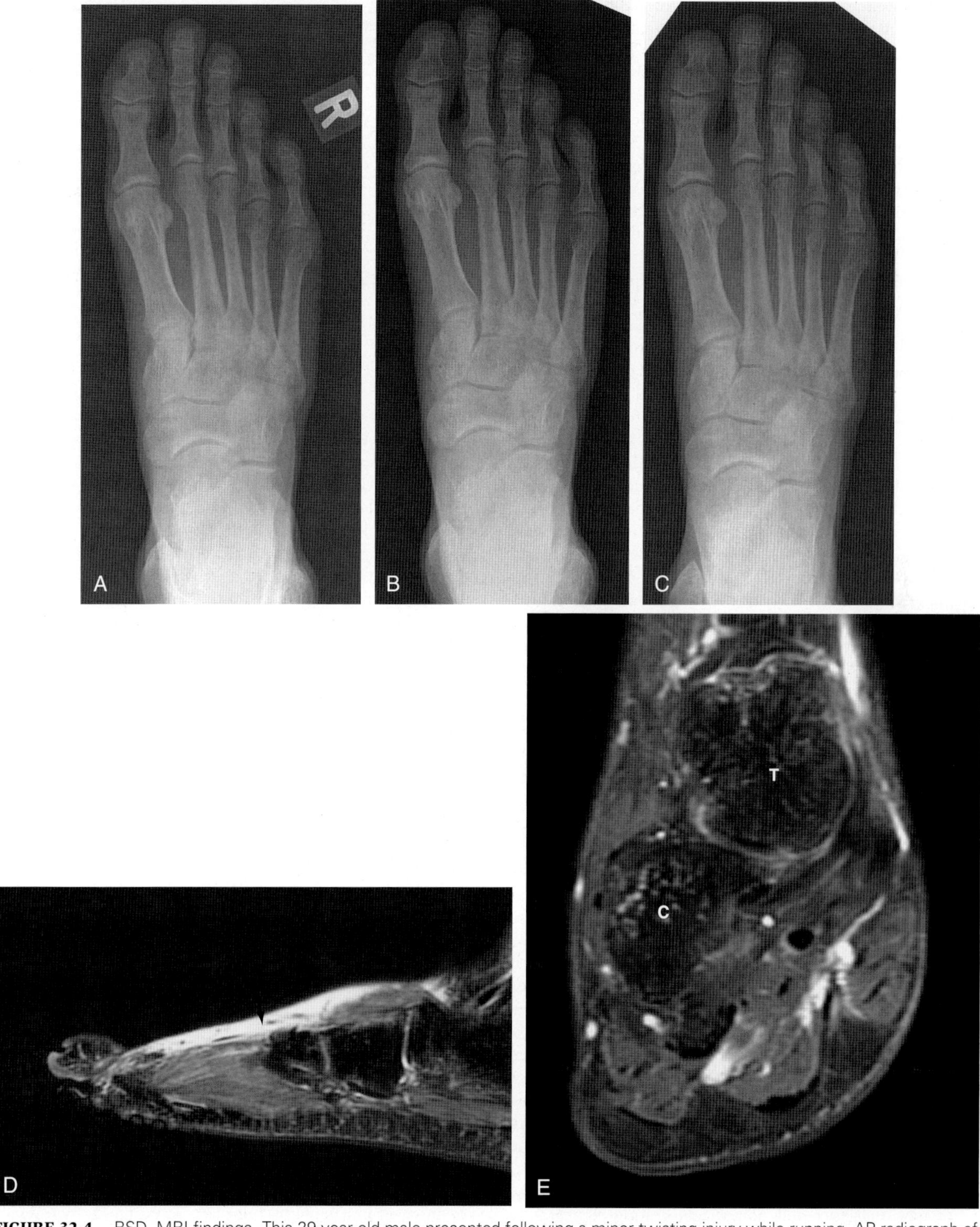

FIGURE 32-4. RSD, MRI findings. This 29-year-old male presented following a minor twisting injury while running. AP radiograph of the foot obtained following the injury **(A)** was normal. One month later **(B)**, and **C,** two months following the injury, there is progressive development of subcortical osteopenia. An MRI was ordered to evaluate for a possible occult stress fracture. **D,** T2-weighted fat suppressed image shows soft-tissue swelling *(arrow)* overlying the dorsal aspect of the foot. A coronal T1 fat-suppressed image post intravenous gadolunium administration **(E)** shows mild soft-tissue enhancement of the plantar aspect of the foot, as well as enhancing areas within, the tarsal bones (*T*, talus; *C*, calcaneus) that correlate with regions of periarticular osteoporosis on the radiographs. Based on these imaging findings and the clinical presentation, the diagnosis of RSD was made. The patient went on to full recovery three months later.

involvement, as well as spread from one part of a joint to another can occur in both disorders.[49] Similar scintigraphic findings are observed on bone scans in the two disorders.[48] Clinical improvement may also occur with sympathetic blocks in both disorders.[47]

A recently proposed hypothesis to explain the bone-marrow edema pattern observed on MRI is the regional accelerated phenomenon (RAP).[51] In this proposed mechanism, areas of normal bone metabolism are rapidly increased to function between 2 and 10 times their normal rate as a response to noxious stimuli. The noxious stimuli may include microtrauma such as microscopic trabecular fractures due to stress or excessive loading of a mildly osteoporotic bone. A prolonged, exaggerated RAP can activate multiple different foci, where the normal bone repair mechanisms are most active, resulting in multifocal disease evidenced by the development of bone marrow edema along with the patient's clinical symptoms.[51] Although there are multiple proposed mechanisms for this disease, a definite consensus is still lacking.

TABLE 32-2. Imaging Findings of RMO

Radiographs	Osteopenia (after 4–8 weeks)
	Cartilage space remains normal
	± wavy periosteal reaction
Scintigraphy	Increased activity on all three phases when disease is active.
	Blood flow and blood pool images may show decreased activity with healing.
MRI	Edema signal (low on T1W and high on T2W images) is seen in the bone marrow.
	Joint effusion.
	No cartilage loss.

Clinical Presentation

Clinically, patients with RMO have a moderate degree of tenderness over the affected joint, a joint effusion, and swelling with preservation of their full range of motion.[46] Patients describe a history of acute or gradually increasing monoarticular joint pain with no related trauma or injury.[47] The pain increases with weight bearing and reaches a maximum at approximately 2 months after the initial presentation.[52-54] Weight-bearing-induced pain often results in a limp. In the ensuing weeks or months after initial presentation, additional joints may become involved. Often this will occur as the symptoms in the originally affected joint are resolving. The time interval varies between recurrences and has been reported as long as up to 2 years after the initial presentation.[51] Usually the process progresses from adjacent joints, with the joint nearest the diseased one becoming the next to be affected. The clinically affected joints may overlap with more than one joint being affected at the same time, and rarely the same joint will be affected recurrently or with different parts of the joint being affected at different time intervals.[55]

An isolated portion of a joint being affected at one time was first described by Lequesne et al.,[52] and was given the name *partial transient osteoporosis.* Two types of partial transient osteoporosis have been described, including the radial type where one or two rays of the hand or foot are involved,[57] and the zonal type.[57,58] In the zonal type, when the knee is involved, the affected portion of the joint will only be either the medial or lateral femoral condyle.[58] Migration of the process to involve the entire joint or to involve another joint is observed. This migration in the zonal pattern resembles the classically described pattern of RMO.[47] Classically described as a disease of the extremities, recent reports have described involvement of the axial skeleton, with associated spinal osteoporosis, which may be advanced and result in collapse of vertebral segments due to insufficiency fractures.[59]

The clinical course can last up to nine months.[52,53] Treatment consists of oral analgesics and non–weight-bearing strategies, as well as watchful waiting. A report has described a relapse of the disease following complete resolution of the initial episode.[60]

Imaging

Radiographs

Radiographs will remain normal within the first several weeks (Table 32-2). Four to eight weeks will be required to see visible changes, following the onset of symptoms,[61] since osteopenia, which has begun with the initial presentation, is not yet severe enough until then for detection.[47] Variable but often severe osteopenia will develop in the affected joint. The osteopenia progresses rapidly, subsequently diminishes, and then appears at other sites. In advanced cases, periarticular osteoporosis can be observed extending a large distance from the joint. Occasionally wavy periosteal bone formation can be seen along the shafts of tubular bones.[47] The joint space is preserved which helps in differentiating this process from the advanced stages of avascular necrosis.[46] Following the resolution of symptoms, bone remineralization occurs spontaneously after a 6-month to 8-month period.[47]

Bone Scintigraphy

Initially in this disease process, there is increased activity in all three phases of the three-phase bone scan. This activity can be appreciated a few days after the onset of the patient's symptoms, but before radiographic changes are evident.[62] As the patient's symptoms improve, the degree of hyperemia to the affected joint decreases, which is reflected as a relative decrease in the amount of activity on the perfusion and blood pool phases of the three-phase bone scan, when compared with the patient's initial examination. There continues to be persistent uptake in the delayed phase of the examination due to the osteoblastic activity.[63] This abnormality may be observed for months after the patient's initial positive examination.

Magnetic Resonance Imaging

A diffuse bone marrow edema pattern can be observed with MRI, which can be detected as soon as 48 hours following the onset of clinical symptoms, similar to the three-phase bone scan. The changes are characterized by a homogeneous, ill defined area of mildly decreased signal on T1-weighted images and high signal on T2-weighted images[64] (Figure 32-5). These signal characteristics are thought to correspond to an increase in free water or edema within the fatty bone marrow. These marrow changes always abut the articular cartilage of the affected joint and extend into the metaphysis where the transition to normal marrow is ill-defined.[63,65] In the femur, the marrow changes are generally seen affecting the head, neck, and intertrochanteric region.[66] In the knee, the changes are observed more frequently in the lateral condyle[67] (Figure 32-6). The tarsal bones are commonly affected, but the metatarsal bones will rarely be involved.[68] A small joint effusion may be observed in the affected joints.[47] Following symptomatic and supportive therapy a regression of the MRI signal abnormalities can be seen without the persistence of identifiable abnormalities within the bone marrow.[69]

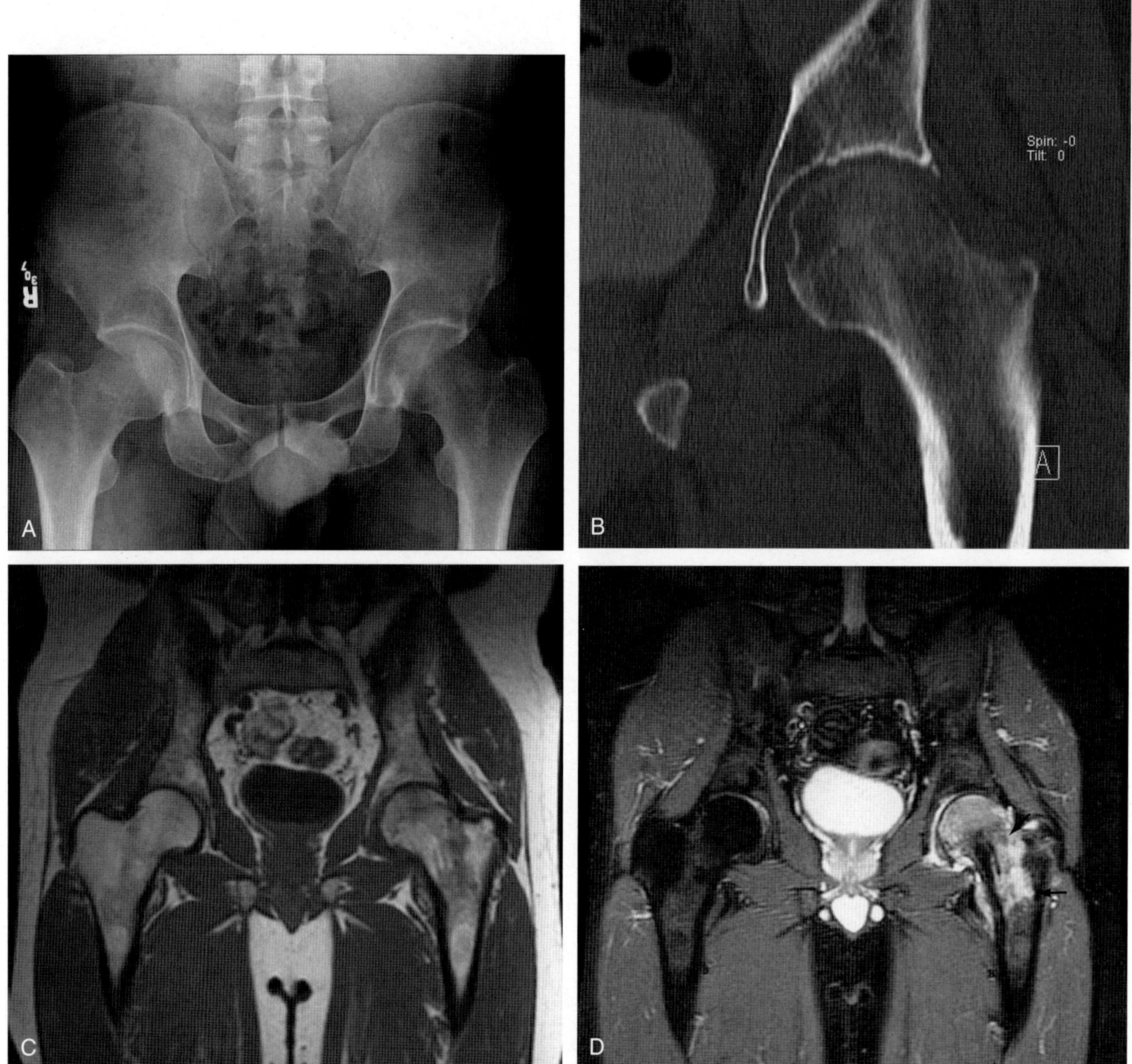

FIGURE 32-5. Regional migratory osteoporosis. Forty-eight-year-old male with an acute onset of left hip pain. Radiographs of the pelvis **(A)** show focal osteopenia involving the left femoral head without associated fracture, sclerosis, subchondral lucency, or osseous collapse to suggest AVN. A CT was performed in further evaluation of this patient **(B)**, confirming focal osteopenia without fracture. MRI of the hips was performed with focal decreased T1 signal within the left femoral head **(C)** with corresponding increased T2 signal **(D)** consistent with the edema associated with regional migratory osteoporosis.

Differential Diagnosis

Differential considerations for migratory periarticular osteoporosis include crystal-induced arthropathy, rheumatoid arthritis, and infectious arthritis.[61] The key finding that differentiates RMO from these other arthritides is the preservation of the joint space in RSD. Other considerations for pain include primary bone tumors, metastatic disease, tuberculosis of the bone, osteomyelitis, multiple myeloma, and metabolic bone disease, but these all can be differentiated from RMO by the characteristic imaging findings, classical clinical presentation, and normal laboratory studies in RSD.[51]

Also included in the differential diagnosis is RSD. This can usually be excluded because patients with RSD will have a preceding history of trauma or prior surgical intervention.[47] When imaging RSD, the bone scan and MRI will have a different pattern of involvement than observed in RMO with alterations in uptake/signal abnormalities in the bone, as well as the regional soft tissues.[61]

Avascular necrosis (AVN)/osteonecrosis in its early phase must be differentiated from RMO since these two entities have very different therapeutic approaches.[61] Avascular necrosis is a progressive condition that will lead to significant joint destruction that ultimately requires surgical intervention and repair, whereas RMO is a treatable condition. In the early stages, these two entities are difficult to differentiate. When patients present early, the radiographs will not be helpful in revealing the underlying pathology.[70]

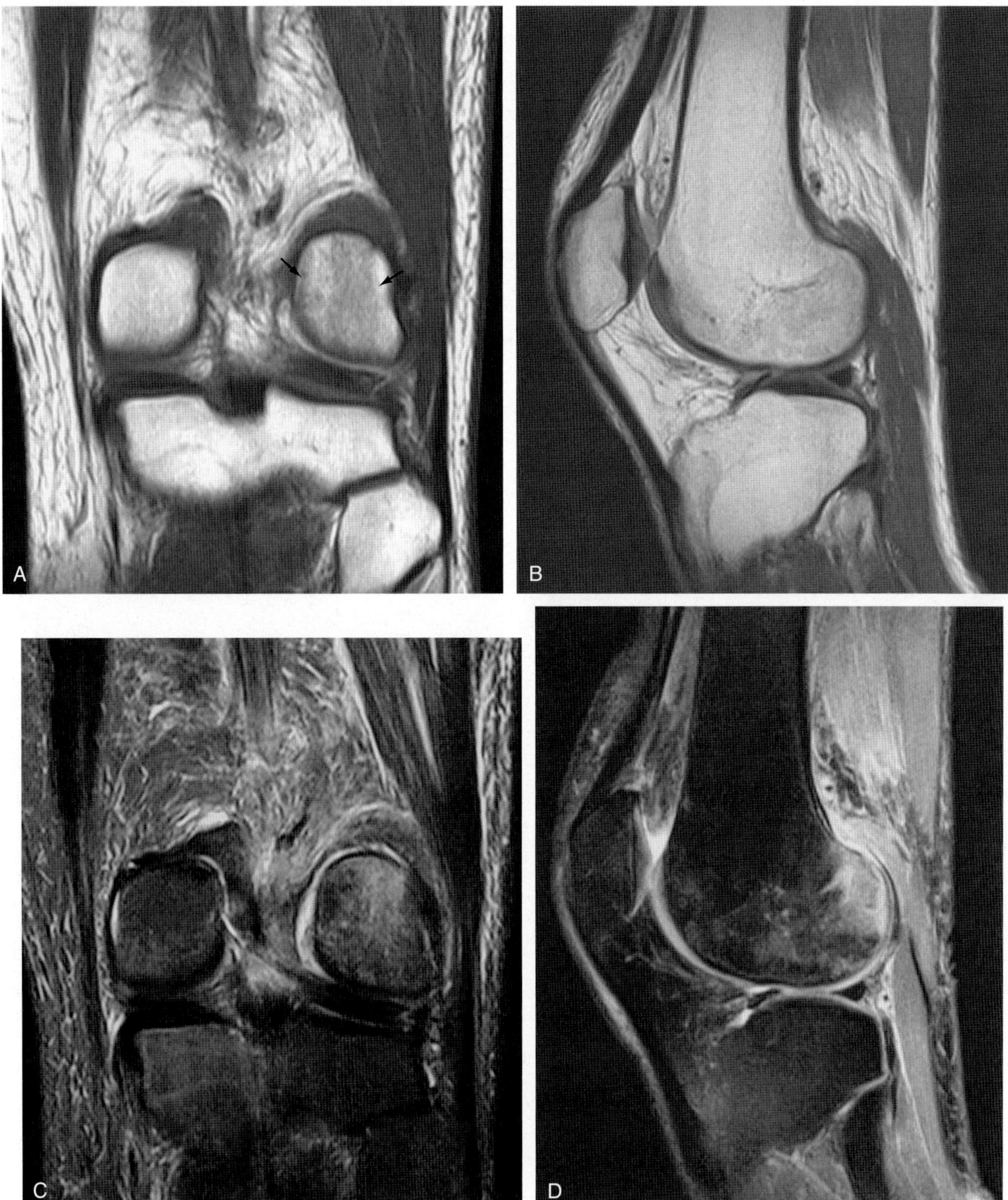

FIGURE 32-6. RMO. This 42-year-old male presented with left lateral knee pain and no known history of knee injury. Three months prior, the patient had a 2-week history of left hip pain that resolved after 2 weeks. An MRI was performed to evaluate for meniscal injury. The menisci were both intact. **A,** coronal and **(B)** sagittal T1-weighted images show replacement of normal fatty marrow in the lateral femoral condyle by poorly defined intermediate signal *(arrows)* consistent with edema. **C,** coronal and **(D)** sagittal T2-weighted images show increased (bright) signal in the lateral femoral condyle. Based on the patient's history and the imaging findings, RMO was the presumed diagnosis.

On bone scintigraphy, the uptake patterns may also be similar in the two conditions.[61] Occasionally in osteonecrosis, the uptake may be less intense and is limited to the affected joint; if a cold spot appeared over the joint, it would be pathognomonic for osteonecrosis and this will never be seen with regional migratory osteoporosis.[61] Above all, the most useful tool in the differentiation of these entities is MRI.[61] Although bone marrow edema may be present in both conditions, the presence of a well-demarcated lesion in the femoral head with a classic "double-line" sign is essentially pathognomonic for osteonecrosis making the distinction from regional migratory osteoporosis straightforward in most cases (Table 32-3).[70]

OSTEOGENESIS IMPERFECTA

Osteogenesis imperfecta is a spectrum of genetic disorders that are characterized by connective tissue defects that affect the osseous structures, their adjacent ligaments, the overlying skin, the sclera, and the dentin.[71] Osteogenesis imperfecta is the most common genetic cause of osteoporosis.[72] In most cases, there is a reduction in the production or the synthesis of normal type I collagen as a result of a mutation in the type I collagen genes (COL1A1 and COL1A2), which are found on chromosome 7.[73] Type I collagen comprises 90% of the organic matrix of bone.[74] Together with type I collagen, the type II and type III forms help comprise the majority of extracellular connective tissues including skin, bones, tendons, ligaments, and cartilage.[74] Cells with this mutation produce a mixture of both normal and abnormal collagen. While a majority of cases arise from this mutation, there are other patients in whom such mutations are absent or a mutation in a different gene is the causative event.[75] Throughout medical history, osteogenesis imperfecta has been known by many different names, including osteopsathyrosis, Vrolik's disease, fragilitas ossium, mollities ossium, Lobstein's disease, and van der Hoeve syndrome.[76]

The severity of this disease varies greatly, ranging from intrauterine fractures resulting in death to very mild forms without fractures.[77] The clinical diagnosis of osteogenesis imperfecta is based primarily upon the presence of osteoporosis with abnormal fragility of the skeleton, blue sclera, dentinogenesis imperfecta (grey teeth), hyperlaxity of the ligaments and skin, hearing impairment, and the presence of Wormian bones on skull radiographs.

TABLE 32-3. Comparison of Imaging Features of Transient Regional Osteoporosis and Osteonecrosis

	Transient Regional Osteoporosis (TOH/RMO)	Osteonecrosis
Affected individuals	Middle-aged males. Pregnant women.	Patients with predisposing causes (e.g., corticosteroids).
Symptoms	Acute onset.	Acute onset.
Radiograph	Normal initially, then osteopenia. Normal cartilage space. 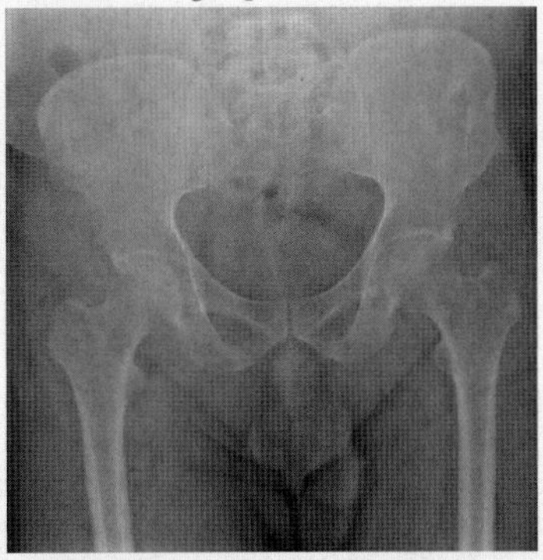	Normal initially. Crescent sign. Eventual collapse and secondary osteoarthritis. 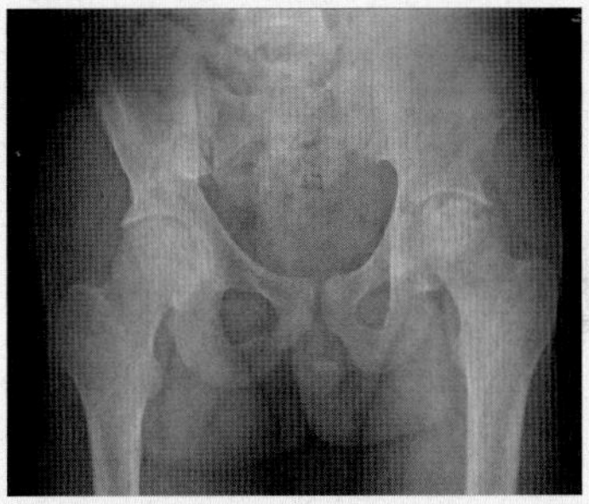
Scan	Increased uptake on all three phases.	May have "cold" area initially. Usually increased uptake on all three phases.
MRI	Edema-like signal (*arrow*). Joint effusion with variable low signal line on T2W sequences. 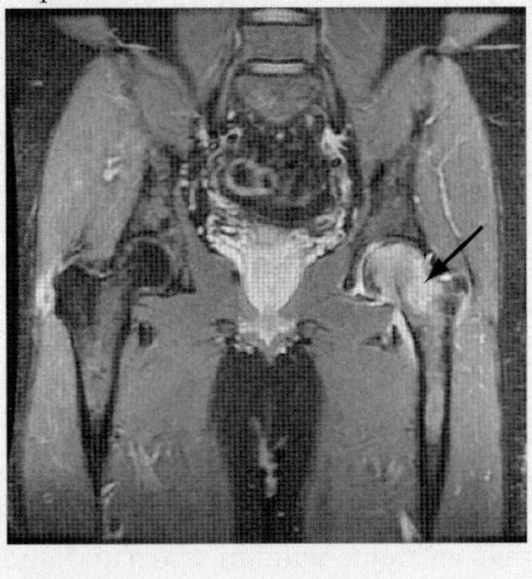	Focal signal abnormalities (*arrow*, with a peripheral rim, double-line sign). Marrow edema-like signal may be present. Late-stage collapse and osteoarthritis 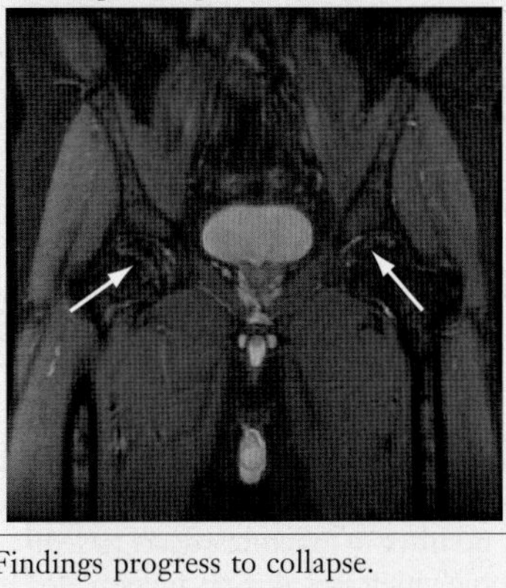
Course	Findings resolve.	Findings progress to collapse.

Wormian bones, named after Ole Worm, Danish physician and anatomist (1588-1654), are intersutural bones in the skull that are seen in osteogenesis imperfecta, as well as in a few other uncommon disorders.

BOX 32-2. Selected Clinical Features of Type I Osteogenesis Imperfecta

- Blue sclerae
- Fractures
- Ligamentous laxity
- +/− dentinogenesis imperfecta
- Thin skin
- Easy bruising
- Hernias
- Mitral valve prolapse, aortic insufficiency

Traditionally, great emphasis has been placed on the presence of blue sclera and dentinogenesis imperfecta as the diagnostic signs, but the limitations of these signs should be understood. Dark or bluish sclera is typical in healthy infants. Dentinogenesis imperfecta is more frequently clinically evident in the primary than in permanent teeth of patients with osteogenesis imperfecta.[78] The clinical hearing loss frequently described is rarely found in the first two decades of life, even though subtle audiometric abnormalities may be identified in a large proportion of children with osteogenesis imperfecta.[79] Almost 50% of patients with osteogenesis imperfecta who are older than 50 years of age report hearing loss with an even higher percentage having abnormal audiometric testing.[79] The diagnosis of osteogenesis imperfecta is straightforward in patients with a family history or in those patients with several "typical" features, but the clinical diagnosis often proves difficult in cases where there are no affected family members and when bone fragility is not associated with obvious extraskeletal manifestations.

The diagnosis of osteogenesis imperfecta depends on characteristic skeletal and extraskeletal manifestations in a patient with a positive family history or by evaluation of the collagen type I gene. In these difficult situations, analysis of the collagen type I gene may be helpful. DNA may also be obtained from the white blood cells, and the coding region of the COL1A1 and COL1A2 genes can be screened for mutations to help to make this diagnosis.[80]

Due to the wide spectrum of the disease and the interfamilial and intrafamilial variability, classification is difficult. One of the first attempts at classification was performed by Looser in 1906, in which he divided the disease into two forms[81]: "congenita" and "tarda," depending on the severity of the presentation. In the congenital form, multiple fractures may occur in utero, whereas in the tarda form, fractures happen at the time of birth or later. This classification is no longer valid because it fails to encompass the vast clinical variability associated with this disorder. Many other attempts at classification have been made, but currently, the most commonly used is the one initially proposed by Sillence in 1979.[82] He initially divided patients into four types (I to IV), although it is now recognized that there are more types of osteogenesis imperfecta.[83-85] This classification system is useful, however, to assess prognosis and help assess the effects of therapeutic interventions.

Osteogenesis imperfecta type I is an autosomal dominant disease that is characterized by blue sclera, increased tendency to sustain fractures, and ligamentous laxity due to the underlying genetic defect in the synthesis of type I collagen. It is the most common, as well as the mildest form of this disease, with 60% of osteogenesis imperfecta patients belonging to this group.[86] There is significant variability in the presentation of these patients, suggesting that there are factors other than just the type and the location of the collagen gene mutation that will influence the clinical phenotype (Box 32-2). In the mild cases, only a few fractures or mild osteopenia will be observed, but in severe cases, numerous fractures will be present. The osseous fragility results in an increase in the number of fractures, especially in the lower extremities. Most patients are of normal height or within two standard deviations of the norm. The observation of fractures is rare in the perinatal period, and they are found most commonly in the period from childhood to puberty. The number of fractures decreases throughout adulthood and then often increases during menopause in women and after the sixth decade in men. These patients also suffer from early hearing loss and maintain blue sclera throughout their life.

An attempt has been made to further subdivide type I based on the presence of dentinogenesis imperfecta. If present, the patient is subclassified as type IB and if absent, type IA.[87] Unfortunately, this classification is controversial because there is no clear cutoff in the spectrum of detinogenesis imperfecta and because of this, detection of cases of mild detinogenesis imperfecta causes difficulty in the assignment of the patient to a specific group.[88] Patients with associated dentinogenesis imperfecta usually have a more severe form of the disease with greater fracture rates and more pronounced growth retardation.[89]

The extraskeletal manifestations of osteogenesis imperfecta type I are found in other collagen-containing tissues such as the sclera, cornea, skin, heart valves, and tendons, which show an overall reduction in the amount and thickness of the collagen. As a result, these patients will present clinically with thin skin, hernias, and joint hypermobility. They have a tendency to bruise and bleed easily due to fragility of the blood vessels.[90] Mitral valve prolapse, aortic valve insufficiency, and even dilation of the aortic root have been reported.[91] Patients with osteogenesis imperfecta type I usually have a normal life span and die of an unrelated illness.[92]

Osteogenesis imperfecta type II is the most severe form of the disease. This subtype is characterized by dwarfism and severe bone deformities.[93] Newborns will have soft calvarial bones, a distinctive triangular face, blue sclera, and a beaked nose. A narrow thorax with short and deformed limbs containing multiple fractures is also observed.[93] Death usually occurs in the neonatal period due to pulmonary infection or cardiac disease with survival beyond this period being extremely rare.[94] Osteogenesis imperfecta type II has also been associated with perivenous microcalcifications and impaired neuronal migration.[95]

Osteogenesis imperfecta type III is observed in approximately 20% of patients with osteogenesis imperfecta.[96] A majority of infants who are born with fractures and deformity who survive the perinatal period belong to this group. Osteogenesis imperfecta type III is usually identified at birth because the intrauterine fractures result in deformities of the long bones and severe skeletal changes including advanced kyphoscoliosis, as well as other thoracic deformities. The long bones are severely bowed and the altered structure of the epiphysis leads to a "popcorn appearance."[97] Most of these patients have intrauterine growth retardation with progressive growth failure continuing throughout childhood. The growth failure is due to the long bone deformities and spinal involvement. These patients exhibit the most dramatic dwarfing of all osteogenesis imperfecta cases.[86] Many of these patients have large, asymmetric heads with the face appearing triangular in shape with an associated underdevelopment of the facial bones.[97] In infancy, the sclera is often pale blue, but regains its normal color by puberty. Dentinogenesis imperfecta is observed in more than 80% of these patients' primary dentition.[98] Early mortality in these patients is due to respiratory illness or to complications from basilar invagination or injury.

Osteogenesis imperfecta type IV is an autosomal dominant form that differs from type I by the patients having normal or slightly grayish sclera, shorter stature, and commonly dentinogenesis imperfecta. The severity of the osseous manifestations is intermediate between osteogenesis imperfecta types I and III. Even though there is no intrauterine growth retardation, postnatal growth velocity is reduced.[99] This group is further subdivided into group A and B according to the presence of dentinogenesis imperfecta, type A if absent and type B if present (as above).[100] There is interfamilial and intrafamilial heterogeneity. A small proportion of these patients will present with fractures at birth. The frequency of fractures is usually greatest in the period from childhood to puberty and then increases once again at menopause in females and in the sixth decade in males, similar to type I. In these patients, new deformities in both the upper and lower extremities will develop during the first 10 years of life.[99] Muscle strength is mainly decreased in the proximal muscles of the upper and lower extremities. Many of these patients will develop the ability to ambulate, but the ability to continue ambulation may be lost due to progressive spinal deformity. In a minority of these patients, there is a progressive kyphoscoliosis that may lead to severe cardiopulmonary, as well as neurological complications.[101] Basilar impression has been observed in 71% of patients with osteogenesis imperfecta type IV B, with 50% showing signs of compression of structures of the posterior fossa, including hypotonia with communicating hydrocephalus.[101] Overall, the life expectancy in this group of patients is only minimally impaired.[92]

Osteogenesis imperfecta type V is characterized by white sclera, moderate to severe bone fragility, and osteopenia with the frequent development of hypertrophic callus with fracture healing. None of these patients has dentinogenesis imperfecta. Fractures usually occur following the initiation of ambulation.[102] In the patients who have a family history of this disorder, there is an autosomal dominant pattern of transmission.[102] Other associated findings include calcification of the interosseous membrane of the forearm and radiodense metaphyseal bands.[75]

Glorieux et al.[85] described another group of eight patients initially diagnosed with type IV who shared unique and common features. In these patients, fractures were initially documented between 4 and 18 months of age. The sclera was white, and dentinogenesis imperfecta was absent. All patients had vertebral compression fractures. This group was defined by the histologic findings in bone, which contained a higher amount of osteoid than usual and had an abnormal pattern of lamellation.[75] This subtype of osteogenesis imperfecta was classified as type VI. It is felt that osteogenesis imperfecta type VI is a moderate to severe form of the disease with accumulation of osteoid due to a mineralization defect with no disturbance of mineral metabolism; the underlying genetic defect remains to be determined. The mode of inheritance remains unknown.

Recently, type VII was described in a community of Native Americans in northern Quebec. Besides the fragility of the bone, rhizomelia is a prominent feature.[103] Unlike other forms of osteogenesis imperfecta, this subtype exhibits an autosomal recessive form of inheritance.[75]

Imaging

Overall, the most characteristic finding on radiographic examination in osteogenesis imperfecta is a diffuse decrease in osseous density involving both the axial and appendicular skeleton[103] (Figure 32-7) (Box 32-3). Of course the degree of this osteopenia is variable across the spectrum of the disease. Due to the underlying deformity in the matrix structure of the collagen and the disordered alignment and binding of mineral salts to the matrix, a rapid loss of bone mass may be observed in middle-aged patients in addition to the underlying osteoporosis.[105]

Fairbank attempted to classify osteogenesis imperfecta patients based on radiographic findings.[106] The group was divided into

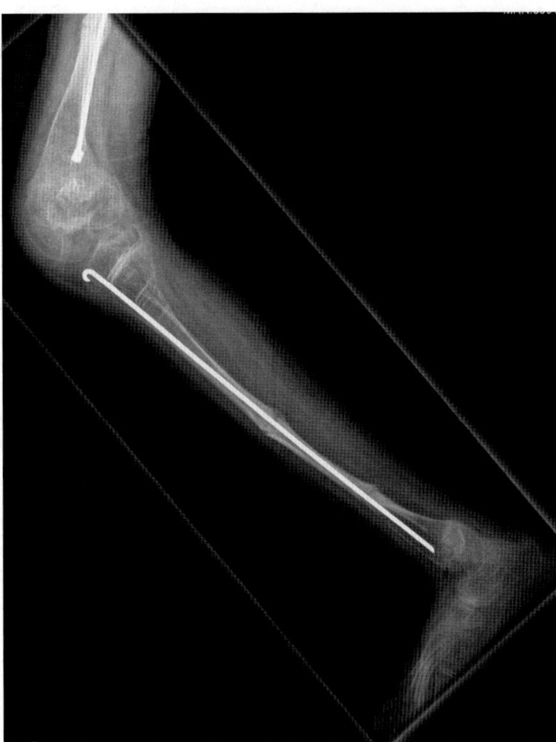

FIGURE 32-7. Osteogenesis imperfecta type 1. A lateral radiograph of the lower leg shows diffuse osteopenia involving the entire lower extremity of this patient. A gracile appearance is seen in the long bones. There are healing fractures in both the femur and tibia. The patient has undergone placement of intramedullary rods to help decrease the amount of osseous deformity and to aid in mobility.

BOX 32-3. Possible Imaging Findings of Osteogenesis Imperfecta

- Osteopenia
- Thin gracile bones
- Short thick bones
- Cystic bone changes
- Wormian bones
- Fractures
- Hyperplastic callus
- Osseous deformities resulting from multiple fractures:
  - Bowing of long bones
  - Radial head dislocations
  - Protrusio acetabuli
  - Coxa valga
  - Genu valgum
- Enlarged sinuses and mastoids
- Skull deformity (platybasia, basilar invagination)
- Kyphoscoliosis, vertebral flattening
- "Popcorn" calcification

three subcategories. The first was patients with thin, gracile bones. A majority of patients belonged to this group, and it included patients classified as Sillence type I and mildly affected type IV. The second group comprised patients with short, thick limbs, which is seen in Sillence types II and III. This is usually associated with micromelia, and overall it carries a poor prognosis. The third category, which included the smallest number of patients, was defined by patients having cystic changes in their extremities. This was seen in the most severely affected patients with flared metaphyses that are hyperlucent and contain coarse trabeculae. Bauze et al. have suggested that the cystic appearance is due to an abnormal stress pattern with resulting altered modeling of bone.[107] As with all classifications systems, difficulties arise in attempting to place a patient in a single distinct category. These groups are not fixed, and during times of active growth, bones may change appearance.[106] For example, patients of the Sillence type II or III who survive the neonatal period may progress from the second category to the first category.

The hallmark of osteogenesis imperfecta is fractures of the extremities. These are most frequently observed in the lower extremity and are transverse in nature.[104] An occasional avulsion fracture may also be observed due to normal muscle stresses at their insertions. Osseous deformities result from multiple fractures, including bowing of the long bones (Figure 32-8), radial head dislocations, protrusio acetabuli, coxa vera, genu valgum, and scoliosis, can all be observed. Micromelia and bowing deformities of the extremities are usually due to multiple fractures that occur during the gestational period[104] (Figure 32-9). The telescoping fractures in the long bones result in limb length discrepancies.[108]

Fracture healing is usually normal, but large amounts of callus, "tumoral callus," and pseudarthrosis can be observed. Tumoral callus must be differentiated from osteosarcoma, which is rarely associated with osteogenesis imperfecta. These two entities may contain many similar radiographic findings. Many authors propose using computed tomography (CT) and/or MRI to better evaluate the lesion and to help to identify a fracture line that would rule out osteosarcoma.[109,110] Occasionally, as observed in Sillence type V patients, excessive callus formation may be present. This will be observed after fracture or surgical intervention. Excessive callus formation has also been observed in association with Sillence types III and IV.[111] Clinically, when this is present, these patients will have low-grade fevers, swelling, and pain associated with tenderness upon palpation at the healing site.[104]

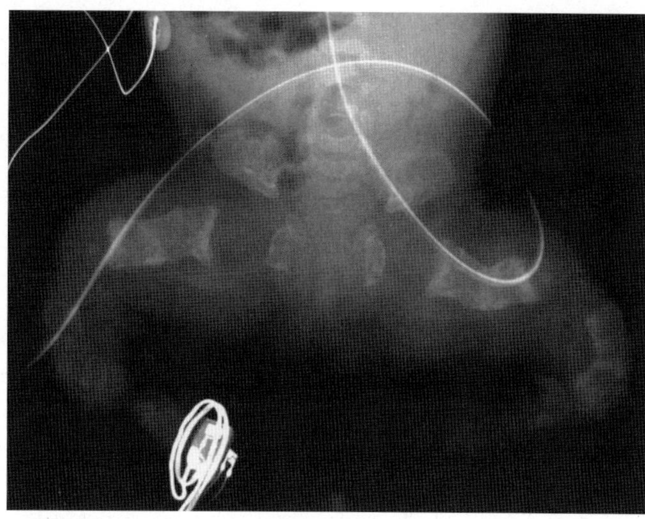

FIGURE 32-9. Osteogenesis imperfecta type II. A radiograph of this newborn with osteogenesis imperfecta type II, shows marked shortening of the long bones of the lower extremities with bowing due to multiple fractures sustained in utero.

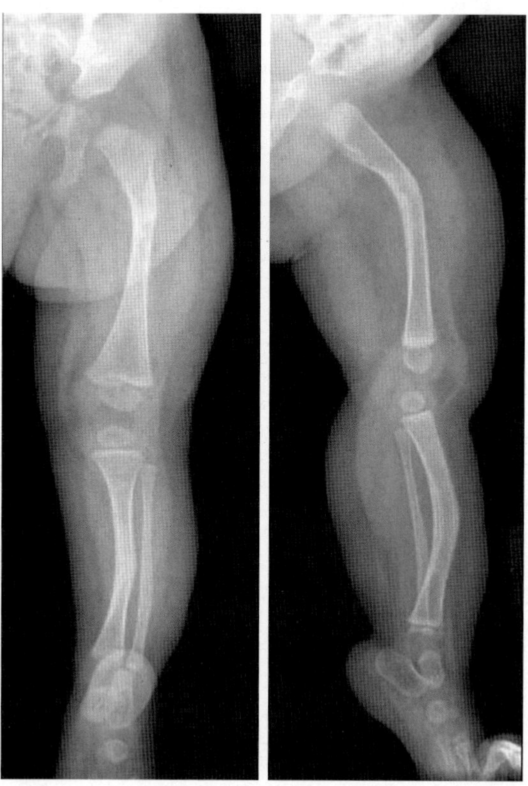

FIGURE 32-8. Osteogenesis imperfecta type I. **A,** Anteroposterior left and **(B)** lateral radiographs of the leg show bowing of the femur and tibia due to multiple healed fractures in this patient with osteogenesis imperfecta.

In children with severe sequelae of osteogenesis imperfecta, the metaphysis or epiphysis of the long bones may contain clusters of scalloped radiolucent areas with sclerotic margins, known as "popcorn calcifications" (Figure 32-10). These are thought to represent detached fragments of the cartilage growth plate.[108] These may first be observed in childhood during active skeletal growth and resolve during adolescence.[108] They are seen in both the epiphysis and metaphysis in close approximation to the growth plate, and their appearance coincides with a variable irregularity or disappearance of the normal horizontal lucency of the growth plate. Popcorn calcifications are seen more frequently in the lower extremities (87%) than the upper extremities.[108]

The joints of the extremities are affected primarily in two ways.[104] The first is due to multiple fractures at the articular surface that result in premature degeneration of the joint. The second is due to ligamentous laxity that results in minor trauma and damage to the hyaline cartilage, which also causes premature degeneration. These sequelae are most commonly seen in Sillence types I and III.[104]

Transient osteoporosis has rarely been observed in patients with osteogenesis imperfecta. Approximately 20 cases have been reported, and this diagnosis should be considered when an osteogenesis imperfecta patient presents with sudden onset of groin or hip pain and a new limp but no visible fracture.[112] Radiographs will show localized osteopenia on examination at least two weeks after the onset of symptoms. Bone scintigraphy will display marked radiotracer accumulation at the affected joint as early as 48 hours after the clinical onset. MRI demonstrates the findings

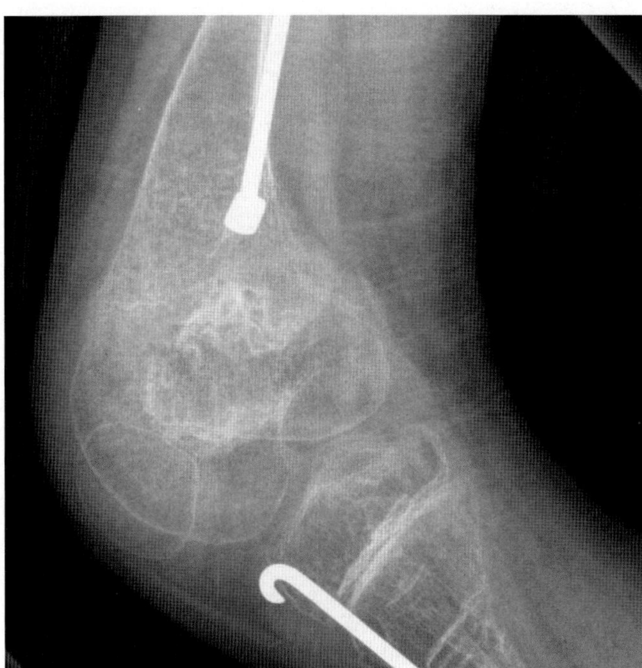

FIGURE 32-10. Osteogenesis imperfecta type I. A lateral radiograph shows multiple small "popcorn calcifications" in the distal femur with blurring and irregularity at the growth plate. This patient has had intramedullary rods placed to help attain greater mobility. (Same patient as in Figure 32-7.)

of edema-like marrow signal around the affected joint and may also be useful by excluding other pathologic processes.[112] These patients may go on to develop a migratory pattern and even have simultaneous or sequential involvement of both hips.[113]

Typical findings observed when evaluating the skull include enlarged frontal and mastoid sinuses with an increase in the number of Wormian bones[71] (Figure 32-11). Wormian bones are small, irregular, intersutural fragments that result from ununited portions of the primary ossification centers of adjacent membranous bones. At least 10 of these fragments must be present and arranged in a mosaic pattern to be considered an abnormal finding.[116] Also frequently observed is platybasia with or without basilar invagination. In basilar invagination, deformity of the skull base may cause impingement on the foramen magnum. On CT or MRI, associated hydrocephalus may also be observed. In patients with premature otosclerosis, thin-section CT will display proliferation of the bony labyrinth that may narrow the middle ear cavity, obliterate the round and oval windows, and envelop the stapes foot plate. Flattening of the cochlea may also be observed.[117] In those patients with dentinogenesis imperfecta, there is a decrease in the junction between the crown and root prior to eruption, as well as absent or enlarged pulp chambers observed on dental radiographs.[104]

Many changes in the spine can be observed. Most commonly, there is flattening of the vertebral bodies, which become biconcave or wedge-shaped anteriorly.[118] In almost 40% of osteogenesis imperfecta patients, severe kyphoscoliosis will be observed.[119] This results from a combination of ligamentous laxity, osteoporosis, and post-traumatic damage to the growth plates, as well as compression fractures. The abnormal spinal curvature begins at a young age and continues to progress throughout childhood and beyond puberty,[119] and when superimposed on multiple rib fractures, may result in a compromise of respiratory function[119] (Figure 32-12). The spinal curvature usually is refractory to

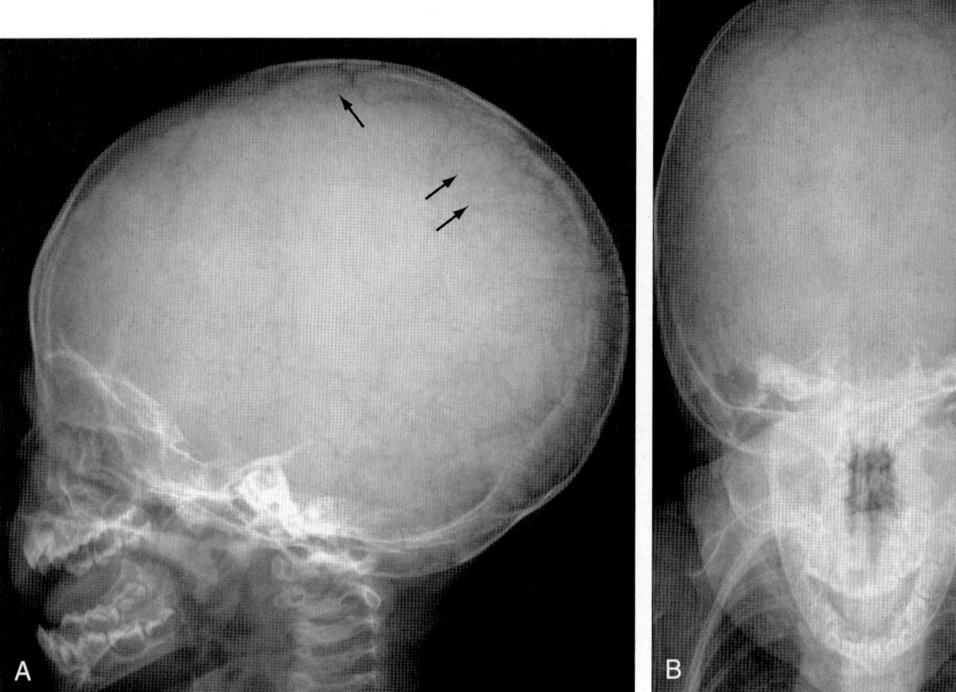

FIGURE 32-11. Osteogenesis imperfecta type I. **A,** lateral and **B,** frontal radiographs of the skull of a neonate with osteogenesis imperfecta illustrate the numerous "Wormian bones" *(arrows)* present within the sutures.

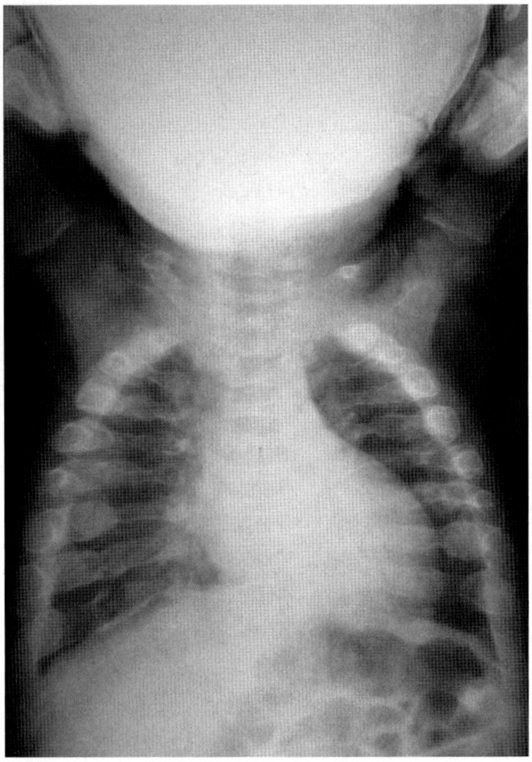

FIGURE 32-12. Osteogenesis imperfecta type I. This neonate with osteogenesis imperfecta presented with difficulty in breathing. The chest radiograph demonstrates widened, irregular ribs due to multiple rib fractures.

bracing, and surgical repair is not usually an option due to the diffusely osteoporotic bone. Surgery is sometimes unavoidable in the most severe cases, due to the severe spinal deformity that interferes with normal respiration and the risk of the patient developing paraplegia.[104]

The pelvis will be narrowed and even triradiate in shape.[75] Protrusion deformities of the acetabula or even shepherd's crook deformities of the proximal femora may be observed. Overall protrusion of the acetabulum is seen in 30% of all patients with osteogenesis imperfecta, more frequently in those type III and IV patients and relatively rarely in type I patients.[108] (Severe pelvic deformities may result from the bilateral protrusion of the acetabulum that could result in a distal colonic obstruction or other nonspecific complaints of abdominal pain.[120] In the soft tissues adjacent to the pelvis, premature vascular calcifications may also be observed.)

On prenatal ultrasound, most cases of severe osteogenesis imperfecta can be detected[93] (Box 32-4).

> Most cases of severe osteogenesis imperfecta can be detected on prenatal ultrasound examination.

Differentiation among specific types is not possible with ultrasound. Munoz et al. first described the sonographic criteria to diagnose osteogenesis imperfecta prenatally.[93] These criteria include the presence of multiple fractures resulting in discontinuity, crumpling, or a "wrinkled" appearance of the long bones, severe demineralization of the calvaria with resulting easy visualization of the intracranial structures, and asymmetric shortening of the femoral length to greater than three standard deviations below the mean for the patient's gestational age. Other described sonographic findings include platyspondyly, "beaded," thickened ribs, a small thoracic circumference, and occasionally Wormian bones.[93] Sonography is useful in determining the fetal prognosis and in planning for delivery.

BOX 32-4. Ultrasound Findings in Intrauterine Osteogenesis Imperfecta

- Multiple fractures resulting in discontinuity, crumpling, or "wrinkled" appearance of the long bones
- Severe osteopenia of the calvaria with resulting easy visualization of the intracranial structures
- Asymmetric shortening of the femoral length to greater than three standard deviations below the mean for the patient's gestational age
- Wormian bones
- Small thoracic circumference
- "Beaded" thickened ribs
- Platyspondyly

Although very nonspecific and controversial in its application to osteogenesis imperfecta, bone mineral density measurements have been used to evaluate disease severity and as a predictor of the long-term functional outcomes for these patients.[121] It also has been used in monitoring therapeutic response in patients treated with bisphosphonates.[122]

Differential Diagnosis

Several primary skeletal disorders may be confused with osteogenesis imperfecta depending upon the amount of osteoporosis. These include idiopathic autosomal recessive hyperphosphatasia (juvenile Paget's disease), hypophosphatasia, Cole-Carpenter syndrome, idiopathic juvenile osteoporosis, and child abuse. Many of these conditions will have altered serum biochemical markers allowing for easy differentiation from osteogenesis imperfecta. Idiopathic autosomal recessive hyperphosphatasia is characterized by a marked increase in the rate of bone turnover and can usually be distinguished from osteogenesis imperfecta by these patients having very high serum alkaline phosphatase activity.[123] Hypophosphatasia also has a variable clinical expression with symptoms ranging from stillbirth without mineralized bone to pathological fractures that develop in adulthood.[124] Radiographically, these patents may have lucent bones and bowing of the extremities with associated metaphyseal changes that resemble rickets.[104] The Cole-Carpenter syndrome, described in only a few patients, is characterized by osteoporosis, short stature, craniosynostosis, and ocular proptosis, but these patients do not possess type 1 collagen mutations. Idiopathic juvenile osteoporosis is transient and usually develops prior to puberty. It is radiographically indistinguishable from osteogenesis imperfecta.[104] Most importantly spontaneous recovery usually occurs in these particular patients.

The other entities presenting with multiple fractures include congenital indifference to pain, scurvy, and Menke's kinky hair syndrome.

> Menke's kinky hair syndrome may mimic nonaccidental trauma but is due to abnormal copper metabolism (possibly decreased absorption) and has clinical manifestations that include brittle, kinky hair, tortuous arteries, seizures, and hypothermia.

The most important entity to exclude is that of the battered child syndrome (nonaccidental trauma). Child abuse is a frequent cause of fractures with the highest incidence during the first year of life.[125] A normal bone density at sites distant from the fractures, as well as a lack of other findings associated with osteogenesis imperfecta (dentinogenesis imperfecta and multiple Wormian bones) should suggest nonaccidental trauma. It is always better to err on the side of safety by recommending a full clinical evaluation of the child to exclude nonaccidental trauma.

It is most important to exclude nonaccidental trauma when evaluating a child with multiple fractures.

Treatment

Physical therapy and orthopedic surgery are the primary modes of treatment in patients with osteogenesis imperfecta.[126] The main goals of physical therapy are to improve mobility and prevent contractures and immobility-induced bone loss.[127] Recently treatment with bisphosphonates has been used to inhibit the function of osteoclasts and improve bone mineral density.[123] These drugs often improve mobility, decrease the patient's pain symptoms, and decrease fracture rates.[122] Unfortunately, many of the long-term outcomes of this medical therapy are unknown. Many new forms of treatment are currently being investigated, including bone marrow transplantation[123] and gene therapy.[127] In 1959, the Sofied procedure (multiple osteotomies and placement of intramedullary rods) was introduced to correct bowing and prevent fractures.[114] This has allowed sustained ambulation in more of these patients.

Osteotomies and intramedullary rodding of the lower extremities may allow ambulation in patients with deformities due to multiple fractures.

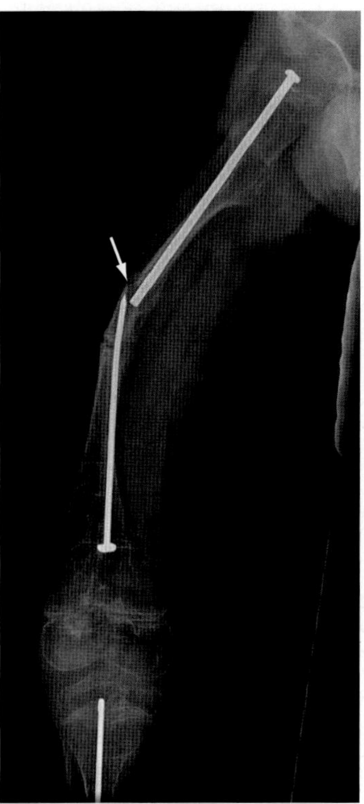

FIGURE 32-13. Osteogenesis imperfecta type I. This patient has outgrown the expandable intramedullary rod with resulting separation at the expansion site. A fracture with angular deformity (*arrow*) is present at the level of the separation. Another healing fracture is seen more distally.

Unfortunately, with this procedure some unique complications may occur, including fractures below or above the level of the intramedullary rod. If one end of the rod is found protruding into the joint, early degenerative changes may develop. The modification to this original procedure, the use of expanding rods, has decreased the frequency of reoperation as the child grows, but many of these complications are still present[87] (Figure 32-13).

References

1. Mitchell SW, Morehouse GR, Keen WW: *Gunshot Wounds and Other Injuries of Nerves*, Philadelphia, 1864, JB Lippincott.
2. Ward WW: Posttraumatic reflex sympathetic dystrophy. In Foy MA, Fagg PS (eds): *Medicolegal Reporting in Orthopaedic Trauma*, New York, 1995, Churchill Livingstone, pp 5.5-05-5.5-08.
3. Resnick D: Osteoporosis. In Resnick D (ed): *Diagnosis of Bone and Joint Disorders*, 4th ed, Philadelphia, 2002, WB Saunders, pp 1798-1804.
4. Stanton-Hicks M, Janig W, Hassenbusch S et al: Reflex sympathetic dystrophy: changing concepts and taxonomy. *Pain* 63:127-133, 1995.
5. Roberst CS, Gleis GE, Seligson D: Diagnosis and treatment of complications. In Browner BD, Levine AM, Jupiter JB et al (eds): *Skeletal Trauma*, 3rd ed, Philadelphia, 2003, Elsevier Science, pp 464-469.
6. Bickerstaff DR, Kqanis JA: Algodystrophy: An under-recognized complication of minor trauma, *Br J Rheumatol* 33:240, 1994.
7. Sarangi PP, Ward AJ, Smith EJ et al: Algodystrophy and osteoporosis after tibial fractures, *J Bone Joint Surg Br* 75:450-452, 1993.
8. Schwartzman RJ, McLellan TL: Reflex sympathetic dystrophy. A review, *Arch Neurol* 44:555, 1987.
9. Kozin R: Reflex sympathetic dystrophy syndrome, *Bull Rheum Dis* 36:1, 1986.
10. Nadel HR, Stilwell ME: Nuclear medicine topics in pediatric musculoskeletal disease: techniques and applications, *Radiol Clin North Am* 39:636-640, 2001.
11. Michaels RM, Sorber JA: Reflex sympathetic dystrophy as a probable paraneoplastic syndrome: Case report and literature review, *Arthritis Rheum* 27:1183, 1984.
12. Taggart AJ, Iverson JMI, Wright V: Shoulder-hand syndrome and symmetrical arthralgia in patients with tubo-ovarian carcinoma, *Ann Rheum Dis* 43:391, 1984.
13. Medsger TA Jr, Dixon JA, Garwood VF: Palmar fasciitis and polyarthritis associated with ovarian carcinoma, *Ann Intern Med* 96:424, 1982.
14. Goldberg E, Dobransky R, Gill R: Reflex sympathetic dystrophy associated with malignancy, *Arthritis Rheum* 26:1079, 1985.
15. Prowse M, Higgs CMB, Forrester-Wood C et al: Reflex sympathetic dystrophy associated with squamous cell carcinoma of the lung, *Ann Rheum Dis* 48:339, 1989.
16. Ameratunga R, Daly M, Caughey DE: Metastatic malignancy associated with reflex sympathetic dystrophy, *J Rheumatol* 16:406, 1989.
17. Cooper DE, DeLee JC, Ramamurthy S: Reflex sympathetic dystrophy of the knee: treatment using continuous epidural anesthesia, *J Bone Joint Surg Am* 71:365, 1989.
18. Niehof SP, Huzgen FJ, von der Weerd RW et al: Thermography imaging during static and controlled thermoregulation in complex regional pain syndrome type I: diagnostic value and involvement of the central sympathetic system, *Bio Med Eng Online* 5:30.
19. Breivik H: Chronic pain and the sympathetic nervous system, *Acta Anesthesiol Scand* 1:131, 1997.
20. Merskey H, Bogduk N (eds): *Classification of Chronic Pain*, Seattle, 1994, IASP Press.
21. Sandroni P, Low PA, Ferrer T et al: Complex region pain syndrome I (CRPS I): prospective study and laboratory evaluation, *Clin J Pain* 14:282-289, 1998.
22. Koch E, Hofer HO, Sialer G et al: Failure of MR Imaging to detect reflex sympathetic dystrophy of the extremities, *AJR Am J Roentgenol* 156:113-115, 1991.
23. Doury P, Dirheimer Y, Pattin S: *Algodystrophy, Berlin*, 1981, Springer-Verlag.
24. Genant HK, Kozin F, Bekerman C et al: The reflex sympathetic dystrophy syndrome, *Radiology* 117:21-32, 1975.
25. Arnstein A: Regional osteoporosis, *Orthop Clin North Am* 3:585-600, 1972.
26. Raj PP, Calodney A: Complex regional pain syndrome (reflex sympathetic dystrophy). In Browner B, Jupiter J, Levine A et al (eds): *Skeletal Trauma*, 2nd ed, Philadelphia, 1998, WB Saunders, pp 589-617.
27. Burkhart JM, Jowsey J: Parathyroid and thyroid hormones in the development of immobilization osteoporosis, *Endocrinology* 81:1053, 1967.
28. Griffiths HJ, Virtama P: Juxta-articular erosions in reflex sympathetic dystrophy, *Acta Radiol* 29:183, 1988.
29. Fahr LM, Sauser DD: Imaging of peripheral nerve lesions, *Orthop Clin North Am* 19: 27, 1988.
30. Doherty M, Watt I, Dippe P: Apparent bone erosions in painful regional osteoporosis, *Rheumatol Rehabil* 19:95, 1980.
31. Doury P, Pattin S, Eulry F et al: Fractures de fatigue du col femoral suivies d'algodystrophie, *Rev Rhum Mal Osteoartic* 54:425, 1987.
32. Kozin F, Genant H, Bekerman C et al: The reflex sympathetic dystrophy syndrome. Clinical and histologic studies: evidence for bilaterality, response to corticosteroids and articular involvement, *Am J Med* 60:321, 1976.
33. Kozin F, Soin JS, Ryan LM et al: Bone scintigraphy in the reflex sympathetic dystrophy syndrome, *Radiology* 138:437, 1981.
34. Holder LE, Mackinnon SE: Reflex sympathetic dystrophy in the hands: clinical and scintigraphic criteria, *Radiology* 152:517, 1984.
35. Genant HK, Bautovich GJ, Singh M et al: Bone-seeking radionuclides: an in vivo study of factors affecting skeletal uptake, *Radiology* 113:373, 1974.

36. Mackinnon SE, Holder LE: The use of three-phase radionuclide bone scanning in the diagnosis of reflex sympathetic dystrophy, *J Hand Surg* 9A:556-562, 1984.
37. Hauzeur J-P: Epiphyseal migration of abnormalities in algodystrophy: the role of bone scintigraphy, *J Rheumatol* 19:1486, 1992.
38. Graif M, Schweitzer ME, Marks B et al: Synovial effusion in reflex sympathetic dystrophy: an additional sign for diagnosis and staging, *Skeletal Radiol* 27:262, 1998.
39. Laxer RM, Allen RC, Malleson PN et al: Technetium-99m methylene diphosphonate bone scans in children with reflex neurovascular dystrophy, *J Pediatr* 106:437, 1985.
40. Schweitzer ME, Mandel S, Schwartzman RJ et al: Reflex sympathetic dystrophy revisited: MR imaging findings before and after infusion of contrast material, *Radiology* 195:211, 1995.
41. Darbois H, Boyer B, Dubayle P et al: Semeiologie IRM de l'algodystrophie du pied, *J Radiol* 80:849, 1999.
42. Intenzo C, Kim S, Millian J et al: Scintigraphic patterns of the reflex sympathetic dystrophy syndrome of the lower extremities, *Clin Nucl Med* 14:657-661, 1989.
43. Berthelot JM: Current management of reflex sympathetic dystrophy syndrome (complex regional pain syndrome type I), *Joint Bone Spine* 73:495-499, 2006.
44. Bennett DS, Brookoff D: Complex regional pain syndromes (reflex sympathetic dystrophy and causalgia) and spinal cord stimulation, *Pain Med* 7S1:S64, 2006.
45. Pertoldi S, Di Benedetto P: Shoulder-hand syndrome after stroke. A complex regional pain syndrome, *EURA Mediophys* 41:283, 2005.
46. Toms AP, Marshall TJ, Becker E et al: Regional migratory osteoporosis: A review illustrated by five cases, *Clin Radiol* 60:425-438, 2005.
47. Resnick D: Osteoporosis. In Resnick D (ed): *Diagnosis of Bone and Joint Disorders*, 4th ed, Philadelphia, 2002, WB Saunders, pp 1847-1851.
48. Duncan H, Frame B, Frost HM et al: Migratory osteolysis of the lower extremities, *Ann Intern Med* 66:1165-1173, 1967.
49. McCord WC, Nies K, Campion DS et al: Regional migratory osteoporosis, *Arthritis Rheum* 21:832-838, 1978.
50. Kaplan SS, Stegman CJ: Transient osteoporosis of the hip. A case report and review of the literature, *J Bone Joint Surg* 73-A:451-455, 1985.
51. Trevisan C, Ortolani S, Monteleone M et al: Regional migratory osteoporosis: a pathogenetic hypothesis based on three cases and a review of the literature, *Clin Rheumatol* 21:418-425, 2002.
52. Lesquesne M: Transient osteoporosis of the hip. A nontraumatic variety of Sudeck's atrophy, *Ann Rheum Dis* 27:463-471, 1968.
53. Duncan H, Frame B, Frost H et al: Regional migratory osteoporosis, *South Med J* 62:41-44, 1969.
54. Swezey RL: Transient osteoporosis of the hip, foot, and knee, *Arthritis Rheum* 13:858-868, 1970.
55. Hofmann S, Engel A, Neuhold A et al: Bone-marrow edema syndrome and transient osteoporosis of the hip: an MRI-controlled study of treatment by core decompression, *J Bone Joint Surg* 75-B:210-216, 1993.
56. Bianchi S, Abdelwahab IF, Garcia J: Partial transient osteoporosis of the foot. Bone marrow edema in 4 cases studied with MRI, *Acta Orthop Scand* 68:577, 1997.
57. Parker RK, Ross Gj, Urso JA: Transient osteoporosis of the knee, *Skeletal Radiol* 26:306, 1997.
58. Wambeek N, Munk PL, Lee MJ et al: Intra-articular regional migratory osteoporosis of the knee, *Skeletal Radiol* 29:97, 2000.
59. Mavichak V, Murray TM, Hodsman AB et al: Regional migratory osteoporosis of the lower extremities with vertebral osteoporosis, *Bone* 7:343, 1986.
60. Wilson AJ, Murphy WA, Hardy DC et al: Transient osteoporosis: transient bone marrow edema? *Radiology* 167:757-760, 1988.
61. Crespo E, Sala D, Crespo R et al: Transient osteoporosis, *Acta Orthop Belg* 67:330-337, 2001.
62. O'Mara RE, Pinals RS: Bone scanning in regional migratory osteoporosis, *Radiology* 97:579-581, 1970.
63. Kim SM, Desai AG, Krakovitz M et al: Scintigraphic evaluation of regional migratory osteoporosis, *Clin Nucl Med* 14:36-39, 1989.
64. Volger III JB, Murphy WA: Bone marrow imaging, *Radiology* 168:679-693, 1988.
65. Eustace S, Keogh C, Blake M et al: MR imaging of bone edema: mechanisms and interpretation, *Clin Radiol* 56:4-12, 2001.
66. Guerra JJ, Steinberg ME: Distinguishing transient osteoporosis from avascular necrosis of the hip, *J Bone Joint Surg Am* 77:616-624, 1995.
67. Rosen RA: Transitory demineralization of the femoral head, *Radiology* 94, 509-512, 1970.
68. Calvo E, Alvarez L, Fernandez-Yruegas D et al: Transient osteoporosis of the foot. Bone marrow edema in 4 cases studies with MRI, *Acta Orthop Scand* 68, 577-580, 1997.
69. Daniel WW, Sanders PC, Alarcon GS: The early diagnosis of transient osteoporosis by magnetic resonance imaging. A case report, *J Bone Joint Surg* 74-A, 1262-1264, 1992.
70. Guerra JJ, Steinberg ME: Distinguishing transient osteoporosis from avascular necrosis of the hip, *J Bone Joint Surg* 77(A):616-624, 1995.
71. Stoltz MR, Dietrich SL, Marshall GJ: Osteogenesis imperfecta perspectives, *Clin Orthop* 242:120-136, 1989.
72. Plotkin H, Rauch F: Pamidronate treatment in severe osteogenesis imperfecta in children under 3 years age, *J Clin Endocrinol Metab* 11:85-90, 2000.
73. Cohn DH, Byers PH: Clinical screening for collagen defects in connective tissue diseases, *Clin Perinatol* 17:793, 1990.
74. Vetter U, Fisher LW, Mintz KP et al: Osteogenesis imperfecta: Changes in noncollagenous proteins in bone, *J Bone Miner Res* 6:501-505, 2000.
75. Roughley PJ, Rauch F, Glorieux FH: Osteogenesis imperfecta—clinical and molecular diversity, *Eur Cells Mater* 5:41-47, 2003.
76. Plotkin H: Syndromes with congenital brittle bones, *BMC Pediatr* 4:16-22, 2004.
77. Shapiro JR, Stover ML, Burn VE et al: An osteopenic nonfracture syndrome with features of mild osteogenesis imperfecta associated with the substitution of a cysteine for glycine at triple helix position 43 in the pro alpha 1 (I) chain of type I collagen, *J Clin Invest* 89:567-573, 1992.
78. Petersen K, Wetzel WE: Recent findings in classification of osteogenesis imperfecta by means of existing dental symptoms, *ASDC J Dent Child* 65:305-309, 1998.
79. Paterson CR, Monk EA, McAllion SJ: How common is hearing impairment in osteogenesis imperfecta? *J Laryngol Otol* 115:280-282, 2001.
80. Korkko J, Ala-Kokko L, De Paepe A et al: Analysis of the COL1A1 and COL1A2 genes by PCR amplification and scanning by conformation-sensitive gel electrophoresis identifies only COL1A1 mutation in 15 patients with osteogenesis imperfecta type I: identification of common sequences of null-allele mutations, *Am J Hum Genet* 62:98-110, 1998.
81. King JD, Boblechko WP: Osteogenesis imperfecta: an orthopedic description and surgical review, *J Bone Joint Surg* 53B:72-89, 1971.
82. Sillence DO, Senn A, Danks DM: Genetic heterogeneity in osteogenesis imperfecta, *J Med Genet* 16:101-116, 1979.
83. Sillence D: Osteogenesis imperfecta 2000, *Bone* 27:4s, 2000.
84. Plotkin H, Primorac D, Rowe D: Osteogenesis imperfecta. In Glorieux F, Pettifor J, Juppner J (eds): *Pediatric Bone Biology and Disease*, San Diego, Calif, 2003, Elsevier Science, pp 443-471.
85. Glorieux FH, Rauch F, Plotkin H et al: Osteogenesis imperfecta type VI: a form of brittle bone disease with a mineralization defect, *J Bone Miner Res* 17:30-38, 2002.
86. Sillence D: Osteogenesis imperfecta: an expanding panorama of variants, *Clin Orthop* 59:11-25, 1981.
87. Edwards MJ, Graham JM Jr: Studies of type I collagen in osteogenesis imperfecta, *J Pediatr* 117:67-72, 1990.
88. Waltimo J, Ojanotko-Harri A, Lukinmaa PL: Mild forms of dentinogenesis imperfecta in association with osteogenesis imperfecta as characterized by light and transmission electron microscopy, *J Oral Pathol Med* 25:256-264, 1996.
89. Petersen K, Wetzel WE: Recent findings in classification of osteogenesis imperfecta by means of existing dental symptoms, *ASDC J Dent Child* 65:305-309, 1998.
90. Evensen SA, Myhre L, Stormorken H: Hemostatic studies in osteogenesis imperfecta, *Scand J Haematol* 33:177-179, 1984.
91. White NJ, Winearls CG, Smith R: Cardiovascular abnormalities in osteogenesis imperfecta, *Am Heart J* 106:1416-1420, 1983.
92. McAllion SJ, Paterson CR: Causes of death in osteogenesis imperfecta, *J Clin Pathol* 49:627-630, 1996.
93. Munoz C, Filly RA, Golbus MS: Osteogenesis imperfecta type II: prenatal sonographic diagnosis, *Radiology* 174:181-185, 1990.
94. Byers PH, Tsiopouras P, Bonadio JF et al: Perinatal lethal osteogenesis imperfecta (OI type II): a biochemically heterogenous disorder usually due to new mutation in the genes for the type I collagen, *Am J Hum Genet* 42:237-248, 1998.
95. Verkh Z, Russel M, Miller CA: Osteogenesis imperfecta type II: microvascular changes in the CNS, *Clin Neuropathol* 14:154-158, 1995.
96. Sillence DO, Barlow KK, Garber AP et al: Osteogenesis imperfecta type II. Delineation of phenotype with reference to genetic heterogeneity, *Am J MedAm J Med Genet* 17:407-423, 1984.
97. Plotkin H: Syndromes with congenital brittle bones, *BMC Pediatr* 4:16-22, 2004.
98. O'Connell AC, Marini JC: Evaluation of oral problems in an osteogenesis imperfecta population, *Oral Surg Oral Med Oral Pathol Oral Radiol Endod* 87:189-196, 1999.
99. Vetter U, Pontz B, Zauner E et al: Osteogenesis imperfecta: a clinical study of the first ten years of life, *Calcif Tissue Int* 50:36-41, 1992.
100. Levin LS, Salinas CF, Jorgenson RJ: Classification of osteogenesis imperfecta by dental characteristics, *Lancet* 1:332-323, 1978.
101. Sillence DO: Craniocervical abnormalities in osteogenesis imperfecta: genetic and molecular correlation, *Pediatr Radiol* 24:427-430, 1994.
102. Glorieux FH, Ranch F, Poltroon H et al: Type V osteogenesis imperfecta: a new form of brittle bone disease, *J Bone Miner Res* 15:1650-1658, 2000.
103. Ward LM, Rauch F, Travers R et al: Osteogenesis imperfecta type VII: an autosomal recessive form of brittle bone disease, *Bone* 31:12-18, 2002.
104. Goldman AB: Heritable diseases of connective tissue, epiphyseal dysplasias, and related conditions. In Resnik D (ed): *Diagnosis of Bone and Joint Disorders*, Philadelphia, 2002, WB Saunders, pp 4398-4409.
105. Gertner JM, Root L: Osteogenesis imperfecta, *Orthop Clin North Am* 21:151-162, 1990.
106. Fairbank T: Atlas of general affectations of the skeleton. Eidenburgh and London, 1951, E.S. Livingstone, pp 1-30.
107. Bauze RJ, Smith R, Francis MJO: A new look at osteogenesis imperfecta, *J Bone Joint Surg Br* 57:2-12, 1975.
108. King JD, Bobechko WP: Osteogenesis imperfecta—an orthopedic description and surgical review, *J Bone Joint Surg* 53B:72-89, 1971.
109. Azouz EM, Fassier F: Hyperplastic callus formation in osteogenesis imperfecta, *Skel Radiol* 26:744-745, 1997. (Letter.)
110. Dobrocky I, Seidl G, Grill F: MRI and CT features of hyperplastic callus in osteogenesis imperfecta tarda, *Eur Radiol* 9:665-668, 1999.
111. Heimert TL, Lin DDM, Yousem DM: Case 48: Osteogenesis imperfecta of the temporal bone, *Radiology* 224:166-170, 2002.
112. Noorda RJ, van der Aa JP, Wuisman PL et al: Transient osteoporosis and osteogenesis imperfecta. A case report, *Clin Orthop* 337:249-255, 1997.
113. Karagkevrekis CB, Ainscow DA: Transient osteoporosis of the hip associated with osteogenesis imperfecta, *J Bone Joint Surg Br* 80:54-55, 1998.

114. Sofield HA, Millar EA: Fragmentation realignment and intramedullary rod fixation of deformities of the long bones in children: a ten-year appraisal, *J Bone Joint Surg Am* 41:1371, 1959.
115. Porat S, Heller E, Seidman DS et al: Functional results of peratoin in osteogenesis imperfecta: elongating and nonelongating rods, *J Pediatr Orthop* 11:200-203, 1991.
116. Cremin B, Goodman H, Spranger J et al: Wormian bones in osteogenesis imperfecta and other diseases, *Skeletal Radiol* 8:35-38, 1982.
117. Tabor EK, Curtin HD, Hirsch BE et al: Osteopenia imperfecta tarda: appearance of the temporal bones at CT, *Radiology* 175:181-183, 1990.
118. Falvo KA, Root L, Bullough PG: Osteogenesis imperfecta: clinical evaluation and management, *J Bone Joint Surg Am* 56:783-793, 1974.
119. Yong-Hing K, MacEwen GE: Scoliosis with osteogenesis imperfecta: results of treatment, *J Bone Joint Surg Br* 64:36-43, 1982.
120. Lee JH, Gamble JG, Moore RE et al: Gastrointestinal problems in patients who have type III osteogenesis imperfecta, *J Bone Joint Surg* 77:1352-1356, 1995.
121. Huang RP, Ambrose CG, Sullivan E et al: Functional significance of bone density measurements in children with osteogenesis imperfecta, *J Bone Joint Surg Am* 88:1324-1330, 2006.
122. Rauch F, Glorieux FH: Osteogenesis imperfecta, current and future medical treatment, *Am J Genet C Semin Med Genet* 139:31-37, 2005.
123. Rauch F, Glorieux FH: Osteogenesis imperfecta, *Lancet* 363:1377-1385, 2004.
124. Whyte MP, Obrecht SE, Finnegan PM et al: Osteoprotegerin deficiency and juvenile Paget's disease, *N Engl J Med* 347:175-184, 2002.
125. Nimkin K, Kleinman PK: Imaging of child abuse, *Radiol Clin North Am* 39:843-864, 2001.
126. Engelbert RH, Pruijs HE, Beemer FA et al: Osteogenesis imperfecta in childhood: treatment strategies, *Arch Phys Med Rehabil* 79:1590-1594, 1998.
127. Pereira RF, O'Hara MD, Laptev AV et al: Marrow stromal cells as a source of progenitor cells for nonhematopoietic tissues in transgenic mice with a phenotype of osteogenesis imperfecta, *Proc Natl Acad Sci U S A* 95:1142-1147, 1998.

CHAPTER 33

Imaging Hyperparathyroidism and Renal Osteodystrophy

D. LEE BENNETT, MD, MA, *and* GEORGES Y. EL-KHOURY, MD

KEY FACTS

- Excessive parathyroid hormone causes increased osteoclastic activity, which leads to bone resorption and replacement with fibrous tissue.
- Patients with primary hyperparathyroidism are usually asymptomatic but have laboratory evidence of hypercalcemia and excessive parathyroid hormone.
- Tc-99m sestamibi SPECT scan and magnetic resonance imaging of the neck are highly reliable in identifying the cause of hyperparathyroidism but are most often used when a patient has had prior neck surgery.
- When minimally invasive parathyroid surgery is to be performed, preoperative tumor localization is indicated.
- When a patient younger than 35 years of age presents with hyperparathyroidism or has a known first-degree relative with MEN type I, screening with appropriate laboratory tests for evidence of pituitary gland tumors, parathyroid adenomas, pancreatic islet cell tumors, and neuroendocrine tumors is indicated.
- Symptoms of advanced hyperparathyroidism include multiple kidney stones, bone pain with localized swelling, anorexia, weight loss, abdominal pain, peptic ulcer disease, and mental status changes of hypercalcemia.
- The earliest radiographic manifestations of hyperparathyroidism are subperiosteal resorption and acro-osteolysis in the fingers.
- A normal hand radiograph in a patient suspected of having advanced hyperparathyroidism effectively excludes the diagnosis.
- Renal osteodystrophy consists of renal failure-induced rickets or osteomalacia, secondary hyperparathyroidism, and soft tissue calcification.
- In renal osteodystrophy, the presence of a rugger jersey spine (osteosclerosis) precludes the diagnosis of aluminum toxicity.

HYPERPARATHYROIDISM

The sine qua non of osseous disease in hyperparathyroidism is resorption of bone with or without formation of brown tumors coupled with replacement of bone by fibrous tissue. Bone resorption occurs due to increased osteoclastic activity caused by excessive parathyroid hormone. In primary hyperparathyroidism, the excessive parathyroid hormone is caused by a solitary parathyroid adenoma in 80% to 85% of cases, hyperplasia in 10% to 15% of cases, multiple adenomas in 3% to 5% of cases, and carcinoma in 1% of cases.[1]

> Primary hyperparathyroidism is usually due to a parathyroid adenoma.

Primary hyperparathyroidism occurs classically in middle-aged and elderly females. Secondary hyperparathyroidism is due to calcium imbalance from chronic renal failure resulting in excessive parathyroid hormone. Pseudohyperparathyroidism occurs due to secretion of a parathyroid hormone-like substance by neoplasms.[2]

Imaging of hyperparathyroidism has undergone a paradigm shift in the last few decades. Before the advent of the automated laboratory chemistry panel in the 1970s and its widespread institution by the 1980s, bone imaging played a role in the diagnosis of primary hyperparathyroidism. In this earlier time period, hyperparathyroid patients presented with hypercalcemic symptoms or constitutional symptoms.[3] If the physician suspected hyperparathyroidism, imaging studies of the bones (a radiographic skeletal survey) were ordered to confirm the diagnosis. After parathyroidectomy, patients were followed up with skeletal surveys to confirm successful treatment as evidenced by the resolution of abnormal imaging findings.

In current medical practice, the typical clinical presentation of a patient with primary hyperparathyroidism is an asymptomatic individual with laboratory evidence of hypercalcemia and excessive parathyroid hormone. Given the current asymptomatic clinical presentation of this disease, both conservative and surgical treatments can be used for hyperparathyroidism. Consensus guidelines for when to use conservative versus surgical treatment have been developed.[4,5]

The role of modern imaging in primary hyperparathyroidism is in preoperative localization of the lesion (i.e., parathyroid adenoma) in patients with any prior neck surgery (failed parathyroid adenoma resection surgery or any other prior neck surgery).

> Imaging studies are appropriate for patients with prior neck surgery and primary hyperparathyroidism.

The preferred imaging techniques for preoperative localization of the parathyroid lesion are both a Tc-99m sestamibi SPECT imaging study and a magnetic resonance image (MRI) of the neck.[6,7] This combination of imaging modalities provides a high success rate of localization (~95% sensitivity and ~98% positive predictive value).[7]

There is currently debate over whether preoperative localization of the parathyroid disease is necessary in the previously unoperated neck. Standard exploratory neck dissection (in the unoperated neck) has a higher success rate for identification of a parathyroid adenoma than imaging localization exams.[8] If the surgeon plans to perform a standard neck dissection for parathyroid disease, then preoperative imaging localization is not recommended.[8-10] However, some surgeons prefer to use minimally invasive neck surgery with a small skin incision over the site of the lesion; in these cases, preoperative imaging localization is mandatory with Tc-99m sestamibi SPECT imaging (with or without computed tomography [CT] image fusion) being the imaging exam of choice.[8-10]

> In patients without prior neck surgery in whom minimally invasive surgery for primary hyperparathyroidism is planned, Technetium-99m sestamibi SPECT scanning (with or without CT image fusion) is necessary for localization of the lesion. In addition, some surgeons will use ultrasound (US) imaging to mark the skin surface entry site immediately prior to the minimally invasive surgery.[8]

Osteoarticular Imaging Features

One should still be familiar with the radiographic osteoarticular findings of hyperparathyroidism, as patients do occasionally present with advanced disease.[11] Radiographically visible osseous resorption can occur at multiple locations such as subperiosteal, endosteal, subchondral, subligamentous, subtendinous, and trabecular[3] (Table 33-1).

The earliest occurrence of subperiosteal resorption occurs along the radial aspect of the middle phalanges of the index and middle fingers.[12] This is seen as bone resorption under the periosteum with cortical tunneling. Grossly, this resembles a long curved erosion along the length of the phalanx with the osseous surface taking on the appearance of toothbrush bristles (Figure 33–1). Acro-osteolysis is also an early finding of bone resorption due to hyperparathyroidism (Figure 33–1). Other common locations for subperiosteal resorption are the ribs, lamina dura of the teeth, and the medial aspect of the long bone metaphyses. Subchondral

TABLE 33–1. Imaging Findings of Primary Hyperparathyroidism

Abnormality	Common Manifestation	Example
Bone resorption		
Subperiosteal, tuft resorption	Lacelike appearance of the radial cortex of the middle phalanges of the index and middle fingers Erosion of tufts of distal phalanges Erosion of medial metaphysis of tibia, humerus or other long bones Rib erosion (superior surface) Absence of lamina dura of the teeth	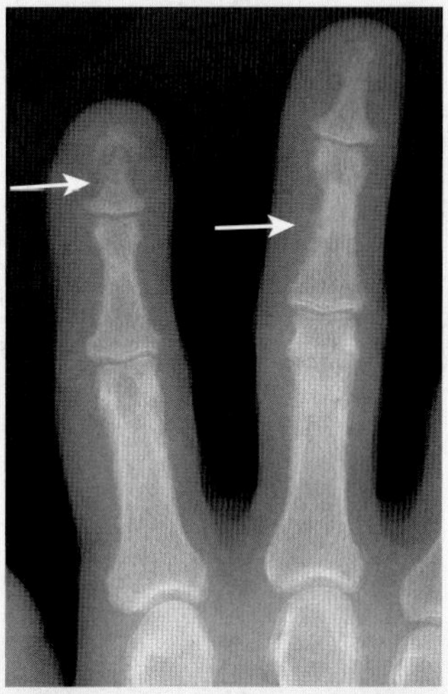 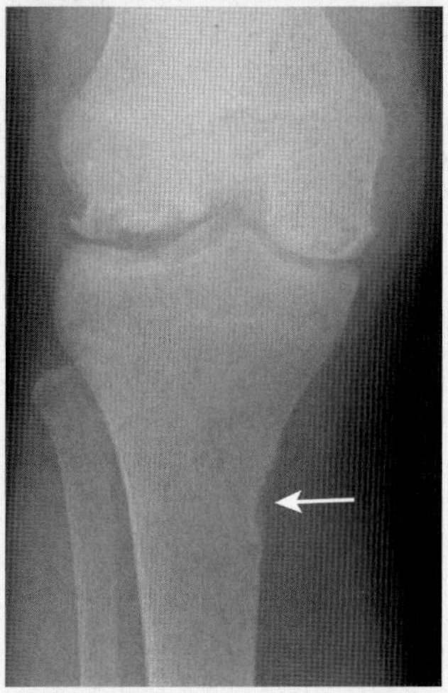

(Continued)

TABLE 33–1. Imaging Findings of Primary Hyperparathyroidism—cont'd.

Abnormality	Common Manifestation	Example
Endosteal, intracortical tunneling		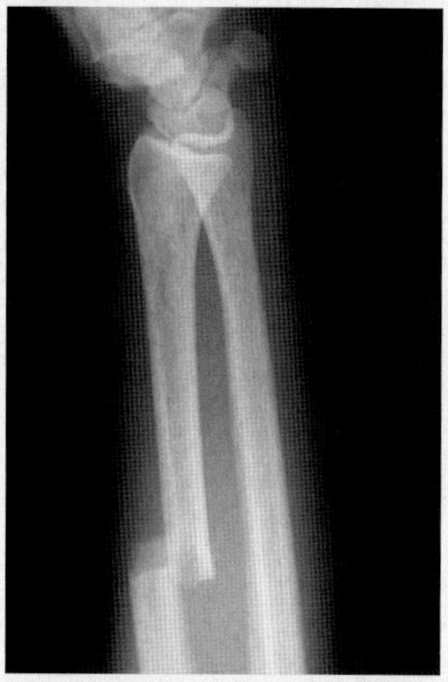
Subchondral	Erosion of sacroiliac, acromioclavicular, sternoclavicular, temporomandibular joints, symphysis pubis, patella	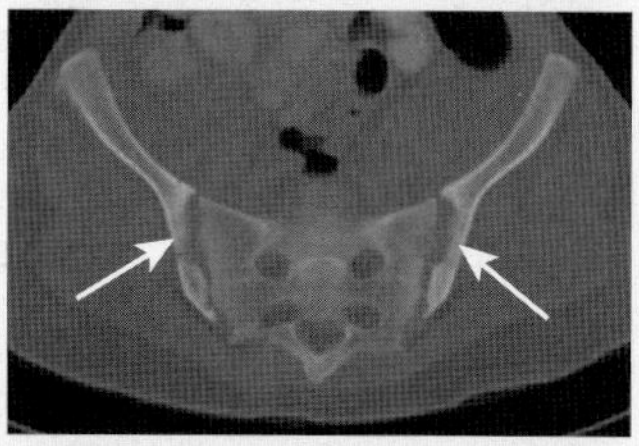
Subligamentous/ subtendinous	Erosion of femoral trochanters and humeral tuberosities, ischial tuberosities, calcaneus, undersurface of distal clavicle	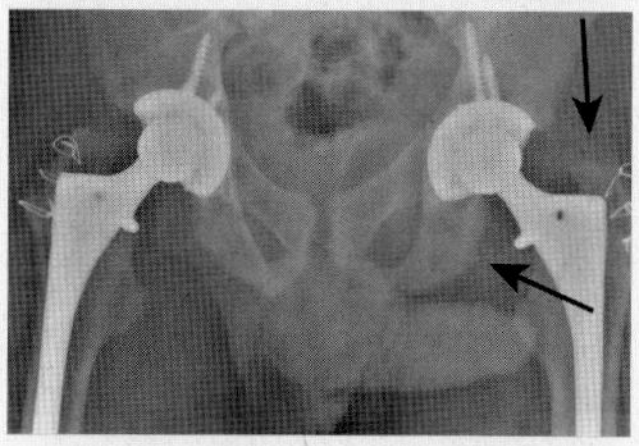 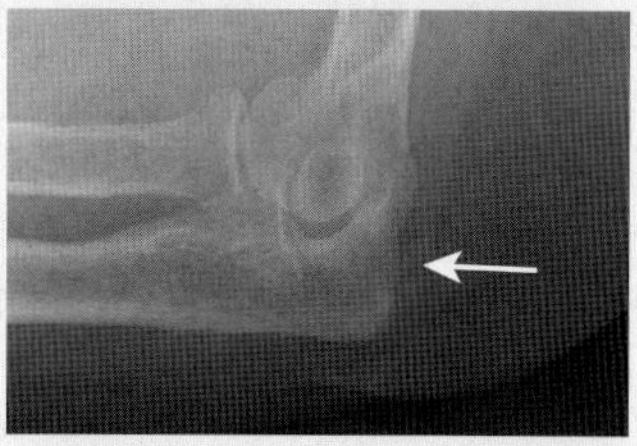
Trabecular	"Salt-and-pepper" skull	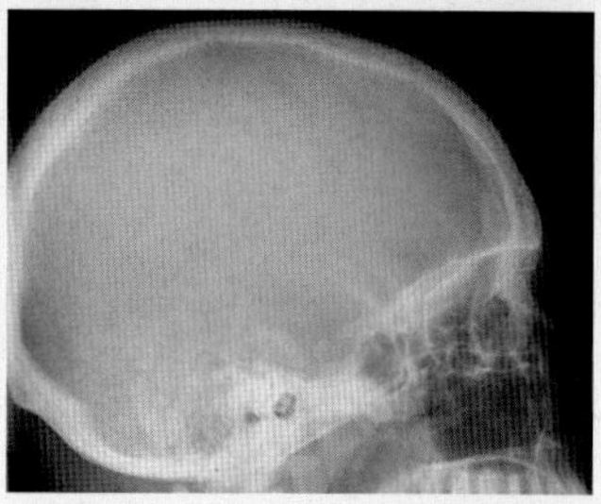

(Continued)

TABLE 33–1. Imaging Findings of Primary Hyperparathyroidism—cont'd.

Abnormality	Common Manifestation	Example
Brown tumors	Lytic lesions	
Chondrocalcinosis	Calcification of articular fibrocartilage and hyaline cartilage	

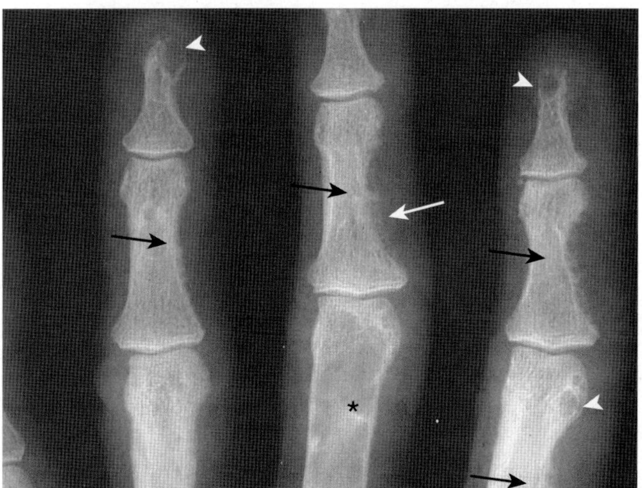

FIGURE 33–1. Subperiosteal resorption. Coned-down posteroanterior radiograph of the hand in a patient with hyperparathyroidism. Subperiosteal resorption can be seen involving the radial margins of the visualized middle phalanges as well as the proximal phalanx of the index finger *(black arrows)*. The classic toothbrush bristle appearance can also be seen *(white arrow)*. Brown tumors are also present *(white arrowheads)*. Incidentally, an enchondroma is also present *(asterisk)*.

bone resorption occurs classically at the sacroiliac joints, acromioclavicular joints, sternoclavicular joints, temporomandibular joints, symphysis pubis, and the patella (Figure 33–2). Subligamentous and subtendinous resorption occurs most commonly at the femoral trochanters, ischial tuberosity, calcaneus, clavicle, and humeral tuberosities (Figure 33–3).[3]

Bone resorption may be responsible for nontraumatic tendon avulsions, particularly at the patellar tendon and quadriceps tendon attachments.

Trabecular resorption is seen classically as the salt-and-pepper appearance to the skull (Figure 33–4).[3]

CT imaging shows the findings seen by radiography but with better detail. There are case reports that describe nonspecific increased signal on T2-weighted magnetic resonance images within the marrow of involved bones.[13] However, MRI is not routinely used to evaluate the osseous changes in hyperparathyroidism.

Brown tumors are so named because of their brown color; this results from blood products.

Brown tumors are essentially osteoclastomas with areas of necrosis and hemorrhage. On radiography, they are geographic lytic lesions. Alone, they are nonspecific in appearance. However, when subperiosteal resorption is present, then the presence of polyostotic, geographic, lytic lesions is nearly pathognomonic for brown tumors (Figures 33–1, 33–4, and 33–5). After resection of the offending parathyroid adenoma, brown tumors can become sclerotic as they heal. When they become sclerotic, they may mimic blastic metastases (Figure 33–6).[3,14] Rarely, a brown tumor can be the initial skeletal finding in hyperparathyroidism (Figure 33–7).[14] Because brown tumors usually contain hemosiderin, their classic MRI appearance is hypointense (dark) signal on both T2-weighted and T1-weighted sequences with blooming artifact on gradient echo sequences.[14] However, if not much hemosiderin is present, brown tumors can be hyperintense on the T2-weighted images.

Finally, chondrocalcinosis (cartilage deposition of calcium pyrophosphate dihydrate crystals) can also be seen with

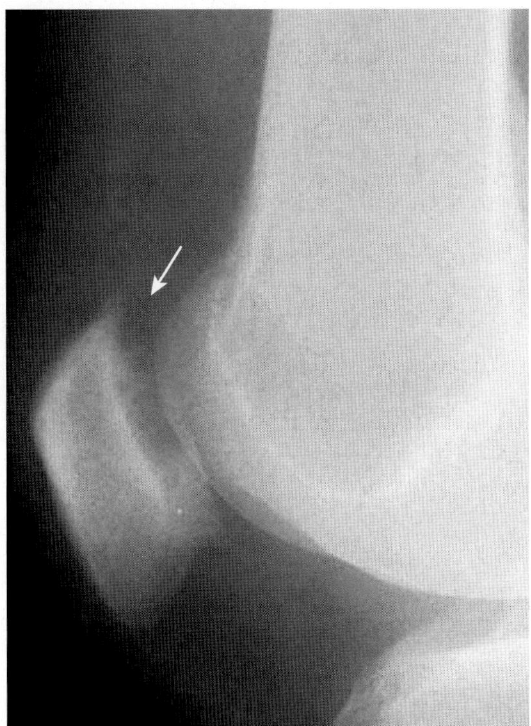

FIGURE 33–2. Subchondral resorption. Lateral radiograph of the knee in a patient with hyperparathyroidism. Subchondral resorption of the patella can be seen *(white arrow).*

hyperparathyroidism. This crystal deposition is most commonly seen on radiographs within the fibrocartilaginous menisci of the knee, the triangular fibrocartilage complex of the wrist, and the fibrocartilaginous disk of the symphysis pubis (Figure 33–8).[3]

Extraarticular Imaging Findings

Extraskeletal imaging of hyperparathyroidism is confined primarily to preoperative localization of the causal parathyroid adenoma. By US, adenomas are classically well-defined, hypoechoic nodules separated from the thyroid gland (Figure 33–9).[15] On CT with intravenous contrast, adenomas are isodense to hypodense relative to the markedly enhancing thyroid gland and hyperdense relative to adjacent fat. The MRI appearance of adenomas is typically that of a mass that is isointense on T1-weighted images, hyperintense on T2-weighted images, and demonstrates enhancement on fat-saturated T1-weighted post-contrast (gadolinium) images. On Tc-99m sestamibi studies, there is retention of activity relative to the thyroid gland (Figure 33–10).[1]

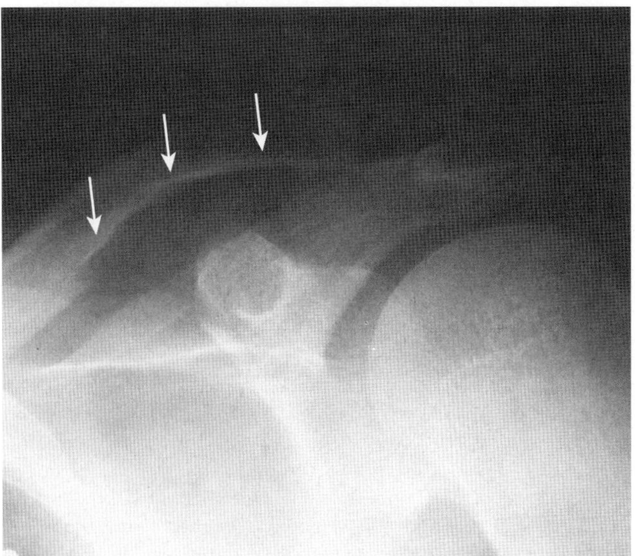

FIGURE 33–3. Subligamentous resorption. Anteroposterior radiograph of the left shoulder in a patient with hyperparathyroidism. Subligamentous resorption of the clavicle at the attachment of the coracoclavicular ligaments is demonstrated *(white arrows).*

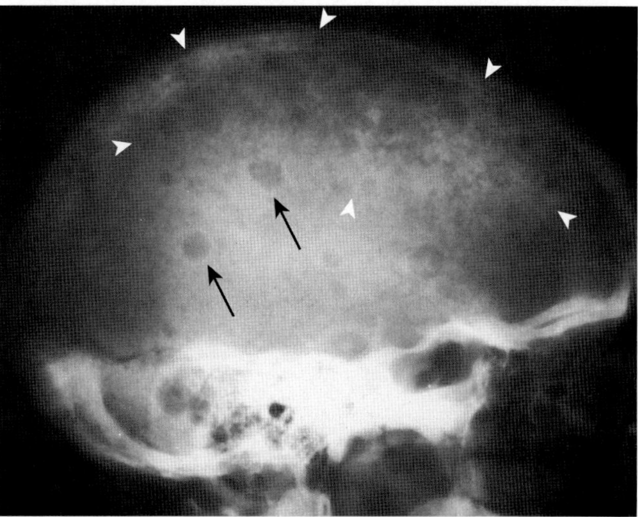

FIGURE 33–4. Salt-and-pepper skull. Lateral radiograph of the skull in a patient with primary hyperparathyroidism. A classic salt-and-pepper appearance indicative of trabecular resorption is seen (*white arrowheads* point out the regions of the salt-and-pepper appearance). Multiple brown tumors are also present *(black arrows).*

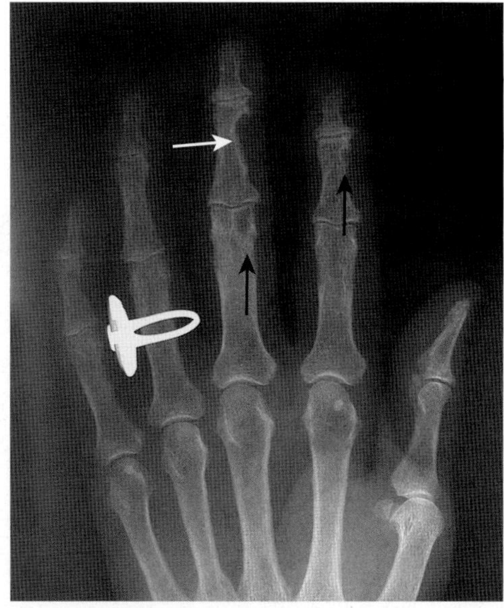

FIGURE 33–5. Subperiosteal resorption and brown tumors. Posteroanterior radiograph of the hand in a patient with hyperparathyroidism. Subperiosteal resorption *(white arrow)* and brown tumors are demonstrated *(black arrows).*

Hyperparathyroidism can also occur in the multiple endocrine neoplasia (MEN) syndromes. MEN type I usually presents as hyperprathyroidism in the second decade of life. The other diseases

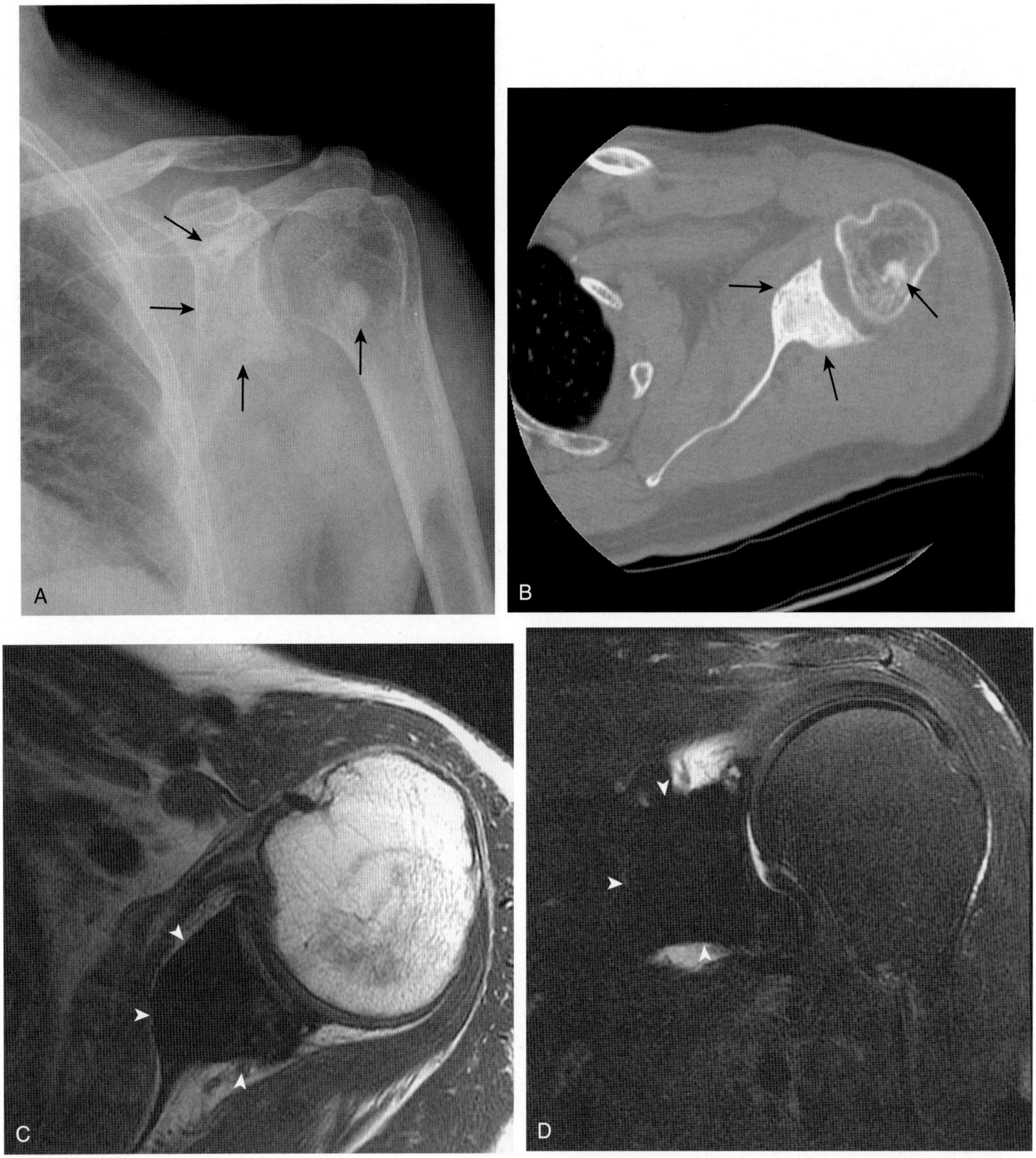

A

B

C

D

FIGURE 33–6. Radiographic and MRI images of a patient with treated hyperparathyroidism and healing brown tumors. **A,** Anteroposterior radiograph of the left shoulder shows two sclerotic lesions that are biopsy-proven healing brown tumors *(black arrows)*. **B,** Transverse CT image of the left shoulder demonstrates the sclerotic appearance that healing brown tumors can have *(black arrows)*. These healing lesions have an imaging appearance similar to that of osteoblastic metastases. The T1-weighted transverse MR image **(C)** of the left shoulder shows the expected low signal intensity of a sclerotic bone lesion *(white arrowheads)*. Sclerotic healing brown tumors will have low signal intensity on both T1-weighted and T2-weighted **(D)** images given their high calcium content. *White arrowheads* point out the healing brown tumor on images **C** and **D**.

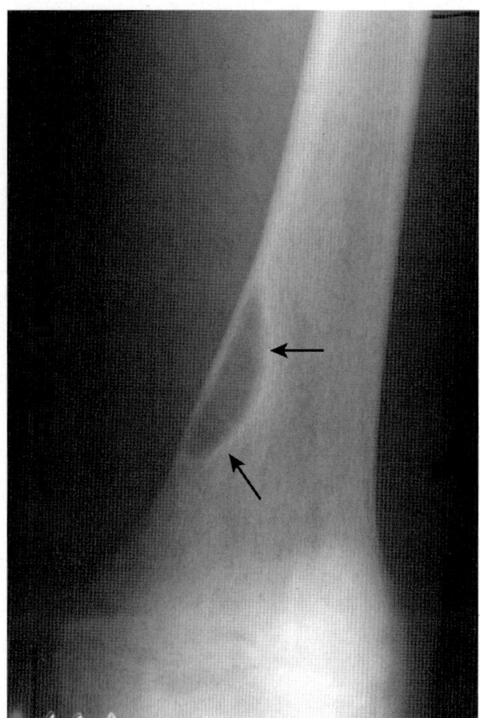

FIGURE 33–7. Anteroposterior radiograph of the knee in a pediatric patient with a brown tumor *(black arrows)*. The radiographic appearance of a brown tumor is nonspecific. However, in this patient with renal disease, the appearance of this lesion led to laboratory tests that revealed hyperparathyroidism. After treatment for hyperparathyroidism, this lesion resolved.

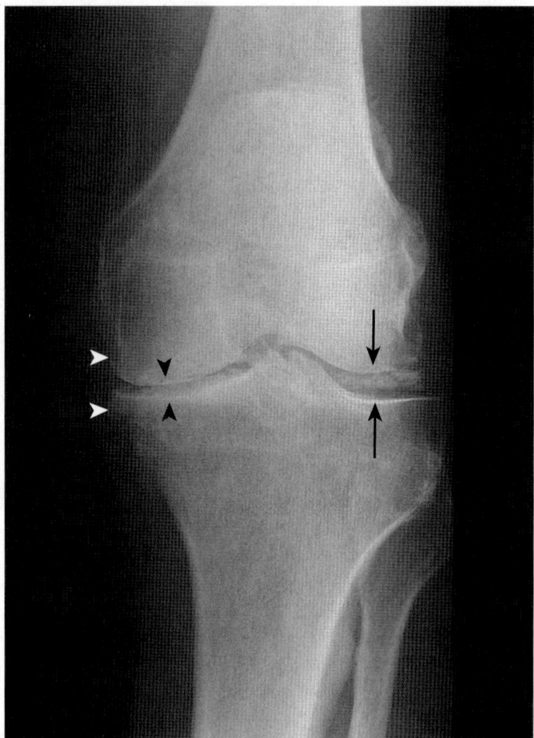

FIGURE 33–8. Chondrocalcinosis. Anteroposterior radiograph of the left knee in a patient with secondary hyperparathyroidism. Calcific density in the lateral meniscus *(black arrows)* is essentially pathognomonic for CPPD crystal deposition. In addition, note the superimposed osteoarthritis as shown by the joint space narrowing *(black arrowheads)* and osteophyte formation *(white arrowheads)*.

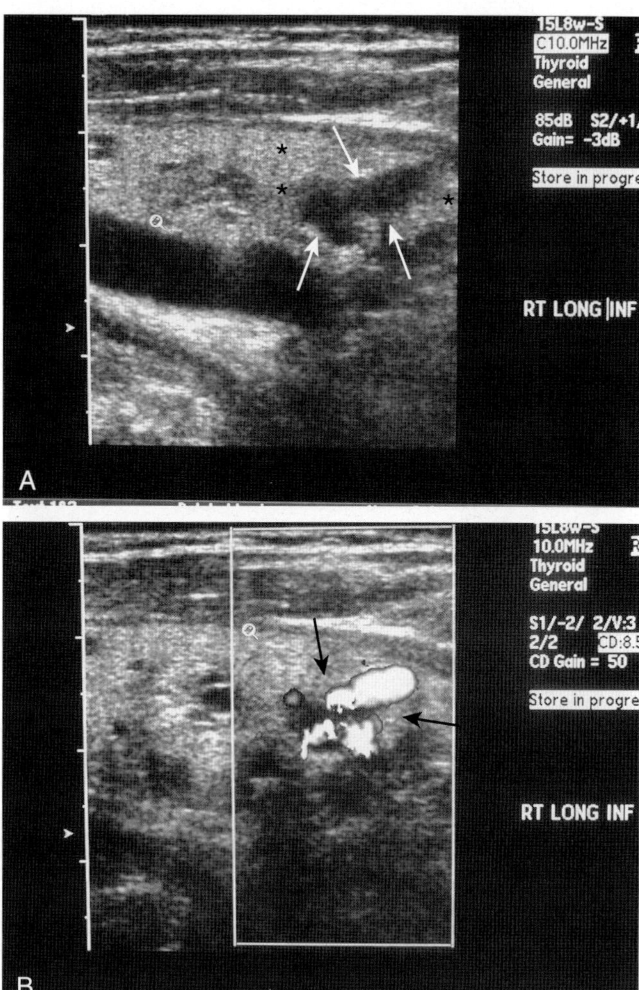

FIGURE 33–9. Ultrasound images of a parathyroid adenoma in a patient with primary hyperparathyroidism. **A,** The lesion is seen to be hypoechoic *(white arrows)* and well demarcated from the surrounding thyroid tissues *(asterisks)*. **B,** Doppler images demonstrate abundant vascularity within the lesion *(black arrows)*.

of MEN type I (pancreatic islet cell tumor, involvement of the pituitary gland, and carcinoid tumor) occur later in life. Medical imaging such as Tc-99m sestamibi, In-111 pentetreotide, and dynamic contrast-enhanced CT scans can be used to evaluate for these extraskeletal lesions. Hyperparathyroidism can also be found in MEN type II syndrome. However, it occurs later in the course of this disease and tends to be milder.

Recommendations

Imaging for preoperative localization of the adenoma is uniformly recommended in patients requiring repeat surgery due to an initially unsuccessful neck exploration for resection of the offending parathyroid gland(s). The most successful preoperative imaging protocol documented is combined Tc-99m sestamibi and contrast enhanced MRI of the neck and upper chest.[7] If preoperative imaging localization is unsuccessful in a previously operated neck, one may have to resort to selective venous catheterization of the neck to obtain blood samples from various veins draining the neck. When a blood sample has a markedly elevated parathyroid hormone level, it suggests the location of the adenoma.[5]

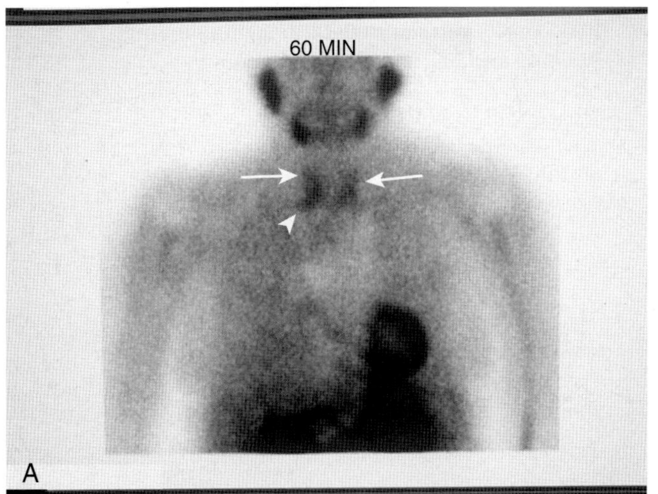

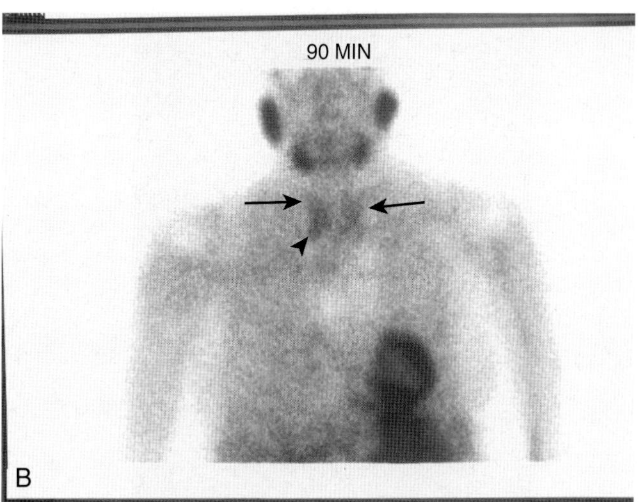

FIGURE 33–10. Tc-99m sestamibi planar images of a parathyroid adenoma in a patient with hyperparathyroidism. The 60-minute **(A)** and 90-minute **(B)** delayed images show preferential washout of activity from the thyroid gland *(arrows)* with relatively persistent activity within the parathyroid adenoma located at the inferior aspect of the thyroid gland *(arrowheads)*.

When minimally invasive surgery is to be performed rather than standard neck dissection surgery, preoperative localization using US or Tc-99m sestamibi is performed. This is so the optimal skin entry incision site can be determined.[8]

When a patient presents with hyperparathyroidism before the age of 35 or has a known first-degree relative with MEN type I, the patient should be screened with appropriate laboratory tests looking for evidence of pituitary gland tumors, parathyroid adenomas, pancreatic islet cell tumors, and neuroendocrine tumors.[16] Appropriate diagnostic imaging should then be guided by the results of the laboratory tests. These would include, but would not be limited to, an MRI of the pituitary gland, Tc-99m sestamibi scintigraphy of the parathyroid glands, high-resolution CT or MRI of the pancreas, and In-111 pentetreotide scintigraphy of the whole body.[16]

Finally, one should still be familiar with the osteoartricular radiographic findings of hyperparathyroidism since patients still present occasionally with advanced disease and bone symptoms. Since the earliest radiographic findings of hyperparathyroidism are subperiosteal resorption of the middle phalanges, one should start with hand radiographs to confirm or rule out the possibility of advanced changes in patients presenting with clinical symptoms of potentially advanced hyperparathyroidism.

> Bone resorption along the radial surface of the middle phalanges of the index and middle fingers is the earliest and most characteristic radiographic feature of hyperparathyroidism.

If the hand radiographs are negative, then the patient does not have advanced hyperparathyroidism.[11,12] Some of the symptoms of advanced hyperparathyroidism are multiple kidney stones, bone pain, soft tissue swelling in the areas of bone pain, anorexia, weight loss, abdominal pain, peptic ulcer disease, and mental status changes of hypercalcemia.

RENAL OSTEODYSTROPHY

In its simplest definition, renal osteodystrophy is the bone disease caused by renal failure induced low levels of 1,25-$(OH)_2$ vitamin D. These low levels result in rickets in children or osteomalacia in adults. Also, the low levels of 1,25-$(OH)_2$ vitamin D result in hypocalcemia, thereby causing secondary hyperparathyroidism. Therefore, renal osteodystrophy is renal failure-induced rickets or osteomalacia and secondary hyperparathyroidism.

Several authors have also included soft tissue calcification as part of the definition of renal osteodystrophy.[17] For purposes of this chapter, we will define renal osteodystrophy as renal failure-induced rickets or osteomalacia, secondary hyperparathyroidism, and soft tissue calcifications. The soft tissue calcifications of renal failure are felt to be a result of an abnormal calcium ion-phosphate ion product.

> The soft tissue calcification in renal osteodystrophy results from a calcium, phosphate ion product greater than 75 mg/dl.[17]

These soft tissue calcifications are primarily composed of calcium hydroxyapatite crystals when they occur in the subcutaneous fat, periarticular tissues, and arterial walls. The visceral (lung, stomach, heart, kidney, and muscle) calcifications of renal failure are amorphous and rarely visible on radiographs.

Many decades ago, renal osteodystrophy was a rare condition given the relatively short life expectancy of patients with chronic renal failure. However, with the advent of dialysis several decades ago, there was an increase in cases of renal osteodystrophy. This was felt to be due to the increasing life span of chronic renal failure patients coupled with a limited understanding of how to medically treat and control calcium and phosphorus imbalances.[18] Since the mid-1970s, renal osteodystrophy has become less common given the improvement in the medical management of patients on chronic dialysis.

In dialysis patients with asymptomatic bone disease, skeletal surveys had been used in the past to document the presence of hyperparathyroidism and rickets prior to the development of useful laboratory tests. Today, radiographic skeletal surveys and more focused radiographs are still used to evaluate dialysis patients presenting with diffuse or focal bone pain.[19,20] In many cases, radiographs can help identify the source of the new pain. Some examples of the imaging features associated with chronic renal disease and dialysis include hyperparathyroidism (the rugger jersey spine finding in the setting of chronic renal failure is pathognomonic for secondary hyperparathyroidism) (Figure 33–11), avascular necrosis of the hip (Figure 33–12), severe progressive spondyloarthropathy of the cervical spine, and amyloid deposition (Box 33-1). Advanced imaging studies such as MRI are also helpful in the diagnosis of avascular necrosis, severe progressive spondyloarthropathy of the cervical spine, amyloid deposition, tendon rupture, and insufficiency fractures.

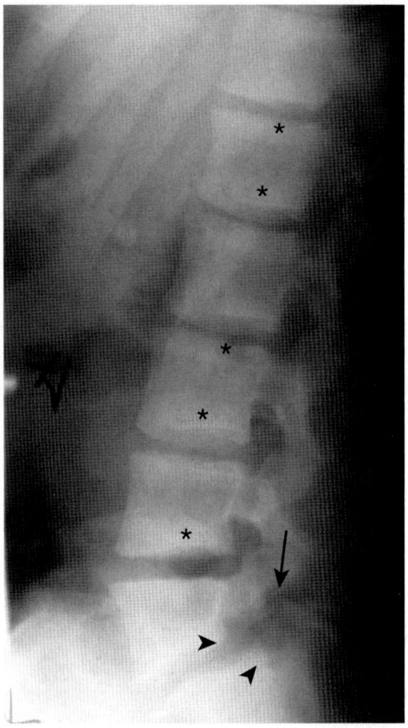

FIGURE 33–11. Rugger jersey spine. Lateral radiograph of the lumbar spine in a renal failure patient with secondary hyperparathyroidism. The osteosclerosis of the vertebral endplates can be seen *(asterisks)*. L5 spondylolysis *(black arrow)* and L5–S1 spondylolisthesis *(black arrowheads)* are also present. When osteosclerosis is present, this rules out clinically significant aluminum toxicity and adynamic bone disease.[20]

BOX 33-1. Musculoskeletal Imaging Findings in Patients on Long-Term Hemodialysis

Hyperparathyroidism
Sclerosis ("rugger jersey spine")
Soft tissue calcification
Amyloid spondylitis (usually cervical spine)
Amyloid arthropathy
Osteomalacia
Insufficiency fractures
Tendon rupture
Aluminum toxicity
Osteonecrosis
Epiphyseal sclerosis

Osteoarticular Imaging Features of Renal Osteodystrophy

The imaging findings of hyperparathyroidism are described in the section on hyperparathyroidism earlier in this chapter. Some differences in imaging findings of secondary as opposed to primary hyperparathyroidism relate to brown tumors, which are more common in primary hyperparathyroidism, as well as cortical tunneling and osteosclerosis (rugger jersey spine), which are more pronounced in secondary hyperparathyroidism.[17]

The radiographic appearance of rickets includes irregular epiphyses adjacent to widened physes with frayed, irregular, cup-shaped metaphyses (Figure 33–13); concave impression of

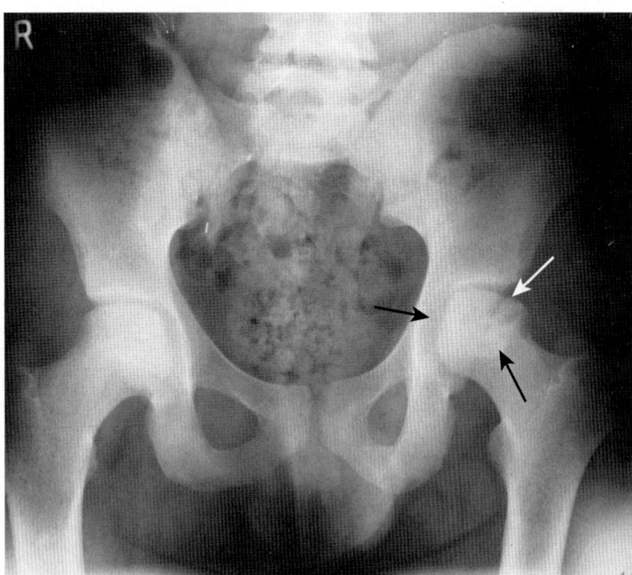

FIGURE 33–12. Anteroposterior radiograph of the pelvis in a renal failure patient with secondary hyperparathyroidism. Diffuse density (osteosclerosis) of the bones is present indicating secondary hyperparathyroidism. Collapse of the left femoral head with patchy sclerosis noted, consistent with avascular necrosis *(arrows)*.

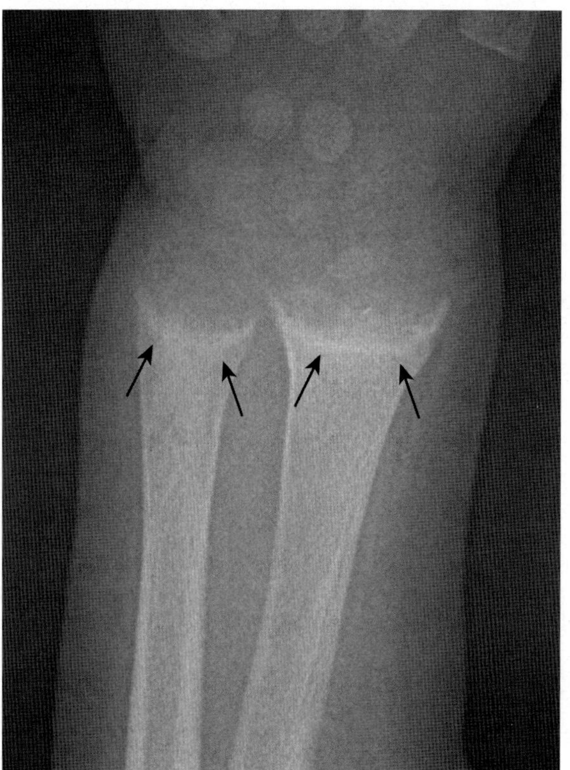

FIGURE 33–13. Posteroanterior radiograph of the wrist in a pediatric patient with renal disease and rickets. The classic frayed, cup-shaped metaphyses of rickets can be seen *(black arrows)*.

the vertebral endplates; irregularity, fraying, and widening at the costochondral junction of the ribs; genu valgum or genu varum; and a delay in bone age (Figures 33–13, 33–14, and 33–15).[3,17]

Rickets is osteomalacia in the immature skeleton.

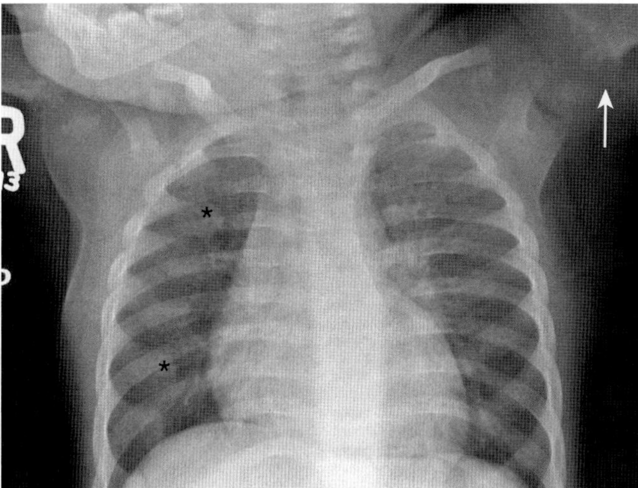

FIGURE 33–14. Anteroposterior radiograph of the chest in a pediatric patient with rickets. The prominence or widening of the ribs at the costochondral junction can be seen *(asterisks)*. Also, note the irregular, frayed appearance to the proximal metaphysis of the left humerus *(white arrow)*.

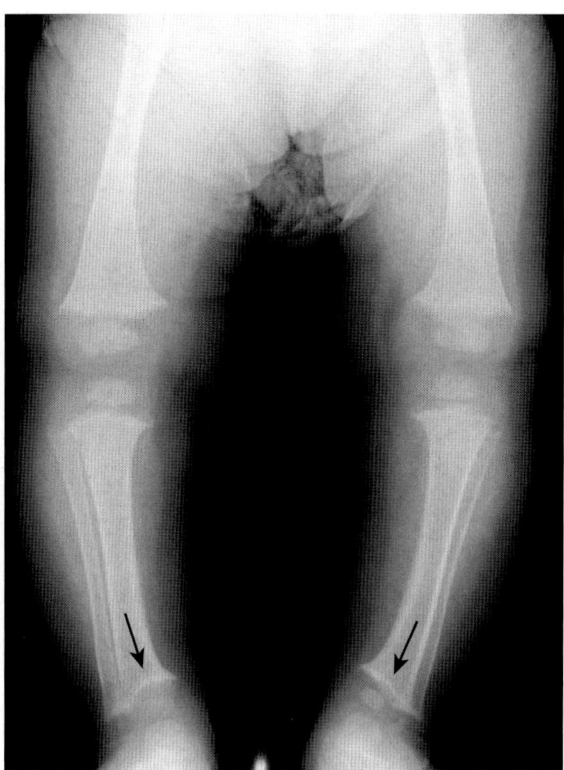

FIGURE 33–15. Anteroposterior radiograph of the lower extremities in a pediatric patient with renal disease and rickets. Note the bowed appearance (genu varum) of the lower extremities with the apex of the bowing centered at the knee joints. The classic frayed, cup-shaped metaphyseal appearance is also demonstrated in the distal tibiae *(black arrows)*.

Osteomalacia is difficult to recognize on radiographs unless Looser's zones are present.

Looser zones are incomplete, often symmetrical fractures that are pathognomonic of osteomalacia.

One can also see a non-specific ill-defined or smudgy appearance to the trabeculae in patients with osteomalacia.[3,17] Looser zones are most commonly seen in the anterior aspect of the upper ribs, the pubic rami, and the femoral necks (Figure 33–16). Other less common locations for Looser's zones are the scapular blades and the diaphyses of long bones (usually the femur) (Figure 33–17).[3,17] Advanced imaging studies such as CT, MRI, and scintigraphy are not used routinely to evaluate osteomalacia.

Soft tissue calcifications in the form of calcium hydroxyapatite can be seen on radiographs. Calcium hydroxyapatite deposits can be seen as calcifications in the subcutaneous fat (including breasts), as clustered calcifications in a periarticular distribution and as vascular calcifications (Figure 33–18).[17]

Calcification in renal osteodystrophy is seen in vessel walls, subcutaneous tissues, and around joints.

The soft tissue calcifications in the subcutaneous fat and about the joints can mimic a tumor on physical exam; the periarticular calcifications can also cause adjacent inflammation mimicking an inflammatory arthritis on physical exam. Radiographs are useful in differentiating between calcification and an actual tumor or between calcification and an inflammatory arthritis. The amorphous visceral calcifications that can occur in renal osteodystrophy are not readily visible on radiographs; however, they can be seen on nuclear medicine bone scans due to increased uptake of the bone scan agent.[21]

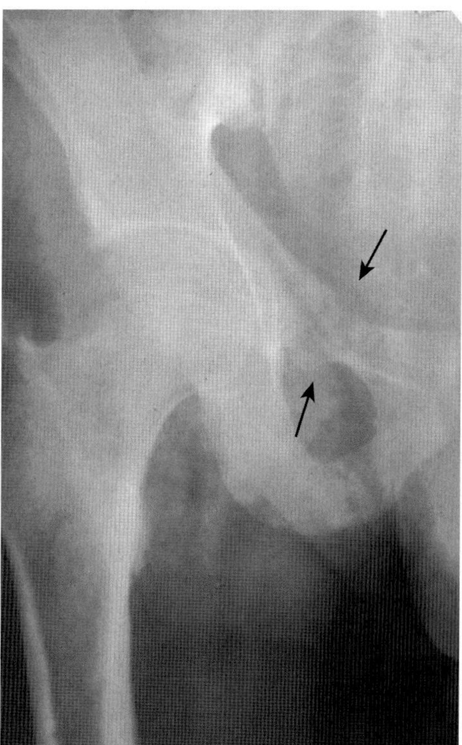

FIGURE 33–16. Looser zone. Anteroposterior radiograph of the right hip in a patient with renal failure and osteomalacia. A Looser zone can be seen at the right superior pubic ramus *(black arrows)*.

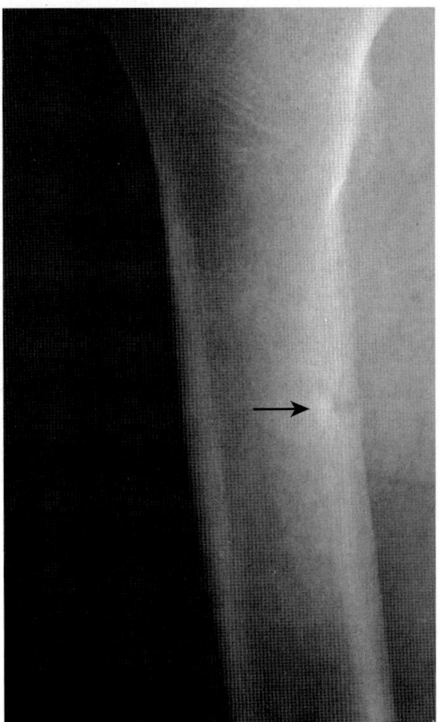

FIGURE 33–17. Looser zone Coned-down anteroposterior view of the right femur. In this patient with renal failure and osteomalacia, one can see a Looser zone at the medial aspect of the right femoral shaft *(black arrow)*.

Imaging Features of Associated Conditions and Complications

In patients on chronic dialysis, amyloid deposition can occur in the soft tissues and bones from circulating β_2-microglobulin. It is rare in patients who have been dialyzed for less than 5 years; however, approximately 80% of patients may be affected by amyloidosis after more than 10 years of hemodialysis.[22] Frequent sites of osteoarticular involvement are the hand, wrist, shoulder, hip, and cervical spine. On radiographs, amyloid will appear as cysts or lytic areas in the bone that are actually pressure erosions from amyloid deposits in the adjacent soft tissues (Figure 33–19).[22] Amyloid involvement in the cervical spine is known as destructive spondyloarthropathy, which radiographically resembles infectious spondylodiskitis.[23,24] MRI is useful in this scenario since it will not demonstrate the characteristic findings of spine infection; instead it will demonstrate low signal intensity on all sequences.[24] Occasionally, biopsy or fine-needle aspiration of the spine may be necessary when the MRI findings are inconclusive for amyloid spondyloarthropathy.[24]

Patients with renal osteodystrophy can also develop azotemic erosive arthropathy of the hands. The erosions can develop at the interphalangeal joints and metacarpophalangeal joints. Cyst-like erosions can also occur in the wrist. Azotemic erosive arthropathy is felt to be multifactorial with amyloid and hyperparathyroidism playing etiologic roles. Most likely, the subchondral erosions are related to secondary hyperparathyroidism and the cyst-like changes are related to amyloid deposition.[17,25] The clinical significance of this erosive arthropathy is felt to be minimal as there is no direct association with symptoms based on the literature.[26]

> Erosive arthropathy in renal disease is probably of minimal clinical significance.

The radiographic severity of this arthropathy is primarily a function of the patient's age and the number of years the patient has been undergoing dialysis.[26] Finally, amyloid deposition in the wrists can lead to carpal tunnel syndrome necessitating surgical decompression (Figure 33–20).[17]

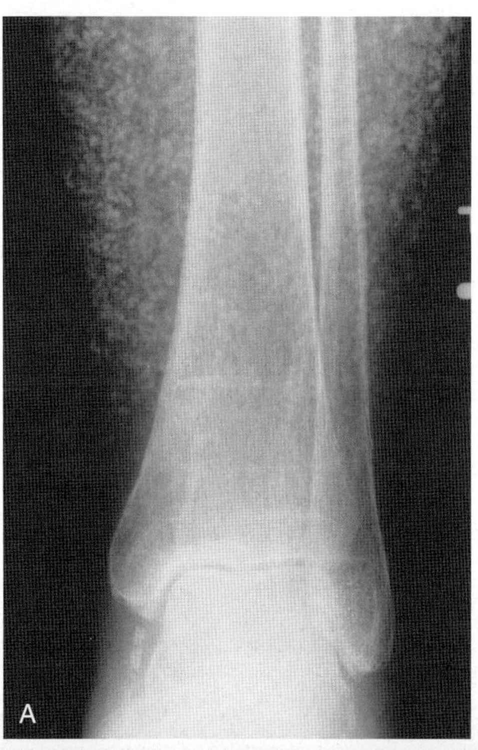

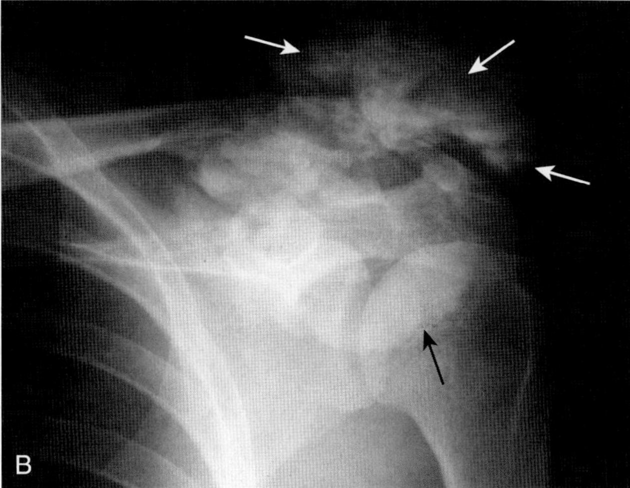

FIGURE 33–18. Images demonstrating soft tissue calcification secondary to renal failure. **A,** On this anteroposterior radiograph of the left ankle, diffuse soft tissue calcifications (calcium hydroxyapatite) can be seen in the subcutaneous fat of the left lower extremity. **B,** This anteroposterior radiograph of the left shoulder demonstrates periarticular soft tissue calcification about the left acromioclavicular joint *(arrows)*. One can see how this type of soft tissue calcification would mimic a tumor on physical exam. Radiographs can help differentiate between a soft tissue mass and periarticular soft tissue calcification.

(Continued)

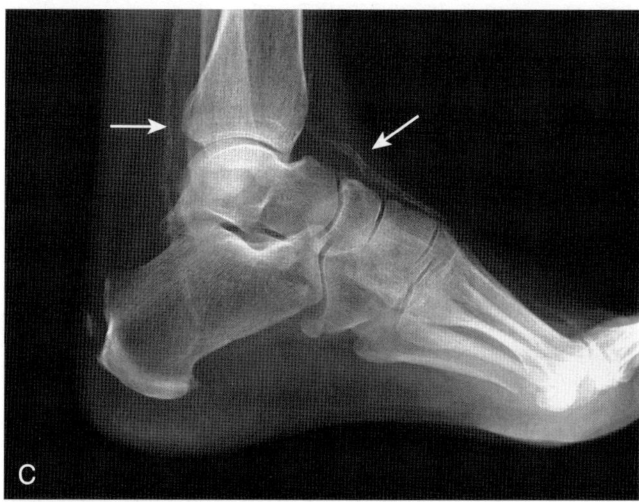

FIGURE 33-18—cont'd. C, Extensive vascular calcifications *(white arrows)* from secondary hyperparathyroidism are seen on this lateral radiograph of the right foot.

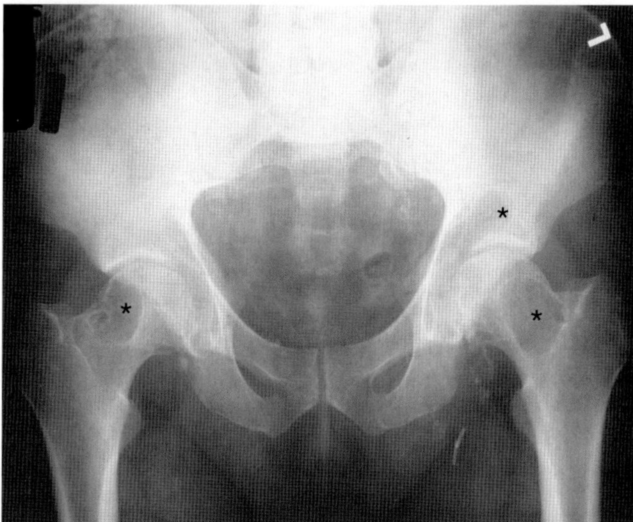

FIGURE 33–19. β2-microglobulin amyloid. Anteroposterior radiograph of the pelvis in a renal failure patient on long-term hemodialysis with bilateral hip pain. This radiograph demonstrates prominent erosions (resembling cyst-like structures) at both hips *(asterisks)*. This appearance is classic for amyloid deposition in a patient on chronic hemodialysis.

Another complication associated with chronic renal failure and its treatment is insufficiency fracture. In some studies, the percentage of chronic renal failure patients with an insufficiency fracture approaches nearly 25%.[17] Given the marked osteopenia that can accompany chronic renal failure, these insufficiency fractures can be radiographically occult; therefore, if the radiographic study is negative and there is continued suspicion of a fracture, MRI is the imaging exam of choice.[27] On MRIs, insufficiency fractures are seen as a band of low signal on T1-weighted images and increased signal on the T2-weighted or STIR images (Figure 33–21).[27] Common locations for insufficiency fractures are the sacrum, pubic bone, femoral neck, tibia, calcaneus, and ribs. A unique insufficiency fracture known as the calcaneal insufficiency avulsion (CIA) fracture is nearly confined to diabetic patients. Although it is felt that diabetic neuropathy is the main causative factor in CIA fractures, a majority of the patients with this fracture also have underlying chronic renal failure. It is felt that the renal failure with its accompanying osseous abnormalities also contributes to the etiology of this fracture (Figure 33–22).[28]

Tendon rupture is a documented complication of renal failure patients on long-term hemodialysis who have lab test evidence of secondary hyperparathyroidism. It occurs typically at the quadriceps, patellar, triceps, and finger tendons.[17] In the lower extremities, the ruptures can be bilateral and simultaneous.[29] Tendon ruptures in hemodialysis patients with secondary hyperparathyroidism most commonly occur in the quadriceps mechanism, with one study reporting that 50% of tendon ruptures in renal failure patients occurred at the quadriceps. If imaging documentation of the tendon rupture or preoperative planning is required, MRI is the imaging modality of choice. MRI can readily demonstrate the location and extent of the injury (Figure 33–23). The likelihood of tendon rupture increases with increased age and with increased number of years on hemodialysis.[29]

Another complication in renal failure is aluminum toxicity. Aluminum toxicity of the bones (also known as adynamic bone disease) has become less common given improvements in the medical management of dialysis patients. Aluminum toxicity cannot be readily diagnosed radiographically as it causes osteopenia, which is a nonspecific radiographic finding. The current reference standard for diagnosing aluminum toxicity of bone is a tetracycline-labeled bone biopsy. This is done typically when indicated by abnormal laboratory tests.

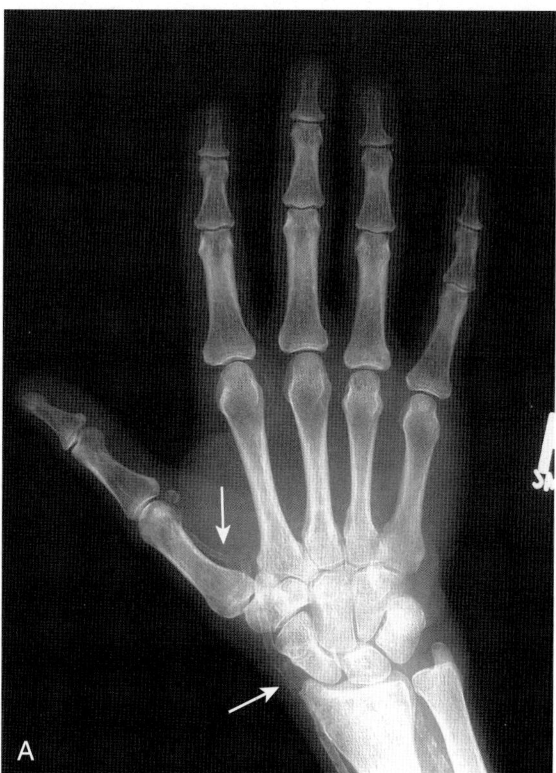

FIGURE 33–20. Images of the right hand and wrist in a patient on long-term hemodialysis with carpal tunnel syndrome. **A,** This posteroanterior radiograph of the right hand demonstrates extensive vascular calcifications *(white arrows)* consistent with a history of renal osteodystrophy.

(Continued)

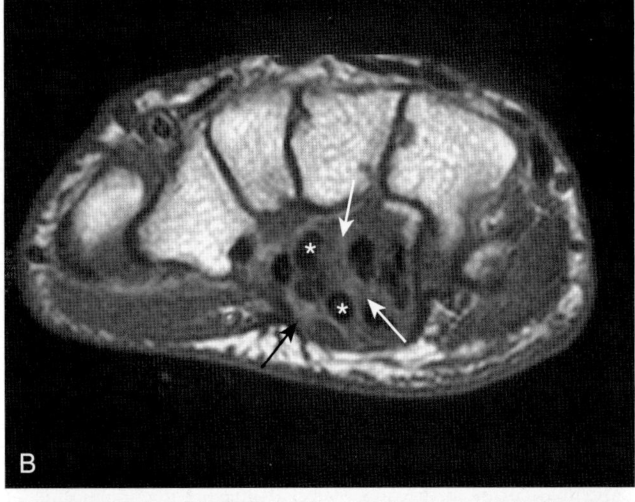

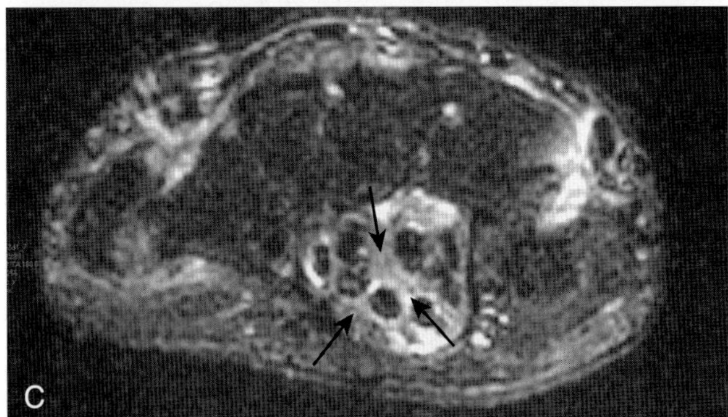

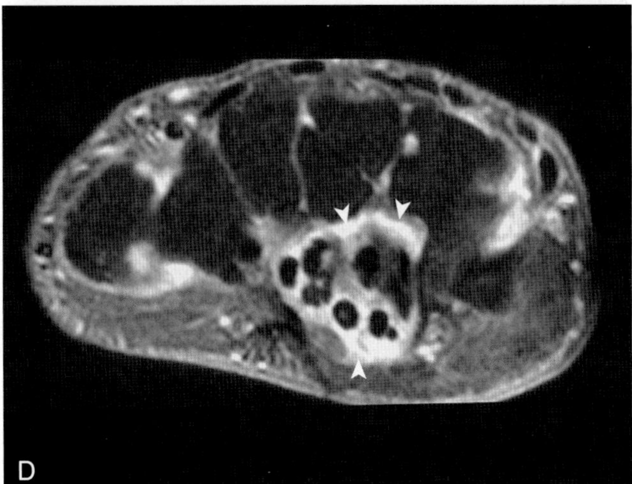

FIGURE 33–20—cont'd. Transverse MRIs that are T1-weighted **(B)**, STIR **(C)**, and post-contrast fat-saturated T1-weighted **(D)** demonstrate tissue within the carpal tunnel surrounding the flexor tendons (the *asterisks* mark a few tendons) that has heterogeneous signal characteristics *(arrows)* and heterogeneous contrast enhancement *(arrowheads)*. This was felt to represent amyloid deposition given the patient's history. Amyloid deposition was confirmed by surgical biopsy during the carpal tunnel release surgery.

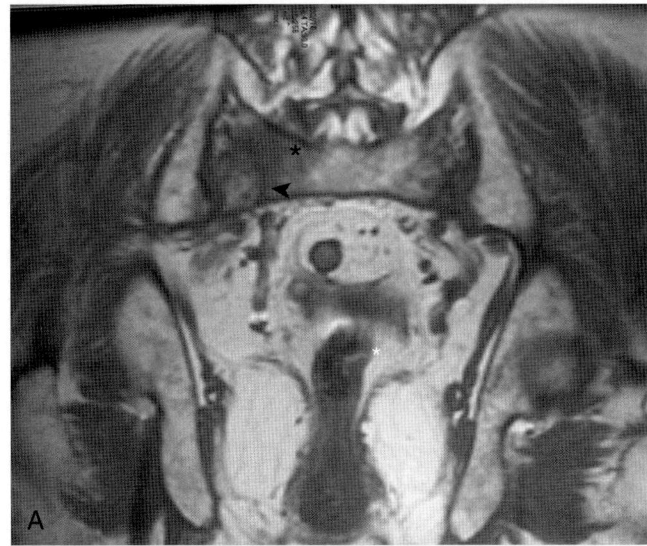

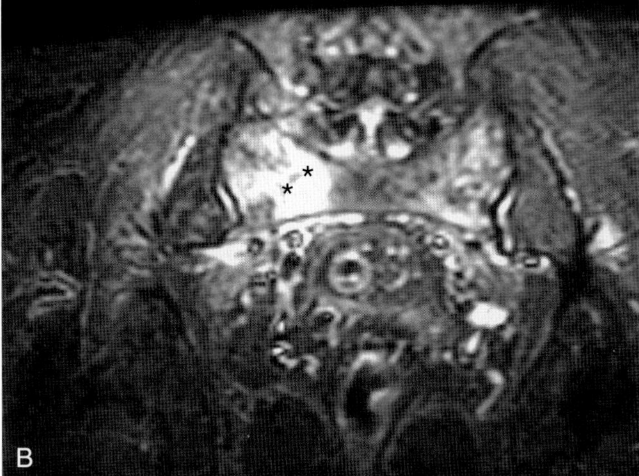

FIGURE 33–21. Insufficiency fracture. Coronal MRIs in a patient with chronic renal failure. **A,** Coronal T1-weighted MR image shows a linear focus of low signal intensity *(black arrowhead)* surrounded by more diffuse area of low signal intensity *(asterisks)*. **B,** Coronal STIR image shows increased signal consistent with edema *(asterisks)* about the insufficiency fracture.

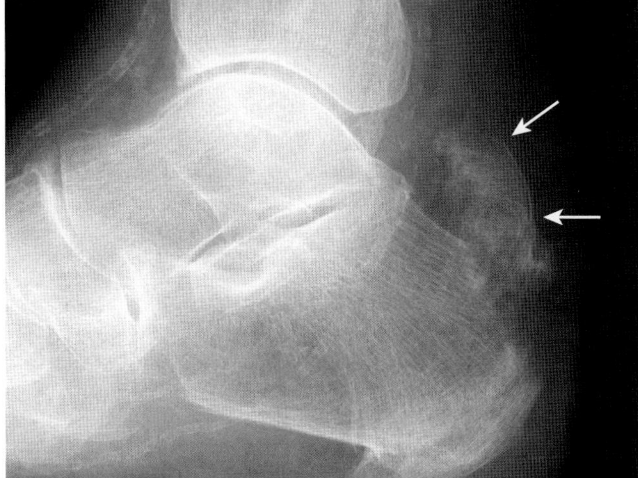

FIGURE 33–22. Calcaneal avulsion fracture. Coned-down lateral view of the right ankle in a patient with chronic renal failure and diabetes. The calcaneal insufficiency avulsion fracture is pointed out by the *white arrows*. Also note the extensive vascular calcifications in this patient with a history of renal osteodystrophy.

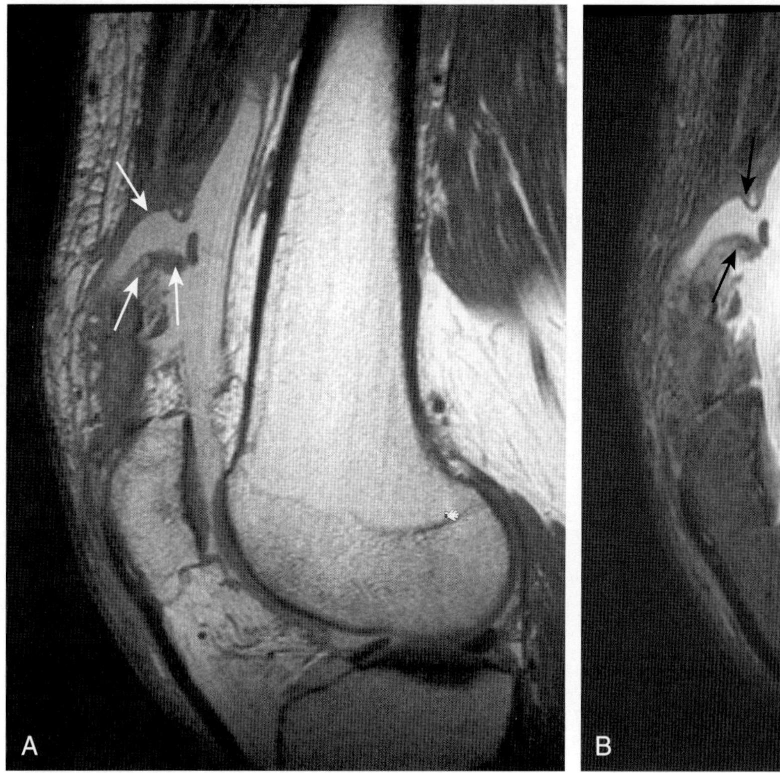

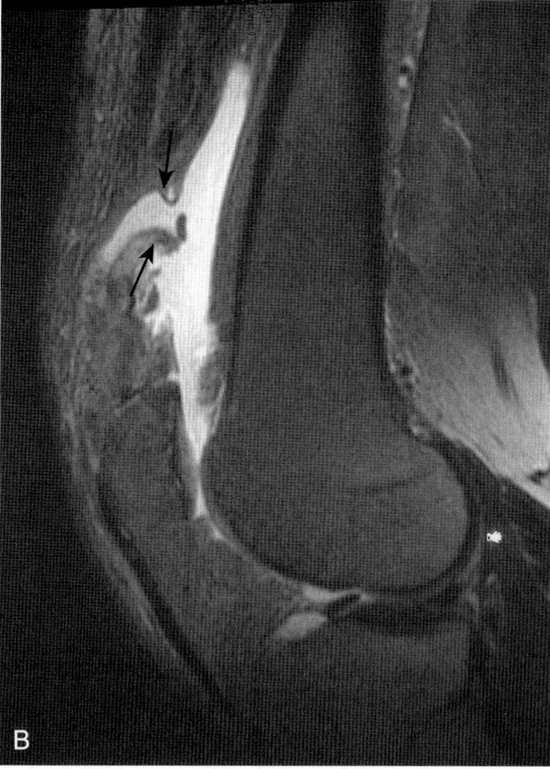

FIGURE 33–23. Quadriceps tendon rupture. Sagittal MRI of the distal left femur in a patient with secondary hyperparathyroidism on long-term hemodialysis. Both the T1-weighted **(A)** and the fat-saturated fast spin echo T2-weighted **(B)** images readily demonstrate the rupture of the quadriceps tendon *(arrows)*.

Recommendations

Radiography is the initial test of choice in patients with new onset of bone pain. In the dialysis patient, diffuse bone pain is caused typically by hyperparathyroidism or aluminum toxicity.[30] A lateral view of the spine is the most helpful initial screen in dialysis patients with new diffuse bone pain because if osteosclerosis (rugger jersey spine) is present, then clinically significant aluminum toxicity is ruled out.[20] However, if the radiograph does not demonstrate osteosclerosis, then the patient may have hyperparathyroidism, aluminum toxicity of bone, or both. In this case, further laboratory tests would be warranted. In a patient with focal pain, radiography of the site of symptoms will help detect hyperparathyroidism, insufficiency fracture, avascular necrosis, soft tissue calcification, or amyloid deposition. If the radiograph is not contributory, then advanced imaging such as MRI would be warranted in the dialysis patient with focal musculoskeletal pain.

References

1. Nguyen BD: Parathyroid imaging with Tc-99m sestamibi planar and SPECT scintigraphy, *Radiographics* 19:601-614, 1999.
2. Sharp CF Jr., Rude RK, Terry R et al: Abnormal bone and parathyroid histology in carcinoma patients with pseudohyperparathyroidism, *Cancer* 49:1449-1455, 1982.
3. Lenchik L, Sartoris DJ: Orthopedic aspects of metabolic bone disease, *Orthop Clin North Am* 29:103-134, 1998.
4. Bilezikian JP, Potts JT Jr, Fuleihan Gel-H et al: Summary statement from a workshop on asymptomatic primary hyperparathyroidism: a perspective for the 21st century, *J Bone Miner Res* 17(Suppl 2):N2-N11, 2002.
5. Bilezikian JP, Potts JT Jr: Asymptomatic primary hyperparathyroidism: new issues and new questions—bridging the past with the future, *J Bone Miner Res* 17(Suppl 2):N57-N67, 2002.
6. Giron J, Ouhayoun E, Dahan M et al: Imaging of hyperparathyroidism: US, CT, MRI and MIBI scintigraphy, *Eur J Radiol* 21:167-173, 1996.
7. Gotway MB, Reddy GP, Webb WR et al: Comparison between MR imaging and 99mTc MIBI scintigraphy in the evaluation of recurrent or persistent hyperparathyroidism, *Radiology* 218:783-790, 2001.
8. Ahuja AT, Wong KT, Ching AS et al: Imaging for primary hyperparathyroidism—what beginners should know, *Clin Radiol* 59:967-976, 2004.
9. Nies C: Primary hyperparathyroidism: is there a role for imaging? (Against), *Eur J Nucl Med Mol Imaging* 31:1324-1326, 2004.
10. Roka R, Pramhas M, Roka S: Primary hyperparathyroidism: is there a role for imaging? (Pro), *Eur J Nucl Med Mol Imaging* 31:1322-1324, 2004.
11. McDonald DK, Parman L, Speights VO Jr: Best cases from the AFIP: primary hyperparathyroidism due to parathyroid adenoma, *Radiographics* 25:829-834, 2005.
12. Ashebu SD, Dahniya MH, Muhtaseb SA et al: Unusual florid skeletal manifestations of primary hyperparathyroidism, *Skeletal Radiol* 31:720-723, 2002.
13. Gerrand C, Griffin AM, White LM et al: Musculoskeletal images. Early bone changes in hyperparathyroidism detected on magnetic resonance imaging, *Can J Surg* 42:330, 1999.
14. Mustonen AO, Kiuru MJ, Stahls A et al: Radicular lower extremity pain as the first symptom of primary hyperparathyroidism, *Skeletal Radiol* 33:467-472, 2004.
15. Gotway MB, Leung JW, Gooding GA et al: Hyperfunctioning parathyroid tissue: spectrum of appearances on noninvasive imaging, *AJR Am J Roentgenol* 179:495-502, 2002.
16. Scarsbrook AF, Thakker RV, Wass JA et al: Multiple endocrine neoplasia: spectrum of radiologic appearances and discussion of a multitechnique imaging approach, *Radiographics* 26:433-451, 2006.
17. Murphey MD, Sartoris DJ, Quale JL et al: Musculoskeletal manifestations of chronic renal insufficiency, *Radiographics* 13:357-379, 1993.
18. Weller M, Edeiken J, Hodes PJ: Renal osteodystrophy, *Am J Roentgenol Radium Ther Nucl Med* 104:354-363, 1968.
19. Adams JE: Renal bone disease: radiological investigation, *Kidney Int* 56(Suppl 73): S38-S41, 1999.
20. Kriegshauser JS, Swee RG, McCarthy JT et al: Aluminum toxicity in patients undergoing dialysis: radiographic findings and prediction of bone biopsy results, *Radiology* 164:399-403, 1987.
21. Taylor RE: Multifactorial uptake of Tc-99m methylene diphosphonate in chronic renal failure, *Clin Nucl Med* 28:939-940, 2003.
22. Cobby MJ, Adler RS, Swartz R et al: Dialysis-related amyloid arthropathy: MR findings in four patients, *AJR Am J Roentgenol* 157:1023-1027, 1991.
23. Naidich JB, Mossey RT, McHeffey-Atkinson B et al: Spondyloarthropathy from long-term hemodialysis, *Radiology* 167:761-764, 1988.
24. Leone A, Sundaram M, Cerase A et al: Destructive spondyloarthropathy of the cervical spine in long-term hemodialyzed patients: a five-year clinical radiological prospective study, *Skeletal Radiol* 30:431-441, 2001.
25. Kamphuis AG, Geerlings W, Hazenberg BP et al: Annual evaluation of hip joints and hands for radiographic signs of A beta 2M-amyloidosis in long-term hemodialysis patients, *Skeletal Radiol* 23:421-427, 1994.

26. Falbo SE, Sundaram M, Ballal S et al: Clinical significance of erosive azotemic osteodystrophy: a prospective masked study, *Skeletal Radiol* 28:86-89, 1999.
27. Manaster BJ, Grossman JW, Dalinka MK et al: Stress/insufficiency fracture, including sacrum, excluding other vertebrae. In *ACR Appropriateness Criteria,* Reston, VA, 2005, American College of Radiology, pp 1-7.
28. Kathol MH, El-Khoury GY, Moore TE et al: Calcaneal insufficiency avulsion fractures in patients with diabetes mellitus, *Radiology* 180:725-729, 1991.
29. Munakata T, Nishida J, Shimamura T et al: Simultaneous avulsion of patellar apexes bilaterally in a hemodialysis patient, *Skeletal Radiol* 24:211-213, 1995.
30. Fournier A, Oprisiu R, Hottelart C et al: Renal osteodystrophy in dialysis patients: diagnosis and treatment, *Artif Organs* 22:530-557, 1998.

CHAPTER 34

Hypoparathyroidism and PTH Resistance

PARHAM PEZESHK, MD, *and* JOHN A. CARRINO, MD, MPH

KEY FACTS

- DiGeorge's syndrome, type I autoimmune polyglandular syndrome, X-linked or autosomally inherited hypoparathyroidism, and PTH gene mutations are the most frequent causes of congenital hypoparathyroidism.
- Pseudohypoparathyroidism (PHP) is an inherited disorder resulting from mutations in the end-organ PTH receptors, leading to PTH resistance.
- Albright hereditary osteodystrophy is a somatic phenotype of PHP characterized by developmental delay, mental retardation, obesity, round face, hypoplastic dentition, short stature, subcutaneous calcifications, brachymetacarpals, and brachymetatarsals (shortening of affected bones).

Hypoparathyroidism, the impaired secretion of parathyroid hormone (PTH) from the parathyroid glands, is the most common cause of hypocalcemia. The inadequate parathormone (PTH) secretion causes failure to mobilize calcium from bone, reabsorb calcium from the distal nephron, or stimulate renal I α-hydroxylase activity. The decreased $1,25[OH]_2$ vitamin D leads to inefficient absorption of calcium from the gut[1] (Figure 34-1). Hypoparathyroidism occurs as a result of congenital (inherited) or acquired (secondary) disorders. DiGeorge's syndrome, type I autoimmune polyglandular syndrome, X-linked or autosomally inherited hypoparathyroidism, and PTH gene mutations are the most frequent causes of congenital hypoparathyroidism. In DiGeorge's syndrome, a defect in the development of the third and fourth pharyngeal pouches leads to agenesis of parathyroid gland. Type I polyglandular syndrome is characterized by hypoparathyroidism, adrenal failure, and mucocutaneous candidiasis and develops from circulating antibodies against parathyroid, thyroid, and adrenal glands. Parathyroid glands are absent in X-linked (or autosomally) inherited hypoparathyroidism. PTH is deficient in PTH gene mutations.[2]

Damage to the parathyroid glands can lead to secondary hypoparathyroidism. Postsurgical hypoparathyroidism is the most frequent cause of prolonged hypocalcemia and is seen after thyroid and other head and neck surgeries. Infiltration of the parathyroid glands may develop subsequent to several disorders including hemochromatosis, thalassemia major (iron overload due to numerous blood transfusions), Wilson's disease, and rarely, metastases. Radiation and radioactive iodine thyroid ablation are other secondary causes.

Pseudohypoparathyroidism (PHP) is an inherited disorder resulting from mutations in the end-organ PTH receptors leading to PTH resistance. Similar to hypoparathyroidism, the ultimate outcome would be the absence of PTH action on end organs. In contrast to hypoparathyroidism, in pseudohypoparathyroidism the serum level of PTH is high due to of the lack of negative feedback on the parathyroid glands. Besides the radiographic manifestations of hypoparathyroidism, specific findings are also noticed in pseudohypoparathyroidism as described below.

IMAGING FEATURES OF HYPOPARATHYROIDISM

Radiographs

Radiography is the most widely used modality to evaluate the skeletal and soft tissue changes of hypoparathyroidism. Localized or diffuse osteosclerosis (increased density of bone tissue) is the most common skeletal finding in hypoparathyroidism. Thickening of the facial bones and cranial vault[3] with a widened diploe are seen. Sutural diastasis may be present as a consequence of increased intracranial pressure.[4] Intracranial calcifications (basal ganglia, falx, and rarely the cerebellum and choroids plexus) occur due to the metabolic abnormality. Calcification of ligaments (e.g., anterior longitudinal ligament and posterior paraspinal ligaments in the spine) and calcifications of muscle insertions (enthesopathy) are features of hypoparathyroidism.[5] Hypoplastic dentition, delayed or failed eruption of the teeth, and a thickened lamina dura (the thin hard layer of bone that lines the socket of a tooth appearing as a white line on radiography) may be observed.[6] Asymptomatic or painful subcutaneous calcifications, particularly around shoulders and hips, can develop. Band-like radiodensities are noticed in the metaphyses of long bones, and sclerosis of the iliac crests and the margins of the vertebral bodies may be present.[5] Premature closure of the physes is another radiographic finding in the developing skeleton.

Rarely, the radiologic changes of ankylosing spondylitis and hypoparathyroidism may resemble each other. However, in the latter, there is no tenderness in the spine and pelvis, and although spinal osteophytes and calcification of spinal ligaments may be seen, the sacroiliac joints are spared.[5]

Ultrasonography

Renal ultrasonography may reveal nephrocalcinosis in the patients receiving treatment due to the resultant calciuria. Therefore, a baseline renal ultrasonogram is recommended prior to the initiation of treatment.

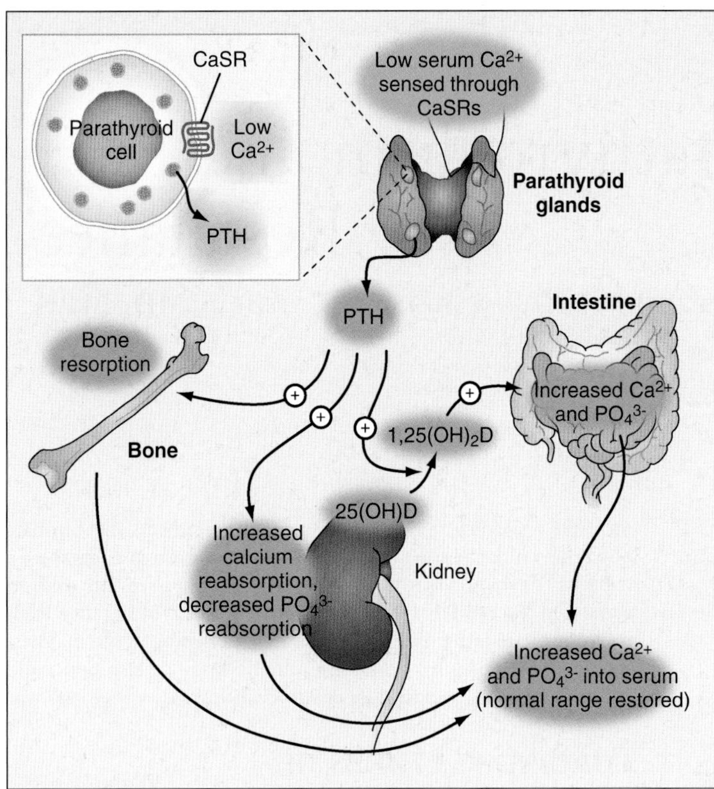

FIGURE 34-1. Control of mineral metabolism by parathyroid hormone. Levels of serum ionized calcium (Ca^{2+}) are tightly controlled through the action of parathyroid hormone (PTH) and 1,25-dihydroxyvitamin D (1,25[OH]$_2$D). Both the rate and magnitude of changes in the serum ionized Ca^{2+} concentration are detected by extracellular calcium-sensing receptors (CaSRs) expressed on parathyroid cells. When ionized Ca^{2+} levels decrease, PTH secretion is triggered. Conversely, when ionized Ca^{2+} levels increase, PTH secretion is suppressed. PTH stimulates bone resorption, which delivers calcium and phosphorus (PO_4^{3-}) into the circulation. In the kidney, PTH stimulates renal reabsorption of calcium and promotes phosphate excretion. PTH also enhances the conversion of 25-hydroxyvitamin D (25[OH]D) to the active vitamin D metabolite 1,25(OH)$_2$D, which increases the transepithelial transport of calcium and PO_4^{3-} through actions in intestinal cells. In concert, these steps restore ionized Ca^{2+} levels to the normal range and, through the actions of PTH and other factors (e.g., fibroblast-derived growth factor 23) in the kidney, reset the level of serum PO_4^{3-} within the normal range. When the actions of PTH are reduced or lost, all subsequent steps in the maintenance of homeostasis are impaired, resulting in hypocalcemia, hyperphosphatemia, and hypercalciuria. (From Shoback D: Hypoparathyroidism, *N Engl J Med,* 359:391, 2008.)

Nephrocalcinosis may develop with treatment of hypoparathyroidism as a consequence of calciuria. A baseline renal ultrasound examination is recommended.

DIFFERENTIAL DIAGNOSES

The radiographic manifestations of hypoparathyroidism may also be seen in a variety of other disorders (Table 34-1).[5,6]

Pseudohypoparathyroidism

Pseudohypoparathyroidism (PHP) is a PTH-resistant disorder resulting from mutations in the end-organ PTH receptors. The ultimate consequence is the inability of PTH to exert its biologic effects, imitating a hypoparathyroid state. Albright hereditary osteodystrophy (AHO) is a somatic phenotype of PHP (type Ia) characterized by developmental delay, mental retardation, obesity, round face, hypoplastic dentition, short stature, subcutaneous calcifications, brachymetacarpals, and brachymetatarsals (shortening of affected bones) (Figures 34-2 and 34-3). Pseudopseudohypoparathyroidism (PPHP) is a disorder characterized by normal calcium homeostasis and biomedical parameters in individuals with the phenotype of AHO.

Radiographic Manifestations

Radiographic evaluation of PHP and PPHP may show bowing of the extremities, premature physeal fusion, calvarial thickening, and soft tissue calcification (Table 34-2). Bone density may be decreased, normal, or increased.[5,6]

Basal ganglia calcification is characteristic of PHP and hypoparathyroidism.

TABLE 34-1. Differential Diagnoses of Radiographic Findings of Hypoparathyroidism

Finding	Differential Diagnoses
Diffuse Osteosclerosis	Paget's disease Pyknodysostosis Hematologic causes: sickle cell anemia, myelofibrosis, mastocytosis, polycythemia vera Neoplasms: myeloma, lymphoma, leukemia, prostate, breast, gastrointestinal tract, bladder Metabolic diseases: primary hyperparathyroidism, familial hypophosphatemic osteomalacia, hypervitaminosis D, fluorosis
Calvarial thickening	Paget's disease, chronic anemias, fibrous dysplasia, Dilantin therapy, fluorosis, and hyperphosphatasia
Basal ganglia calcification	Carbon-monoxide exposure Fahr syndrome (ferrocalcinosis) Toxoplasmosis and cytomegalic inclusion disease Radiation therapy
Hypoplastic dentition	Certain congenital syndromes, hypothyroidism, hypopituitarism
Subcutaneous calcification	Renal osteodystrophy, hypervitaminosis D, milk-alkali syndrome, collagen vascular disease

Features such as exostoses and shortening of metacarpal and metatarsal bones are prominent in PHP and PPHP but not in hypoparathyroidism. Exostoses (formation of new bone on the surface of a bone showing cortical and medullary continuity with underlying bone) project at right angles to the cortex rather than away from the joint as seen in the usual exostosis. Exostoses

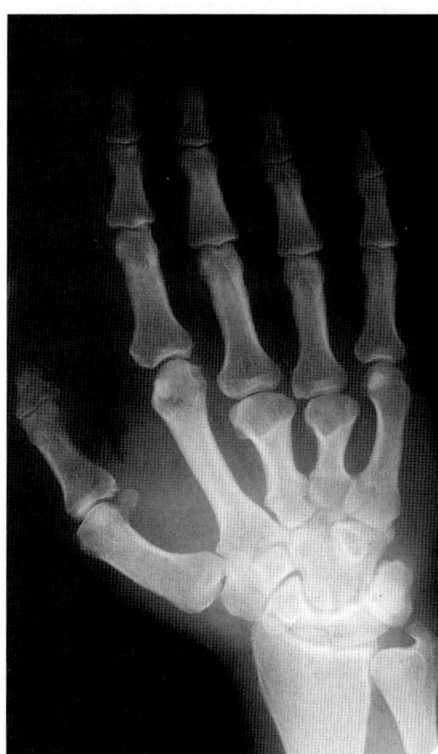

FIGURE 34-2. Pseudohypoparathyroidism. Posteroanterior hand radiograph shows metacarpal shortening of the middle and ring fingers.

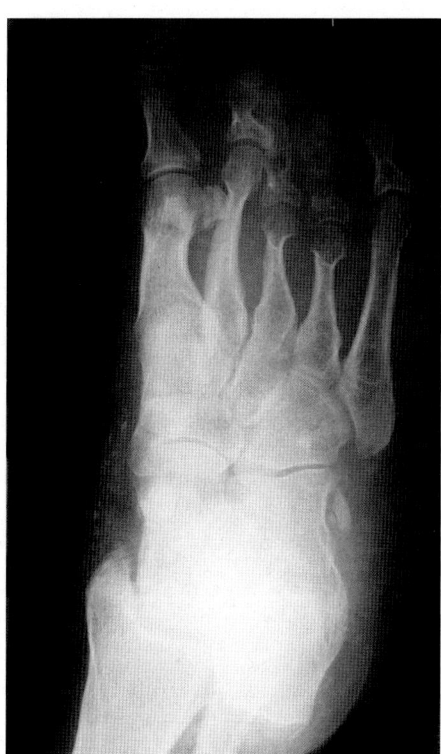

FIGURE 34-3. Pseudohypoparathyroidism. Oblique foot radiograph shows shortening of the first, third, and fourth metatarsal bones. The phalanges appear wide and short. Subcutaneous soft tissue calcifications are present.

TABLE 34-2. Radiographic Findings of PHP and PPHP

PHP	PPHP
Basal ganglia calcification	
Bowing of the extremities	Bowing of the extremities
Premature physeal fusion	Premature physeal fusion
Calvarial thickening	Calvarial thickening
Soft tissue calcification	Soft tissue calcification
Exostoses	Exostoses

associated with PHP or PPHP are broadbased and mostly present in the mid-shafts of tubular bones.[6] Metacarpal shortening is usually seen in the first, fourth, and fifth digits. The phalanges may be wide and short, and the first metacarpal bone may appear excessively curved and wide.[5] Metatarsal shortening frequently develops in the first and fourth digits. As a result of short metacarpal bones, a positive "metacarpal sign" may be found. In normal subjects, a line that is drawn tangentially to the heads of the fifth and fourth metacarpal bones does not cross the third metacarpal bone or just meets its articular surface. In PHP and PPHP, this line crosses the third metacarpal bone due to the shortening of the fourth and fifth metacarpal bones (a positive "metacarpal sign"). However, if the third metacarpal bone is also shortened, this sign may not be observed. A positive metacarpal sign is not specific for PHP and PPHP and can be seen in other conditions producing short metacarpals such as Turner's syndrome, sickle cell anemia with infarction, juvenile chronic arthritis with early epiphyseal closure, neonatal hyperthyroidism, and trauma. Radiographic changes in the hands are almost similar in PHP and PPHP, though the short distal phalanges are more frequent in the former while shorter metacarpals are more commonly seen in the latter.[7]

> A positive metacarpal sign is not specific for PHP and PPHP and can be seen in other conditions producing short metacarpals.

Radiographs may also demonstrate calcification of the posterior longitudinal ligament of the cervical spine. The findings of hyperparathyroidism (e.g., subperiosteal) may coexist with PHP and PPHP.[4] Pseudohypo-hyperparathyroidism is a rare variant of PHP characterized by a normal skeletal response but unresponsive kidneys to PTH. In this condition, the skeletal radiographic features of hyperparathyroidism may coexist with those of hypoparathyroidism.[5,8]

REFERENCES

1. Shoback D: Hypoparathyroidism, *N Engl J Med* 359:391-403, 2008.
2. Bringhurst FR, Demay MB, Kronenberg HM: Hormones and disorders of mineral metabolism, In Larsen PR (ed): *Williams Textbook of Endocrinology*, 10th ed, Philadelphia, 2003, Saunders, pp 1303-1372.
3. Goldman R, Reynolds JL, Cummings HR et al: Familial hypoparathyroidism; report of a case, *J Am Med Assoc* 150:1104-1106, 1952.
4. Strom L, Winberg GJ: Idiopathic hypoparathyroidism, *Acta Paediatr* 43:574-581, 1954.
5. Resnick D: Parathyroid disorders and renal osteodystrophy. In Resnick D (ed): *Diagnosis of Bone and Joint Disorders*, 4th ed, Philadelphia, 2002, Saunders, pp 2043-2111.
6. Vogler JB III, Kim JH: Metabolic and endocrine disease of the skeleton. In Grainger RG, Allison DJ, Adam A et al (eds): *Grainger & Allison's Diagnostic Radiology: A Textbook of Medical Imaging*, 4th ed, Churchill Livingstone, 2001, pp 1925-1966.
7. Poznanski AK, Werder EA, Giedion A et al: The pattern of shortening of the bones of the hand in PHP and PPHP—a comparison with brachydactyly E, Turner Syndrome, and acrodysostosis, *Radiology* 123:707-718, 1977.
8. Hall FM, Segall-Blank M, Genant HK et al: Pseudohypoparathyroidism presenting as renal osteodystrophy, *Skel Radiol* 6:43-46, 1981.

CHAPTER 35

Rickets and Osteomalacia

PARHAM PEZESHK, MD, *and* JOHN A. CARRINO, MD, MPH

KEY FACTS

- Rickets and osteomalacia result from inadequate or delayed mineralization of newly synthesized organic matrix (osteoid) in mature bone (osteomalacia) or growing bone (rickets).
- The causes of rickets and osteomalacia fall into three main categories: (1) abnormalities of vitamin D metabolism, (2) abnormalities of calcium and phosphorus metabolism, and (3) disorders with a radiographic appearance of rickets and osteomalacia with no primary abnormalities in vitamin D or mineral metabolism.
- Looser zones are perpendicular areas of lucency with adjacent sclerosis that are often symmetrical, involve the pelvis, proximal femurs, scapulae, and ribs, and are typical features of osteomalacia.
- Hereditary causes of Vitamin D–dependent rickets are type I (pseudovitamin D–deficiency rickets) due to a deficiency in the production or activity of 1α-hydroxylase and type II (also known as hereditary vitamin D–resistant rickets).

Rickets and osteomalacia describe a spectrum of metabolic disorders with similar histopathologic and radiologic abnormalities, which result from inadequate or delayed mineralization of newly synthesized organic matrix (osteoid) in mature bone (osteomalacia) or growing bone (rickets). In other words, rickets and osteomalacia reflect the same disease process with different ages of onset.

1,25-dihydroxyvitamin D (1,25[OH]$_2$D) is a steroid hormone that plays the major role in the homeostasis of calcium and phosphorus, as well as mineralization of bones. Vitamin D_2 (plant source) and vitamin D_3 (animal source) are two prohormonal forms of 1,25(OH)$_2$D that should undergo hydroxylation in both the liver and kidney to become active. The major source of vitamin D in most people is supplied from conversion of 7-dehydrocholesterol in the skin to vitamin D_3 on exposure to the ultraviolet radiation in sunlight.[1] Season, latitude, time of day, clothing, and sunscreen use are some of the factors that may affect UV exposure.[2,3] Dietary sources of vitamin D such as fish oil and fortified foods are of secondary importance. Whatever the source, vitamin D as a prohormone undergoes two sequential hydroxylations to become biologically active. The first hydroxylation occurs in liver by 25-hydroxylase, a reaction that is not rigidly regulated. The resultant product, 25-hydroxyvitamin D (25-OH-D), is the major circulating and storage form of vitamin D and a reliable indicator to assess vitamin D status. 25-OH-D is hydroxylated in the kidney by 1α-hydroxylase to produce the physiologically active 1,25(OH)$_2$D. This step is tightly regulated by PTH, calcium, phosphorus, and 1,25(OH)$_2$D.[4]

The main target organs of 1,25(OH)$_2$D are the intestine and bone, although the kidney and parathyroid glands have also been shown to be sites of action. In the intestine, 1,25(OH)$_2$D increases the absorption of calcium and phosphorus.[5,6] 1,25(OH)$_2$D has two actions on the bone that may seem diametrically opposed. In the presence of PTH, it stimulates osteoclastic osteolysis, which results in release and mobilization of calcium and phosphorus from previously formed bones.[6-8] 1,25(OH)$_2$D also promotes mineralization of organic matrix by maintenance of adequate serum calcium and phosphorus or by exerting a direct effect on the bone (or both).[9] This dual action plays a major role in the homeostasis of calcium and phosphorus by the skeleton. 1,25(OH)$_2$D also increases the resorption of phosphate in the renal tubules and suppresses the secretion of PTH from the parathyroid glands by a negative feedback loop.

The causes of rickets and osteomalacia fall into three main categories: (1) abnormalities of vitamin D metabolism, (2) abnormalities of calcium and phosphorus metabolism, and (3) a group of disorders with a radiographic appearance of rickets and osteomalacia with no primary abnormalities in vitamin D or mineral metabolism.[10] The etiologic factors may be acquired or inherited. Any factor that interferes with the steps in the sequence of vitamin D metabolism (intake, UV conversion of prohormone in the skin, hydroxylation in liver or kidney, and end-organ resistance due to receptor defects) can result in osteomalacia and rickets. Due to fortification of many foods with vitamin D, the incidence of inadequate intake of this vitamin is lower in the United States than in other countries. Vitamin D deficiency is mostly the combined consequence of low dietary intake (or malabsorption) and decreased biosynthesis of vitamin D in the skin following deficient sun exposure.[11,12] Disorders of the pancreas and hepatobiliary system, as well as small-intestine malabsorptive states such as celiac disease, regional enteritis, and bypass surgery can result in vitamin D malabsorption and deficiency.[13,14] Abnormalities in the hydroxylation of provitamin D3 in liver and kidney can also lead to osteomalacia and rickets. While dysfunction of 25-hydroxylase following severe liver disease or isoniazide treatment is an infrequent cause of vitamin D deficiency, impaired 1α-hydroxylase is common in patients with advanced renal disease.[6] The resultant hypocalcemia following low vitamin D and phosphate retention in chronic renal failure results in secondary hyperparathyroidism, which increases calcium and phosphate release from the skeleton leading to osteomalacia and osteopenia. As phosphate retention advances, the calcium phosphate product (Ca × P) increases, resulting in calcification of soft tissues that can be detected radiographically.

OSTEOARTICULAR IMAGING FEATURES

Radiographs

Having a common pathophysiologic basis resulting in histologic and gross morphologic changes, rickets and osteomalacia have similar radiologic manifestations. However, there are some characteristic radiographic changes that can help in the diagnosis of select diseases.

Rickets

The clinical and radiographic manifestations of rickets depend on the age at which it occurs and the severity of the vitamin D deficiency; most severe changes occur if they coincide with a period of rapid growth. Retardation in body growth and generalized osteopenia owing to decreased mineralization of bones are seen.[12] Chaotic proliferation of cartilaginous cells in the zone of maturation of the epiphyseal plate results in a bulky mass of cells in both the longitudinal and latitudinal axes in the poorly mineralized metaphysis.

The earliest radiographic finding of rickets consists of slight axial widening at the growth plate[15] followed by a decrease in the density of the metaphyseal side of the growth plate (zone of provisional calcification).[9] With progression of the disease, the widening of the growth plate increases and the zone of provisional calcification becomes irregular.[16] Fraying and disorganization of the spongy bone in the metaphysis occurs.[9] As the bulk of cell mass increases, it protrudes into the nonmineralized and weakened metaphyseal end, resulting in widening and cupping of the metaphyses.[10,12,17] These are the characteristic radiologic findings of rickets (Figure 35-1) (Box 35-1). The radiographic changes of rickets are best seen in the regions with the most active growth. In decreasing order, the regions with the highest rate of growth and radiographic yield are costochondral junctions of the middle ribs, the distal femur, the proximal portion of the humerus, both ends of the tibia, and the distal ends of the ulna and radius. Because of the faster growth of distal ulna, radiographic evaluation of the ulna is more sensitive for detecting rickets than is evaluation of the distal radius.[9] However, low production of osteoid following severe malnutrition can mask the radiographic signs of rickets.[18,19]

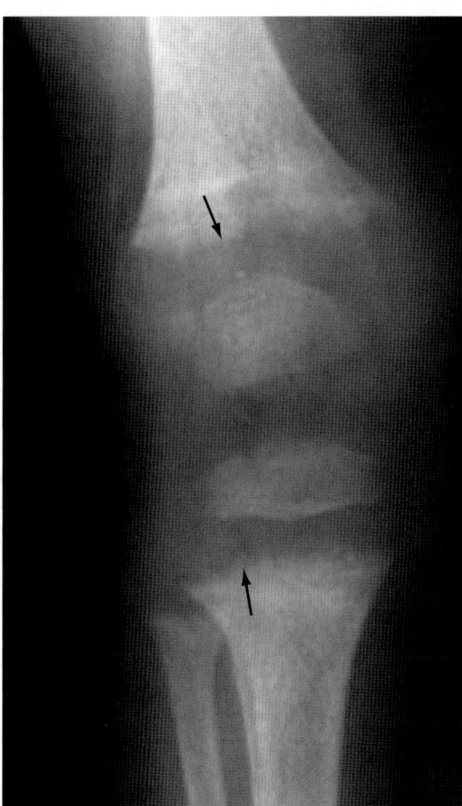

FIGURE 35-1. Rickets. Anteroposterior radiograph of the knee in an infant shows widening of the physes *(arrows)* and irregularity of the zone of provisional calcification (frayed metaphyses).

BOX 35-1. Radiographic Features of Rickets

- Widening of the growth plates
- Irregularity or loss of the sclerotic zone of provisional calcification
- Widening and cupping of the metaphysis
- Skull deformities (infancy)
- Bowing deformities
- Greenstick fractures
- Rachitic rosary
- Pectus carinatum
- Scoliosis, ballooned disks
- Triradiate pelvis
- Slipped capital femoral epiphysis

> Not all regions of the skeleton are affected equally in rickets. The radiographic changes are best seen in the regions with the most active growth such as the knees, proximal humeri, and wrists.

It has been shown that the head deformity of rickets occurs in the first months of life.[20] The incessant overproduction and accumulation of osteoid in the frontal and parietal regions results in the prominence of frontal bones (frontal bossing), and flattening of the posterior skull, basilar invagination, and squared appearance of the skull (known as craniotabes or caput quadratum). During infancy and childhood, the long bones develop deformities both at the shaft-cartilage junction and in the diaphyses (bowing), with the weight-bearing limbs being most severely affected. While forearm deformities develop in crawling children, genu varum ("bow legs") or genu valgum ("knock knees") is seen in toddlers.[12] Anterior bowing of the tibia (saber shin deformity) may also occur. Greenstick fractures may occur in the weakened long bones with no clinical symptoms, and the callus may be observed on radiographic images. There may be a delay in the eruption of the teeth with defects and hypoplasia of enamel resulting in caries. The deposition of newly formed uncalcified osteoid at the junction of the bone shafts and cartilage can lead to swelling about the joints and bead-like rounded knobs at the costochondral junctions of the middle ribs (rachitic rosary). A semicoronal impression (Harrison's groove) may be seen over the abdomen at the level of the insertion of the diaphragm, resulting from pulling on the weakened ribs by the diaphragm during inspiration. The sternum may appear prominent and project anteriorly (pigeon breast deformity or pectus carinatum).[21]

As age increases, weight bearing results in the development of scoliosis and, coupled with bending of the long bones, leads to a decrease in height. The intervertebral disk spaces expand, and concave impressions are formed on endplate surfaces of vertebral bodies, giving them a biconcave appearance.[9,17] A promontory can be seen following the intrusion of the spine into the soft pelvis, producing a triradiate configuration. The anteroposterior diameter of the pelvis may diminish as a result of scoliosis. Slipped capital femoral epiphyses may also be noted on radiographic images.[17]

It takes several months for the osseous changes of vitamin D–deficiency rickets to be apparent radiographically. Although rickets may arise within 2 months in breast-fed infants of vitamin D–deficient mothers, it usually develops toward the end of the first year and during the second year of life.[21]

Rickets usually develops toward the end of the first year and during the second year of life.

Osteomalacia

Osteopenia, a decrease in the radiographic bone density, is a general and nonspecific finding in osteomalacia. A coarsened and indistinct trabecular pattern with "fuzzy" or unsharp margins is seen, which can be useful in differentiation of osteomalacia from osteoporosis.[9,17] Skull, spine, long bones, and pelvis may develop the deformities discussed in rickets (Box 35-2).

Looser zones or pseudofractures, the classic radiographic findings of osteomalacia are radiolucent bands perpendicular to the cortex that incompletely span the diameter of the bone. Mild to moderate sclerosis may be seen at the margins of these pseudofractures. Looser zones result from the focal deposition of uncalcified osteoid and may precede other radiographic changes.[15,18] They are seen in characteristic sites such as the femoral neck (Figures 35-2 and 35-3) below the lesser trochanter (subtrochantric region), the superior and inferior pubic rami, and the axillary margins of the scapula, ribs, and posterior margins of the proximal ulnae. Complete fractures may occur in the weakened areas. Pseudofractures typically appear bilateral and symmetric, which is another characteristic sign of osteomalacia and may be easily missed at early stages.[12,22] Similar radiolucent areas may also be observed in Paget's disease, fibrous dysplasia,[9,17] and rarely osteoporosis.[23] In contrast to the pseudofractures of osteomalacia, the fractures in Paget's disease and fibrous dysplasia are confined to the affected bone and do not have a generalized pattern. At the early stages, Looser zones may be easily missed, and a bone scan can show regions of cortical abnormality that ultimately develop into Looser zones.[12]

BOX 35-2. Imaging Features of Osteomalacia

Decreased bone density
Blurring of trabeculae
Bone deformity (e.g., bowing)
Looser zones

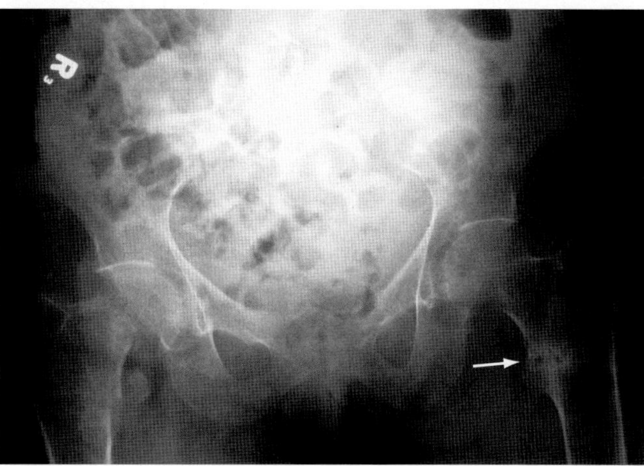

FIGURE 35-3. Osteomalacia in a patient with sprue. An anteroposterior view of the pelvis shows an avulsion fracture of the right lesser trochanter and a Looser zone *(arrow)* in the left femur. There is markedly reduced bone density.

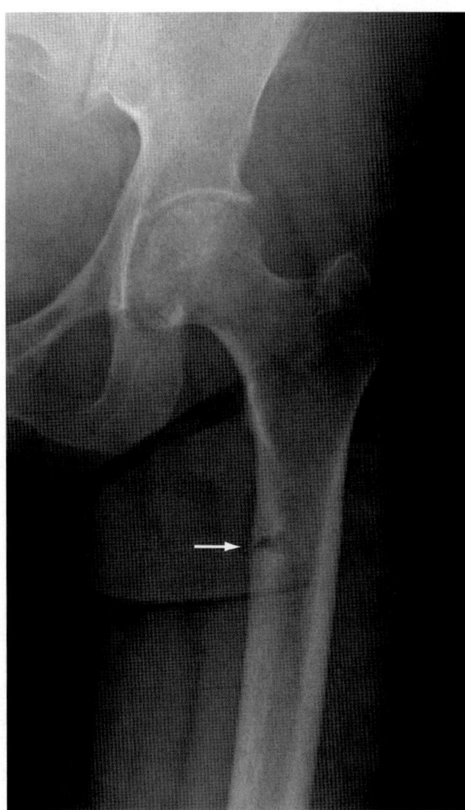

FIGURE 35-2. Osteomalacia: Looser zones (pseudofractures). Anteroposterior radiograph of the left hip shows a radiolucent band perpendicular to the cortex that incompletely spans the bone diameter *(arrow)*. Mild to moderate sclerosis is seen parallel to the margins. The subtrochantric region is a characteristic location. A healing fracture of the superior pubic ramus is also noted.

Computed Tomography

Computed tomography can help in the evaluation of fractures in rickets and osteomalacia. It is also more accurate than radiography in evaluating bone density.

Magnetic Resonance Imaging

Magnetic resonance imaging may be useful in the detection of Looser zones and the widened physes in rickets.

Scintigraphy

As Looser zones may be difficult to identify in their early stages on radiographs, bone scintigraphy may be helpful because it is more likely to show cortical infractions that later develop into Looser zones.[12] Bone scans using 99 mTC-methylene diphosphonate (MDP) may demonstrate symmetric, bilateral sites of increased uptake in the characteristic locations for Looser zones.[24] These sites may show a "flare" response following initiation of treatment of osteomalacia, which is speculated to be the result of osteoblastic activity occurring during the course of treatment, and should not be considered as a poor prognostic sign.

Ultrasonography

Ultrasonography is helpful to identify the presence and severity of slipped capital femoral epiphyses in children. This is a potential complication of rickets.

SOME SPECIFIC CAUSES OF OSTEOMALACIA AND RICKETS

Renal Osteodystrophy (Uremic Osteopathy)

Chronic renal failure affects bone and calcium metabolism by two main mechanisms: secondary hyperparathyroidism and abnormal metabolism of vitamin D. The hypocalcemia that primarily results from phosphate retention provokes increased secretion of PTH (parathyroid hormone). Synthesis of $1,25(OH)_2D$ declines subsequent to phosphate retention and the reduced renal mass, exacerbating the secondary hyperparathyroidism by decreasing the negative feedback suppression.

Radiographic findings of chronic renal failure are seen both in bones and soft tissues (Table 35-1). Changes in bones include rickets, osteomalacia, and osteosclerosis. Rickets may be the first presentation of chronic renal failure in children. Symmetric slipped capital femoral epiphyses are seen in contrast to the asymmetry of idiopathic slipped capital femoral epiphyses. Osteitis fibrosa cystica (hyperparathyroid changes in bone) may also be seen.

The earliest radiographic finding of hyperparathyroidism in adults is subperiosteal resorption of bone on the radial aspects of the middle phalanges of the index and long fingers of the hands, as well as the cortical bone of the distal phalanges (Figure 35-4). Due to increased porosity, the cortical outline may appear blurred and lamellated. As the disease progresses, subperiosteal resorption is observed in the other bones such as the medial aspects of the proximal tibias (Figure 35-5) and the medial margins of the femoral necks. Subtendinous and subligamentous bone resorption are characteristically found at the insertion of the plantar aponeurosis on the calcaneus, the femoral trochanters, ischial and humeral tuberosities, and the triceps insertion on the olecranon. Subchondral bone resorption may be seen in the symphysis pubis (Figure 35-6), sacroiliac joints (Figure 35-7), distal

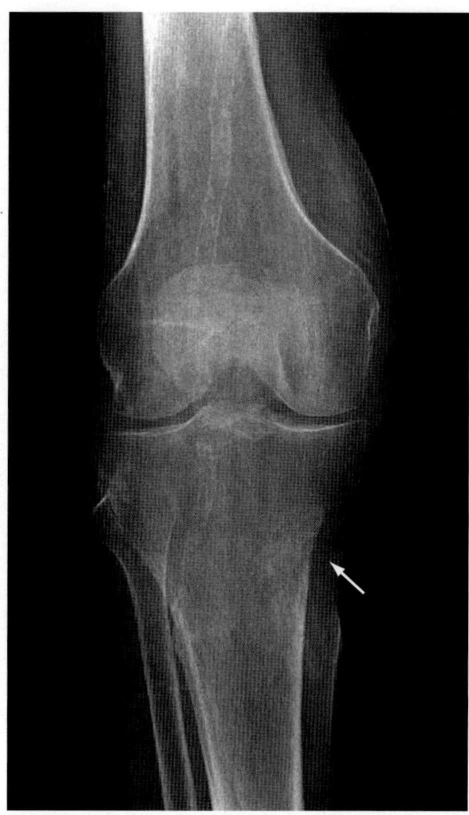

FIGURE 35-5. Renal osteodystrophy: secondary hyperparathyroidism. Anteroposterior radiograph of the knee shows subperiosteal resorption of bone along the medial aspect of the proximal medial tibial metaphysis *(arrow)*.

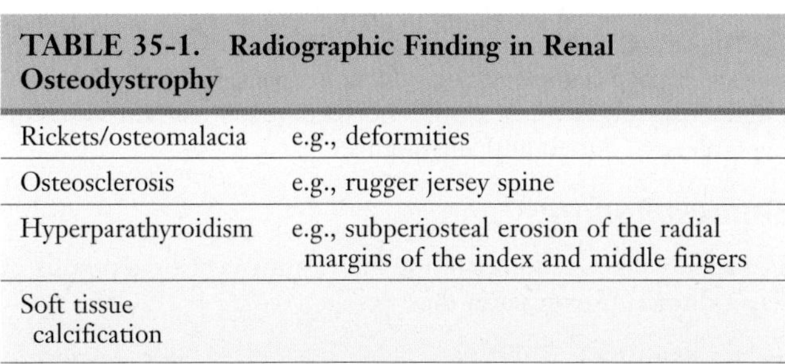

TABLE 35-1. Radiographic Finding in Renal Osteodystrophy

Rickets/osteomalacia	e.g., deformities
Osteosclerosis	e.g., rugger jersey spine
Hyperparathyroidism	e.g., subperiosteal erosion of the radial margins of the index and middle fingers
Soft tissue calcification	

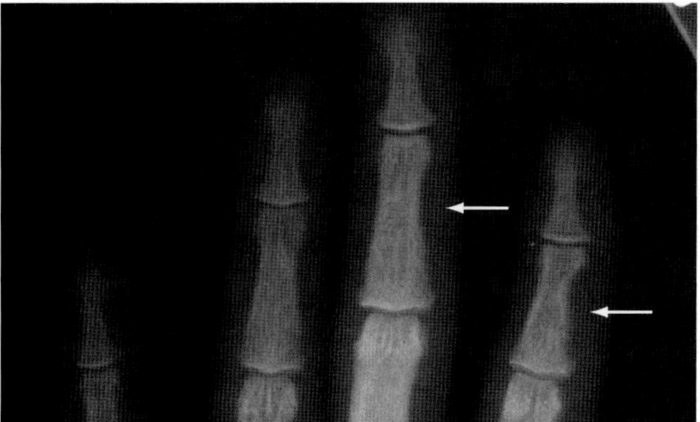

FIGURE 35-4. Renal osteodystrophy: secondary hyperparathyroidism. Posteroanterior radiograph of the hand shows subperiosteal resorption of bone along the radial aspects of the middle phalanges of the index and long fingers *(arrows)*.

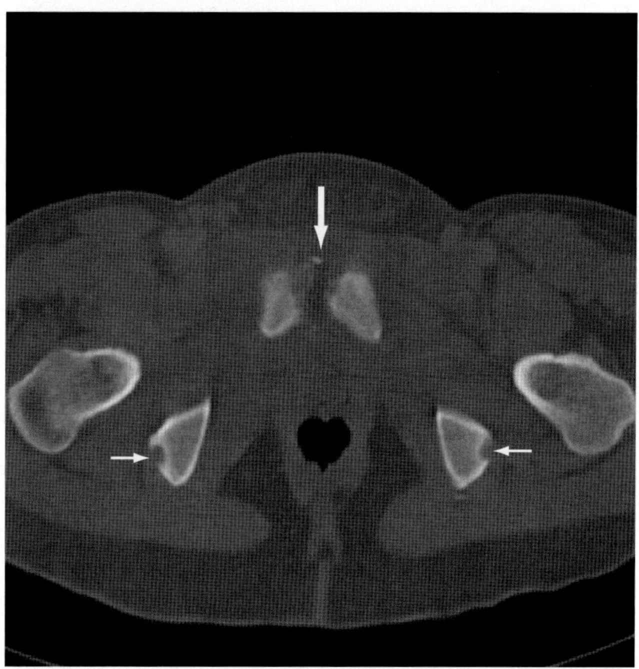

FIGURE 35-6. Renal osteodystrophy: secondary hyperparathyroidism. Axial CT image shows subchondral bone resorption of the pubic symphysis *(large arrow)* and subenthesial resorption of the ischial tuberosities at the hamstring attachment sites *(small arrows)*.

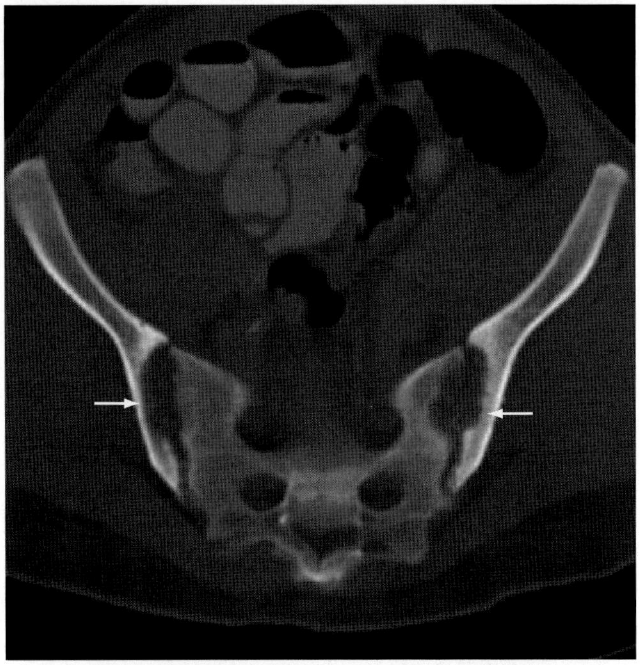

FIGURE 35-7. Renal osteodystrophy: secondary hyperparathyroidism. Axial CT image shows subchondral bone resorption of the sacroiliac joints *(arrows)*.

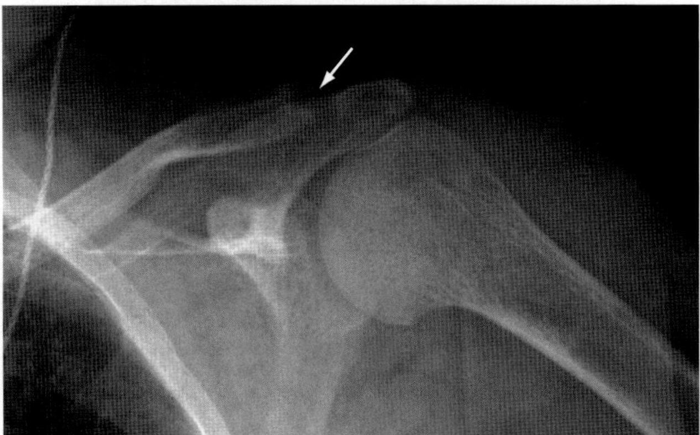

FIGURE 35-8. Renal osteodystrophy. Anteroposterior radiograph of the shoulder shows secondary hyperparathyroidism with subchondral bone resorption of the distal clavicle *(arrow)* and the undersurface of the clavicle at the attachment site of the coracoclavicular ligaments.

clavicles (Figure 35-8). Resorption occurs at the proximal medial cortical surface of long bones, and the lamina dura of the mandible. Fibrous replacement following the subchondral resorption of bone can result in widening of acromioclavicular and sacroiliac joints as well as symphysis pubis.[25] Intracortical tunneling (resorption) occurs in long and tubular bones following secondary hyperparathyroidism. Decreased bone density due to loss of secondary trabeculae results in a coarsened appearance of the bone and lucent striations through the cortex parallel to the shaft. It can be observed in phalanges and metacarpals by high-resolution magnification techniques. Intracortical tunneling is more common than pseudofractures in radiographs and is a sensitive (but not specific) radiographic finding in osteomalacia.[17]

Osteoclastomas (brown tumors) result from the secondary hyperparathyroidism in renal failure and are solitary or multifocal lytic lesions with well-defined margins. Brown tumors (osteoclastomas) are features of hyperparathyroidism (especially primary hyperparathyroidism) and are so named because of the chronic hemorrhage that results in a brown coloration. They can be found in any bone of the body, however are mostly seen in mandible, pelvis, ribs, and femurs. They often resemble true neoplasms and resolve or become sclerotic with treatment of the underlying hyperparathyroidism.[17] Deposition of calcium in the excessive osteoid results in areas of osteosclerosis (increased density) in some patients. Osteosclerosis subjacent to the vertebral body end-plates leads to an appearance of alternating bands of decreased and increased density, a characteristic appearance known as "rugger-jersey" spine.

As the serum calcium × phosphate product increases following phosphate retention, calcium precipitation occurs and results in calcifications of visceral (typically kidneys and lungs) and nonvisceral soft tissues.[26,27] Amorphous calcium may accumulate in periarticular regions, seen as single or multiple deposits on radiographs sometimes with fluid/calcium levels.

Drug-Induced Rickets and Osteomalacia

Some medications have been shown to interfere with bone metabolism resulting in rickets and osteomalacia and their radiographic findings. Several of the medications are discussed below.

Anticonvulsants

Prolonged treatment with anticonvulsants such as carbamazepine, phenytoin, phenobarbital, and primidone may result in rickets and osteomalacia. These drugs not only increase the catabolism of vitamin D by induction of liver enzymes but also decrease vitamin D and calcium absorption from the intestines. Rachitic changes can be seen in children as early as 2 years following initiation of treatment. Maintenance of long-term phenytoin may cause diffuse calvarial thickening with involvement of the diploic space. The severity of thickening depends on the duration and dosage of the drug, as well as the age at which therapy was started.[28] Acetazolamide accentuates osteomalacia and rickets by increasing excretion of calcium and phosphorus following renal tubular acidosis.[29] High doses of calcium should be used to correct the resultant hypocalcemia due to anticonvulsants.

Diphosphonates

In patients taking etidronate for the treatment of osteoporosis or Paget disease, osteomalacia may develop.

Deferoxamine

High doses of subcutaneous deferoxamine in thalassemic patients younger than 3 years of age, in whom iron overload has not been established, can cause rickets. Radiographs may show loss of height of the thoracic and lumbar vertebral bodies, as well as thickening and irregularity of the metaphyseal lines. Distal parts of the ulna and radius are the first areas that show the changes, followed by humerus, femur, tibia, and fibula. Small lucencies with sclerotic margins may be noted in the metaphyses. Deferoxamine-induced, long-bone changes have been reported in some thalassemic patients receiving hypertransfusion and chelation, and in patients on chelation therapy at doses of less than 50 mg/kg/day.[30] MRI of the knee in these patients has revealed changes such as physeal widening, blurring of the physeal–metaphyseal junction, and hyperintense areas in the metaphyses, as well as metadiaphyseal, epiphyseal, and patellar lesions.

Ifosfamide

A derivative of cyclophosphamide, ifosfamide is used in the treatment of malignancies. As it is a nephrotoxic agent, ifosfamide can increase excretion of phosphate due to renal tubular damage (producing hypophosphatemic rickets). Oral phosphate after cessation of ifosfamide resolves the condition.

Aluminum

In patients with chronic renal failure, aluminum toxicity may occur following dialysis or by taking phosphate binders that contain aluminum. Osteopenia and multiple fractures (often more than three) are found on radiographs. The fractures tend to occur in ribs and vertebrae. Fractures of the second, third, and fourth ribs, which are almost always pathologic, are characteristic of this condition. Subperiosteal resorption is less observed in aluminum toxicity compared to patients without the disorder. Nontraumatic, isolated fractures with no evidence of healing may be seen in long bones and should raise the suspicion of aluminum-induced osteomalacia in a uremic patient undergoing dialysis. Aluminum toxicity in children results in rickets with osteopenia, pathologic fractures, and rachitic changes at the physes.

Other Medications

There are several medications that are less commonly associated with rickets and osteomalacia. Rifampin, a first-line antituberculosis agent, can diminish the serum level of 25-OH-D by induction of liver enzymes.[31] Cholestyramine interferes with intestinal absorption of fat-soluble vitamins including vitamin D and increases the risk of osteomalacia.[32] The phytic acid present in cereals can decrease intestinal absorption of calcium by binding to it.

Hereditary Vitamin D–Dependent Rickets

This autosomal recessive disorder has two types: type I (pseudovitamin D–deficiency rickets) and type II (also known as hereditary hypocalcemic vitamin D–resistant rickets or hereditary $1,25[OH]_2D$-resistant rickets).The biochemical and radiographic manifestations of type I are similar to vitamin D–deficiency rickets (low calcium, phosphorus, and $1,25[OH]_2D$ level with secondary hyperparathyroidism) and results from a deficiency in the production or activity of 1α-hydroxylase in kidneys. In contrast to vitamin D–deficiency rickets, symptoms may appear early (by 3 months of age), and by the end of the first year most patients are symptomatic. Rachitic changes in the bones may be progressive and severe with pathologic fractures. Type II results from a defect in the vitamin D receptor leading to end-organ resistance. In contrast to type I, the serum level of $1,25[OH]_2D$ is high. Rachitic changes and bowing of the extremities may also be severe in type II.

Hypophosphatemic Rickets

Rickets and osteomalacia due to X-linked hypophosphatemia (also known as hypophosphatemic vitamin D–resistant rickets and familial vitamin D–resistant rickets) are characterized by a low rate of phosphate reabsorption in the proximal renal tubules. In X-linked hypophosphatemia, which is a dominant trait, rickets usually appears between 12 and 18 months of age (Figure 35-9). Patients are stocky and short with bowlegs and may develop spontaneous dental abscesses in the absence of dental caries. Skull deformity may occur following the premature fusion of the cranial sutures and can lead to increased intracranial pressure.

Bowing of the long bones is more prominent in the lower limbs, and radiographs show thick cortices and coarse trabeculae, which are exacerbated with increasing age. By adulthood, radiographs reveal the characteristic finding of a generalized increment in bone density, particularly in the axial skeleton. Enthesopathic changes (calcification and ossification at the sites of musculotendinous insertion) are unique features of this type of osteomalacia. These changes occur in the anulus fibrous, paravertebral ligaments, and capsules of appendicular and apophyseal (facet) joints. Radiographic changes in the axial skeleton may mimic ankylosing spondylitis; however, bone erosions are absent in the sacroiliac joints with X-linked hypophosphatemia.

Multiple sites of calcification and bone formation may be seen throughout the skeleton and ligament attachments. The radiographic manifestations of this disorder are characteristic and distinctive (Box 35-3) (Figure 35-9).

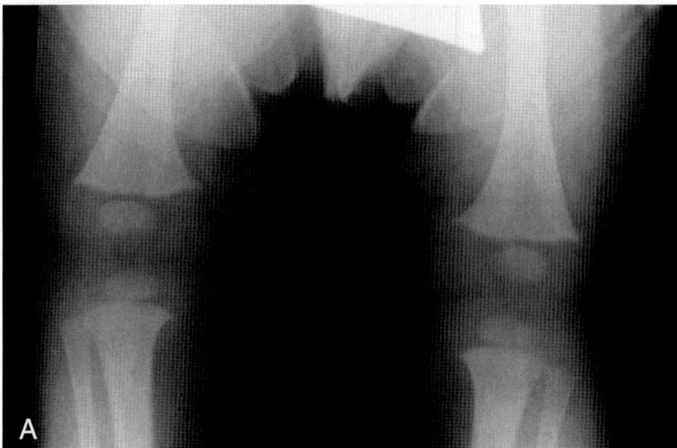

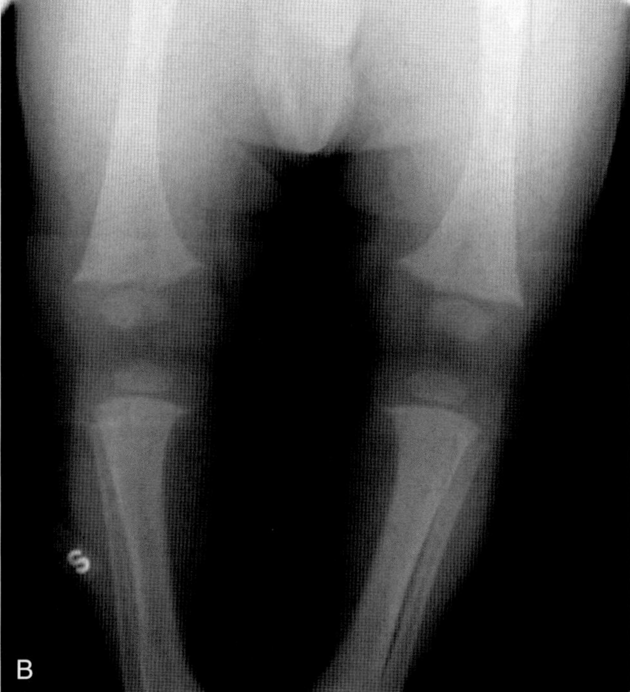

FIGURE 35-9. Hypophosphatemic vitamin D–resistant rickets. **A,** This boy was first discovered to have hereditary hypophosphatemic Vitamin D-resistant rickets at 8 months of age. He had a family history of rickets, a low serum phosphate, and rachitic changes in the knees at that time. **B,** At 10 months, there is additional irregularity of the growth plates.

(Continued)

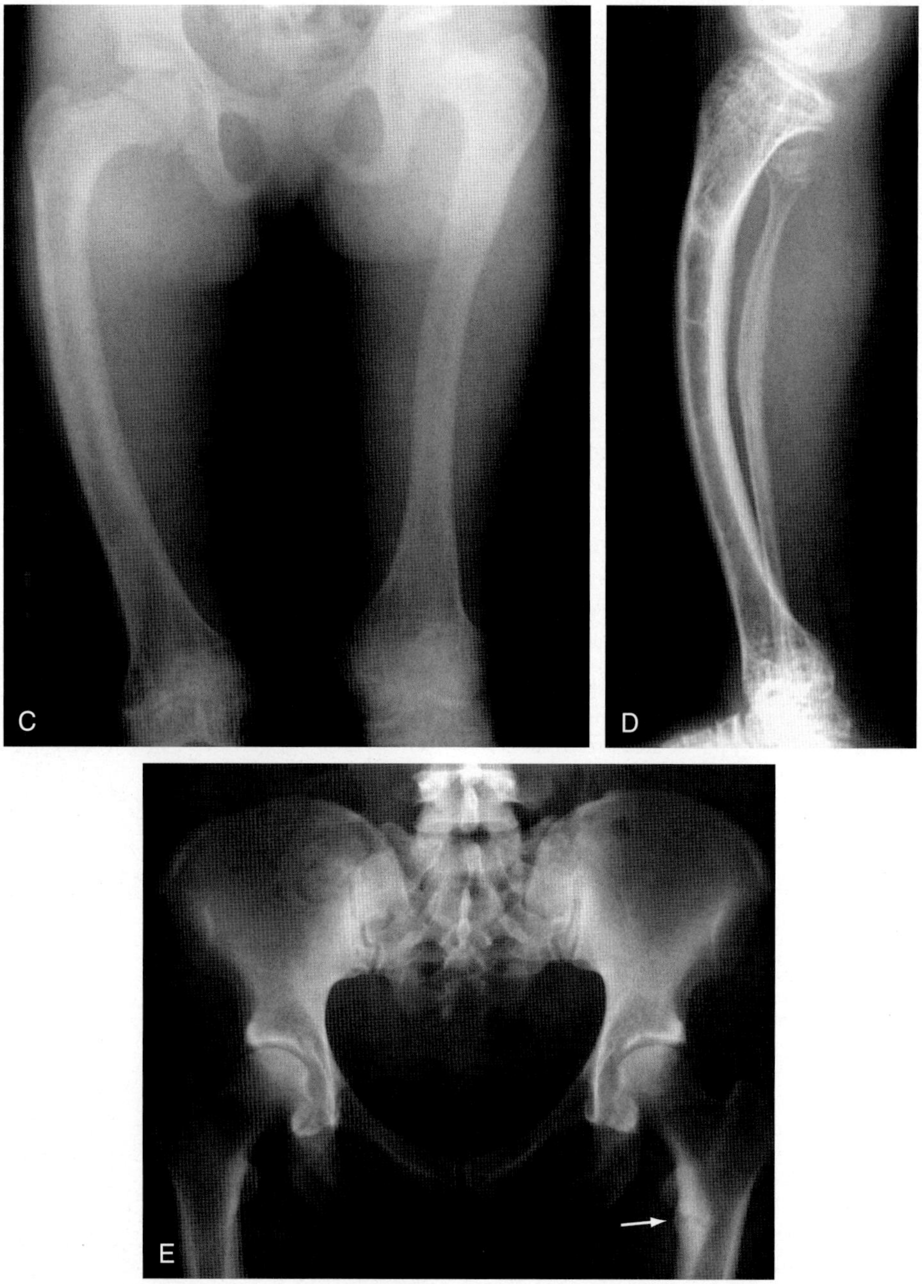

FIGURE 35-9—cont'd. **C,** This 14-year-old girl had been treated with vitamin D for hypophosphatemic rickets. Anteroposterior view of the femurs and **(D)** lateral radiograph of the tibia show residual bowing deformity. **E,** An anteroposterior radiograph of the pelvis in another patient shows a Looser zone in the left femur *(arrow)*. The bones are relatively dense. Figures A, B, C, and D courtesy of Dr. Jeanne Chow, Children's Hospital, Boston, MA.

Tumor-Associated Rickets and Osteomalacia

This hypophosphatemic hyperphosphaturic form of rickets is seen in several benign fibrous and mesenchymal tumors, including sclerosing angioma, benign angiofibroma, hemangiopericytoma, soft-parts chondromalike tumor, giant cell tumor of bone, fibrous dysplasia, and neurofibromatosis.[10,33,34] Breast carcinoma, chronic lymphocytic leukemia, multiple myeloma, prostate carcinoma, oat cell carcinoma, and linear nevus sebaceous syndrome have also been associated with this condition.[34-36]

A humoral factor secreted by the tumors increases renal loss of phosphate and lowers the synthesis of $1,25(OH)_2D$. The serum $1,25(OH)_2D$ and phosphate are low, but normal PTH and calcium levels are present. Compared to other causes of osteomalacia, osteopenia is usually more conspicuous in tumor-associated osteomalacia. Recurrent fractures may occur. As tumors are usually small and present in obscure areas, the identification of tumor

BOX 35-3. Radiographic Features of X-linked Hypophosphatemic Rickets

Appears at 1 to 1½ years
Premature fusion of cranial sutures
Bowing of long bones
Thick cortices, increased bone density
Looser zones
Enthesopathy with calcification of annulus fibrosis, paraspinal ligaments, apophyseal joints

location is difficult. The isotopic somatostatin-receptor scan has shown improvement in the detection of tumors associated with this condition. (See also Chapter 36 for a more complete discussion of this condition.)

References

1. Holick MF: Sunlight and vitamin D for bone health and prevention of autoimmune diseases, cancers, and cardiovascular disease, *Am J Clin Nutr* 80:1678S-1688S, 2004.
2. Holick MF: Vitamin D: a millennium perspective, *J Cell Biochem* 88:296-307, 2003.
3. Holick MF: McCollum Award Lecture, 1994: Vitamin D—new horizons for the 21st century, *Am J Clin Nutr* 60:619-630, 1994.
4. Bringhurst FR, Demay MB, Kronenberg HM: Hormones and disorders of mineral metabolism. In Larsen PR, Kronenberg HM, Melmed S et al (eds): *Williams Textbook of Endocrinology*, 10th ed, Philadelphia, 2003, Saunders, pp 1303-1372.
5. Norman AW: Intestinal calcium absorption: a vitamin D-hormone-mediated adaptive response, *Am J Clin Nutr* 51:290-300, 1990.
6. DeLuca HF: The kidney as an endocrine organ for the production of 1,25-dihydroxy-vitamin D 3, a calcium-mobilizing hormone, *N Engl J Med* 289:359-365, 1973.
7. Garabedian M, Tanaka Y, Holick MF et al: Response of intestinal calcium transport and bone calcium mobilization to 1,25 dihydroxyvitamin D3 in thyroparathyroidectomized rats, *Endocrinology* 94:1022-1027, 1974.
8. Rasmussen H, Bordier P, Kurokawa K et al: Hormonal control of skeletal and mineral homeostasis, *Am J Med* 56:751-758, 1974.
9. Pitt MJ: Rickets and osteomalacia. In Resnick D (ed): *Diagnosis of Bone and Joint Disorders*, 4th ed, Philadelphia, 2002, Saunders, pp 1901-1945.
10. Mughal Z: Rickets in childhood, *Semin Musculoskelet Radiol* 6:183-190, 2002.
11. Raisz LG, Kream BE, Lorenzo JA: Metabolic bone disease. In Larsen PR, Kronenberg HM, Melmed S et al (eds): *Williams Textbook of Endocrinology*, 10th ed, Philadelphia, 2003, Saunders, pp 1373-1411.
12. Berry JL, Davies M, Mee AP: Vitamin D metabolism, rickets, and osteomalacia, *Semin Musculoskelet Radiol* 6:173-182, 2002.
13. Sitrin M, Meredith S, Rosenberg IH: Vitamin D deficiency and bone disease in gastrointestinal disorders, *Arch Intern Med* 138:886-888, 1978.
14. Franck WA, Hoffman GS, Davis JS et al: Osteomalacia and weakness complicating jejunoileal bypass, *J Rheumatol* 6:51-56, 1979.
15. Steinbach HL, Noetzli M: Roentgen appearance of the skeleton in osteomalacia and rickets, *Am J Roentgenol Radium Ther Nucl Med* 91:955-972, 1964.
16. Caffey J: *Pediatric X-ray Diagnosis*, vols 1, 2, 6th ed, Chicago, 1972, Year Book.
17. Vogler JB III, Kim JH: Metabolic and endocrine disease of the skeleton. In Grainger RG, Allison DJ, Adam A et al (eds): *Grainger & Allison's Diagnostic Radiology: A Textbook of Medical Imaging*, 4th ed, London, 2001, Churchill Livingstone, pp 1933-1934.
18. McKenna MJ, Kleerekoper M, Ellis BI et al: Atypical insufficiency fractures confused with Looser zones of osteomalacia, *Bone* 8:71-78, 1987.
19. Salimpour R: Rickets in Tehran. Study of 200 cases, *Arch Dis Child* 50:63-66, 1975.
20. Park EA: The Blackader lecture on some aspects of rickets. *Can Med Assoc J* 26:3, 1932.
21. Heird WC: Vitamin deficiencies and excesses. In Behrman RE, Kliegman RM, Jenson HB (eds): *Nelson Textbook of Pediatrics*, 17th ed, Philadelphia, 2004, WB Saunders, pp 177-190.
22. Steinbach HL, Kolb FO, Gilfillan R: A mechanism of the production of pseudofractures in osteomalacia (Milkman's syndrome), *Radiology* 62:388-395, 1954.
23. Perry HM III, Weinstein RS, Teitelbaum SL et al: Pseudofractures in the absence of osteomalacia, *Skeletal Radiol* 8:17-19, 1982.
24. Akaki S, Ida K, Kanazawa S et al: Flare response seen in therapy for osteomalacia, *J Nucl Med* 39:2095-2097, 1998.
25. Reynolds WA, Karo JJ: Radiologic diagnosis of metabolic bone disease, *Orthop Clin North Am* 3:521-543, 1972.
26. Parfitt AM: Soft-tissue calcification in uremia, *Arch Intern Med* 124:544-556, 1969.
27. Parfitt AM, Massry SG, Winfield AC et al: Disordered calcium and phosphorus metabolism during maintenance hemodialysis. Correlation of clinical, roentgenographic and biochemical changes, *Am J Med* 51:319-330, 1971.
28. Stamp TCB: Drug and chemical-induced rickets (and osteomalacia). In Preger L (ed): *Induced Disease—Drug, Irradiation, Occupation*, New York, 1980, Grune & Stratton, pp 27-43.
29. Mallette LE: Acetazolamide-accelerated anticonvulsant osteomalacia, *Arch Intern Med* 137:1013-1017, 1977.
30. Chan Y, Li C, Chu WC et al: Deferoxamine-induced bone dysplasia in the distal femur and patella of pediatric patients and young adults: MR imaging appearance. *AJR Am J Roentgenol* 175:1561-1566, 2000.
31. Brodie MJ, Boobis AR, Dollery CT et al: Rifampicin and vitamin D metabolism. *Clin Pharmacol Ther* 27:810-814, 1980.
32. Heaton KW, Lever JV, Barnard D: Osteomalacia associated with cholestyramine therapy for postileectomy diarrhea, *Gastroenterology* 62:642-646, 1972.
33. Renton P: Radiology of rickets, osteomalacia and hyperparathyroidism, *Hosp Med* 59:399-403, 1998.
34. Drezner MK: Tumor-induced rickets and osteomalacia. In Favus MJ (ed): *Primer on the Metabolic Bone Diseases and Disorders of Mineral Metabolism*, 3rd ed, Philadelphia, 1996, Lippincott Williams & Wilkins, pp 319-325.
35. Hosking DJ, Chamberlain MJ, Shortland-Webb WR: Osteomalacia and carcinoma of prostate with major redistribution of skeletal calcium, *Br J Radiol* 48:451-456, 1975.
36. McClure J, Smith PS: Oncogenic osteomalacia. *J Clin Pathol* 40:446-453, 1987.

CHAPTER 36

Oncogenic Osteomalacia

FRIEDA FELDMAN, MD, FACR

KEY FACTS

- Osteomalacia resulting from the presence of a bone or soft tissue lesion or tumor is known as oncogenic osteomalacia or tumor-induced osteomalacia (TIO).
- Adults are usually affected with nonspecific complaints such as bone and muscle pain, weakness, fatigue, and recurrent fractures.
- Hypophosphatemia, hyperphosphaturia, low 1,25-dihydroxy–vitamin D, normal serum calcium, and normal PTH levels are noted.
- Radiographs are the primary imaging method for identifying osteomalacia.
- Additional studies may be necessary to identify the causative, lesion.
- Prompt remission of symptoms and biochemical abnormalities follow successful lesion excision.

Osteomalacia, a common metabolic disease, has multiple familiar and a few less well-appreciated etiologies. One of the latter, known as oncogenic, paraneoplastic, oncogenous, or tumor-induced osteomalacia (TIO), is regarded as relatively rare with fewer than 150 reported cases. It has been clinically underestimated as a distinct entity since it shares osteomalacia, a nonspecific endpoint, with other commoner etiologies. McCance first considered a coexistent bone lesion as a cause of TIO.[1] Hauge then suspected, and Prader proved, the link between a tumor and osteomalacia.[2] To date, understanding of the pathogenesis and mechanisms associated with TIO is still evolving.

This review aims to provide evidence to medical generalists as well as specialists for considering TIO as a possible cause when classic etiologies for osteomalacia are absent. Biochemical, physiologic, genetic, and imaging criteria will be summarized to enable more fruitful investigations leading to recognition and documentation of TIO in both children and adults.

CLINICAL FEATURES

TIO has a male-to-female ratio of 1.2:1 and affects individuals aged 5 to 75 years. It usually occurs in adults over age 30[3] with nonspecific complaints such as bone and muscle pain, weakness, fatigue, and recurrent fractures, often attributed to osteoporosis. Children may present with gait disturbances, growth retardation, modeling deformities, and abnormal physes that, when recognized as rickets, lack a confirmed cause (Box 36-1). Symptoms may be delayed, gradual, or precede the awareness of osteomalacia. Conversely, when osteomalacia is recognized, coexistent lesions may not be held responsible because most are familiar as independent entities. As a result, TIO has remained clinically elusive for several months to 20 years.[4,5] Moreover, even when a coexistent lesion is considered, TIO remains a presumptive diagnosis until removal of the lesion is followed by prompt remission of all symptoms and biochemical aberrations. This healing may occur within hours to days (Figure 36-1).

Lesions Responsible for TIO

Responsible benign or malignant primary and non-neoplastic TIO lesions occur in bones or soft tissues with approximately equal incidence. The most frequent bone sites are long bones, that is, femora or tibias. The next most frequent loci are in the craniofacial bones. Similar anatomic distributions are noted for the 50% of TIO lesions involving soft tissues.

Although diverse and unrelated, 70% to 80% of TIO lesions have been described as mesenchymal. Others histologically characterize 40% as "vascular," with hemangiopericytoma representing 50% of vascular and 20% of all TIO lesions.

Hemangiopericytoma causes 20% of all cases of TIO.

Another large group described as "fibrohistiocytic and giant-cell lesions" contain prominent vasculature with less frequent osseous, cartilaginous, and neurologic components, while a third, with no clear-cut characteristics have been termed "mixed fibrovascular or mesenchymal."[6]

For convenience, known causative lesions have been grouped according to their predominant histologic features (Box 36-2). While most often these lesions occur independently, all have been associated with the TIO syndrome.[3,6-18] Nevertheless, none differ histologically, ultrastructurally, or immunohistochemically from their independent counterparts that have no TIO association.[6] Most are small (0.5 to 15 cm), may grow slowly, or present prior to clinical complaints or establishment of osteomalacia. Consequently, coexistent biochemical and metabolic stigmata in general and osteomalacia in particular must be considered to determine their role.

BIOCHEMICAL AND PATHOPHYSIOLOGIC ASPECTS OF TIO

Phosphorus homeostasis is normally maintained by intestinal absorption interacting with intracellular and bone storage pools. It is vital for normal skeletal development and mineralization but is principally regulated by the kidney. Hypophosphatemia normally stimulates phosphorus proximal renal tubular reabsorption, calcitriol synthesis via 25-hydroxy–vitamin D-1 alpha-hydroxylase, with intestinal calcium and phosphorus absorption and

BOX 36-1. Possible Clinical Manifestations of Tumor-Induced Osteomalacia

Bone and muscle pain
Weakness
Fatigue
Recurrent fractures
Gait disturbances
Growth retardation
Bony modeling deformities on radiographs
Rickets on radiographs

mobilization from bone. However, the classic PTH-vitamin D axis fails to explain all facets of phosphorus homeostasis.[4,5,19,20] While PTH does help regulate phosphorus reabsorption, it chiefly maintains calcium homeostasis, with recent investigators continuing to identify additional important regulators.[21-39]

The biochemical aberrations of TIO are caused by phosphorus wasting and abnormal vitamin D metabolism.

> TIO is manifested chemically by hypophosphatemia, hyperphosphaturia, low calcitriol (1,25-dihydroxy–vitamin D), normal serum calcium, and normal PTH levels.

Phosphorus wasting is caused by the inhibition of renal proximal tubular phosphorus reabsorption. Abnormal vitamin D metabolism prevents the compensatory rise in calcitriol (1,25-dihydroxy–vitamin D) normally stimulated by hypophosphatemia due to inhibition of the 1-alpha–hydroxylase enzyme by humoral factors.

TIO is diagnosed by identifying a lesion producing such a factor with resultant typical biochemical abnormalities (Table 36-1) (Box 36-3) with remission of the syndrome after its complete removal. However, diagnosis may be hampered or delayed since serum phosphorus determinations are not routinely included in standard laboratory metabolic profiles and must be specifically requested. Other conditions simulating TIO must also be excluded.

OTHER DIAGNOSTIC CONSIDERATIONS

TIO may be biochemically indistinguishable from X-linked hypophosphatemic rickets (XLHR), autosomal dominant hypophosphatemic rickets (ADHR), and hereditary hypophosphatemic rickets. The latter is distinguished from XLHR and ADHR by hypercalciuria and elevated serum calcitriol (see Table 36-1) (see Box 36-3).[5,21,36-39] However, XLHR and ADHR typically involve children and have occasional delayed age onset, while XLHR is associated with osteosclerosis, calcified entheses, infrequent fractures, and no muscle weakness.[21] Other renal phosphate wasting syndromes, such as Fanconi syndrome, multiple myeloma, Wilson disease, and cystinosis, display more global renal tubular defects causing hypercalciuria, elevated serum calcitriol, amino-aciduria, glycosuria, and renal tubular acidosis.[4] Chemotherapeutic agents, such as ifosfamide, may also be nephrotoxic with more global biochemical aberrations, again excluding TIO.[40]

EXPERIMENTAL EVIDENCE FOR A HUMORAL SUBSTANCE

Biochemical aberrations produced by TIO lesions have been attributed to a humoral factor or factors initially referred to as phosphatonin.[4,21,22,27,32,39] Animals injected with tumor extracts

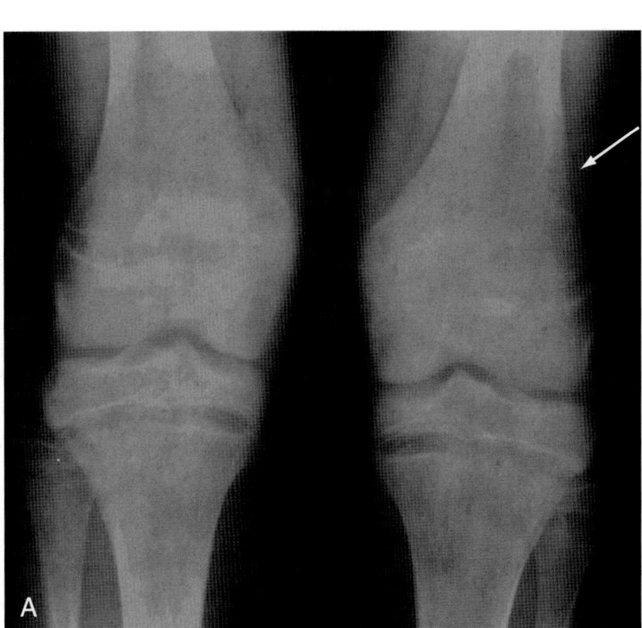

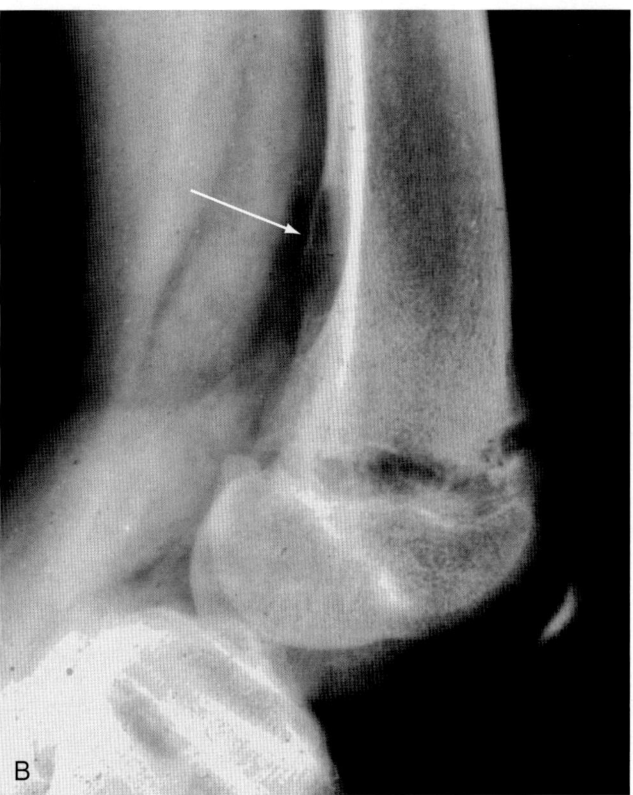

FIGURE 36-1. Teen-aged girl referred by her pediatrician for several months of severe generalized pain with unknown cause. Preoperative radiographs: **A,** Anteroposterior view of both knees. **B,** Lateral view of left knee.

(Continued)

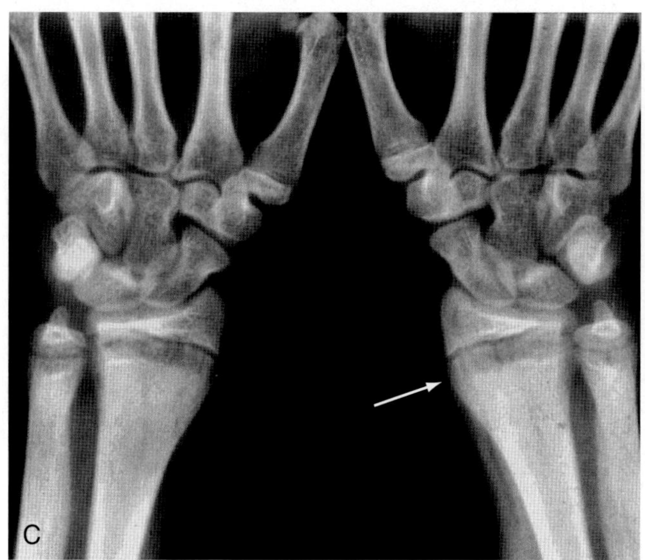

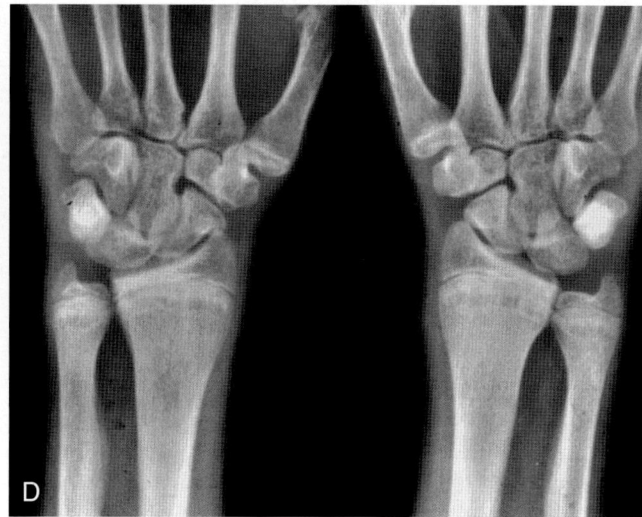

FIGURE 36-1—cont'd. **C,** Posteroanterior view of both wrists. All reveal classic stigmata of rickets—generalized osteopenia, coarsened trabecular pattern, and abnormally wide radiolucent physes in wrists *(arrow)* and distal femora. A posterolateral, benign cortical defect was noted in the left femoral metaphysis *(arrows in A and B)*. **D,** A postoperative radiograph, of both wrists 3 weeks after cortical defect excision show nearly completely remineralized physes. Clinical symptoms and abnormal biochemistries (see Box 36-2) regressed within days.

BOX 36-2. Tumor-Induced Osteomalacia: Previous Causative Lesions, Predominant Histology

GROUP 1[a] VASCULAR
Hemangiopericytoma
Hemangioma
Hemangioendothelioma
Angiosarcoma

GROUP 2[b] FIBROCYTIC
Nonossifying fibroma
Malignant fibrous histiocytoma
Neurofibromatosis
Polyostotic fibrous dysplasia
Fibrous xanthoma

GROUP 3[b] GIANT CELL
Bone
Primary giant cell tumor
Giant-cell reparative granuloma
Giant-cell rich malignant fibrous histiocytoma
Soft tissue
Pigmented villonodular synovitis

GROUP 4 BONE/CARTILAGE/EPITHELIAL
Osteoblastoma
Osteosarcoma
Chondroma
Mesenchymal chondrosarcoma
Breast carcinoma
Prostatic carcinoma

GROUP 5 UNCLEAR CLASSIFICATION
"Vascular" fibrous histiocytoma
Malignant mesenchymal tumors
Undifferentiated sarcomas

[a]Group 1 most common.
[b]Groups 2 and 3 are the next most common.

or transplanted cells from TIO lesions inhibit phosphorus transport in vitro[7,22,23] and produce phosphaturia and hypophosphatemia in vivo.

Tissue culture media derived from them also inhibit phosphate uptake in opossum kidneys whose proximal tubules, as in humans, normally reabsorb phosphate.[25] A humoral substance in cultured kidney cells, with other factors, also inhibits 1-alpha–hydroxylase enzyme with resultant serum 1,25-dihyroxy–vitamin D reduction.[4,7]

While slow growth and loss of humoral activity in tissue cultures have heretofore hampered phosphatonin investigations, recent strategy has centered on analyzing gene expression profiles of TIO lesions.[5,26,29-39] One of several genes involved in producing a phosphaturic substance has been identified as FGF23 of the fibroblast growth family.[5,8,28,34,35] It inhibits phosphorus transport in cultured renal proximal tubular epithelium, reduces serum phosphorus, and increases its excretion in injected mice who become hypophosphatemic when chronically exposed.[27] Conversely, FGF23-deficient mice exhibit hyperphosphatemia, hypercalcemia, elevated calcitriol, growth retardation, and premature death.[29] While low FGF23 levels may be found in normal human tissues and serum and are occasionally slightly higher in polyostotic fibrous dysplasia,[8] FGF23 is most highly expressed in TIO tumors.[27] It may also operate in XLH due to a mutation in the PHEX gene, which encodes endopeptidase whose lost activity leads to phosphorus wasting. FGF23 has been cited as a substrate for PHEX with resultant failure of FGF23 cleavage said to enhance

TABLE 36-1. TIO: Distinguishing Biochemical Features

Condition	Serum Phosphate	Urinary Phosphate	Serum Calcium	Urine Calcium	PTH	Di OH Vitamin D	Other
TIO	Low[a]	High[b]	Normal		Normal	Low[c]	
XLHR	Low	High	Normal		Normal	Low	Children, osteosclerosis, calcified entheses Infrequent fractures, no muscle weakness
ADHR	Low	High	Normal		Normal	Low	Children
Hereditary hypophosphatemic rickets				Increased		Elevated	

[a]Due to decreased proximal tubular reabsorption.
[b]Due to increased P excretion.
[c]Due to inhibition of 1-alpha-hydroxylase.
ADHR, autosomal dominant hypophosphatemic rickets; *TIO*, tumor induced osteomalacia; *XLHR*, X-linked hypophosphatemic rickets.

BOX 36-3. Features Supporting Diagnosis of TIO

1. Biochemical Screening
   Serum P, Ca+, alkaline phosphatase, Creatinine, Intact PTH, 1,25-dihydroxy–vitamin D (calciferol), Fasting P, Urine Fasting 2 hr P, Creatinine, Ca, Amino acid, Glucose
2. Previously normal serum P
3. No family history of bone or mineral disorder, such as inherited hypophosphatemic rickets
4. Adult-onset progressive pain, weakness, multiple fractures without trauma
5. Symptoms more severe than other renal-phosphate wasting syndromes
6. Gene mutations—defective
   PHEX: P-regulating gene—homologies to endopeptidases on X chromosome as in XLHR–X-linked hypophosphatemic rickets
   FGF-23—Autosomal dominant hypophosphatemic rickets—ADHR; XLHR and ADHR both have family history, short stature, may have adult onset
   NPT2—Major Na-P cotransporters in proximal renal tubule; hypophosphatemia with increased Ca and calcitriol
7. Exclude
   a. Other renal-tubular P-wasting syndromes:
      Fanconi syndrome, myeloma, Wilson's disease, cystinosis, more global tubular dysfunction, enzyme deficiencies, hypophosphatasemia, mineralization inhibitors, Al, Fl, bisphosphonates, Cadmium, Ca deficiency + hypophosphatemia
   b. Drug nephrotoxicity
   c. Ifosfamide (RX of solid tumors): hypophosphatemia + global tubular dysfunction
8. Bone histomorphology:
   Biopsy posttetracycline labeling shows osteomalacia
   Increased unmineralized bone or osteoid surfaces
   Increased mineralization time—distance between 2 tetracycline labels
9. Suspicious causative lesion
   Detect: Serial physical examination or imaging
   Document: Humoral factor production by venous assay
   Remove: Resultant complete symptomatic and biochemical remission

its activity.[4,36-38] FGF 23 plays a role in several distinct disorders of renal P wasting.

1. In TIO tumors, strong expression of FGF23 inhibits phosphorus reabsorption by proximal renal tubules and down-regulates 25-hydroxy–vitamin D-1 alpha-hydroxylase with resultant hypophosphatemia and osteomalacia.
2. In ADHR, FGF23 gene mutation enhances its biologic activity by becoming resistant to proteolytic cleavage, again resulting in hypophosphatemic rickets.
3. In XLH, the PHEX mutation directly or indirectly increases circulatory FGF23, similarly interfering with proximal renal tubular phosphaturic activity. FGF23 is not the only factor in TIO tumors that may affect renal phosphate handling and bone mineralization. Another phosphatonin candidate due to mutations in NPT2, a major sodium-phosphate cotransporter in renal proximal tubules that reabsorbs up to 85% of glomerular filtered phosphorous, has been proposed as a new hypophosphatemic disorder. However, hypercalciuria and elevated calcitriol distinguish it from TIO.[33]

IMAGING

Radiologists may be the first or last to raise the possibility of TIO since osteomalacia, the imaging manifestation of its endpoint, may be initially reflected or incidentally noted on images of the musculoskeletal system. However, its nonspecific, clinically overlapping presentations potentially involve a variety of physicians who may be originally consulted, including family practitioners, orthopedists, endocrinologists, neurologists, and if the cause remains obscure, psychiatrists. The selection of an imaging modality is thereby tempered by the training and familiarity of referring physicians with the bonanza of currently available technologies.

Unfortunately, the increasing and often exclusive reliance on computed tomography (CT), magnetic resonance imaging

(MRI), or positron emission tomography (PET) as the initial or sole imaging study has led to the underappreciation of TIO and the underutilization of radiographs, which remain the best primary modality for recognizing osteomalacia. Long-established radiographic stigmata such as generalized osteopenia, modeling deformities, trabecular and cortical alterations, and insufficiency fractures often appear on a single radiograph (Figure 36-2, *A* to *C*). Simultaneously included large anatomic areas on a radiograph of the bony pelvis may contain several telltale clues (Figure 36-3). Among them are "Looser zones" whose wide, relatively radiolucent, unmineralized osteoid seams, often bordered by indistinct, incompetent callus, represent a specific type of insufficiency fracture that serves to reinforce a diagnosis of osteomalacia (see Figure 36-3). Long bones (Figure 36-4), vertebra, ribs, and particularly scapulas, usually visible on a single chest radiograph, often reveal the classic "signature" of osteomalacia (see Figure 36-2). Pelvic and chest radiographs are, in fact, the two most revealing diagnostic imaging studies. Conversely, it is difficult, if not impossible, to appreciate these hallmarks as osteomalacic stigmata per se on MRI or CT, which are further limited by small fields of view on studies ordered for specific sites (see Figure 36-4).

MRI is justifiably the modality of choice for documenting occult or subtle focal fractures. It does so earliest, most efficiently, and most accurately, since it best depicts their extent compared to bone scans or CT. However, although better defined, fractures are seen in isolation and usually not categorized, such as insufficiency versus stress-related fractures,[41] both of which may be attributed to other causes (Figure 36-5).

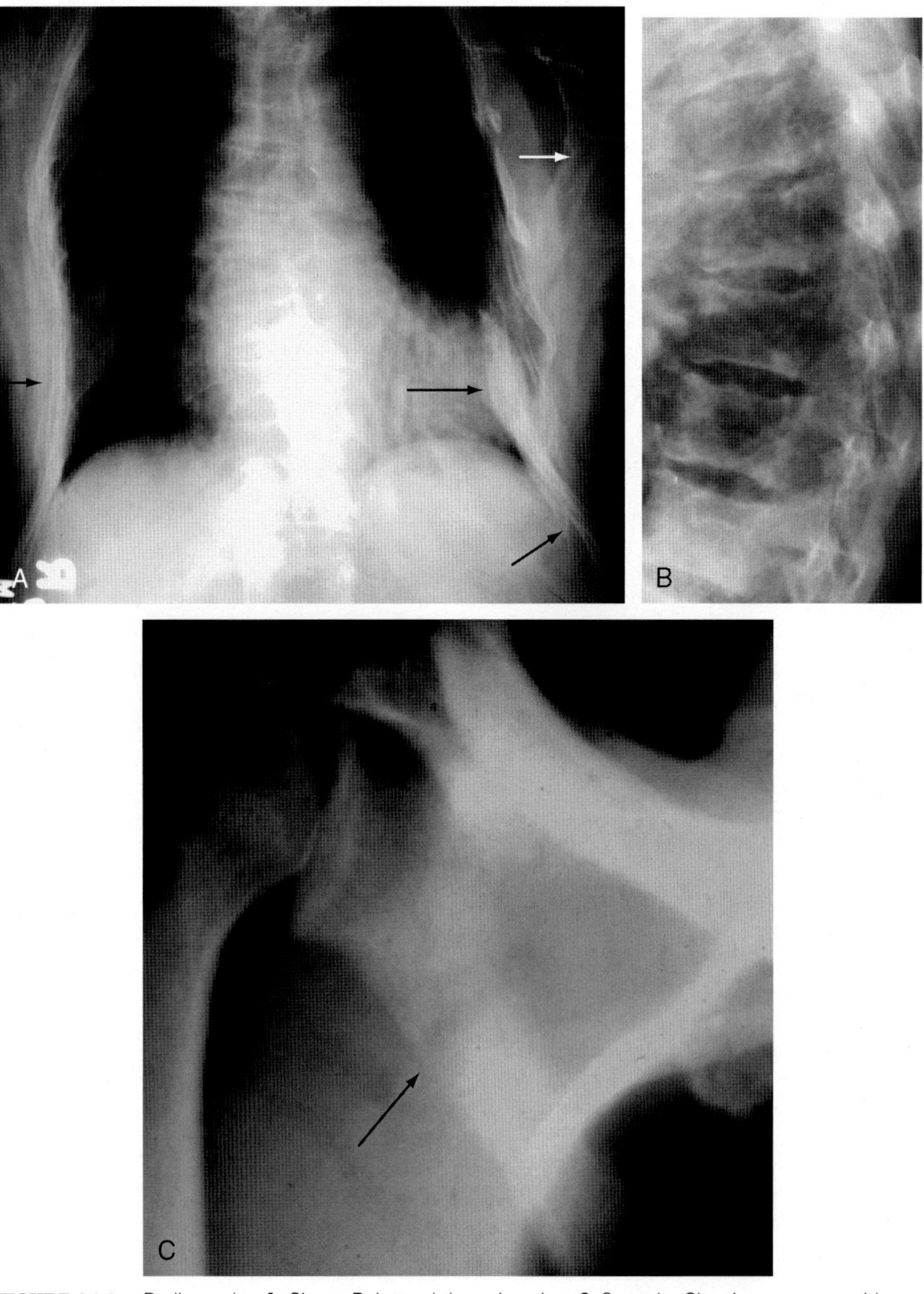

FIGURE 36-2. Radiographs. **A,** Chest. **B,** Lateral thoracic spine. **C,** Scapula. Classic roentgen evidence of osteomalacia are seen. Generalized osteopenia and a medially, curvilinearly collapsed "bell-shaped" rib cage *(black arrows in A)*. Indistinct cortices, coarsened vertebral trabeculae, and subtle biconcave end plates **(B)**. Insufficiency fracture at right angles to scapular cortex (Looser zone) *(white arrow in A and black arrow in C)*.

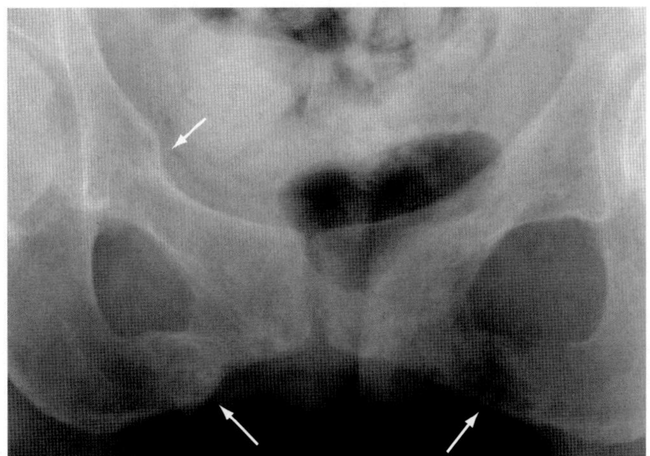

FIGURE 36-3. Osteomalacia. Anteroposterior pelvic radiograph—coned down view. Shows indistinct cortices with acute and chronic insufficiency fractures (Looser zones) in right superior pubic ramus and both ischia in different stages of repair *(arrows).*

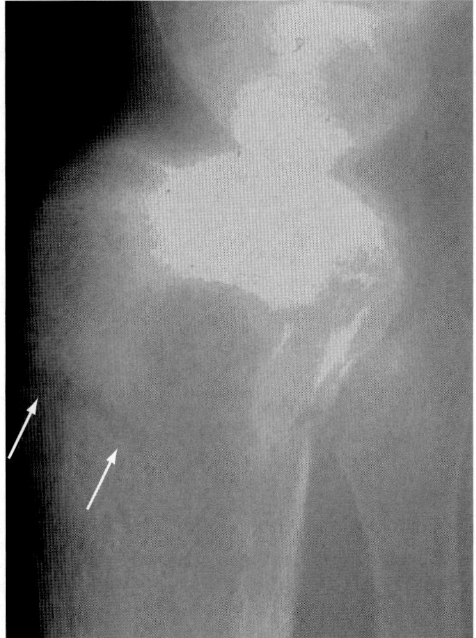

FIGURE 36-4. Osteomalacia. Lateral radiograph proximal tibia. Osteomalacic stigmata in a favored long-bone, lower-extremity site include severe osteopenia, barely distinguishable bony architecture, and a subtle insufficiency fracture at right angles to anterior cortex *(arrows).*

Osteopenia and bone quality in general and osteomalacia in particular are not well appreciated on any of the imaging modalities favored for documenting fractures, that is, bone scans, CT, or MRI. They therefore do not uniformly elicit suspicion or lead to further investigation for causative factors, particularly in older osteoporotic patients. Moreover, while MRI is still the modality of choice for documenting occult or clinically unappreciated soft tissue masses and has the further advantage of simultaneously visualizing bone lesions in inaccessible or unexpected sites (see Figures 36-5 and 36-6, *F*), such lesions are depicted in isolation. In fact, neither may be culpable since all may exist independently and not be associated with TIO.

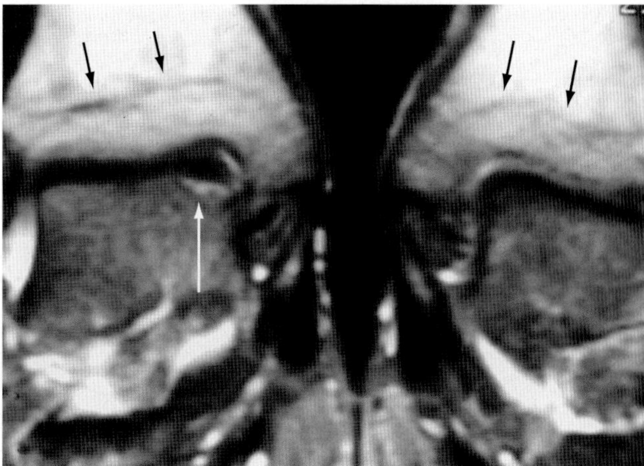

FIGURE 36-5. A middle-aged man presented with chronic ankle pain, no history of trauma or sports-related injury, and hypophosphatemic osteomalacia. MR coronal proton-density image of both ankles. Linear, transverse low signal foci in tibial metaphyses *(black arrows)* and an osteochondral fracture in right medial talar dome *(white arrow)* represent insufficiency fractures due to a small, soft tissue fibrovascular lesion in the right extremity.

Consequently, whole-body MRI, CT, or PET, while potentially revealing occult benign or malignant responsible lesions, may also delineate unrelated and irrelevant lesions with no pathologic or clinical significance and at great expense.[34,42-45] Radiographic skeletal surveys are another whole-body alternative, but they have the same drawbacks, especially in children in view of radiation exposure. Its selection as a search modality must therefore be carefully considered in terms of patient age and the fact that it may not be as rewarding in detecting involved soft tissue lesions.

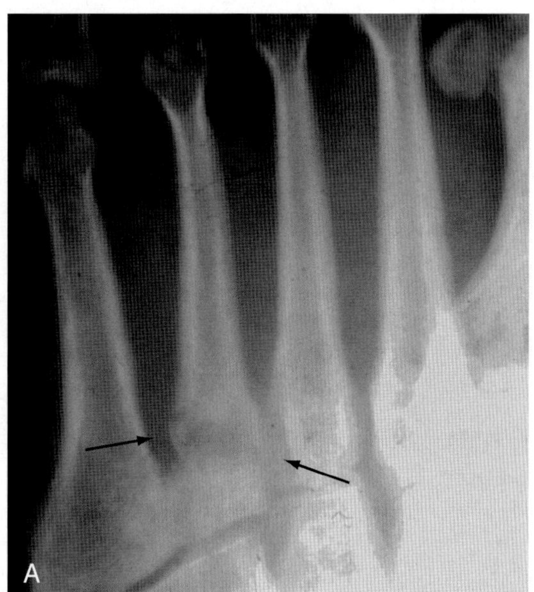

FIGURE 36-6. Multiple sequential images of a 45-year-old man with weakness and progressive pain in the chest and upper and lower extremities show insufficiency fractures at multiple sites. **A,** Oblique radiograph of the left foot shows a large, radiolucent zone at the base of the fourth metatarsal with no evidence of callus *(arrows).*

(Continued)

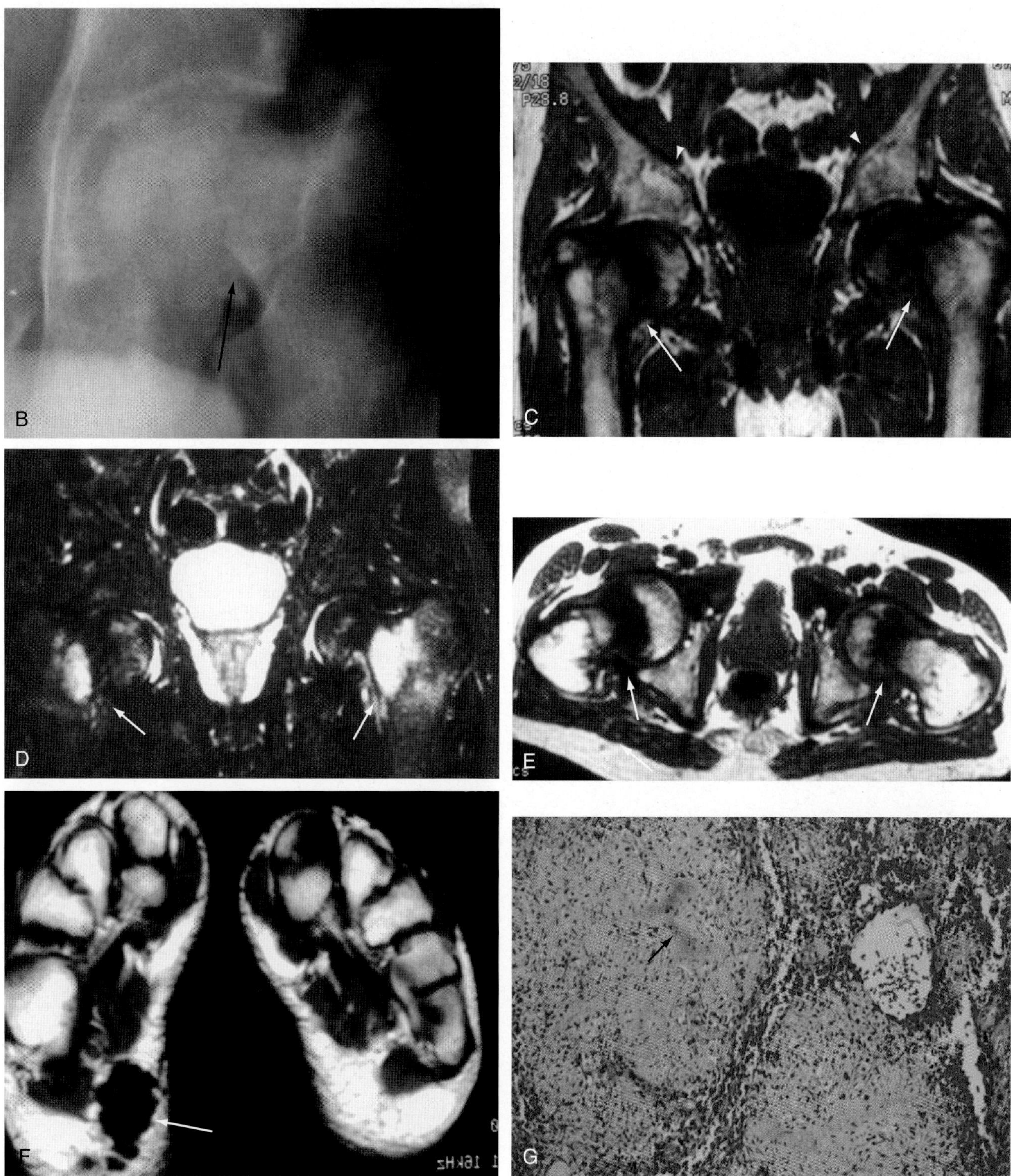

FIGURE 36-6—cont'd. B, Anteroposterior view of the left hip reveals marked osteopenia, a mottled trabecular pattern and a left proximal femoral varus deformity due to an unhealed insufficiency fracture *(arrow)*. **C,** Preoperative pelvis MRI coronal T1-weighted image reveals wide, bilateral, femoral neck signal voids *(white arrows)* due to zones of unmineralized osteoid and lamellar bone. Note contracted, triradiate pelvis and acetabular insufficiency fractures *(arrowheads)*. **D,** Preoperative pelvis coronal T2-weighted fat-suppressed MRI. Increased signal intensity denotes proximal femoral insufficiency fractures with surrounding edema *(arrows)*. **E,** Preoperative MR axial T1-weighted image again shows large signal voids in deformed, fractured femoral necks *(arrows)*. **F,** Preoperative MRI of both feet, axial T1-weighted image. Physical examination *(after C to E)* revealed a focal nodule in the sole of the right foot that MRI defined as an irregularly shaped 2 × 2 × 1-cm signal void *(arrow)* in the right medial plantar soft tissue which proved to be the TIO responsible lesion. **G,** Histologic specimen of the excised mass in **F** revealed spindle-shaped cells with small nuclei, vascular channels, and cartilage foci *(arrows)* indicative of mesenchymal origin with giant cells and a reticulin network in some sections.

(Continued)

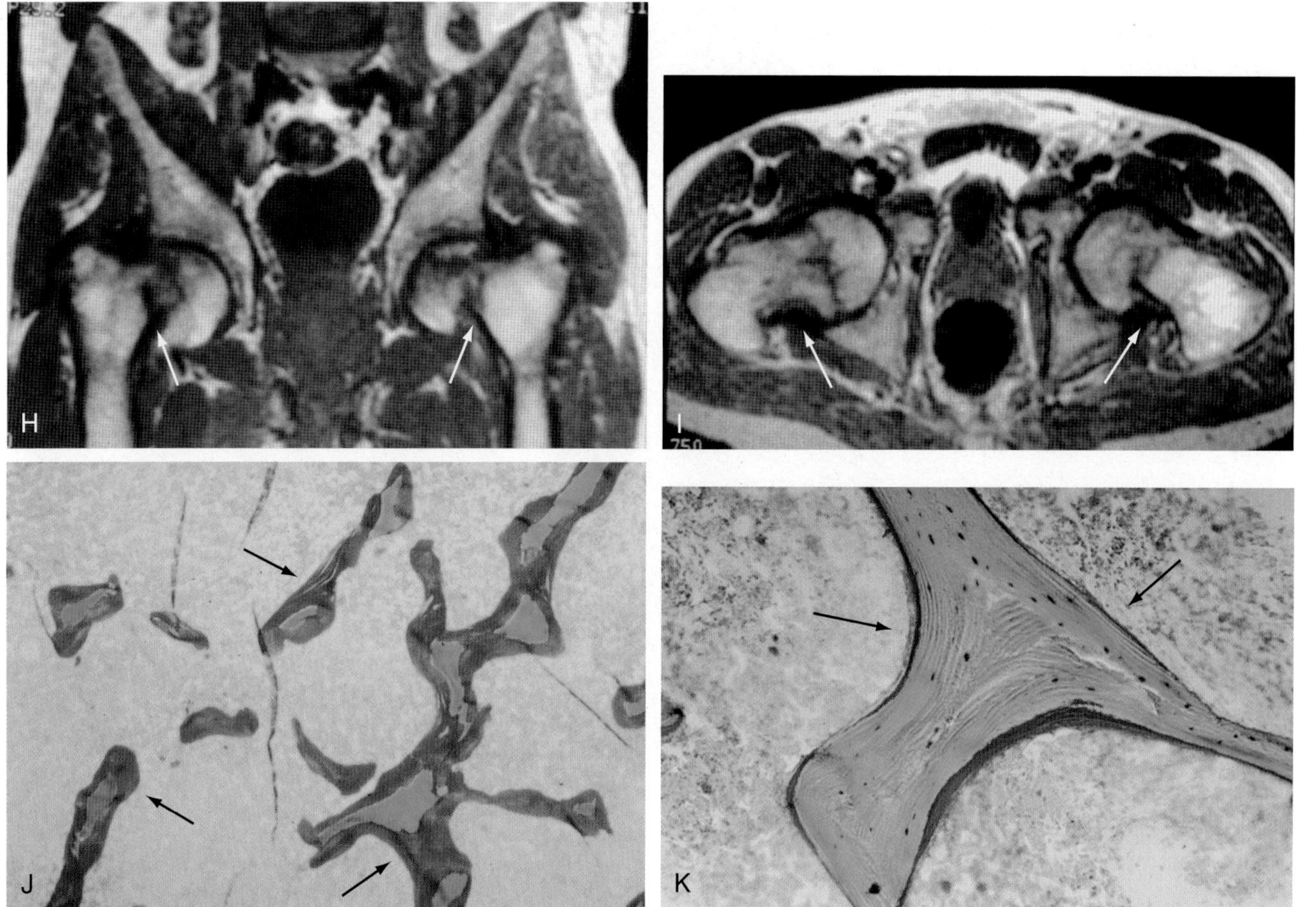

FIGURE 36-6—cont'd. Postoperative pelvic MRI coronal T1-weighted images **(H)** and postoperative pelvic MRI axial T1-weighted **(I)** images show increasingly uniform marrow signal compared with preoperative signal voids *(C to E)* due to remineralizing osteoid *(white arrows)*. The contracted pelvis and protrusio acetabula are still evident, but acetabular fractures are less well defined due to partial healing. The patient's biochemistries and symptoms improved 16 hours postsurgery. Tubular phosphorus resorption normalized in a day and he was asymptomatic at 2-year follow-up. **J,** Preoperative iliac crest biopsy. Photomicrograph at low power (42× reduced 30%) shows severe osteomalacia with increased osteoid volume, surface, and thickness with marked reduction in calcification rate *(arrows)*. Note the thin central trabecula. **K,** Postoperative iliac crest biopsy.

Technetium (Tc-99m) bone scans, while also able to document diffuse skeletal uptake of multiple synchronous or solitary fractures with radionuclide concentration, are again nonspecific (Figure 36-7). Octreotide scans with a radiolabeled somatostatin analog (In111-pentetreotide) may more efficiently target mesenchymal tumors if they express somatostatin receptors (SSTRs).[46,47] Octreotide has also been used for treatment of a variety of lesions since SSTRs are not limited to those producing TIO.[48] Conversely, other TIO lesions may not express them at all so that biochemical confirmation is always necessary before undertaking exhaustive imaging or other avenues of investigation.

PET is also able to document multiple bone and soft tissue lesions simultaneously as in MRI, but it has the additional ability of separating benign from malignant lesions.[45] Pitfalls, just as in whole-body MRI or CT include the considerations that, although positive on PET scans, lesions may exist independently without being TIO producers (see Box 36-1), they may be benign and hypermetabolic (i.e., false-positive inflammatory, giant cell-rich), or they may be benign and hypometabolic. Benign lesions may also not concentrate radionuclides at all, while very small lesions may not be visualized.[45] However, PET uniquely provides the added parameter of metabolic activity, which can be visualized and quantified.

The refined anatomic detail of PET/CT has also improved lesion localization so as to better direct biopsy and enhance its accuracy. Difficulties shared by all imaging modalities include TIO lesions that are slow growing, small, and not resolvable or obscured by volume averaging. They may also occur in unexpected (see Figure 36-6, *F*) or difficult-to-appreciate or access sites on physical examination, such as retroperitoneal, craniofacial, and nasopharyngeal regions, with the latter representing the most common locus for TIO lesions.

Recently, both indirect and direct methods of substantiating the existence of TIO lesions have been reported, including serum assays for FGF23, which is highly expressed in TIO lesions.[35] Another recently advocated approach when a suspicious mass is noted is to cannulate its venous outflow to directly measure its FGF23 content.[49] The latter, in particular, may represent a means of avoiding unnecessary and unrewarding multiple excisions. Conclusive evidence that a specific lesion is culpable further lies in prompt symptomatic relief and elimination of all biochemical abnormalities after its removal.

Prompt symptomatic relief and elimination of all biochemical abnormalities are noted after removal of the causative lesion. Both techniques show promise.

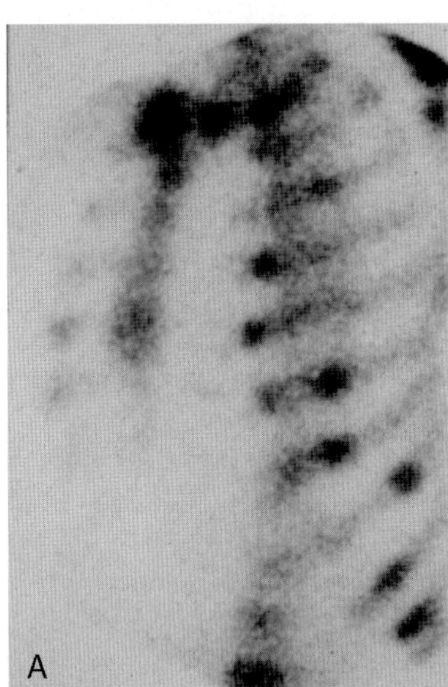

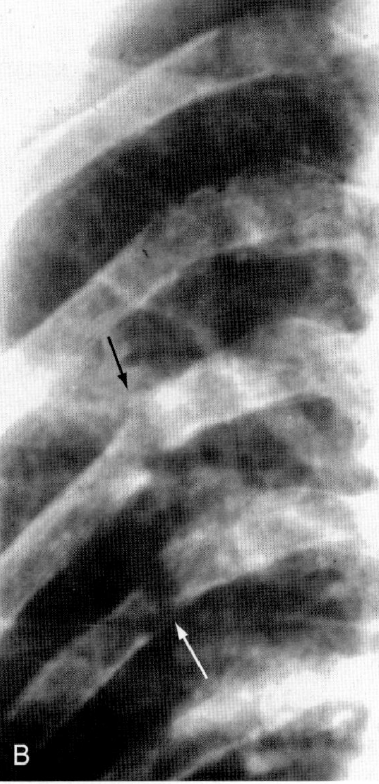

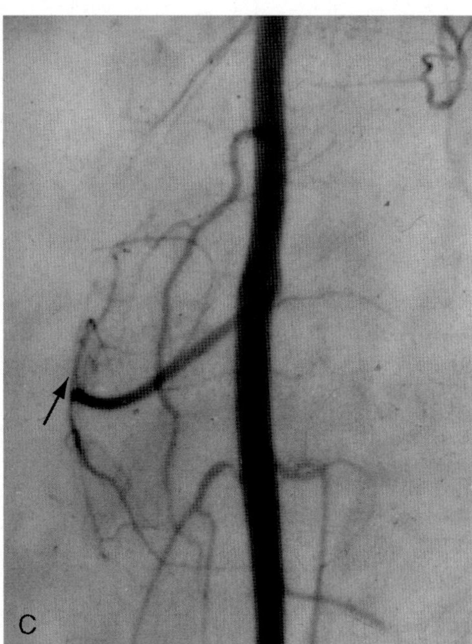

FIGURE 36-7. A 47-year-old "outdoors man" who lived in a sunny climate had progressive bone pain with no known cause. **A,** Bone scan showed radionuclide concentration in multiple thoracic and shoulder girdle sites. **B,** Radiographic detail of rib cage shows multiple, unhealed rib fractures separated by wide lucent zones *(arrows)* due to unmineralized lamellar bone and no evidence of callus. **C,** Angiogram of the thigh. A small soft-tissue mass ignored by the patient for "some time" appears as a punctuate hypervascular mass *(arrow)* histologically diagnosed as a small hemangioma. After excision, all biochemical and clinical aberrations were resolved.

Physicians, including radiologists, should to be aware of the variety of lesions known to cause hypophosphatemic vitamin D-refractory states. History, physical examination, and specific biochemical determinations are mandatory. The plethora of techniques now part of the imaging armamentarium, whether used singly or together, must be selected in proper sequence with individual patients and particular circumstances in mind.

While radiographs, particularly of the chest and pelvis often hold a key to recognizing osteomalacia per se, supplementary imaging such as radionuclide scanning (including PET), MRI, or CT when undertaken, must be appropriately tailored to the individual patient. Imaging choices for exploring the whole body may also include skeletal surveys with the proviso that the latter are more suitable for characterizing bone lesions. Whole-body MRI, CT, and skeletal surveys are also not as efficient as PET in separating benign from malignant lesions. Histomorphology (see Figure 36-6, *J* and *K*) is another means of establishing the sentinel but nonspecific finding of osteomalacia, which may be attributable to such common etiologies as renal disease. Renal disease, in turn, may be genetic or hereditary or secondary to inflammatory, endocrine, or metabolic diseases such as diabetes or parathyroid aberrations.[19] Other diverse causes include alcoholism, myeloma, and toxic therapeutic or industrial chemical agents.

SUMMARY

TIO is distinguishable from most common forms of osteomalacia by appropriate biochemistries that typically reveal hypophosphatemia, hyperphosphaturia, low calcitriol (1,25-dihydroxy–vitamin D), normal serum calcium, and intact PTH levels. While several humeral substances have been identified as causative, investigators continue to reveal new initial or interim factors. A permanent cure depends on complete elimination of a causative lesion with observed complete resolution of all clinical and biochemical aberrations. Continuing or recurrent symptoms after removal signify incorrect identification or incomplete ablation of a causative lesion. Uninformed and, therefore, often inappropriate treatment, such as administration of calciferol in TIO, may lead to symptomatic relief in some instances, but it is usually temporary and uniformly unsuccessful.

Imaging, along with other methodologies, if well considered and well planned, has a complementary role in detecting initial and residual, as well as unsuspected multiple lesions.

References

1. McCance RA: Osteomalacia with Looser's nodes (Milkman's syndrome) due to a raised resistance to vitamin D acquired about the age of 15 years, *Q J Med* 16:33-46, 1947.
2. Prader VA, Illig R, Vehlinger E, et al: Rachitis infolge, knochen tumors, *Helv Paediatr Acta* 14:554-565, 1959.
3. Sundaram M, McCarthy EF: Oncogenic osteomalacia, 29:117-124, 2000.
4. Jan de Beur SM: Tumor induced osteomalacia, *J Am Med Assoc* 294:1250-1267, 2005.
5. Jan de Beur SM, Levine MA: Molecular pathogenesis of hypophosphatemic rickets, *J Clin Endocrinol Metab* 87:2467-2473, 2002.
6. Dorfman H, Czerniak B: *Bone Tumors,* St Louis, 1998, Mosby.
7. Miyauchi A, Fukase M, Tsutsumi M et al: Hemangiopericytoma-induced osteomalacia: tumor transplantation in nude mice causes hypophosphatemia and tumor extract inhibit renal 25-hydroxyvitamin D 1 alpha activity, *J Clin Endocrinol Metab* 67:46-53, 1988.
8. Riminucci M, Collins MT, Fedarko NS et al: FGF23 in fibrous dysplasia of bone and its relationship to renal phosphate wasting, *J Clin Invest* 112:683-692, 2003.
9. Martini A, Notarangelo LD, Barberis L et al: Acquired vitamin-D resistant rickets caused by prolonged latency in appearance of bone tumor, *Am J Dis Child* 137:1025-1026, 1983.
10. Nomura G, Koshino Y, Morimoto H et al: Vitamin D resistant hypophosphatemic osteomalacia associated with osteosarcoma of the mandible: report of a case. *Japn J Med* 21:35-39, 1981.

11. Park YK, Unni KK, Beabout JW et al: Oncogenic osteomalacia: a clinicopathologic study of 17 bone lesions, *J Korean Med Sci* 9:289-298, 1994.
12. Aschinberg LC, Solomon LM, Zeis PM et al: Vitamin D resistant rickets associated with epidermal nevus syndrome: demonstration of a phosphaturic substance in dermal lesions, *J Pediatr* 91:56-60, 1977.
13. Leehey DJ, Ing TS, Daugirdas JT: Fanconi syndrome associate with a non-ossifying fibroma of bone, *Am J Med* 78:708-710, 1985.
14. Nitzan DW, Marmary Y, Azaz B: Mandibular tumor-induced muscular weakness and osteomalacia, *Oral Surg Oral Med Oral Pathol* 52:253-256, 1981.
15. Prowse M, Brooks PM: Oncogenic hypophosphatemic osteomalacia associated with a giant cell tumour of a tendon sheath, *Aust N Z J Med* 17:330-332, 1987.
16. Renton P, Shaw DG: Hypophosphatemic osteomalacia secondary to vascular tumors of bone and soft tissue, *Skeletal Radiol* 1:21-24, 1976.
17. Shenker Y, Grekin RJ: Oncogenic osteomalacia, *Isr J Med Sci* 20:739-741, 1984.
18. Turner ML, Dalinka MK: Osteomalacia: uncommon causes, *AJR Am J Roentgenol* 133:539-540, 1979.
19. Feldman F: Skeletal manifestations of ectopic or inappropriate endocrine and metabolic syndromes, *Radiol Clin North Am* 29:119-134, 1991.
20. Popovtzer MM: Tumor-induced hypophosphatemic osteomalacia (TIO): evidence for a phosphaturic cyclic AMP-independent action of tumor extract. *Clin Res* 29:418A, 1981.
21. Econs MJ, Drezner MK: Tumor induced osteomalacia unveiling a new hormone, *N Engl J Med* 330:1679-1681, 1994.
22. Cai Q, Hodgson SF, Kao PC et al: Brief report: inhibition of renal phosphate transport by a tumor product in a patient with oncogenic osteomalacia, *N Engl J Med* 330:16450-1649, 1994.
23. Wilkins GE, Granleese S, Hegele RG: Oncogenic osteomalacia: evidence for a humoral phosphaturic factor, *J Clin Endocrinol Metab* 30:1628-1634, 1995.
24. Rowe PS, Ong AC, Cockerill FJ, et al: Candidate 56 and 58 kDa protein(s) responsible for mediating the renal defects in oncogenic hypophosphatemic osteomalacia, *Bone* 18:159-169,1996.
25. Jonnson K, Mannstadt M, Miyauchi A et al: Extracts from tumors causing oncogenic osteomalacia inhibit phosphate uptake in opossum kidney cells, *J Endocrinol* 169:613-620, 2001.
26. Rowe PS, de Zoysa PA, Dong R et al: MEPE, a new gene expressed in bone marrow and tumors causing osteomalacia, *Genomics* 67:54-68, 2000.
27. Schiavi SC, Moe OW: Phosphatonins: a new class of phosphate regulating proteins, *Curr Opin Nephrol Hypertens* 11:423-430, 2002.
28. Shimada T, Muzutani S, Muto T et al: Cloning and characterization of FGF23 as a causative factor of tumor-induced osteomalacia, *Proc Natl Acad Sci USA* 98:6500-6505, 2001.
29. Sitaria D, Razzaque M, Hesse M et al: Homozygous ablation of fibroblast growth factor-23 results in hyperphosphatemia and impaired skeletogenesis, and reverses hypophosphatemia in PHEX-deficient mice, *Matrix Biol* 23:421-432, 2004.
30. Berndt T, Craig TA, Bowe AE et al: Frizzled related protein 4 is a potent phosphaturic agent, *J Clin Invest* 112:785-794, 2003.
31. Gowen LC, Petersen DN, Mansolf AL et al: Targeted disruption of the osteoblast/osteocyte factor 45 gene (OF45) results in increased bone formation and bone mass, *J Biol Chem* 278:1998-2007, 2003.
32. Rowe PS, Kumagai Y, Gutierrez G, et al: MEPE has the properties of an osteoblastic phosphatonin and minhibin, *Bone* 34:303-319, 2004.
33. Prie D, Huart V, Barkow N et al: Nephrolithiasis and osteoporosis associated with hypophosphatemia caused by mutations in the type 2a sodium phosphate cotransporter, *N Engl J Med* 347:983-991, 2002.
34. Dupond JL, Mahammedi H, Prie D et al: Oncogenic osteomalacia: diagnostic importance of fibroblast growth factor 23 and F-18 fluorodeoxyglucose PET/CT scan for the diagnosis and follow-up in one case, 36:375-378, 2005.
35. Yamazaki Y, Okazaki R, Shibata M et al: Increased circulatory level of biologically active full-length FGF-23 in patients with hypophosphatemic rickets/osteomalacia, *J Clin Endocrinol Metab* 87:4957-4960, 2002.
36. The HYP Consortium: A gene (PEX) with homologies to endopeptidases is mutated in patients with X-linked hypophosphatemic rickets. *Nat Genet* 11:130-136, 1995.
37. Holm IA, Huang X, Kunkel LM: Mutational analysis of the PEX gene in patients with X-linked hypophosphatemic rickets, *Am J Hum Genet* 60:790-797, 1997.
38. Nelson AE, Mason RS, Robinson BG: The PEX gene: not a simple answer for X-linked hypophosphataemic rickets and oncogenic osteomalacia, *Mol Cell Endocrinol* 132:1-5, 1997.
39. Nesbitt T, Drezner MK: Hepatocyte production of phosphatonin in HYP mice, *J Bone Miner Res* (Suppl 1):S136, 1996.
40. Pitt MJ: Rickets and osteomalacia. In Resnick D (ed): *Diagnosis of Bone and Joint Disorders*, 4th ed, Philadelphia, 2002, WB Saunders, pp 1901-1945.
41. Ohashi K, Ohnishi T, Ishikawa T et al: Oncogenic osteomalacia presenting as bilateral stress fractures of the tibia, *Skel Radiol* 28:46-49, 1999.
42. Avila NA, Skarulis M, Rubino DM et al: Oncogenic osteomalacia: lesion detection by MR skeletal survey, *AJR Am J Roentgenol* 167:343-345, 1996.
43. Fukumoto S, Takeuchi Y, Nagano A et al: Diagnostic utility of magnetic resonance imaging skeletal survey in a patient with oncogenic osteomalacia, *Bone* 25:357-375, 1990.
44. Imanishi Y, Nakatsuka K, Nakayama T et al: False positive MRI skeletal survey in a patient with sporadic hypophosphatemic osteomalacia, *J Bone Miner Metab* 21:57-59, 2003.
45. Feldman F, Van Heertum R, Manoj C: 18 FDG Pet scanning of benign & malignant musculoskeletal lesions, *Skel Radiol* 32:201-208, 2003.
46. Jan de Beur SM, Streeten EA, Civelek AC et al: Localization of mesenchymal tumors causing oncogenic osteomalacia with somatostatin receptor imaging, *Lancet* 359:761-763, 2002.
47. Rhee Y, Lee JD, Shin KH et al: Oncogenic osteomalacia associated with mesenchymal tumor detected by indium-111 octreotide scintigraphy, *Clin Endocrinol* 54:551-554, 2001.
48. Seufert J, Ebert K, Muller J et al: Octreotide therapy for tumor-induced osteomalacia, *N Engl J Med* 345:1883-1888, 2001.
49. Takeuchi Y, Suzuki H, Ogura S et al: Venous sampling for fibroblast growth factor-23 confirms preoperative diagnosis of tumor-induced osteomalacia, *J Clin Endocrinol Metab* 889:3979-3982, 2004.

CHAPTER 37

Hypophosphatasia

PARHAM PEZESHK, MD, *and* JOHN A. CARRINO, MD, MPH

KEY FACTS

- Hypophosphatasia is an autosomal recessive disorder.
- Radiographic findings of osteomalacia or rickets are present without abnormalities of vitamin D metabolism.
- High levels of phosphoethanolamine are noted in the blood and urine.
- In the neonatal form, transverse bony spurs (Bowdler spurs) may be present under skin dimpling.
- Craniosynostosis may result in a small skull.
- In contrast to most causes of osteomalacia in which Looser zones appear in the inner cortex, hypophosphatasia presents with Looser zones in the outer cortex of long bones.

Hypophosphatasia, an autosomal recessive disorder, is one of the rare syndromes in which the radiographic findings of osteomalacia or rickets are present in the absence of abnormalities of vitamin D metabolism. Serum levels of calcium and phosphate are high or normal. The serum alkaline phosphatase is low and there are abnormal amounts of phosphoethanolamine in the urine and blood.[3]

MUSCULOSKELETAL FINDINGS

The severity of radiologic findings depends on the age of presentation and increases as the disease presents in younger ages.[1] Radiographs show generalized osteopenia with a coarse trabecular pattern, healing or non-healing fractures, bowing deformities (especially involving the tibiae), chondrocalcinosis, craniosynostosis (resulting in a small skull), early loss of deciduous teeth, and subperiosteal bone formation. In the neonatal form, transverse bony spurs from the radius, ulna, and fibula (Bowdler spurs) may be present under skin dimpling.

Severe osteopenia is observed in the calvarium; however, the appearance of the skull base is more normal. Cranial sutures may appear widened due to undermineralization.

Growth plate changes resemble those seen in rickets with characteristic irregular and prominent tongue-like radiolucent extensions into the metaphyses of the distal femurs, proximal humeri, epiphyses, and carpal bones.[2,3]

Fractures occur following minor trauma, and minimal callus may be seen with delayed healing.[4] In contrast to most causes of pure vitamin D-deficient osteomalacia in which Looser zones involve the inner cortex, hypophosphatasia presents with Looser zones in the outer cortex of long bones. Multiple rib fractures and abnormal appearance of the distal phalanges are other radiographic manifestations.[3]

Tendinous and ligamentous insertions in the paravertebral regions may show ossification.

SYSTEMIC IMAGING FEATURES

Nephrocalcinosis may develop subsequent to hypercalciuria.

REFERENCES

1. Berry JL, Davies M, Mee AP: Vitamin D metabolism, rickets, and osteomalacia, *Semin Musculoskelet Radiol* 6:173-182, 2002.
2. Pitt MJ: Rickets and osteomalacia. In Resnick D (ed): *Diagnosis of Bone and Joint Disorders*, 4th ed, New York, 2002, W B Saunders, pp 1901–1945.
3. Herman TE, McAlister WH: Inherited diseases of bone density in children, *Radiol Clin North Am* 29:149-164, 1991.
4. Anderton JM: Orthopaedic problems in adult hypophosphatasia: a report of two cases. *J Bone Joint Surg Br* 61:82-84, 1979.

CHAPTER 38

Fanconi Syndrome and Renal Tubular Acidosis

Parham Pezeshk, MD, *and* John Carrino, MD, MPH

Key Facts

- Fanconi syndrome and renal tubular acidosis are infrequent causes of osteomalacia and rickets.
- Imaging manifestations include nephrocalcinosis.

FANCONI SYNDROME

Fanconi syndrome includes a heterogeneous group of disorders characterized by a defect in transport capacity of the proximal tubules that results in impaired reabsorption of glucose, calcium, phosphate, amino acids, bicarbonate, uric acid, and organic acids. Excretion of low-molecular-weight proteins (< 50,000 Da), magnesium, sodium, and potassium are also increased.[1,2] Various familial and acquired disorders contribute to the pathogenesis of this syndrome, ultimately resulting in injury to the proximal tubules. The most common causes of Fanconi syndrome in adults and children are light-chain myeloma and cystinosis (autosomal-recessive cystine storage disease), respectively.[3] This syndrome has also been seen in vitamin D deficiency.[4] Box 38-1 presents selected causes of Fanconi syndrome.

Affected children present with polyuria, polydipsia, and dehydration following the loss of significant amounts of solutes and water. Growth failure is a striking clinical feature of this syndrome. Excessive urinary loss of calcium and phosphorus in conjunction with the defect in vitamin D metabolism can result in rickets in children and osteomalacia in adults. Serum level of $1,25(OH)_2D$ is low or normal but not increased as expected in the course of hypophosphatemia and secondary hyperparathyroidism.[5] Decreased levels of $1,25(OH)_2D$ may be related to the defect in the hydroxylation of 25-OH-D into its active form following damage to the proximal tubules, which contain 1-α-hydroxylase. In contrast, it has also been shown that the defect in the hydroxylation of 25-OH-D ensues only when renal insufficiency occurs.[6] Hepatic damage and cirrhosis occur as a result of some causes of Fanconi sundrome.

A dysfunction of proximal tubules resembling Fanconi syndrome is seen in vitamin D deficiency and is resolved with vitamin D supplements. Persistent phosphaturia is a major factor in the development and maintenance of rickets and osteomalacia.[1] Moreover, osteonecrosis may occur as a result of longstanding Fanconi syndrome.[7] Imaging studies may reveal nephrocalcinosis as a result of hypercalciuria, which is common particularly when Wilson's disease is the cause of Fanconi syndrome.

BOX 38-1. Hereditary and Acquired Causes of Fanconi Syndrome

INHERITED
Galactosemia
Cystinosis
Hereditary fructose intolerance
Glycogen storage disease
Wilson's disease
Tyrosinosis (tyrosinemia, type I)

ACQUIRED
Amyloidosis
Multiple myeloma
Nephrotic syndrome
Heavy metal exposure (lead, mercury)
Malignancy
Vitamin D deficiency
Medications (aminoglycosides, valproic acid, ifosfamide, outdated tetracycline, cis-platinum)
Glue sniffing (toluene inhalation)

RENAL TUBULAR ACIDOSIS

Renal tubular acidosis (RTA) reduces the capability of the kidneys to reabsorb bicarbonate. The reduction of bicarbonate reabsorption and the inability to secrete hydrogen ions (H^+) by the tubules result in systemic metabolic acidosis. Currently, RTA is classified into three types: RTA type I (distal tubular H^+ ion gradient form), RTA type II (proximal tubular bicarbonate wasting form), and RTA type IV (hyperkalemic form). The RTA type III is no longer applied and is considered a hybrid of types I and II. Urinary loss of bicarbonate is highest in type II and lowest in type IV. RTA type I rarely leads to rickets and osteomalacia; however, imaging studies of patients with this type of RTA may show bone erosion as a result of calcium release from bones due to systemic metabolic acidosis.

In RTA type II, osteomalacia and rickets are common findings. Nephrocalcinosis and hypercalciuria are less often seen as compared to RTA type I because acidic urine prevents deposition of calcium phosphate in RTA type II. Renal osteodystrophy can be observed as renal insufficiency progresses in RTA type IV.[8]

REFERENCES

1. Chesney RW: Fanconi syndrome and renal tubular acidosis. In Favus MJ, Christakos S (eds): *Primer on the Metabolic Bone Diseases and Disorders of Mineral Metabolism*, 3rd ed, Philadelphia, 1996, Lippincott Williams & Wilkins, pp 328-333.
2. Chesney RW, Jones DP: Renal tubular syndromes. In Gonick HC (ed): *Current Nephrology*, vol 19, Chicago, 1995, Mosby Yearbook, pp 1-34.
3. Brewer ED: The Fanconi syndrome: clinical disorders. In Gonick HC, Buckalew VW (eds): *Renal Tubular Disorders*, New York, 1985, Marcel Dekker, 475-544.
4. Chesney RW, Harrison HE: Fanconi syndrome following bowel surgery and hepatitis reversed by 25-hydroxycholecalciferol, *J Pediatrics* 86:857-861, 1975.
5. Baran DT, March TW: Evidence for a defect in vitamin D metabolism in a patient with incomplete Fanconi syndrome, *J Clin Endocrinol Metab* 59:998-1001, 1984.
6. Steinberg R, Chesney RW, Schulman J et al: Circulating vitamin D metabolites in nephropathic cystinosis, *J Pediatrics* 120:592-594, 1983.
7. Gaucher A, Thomas JL, Netter P et al: Osteomalacia, pseudosacroiliitis and necrosis of the femoral heads in Fanconi syndrome in an adult, *J Rheumatol* 8:512-515, 1981.
8. Chesney RW: Fanconi syndrome and renal tubular acidosis. In Favus MJ (ed): *Primer on the Metabolic Bone Diseases and Disorders of Mineral Metabolism*, 3rd ed, Philadelphia, 1996, Lippincott-Raven, pp 328-333.

CHAPTER 39

Soft Tissue Calcification and Ossification

Arthur H. Newberg, MD, FACR

Key Facts

- Soft tissue calcifications appear on radiographs as punctuate, circular, linear, or plaque-like radio-dense areas. Often these calcifications, by their appearance and location, can provide clues to an associated medical disorder.
- Calcific tendinitis (hydroxyapatite deposition disease) is most commonly located in the supraspinatus tendon of the shoulder. It may be asymptomatic or may result in severe pain, erythema, swelling, painful range of motion, and fever.
- Tumoral calcinosis is a condition usually affecting dark-skinned people. It is characterized by prominent periarticular calcified masses around large joints, especially the hips. Large amorphous masses containing fluid-calcium levels are identified, especially on cross-sectional imaging.
- Myositis ossificans is a localized form of post-traumatic heterotopic calcification and ossification that occurs in a traumatized muscle, particularly in the anterior thigh. The mass characteristically matures from the periphery to the center; a rim of calcification is seen by 6 to 8 weeks and is separate from the underlying bone.
- Fibrodysplasia ossificans progressiva is a very rare condition presenting in childhood, characterized by painful soft tissue masses that progress to sheets and struts of ossification that bridge joints. These ossific bands eventually result in severely limited mobility and diminished chest wall excursion, leading to early death.

The radiographic detection of calcification and ossification in the soft tissues often provides an important clue to the correct clinical diagnosis. Soft tissue calcifications appear as irregular punctuate, circular, linear, or plaque-like radio-dense areas that do not possess a trabecular or cortical structure. The location of soft tissue calcifications is of importance in narrowing the differential diagnostic considerations.

Soft tissue calcifications that occur in tendons or bursae suggest hydroxyapatite deposition disease or calcium pyrophosphate deposition disease. Calcification in lymph nodes may indicate granulomatous infection such as tuberculosis. Arterial calcification is seen in renal osteodystrophy, diabetes mellitus, and hypervitaminosis D. Calcified nerves are a hallmark of leprosy. Chondrocalcinosis has a long list of causes including hemochromatosis, primary hyperparathyroidism, and Wilson's disease, among others. Multiple calcified intervertebral disks suggest alkaptonuria. Soft tissue calcification of the fingertips is characteristic of collagen vascular disorders, especially the scleroderma variant known as CREST (calcinosis, Raynaud's, esophageal dysmotility, sclerodactyly, and telangiectasias). Calcification of the pinna of the ear may raise suspicion for endocrine disorders or previous thermal trauma. Multiple calcifications in the muscles may suggest parasite or worm infestation (Figure 39-1).

Soft tissue ossification may occur in neurologic diseases, physical and thermal trauma, venous insufficiency, neoplasms such as soft tissue osteosarcoma, myositis ossificans (MO) progressiva, melorrheostosis, and in surgical scars.[1]

Generally, the work-up of a patient with soft tissue calcifications includes measurements of serum calcium, serum phosphate, PTH levels, calcitonin measurement, 24-hour urinary calcium, and phosphorus.[2] The evaluation of cartilage calcification (chondrocalcinosis) may include measurement of serum iron, total iron binding capacity, ferritin, parathyroid hormone, and thyroid function studies.

HYDROXYAPATITE DEPOSITION DISEASE (CALCIFIC TENDINITIS, CALCIFIC PERIARTHRITIS)

Hydroxyapatite crystal deposition disease (HADD) is a crystal-induced arthropathy in which there is deposition of hydroxyapatite crystals in the paraarticular soft tissues resulting in tendinitis and bursitis.[3] It may occur as a primary idiopathic phenomenon or be secondary to other disease states. Thus, HADD may also be seen in patients with connective tissue disorders such as scleroderma, secondary hyperparathyroidism, or osteoarthritis. More than 30% of patients with insulin-dependent diabetes mellitus may develop asymptomatic tendon calcification.[4]

HADD is characterized by the presence of basic calcium phosphate crystals—predominantly hydroxyapatite in the periarticular soft tissue, especially the tendons (Figure 39-2). Since the actual deposition may occur in the tendon, bursa, or joint capsule, the term *periarthritis,* rather than *peritendinitis* is preferred.[5] Macroscopically, HADD appears as calcified amorphous material with a "milky" or "cheesy" consistency in the paraarticular fibrous connective tissue.[3] HA crystals vary in size from 100 to 200 nm and are too small to be seen with ordinary polarized light microscopy.

A continuum of abnormalities ranging from monarticular periarthritis to polyarticular disease to joint destruction may occur.[5]

The peak incidence of calcific tendinitis occurs in the fourth to sixth decades of life. It is responsible for almost 50% of all shoulder pain.[6] Calcification about the shoulder is seen in

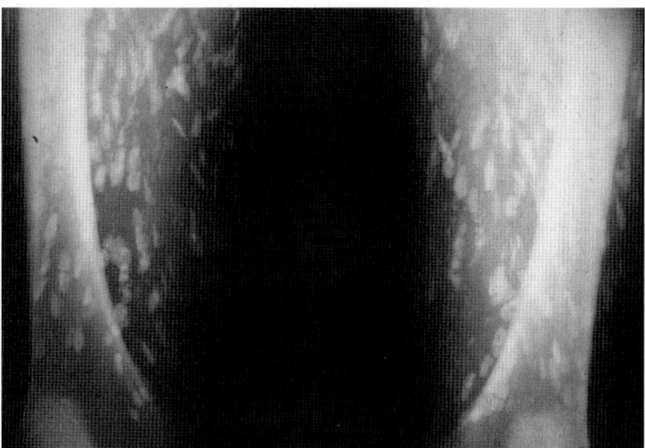

FIGURE 39-1. Cysticercosis. Radiograph of both thighs demonstrates a multitude of soft-tissue intramuscular oval densities characteristic of the calcified larvae in tapeworm infestation.

approximately 3% of adults, although most cases discovered on radiographs are asymptomatic.[7]

Calcific tendinitis most commonly affects the tendons about the shoulder. In addition, the tendons of the gluteus maximus, rectus femoris, vastus lateralis, quadriceps, pectoralis major, deltoid, and adductor magnus, as well as tendons of the wrist, hand, neck, and ankle may be affected.

> Although most frequent in the shoulder, calcific tendinitis may affect many different tendons, including the gluteus maximus insertion and the longus colli in the neck.

In the shoulder, the most common tendon involved is the supraspinatus, and a site 1.5 cm proximal to its insertion on the greater tuberosity is the most common area of that tendon to

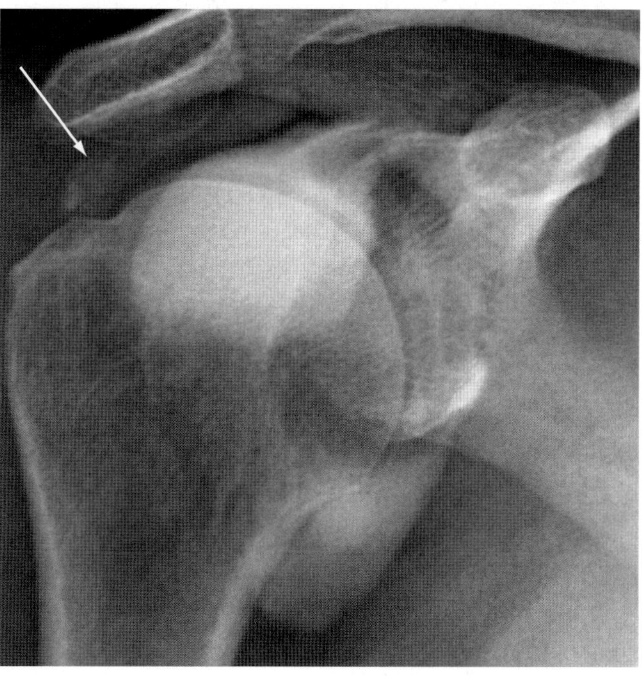

FIGURE 39-3. Calcific tendinitis. Fluoroscopic external rotation view of the right shoulder taken during a shoulder arthrogram injection demonstrates an area of oblong amorphous calcification in the expected location of the distal supraspinatus tendon *(arrow)*.

be affected.[8] This portion of the tendon has been shown to be subject to hypoxic and mechanical stress and is termed the *critical zone.* These stresses may incite events leading to fibrocartilage transformation followed by calcification[1] (Figure 39-3). Resorption of the calcification (the resorptive phase) produces extreme pain that may become incapacitating. This acute pain, which can mimic septic arthritis, may be due to increased intratendinous

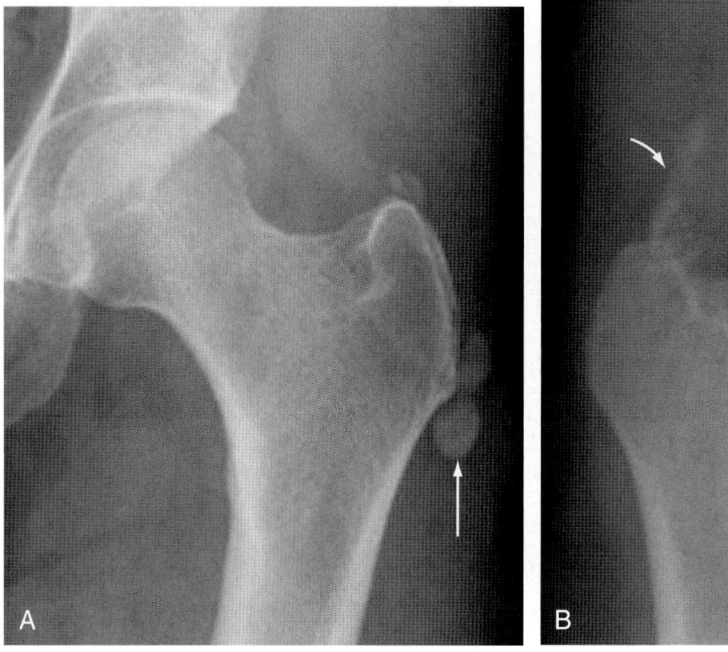

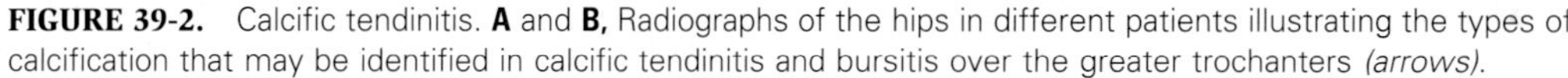

FIGURE 39-2. Calcific tendinitis. **A** and **B,** Radiographs of the hips in different patients illustrating the types of calcification that may be identified in calcific tendinitis and bursitis over the greater trochanters *(arrows)*.

TABLE 39-1. Stages of Supraspinatus Tendinitis

Stage	Histologic Findings	Clinical Findings	Radiographic Findings
Precalcific	Fibrocartilage transformation of the "critical zone"	Symptomatic or asymptomatic	None
Calcific: formative	Fibrocartilage replaced by calcific deposit		Homogeneous well-defined calcification
Calcific: resorptive	Macrophages and giant cells resorb the calcification.	Acute symptoms	Amorphous, less dense, ill-defined calcification. Soft tissue swelling
Postcalcific	Calcification has been resorbed and the defect fills with collagen	Chronic pain until new collagen is aligned with long axis of tendon	None

Information from Kraemer E, El-Khoury G: Atypical calcific tendinitis with cortical erosions. *Skel Radiol* 29:690-696, 2000.

pressure.[8] Acutely, erythema, swelling, painful range of motion, and fever may be noted. Finally, in the postcalcific phase, the calcific deposit has been phagocytized, and the void is rapidly replaced by granulation tissue. The chronic pain of the postcalcific stage is thought to last until the newly synthesized collagen fibers align themselves along the axis of the tendon (Table 39-1).

Hydroxyapatite deposits are seen on radiographs as homogeneous, amorphous densities without trabeculation. They are variable in size and their margins may be smooth and well-defined or ill-defined (Figure 39-4).

Well-defined dense calcifications are usually chronic and may be incidental findings, whereas poorly defined, less dense calcifications correlate with acute symptoms.

Calcific tendinitis of the supraspinatus tendon is best visualized on external rotation views of the affected shoulder. As the shoulder is rotated internally, the calcifications move medially, so that the calcific deposits may project over the humeral head making them more difficult to identify.

In patients with radiographically demonstrated supraspinatus calcification, it is estimated that fewer than 10% will ever develop symptoms of acute calcific tendinitis.[5]

Subscapularis calcific tendinitis may be more difficult to see on routine radiographs of the shoulder because the calcification can be obscured by overlying bone (Figure 39-5). An axillary view is helpful. Calcific deposits due to HADD may enlarge, decrease, disperse, or completely resolve with time.

The diagnosis of calcific tendinitis is usually made clinically and can be confirmed on appropriate radiographs.

Patients with acute calcific tendinitis present with severe pain involving the affected joint. There may be intense soft tissue swelling and warmth mimicking infection.

Occasionally computed tomography (CT) is used, especially when the calcium is atypical or there is concern for cortical involvement. The use of magnetic resonance imaging (MRI) is limited and may actually be confusing as the presence of soft tissue and osseous edema may raise the suspicion of infection or neoplasm. On MRIs, the calcification appears as areas of decreased signal intensity on T1-weighted images, whereas T2-weighted images may show increased signal corresponding to edema surrounding the low signal calcific deposit (Figure 39-6).

Acute calcific periarthritis of the hand mainly affects women (5:1) in the premenopausal age group. In the wrist, the distal flexor carpi ulnaris tendon is the most common location of calcific tendinitis. This may be a cause of volar wrist pain and marked associated soft tissue swelling. The calcification is best seen on a carpal tunnel

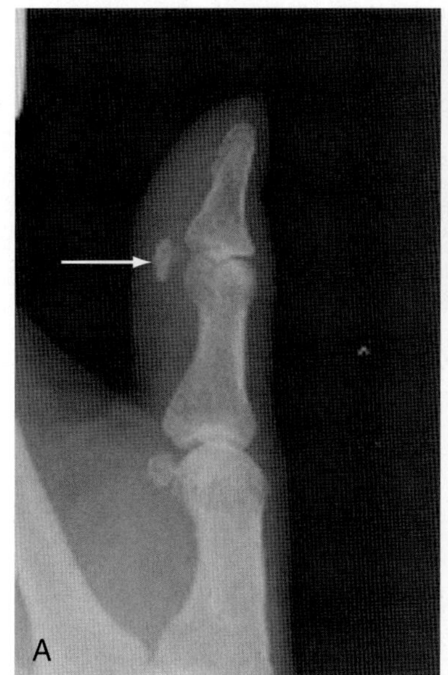

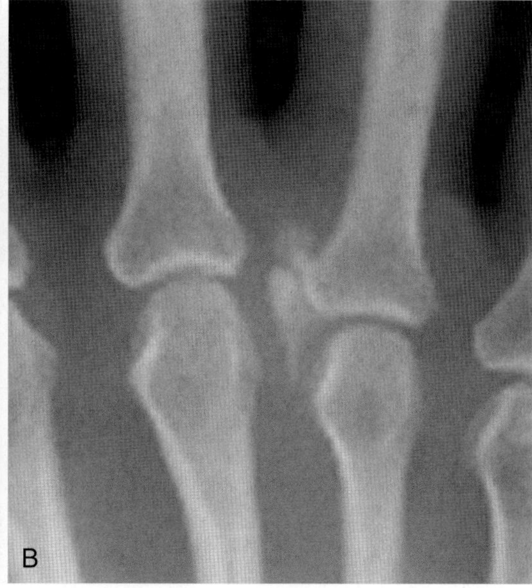

FIGURE 39-4. Acute calcific periarthritis (**A** and **B**). Two patients presenting with severe acute onset of joint pain demonstrate calcific deposits in a periarticular distribution *(arrow)*. After treatment these calcifications may promptly resorb.

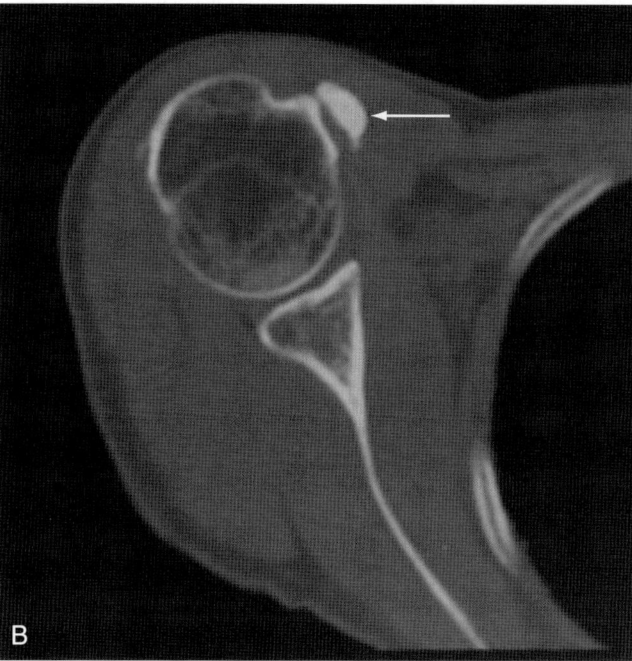

FIGURE 39-5. Subscapularis calcific tendinitis. **A**, Anteroposterior radiograph of the right shoulder demonstrates increased density overlying the humeral head *(arrow)*. It is difficult to be certain as to the exact location of this calcification. **B**, Axial CT scan image of the right shoulder shows the calcification to be located at the distal insertion site of the subscapularis tendon into the lesser tuberosity of the humeral head *(arrow)*.

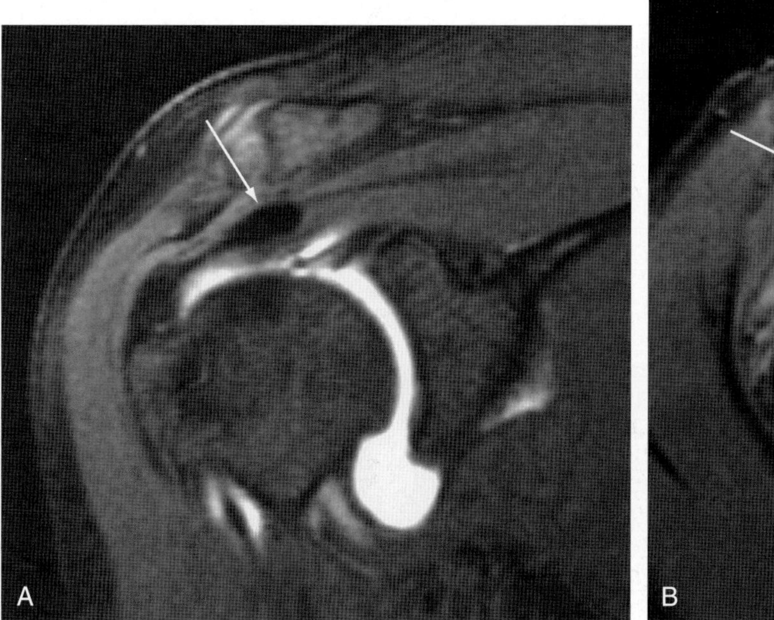

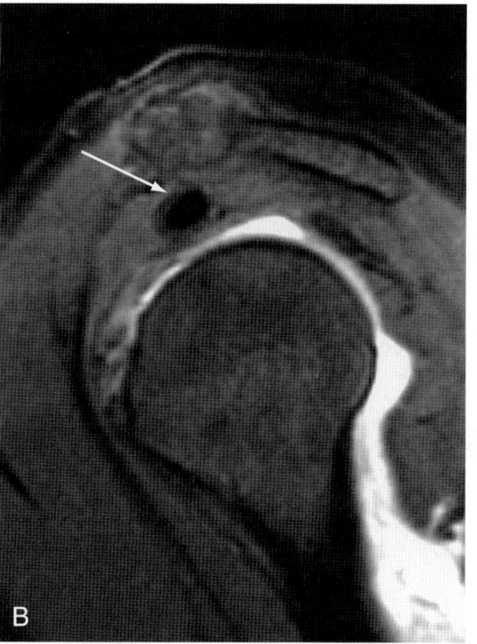

FIGURE 39-6. MRI of calcific tendinitis. Coronal **(A)** and sagittal **(B)** oblique T1 fat-suppressed images from an MR arthrogram with intraarticular gadolinium of the right shoulder demonstrates an elongated low signal focus in the supraspinatus tendon representing calcific tendinitis *(arrows)*.

view, semi-supinated oblique view of the wrist, or can be readily identified on axial noncontrast CT scans (Figure 39-7).

In the neck, calcification may affect the longus colli muscle, whose primary function is neck flexion. Calcification of the longus colli is best seen on well-positioned lateral cervical spine radiographs, where the calcification is seen just anterior to C1 or occasionally C2. CT confirms calcification at the C1-C2 level and the accompanying soft tissue swelling. MRI may demonstrate prevertebral increased signal on T2-weighted images due to muscle swelling.

> Calcific tendinitis of the longus colli muscle can produce odynophagia, dysphagia, and fever in older patients. The correct diagnosis can often be made on radiographs.

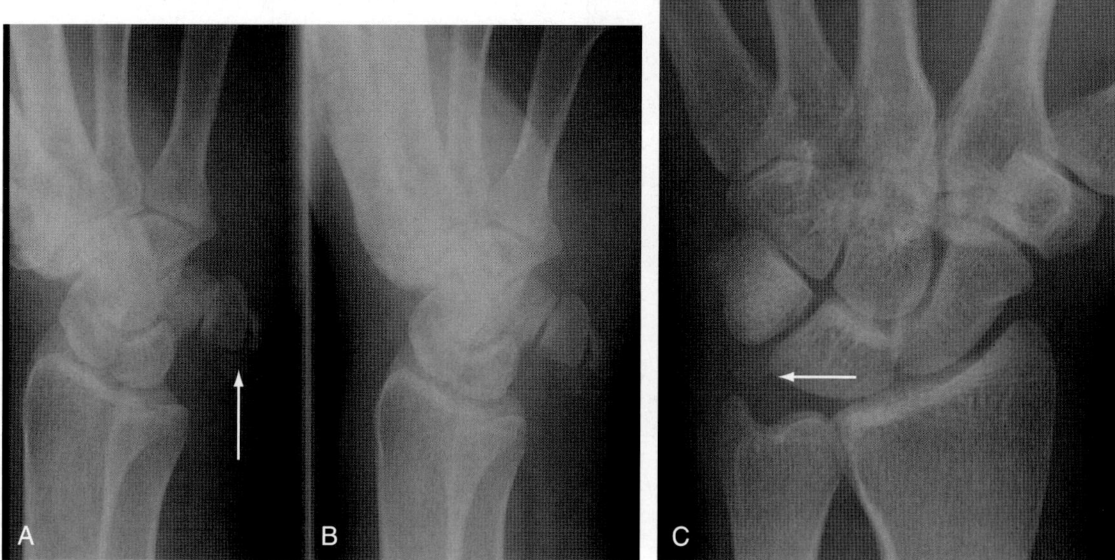

FIGURE 39-7. Flexor carpi ulnaris (FCU) calcific tendinitis. **A, B,** Semisupinated and **C,** posteroanterior radiographs of the left wrist show a density in the soft tissues adjacent to the pisiform representing calcification in the distal FCU tendon *(arrows)*.

Calcific tendinitis of the distal insertion of the gluteus maximus may present with a painful upper posterior thigh. Most of the fibers of the gluteus maximus insert on the iliotibial tract of the tensor fascia lata, dorsal and distal to the greater trochanter, but some insert on the gluteal tubercle of the posterior lateral upper femoral shaft (part of the linea aspera). Calcification that occurs here can be difficult to detect. The calcium will overlie the upper femoral shaft on an anteroposterior radiograph, and therefore may be best seen on a frog lateral radiograph or even more easily on axial CT images (Figure 39-8). The pain associated with calcium in this location may mimic radicular pain. In addition, posterior femoral cortical erosion adjacent to the calcification has been noted in some cases (Figure 39-9).

Cortical bone erosion has been observed in calcific tendinitis,[9,10] although bone destruction is not generally considered to be a feature of the disorder. Calcific tendinitis with bone erosion is most commonly observed in the femur (40%) and the humeral head (40%).[9] Hayes et al.[10] presented five cases; two involved the pectoralis major insertion, two involved the gluteus maximus insertion, and one the adductor magnus insertion. Bone resorption may reflect increased local vascularity and active inflammation at the tendon insertion. Alternatively, it may be caused by local pressure from the calcium deposit[10] (Figure 39-10).

Cortical erosion is the most common manifestation of osseous involvement (78% of cases), but bone marrow involvement has been demonstrated in 18 of 50 cases (36%)[9]; (61%) involving the greater or lesser tuberosities of the humeral head.[9] When calcific tendinitis presents with osseous destruction, bone marrow signal changes on MRI, and soft tissue calcification, there may be confusion with neoplasm both radiographically and pathologically.

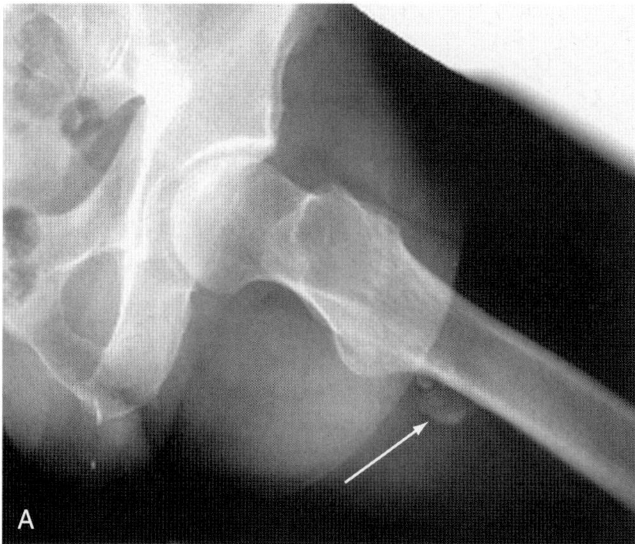

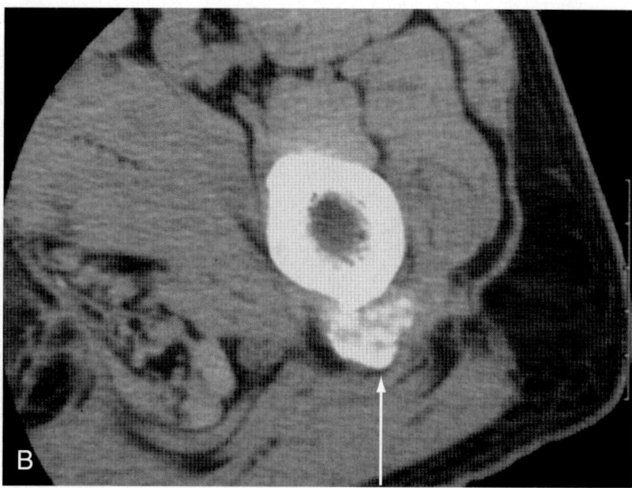

FIGURE 39-8. Gluteus maximus calcific tendinitis. Frog leg lateral radiograph **(A)** and axial CT image **(B)** of the left hip demonstrate amorphous calcification *(arrows)* located posterior to the proximal femur at the insertion of the lower fibers of the gluteus maximus tendon in this patient with upper posterior thigh pain.

FIGURE 39-9. Bone erosion by hydroxyapatite. Axial T1-weighted MRI of the upper thighs demonstrates an isointense mass posterior to the left femur *(curved arrow).* Within the mass are a few low signal flecks of calcification. There is also subtle thinning of the adjacent posterior femoral cortex caused by erosion from the calcific mass *(arrow)*.

> Calcific tendinitis may be associated with adjacent cortical erosion and marrow changes causing confusion with neoplasm. A comet-tail appearance of the calcification, present in calcific tendinitis, may suggest the correct diagnosis.

The main differential diagnosis for the acute symptoms of calcific tendinitis at presentation is infection or crystal induced arthritis, such as gout, especially if the area of involvement is near a joint.[11] Rarely, acute attacks can occur at multiple sites.[12] The differential diagnosis of radiographically demonstrated periarticular calcification due to HADD includes calcium pyrophosphate deposition disease (CPPD), metastatic calcification, connective tissue diseases, accessory ossicles (a normal variant), and soft tissue tumors containing calcium.[13]

Milwaukee Shoulder

Milwaukee shoulder[14] is a destructive arthropathy of the shoulder associated with chronic tears of the rotator cuff and joint effusions containing hydroxyapatite. Milwaukee shoulder most commonly affects elderly women. In addition to HA crystals, calcium pyrophosphate crystals are also frequently identified in the joint fluid. Radiographically, one can identify glenohumeral degenerative changes, soft tissue calcification, loose bodies, which will present as filling defects during arthrography, joint instability, rotator cuff tear, and soft tissue swelling.[11] Many patients also have a severe destructive arthropathy of the knees.

Calcinosis Universalis

Idiopathic calcinosis universalis is of unknown etiology and affects infants and children. Calcium phosphate and calcium carbonate are deposited about normal fat cells. There is a foreign body reaction. Serum calcium and phosphorus levels are normal. Discrete conglomerates of calcium are arranged in longitudinal bands. The major differential diagnosis includes dermatomyositis and hyperparathyroidism.

Tumoral Calcinosis

The term *tumoral calcinosis* has been used liberally to describe any massive collection of periarticular calcification, although the term actually refers to a hereditary condition associated with massive periarticular calcification (Figure 39-11). The inheritance of the latter condition is autosomal dominant with variable expressivity[15,16]; it may be related to an inborn error of phosphorus metabolism. Patients have slightly raised levels of urinary hydroxyproline, reduced fractional phosphate excretion, increased 1,25-dihydroxy–vitamin D formation, and a normal dynamic response to parathormone and hyperphosphatemia.[16] Some patients may have an elevated level of serum

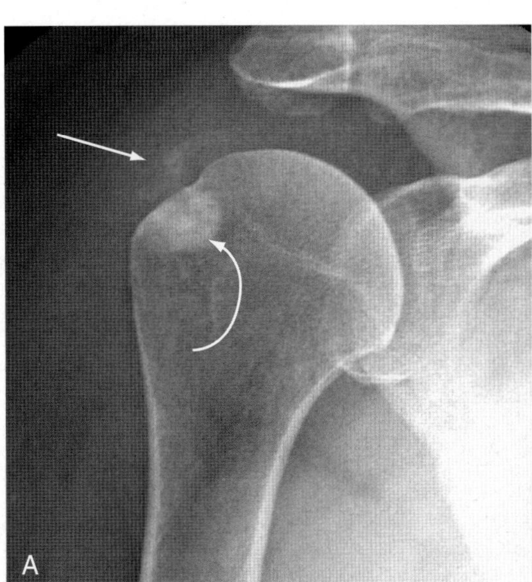

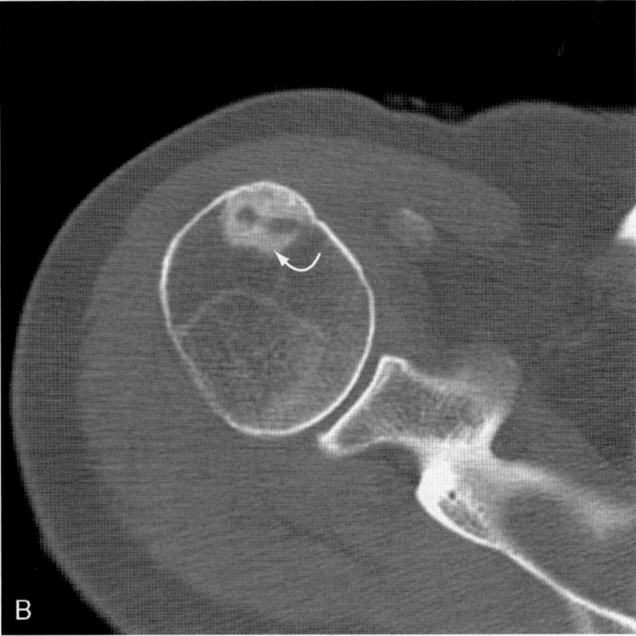

FIGURE 39-10. Calcific tendinitis with erosion into bone. Middle-aged woman presenting with severe pain in the right shoulder. **A**, Anteroposterior radiograph of the right shoulder demonstrates amorphous soft tissue calcium *(arrow)*, in the expected location of the supraspinatus tendon. There is also increased density in the greater tuberosity *(curved arrow)* representing erosion of calcium into the bone.

(Continued)

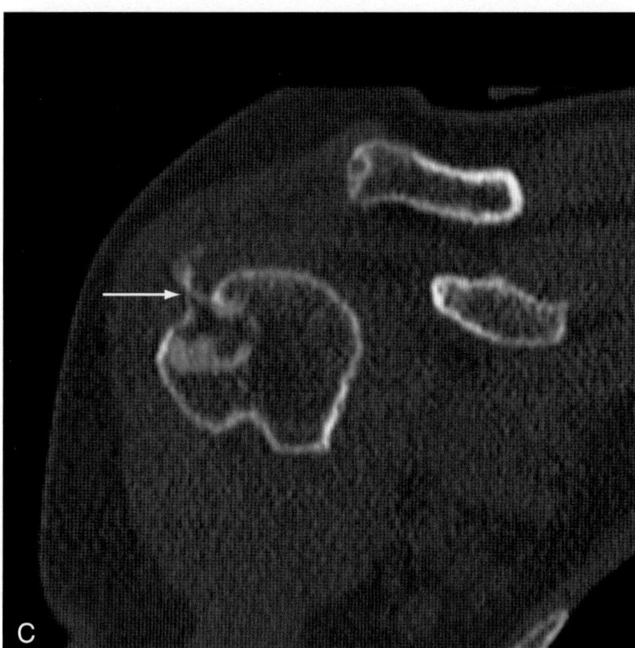

FIGURE 39-10—cont'd. **B**, Axial CT image and **(C)** coronal reformatted image demonstrates the communication *(arrow)* between the soft tissue calcification and the intraosseous extension of the calcification *(curved arrow in* B*)*.

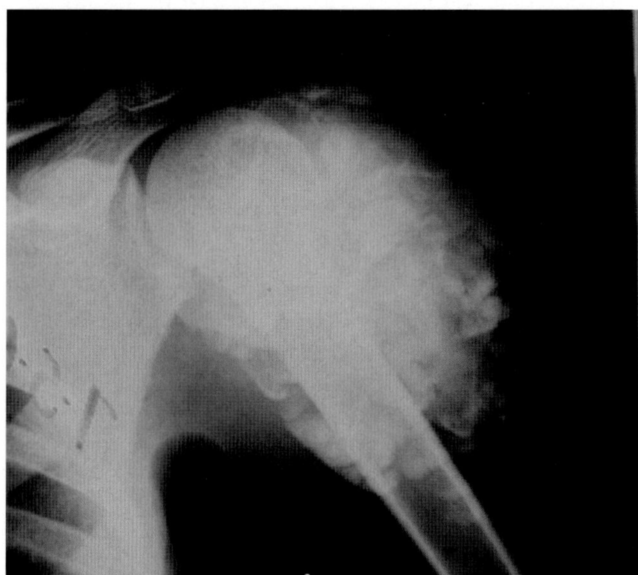

FIGURE 39-11. Tumoral calcinosis. Upright radiograph of the left shoulder reveals a large mass of calcification surrounding the upper humerus. The radiograph suggests that these masses are homogeneous and possibly have a liquid component as fluid levels can be seen.

phosphorus. However, serum calcium, parathyroid hormone, renal function, and alkaline phosphatase are normal.

Tumoral calcinosis can be idiopathic but is more commonly associated with abnormal phosphate metabolism with a high calcium-phosphate product (above 75 mg/100 mL) often due to secondary hyperparathyroidism.[17] The resulting hyperphosphatemia and hypervitaminosis D may stimulate the formation of extracellular matrix vesicles in the synovial bursae, marrow, dental pulp, and so on, inducing mineralization in the form of hydroxyapatite crystals. This calcium deposition may elicit the typical granulomatous reaction of tumoral calcinosis.[15]

Hereditary tumoral calcinosis is an uncommon disorder characterized by prominent periarticular calcified masses especially around large joints such as the hip, shoulder, and elbow, as well as the foot and wrist. Early and small lesions may be distinctively located in regions known to be occupied by bursae. The masses are most often distributed along the extensor surfaces of large joints. Hereditary tumoral calcinosis usually occurs in the second and third decades, is more common in men than women, and has a predilection for dark-skinned people and peoples from tropical climates. Tumoral calcinosis has also been described in association with Down syndrome. The patients present with firm, tumor-like, painless swellings that are shown on radiographs to be well-demarcated masses of calcium about articulations. The lesions grow slowly and can become quite large. These calcific masses are not painful, but in late stages, ulceration of the skin may occur. The lesions contain white to pale yellow, chalky material identified as calcium hydroxyapatite crystals with amorphous calcium carbonate and calcium phosphate. Histologically, the lesions contain epithelioid elements and multinucleated giant cells surrounding the calcified granules.[16]

Tumoral calcinosis may appear as a dense calcified mass that is homogeneous except for a "chicken wire" pattern of lucencies that correlate histologically to thin fibrous septae.[17] One may see fluid levels on radiographs, CT, or MRI. Computed tomography shows the sedimentation sign—amorphous, cystic, multilobulated masses with fluid-calcium levels (Figure 39-12). The fluid-calcium levels are due to a semifluid calcified material, similar to milk of calcium bile, with mineral pooling in dependent areas.[17] There is usually an absence of bone erosion, but smooth osseous erosions may occur.[17]

Use of MR imaging in tumoral calcinosis is rare; however, in one study, T2-weighted axial images demonstrated these masses to be nonhomogeneous but mostly high in signal intensity. The calcification, however, will show low signal intensity related to the long T1 of calcium.[15]

Other areas that have been affected in tumoral calcinosis include rare involvement of the bone marrow, dural calcification, calcification of articular cartilage, dental abnormalities, and CPPD-like changes in the hands.[15] Another rare component of this syndrome includes features that resemble pseudoxanthoma elasticum, including skin calcifications, vascular calcifications, and angioid streaks of the retina.[15]

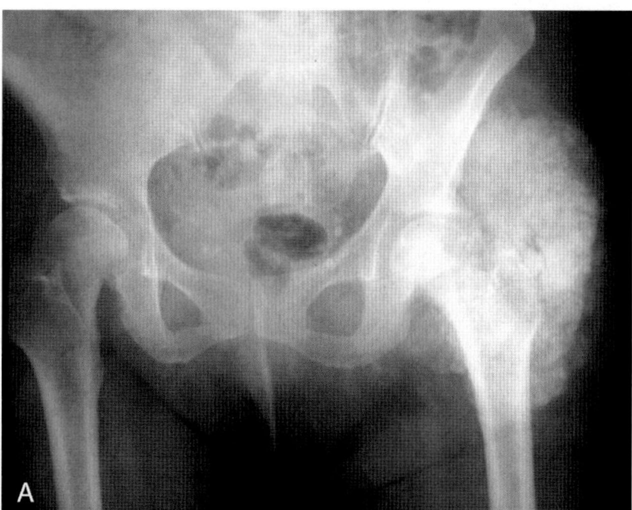

FIGURE 39-12. Tumoral calcinosis. **A,** Radiograph of the pelvis demonstrates an amorphous large calcific mass surrounding the left hip.

(Continued)

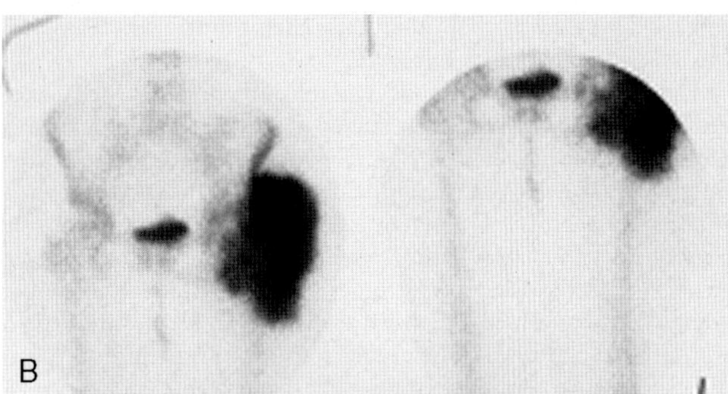

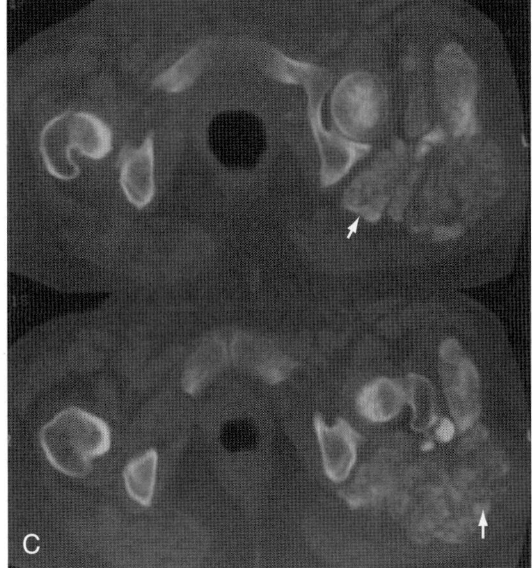

FIGURE 39-12—cont'd. **B,** Radionuclide bone scan shows intense radiotracer uptake in the soft tissues around the left hip. **C,** Axial CT scans show the amorphous calcific masses are separate from the underlying bone. There is a suggestion of a few fluid-fluid levels *(arrows)*. (Courtesy of Lee Katz, MD, New Haven, Conn.)

TABLE 39-2. Conditions Causing Soft Tissue Calcification or Ossification

Cause	Examples
Metabolic	Gout, HADD, sarcoid, hypercalcemia, chronic renal failure
Dystrophic	Connective tissue diseases, scleroderma, MCTD, dermatomyositis, SLE
Metaplastic	Synovial osteochondromatosis
Degenerative	CPPD, calcific tendinitis
Idiopathic	
Neoplasms	Osteosarcoma, chondrosarcoma, synovial sarcoma

The differential diagnosis of tumoral calcinosis is extensive and includes processes that produce soft tissue calcification and ossification (Table 39-2). In one series, 3 of 12 cases of tumoral calcinosis were initially thought to be either osteosarcoma or chondrosarcoma.[17] Additional differentials include neuropathic joints, HADD, hyperparathyroidism, hypervitaminosis D, and gout.[17] Tumoral calcinosis is often a diagnosis of exclusion.

Connective Tissue Disorders

Scleroderma is an uncommon connective tissue disorder. When there is scleroderma in association with systemic involvement, it is known as progressive systemic sclerosis. Skin changes are often the most characteristic clinical feature and virtually all patients have Raynaud's phenomenon. Early edema is later replaced by rigid and thick skin. Small or large calcifications later develop in the subcutaneous tissues; more commonly in women (Figure 39-13). These calcific masses can ulcerate onto the skin surface, particularly of the fingertips, and around bony protuberances. Scleroderma is characterized by flexion contractures, soft tissue atrophy, distal finger tuft

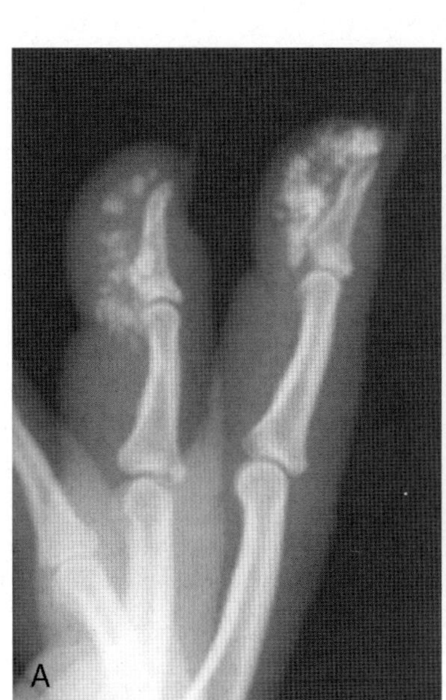

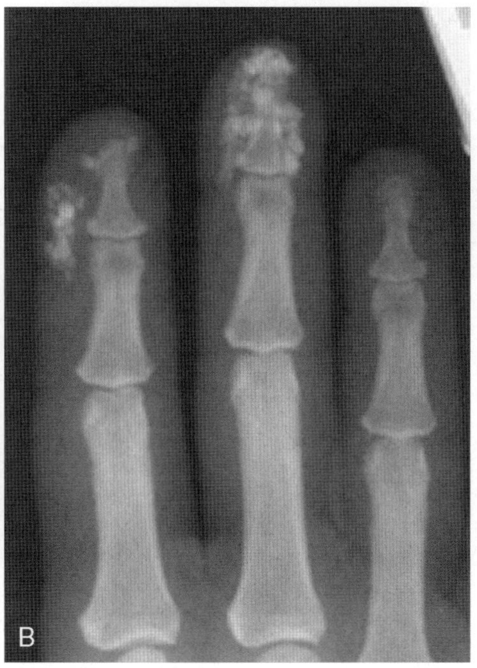

FIGURE 39-13. Scleroderma. Lateral (**A**) and PA (**B**) radiographs demonstrate amorphous calcification in the soft tissues of the distal phalanges in two adjacent digits.

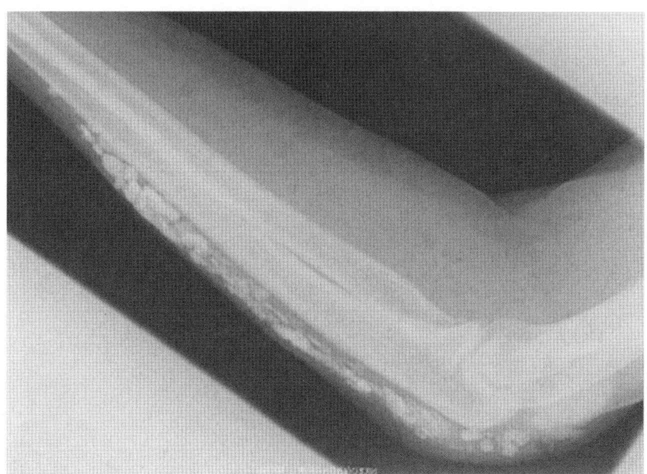

FIGURE 39-14. Scleroderma. Lateral radiograph of the forearm demonstrates calcifications along the extensor surface of the forearm.

resorption, and systemic manifestations such as those due to cardiac, pulmonary, and renal or gastrointestinal involvement.

Soft tissue calcifications are a hallmark of the disease, and these occur especially in the hands, forearms, elbows, axillae, face, pelvis, and hips (Figure 39-14).[18] In one study of 55 patients with scleroderma, calcium deposition was seen in 14 patients.[19] The calcifications that are observed in scleroderma are dystrophic in origin, reflecting a response to tissue damage. The exact mechanism producing soft tissue calcification is unclear but probably includes trauma and local tissue factors such as ischemia. Thus, they are most frequently seen in the fingers, especially in the fingertips (Figure 39-15).

Patients with CREST syndrome (calcinosis, Raynaud's, esophageal dysmotility, sclerodactyly, and telangiectasia) may have prominent calcification.

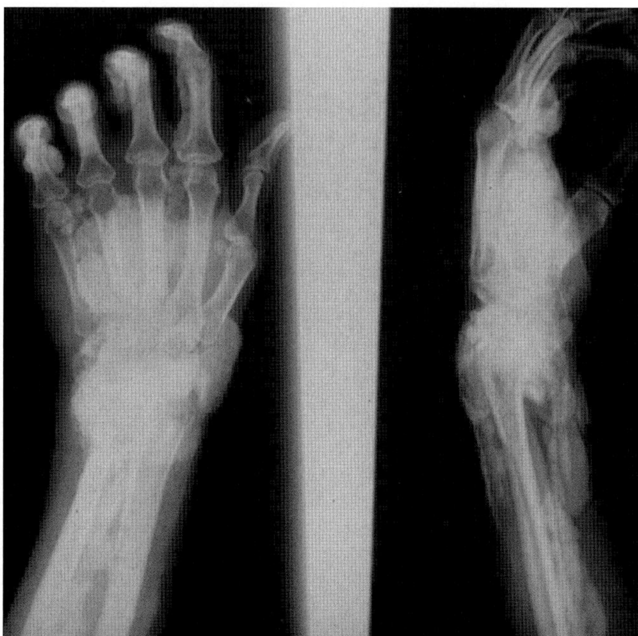

FIGURE 39-15. Scleroderma. Posteroanterior and lateral radiographs of the hand and wrist show extensive soft tissue calcific masses and subcutaneous calcific deposits in a patient with severe scleroderma.

BOX 39-1. Radiographic Features in the Hands of Scleroderma

- Distal phalangeal tuft bone loss
- Distal soft tissue atrophy
- Distal soft tissue calcification
- Erosion of thumb carpometacarpal
- Distal phalangeal sclerosis
- Joint erosion that may mimic rheumatoid arthritis

Other characteristic features of scleroderma in the fingers include terminal tuft resorption (acro-osteolysis), distal soft tissue atrophy, joint erosions, terminal phalangeal sclerosis, and capsular calcification. Scleroderma also has a predilection for the thumb carpometacarpal joint. This joint may present with osseous erosion, radial subluxation of the base of the thumb metacarpal, and intraarticular calcification[20] (Box 39-1).

Patients with systemic lupus erythematosus (SLE) may also demonstrate soft tissue calcification. These calcifications are often diffuse, linear, streaky, or nodular conglomerates, or a combination of these in the subcutaneous and deeper tissues, especially in the lower extremities.[21] In late-onset SLE, that is, after age 50, calcification in the soft tissues seems to be a less common finding.[22-24]

Mixed connective tissue disease (MCTD) represents an overlap syndrome combining features of scleroderma, SLE, polymyositis, and rheumatoid arthritis.[25,26] The clinical entity is characterized serologically by an antibody to the ribonucleoprotein component (RNP) of extractable nuclear antigen (ENA).[27] Patients with MCTD have a high frequency of Raynaud's syndrome, swollen hands, sclerodactyly, arthritis, polymyositis, and interstitial lung disease.[26] Similar to other connective tissue diseases, it shows a 9:1 female predominance. Patients with MCTD may show periarticular and fingertip calcifications, and radiologic evidence of esophageal dysmotility has been recognized in more than 50% of patients. The prognosis in MCTD is variable, and it may evolve into scleroderma or SLE.

The clinical features of MCTD, their relationship to antibodies to U1-RNP, and whether they constitute a distinct entity are still debated.[26]

Dermatomyositis and polymyositis are disorders of striated muscle characterized by diffuse inflammation and degeneration (Figure 39-16). The most constant clinical finding in these patients is muscular weakness. Dermatomyositis, especially in its childhood form, has an insidious onset with muscle pain, cramps, tenderness, limitation of motion, and periarticular edema. It is more common in girls, and fever, weight loss, and malaise may be apparent. Soft tissue calcifications develop two to three times more commonly in children than in adults[28] (Figures 39-17 and 39-18). Calcifications have been reported in 25% to 50% of juvenile dermatomyositis patients.[29] Small or large calcifications are seen, especially in the muscular fascial planes, although subcutaneous calcifications resembling those seen in scleroderma remain a common finding (Figure 39-19). These soft tissue calcifications may progress with increased duration of the disease.

Calcifications in dermatomyositis are more frequent in children and typically are located in the muscular fascial planes.

MYOSITIS OSSIFICANS

MO circumscripta (or traumatica) refers to the localized formation of non-neoplastic heterotopic bone and cartilage in the soft tissues

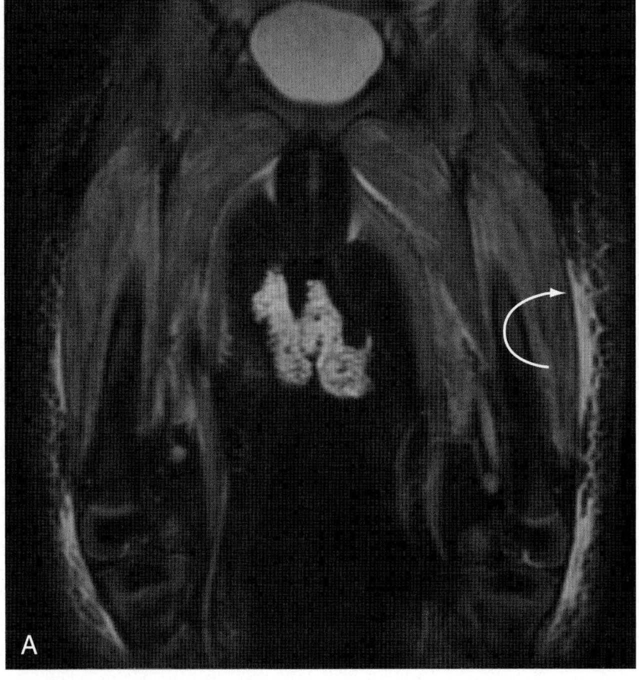

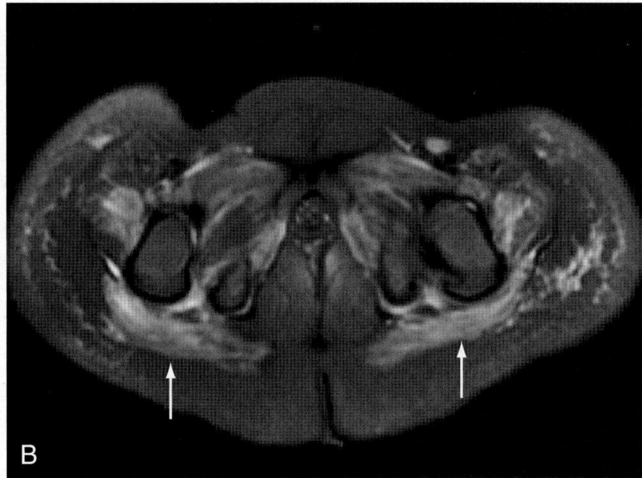

FIGURE 39-16. Dermatomyositis. **(A)** Coronal FSEIR and **(B)** axial FSE T2-weighted image with fat saturation of the pelvis and hips illustrate both subcutaneous edema *(curved arrow)* as well as diffuse muscle edema characterized by increased muscle signal intensity *(arrows)*. (Courtesy of Tal Laor, MD, Cincinnati, Ohio.)

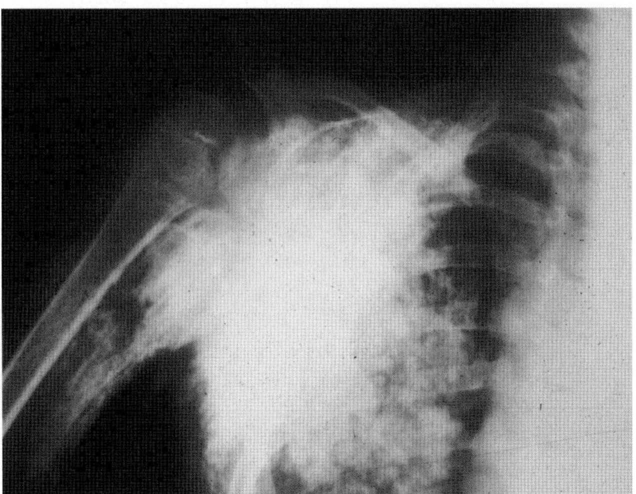

FIGURE 39-17. Dermatomyositis. Radiograph of a 5-year-old child with painful extensive soft-tissue calcification of the shoulder girdle.

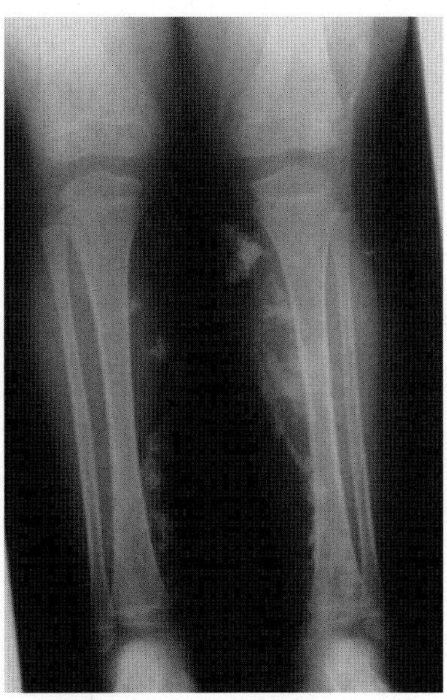

FIGURE 39-18. Dermatomyositis. Radiograph of the same 5-year-old girl with mottled calcific deposits of the soft tissues of the legs.

in or adjacent to muscle and in proximity to bone. Most cases are related to a single episode of severe trauma or repeated minor trauma. MO is more frequent in areas prone to direct trauma such as the elbow, thigh, buttocks, and less often the calf and upper arm.

MO circumscripta results from post-traumatic hemorrhage followed by fibrosis and granulation tissue formation. Although MO may develop spontaneously, the process is initiated by trauma in 60% to 75% of cases.[30] The frequency of MO has not been well documented, although after a direct blow to a muscle, the incidence has been reported as 9% to 17%.[31] The incidence is also thought to be related to the severity of the injury.

The term *myositis ossificans* is really a misnomer in that no primary inflammation of skeletal muscle is associated with the process.[32] Synonyms for MO include pseudomalignant osseous tumor of soft tissue and heterotopic bone.

Radiographs in patients with MO show faint calcification within 2 to 6 weeks after the onset of symptoms (Table 39-3). A sharply circumscribed mass is usually apparent by 6 to 8 weeks, although it may be seen much earlier.

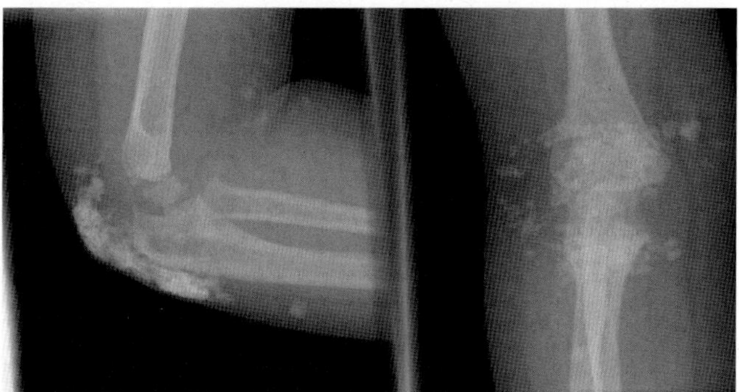

FIGURE 39-19. Dermatomyositis. Anteroposterior and lateral radiographs of the elbow in a young child with characteristic calcifications of juvenile dermatomyositis. (Courtesy of Tal Laor, MD, Cincinnati, Ohio.)

TABLE 39-3. Radiographic Features of Myositis Ossificans

Initially	Nonspecific soft tissue mass
2 to 6 weeks	Calcification appears
6 to 8 weeks	Peripheral rim of calcification/ossification with more lucent center Lucent zone between cortex and lesion Center of lesion ossifies last
5 to 6 months	Lesion may become smaller with time
Years	Residual cortical thickening or bone spicule

Calcifications occur within 2 to 6 weeks after the onset of symptoms. Absence of calcification at this time makes the diagnosis of MO less likely.

The mineralization shows a characteristic zonal pattern, that is, mineralization is denser at the periphery of the lesion (Figure 39-20). Floccular calcifications can be recognized on radiographs by the third week, although the appearance time may vary from 2 to 6 weeks. At 6 to 8 weeks, a lacy pattern of new bone becomes sharply circumscribed at the periphery by a cortex[33] (Figure 39-21).

Tumors such as osteogenic sarcoma display calcification that is denser centrally, whereas MO typically exhibits calcification that is more dense peripherally.

By 5 to 6 months, the mass becomes smaller and more mature. Often after a year or so, the firm mass becomes smaller and, rarely, it may disappear completely. Years after onset, the only residuum of MO may be focally thickened underlying bony cortex or a spicule of bone arising from the cortex that may mimic a solitary osteochondroma (Figure 39-22).

The radiologic findings parallel the histologic pattern of maturation. Early on there is muscle necrosis and hemorrhage. At this time, the radiograph may demonstrate soft tissue swelling. There is often pain, warmth, and edema in the affected surrounding soft tissues. After about 6 weeks, a centrifugal pattern of maturation is evident with the lesion more mature in the periphery and immature in the center. This maturation is responsible for the presence of the calcification in the lesion; the diagnosis of MO is based on the recognition of a peripheral rim of calcification and ossification about a more lucent center (Figure 39-23). A radiolucent band or zone between the lesion and subjacent cortex is a very important finding. This finding allows differentiation from parosteal osteosarcoma. The peripheral shell of maturing bone exists about a soft cellular center and maturation proceeds in a centrifugal fashion with the center of the lesion being the last to ossify.[34] Cartilage may form leading to enchondral bone formation or alternatively, the fibrous tissue may calcify followed by ossification.

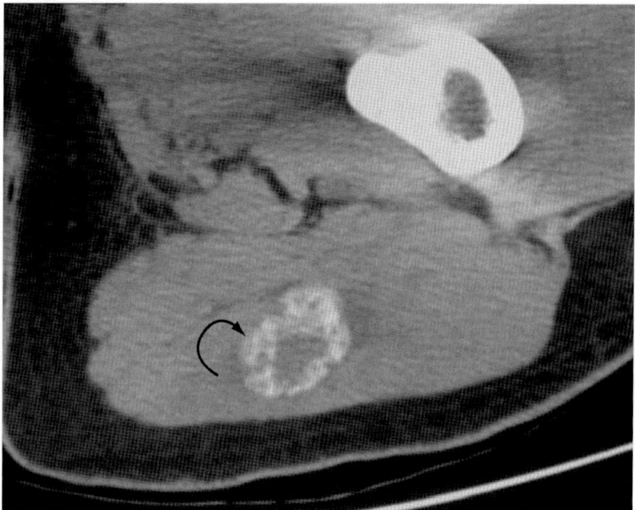

FIGURE 39-20. Myositis ossificans. Axial CT scan of the left hip shows that a mass in the buttock was due to a calcified lesion in the gluteus maximus muscle. The maturing peripheral calcification surrounds a more lucent area of lower central attenuation *(curved arrow)*. This appearance is characteristic of MO circumscripta.

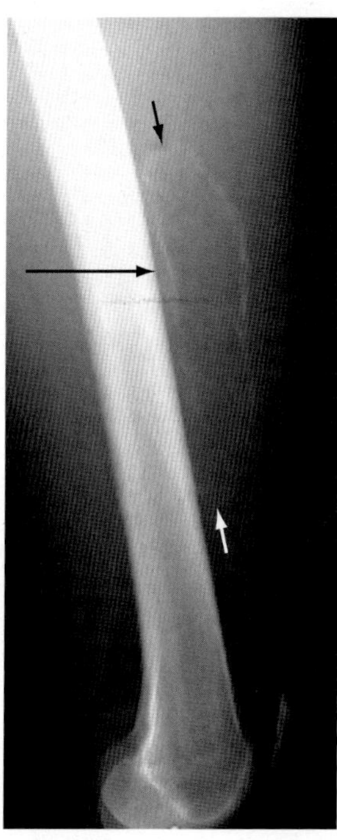

FIGURE 39-21. Myositis ossificans. Lateral radiograph of the femur in a hockey player who had sustained severe anterior thigh trauma several months earlier. A shell of calcification (*arrows*) surrounds the radiolucent mass. Note that the lesion is separate from the underlying femoral cortex.

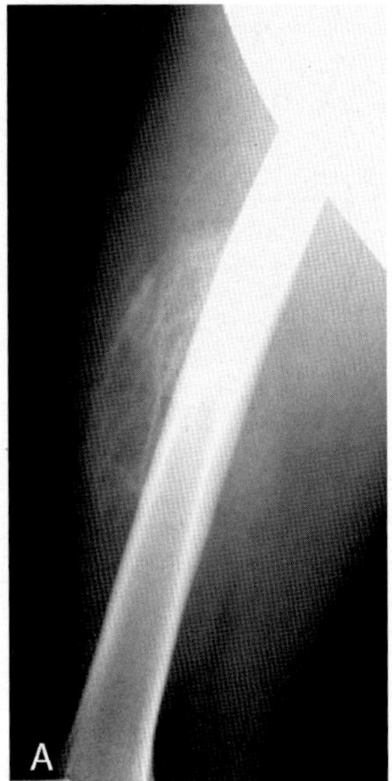

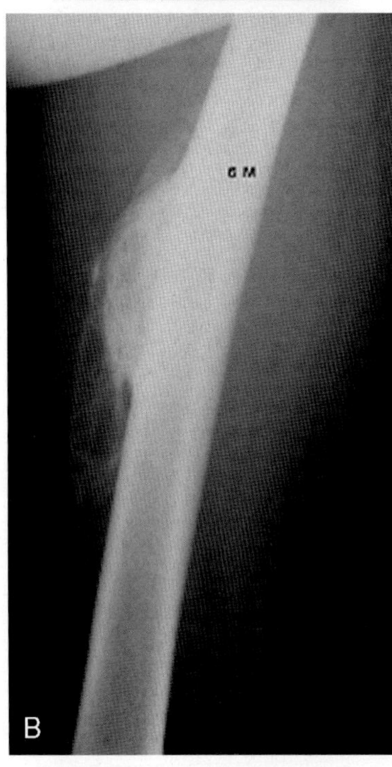

FIGURE 39-22. Myositis ossificans. **(A)** Lateral radiographs of the femur demonstrates sheets of ossification anterior to the femur. The periphery shows well-defined calcification. **(B)** Follow-up lateral radiograph 6 months later shows a bony mass that has matured, flattened out, and incorporated into the anterior femoral cortex. This is the natural history of MO.

The histologic features reflect the maturation process described above. Early on, there are very cellular sheets of plump fibroblasts and mitotic figures are numerous. As early as 1 week after a mass is palpable, seams of osteoid appear in the peripheral portions of the mass. Because of dense cellularity and osteoid production, lesions at this early stage of evolution have been called *pseudomalignant osseous tumors of soft tissue.*[30]

Pathologically, there are three distinct zones. The central zone contains fibroblasts with hemorrhage and necrosis, corresponding to the lucent central region seen radiographically and on computed tomographic images. A middle zone with numerous osteoblasts and immature bone is present around the core.

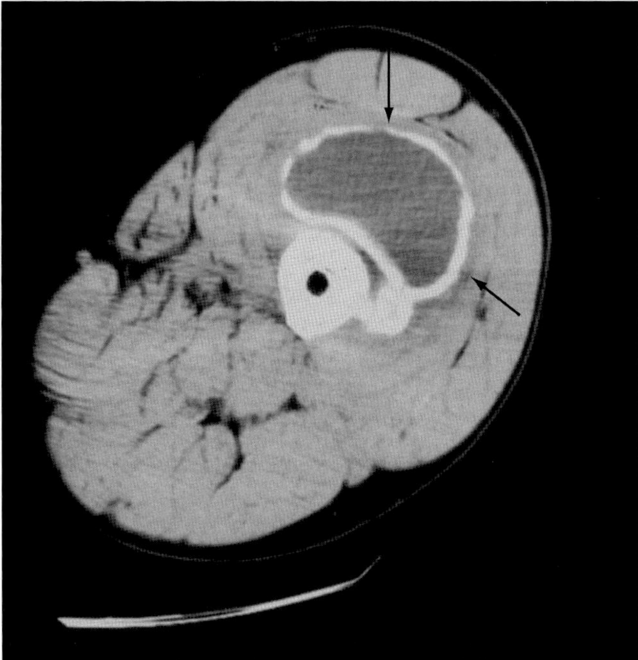

FIGURE 39-23. Myositis ossificans. Axial CT of early MO of the thigh. A thin rim of calcification *(arrows)* within the vastus intermedius muscle surrounds a fluid density center. The mass is separate from the underlying femoral cortex.

Biopsy of early MO is not advisable because the results of biopsy of any of these three zones can lead to a mistaken histologic diagnosis of sarcoma because of the cellular proliferation with central hemorrhage and necrosis. The outermost layer in MO consists of mature bony trabeculae that are well demarcated from surrounding connective tissue.

> Biopsy of early MO may erroneously lead to a diagnosis of malignancy, especially if the central portion of the lesion is sampled. Demonstration of the zonal pattern of increasing maturation peripherally can lead to the correct diagnosis.

The differential diagnosis of early MO includes tumors that may produce secondary changes in neighboring bones such as cortical erosion, periosteal reaction, and medullary destruction, and these include extraosseous osteosarcoma, chondrosarcoma, parosteal osteosarcoma, periosteal osteosarcoma, and synovial sarcoma, as well as osteochondroma, osteoma, and juxtacortical chondroma. On cross-sectional imaging, muscle fibers and the soft tissue structures surrounding the MO lesion may be compressed, but there is no evidence of invasion.

Magnetic Resonance Imaging in MO

Early and intermediate lesions demonstrate a nonhomogeneous soft tissue mass with increased T2 signal intensity and extensive diffuse surrounding soft tissue edema[35] (Figure 39-24). The T1-weighted sequence may be normal. The lesion may be isointense to surrounding muscle. Often the only recognizable T1 abnormality is a mass effect displacing the fascial planes. Muscle edema manifests as poorly defined increased signal intensity on T2-weighted images superimposed on an otherwise normal appearance of the involved muscle. The soft tissue mass is nonspecific and may be indistinguishable from a sarcoma.

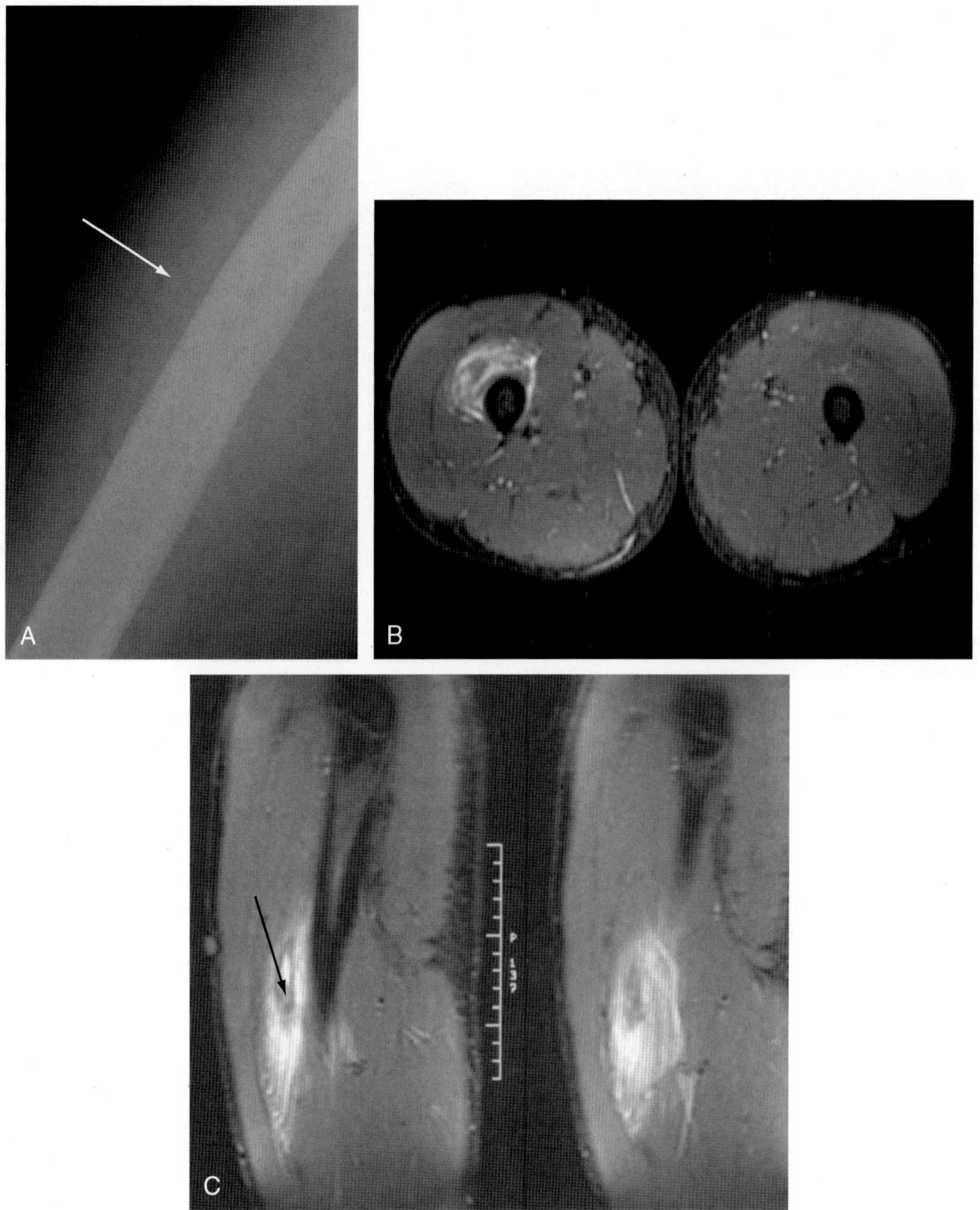

FIGURE 39-24. Myositis ossificans. Sixteen-year-old boy following a basketball injury to the anterior thigh. **(A)** Faint soft-tissue calcification is present in the anterior thigh soft tissues *(arrow)*. **(B)** Axial fat suppressed T2-weighted image demonstrates high signal intensity representing edema and hemorrhage in the vastus intermedius. **(C)** Sagittal T2-weighted, fat-suppressed images demonstrate high signal in the muscle representing hemorrhage and edema, and a central focus of lower signal intensity representing early calcification *(arrow)*.

MO will show enhancement following the administration of intravenous gadolinium. An important limitation of MRI is its relative inability to detect soft tissue calcification.[36] The areas of T2 increased signal intensity seen centrally within the early lesions are probably related to the extremely cellular central areas of proliferating fibroblasts and myofibroblasts within a myxoid stroma or extracellular matrix.[32]

Mature or late lesions show a well-defined inhomogeneous mass with signal characteristics similar to fat on both T1 and T2 pulse sequences. On all pulse sequences, a rim of decreased signal intensity surrounds the lesion[32] (Figure 39-25).

The differential diagnosis of the MRI findings in MO depends on the stage at which the lesion is imaged. Early lesions with surrounding edema could suggest abscess, hematoma, or rhabdomyolysis. When minimal mineralization is present the differential includes synovial sarcoma, rhabdomyosarcoma, and malignant fibrous histiocytoma. In the mature stage, differential considerations include parosteal osteosarcoma, extraskeletal osteosarcoma, and chondrosarcoma.[36]

Ultrasound of the early lesions of MO demonstrates an oval, hypoechoic mass with a central reflective core, the so-called *zone phenomenon.* One may also see a well-circumscribed, homogeneous or heterogeneous hypoechoic mass with scattered internal calcifications.

Surgery for removal of the heterotopic bone should not be considered for at least 1 year following the episode of trauma or when

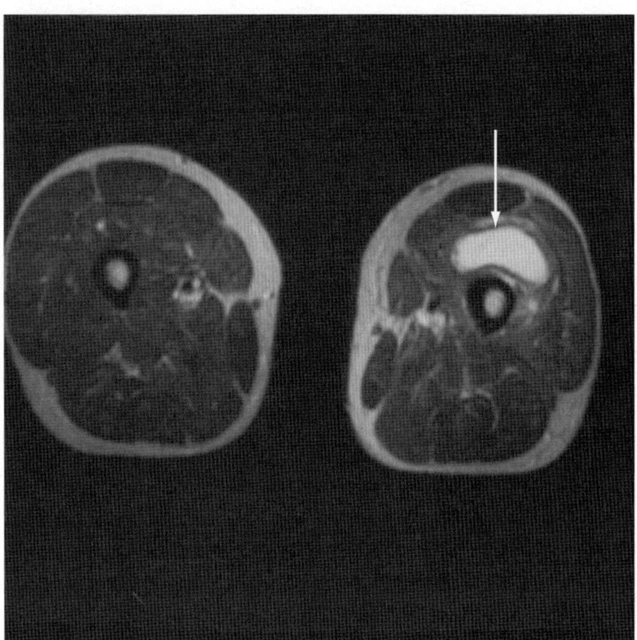

FIGURE 39-25. Myositis ossificans. Axial T2-weighted MRI of the mid-thigh shows high T2 signal in the central portion of an area of MO *(arrow)*. The low signal rim is consistent with calcification. This MRI is comparable to the CT image in Figure 39-23.

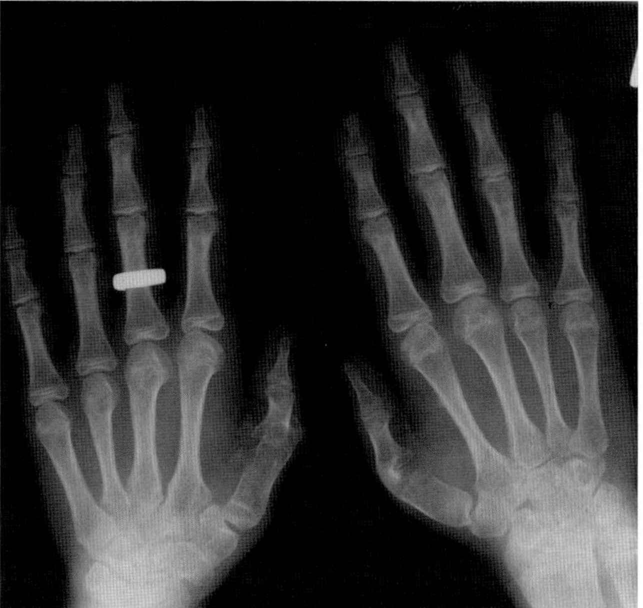

FIGURE 39-26. Fibrodysplasia ossificans progressiva. Posteroanterior radiograph of both hands demonstrates the typical congenital anomaly of the thumbs that may be seen in FOP. Both the thumb metacarpals and proximal phalanges are abnormal in their morphology.

the bone has fully matured, which is 12 to 24 months after the start of the symptoms, as the excision of immature bone often results in local recurrence.[37]

FIBRODYSPLASIA OSSIFICANS PROGRESSIVA (MYOSITIS OSSIFICANS PROGRESSIVA)

Fibrodysplasia ossificans progressiva (FOP) is a rare entity (only 400 cases in the United States) characterized by the development of nodular painful soft tissue masses that begin in early childhood. Inflammatory foci appear and proliferate in fibrous tissue. Extensive heterotopic ossification progressively develops at multiple periarticular sites and eventually causes complete immobilization ("stone man disease"). It arises by spontaneous mutation and has no gender or race/ethnic predilection.[30] Heterotopic ossification usually begins in the first decade at about 3 years of age.

The development of the lesions in FOP occurs in an orderly fashion. First, there is an inflammatory reaction in the injured soft tissues. There is muscular degeneration and lymphoid infiltrate. This is followed by proliferation of a highly vascular fibrous tissue in which bone morphogenetic proteins (BMPs) 2 and 4 have been demonstrated. Lymphocytes overexpressing BMP4 may be recruited in response to trivial trauma, resulting in high local concentrations of BMP4, and subsequently, binding of collagen IV, endothelial cells, and muscle cells to BMP4 may result in the development and proliferation of fibroblasts and in the occurrence of cellular events leading to enchondral ossification.[38] Osteoid then forms in this fibroblastic stroma. In addition, hyaline cartilage, which is undergoing endochondral ossification, is abundant in FOP. Endochondral ossification appears to be the principal mechanism of bone formation in FOP.[30]

FOP initially presents in the upper back with a palpable soft tissue mass. Lesions develop from cranial to caudad and from the axial to the appendicular skeleton. By the third decade, most patients are severely crippled with extensive periarticular ossification. Up until now, most patients died in their third or fourth decade from pneumonia.

This condition has a high association with other congenital abnormalities of the thumb and great toe (Figure 39-26). FOP is associated with short great toes due to synostoses or deformities of the phalanges, and hallux valgus has been observed.[39,40]

> The diagnosis of FOP may be suggested by the presence of short great toes and thumbs.

Radiographs early on may be negative, but with time there is development of long bands of soft tissue ossification. These sheets of ossified tissue are seen along the chest wall and abdominal wall (Figure 39-27). They may extend to bridge articulations leading to contractures and ankylosis. Cervical spine radiographs show posterior bands of ossification. In addition, the cervical vertebrae are taller than they are wide and the neural arches may be fused[38] (Figure 39-28). As the chest becomes encased in these bony strands, respiratory function is severely compromised. Ossification of the intercostal spaces produces a restrictive ventilatory deficit, while ossification of the temporomandibular joints can make eating so difficult that severe weight loss develops. The early use of CT is valuable, as the ossification may be apparent on CT prior to its appearance on radiographs.[41]

MRI of early soft tissue masses shows high T2 and STIR signal intensity involving muscles and fascial planes. This high signal intensity is probably due to edema, which is thought to be secondary to fibroblast proliferation.[42]

The early lesions are multifocal, interconnecting nodules composed of spindle-shaped fibroblast-like cells in a distinctive connective tissue matrix, with centrally located osseous spicules. Later lesions are composed of mature lamellar bone with adipose and hematopoietic tissue in the cancellous spaces and a rim of fibroblast-like cells is lacking.[43]

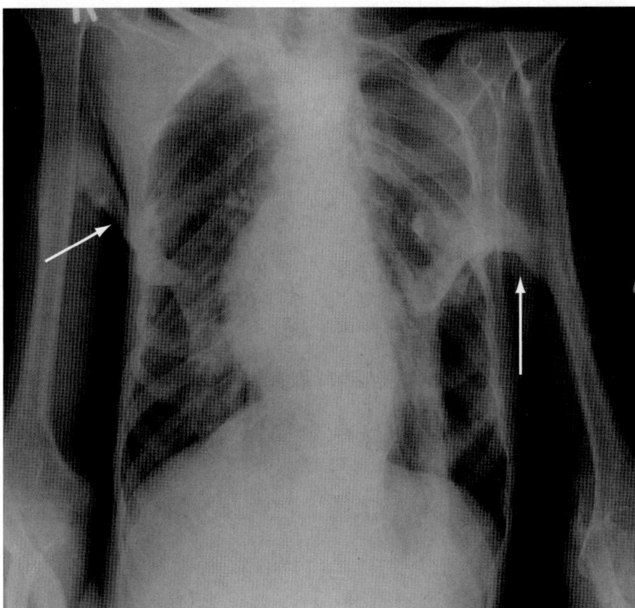

FIGURE 39-27. Fibrodysplasia ossificans progressiva. Posteroanterior chest radiograph shows thick, dense bands of ossification extending from the humeri to the chest wall *(arrows)*. These ossific struts severely limit respiratory excursion leading to respiratory compromise. The cachexia of the patient is suggested by the decreased chest wall fat.

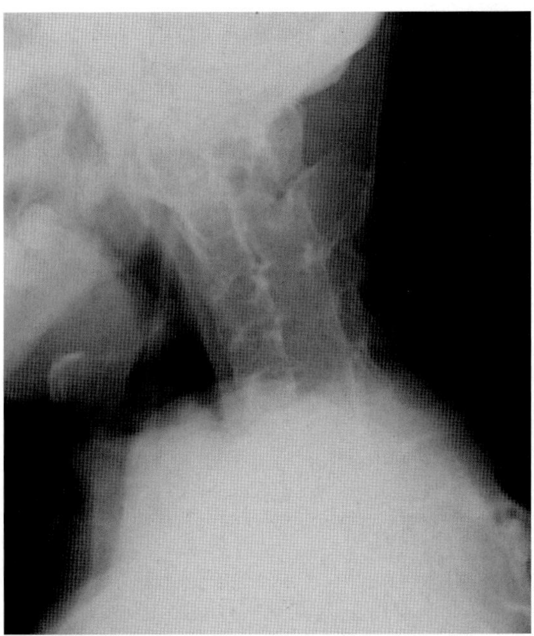

FIGURE 39-28. Fibrodysplasia ossificans progressiva. Lateral cervical spine radiograph demonstrates fusion of the posterior elements throughout the length of the spine.

SUMMARY

The radiographic appearance of soft tissue calcifications and ossification represents a spectrum of findings, locations, and differential diagnostic possibilities. Often the location, appearance, patient age and gender, and other factors help in diagnosing the underlying medical disorder. Utilization of all the various imaging modalities in today's modern radiology department is useful in the diagnostic workup of a patient with soft tissue calcifications or ossification, but often the diagnosis depends on the typical appearance on radiographs.

REFERENCES

1. Resnick D: *Diagnosis of Bone and Joint Disorders*, 4th ed, Philadelphia, 2002, WB Saunders, pp 5(84):4635-4641.
2. Hussmann J, Russell R, Kucan J et al: Soft-tissue calcifications: differential diagnosis and therapeutic approaches, *Ann Plast Surg* 34:138-147, 1995.
3. Garcia G, McCord G, Kumar R: Hydroxyapatite crystal deposition disease, *Semin Musculoskel Radiol* 7:187-193, 2003.
4. Hurt G, Baker C: Calcific tendinitis of the shoulder, *Orthop Clin North Am* 34:567-575, 2003.
5. Bonavita J, Dalinkja M, Schumacher H: Hydroxyapatite deposition disease, *Radiology* 134:621-625, 1980.
6. Holt P, Keats T: Calcific tendinitis: a review of the usual and unusual, *Skeletal Radiol* 22:1-9, 1993.
7. Hayes C, Conway W: Calcium hydroxyapatite deposition disease, *RadioGraphics* 10:1031-1048, 1990.
8. Kraemer E, El-Khoury G: Atypical calcific tendinitis with cortical erosions, *Skeletal Radiol* 29:690-696, 2000.
9. Flemming D, Murphey M, Shekitka K et al: Osseous involvement in calcific tendinitis: a retrospective review of 50 cases, *AJR Am J Roentgenol* 181:965-972, 2003.
10. Hayes C, Rosenthal D, Plata M et al: Calcific tendinitis in unusual sites associated with cortical bone erosion, *AJR Am J Roentgenol* 149:967-970, 1987.
11. Arandas F, Santos F, deSouza S et al: Acute calcific periarthritis of the hand, *J Clin Rheumatol* 4:223-224, 2005.
12. Pinals R, Short C: Calcific periarthritis involving multiple sites, *Arthritis Rheum* 9:566-574, 1966.
13. Resnick D: *Diagnosis of Bone and Joint Disorders*, 4th ed, Philadelphia, 2002, WB Saunders, pp 2(40):1645-1646.
14. McCarty D, Halverson P, Carrera G et al: "Milwaukee shoulder"—association of microspheroids containing hydroxyapatite crystals, active collagenase, and neutral protease with rotator cuff defects. I. Clinical aspects, *Arthritis Rheum* 24:464-473, 1981.
15. Martinez S, Vogler J, Harrelson J et al: Imaging of tumoral calcinosis: new observations, *Radiology* 174:215-222, 1990.
16. Olsen K, Chew F: Tumoral calcinosis: pearls, polemics, and alternative possibilities, *Radiographics* 26:871-885, 2006.
17. Steinbach L, Johnston J, Tepper E et al: Tumoral calcinosis: radiologic-pathologic correlation, *Skeletal Radiol* 24:573-578, 1995.
18. Resnick D, Scavulli J, Goergen T et al: Intra-articular calcification in scleroderma, *Radiology* 124:685-688, 1977.
19. Bassett L, Blocka K, Furst D et al: Skeletal findings in progressiva systemic sclerosis (scleroderma), *AJR Am J Roentgenol* 136:1121-1126, 1981.
20. Resnick D, Greenway G, Vint V et al: Selective involvement of the first carpometacarpal joint in scleroderma, *AJR Am J Roentgenol* 131:283-286, 1978.
21. Budin J, Feldman F: Soft tissue calcifications in systemic lupus erythematosus, *AJR Am J Roentgenol* 124:358-364, 1975.
22. Braunstein E, Weissman B, Sosman J et al: Radiologic findings in late-onset systemic lupus erythematosus, *AJR Am J Roentgenol* 140:587-589, 1983.
23. Lalani T, Kanne J, Hatfield G et al:. Imaging findings in systemic lupus erythematosus, *RadioGraphics* 24:1069-1086, 2004.
24. Weissman B, Rappaport A, Sosman L et al:. Radiographic findings in patients with systemic lupus erythematosis, *Radiology* 126:313-317, 1978.
25. Udoff E, Genant H, Kozin F et al: Mixed connective tissue disease: the spectrum of radiographic manifestations, *Radiology* 124:613-618, 1977.
26. Venables P: Mixed connective tissue disease, *Lupus* 15:132-137, 2006.
27. Silver T, Farber S, Bole G et al: Radiological features of mixed connective tissue disease and scleroderma–systemic lupus erythematosus overlap, *Radiology* 120:269-275, 1976.
28. Steiner R, Glassman L, Schwartz M et al: The radiological findings in dermatomyositis of childhood, *Radiology* 11:385-393, 1974.
29. Eddy M, Leelawattana R, McAlister W et al: Calcinosis universalis complicating juvenile dermatomyositis: resolution during probenecid therapy, *J Clin Endocrinol Metab* 82:3536-3542, 1997.
30. McCarthy E, Sundaram M: Heterotopic ossification: a review, *Skeletal Radiol* 34:609-619, 2005.
31. Beiner J, Jokl P: Muscle contusion injury and myositis ossificans traumatica, *Clin Orthop Rel Res* 403S:110-119, 2002.
32. Kransdorf M, Meis J, Jelinek J: Myositis ossificans: MR appearance with radiologic-pathologic correlation, *AJR Am J Roentgenol* 157:1243-1248, 1991.
33. Amendola M, Glazer G, Agha F et al: Myositis ossificans circumscripta: computed tomographic diagnosis, *Radiology* 149:775-779, 1983.
34. Resnick D: *Diagnosis of Bone and Joint Disorders*, 4th ed, Philadelphia, 2002, WB Saunders, pp 5(84-85):4643-4652, 4727-4730.
35. Elsayes K, Lammie M, Shariff A et al: Value of magnetic resonance imaging in muscle trauma, *Curr Probl Diagn Radiol* 35:206-212, 2006.
36. Parikh J, Hyare H, Saifuddin A: The imaging features of post-traumatic myositis ossificans, with emphasis on MRI, *Clin Radiol* 57:1058-1066, 2002.

37. Jarvinen T, Jarvinen TL, Kaarianen M et al: Muscle injuries: biology and treatment, *Am J Sports Med* 33:745-764, 2005.
38. Job-Deslandre C: Inherited ossifying diseases, *J Bone Spine* 71:98-101, 2004.
39. Harrison R, Pitcher J, Mizel M et al: The radiographic morphology of foot deformities in patients with fibrodysplasia ossificans progressiva, *Foot Ankle Int* 26:937-941, 2005.
40. Connor J, Evans D: Fibrodysplasia ossificans progressiva. The clinical features and natural history of 34 patients, *J Bone Joint Surg Br* 64B:76-83, 1982.
41. Reinig J, Hill S, Fang M et al: Fibrodysplasia ossificans progressiva. CT appearance, *Radiology* 159:153-157, 1986.
42. Merchant R, Sainani N, Lawande M et al: Pre- and post-therapy MR imaging in fibrodysplasia ossificans progressiva, *Pediatr Radiol* 36:1108-1111, 2006.
43. Resnick D: *Diagnosis of Bone and Joint Disorders*, 4th ed, Philadelphia, 2002, WB Saunders, pp 5(80):4409-4415.

Section IV

Interventions

CHAPTER 40

Percutaneous Spine Interventions: Discography, Injection Procedures (Epidural Corticosteroids and Facet Joint and Sacroiliac Joint Injections), and Vertebral Augmentation (Vertebroplasty and Kyphoplasty)

TARAK H. PATEL, MD, *and* JOHN A. CARRINO, MD, MPH

KEY FACTS

- Spine injection procedures can be helpful in localizing pain to a particular source (nociceptor) and in treating symptoms.
- Careful image guidance is necessary to optimize results and minimize complications.
- Vertebroplasty and kyphoplasty have both shown good pain relief and improved function with minimal complication rates in appropriately selected patients.
- Kyphoplasty (balloon-assisted vertebroplasty) is a percutaneous procedure in which an inflatable bone tamp is used to create a void in an attempt to restore lost vertebral body height before cement is injected.

Neck, dorsal spine, and lower back pain are extremely common, and the majority of the population will have activity-limiting pain at some point in their life. Percutaneous spine interventions in conjunction with other modalities of therapy (e.g., physiotherapy) can provide symptomatic relief and facilitate functional restoration for select patients with these conditions. This chapter discusses several image-guided spine interventions. Pertinent anatomy and technical aspects, as well as a discussion of safety considerations will be presented in the context of current concepts of painful spine syndromes.

DISCOGRAPHY

Overview and General Considerations

There is anatomic evidence and hence concept validity that the disk can be a source of pain (nociceptor) because of the innervation that exists along the outer anulus from the ventral nerve roots that provide branches anteriorly (grey ramus communicans) and posteriorly (sinu-vertebral nerve).[1] This is best established in the lumbar region. However, there are many other structures in and around the spine that may be nociceptors, and it is often difficult for the clinician to differentiate among these potential sources of pain or, when there are multiple causes, to determine which is the primary inciting source. The numerous pain sources have a variety of clinical expressions that overlap with each other and with other disorders as well.

> Discography is the injection of contrast material into a disk with monitoring of any symptoms produced and analysis of contrast distribution on imaging (e.g., CT).

While the concept of discogenic pain represents a reasonable paradigm, poorly performed discography can be confusing rather than helpful. Currently, the primary purpose for discography is for documentation of the disk as a pain source.[2] For patients whose symptomatology is predominately axial, nonmyelopathic, and nonradicular, imaging may be insufficient or equivocal for determining the nature, location, and extent of symptomatic abnormalities. Moreover, imaging reveals asymptomatic abnormalities in a substantial proportion of patients.

Demand for discography is increasing as a diagnostic tool to determine levels of pain generation for patients who are being considered for surgical management (e.g., interbody arthrodesis) or other procedures. Degenerated disks may be relatively motionless, and the source of pain may be at the relatively normal-appearing or less degenerated-appearing levels above or below due to abnormal biomechanics at these levels. Surgeons concerned with limiting the extent of fusion are interested in obtaining added evidence beyond magnetic resonance imaging (MRI) abnormalities to document what intervertebral disk levels are contributing to the painful syndrome.

Interpretation of a discogram includes both morphologic and functional evaluation. The functional evaluation is more important because MRI is well suited for characterization of morphologic findings. The tenet of discography is that injection into the disks and subsequent increased intradiscal pressure will elicit a concordant pain response (one that mimics the patient's typical pain) if that disk is a pain generator. A scale of subjective pain severity from 0 (no pain) to 10 (maximal pain) can be determined during the procedure by asking the patient to relate what their level of pain is during each injection. The patient is also asked whether the pain mimics their typical pain (i.e., "concordant"). In order to evaluate the patient's pain response more objectively, multiple vertebral levels around the suspected pain generator are injected during the procedure; the patient is not told which level is being injected or when the injection is starting. It is important to establish a "reference level," or relatively pain-free level with injection. For discography to be considered positive, there should be at least one reference level, which is defined by the absence of pain or lack of concordant symptoms upon injection. An unquestionably positive discogram consists of a single concordantly symptomatic disk with control disks above and below that level (except at the lumbosacral junction or in the cervical spine). Optimal benefit results when one or two levels demonstrate a highly concordant pain response, with a relatively pain-free adjacent reference level(s). If all levels are painful, a limited fusion may not result in patient satisfaction and can suggest to the surgeon that continued medical management instead of surgery might be the best course.

> Injection into the disks and subsequent increased intradiscal pressure will elicit a concordant pain response (one that mimics the patient's typical pain) if that disk is a pain generator.

Guidance for needle placement should be performed with a C-arm, floating image intensifier, or biplane fluoroscopy. Patients must be informed ahead of time that the purpose of the procedure is to generate a pain response, which in some circumstances can be severe. Complications include persistent pain, infection, bleeding, and injury to exiting nerve roots. Antibiotics should always be administered, whether intravenous or intradiscal.[3] A small dose of short-acting anesthetic (e.g., fentanyl) or anxiolytic (e.g., midazolam) may be administered but can potentially blunt a positive response. Information assessed and recorded should include the volume of contrast-injected, pain response with particular emphasis on its location and concordance to clinical symptomatology, and the pattern of contrast distribution. Computed tomography (CT) imaging may be used to complement projectional imaging techniques, and grading systems are available to characterize internal disk derangement. CT allows additional information regarding the location of an anular abnormality to be gleaned.

Classifying patients based on the results of pressure-controlled manometric discography can be clinically relevant. This technique may help stratify patients into categories that identify patients who are more likely to improve from interbody fusions.[4] Less invasive forms of intradiscal therapy (e.g., percutaneous disk decompression) that are evolving may also make discography increasingly valuable. Discography techniques therefore are important for the next generation of minimally invasive intradiscal therapies.

Cervical Spine Technique

The complication rate and false positive rates of cervical discography appear to be higher than lumbar discography, and its use is limited relative to lumbar discography. Cervical discography is performed using an anterolateral approach. The patient position is supine with a small rolled towel between the scapulae to extend the neck and a small pillow under the neck itself for comfort. Disk puncture can be accomplished using anteroposterior imaging for frontal visualization. An alternative technique is to use an oblique projection similar to cervical transforaminal injections. With this technique, the needle is directed down the beam just anterior to the uncinate process to achieve disk puncture. The adult cervical disk normally accepts a volume of less than 0.5 cc. Usually, a 25-gauge single needle approach will suffice. As mentioned, the lateral and posterolateral portions of the cervical disk anulus are relatively attenuated. This results in clefts (joints of Lushka) that communicate with the disk, which are unique to the cervical spine. Opacification of these regions in patients aged more than 20 years should not be confused with degenerative disk disease based on this morphologic finding alone (Figure 40-1, *A*).

Thoracic Spine Technique

Thoracic spine discography can be performed in the prone or prone semi-oblique 45-degree position (using a wedge) with the less painful side up. The C-arm is rotated to the side of injection until a lucent zone directly in line with the beam is seen projecting over the thoracic disk. The needle should enter the disk lateral to the interpediculate line and medial to the costovertebral joints in order to avoid potential complications such as accidental puncture of the lung or thecal sac. This procedure is often done as a single-needle technique (23 or 22 gauge). The thoracic disk normally accepts a small volume of injectant, less than 1.0 cc. Fluoroscopic images may be difficult to interpret because of the superimposition of osseous structures (Figure 40-1, *B*), difficulty obtaining a true lateral projection, and presence of only a small amount of injected contrast. Therefore, postdiscography CT imaging is often a useful adjunct to delineate internal disk derangement (IDDs) and herniated nucleated pulposus (Figure 40-2, *A*).

Lumbar Spine Technique

The technique for lumbar injection is a posterolateral extradural approach. Levels for injection are chosen based on imaging findings and clinical exam. The most common levels are L3-L4, L4-L5, and L5-S1. The patient is positioned in a prone or a prone-oblique position (with the less painful side up). Each level is set up fluoroscopically so that the disk is parallel to the beam and obliqued so that the superior articular process of the overlying facet joint is slightly posterior to the center of the end plate (30% to 50% zone). The needle is advanced along the x-ray beam toward the disk, past the anterior margin of the superior articular process. A single-needle or coaxial technique is used to place the discography needles in each disk. The coaxial technique may reduce the risk of infection and allows one to redirect the inner needle if needed. The larger outer needle allows rapid positioning at the disk margin, with a small-gauge needle used to penetrate the anular fibers. The L5-S1 disk may be located below the pelvic rim, and can be difficult to access making this coaxial technique helpful. Generally, the x-ray beam is oriented with more caudal angulation than used for the higher levels and is rotated to open a small triangle of access over the iliac crest. Positioning of all needles during placement is checked frequently in the plane along the trajectory of the needle and is supplemented with the anteroposterior and lateral planes as the tip approximates the disk. The tip of the inner needle should be positioned as close as possible to the center of the disk, so that injection is into the nucleus pulposus instead of the innervated annular fibers, which can result in a false-positive pain response. After all needles are placed, typically 1 to 3 cc of contrast (mixed with antibiotic) is injected at each level, with fluoroscopic monitoring and assessment of any pain elicited. A morphologically normal disk demonstrates a central globule of contrast collection or "hamburger bun" configuration and degeneration is indicated by a horizontal, linear distribution of contrast (Figure 40-1, *C*). An anular tear is diagnosed if contrast extends into the periphery of the disk in the expected region of the anular fibers (Figure 40-2, *B*).

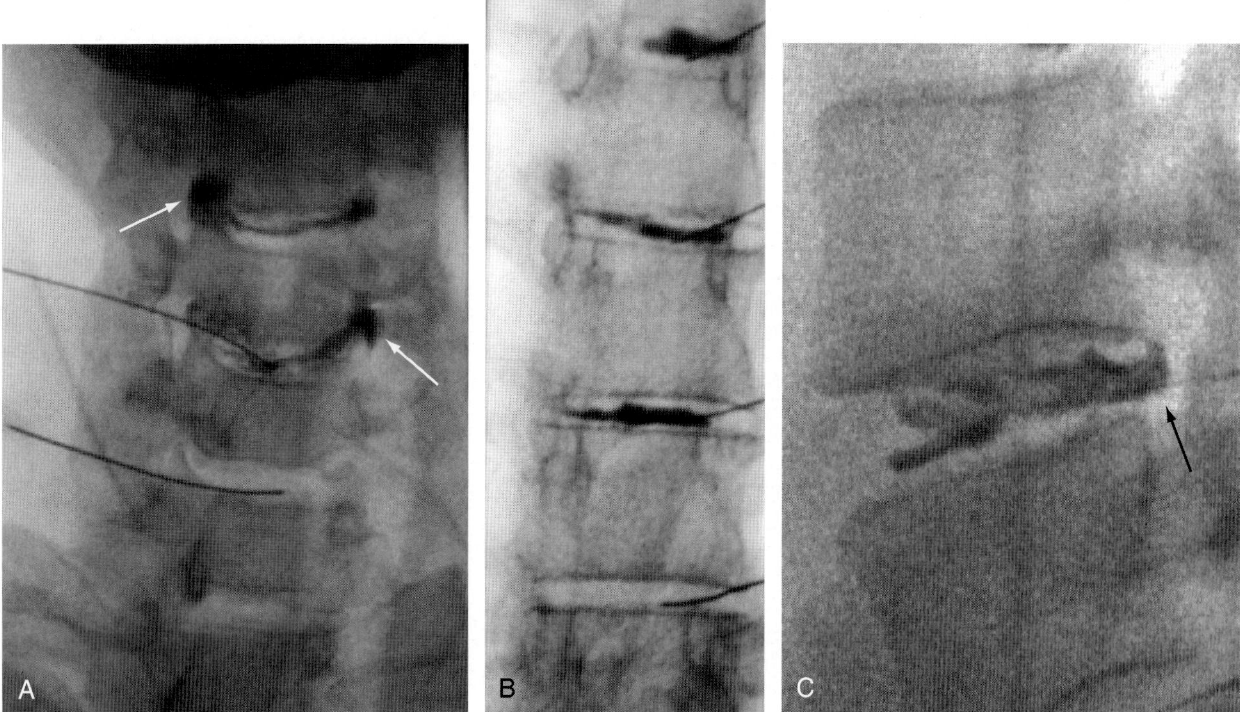

FIGURE 40-1. Discography. **A,** Cervical morphology: anteroposterior fluoroscopic image shows spinal needles at two levels. There is contrast material (black) opacifying the nucleus pulposus at two levels with extension posterolaterally into the uncovertebral articulations *(arrows)*. **B,** Thoracic anteroposterior fluoroscopic image shows contrast opacifying the intervertebral disks. Distinguishing normal from abnormal morphology is often difficult in this region. **C,** Lumbar discogram showing internal disk derangement (IDD) and degenerative disk disease (DDD) are indicated by a horizontal, irregular linear distribution of contrast. Anular fissure is identified by contrast extending beyond the expected confines of the nucleus pulposus and into the region of the annulus *(arrow)*.

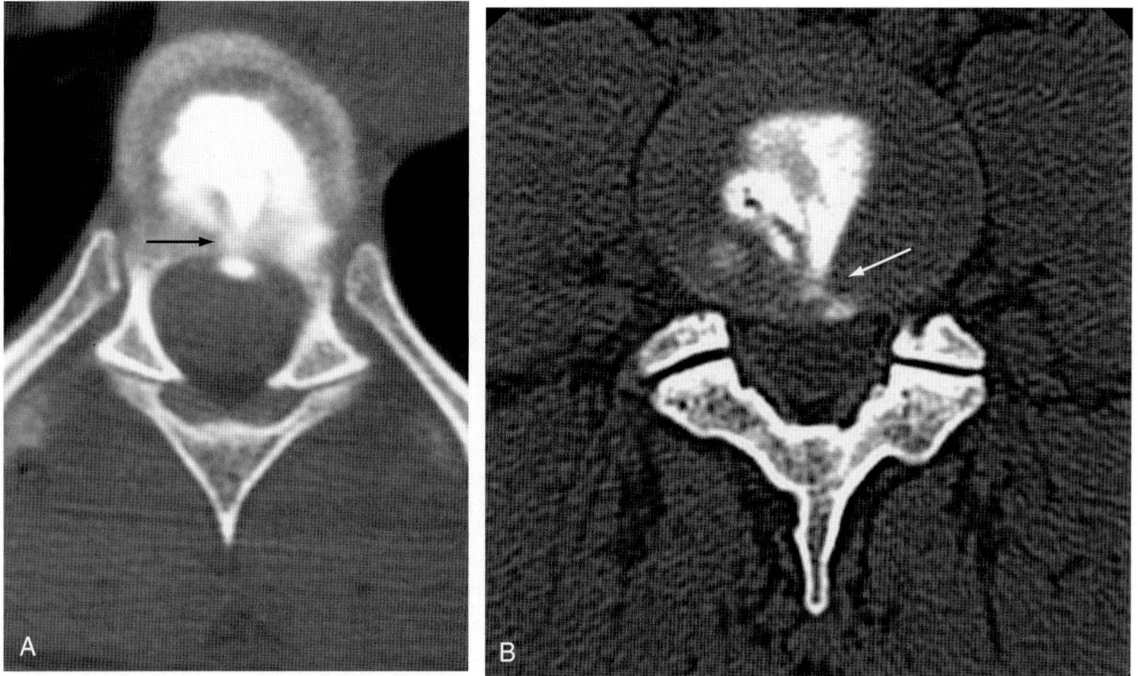

FIGURE 40-2. CT characterization of disk morphology **A,** Thoracic spine: Axial CT image shows contrast opacifying a peripheral anular tear *(arrow)* and extending posteriorly into a focal central herniation. **B,** Lumbar Spine: Contrast material is noted within the nucleus pulposus, but also extends in a radial fashion posteriorly beyond the expected confines of the nucleus pulposus into the region of the anulus fibrosis *(arrow)*.

EPIDURAL INJECTIONS

Overview and General Considerations

Degenerative disk disease is a common cause of back pain, with or without radicular symptoms. Disk material that extends from its normal position can compress nerve roots, the dorsal root ganglion, or proximal segmental nerve, all of which can cause pain. Disk-based inflammation can also cause pain, which is thought to be due to inflammatory mediators such as phospholipase A2 and others. Disk herniations tend to shrink over time, which can relieve compressive nerve pain, but the injection of corticosteroid can decrease inflammatory mediator-based pain and radiculopathy. Epidural injection is most commonly requested for the lumbar or cervical region.

There is high-quality evidence that lumbar transforaminal epidural corticosteroid injection (ESI) is also useful for lower-extremity radicular pain.[5] However, with regard to axial low-back pain, there is evidence that interlaminar ESI is not useful.[6]

The patient's pain is estimated with a visual analog scale prior to and following the procedure. The dictated report should include the degree of pain relief and a statement whether relief of the typical pain was complete, partial, or none. This immediate symptomatic improvement is due to the anesthetic component of the injectate (referred to as the "anesthetic phase"). The corticosteroid effect takes several days to initiate and is typically assessed at 1 to 2 weeks postinjection. The duration of effect is variable. For lumbar injections, the patient must be watched, and ambulation should begin with assistance since both motor and sensory block often occur, and the patient may comment on slight difficulty with ambulation.

> Following epidural injection, immediate symptomatic improvement is due to the anesthetic component of the injectate. The corticosteroid effect takes several days to initiate and is typically assessed at 1 to 2 weeks postinjection.

Cervical Spine Technique

For cervical nonselective epidural corticosteroid injection, a paramedian interlaminar approach is commonly used. The needle is advanced at the C7-T1 interspace, where capacity of the spinal canal is more generous, and the cord is positioned anteriorly in the thecal sac. Improved efficacy for injection at a higher level has not been proven, even if the likely pain generator is higher, and the risks are increased at higher levels. A paramedian approach allows the physician to determine appropriate needle depth by touching the lamina and then walking off the edge toward the epidural space. This detail should be stressed: The epidural space is much closer to the adjacent lamina in the cervical spine, and therefore placing the needle too deep with dural puncture is more likely. The lateral projection is also used to visualize the needle and prevent passing the spinolaminar line. The injection is similar to the lumbar spine. If the needle appears to be too deep and potentially within the spinal cord substance, then no injection should be performed because this will cause more neurologic damage than just the needlestick itself.

For cervical transforaminal or selective segmental nerve block, the patient is placed supine with the head turned away from the affected side. The C-arm should be positioned so that a good view of the foramen is obtained, and the target zone of the needle tip must be in the posterior inferior corner of that foramen. To determine depth, the C-arm is moved to an anteroposterior position for that level of the spine, accommodating the rotated head position, and the needle should be advanced no more than midway across the articular pillar in this view (50% zone). This zone is identified as the midpoint between a line formed by the uncinate process and the lateral margin of the lateral masses. Using sterile technique after cutaneous local anesthesia, a 25-gauge needle (2.5 or 3.5 in) is directed toward the posterior inferior portion of the target foramen under oblique fluoroscopic control. The vertebral artery runs along the anterior aspect of the foramen just behind (posterolateral to) the uncinate process. In addition, there is a wide array of cervical medullary and segmental arteries in and about the foramen with the least density being in the target zone. Injection of a small amount of contrast should show epiradicular and epidural opacification without vascular uptake (Figure 40-3, *A*). There are several case reports of spinal cord infarction with transforaminal cervical injections; the etiology is felt to be an embolic event from particulate material injected within a cervical medullary artery or branch. In order to minimize this complication, the following technique modifications are suggested: use of digital subtraction angiography during contrast injection to identify spinal artery opacification; if no vascular uptake is identified then perform a test injection of a small bolus of local anesthetic and test the patient for sensory or motor changes; and use of a nonparticulate corticosteroid preparation (dexamethasone).

Thoracic Spine Technique

Thoracic selective injections are performed with the patient in the prone position. The x-ray beam is tilted laterally such that a window is created allowing access between the facet joint, pedicle, transverse process, and rib, similar to the projection for thoracic discography. The beam is tilted craniocaudally such that it is directed "down the barrel" of the pedicle, the lower margin of which is about halfway between the end plates. The area is prepped and draped, the skin entry site is localized fluoroscopically, and subcutaneous short-acting anesthetic is administered. Deeper anesthetic is administered along the angle of the x-ray beam. Next, a 22- to 25-gauge spinal needle is advanced inferior to the pedicle through the aforementioned window until the posterolateral vertebral body is reached or radicular pain is perceived. If there is severe radicular pain, the needle should be repositioned. Care must be taken to avoid the pleural margin more laterally, which is easily visualized fluoroscopically. The needle should not be advanced more medial than the medial margin of the pedicle, which forms the border of the spinal canal.

If there is any blood return from the needle, the tip should immediately be repositioned; in the thoracic spine, especially from T7 to T9, small arterial feeders to the spinal cord can extend through the superior aspect of the neural foramen. Injection of air, short-acting anesthetic, or particulate corticosteroid into these branches has the potential to cause cord infarction. For this reason we also position the needle more inferiorly within the neural foramen, since the feeding vessels run just below the pedicle. Next, contrast injection is performed to verify satisfactory positioning. The injected contrast should extend centrally into the lateral epidural space of the spinal canal and peripherally around the nerve root. If there is vascular opacification, the needle should be repositioned. If the patient complains of acute onset of severe radicular pain immediately upon injection, an intraneural injection may have occurred; injection should be stopped immediately, and the needle should be repositioned. After proper positioning is verified, the anesthetic and corticosteroid mixture is injected with periodic fluoroscopic observation.

Lumbar Spine Technique

The lumbar epidural space can be approached in three ways, caudally: dorsally via an interlaminar or interspinous approach, and via the spinal foramen at a particular level. For the caudal approach, the fact that the thecal sac ends at the S2 level is

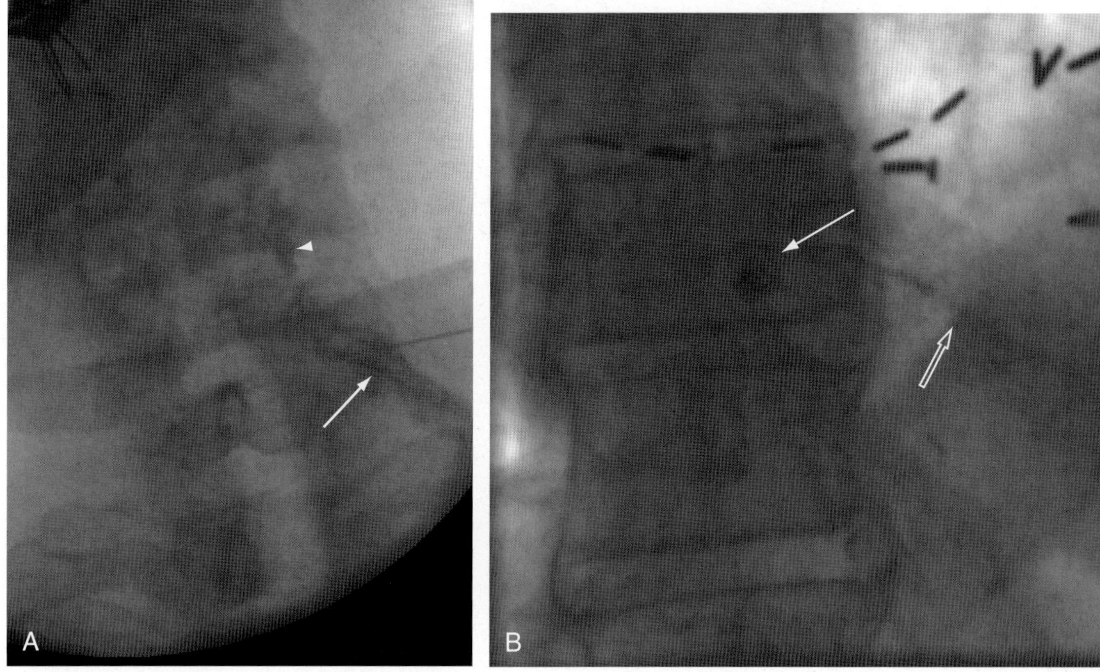

FIGURE 40-3. Epidural (transforaminal). **A,** Cervical: Supine anteroposterior fluoroscopic image shows the needle projected over the left lateral mass at the C6-C7 level. Contrast material spread is noted in an epiradicular *(arrow)* and epidural *(arrowhead)* distribution. **B,** Lumbar: Prone angled posteroanterior fluoroscopic image centered at the thoracolumbar junction shows the needle tip *(arrow)* projected at the inferior margin of the left T_{11} pedicle. Contrast material spread is noted in an epiradicular *(open arrow)* and epidural distribution.

advantageous because a needle placed through the sacral hiatus is less likely to penetrate the thecal sac than when approached with the other methods.[7] To perform a caudal block, the patient is placed prone on the table, and the low back is prepped and draped in sterile fashion. The sacral hiatus is palpated, identified on anteroposterior and lateral fluoroscopy, and then marked. Care should be made to adequately anesthetize the overlying skin, subcutaneous tissue, and periosteum, as this is a sensitive area for many patients. A 22-gauge spinal needle, straight or curved at the tip, is inserted into the sacral canal, which is confirmed with lateral fluoroscopy to ensure neither dorsal nor ventral needle position. The needle should not be advanced above the S2-S3 disk to minimize risk of dural puncture. Review of MRI is useful to ascertain that dural ectasia with multiple perineural (Tarlov) cysts does not exist. Injection of contrast material is indicated to confirm typical sacral epidurogram, and lack of intravascular uptake (Figure 40-4). A combination of local anesthetic and corticosteroid is injected (usually about a 3-cc volume), followed by 3 to 5 cc of saline. When dural puncture occurs with a caudal approach, a low thecal sac is usually present.

The interlaminar approach is performed with the patient prone. Fluoroscopy is used to visualize the interlaminar space one interspace above or below the most likely pain-generating level. Some physicians inject at the most symptomatic level, but if there is stenosis due to a disk bulge, the injectate can transiently raise intrathecal pressure and be uncomfortable for the patient. The needle is advanced to the inferior margin of the lamina of the vertebra above the target space. The lateral projection is used to confirm that the needle tip is located in the region of the dorsal epidural space. A blunt-tipped needle is preferred by some operators for the procedure. The needle is walked off the lamina into the interlaminar space and slowly advanced into the epidural space. To determine when the epidural space is entered, some physicians advocate continuous light pressure on a glass syringe connected to the needle, detecting loss of resistance. An alternative is to use a low-friction plastic or glass syringe and connecting tube filled almost to the end with contrast. A small quantity of air is left within the tubing when connected to the needle. Slight ballottement on the syringe plunger will cause the meniscus between the air and contrast in the tubing to "bounce" when resistance at the needle tip is present. As the epidural space is entered, the resistance decreases and the meniscus "jumps" forward. The contrast can then be injected to confirm under direct visualization that the needle is within the epidural space. Ideally, the contrast material and injectate should reach the ventral epidural space to theoretically maximize effectiveness. If the dura is punctured, the procedure can be performed at another site and the patient counseled for the risk of headache.

The transforaminal ESI has the intuitive advantage of a more targeted placement of the corticosteroid and anesthetic if injected. The risk of an intradural injection is much lower, but there is an increased possibility of nerve stimulation and pain during the procedure. This can be minimized by careful needle placement. For this technique, the patient is prone so the intervertebral disk of interest is profiled and the image intensifier rotated to access the foramen of the affected level. This is best done by projecting the ring shadow of the pedicle in the upper portion of the vertebral body using an obliquity that allows needle passage lateral to the lamina and under the transverse process. The needle is advanced to a level just under the pedicle at the 6-o'clock position into the "safe triangle."[8] If the needle comes in proximity to the nerve, the patient can be asked if the sensation follows her or his typical radicular distribution, although the sensation itself will likely be different from their typical pain. Injection of a small amount of contrast can confirm both epidural and epiradicular spread (see Figure 40-3, *B*); corticosteroid with anesthetic can then be injected. This is very similar to selective nerve blockade.

Selective segmental nerve blockade (SNRB) is a procedure very similar to transforaminal epidural corticosteroid injection (some use these terms synonymously). SNRB is usually performed as a

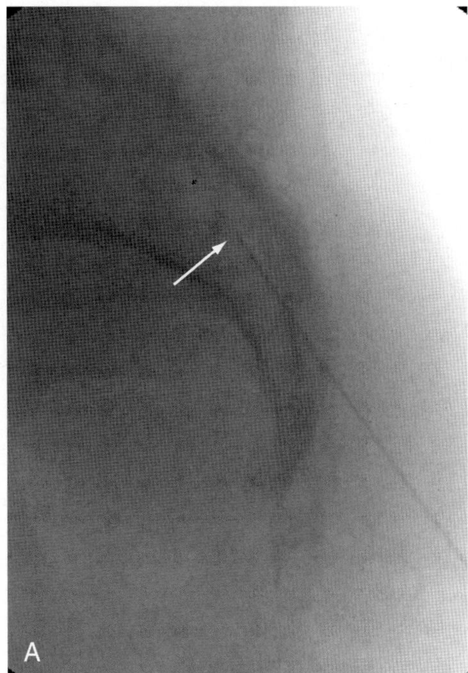

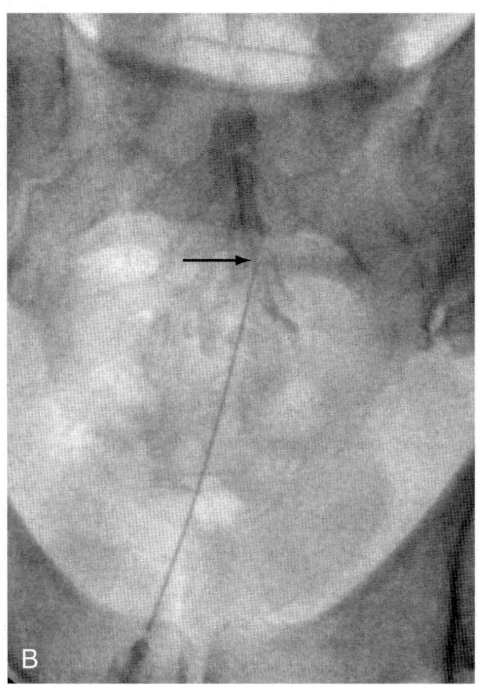

FIGURE 40-4. Epidural (caudal). **A,** Lateral fluoroscopic image shows the needle *(arrow)* that has entered the spinal canal via the sacral hiatus. **B,** Anteroposterior fluoroscopic image shows the needle in place at the S2-S3 level *(arrow)*. Contrast material demonstrates epidural opacification.

diagnostic test, but therapeutic injection of corticosteroid is sometimes performed as well. The value of selective nerve blocks is in identifying a particular level as a pain generator.[9] A block that does not relieve the patient's pain is a strong negative predictor for subsequent surgical benefit.[10] Surgeons might request sequential blocks spaced over time to fully elucidate a patient's pain generators prior to surgical intervention. That level is targeted with an oblique fluoroscopic approach similar to a transforaminal ESI. With ESI, the "safe triangle" is targeted, compared to SNRB in which the needle is directed slightly lower, just anterior and below the pedicle to approach the postganglionic nerve as it descends and traverses the vertebral body. The goal is to minimally touch the tissue adjacent to the nerve root to elicit a radicular sensation. The patient is asked if that sensation follows their typical pain pattern. If it is a portion of the pattern or all of it, the block is carried out. If the sensation is in a completely different distribution than typical pain, then that level may be blocked with an anticipated negative result or a block one level above or below may be considered.

Targeted epidural corticosteroid injections are most likely to benefit those patients whose imaging studies correlate in a neuroanatomic fashion with their clinical examination findings.

In addition, these findings may also be helpful in assessing patients for surgery; if there is clinical improvement noted following an ESI procedure, even for a brief period, this may confirm to the clinician that the site of pain generation in the spine has been identified.

FACET JOINT INJECTION

Overview and General Considerations

The facet joints have been implicated as nociceptors in the cervical, thoracic, and lumbar spine to varying degrees. Similar to other joints in the spine, the imaging manifestations of degenerative joint disease (i.e., osteoarthritis for synovial joints) do not correlate well with symptomatology. Intraarticular injections or nerve blocks have served as tools for diagnosing "facet syndrome." To effectively "block" a particular facet joint, two nerves (regions) must be injected because of the dual segmental innervation. The indications for facet joint injections are axial pain, referred pain, or putative implication that this joint is contributing to a spine pain syndrome. Pain maps have been generated in the cervical, thoracic, and lumbar regions for correlation.

The complications of facet joint injections are typically minimal. Because of its posterior location there is less likelihood of collateral damage to the exiting nerve roots and spinal cord. Spinal blocks from intrathecal needle positioning are also uncommon.

Cervical Spine Technique

For cervical-spine-facet joint injections, the approach may be posterior, lateral, or using a pillar-type projection.[11] The patient is placed in the supine or decubitus position for the lateral approach or prone position with the head turned away from the affected side. These injections are best performed under C-arm fluoroscopy. Because at the C2-C3 level the facet joint slopes inferiorly at its posterior and medial aspect, special projections are used. One option is to rotate the x-ray tube cephalad until the joint is profiled. Another option is to rotate the x-ray tube to the patient's rear (posteriorly) to bring the posterolateral aspect of the joint into profile. For the C3-C6 levels, a lateral approach is advocated. The target zone is the mid-portion of the joint along its lateral margin. If the x-ray tube is rotated close to a true lateral, this will profile the joint margins. The left and right joints might be nearly superimposed, and slight rotation of the C-arm may be performed to determine which is the appropriate side (e.g., the closest). However, if truly superimposed then the targeting should be similar despite the side and should not be problematic. Contrast injection is typically 0.1 to 0.3 mL so as not to rupture the joint capsule prior to anesthetic/corticosteroid administration (Figure 40-5, *A*).

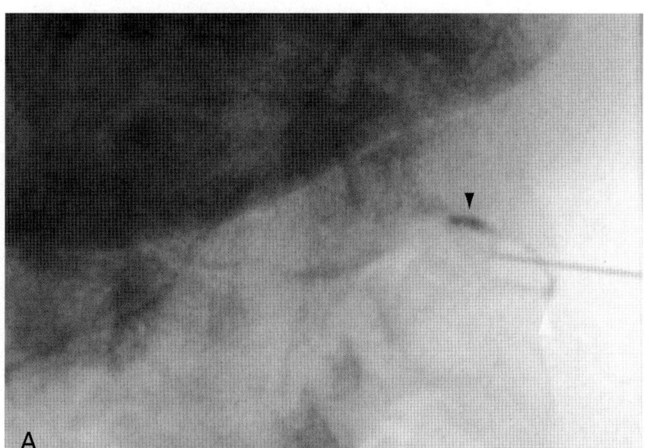

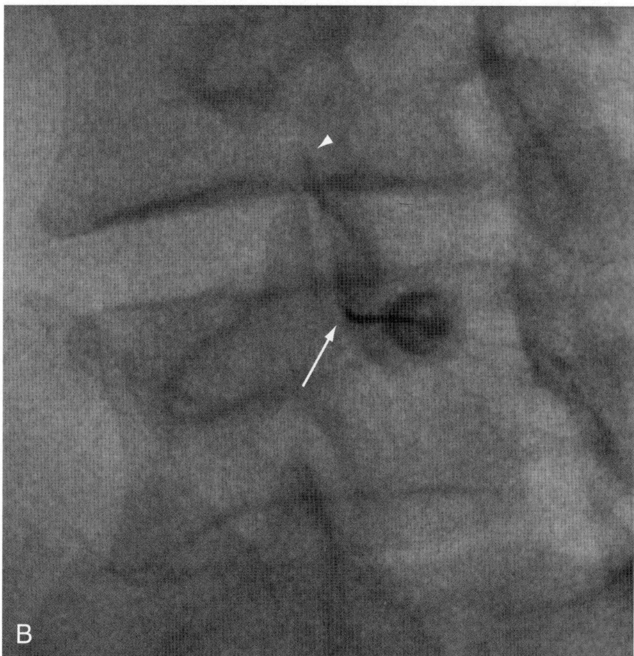

FIGURE 40-5. Facet joint injection. **A,** Cervical: Supine anteroposterior fluoroscopic image shows needle projected within the left C4-C5 facet joint. Contrast material injection shows normal arthrogram with ring-like opacification *(arrowhead)* indicative of an intra-articular location. **B,** Lumbar: Prone oblique fluoroscopic image shows the needle tip projected over the inferior recess *(arrow)* of the left L4-L5 facet joint. Contrast material shows a slit-like arthrogram and contrast material collecting in the superior joint recess *(arrowhead)*.

Lumbar Spine Technique

Numerous technical descriptions exist for lumbar facet joint injections performed under CT or fluoroscopic guidance. Some prefer the CT technique because the posterior joint space can be readily identified. The anatomy of the lumbar facet joints is such that there is a C-shaped auricular curve from anterior to posterior, which is variable. There are two main fluoroscopic techniques used for accessing the lumbar facet joints: oblique and posterior. In both approaches the patient is prone on a radiolucent table with pillows or cushions underneath the abdomen to decrease the lumbar lordosis and increase the size of the inferior recess.

In the oblique approach, the C-arm is started in the posteroanterior projection and centered over the joint of interest. While using continuous fluoroscopy, the tube is rotated toward the lateral direction until the first profile of the articular margins (as defined by sclerotic lines) is encountered. This should be the posterior joint space. Note that the traditional 45-degree oblique position ("Scotty dog") profiles the anterior aspect of the joint (anterior joint space) but is not necessarily the correct target in many patients. If one simply positions at this designated angle without observing for the most posterior portion of the joint, then the needle will not be able to access the joint because of bone. This approach is also problematic for lumbar facet joints with prominent osteophytosis. However, one can use the inferior recess to access the facet joint from an oblique or posterior projection.

In the posterior approach, the x-ray tube is left in a vertical position centered over the level of interest.[12] The goal is to access the inferior joint recess. The target zone is just below the superior articular process along its inferomedial aspect. Often the landmarks of the superior articular process are not well visualized and an alternative target zone is just above the pedicle of the lower segment at its superomedial aspect. The skin is marked, and the needle is placed straight down until the bone is encountered. Once the needle encounters the bone, passage into the joint is often perceived as a "pop" or loss of resistance as the tip passes through the capsule.

With either the oblique or posterior technique, a facet joint arthrogram should be obtained with the installation of a small amount (0.5 cc) of contrast material. The arthrogram may be ovoid or linear depending on the projection, and there is often flow into the superior recess (Figure 40-5, *B*). Often the posteroanterior projection is sufficient and no other deviation of the fluoroscope is needed to visualize the arthrogram. If a pars defect (spondylolysis) is present, it is often opacified by injecting the facet joint.

Both intraarticular injections and anesthetic medial branch blocks are considered primarily diagnostic tests. The false positive rate of uncontrolled blocks approaches 38% with a positive predictive value of only 31% when compared to a more rigorous diagnostic algorithm of sequential blocks with anesthetics of various durations for comparative and confirmatory blocks.[13] Studies show that the long-term effects for pain reduction are limited. This is true in both the cervical[14] and lumbar regions.[15] Procedures encompassing nerve ablations are useful to provide more lasting reduction of symptoms.[16]

SACROILIAC JOINT INJECTION

Overview and General Considerations

The sacroiliac (SI) joint can be a primary source of low back pain. More often, it is a secondary site or part of a multifactorial syndrome from dysfunction elsewhere in the spine. SI joint injections provide diagnostic information and may be potentially therapeutic in certain circumstances. The SI joint has a diffuse innervation pattern without a fixed course for the efferent nerves. Therefore there is no effective nerve block for the SI joint and only intraarticular injections can selectively anesthetize the SI joint. It has also been postulated that some of the pain mediated from the SI joint may be via communication with adjacent nerve structures. Fortin et al.[17] found five principal patterns of extracapsular contrast extravasation with three of these patterns exhibiting a potential pathway of communication between the SI joint and nearby neural structures. These included posterior extension into the dorsal sacral foramina, superior recess extravasation at the sacral alar level to the fifth lumbar epiradicular sheath, and ventral leakage to the lumbosacral plexus. They present the concept that inflammatory mediators could leak from the SI joint along these pathways and cause irritation of adjacent neurologic structures, which could, in part, explain how SI joint dysfunction may manifest as lower-extremity symptoms. Nevertheless, this does not negate the potential for pain mediation via direct subchondral bone irritation through cartilage loss, altered biomechanics, and marrow edema as it occurs in other synovial type articulations. Pain referral maps have been successfully produced using intraarticular injections in asymptomatic people.[18] In one study, a physical exam immediately after SI joint injection revealed an area of buttock hypesthesia extending about 10 cm caudally and 3 cm laterally from the posterior superior iliac spine. This map would explain the referral distribution based on primary SI joint pathology. Therefore, the indications for SI joint injection are to identify, diagnose, or treat pain putatively to be of SI joint origin. There is good evidence from several trials[19–22] for using SI joint injection to treat inflammatory spondyloarthropathies that have SI joint involvement. The data on the efficacy of corticosteroid intraarticular injections for mechanical somatic dysfunction are conflicting.

> The indications for SI joint injection are to identify, diagnose, or treat pain thought to be of SI joint origin. There is good evidence for using SI joint injection to treat inflammatory spondyloarthropathies that have SI joint involvement.

SI Joint Injection Technique

The SI joint may be injected under fluoroscopic or cross-sectional imaging guidance. A number of fluoroscopic or C-arm guided techniques have been described.[23] MRI has been used for guidance, but CT is used most commonly. Learning fluoroscopic techniques is more challenging than performing the technique under CT guidance. However, once fluoroscopic techniques are mastered, they may be faster than with CT guidance, and the decision for the type of imaging guidance is ultimately based mainly on operator's preference. In all of these techniques, SI joint arthrography is performed to confirm an intraarticular location. Often a small inferior caudal recess is opacified with a variable portion of the synovial joint. It is uncommon to opacify the entire SI joint. Also common in most techniques is that the needle encounters the sacral side while the operator is avoiding being too low or too lateral because of the proximity of the sciatic notch (sciatic nerve). From here the needle is guided into the joint until one feels a depression or a "pop," and then advancing it 1 to 2 mm. When the inferior joint is not accessible under fluoroscopy, most would advocate injecting the mid portion of the joint, which is more cephalad. Alternatively, a cross-sectional imaging technique can be used if attempts using fluoroscopy are not adequate. The maximum volume of contrast injected should be between 0.3 and 1.0 mL. This is to allow enough residual volume within the joint for anesthetic injection. In a small number of patients, it may be impossible to obtain an arthrogram. Other flow patterns to be cognizant of are venous or extracapsular opacification. With venous opacification small tributaries are identified flowing away from the SI joint. Extracapsular injections are characterized by irregular collections. These may occur concurrently with an intraarticular injection. The needle tip may be advanced or rotated slightly in this circumstance. In order to best visualize the arthrogram, an anteroposterior or slight oblique projection can be used to profile the structures of interest (Figure 40-6).

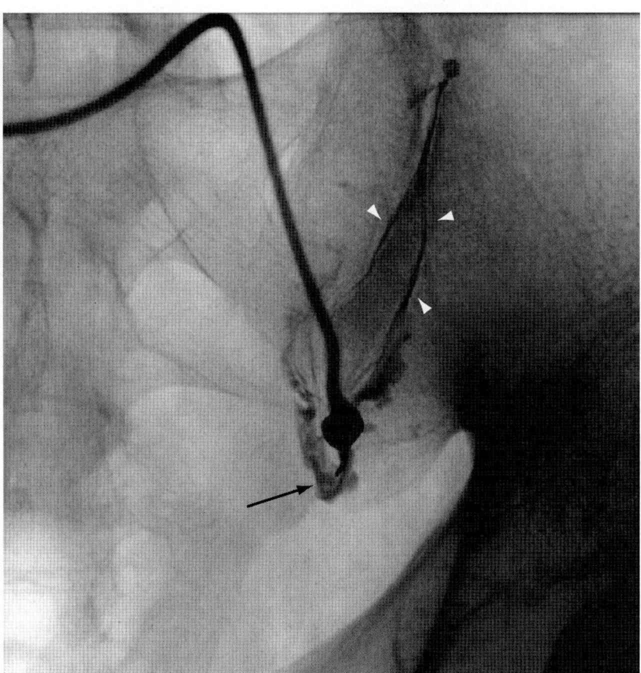

FIGURE 40-6. Sacroiliac joint: Prone angled oblique fluoroscopic image shows the needle tip projected over the inferior aspect of the sacroiliac joint *(arrow)*. Contrast material shows two linear intraarticular collections *(arrowheads)* reflecting the curved nature of the sacroiliac joint.

The interpretation of this procedure (similar to ESI) is based primarily upon pain relief and not the provocative aspect. Concordant pain production during SI joint injection is not validated as a diagnostic test confirming pain of SI joint origin. Practically, the assessment should be before the injection, immediately subsequent and approximately 15 to 30 minutes after the injection. The anesthetic response is most often assessed using a visual analog scale (VAS) and/or percentage of pain relieved. The result is considered positive (good) if greater than 75% of pain is relieved and negative if less than 50% of the pain is relieved. Pain relief may not be expected to be total because the SI joint is usually only one component of a multifactorial reason for back pain. However, when there is complete relief regionally in an area that corresponds to the SI joint distribution, the SI joint is established as the nociceptor.

VERTEBRAL AUGMENTATION (VERTEBROPLASTY/KYPHOPLASTY)

Overview and General Considerations

Painful nontraumatic vertebral fractures related to osteoporosis or neoplasms are common and can be associated with a significant morbidity to both the patient and society. Based on clinical experience and numerous case series, image-guided therapy using minimally invasive percutaneous techniques in the form of vertebroplasty and kyphoplasty (balloon-assisted vertebroplasty) have both shown good pain relief and improved function with minimal complication rates in appropriately selected patients. Osteoporotic compression fractures do better with respect to pain management than do fractures resulting from metastatic disease. Vertebral augmentation has become an essential component of the current treatment paradigm and will likely continue to serve an important therapeutic role for painful vertebral fractures and neoplasms.

Osteoporotic compression fractures can be associated with prolonged pain and spine deformity. Although conservative management may be adequate for pain relief in a majority of the cases, some patients experience limiting pain. Furthermore, the ensuing spinal deformity from the collapsed vertebral body may result in a severe deterioration of the quality of life of elderly individuals. The application of traditional surgical techniques with conventional spinal instrumentation is often fraught with problems such as hardware migration, screw pullout, or lack of rigid stability due to the poor bone quality related to underlying osteoporosis. Therefore the majority of patients are treated nonoperatively even in the presence of a progressive spinal deformity. Although many patients respond to nonoperative intervention, a subset of them will develop worsening or chronic severe pain, discomfort, and disability that affect their overall level of function. Medical pain management is also associated with increased pharmacologic side effects in this predominantly elderly population with a restricted physiologic reserve. In addition, some patients go on to develop a deformity that can compromise pulmonary and gastrointestinal functioning whether or not the fracture pain resolves. The sometimes less-than-effective nonoperative treatment and risks of traditional spine instrumentation have been the impetus to use minimally invasive treatment methods. Surgery is usually reserved for patients with compression of neural elements or compressive symptoms with neurologic deficits.

Percutaneous vertebral augmentation has been advocated as a technique to address pain related to a compromised vertebra either from an osteoporotic fracture or neoplasm. The intravertebral injection of acrylic resin cement is felt to stabilize the fracture site and thus reduce pain. However, vertebroplasty does not aim at restoring height and ultimately preventing spinal deformity. The ideal minimally invasive intervention should be designed to not only treat the present pain and discomfort from the compressed vertebrae but also to change the natural history of continued compression of the vertebra and future compression of adjacent vertebrae from altered spinal biomechanics. This was part of the impetus to develop kyphoplasty (balloon-assisted vertebroplasty), a percutaneous procedure where an inflatable bone tamp is used to create a void in order to attempt to restore lost vertebral body height before the injection of cement.

Indications, Technique, and Potential Complications

The primary indication for performing vertebral augmentation is to manage the pain related to nontraumatic benign or neoplasm associated vertebral fractures. The primary goals in osteoporosis are pain relief, prevention of further deformity, and restoration of vertebral body height if possible. A secondary indication is the management of benign or malignant neoplasms affecting the vertebrae (aggressive hemangioma, metastasis, and myeloma). For neoplasm, the indications are somewhat broader and the procedure may be done for pain management or stabilization. In the context of neoplasms, the indications also include treatment of osteolytic lesions undergoing chemotherapy or radiotherapy that may collapse if substantial tumor necrosis is achieved.

> The primary indication for performing vertebral augmentation is to manage the pain related to nontraumatic benign or neoplasm-related vertebral fractures. Patients with osteoporosis who respond best to vertebral augmentation have only one or two new fractures that are not severely compressed and have had a fracture for less than 12 months. Chronic lesions may also respond.

The patients with osteoporosis who seem to respond best to vertebral augmentation are ones that have only one or two new fractures that are not severely compressed and have had a fracture for less than 12 months, although more chronic lesions do also respond. Patients who are likely to benefit have fracture(s) that demonstrate bone marrow edema on MRI or radiotracer uptake on a nuclear medicine bone scintigram.

> Patients who are likely to benefit have fracture(s) that demonstrate bone marrow edema on MRI or radiotracer uptake on a nuclear medicine bone scan.

The patient should be in significant pain, and the pain from the fracture should alter their lifestyle. The benign neoplasms most commonly treated are hemangiomas (a vascular tumor composed of endothelial cells). While hemangiomas have a benign histology they may exhibit an aggressive growth pattern and come to clinical attention because of axial pain or compressive symptoms (so called *aggressive hemangioma*). Vertebral augmentation consolidates the vertebral body and reduces the risk of hemorrhage. In this fashion, vertebral augmentation is another adjuvant treatment similar to intralesional sclerosis or preoperative embolotherapy. The malignant neoplasms most commonly treated are metastases. Vertebral augmentation is efficacious in treating osseous vertebral metastases that result in pain or instability providing immediate and long-term pain relief and contributing to spinal stabilization.[24] Vertebral augmentation is not an ablative procedure, but the resultant structural bone reinforcement may produce the analgesia. The mechanism of effect is most likely related to increased strength and stiffness and not to a thermal ablative phenomenon.[25] A secondary role has been to allow other therapies such as radiotherapy or surgical resection and fixation to ensue while minimizing the risk of further collapse or fracture. Therefore if a spinal stabilization procedure is contemplated, preoperative vertebroplasty may be indicated.

Multiple myeloma is a plasma cell dyscrasia and is the most common primary bone neoplasm in the over 40-year-old age group. The myeloma cells physically displace the bone structure and secrete a chemical that destroys bone. This bone destruction results in bone pain, bone fractures, and hypercalcemia. There are several musculoskeletal manifestations. In the axial skeleton, myeloma is associated with compression deformities but not necessarily from focally destructive lesions. There is no correlation between the preexistence of focal vertebral marrow lesions detected with MRI and the subsequent development of vertebral fractures.[26] These patients can develop kyphotic deformities despite treatment, which may be painful and impact quality of life. Therefore vertebral augmentation goals should also be directed at correcting the deformity.

Marked vertebral body compression (i.e., the vertebral body height is smaller than the sagittal pedicle height) and vertebra plana (height loss greater than two-thirds of the original vertebral body height) make it technically challenging to place a cannula within the vertebra and has therefore been considered a relative contraindication to vertebral augmentation. However, there is evidence from case series that this population can also derive adequate pain management and this treatment should not necessarily be withheld.[27] Needle placement does require some additional expertise; smaller diameter needles (13 gauge) and judicious cement injection are advocated because pain relief is not necessarily correlated with amount of cement or proportion of vertebral filling. In patients who have a pseudoarthrosis as manifested by an intravertebral vacuum cleft,[28] some advocate filling of the cleft with cement to maximize stabilization of the fracture fragments.[29] Attempting to obtain some cephalocaudal vertebral filling is also felt to be important, but a paramount goal should be to minimize complications.

Preevaluation imaging should nominally consist of a morphologic technique and a physiologic technique that can demonstrate an incompletely healed (i.e., "active") fracture, but there are certainly many contexts where additional imaging may be useful. Other goals are to detect neoplastic involvement and assess the degree of associated degenerative disease. Radiography is useful for showing the degree of collapse. The age of the compression fracture is less important than the presence of bone marrow edema on MRI and is relevant for people who have had symptoms for months or years. If MRI is contraindicated, then scintigraphy can be used as a substitute to show physiologic activity related to an incompletely healed fracture. There are data showing that increased activity (if localized to the vertebral body) is highly predictive of positive clinical response to vertebral augmentation.[30] Computed Tomography (CT) imaging is useful as a morphologic adjunct to scintigraphy and in neoplasms to delineate areas of osteolysis, show cortical interruption, and quantify the degree of osseous retropulsion.

> If MRI is contraindicated, then scintigraphy can be used as a substitute to show physiologic activity related to an incompletely healed fracture.

Concordant pain has been considered an important criterion for determining those patients with benign fractures who will respond to augmentation. The back is percussed and palpated over the spinous processes marking the areas of tenderness. A physical examination under fluoroscopy may be performed to determine if the patient's symptoms are concordant with the level of the active compression fracture on MRI. The patient also assumes any position that triggers the pain, and the painful site is marked. If the pain corresponds to the fractured level (usually within one vertebral level above or below), then the symptoms are likely to be amenable to treatment at that vertebral level. This evaluation is less reliable for lesions related to neoplasm without fracture.

> If the pain corresponds to the fracture level (usually within one vertebral level above or below), then the symptoms are likely to be amenable to treatment at that vertebral level.

Detailed technical descriptions are available.[31-36] The technique for vertebral augmentation entails penetration of the involved vertebra(e) followed by injection of a cement or another reinforcing substance into the vertebral body (Figure 40-7, *A* and *B*). The cement may be injected with or without the creation of a void and some height restoration. Techniques that employ an inflatable balloon tamp are known as kyphoplasty or balloon-assisted vertebroplasty (Figure 40-7, *C* and *D*).

The image guidance modalities used are either fluoroscopy or CT, with or without CT fluoroscopy. Needle placement may be transpedicular or extrapedicular. The traditional mode for both vertebroplasty and kyphoplasty has been to perform a two-needle bipedicular technique. However, unipedicular or unilateral extrapedicular injections can also result in substantial vertebral reinforcement when adequate volumes of cement are injected resulting in a similar distribution to bilateral injections.

Kyphoplasty can be accomplished using a modified vertebroplasty technique. The position of the inflatable bone tamp (balloon) is identified by distal and proximal radiographic markers. The balloon should reside in the anterior half of the vertebral body. The balloon(s) are then inflated with contrast material, elevating the end plates in an attempt to restore vertebral body height. For patients with a history of severe contrast allergic reaction, gadolinium should be employed because there is a possibility of balloon rupture during the course of intravertebral inflation, and thus contrast could gain intravascular access from a leak into the basivertebral venous plexus. The endpoint of balloon inflation occurs when (1) adequate reduction of the compression fracture is accomplished, (2) maximum inflation pressure is reached, (3) proximity of the bone tamp to one of the cortices, or (4) maximum inflation volumes are achieved. Higher pressures are generally needed for more dense bone as well as for subacute fractures, while low pressures are commonly necessary in less dense bone and more acute fractures. The operator must be vigilant in detecting any evidence of a cortical breach or leakage of any contrast material from the balloon. Once the endpoint is achieved, the bone tamp is deflated and removed. For more acute fractures, the balloons may be deflated on only one side to prevent the loss of reduction. The cavity created by kyphoplasty can often be identified as a lucent region on fluoroscopic imaging; this area is then filled with cement.

Specific technical considerations for metastatic neoplastic lesions include needle placement, cement volume, and adjuvant therapy. Needle placement is similar to osteoporosis cases (transpedicular or parapedicular approach) and not necessarily altered based on lesion location. Often the needle may be placed in normal non–tumor-infiltrated bone. The goal in the cement application is to obtain craniocaudal filling (attempting to get superior to inferior end-plate filling) that crosses the midline transversely providing a strut. The cement may fill part of the tumor. However, attempting to fill the whole tumor may not be advisable if there is posterior cortical disruption or a significant extraosseous component. Thus this may be difficult or impossible to accomplish, and there is a risk that the neoplastic tissue would be displaced into the canal causing a symptomatic stenosis, which may require surgical debulking. It is believed that the tumor is killed within 2 mm of the cement from the exothermic reaction. Thus if filling of the tumor is not achieved during the procedure, then adjuvant therapy (surgery, chemotherapy, or radiotherapy) should be performed (or at least considered) so that entire tumor kill can be achieved.

The common component for the majority of vertebral augmentation procedures currently performed is the instillation of acrylic resin cement into the vertebral body. There are several issues related to the cement, including what agent to use, how much, and how to apply it. The bone cement most commonly used is some form of polymethylmethacrylate (PMMA). Implant material is an active area of development. The most salient considerations for choice of an agent include ability to increase vertebral strength and stiffness, visibility under fluoroscopy, ease of cement flow, and simplicity of use. The cement flow needs to be carefully monitored, and the injection should cease if there is resistance or cement approaches the posterior vertebral margin.

Fortunately, major complications of vertebral augmentation are uncommon. Minor nonclinically significant complications do occur and are most often related to extraosseous cement leakage. The potential complications for kyphoplasty and vertebroplasty are similar and include cement extravasation and pulmonary embolism. The incidence of epidural leakage is related to the amount of injected cement and vertebral level with a higher incidence of leakage when more cement is injected and when injecting vertebrae above T7.[37] The clinical significance of extraosseous cement is less important than previously felt. Small to moderate amounts of cement may leak outside bone with no significant effect on therapeutic success.[38] Overall, there is a high technical success rate reported for accomplishing vertebral augmentation with minimal complications by experienced operators.

Clinical Experience

Overall, postvertebral augmentation patients with osteoporosis have done well with respect to pain management, and this therapeutic response has led to the popularity of these procedures.[39] Several studies have been performed and uniformly report good pain relief, reduced requirements for analgesics, and improved

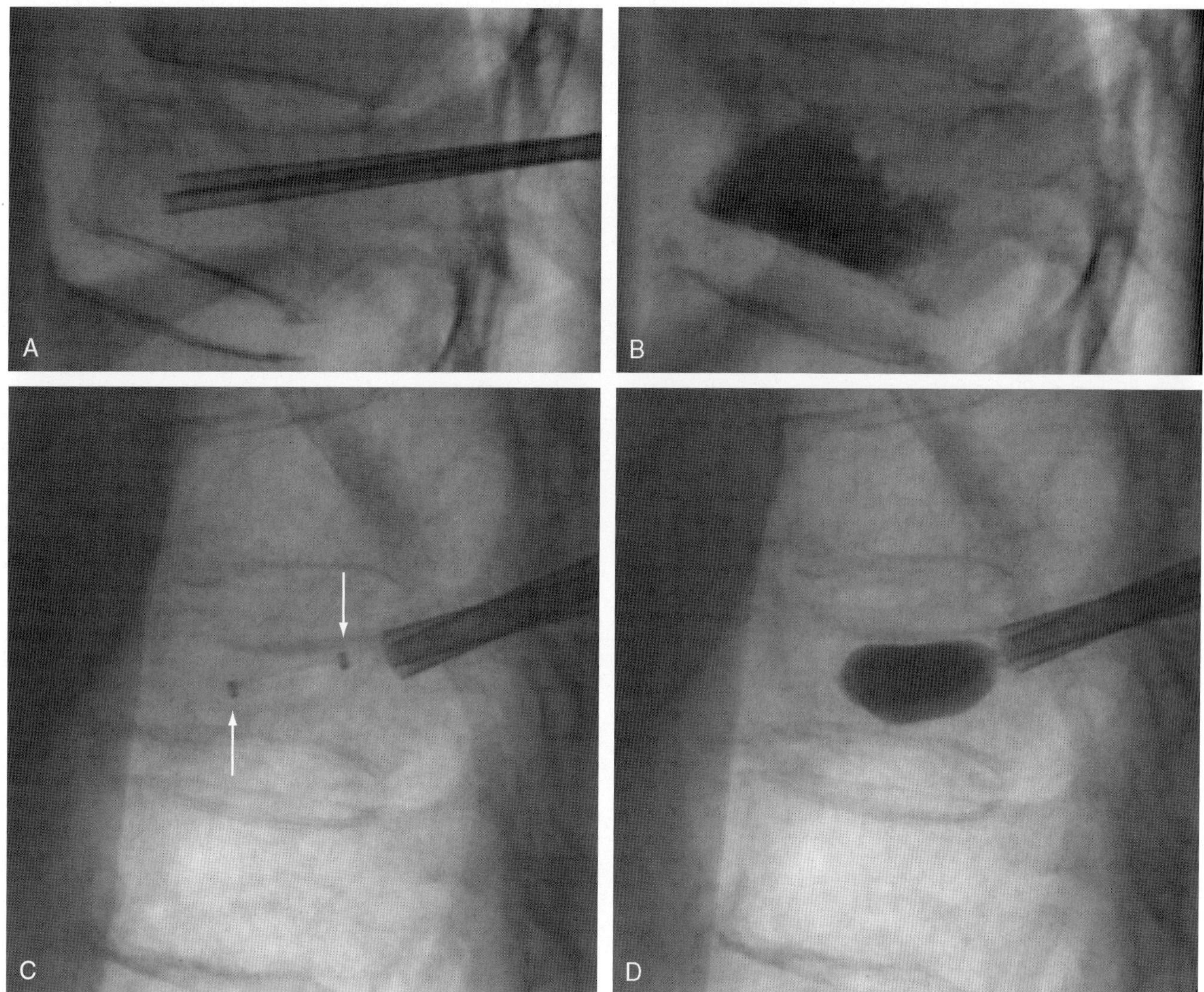

FIGURE 40-7. Vertebral augmentation. **A,** Vertebroplasty: Lateral fluoroscopic image shows needle tips projected in the anterior third of a moderately compressed vertebral body. **B,** Vertebroplasty: Lateral fluoroscopic image shows cement distribution postinjection with filling of the trabecular interstices of the anterior 75% of the vertebral body without evidence of extraosseous extent. **C,** Balloon-assisted vertebroplasty (kyphoplasty): Lateral fluoroscopic image shows the inflatable bone tamp placed through a working cannula with radiopaque markers denoting the balloon's longitudinal extent distally and proximally *(arrows)*. **D,** Lateral fluoroscopic image shows balloon inflation with end plate elevation and partial height restoration.

functional mobility following vertebroplasty.[40-42] Literature reviews are available summarizing the reports of numerous case series documenting pain relief from these procedures in 67% to 100% of cases.[43] Prospective noncontrolled trials report pain reduction in a high proportion of patients in the short term[44] and in the longer term (15 to 18 months) with high patient satisfaction.[45] In a nonrandomized trial, when compared with conservative therapy, percutaneous vertebroplasty resulted in prompt pain relief and rapid rehabilitation within 24 hours, but clinical outcomes were similar at 6 weeks and 6 to 12 months.[46] There is also evidence that for kyphoplasty, the pain benefits persist at 1-year posttreatment.[47] Durable results have been documented in vertebroplasty for up to 4 years.[48] Long-term pain management and mechanical and physiological benefits have not yet been demonstrated. Vertebroplasty is also efficacious therapy for relief of pain and improvement in mobility for chronic fractures (benefit is not fracture age dependent) provided the fracture is high in signal on T2-weighted images or shows increased uptake on bone scan.[49] The growing consensus is that kyphoplasty and vertebroplasty are felt to be safe and effective and have a useful role in the treatment of painful osteoporotic vertebral compression fractures that do not respond to conventional treatments.[50] There are no accepted criteria indicating when to perform one type of vertebral augmentation over another. Both vertebroplasty and kyphoplasty are undergoing technical developments and improvements. It is likely that both techniques and probably new ones will have a role in vertebral and other bone augmentation applications.

There are no accepted criteria as to when to perform one type of vertebral augmentation procedure over another.

CONCLUSION

In this chapter, the indications, contraindications, rationale, technique, and clinical experience for performing discography, epidural corticosteroid injection, selective nerve blockade, SI joint injection, facet joint injection, and vertebral augmentation were reviewed. Spine injections are an important component of a comprehensive management approach to chronic spine pain syndromes for establishing a diagnosis, directing therapy, and facilitating rehabilitation. The decision to perform spine procedures should be made by a spine specialist or a multidisciplinary team because the choice between medical treatment, injections, surgery, or a combination thereof depends on a number of factors. Spine injections should be viewed as only one component of a comprehensive program to manage disorders affecting the axial skeleton. However, it is meticulous attention to technique that makes percutaneous spine injections safe and successful procedures.

REFERENCES

1. Bogduk N: *Clinical Anatomy of the Lumbar Spine and Sacrum,* New York, 1997, Churchill Livingstone.
2. Guyer RD, Ohnmeiss DD: Contemporary concepts in spine care. Lumbar discography: position statement from the North American Spine Society, *Spine* 20:2048-2059, 1995.
3. Osti OL, Fraser RD, Vernon-Roberts B: Discitis after discography. The role of prophylactic antibiotics, *J Bone Joint Surg Br* 72:271-274, 1990.
4. Derby R, Howard MW, Grant JM, et al: The ability of pressure-controlled discography to predict surgical and nonsurgical outcomes, *Spine* 24:364-371, 1999.
5. Rapp SE, Haselkorn JK, Elam K, et al: Epidural steroid injection in the treatment of low back pain: a meta-analysis, *Anesthesiology* 81:A923, 1994.
6. Carette S, Leclaire R, Marcoux S, et al: Epidural corticosteroid injections for sciatica due to herniated nucleus pulposus, *N Engl J Med* 336:1634-1640, 1997.
7. Berg TD, El-Khoury GY: Epidurography and epidural steroid injections. In Williams AL, Murtagh FR (eds), *Handbook of Diagnostic and Therapeutic Spine Procedures,* St. Louis, 2002, Mosby, pp 1-18.
8. Bogduk N, Aprill C, Derby R: Epidural steroid injections. In White AH, Schofferman J (eds), *Spinal Care Diagnosis and Treatment,* St. Louis, 1995, Mosby, pp 322-344.
9. Wagner AL, Mrutagh FR: Selective nerve root blocks, *Tech Vasc Interv Radiol* 5:194-200, 2002.
10. Derby R, Kine G, Saal JA, et al: Response to steroid and duration of radicular pain as predictors of surgical outcome, *Spine* 17:S176-S183, 1992.
11. Silbergleit R, Mehta BA, Sanders WP, et al: Imaging-guided injection techniques with fluoroscopy and CT for spinal pain management, *Radiographics* 21:927-939, 2001.
12. Sarazin L, Chevrot A, Pessis E, et al: Lumbar facet joint arthrography with the posterior approach, *Radiographics* 19:93-104, 1999.
13. Schwarzer AC, Aprill CN, Derby R, et al: The false-positive rate of uncontrolled diagnostic blocks of the lumbar zygapophysial joints, *Pain* 58:195-200, 1994.
14. Barnsley L, Lord SM, Wallis BJ, et al: Lack of effect of intraarticular corticosteroids for chronic pain in the cervical zygapophyseal joints, *N Engl J Med* 330:1047-1050, 1994.
15. Carette S, Marcoux S, Truchon R, et al: A controlled trial of corticosteroid injections into facet joints for chronic low back pain, *N Engl J Med* 325:1002-1007, 1991.
16. Lord SM, Barnsley L, Wallis BJ, et al: Percutaneous radio-frequency neurotomy for chronic cervical zygapophyseal-joint pain, *N Engl J Med* 335:1721-1726, 1996.
17. Fortin JD, Washington WJ, Falco FJ: Three pathways between the sacroiliac joint and neural structures, *AJNR Am J Neuroradiol* 20:1409-1434, 1999.
18. Fortin JD, Dwyer AP, West S, et al: Sacroiliac joint: pain referral maps upon applying a new injection/arthrography technique. Part I: Asymptomatic volunteers, *Spine* 19:1475-1482, 1994.
19. Maugars Y, Mathis C, Berthelot JM, et al: Assessment of the efficacy of sacroiliac corticosteroid injections in spondyloarthropathies: a double-blind study, *Br J Rheumatol* 35:767-770, 1996.
20. Braun J, Bollow M, Seyrekbasan F, et al: Computed tomography guided corticosteroid injection of the sacroiliac joint in patients with spondyloarthropathy with sacroiliitis: clinical outcome and followup by dynamic magnetic resonance imaging, *J Rheumatol* 23:659-664, 1996.
21. Bollow M, Braun J, Taupitz M, et al: CT-guided intraarticular corticosteroid injection into the sacroiliac joints in patients with spondyloarthropathy: indication and follow-up with contrast-enhanced MRI, *J Comput Assist Tomogr* 20:512-521, 1996.
22. Hanly JG, Mitchell M, MacMillan L, et al: Efficacy of sacroiliac corticosteroid injections in patients with inflammatory spondyloarthropathy: results of a 6 month controlled study, *J Rheumatol* 27:719-722, 2000.
23. Dussault RG, Kaplan PA, Anderson MW: Fluoroscopy-guided sacroiliac joint injections, *Radiology* 214:273-277, 2000.
24. Weill A, Chiras J, Simon JM, et al: Spinal metastases: indications for and results of percutaneous injection of acrylic surgical cement, *Radiology* 199:241-247, 1996.
25. Deramond H, Wright NT, Belkoff SM: Temperature elevation caused by bone cement polymerization during vertebroplasty, *Bone* 25(2 Suppl):17S-21S, 1999.
26. Lecouvet FE, Vande Berg BC, Michaux L, et al: Development of vertebral fractures in patients with multiple myeloma: does MRI enable recognition of vertebrae that will collapse? *J Comput Assist Tomogr* 22:430-436, 1998.
27. Peh WC, Gilula LA, Peck DD: Percutaneous vertebroplasty for severe osteoporotic vertebral body compression fractures, *Radiology* 223:121-126, 2002.
28. Peh WC, Gelbart MS, Gilula LA, et al: Percutaneous vertebroplasty: treatment of painful vertebral compression fractures with intraosseous vacuum phenomena, *AJR Am J Roentgenol* 180:1411-1417, 2003.
29. Lane JI, Maus TP, Wald JT, et al: Intravertebral clefts opacified during vertebroplasty: pathogenesis, technical implications, and prognostic significance, *AJNR Am J Neuroradiol* 23:1642-1646, 2002.
30. Maynard AS, Jensen ME, Schweickert PA, et al: Value of bone scan imaging in predicting pain relief from percutaneous vertebroplasty in osteoporotic vertebral fractures, *AJNR Am J Neuroradiol* 21:1807-1812, 2000.
31. Jensen ME, Evans AJ, Mathis JM, et al: Percutaneous polymethylmethacrylate vertebroplasty in the treatment of osteoporotic vertebral body compression fractures: technical aspects, *AJNR Am J Neuroradiol*18:1897-1904, 1997.
32. Deramond H, Depriester C, Galibert P, et al: Percutaneous vertebroplasty with polymethylmethacrylate. Technique, indications, and results, *Radiol Clin North Am* 36:533-546, 1998.
33. Ahrar K, Schomer DF, Wallace MJ: Kyphoplasty for the treatment of vertebral compression fractures, *Semin Interven Radiol* 19:235-243, 2002.
34. Ortiz AO, Zoarski GH, Beckerman M: Kyphoplasty, *Tech Vasc Interv Radiol* 5:239-249, 2002.
35. Peh WC, Gilula LA: Percutaneous vertebroplasty: indications, contraindications, and technique, *Br J Radiol* 76:69-75, 2003.
36. Mathis JM, Wong W: Percutaneous vertebroplasty: technical considerations, *J Vasc Interv Radiol* 14:953-960, 2003.
37. Ryu KS, Park CK, Kim MC, et al: Dose-dependent epidural leakage of polymethylmethacrylate after percutaneous vertebroplasty in patients with osteoporotic vertebral compression fractures, *J Neurosurg* 96(1 Suppl):56-61, 2002.
38. Hodler J, Peck D, Gilula LA: Midterm outcome after vertebroplasty: predictive value of technical and patient-related factors, *Radiology* 227:662-668, 2003.
39. Phillips FM: Minimally invasive treatments of osteoporotic vertebral compression fractures, *Spine*28(15):S45-S53, 2003.
40. Cyteval C, Sarrabere MP, Roux JO, et al: Acute osteoporotic vertebral collapse: open study on percutaneous injection of acrylic surgical cement in 20 patients, *AJR Am J Roentgenol* 173:1685-1690, 1999.
41. Cortet B, Cotten A, Boutry N, et al: Percutaneous vertebroplasty in the treatment of osteoporotic vertebral compression fractures: an open prospective study, *J Rheumatol* 26:2222-2228, 1999.
42. Evans AJ, Jensen ME, Kip KE, et al: Vertebral compression fractures: pain reduction and improvement in functional mobility after percutaneous polymethylmethacrylate vertebroplasty retrospective report of 245 cases, *Radiology* 226:366-372, 2003.
43. Watts NB, Harris ST, Genant HK: Treatment of painful osteoporotic vertebral fractures with percutaneous vertebroplasty or kyphoplasty, *Osteoporos Int;* 12:429-437, 2001.
44. McGraw JK, Lippert JA, Minkus KD, et al: Prospective evaluation of pain relief in 100 patients undergoing percutaneous vertebroplasty: results and follow-up, *J Vasc Interv Radiol* 13:883-886, 2002.
45. Zoarski GH, Snow P, Olan WJ, et al: Percutaneous vertebroplasty for osteoporotic compression fractures: quantitative prospective evaluation of long-term outcomes, *J Vasc Interv Radiol* 13:139-148, 2002.
46. Diamond TH, Champion B, Clark WA: Management of acute osteoporotic vertebral fractures: a nonrandomized trial comparing percutaneous vertebroplasty with conservative therapy, *Am J Med* 114:257-265, 2003.
47. Coumans JV, Reinhardt MK, Lieberman IH: Kyphoplasty for vertebral compression fractures: 1-year clinical outcomes from a prospective study, *J Neurosurg* 99 (1 Suppl):44-50, 2003.
48. Grados F, Depriester C, Cayrolle G, et al: Long-term observations of vertebral osteoporotic fractures treated by percutaneous vertebroplasty, *Rheumatology (Oxford)* 39 (12):1410-1414, 2000.
49. Kaufmann TJ, Jensen ME, Schweickert PA, et al: Age of fracture and clinical outcomes of percutaneous vertebroplasty, *AJNR Am J Neuroradiol* 22:1860-1863, 2001.
50. Garfin SR, Yuan HA, Reiley MA: New technologies in spine: kyphoplasty and vertebroplasty for the treatment of painful osteoporotic compression fractures, *Spine* 26:1511-1515, 2001.

CHAPTER 41

Bone Disease Following Organ Transplantation

RAUL GALVEZ-TREVINO, MD, CAROLYN BOLTIN, MD, PARHAM PEZESHK, MD, and ANIL K. CHANDRAKER, MB, FRCP

KEY FACTS

- Musculoskeletal complications may occur following otherwise successful renal, cardiac, or lung transplantation and may result in a diminished quality of life.
- Hyperparathyroidism may persist after renal transplantation and parathyroidectomy becomes necessary in a small percentage of cases.
- Osteoporosis is a frequent complication in post-transplant patients. It is estimated that over 40% of renal transplant recipients followed more than 5 years suffer an osteoporotic fracture.
- Gout occurs in up to 7.6% of renal transplant patients.
- Post-transplant bone-marrow edema syndrome is a cause of severe bilateral distal lower extremity pain in transplant recipients. This syndrome usually occurs early in the clinical course. Its cause is uncertain. Bone marrow edema and, in some cases, insufficiency fractures, are demonstrated on magnetic resonance imaging.
- Pretransplantation bone loss is an important predictor of post-transplantation fracture risk. To prevent the development of post-transplantation osteoporosis, attention should be focused on optimizing bone metabolism and bone mass prior to transplantation.
- Osteonecrosis has become less frequent after transplantation owing to changes in immunotherapy.

The modern era of organ transplantation began in 1954 with the successful transplantation of a kidney from one brother to his twin at the Brigham and Women's Hospital in Boston, Massachusetts.[1] Now, more than 25,000 solid organ transplants are performed yearly in the United States and the types of organs and tissues transplanted are increasing.[1] The advances in transplantation have led to a corresponding need for imaging of these patients after surgery. This chapter reviews the major musculoskeletal complications that may occur following renal, lung, or cardiac transplantation. Selected treatment options are mentioned, but the reader is referred to other sources for detailed treatment plans.

Organ transplantation is the optimal form of therapy for those with many forms of irreversible chronic diseases such as chronic renal disease, hepatic failure, cystic fibrosis (CF), chronic obstructive pulmonary disease (COPD), and congestive heart failure. Advances in immunosuppressive medications have improved allograft function over the last several decades and have significantly increased survival. The cost of containing once life-threatening complications such as rejection has been the increase in side effects, including metabolic bone disease, resulting from immunosuppressive medications.

Post-transplantation bone disease is a generic term referring to the spectrum of transplantation-related disorders of bone metabolism and function. The most important of these skeletal complications are the development of osteoporosis and related fractures, osteonecrosis (avascular necrosis), and diffuse bone pain. The importance of bone-related complications after organ transplantation was directly assessed by Navasa et al.[2] His results underline the clinical and socioeconomic relevance of transplantation-related bone disorders, proving that these have a detrimental effect on the quality of life of patients by causing pain, imposing limitations in activities of daily living, and producing emotional stress. These individual effects also create a significant burden on the public health system due to the direct and indirect costs of treatment.[3]

Bone disorders related to organ transplantation have similar pathophysiologic mechanisms, leading to common endpoints such as osteoporosis (Box 41-1). However, each organ has unique epidemiologic characteristics and specific risk factors that can be highlighted.

In liver diseases, the development of fractures has been a long-recognized clinical complication. Interestingly, the prevalence of fracture after liver transplantation is markedly higher among patients with cholestatic diseases (6%), such as primary biliary cirrhosis (PBC) and primary sclerosing cholangitis (PSC), than it is after hepatitis or other liver diseases (1%).[3]

Patients with chronic heart failure have been found to have increased risk of low bone mass attributed to multiple factors including prolonged immobility, anorexia, hypogonadism, the use of loop diuretics, and vitamin D deficiency. Additionally, a trend has been noted for a higher rate of incident vertebral fractures among patients with ischemic cardiomyopathy, in comparison to those with dilated cardiomyopathy or other cardiac diseases, suggesting that vascular changes due to atherosclerosis may also be related to bone metabolic alterations and increased risk of osteoporosis.[4]

Patients with chronic lung disease have a significantly increased risk of low bone mass and osteoporosis before transplantation. These are secondary to pre transplant exposure to glucocorticoids and a high prevalence of vitamin D deficiency, which has been found in up to 36% of patients with CF, and in 20% of patients with other pulmonary diseases[5] (see Box 41-1).

BOX 41-1. Factors Predisposing to Osteoporosis in Transplant Recipients

- Older age
- Calcium deficiency
- Vitamin D deficiency
- Inactivity
- Excessive alcohol/tobacco
- Medicines (loop diuretics, anticoagulants, glucocorticoids)
- Renal or liver failure
- Immunosuppression

Patients with severe chronic kidney disease who undergo renal transplantation now have 1-year survival exceeding 90%. Improving the long-term quality of life for renal transplant patients, including the prevention and treatment of bone-related disorders has become a major goal in the post-transplantation period. The risk factors for developing transplant-related bone disease are multiple in nephropathic patients. The most important is renal osteodystrophy, followed by secondary hyperparathyroidism, osteomalacia, adynamic bone disease, aluminum bone disease or β_2-microglobulin amyloidosis, all contributing to distortion of osseous architecture and increased risk for fractures and bone pain (Figure 41-1).

MECHANISMS

In organ transplantation, the primary goal is to prevent or inhibit donor-organ rejection by the recipient's immune system. This has been achieved through the administration of immunosuppressants, of which the most used and best understood are glucocorticoids.

Unfortunately, there is strong indirect evidence that glucocorticoid therapy is one of the major etiologic factors for the development of severe post-transplantation osteoporosis.[6] The first 6 months after transplantation is the period with the highest rate of bone loss and the highest incidence of fractures; it is also the time interval in which the highest doses of glucocorticoids are administered. Several studies on dynamic changes of bone mass after liver transplantation support the observation that bone loss after transplantation predominantly occurs during the first 6 months, with a more variable course afterward, resulting in recovery of some bone mass. Porayko et al. reported that fractures occurred predominantly within a short time period after transplantation: 57% of the fractures occurred within the first 6 months, 24% between 6 and 12 months, and only 19% developed more than 12 months after transplantation.[7]

> Bone loss after transplantation occurs predominantly during the first 6 months when corticosteroid doses are highest.

It has been suggested that initially, increased bone resorption after transplantation may be related to the effect that glucocorticoids exert on the synthesis of osteoprotegerin (OPG), decreasing its expression by osteoblasts leading to increased bone resorption.[8] Osteoprotegerin is a decoy receptor for the RANK ligand (RANKL) and is produced by several cell types including osteoblasts and arterial cells. OPG blocks the RANK-RANKL signaling pathway, inhibiting osteoclastogenesis and osteoclast function resulting in a decrease in bone turnover. Hofbauer et al. assessed the effects of glucocorticoids on OPG and RANKL expression in human osteoblastic lineage cells, and found that dexamethasone inhibited OPG and stimulated RANKL production by osteoblastic lineage cells, indicating a potential mechanism for glucocorticoid-induced bone loss with further evidence suggesting that OPG has a role in the development of post-transplantation osteoporosis.

> In early phases, when corticosteroid doses are high, there is suppression of osteoblastic-mediated bone formation and an increase in osteoclastic bone resorption. Later, when corticosteroid doses are low, there is an increase in bone formation with recoupling of bone remodeling.

Another category of widely used immunosuppressants are the calcineurin inhibitors cyclosporine (CsA) and tacrolimus. These drugs have a significant impact on preventing organ rejection and preserving life. One of the drawbacks to their use, however, is their propensity to cause rapid and profound bone loss. CsA and tacrolimus are inhibitors of calcineurin. They require binding to intracellular proteins—CsA to cyclophilins and tacrolimus to

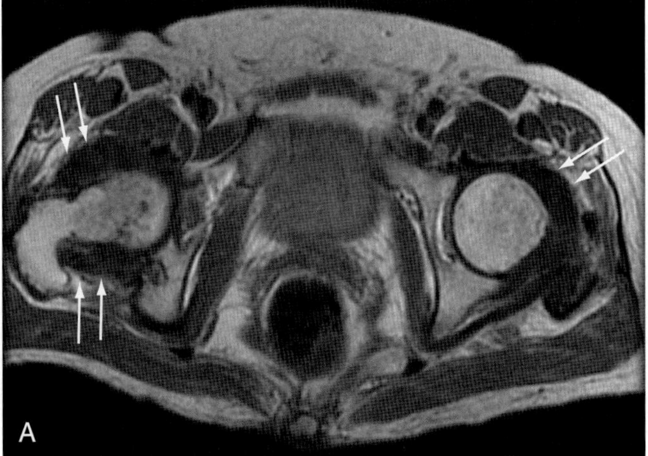

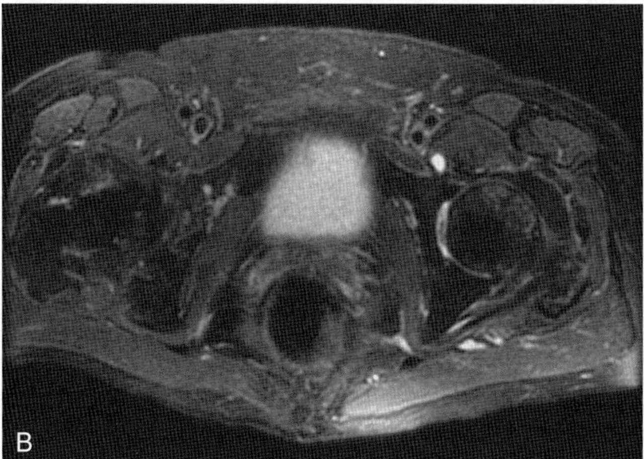

FIGURE 41-1. Beta 2 microglobulin amyloid. This 71-year-old woman complained of left hip pain 16 months after renal transplantation. **A,** T1W axial image of the hips shows intermediate signal tissue *(arrows)* distending the hip joints bilaterally. **B,** Axial STIR image at the same level as **A** shows that the tissue distending the hips is low in signal. A small amount of bright joint fluid is also present.

FK binding proteins. The resulting complexes inhibit the intracellular phosphatase calcineurin, which prevents transcription of T-lymphocyte cytokine genes and genes that control membrane molecules such as CD40 ligand. Calcineurin is a serine-threonine phosphatase that is uniquely regulated by calcium and calmodulin. Calcineurin interacts with nuclear factor of activated T cells (NF-AT), which constitute a family of transcription factors necessary for activation of genes involved in the inflammatory and immune system. Thus, inhibiting calcineurin, CsA and tacrolimus prevents activation of NF-AT with consequent inhibition of growth and differentiation of T lymphocytes critical to the immune response.[9]

It has become evident that T cells are implicated in bone remodeling and that they appear to be a prerequisite for the development of CsA-induced osteopenia. T-lymphocyte numbers and subsets are altered, and decreased T-lymphocyte populations have been associated with increased osteoclast formation, producing increased bone turnover with predominant resorption over formation resulting in a decreased bone mineral density (BMD). Calcineurin promotes T-cell growth and differentiation, which induces osteoblast activation.[10]

Guo et al. proposed a model in which bone loss after transplantation results from an increase in the rate of bone turnover in association with remodeling imbalance.[11] This imbalance is in part a consequence of the inhibition of bone formation by glucocorticoids, and it is likely that this is a result of an increase in the rate of osteoblast apoptosis. This model applies to the early post-transplantation period, since the later phase of transplantation-related bone loss does not include the effects of glucocorticoids.

> Doses of corticosteroids are usually sharply reduced after the first 6 months and may be stopped 1 to 2 years after surgery.[12]

> Proposed mechanisms to explain elevated bone turnover late after transplantation involve a decrease in glomerular filtration rate and subsequent elevation in creatinine resulting in an increase in osteocalcin, a persistently elevated PTH, as well as changes in serum calcium and decrease in calcitriol.[11,13,14]

The increase in bone turnover after transplantation may result from a number of factors, including hypogonadism, immunosuppressants such as cyclosporine, and increased parathyroid hormone (PTH) secretion.[11] Hypogonadism is most marked in men during the first few months after transplantation. This time course would be consistent with an effect of glucocorticoids, which suppress testosterone by a direct effect on the testis and by inhibiting the secretion of gonadotrophins. There is also a decrease in the production of adrenal androgens, as shown by a decrease in dehydroepiandrosterone sulfate (DHEA-S), resulting from adrenal suppression by glucocorticoids. Testosterone has direct effects on bone formation and resorption, but more importantly, it acts as a substrate for the production of estrogen (by aromatase) and hence inhibits bone resorption. Thus, low levels of testosterone (and DHEA-S) might be expected to increase bone turnover and cause a relative reduction in bone formation.[15] The increase in PTH is multifactorial. PTH increase may be secondary to decreased renal function prior to transplant. PTH increase may be related in part to the inhibition of intestinal calcium absorption secondary to high-dose glucocorticoids and a decline in synthesis of calcitriol that is associated with renal impairment.[16,17] Although excellent immunosuppressive drugs, cyclosporine, and tacrolimus are well known to cause renal toxicity in a dose-dependent fashion.

SKELETAL PRETRANSPLANT ASSESSMENT AND TREATMENT

Optimization of skeletal health should be a priority in patients awaiting a solid organ transplant. The assessment at or around the time of transplantation should include a complete clinical evaluation with focus on any history for remote or current fractures, oligomenorrhea, and a nutritional evaluation, with estimation of calcium intake.

Laboratory tests should include a comprehensive chemistry panel with serum phosphate, liver function tests, thyroid function, 25(OH) vitamin D, testosterone in males, and estrogen in females.[4] In patients with renal failure, there should also be measurement of parathyroid hormone, which can be used as a surrogate for bone turnover. Low parathyroid hormone may predict low bone turnover and bisphosphonates have more potential to do harm in this subgroup.[18] Urinary 24-hour calcium levels to assess for hypercalciuria could be helpful. Hypercalciuria predisposes to osteoporosis, and could be improved with thiazides which reduce urinary calcium losses.[19]

A skeletal imaging file comprising anteroposterior and lateral radiographs of the thoracic and lumbar spine and DXA BMD measurements of the lumbar spine, hip, and the radius are suggested. The addition of the forearm measurement provides assessment of cortical bone density that may be affected by bone loss in hyperparathyroidism. The other sites allow assessment of trabecular bone that are especially sensitive to bone loss leading to osteoporosis.

A nutrition plan should be tailored to provide adequate calories and protein with avoidance of excess magnesium. The adjustment of calcium supplements should consider the urine calcium and PTH. The active metabolites of vitamin D are reserved for patients with malabsorption and secondary hyperparathyroidism; otherwise, 400 to 1000 IU per day of cholecalciferol are commonly administered doses.[12]

Implementing an exercise program might be challenging or not even feasible, but this should be a goal in the post-transplant stage. Evidence from two small prospective randomized trials in cardiac transplant patients and one involving lung transplant recipients showed that resistance training restored BMD toward pretransplantation levels more rapidly and in conjunction with alendronate, was more effective that alendronate alone.[20,21]

> An exercise program, if possible, is helpful in the post-transplant patient.

Pretransplant medication optimization and risk factor modification are important strategies while patients await the procedure. Adjustment and whenever possible replacement of osseous-wasting medications, such as loop diuretics for thiazides and glucocorticoid dose reduction, should be considered (see Box 41-1). Patients should be advised about avoidance of alcoholic beverages and they should eliminate any tobacco use.[4]

BONE DISEASE FOLLOWING RENAL TRANSPLANTATION

Renal osteodystrophy, the skeletal complication of end-stage renal disease, is a multifactorial disorder[22] with complex manifestations. The constellation of findings includes those due to secondary hyperparathyroidism (osteoclastic bone resorption leading to subperiosteal resorption and brown tumors), osteosclerosis, osteomalacia, osteoporosis, and soft tissue and vascular calcification).[23] As management of chronic renal disease continues to improve, the prevalence of radiologic changes of renal osteodystrophy is decreasing. For example, prior to the 1970s, when vitamin D metabolism was less well understood, deficiency in 1,25$(OH)_2$D due to renal insufficiency, which leads to defective mineralization of osteoid, was a common cause of rickets in the immature skeleton and osteomalacia in the mature skeleton. With improved vitamin D compounds, rickets and severe osteomalacia are now seen less frequently.[19]

Renal osteodystrophy refers to the bone disease seen in patients with chronic renal failure and consists of hyperparathyroidism, osteomalacia, osteosclerosis, osteoporosis, and soft tissue and vascular calcification.

Renal transplantation has become an effective treatment modality for end-stage renal disease and largely restores renal function. Consequently, some of the characteristic findings of renal osteodystrophy may no longer be seen in the post-transplant population, these patients experience persistent abnormalities of mineral metabolism. In addition, pretransplant renal osteodystrophy can significantly contribute to the maintenance or development of post-transplant alterations of bone remodeling.[24] Also, due to glucocorticoid therapy as well as other immunosuppressive drugs such as cyclosporine, tacrolimus, azathioprine, and rapamycin,[25] renal transplant recipients are at significantly increased risk for a wide range of post-transplant bone complications.

Persistent Hyperparathyroidism

Secondary hyperparathyroidism is associated with increased bone turnover and decreased overall bone density. Excess parathyroid hormone affects the ratio of osteoclasts, osteoblasts, and osteocytes,[23] leading to increased osteoclastic bone resorption.[26] After successful kidney transplantation, biochemical evidence of hyperparathyroidism persists in approximately 30% to 50% of recipients.[27] The increases in PTH may be due in part to a large glandular mass of parathyroid cells that develops during chronic renal disease and persists after renal transplantation (tertiary hyperparathyroidism).[28]

Tertiary hyperparathyroidism is characterized by relatively autonomous parathyroid function and hypercalcemia that may occur in patients with chronic renal failure and longstanding secondary hyperparathyroidism.

As in native kidney disease, some patients may develop de novo secondary hyperparathyroidism after kidney transplantation resulting from progressive functional decline of the transplanted kidney. Persistent elevations in the levels of PTH have also been associated with a longer duration of dialysis prior to transplantion.[24] Increased serum levels of PTH are regularly found until 6 months after renal transplantation. After 1 year, levels greater than twice the normal are present in more than 50% of patients, and after 2 years in 27% of patients.[25] Approximately 5% of these patients will require parathyroidectomy to alleviate the symptoms of hyperparathyroidism.[28]

The most common radiographic feature of hyperparathyroidism is bone resorption. The resorption occurs under the periosteum, or involves the cortex, subchondral bone, trabecular bone, endosteum, or ligament insertions.[22] These erosions usually occur at characteristic locations: juxta-articular, tendon/ligament insertions, skull vault, outer ends of clavicles, metaphysis, iliac margins of the sacroiliac joints, and most often, in the hands along the radial margins of the middle phalanges of the index and middle fingers. Erosions of the terminal phalanges (acro-osteolysis) may also occur.[26]

Subperiosteal bone erosion along the radial aspects of the index- and middle-finger middle phalanges and erosion of the cortices of the terminal tufts are characteristic features of hyperparathyroidism.

Osteoclastomas or brown tumors are caused by excessive osteoclastic resorption and localized replacement of bone by vascularized fibrous tissue. Cystic changes may occur due to necrosis.[23] Parathyroid hormone stimulation of osteoblasts may result in periosteal new bone formation. Hyperparathyroidism also leads to osteosclerosis caused by excess accumulation of poorly mineralized osteoid or due to an exaggerated osteoblastic response following bone resorption. Increase in bone density is usually localized to the axial skeleton where the mid-portion of the vertebral bodies are normal in density while the endplates become sclerotic, producing an appearance termed the "rugger-jersey" spine. These radiologic findings of hyperparathyroidism are typical of pretransplant renal osteodystrophy but can be seen in post-transplant patients as well. Periostitis is a rare finding that is most commonly associated with severe disease. This can be seen paralleling the humeri, femurs, tibiae, radii, ulnae, metacarpals, metatarsals, phalanges, and the pubic rami along the iliopectineal line.[23]

Additionally and most importantly, elevated rates of bone turnover and excessive bone resorption due to secondary hyperparathyroidism in the post-transplant patient may be one of several important contributing factors to progressive loss of bone mass and increased fracture risk.[29]

Osteoporosis

Trabecular bone biopsies of post-transplant patients reveal many factors contributing to decreased BMD and subsequent increased fracture risk.[27] Of the spectrum of metabolic bone abnormalities, osteoporosis is one of the most prominent findings in post-transplant patients.

Osteoporosis is defined by the World Health Organization as a progressive systemic disease characterized by low bone density and microarchitectural deterioration of bone tissue, with a consequent increase in bone fragility and susceptibility to fracture.[30]

Estimated rates of bone loss are reported of up to 6.8% during the first year after transplantation.[25] While some studies suggest this early rapid bone loss is a transient phenomenon, more recent data suggest bone loss continues after the first transplant year with ongoing bone loss found in up to 88% of long-term renal transplant patients with stable renal function.[29] Rapid bone loss within the first 6 to 12 months following renal transplantation is thought to be due primarily to corticosteroid use and the resulting low bone turnover.[31] Immunosuppressive agents used to prevent rejection including cyclosporine A and tacrolimus are now believed to be important risk factors for osteoporosis as well. Both these drugs are shown to cause high-turnover bone loss in animal studies thought to be mediated by cytokines IL-1 and IL-6, which play a major role in the bone resorptive process.

In the initial post-transplant period, when doses of glucocorticoids are high, the corticosteroid effect may predominate, leading to a low bone turnover state. After the first year, maintenance glucocorticoids are relatively low which may allow the high-turnover state induced by cyclosporine or tacrolimus to predominate.[29]

Decreased BMD places transplant patients at a high risk for fractures particularly involving vertebral bodies, ribs and hips, areas rich in trabecular bone. It is estimated that approximately 44% of patients who are at least 5 years post-transplant suffer from osteoporosis-related fractures.[27] Relative to patients with impaired renal function undergoing dialysis, renal transplantation is associated with a 34% greater risk of hip fracture up to 630 days following the transplant.[32]

Renal transplant patients are at risk for osteoporotic fractures in areas of predominantly trabecular bone, such as the vertebral bodies, ribs, and hips.

The spine and proximal femur are two sites rich in trabecular bone and, therefore, most at risk for osteoporotic fracture. Radiographically, osteoporotic bone demonstrates decreased density with relatively thin cortices and a reduced number of trabeculae. In the spine, there is predominant loss of transverse trabeculae and prominence of vertical trabeculae producing a striated appearance. Vertebral deformities are described as biconcave, crush or wedge deformity.[33] These fractures may be detected on radiographs, however, their chronicity may be difficult to determine. Magnetic resonance imaging (MRI) with fluid-sensitive sequences can help differentiate acute from chronic osteoporotic fractures, with acute fractures demonstrating bone marrow edema on fluid-sensitive sequences and increased signal on diffusion-weighted sequences if obtained.

Acute osteoporotic fractures will exhibit edema signal on fluid-sensitive MRI sequences.

Similarly, if radiographs are indeterminate in cases of suspected hip fracture, MRI is a useful next step. Hip fractures that are occult on radiographs, may demonstrate a linear low signal fracture line on T1 or proton-density MRI sequences with accompanying bone marrow edema on fluid-sensitive sequences indicating acute fracture. If MRI cannot be obtained, radionuclide scintigraphy can be diagnostic by demonstrating increased radiotracer uptake in the area of suspected fracture.

Quantitative measurement of BMD is recommended to assess patient risk and plan any necessary treatment. Dual-energy x-ray absorptiometry (DXA scanning) can be performed in clinically relevant sites such as the lumbar spine, proximal femur, and forearm. Quantitative computed tomography (QCT) is a technology that is most often performed for assessment of spine density.[26] The National Kidney Foundation recommends DXA scanning at the time of renal transplantation and at 6 months, 1 year, and 2 years post-transplant.[27] In patients with a "rugger jersey" pattern of vertebral sclerosis from renal osteodystrophy, examination of the spine may be of limited benefit.

DXA scanning is recommended at the time of renal transplantation and at 6 months, 1 year, and 2 years after renal transplantation.

In patients with significantly low bone-mineral density, antiresorptive drugs including bisphosphonates or calcitonin have been suggested depending on the clinical picture and renal function. There is concern that bisphosphonates may lead to adynamic bone disease, however, and some authors use them only for the first postoperative year.[34] Low doses of active vitamin D derivatives and calcium via calcium carbonate have also been shown to prevent bone loss in the lumbar spine and proximal femur when given for the first 6 months after transplantation.[25] Other preventive measures to reduce the risk of osteoporotic fracture include the use of low corticosteroid doses for a limited time in the pretransplant period in patients with end-stage renal disease (ESRD) awaiting transplantation, 30 minutes of vigorous daily physical exercise, limiting alcohol or nicotine consumption, and treating non–transplant-associated risk factors for osteoporosis.[25]

Post-Transplant, Distal-Limb, Bone-Marrow Edema Syndrome

Debilitating musculoskeletal pain is seen in up to one-third of patients following renal transplantation.[35] Osteoporosis related fractures caused by immunosuppressive therapy with corticosteroids have been recognized as the most common causative factor producing bone pain after transplantation.

Debilitating musculoskeletal pain is seen in up to one-third of patients following renal transplantation.

In the last decade, however, an unusual pain syndrome in the lower limbs has been reported with increasing frequency. Symptoms are characterized by episodes of severe bilateral distal lower limb pain occurring within the first 2 years after transplantation with most episodes occurring in the first several months after surgery and persisting for weeks to months.[36] Patients describe worsening pain with physical stress such as walking. Patients also have elevation in their serum alkaline phosphatase. The first description of this entity relating the pain syndrome to cyclosporine therapy in renal-transplant recipients was reported by Lucas et al. in 1991.[35] Since then, the symptoms have been found most commonly in patients treated with cyclosporine and tacrolimus, and the syndrome is frequently referred to as calcineurin-inhibitor–induced pain syndrome (CIPS). However, recently cases have been reported in patients not on calcineurin inhibitors leading to renaming of the condition as post-transplant, distal-limb, bone marrow edema syndrome. While the pathogenesis is still uncertain, post-transplant, distal-limb bone marrow edema is often associated with high calcineurin-inhibitor levels and reduction of calcineurin-inhibitor doses or other immunosuppressive drugs has been shown to alleviate symptoms.[35] One hypothesis points to a calcineurin-inhibitor–induced vasculitis leading to increased bone perfusion and permeability, ultimately resulting in bone marrow edema and pain.[35] Microscopic fractures with marrow edema and alterations of pain threshold have also been suggested as possible etiologies.[25]

CIPS (calcineurin-inhibitor–induced pain syndrome), also called "post-transplant, distal-limb, bone marrow edema syndrome" refers to bone pain that occurs in the distal lower limbs of patients after transplantation.

Radiographic findings of post-transplant, distal-limb, bone marrow edema syndrome include a normal initial appearance or nonspecific diffuse or patchy osteoporosis. Bone scintigraphy demonstrates increased radiotracer uptake on all three phases of the bone scan with an unusually symmetric accumulation of tracer on the late phase in the clinically affected areas.[36] MRI findings can be striking with patchy bone marrow edema (poorly defined low-signal intensity on T1-weighted MRI sequences and high-signal intensity on T2-weighted sequences), which can include the entire involved bone,[36] and may extend from the epiphyseal to the metaphyseal regions of long bones.[37] Insufficiency fractures (low-signal lines within the edematous regions) may also be present (Figure 41-2).

The differential diagnosis for post-transplant musculoskeletal pain is extensive. An algorithmic approach can be helpful to

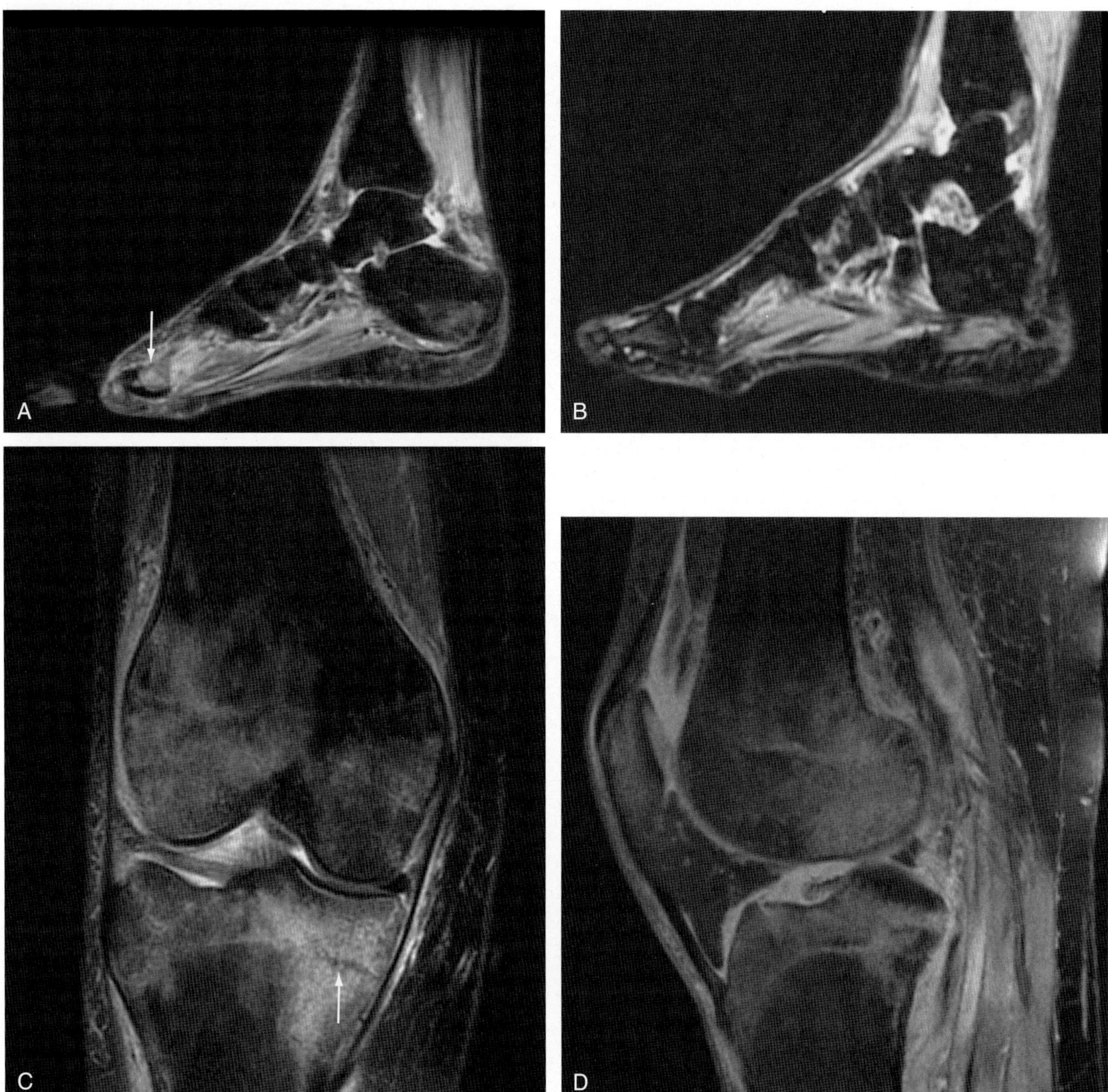

FIGURE 41-2. Post-transplant distal limb bone marrow edema syndrome. Fifty-three-year-old woman 11 months after renal transplantation, taking tacrolimus. **A,** Sagittal STIR image of the foot shows increased signal in the first metatarsal head *(arrow)*. There is bright edema signal in the adjacent soft tissues. **B,** Sagittal STIR image obtained at a slightly different level than **A,** after symptoms subsided, shows return of normal low signal fat in the medullary cavity of the first metatarsal. **C,** Coronal STIR MRI shows increased (bright) signal replacing the normally low signal *(dark)* marrow. The bright signal is consistent with edema. A low signal line suggests an insufficiency fracture *(arrow)*. There is also soft tissue edema. **D,** The sagittal STIR MRI shows similar bone-marrow edema-like signal. There is a joint effusion.

(Continued)

determine the next appropriate diagnostic step by first assessing the clinical picture and separating symptoms into unilateral versus bilateral lower extremity pain as outlined by Wolfgang et al. in Figure 41-3.

Gout, fracture, and Morton's neuroma are important causes of unilateral symptoms to exclude. Reflex sympathetic dystrophy is often asymmetrical. Bilateral symmetrical bone pain can be caused by polyneuropathy, hyperparathyroidism, and osteonecrosis (avascular necrosis). The MRI appearance can help differentiate bone marrow edema syndrome from these other causes of symmetric musculoskeletal pain. For example, the typical changes of avascular necrosis on MRI include a focal lesion outlined by a "double-line sign" (serpentine increased signal on T2-weighted sequences in conjunction with a more peripheral thin, serpentine low-signal line). This sign is not demonstrated in patients with bone marrow edema syndrome.[37] The clinical findings of weight-bearing pain, commonly localized to the hip with a history of corticosteroid treatment, is also suggestive of avascular necrosis.[35] However, bone marrow edema itself is a nonspecific finding and only when associated with bilateral lower limb pain, an otherwise near normal

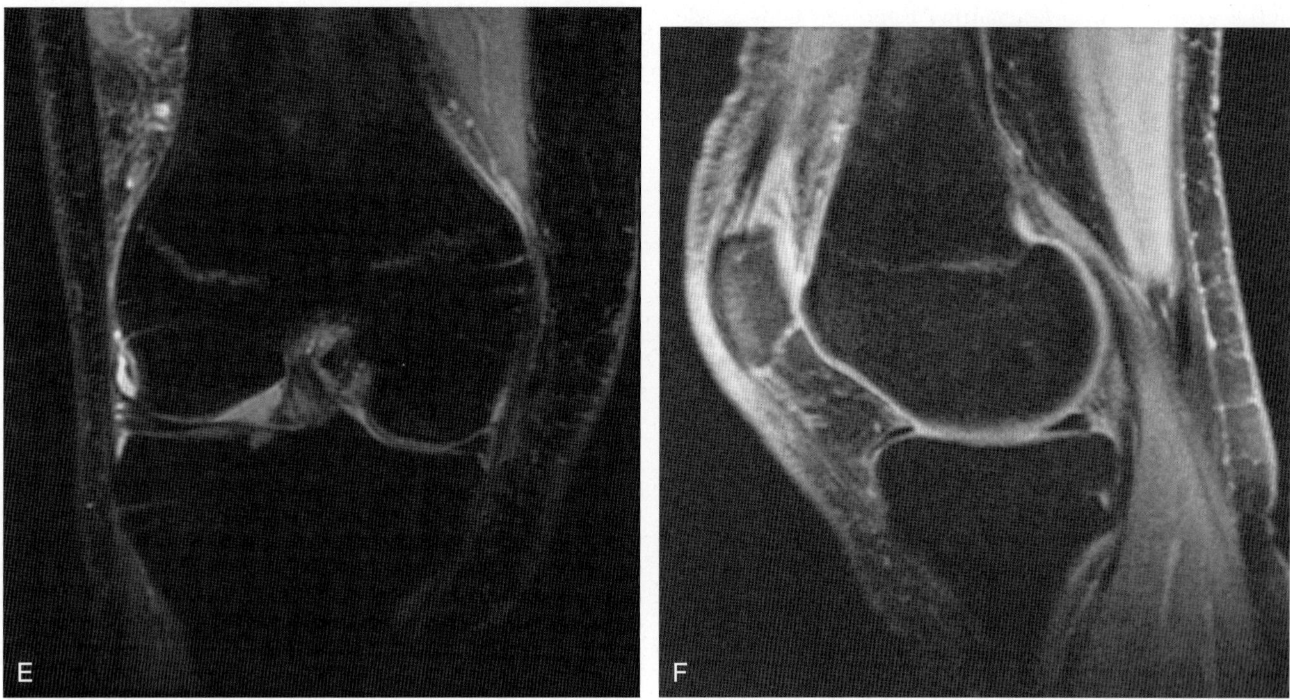

FIGURE 41-2—cont'd. **E,** Coronal STIR image 6 months later shows return to normal signal intensity in the femur and tibia. **F,** The sagittal STIR image shows the decreased effusion.

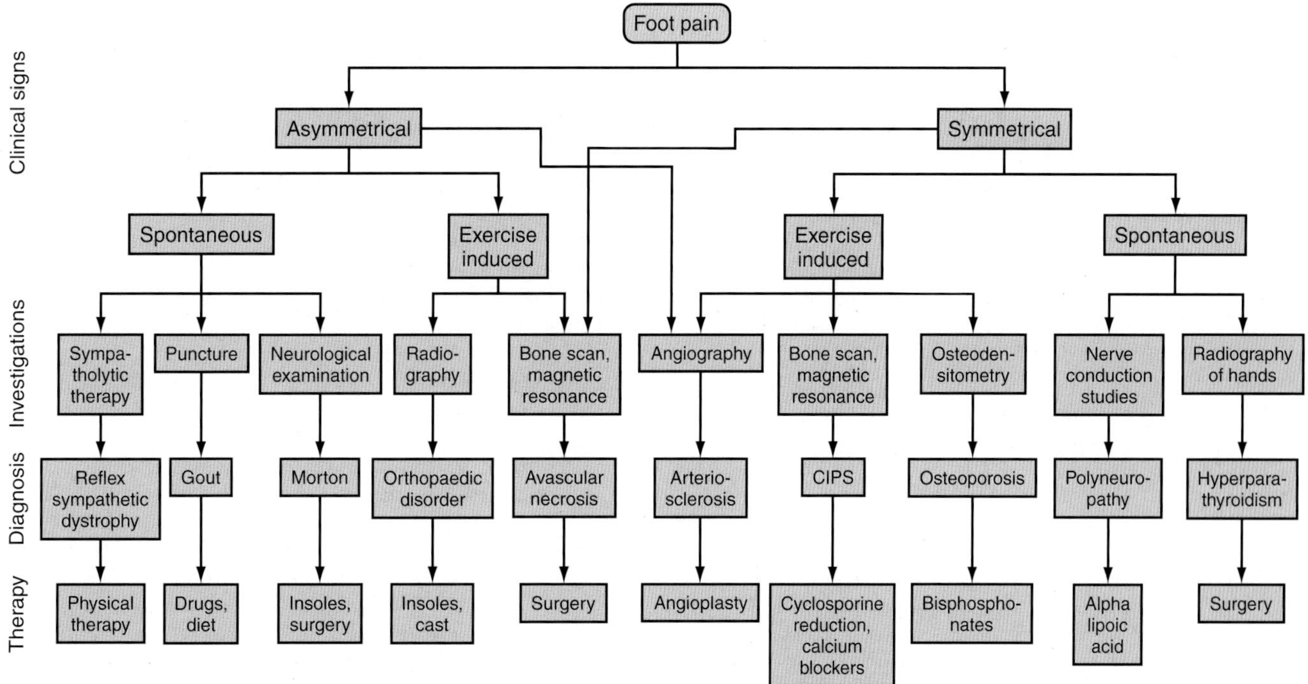

FIGURE 41-3. Diagnostic and therapeutic algorithm of foot pain in post transplantation patients. From Wolfgang, by permission.

physical examination, low cumulative corticosteroid doses and high cyclosporine or tacrolimus levels in a postrenal transplant patient can the diagnosis of post-transplant, distal-limb bone marrow edema be suggested.[36]

Reduction of cyclosporine or tacrolimus or other immunosuppressive doses generally provides symptomatic relief within 3 months[37] with eventual resolution of MRI changes as well. Calcium channel blockers such as nifedipine or nitrendipine or the synthetic analog of prostacyclin PGI_2, iloprost, have been suggested to hasten pain relief and provide a prophylactic effect. Leg rest and elevation are recommended.[35]

Osteonecrosis (Avascular Necrosis)

As previously suggested, avascular necrosis (osteonecrosis) is an important cause of musculoskeletal pain complicating the care of renal transplant recipients. Avascular necrosis most commonly occurs in the femoral heads but can be seen with frequency in the knees, humeral heads, femoral condyles, capitella, tali, and carpal bones. Bilateral lesions are identified in up to half of presenting patients.[38] The prevalence of osteonecrosis of the femoral head has decreased in recent years from approximately 20% to 5%.[39] This is primarily due to reduction in corticosteroid dosing with the availability of corticosteroid-sparing anticalcineurin agents.[40] In addition to corticosteroids, other proposed causative factors of avascular necrosis include post-transplant body-weight gain,[41] long duration of pretransplant dialysis, liver disease and secondary hyperparathyroidism,[42] blood urea nitrogen level, and hypofibrinolysis.[43]

Radiographic signs of osteonecrosis within the femoral or humeral head include a thin fracture line within the subchondral bone parallel to the articular surface representing an osteochondral fracture (the "crescent sign") and sclerosis or osteopenia of the femoral head bordered by a sclerotic line. (See chapter 16 on avascular necrosis for greater detail.) Later, collapse of the articular surface with flattening and irregularity of the underlying bone is seen as the lesion progresses. Within the knee, osteonecrosis often involves the weight-bearing portion of the femoral condyles; irregularity, sclerosis, and subchondral fracture with separate bone fragments can be seen.[44] Radiographic evaluation may be normal at the early stages, however. Therefore, magnetic resonance imaging is recommended for patients with persistent hip, knee, or shoulder pain in order to detect early disease. Once the radiograph shows flattening or cartilage space narrowing, treatment options are limited to total joint arthroplasty.[38]

MRI findings of avascular necrosis include crescentic areas of low signal intensity along the weight-bearing portion of the femoral head and collapse of the femoral head.[42] The previously described "double-line sign" refers to a dark band with a high-signal-intensity inner margin on T2-weighted MR images. The dark line represents the demarcation between necrotic and viable bone, edged by an inner hyperintense rim of granulation tissue and is seen in up to 80% of patients with avascular necrosis (Figure 41-4).[45]

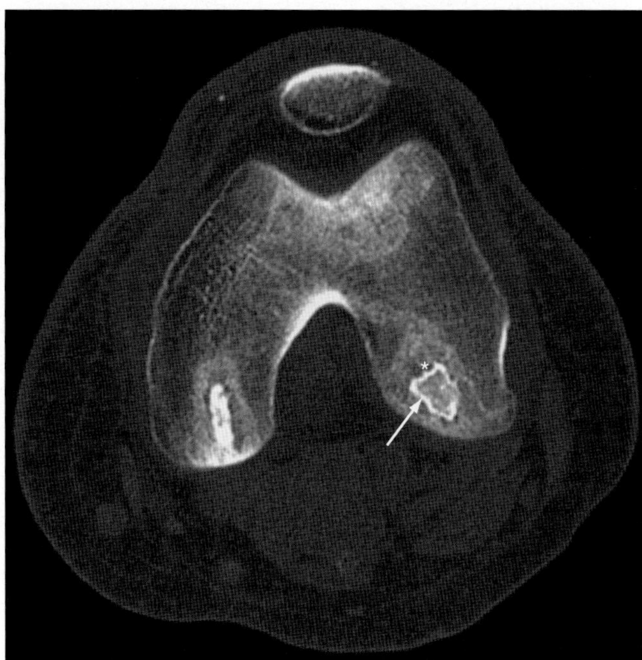

FIGURE 41-4. CT of infarction. This 50-year-old woman underwent lung transplantation many years before and renal transplantation in 2003. An axial CT scan through the femoral condyles shows characteristic findings of marrow infarction with a serpentine zone of sclerosis *(arrow)* in each femoral condyle. Adjacent lucency *(asterisk)* is likely granulation tissue, which is bordered by another thin dense line.

Renal Transplant–Associated Gout

The development of new-onset gout following renal transplantation is not uncommon, occurring in up to 7.6% of patients 3 years after transplant.[46] The painful symptoms of gout can be debilitating. In addition, gout is associated with an increased risk of graft loss and even death in the post-transplant population.[46]

Gout is caused by an inflammatory reaction to monosodium urate crystals in joint fluid and periarticular tissue. Increased production of uric acid or reduced excretion can predispose to gout with a concentration of uric acid over 7 mg/dl favoring the spontaneous crystallization of monosodium urate. Cyclosporine leads to a reduction in renal urate clearance, and the resulting hyperuricemia may be the most important risk factor for the development of gout in this population.[47] Calcineurin inhibitors such as tacrolimus have also been found to cause hyperuricemia; however, patients receiving cyclosporine are at a significantly higher risk for developing gout than patients prescribed tacrolimus.[46] Post-transplant renal insufficiency has also been identified as an independent risk factor for new-onset gout due to the subsequent hyperuricemia caused by renal insufficiency.[46]

> New-onset gout is not uncommon following renal transplantation.

The symptoms of gout may manifest within months to years following transplantation and can present as either monoarticular or oligoarticular disease. As in the general population, gout is typically seen in the first metatarsophalangeal joint as well as the wrists, knees, and elbows. On radiographs, osseous lesions are classically described as punched-out lytic lesions with an overhanging margin.[48] Soft tissue tophi are present adjacent to the erosions. More proximal distribution of gouty arthritis involving the hips, shoulders, and sacroiliac joints has also been described in post-transplant patients as well as extra-articular presentations including tenosynovitis of the dorsum of the foot and ankle.[47]

Uric-acid–lowering therapy should be initiated in post-transplant patients suffering from gout and in patients with a history of hyperuricemia or gout at the time of transplantation once cyclosporine has been initiated. Treatment options are similar to those in the general population with close monitoring of renal function in the post-transplant group as well as attention to increased risk of certain drug-related complications such as the increased risk of neuropathy, a side effect of colchicine, in post-transplant patients.[47]

BONE DISEASE FOLLOWING LIVER TRANSPLANTATION

In the past two decades, liver transplantation has become an established and effective therapy for end-stage liver diseases. Survival probability averaged 82% in the United States from 2002 to 2004 for all causes, reaching over 90% for cholestatic diseases such as primary biliary cirrhosis (PBC), and remains high at 3 years with a 72.5% graft survival rate.[49] Long-term complications not related to graft dysfunction have become more relevant as patients not only live longer, but pursue a higher quality of life. Among these, the most important extrahepatic complication following hepatic transplantation is bone disease, characterized by bone pain, osteoporosis, avascular necrosis, and fractures.[2,50,51]

In the study of Navasa et al., bone pain occurred in 58% of liver transplant recipients, and was one of the most important factors leading to a decrease in the perception of life quality.[2] Since then, multiple studies have identified osseous disease as a major burden in the recovery of patients after undergoing solid-organ transplantation.[16,52-56]

Risk Factors and Predictors of Fracture

At the beginning of the 1990s, it was noticed by Porayko et al. and Eastell et al. that patients with cholestatic diseases carried a higher risk for fractures than patients with other liver diseases such as alcoholic cirrhosis or infectious hepatitis, such as hepatitis B (HBV) and hepatitis C (HCV).[7,57] Further studies reported that patients with primary sclerosing cholangitis (PSC) and PBC had lower BMD than those with noncholestatic diseases.[51] Low BMD was one of the first risk factors identified in a group of patients more likely to suffer a fracture. Long-term immobilization, hypogonadism, malnutrition, and previous osteodystrophy were subsequently found to be additional characteristics present in liver recipient patients that placed them at greater risk for bone disease.[3] In addition, women requiring a liver transplant develop more fractures than men. This has been associated with the lower weight and decreased BMD seen in this patient population. As for osteoporosis, no statistically significant difference has been found thus far between the genders.[3,50]

Age at transplant has had a mixed association with the risk of fractures and osteoporosis development. No difference was found among age groups in patients with osteoporosis. However, menopausal status was found to be of greater significance among women with osteoporosis, compared to those with osteopenia or normal BMD. Thus, fewer fractures were present in the premenopausal (13.3%) versus postmenopausal patients (36.6%) after liver transplantation.[3] The risk of fracture increased by 7% with every 5-year increase in the post-transplant stage (regardless of the gender or menopausal status), but this did not reach statistical significance.[50]

Post-Transplantation Fracture Risk

The various immunosuppressive regimens have been among the post-transplantation factors that contribute to fracture risk. When studying groups of patients taking glucocorticoids versus cyclosporine, who had presented with fracture, no significant difference was found on daily or cumulative dosages of either immunosuppressive regime.[7,50,57] However, there has been a difference reported among the fracture rate of patients receiving tacrolimus versus cyclosporin, with the former having lower fracture rates than the latter (5% versus 20%).[50] Although appealing, this effect has not been constant and further studies are warranted to assess whether patients receiving tacrolimus will have a lower rate of bone complications, without compromising allograft function. The effect of other newer immunosuppressants, such as sirolimus or mycophenolate mofetil, on fracture incidence has not yet been established and, although currently in use, their effect on bone metabolism remains to be elucidated.[58,59]

As with renal transplantation, the highest rate of bone loss and the highest incidence of fractures occurs in the first 4 to 6 months following transplantation. This is also the time interval in which the highest dosages of glucocorticoids are used. Multiple studies have found a direct relationship between glucocorticoid dosages and changes in bone mass.[60,61] Thereafter, it appears that bone density starts to recover and may reach pretransplant levels at the end of the first year.[2,50] In the first transplant year, fracture incidence was estimated at 22%.[16] By the second and third years, the fracture prevalence reaches up to 27% and 33%, respectively.[62,63]

The fracture pattern and distribution are similar to those of postmenopausal osteoporosis: most wedge fractures were found in the thoracic spine and in the first lumbar vertebra, and most biconcave fractures were present in the lumbar spine. Besides the vertebral fractures, 7% of patients experienced nonvertebral fractures.[50] One-third of patients with a fracture suffered multiple fractures. No bone necrosis was found in liver transplant recipients.[50] A similar rate of nonvertebral fractures was described within a small group of patients after liver transplantation,[64] in which 6% (3 of 49 patients) suffered a limb fracture, but only 4% (2 of 49 patients) suffered a vertebral fracture within 2 years of follow-up after transplantation.

Prevention

After transplantation, regimens for prevention of fractures and osteoporosis have traditionally included supplementation of calcium (1000 mg/day) and vitamin D (400 to 1000 IU/day). Androgenic/estrogen hormone replacement, sodium fluoride, calcitonin, or bisphosphonates have been used with mixed responses, and further evaluation and follow-up are needed to assess their specific benefit. All patients scheduled for liver transplantation must be considered at high risk for developing incident fractures after transplantation.

BONE DISEASE FOLLOWING CARDIAC TRANSPLANTATION

There were 2016 heart transplants performed in the United States in 2004.[65] As of July 15, 2005, the 1-year survival rate for males and females was 86.4% and 84.6%, respectively, and it approached 72% and 68.5% at 5 years.[65] Compared to other solid organ transplants, heart transplant recipients have remarkable short- and long-term survival rates, making transplantation a well-established therapy for end-stage heart disease.

The current immunosuppressive regimes and the predisposing risk factors particular to cardiac conditions put these transplant patients at increased risk for osteoporosis, fractures and bone pain. As with other transplant recipients, these complications can significantly affect the quality of life and have become a management challenge.

Pretransplant Assessment and Risk Factors

Cardiac patients are usually exposed to loop diuretics, heparin, or warfarin, and have poor mobility and reduced levels of vitamin D. Each of these factors has proved to increase the risk for osteoporosis and subsequent fractures. Furosemide can cause prerenal azotemia and renal insufficiency, which are related to decreased 1-alpha hydroxylase activity and reduced synthesis of vitamin D, as well as hyperparathyroidism.[2] In addition to this, loop diuretics increase urinary calcium loss and have been associated with increased fracture risk.[66,67] Long-term use of anticoagulants, either heparin or warfarin, could also contribute to bone loss and has been linked to vertebral fractures.[68-70] Warfarin, in particular, blocks vitamin K–dependent gamma carboxylation of osteocalcin and affects its binding to calcium.[70] This risk factor was corroborated in the study of Caraballo et al. where long-term exposure to oral anticoagulation was an independent predictor of vertebral and rib fractures.[54,71]

It is known that immobility and physical inactivity may lead not only to decreased bone remodeling and osteopenia, but also to less sunlight exposure with consequent low 25-OHD levels, therefore putting these patients at an increased risk for osteopenia, osteoporosis, and osteomalacia. Vitamin D deficiency, as summarized by Holick, causes osteopenia precipitates and exacerbates osteoporosis, causes the painful bone disease osteomalacia, and increases muscle weakness, which worsens the risk of falls and fractures.[72] Evaluations of BMD in patients with severe congestive heart failure have proved that low BMD is significant in this patient population with osteopenia and osteoporosis present in 43% and 7% of patients, respectively.[5,73]

Post-Transplantation Bone Disease

During the first year after heart transplantation, the reported bone loss of nearly 10%[74] is high compared with a mean bone loss of 0.53% per year for healthy women and 0.3% for healthy men[75,76] (Figure 41-5). Two to 4 years after transplantation, 28% of cardiac recipients treated with 1000 mg/day of calcium and 50,000 IU/week of vitamin D had documented lumbar spine osteoporosis.[50] In untreated patients, the rate was 41%.[77] The prevalence of vertebral fractures in this transplant population is 22% to 42%[77] with an incidence ranging from 15% to 36% in the first year[50,74,78] (Figure 41-6). After that, the rates decrease or remain constant

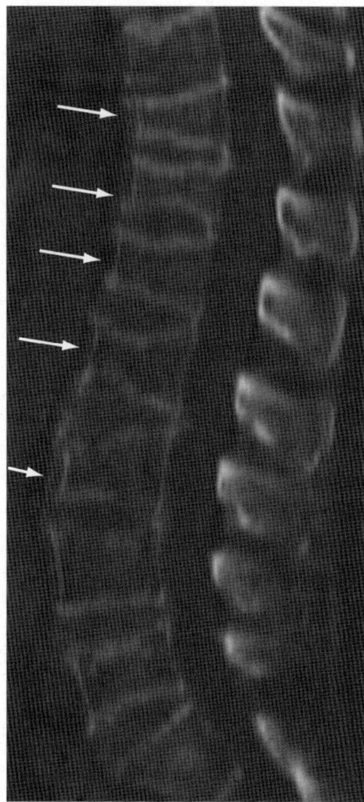

FIGURE 41-5. CT demonstrating compression fractures after heart transplantation. This 67-year-old woman presented with back pain 7 months after heart transplantation. The sagittal, reformatted CT scan shows multiple vertebral fractures *(arrows)*. The prominent sclerosis of each endplate is a finding seen in healing fractures occurring in patients on corticosteroids.

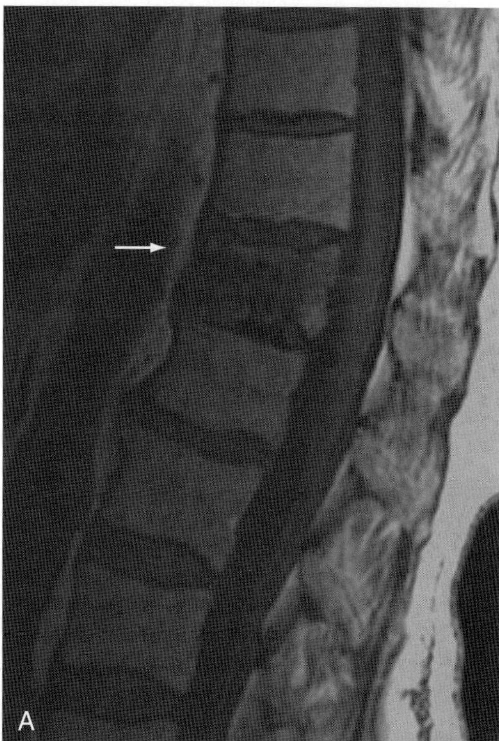

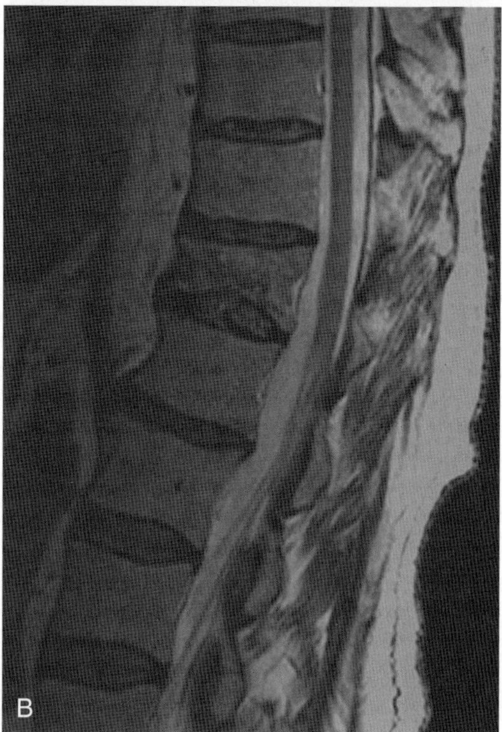

FIGURE 41-6. MRI demonstrating compression fracture after heart transplantation. This 68-year-old man presented with mid-back pain 6 months after heart transplantation. **A,** Sagittal T1W MRI shows compression of the T12 vertebral body *(arrow)*. **B,** Sagittal T2W MRI shows some edema posteriorly in the vertebral body and low signal anteriorly that may be due to the trabecular impaction.

with one-third of patients sustaining vertebral fractures by the end of the third year following transplantation.[50]

When the pretransplantation risk factors are reviewed, a lumbar spine bone mineral density (BMD) T score of less than –1 and older age confer a greater risk of vertebral fracture over a mean follow-up time of 3.7 years.[50] The relationship between fracture incidence and femoral neck BMD and age holds only for women. In male patients, those who fractured sustained significant bone loss at the femoral neck in the first 6 months.[78]

The biochemical evidence of abnormal bone turnover has been studied and two distinct phases are characteristic. An early period of rapid bone loss occurs in the first 6 months during which there is decreased bone formation and increased bone resorption.

In a cross-sectional study where patients were assessed 28 months after heart transplantation, serum osteocalcin levels were increased.[79] The authors considered the biochemical pattern to be uncharacteristic of corticosteroid-induced osteoporosis and speculated on the presence of accelerated bone loss. A few years later, the same group found biochemical evidence of suppressed bone formation and increased bone resorption during the first 6 months after transplantation.[80] Another study demonstrated that by 6 to 12 months, bone formation matched resorption in a high-turnover state.[15] Either secondary hyperparathyroidism of unknown origin or a deleterious effect of cyclosporine may be responsible for the sustained increase in bone turnover.[81]

Another investigated theory was bone loss caused by accelerated bone turnover and hypogonadism since some studies found hypogonadism in male heart transplant recipients.[11,15] Percentages of male heart transplant recipients with hypogonadism vary between 20%[19] and 52%.[82] Decreased serum testosterone early after transplantation with a later return to baseline values has been reported.[80]

Impaired renal function is observed frequently in patients after heart transplantation. One study found renal failure in 50% of its heart transplant recipients.[77] After cardiac transplantation, acute renal failure necessitating hemodialysis portends a poor outcome[83] and a higher likelihood of osseous adverse events.

There is a strong association between the development of avascular necrosis (AVN) in cardiac transplant recipients and the amount of parenterally administered high-dose corticosteroids. AVN mostly affects the femoral head as occurs in renal transplantation, however, AVN is less frequent following cardiac transplantation than after renal transplantation[84] (Figure 41-7).

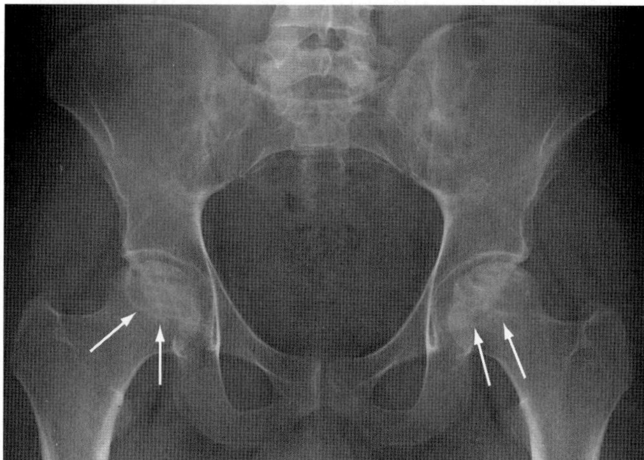

FIGURE 41-7. Bilateral avascular necrosis after heart transplantation. Twenty-one-year-old man at 27 months after heart transplantation. This anteroposterior view of both hips shows the characteristic features of avascular necrosis. The areas of lucency are delimited by a thin sclerotic reactive zone *(arrows)*. There is slight irregularity of the femoral heads bilaterally indicating early collapse.

The risk of gout is increased in cyclosporine-treated heart transplant recipients, and almost 10% of the men in this population develop gout after transplantation[85] (Figures 41-8 and 41-9).

BONE DISEASE FOLLOWING LUNG TRANSPLANTATION

The first human lung transplant was performed by James Hardy at the University of Mississippi in 1963 for an isolated cancer of the lung. The patient lived for 18 days and died of kidney failure.

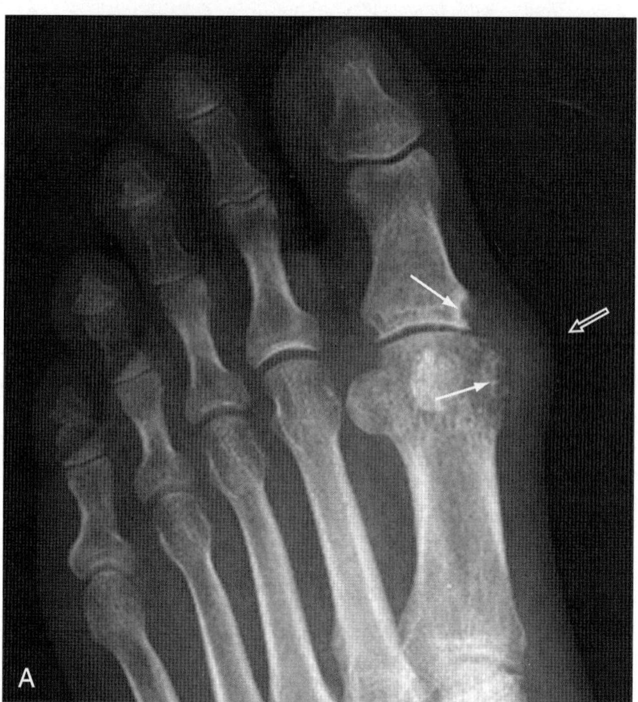

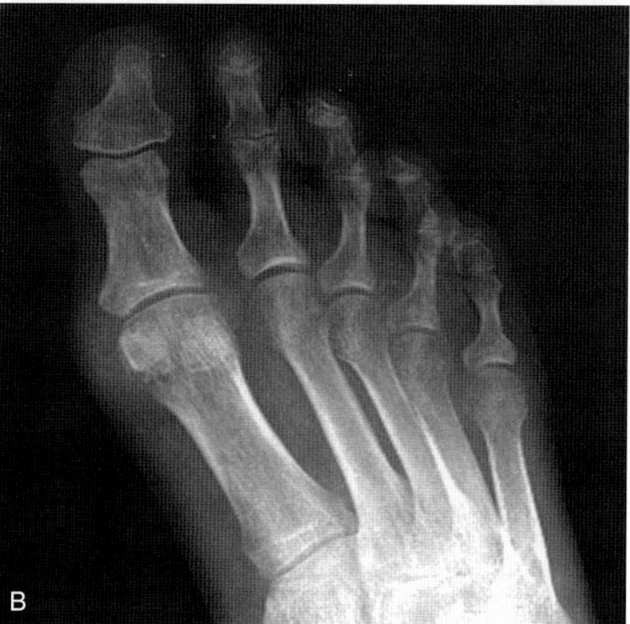

FIGURE 41-8. Gout after heart transplantation. This 55-year-old man was undergoing pretransplant care for heart transplantation. **A,** An anteroposterior oblique view of the left forefoot shows focal swelling (tophus, *open arrow*) at the great toe metatarsophalangeal (MTP) joint with accompanying erosion *(arrows)* consistent with gout. **B,** There is swelling over the right great toe MTP as well.

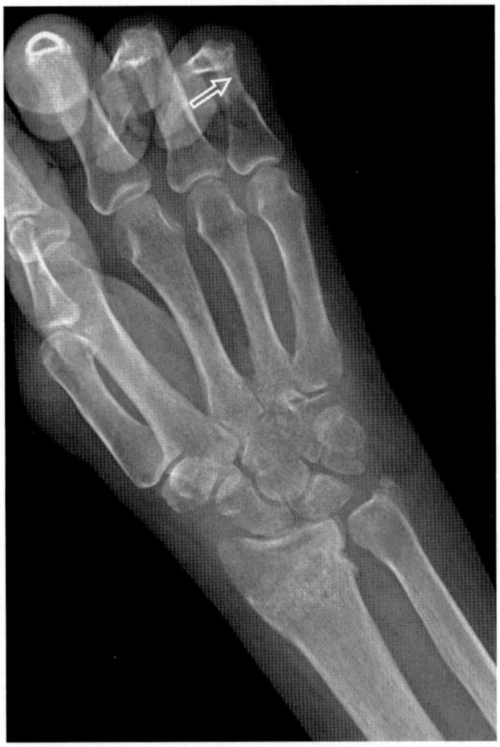

FIGURE 41-9. Gout after heart transplantation. Fifty-two-year-old man 15 years after heart transplantation. Wrist pain developed during treatment of a wrist fracture. A posteroanterior view of the hand and wrist shows a calcified tophus. There is swelling and erosion *(open arrow)* of the fifth-finger proximal interphalangeal joint and the base of the fifth metacarpal. The radiocarpal joint is mildly narrow. Fractures are present of the distal radius and ulnar styloid.

Between 1963 and 1980, about 44 transplants were performed at medical centers around the world with no real success. Most of these transplants were performed on debilitated patients as "rescue" attempts after they became ventilator-dependent. Only two recipients lived longer than 1 month. This disappointing start contributed to a halt in lung transplantation until cyclosporine was introduced in the early 1980s. Heart–lung transplantation was performed successfully in 1981 at Stanford University and became the only option for lung transplantation until lung transplantation became commonplace in the late 1980s.

The first lung transplant associated with prolonged postoperative survival was performed by Joel Cooper at the Toronto General Hospital in 1983. The patient received a right lung transplant for idiopathic pulmonary fibrosis (IPF) and survived for over 6.5 years before succumbing to renal failure. In 1986, Cooper performed the first successful double lung transplant.[86]

The 40th anniversary of the first human lung transplant was celebrated in 2003, with more than 3000 heart–lung transplants and more than 17,000 lung transplants performed in that period.

Survival rates for lung transplant are 84% at 3 months, 74% at 1 year, 58% at 3 years, and 47% at 5 years.[87] These numbers reflect the great challenge that a pulmonary transplant represents, although since 1963, great advances have been made providing patients improved exercise tolerance and quality of life.

Patients with COPD, IPF, and CF represent the leading candidates for lung transplantation in adults. They are usually between the ages of 50 and 64 years and most of them have been exposed chronically to corticosteroids and have had low physical activity. Bone loss and osteoporosis are highly prevalent and have been studied in more detail than in any other type of organ transplantation.

Standard immunosuppression includes calcineurin inhibitors, azathioprine and corticosteroids with an extremely aggressive regime after lung transplantation because the lung is considered a strongly immunogenic organ. This regime has improved the control over acute and chronic rejection, but favors the onset of complications, such as renal dysfunction. Renal dysfunction is the second most common life-threatening factor, after systemic hypertension, that occurs in lung transplant recipients. Up to 30% of lung transplant patients show renal impairment and up to 28.9% of patients require dialysis or renal transplant.[87,88]

Bone Mass Density and Pretransplantation Fracture Prevalence

The percentage of patients with normal BMD prior to lung transplantation is low, ranging from 15% to 25%, and 30% to 60% have osteoporosis.[89-92] Other associated factors that put recipients of lung transplant at risk for fractures are vitamin D deficiency, which has been observed in 20% to 36% of patients.[93]

A few studies have assessed fractures before transplantation. Shane et al.[94] found that vertebral fractures were present before transplantation in only 2 of 30 (6.7%) patients, while Cahill et al.[91] found a higher rate of prevalent vertebral or hip fractures (29%). A similar high rate of prevalent fractures was described by Aris et al.,[96] who found vertebral or rib fractures in 11 of 34 (32%) patients before lung transplantation.

Osteoporosis and Fractures Post-Transplantation

In one series, at 1 year after the procedure, 37% of lung transplant patients sustained a fracture.[94] This in spite of being treated with calcium and vitamin D supplementation. The most prevalent sites were vertebral, rib, and sacral fractures and the average time to first fracture was about 4 to 5 months after transplantation[94] (Figures 41-10 through 41-15). Surprisingly, the rate of bone loss was relatively low (1.3% to 2.8% in the lumbar spine and femoral neck), and the number of fractures was strongly predicted by the time patients had been on glucocorticoids and the preprocedure BMD.

Other studies[91,93,96] have shown that patients treated with IV pamidronate only had a 5% to 19% fracture incidence, independent of their BMD value before transplantation. In these populations, subjects also received calcium and vitamin D supplementation, and HRT was given in cases of recognized hypogonadism. After the intervention, the BMD remained stable or increased in 76% (16 of 21) of the patients at 1 year.

Shane et al. found that the mean duration of glucocorticoid use was 4.9 years in fractured patients and 1.3 years in patients without fractures.[89] Furthermore, markers of bone turnover at baseline were higher in patients with fractures. There were no differences in fractures with respect to age, rates of bone loss, rejection episodes, or glucocorticoid dosages after transplantation.[94]

A high incident rate of compression vertebral and nonvertebral fractures is seen among untreated lung-transplant patients. This, as well as the prevalent preprocedural low bone density, highlight the importance of identifying these potential risk factors, as key

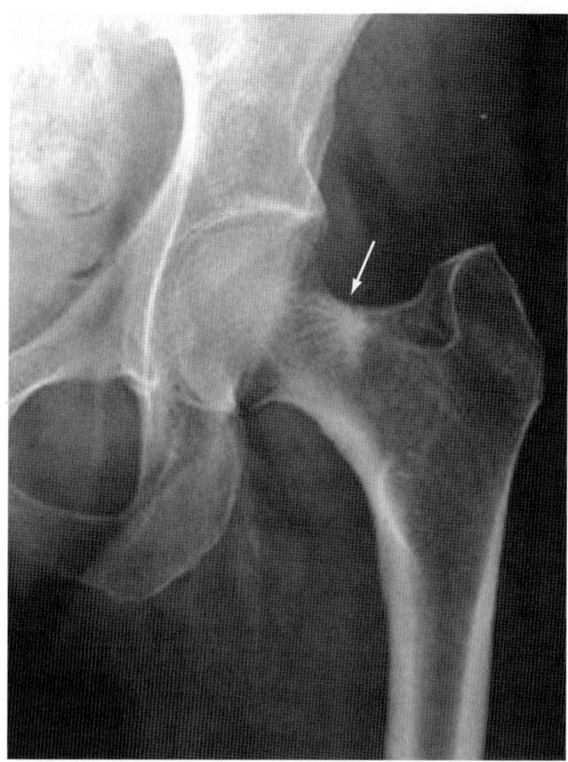

FIGURE 41-10. Femoral neck insufficiency fracture after lung transplantation. This 46-year-old woman developed inability to bear weight 9 years after a lung transplant. An anteroposterior view of the left hip shows a small linear area of lucency with adjacent sclerosis *(arrow)*. The location of this insufficiency fracture on the tension side of the bone is uncommon. (Courtesy of Anne L. Fuhlbrigge, MD.)

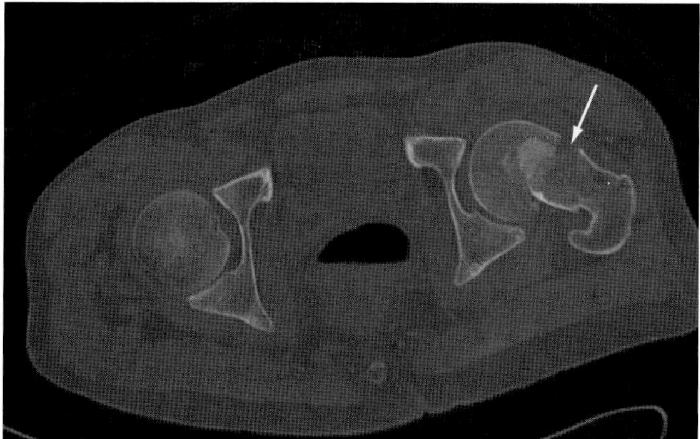

FIGURE 41-11. Femoral neck fracture in a lung transplant recipient. This 30-year-old man suffered a seizure and possible trauma, 6 months after lung transplantation. Axial CT image shows a complete fracture through the subcapital region of the left femur *(arrow)*. (Courtesy of Anne L. Fuhlbrigge, MD.)

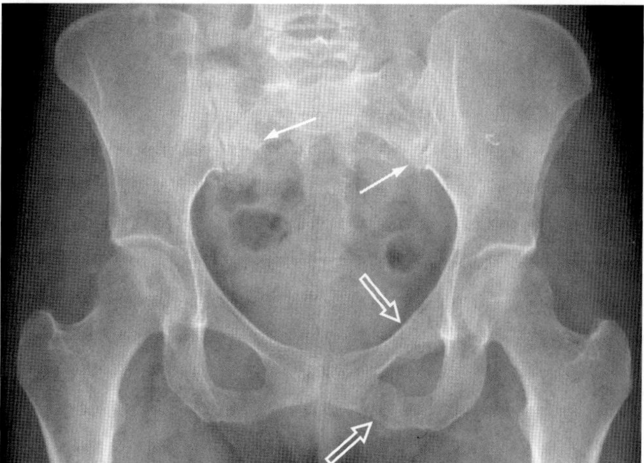

FIGURE 41-12. Sacral and pelvic insufficiency fractures after lung transplantation. This 50-year-old woman complained of left hip pain 7 months after lung transplantation. The anteroposterior view of the pelvis shows healing fractures of the left superior and inferior pubic rami *(open arrows)*. The sclerotic band-like densities in the sacrum *(arrows)* are due to healing insufficiency fractures. (Courtesy of Anne L. Fuhlbrigge, MD.)

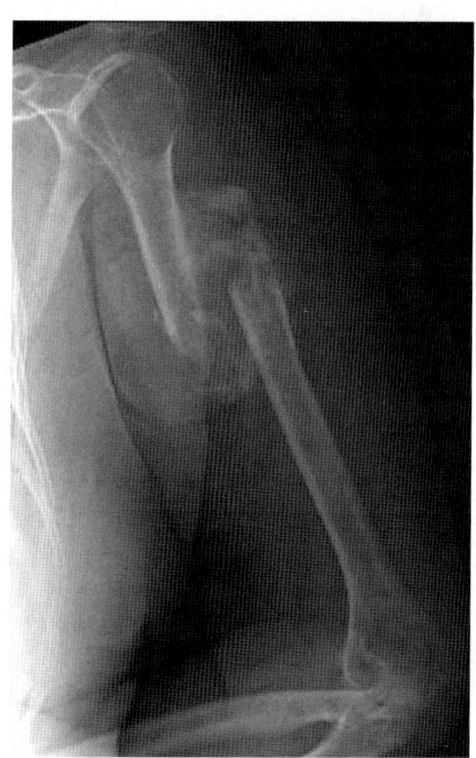

FIGURE 41-13. Humeral fracture after lung transplantation. This 61-year-old woman with osteoporosis suffered a humeral fracture 2 years after lung transplantation. The opacities in the native lung are a consequence of interstitial lung disease. (Courtesy of Anne L. Fuhlbrigge, MD.)

elements in the prevention of post-transplant axial and appendicular skeletal fractures.

There is evidence from the Vautour population-based study[97] of renal transplant recipients that long-term risk of fractures remains markedly increased over 10 or more years after transplantation. There are no comparable data on long-term risk in patients after liver, cardiac, or lung transplantation. Long-term bone density and fracture outcomes need to be studied to help evaluate the use of preventive and therapeutic strategies, and to clarify the necessity and efficacy of long-term therapeutic interventions after transplantation.

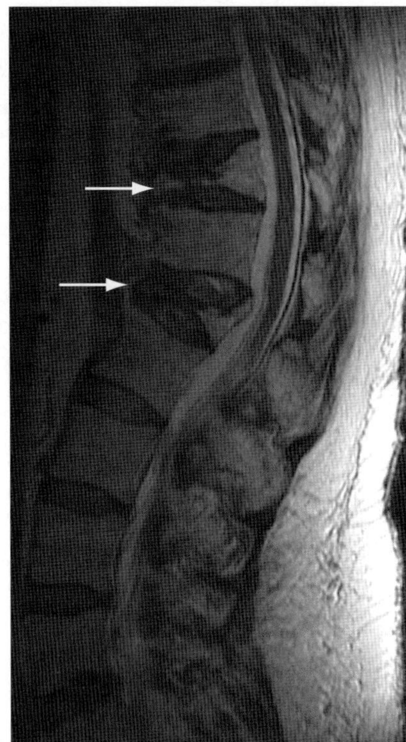

FIGURE 41-14. Compression fracture after lung transplant. Fifty-four-year-old man with low back pain 8 years after lung transplantation. Sagittal T1W MRI of the thoracolumbar spine shows the compression deformities *(arrows)* of T11 and L1. The normal fat signal of the vertebrae excludes metastatic disease.

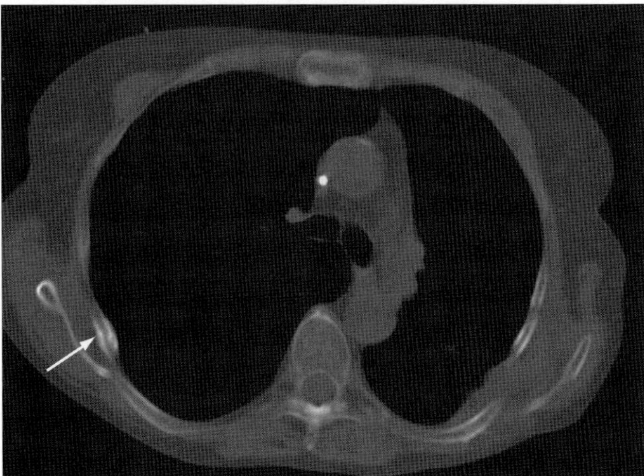

FIGURE 41-15. Rib fracture after lung transplantation. This 56-year-old women underwent a left-sided lung transplant. Four years after surgery, a right-sided rib fracture is noted *(arrow)* on follow-up CT scan. The large emphysematous right lung is contrasted with the transplanted left side. (Courtesy of Anne L. Fuhlbrigge, MD.)

REFERENCES

1. Collins J: Letter from the editor: the history and future of transplantation, *Semin Roentgenol* 41:2-3, 2006.
2. Navasa M et al: Quality of life, major medical complications and hospital service utilization in patients with primary biliary cirrhosis after liver transplantation, *J Hepatol* 25:129-134, 1996.
3. Navasa M et al: Bone fractures in liver transplant patients, *Br J Rheumatol* 33:52-55, 1994.
4. Stempfle HU et al: Prevention of osteoporosis after cardiac transplantation: a prospective, longitudinal, randomized, double-blind trial with calcitriol, *Transplantation* 68:523-530, 1999.
5. Shane E et al: Bone mass, vitamin D deficiency, and hyperparathyroidism in congestive heart failure, *Am J Med* 103:197-207, 1997. [See comment.]
6. Briner VA et al: Prevention of cancellous bone loss but persistence of renal bone disease despite normal 1,25 vitamin D levels two years after kidney transplantation, *Transplantation* 59:1393-1400, 1995.
7. Porayko MK et al: Bone disease in liver transplant recipients: incidence, timing, and risk factors, *Transplant Proc* 23:1462-1465, 1991.
8. Hofbauer LC: Pathophysiology of RANK ligand (RANKL) and osteoprotegerin (OPG), *Ann Endocrinologie* 67:139-141, 2006.
9. Katz I et al: Influence of age on cyclosporin A-induced alterations in bone mineral metabolism in the rat in vivo, *J Bone Miner Res* 9:59-67, 1994.
10. Buchinsky FJ et al: T lymphocytes play a critical role in the development of cyclosporin A-induced osteopenia, *Endocrinology* 137:2278-2285, 1996.
11. Guo CY et al: Mechanisms of bone loss after cardiac transplantation, *Bone* 22:267-271, 1998.
12. Cohen A, Sambrook P, Shane E: Management of bone loss after organ transplantation, *J Bone Miner Res* 19:1919-1932, 2004. [See comment.]
13. Myers BD et al: The long-term course of cyclosporine-associated chronic nephropathy, *Kidney Int* 33:590-600, 1988.
14. Bertani T et al: Nature and extent of glomerular injury induced by cyclosporine in heart transplant patients, *Kidney Int* 40:243-250, 1991.
15. Sambrook PN et al: Mechanisms of rapid bone loss following cardiac transplantation, *Osteoporos Int* 4:273-276, 1994.
16. Compston JE: Osteoporosis after liver transplantation, *Liver Transplant* 9:321-330, 2003.
17. Brandenberger G et al: Parathyroid function in cardiac transplant patients: evaluation during physical exercise, *Eur J Appl Physiol Occup Physiol* 70:401-406, 1995.
18. Finkelstein JS et al: The effects of parathyroid hormone, alendronate, or both in men with osteoporosis, *N Engl J Med* 349:1216-1226, 2003. [See comment.]
19. Adams JS, Song CF, Kantorovich V: Rapid recovery of bone mass in hypercalciuric, osteoporotic men treated with hydrochlorothiazide, *Ann Intern Med* 130:658-660, 1999.
20. Braith RW et al: Resistance exercise training and alendronate reverse glucocorticoid-induced osteoporosis in heart transplant recipients, *J Heart Lung Transplant* 22:1082-1090, 2003.
21. Mitchell MJ et al: Resistance training prevents vertebral osteoporosis in lung transplant recipients, *Transplantation* 76:557-562, 2003.
22. Hruska KA, Teitelbaum SL: Renal osteodystrophy, *N Engl J Med* 333:166-174, 1995. [See comment.]
23. Murphey MD et al: Musculoskeletal manifestations of chronic renal insufficiency, *Radiographics* 13:357-379, 1993.
24. Bellorin-Font E et al: Bone remodeling after renal transplantation, *Kidney Int Suppl* 2003:S125-S128, 2003.
25. Sperschneider H, Stein G: Bone disease after renal transplantation, *Nephrol Dialysis Transplant* 18:874-877, 2003.
26. Adams JE: Renal bone disease: radiological investigation, *Kidney Int Suppl* 73: S38-S41, 1999.
27. Saab G et al: Post-Transplant Osteodystrophy in the Era of the K/DOQI Guidelines for Dialysis and Transplantation, 2003.
28. National Kidney Foundation: Advisory on KDOQI Clinical Practice Guidelines in Chronic Kidney Disease.
29. Cayco AV et al: Posttransplant bone disease: evidence for a high bone resorption state, *Transplantation* 70:1722-1728, 2000.
30. Genant HK et al: Interim report and recommendations of the World Health Organization Task Force for Osteoporosis, *Osteoporos Int* 10:259-264, 1999.
31. Julian BA et al: Rapid loss of vertebral mineral density after renal transplantation, *N Engl J Med* 325:544-550, 1991.
32. Ball AM et al: Risk of hip fracture among dialysis and renal transplant recipients, *J Am Med Assoc* 288:3014-3018, 2002.
33. Genant HK et al: Vertebral fracture assessment using a semiquantitative technique, *J Bone Miner Res* 8:1137-1148, 1993.
34. Kulak C et al: Transplantation osteoporosis, *Arq Bras Endocinol Metabol* 50:783-792, 2006.
35. Grotz WH et al: Calcineurin-inhibitor induced pain syndrome (CIPS): a severe disabling complication after organ transplantation, *Transplant Int* 14:16-23, 2001.
36. Hetzel GR et al: Post-transplant distal-limb bone-marrow oedema: MR imaging and therapeutic considerations, *Nephrol Dialysis Transplant* 15:1859-1864, 2000.
37. Coates PT et al: Transient bone marrow edema in renal transplantation: a distinct post-transplantation syndrome with a characteristic MRI appearance, *Am J Transplant* 2:467-470, 2002. [See comment.]
38. Mulliken BD et al: Prevalence of previously undetected osteonecrosis of the femoral head in renal transplant recipients, *Radiology* 192:831-834, 1994.
39. Torres A, Lorenzo V, Salido E: Calcium metabolism and skeletal problems after transplantation, *J Am Soc Nephrol* 13:551-558, 2002.
40. Miyanishi K et al: Effects of cyclosporin A on the development of osteonecrosis in rabbits, *Acta Orthopaedica* 77:813-819, 2006.
41. Tang S et al: Risk factors for avascular bone necrosis after renal transplantation, *Transplant Proc* 32:1873-1875, 2000.
42. Kopecky KK et al: Apparent avascular necrosis of the hip: appearance and spontaneous resolution of MR findings in renal allograft recipients, *Radiology* 179:523-527, 1991.

43. Helenius I et al: Incidence and predictors of fractures in children after solid organ transplantation: a 5-year prospective, population-based study, *J Bone Miner Res* 21:380-387, 2006.
44. Levine E et al: Osteonecrosis following renal transplantation, *AJR Am J Roentgenol* 128:985-991, 1977.
45. Glickstein MF et al: Avascular necrosis versus other diseases of the hip: sensitivity of MR imaging, *Radiology* 169:213-215, 1988.
46. Abbott KC et al: New-onset gout after kidney transplantation: incidence, risk factors and implications, *Transplantation* 80:1383-1391, 2005.
47. Clive DM: Renal transplant-associated hyperuricemia and gout, *J Am Soc Nephrol* 11:974-979, 2000.
48. Martel W: The overhanging margin of bone: a roentgenologic manifestation of gout, *Radiology* 91:755-756, 1968.
49. Scientific Registry of Transplant Recipients: http://www.ustransplant.org/csr/current/nats.aspx, accessed 1/30/2006.
50. Leidig-Bruckner G et al: Frequency and predictors of osteoporotic fractures after cardiac or liver transplantation: a follow-up study, *Lancet* 357:342-347, 2001. [See comment.]
51. Ninkovic M et al: High prevalence of osteoporosis in patients with chronic liver disease prior to liver transplantation, *Calcif Tissue Int* 69:321-326, 2001.
52. Stellon AJ et al: Lack of osteomalacia in chronic cholestatic liver disease, *Bone* 7:181-185, 1986.
53. Bonkovsky HL et al: Prevalence and prediction of osteopenia in chronic liver disease, *Hepatology* 12:273-280, 1990.
54. Diamond T et al: Osteoporosis and skeletal fractures in chronic liver disease, *Gut* 31:82-87, 1990.
55. Abdelhadi M et al: Bone mineral status in end-stage liver disease and the effect of liver transplantation, *Scand J Gastroenterol* 30:1210-1215, 1995.
56. Hay JE: Bone disease in cholestatic liver disease, *Gastroenterology* 108:276-283, 1995.
57. Eastell R et al: Rates of vertebral bone loss before and after liver transplantation in women with primary biliary cirrhosis, *Hepatology* 14:296-300, 1991.
58. Jain A et al: Intravenous mycophenolate mofetil with low-dose oral tacrolimus and steroid induction for live donor liver transplantation, *Exp Clin Transplant* 3:361-365, 2005.
59. Zaghla H et al: A comparison of sirolimus vs. calcineurin inhibitor-based immunosuppressive therapies in liver transplantation, *Aliment Pharmacol Ther* 23:513-520, 2006.
60. Monegal A et al: Bone disease after liver transplantation: a long-term prospective study of bone mass changes, hormonal status and histomorphometric characteristics, *Osteoporos Int* 12:484-492, 2001.
61. Guthery SL et al: Bone mineral density in long-term survivors following pediatric liver transplantation, *Liver Transplant* 9:365-370, 2003.
62. Carey EJ et al: Osteopenia and osteoporosis in patients with end-stage liver disease caused by hepatitis C and alcoholic liver disease: not just a cholestatic problem, *Liver Transplant* 9:1166-1173, 2003.
63. Bjoro K et al: Secondary osteoporosis in liver transplant recipients: a longitudinal study in patients with and without cholestatic liver disease, *Scand J Gastroenterol* 38:320-327, 2003.
64. Ramsey-Goldman R et al: Increased risk of fracture in patients receiving solid organ transplants, *J Bone Miner Res* 14:456-463, 1999.
65. American Heart Association: www.americanheart.org/presenter.jthml?identifier=4588.
66. Nishio K et al: Congestive heart failure is associated with the rate of bone loss, *J Intern Med* 253:439-446, 2003.
67. Heidrich FE, Stergachis A, Gross KM: Diuretic drug use and the risk for hip fracture, *Ann Intern Med* 115:1-6, 1991. [See comment.]
68. Dahlman TC, Sjoberg HE, Ringertz H: Bone mineral density during long-term prophylaxis with heparin in pregnancy, *Am J Obstet Gynecol* 170:1315-1320, 1994.
69. Dahlman TC: Osteoporotic fractures and the recurrence of thromboembolism during pregnancy and the puerperium in 184 women undergoing thromboprophylaxis with heparin, *Am J Obstet Gynecol* 168:1265-1270, 1993.
70. Rosen H: Drugs that affect bone metabolism, *UpToDate.*
71. Caraballo PJ et al: Long-term use of oral anticoagulants and the risk of fracture, *Arch Intern Med* 159:1750-1756, 1999.
72. Holick MF: The role of vitamin D for bone health and fracture prevention *Curr Osteoporo Rep* 4:96-102, 2006.
73. Kerschan-Schindl K et al: Pathogenesis of bone loss in heart transplant candidates and recipients, *J Heart Lung Transplant* 22:843-850, 2003.
74. Van Cleemput J et al: Timing and quantification of bone loss in cardiac transplant recipients, *Transplant Int* 8:196-200, 1995.
75. Rico H et al: Age- and weight-related changes in total body bone mineral in men, *Miner Electrolyte Metab* 17:321-323, 1991.
76. Grampp S et al: Comparisons of noninvasive bone mineral measurements in assessing age-related loss, fracture discrimination, and diagnostic classification, *J Bone Miner Res* 12:697-711, 1997. [See comment.]
77. Glendenning P et al: High prevalence of osteoporosis in cardiac transplant recipients and discordance between biochemical turnover markers and bone histomorphometry, *Clin Endocrinol* 50:347-355, 1999.
78. Shane E et al: Fracture after cardiac transplantation: a prospective longitudinal study, *J Clin Endocrinol Metab* 81:1740-1746, 1996.
79. Shane E et al: Osteoporosis after cardiac transplantation, *Am J Med* 94:257-264, 1993.
80. Shane E et al: Bone loss and turnover after cardiac transplantation, *J Clin Endocrinol Metab* 82:1497-1506, 1997.
81. Thiebaud D et al: Cyclosporine induces high bone turnover and may contribute to bone loss after heart transplantation, *Eur J Clin Invest* 26:549-555, 1996.
82. Muchmore JS et al: Prevention of loss of vertebral bone density in heart transplant patients, *J Heart Lung Transplant* 11:959-963; discussion 963–964, 1992.
83. Canver CC, Heisey DM, Nichols RD: Acute renal failure requiring hemodialysis immediately after heart transplantation portends a poor outcome, *J Cardiovasc Surg* 41:203-206, 2000.
84. Bradbury G et al: Avascular necrosis of bone after cardiac transplantation. Prevalence and relationship to administration and dosage of steroids, *J Bone Joint Surg Am* 76:1385-1388, 1994.
85. Burack DA et al: Hyperuricemia and gout among heart transplant recipients receiving cyclosporine, *Am J Med* 92:141-146, 1992. [See comment.]
86. Hakim N, Vassilios E: *History of Organ and Cell Transplantation,* River Edge, NJ, 2003, Imperial College Press.
87. The Registry of the International Society for Heart and Lung Transplantation. *J Heart Lung Transplant* 23:805-815, 2004.
88. Ojo AO et al: Chronic renal failure after transplantation of a nonrenal organ, *N Engl J Med* 349:931-940, 2003. [See comment.]
89. Shane E et al: Osteoporosis in lung transplantation candidates with end-stage pulmonary disease, *Am J Med* 101:262-269, 1996. [See comment.]
90. Aris RM et al: Adverse alterations in bone metabolism are associated with lung infection in adults with cystic fibrosis, *Am J Respir Crit Care Med* 162:1674-1678, 2000.
91. Cahill BC et al: Prevention of bone loss and fracture after lung transplantation: a pilot study, *Transplantation* 72:1251-1255, 2001.
92. Tschopp O et al: Osteoporosis before lung transplantation: association with low body mass index, but not with underlying disease, *Am J Transplant* 2:167-172, 2002.
93. Ferrari SL et al: Osteoporosis in patients undergoing lung transplantation, *Eur Respir J* 9:2378-2382, 1996.
94. Shane E et al: Bone loss and fracture after lung transplantation, *Transplantation* 68:220-227, 1999.
95. Spira A et al: Osteoporosis and lung transplantation: a prospective study, *Chest* 117:476-481, 2000.
96. Aris RM et al: Efficacy of pamidronate for osteoporosis in patients with cystic fibrosis following lung transplantation, *Am J Respir Crit Care Med* 162:941-946, 2000.
97. Vautour LM et al: Long-term fracture risk following renal transplantation: a population-based study, *Osteoporos Int* 15:160-167, 2004.

Glossary

Accuracy—Calculated as true positives + true negatives / true positive + false positives + true negative + false negatives. Accuracy describes how well the test identifies all people with and without a condition.

ADC—Apparent diffusion coefficient. An ADC map shows apparent diffusion coefficients of diffusion-weighted images.

Arthrography—Injection of contrast into a joint to study the articular structures. This is often followed by radiographs, MRI (MR arthrography), or CT (CT arthrography).

Brown tumors (osteoclastomas)—Lytic lesions seen in hyperparathyroidism (usually primary hyperparathyroidism). The lesions contain osteoclasts and fibrous tissue and are brown in color due to hemorrhage and hemosiderin accumulation.

Bursa—Synovial-lined structure that lies between a tendon and an adjacent bony prominence. Adventitial bursae may develop at sites of friction.

Calcific tendinitis—Calcium hydroxyapatite deposited within a tendon. It may or may not be symptomatic.

Charcot joint—Also called *neuropathic joint.* Charcot described the association of loss of sensation and arthropathy.

CNR—Contrast-to-noise ratio.

Constrained prostheses—Constrained prostheses, such as a hinge or rotating hinge prostheses, provide varying degrees of stability. See also *Unconstrained prostheses.*

CPPD—Calcium pyrophosphate dihydrate deposition disease. This has various clinical manifestations, including, "pseudogout."

DESS—Dual echo steady state MRI sequence.

dGEMRIC—Delayed gadolinium-enhanced magnetic resonance imaging of cartilage. This technique provides an estimate of joint cartilage glycosaminoglycan (GAG) content by T1-relaxation time measurements after penetration of cartilage by the intravenously injected hydrophilic contrast agent gadolinium-DTPA(2-).

Entheses—The sites of attachment of ligaments or tendons to bone.

Enthesitis—Inflammation at sites of ligament or tendon attachment to bone.

Fat suppression—A set of MRI techniques that attempts to eliminate bright MRI signal from fat in order to aid visualization of subtle underlying features, such as contrast enhancement.*

Field strength—Static magnetic field within the scanner, measured in Tesla. Magnet field strength may be high-field ($\geq$ 1.0T), mid-field (0.5T-1.0T), or low-field ($<$ 0.5T).**

FOV—Field of view. The distance of anatomic coverage in a given imaging direction, determined in part by the size of the radiofrequency coil being used.**

FSE—Fast spin echo.

Gadolinium (Gd)—Paramagnetic contrast agent used in MRI. The most commonly used contrast agents are gadolinium chelates, which shorten the spin-lattice relaxation times (T1) of tissues.**

GRE—Gradient echo. A category of MRI pulse sequences that is particularly sensitive to magnetic field inhomogeneities. These are rapid sequences and are often used to create volumetric 3-dimensional image data to visualize dynamic processes such as transient contrast enhancement.*

HADD—Hydroxyapatite deposition disease. Also called *calcific tendinitis.*

Hertz—A unit of frequency.

Hounsfield units—Named after Sir Godfrey Hounsfield, one of the Nobel laureates responsible for the development of the CT scanner.

Indirect arthrography—Arthrography performed using intravenous rather than intraarticular injection of gadolinium. Contrast injected intravenously enters the joint through diffusion.

Insufficiency fracture—Fracture occurring in abnormal bone (e.g., osteoporosis) subjected to normal stress.

Isotropic imaging—Image in which all dimensions of the volume elements (voxels) are the same size. This allows images to be obtained in any plane without degradation.

Involucrum—Periosteal new bone surrounding dead bone (sequestrum) in chronic osteomyelitis.

Looser zone—An incomplete fracture seen in osteomalacia.

Low-field magnet—Usually $<$ 0.5T. See also *Field strength.*

Magic angle artifact—Increased signal in a structure such as a tendon that lies at approximately 54.7 degrees to the main magnetic field on short TE sequences. This artifact may simulate a tear or tendinosis.

Matrix—The number of in-plane pixels along each given image direction. In combination with FOV, determines the in-plane image resolution.**

MDCT—Multidetector CT.

MPR—Multiplanar reformatted (images).

Microbubble (intravascular microbubble contrast)—Technique used to improve Doppler signal intensity.

NPV—Negative predictive value. The probability that the patient will not have the disease when the test is negative (true negatives / true negatives + false negatives)

NSF/NFD—Nephrogenic systemic fibrosis/nephrogenic fibrosing dermopathy. A condition causing skin thickening and sometimes systemic manifestations or death that may rarely be seen in patients with renal disease receiving gadolinium contrast.

Osteonecrosis—Synonymous with avascular necrosis AVN.

Osteopenia—A general term applied to decreased bone density as seen on radiographs. Also a more specific term applied to bone mineral density measurements that are decreased but not as severely as in osteoporosis. Used to designate bone mineral density measurements between 1 and –2.5 standard deviations below peak bone mass.

Pixel—Picture element.

PPV—Positive predictive value. Calculated as true positives / true positives + false positives. The probability that a patient with a positive test has the condition.

Pulse sequences—Timing of MRI parameters (radiofrequency pulse strength and spacing, magnetic field gradients, and signal collection) used to create MR images with varying degrees of tissue contrast.**

Scintigraphy—The use of radioisotopes to image the body.

Sensitivity—Probability of a positive test among patients with the disease. Calculated as true positive / true positive + false negative. A sensitive test rules out disease when negative.

Sequestrum—Dead bone usually resulting from osteomyelitis.

SNR—Signal-to-noise ratio.

Sonographer—Ultrasound technologist.

Spatial resolution—Definition of the smallest structures that can be differentiated on an image, generally related to pixel or voxel dimensions, although voxels can be interpolated to artificially increase display resolution from the true image resolution. True in-plane resolution equals field of view divided by matrix.**

Specificity—The probability of a negative test among patients without a disease. Calculated as true negative / true negative + false positive. A very specific test rules in disease when positive.

STIR—Short-tau inversion recovery. A particularly robust MRI fat suppression technique. This relies on the short T1-relaxation time of fat to selectively eliminate MRI signal from fat.*

T1—Intrinsic tissue. Dependent "longitudinal" relaxation time of equilibrium magnetization along the axis of the MRI scanner. Equilibrium magnetization (from which the MRI signal is later formed) is restored by T1 relaxation, rapidly for fat, but more slowly for water.*

T1-weighted—Images that create contrast between tissues based on their different intrinsic T1 relaxation rates.*

T2—Intrinsic tissue-dependent "transverse" relaxation time of MRI, governing the decay of MRI signal. Once magnetization is formed in the "transverse" plane perpendicular to the long axis of the scanner, it decays exponentially with T2 relaxation, rapidly for fat, but more slowly for water.*

T2-weighted—Images that create contrast between tissues based on their different intrinsic T2 relaxation rates.*

TE—Echo time. An MRI parameter that can be adjusted to control image contrast, particularly T2-weighted contrast. Changing TE permits different amounts of T2 relaxation to occur for different tissues, so appropriate TE selection can maximize T2-weighted contrast based on the different intrinsic T2 relaxation rates of the tissues.*

Tear—Tendon tears are categorized as 1.) enlarged and heterogeneous, 2.) thinned, and 3.) completely ruptured.

Tendinopathy—Clinical term referring to tendon pain, swelling, and impaired function.

Tendinosis—Intrasubstance tendon degeneration. May be symptomatic.

Tenosynovitis—Fluid or synovial thickening within the tenosynovial lining.

Tesla (T)—Unit of magnetic field strength. One Tesla equals 10,000 gauss. (Earth's magnetic field strength is 0.5 gauss.) **

TR—Repetition time. An MRI parameter that can be adjusted to control image contrast, particularly T1-weighted contrast. Changing TR permits different amounts of T1 relaxation to occur for different tissues, so appropriate TR selection can maximize T1-weighted contrast based on the different intrinsic T1 relaxation rates of the tissues.*

Unconstrained prostheses—Unconstrained prostheses provide little or no constraint (limitation) to motion and depend on having intact (or reconstructed) ligaments to maintain stability.

Voxel—Volume element, the 3-dimensional size of each point in an image, generally determined by two in-plane pixel dimensions (in turn determined by FOV and matrix) and the slice thickness.**

---

*Information is provided by Aaron D Sodickson, MD, PhD (Brigham and Women's Hospital, Boston, MA).

**Prior publication of these terms in Cohen S, American College of Rheumatology Extremity Magnetic Resonance Imaging Task Force: Extremity magnetic resonance imaging in rheumatoid arthritis: Report of the American College of Rheumatology Extremity Magnetic Resonance imaging Task Force, *Arth & Rheum* 54:1034-1037, 2006.

INDEX

Note: Page numbers followed by *f* indicate figures; *t* indicate tables; *b* indicate boxes; and page numbers in bold indicate chapters.

B

D

E

H

M

N

Q

R

S

U

V

W

X

Z